Moss' Heart Disease in Infants, Children, and Adolescents

3rd Edition

Moss' Heart Disease in Infants, Children, and Adolescents

3rd Edition

Edited by

Forrest H. Adams, M.D.

Professor of Pediatrics Emeritus
Former Head, Division of Cardiology
Department of Pediatrics
University of California, Los Angeles School of Medicine
Los Angeles, California

George C. Emmanouilides, M.D.

Professor of Pediatrics
University of California, Los Angeles School of Medicine
Chief, Division of Pediatric Cardiology
Harbor University of California, Los Angeles Medical Center
Torrance, California

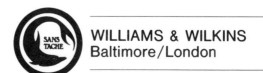

WILLIAMS & WILKINS
Baltimore/London

Made in the United States of America

First Edition, 1968
Second Edition, 1977
  Reprinted 1978, 1979

Library of Congress Cataloging in Publication Data

Heart disease in infants, children, and adolescents. Moss' Heart disease in infants, children, and adolescents.

  Includes index.
  1. Heart—Diseases. 2. Pediatric cardiology. I. Moss, Arthur J. II. Adams, Forrest H. III. Emmanouilides, George C. IV. Title. [DNLM: 1. Heart diseases—In adolescence. 2. Heart diseases—In infancy and childhood. WS 290 H436]
RJ421.H38 1982   618.92′12   82-4952
ISBN 0-683-00051-9   AACR2

Composed and printed at
Waverly Press, Inc.
Mt. Royal and Guilford Aves.
Baltimore, MD 21202, U.S.A.

Title Page for the First Edition

HEART DISEASE IN INFANTS, CHILDREN, AND ADOLESCENTS

edited by

Arthur J. Moss, M.D.

PROFESSOR AND CHAIRMAN,
DEPARTMENT OF PEDIATRICS,
UCLA SCHOOL OF MEDICINE, LOS ANGELES, CALIFORNIA

Forrest H. Adams, M.D.

PROFESSOR OF PEDIATRICS,
HEAD, DIVISION OF CARDIOLOGY, DEPARTMENT OF PEDIATRICS,
UCLA SCHOOL OF MEDICINE, LOS ANGELES, CALIFORNIA

with 73 contributors

...IN AN ABUNDANCE
OF COUNSELORS THERE IS SAFETY.

Proverbs, 11:14

BALTIMORE 1968 • THE WILLIAMS & WILKINS CO.

Preface

The need for a third edition of this book has been dictated by the fact that the previous edition was well received, and reprinting of the second edition would have been inappropriate in view of the more recent strides made in the diagnosis and treatment of heart disease in the young.

As with the previous editions, the multicontributor approach has been utilized. Cardiology, as it applies to the young, has become a complex discipline. Its communication to the interested student and professional is almost impossible to be rendered by one or two individuals who could be considered masters in all areas of the field. Thus, the help of more than 80 contributors from 35 cardiac centers has been solicited to accomplish this task. These contributors have been selected primarily for their expertise in the respective areas, and their cooperation and willingness to participate in this effort are well appreciated.

With the recent application of two-dimensional echocardiography, especially in the diagnosis of congenital heart disease, it became necessary to include, as much as possible, information pertaining to this most useful noninvasive technique. A number of new contributors have been recruited and a few new chapters have been added.

The general layout of the book has been preserved with sections on general cardiology, congenital defects, infectious diseases, metabolic and degenerative diseases, and special problems.

In the section of general cardiology, the chapters on electrocardiography and vectorcardiography have been combined into one, the chapter on echocardiography has been expanded to include the two-dimensional technique, and new chapters on nuclear cardiology and exercise testing have been added. The chapters of the other sections have been updated or rewritten in order to incorporate available two-dimensional echocardiographic data and new medical and surgical modes of treatment. A new chapter on cardiomyopathies has replaced the previous one on endocardial fibroelastosis.

The reader should recognize that although much of the material presented is based on original observations made by the contributors themselves, for reasons of uniformity of presentation some editing of the material was necessary. For this reason, we ask the forgiveness of the contributors for intruding on their literary styles. Unfortunately, an unavoidable imbalance among chapters may be evident, but we purposely did not attempt to restrict the length of a chapter according to its significance.

Some chapters on rare malformations of the heart are "classics" not found in any other textbook on heart disease of the young.

When controversial issues are discussed, attempts were made not to suppress or eliminate them but to let the reader become aware of them and decide for himself. We made an attempt to cover as many areas as possible on the subject of heart disease in infants, children and adolescents, and we believe that very few, if any, subjects of current interest and value were missed.

We would like to make certain acknowledgements, primarily to the contributors. We are most grateful to them for their willingness to participate in this venture in spite of their busy schedules. To their and our secretaries, who spent many hours typing and retyping manuscripts, we wish to express our deep appreciation. Finally, we are very grateful to the publisher, Williams & Wilkins, whose continuing encouragement and help made this book possible.

FORREST H. ADAMS, M.D.
GEORGE C. EMMANOUILIDES, M.D.
January, 1983

Contributors

Forrest H. Adams, M.D.
Professor of Pediatrics Emeritus
Former Head, Division of Cardiology
Department of Pediatrics
UCLA School of Medicine
Los Angeles, California

Robert H. Anderson, M.D.
Professor in Pediatric Morphology
Joseph Levy Foundation
Cardiothoracic Institute
Brompton Hospital
London, England

Lionel M. Bargeron, Jr., M.D.
Professor of Pediatrics and Pediatric Cardiology
University of Alabama
Birmingham, Alabama

David Baum, M.D.
Professor, Department of Pediatrics
Chief, Division of Pediatric Cardiology
Stanford University Medical Center
Stanford, California

Barry G. Baylen, M.D.
Assistant Professor of Pediatrics
UCLA School of Medicine
Harbor-UCLA Medical Center
Torrance, California

Harvey W. Bender, M.D.
Professor of Surgery
Chairman, Department of Cardiac and Thoracic Surgery
Vanderbilt University Medical Center
Nashville, Tennessee

Lee N. Benson, M.D.
Adjunct Assistant Professor, Department of Pediatrics
UCLA School of Medicine
Center for Health Sciences
Los Angeles, California

Joan L. Caddell, M.D.
Research Professor,
Department of Pediatrics/Adolescent Medicine
St. Louis University
St. Louis, Missouri

Guy A. Carter, M.D.
Associate Professor, Department of Pediatrics
Chief, Division of Pediatric Cardiology
University of South Dakota School of Medicine
Sioux Falls, South Dakota

J. Michael Criley, M.D.
Professor of Medicine and Radiological Sciences
UCLA School of Medicine
Chief, Division of Cardiology
Harbor-UCLA Medical Center
Torrance, California

Gordon K. Danielson, M.D.
Consultant, Division of Thoracic and Cardiovascular
    Surgery
Mayo Clinic
Professor of Surgery
Mayo Medical School
Rochester, Minnesota

Macdonald Dick, II, M.D.
Associate Professor of Pediatrics
The University of Michigan Medical School
C. S. Mott Children's Hospital
Ann Arbor, Michigan

Jesse E. Edwards, M.D.
Senior Consultant in Anatomic Pathology
United Hospitals of St. Paul
St. Paul, Minnesota
Professor of Pathology
University of Minnesota
Minneapolis, Minnesota

William D. Edwards, M.D.
Consultant, Department of Anatomic Pathology
Mayo Clinic and Mayo Foundation
Assistant Professor of Pathology
Mayo Medical School
Rochester, Minnesota

Larry P. Elliott, M.D.
Professor and Chairman
Department of Radiology
Georgetown University
Washington, D.C.

George C. Emmanouilides, M.D.
Professor of Pediatrics
UCLA School of Medicine
Chief, Division of Pediatric Cardiology
Harbor-UCLA Medical Center
Torrance, California

Mary Allen Engle, M.D.
Stavros S. Niarchos Professor of Pediatric Cardiology
Professor of Pediatrics
Director of Pediatric Cardiology
The New York Hospital-Cornell Medical Center
New York, New York

Robert H. Feldt, M.D.
Consultant, Division of Pediatric Cardiology
Mayo Clinic and Mayo Foundation
Professor of Pediatrics
Mayo Medical School
Rochester, Minnesota

Robert M. Freedom, M.D.
Professor of Paediatrics and Pathology
The University of Toronto, Faculty of Medicine
Director, Cardiovascular Pathology Registry
The Hospital for Sick Children
Toronto, Canada

William F. Friedman, M.D.
J. H. Nicholson Professor of Pediatric Cardiology
Chairman, Department of Pediatrics
UCLA School of Medicine
Center for Health Sciences
Los Angeles, California

Valentin Fuster, M.D.
Arthur and Hilda Master Professor of Medicine
Director, Division of Cardiology
Mount Sinai Medical Center
New York, New York

Arthur Garson, Jr., M.D.
Associate Professor of Pediatrics and Medicine
Baylor College of Medicine
Director of Electrocardiography Laboratory
Texas Children's Hospital
Houston, Texas

Welton M. Gersony, M.D.
Professor of Pediatrics
College of Physicians & Surgeons of Columbia University
Director, Division of Pediatric Cardiology
Department of Pediatrics
Babies Hospital at Columbia Presbyterian Medical Center
New York, New York

Paul C. Gillette, M.D.
Professor of Pediatrics and Associate Professor of Experimental Medicine
Baylor College of Medicine
Director of Clinical Electrophysiology and Pacing
Texas Children's Hospital
Houston, Texas

Thomas P. Graham, Jr., M.D.
Professor of Pediatrics and Director of the Division of Pediatric Cardiology
Vanderbilt University Medical Center
Nashville, Tennessee

F. Acerete Guillén, M.D.
Chief of Section of Pediatric Cardiology
Centro Especial Ramon y Cajal
Madrid, Spain

Warren G. Guntheroth, M.D.
Professor of Pediatrics
Head, Division of Pediatric Cardiology
University of Washington School of Medicine
Seattle, Washington

Donald J. Hagler, M.D.
Consultant, Division of Pediatric Cardiology
Mayo Clinic and Mayo Foundation
Associate Professor of Pediatrics
Mayo Medical School
Rochester, Minnesota

Lulu M. Haroutunian, M.D. (deceased)
Assistant Professor of Pediatrics and Medicine
Johns Hopkins University and Hospital
Baltimore, Maryland

Michael A. Heymann, M.D.
Professor of Pediatrics and Obstetrics, Gynecology, and Reproductive Sciences
Senior Staff Member, Cardiovascular Research Institute
University of California-San Francisco
San Francisco, California

Roger A. Hurwitz, M.D.
Professor of Pediatrics
University of Indiana Medical Center
Indianapolis, Indiana

Fredrick W. James, M.D.
Professor of Pediatrics
University of Cincinnati College of Medicine
Head, Exercise Laboratory
Division of Cardiology
Children's Hospital Medical Center
Cincinnati, Ohio

Jay M. Jarmakani, M.D.
Professor of Pediatrics (Cardiology)
Director, Cardiopulmonary Laboratory
UCLA School of Medicine
Los Angeles, California

M. Quero Jiménez, M.D.
Chief of the Service of Pediatric Cardiology
Centro Especial Ramon y Cajal
Madrid, Spain

Edward L. Kaplan, M.D.
Professor of Pediatrics
University of Minnesota
Minneapolis, Minnesota

Samuel Kaplan, M.D.
Professor of Pediatrics and Medicine
University of Cincinnati College of Medicine
Director, Division of Cardiology
Children's Hospital Medical Center
Cincinnati, Ohio

Isamu Kawabori, M.D.
Associate Professor
Department of Pediatrics (Cardiology)
University of Washington School of Medicine
Seattle, Washington

James K. Kirklin, M.D.
Assistant Professor of Surgery
Division of Cardiac Surgery
University of Alabama
Birmingham, Alabama

Ronald M. Lauer, M.D.
Professor of Pediatrics
University of Iowa
Iowa City, Iowa

Martin H. Lees, M.D.
Professor of Pediatrics
Director of Pediatric Cardiology
University of Oregon Health Sciences Center
Portland, Oregon

Jerome Liebman, M.D.
Professor of Pediatrics
Case Western Reserve University School of Medicine
Division of Pediatric Cardiology
Rainbow Babies and Children's Hospital
Cleveland, Ohio

Jennifer M. H. Loggie, M.D.
Professor of Pediatrics
University of Cincinnati
The Children's Hospital Research Foundation
Cincinnati, Ohio

Russell V. Lucas, Jr., M.D.
Professor of Pediatrics
University of Minnesota
Minneapolis, Minnesota

Paul R. Lurie, M.D.
Emeritus Professor of Pediatrics
University of Southern California School of Medicine
Formerly Head, Division of Cardiology
Children's Hospital of Los Angeles
Los Angeles, California

Douglas D. Mair, M.D.
Consultant, Division of Pediatric Cardiology
Mayo Clinic and Mayo Foundation
Professor of Pediatrics
Mayo Medical School
Rochester, Minnesota

Barry J. Maron, M.D.
Senior Investigator
Cardiology Branch
National Heart, Lung, and Blood Institute
Bethesda, Maryland

Rumiko Matsuoka, M.D.
Childrens' Hospital Medical Center
Harvard Medical School
Boston, Massachusetts

Dan G. McNamara, M.D.
The Lillie Frank Abercrombie Section of Cardiology
Professor, Department of Pediatrics
Baylor College of Medicine and Texas Children's Hospital
Houston, Texas

Richard A. Meyer, M.D.
Professor of Pediatrics
University of Cincinnati College of Medicine
Division of Cardiology
Children's Hospital Medical Center
Cincinnati, Ohio

James H. Moller, M.D.
Professor of Pediatrics
University of Minnesota
Minneapolis, Minnesota

Catherine A. Neill, M.D.
Associate Professor of Pediatrics and Cardiology
Johns Hopkins University and Hospital
Baltimore, Maryland

Ronald J. Nelson, M.D.
Professor of Surgery
UCLA School of Medicine
Chief, Cardiovascular and Thoracic Surgery
Harbor-UCLA Medical Center
Torrance, California

James J. Nora, M.D., M.P.H.
Professor of Pediatrics, Genetics, and Preventative Medicine
Director of Preventative Cardiology
University of Colorado School of Medicine
Director, Human Genetics Institute
Rose Medical Center
Denver, Colorado

George R. Noren, M.D.
Assistant Chief of Pediatrics
Hennepin County Medical Center
Associate Professor of Pediatrics
University Minnesota
Minneapolis, Minnesota

Milton H. Paul, M.D.
Director, Division of Cardiology
The Willis J. Potts Children's Heart Center
The Children's Memorial Hospital
Professor of Pediatrics
Northwestern University Medical School
Chicago, Illinois

Mary Ella Mascia Pierpont, Ph.D., M.D.
Assistant Professor of Pediatrics
University of Minnesota
Minneapolis, Minnesota

Robert Plonsey, Ph.D.
Professor of Bioengineering
Director, Department of Bioengineering
Case Western Reserve University
Cleveland, Ohio

Co-burn J. Porter, M.D.
Assistant Professor
The Lillie Frank Abercrombie Section of Cardiology
Department of Pediatrics
Baylor College of Medicine
Texas Children's Hospital
Houston, Texas

Francisco J. Puga, M.D.
Consultant, Section of Thoracic, Cardiovascular, Vascular and General Surgery
Mayo Clinic and Mayo Foundation
Assistant Professor of Surgery
Mayo Medical School
Rochester, Minnesota

Marlene Rabinovitch, M.D.
Assistant Professor of Pediatrics
Harvard Medical School
Associate in Cardiology
Children's Hospital Medical Center
Boston, Massachusetts
The Hospital for Sick Children
Toronto, Ontario, Canada

Thomas A. Riemenschneider, M.D.
Professor and Chief
Division of Pediatric Cardiology
Department of Pediatrics
Case Western Reserve University School of Medicine
Rainbow Babies and Children's Hospital
Cleveland, Ohio

Donald G. Ritter, M.D.
Chairman, Division of Pediatric Cardiology
Mayo Clinic and Mayo Foundation
Professor of Pediatrics
Mayo Medical School
Rochester, Minnesota

Amnon Rosenthal, M.D.
Professor of Pediatrics
The University of Michigan Medical School
C. S. Mott Children's Hospital
Ann Arbor, Michigan

Herbert D. Ruttenberg, M.D.
Professor of Pediatrics
Chief, Division of Pediatric Cardiology
University of Utah School of Medicine
Salt Lake City, Utah

Gerald L. Schiebler, M.D.
Professor and Chairman
Department of Pediatrics
University of Florida
Gainesville, Florida

James B. Seward, M.D.
Consultant, Division of Cardiovascular Diseases and Internal Medicine and Division of Pediatric Cardiology
Mayo Clinic and Mayo Foundation
Associate Professor of Medicine and Pediatrics
Mayo Medical School
Rochester, Minnesota

Stanford T. Shulman, M.D.
Professor of Pediatrics
Northwestern University Medical School
The Children's Memorial Hospital
Chicago, Illinois

Norman J. Sissman, M.D.
Professor of Pediatrics
Director of Pediatric Cardiology
Rutgers Medical School
New Brunswick, New Jersey

Madison S. Spach, M.D.
Professor and Chief Division of Pediatric Cardiology
Department of Pediatrics
Duke University Medical Center
Durham, North Carolina

Nancy A. Staley, M.D.
Director, Clinical Electron Microscopy Laboratory
Department of Pathology
Veterans Administration Hospital
Assistant Professor
University of Minnesota
Minneapolis, Minnesota

Cecille O. Sunderland, M.D.
Professor of Pediatrics (Pediatric Cardiology)
University of Oregon Health Sciences Center
Portland, Oregon

Norman S. Talner, M.D.
Professor of Pediatrics and Diagnostic Radiology
Director of Pediatric Cardiology
Yale University School of Medicine
New Haven, Connecticut

Masato Takahashi, M.D.
Associate Professor of Pediatrics
University of Southern California School of Medicine
Childrens Hospital of Los Angeles
Los Angeles, California

S. T. Treves, M.D.
Director, Division of Nuclear Medicine
Associate Professor of Radiology
Harvard Medical School
The Children's Hospital Medical Center
Boston, Massachusetts

Lodewyk H. S. Van Mierop, M.D.
Professor of Pediatrics (Cardiology) and Pathology
Graduate Research Professor
College of Medicine
University of Florida
Gainesville, Florida

Richard Van Praagh, M.D.
Professor of Pathology and Research Associate in Cardiology
Harvard Medical School
Children's Hospital Medical Center
Boston, Massachusetts

Stella Van Praagh, M.D.
Assistant Professor of Pathology and Associate in Cardiology
Harvard Medical School
Children's Hospital Medical Center
Boston, Massachusetts

Benjamin E. Victorica, M.D.
Professor of Pediatrics
University of Florida College of Medicine
Gainesville, Florida

Lewis H. Wannamaker, M.D.
Professor of Pediatrics and of Microbiology
University of Minnesota
Minneapolis, Minnesota
Career Investigator of the American Heart Association

William H. Weidman, M.D.
Consultant, Division of Pediatric Cardiology
Mayo Clinic and Mayo Foundation
Professor of Pediatrics
Mayo Medical School
Rochester, Minnesota

Paul M. Weinberg, M.D.
Director, Cardiac Registry
The Children's Hospital of Philadelphia
Assistant Professor Pediatric (Cardiology) and Consultant
    of Pathology
University of Pennsylvania School of Medicine
Philadelphia, Pennsylvania

Contents

Part 3: Infectious Diseases

Part 4: Connective Tissue: Metabolic and Degenerative Diseases

Part 5: Special Problems

Part 6

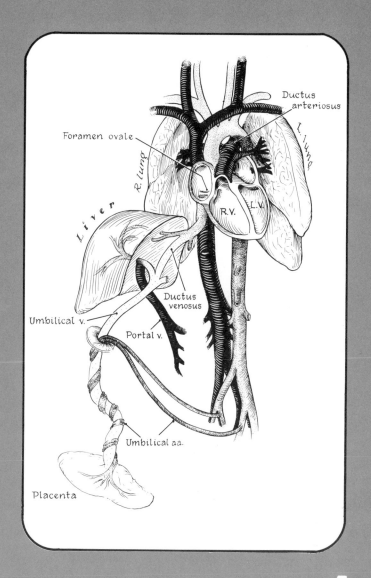

Ductus arteriosus

Foramen ovale

L. lung

R. lung

L i v e r

R.V.

L.V.

Ductus venosus

Umbilical v.

Portal v.

Umbilical aa.

Placenta

Part 1
GENERAL
CARDIOLOGY

1

Etiologic Aspects of Heart Diseases

James J. Nora, M.D.

Cardiovascular diseases of all types are familial. However, when discussing etiology it is useful to talk of genetic epidemiology rather than just genetics to emphasize the important contributions of both heredity and environment to causation.[14, 16] The major focus of this book and the presentation in this chapter is on congenital heart diseases, but the other three major categories of cardiovascular diseases, atherosclerosis, hypertension, and rheumatic fever will benefit from an etiologic overview. Figure 1.1 places these four categories on a continuum between heredity and environment with everything but rheumatic fever clustering in the middle. Rheumatic fever may have a very strong genetic basis, but of course, requires the essential environmental interaction with the group A beta hemolytic streptococcus.

CONGENITAL HEART DISEASES

The majority of studies attempting to define the causes of congenital heart diseases have taken place during the past two decades.[1, 2, 5, 6, 8–10, 13, 15, 16] Table 1.1 summarizes the etiologic subgroups from our patient experience. Approximately 8% of our congenital heart patients have an etiologic basis which is attributable to genetic factors with very little contribution from the environment; about 2% have an environmental etiology with little if any genetic contribution; but the great majority of our patients (approximately 90%) are best explained by a genetic-environmental interaction (multifactorial inheritance),[10] in which the genetic and environmental contributions are of comparable importance. These subgroups will be discussed at greater length in sections that follow.

PRIMARILY GENETIC FACTORS

CHROMOSOMAL CAUSES

Gross chromosomal anomalies exist in about 5% of the patients with congenital heart disease we have seen. On the other hand, studies have failed to demonstrate chromosomal anomalies in patients with congenital heart defects (both familial and nonfamilial cases) which were not part of a syndrome.[2, 10] It may become apparent through the use of newer methods of chromosomal study that some familial cases of congenital heart disease will be associated with minor chromosomal aberrations. However, even a minor anomaly of a chromosome affects many gene loci and would be likely to cause abnormalities of other structures in addition to the heart. Certainly this is true of gross chromosomal disorders in which the addition or subtraction of hundreds of genes causes developmental confusion in many systems and produces a syndrome.

The picture, then, that one should have in mind for a congenital heart defect associated with a chromosomal anomaly is a syndrome. Table 1.2 lists a selection of chromosomal syndromes known to be associated with congenital heart defects, the frequency of the association, and the three most common cardiovascular malformations found with each chromosomal anomaly. There have been a number of anomalies described in C group chromosomes—trisomies, partial trisomies, deletions, and mosaicism. Since the heart lesions that have been described are similar, all of these chromosomal disorders are grouped together.

With the exception of the XO Turner syndrome and XXXXY syndrome, the most common defect in the general population is also the most common defect in the various chromosomal syndromes (actually ventricular septal defect (VSD) and atrioventricular canal are about equally common in 21 trisomy). The XO Turner and XXXXY syndromes are the only sex chromosomal syndromes represented in Table 1.2. There seems to be very little increase in frequency of association of cardiovascular disorders with XXY Klinefelter, XYY, and XXX syndromes. There are very few cases of XXXXX, but patent ductus arteriosus (PDA) has been reported. Some workers have tried to define a role for the X chromosome in patent ductus arteriosus production, since the frequency in females is twice as high as in males. Patients with Turner syndrome are "deficient" in X chromosomes, and most often have the "male-associated" coarctation of the aorta; whereas the XXXXY patients with three extra X chromosomes have the "female-associated" disorder, PDA. How this relates precisely to morphogenesis of the cardiovascular system remains to be demonstrated.

Counseling Situations

The counseling in families with a child with congenital heart disease and a chromosomal anomaly is usually undertaken by a clinical geneticist. The recurrence risk of the heart lesions is related to the recurrence risk of the chromosomal anomaly. There is a higher frequency of nondisjunction following the birth of a child with a trisomy and familial translocations. Amniocentesis may be required in subsequent pregnancies to provide optimal information for recurrence risks.

Clinical Example. At 4 months of age this infant male was referred to our cardiology service because of the presence of a heart murmur. It was clear that the patient had Down's syndrome, although this diagnosis had not been previously called to the attention of the parents. The murmur was compatible with VSD as was the electrocardiogram which showed biventricular hypertrophy with an axis of +120°. The parents wanted to discuss the chance of heart disease recurring, but we felt it was important to lead into this gradually through a series of sessions in which the diagnosis of Down's syndrome had to be revealed with caution and understanding. The mother was 23 and the father 25 years old. This was their firstborn and they wanted more children. Inherited translocations are most common in younger mothers, but are still relatively rare. Only one in 50 infants born to mothers under 30 years of age have inherited translocations, yet this infant had an unbalanced translocation inherited from his phenotypically normal mother who was a balanced translocation carrier. The empiric data show that between 6 and 20% of the offspring of mothers with balanced D/G translocation have unbalanced translocation Down's syndrome (less than

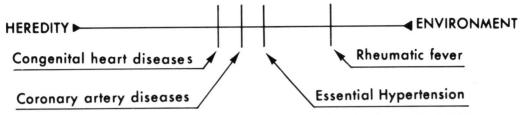

Fig. 1.1 Cardiovascular disease in the continuum of genetic and environmental influences.

TABLE 1.1 ETIOLOGIC BASIS OF CONGENITAL HEART DISEASES

Primary genetic factors	
Chromosomal	5%
Single mutant gene	3%
Primarily environmental factors	
Rubella	≈1%
Other	≈1%
Genetic-environmental interaction	
(Multifactorial inheritance)	≈90%

TABLE 1.2 CONGENITAL HEART DISEASE (CHD) IN SELECTED CHROMOSOMAL ABERRATIONS

Population Studied	Incidence of CHD (%)	Most Common Lesions 1	2	3
General population	1	VSD	PDA	ASD
4p−	40	VSD	ASD	PDA
5p− (Cri-du-chat)	25	VSD	PDA	ASD
C group anomalies	25–50	VSD	PDA	
13 trisomy	90	VSD	PDA	Dext[a]
13q−	50	VSD		
18 Trisomy	99+	VSD	PDA	PS
18q−	50	VSD		
21 trisomy	50	VSD	AV canal	ASD
XO Turner	35	CA	AS	ASD
XXXXY	14	PDA	ASD	

[a] Abbreviations used are: Dext, Dextroversion; CA, coarctation of aorta; AS, aortic stenosis; AV, atrioventricular.

would be predicted on cytologic grounds). We round the data off and give a 15% recurrence risk. Our counseling in this situation emphasized the need for amniocentesis if future pregnancies were to be considered to determine whether or not the fetus had an unbalanced translocation.

SINGLE MUTANT GENE CAUSES

As in chromosomal causes of cardiovascular diseases, the picture one should have a single mutant gene causes is also that of a syndrome. There are exceptions, and these will be discussed first.

Idiopathic hypertrophic subaortic stenosis is a dominantly inherited abiotrophy, the earliest diagnostic manifestations of which may be detected by echocardiography. It is not a cardiac maldevelopment as such, but a progressive disease of the myocardium. The gene for this disorder has been provisionally located on chromosome 6. Also provisionally assigned to chromosome 6 is the gene for the uncommon dominantly inherited form of atrial septal defect (ASD). Please note that the great majority of cases of ASD are not caused by single mutant genes, but are in the mode of multifactorial inheritance. There are also clearly autosomal dominant and recessive forms of conduction defects as well

as the possibility that other structural defects that are usually attributed to multifactorial inheritance may, in some families, follow a Mendelian pattern.

Since many genes are required in cardiac organogenesis, if one mutant gene is going to produce cardiac maldevelopment it should be a gene of large effect. In general, genes of large effect influence the development of more than one structure—thus the expectation of a syndrome rather than a discrete cardiac anomaly. But many of us working in the area of etiology of congenital heart diseases have seen and reported families with three generations of discrete congenital heart lesions, most often ASD. On closer scrutiny, some members of these families had associated minor anomalies of the hands, which could lead one to diagnose the dominantly inherited Holt-Oram syndrome. In some families no skeletal anomalies are apparent nor is there evidence of prolonged P-R interval. From the point of view of genetic counseling, the practical consideration in such infrequently encountered families, demonstrating direct inheritance through three generations, is that the recurrence risk is high—whether one categorizes the family as an autosomal dominant or a type C multifactorial inheritance family (to be discussed in the next section). A counseling example of this problem will be provided later in this section.

It is essential to recognize families in which the congenital heart defects are transmitted by Mendelian inheritance, because their risks are much higher than the usual families demonstrating multifactorial inheritance. It is typical that a congenital heart anomaly caused by a single mutant gene will be found as part of a syndrome and will have a 25% recurrence risk *of the syndrome* if the gene is recessive and a 50% recurrence risk if the gene is dominant. Congenital heart disease may not be present in everyone affected with the syndrome as will be demonstrated in the counseling examples which follow.

Tables 1.3 to 1.5 list some of the single mutant gene syndromes which have cardiovascular disease as part of the syndrome in a variable percentage of cases. The frequency of cardiovascular involvement as a part of the syndromes may range from 5 to almost 100%. We have tried to select syndromes which have a high enough recurrence risk of heart disease within the syndrome to warrant counseling for that specific problem.

Counseling Situations

Frequently it will be beneficial to consult with a clinical geneticist in counseling situations involving syndromes. Expertise in cardiovascular diagnosis does not necessarily imply similar expertise in the diagnosis of syndromes. However, there are clinical problems encountered with such frequency by pediatric cardiologists that the involvement of a geneticist is superfluous.

Clinical Example 1. A recently married young woman with ASD has only one sibling, and this sibling also has ASD. Their mother has ASD as well. The young woman wants to start her family and wants to know the risk of her child having ASD. The recurrence risk, shown in Table 1.6 is 2.5%, given only one first-degree relative with the heart defect.[15] The young woman seeking

TABLE 1.3   AUTOSOMAL RECESSIVE SYNDROMES WITH ASSOCIATED CARDIOVASCULAR ABNORMALITIES

Syndrome	Abnormality
Adrenogenital (21 and 3)	Hyperkalemia, broad QRS, arrhythmias
Alkaptonuria	Atherosclerosis, valve disease
Carpenter	PDA
Conradi	VSD, PDA
Cockayne	Accelerated atherosclerosis
Cutis laxa	Pulmonary hypertension, peripheral pulmonary artery stenosis
Cystic fibrosis	Cor pulmonale
Ellis-van Creveld	ASD, most commonly single atrium, and other CHD[a]
Friedreich ataxia	Myocardiopathy
Glycogenosis IIa, IIIa, and IV	Myocardiopathy
Homocystinuria	Coronary and other vascular thromboses
Jervell-Lange-Nielsen	Prolonged QT, sudden death
Laurence-Moon-Biedl	VSD and other CHD
Mucolipidosis III	Aortic valve disease
Mucopolysaccharidosis (MPS) IH (Hurler)	Coronary artery disease, aortic and MI
MPS IS (Scheie), MPS IV (Morquio) MPS VI (Maroteaux-Lamy)	Aortic valve disease, coronary artery disease
Osteogenesis imperfecta	Aortic valve disease
Progeria	Accelerated atherosclerosis
Pseudo-xanthoma elasticum	Coronary insufficiency, MI, hypertension
Riley-Day	Episodic hypertension, postural hypotension
Refsum's	Atrioventricular (AV) conduction defects
Seckel	VSD, PDA
Sickle cell disease	Myocardiopathy, MI
Smith-Lemli-Opitz	VSD, PDA, and other CHD
Thrombocytopenia and absent radius (TAR)	ASD, TF, dextrocardia
Thalassemia major	Myocardiopathy
Weill-Marchesani	PDA
Werner's	Vascular sclerosis

[a] Abbreviations used are CHD, congenital heart disease; MI, mitral insufficiency; TF, telralogy of Fallot.

TABLE 1.4   AUTOSOMAL DOMINANT SYNDROMES WITH ASSOCIATED CARDIOVASCULAR ABNORMALITIES

Syndrome	Abnormality
Apert	VSD, TF
Crouzon	PDA, CA
Ehlers-Danlos	Rupture of large blood vessels, e.g., carotids, dissecting aneurysms of the aorta
Familial periodic paralysis	Hypokalemia, supraventricular tachycardia
Forney	MI
Holt-Oram	ASD, VSD
Idiopathic hypertrophic subaortic stenosis (IHSS)	Subaortic muscular hypertrophy
Leopard	PS[a], prolonged P-R interval, abnormal p waves
Lymphedema (Milroy and Meige)	Lymphedema
Marfan	Great artery aneurysms, AI, MI
Myotonic-dystrophy (Steinert)	Myocardiopathy
Neurofibromatosis	PS, pheochromocytoma with hypertension, CA
Noonan	PS, ASD, IHSS
Osler-Weber-Rendu	Multiple telangiectasias, pulmonary arteriovenous fistulas
Osteogenesis imperfecta	AI
Romano-Ward	Prolonged Q-T, sudden death
Treacher Collins	VSD, PDA, ASD
Tuberous sclerosis	Myocardial rhabdomyoma
Von Hippel-Lindau	Hemangiomas, pheochromocytoma with hypertension

[a] Abbreviations used are: PS, pulmonary stenosis; AI, aortic insufficiency.

TABLE 1.5   X-LINKED RECESSIVE AND DOMINANT (R AND D) SYNDROMES WITH ASSOCIATED CARDIOVASCULAR ABNORMALITIES

Syndrome	Abnormality
MPS II (Hunter) (X-R)	Coronary artery disease, valve disease
Muscular dystrophy (Duchenne) (X-R)	Myocardiopathy
Muscular dystrophy (Dreifuss) (X-R)	Myocardiopathy
Incontinentia pigmenti, (X-D)	Patent ductus arteriosus
Goltz (X-D)	Occasional congenital heart defects, telangiectasia

counseling is the only first-degree relative with ASD, as far as her prospective baby is concerned. Her husband is free of heart disease and they have no other children. The young woman has no stigmata of Holt-Oram syndrome, no prolongation of the P-R interval, and her mother and sister, who are not available for examination, are reported to be free of limb anomalies.

First, should the young woman receive low-risk or high-risk counseling? Clearly, there are too many close relatives with ASD to consider that she has a low risk for her offspring. Is she a member of a family with autosomal dominant transmission of the heart defect? Possibly. And it is also possible that if we had examined her mother closely, we would find that she has some proximal displacement of her thumb (Holt-Oram). But even in the absence of associated anomalies, this should be considered a high-risk family, and we would suggest a 50% recurrence risk. We might, in the absence of associated abnormalities, prefer a type C multifactorial inheritance designation to autosomal dominant inheritance. However, this is academic. What is important is to recognize from the high frequency of disease in close relatives that this should prove to be a high-risk family.

Clinical Example 2. This short, bright-looking 5-year-old girl with long blonde hair and a somewhat unusual facies has clinical evidence of pulmonic stenosis. When her hair was drawn back it was observed that her ears were low-set and her neck was slightly webbed. A number of other stigmata plus a positive buccal smear helped establish the diagnosis of Noonan syndrome. On closer inspection it was noted that her mother was also quite short and wore her long hair loosely to cover prominent ears and minimal webbing of the neck. The mother and child had the same syndrome. There were no other children and there had been two miscarriages since the birth of this little girl. Whereas the child had severe pulmonary valve stenosis and an ASD, the mother had no heart murmur to suggest the presence of a cardiac anomaly. However, echocardiography revealed a thickened left ventricle (LV) with a septal/LV wall ratio of 1.7:1.

The family was counseled that the recurrence risk for the autosomal dominant Noonan syndrome was one in two and that approximately one-half of the patients with the syndrome have cardiovascular involvement.[15] Therefore the chance that the next child would have heart disease was $\frac{1}{2} \times \frac{1}{2}$ or $\frac{1}{4}$. It was emphasized that the heart disease could vary from a defect severe enough to require surgery (as in the child) to an abnormality so mild as to produce no symptoms (as in the mother).

There are differences in philosophy of genetic counseling. The usual approach is to present the risks objectively and to allow the decision regarding future children to be made by the family.[13, 15] Some families elect to accept high risks and others refuse to accept even low risks. As for the high-risk situations presented here, the family with ASD in two generations opted for pregnancy. Their first child was a boy free of heart disease and their second was a girl with atrial and ventricular septal defects. Following the birth of the second child the family decided against having further children. In the Noonan family, a decision against future pregnancies was made at the counseling session.

PRIMARILY ENVIRONMENTAL FACTORS

Recently we have had to add this category to our classification, as our thinking has been modified over the years. In the past we were willing to lump these cases in the multifactorial inheritance group, while acknowledging that the environmental considerably outweighed the genetic contribution.

RUBELLA

We have evidence that rarely is there a positive family history in some cases of VSD and PDA in the rubella syndrome. However, the majority of cases of PDA and all cases we have investigated of peripheral pulmonary artery stenosis are without a positive family history, making us feel that the genetic contribution is negligible.[13]

The percentage of patients who have rubella syndrome varies with time and place. During the rubella pandemic of 1964–1965, 2 to 3% of our pediatric cardiovascular patients in Houston had rubella syndrome. Reviewing the etiologies in the multicenter Natural History Study, we found that 2% of pulmonary valve stenosis patients enrolled in the study in the 1960's had rubella syndrome. In 1977, in Denver, far fewer than 1% of our patients had rubella syndrome. Now, we are inclined to use 1% as representative of rubella syndrome as a cause of congenital cardiovascular disease in children.

OTHER

A recent cause of cardiovascular disease that is essentially environmental (but postnatal environmental) is the aggressive perinatal care of premature infants leading to a frequency of PDA in high-risk premature nurseries that varies from 20 to 50%.

There are other prenatal environmental triggers which may not require a significant genetic predisposition. Thalidomide is a case in point. Perhaps cytomegalovirus and lithium chloride may prove to be teratogenic without requiring an important polygenic predisposition in the host. We can only estimate at this time that approximately 1% of congenital heart disease fall in this category.

GENETIC-ENVIRONMENTAL INTERACTION
MULTIFACTORIAL INHERITANCE

The majority of cases of congenital heart disease fall into this category of etiology. The situations in which the factors are primarily genetic or primarily environmental are uncommon. It is the situation in which there is a hereditary predisposition to cardiovascular maldevelopment which interacts with an environmental trigger (e.g., virus or drug) at the vulnerable period of cardiogenesis that appears to be the etiologic basis for most congenital cardiovascular anomalies.

This is called multifactorial inheritance which should *not* be taken as a vague, nonspecific category, meaning only "many factors." It is a specific mode of inheritance just as Mendelian inheritance is. There are mathematical models of multifactorial inheritance which vary from relatively simple ones to quite complex ones. The essential ingredients are that: the individual must be genetically predisposed to cardiovascular maldevelopment; there must also be a genetic predisposition to react adversely to the environmental teratogen; and the environmental insult must occur at the vulnerable period of cardiac development very early in pregnancy.

We have used a construction metaphor to illustrate how we visualize the development of the heart.[13] Consider that it requires the products of a lot of different genes to build a ventricular septum—genes-specifying structural proteins, genes-specifying enzymes— and there is a precise timetable which must be followed. The correct building blocks must be laid in the correct sequence and speed. The contribution from the endocardial cushions, conus, and ventricular septum must arrive at precisely the correct time for the ventricular septum to close. But if, for example, the contribution from the endocardial cushions is a little late in arriving or there are some minor deficiencies of building blocks, the septum will not close completely. The threshold from normal and abnormal development has been crossed. This is probably what happens in cardiac maldevelopment of the multifactorial inheritance mode. There is a precarious balance of many genes which individually may be normal. This balance may be influenced by environmental triggers producing acceleration or delay of primary gene products, thus throwing off the schedule of orderly development.

Figure 1.2 illustrates this concept in terms of polygenic predisposition and developmental thresholds and shows that in some families there is no predisposition to congenital heart disease. Even the addition of strong environmental teratogens cannot push the threshold far enough to the left to produce cardiovascular maldevelopment (see type A family).

The next curve is that of the typical family with congenital heart disease as it presents itself in the counseling situation, the type B family in which there is one first-degree relative with a cardiovascular anomaly (e.g., a previously affected child). This family is established as having a genetic predisposition. The addition of an environmental trigger upsets the precarious balance, and maldevelopment may result. The recurrence risks when there is only one affected first-degree relative are given in Table 1.7. The figure to remember for the range of recurrence risk is 1 to 4%; the more common the heart defect, the more likely it is to recur. So VSD would be more likely to recur in a family than tricuspid atresia.

In Tables 1.6 and 1.7, in contrast to the previous edition in which only personal or single series data were offered, the suggested recurrence risk figures in the far column to the right are combined from many series in the literature. In most cases the figures from our own series and the combined series are very close. We now use the recurrence risk data from the combined series.

The next point of counseling information is that the risk in multifactorial inheritance increases rapidly with the number of affected first-degree relatives. If there are two affected

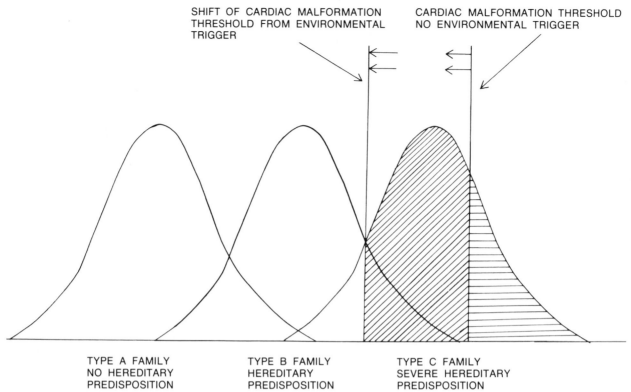

SHIFT OF CARDIAC MALFORMATION
THRESHOLD FROM ENVIRONMENTAL
TRIGGER

CARDIAC MALFORMATION THRESHOLD
NO ENVIRONMENTAL TRIGGER

TYPE A FAMILY
NO HEREDITARY
PREDISPOSITION

TYPE B FAMILY
HEREDITARY
PREDISPOSITION

TYPE C FAMILY
SEVERE HEREDITARY
PREDISPOSITION

Fig. 1.2 Three hypothetical curves of polygenic predisposition to congenital heart disease and the threshold of environmental influence. Moving the threshold to the left by introducing an environmental teratogen produces congenital cardiac maldevelopment in a small percentage of patients in the usual low-risk type B family, in a high percentage of patients in the uncommon high-risk type C family, and does not cause congenital heart disease in the type A family which has no genetic predisposition. The genetic component in the high-risk type C family is so great that an environmental trigger may not be required to produce maldevelopment in a proportion of cases.

TABLE 1.6   AFFECTED OFFSPRING: GIVEN ONE PARENT WITH A CONGENITAL HEART DEFECT: PERSONAL SERIES AND SUGGESTED RISK FROM COMBINED DATA[a]

Anomaly	No. Offspring	%	Suggested Risk %
VSD	7/174	4	4
PDA	6/139	4.3	4
ASD	5/199	2.5	2.5
TF	6/141	4.2	4
PS	4/111	3.6	3.5
CA	7/253	2.7	2
AS	4/103	3.9	4

[a] From J. J. Nora and A. H. Nora.[15]

TABLE 1.7   RECURRENCE RISKS GIVEN ONE SIBLING WHO HAS A CARDIOVASCULAR ANOMALY: PERSONAL SERIES AND SUGGESTED RISKS DERIVED FROM COMBINED DATA[a]

Anomaly	Probands	Affected No.	Sibling %	Suggested Risk %
VSD	306	28/672	4.2	3
PDA	220	18/516	3.5	3
ASD	172	11/380	2.9	2.5
TF	180	11/366	3.0	2.5
PS	166	10/375	2.7	2
CA	131	5/281	1.8	2
AS	155	8/361	2.2	2
TGA	116	4/229	1.7	2
AV canal	73	4/151	2.6	2
EFE[b]	119	11/286	3.8	4
TA	52	1/98	1.0	1
Ebstein's anomaly	47	1/105	1.0	1
Truncus arteriosus	43	1/86	1.2	1
PA	36	1/80	1.3	1
Hypoplastic left heart	164	8/370	2.2	2

[a] From J. J. Nora, and A. H. Nora.[15]

[b] EFE, endocardial fibroelastosis; TA, tricuspid atresia.

first-degree relatives, the risk is approximately tripled. To illustrate, if there has been only one child with a VSD the risk to the next child is approximately 5%, but if there have been two children or a parent and one child, the risk to the next child is approximately 15%.

This leads to the rare, unfortunate type of family we have called the type C family. Here the genetic balance is so precarious that the majority of first-degree relatives will have cardiac maldevelopment—probably even without much insult from the environment. The risk becomes higher even than in Mendelian inheritance. In autosomal recessive inheritance, the risk is fixed at 25%, and in dominant inheritance at 50%; but in multifactorial inheritance, the risk may exceed 50%. We have had the experience of working with many of these families and have concluded that if there are three affected first-degree relatives, the family should be

considered type C, and the recurrence risk may be higher than Mendelian risks.

In summary, the risk of congenital heart disease in subsequent pregnancies after the birth of an affected child with no affected parent is approximately 1 to 4%, depending on how common the heart defect is. If there are two affected first-degree relatives, the risk is tripled. If there are three affected first-degree relatives, the family is probably a type C with a very high recurrence risk. These factors apply to the majority of counseling situations.

RISKS TO OFFSPRING OF AN AFFECTED PARENT

We are gradually accumulating data to answer the inevitable questions of our congenital heart patients as they grow to maturity and wish to make plans for families of their own. What are the chances that their children will have congenital heart disease? Much of what has been discussed previously applies here as well. It is certainly important in accumulating risk figures to be precise in the categorization of the etiologic modes and the specific lesions involved. To say that X% of the children of adults who have congenital heart disease also have congenital heart disease is meaningless at best and misleading at worst. An adult with pulmonic stenosis, who has no syndrome and no affected children, has a risk of 3% recurrence in the next child. If the adult has Noonan syndrome, the risk is 50% that the next child will have the syndrome, and 25% that there will be heart disease (most often pulmonic stenosis). One simply cannot mix the Mendelian and multifactorial inheritance patients. They have separate risks.

Table 1.6 displays suggested recurrence risks given one parent with a congenital heart defect. As in Table 1.7, the combined series is contrasted with our personal and single series data and is recommended for more definitive counseling. The specific anomalies are the seven most common malformations compatible with survival to a reproductive age. Care has been taken to eliminate families showing Mendelian inheritance, since the one in four and one in two risks for this type of inheritance are well known, and to mix Mendelian and multifactorial cases would give incorrect recurrence risks for both modes of inheritance. It is the multifactorial inheritance risks that need to be developed, and these are shown in Table 1.6.

We have had an example in which both parents had congenital heart defects; one had VSD and the other had AS. These young people married after becoming acquainted on our service over the years of diagnostic evaluation, surgery, and postsurgical examinations. We are concerned about patients with the same congenital heart lesion marrying, on the grounds that children of such a marriage will start with the relatively high risk of two affected first-degree relatives. We also are concerned, but to a lesser degree, about marriages between individuals with different, and generally unrelated, cardiovascular defects, because of the possibility of a shared predisposition to maldevelopment, particularly of the cardiovascular system which may yield a higher but still undetermined risk of cardiac defects. This young couple has so far had only one child, and the child shows no evidence of heart disease.

ENVIRONMENTAL CONTRIBUTION TO THE GENETIC-ENVIRONMENTAL INTERACTION

The importance of the environmental contribution to the production of a congenital heart defect is becoming more clearly established as evidence rapidly accumulates. We are able to identify potentially teratogenic exposures to mothers of over half of our congenital heart patients. Proving that these "potential" teratogens are the environmental triggers is another story. A respiratory infection or "flu" in the first weeks of pregnancy may or may not have played a role. The probability that the infection was etiologic may be increased by demonstrating antiheart IgM—but definitive proof is still lacking. Table 1.8 lists agents which are clearly established or highly suspected of being associated with cardiovascular maldevelopment. As stated earlier, rubella and thalidomide appear to require very little interaction with a genetic predisposition. Better models for genetic-environmental interaction may be Coxsackie B and dextroamphetamine, which produce a lower frequency of cardiovascular malformations and, in the case of dextroamphetamine, clearly works with a genetic predisposition.[15]

There are probably a large number of teratogens, taken singly or in combination, which act as environmental triggers under the proper circumstances. The proper circumstances are: the subject is predisposed to the malformation (a type B or type C family); the subject is predisposed to react adversely to a given environmental agent; and the teratogenic exposure is at the vulnerable period of cardiogenesis. In addition, the typical teratogenic exposure is usually of short duration. A long exposure will frequently kill a susceptible fetus or not harm a fetus that is not susceptible.

The dangerous period for exposure to cardiac teratogens is early in pregnancy, just at the time a woman is beginning to wonder whether or not she is pregnant. Table 1.9 shows what we consider the limits and the most sensitive periods of vulnerability of the developing heart to teratogens. From the thalidomide data of Lenz[7] and from our own dextroamphetamine data,[13] it would appear that an effective teratogenic insult occurs between 1 and 2 weeks before the completion of the embryologic event. Therefore, when trying to decide on the role a teratogen might have played in the etiology of transposition of the great arteries, it could not be implicated if the exposure occurred after the 34th day and would not be likely to be responsible if it occurred after the 22nd day. The prime time for exposure would be day 20.

Given the right combination of predisposition to a heart defect and exposure at the vulnerable period of cardiac development, it is likely that a large number of drugs may be teratogenic. When dealing with a pregnancy in a family

TABLE 1.8   SELECTION OF POTENTIAL CARDIOVASCULAR TERATOGENS

Potential Teratogens	Frequency of CV Disease	Most Common Malformations
Drugs		
Alcohol	25–30%	VSD, PDA, ASD
Amphetamines	?5%	VSD, PDA, ASD, TGA
Anticonvulsants		
Hydantoin	2–3%	PS, AS, CA, PDA
Trimethadione	15–30%	TGA, TF, HLHS[a]
Chemotherapy	?5%	PS, AS, VSD, ASD
Lithium	10%	Ebstein, TA, ASD
Sex hormones	2–4%	VSD, TGA, TF
Thalidomide	5–10%	TF, VSD, ASD, truncus arteriosus
Infections		
Rubella	35%	Peripheral pulmonary artery stenosis, PDA, VSD, ASD
Maternal conditions		
Diabetes	3–5%	TGA, VSD, CA
	30–50%	Cardiomegaly and cardiomyopathy
Lupus	?	Heart block
Phenylketonuria	25–50%	TF, VSD, ASD

[a] HLHS, hypoplastic left heart.

TABLE 1.9   PRESUMED VULNERABLE PERIOD FOR TERATOGENIC INFLUENCE ON CARDIOVASCULAR DEVELOPMENT

Abnormality	Embryonic Event Completed (days)	Limits of Vulnerable Period	Most Sensitive Vulnerable Period (days)
Truncoconal septation	34	14–34	18–29
Endocardial cushions	38	14–38	18–33
Ventricular septum	38–44	14–44	18–39
Atrial septum secundum	55	14–55	18–50
Semilunar valves	55	14–?	18–50
Patent ductus arteriosus		14–?	18–60
Coarctation of aorta		14–?	18–60

having a first-degree relative with a congenital heart disease, indiscriminate use of drugs should be avoided.

Certainly drugs that have come under strong suspicion of a teratogenic role with regard to the heart should be considered guilty until proved innocent. It is clear that some drugs, including those strongly suspected of teratogenicity, cannot be eliminated from the regimens of pregnant women who require them. Other drugs, such as dextroamphetamine and progestogen pregnancy tests can be completely removed.

SPECIFIC COUNSELING SITUATIONS

Three families each presenting with a child with ventricular septal defect (VSD) will be discussed to illustrate the approaches to patients with different risks and/or etiologic mechanisms for the same cardiovascular malformation.

Clinical Example 1

This 13-month-old girl has been followed by our service since early infancy. Her clinical findings have been consistent with the diagnosis of a moderate-sized VSD without significant pulmonary hypertension. Her major problem has been a failure to grow satisfactorily despite medical management with digitalis and careful attention to caloric and sodium intake. Cardiac catheterization confirmed the diagnosis of VSD and revealed a shunt of almost equal magnitude at the atrial level. Pulmonary artery systolic pressure was 40 mm Hg, pulmonary arteriolar resistance was 2 units, and the total left to right shunt was 3 to 1. This child weighed 8 lbs at birth, 13 lbs at 8 months of age, and 14 lbs at 13 months of age. The options regarding early surgical intervention versus continued efforts at longer term medical management were discussed, and the decision for early surgery was made.

The parents had many questions about the cause of the heart defect and the possibility of recurrence. This was their only child; they wanted to increase their family soon, and they were aware of similar congenital heart disease in a first cousin. The pedigree is shown in Figure 1.3, and a positive teratogenic history had been obtained earlier as part of our routine evaluation. Maternal exposures to potential teratogens in the first weeks of pregnancy were many—including analgesics, decongestants, antihistamines, and antinausea medications.

The genetic history revealed no other first-degree relative with a congenital heart defect, only the cousin who apparently had VSD and pulmonic stenosis. In the framework of the type A, B, and C families shown in Figure 1.2, where would this family fall? Since there obviously is congenital heart disease in the family, it is not type A. And since there are not three or more affected *first-degree* relatives, the family is not type C. This is clearly the most common type of family and counseling situation we encounter in congenital heart disease, a type B family with one affected first-degree relative.

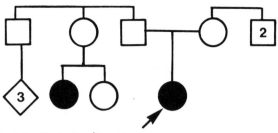

Fig. 1.3 Typical family with the common, low-risk type B predisposition to congenital heart disease (see text).

What is the recurrence risk? The range is 1 to 5% for all congenital heart lesions. The more common the defect, the higher is the risk. Ventricular septal defect, which appears to be the main lesions in this family, is the most common congenital heart anomaly. Therefore, without looking at Table 1.6 one would know that the recurrence risk is approximately 5%. But feel free to refer to Table 1.6 to confirm the risk. This family has not had another child, but on the basis of the predicted low recurrence risk they have decided to have a child in the near future.

Clinical Example 2

The family in Figure 1.4 represents a typical type C family with ventricular septal defects.[13, 15] Because there are at least three affected first-degree relatives, the recurrence risk may be predicted from what has already been experienced in this family. There have been 10 pregnancies; these include four stillbirths, and six livebirths. Five of the liveborn infants had VSD, and one died early of his disease. It is unusual to have such a large history of previous pregnancies on which to make predictions. Rather than counsel that a type C family has a "high" recurrence risk, one can base the counseling on what has already happened in this family: 10 pregnancies producing only one normal child, giving a 90% recurrence risk. An environmental contribution to this situation may be postulated. The family resided at an altitude of 7000 feet. Leaving their residence and business for a lower altitude did not seem possible. The surgical repair of the child with severe disease was highly satisfactory. On religious grounds the family did not consider abrogating future pregnancies.

Clinical Example 3

An infant presented to our service at 1 day of age in severe heart failure. Cardiac catheterization confirmed the clinical diagnosis of Ebstein's anomaly. There was no history of congenital heart disease in the family, but the mother volunteered that she had taken lithium chloride during her pregnancy for a manicdepressive disorder. We immediately remembered another case of an association of maternal exposure to lithium chloride and Ebstein's anomaly in our series. We then reviewed all of the teratogenic histories we had taken during the time period that these two cases were ascertained. In 733 teratogenic histories there were only two recorded maternal exposures to lithium chloride and in both cases the infant had Ebstein's anomaly. We have combined our cases with those recorded in the Lithium Registry of exposures to this agent during pregnancy.[18] The most recent summary of this experience is that of 141 maternal exposures to lithium chloride there have been 12 cases (8.5%) of congenital heart disease, 4 of which have been the relatively rare Ebstein's anomaly.

Our present assessment is that these cases belong in the category of genetic-environmental interaction because the frequency of malformations, while high, does not reach the level found in the thalidomide and rubella syndromes. Our counseling was that the recurrence risk for Ebstein's anomaly should only be approximately 1% *if* lithium were not consumed during the next pregnancy. Our major emphasis in this counseling situation was on the avoidance of a

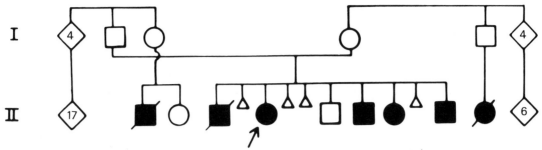

Fig. 1.4 Typical family with the uncommon high-risk type C predisposition to congenital heart disease (see text).

teratogen demonstrated to be associated with cardiac malformations. The mother no longer requires lithium and has stated that she will not take the drug during any subsequent pregnancy.

THE CHILD AT RISK OF ATHEROSCLEROSIS AS AN ADULT

Approximately 1% of individuals in American populations have a single gene hyperlipoproteinemia[15]; however, atherosclerotic disease is responsible for almost half of deaths in the United States. Clearly, the vast majority of these deaths result from a complex process in which heredity and environment interact as is shown in Figure 1.5. The most important single risk factor in our studies is early onset coronary heart disease in a first-degree relative (e.g., parent, sibling, child) less than 55 years of age.[14] About 20% of individuals with coronary disease beginning before age 55 have a single gene form of hyperlipoproteinemia.[4] In a study of the Mormon pedigrees in Utah, 85% of coronary heart disease clusters in only 16% of families.[22] We have calculated the heritability of early onset coronary heart disease at 63%—and if one excludes the single gene forms of the disease, the heritability still remains high at 57%.[14].

Our estimates are that at least 10% of individuals are at high genetic risk of early onset coronary heart disease.[11] There is possibly an equal percentage of individuals who have very low susceptibility to atherosclerotic vascular disease. One factor in low susceptibility may reside in the tissue type HLA-DR4.[12] The remaining 80% of the population is at intermediate risk. In this intermediate risk category environmental factors, such as diet, smoking, and aerobic exercise, may be manipulated with a very high expectation of success. Even within the high risk category of 10% of the population, environmental manipulation will reduce lipid elevations to acceptable levels in 9 of 10 individuals. In the high-risk group, the diets have to be more restrictive and the commitment to aerobic exercise more profound, but preventive programs without pharmacologic or surgical intervention are promising for all but that 1% of the population who have the single gene hyperlipoproteinemias.

The single gene hyperlipoproteinemias are most readily recognized by family studies.[11, 12, 14] Within such families there are clearly two populations of cholesterol values. Affected adults will have cholesterol determinations ranging from 270 to 350 mg/dl. Unaffected adults will usually be below 220. Affected children will usually have values above 240. Unaffected children will usually be below 190. The polygenic forms of the hyperlipidemia will follow a normal distribution curve around a mean of about 250 in adults and 220 in children. So there are two population curves in the single gene families and one curve in the polygenic families.

Another way to distinguish between the single gene abnormalities is the poor response to diet as compared with the polygenic form of hyperlipoproteinemia. However, for

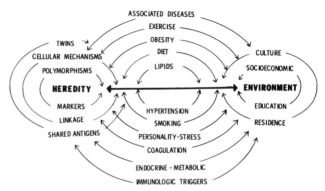

Fig. 1.5 The genetic-environmental interaction underlying atherosclerosis.

preschool children we usually favor diet alone, even if control is less than optimal. For school-age children and beyond, resins and nicotinic acid, each in as low a dose as possible, may be used to supplement strict diet in the single gene heterozygote. For the homozygote (type IIa) who runs cholesterol levels in the vicinity of 1000 mg/dl, early aggressive surgical intervention must be considered. We have seen children as young as 18 months of age suffer fatal myocardial infarction. The most effective surgical intervention in our experience for those with the double dose of the gene for the particularly disastrous type IIa familial hypercholesterolemia is portacaval shunt.[15]

It is of interest that the gene for familial hypercholesterolemia may be closely linked to the HLA genes in the major histocompatibility complex. Certainly the data from that 1% of the population that has the single mutant gene forms of hyperlipoproteinemia has proved most informative in our understanding cellular mechanisms of regulation. The membrane receptors for lipoprotein and the interaction with HMG CoA reductase have provided a model for our investigation of complex metabolic processes.[4] Portacaval shunts for the type IIa homozygote represents perhaps the first exploratory effort in metabolic surgery.[15]

What we must bear in mind, however, is that as exciting as these advances are, they are not relevant to the vast majority of children at risk of atherosclerosis as adults. For this significant percentage of the pediatric population, there are effective means of identifying in early childhood those at risk and instituting preventive programs[12] that should prove highly effective in forestalling early onset coronary disease, while promoting the possibility of normal life and life expectancy. The approach is a direct attack on the specific risk factors that can be identified in the child and in his family. The earlier an appropriate preventive program is instituted, the more effective one would predict it should be. Hypercholesterolemia begins to track after 4 months of age and certainly before 2 years of age.[3] Dietary management is appropriate in the preschool child and beyond. The commitment to aerobic exercise, abrogation of smoking, blood pressure control, and encouragement of type B behavior patterns is also effectively established in childhood.[11, 12]

ESSENTIAL HYPERTENSION

The genetic basis of essential (primary) hypertension has been rather vigorously debated over the past 2 decades, with Pickering[19] and his group advocating the polygenic nature of the hereditary predisposition and Platt[20] defending the concept that major genes were responsible. A position of accommodation has been reached in the minds of many investigators. The large effect of a major gene and the additive small effects of many genes may operate at the hereditary pole of the continuum in Figure 1.1. The interacting environmental factors of concern are salt and stress. The striking familial nature of essential hypertension is such that we hesitate to diagnose primary hypertension in a young person unless there is a positive family history.

Many questions regarding the diagnosis and treatment of primary and secondary hypertension in pediatric patients are approached in the chapter in this volume on hypertension. What has become apparent from both the study of animal models and human subjects is that the earlier preventive and therapeutic interventions are instituted the more successful are the outcomes.

RHEUMATIC FEVER

It is ironic that the major cardiovascular disease most dependent on an environmental factor is the first one that was subjected to a systematic genetic analysis.[23] Before the etiologic role of the streptococcus was widely accepted, the possibilities of autosomal dominant, recessive, and X-linked inheritance of rheumatic fever were tested, and the conclusion was reached that the susceptibility to rheumatic fever was transmitted as an autosomal recessive trait. For several years after group A beta hemolytic streptococcal infections were clearly implicated in the etiology of rheumatic fever, the proponents of genetic susceptibility continued to promote the hypothesis of genetic susceptibility. Eventually, even the strongest advocates of the hereditary basis of rheumatic fever were no longer heard. Now, from what we are learning about the susceptibility to autoimmune disease as it relates to histocompatibility, HLA loci, specific HLA antigens, and linkage disequilibrium, it may be that the hypothesis of some type of genetic susceptibility had merit after all. Our own unpublished preliminary investigations are compatible with the idea of HLA-associated susceptibility.

REFERENCES

1. Anders, J. M., Moores, E. C., and Emanuel, R.: Chromosome studies in 156 patients with congenital heart disease. Br. Heart J. 27:756–765, 1965.
2. Anderson, R. C.: Causative factors underlying congenital heart malformations. I. Patent ductus arteriosus. Pediatrics 14:143–151, 1954.
3. Darmady, J. M., Fosbrooke, A. S., and Lloyd, J. K.: Prospective study of serum cholesterol levels during first year of life. Br. Med. J. 2:685–687, 1972.
4. Fredrickson, D. S., Goldstein, J. L., and Brown, M. S.: The familial hyperlipoproteinemias. In The Metabolic Basis of Inherited Disease, 3rd ed., edited by J. S. Stanbury, J. B. Wyngaarden, and D. S. Fredrickson. McGraw-Hill, New York, 1978.
5. Fuhrmann, W.: Genetische und peristatische Urasachen angeborener Angiokardiopathien, Ergeb. Inn. Med. Kinderheilkd. 18:47–115, 1962.
6. Lamy, M., DeGrouchy, J., and Schweisguth, O.: Genetic and non-genetic factors in the etiology of congenital heart disease: A study of 1188 cases. Am. J. Hum. Genet. 9:17–41, 1957.
7. Lenz, W., and Knapp, K.: Die Thalidomid-

Embryopathie. Dtsch. Med. Wochenschr. 87:1232–1242, 1962.
8. McKeown, T., MacMahon, B., and Parson, C. G.: The familial incidence of congenital malformations of the heart. Br. Heart J. 15:273–277, 1953.
9. McKusick, V. A.: A genetic view of cardiovascular disease. Circulation 30:326–357, 1964.
10. Nora, J. J.: Multifactorial inheritance hypothesis for the etiology of congenital heart diseases: The genetic environmental interaction. Circulation 38:604–617, 1968.
11. Nora, J. J.: The Whole Heart Book. Holt, Rinehart and Winston, New York, 1980.
12. Nora, J. J.: Identifying the child at risk of coronary disease as an adult: A strategy for prevention. J. Pediatr. 97:706–714, 1980.
13. Nora, J. J., and Fraser, F. C.: Medical Genetics: Principles and Practice, 2nd ed. Lea & Febiger, Philadelphia, 1981.
14. Nora, J. J., Lortscher, R. H., Spangler, R. D., Nora, A. H., and Kimberling, W. J.: Genetic-epidemiologic study of early-onset ischaemic heart disease. Circulation 61:503–508, 1980.
15. Nora, J. J., and Nora, A. H.: Genetics and Counseling in Cardiovascular Diseases. Charles C Thomas, Springfield, Ill., 1978.

16. Nora, J. J., and Nora, A. H.: The evolution of specific genetic and environmental counseling in congenital heart diseases. Circulation 57:203–213, 1978.
17. Nora, J. J., Nora, A. H., Sinha, A. K., Spangler, R. D., and Lubs, H. A.: The Ullrich-Noonan syndrome (Turner phenotype). Am. J. Dis. Child 127:48–55, 1974.
18. Nora, J. J., Nora, A. H., and Toews, W. H.: Lithium, Ebsteins anomaly, and other congenital heart defects. Lancet 2:594–595, 1974.
19. Pickering, G. W.: High Blood Pressure, 2nd ed. Churchill, London, 1968.
20. Platt, R.: The natural history and epidemiology of essential hypertension. Practitioner 193:5, 1964.
21. Polani, P. E., and Campbell, M.: An aetiological study of congenital heart disease. Ann. Hum. Genet. 19:209–230, 1955.
22. Williams, R., Skolnick, M., Carmelli, D., Maness, A. T., Hunt, S. C., Sasstedt, S., Reiber, G. E., and Jones, R. K.: Utah pedigree studies: Preliminary data for premature male CHD deaths. Prog. Clin. Biol. Res. 32:711–729, 1979.
23. Wilson, M. G., and Schweitzer, M. D.: Rheumatic fever as a familial disease. J. Clin. Invest. 16:555–565, 1937.

2

Fetal and Neonatal Circulations

Forrest H. Adams, M.D.

Knowledge regarding the status of the normal fetal and neonatal circulation is essential not only because it helps to put cardiovascular disease in proper perspective, but also because it provides the necessary information that will permit advances in diagnosis and treatment of cardiovascular diseases. This is particularly true for the neonatal period. Since a significant percentage of infants born with heart disease succumb during the first months of life,[1, 41] efforts should be directed toward resolving this problem in infancy. Furthermore, such knowledge is important for a better understanding of the effects of postnatal circulatory adjustments in congenital heart disease.[55]

FETAL CIRCULATION

Physiologic studies of the human fetal circulation are so few that most of our current ideas are necessarily inferred from physiologic investigations in other mammals such as sheep or from autopsy examination of human fetal material. The recent literature on the fetal and neonatal pulmonary circulation has been extensively reviewed.[56]

SPECIAL FEATURES OF THE FETAL CIRCULATION

There are some aspects of the fetal circulation that make it quite different from the neonatal or adult circulation. These are:

1. Intra- and extracardiac shunts are present.
2. The two ventricles work in parallel rather than in series.
3. The right ventricle pumps against a higher resistance than the left ventricle.
4. Blood flow to the lung is only a fraction of the right ventricular output.
5. The lung extracts oxygen from the blood instead of providing oxygen for it.
6. The lung continually secretes a fluid into the respiratory passages.
7. The liver is the first organ to receive maternal substances, such as oxygen, glucose, amino acids, etc.
8. The placenta is the major route of gas exchange, excretion, and acquisition of essential fetal chemicals.
9. The placenta provides a low resistance circuit.

As early as 1628, William Harvey[27] described some of the anatomic and functional differences between the fetal and adult circulation. Only recently have we been able to quantitate some aspects of the various parameters, but this has been accomplished mainly in the animal and not in the human fetus.[14, 57, 58]

COURSE OF THE FETAL CIRCULATION

In a description of the course of the fetal circulation, it is only proper to begin with the placenta (Greek ΠΛΑΚΟΥΣ equals pancake). Here the fetus exchanges his metabolic end products for new sources of energy and metabolism such as oxygen, glucose, amino acids, fatty acids, fluids, and electrolytes. As shown in Figure 2.1, the nutritious material is collected from the placenta and proceeds up the umbilical vein to the fetus. Under normal circumstances, a significant proportion of the blood (50%) carrying these substances perfuses the liver parenchyma and then proceeds to the inferior vena cava via the hepatic veins. Another portion bypasses the liver via the ductus venosus and empties directly into the inferior vena cava. The exact physiologic significance of the ductus venosus is not yet clearly understood nor are the factors that control the flow of blood through it.[38] Apparently, not all species of mammals possess this structure at maturity. It is likely that control of the flow of blood through the liver is regulated by constriction and dilatation of the ductus venosus. It is also likely that disturbances of blood flow through it will be demonstrated in pathologic states in the future.

The blood returning via the umbilical vein empties into the inferior vena cava and joins the blood, which returns from the lower half of the body. Approximately one-third of the inferior vena caval blood passes through the foramen ovale into the left atrium, left ventricle, and ascending aorta. The remaining two-thirds goes into the right atrium, right ventricle, and pulmonary artery. The separation of the inferior vena caval blood stream into two parts is accomplished by the special anatomic relationship between the inferior vena cava, the two atria, and the foramen ovale. The entrance of the inferior vena cava is in line with the free edge of the interatrial septum (crista dividens), and thus there is direct functional communication between the cava and both atria.

Most of the blood returning from the upper part of the body via the superior vena cava empties into the right atrium and then passes into the right ventricle and pulmonary artery. The blood from the coronary sinus also follows a similar route. The output of the right ventricle goes in part to the lung, and the remainder passes through the ductus arteriosus into the descending aorta where it is joined by that blood ejected from the left ventricle through the aortic arch.

Although it is sometimes hazardous to apply information obtained from animal investigations directly to man, this appears warranted in regards to the course of the fetal circulation. Lind et al.[38] have summarized their findings obtained over many years on human fetuses delivered at the time of legal abortion by cesarean section, and in all essential respects the course is identical to that present in animals. The major criticism of these human investigations is the poor physiologic status of the fetus at the time the investigations were performed.[59] This no doubt affected the amount and distribution of blood flow to the various regions of the body.

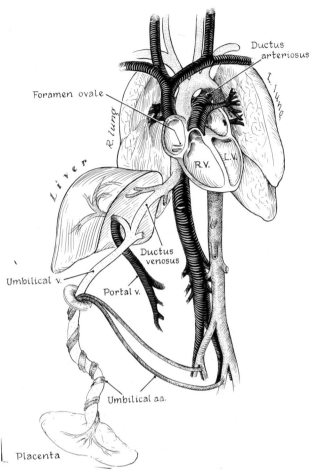

Fig. 2.1 Human fetal circulation. Intensity of dots within vessels indicates degree of oxygen desaturation of hemoglobin. Note possible course of blood from the placenta through the liver or through the ductus venosus to the inferior vena cava, and then to the heart. Note major sites of mixing of blood streams of varying oxygen content: portal vein, hepatic vein, inferior vena cava, foramen ovale, and ductus arteriosus.

FETAL CARDIAC OUTPUT AND RELATIVE REGIONAL FLOWS

Uterine blood flow and umbilical blood flow in the human seem to increase in a linear fashion throughout pregnancy. If certain assumptions are made, the effective cardiac output of the human fetus *in utero* is approximately 200 ml/kg/minute.[9] This estimate is not too dissimilar from the value of 164 ml/kg/minute obtained on normal newborn infants.[5, 19, 22]

Although the *course* of the flow of blood through the fetus is agreed upon by most investigators, the *relative flows* to the organs and regions of the body is not agreed upon. Differences in techniques used probably account for the variations in the results observed. It is the author's opinion that the radionuclide-labeled microsphere technique[57] in chronically instrumental fetal lambs probably gives the best static answers, but phasic changes are known to occur when electromagnetic flowmeters are used.[37]

In the term fetal lamb,[29, 58] 70% of the combined ventricular output goes to the lower part of the body and placenta, 20% to the upper body, 7% to the lungs, and 3% to the coronary arteries, as shown in Figure 2.2. Essentially, all the blood from the superior vena cava, from the coronary sinus, and about 60% from the inferior vena cava enters into the right atrium and then the right ventricle. About 67% of the

combined output is ejected by the right ventricle, and only 33% is ejected by the left ventricle.[58] As would be expected, the combined ventricular output increases with gestational age, but the proportions distributed to the organs change.[58] There is a gradual reduction in the percentage distributed to the placenta, and there is an increase in the percentage going to the brain, lungs, and gastrointestinal tract.

FETAL PULMONARY CIRCULATION

Although the pressures in the pulmonary artery and the aorta are nearly identical, the high pulmonary vascular resistance forces most of the right ventricular output through the ductus arteriosus into the descending aorta.[29, 56] Even so, prostaglandins, their inhibitors, and oxygen affect the contractile state of the fetal ductus arteriosus.[26, 34, 56]

The site of the high pulmonary vascular resistance in the fetal lung and the various factors that influence it are not completely understood at this time.[56] The regulation of pulmonary blood flow is probably under neurohumoral control, although mechanical and physical factors must also be considered.[14, 56] Epinephrine and norepinephrine cause pulmonary vasoconstriction. On the other hand, bradykinin, oxygen, acetylcholine, histamine, and isoproterenol produce pulmonary vasodilation.[14, 56] Fetal hypoxia causes pulmonary vasoconstriction,[14, 56] and the response to hypoxia increases with advancing gestation.[37]

An important point to consider is the significance of the blood flow to the lungs at a time when they are not actively involved in gas exchange, since the placenta performs this function for the fetus. Dawes[14] has found that the fetal lamb lung extracts about 1.6 ml of oxygen per 100 ml of blood flow. This indicates that the fetal lungs are metabolically active. Part of the metabolism is undoubtedly concerned with the growth of lung tissue itself. However, we also know that the fetal lung continually produces a fluid with a special chemical composition which, near term, contains increasing amounts of surfactant.[3] This special fluid distends the poten-

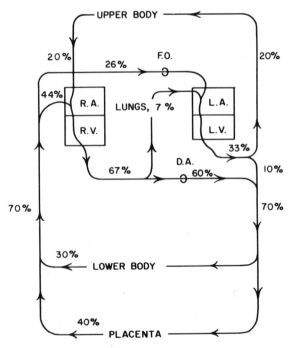

Fig. 2.2 Relative distribution of blood flow in the sheep fetus, given as percentages of the combined ventricular outputs. *F. O.*, foramen ovale; *D.A.*, ductus arteriosus. (Modified from M. A. Heymann and A. M. Rudolph.[29])

tial air spaces and is periodically discharged into the nose, throat, and amniotic cavity.[6] Following birth, all the fluid in the potential air spaces must be removed before normal gas exchange can occur. Studies in full-term newborn rabbits show that the fluid disappears slowly over a period of several days, initially more rapidly in those delivered vaginally as compared with those delivered by cesarean section.[7]

FETAL CARDIOVASCULAR REFLEXES

It was once believed that the fetus has a deficiency of autonomic nervous control. Recent studies show this not to be so. Stimulation of the carotid sinus or the peripheral end of the vagus nerve causes profound bradycardia.[14] Acute artificial elevation of the fetal lamb blood pressure produces the characteristic barostatic response seen in the adult.[4] Clinical factors known to affect the fetal heart rate which probably involve cardiovascular reflexes are: compression of the fetal skull, strong uterine contractions, maternal exercise, and smoking.[2] Finally, the fetal blood pressure in several animal species is known to rise during the course of gestation.[14]

FETAL ELECTROCARDIOGRAM

It is possible to record the fetal electrocardiogram if special instrumentation is used and care is taken with the placement of electrodes. Most investigators have used the electrocardiogram to determine evidence and signs of "fetal distress," but thus far it has proved to give only a crude estimate. The technique permits an accurate determination of the variation of the heart rate throughout pregnancy and labor as well as the amplitude and duration of the various electrical events. Congenital heart block, multiple pregnancy, and the position of the fetus can also be determined by its use.

Recently, M-mode and real-time two dimensional echocardiographic imaging techniques have been used to assess the structure and rhythm of the developing human heart.[32] Their value as an aid in the management of pregnancy and delivery remains to be demonstrated.

FETAL CARDIOVASCULAR ANATOMY

Placental Pathology

Placental insufficiency may be a major cause of "fetal distress." Infants born malnourished and retarded in growth may have been exposed to a prolonged period of intrauterine deprivation. Frequently, the placenta is small in size, and both gross and microscopic lesions such as microinfarcts and avascular villi are present.

The occurrence of a single umbilical artery is associated with a high incidence (50%) of major anomalies. It occurs in 1% of all births and 7% of twin pregnancies.[11]

In the intrauterine parabiotic syndrome, a transfer of blood between twins occurs through arteriovenous anastomoses in the placenta. Thus, one twin becomes polycythemic and the other anemic. Other differences occur as well.[46]

Heart

There are histologic differences in the amount of contractile tissue obtained from fetal, neonatal, and adult hearts. Friedman[20] has shown in sheep that these differences are associated with functional effects in that the fetal myocardium develops greater tension at rest and less active tension with contraction. Thus, the fetal heart is less compliant than that of the adult.

In some animal species, the sympathetic innervation of the heart is poorly developed in the fetus.[20] Its status in humans is uncertain at the present time.

The absolute and relative weights of the two ventricles have been determined during fetal life.[15] Prior to the 24th week, the left ventricle is usually heavier than the right. After about the 28th week of gestation, the right ventricle weighs more than the left. Quantitative measurements of the fetal coronary arteries, including the external diameter, medial thickness, and intimal thickness, show that all increase with age, with males having higher values than females at the same age.[48]

Pulmonary Artery and Aorta

The greater muscularity of the small pulmonary arteries during fetal life[13] has been invoked as the mechanism for the high pulmonary vascular resistance in the fetus. Recent studies suggest that normally there is no change during fetal life in the thickness of the muscular layers of these arteries in either the human[30] or the lamb.[36] However, factors that cause an increase in pulmonary hypertension during fetal life[34] seem to result in an increase in the muscle layers[26, 35] and may be a possible cause of persistent fetal circulation (PFC) in the newborn.[26, 35] The role of the "stretch" induced pulmonary hypertension in PFC remains to be elucidated.[10]

The fetal pulmonary artery has an elastic tissue configuration similar to that observed in the ascending aorta.[28] From about the 4th fetal month, the thickness of the fibers increases, their tortuosity decreases, and a well-defined parallel disposition is noticeable. In the last 3 months of prenatal life, the elastic configuration of the pulmonary artery and aorta is similar to that of the newborn infant. After birth, a transition occurs in this configuration which seems to take several months. It is postulated that the microscopic findings in the pulmonary artery are related to the pulmonary artery pressure and resistance. It is of particular interest that in those individuals living above 13,250 feet, the elastic tissue configuration of the pulmonary artery maintains the "aortic" type up to 9 years of age.[60] It is also known that children living at high altitudes maintain a certain degree of pulmonary hypertension.[61]

NEONATAL CIRCULATION

Two very important events take place immediately following birth. First, the infant takes his first breath of air, and second, the infant is separated from the placenta. For these and other reasons, the infant's circulation changes drastically at birth, but it does not immediately acquire the adult pattern, so the term neonatal or transitional circulation has been applied.

SPECIAL FEATURES OF THE NEONATAL CIRCULATION

Immediately after delivery, the cardiovascular system of the infant changes in the following ways:

1. The pulmonary vascular resistance decreases.
2. The pulmonary blood flow increases.
3. The systemic vascular resistance increases.
4. The blood flow through the ductus arteriosus becomes primarily left to right.
5. The foramen ovale closes.

The factor or factors that cause the infant to take his first breath are not yet clearly understood. Until he breathes, hypoxemia, hypercarbia, and acidosis are progressive. All three of these changes should act as a stimulus to breathing, yet often it is delayed. The possibility also exists that the compression of the chest during vaginal delivery might be followed by an elastic recoil which would initiate the first breath. Even though the infant's thoracic cage is considerably compressed, the intrathoracic pressure increasing to 50 to 100 cm of H_2O during its passage through the birth canal, an elastic recoil does not occur, and the first breath is unrelated to it.[31] Another factor that might play a role in initiating respiration is the increase in the number of sensory impulses which stimulate the neonate's central nervous system. The sudden change in environmental temperature, the change from a condition of relative weightlessness *in utero*, and the stimulation of the skin, all rudely awaken the sleeping newborn.

COURSE OF NEONATAL CIRCULATION

As soon as the infant is separated from the placenta, the systemic blood pressure increases temporarily due to the removal of this low resistance part of his circulation. With the first breath, pulmonary blood flow increases greatly, mainly due to a reduction in pulmonary vascular resistance, probably due to the combined effects of increased arterial partial pressure of oxygen and release of bradykinin.[14, 40] The role of prostaglandins remains unclear at present.[56]

With the simultaneous decrease in pulmonary vascular resistance and the increase in systemic vascular resistance, the blood flows through the ductus arteriosus from the aorta into the pulmonary artery. During the first few hours of extrauterine life, the left to right shunt through the ductus arteriosus is 30 to 50% of the left ventricular output. Thus, the amount of blood returning to the heart via the pulmonary veins is much greater than that of the fetal circulation. This distends the left atrium and increases the left atrial pressure, which in turn assists in the functional closure of the foramen ovale.

CLOSURE OF THE FORAMEN OVALE

Functional closure of the foramen ovale is incomplete immediately after birth. Right to left shunting through it has been reported in 50% of babies during crying up to 8 days of age.[52] As seen in Figure 2.3, probe patency of the

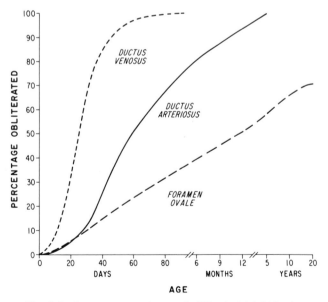

Fig. 2.3 Average percentages of obliterated fetal blood passages according to age. (Modified from R. E. Scammon and E. H. Norris.[62]) (Reproduced with permission from F. H. Adams: *Heart and Circulation in the Newborn and Infants*, edited by D. E. Cassels. Grune & Stratton, New York, 1966.

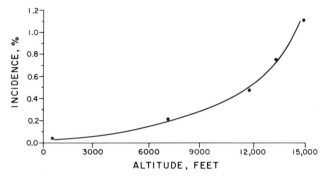

Fig. 2.4 Incidence of patent ductus arteriosus occurring in infants born at increasing altitudes. Modified from D. Penaloza *et al.*[50] Note that the incidence at 15,000 feet is almost 30 times that at sea level. (Reproduced with permission from F. H. Adams: *Heart and Circulation in the Newborn and Infants*, edited by D. E. Cassels. Grune & Stratton, New York, 1966.)

foramen ovale exists in 50% of individuals up to 5 years of age and in more than 25% over 20 years of age.[62] The foramen rarely closes prematurely *in utero*. When this happens, the infant develops right-sided cardiomegaly before birth and generally shows early signs of heart failure.[47]

CLOSURE OF THE DUCTUS ARTERIOSUS

During the early hours of life, a right to left, bidirectional, or left to right shunt may occur, depending upon a number of factors.[5, 43, 44, 53] A left to right shunt through the ductus arteriosus generally persists for 15 to 20 hours after birth, but it may last for several days.

A right to left or bidirectional shunt through the ductus arteriosus is uncommon in healthy infants and persists for only 1 hour after birth. Hypoxemia will produce or increase a right to left shunt. Thus, it is not surprising that persistent patency of the ductus arteriosus is found in those situations known to be associated with hypoxemia such as: neonatal distress,[54] prematurity,[51] and infants born at high altitidue.[50] As seen in Figure 2.4, the incidence at 15,000 feet altitude is almost 30 times that at sea level. Administration of 100% oxygen to infants under 15 hours of age will constrict the ductus, and 13% oxygen will cause it to dilate.[43] These responses are most pronounced during the first 3 hours of life.

The basic physiology of the various factors that control the ductus arteriosus is contained in an extensive review,[29] as well as in Chapter 11. The most important factor for closure is the constrictor effect of increased oxygen tension in the arterial blood. This response seems to be related to fetal age in that the response is stronger and occurs at lower oxygen tensions as the fetus approaches term. In term fetal lambs, the ductus arteriosus constricts strongly at an arterial pO_2 of 40 to 60 mm Hg.[64]

Studies on the isolated ductus arteriosus obtained from fetal lambs and guinea pigs show similar responses to variation in oxygen concentration.[33] These were independent of pH and CO_2 content within wide limits and were not abolished by high concentrations of cyanide. Epinephrine, norepinephrine, and acetylcholine also caused the ductus to contract, and these reactions could be abolished by either dibenamine or by atropine without affecting the response to oxygen. Bradykinin and prostaglandin inhibitors are also constrictors of the ductus.[29]

The role of the autonomic nervous system in closure of the ductus needs further research. Both sympathetic and parasympathetic nerve fibers are known to be present in the ductus in humans and some animal species.[29] Furthermore, their chemical mediators are known to be capable of constricting the ductus, and the effects of these mediators plus oxygen have been shown to be additive.[39]

Anatomic closure of the ductus arteriosus may begin soon after birth but, as shown in Figure 2.3, it is not obliterated in the majority of infants until several months of age, and in some not until a year of age.[62] Figure 2.5 shows the nature of the obliterative changes described by Gérard in 1900.[21] In the central portion, the obliteration occurs mainly by muscular contraction, whereas at either end a pad-like thickening of the intima and media occurs. The pads meet and coalesce in the center. Thrombosis occurs in the midportion. Recent histological studies on the ductus arteriosus would indicate that there are stages of maturation during gestation, and that those infants and children with a persistent ductus have a histological appearance which most resembles an immature ductus normally seen during the second and third trimesters of pregnancy.[23]

CARDIAC OUTPUT

The cardiac output immediately following birth is influenced by a number of critical factors such as: the degree of maternal anesthesia or analgesia; the nature of the delivery; early vs. late clamping of the umbilical cord; environmental conditions; body temperature; and the magnitude of intra- and extracardiac shunts. As shown in Table 2.1, the mean systemic blood flow ranges from 2.3 to 3.1 liters/minute/m² of body surface, depending upon the investigator and the techniques used.[5, 19, 22, 53] Babies born by the vaginal route have slightly higher outputs than those delivered by cesarean section.[22] The stroke volume of the newborn is approximately 4 cc.

OTHER ASPECTS OF CARDIAC FUNCTION

The transverse diameter of the heart of mature healthy infants is larger in those subjected to stripping of the umbilical cord or to asphyxiation, and the effects are additive.[12] This is probably due to the increased blood volume given to or withheld from the infant by early or late clamping of the

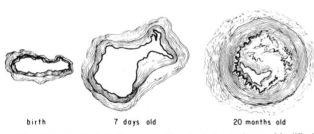

birth   7 days old   20 months old

Fig. 2.5 Postnatal changes in the ductus arteriosus. Modified from Gérard.[21] (Reproduced with permission from F. H. Adams: *Heart and Circulation in the Newborn and Infant*, edited by D. E. Cassels. Grune & Stratton, New York, 1966.)

umbilical cord.[63] Delayed clamping of the cord also has the effect of producing infants with higher blood pressures and higher respiratory rates for the first 24 hours of life.[8, 49]

Using indirect methods, the isovolumic contraction and ejection times of the left ventricle have been determined.[24] Initially, the isovolumic contraction time is prolonged, but after several days of age it approaches normal values for childhood. This implies improvement in the contractility of the heart, which in turn might be related to alterations in catecholamine metabolism.

Echographic techniques can also be used to measure both right and left ventricular function in neonates.[25] Normal values have been established, and it is anticipated that the technique will be helpful in the management of certain neonatal cardiovascular problems.

PULMONARY AND SYSTEMIC ARTERIAL PRESSURES

Pulmonary arterial pressure does not fall abruptly after the establishment of respiration, even though there is a marked decrease in pulmonary vascular resistance. This helps to explain why the shunt through the ductus arteriosus may occasionally be right to left or bidirectional for the 1st hour after birth of the infant. As shown in Figure 2.6, the mean systolic pressure approximates that in the aorta during the first few hours of life and is accompanied by a drop in diastolic pressure. The mean pulmonary arterial pressure approaches the 50% value of mean systemic pressure by the end of the 1st day.[18] Normal adult values for pulmonary arterial pressure probably are not reached for several days or weeks. The factors contributing to the elevated pulmonary pressure and resistance are likely a combination of the following:

1. Pulmonary vasoconstriction due to hypoxemia and acidosis.
2. Increased pulmonary blood flow due to the left to right shunt through the ductus arteriosus.
3. The reduced volume of the pulmonary vascular bed due to the presence of medial hypertrophy of the small pulmonary arteries.
4. Delayed clamping of the umbilical cord.

The gradual decrease in pulmonary arterial pressure and vascular resistance over the next few weeks of life is most likely the result of involutionary changes in the wall of the small pulmonary arteries. Infants born at high altitude tend to maintain some degree of pulmonary hypertension, and histologic examination of their pulmonary arterioles shows a tendency toward persistence of the fetal pattern.

CARDIOVASCULAR REFLEXES

Since the fetus possesses many of the known cardiovascular reflexes, it is not surprising that the neonate does also. The barostatic receptors are active in the newborn infant. Both the premature and the full-term infant respond to the cold pressor test and postural tilting, indicating the presence of vasomotor regulatory mechanisms.[42]

TABLE 2.1 CARDIAC OUTPUT AND PULMONARY BLOOD FLOW OF THE NEWBORN INFANT

Author and Year	No. of Infants	Age of Infants	Systemic Blood Flow (liters/min/m²)		Pulmonary Blood Flow (liters/min/m²)		Left to Right Shunt (%)	Method of Study
			Average	Range	Average	Range		
Prec and Cassels[53]	10	2–26 hr	2.5	0.9–3.7	2.5	0.9–3.7	0	Indicator dilution
Adams and Lind[5]	10	7 hr–14 days	2.3	1.1–4.2	3.2	1.5–5.9	0–59	Fick
Gessner et al.[22]	14	1 hr	2.6	2.9–3.4	4.0	2.8–5.4	28–49	Indicator dilution
Emmanouilides et al.[19]	23	6–35 hr	3.1	1.4–5.1	4.1	1.6–6.3	0–44	Indicator dilution

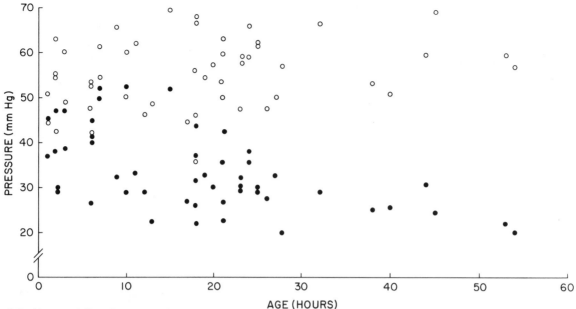

Fig. 2.6　Mean systolic pulmonary and systemic arterial pressures in normal infants according to age after birth. ●, pulmonary artery; ○, aorta. (Reproduced with permission from G. C. Emmanouilides et al.[18])

ELECTROCARDIOGRAM

No change occurs in the electrocardiogram in normal infants after the first breath. Those infants who experience difficulty in establishing respiration show a greater deviation of the electrical axis to the right. The postnatal hemodynamic changes are reflected in the electrocardiogram of the normal newborn infant.[17] Upright T waves in the right precordial leads are associated with significantly higher pulmonary arterial pressures. A R/S ratio less than one in the right precordial leads is observed only in infants with left to right shunts through the ductus arteriosus, whereas a R/S ratio of more than one in V_6 is associated with a lower pulmonary to systemic arterial pressure ratio.

CARDIOVASCULAR ANATOMY

The changes in the small pulmonary and systemic arterial beds of normal infants follow a distinct pattern.[45] Hypoxemia, however, seems to arrest the relative involution of smooth muscle in the pulmonary arterial bed. After birth, the muscle mass in the systemic bed continues to increase while the pulmonary mass undergoes a relative decrease. As stated earlier, at birth, the right ventricle weighs more than the left, but this is reversed by 4 weeks of age.[16]

CLINICAL IMPLICATIONS

The majority of congenital heart lesions seen in infancy and childhood create no serious problem for the infant during intrauterine life. This is because both ventricles work in parallel and unless the lesion, usually a stenosis, is very extreme, the output of the nonobstructed ventricle can take over for the other. Intrauterine heart failure is rarely observed. When it occurs, it is usually associated with prenatal narrowing or closure of the foramen ovale or with intrauterine tachycardia.

Theoretically, severe coarctation of the aorta of the adult or abdominal type should be incompatible with normal intrauterine life (unless early and extensive collateral blood flow develops) since the fetus is entirely dependent upon a large blood flow to the placenta via the aorta.

Lesions such as ventricular septal defect, atrial septal defect, tetralogy of Fallot, and transposition of the great arteries are compatible with normal intrauterine existence. Immediately following birth, the likelihood of cardiac failure developing in an infant with a left to right shunt is largely dependent upon the rapidity with which the pulmonary vascular resistance falls, and on the ability of the left ventricle to adjust to an increased volume. With a large ventricular septal defect, a rapid postnatal decrease in pulmonary vascular resistance will allow a large left to right shunt with volume overload of the left ventricle which may lead to cardiac failure. Fortunately, however, a large communication between the pulmonary and systemic circulations appears to alter the rate of the involution of the pulmonary vessels, and this slower reduction of pulmonary vascular resistance may act as a protective mechanism against the early development of left heart failure. This may explain why many infants with a ventricular septal defect or a patent ductus arteriosus usually do not manifest heart failure for several weeks after birth. The reason some infants with lesions identical in size and location develop heart failure early and others do not is not entirely clear at this time. It may in part be due to the status of the catecholamine metabolism of the infant, since catecholamines are known to affect myocardial function.[55]

REFERENCES

1. Adams, F. H.: The early definitive diagnosis of patients with congenital heart disease. J. Pediatr. 52:202, 1957.
2. Adams, F. H.: Fetal and neonatal cardiovascular and pulmonary function. Annu. Rev. Physiol. 27:257, 1965.
3. Adams, F. H.: Functional development of the fetal lung. J. Pediatr. 68:794, 1966.
4. Adams, F. H., Assali, N., Cushman, M., and Westersten, A.: Inter-relationships of maternal and fetal circulations. I. Flow pressure responses to vasoactive drugs in sheep. Pediatrics 27:627, 1961.
5. Adams, F. H., and Lind, J.: Physiologic studies on the cardiovascular status of normal newborn infants (with special reference to the ductus arteriosus). Pediatrics 19:431, 1957.
6. Adams, F. H., Latta, H., El-Salawy, A., and Nozaki, M.: The expanded lung of the term fetus. J. Pediatr. 75:59, 1969.
7. Adams, F. H., Yanagisawa, M., Kuzela, D., and Martinek, H.: The disappearance of fetal lung fluid following birth. J. Pediatr., 78:837, 1971.
8. Arcilla, R. A., Oh, W., Lind, J., and Gessner, I.

H.: Pulmonary arterial pressures of newborn infants born with early and late clamping of the cord. Acta Paediatr. Scand. 55:305, 1966.

9. Assali, N. S., Rauramo, L., and Peltonen, T.: Measurement of uterine blood flow and uterine metabolism. VIII. Uterine and fetal blood flow and oxygen consumption in early human pregnancy. Am. J. Obstet. Gynecol. 79:86, 1960.

10. Baylen, B. G., Emmanouilides, G. C., Juratsch, C. E., Yoshida, Y., French, W. J., and Criley, J. M.: Main pulmonary artery distention: A potential mechanism for acute pulmonary hypertension in the human newborn infant. J. Pediatr. 96:540, 1980.

11. Bourne, G. L., and Benirschke, K.: Absent umbilical artery. Arch. Dis. Child. 35:534, 1960.

12. Burnard, E. D., and James, L. S.: Radiographic heart size in apparently healthy newborn infants: Clinical and biochemical correlations. Pediatrics 27:726, 1961.

13. Civin, W. R., and Edwards, J. E.: The postnatal structural changes in the intrapulmonary arteries and arterioles. Arch. Pathol. 51:192, 1951.

14. Dawes, G. S.: Foetal and Neonatal Physiology. Chicago, Year Book Medical Publishers, 1968.

15. Emery, J. L., and MacDonald, M. S.: The weight of the ventricles in the later weeks of intra-uterine life. Br. Heart J. 22:563, 1960.

16. Emery, J. L., and Mithal, A.: Weights of cardiac ventricles at and after birth. Br. Heart J. 23:313, 1961.

17. Emmanouilides, G. C., Moss, A. J., and Adams, F. H.: The electrocardiogram in normal newborn infants: Correlation with hemodynamic observations. J. Pediatr. 67:578, 1965.

18. Emmanouilides, G. C., Moss, A. J., Duffie, E. R., Jr., and Adams, F. H.: Pulmonary arterial pressure changes in human newborn infants from birth to 3 days of age. J. Pediatr. 65:327, 1964.

19. Emmanouilides, G. C., Moss, A. J., Monset-Couchard, M., Marcano, B. A., and Rzeznic, B.: Cardiac output in newborn infants. Biol. Neonate 15:186, 1970.

20. Friedman, W. F.: The intrinsic physiologic properties of the developing heart, In Neonatal Heart Disease, edited by W. F. Friedman, M. Lesch, and E. Sonnenblick, New York: Grune & Stratton, 1973, pp. 21–49.

21. Gérard, G.: De l'obliteration du canal arterial. Les theories et les faits. J. Anat. Physiol. (Paris) 36:323, 1900.

22. Gessner, I., Krovetz, L. J., Benson, R. W., Prystowsky, H., Stenger, V., and Eitzman, D. V.: Hemodynamic adaptations in the newborn infant. Pediatrics 36:752, 1965.

23. Gittenberger-De Groot, A. C., Moulaert, A. J. M., and Hitchcock, J. F. Histology of the persistent ductus arteriosus in cases of congenital rubella. Circulation 62:183, 1980.

24. Graser, F., and Berger, H.: Der zeitliche Verlauf der Herzkontraktion bei neugeborenen und jugen Säuglingen. Monatschr. Kinderheilkd. 109:532, 1961.

25. Halliday, H., Hirshfeld, S., Riggs, T., Liebman, J., and Fanaroff, A.: Echographic ventricular systolic time intervals in normal term and premature neonates. Pediatrics 62:317, 1978.

26. Harker, L. C., Kirkpatrick, S. E., Friedman, W. F., and Bloor, C. M.: Effects of indomethacin on fetal rat lungs: A possible cause of persistent fetal circulation. Pediat. Res. 15:147,

1981.

27. Harvey, W.: Anatomical Studies on the Motion of the Heart and Blood (Exercitatio Anatomica de Motu Cordis et Sanguinis in Animalibus), the Leake Translation, 3rd ed. Springfield, Ill.: Charles C Thomas, 1949, pp. 54 and 119.

28. Heath, D., Wood, E. H., DuShane, J. W., and Edwards, J. E.: The structure of the pulmonary trunk at different ages and in cases of pulmonary hypertension and pulmonary stenosis. J. Pathol. Bacteriol. 77:443, 1959.

29. Heymann, M. A., and Rudolph, A. M.: Control of the ductus arteriosus. Physiol. Rev. 55:62, 1975.

30. Hislop, A., and Reid, L.: Intrapulmonary arterial development during fetal life—Branching pattern and structures. J. Anat. 113:35, 1972.

31. Karlberg, P., Adams, F. H., Guebelle, F., and Wallgren, G.: Alteration of the infant's thorax during vaginal delivery. Acta Obstet. Gynecol. Scand. 41:223, 1962.

32. Kleinman, C. S., Hobbins, J. C., Jaffe, C. C., Lynch, D. C., and Talner, N. S.: Echocardiographic studies of the human fetus: Prenatal diagnosis of congenital heart disease and cardiac dysrhythmias. Pediatrics 65:1059, 1980.

33. Kovalcik, V.: The response of the isolated ductus arteriosus to oxygen and anoxia. J. Physiol. 169:185, 1963.

34. Levin, D. L., Fixler, D., Morriss, F. C., and Tyson, J.: Morphological analysis of the pulmonary vascular bed in infants exposed *in utero* to prostaglandin synthetase inhibitors. J. Pediatr. 92:478, 1978.

35. Levin, D. L., Hyman, A. I., Heymann, M. A., and Rudolph, A. M.: Fetal hypertension and the development of increased pulmonary vascular smooth muscle. J. Pediatr 92:265, 1978.

36. Levin, D. L., Rudolph, A. M., Heymann, M. A., and Phibbs, R. H.: Morphological development of the pulmonary vascular bed in fetal lambs. Circulation 53:144, 1976.

37. Lewis, A. B., Heymann, M. A., and Rudolph, A. M.: Gestational changes in pulmonary vascular responses in fetal lambs *in utero*. Circ. Res. 39:536, 1976.

38. Lind, J., Stern, L., and Wegelius, C.: Human Foetal and Neonatal Circulation, Charles C Thomas, Springfield, Ill., 1964, p. 10.

39. McMurphy, D. M., Heymann, M. A., Rudolph, A. M., and Melmon, K. L.: Developmental changes in constriction of the ductus arteriosus: Responses to oxygen and vasoactive agents in the isolated ductus arteriosus of the fetal lamb. Pediatr. Res. 6:231, 1972.

40. Melmon, K. L., Cline, M. J., Hughes, T., and Nies, A. S.: Kinins: Possible mediators of neonatal circulatory changes in man. J. Clin. Invest. 47:1295, 1968.

41. Mitchell, S. C., Korones, S. B., and Berendes, H. W.: Congenital heart disease in 56, 109 births. Circulation 43:323, 1971.

42. Moss, A. J., Duffie, E. R., Jr., and Emmanouilides, G. C.: Blood pressure and vasomotor reflexes in the newborn infant. Pediatrics 32:175, 1963.

43. Moss, A. J., Emmanouilides, G. C., Adams, F. H., and Chuang, K.: The effect of hypoxia and status of ductus arteriosus on acid-base balance in newborn infants. J. Pediatr. 65:819, 1964.

44. Moss, A. J., Emmanouilides, G. C., and Duffie, E. R., Jr.: Closure of the ductus arteriosus in

the newborn infant. Pediatrics 32:25, 1963.

45. Naeye, R. L.: Arterial changes during the perinatal period. Arch. Pathol. 71:121, 1961.

46. Naeye, R. L.: Human intrauterine parabiotic syndrome and its complications. N. Engl. J. Med. 268:804, 1963.

47. Naeye, R. L., and Blanc, W. A.: Prenatal narrowing or closure of the foramen ovale. Circulation 30:736, 1964.

48. Neufeld, H. H., Wagenvoort, C. A., and Edwards, J. E.: Coronary arteries in fetuses, infants, juveniles, and young adults. Lab. Invest. 11:837, 1962.

49. Oh, W., Lind, J., and Gessner, I. H.: The circulatory and respiratory adaptation to early and late cord clamping in newborn infants. Acta Paediatr. Scand. 55:17, 1966.

50. Penaloza, D., Arias-Stella, J., Sime, F., Recauarreu, S., and Marticorena, E.: The heart and pulmonary circulation in children at high altitudes: Physiological, anatomical, and clinical observations. Pediatrics 34:568, 1964.

51. Powell, M. L.: Patent ductus arteriosus in premature infants. Med. J. Aust. 2:58, 1963.

52. Prec, K. J., and Cassels, D. E.: Oximeter studies in newborn infants during crying. Pediatrics 9:756, 1952.

53. Prec, K. J., and Cassels, D. E.: Dye dilution curves and cardiac output in newborn infants. Circulation 11:789, 1955.

54. Record, R. G., and McKeown, T.: Observations relating to the aetiology of patent ductus arteriosus. Br. Heart J. 15:376, 1953.

55. Rudolph, A. M.: The changes in the circulation after birth: Their importance in congenital heart disease. Circulation 41:343, 1970.

56. Rudolph, A. M.: Fetal and neonatal pulmonary circulation. Annu. Rev. Physiol. 41:383, 1979.

57. Rudolph, A. M., and Heymann, M. A.: The circulation of the fetus in utero: Methods for studying distribution of blood flow, cardiac output, and organ blood flow. Circ. Res. 21:163, 1967.

58. Rudolph, A. M., and Heymann, M. A.: Circulatory changes with growth in the fetal lamb. Circ. Res. 26:289, 1970.

59. Rudolph, A. M., Heymann, M. A., Teramo, K. A. W., Barrett, C. T., and Räihä, N.: Studies on the circulation of the previable human fetus. Pediatr. Res. 5:452, 1971.

60. Saldana, M., and Arias-Stella, J.: Studies on the structure of the pulmonary trunk. II. The evolution of the elastic configuration of the pulmonary trunk in people native to high altitudes. Circulation 27:1094, 1963.

61. Saldena, M., and Arias-Stella, J.: Studies on the structure of the pulmonary trunk. III. The thickness of the media of the pulmonary trunk and ascending aorta in high altitude natives. Circulation 27:1101, 1963.

62. Scammon, R. E., and Norris, E. H.: On the time of the postnatal obliteration of the fetal blood passages (foramen ovale, ductus arteriosus, ductus venosus). Anat. Rec. 15:165, 1918.

63. Sisson, T. R. C., and Whalen, L. E.: The blood volume of infants. III. Alterations in the first hours after birth. J. Pediatr. 56:43, 1960.

64. Zapol, W. M., Kolobow, T. Doppman, J., and Pierce, J. E.: Response of ductus arteriosus and pulmonary blood flow to blood oxygen tension in immersed lamb fetuses perfused through an artificial placenta. J. Thorac. Cardiovascular Surg. 61:891, 1971.

3

Electrocardiography

Jerome Liebman, M.D., and Robert Plonsey, Ph.D.

In this textbook, the traditional separation of standard electrocardiography and vectorcardiography will not be made, for the separation is artificial and the principles of interpretation are the same. In vectorcardiography, the resultant of two scalar leads is continuously recorded on an X-Y oscilloscope or plotter to form a vector loop. In electrocardiography, the recordings are scalar projections of the cardiac vectors, distorted by proximity and multiple other factors. There have been large numbers of electrocardiographic lead systems developed with great variation in the information obtained about cardiac electrical activity. Standard electrocardiography includes three of these lead systems, the limb leads of Einthoven,[1, 2] the augmented limb leads of Goldberger,[3] and the chest leads of Wilson.[4] All use scalar representations, although it should be recalled that the tetrahedron lead system of vectorcardiography uses leads I and AVF for its frontal plane. Furthermore, the X, Y, and Z scalars of the so-called orthogonal vectorcardiographic lead systems are readily recorded.

This chapter provides a description of clinical electrocardiography and vectorcardiography with emphasis on infants, children, and adolescents. Early sections introduce basic principles of cardiac electrophysiology on which the subsequent sections are based.

ELECTROPHYSIOLOGY

EXCITABLE CARDIAC CELLS

The excitation mechanism of all types of excitable cells (cardiac muscle, skeletal muscle, nerve) appears to be very similar. The fascinating history of the development of knowledge of the action potential of the myocardial cell will not be discussed, but it is worth reading.[5, 6] For details of intracellular microelectrode recording of cardiac cells, the reader is referred to many excellent discussions and reviews.[7-13] The intracellular potentials are directly related to the flow of electrolytes across the cell membrane.[14-22] The excitation process is based upon the triggering of a rapid increase in the selective permeability of the membrane to sodium and on the unequal ionic composition of intra- and extracellular space. Regarding the latter, Table 3.1 gives the major ionic constituents of the intracellular and extracellular medium of cardiac tissue. One notes that in the intracellular region potassium is high in concentration and sodium low in concentration, and just the reverse is true in the extracellular medium. Because the membrane has a high resting potassium permeability, this ion dominates the character of the resting condition. In particular, the potassium cation will diffuse out of the cell (from high to low concentration) leaving the inner membrane negatively charged relative to the positive charge on the outer membrane. The resting transmembrane potential is therefore negative (inside negative relative to the outside) and constitutes an inward electrical force on potassium which equilibrates the outward diffusional force. This equilibrium condition is described by the potassium Nernst potential:

$$V_m = V_K = 60 \log_{10} [K]_o/[K]_i \text{ mv}$$

where V_m is the transmembrane potential, $[K]_o$ is the extracellular

potassium concentration, $[K]_i$ the intracellular potassium concentration, and V_K is the potassium equilibrium Nernst potential. For the values given in Table 3.1, $V_K = 60 \log (4/140) = -92.6$ mv, and this will approximate the resting transmembrane potential.

A transthreshold stimulus initiates a regenerative process in which the sodium permeability increases by several orders of magnitude. As a consequence the sodium ion dominates all others with regard to transmembrane flux, and the membrane potential quickly moves toward the sodium equilibrium Nernst potential. In this case, since the extracellular sodium concentration is much greater than the intracellular, sodium diffusion is necessarily inward in contrast to outward for potassium. Consequently, equilibrium is established when the intracellular potential is positive relative to the extracellular, since such polarity constitutes an outward electric field that balances the inward diffusional force. The sodium Nernst potential, using the data in Table 3.1, is given by

$$V_{Na} = 60 \log_{10} ([Na]_o/Na]_i) = 60 \log_{10} (140/10) = 69 \text{ mv}$$

and the peak of the action potential approaches this value.

Following depolarization sodium conductivity is rapidly inactivated while potassium conductances increase. The result is a reduction of sodium influx coupled with an increasing potassium efflux, as a consequence of which the transmembrane potential becomes more negative until the cell recovers its initial values. Cardiac repolarization is of long duration (approximately 300 msec) in contrast to nerve or skeletal muscle where the duration is only a few milliseconds.

The unequal chemical composition of intracellular and extracellular space is seen to play a vital role in the generation of the action potential through the diffusional forces they create. During activation, sodium ions move into the cell; recovery involves a restoration of the dominant potassium permeability, and a consequent potassium efflux is associated with recovery. These ion movements are in such a direction as to tend to equalize the unbalanced sodium and potassium distribution between intracellular and extracellular space. Restoration of baseline concentrations requires a reverse ion movement against the passive gradients—requiring the expenditure of energy. Such is provided by the sodium/potassium *pump* which is operated by the splitting of ATP. Since, for each mole of ATP, 3 sodium moles are moved out while 2 potassium moles are moved in, a net contribution to the transmembrane current of 1 mole results. This *electrogenic* current must be considered when examining the action potential quantitatively[23] (Table 3.1).

Typical cardiac action potential wave forms are shown in Figure 3.1. The most striking characteristic of the ventricular (working) muscle is the long *plateau*, which has already been noted as distinguishing cardiac tissue from all other excitable tissue. The electrophysiological basis for the plateau is controversial, but many assert it to be a combination of residual sodium influx, calcium influx, and several slow potassium efflux components that require several hundred milliseconds to fully develop and restore resting conditions.[24] During the plateau an influx-efflux balance maintains the transmembrane potential relatively constant. Recent work emphasizes the importance of including the electrogenic currents and suggests that possibly a simpler explanation for cardiac repolarization is possible when the properties of the pump current are taken into account.

18

TABLE 3.1   IONIC COMPOSITION FOR CARDIAC CELLS (mM/LITER)

Ion Type	Intracellular	Extracellular
Na^+	10	140
K^+	140	4
Ca^{2+}	0.0001	2
Cl^-	30	140
$A^{-\ a}$	120	8

[a] Nondiffusable anion; required for electroneutrality.

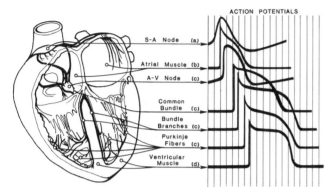

Fig. 3.1 Typical intracellular action potential wave forms for (a) pacemaker cells (S-A node), (b) atrial cells, (c) His-Purkinje system, and (d) ventricular cells. (Adapted from an original painting by Frank H. Netter, M.D. From The Ciba Collection of Medical Illustrations, copyright by CIBA Pharmaceutical Company, division of CIBA-GEIGY Corporation, Vol. 5, The Heart, 1969.)

In addition to the ventricular cells, other specialized cells of the heart can be identified with different electrophysiological behavior. For example, the Purkinje fiber action potential described in Figure 3.1 is similar to that of the ventricular cell except for a characteristic initial rapid repolarization. The atrial muscle has a shorter duration but is otherwise similar to the ventricle. The cells in the sinus node have an unusual property in that they do not maintain a resting potential. Instead, there is a slow spontaneous depolarization which, when threshold is reached, leads to the firing of an action potential. The result is a rhythmic behavior which is conveyed throughout the heart. Such cells are described as *pacemaker cells*.

ACTIVATION OF THE HEART

In the previous section, the cardiac action potential and its electrophysiological origin was briefly described. It was also noted that the action potential from each of the different specialized cardiac fibers is different, accounting for differences in function. In this section, we consider the detailed electrical behavior of the heart throughout the heart cycle.

The sinus venosus, in man as well as in many animals, is the primitive cardiac pacemaker.[25] In man, the area of the sinus venosus becomes incorporated into the regions of the ostia of the two venae cavae, coronary sinus, sinus intercavarum, Eustachian ridge, and most of the intraatrial septum. Included are the sinus node and the specialized conduction tissue, the three internodal tracts.

The sinus node normally initiates cardiac activity. It is a small structure, $15 \times 5 \times 1.5$ mm, situated at the lateral margin of the superior vena cava-right atrial junction.[26-28] Numerous ganglion cells are seen in the vicinity, and nerve fibers are evident in the substance of the node itself. At birth, parasympathetic innervation of the heart is almost completed, whereas sympathetic innervation is not functional until several months after birth.[29-31] In the newborn, there is a small amount of collagen, but with aging a dense collagen network develops. The primary cells of the node are the P cells and transitional cells, with the former more common with increasing

age. The P cells occur in groups centrally located near the sinus node's nutrient artery. They are pale, round, primitive-appearing cells which connect only with other P cells or transitional cells. The transitional cells are small and slender and longitudinally arranged. They connect peripherally with other transitional cells and with Purkinje cells, which appear to mark the beginning of the internodal and interatrial tracts.

Until recently, tradition had agreed that there are specific pathways of conduction in the ventricles, but that conduction through the atrium was "syncytial" in nature without specific pathways.[32-34] Nonetheless, such pathways were suggested more than 60 years ago.[35-37] The great discussions of the early 1920s between Eyster and Meek,[38] who gave evidence for internodal tracts, and Sir Thomas Lewis,[33, 39] who believed in the concept of atrial depolarization occurring as an enlarging circle of excitation originating at the sinus node, ended with virtually all cardiologists and physiologists agreeing with Lewis. However, in the decade of the 1960s, a series of landmark anatomic observations by James,[40-42] associated with considerable electrophysiological confirmation,[43-46] brought back the concept of internodal tracts. The tracts have been described by others as well.[47, 48] Most cardiologists and electrophysiologists believe James to be substantially correct, but distinguished workers, including Spach,[49] Scher,[50] Janse,[51] and Anderson[52] disagree. In an exhaustive review by Janse and Anderson,[53] the concept is entirely disclaimed.

According to James[28, 40-42], there are three connecting pathways between the sinus node and the atrioventricular (AV) node. They were described partially by Wenckebach,[36] Thorel,[37] and Bachmann.[35] The fibers destined for Bachmann's bundle (anterior interatrial myocardial band) and for the anterior internodal pathway exit together from the anterior margin of the sinus node. They then course leftward and anterior to the superior vena cava. The Bachmann bundle continues beyond the interatrial septum, posterior to the aorta, into the left atrium, while the anterior internodal pathway curves downward into the anterior portion of the interatrial septum, gradually coursing posteriorly to reach the crest of the AV node. The middle internodal pathway exits from the sinus node to course posterior to the superior vena cava in the sinus intercavarum.[36] It then enters the interatrial septum, where it travels just anterior to the limbus of the septum ovale to merge with the anterior internodal pathway before reaching the crest of the AV node. The posterior internodal pathway exits from the sinus node at its posterior margin to run in the crista terminalis.[37] It then curves beneath the inferior vena cava, enters the Eustachian ridge, and courses over the top of the coronary sinus toward the posterior margin of the AV node.

The majority of the fibers from the posterior internodal pathway bypass the bulk of the AV node, travelling between it and the right atrial endocardium to enter the node near its junction with the His bundle, while some of these fibers end blindly in the tricuspid ring. Some of the posterior internodal fibers join with those of the anterior and middle pathways at the crest of the AV node, and a few from the latter two pathways bypass the crest of the AV node to join it more anteriorly. Therefore, there are multiple interconnections among all three internodal tracts in the region of the AV node.

According to Sherf and James,[28] these pathways are composed of six different kinds of cells including a myofibril-rich cell not distinguishable from working myocardial cells and a myofibril-poor cell resembling Purkinje cells. There are also two types of transitional cells, a complex ameboid cell seen only in the Eustachian ridge, and P cells similar to those found in the AV node. There is no sheath separating the internodal tracts from contractile atrium, so that conduction laterally is present at all levels.

Electrophysiological evidence is strong that the Purkinje cells in the internodal tracts have automatic properties and that conduction is more rapid than in regular atrial myocardium. Despite the reasonable doubts expressed by Janse and Anderson,[53] most electrophysiologic and anatomic evidence is confirmatory.

The AV node is located in the lower atrial septum, just above the septal leaflet of the tricuspid valve, just anterior to the coronary sinus, and with its left surface touching the mitral annulus. It is made up of a few P cells in the center and a preponderance of interweaving transitional cells. Anderson and Taylor,[52] however, describe no P cells. Posterior to the node are many ganglia and nerve endings.

Anterior and inferior to the AV node is the bundle of His, composed mainly of parallel longitudinal rows of Purkinje fibers separated by thin cylinders of collagen. In fetal life and in the newborn period, the AV node and His bundle are frequently connected to the crest of the ventricular septum by the paraspecific fibers of Mahaim.[56] With aging, the Mahaim connections become less prevalent.[42]

The AV node and His bundle of the newborn are relatively large at birth with irregular surfaces which extend on the left into the mitral annulus and central fibrous body. After birth, the left side gradually resorbs and smooths out, but it may take a year before the adult size and shape are present.[42, 57]

After the common bundle of His penetrates the central fibrous body to reach the crest of the muscular interventricular (IV) septum, it continues anteriorly below or in the anterior margin of the membranous IV septum.[32, 58-62] In 75 to 80% of human hearts, the anterior His bundle runs along the left side of the crest of the muscular IV septum, thereby providing a relatively wide origin for the left bundle branch. In the remaining 20 to 25%, however, the anterior His bundle travels along the right side of the crest of the muscular IV septum. In these hearts, the His bundle connects to the left bundle branch by a narrow stem less then 1 millimeter in size.[58-62]

Regardless of the width of its origin, the left bundle branch fans out over the left septal surface forming multiple fiber groups with variable separation from one another. There is great variability in the normal anatomy of the left bundle branch system from one heart to the next.

Thus in some hearts, the right bundle and left anterior branch originate together, with the left posterior branch clearly separate.[63] In other hearts, the left bundle originates as a "fan" with no clear origin.[64] Finally, Kulbertus[65, 66] believes that there are three distinct portions to the left bundle: the left anterior, the left posterior, and a shorter left middle branch.

The proximal third of the right bundle branch may have a short intramyocardial course before reaching the right IV septal subendocardium, or it may be subendocardial from its beginning. The middle third is characteristically intramyocardial, and the distal third courses through the moderator band to reach the base of the papillary muscle of the right ventricle.[67] In most human hearts, the right bundle branch does not divide before reaching the anterior papillary muscle.

The posterior branch of the left bundle is the largest and extends posteriorly to terminate in the posterior papillary muscle. The left anterior branch extends anteriorly to terminate in the anterior papillary muscle. Kulbertus' middle branch apparently does not extend as far into the left ventricle as do the anterior and posterior. These bundles are rich in Purkinje cells but make no contact with the ventricular muscle, since they are enveloped in a sheath of connective tissue. However, there are multiple fine branches which form an endocardial network most widespread in the central and apical portions of the right and particularly left ventricular free walls. The apices, as well as the middle and inferior septum, are richly endowed with Purkinje spread; but in the posterobasal free wall and upper septum, branches are sparse.

EXCITATION PATHWAYS

In the atria, excitation normally begins in the area of the atrium near the connections to the internodal tracts. As conduction passes down the tracts to the AV node, there is extension to the atrial muscle laterally. Since the anterior internodal tract has a branch to

the left atrium, much of the right atrium is activated prior to the onset of activation in the left atrium.

Ventricular excitation begins on both septal surfaces, although a bit earlier on the left.[50, 68-74] The left posterior branch of the left bundle stimulates the left posterior portion of the septum as well as the posterior portion of the free wall of the left ventricle near the septum.[70] It is not the entire septum that demonstrates excitation, but a broad, and relatively well delineated area about one-half to two-thirds the distance down the septum near the termination of the left posterior bundle branch consistent with the anatomy described above. On the right side, activation of the septum begins a little more inferior, after the base of the anterior papillary muscle. However, via connections through several branches in the moderator band, it is now believed that right-sided excitation is even earlier at the endocardium.[67, 70] The entire endocardium then activates,[67] including the apices,[75] though the anterior ventricles appear to be dominant. Almost as soon as septal activation begins, it also slowly begins to depolarize up the septum. Although posterior spread in the left ventricle begins relatively early in the cycle, most of the left ventricle remains to be depolarized after apical depolarization is completed. After the apical myocardium has been excited, much of the remainder of the excitation wave is outward. The lateral walls of both ventricles are depolarized at about the same time, but possibly because most of the experiments have been done with adult dogs, in which the left ventricle is thicker than the right, the right ventricle's activity in this area is completed well before the left. The final areas to be depolarized are the posterior left ventricle, followed by the posterobasal left ventricle and the superior septum. However, recent data utilizing body surface potential maps in children have indicated that any of four areas of the normal child's heart may be the last to depolarize. These are the right ventricular infundibulum, the superior septum, the posterobasal left ventricle, and occasionally the posterior left ventricle.[76] Sometimes two or three complete depolarizations simultaneously. It is important to note that there is less Purkinje tissue on the right side of the septum than on the left, resulting in the right side of the upper septum being depolarized from left to right.

Durrer et al.,[77] studying epicardial breakthrough and using the resuscitated fetal heart of the human, have confirmed the animal work. The earliest epicardial excitation wave was determined to be the region of attachment of the right ventricular anterior papillary muscle. Spread was then radial and simultaneous in two waves. One was across the left ventricle toward the posterobasal region; another was across the right ventricle toward the same region. A double envelopment of the epicardial surface results. A more detailed activation analysis was provided by the classic data of the resuscitated normal adult human heart.[70] In a later section, the above details will be summarized and explained in relation to the genesis of the resulting electrocardiogram.

CELL TO CELL CONDUCTION

Electron microscopy has shown that a membrane completely surrounds every cardiac cell, and studies of its electrophysiology have shown that this membrane has a very high electrical resistance.[79] At the ends of each cardiac cell, the abutment of opposing cellular membranes give rise to a structure called the intercalated disk. The disk is the location of several types of specialized junctions, including the gap junction, which is believed to provide intercellular electrical paths of extremely low resistance. Each cell connects with one to two other cells, providing numerous branching arrangements.

Electrical activity initiated in ventricular working fibers by the conduction tissue will spread contiguously in all directions. However, since the low resistance junctions are mainly found at the ends of cells, propagation along the cardiac fibers is more rapid than in the transverse direction, which depends on a zigzag pathway in order to utilize the end-to-end communicating structures. The greater number of junctions encountered by action currents in the transverse direction relative to that in the longitudinal direction is also a factor in explaining the slower transverse velocity—since a time delay is associated with propagation across each junction. The ease with which excitation spreads from cell to cell in all directions in cardiac tissue is the basis for characterizing the heart as an electrical *syncytium.*

From a macroscopic point of view, the cardiac muscle fibers encircle each cavity, but also spiral in their circular course. A "through the wall" block of tissue, if sectioned from endocardium to epicardium, shows a continuous change in fiber angle. The angle is circumferential at midwall and at "5 o'clock" epicardially and "1 o'clock" endocardially. Because the conduction system tends to initiate activity across a broad endocardial region, the spread of activation tends to go from endocardium to epicardium in a cross-fiber direction. This tendency is enhanced by the effect of the anisotropic velocity itself which causes the excitation front to orient itself in the slow direction. This consequence is one of the conclusions of a computer simulation study of anisotropic cardiac tissue.[80]

EXCITABLE CELLS AS ELECTRICAL GENERATORS

Most cells of the heart are working atrial or ventricular cells, each one of which is capable of being activated.[81, 82] When a cardiac cell is subjected to a transthreshold stimulus, the ensuing events are as described earlier—the membrane permeability to sodium increases greatly, a sodium influx occurs, and the intracellular potential increases until it reaches a peak positive value approaching the sodium Nernst potential. Because the tissues of the body are good electrical conductors, the disturbed electrical condition in the cell undergoing activation causes the flow of currents between the cell and all points of the body, although the current strength diminishes as the distance from the active cell(s) increases. The cell, in effect behaves like a battery and since it is immersed in a conducting medium causes a flow of current throughout that medium. This electrical disturbance extends, in particular, to points on the body surface where the associated electrical potentials can be measured by a sensitive voltmeter. The collective effect of *action currents* from all active cells in the heart when viewed at the body surface constitutes the *electrocardiogram*, which is the temporal variation in potential of the body surface due to electrical activity in the heart.

If a commercial battery is submerged in a conducting electrolyte, current will flow from the positive to the negative terminal. The "strength" of the current depends on the EMF (voltage) of the battery and the resistivity of the medium. If the positive (source) and negative (sink) terminals are close together, the current flow field that results is characteristic of a *dipole field*, illustrated in Figure 3.2. The term "dipole" refers to the source-sink combination. Since the resultant field depends on the source-sink *orientation* as well as magnitude, a *vector* is required to describe a dipole. By convention, the vector direction points from the negative to the positive pole. When examining such a current flow field, one notes that at a given distance from the dipole, the maximum voltage is found along the dipole axis (either positive or negative), while at points perpendicular to the dipole axis, the voltage is zero. For points closer to the positive pole of the dipole, the voltage is positive, while at those closer to the negative pole, the voltage is negative.

If the conducting medium contains more than one battery, then the resulting current and potential pattern can be found by summing the contributions from each battery acting separately (this is the *principle of superposition*). If two batteries are very close together, then their effect is equivalent to that from a single battery which is the combination of the two. Note, however, that the sum of two such dipole sources (batteries) is not algebraic, since each has a direction as well as magnitude and the law of *vector* addition must be applied. Since each cardiac cell acts as a dipole the contribution from a group of cells which are sufficiently close together can be considered as arising from a single resultant dipole.

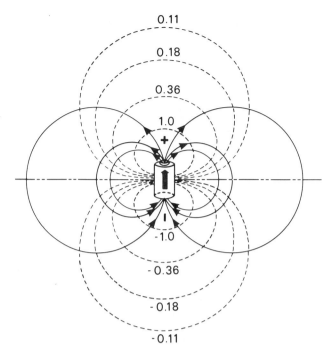

Fig. 3.2 A dry cell battery is submerged in a conducting fluid. Current flows out of the positive terminal and returns to the negative terminal along the paths shown. The vector (*circular arrow*) shows the orientation of the battery and, correspondingly, of the field. Under these conditions, since the battery provides a source-sink combination it is characterized as a dipole. The vector representing this (dipole) property of the battery has orientation (from negative to positive within the battery) and magnitude (strength of the dipole related to the battery electromotive force). Several interrupted lines of equipotential, and their relative values, are shown. This physical example is analogous to the electrocardiographic situation. In the latter case, the active muscle in the heart constitutes the dipole generator. Current flows away from the positive region (leaves the heart) into the torso volume conductor and returns to the negative region of the heart. Since the region of activity shifts from moment to moment, the dipole characterizing it is continually changing orientation and magnitude, and the current flow field and associated surface potentials change concomitantly. (Reproduced with permission from J. Liebman and R. Plonsey[83] and from the publisher, S. Karger, Basel, Switzerland.)

Measurement of electrocardiograms involves connecting electrodes to the torso at specific anatomic landmarks and recording the voltage between such points. A particular pair of electrodes is referred to as a *lead*. For example, if we put an electrode on the tip of the right ear and another on the left big toe, and if we attach these electrodes to the proper recording system, an electrocardiogram will result. We will have recorded the voltage of a lead, *but what will the lead voltage mean?* Ideally, we should know exactly what that lead reflects in terms of cardiac electrical activity. We shall discuss lead properties in a subsequent section.

The term *vector* has already been used; it is a quantity defined by magnitude and direction. Vector quantities are often contrasted to scalar quantities, which have magnitude only. When vectors have a common origin or are close together they can be summed. The law of vector summation is called the *parallelogram law* and is illustrated in Figure 3.3.

As we see, the procedure is to construct a parallelogram with the two component vectors to be summed ($\bar{A}$ and $\bar{B}$) as adjacent sides. The *resultant* ($\bar{C}$) is the diagonal of the parallelogram. If there are more than two vectors, the resultant of any two is combined with a third. Its resultant is then combined with a fourth vector, etc., so that only one net resultant remains. One can prove that the resultant

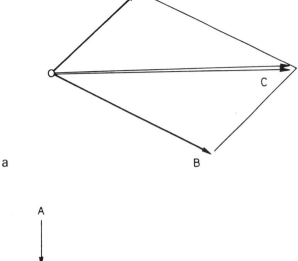

a

b

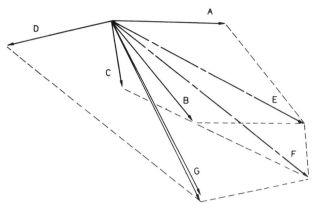

Fig. 3.4 The sum of vectors A + B + C + D is carried out by successive application of the parallelogram principle. Here A and B are summed to produce the resultant E. Then E is combined with C to yield F. The sum of F and D is G which is the resultant of the original vectors, i.e., A + B + C + D = G. (Reproduced with permission from J. Liebman and R. Plonsey[83] and from the publisher, S. Karger, Basel, Switzerland.)

Fig. 3.3 (*a*) Parallelogram law of vector addition, A + B = C. The component vectors A and B are acting at a common origin. By considering them to be adjacent sides of a parallelogram and constructing the diagonal their resultant C is obtained. (*b*) If A and B are not acting at the same point (or reasonably close together) the parallelogram law does not apply. Here A and B are equal and opposite forces. If one ignores their separation the conclusion is that the propeller is at rest (in equilibrium), whereas these forces will actually produce rotation. (Reproduced with permission from J. Liebman and R. Plonsey[83] and the publisher, S. Karger, Basel, Switzerland.)

is independent of the order of combining constituent vectors. In Figure 3.4, the resultant of several multiple vectors is depicted. Just as vectors may be combined, so also can a vector be resolved into components, as, for example, along three mutually perpendicular directions. In rectangular coordinates these directions are labeled X, Y, and Z and the components of a spatial vector $\bar{A}$ are simple A_x, A_y, and A_z. Such a procedure is shown in Figure 3.5. If the parallelogram law is applied to these vector components, it is confirmed that their sum equals the original vector.

Assuming that all active cells in the heart at each instant are reasonably close together, then a single net dipole is an adequate description of the heart as a generator. The net vector is referred to as the *heart vector* or *cardiac vector*; its magnitude and orientation vary as a function of time throughout the heart cycle corresponding to the activation of different regions of the myocardium. The behavior of the heart vector as a function of time can be described by its components along the X (right-left), Y (superior-inferior), and Z (anterior-posterior) cardiac axes. The latter constitute three scalar electrocardiograms.

The actual time varying voltage that is recorded by a particular lead depends on the time course of the heart vector, and, in addition, depends on the specific geometrical relationship of the heart, torso, and lead. The latter factors contribute to a vector known as the *lead vector*, and this has the property that the corresponding lead voltage is proportional to the projection of the heart vector on the lead vector. Since the lead vector depends only on the geometry, it is essentially fixed in time. Consequently, the time variation in the

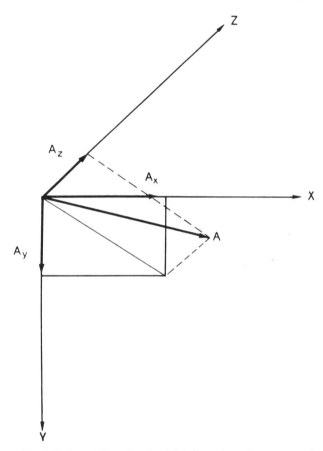

Fig. 3.5 Resolution of vector A into its rectangular components Ax, Ay, and Az along the X, Y, Z coordinate axes. The latter have been drawn following electrocardiographic convention. (Reproduced with permission from J. Liebman and R. Plonsey[83] and from the publisher, S. Karger, Basel, Switzerland.)

lead voltage depends on the changing projection of the heart vector on the corresponding lead vector. These relationships constitute the fundamental basis for electrocardiographic reconstruction of cardiac activity. It is illustrated further in Figure 3.6.

A crude approximation to the lead vector orientation is that it runs parallel to the line connecting the two electrodes. Thus, if one

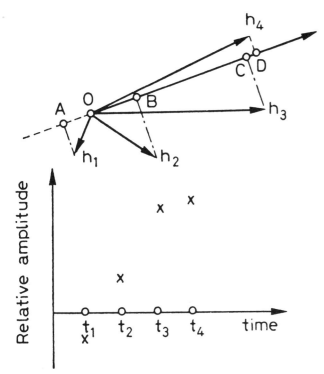

Fig. 3.6 The vectors h_1, h_2, h_3, and h_4 represent the cardiac vector at four successive instants of time t_1, t_2, t_3, and t_4, respectively. The lead vector for lead I is also shown. It does not vary with time since it depends only on the torso-heart geometry and the lead placement. The actual voltage measured by the instrument, when connected to lead I electrodes, at each instant of time is proportional to the projection of the heart vector at that instant on the lead vector. Thus, at t_1 the projection of H_1 on lead I is OA, at t_2 it is OB, at t_3 OC, and at t_4 OD. Note how both magnitude and orientation of the heart vector are important in this determination. A plot of the relative amplitude is given in the figure. As noted, the lead voltage is proportional to the projection of the heart vector on the lead vector. The actual value of lead voltage is found by multiplying the projection by the magnitude of the lead vector. In this way, both the strength as well as the direction of the lead vector enters into the final determination of lead voltage. (Reproduced with permission from J. Liebman and R. Plonsey[83] and from the publisher, S. Karger, Basel, Switzerland.)

electrode is attached to the left arm and the other to the right arm, an approximate horizontal (X axis) lead vector is formed. This lead (lead I) should respond to the X component of the heart vector (positive from right to left) but not the Y and Z components. The latter components are orthogonal (perpendicular) to an X-directed lead and, therefore, yield no voltage in that particular lead. Cardiac vectors to the left produce, accordingly, positive deflections in lead 1, while cardiac vectors to the right produce negative deflections in lead 1. The Einthoven equilateral triangle is an idealized view of the lead vectors associated with the limb leads as being equal in magnitude and at an angle of 60° from one another. It is known that this is a crude approximation; more will be provided on this subject in a later section.

When a particular lead is used, the interpretation of the ensuing electrocardiogram depends on how accurate its lead vector can be specified a priori and how well the heart vector approximates the distributed electrical dipole sources in the heart. *For standard electrocardiography the aforementioned interpretations are generally poor.* Only under very ideal conditions would, for example, the lead vector correspond to the direction from one electrode to the other. The body shape and internal inhomogeneities combine to "distort" the idealized lead vector orientation.

Regarding the single dipole representation of the heart's electrical

activity, this is a great oversimplification.[84–88] As noted, such an approximation requires that the cellular dipole elements be close together. The measure of "closeness" is that the distance between dipoles be small compared to their distance to the electrocardiographic electrodes. However, since the heart is very large in relation to the chest, especially in infants and in pathologic situations,[89] this approximation is a poor one.[90, 91] The larger the heart in relation to the chest and the closer the heart to the chest electrodes, the greater is the observed deviation of the heart from "dipolarity." This is sometimes described as a *proximity effect*,[92] and it distorts the lead voltage from being a projection of a simple cardiac vector. When Wilson *et al.*[4, 93, 94] developed the chest lead system of electrocardiography, the concept was that the specific chest electrode would reflect activity of the heart muscle just under that electrode. We know that such is not true but that every scalar potential reflects the sum total of electrical activity from everywhere in the heart. However, the lead weighs each source component differently according to location and distance and does favor the closer elements.[93] Obviously, this proximity effect occurs most when the heart is large in relation to the chest, and especially in the right chest leads.

As a consequence of the conduction system, separate heart regions which are widely apart can be simultaneously active. In such a case, each region may itself be well represented by a single dipole, but the combination cannot be regarded as dipolar. In such a circumstance, the heart is said to be *nondipolar*, and the single heart vector will be a very poor approximation to the cardiac activity.

The effect of inhomogeneities was mentioned briefly above. These cause the torso currents to differ from what they would be under homogeneous conditions. Major contributions arise from intracavitary blood, lungs, and surface muscle. These inhomogeneities vary from patient to patient. A fine example is provided in cystic fibrosis,[95] wherein, because of air trapping anteriorly, the cardiac vector is projected far posteriorly. This abnormally posterior vector is ascribed to increased resistance anteriorly. It is the lead vector which is affected by the presence of inhomogeneities.

An idealized model of the electrocardiographic volume conductor which nevertheless permits a consideration of the major inhomogeneities consists of a spherical "heart" eccentrically located in a spherical "torso." This is described in Figure 3.7. The (single chamber) heart consists of concentric regions of different conductivity, each representing blood, muscle, and pericardium, while the torso is similarly constituted of lung, surface muscle, and fat. The source is a concentric double layer in the heart muscle. This model was investigated mathematically by Rudy *et al.*[96] Some important conclusions are:

1. The effect of many regions of different conductivity requires that they be considered simultaneously because there can be significant interactions. For example, the "Brody effect" (an enhance-

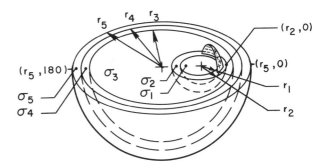

Fig. 3.7 The eccentric spherical model of the inhomogeneous torso. The double layer source is marked by + and − signs on its positive and negative surfaces, respectively. The region with conductivity σ_1 is the intracavitary blood; σ_2, heart muscle; σ_3, lungs; σ_4, muscle; and σ_5, the surface fat.

ment of the potential from radial dipoles and a reduction in potential from tangential dipoles due to intracavitary blood) is substantially diminished due to the interaction of the effect of the blood cavity with other inhomogeneities (i.e., the effect of the blood alone, assuming all else to be homogeneous at the conductivity of heart muscle, is a surface potential enhancement of 72%, but if all inhomogeneities are chosen at physiological values the enhancement is only 46%).

2. The effect of lung conductivity in the presence of surface muscle and fat is to cause a reduction in surface potential at *both* low and high lung conductivity. (A clinical manifestation involving reduced conductivity is the air trapping associated with obstructive lung disease, and in this case the skeletal muscle layer plays an important role in controlling the surface potential. On the other hand, high conductivity blood serum in the lungs will also decrease the surface potential. The highest surface potential apparently results for parameters lying in the physiological range.)

3. For decreasing hematocrit (increasing blood conductivity) there is an increase in surface potential due to the enhanced Brody effect. Similarly, potentials should be reduced by polycythemia.

4. Low skeletal muscle conductivity enhances the surface potential, and this is verified in the case of Pompe's disease.

5. The effect of obesity, when simulated by an increased thickness of subcutaneous fat, does not significantly affect the surface potential magnitude. This factor is sometimes incorrectly invoked to explain the difference in potential between the teenage boy and girl population.

6. An increase in the thickness of the myocardium at the expense of the blood cavity causes a decrease in surface potential.

7. Dilatation, per se, causes a greater increase in potential than does an increase in myocardial thickness due to an increase in the area of the source.

Clear documentation of the nondipolar behavior of the heart comes from the measurement of electrocardiograms at many body surface sites simultaneously. The potentials thus obtained are usually presented graphically in the form of isopotential "maps." The measurement of such maps based on potentials at up to 250 points became practical only in recent years as a result of the availability of inexpensive integrated circuits which are necessary for multichannel amplification and time multiplexing of a very large number of electrocardiographic channels.[97] An example is shown in Figure 3.8. This normal body surface potential map reveals two negative peaks and clearly could not arise from a single dipole source. An advantage in recording high density leads on the torso is the preservation of all details in the electrical potential pattern, which can be expected to have a useful diagnostic value.

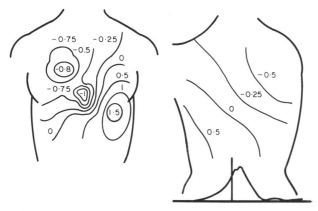

Fig. 3.8 Distribution of equipotential lines on the thoracic surface of a human at the time indicated by the vertical line intersecting the enlarged QRS complex at the lower right of the figure. Two separate minimums are present. The presence of the *saddle* has frequently been associated with right ventricular breakthrough.

In spite of the problems noted above, an increasing body of knowledge regarding the electrocardiogram and its clinical and biophysical significance has evolved based on research on cellular electrophysiology, activation of cardiac tissue, and correlations with clinical cardiology. The recent utilization of mathematical models has contributed to a quantitative understanding of electrocardiography and also serves as a general framework for the interpretation of experimental observations. The ready availability of high speed computers makes feasible even more complex models which are capable of reflecting the fine details of source generation, inhomogeneities, and body shape[98]; the result is a truly deterministic association of source and electrocardiographic field.

ACTIVATION SOURCES

In this section we will take a closer look at the electrical sources generated by activation of the heart. Our knowledge of the activation sequence comes from intramural measurements with specially designed *needle electrodes*. Each needle consists of perhaps 15 separate electrodes spaced at from 0.5 to 1 mm apart along the needle axis. Numerous such needles are inserted through the heart of an experimental animal so that simultaneous electrical potentials at a large number of intramural sites are available.

If one defines a surface which passes through all cells in the heart which are just on the verge of undergoing depolarization at some given instant of time, then, by virtue of being isochronous, the surface is referred to as an isochrone. Such a surface can be thought of as being initiated by the specialized conduction system in the ventricles; it subsequently propagates in a fairly uniform way from activated to contiguous resting tissue. A number of such surfaces may exist simultaneously, since there are numerous Purkinje terminations in different parts of the heart that initiate activity in separate regions. These waves of excitation will propagate until they collide with other waves or run out of tissue. It turns out that the action currents associated with the depolarizing cells that lie behind the isochrones appear to arise from a layer of dipoles spread over the isochronal surfaces (oriented in the direction of the advancing wavefronts). Thus, the *electrical sources* associated with cardiac activation are dipole layers (double layers) lying at each isochrone surface. Therefore, the isochrone not only describes the advancing cardiac wave front but is the site for the cardiac double layer sources.

As a double layer of activation approaches an intramural electrode, an increasing positive potential is detected which reaches its maximum when the wave front is at the recording electrode. As it passes across the electrode the polarity changes rapidly and becomes maximally negative as the negative side of the double layer is "viewed" by the recording electrode. The negative potential then diminishes to zero as the dipole layer recedes. The rapid deflection from positive to negative is known as the *intrinsic deflection* and serves as a temporal marker for the passage of activation across the site of the electrode. By recording the time of the intrinsic deflection at the many electrode sites, using a system of needle electrodes, the isochronal surfaces are obtained.[22]

The distribution of isochrones, hence of dipole layers, is fairly complex. One can replace each small region of double layer with a single dipole as a simplifying approximation. If the region is small, the approximation is satisfactory but for large regions the approximation is necessarily degraded. In Figure 3.9, we describe an approximation to the actual dipole layers in the heart by 10 to 20 discrete dipoles which are also shown summed to form a single net dipole (the heart vector). One can appreciate by this procedure, which passes from the exact, detailed, distributed dipole source layers to a multiple dipole distribution to a single dipole representation, successive levels of increasing approximation.

In spite of the approximation involved, the net heart vector arises from the activation isochrones and hence reflects, at least in a gross sense, the cardiac excitation sequence (Fig. 3.10). The locus of the tip of the cardiac vector sweeps out a *vector loop* in space; one object of vectorcardiography is to reconstruct this loop from surface potential measurements, but the main goal is to interpret the genesis of a particular loop in terms of a possible electrophysiological (actually clinical) origin. A strength of this approach is that fundamental principles of cardiac electrophysiology (in particular the activation sequence) accounts for the resulting vector loop ("forward problem"). On the other hand, the vector loop, based as it is on the single fixed heart dipole, fails to utilize any information associated with the *distribution* of the dipole elements, and consequently since more than one activation pattern could account for a particular vector loop, the measured vector loop does not have a unique *electrophysiological* interpretation (inverse problem). Fortunately, while there may be no unique electrophysiological solution, the clinical implications may be quite definite.

Some efforts have been made to model the heart as a multiple dipole distribution using from 9 to 15 dipoles. The advantage of such a model is the direct regional information associated with each dipole. For example, the presence of an infarct in a region would be reflected in a diminished dipole strength assigned to that region. The problem with this model is that a given surface potential distribution yields ambiguous multiple dipole distributions. While this approach to date has been equivocal, it has been utilized to evaluate left ventricular hypertrophy with considerable accuracy.[99]

LEAD VECTORS

We have noted that the lead vector for a given lead is a fixed vector and that the lead voltage is proportional to the projection of the heart vector on the lead vector. The orientation of the lead vector depends on the geometry of the leads, the presumed location of the heart vector, and the body shape and other inhomogeneities.

The direction of the lead vector is approximately along a line which joins the electrodes forming the leads. For the limb leads, V_I is approximately right to left, V_{II} approximately superior to inferior and leftward at a 60° angle, while V_{III} is approximately superior to inferior and rightward at a 60° angle. In fact, these lead vectors form an equilateral triangle.[100] By using an electrolytic tank, Burger[101] measured the actual lead vectors. These form a scalene, rather than equilateral, triangle. Furthermore, the limb lead vectors do not lie ideally in the frontal plane but have some front-to-back component. In Figure 3.11, we show the idealized Einthoven triangle

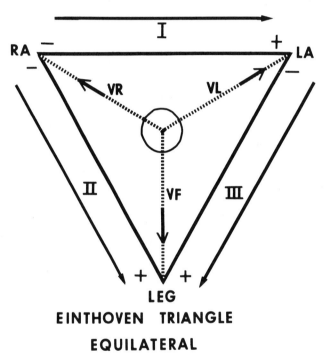

EINTHOVEN TRIANGLE

EQUILATERAL

Fig. 3.11 The Einthoven triangle. Note that it is equilateral, implying that the magnitude of leads I, II, and III are equal, as are VR, VL, and VF. The *arrow* in the perimeter indicates the direction of the vector. It is to the left in lead I and toward the foot in leads II and III.

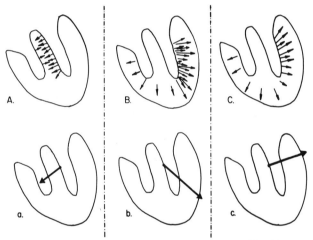

Fig. 3.9 *A, B,* and *C* represent early, mid, and late instants during ventricular depolarization. The dipoles formed are represented by dipole vectors (*small arrows*). In *a, b,* and *c,* the *large arrows* are the corresponding instantaneous resultant vectors. Each represents the average of all the dipole vectors formed in that instant, and each indicates the average magnitude, orientation, and direction of all the forces developed.

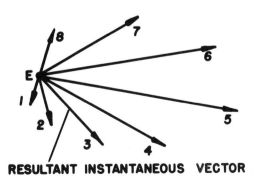

RESULTANT INSTANTANEOUS VECTOR

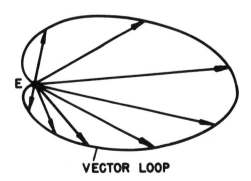

VECTOR LOOP

Fig. 3.10 (*Left*) Representative sequential instantaneous resultant vectors formed during ventricular depolarization. Vector 1 represents the average magnitude, orientation, and polarity of all the vectors formed during septal activation. The other vectors reflect the successive balance of forces as the path of activation sweeps through the ventricles. (*Right*) QRS vector loop formed by drawing a line to connect the heads of all the resultant vectors.

and the contrasting, more realistic, Burger triangle is shown in Figure 3.12.

If the right arm, left arm, and left leg are each connected to a common point through a 5K resistor, then the potential at the common point will be the average of the extremities (Fig. 3.13). Wilson suggested that this ought to be a *zero potential*, a neutral reference, and this has come to be accepted and used as a zero reference. In fact, it is possible to make a strong case for a zero reference being an average of potentials over the entire body surface,[102] but Wilson's *Central Terminal* does not differ greatly and is obviously much simpler to obtain. It is conventional to derive the precordial leads relative to the Central Terminal, and, in this case, the lead vector for each precordial lead is approximately in the direction from the torso center out to the electrode position on the thorax.

Assuming that the vector loop is known, then the scalar electrocardiographic leads can be obtained by projecting the heart vector on the lead vector for the scalar lead. This could be the lead vector corresponding to the limb leads or the lead vector associated with the precordial unipolar leads (i.e., relative to the Wilson Central Terminal). An example of such a resolved scalar lead derived from the vector loop for the lead V_6 is shown in Figure 3.14. Since the lead vector in this case is approximately from left to right, a positive lead voltage is obtained when the heart vector points to the left into the stippled space while a negative projection arises when the heart vector is oriented to the right into the clear space. In this case, the vertical line separates positive from negative lead voltages.

Just as the vector loop can be resolved into lead voltages, the reverse process whereby lead voltages are composed into a vector loop can be performed. In fact, one can identify, from the direction of their respective lead vectors, that V_5 would measure the x component of the heart vector, V2 the z component, and AVF the y component. The quality of these transformations is quite variable, since the lead vectors on which they depend are very sensitive to body shape and inhomogeneity. In addition, while the orientation of the lead vector may be correct, its relative magnitude may be incorrect (e.g., while the lead vectors of V2, V5, AVF may be orthogonal, their strengths may be unequal, hence resulting in a distorted heart vector). In the next section, we present several

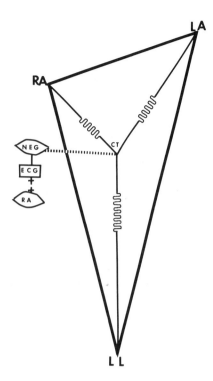

LEAD VR - WILSON

Fig. 3.13 Representation of the use of Wilson's central terminal to take lead VR. Each extremity is connected to the central terminal through a 5000-ohm resistor, and the central terminal (*CT*) is connected to the negative terminal of the galvanometer. The right arm electrode is connected to the positive pole of the galvanometer as well as to the central terminal.

vector lead systems that were designed to avoid some of these shortcomings.

One must also bear in mind that the notion of a heart vector and the vector loop representation of cardiac activity is an approximation. Consequently, the expected behavior, such as described in this section, which depends on this assumption, may be poorly fulfilled. In fact, an increasing interest is developing in the use of *body surface potential mapping*, where the potentials over the entire thorax are measured and displayed in the form of isopotential maps. Some leaders in the area, Taccardi[97, 103, 104] and Spach and Barr,[102, 105] believe that some form of surface mapping technology has a good chance to become the standard "lead system" for electrocardiography. The body of knowledge necessary to settle the issue is not yet available, but the authors' opinion is that we have no choice at the present time but to continue searching for the best orthogonal system and best measurements, while doing research with body surface potential maps. Correlative data with orthogonal lead systems in our laboratory[95, 107–110] have been superior to that of standard electrocardiography, and the latter's diagnostic ability is considerably improved when interpreting each lead as being a reflection of the entire cardiac vector.

CORRECTED ORTHOGONAL LEADS

As we have seen, the actual cardiac sources are distributions of dipoles which, during activation, lie along the isochrones. The heart vector has been described as only an approximation of the resultant vector, as if all distributed dipoles had a common origin. Recognizing the limitation of the net heart vector as representing distributed cardiac activity, it nevertheless has proved to be a valuable parameter in electrocardiography. One can show that it is the *leading term* in a series of multipoles; the higher terms constitute corrections

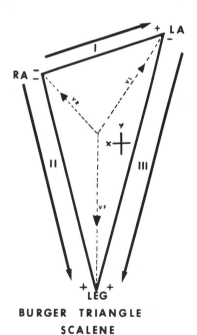

BURGER TRIANGLE

SCALENE

Fig. 3.12 Burger's scalene triangle. Note that lead I is smaller than leads II and III, and that lead III is larger than lead II. Note how poor an X axis lead I must be.

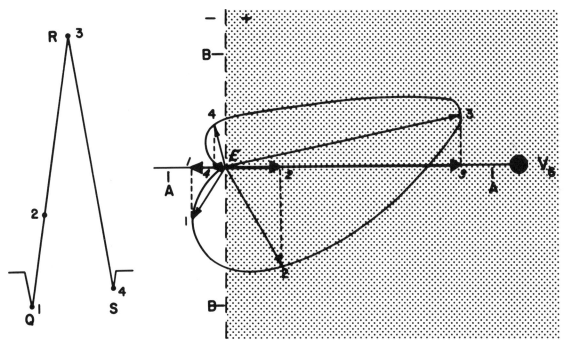

Fig. 3.14 Derivation of QRS in lead V₆ from horizontal plane projection of QRS vector loop. Lead axis of V₆ (AA) is drawn through E point, and perpendicular to it BB is constructed. Points on QRS complex, to left, are derived from component vectors.

which may or may not be of clinical importance. One can view the goal of electrocardiographic measurement as the obtaining of the heart vector. This, in turn, requires the design of a lead system that responds to elemental dipole sources without regard to their location within the heart. That this property is necessary is implied by the definition of the net heart vector as arising from the vector sum of all elements regarded as having a common origin. It is further necessary that a lead system accomplish this goal, regardless of the body shape and internal inhomogeneities of the patient. The concept used in the development of the orthogonal or "corrected" lead systems was the need to penetrate the heart in parallel and uniform flow lines.[81, 101, 111–116]. Obviously these goals can be achieved only approximately.

The purposeful development of lead systems for the measurement of the heart dipole has utilized multiple body electrodes and normalizing resistor networks. The purpose of using this complexity is to ensure that the lead vector for the system is the same throughout the heart and to ensure that the orientation of the lead vectors is along the appropriate coordinate axes. Since the approach is to measure separately the X, Y, and Z component of the heart vector, it is important that the same scale factor be inherent for each scalar component. One very successful system is the Frank lead system[117, 118]; here the resistor network is a means of adjusting the relative scalar component strengths so that a unit X, Y, or Z dipole will each generate the same signal amplitude. The positioning and use of multiple electrodes is to achieve uniform sensitivity and accurate direction.

The larger the number of electrodes utilized, the more nearly ideal can the lead system be made. Since there are three independent axis orientations, a minimum of three electrodes are required. Additional electrodes can improve performance. The number of electrodes used in a lead system is limited by the practicality of diminishing improvement in quality with each new electrode. In all these matters, compromise and tradeoff are necessary. A lead system which has the above properties in a more or less satisfactory performance is known as a *corrected orthogonal lead system*. At present, the Frank[117] system and McFee-Parungao[119] system are the major such vectorcardiographic systems with satisfactory perform-

ance. Systems with larger numbers of electrodes have rarely been tested in laboratories other than where they were developed.

RECOVERY

The previous sections of this chapter have stressed, mainly, cardiac activation. We have seen that this is a propagated phenomena initiated in the atria by pacemaker cells of the sinus node and in the ventricles by the conduction system. It is characterized by contiguous propagation within the atrial and ventricular working cells and can be described by a sequence of isochrones at the boundary of the surface of just activating cells. We have noted that the isochrones are the site of action currents responsible for the surface electrocardiographic P and QRS electrocardiograms and that these sources behave as dipole moment densities at the isochronous surfaces.

The activation double layer sources are actually not an infinitely thin layer but occupy a rather thin volume. This volume is defined by the collection of cells which at any instant of time are undergoing activation. Considering the rising phase of the cardiac action potential to have a duration of 1 msec and the propagation velocity of the isochrone to be around 50 cm/second means that a region of cells (50 cm/second × 1 msec = 0.5 mm thick) constitutes the active source region. This region lies just behind the isochronal surfaces. Since this is quite thin one can regard the dipole source density as being infinitely thin (a true dipole or double-layer). Considering the ventricle to be 1 cm thick means that around 5% of the cells of the heart are undergoing activity at any moment during the QRS.

We know that when all the cells in a region are at rest, they generate no action currents and hence do not constitute a *source* for electrocardiographic potentials. But, when adjoining cells are at different potentials due to being in a different activation phase, they then contribute action currents and constitute a dipole source. The propagation of activity ensures that cells lying between the leading edge of the isochrones (cells just being activated) and trailing edge of isochrones (cells just entering the plateau) will show a pattern of uniform progression of activation phase, hence the site of the dipole source described above.

Recovery consumes from 100 to 300 msec, and hence *all* the cells in the heart can be undergoing recovery for a substantial period of time. Whether or not adjoining cells are in a different phase depends on the order in which they were activated, inherent differences in action potential duration (epicardial cells tend to repolarize sooner than endocardial cells, though endocardial cells are activated earlier[120]), and cell to cell influence in recovery. The result is a greater degree of complexity in accounting for cardiac sources during recovery than for activation. Suffice it to say that dipole sources are associated with the *spatial* distribution in the transmembrane action potential of all cells in the heart; the source strength density is much less than for activation but is persistent for a much greater time and occupies a much larger volume. The earlier recovery of epicardial cells means that they can be just fully recovered, while the endocardial cells are not recovered. This is equivalent to the situation during activation, where the subepicardial layer may be depolarizing while the epicardium is still at rest. The direction of the force is consequently outward in both activation and recovery and explains why both the QRS vector and the T vector are directed relatively near to each other in normals. If the T wave were exactly propagated then the polarity would be reversed.

As with activation, one can sum the dipole source elements throughout the heart during recovery and obtain a net heart vector. And one can plot the locus of the tip of this vector through the period of recovery. The interpretation in terms of underlying electrophysiology is much more complicated than for activation, and, in fact, there exists no simple account. In fact, one has recourse at this time only to rather recent and sophisticated models to account for the specific wave form of the T wave based on an electrophysiological model with realistic properties.

If the activation pattern were changed, as the result of an ectopic stimulus, then both the QRS and T wave would be affected. But, if the cells retain the same action potential duration, then, as was shown by Wilson, the sum of the area under the QRS plus T is unchanged. The change in A_{QRS} is just balanced by the change in A_T. Wilson[121] called the combined area, A_{QRST}, the *ventricular gradient*. And, since it is relatively insensitive to the activation sequence, it is mainly sensitive to recovery and as such should be a useful tool in examining recovery. Abildskov *et al.*[122] have produced additional experimental evidence in support of Wilson's thesis. They have, in addition, suggested that A_{QRST} might be useful in looking for "disparity in recovery"[123] which they believe to be a condition which predisposes for reentry and dysrhythmia. The properties of the ventricular gradient are still somewhat controversial, and the dysrhythmia index of Abildskov is yet to be supported by definitive experiments.

INSTRUMENTATION

The first representation of the resultant of the human heart's electrical activity was in 1889 by Waller,[124] who used a modification of Lippmann's capillary electrometer.[125] The instrument was sensitive but sluggish. By 1903, Einthoven[126] had adapted the string galvanometer to develop the modern electrocardiograph; and in 1913[2] it appeared in almost final form. Many modifications appeared in the next quarter century,[127] the most important being the amplified mirror galvanometer. After World War II, direct writing, hot stylus, instruments appeared, resulting in a decrease in detail, accuracy, and frequency response, but in great convenience.

All leads utilized to represent the heart's electrical activity are bipolar, although all leads other than Einthoven's original standard limb leads have been erroneously called unipolar. Each lead must have one connection to the positive terminal and another to the negative terminal of the galvanometer, or other suitable voltage-measuring instrument. Each recorded bipolar lead represents a difference in potential between two points. In the case of the string galvanometer, the two electrode wire connections terminate a very fine gold- or platinum-plated quartz filament. The fine string is suspended under just the proper amount of tension in the field of a powerful magnet, and when the heart's electrical current passes through, it creates a magnetic field of its own. The filament is thus made to move in a direction perpendicular to the field of the magnet. A recording of these delicate movements is made by focusing a beam of light on the string and projecting the interrupted beam onto moving photographic paper. This sensitive instrument required great care in application of the skin electrodes, for the apparatus provided little resistance to flow in comparison to the naturally high impedance at the interface of electrode and skin. To obtain the relatively high frequency response the machine was capable of, and without distortion, the skin had to be vigorously rubbed with special pastes to ensure that polarization effects were negligible, and that skin resistance was kept low.[127]

The development of vacuum-tube amplifiers allowed an electrocardiograph which drew only minimal current from the patient and made skin resistance much less important. At the same time, the string was replaced by a coil and put between the poles of a stronger magnet to which was attached a mirror. The electrical forces from the body were amplified and passed through the coil, which was thus caused to rotate. Light was focused on the mirror, and the reflection from the magnetized rotating coil was passed onto the moving photographic paper. The amplified mirror galvanometer type of instrument was less sensitive than the string galvanometer, but provided a higher frequency response, that is, up to 800 Hz.

Smaller direct writing instruments became possible with the use of smaller and more powerful permanent magnets and better vacuum tubes. The advent of solid state electronics provided even greater advantages so that the instrumentation field is constantly changing. The amplifier must be sufficiently strong to increase the recording of the heart's potentials enough to mechanically move a writing stylus attached to a conducting unit between the poles of a magnet. The use of high impedance "buffer" amplifiers between the electrode and the resistor network has now made skin resistance problems minimal, since changes in skin resistance will be trivial compared to the interposed high impedance.[128] A recent advance is that of active electrodes with no need for paste and with built-in buffer amplifiers on each electrode. These electrodes are impedance transformers with high input impedance and low output impedance.[129] This type of advance has allowed high frequency multichannel recordings with insignificant distortion.

Most direct writing instruments in use today continue to have deficiencies. The fine papers of Lepeschkin[127] and Dower[130] almost 20 years ago remain pertinent. The majority of instruments in use are single channel, allowing only one lead to be recorded at a time. Most such recorders use a heated stylus system with waxed carbon paper, inherently a low frequency response system. There are direct writing instruments, however, which allow a very high frequency response. One type uses a fine glass capillary mounted on a wire loop in the center of the magnet, but of increasing popularity is that which writes with a fine jet of quick drying ink and provides six simultaneous channels with a frequency response of 700 Hz.

Thomas[131] makes the important distinction between "frequency response" and "frequency content." The recording device has a frequency response, but the electrocardiographic signals being recorded have "frequency content" or "frequency components." Though some very high frequency components of the electrocardiogram may be important,[132-134] most agree that the important high frequency diagnostic components are not above 100 to 125 Hz.[135, 136] However, Thomas' experiments clearly demonstrate that in order to ensure that these frequency components will be measured, the recorder's measurement system frequency response must usually exceed 200 Hz. Most single channel direct writer recorders in operation today cannot measure a frequency above 80 Hz, and after short use are often tested as low as 40 Hz. In Dower's[130] extensive tests, each direct writing machine tested differently and variably, depending upon the speed of inscription of the recording.

Recently, the American Heart Association has raised its required upper cutoff frequency to 100 Hz, and many manufacturers are now providing simultaneous three channel machines with a 125 Hz cutoff frequency. However, this improvement is still not satisfactory; for in our studies, the QRS voltages will be higher when the electrocardiograph has a capability of more than 200 Hz at the high end. Most manufacturers deliver a satisfactory low frequency response cutoff of 0.5 Hz, so that the ST segments are satisfactory. Nonetheless, because of the inadequate high frequency response of most instruments in use, two sets of voltage standards are necessary. Ziegler's[137] classic early data for children were obtained with an optical recorder which had a frequency response of 700 Hz. One set of standards must be used for such tracings, while another set of standards must be used for low frequency tracings. Most orthogonal electrocardiographic data, however, have been recorded with high frequency vectorcardiography machines.

LEAD PLACEMENT

In standard electrocardiography, the lead placement attempts to represent the frontal plane (limb leads) and the horizontal plane (chest leads). The sequential plane is not recorded as completely, although, obviously, the superior-inferior forces of the frontal plane and the anterior-posterior forces of the horizontal plane can be utilized in constructing the sagittal plane. The limb lead electrodes are placed on the right arm, left arm, and left leg, with a ground electrode on the right leg. Since the extremities are relatively distant from the heart, and are long compared to their cross-section, little current flows into and out of them, making them relatively equipotential. Consequently, an electrode can be placed anywhere along the extremity with similar effect.

The so-called "unipolar" limb leads involve the use of Wilson's central terminal (Fig. 3.13).[93, 138, 139] The Wilson central terminal is connected to the negative pole of the galvanometer, while the electrodes on the extremity are connected to the positive pole. Voltages recorded in this way are denoted VR, VL, and VF. With this method the voltages were too low. A 50% increase in amplitude was obtained by Goldberger's simple and clever modification, in which the central terminal connection to the extremity on which the exploring electrode lies, is disconnected. For example, when VR is to be recorded, the connection from the right arm to the negative central terminal is disconnected, leaving only the connection to the left arm and left leg. Because of the increase in voltage, the lead is called augmented VR, or AVR. The same technique is used for AVL and AVF. The so-called "unipolar" chest leads use the Wilson central terminal without augmentation, connecting the negative voltmeter input to the Wilson terminal, while the positive input is connected to electrodes on the chest.

The standard chest leads are:

V1, fourth intercostal space, right parasternal line.

V2, fourth intercostal space, left parasternal line.

V3, between fourth and fifth intercostal space, exactly midway between V2 and V4.

V4, fifth intercostal space, at left midclavicular line.

V5, same transverse level as V4 (not along intercostal space) t left anterior axillary line.

V6, same transverse level as V4 and V5, at left midaxillary line. In addition, as a routine, V3R or V4R is strongly recommended. V4R is the lead most commonly used.

V4R, fifth intercostal space, at right midclavicular line.

V7, same transverse level as V4, V5, and V6, at left posterior axillary line.

V8, same transverse level as V4, V5, V6, and V7, at tip of left scapula.

When dextrocardia is present, equivalent right chest leads should be taken, but the limb leads should not be altered. *Unlike the situation in the limb leads, one cannot be too strong in urging*

extreme accuracy in the placement of the chest leads. Minor electrode misplacement may cause considerable change.

The orthogonal lead system of Frank utilizes just seven electrodes, named I, E, C, A, M, F, and H. After much work attempting to find a different and appropriate electrode position for each patient, it was finally determined that the 5th intercostal space was appropriate. However, this appears to be better for the patient standing; Langner[140] later determined that the 4th intercostal space was more appropriate with the patient recumbent. There is dispute over this, but the 4th intercostal space is used by most, including our laboratory. Electrode placements are:

I, right midaxillary line in the 4th intercostal space

A, left midaxillary line in the 4th intercostal space

E, over the sternum (midline) in the 4th intercostal space

C, 45° angle between A and E in the 4th intercostal space

M, over spin (midline) in the 4th intercostal space

H, back of neck, 1 cm to the right of the midline

F, Left leg

The X lead (X axis) is from electrodes A + C + E

The Y lead (Y axis) is from electrodes H − F + M

The Z lead (Z axis) is from electrodes A + C + E + I + M

The orthogonal lead system of McFee-Parungao utilizes nine electrodes.[119]

STANDARD PROCEDURE FOR OBTAINING SCALAR ELECTROCARDIOGRAM

Machines utilizing buffer amplifiers are essential. Proper preparation of the skin to lower skin resistance is essential, unless the electrocardiograph has *very high impedance* buffer amplifiers or dry active electrodes with built-in buffer amplifiers.[128] The use of water or saline instead of rubbed-on electrode paste when standard electrodes are used will lead to erratic and erroneous voltages.

The electrocardiograph machine should have a frequency response of at least 200 Hz.

Time must be taken to place the electrodes on the chest accurately. Time and patience and kindness are necessary with the infant and young child. Fewer electrocardiograms can be taken per day in a pediatric laboratory than in an adult laboratory.

Simultaneous recording of at least three leads is highly desirable. If three or four leads are taken simultaneously, those recommended are: I, II, and III; AVR, AVL, and AVF; V4R, V2, and V5; V1, V4, and V6; and II, V1, V2, and V5 at double speed and double standardization for P wave analysis.

NOMENCLATURE

The sinus node's electrical activity is not represented in the electrocardiogram, the first deflection being that due to depolarization of the atrium. This is the P wave (Fig. 3.15). Repolarization of the atrium, the Ta, is usually partially buried in the QRS deflection and may or may not be seen. If visible, the repolarization wave is usually seen to be opposite in direction from that of the P wave and may also begin before depolarization has been completed. Consequently, the height, or magnitude, of the P wave should always be measured from the isoelectric line at the onset, not at the end, of the deflection. Depolarization of the atrioventricular node is not recorded on the surface electrocardiogram, the next deflection in the diagram being due to depolarization of the ventricle, the QRS. The interval between the onset of the P wave and the onset of the QRS is called the PR interval, and the interval between the end of the P wave and the onset of the QRS is called the PR segment. Nomenclature for the QRS is very specific: The Q wave is the first downward deflection before an upward deflection. The R wave is the first upward deflection. The S wave is the first downward deflection after an upward deflection. Secondary R and S deflections are termed R′ and S′ waves, respectively. Tertiary R and S deflec-

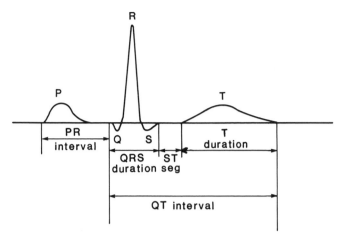

Fig. 3.15 Nomenclature for the standard scalar electrocardiogram.

tions are termed R″ and S″ waves, respectively. Small deflections, generally under 5 mm, are usually written in lower case letters, q, r, and s.

Repolarization of the ventricles is represented by the ST segment and the T wave, the latter being the next major deflection after the QRS. The junction between the end of ventricular depolarization and the beginning of the ST segments is the J point. The interval between the end of the QRS and the onset of the T wave is the ST segment.

The QT interval is the period between the onset of the QRS and the end of the T wave. The U wave, often barely perceptible, is the final deflection occurring between the T and the P wave. For purposes of timing the various deflections, as well as for measuring the heart rate, the electrocardiographic paper is divided into specific intervals. With the most commonly used machines, recording at 25 mm/second, there are heavy vertical lines 0.2 second apart. These are further divided into time lines 0.04 second apart. At least part of the tracing should be recorded at 50 mm/second for better delineation and timing. Also present are horizontal lines 1 mm apart. At full standardization (10 mm = 1 mv), each millimeter deflection represents a magnitude of 0.1 mv.

STANDARD PROCEDURE FOR OBTAINING ORTHOGONAL ELECTROCARDIOGRAM WITH VECTORCARDIOGRAPHIC DISPLAYS

The principles described above for standard electrocardiography are the same as for orthogonal electrocardiography with vector displays, but in the past 25 years, since the methodology became popular, there has been considerable change. Originally, the loops had to be photographed directly from the oscilloscope, with the vectorcardiographer having to use great skill in photographing P, QRS, and T loops separately or together directly from the oscilloscope. Later, the technique of trace shifting became available, whereby the loops were photographed while a strip chart paper was moving. This allowed separation of the QRS from the T, for analysis of the initial QRS away from a fuzzy E point. Nowadays, the simultaneous X, Y, Z scalars can be recorded together with each of the three planes utilizing a memory tape. Any portion of the P, QRS, or T desired for analysis can be readily recorded.

NOMENCLATURE

Standard procedure for orthogonal electrocardiography is to record three scalars, the X, Y, and Z. These scalars represent, respectively, the right-left forces (X axis), the superior-inferior forces (Y

axis), and the anterior-posterior (Z axis). These scalars are written exactly as the scalars of standard electrocardiography, and the nomenclature for these scalars is also exactly the same. The X and Z axes, when recorded together, give us the resultant of the two axes, the horizontal plane. The X and Y axes, when recorded together, give us the frontal plane; and the Y and Z axes, when recorded together, give us the sagittal plane. In Figure 3.16, a diagram of a typical normal horizontal (XZ) plane is depicted. Though many "vectorcardiographers" utilize such terms as Q loop, R loop, S loop, etc., we prefer to think vectorially, and, if possible, spatially. Therefore, the terminology for the horizontal plane is as depicted: Initial X right (maximal initial projection to the right); Z anterior (maximal anterior projection); X left (maximal leftward projection); Z posterior (maximal posterior projection); terminal X right (maximal terminal rightward projection and maximal vector in the horizontal plane). To measure the mean vector *exactly* requires a planimeter or a computer and is neither practical nor useful. The frontal plane, made up of X and Y axes, allows the additional measurements of initial Y superior (maximal initial projection superior) and terminal Y superior (maximal terminal projection superior), as well as Y inferior (maximal inferior projection). The sagittal (YZ) plane is not essential, since all the information is in the horizontal and frontal planes. Spatial vectors can also be measured utilizing the formula, maximal spatial vector (MSV) = $\sqrt{X^2 + Y^2 + Z^2}$. In making such a measurement, an automated computerized system can be used, or, if done by hand, a system for simultaneous recording of the three timed loops is easy to utilize. Relatively inexpensive vector records are readily available, which record the loops simultaneously, then, by virtue of a memory tape, slowly inscribe each loop, blanked at 2-msec intervals. This allows easy calculation of the maximal spatial vector, particularly since the X, Y, Z scalars are also recorded simultaneously as a check. Some recorders can record the X, Y, Z scalars at very fast speed, therefore allowing calculation of the maximal spatial vector utilizing no tools other than a transparent ruler and a pencil.[142] The calculation of the maximal spatial vector to the left (MSVL) or maximal spatial vector to the right (MSVR) gives us another tool for interpretation of atrial or ventricular hypertrophy. It should be clear that the maximal vector in *each* plane must not be used for calculation of the MSV. An erroneously high result will occur.

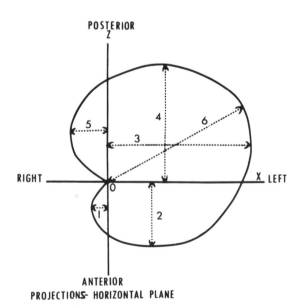

Fig. 3.16 Typical normal horizontal plane of a child after infancy to help define easily measured parameters: (*1*) initial X right, (*2*) Z anterior, (*3*) X left, (*4*) Z posterior, (*5*) terminal X right, and (*6*) maximal vector.

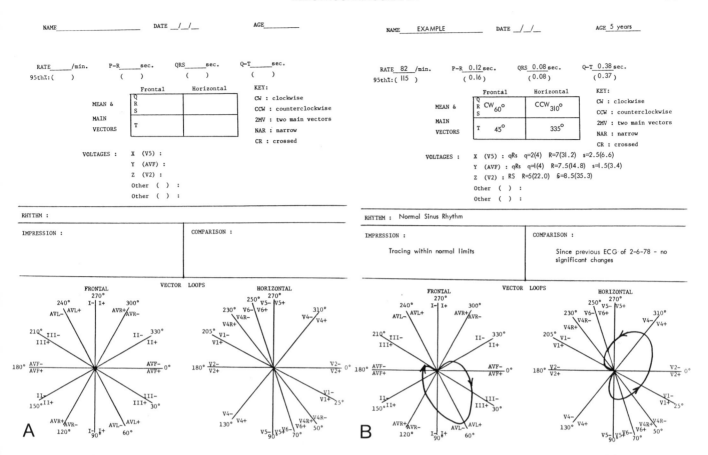

Fig. 3.17   (*A*) Data sheet used for standard ECG. (*B*) Sample ECG data sheet derived from a hypothetical ECG.

METHODOLOGY FOR INTERPRETATION

The interpretation of the standard electrocardiogram (ECG) demands development of a methodology implementing certain routines which provide standardization and completeness. Terminology must be based upon appropriate principles. Though clearly there are many areas of interpretation where little is understood, pattern reading is not generally reliable, is not much fun, and does not allow attempting to "figure things out" when something unusual presents itself. The electrocardiographer must try to determine what is being depolarized and when. He must also have available the quantitative limits for specific leads and utilize these numbers within the guidelines of proper statistics.[143]

Figure 3.17 is a sample ECG data sheet from a hypothetical standard electrocardiogram, while Figure 3.18 is a sample VCG data sheet (orthogonal ECG with vector display).

As an aid to determining the sequence of activation, construction of the vector loop is very useful and frequently essential. The frontal plane loop has been constructed by many electrocardiographers for many years,[144] and the first vector loops recorded in this country from leads I and AVF were by Wilson.[145] We have learned that construction of the horizontal plane vector is much more useful, even though proximity effects for standard electrocardiography may lead to difficulties in the reconstruction. We will not discuss in depth whether standard electrocardiography with its vector interpretation is more or less accurate than is orthogonal electrocardiography with vector display. However, there is no question that the actual vector display, with its accurate electronic construction from the X, Y, Z scalars, can inherently make the information more readily attainable—particularly for subtle and even manifest conduction abnormalities.

FRONTAL PLANE

The six limb leads have traditionally been used to make up a hexaxial system 30° from one another (Fig. 3.19), though we realize the inadequacies from Burger's data (Fig. 3.12), particularly in lead I, where superior-inferior forces markedly distort. Burger's scalene triangle also teaches us that the magnitudes of leads II, III, and AVF are much larger than those of leads I, AVR, and AVL. Lead AVF, however, is considered a good Y axis.[90] In Figure 3.17, the same hexaxial reference frame was redone with the perpendiculars to the leads for easier understanding. Therefore, considering lead I, for example, if any electrocardiographic point in time is to the left, it will lie on the 0° side of the 90 to 270° line (the lead I perpendicular); and if any point is to the right, it will lie on the 180° side of the lead I perpendicular. By the same token, considering lead AVF, if any electrocardiographic point in time is inferior, it will lie on the 90° side of the 0 to 180° line (the lead AVF perpendicular); and, if any point is superior, it will lie on the 270° side of the lead AVF perpendicular. The same principles are used for leads AVL and AVF and, of course, leads II and III, if necessary. In such a manner, a relatively accurate vector loop for the frontal plane can be drawn. We usually draw the loop *before* estimating the mean vector, since the analysis of the loop per se and maximal vectors are more instructive than is the estimation of the mean vector (formerly called "the axis"). The inscription of the QRS vector begins with the determination of the "initial forces." Figure 3.20*A* represents a segment from an enlarged idealized six-channel standard ECG. The initial QRS is negative in AVF (q wave) and positive in lead I (R wave) putting the resultant in the left upper quadrant (Fig. 3.20*B*). For further delineation, leads II and AVR are examined. Since both are negative, the initial QRS vector is between 300 and 330° (Fig.

	FRANK			MCFEE		
	F	S	H	F	S	H
DIRECTION OF QRS LOOP						
INITIAL QRS						
TERMINAL QRS						
MAXIMUM QRS VECTOR						
MAXIMUM T. VECTOR						
MSV TO LEFT						
MSV TO RIGHT						
EST. LV OR RV PEAK PR.						

MAXIMAL VECTORS		
X TO L	( ) mv.	( ) mv.
INITIAL X TO R	( ) mv.	( ) mv.
TERM. X TO R	( ) mv.	( ) mv.
INITIAL Y TO S	( ) mv.	( ) mv.
TERMINAL Y TO S	( ) mv.	( ) mv.
Y TO I	( ) mv.	( ) mv.
Z TO A	( ) mv.	( ) mv.
Z TO P	( ) mv.	( ) mv.
TERMINAL X RIGHT / X LEFT	( )	( )
Y TERMINAL SUP. / INF	( )	( )
Z-A / Z-P	( )	( )

IMPRESSION:

COMPARISON:

Fig. 3.18 Form for insertion of measurements and interpretation for orthogonal ECG with vector display.

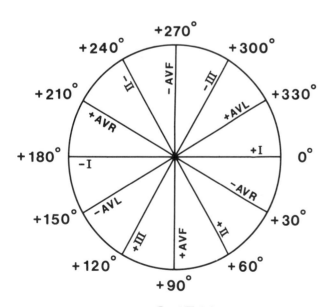

FRONTAL

Fig. 3.19 Reference frame for the frontal plane according to Einthoven's equilateral triangle. The lines are drawn through the center to the negative terminus of each lead. Thus the 360° is divided into multiple 30° sections.

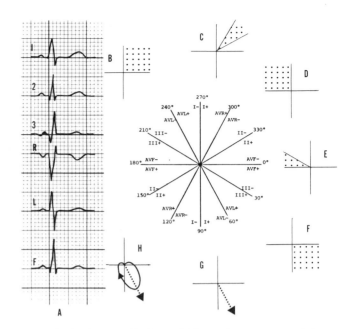

Fig. 3.20 See text. (A) Single QRS complex from a frontal plane simultaneous six-channel ECG. (B) Quadrant to the initial forces. (C) Angle of the initial forces. (D) Quadrant of the terminal forces. (E) Angle of the terminal forces. (F) Quadrant of the mean vector. (G) Angle of the mean vector. (H) Frontal plane QRS vector loop.

3.20C). If one wishes to determine the terminal vector and then the mean vector, one can proceed as in 3.20D to G. Leads I and AVF both terminate negatively (to the right and superior), resulting in a terminal vector in the right upper quadrant. Since lead III terminates positive and lead AVL negative, the terminal vector is between 180 and 210° (Fig. 3.20E). The mean QRS vector can now readily be determined by looking at leads I and AVF. Both are mainly positive, putting the vector between 0 and 90° (Fig. 3.20F). Since lead III is positive, the vector is between 30 and 90°. Since AVL is isoelectric, the mean vector is approximately 60° (Fig. 3.20G). The approximate loop is in Figure 3.20H and is clearly inscribed clockwise. Figure 3.21 is an enlargement of lead I, AVF, and AVL to better represent the simultaneous timing of events. As can be seen, the Q wave of AVF in this case occupies the first 0.01 seconds of the QRS complex. In that period of time, lead I is approaching approximately one-third of its maximal positive voltage, resulting in the inscription of section a of the QRS loop. At 0.03 seconds, lead I has obtained its maximal positive deflection (b) At 0.04 seconds, AVF is maximally positive and lead I is less positive (c). At 0.05 seconds, lead I is at zero and AVF is less positive (d). When AVF has become zero, at 0.07 seconds, lead I is maximally negative (e). During the last 0.01 seconds, both leads I and AVF are negative before returning to zero (f). The simultaneous registration of lead AVL revealed that the first 0.04 seconds were positive and the second 0.04 seconds were negative. The QRS frontal plane vector loop determined above is now drawn in the bottom left hand corner of the ECG data sheet (Fig. 3.17) and CW 60° is written into the box provided.

HORIZONTAL PLANE

The horizontal plane vector loop is determined in the same way as that in the frontal plane, with leads V2 and V5 utilized as were leads I and AVF. Other leads will always be needed as well, V4R being particularly useful as a starting point, unless the voltages are very low. Figure 3.22A represents a segment from an idealized six-channel standard ECG. In each of the lettered segments B through H the horizontal line is the line perpendicular to lead V2, while the vertical line is the line perpendicular to lead V5. Since the initial

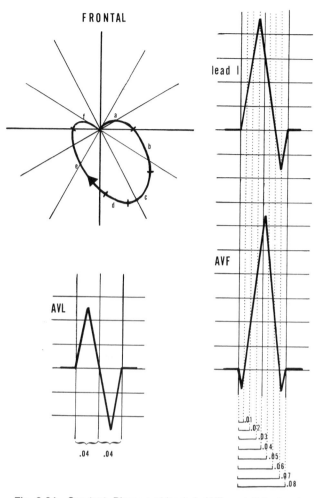

FRONTAL

lead I

AVF

AVL

.04   .04

.01
.02
.03
.04
.05
.06
.07
.08

Fig. 3.21 See text. Blow-up of leads I, AVF, and AVL showing timing of simultaneous events: *a* (0 to 0.01 sec), *b* (0.01 to 0.03 sec), *c* (0.03 to 0.04 sec), *d* (0.045 to 0.055 sec), *e* (0.055 to 0.07 sec), and *f* (0.07 to 0.08 sec).

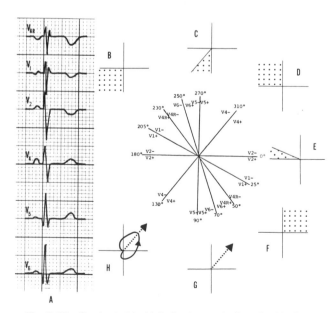

Fig. 3.22 See text. *A* to *H* similar to events described in Figure 3.20, but with horizontal plane leads.

QRS is to the right, negative in V5 and positive in V2, the initial QRS is between 90 and 180° (Fig. 3.22*B*). Because V4 begins upright, the initial QRS angle is between 90 and 130° (Fig. 3.22*C*). If one then wishes to determine the terminal vectors and then the mean vector, one can proceed as in Figure 3.22*D* to *G*. Leads V5 and V6 both terminate negatively, to the right and posterior, resulting in a terminal vector in the right upper quadrant (Fig. 3.22*D*). Since V6 terminates negative, V2 terminates negative, and V1 terminates positive (r'), the terminal vector is between 180 and 205° (Fig. 3.22*E*). In drawing out the vector loop (3.22*H* is approximate), the maximal vector and the mean vector (3.22*G*) are seen to be approximately the same at 310°. The loop is inscribed counterclockwise, so that CCW 310° is written into the box provided in Figure 3.17.

Accurate interpretation of the standard ECG not only relies on comparisons of voltages, rates, intervals, etc. with normals, but also on estimation of whether the orientation of the loop is within the normal range for the age (Fig. 3.23).

At this juncture, it is desirable to indicate the use of vector concepts utilizing tracings of real children. First, we show a Frank system vectorcardiogram of a normal 14-year-old with its three component scalars and the horizontal (XZ), sagittal (YZ), and frontal (XY) planes (Fig. 3.24). Now let us analyze the vector loop as well as the X and Z leads in relation to the sequence of ventricular depolarization. As previously described, there are four major areas which take part in initial depolarization, but in the normal older child, the most important is that due to activation of the left side of the septum. The vector from this area far outweighs the other vectors, and since activation begins on the left posterior part of the septum and the septum is obliquely placed, the initial QRS vector is to the right and anterior. The anterior part of the right ventricle, near the anterior papillary muscle, continues activating after which

AGE	FRONTAL	HORIZONTAL
0-24 Hours		
1 Week		
1 Month		
2 Months		
6 Months		
6 Years		

Fig. 3.23 Diagrammatic estimates of normal frontal and horizontal plane vector loops for various ages. *Solid lines*, QRS loop; *dashed lines*, T loop.

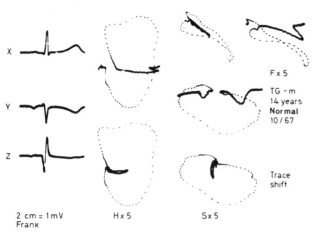

Fig. 3.24 A 14-year-old boy's normal Frank system vectorcardiogram with X, Y, and Z simultaneous scalar components. The horizontal plane (*H*) is at 5 cm = 1 mV as are the sagittal (*S*) and frontal (*F*) planes. The H plane includes the X and Z axes, the S plane the Y and Z axes, and the F plane the Y and X axes. Each "loop" consists of the terminus of consecutive vectors at 0.001 second. The vectors of the H plane cause a counterclockwise loop, the S plane a counterclockwise loop, and the F plane a narrow clockwise loop. Each "dot" (the terminus) is comma-shaped with the sharp end leading, so that the direction of the vector "loop" can be determined. By analyzing the vector at each instant of time, we are able to estimate the vector of everything being activated at each instant of time. Each loop has an accompanying loop where the paper has been moved as the trace is being developed. This "trace shift" allows delineating of the initial QRS vectors. Each loop also has a smaller, more slowly inscribed T wave. (Reproduced with permission from J. Liebman and R. Plonsey[83] and from the publisher, S. Karger, Basel, Switzerland.)

the anterior portions of each ventricle are prominent. By the time both ventricular free walls are activating, the vector is to the left as well as anterior, because the left ventricle is thicker than the right. At the time both lateral portions are depolarized, the vector is well to the left, since the free wall of the left ventricle is thicker than that of the right ventricle. The vector is then directed posterior, because both portions of the ventricles are depolarized. Finally, the terminal heart vector is slightly to the right, since two of the last portions to be depolarized, the superior septum and posterobasal left ventricle, are slightly to the right of the area where initial septal activation took place. The right ventricular outflow tract may also be depolarized during that last period, and this is also slightly to the right of where initial activation took place. It is obvious that during the entire time the vector is to the left, the right ventricle is being depolarized as well as the left. Had the right ventricle been thicker, the cardiac vector would have been less to the left and less posterior. In fact, had the right ventricle been much thicker, certain portions of the vector at those times might have been anterior and to the right. Had the left ventricle been thicker than normal, it is obvious that the sum total of electrical activity, during the times the ventricular free wall was being activated, might be even more to the left and posterior.

There is nothing magical, however, about seeing a vector loop as electronically constructed. As mentioned above, it is our policy in analyzing the standard electrocardiogram: to construct the vector; to measure the magnitudes of the X, Y, and Z axes; to measure any other leads which appear to be abnormal; to determine what is being depolarized and when; and to attempt to visualize what must be the pathology to cause that vector.

We will now show three standard electrocardiograms and demonstrate the method of analysis. In each case, the full standard electrocardiogram is shown, plus a blow-up of leads V4R, V2, and V5. Leads V2 and V5 are approximations of the Z and X axes,

respectively, while lead V4R almost bisects the other two axes. Therefore, an approximate construction of the horizontal plane vector is possible and is depicted.

In Figures 3.25*A* and *B*, the activation sequence is quite normal for a teenager, though the maximal magnitude on the X and Z axes are much greater than normal. During the entire time that the free walls of the right and left ventricles are being depolarized, the vector is more to the left and posterior than normal. Therefore, left ventricular hypertrophy is diagnosed.

In Figures 3.26*A* and *B*, the activation sequence is not normal. The vector originates directly to the left. Many conditions may cause this, including, naturally, left bundle branch block. However, fibrosis of the left side of the septum, left posterior free wall hypertrophy, and severe right ventricular hypertrophy can also all cause the initial QRS vector to originate directly to the left. It is important that at the time the posterior free walls of each ventricle are depolarized, the vector is less posterior than average. Finally, the terminal right ward vector is of considerable duration. An actual vectorcardiogram would probably rule out terminal slowing, and thus, right bundle branch block. Right ventricular hypertrophy is diagnosed. Please note that after the first three timed points, lead V4R is always positive, and this does not fit with leads V2 and V5. Clearly, lead V4R is demonstrating considerable proximity effect; therefore, that lead cannot be utilized in constructing the vector. The latter phenomenon is very common.

In Figures 3.27*A* and *B*, the activation sequence is also abnormal. The initial vector is almost to the left. After point 3, the vectors are anterior instead of posterior, so that the "loop" has to become clockwise in orientation. Therefore, the free wall of the right ventricle must be very thick to cause the vectors to be anterior first to the left, and then to the right. Right ventricular hypertrophy is the diagnosis.

THE NORMAL ELECTROCARDIOGRAM

The interpretation of the electrocardiogram in any lead system requires knowledge of the normal standards for that age and system. The large amount of data necessary to develop appropriate statistics at each age group from the prematurely born baby to late adolescence has not yet been obtained. Furthermore, for standard electrocardiography, separate standards must be available for QRS tracings taken with a low frequency response (most instruments in use today) and those with a high frequency response (photographic or jet writers). Other aspects of incompleteness come about because percentiles could not be developed from all the linear data in the literature and because inappropriate linear analyses were often utilized for angular data. In evaluating biological data, it is desirable to determine two standard deviations around the mean. Normal electrocardiographic data, however, may show significant skewing, so that two standard deviations from the mean may exceed the maximum or be less than the minimum. Consequently, percentiles are desirable, with the 5th and 95th percentiles (or 2 ½ and 97 ½) as an indicator of low or high limits of normal. Another caution that should be taken is using circular or spherical statistics for angular data.[147-150]

It is beyond the scope of this chapter to include all the meaningful tabular normal data available, but the reader is referred to the recent publication,[151] which includes 105 tables.

The information from Ziegler's[137] classic monograph was derived from high frequency optical recorders and provides the base for much of the tabular data for high frequency standard electrocardiography, reanalyzed using appropriate statistics as much as possible. The recent excellent standard electrocardiographic high frequency data of Davignon *et al.*[152] is for Caucasians, and because of space considerations

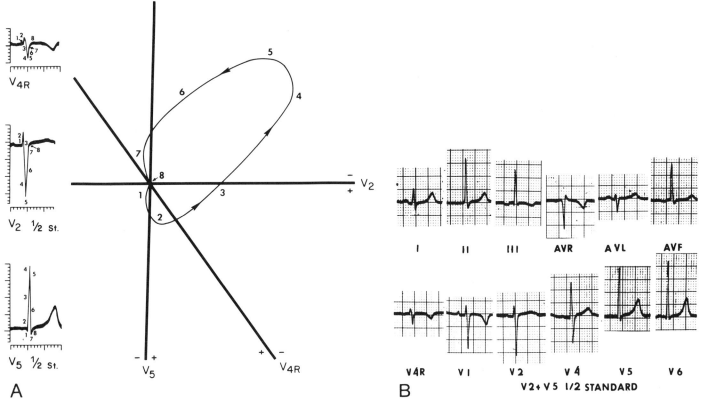

Fig. 3.25 (A) A blow-up of leads V4R, V2, and V5 of a 16-year-old with left ventricular hypertrophy. At eight consecutive instants of time, a vector is projected on the leads (perpendiculars to the leads are depicted). The terminus of each vector forms a "loop." The activation sequence is normal, but the vectors during activation of the free walls of the right and left ventricle are abnormally to the left and posterior. (B) Full standard ECG of A. (Reproduced with permission from J. Liebman and R. Plonsey[83] and from the publisher, S. Karger, Basel, Switzerland.)

is not included in this chapter. Much of the low frequency tabular data is from a regrouping and reanalysis of the data of Namin and Miller[153] and Alimurung et al.[154] Our own data[155, 156] have been added to each group in specific instances. The grouped tables include an unknown mixture of white and black children. In orthogonal electrocardiography, Frank and McFee-Parungao, most of the data available after infancy are from our own laboratory[157-159] and are approximately equal in numbers of blacks and whites. The newborn and infant data of Guller,[160] Namin,[161] and Namin and D'Cruz[162] fill in some of the gaps, and the data from the atria of Ferrer and Ellison[163] are included. For more complete information, the previously mentioned 105 tables are available,[151] as is a selected additional reference list.[164-178]

HEART RATE

The newborn's heart rate is less at birth than at 1 month, after which there is a gradual decrease. The premature infant's heart rate in the first week is higher than that of the full term.

P WAVE AMPLITUDE

The 95th percentile in lead II is 0.2 mv for prematures, approximately 0.25 mv for newborns to children 12 years old, and 0.20 mv for teenagers. Approximate standards for voltage anterior and posterior are not available.

P WAVE DURATION

The average P duration is slightly greater at 0 to 24 hours (0.051 seconds) than at 1 to 7 days (0.046 seconds). From

then on, there is a gradual increase until that of teenagers at 0.081 seconds. Unfortunately, there are no good data for the parts of the P wave, P initial (P_I), P terminal (P_T), time between anterior and posterior peaks, and ratio of P wave duration to the duration of the PQ segment (Macruz index).

PR INTERVAL

The PR interval increases with increasing age, but the exhaustive study of McCammon showed no relationship to heart rate. He also demonstrated the striking stability of the well child's PR interval.

QRS DURATION

There is an increase with increasing age, the duration being particularly low in the premature infant where the mean is 0.03 and the 95th percentile is 0.04. In full terms, Ziegler's data demonstrates a greater mean duration (0.065 second) at 24 hours than at 1 to 7 days (0.056).

QRS MAGNITUDES

The normal newborn has very low voltages (even lower in the premature) with potential gradually increasing until 2 to 3 months of age. With the onset of puberty, magnitudes once again diminish, more in females than males. The onset of the decrease occurs earlier in the female than the male.

The Q wave voltages are not included in the tables (except for the adolescents), but are given here because of their importance in specific leads (AVF, V5, V6). All figures are

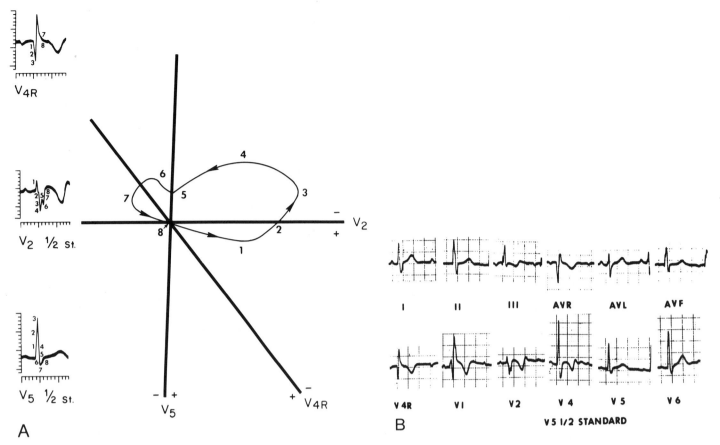

Fig. 3.26 (*A*) A blow-up of leads V_{4R}, V₂, and V₅ of a 5-year-old with mild right ventricular hypertrophy. At eight consecutive instants of time, a vector is projected on the leads. The activation sequence is very abnormal. The initial vector is to the left, the vectors during the midportion are less posterior than average, and the duration that the vector is rightward is abnormal. Note also that there is a considerable proximity effect in lead V_{4R} which must be deleted in constructing the vector. (*B*) Full standard ECG of *A*. (Reproduced with permission from J. Liebman and R. Plonsey[83] and from the publisher, S. Karger, Basel, Switzerland.)

for the 95th percentile:

High frequency recorders (Ziegler)
  AVF: Up to age 6 months, 4 mm; 6 months to 3 years, 5 mm;
    remainder of childhood, 4 mm.
  V5: Up to age 3 years, 5 mm; remainder of childhood, 4 mm.
  V6: Up to age 3 months, 4 mm; up to age 12 years, 4 mm;
    teenage, 2.5 mm.
Low frequency records (Alimurung)
  AVF: Up to age 9 months, 3.5 mm; 10 to 24 months, 3.5 mm;
    2 to 5 years, 1.7 mm; over 5 years, 1.8 mm.
  V5: Up to age 9 months, 3.0 mm; 10 to 24 months, 4.0 mm;
    2 to 5 years, 1.7 mm; over 5 years, 1.8 mm.
  V6: Up to age 9 months, 2.3 mm; 10 to 24 months, 2.5 mm;
    2 to 5 years, 2.8 mm; over 5 years, 2.3 mm.

QRS MEAN VECTOR

The prevalent direction in the frontal plane at 0 to 24 hours is 135°, with the 95th percentile at 180°. There is rapid change to the left by 3 to 6 months and onward, when the prevalent direction is 65°, and the 95th percentile is 80 to 100°. Data for the horizontal plane is available only for the premature infant and the adolescent, but the trend is from right and anterior to left and posterior. Of greater diagnostic value are maximal, or main, vectors, for which adequate data are also not available. In the premature infant, for example, the prevalent direction is 74°, but 16 of the 74 infants had a second main vector at 239°.

ST SEGMENT

Slight elevations of the ST segment followed by a sloping decrease before the T wave rise are very common, particularly in the mid- and left precordial leads, but also in II, III, and AVF. This is normal, and has been called early repolarization. That term is a misnomer, for repolarization begins in each cell as soon as depolarization ends. However, in the chimpanzee, Spach's group[105] has documented repolarization in the last 40% of the QRS. We have also seen repolarization in normal children's body surface potential maps before the end of the QRS.[106] True ST segment elevation is considered allowable for up to 2 mm in the chest leads and 1 mm in the limb leads.

QT INTERVAL

This interval has traditionally been corrected for the heart rate. We have not chosen to measure the relatively cumbersome $QTC = $ actual $QT/\sqrt{R\text{-}R}$ or the QT ratio = actual $QT/0.40 \sqrt{R\text{-}R}$, for we have found most satisfactory the use of the ruler made by Bowen and Company, Bethesda, Md. Normality has been judged if the QT interval falls within 0.03 second of that expected for the heart rate. Recently, both Simonson *et al.*[179] and McCammon[180] have stated that the QT was only partially dependent on rate and that the various corrected QT intervals were quite useless. Fluctuations were so wide that in at least 25%, the upper limits of normal extended past the previously considered top normal.

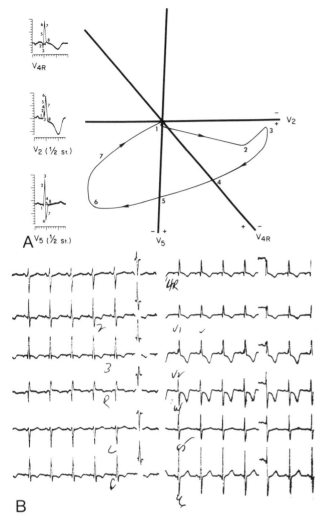

Fig. 3.27 (*A*) A blow-up of leads V₄ᵣ, V₂, and V₅ of an 8-year-old with right ventricular hypertrophy. At eight consecutive instants of time, a vector is projected on the leads. The activation sequence is very abnormal. The initial vector is almost to the left, though points 2 and 3 are normal. However, all points after that are anterior, with the late points also to the right. In an 8-year-old child, right ventricular hypertrophy is diagnosed. (*B*) Full standard ECG of *A*. (Reproduced with permission from J. Liebman and R. Plonsey[83] and from the publisher, S. Karger, Basel, Switzerland.)

T WAVE MEAN VECTORS

The data for the normal direction of the T vector in the first 3 days of life will be described later. Before the end of the first week, the mean T vector is to the left, posterior and anterior. The prevalent direction in the horizontal plane is at 310°, in the frontal plane at 40°. From then on there is very gradual change,[181–183] eventually becoming anterior during teenage or young adulthood, occasionally also becoming superior by then.

QRS-T ANGLE (ALSO ANGULAR DEVIATION OF T FROM QRS)

The differences between the mean vectors of the QRS and T are very great in early infancy. By 3 months, the mean QRS-T angle in the frontal plane is 30°. From 3 to 6 months, an angle of 75° in the frontal plane is considered abnormal; after that, the upper limit is 60°. Normal data for the

horizontal plane are not available for standard electrocardiography, but the angle is somewhat wider. With increasing age, the angular deviation of T from QRS in the horizontal plane narrows, the T vector becomes less posterior, and the mean QRS vector becomes more posterior. A more meaningful statistic than QRS-T angle is the angular deviation of T from QRS. This is a clockwise deviation from 1 to 359° (the latter being a T that is 1° counterclockwise from QRS). Data is available only for adolescents.

NORMAL VALUES (FRANK SYSTEM ORTHOGONAL ELECTROCARDIOGRAPHY) ATRIAL MEASURES

The normal values necessary for interpretation of atrial hypertrophy are much more available in orthogonal electrocardiography than in standard electrocardiography. The data is from the work of Ferrer and Ellison.[163] The normal values necessary for evaluation of newborns are also more available in orthogonal electrocardiography than in standard electrocardiography, because of the data of Guller *et al.*[160] at 1 to 72 hours on large numbers of normal babies. This newborn data is supplemented by the previously available data by Namin *et al.*,[161] which spans the period between the newborn and age 18 months.

Data on older children, from ages 2 to 19 years, have been exhaustively done for both the McFee-Parungao and Frank systems. The entire collection of data, as well as that for the premature infant, has been included in the recently published book.[57]

NORMAL PROGRESSION OF THE ELECTROCARDIOGRAM FROM INFANCY

The newborn's right ventricular dominance, as compared to the adult's, is well known,[161, 107] but it includes extreme variability. The latter is so even if we exclude the premature infant, in whom it has been demonstrated that the pulmonary arteriolar muscle mass is less.[192] The right ventricle is less thick,[193] and the vectorcardiogram shows less right ventricular hypertrophy.[194] At 30 weeks of gestation, the left ventricle is thicker than the right, is about the same thickness as the right ventricle at 32 to 35 weeks, and reaches newborn values at about 36 weeks. From then on, the RV/LV weight ratio averages 1.3:1.[195]

In the first few days after birth, there are rapid hemodynamic changes, which have not been demonstrated to affect the QRS of the electrocardiogram,[107] but there are profound T wave changes. The report of Hait and Gasul[183] demonstrates these changes. Three distinct phases were delineated: birth (0 to 5 min), T vector to left and anterior; transient phase (defined as that time during which the T waves reached their maximal rightward and anterior displacement 1 to 6 hours after birth); and restitution phase, to left and usually posterior (this phase usually takes 3 days to complete, but by 7 days the T vector should be posterior). These data have been confirmed by Castellanos *et al.*[181] and by Hänninen.[176]

In standard electrocardiography, in the first 3 days of life, the majority of horizontal plane vectors will be inscribed clockwise, although a number will be inscribed so that there are narrow or figure of eight loops with two main vectors. A small number will even be counterclockwise, though they will be narrow. In the Frank vectorcardiogram, our data agree with those of Namin *et al.*,[161] Hänninen,[176] and Guller *et al.*,[175] where approximately 60% are clockwise, 15% are counterclockwise, and 25% have two main vectors. The numbers in each study are few, so that the exact percentages are not meaningful statistically; however, the trends are clear. By 6 weeks of age and surely by 2 months of age, the horizontal plane vector is always counterclockwise, though there may be a small terminal right posterior "tail" which rotates clockwise. Though this horizontal plane vector is now counterclockwise, and though the left ventricular to right ventricular ratio is beginning to approach adult levels, the body of the vector will be mainly anterior in the first 6 months, but will not become a mainly posterior vector until ages 1 to 2. Until school age, the change is very gradual, but a prominent anterior projection in the preschool child can be depended upon, presumably due to the proximity effect. Throughout childhood, this anterior projection gradually decreases both in its magnitude and in the relative amount of the early QRS duration that is anterior.

The premature infant would be expected to demonstrate less right ventricular dominance than does a full-term baby, and this expectation has been confirmed for both the standard electrocardiogram and the Frank system.

The frontal plane rotation has not proved diagnostically useful. In infancy, it is almost always inscribed clockwise, and even late in childhood, in the Frank system, the frontal plane is clockwise 85% of the time.

The QRS voltage is known to be low in the newborn, for reasons quite unclear, not reaching peak voltage until ages 2 to 3 months. The premature infant's QRS voltage is even lower. By age 2 to 3 months, however, the electrocardiogram of the premature infant is not different from that of the full-term baby, either in rotation or activation sequence.

The initial QRS vector is also different in newborns from that in children later in life. An initial QRS vector to the left is unusual in the older child, yet it is not at all rare in full-term babies. Presumably, this is due to the newborn's right ventricular dominance. In the premature infant, the initial QRS is less likely to be directed leftward.

The vector loop in the newborn and through much of the first month is mainly anterior rather than terminal rightward during the right ventricular dominance period. When there is less right ventricular dominance, the orientation is often anterior-posterior. The voltages to the left and right appear to be unduly diminished.

THE ABNORMAL ELECTROCARDIOGRAM

ATRIAL HYPERTROPHY

The sinus and AV nodes contribute no voltage to the external electrocardiogram, and the atrial wave is of small magnitude. This not only contributes to the difficulty in diagnosis of dysrhythmias, but also to the diagnosis of atrial hypertrophy. Furthermore, the timed sequence of depolarization is incompletely known. The right atrium begins activation well before the left atrium, beginning very superior and to the right. The direction of activation must be entirely to the left and inferior. Since the sinus node is also quite posterior, initial activation is anterior. Activation of the left atrium is by way of Bachmann's bundle, also anterior (and superior), so left atrial activation also begins anterior. Peuch,[184, 185] for diagnostic purposes, has divided the left atrium into thirds, the first third mainly being due to the right atrium, the final third mainly being due to the left atrium, and the middle third encompassing both atria. Ferrer and Ellison[163] reanalyzed the activation data for the dog atria of Spach's group[49, 186] and determined that the first 36 to 40% of the P duration was due to right atrial activation, that the right atrium was finishing and left atrium beginning at 49 to 53%, and that at 69 to 86% of the P duration, the major areas of the left atrium were being activated. Durrer's

reperfused human atria demonstrated similar behavior. In the human high quality surface electrocardiogram, the three areas cannot be recognized, but two areas are clear.

Interpretation of hypertrophy or enlargement (we cannot distinguish them) must come from increased voltage in specific directions and specific increases in duration. There is no single methodology or parameter which is totally reliable, but simultaneous high gain leads are extremely useful (Fig. 3.28).

STANDARD ELECTROCARDIOGRAPHY

Specific Voltage Increase

Increased magnitude inferior of first portion of P (lead II, because activation is along the lead II axis) indicates right

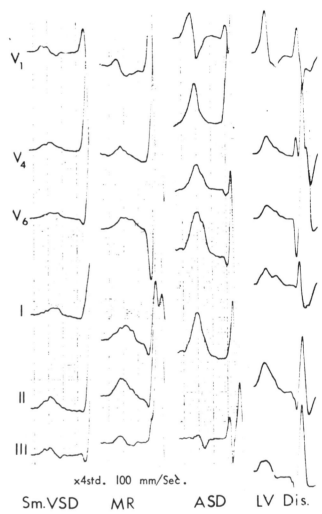

Fig. 3.28 Four representative electrocardiograms for P wave analysis. The simultaneous tracings of leads V₁, V₄, V₆, I, II, and III are recorded at four times standard and 100 mm/second. In the first tracing of a patient with a small ventricular septal defect (*Sm. VSD*), the P waves are normal. In the second patient with mitral regurgitation (*MR*), the second portion of the P wave is very prolonged, indicative of left atrial hypertrophy. In the third tracing of a patient with atrial septal defect (*ASD*), the first portion of the P wave has very high voltage anterior and inferior, indicative of right atrial hypertrophy. In the fourth electrocardiogram from a patient with left ventricular cardiomyopathy (*LV Dis*), the first portion has a large voltage anterior and inferior, indicative of right atrial hypertrophy, while the second portion is very prolonged, indicative of left atrial hypertrophy. Thus, there is combined atrial hypertrophy.

atrial hypertrophy (RAH). Increased magnitude anterior of first portion of P (V1, V2) indicates RAH. Note that it is not rare to have V1 entirely negative and of large magnitude in RAH, if the first portion of V2 is anterior. Increased magnitude posterior of second portion of P (V1, V2) is said to be a good criterion for left atrial hypertrophy (LAH). This is only a fair criterion in our experience.

P Terminal Forces

P terminal forces act as a measurement for determining LAH and give weight to both an increased duration of the second portion of the P wave in V1 and an increased magnitude negative of the second portion. The average for adults[187] is −0.01 with a 95% confidence interval of +0.01 to −0.03. It has been shown to be useful in adults,[188] but normal data for children are not available.

Time between Anterior and Posterior Peaks

On occasion, this is a valuable adjunct. In infants, the peaks are usually not more than 0.02 second apart, and in adolescents, they rarely exceed 0.04 second. In general, the longer the time interval between peaks, the more likely is LAH. This can also be a help in combined atrial hypertrophy (CAH), for if RAH is obvious and the peaks are far apart, additional LAH is likely.

Increased duration of P wave, with second portion of particularly long duration indicates LAH. Simultaneous high quality tracings are necessary for proper interpretation. Increased duration of the first portion, due to RAH, is difficult to recognize.

Increased ratio of P duration/PQ segment (Macruz Index)[189] indicates LAH. This could be a good criterion but, unfortunately, no normal data are available for children.

Orthogonal Electrocardiography

An exhaustive study of parameters has been done by Ferrer and Ellison.[163, 190] The authors' best criteria for RAH were the magnitudes of Z anterior and SVA (spatial voltage at time of maximal anterior). The best criteria for LAH were the magnitudes of Z posterior and SVP (spatial voltage at time of maximal posterior). In the exhaustive study of Ishikawa et al.,[191] the best criteria for LAH were the P duration, and a modification of the P terminal force.

VENTRICULAR HYPERTROPHY

Because of the wide variation of normal even within each specific age group, the diagnosis of normality can sometimes be difficult.[196–201] There are some electrocardiographers who refuse to use voltage criteria because of fear of an occasional false negative. On the other hand, without the use of the normal standards, hypertrophy will frequently be missed. Furthermore, the voltage criteria should not be used de novo; they should be utilized along with our increasing knowledge of the pathways of activation and of vector analysis. The electrical patterns generated by active cardiac cells are reflected reasonably well in the heart's surface but become smoothed out when viewed at the body surface. Consequently, the problems of interpretation involve recovery of details that have tended to be "washed out." Other factors that tend to distort the pattern at the body surface are the internal electrical inhomogeneities and assymetrical geometry (proximity). We believe that the recent and continued work of Rudy et al.[96, 202, 204] on these subjects will prove extremely useful.

We have previously delineated many of the inherent difficulties in interpretation of hypertrophy in simple terms.[83]

Though vector principles are paramount, the closer the heart is to the chest electrodes, the greater is the voltage generated by those leads. This proximity effect, particularly important in infants and those with large hearts, may cause an unequal emphasis on the magnitude of the voltage in some leads and not others. Thus, the lead voltage will be distorted from being a projection of a simple (dipole) cardiac vector. When Wilson[4, 93, 94] developed the chest lead system, the concept was that the specific chest electrode would reflect activity of the heart muscle just under the electrode. We know that this is not true, but that every scalar potential reflects the sum total of electrical activity from everywhere in the heart distorted by that proximity and by much else. Apparently, the right chest lead voltage may be particularly distorted by proximity.

Because the heart is in the left chest, Burger[101, 111, 112] was able to demonstrate that the Einthoven equilateral triangle was actually scalene. Thus, lead I is not a very good X axis. The projection of the cardiac vector on the right-left X axis causes superior-inferior distortion so that whereas a more accurate X axis (lead V5) may show a qR with little or no S wave, lead I may show a qRs with the S wave varying from being small to being even larger than the R wave.

Rudy's data also helps us to explain why a thickly muscled hypoplastic right ventricle provides very little surface voltage, while a thin-walled very dilated ventricle may produce considerable surface voltage. Air in the chest anteriorly and laterally, as in a patient with severe cystic fibrosis, causes decreased voltage anteriorly and laterally. The result is an abnormally posterior vector not due to hypertrophy. Another example is the patient with dilatation of the heart, a large blood-filled cardiac chamber, and a ventricular source close to the chest wall. The voltage in such a case is expected to be high, but with the onset of left-sided heart failure, the lung fluid modifies the effect of the lungs to decrease voltage.

In a discussion of hypertrophy as previously described, it is more difficult to relate the morphology of the T wave to cardiac electrophysiology than it is for the QRS. The T wave, in the normal, is not propagated; the entire heart contributes as an active source for a prolonged period. In contrast, during activation, the cardiac sources are well defined and are limited to relatively narrow regions at each instant of time. In studies of *normal* children's orthogonal electrocardiograms, there was no correlation between the spatial orientation of the QRS and T.[205] However, in our data on *abnormal* hearts, there was a definite relationship.

A few final comments are in order before describing the criteria for interpretation of ventricular hypertrophy. A number of commonly used criteria and terms have been deliberately avoided.

Ventricular Activation Time and the Intrinsicoid Deflection

There is no theoretical basis for the use of ventricular activation and the intrinsicoid deflection, for the only situation in which the intrinsicoid deflection is evident is the electrocardiogram from an isolated cell. The left chest leads are not left ventricular leads; they reflect the cardiac vector from the entire heart.

Cardiac Position

A "vertical" heart is diagnosed when the frontal plane "axis" is toward plus 90°. A "horizontal" heart is diagnosed when the frontal plane "axis" is toward 0°. One is, therefore, merely determining the mean vector as seen in the limb leads. The anatomy of the heart is not related. The terms are useless.

Axis

The only axes used in this chapter are the X, Y, and Z axes, indicative of left-right, inferior-superior, and anterior-posterior directions. The commonly used term "axis" indicates a mean vector. The terms right axis deviation and left axis deviation are not useful. We must realize that the term "marked left axis deviation" is indicative of an abnormally superior vector.[206] That vector is often more to the right than normal.

Anatomic Rotation

Clockwise and counterclockwise rotations are often used to imply anatomic rotation of the heart.[207] For example, right ventricular hypertrophy was said to cause clockwise rotation. Thus, more of the right ventricle faced the chest, causing taller R waves in the right chest leads, with a later progression to rS complexes over the left chest leads. Unfortunately, x-ray, angiogram, and autopsy data have not confirmed this,

other than perhaps a small amount of rotation of the septum in the presence of marked dilatation of the right ventricle.

LEFT VENTRICULAR HYPERTROPHY (LVH)

Inscription of Vector Loops

The activation sequence may be exactly as normal, so that a counterclockwise horizontal plane vector loop is present. In the frontal plane, however, the loop usually remains clockwise, with a counterclockwise loop being only slightly more common in LVH than in the normal. If the frontal plane loop is counterclockwise, begins inferior, and is mainly superior, then the diagnosis is "abnormally superior vector," and is likely to indicate either left anterior division block or an endocardial cushion defect (Fig. 3.29).[206, 208, 209] In the newborns, a wide open counterclockwise horizontal plane loop is indicative of LVH, though a counterclockwise narrow loop may be normal. The latter usually will be prominent anterior and posterior, terminally well to the right, and

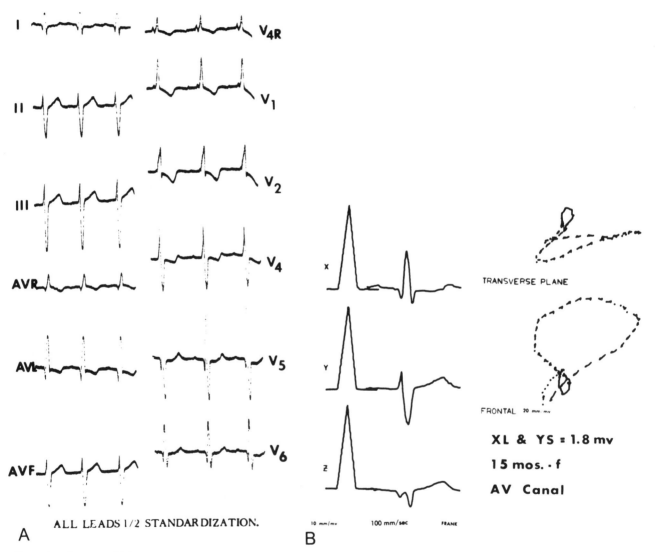

Fig. 3.29 Standard ECG with simultaneous leads (A) and Frank VCG (B) of 15-month-old with intermediate form of endocardial cushion defect (partial AV canal). Both lead systems in this case are remarkably similar except that, the voltages in the standard ECG are much greater. There is an "abnormally superior vector" and combined ventricular hypertrophy. The transverse loop is narrow and mainly clockwise, and entirely anterior. The X left is above normal, giving the diagnosis of additional LVH.

minimally to the left. In the premature, even a wide open counterclockwise loop may be normal.

Increased Magnitude of Posterior Vector (Increased Z Posterior)

The abnormally posterior vector is probably the best single criterion for LVH (Fig. 3.30). Occasionally, very severe right ventricular hypertrophy (RVH) can be associated with a horizontal plane vector which swings to the right and posterior very quickly, with the magnitude posterior very great. In such circumstances, a common error is to diagnose combined ventricular hypertrophy (CVH). A top normal Z posterior together with a top normal X left may indicate a very wide open vector loop and should also suggest LVH. This same wide open loop may cause the projection of R in V6 to be as tall or taller than V5. A top normal Z posterior together with a quite small X left may be part of an abnormally posterior horizontal plane angle and is suggestive of LVH.

If the posterior vector is also very far to the right, it may

indicate additional RVH but, more likely, there is postero-basal LVH as part of the pure LVH.

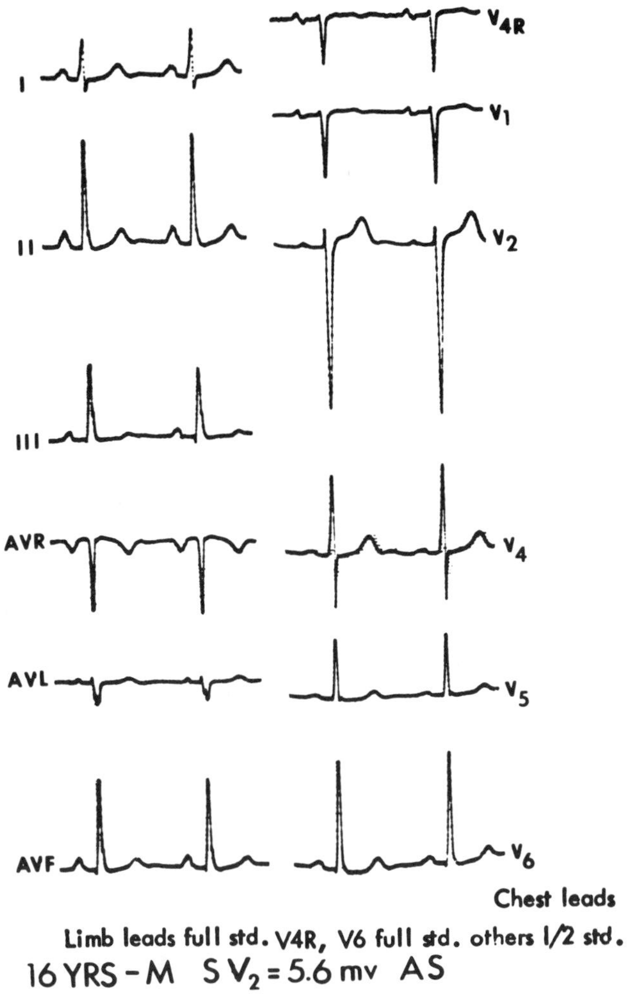

Increased Magnitude of Leftward Vector (Increased X Left, Tall R V5)

This is a very good sign of LVH. If the R in V6 is also above normal, the vector loop is very broad, so that LVH is more certain.

Increased Magnitude of Inferior Vector (Increased Y Inferior, Tall R in AVF)

If the horizontal plane is activated normally, LVH should be suggested since the left ventricle is a more inferior structure than is the right ventricle. However, marked RVH can also cause an inferior vector, so that combined ventricular hypertrophy must not be diagnosed if the horizontal plane clearly indicates RVH.

Initial QRS of Large Magnitude to the Right and Anterior (Deep Q in V5, Tall R in V1,V2 of Brief Duration) (Fig. 3.31)

This recording is believed to usually be caused by hypertrophy of the left side of the septum. A large initial Y superior (deep q in AVF) may also be present, presumably due to activation of the thick wall up the septum. The diagnosis, however, is left septal hypertrophy, not LVH, though there may be other criteria for LVH.

Initial QRS to the Left[210] (No Initial X Right, No q in V5) (Fig. 3.30)

In the presence of LVH, an initial QRS to the left and anterior indicates greater severity, presumably due mainly to hypertrophy of the free wall of the left ventricle at the left posterior portion of the septum where ventricular activation begins.[70]

Decreased ratio of the magnitude of Z anterior to Z posterior is a good criterion, especially useful in the presence of low voltage.

Increased magnitude R in AVL is a good criterion unless there is an abnormally superior vector.

Increased magnitude of the maximal spatial vector to the left. MSVL = $\sqrt{X^2 + Y^2 + Z^2}$ of the leftward vector. This is an excellent criterion. It has been used as a specific criterion of hemodynamic events, such as the left ventricular peak pressure in valvular aortic stenosis.

QRS vector becoming posterior very rapidly is a good criterion, with the major differential that of isolated anterior myocardial infarction which is rare in children.

Main vector abnormally posterior is a good criterion and is better than mean vector abnormally posterior.

Frontal plane abnormally to the left (not superior) is a fair criterion.

ST and T abnormalities are nonspecific, but in the presence of known LVH, a wide deviation of T from QRS will indicate greater severity. When LVH is severe, the T vector is more anterior and less to the left, causing the Z anterior to be greater (taller T's in V1, V2) and the Z posterior to be smaller (smaller voltage in V5,V6). In even severer cases, the T vector is anterior and to the right, so that V5 and V6 are inverted. In maximal severity, the deviation of T from QRS may approach 180°. Also, there may be depression of the ST in the X leads (V5,V6) and anterior elevation in the Z leads (V1,V2), presumably because of inadequate perfusion of the ventricular muscle (Fig. 3.32).

Tall T waves in the left chest leads can also be part of

Chest leads

Limb leads full std. V4R, V6 full std. others 1/2 std.

16 YRS - M   S V2 = 5.6 mv   AS

Fig. 3.30 Standard ECG of a 16-year-old with severe aortic stenosis (*AS*). There is marked LVH with an abnormally posterior vector and mild ST segment abnormality. Note that the QRS moves posterior *very* quickly. Note also that V6 magnitude is at least as great as that of V5, a sign of LVH in its own right, for it indicates that the vector is remaining far to the left for a long time without conduction abnormality.

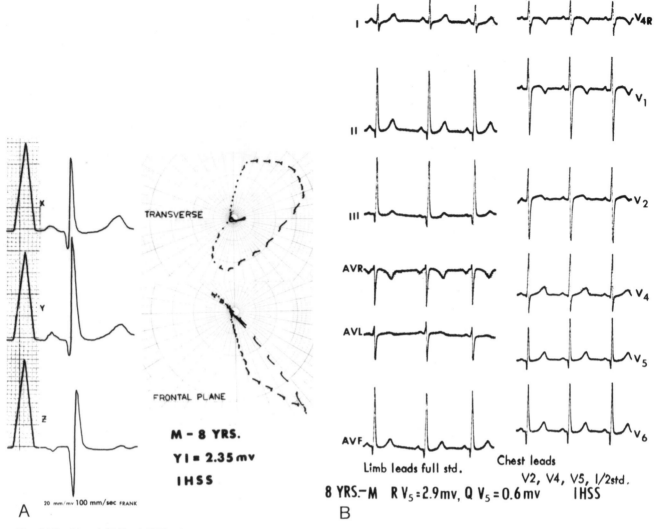

Fig. 3.31 (*A* and *B*) Frank VCG of an 8-year-old with idiopathic hypertrophic subaortic stenosis (IHSS). Note the large initial QRS vector to the right and anterior of left septal hypertrophy. In the standard ECG, the same is documented. LVH is also present.

LVH without an indication of severity. This was once believed to be part of the "diastolic overloading pattern," but it is now known not to be the case.

RIGHT VENTRICULAR HYPERTROPHY (RVH)

Inscription of Vector Loops

In the diagnosis of RVH, analysis of the activation sequence of the vector loop at each instant of time will help delineate deviation from normal. Therefore, as the right and left ventricular free walls begin depolarizing, a vector that is less leftward and/or posterior than normal at succeeding instants of time may cause the direction of inscription to be different from normal. With mild RVH, the main vector may be normally counterclockwise and posterior with a prominent terminal vector to the right. However, with increasing RVH, the vector loop may be less posterior and eventually may cross and/or be narrow; with severe RVH, it may be clockwise.

Since there is a spectrum of RVH as severity increases, it is not useful to describe types of RVH, nor is it useful to diagnose volume overload vs. pressure overload on the basis of the type of activation sequence. Criteria that have been developed to separate volume from pressure overload most

likely indicate differences in severity. A newborn provides a distinct problem in diagnosing RVH on the basis of activation sequences, since, in the latter, a clockwise-directed horizontal plane vector loop is the norm. As the weeks after birth increase, however, RVH becomes more readily diagnosable on the basis of activation sequences.

Increased Magnitude of the Terminal Rightward Vector (Increased Terminal X Axis to the Right, Deep S V5)

This is probably the single most sensitive criterion for RVH. To be certain of its reliability, a deep S in V6 is helpful. An increase in the terminal X to the right in lead I (S lead I) is also helpful, but the latter, by itself, is not useful. If a deep S is seen in lead I without other evidence of RVH, it should be ignored. An isolated S wave in lead I is frequently a distortion by inferior forces.

A large terminal X to the right (S in V5) may or may not be associated with a terminal R wave in lead V4R or V1, for unless the magnitude is great, the terminal vector must extend well anterior to cross the perpendicular to lead V4R and especially lead V1. Because of large variation in how far posterior the main body of the vector "loop" projects, as well as how anterior the most rightward portion of the terminal

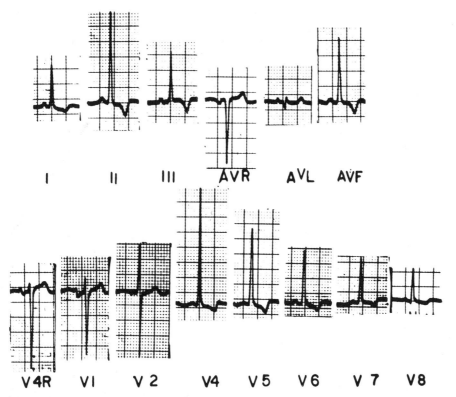

Fig. 3.32 Severe left ventricular hypertrophy in an 8-year-old with severe aortic stenosis. The projection is very far posterior, but, more important, the QRS-T angle is markedly discordant.

vector extends, it is difficult to correlate the magnitude of the terminal R. This helps explain the normal variant rsr' in the right chest leads, particularly when there is not a deep S in V5 and V6, and when the S (Z axis posterior) in V2 is relatively small. The deeper the S in V2, the more significant is the r' as an indicator of RVH. A special problem exists in the presence of an abnormally posterior vector, as seen in LVH, or as part of obstructive emphysema in cystic fibrosis. In such cases, it is common for the vector to be so far posterior that a large terminal vector to the right does not project onto leads V4R or V1 for the reasons described previously. In cystic fibrosis, this large terminal to the right is sometimes seen only in the orthogonal vectorcardiogram, not in the standard electrocardiogram, presumably because of air in the chest laterally.

There are times when in the right chest leads, there is a small voltage but definite terminal R in V4R and/or V1 without a deep S in V5. This is likely to represent a proximity effect and is usually a normal variant. Despite the fact that it represents a proximity effect, it may also be the only clue that leads to a diagnosis of RVH. An orthogonal electrocardiogram with a vector display will usually help delineate the issue as to whether RVH is present.

Increased Magnitude Anterior (Increased Z Anterior, Tall R in V1, V2, and Prominent Terminal R in V4R and V1)

The criterion is reliable, but particularly for a tall initial R, one must be very careful to make sure that the R is not a brief spike of less than 0.03 seconds. In such cases, there may be no RVH, but a proximity effect. Obviously, in cases of prominent terminal R in V1, there may be confusion with partial right bundle branch block and normal variants. A vectorcardiogram may be necessary to distinguish the two.

Increased Magnitude Posterior (Increased Z Posterior, Deep S1, V1, V2)

In very severe RVH, the horizontal plane vector may be clockwise, with the main vector well to the right and posterior.[211] In standard electrocardiography, there may even be an rS in V1, although V4R would likely demonstrate a tall R. Without V4R, and if the vector loop had not been drawn, the diagnosis of LVH might have been made erroneously.

Increased Magnitude Inferior (Increased Y Inferior, Increased R in AVF)

In the presence of marked RVH, an increased magnitude inferior does not indicate additional LVH.

Initial QRS to the Left and Anterior, Occasionally Posterior[210, 212]

In the presence of other signs of RVH, this initial leftward vector is an indicator of increased severity. If the vector is not very anterior, there may be a qR in V4R and even V1, and if the vector is posterior, the Z lead will be initially posterior with the main vector anterior (qR in lead V2). In severe pulmonic stenosis, especially in the McFee-Parungao system, an initial vector to the left is sometimes associated with suprasystemic right ventricular pressure. In cystic fibrosis with cor pulmonale, the initial QRS also averages further to the left than the normal. It is uncommon for a normal older child to have an initial QRS to the left, but it is normal in 5% of prematures and 10% of full-term babies.

An important differential is that of ventricular inversion where the initial QRS vector is well to the left and is either anterior or posterior. One possible clue to differentiation is the high frequency of a large magnitude initial Y superior vector (large q in AVF) in ventricular inversion because of the different orientation of the septum. The explanations as to why the initial vector is to the left in severe RVH are that the right septum is thicker than normal, and the inferior portion of the right ventricle, known to be depolarized very early, may actually be to the left of the area of the septum where depolarization begins. Rotation of the septum in a clockwise direction may also contribute, but this rotation is seen more in dilated right ventricles, where the initial QRS to the left is less common.

Increased Ratio of Magnitude of Z Anterior/Z Posterior and Increased Ratio of Magnitude of X Terminal Right/X Left

These are good criteria, especially in the presence of low voltage.

Increased Magnitude of Terminal R in AVR

This is a reliable but not very sensitive criterion, for the diagnosis of RVH or advanced RBBB is usually obvious from other evidence.

Increased Magnitude of the Maximal Spatial Vector to the Right $(MSVR) = \sqrt{X^2 + Y^2 + Z^2}$ of the Terminal Rightward Vector

This is an excellent criterion. It has been used for pulmonic stenosis as a predictor of right ventricular pressure with approximately the same success as the MSVL for aortic stenosis.

Main Vector Either Abnormally Anterior or to the Right

The use of main vectors has much more of a scientific basis than does the use of mean vectors, for, in so doing, the interpreter is considering activation sequences. Of particular interest are cases where there are two main vectors. The first may be to the left and anterior, the second (terminal) to the right and posterior. If the first vector is also abnormally to the left, then additional LVH is present.

ST and T Abnormality

An anterior leftward T vector after 72 hours of age (T upright V4R, V1 and V2, as well as V5,V6) is an indication of RVH. It is quite reliable and not related to severity. If the T vector is anterior and to the right, then there may be severe LVH. An abnormally posterior T vector is an indication of severity. Severity is even greater if the T vector is to the right as well (inverted V5). The deviation of T from QRS appears to be greater in the horizontal than the frontal plane. In cases of severe RVH, the rotation of the T loop will be opposite from normal. With severe RVH, ST segment abnormality may occur, though it is not as common nor as extensive as in severe LVH. The abnormality is posterior and to the left, so that it will be recognized in standard electrocardiography as depression in the right chest leads.

COMBINED VENTRICULAR HYPERTROPHY (CVH)

Combined ventricular hypertrophy is more difficult to diagnose than is isolated hypertrophy. Often only one of the ventricles can be definitely diagnosed as being hypertrophied while, on occasion, there may be so much cancellation that the electrocardiogram may be interpreted as normal.

Inscription of Vector Loops

The activation sequence may be normal, with a wholly counterclockwise loop, with large leftward and/or posterior projections, so that pure LVH is the diagnosis. However, if the anterior projection is also very large and the anterior projection is prolonged, then CVH can be diagnosed. If the activation sequence is normal, but there is a large terminal vector to the right, CVH may be present, but if the vector is abnormally posterior, the large terminal vector to the right may be part of posterobasal LVH, rather than CVH. If the activation sequence causes a wholly clockwise vector loop, pure severe RVH is the diagnosis. However, if the vector is also abnormally to the left, CVH may be diagnosed. On the other hand, if in the presence of the wholly clockwise vector loop there is a large terminal rightward posterior projection, the abnormally posterior vector does not indicate additional LVH. The diagnosis remains pure and usually severe RVH. If the direction of inscription is such that there are two main vectors, CVH must be considered. The most common situation is that of the first main vector to the left and anterior and a terminal vector to the right and posterior (Fig. 3.33). The most common rotation would be that of an initial counterclockwise vector to the left and anterior and a terminal clockwise vector to the right and posterior. In this situation, RVH is definite. If the leftward vector projects abnormally to the left, there is additional LVH. If the terminal vector is abnormally posterior, additional LVH is also possible on that basis, but less definitely. Two main vectors, of course, are normal early in infancy as part of the change from the normal right ventricular dominance to left ventricular dominance, so that CVH may be more difficult to diagnose in the first months of life.

Increased Magnitude Posteriorly and/or to the Left, along with a Large Terminal Vector to the Right

These provide excellent criteria, but the large terminal vector to the right may be part of posterobasal LVH, so that only LVH is present. In standard electrocardiography, a terminal R in V4R and V1 may not be present, for in the presence of an abnormally posterior vector, a large terminal

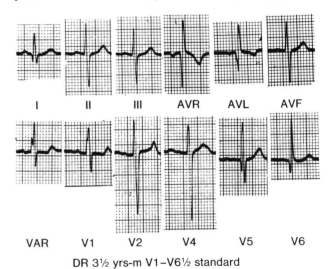

DR 3½ yrs-m V1–V6½ standard

Fig. 3.33 Standard electrocardiogram (leads not simultaneous and low frequency response) in a 3-year-old with a large VSD. There is a prolonged and prominent anterior projection as well as large leftward and posterior projections, the former being manifested mainly in the broad leftward projection so that V₅ is greater than V₅. There is a large initial QRS to the right and anterior of left septal hypertrophy, and there is combined ventricular hypertrophy. There is not an "abnormally superior vector," but the terminal vector is abnormally superior and presumably associated with hypertrophy of the superior portion of the septum and posterobasal LVH. The R wave in AVL is tall, but partly because the vector is superior.

rightward vector may not cross the perpendiculars to the projections of leads V4R and V1.

Increased Magnitude Anteriorly along with Definite Evidence for LVH

One must be careful that left septal hypertrophy has not been responsible for a brief duration rightward anterior vector reflected in a tall positive spike in V1, V2.

An Increased Magnitude Inferior Vector (Increased Y Inferior, Tall R in AVF) in the Presence of RVH

If there is good left ventricular potential, as seen in the chest leads, additional LVH is possible. However, if there is severe RVH, the increased magnitude of the Y inferior is part of the RVH. Tetralogy of Fallot, for example, is often associated with a tall R in AVF (increased Y inferior).

Katz-Wachtel Phenomenon

This is a "pattern" (patterns are not generally useful), but the Katz-Wachtel pattern is commonly read in infancy. However, when activation sequences and vector loops are considered, it becomes obvious that such "pattern reading" concepts are not necessary. The phenomenon is that of tall R and deep S waves in the midprecordial leads, particularly in association with tall R and S waves in two of the three bipolar standard limb leads. Namin and Miller[153] report that R + S in any midprecordial lead over 60 mm suggests CVH. There are usually two main vectors in the horizontal plane, although there can be a wide open counterclockwise horizontal plane vector with the first vector far anterior and the second vector far posterior.

Mean QRS Vector to the Right in the Frontal Plane in the Presence of Definite LVH in the Horizontal Plane

This is unreliable unless the mean vector is very far to the right, because of the potential artifact of the poor X axis in the frontal plane of standard electrocardiography.

Clockwise Rotation of the Frontal Plane in the Presence of Definite LVH in the Horizontal Plane

This is not an indication of CVH, for the clockwise frontal plane vector is present in the majority of children with LVH.

Mean QRS Vector to the Left in the Frontal Plane in the Presence of Definite RVH

Usually, such a vector will rotate counterclockwise. This is not a good sign unless there is increased magnitude of the X axis to the left in the frontal plane (tall R in lead I) or R in AVL is abnormally tall. Even the latter is not very reliable, for when the mean vector in the frontal plane is abnormally to the left, the projection in lead AVL may cause the R wave to be increased in magnitude.

An Abnormally Superior Vector in the Presence of RVH

This is not a sign of CVH, with the abnormal superior vector being a manifestation of a conduction defect. The abnormally superior vector can also cause a tall R to project on lead I and/or AVL, so the latter can also not be used to diagnose CVH.

Definite Hypertrophy of One Ventricle, with Suggested Evidence for the Other

This is a nonspecific statement, but is an overlap of much that has been said above.

VENTRICULAR CONDUCTION ABNORMALITIES

There remains considerable interest and controversy related to ventricular conduction abnormalities. Recently, there has been a great help in their categorization with a classification by Dr. Maurice Rosenbaum.[213, 214] We have suggested a modification of the Rosenbaum classification:

1. Advanced right bundle branch block RBBB) (proximal).
2. Advanced RBBB (distal).
3. Partial RBBB.
4. Terminal right ventricular conduction delay.
5. Advanced left bundle branch block (LBBB) (predivisional).
6. Partial LBBB.
7. Left anterior division block.
8. Abnormally superior vector.
9. Left posterior division block.
10. Divisional LBBB, or simultaneous left anterior and left posterior division block.
11. RBBB with left anterior division block.
12. RBBB with left posterior division block.
13. LBBB with an abnormally superior vector.
14. LBBB with left posterior division block.
15. Advanced bilateral bundle branch block, or simultaneous block in both proximal bundle branches.
16. Advanced trifascicular block (simultaneous block in the proximal right bundle branch plus each of the two divisions of the left bundle branch).
17. Functional "bundle branch blocks" associated with premature beats, tachycardias, and bradycardias.

In this brief discussion, not all 17 varieties will be discussed; the interested reader is referred to a more detailed publication.[215]

RIGHT BUNDLE BRANCH BLOCK

At the present state of our knowledge, advanced proximal and distal right bundle branch block (RBBB) cannot be distinguished from the surface electrocardiogram. Information about the activation sequence in proximal RBBB comes mainly from dog experiments,[67, 216] but can be fairly well confirmed by effects of various injuries to human hearts during surgery as well as due to disease.[217-220] Though there may be differences in experimental and clinical lesions, the effect is delayed activation of the right ventricle (Fig. 3.34). The duration of the QRS is significantly greater than normal. The standard definitions dictate that the QRS duration must be at least 0.12 second. However, experimental data indicate that advanced RBBB can have a lesser duration than 0.12 second, even in adults, and surely in children. In ages where the normal QRS duration is less than in adults, the duration in RBBB can be less.

The specific duration to the right is of major importance in diagnosing RBBB. In the normal child, the duration right is 0.20 ± 0.12 SD. The ratio of duration right over total duration is greater in the younger age groups at 0.32 ± 0.11 at age 2 to 5 years, 0.30 ± 0.14 at age 6 years, and 0.25 ± 0.14 at ages 11 to 19 years. Data for under age 2 years are not available. In the normal, terminal slowing of the loop in the last 0.10 second is normal, but in RBBB, terminal slowing begins shortly after the vector loop has reached the right.

Activation begins normally, initiated as usual by the left posterior division of the left bundle. The opposing forces, from base of right anterior papillary muscle and right septum,[67] are not present, so that the initial vector has its normal orientation to the right, anterior and superior and may be of greater magnitude than normal. The septum

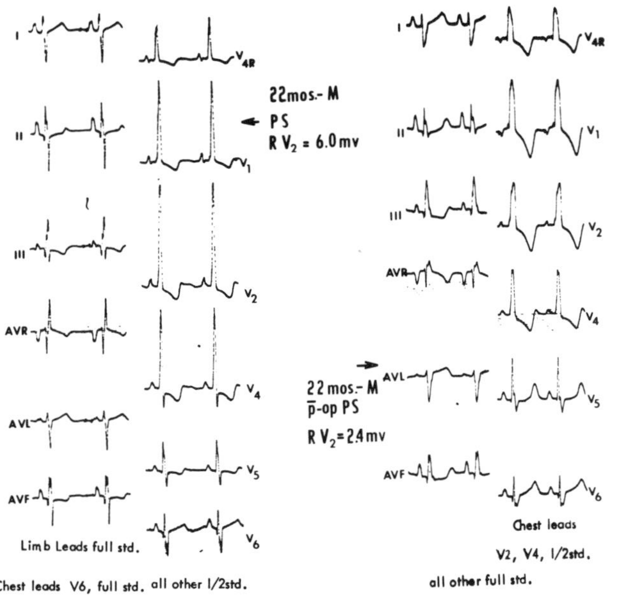

Fig. 3.34 Two standard electrocardiograms (ECGs) with simultaneous leads and high frequency response of a 22-month-old. There was severe pulmonic stenosis (*PS*) with the right ventricular pressure suprasystemic. Immediately after surgery, RBBB was present (which, a few years later, completely resolved). It is presumed that proximal RBBB had *not* been present. There is RAH in each ECG, less so post-op, where the initial portion of the P is no longer upright in lead V$_1$. The RVH pre-op is extremely severe, including a T vector far posterior and to the right. After surgery, there is advanced RBBB. The T vector is even further posterior, but no longer to the right, and the height of the R has decreased from 6.0 to 2.4 mv.

depolarizes slowly, and it takes a long time before the right ventricle begins its depolarization, so that in the first portion of the QRS, the left ventricle is dominant, often causing a very large leftward vector. Continued activation of the septum along with the anterior portion of the left ventricle often causes the QRS not to come very far posterior or to come posterior at all, despite the left ventricular dominance. The right ventricle begins depolarization late, along a broad septal front, and by the time the posterior portion of the left ventricle is being depolarized there is a slow posterior to anterior spread across that septal front, contributing to the frequent lack of a large posterior vector. The strong and broad septal posterior and anterior forces may even cause the vector loop to be directed clockwise. The right ventricle begins its activation, also on a broad front, after most of the left ventricle has completed its normal activation. From then on, transmission through the right ventricle is very slow, by direct muscle cell to muscle cell conduction, rather than via the Purkinje system. Consequently, there is a slowly inscribed terminal vector of long duration and frequently of large magnitude. This terminal vector usually begins inferior, posterior, and to the right, but terminates anterior and superior. Occasionally, the vector terminates posterior in advanced RBBB, but more often in partial RBBB.

Repolarization is of interest since it is likely to be propagated unlike the normal. Left ventricular repolarization is expected to be near completion before right ventricular repolarization begins. Therefore, the T direction is expected to be 180° away from the terminal QRS (right ventricular depolarization).

PARTIAL RBBB

There is no argument about the fact that not all RBBB is complete. That is why the term RBBB rather than complete

RBBB is used. Therefore, since it is accepted that there are varying degrees of RBBB, so that obviously some RBBB is incomplete, it may be confusing to the reader that the authors do not use the term "incomplete RBBB." The reasons are many, including the fact that the term has represented a wastebasket diagnosis for many years, made whenever there was an "rsr' pattern" in the right chest leads. The terminal r or R appears in lead V1 whenever the projection of the cardiac vector crosses the line perpendicular to the V1 lead vector. Such can occur in RBBB of various degree, in right ventricular hypertrophy, with and without terminal right conduction delay, and in normal patients whose terminal right vector is slightly more to the right than average, or normally to the right but slightly less posterior than average. A low voltage rsr' in V4R and sometimes V1 is also common in normals, presumed to be due to proximity effect.

When one adds the fact that an anatomical basis for incomplete RBBB has never been found, then the diagnosis is seen clearly to be useless.

Nonetheless, it should be reiterated that partial RBBB can occur. A cardiac catheter placed in the right ventricular outflow tract may suddenly or gradually cause a prominent slowly conducted terminal vector to the right and anterior and, usually when the catheter is removed, the RBBB gradually decreases, with less and less terminal slowing and lower and lower magnitude to the right and anterior. Obviously, then, partial RBBB is an entity which probably occurs in clinical (noncatheter-induced) states as well. The term incomplete RBBB really has the same meaning, but for the reasons described above, partial RBBB is a better term. The next question is: Can the diagnosis be made with certainty on the basis of obvious terminal slowing, less than in the advanced form, and with no evidence of abnormality in the early vectors? The answer is possibly, and more definitely only if the RBBB was previously more advanced. Sometimes in RBBB the vector does not terminate anterior, remaining posterior. This is another clue to partial RBBB, although a terminal anterior vector may occur here as well.

TERMINAL RIGHT VENTRICULAR CONDUCTION DELAY

This is a definite entity and is usually part of right ventricular hypertrophy with dilatation. In pediatrics, it is seen most commonly in cases of volume overload, such as atrial septal defect and pulmonary and tricuspid insufficiency. The electrocardiographic diagnosis is made in the presence of clear-cut RVH with a mild to moderate increase in terminal right slowing. The vector can terminate anterior or posterior, depending upon the amount of hypertrophy, and usually ends with a small terminal superior vector, consistent, on body surface maps, with prolonged depolarization of the right ventricular outflow tract. If the terminal vector is not very far to the right and/or is relatively posterior, there will not be a terminal r or R' in lead V1 or V4R. Most of the time, the latter is expected. RVH without volume overload may also be associated with some terminal slowing, as in some patients with mild to moderate pulmonic stenosis.

ADVANCED LEFT BUNDLE BRANCH BLOCK

Although most information about activation in LBBB is from dog experiments, there is increasing information about activation in humans.[221, 222] Most is about early activation, but there is also evidence that activation is abnormal in the mid and late portions of the QRS. As in RBBB, there may be differences in experimental and clinical lesions, but the effect is delayed activation of the left ventricle.

The duration of the QRS is significantly greater than

normal, usually being wider than in RBBB, so that in young children, the duration is usually greater than 0.12 second. Commonly, 0.14 second and more are recognized (Fig. 3.35).

Activation in LBBB begins by way of the right bundle, over an area one-half to two-thirds of the way down the septum. Conduction across the septum is to the left very slowly, as is conduction up the septum (responsible in the normal for the initial superior QRS vector). Conduction in the right ventricle, which begins at the endocardium extends anteriorly and inferiorly. Although depolarization of the septum is believed to travel posterior from its origin, the simultaneous right ventricular activation appears to exert a strong influence on the vector. Therefore, in LBBB, the initial QRS is to the left, usually anterior and inferior. However, by 0.02 second, the vector is usually posterior. The inscription is slow and, as the left ventricle is reached, does not speed up much. If the right ventricle is normally thin, the thicker septum and then the left ventricle outbalance it, keeping the vector always to the left. Depolarization in the septum appears to be by muscle cell to muscle cell. Once the left ventricle is reached, with its rich Purkinje network, it would be expected that activation would be fast, but it is still slow and, in the midportion of the QRS, becomes very slow. Activation is apparently by way of cell to cell conduction, not by way of the Purkinje system. Furthermore, it is likely that activation of the posterobasal left ventricle precedes that of the lateral and anterior walls. At the time of its maximal posterior projection, activation is very abnormal and is extremely slow. Consequently, there is usually a very large magnitude posterior vector which reaches its peak relatively early, followed by a slowly inscribed vector remaining well posterior, for a long period of time. Since the lateral ventricle is mostly depolarized after the posterobasal left ventricle, the vector loop must be inscribed either crossed or clockwise. The X lead scalar (V5, V6) will then usually not be of large magnitude but will have in its midportion a slurring or a dip.

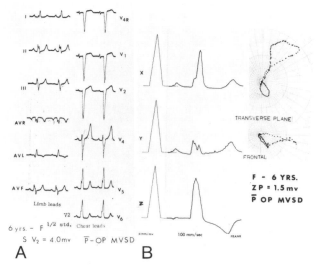

Fig. 3.35 Standard ECG and Frank VCG of a 6-year-old operated upon 6 months previously for multiple muscular VSDs and removal of pulmonary artery band. The approach to the VSDs had been via the left ventricle. The initial QRS is to the left and slightly anterior, after which the vector transverses posterior very rapidly. Most of the QRS, including the midportion, is slowly inscribed. The QRS is crossed, but is mainly inscribed clockwise. The diagnosis of advanced left bundle branch block (LBBB) can be strongly suspected from the standard ECG as well as the VCG, because of the "midpoint" changes of direction in the QRS as recognized in the standard ECG by the notches. Note that the voltages in the standard ECG are much greater than in the VCG. This is typical.

As in advanced RBBB, repolarization is more related to depolarization than in the normal. The T vector is opposite in direction to the main QRS vector (left and posterior), so that it is to the right and anterior.

PARTIAL LBBB

The use of the term partial rather than incomplete LBBB is merely to be consistent with the right-sided terminology. Once again a specific anatomical abnormality has not been documented, though, as in advanced LBBB, left ventricular disease is usually expected. We have seen few patients with congenital LBBB. The majority seen in children occur either as part of left ventricular cardiomyopathy or, more commonly, as a result of left ventricular outflow surgery.

The diagnosis is made on the same grounds as in advanced LBBB, except that the QRS is not as prolonged, particularly in the mid- and left portions. However, the activation sequence is the same, so that all else in the QRS of both the vectors and scalars is the same. Depending upon the degree of LBBB, the ST and T abnormalities are less.

A common error in diagnosis is not to realize that severe LVH can be associated with an initial QRS to the left. That initial vector is presumably due to marked hypertrophy of the posterior free wall of the left ventricle near the septum in the presence of the normal left to right activation of the septum. In severe LVH, marked midportion slowing is not expected, nor is the crossed or clockwise direction of inscription. There may be difficulties in diagnosis, however, when severe LVH is associated with intraventricular conduction abnormality. Since ST and T abnormality may also be present in severe LVH, the distinction between severe LVH and partial LBBB may be difficult.

LEFT ANTERIOR DIVISION BLOCK

Although it is believed that the initial activation of the septum is mainly in the posterior paraseptal area, half to two-thirds of the way down via the posterior division of the left bundle, there is indirect evidence that the nearby anterior paraseptal and midseptal regions are activated as well.[65] These would be by way of the left anterior division and a middle branch of the left bundle. There is considerable human variation, but under any circumstance, if the left posterior division does not begin excitation alone, it contributes to most of it. Consequently, in left anterior division block, initial depolarization appears to be close to normal, with one very important difference. The contribution from the anterior division appears in the normal to contribute much of the initial superior depolarization. Therefore, in left anterior division block, the initial QRS is inferiorly directed rather than superiorly, as in almost all normal children.

According to Rosenbaum,[223] initial activation of the ventricular walls is changed, with the left posteroinferior wall beginning its depolarization before the anterior superior. However, the Purkinje networks of the two distal divisions of the left bundle are well interconnected. Therefore, the anterosuperior wall begins activation after only a very short delay so that the QRS duration is only minimally increased, if at all. Clearly, though, the method of activation has been altered, so that not only is the superior portion of the QRS activated last, but also it appears to take a long time to complete that activation. Consequently, as in advanced RBBB and LBBB, it appears that the conduction in the delayed portion of the heart is more by muscle cell to muscle cell conduction than via the usual Purkinje spread. All of the above gives us clues to why most of the vector is superior in left anterior division block, but the explanation is not fully satisfactory.

The diagnosis is easily made by an initial inferior vector, followed by most of the remainder of the vector, which is abnormally superior.[206, 208] As would be predicted, the direction of the frontal plane vector loop is counterclockwise. There is often, in standard electrocardiography, an unexplained terminal S wave, presumably because of distortion of the X axis (lead I) by superior-inferior forces. The horizontal plane is not significantly affected by left anterior division block so that right ventricular hypertrophy can be diagnosed using the usual standards. Left ventricular hypertrophy can also be diagnosed using the same standards, except that the abnormally superior vector necessarily increases the magnitude of the R wave in AVL, negating the use of the latter.

ABNORMALLY SUPERIOR VECTOR

The electrocardiographic diagnosis of an abnormally superior vector is made the same way as in left anterior division block, except that in the former, the patient seems to be born with it. In fact, the appropriate diagnosis for both is "abnormally superior vector" except that when it appears to be acquired, the reader should probably add "probably due to left anterior division block." Left axis deviation is a particularly bad term because in an abnormally superior vector, the vector is usually more to the right than normal.

In children, an abnormally superior vector almost invariably indicates an endocardial cushion defect, wherein the abnormally superior vector appears to be due to an associated congenital anomaly of conduction related to the left anterior division. Other lesions may be associated with an abnormally superior vector, including double outlet right ventricle, transposition of the great arteries with a large ventricular septal defect (Fig. 3.36), and hypoplastic right ventricle syndrome with tricuspid atresia. The latter, also, is associated with ventricular septal defects in the posterior endocardial cushion position. The hypoplastic right ventricle syndrome is of particular interest, because when it is associated with D-transposition of the great arteries, the vector is inferior because the ventricular septal defect is not in the endocardial cushion position, and when the hypoplastic right ventricle is associated with pulmonary atresia, the vector is also inferior since there is no ventricular septal defect. On occasion, classical tricuspid atresia is associated with an inferior vector. When this occurs, we have observed an anterior ventricular septal defect. One condition, in which a straightforward abnormally superior vector may be seen, without definite explanation, is the Noonan syndrome. The latter is usually associated with right-sided lesions, particularly pulmonic stenosis, although there is some evidence that Noonan syndrome may be associated with abnormalities of left ventricular contraction.

NONSPECIFIC INTRAVENTRICULAR BLOCK

All of the conduction abnormalities as described in the modified classification are specific. The diagnosis of nonspecific intraventricular conduction defect is necessary, implying abnormalities of cell to cell conduction due to generalized disease. Included are myocarditis, diseases due to abnormalities of coronary flow, including anatomical problems, and poor perfusion in severe aortic stenosis with fibrosis. A patient recovering from a shock state may also manifest nonspecific intraventricular conduction defects, as may patients with quinidine toxicity and severe hyperkalemia.

The manifestations of the intraventricular conduction abnormalities vary, but the hallmark is nonspecific slowing of conduction, including the midportion of the QRS. Obviously,

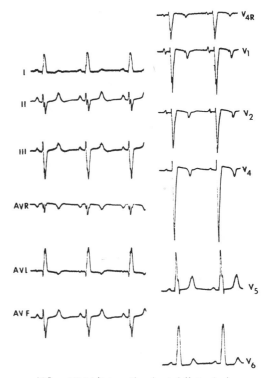

V 2 and V 4 1/2 st., other leads full standard

2 yrs. –F   S V₂ =3.8mv S V₄ = 6.2mv Transpo c̄ PS p̄op

Fig. 3.36 Standard ECG of a 2-year-old with transposition of the great arteries, a large VSD in the endocardial cushion area, and pulmonic stenosis. The typical abnormally superior vector had been present prior to surgery. A Mustard operation was done, the VSD was closed from the right ventricle, and the pulmonic stenosis was left alone.

this diagnosis involves a widening of the QRS which may be recognized in standard electrocardiography, but a vectorcardiographic display may be essential for proper interpretation. ST and T abnormalities will also vary and in mild cases may not be evident. However, in major intraventricular abnormalities, ST and T abnormalities are usually marked.

ST AND T ABNORMALITIES DUE TO VARIOUS PRIMARY CAUSES

Electrolyte Abnormalities

Although the electrocardiogram is useful in evaluating patients with electrolyte abnormalities, the changes from normal may be nonspecific. Clear specificity is sometimes present only in animal experiments. It should be recognized that although the entire body's cellular abnormalities are at issue, the cell most available for scrutiny is the cardiac cell. The surface electrocardiogram is, therefore, the tool that gives us insight into what is happening in the entire body. However, even in situations where we know that the electrocardiogram has been relatively specific (high potassium, low calcium), the complicating effects of sodium chloride, bicarbonate, magnesium, acidosis, alkalosis, dehydration, and other metabolic disturbances often confuse the issue.[224, 225] Two patients with serum potassium levels of 7 mEq/liter may have quite different electrocardiograms, one having tall peaked T waves, while another is nearly normal. Almost certainly, the patient whose electrocardiogram is nearly normal is much less at acute risk of the detrimental effects of hyperkalemia than is the patient whose electrocardiogram

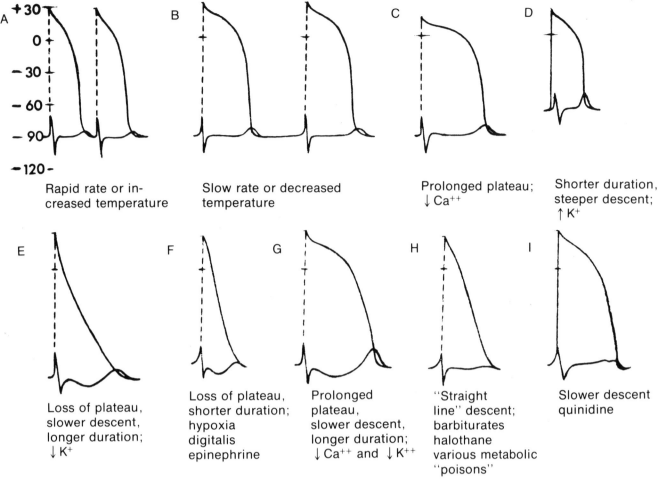

A	B	C	D
Rapid rate or increased temperature	Slow rate or decreased temperature	Prolonged plateau; ↓ Ca++	Shorter duration, steeper descent; ↑ K+

E	F	G	H	I
Loss of plateau, slower descent, longer duration; ↓ K+	Loss of plateau, shorter duration; hypoxia digitalis epinephrine	Prolonged plateau, slower descent, longer duration; ↓ Ca++ and ↓ K++	"Straight line" descent; barbiturates halothane various metabolic "poisons"	Slower descent quinidine

Fig. 3.37 *(A-I)* Diagrammatic presentation of the relation between the ventricular transmembrane action potential and the electrocardiogram. Effect of various factors which alter the duration and velocity of repolarization. The scale at the *top left* represents amplitude in millivolts. The *solid line* representing the upstroke of the action potential in D and I indicates the decreased velocity of depolarization in hyperkalemia and with quinidine. (Reproduced with permission from B. Surawicz.[225] Copyrighted by Medical Arts Publishing Foundation, Houston, 1966.)

demonstrates tall peaked T waves. Therefore, the physician concerned with a patient whose serum potassium level is high is not obtaining all the information available when serum potassiums are measured and electrocardiograms are not being recorded. The reader is referred to two excellent reviews on the subject by Surawicz[226] and Fisch *et al.*[227] The diagrammatic representations of various primary abnormalities by Surawicz is excellent (Fig. 3.37).

The magnitude of the resting transmembrane potential has been shown to be roughly predictable on the basis of the Nernst equation. The resting transmembrane potential, therefore, is dependent upon the ratio of intracellular to extracellular potassium concentrations—an increase in extracellular potassium decreasing the potential and a decrease in extracellular potassium increasing the potential. (An increased transmembrane potential is more negative.) Phases 0, 1, 2, 3, and 4 of the transmembrane potential are differently affected by different electrolytes. Thus, sodium is most important in phase 0, calcium in phase 2, potassium in phase 3, and greater complexity in phase 1, and phase 4.

Although it is instructive to think of the surface electrocardiogram in relation to transmembrane potentials, it must be recognized that the transmembrane potentials are cellular in origin and the surface electrocardiogram is far removed. The known information has never been gathered and summarized better than Surawicz,[225] although there are many

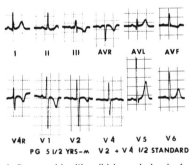

Fig. 3.38 A 5-year-old with mild hyperkalemia (serum potassium 7.0 mEq/liter). The tall T wave in lead V5 is characteristic, but it could also be normal, and could also be part of left ventricular hypertrophy.

valuable papers relating the seriousness of the myocardial metabolic effects with electrocardiography.[229–233]

The electrolyte about which most is known is potassium. Usually, the first effect of high serum potassium is to increase the slope of phase 3 of the transmembrane potential. Since phase 3 is largely responsible for the T wave, the latter becomes taller and relatively narrow, which is especially well seen in the left chest leads (Fig. 3.38). In mild cases of hyperkalemia, a normally tall T or a tall T associated with left ventricular hypertrophy may be similar. With increasing severity, the membrane's resting potential decreases, resulting in a decrease in upstroke velocity of the action potential. Intraventricular conduction is, therefore, slowed, and the QRS is widened.

Transmission of excitation along atrial and atrioventricular pathways is dependent upon potassium, with the propagation velocity increasing with increasing concentrations until an optimum is reached—after which, the propagation velocity decreases. With increasing hyperkalemia, the P-R interval lengthens, and the P wave duration increases. This is followed by a decrease in the P wave amplitude, a very bad sign, for rapid and complete cessation of all atrial activity is likely to follow. Excitability of atrial fibers is abolished at a lower [K]$^+$ concentration than is ventricular excitability, but by this time the QRS duration has increased so much that it has blended into the T, causing a "sine wave effect." The electrocardiogram is now reminiscent of that seen in the "dying heart" from any cause. However, even at this stage, with very irregular ventricular activity, therapy of the hyperkalemia can rapidly bring about a normal electrocardiogram. Therefore, in the presence of a known potential for an elevated serum potassium, monitoring the electrocardiogram can be essential, even life saving. Low serum sodium and low serum calcium, both of which can be seen in association with the hyperkalemia of renal disease, may make the high [K]$^+$ electrocardiogram worse. The administration of sodium and calcium may revert the electrocardiogram towards normal.

In an interesting series of experiments by Roberts and Magida,[234] the hyperkalemia electrocardiogram was obtained in the presence of a normal [K]$^+$ by creating severe acidosis below pH 7.0 with rapid infusion of ammonium chloride, hydrochloric acid, or sulfuric acid. Such an electrocardiogram was not seen in the presence of respiratory acidosis to a similar pH level.

Hypokalemia is more difficult to definitely recognize electrocardiographically. Unlike hyperkalemia, the stepwise change in the electrocardiogram cannot be demonstrated in clinical situations. The electrocardiogram will not be helpful until a level below 3.0 mEq/liter is recorded, and not definitely until a level of 2.7 mEq/liter is reached.

The cardiac cellular transmembrane potential is quite striking in the presence of low potassium levels, with shortening and eventual disappearance of phase 2 coincident with a lengthening of phase 3. Therefore, there is a depression of the ST segment with T vector abnormality. The ventricular Purkinje cells appear to be particularly affected, so that there is a prominent U wave. The QT interval may be increased very little, but there is a prolonged QU. With a prominent U wave, the T and U are fused. The duration of repolarization of the presumed Purkinje cells may be so prolonged in the presence of low [K]$^+$ that when the refractory period is over, repolarization is not completed. Consequently, in severe cases, ectopic beats may occur. This late sign, together with aberrancy of ventricular conduction, may indicate imminent ventricular fibrillation. Roberts and Magida[234] have shown in acute experiments in dogs that the electrocardiographic effects of low potassium are more severe when plasma pH and bicarbonate are increased as well. Furthermore, marked increases of pH, bicarbonate, and sodium without an elevation of potassium could experimentally simulate the low [K]$^+$ electrocardiogram without a change in [K]$^+$. Respiratory alkalosis, however, produced no significant change in the electrocardiogram. We have seen an unusual child with a serum sodium of 199 mEq/liter and a near normal pH who demonstrated an electrocardiogram indistinguishable from that of hypokalemia (Fig. 3.39), al-

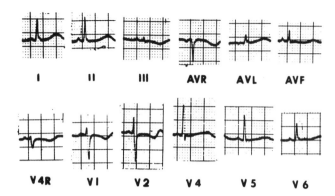

Fig. 3.39 Standard electrocardiogram of a 12-year-old with a serum sodium of 199 mEq/liter, a normal potassium, and a normal pH. This tracing is indistinguishable from that of hypokalemia. The QT interval is normal, and the U wave has appeared to "prolong" the QT in leads V4 and V5. With treatment the serum sodium returned to normal, as did the electrocardiogram.

though usually the changes in [Na]$^+$ needed to change the electrocardiogram are not compatible with life.

Calcium's effect on the transmembrane potential is mainly in phase 2, with hypercalcemia shortening it and hypocalcemia increasing it. Consequently, the major electrocardiographic change is that of a shortening of the ST segment in the presence of high calcium and a lengthening of the ST segment with low calcium. In our experience, the electrocardiogram has not been very helpful in predicting high calcium, for the very high concentrations necessary are rarely seen clinically. In hypocalcemia, it has been an excellent tool (Fig. 3.40). The ST segment is not only lengthened, but it is flat. Since phase 3 is not affected by calcium, the T wave is not changed. When calcium deficiency is present and a prominent U wave is seen along with a prolonged QT with flat ST segment and small T, additional hypokalemia can be diagnosed. Calcium deficiency plus hyperkalemia can also be seen clinically, and they should be suspected when the flat prolonged ST segment is recognized along with a tall peaked T. The effects of high potassium, however, usually obscure the effects of low calcium.

Magnesium deficiency has become a clinical problem of great importance for transport of [K]$^+$, and [Na]$^+$ across the cell membrane appears to require the presence of magnesium ion. The effects on the electrolyte complicate the classical effects of [K]$^+$ described above.[235]

Drugs

Digitalis effects are varied and complex and are not very specific or reliably present. Furthermore, the effects may be more evident on the already abnormal electrocardiogram than on the normal one, making the interpretation more uncertain. Short of manifest toxicity, the electrocardiogram cannot be used to help determine whether enough digitalis has been given. Large doses may cause little effect, and small doses may cause considerable ST and T abnormality. The classical experiments of Hoffman and Singer[236] help us to understand some of the findings. Small doses may prolong the action potential by lengthening phase 3, but with increasing doses, the action potential is decreased by shortening phase 2, often by a marked degree. Though it is not often appreciated, very large doses, according to their experiments, may even shorten phase 3. The classical digitalis effect is that of a shortening of the QT interval with the earliest visible part of the ST segment sharply depressed (Fig. 3.41). This is the J point. The depression will usually be most

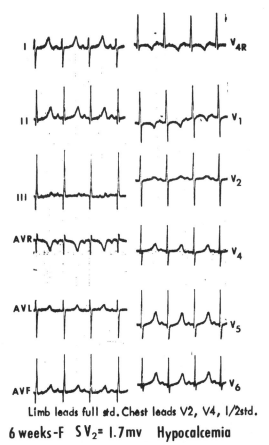

Limb leads full std. Chest leads V2, V4, 1/2std.

6 weeks-F SV₂= 1.7mv Hypocalcemia

Fig. 3.40 Standard electrocardiogram of a 6 week old with the Di George syndrome, right ventricular hypertrophy, and hypocalcemia. Note that the ST segment is lengthened and somewhat flat. The T waves are normal.

obvious in leads where the QRS is upright. Because of effects on phase 3 as well as phase 2, the entire ST segment, including the T, may be affected. Therefore, the T vector may be directed oppositely from the QRS, although frequently it is normal. The exact mechanisms for the effects of digitalis can only be postulated. Experiments in isolated dog Purkinje fibers do not tell the whole story. The newer concepts of repolarization, as previously discussed, indicate that the duration of transmembrane potentials is different in different parts of the myocardium, so that digitalis could be affecting different ventricular myocardial tissues differently.

Quinidine and procainamide both prolong phase 3 of the action potential. Most of the time, a prolonged QT is not recognized, but it can be present. The ST segment and the T wave will not be otherwise changed. The prolonged QT does not necessarily indicate too much quinidine, although it is an extremely important finding, for it may rarely allow a premature ventricular beat to fall on the vulnerable portion of the T. A ventricular dysrhythmia may result. Patients receiving both digitalis and quinidine may have an electrocardiogram that is difficult to distinguish from that due to hypokalemia.

Propranolol may decrease the action potential duration, probably at both phases 2 and 3, so that there is a short QT. The ST segment and T wave are not otherwise changed. Propranolol's effect on the ST segment cannot be due to interference with catecholamines, since the latter also tend to shorten the QT interval.

Diphenlylhydantoin shortens the QT, but the effect is minimal. The ST segment and T wave are not otherwise changed.

Neurological Abnormality

The ST and T changes in neurological abnormality, particularly subarachnoid hemorrhage, but other nonspecific problems as well have been well known for many years. The explanation had always been elusive, but now there are many clues. The concept of repolarization in the endocardium was explained on the basis that the action potential duration is different in different portions of the heart.[233, 238] Therefore, although depolarization begins in the endocardium, a late onset depolarization near the epicardium may have a shorter duration so that repolarization is completed in the epicardium before the endocardium.

The ST and T direction is, therefore, normally similar to that of the QRS, whereas it would be opposite if the duration of the action potential in the epicardium were the same as that in the endocardium. It is now also known that various autonomic influences may change the action potential duration. Stimulation of the left stellate ganglion causes a prolonged QT interval, whereas stimulation of the right stellate ganglion may cause a short QT interval.[239] These and other autonomic influences on the action potential du-

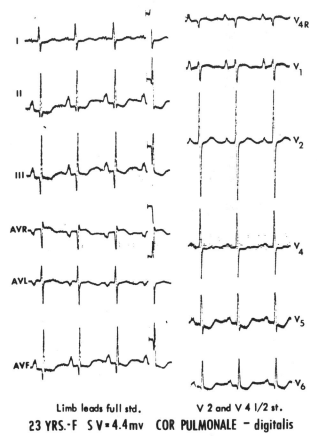

Limb leads full std.   V 2 and V 4 1/2 st.

23 YRS.-F SV=4.4mv COR PULMONALE – digitalis

Fig. 3.41 Standard electrocardiogram of a 23-year-old with cystic fibrosis and an abnormally posterior vector associated with high residual volume. There is right atrial hypertrophy and possible right ventricular hypertrophy. Because of heart failure, digitalis was given. Note that the J point is sharply depressed in leads II, III, AVF, V5, V6, typical of digitalis effect. Prior to digitalization, the ST segments were normal. Note also that the digitalis has not changed the direction of the T vector.

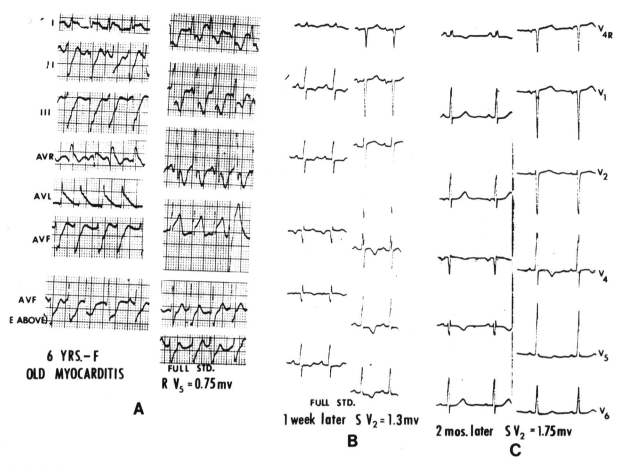

Fig. 3.42 Three standard electrocardiograms of a 6 year old in acute respiratory distress, hypotensive, and with myocarditis. The first tracing (*A*) is not taken with simultaneously recorded leads. The voltages are very low, and there is some ventricular conduction abnormality as well as marked ST segment nonspecific intraventricular conduction abnormality. One week later (*B*), with the child only on digitalis, the QRS voltages are still low, there is minimal J point depression, and the T vector is to the right and anterior (compared to a leftward posterior QRS vector). Two months later (*C*), with the patient still on digitalis, the ST-T abnormality is minimal.

ration (such as from the hypothalamus) are now believed to be part of the genesis of the ST and T abnormality of various central nervous system disorders.[240] Implications should also be evident related to treatment of the prolonged QT syndrome.[241] The so-called neurogenic T wave is large and prolonged, often in the opposite direction from the QRS and usually associated with a prolonged QT and prominent U wave. However, as would be predicted from the above, there is extreme variability from the striking "neurogenic" T wave syndrome to minimal ST and T abnormality.[242, 243]

Myocarditis

The diagnosis is made on clinical grounds, not on the basis of a specific electrocardiogram. Usually, the QRS is not involved, but the ST and T abnormality, though sometimes very severe, is not specific (Fig. 3.42). The findings may be identical with those of acute pericarditis, may simulate acute myocardial infarction, may show severe intraventricular conduction abnormality, or may be trivial. The myocarditis associated with juvenile rheumatoid arthritis may cause a low voltage, particularly of the T waves.

Rhythm and conduction abnormalities, including AV junctional rhythm with AV dissociation, various types of AV block, and bundle branch block, are common. Diphtheria provides an excellent specific example of the latter,[244] but such events occur in any type of myocarditis.

Pericarditis

In the acute form, the electrocardiogram is essentially that of a subepicardial myocarditis. If the entire cardiac surface is involved, there could be elevated ST segments in virtually every lead, though usually not in the right chest leads. If only a portion of the heart is involved, that portion will project onto the surface to cause elevation in only a few leads. The T wave in the early period will be in the same direction as before the pericarditis but may be of larger magnitude. Later, during recovery, the ST segments return to normal, but the direction of the T may be different from normal for a number of weeks, presumably because of localized increases in duration of the action potential.[245-247]

Both myocarditis and pericarditis can be associated with a generalized low voltage, the former because of destruction of so much myocardial tissue and the latter because of pericardial effusion.

Prolapsed Mitral Valve

Another example of a primary T and U abnormality is that of the syndrome of prolapsed mitral valve, which we first described in female children as being possibly due to papillary muscle dysfunction.[248] The T vectors may be superior, may be to the right, and/or may be quite anterior. A short time later they may change completely. There fre-

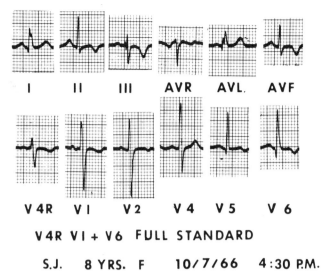

I   II   III   AVR   AVL.   AVF

V 4R   V I   V 2   V 4   V 5   V 6

V4R VI + V6   FULL STANDARD

S.J.   8 YRS.   F   10/7/66   4:30 P.M.

Fig. 3.43 Standard ECG of an 8-year-old with prolapsed mitral valve. In the long strips, there was a very prominent U wave, but the abnormally superior and rightward T vector is particularly striking. This child was admitted for inguinal hernia surgery; and under anesthesia, the T waves changed from being inferior and leftward, so that the anesthesiologists were concerned about the possibilities of myocardial infarction. This child had cardiac catheterization, which confirmed the prolapsed posterior leaflet of the mitral valve, the trivial mitral regurgitation, and the normal coronary arteries. (Reproduced with permission from V. V. Sreenivasan et al.[248])

quently is a prominent U wave (Fig. 3.43). There are many reasons for the interest in this syndrome, but for our purposes here, it should be clear that there are localized areas of the ventricle where the duration of the transmembrane potential is of strikingly different length from other areas. The result is a difference in T direction from normal as well as the frequently prominent U wave. Clearly, also, these directions often change back and forth between abnormality and normality for reasons which are not clear.

Early Repolarization

The term is a misnomer since repolarization in every cell begins as soon as depolarization is completed. Furthermore, in our body surface maps in humans,[106] as well as in Spach's epicardial maps in chimpanzees,[105] the ST segment is frequently present before the end of the QRS. In fact, in Spach's studies, the ST segment may be present in the last 40% of the QRS. Nonetheless, the term has persisted to explain a normal variant, since in many people, especially adolescent males,[249] there is clear-cut ST segment elevation followed by

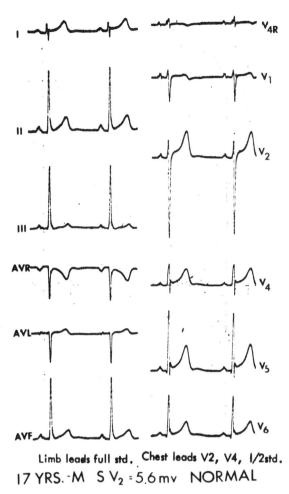

Limb leads full std. Chest leads V2, V4, 1/2std.
17 YRS. - M   S V₂ = 5.6 mv   NORMAL

Fig. 3.44 Standard ECG of a 17-year-old normal black male. Note the so-called normal variant of "early repolarization." The etiology of this "pattern" is not known, for repolarization begins in all normal people well before the QRS ends. This normal variant is recognized in that the early ST segment, although arising high in the QRS, comes back toward the baseline before gradually becoming the T wave. This "pattern" of early repolarization is noted more in adolescents than preadolescents. (Note the extremely large magnitude in this normal teenager, a finding well known in many blacks, for reasons not known. The vector is far posterior, so that LVH must be diagnosed.)

a downward concavity before the onset of a normal T wave (Fig. 3.44). The leads most commonly demonstrating this normal variant are the left chest and leads II, III, and AVF.

REFERENCES

1. Einthoven, W.: Die galvanometrische Registrirung des menschlichen Elektrokardiogramms, zugleich eine Berurtheilung der Anwendung des capillar Elektrometers in der Physiologie. Pfluegers Arch. Ges. Physiol. 99:472, 1903.
2. Einthoven, W., Fahr, G., and de Waart, A.: Ueber die Richtung und die Manifeste Grosse der Potentialschwankugen in menschlichen Herzen und uber den Einfluse der Herzlage auf die Form des Elektrokardiogramms. Pfluegers Arch. Ges. Physiol. 150:275, 1913.
3. Goldberger, E.: A simple indifferent, electrocardiographic electrode of zero potential and

a technique of obtaining augmented, unipolar, extremity leads. Am. Heart J. 23:483, 1942.
4. Wilson, F. N., Johnston, F. D., Rosenbaum, F. F., Erlanger, H., Kossman, C. E., Hecht, H., Cotrim, N., de Oliveira, R. M., Scarsi, R., and Barker, P. S.: The precordial electrocardiogram. Am. Heart J. 27:19, 1944.
5. Burch, G. E., and DePasquale, N. P.: A History of Electrocardiography. Year Book Medical Publishers, Chicago, 1964.
6. Katz, L. N., and Hellerstein, H. K.: Electrocardiography. In Circulation of the Blood: Man and Ideas, edited by A. F. Fishman and

D. W. Richards. Oxford University Press, New York, 1964.
7. Draper, M. H., and Weidmann, S.: Cardiac resting and action potentials recorded with an intracellular electrode. J. Physiol. (Lond.) 115:74, 1951.
8. Grundfest, H.: General introduction of membrane physiology. In Electrophysiology of the Heart, edited by B. Taccardi and G. Marchetti. Pergamon Press, London, 1965.
9. Hecht, H. H. (ed.): Electrophysiology of the heart. Ann. N.Y. Acad. Sci. 65:653, 1957.
10. Hecht, H. H.: Some observations and theories concerning the electrical behavior of heart

muscle. Am. J. Med. 30:720, 1961.
11. Hoffman, B. F., and Cranefield, P. F.: Electrophysiology of the Heart. McGraw-Hill, New York, 1960.
12. Hoffman, B. F., and Cranefield, P. F.: The physiological basis of cardiac arrhythmias. Am. J. Med. 37:670, 1964.
13. Weidmann, S.: Ionic movements underlying the cardiac action potential. Am. Heart J. 61:298, 1961.
14. Plonsey, R.: Biolectric Phenomena. McGraw-Hill, New York, 1969.
15. Briller, S. A.: Ionic exchanges and cardiac action potential in relation to the electrocardiogram. Prog. Cardiovasc. Dis. 2:207, 1959.
16. Conn, H. L., and Wood, J. C.: Cation exchanges in the heart: Relation to the cardiac action potential. J. Clin. Invest. 37:885, 1958.
17. Hodgkin, A. L.: The ionic basis of electrical activity in nerve and muscle. Biol. Rev. 26:339, 1951.
18. Page, E.: The electrical potential difference across the cell membrane of heart muscle. Circulation 26:583, 1962.
19. Reynolds, E. W., Jr.: Ionic transfer in cardiac muscle: An explanation of cardiac electrical activity. Am. Heart J. 67:693, 1964.
20. Weidmann, S.: Electrophysiologie de Herzmuskelfaser. Hans Huber, Bern, 1956.
21. Woodbury, J. W.: Cellular electrophysiology of the heart. In Handbook of Physiology, Vol. 1, edited by W. F. Hamilton and P. Dow. American Physiological Society, Bethesda, Md., 1962.
22. Plonsey, R.: Biophysical basis for electrocardiography. In Pediatric Electrocardiography, edited by J. Liebman, R. Plonsey, and P. Gillette. Williams & Wilkins, Baltimore, 1982.
23. Johnson, E. A.: The genesis of the cardiac action potential: Chemical and electrical considerations. Proc. Aust. Physiol. Pharmacol. Soc. 10:59, 1979.
24. Beeter, G. W., and Reuter, H.: Reconstruction of the action potential of ventricular myocardial fibers. J. Physiol. 268:177, 1977.
25. James, T. N., and Sherf, L.: Specialized tissues and preferential conduction in the atria of the heart. Am. J. Cardiol. 28:414, 1971.
26. James, T. N.: Anatomy of the human sinus anode. Anat. Rec. 141:109, 1961.
27. James, T. N., Sherf, L., Fine, G., and Morales, A. R.: Comparative ultrastructure of the sinus node in man and dog. Circulation 34:139, 1966.
28. Sherf, L., and James, T. N.: Fine structure of cells and their histologic organization within internodal pathways of the heart. Clinical and electrocardiographic implications. Am. J. Cardiol. 44:345, 1979.
29. Friedman, W. F., Pool, P. E., Jacobowitz, D., Seagram, S. C., and Braunwald, E.: Sympathetic innervation of the developing rabbit heart: Biochemical and histochemical comparisons of fetal, neonatal and adult myocardium. Circ. Res. 23:25, 1968.
30. Navaratnam, V.: The ontogenesis of cholinesterase activity within the heart and cardiac ganglia in man, rat, rabbit and guinea pig. J. Anat. 99:459, 1967.
31. Freidman, W. F.: Intrinsic physiologic properties of the developing heart. Prog. Cardiovasc. Dis. 15:87, 1972.
32. Lev, M.: The conduction system. In Pathology of the Heart, edited by S. E. Gould, Chap. 4. Charles C Thomas, Springfield, Ill., 1960.
33. Lewis, T., Meakins, J., and White, P. D.: The excitatory process in the dog's heart. I. The auricles. Philos. Trans. R. Soc. Lond. (Biol. Sci.) 205:375, 1914.
34. Truex, R. C.: Comparative anatomy and functional considerations of the cardiac conduction system. In The Specialized Tissues of the Heart, edited by A. Paes de Carvalho et al. Elsevier, Amsterdam, 1962.

35. Bachmann, G.: The inter-auricular time interval. Am. J. Physiol. 41:309, 1916.
36. Wenckebach, K. F.: Beitrage zur Kenntnis der menschlichen Herztatigkeit. Arch. Anat. Physiol. 3:53, 1908.
37. Thorel, C.: Ueber den Aufbau des Sinusknotens und seine Verbindung mit der Cava Superior und den Wenkebachschen Bundeln. Munch. Med. Wochenschr. 57:183, 1910.
38. Eyster, J. A. E., and Meek, W. J.: Experiments on the origin and conduction of the heart beat. IX. Sino-ventricular conduction. Am. J. Physiol. 61:130, 1922.
39. Lewis, T.: Mechanisms and Graphic Registration of the Heart Beat, 3rd. ed. Shaw and Sons, London, 1925.
40. James, T. N.: The connecting pathways between the sinus and AV node and between the right and left atria in the human heart. Am. Heart J. 66:498, 1963.
41. James, T. N., and Sherf, L.: Specialized tissues and preferential conduction in the atria of the heart. Am. J. Cardiol. 28:414, 1971.
42. Massing, G. K., and James, T. N.: Anatomical configuration of the His bundle and proximal bundle branches in the human heart. Circulation 44(Suppl. 2):64, 1971.
43. Paes de Carvalho, A., and Langan, W. B.: Influence of extracellular potassium levels on atrioventricular transmission. Am. J. Physiol. 205:375, 1963.
44. Vassale, M., Greenspan, K., Jomain, S., and Hoffman, B. F.: Effects of potassium on automaticity and conduction of canine hearts. Am. J. Physiol. 207:334, 1964.
45. Wagner, M. L., Lazzara, R., Weiss, R. M., and Hoffman, B. F.: Specialized conducting fibers in the interatrial band. Circ. Res. 18:502, 1966.
46. Yamada, K., Horiba, M., Sakaida, Y., Okajima, M., Horibe, H., Muraki, H., Kobayashi, T., Miyauchi, A., Oishi, H., Nonagawa, A., Ishikawa, K., and Toyawa, J.: Origination and transmission of impulse in the auricle. Jpn. Heart J. 6:71, 1965.
47. Merideth, J., and Titus, J. L.: The anatomic atrial connections between sinus and AV node. Circulation 37:566, 1968.
48. Waldo, A. L., Bush, J. L., Jr., Gelband, H., Zorn, G. L., Vitikainen, K. J., and Hoffman, B. F.: Effects on the canine P wave in discrete lesions in the specialized atrial tracts. Circ. Res. 29:452, 1971.
49. Spach, M. D., King, T. D., Barr, R. C., Boaz, D. E., Morrow, M. N., and Herman-Giddens, S.: Electrical potential distribution surrounding the atria during depolarization and repolarization in the dog. Circ. Res. 24:857, 1969.
50. Scher, A. M., and Spach, M. S.: Cardiac depolarization and repolarization and the electrocardiogram. In Handbook of Physiology: Section 2: The Cardiovascular System, Vol. 1, The Heart, edited by R. M. Berne, N. Sperelakis, and S. R. Geiger, Chap. 9. Bethesda, Md., American Physiological Society, 1979, pp. 357–392.
51. Janse, M. K., Anderson, R. H., von Capelle, F. J., and Durrer, D.: A combined electrophysiological and anatomical study of the human fetal heart. Am. Heart J. 91:556, 1976.
52. Anderson, R. H., and Taylor, I. M.: Development of the atrioventricular specialized tissue in human heart. Br. Heart J. 34:1205, 1972.
53. Janse, M. J., and Anderson, R. H.: Specialized internodal atrial pathways, fact or fiction. Eur. J. Cardiol. 2:117, 1974.
54. James, T. N.: Morphology of the human atrio-ventricular node, with remarks pertinent to its electrophysiology. Am. Heart J. 62:656, 1961.
55. James, T. N., and Sherf, L.: Ultrastructure of the human A-V node. Circulation 37:1049, 1968.
56. Mahaim, I.: Kent's fibers and the A-V specific

conduction through the upper connections of the bundle of His-Tawara. Am. Heart J. 33:651, 1947.
57. Liebman, J.: Anatomy of the cardiac conduction system. In Pediatric Electrocardiography, edited by J. Liebman, R. Plonsey, and P. Gillette, Chap. 2. Williams & Wilkins, Baltimore, 1982, pp. 16–20.
58. James, T. N., and Sherf, L.: Fine structure of the His bundle. Circulation 44:9, 1971.
59. Lev, M.: The anatomic basis for disturbances in conduction and cardiac arrhythmias. Prog. Cardiovasc. Dis. 2:360, 1960.
60. Reemtsma, K., and Copenhaver, W. M.: Anatomic studies of the cardiac conduction system in congenital malformation of the heart. Circulation 17:271, 1958.
61. Truex, R. C., and Bishof, J. K.: Conduction system in human hearts with interventricular septal defects. J. Thorac. Cardiovasc. Surg. 35:421, 1958.
62. Truex, R. C., and Smythe, M. Q.: Recent observations on the human cardiac conduction system, with special considerations of the atrioventricular node and bundle. In Electrophysiology of the Heart, edited by B. Taccardi and G. Marchetti. Pergamon Press, London, 1965.
63. Rosenbaum, M. B., Elizari, M. V., and Lazzara, J. O.: The hemiblocks. Tampa Tracings, Oldsmar, Fla., 1970.
64. Massing, G. K., and James, T. N.: Anatomical configuration of the His bundle and proximal bundle branches in the human heart. Circulation 44(Suppl. 2):64, 1971.
65. Kulbertus, H. E., and Demmling, J. C.: Pathological findings in patients with left anterior hemiblock. In Vectorcardiography 3, edited by I. Hoffman and R. I. Hamby. North-Holland, Amsterdam, 1976.
66. Kulbertus, H. E.: Advances in the understanding of conduction disturbances. Eur. J. Cardiol. 8:271, 1978.
67. Myerburg, R. H., Nilsson, K., and Gelband, H.: Physiology of canine intraventricular conduction and endocardial excitation. Circ. Res. 30:217, 1972.
68. Amer, N. S., Stuckey, J. H., Hoffman, B. F., Cappelletti, R. R., and Domingo, R. T.: Activation of the interventricular septal myocardium studied during cardiopulmonary bypass. Am. Heart J. 59:224, 1960.
69. Durrer, D.: Electrical aspects of human cardiac activity: A clinical-physiological approach to excitation and stimulation. Cardiovasc. Res. 2:5, 1968.
70. Durrer, D., Van Dorn, R. T., Freud, G. E., Janse, M. J., Meijler, F. L., and Arzbaecher, R. C.: Total excitation of the isolated human heart. Circulation 45:899, 1970.
71. Schaefer, H.: The general order of excitation and of recovery. Ann. N.Y. Acad. Sci. 65:743, 1957.
72. Scher, A. M., and Young, A. C.: The pathway of ventricular depolarization in the dog. Circ. Res. 4:461, 1956.
73. Scher, A. M.: Excitation of the heart. In Handbook of Physiology, Vol. 1., edited by W. F. Hamilton and P. Dow. American Physiological Society, Bethesda, Md., 1962.
74. Scher, A. M.: The sequence of ventricular excitation. Am. J. Cardiol. 14:287, 1964.
75. Durrer, D., and Van Der Twill, L. H.: Excitation of the left ventricular free wall of the dog and goat. Ann. N.Y. Acad. Sci. 65:779, 1957.
76. Liebman, J., Thomas, C., Rudy, Y., and Plonsey, R.: Variations of body surface potential maps (QRS) in normal children. J. Electrocardiol. 14:249, 1981.
77. Durrer, D., Buller, J., Graaff, P., Lo, G. I., and Meyler, F. L.: Epicardial excitation pattern as observed in the isolated revived and perfused fetal human heart. Circ. Res. 9:29,

1961.

78. Crill, W. E., and Woodbury, J. W.: On the problem of impulse conduction in the atrium. Nervous inhibitions. Proceedings of the Second Friday Harbor Symposium, edited by E. Florey. Pergamon Press, London, 1961, p. 124.

79. Weidmann, W.: The functional significance of the intercalated disks. In Electrophysiology of the Heart, edited by B. Taccardi and G. Marchetti. Pergamon Press, London, 1965.

80. Eifler, W., and Plonsey, R.: A cellular model for the simulation of activation in the ventricular myocardium. J. Electrocardiol. 8:117, 1975.

81. Frank, E., Kay, C. F., Serden, G. E., and Keisman, R. A.: A new quantitative basis for electrocardiographic theory: The normal QRS complex. Circulation 12:406, 1955.

82. Gelertner, H. L., and Swihart, J. C.: Numerical computations of body-surface potentials produced by an arbitrary distribution of generators in the heart. In Electrophysiology of the Heart, edited by B. Taccardi and G. Marchetti. Pergamon Press, London, 1965.

83. Liebman, J., and Plonsey, R.: Basic principles for understanding electrocardiography. Paediatrician 2:251, 1973.

84. Plonsey, R.: Limitations on the equivalent cardiac generator (abstr.). Circulation 32:172, 1965.

85. Helm, R. A.: The lead vectors of multiple dipoles located on an electrically homogeneous circular lamina. Am. Heart J. 50:883, 1955.

86. Helm, R. A.: Theory of vectorcardiography: A review of fundamental concepts. Am. Heart J. 49:135, 1965.

87. Okada, R. H.: An experimental study of multiple dipole potentials and the effects of inhomogeneities in volume conductors. Am. Heart J. 54:567, 1957.

88. Plonsey, R.: Factors which contribute to the dipolarity of the cardiac source. In Vectorcardiography, 2nd ed., edited by I. Hoffman. North-Holland Publishing Co., Amsterdam, 1971, pp. 66–71.

89. Gamboa, R.: Applicability of the axial lead system to infants and children. Am. J. Cardiol. 18:690, 1966.

90. Brody, D. A., and Arzbaecher, R. C.: Intrinsic properties of uncorrected and highly corrected leads. Circulation 34:638, 1966.

91. Schaefer, H., and Haas, H. G.: Electrocardiography. In Handbook of Physiology, Vol. 1, edited by W. F. Hamilton and P. Dow. American Physiological Society, Bethesda, Md., 1962.

92. Brody, D. A., and Copeland, G. D.: Electrocardiographic cancellation: Some observations concerning the "nondipolar" fraction of precordial electrocardiogram. Am. Heart J. 56:381, 1958.

93. Wilson, F. N., Johnston, F. D., and Hill, I. G. W.: The interpretation of the galvanometric curves obtained when one electrode is distant from the heart and the other near or in contact with the ventricular surface. Part II. Observations in the mammalian heart. Am. Heart J. 10:176, 1934.

94. Wilson, F. N., Johnston, F. D., Rosenbaum, F. F., and Barker, P. S.: On Einthoven's triangle, the theory of unipolar electrocardiographic leads, and the interpretation of the precordial electrocardiogram. Am. Heart J. 32:277, 1946.

95. Liebman, J., Doershuk, C., Rapp, C., and Matthews, L. W.: The vectorcardiogram in cystic fibrosis: Diagnostic significance and correlation with pulmonary function tests. Circulation 35:552, 1967.

96. Rudy, Y., Plonsey, R., and Liebman, J.: The effects of variations in conductivity and geometrical parameters on the electrocardiogram, using an eccentric spheres model. Circ. Res. 44:104, 1979.

97. Taccardi, B., deAmbroggi, L., and Viganotti, C.: Body surface mapping of heart potentials. In Theoretical Basis for Electrocardiography, edited by C. V. Nelson and D. B. Geselowitz. Claredon Press, Oxford, 1976, pp. 436–466.

98. Miller, W. T., and Geselowitz, D. B.: Simulation studies of the electrocardiogram. Circ. Res. 43:301, 1978.

99. Holt, J. H., Barnard, A. C. L., Lynn, M. S., and Svendson, P.: A study of the human heart as a multiple dipole electrical source. Circulation 40:687, 1969.

100. Einthoven, W., Fahr, G., and de Waart, A.: On the direction and manifest size of the variations of the potential in the human heart and on the influence of the position of the heart on the electrocardiograph (translated by H. E. Hoff and P. Sekelj). Am. Heart J. 40:163, 1950.

101. Burger, H. C., and Van Milaan, J. B.: Heart-vector and leads. Part II. Br. Heart J. 9:154, 1947.

102. Spach, M. S., Silberberg, W. P., Boineau, J. P., Barr, R. C., Long, E. C., Gallie, T. M., Gabor, J. B., and Wallace, A. G.: Body surface isopotential maps in normal children, ages 4–14 years. Am. Heart J. 72:640, 1966.

103. Taccardi, B.: Distribution of heart potentials on the thoracic surface of normal human subjects. Circ. Res. 12:341, 1963.

104. Taccardi, B.: Multipolar distribution of cardiac potentials in body surface mapping. In Electrical Activity of the Heart, edited by B. Taccardi. Charles C Thomas, Springfield, Ill., 1971, pp. 37–52.

105. Spach, M. S., Barr, R. C., Lanning, C. F., and Tucek, P. C.: Origin of body surface QRS and T wave potentials from epicardial potential distributions in the intact chimpanzee. Circulation 55:268, 1977.

106. Barr, R. C., and Spach, M. S.: Physiologic correlates and clinical comparisons of isopotential surface maps with other electrocardiographic methods. In Advances in Electrocardiography, edited by R. C. Schlant and J. W. Hurst. Grune & Stratton, New York, 1972, pp. 27–36.

107. Liebman, J.: The normal electrocardiogram in newborns and infants (a critical review). In Electrocardiography in Infants and Children, edited by D. E. Cassels and R. F. Ziegler. Grune & Stratton, New York, 1966.

108. Liebman, J.: The relationship of the standard electrocardiogram to the vectorcardiogram. In Electrocardiography in Infants and Children, edited by D. E. Cassels and R. F. Ziegler. Grune & Stratton, New York, 1966.

109. Lee, M. H., Liebman, J., and Mackay, W.: Orthogonal electrocardiograph correlative study of 100 children with pure cardiac defects. In Vectorcardiography 3, edited by I. Hoffman and R. I. Hamby. North-Holland Publishing Co., Amsterdam, 1976, p. 181.

110. Ng, M., Liebman, J., Anslovar, J., and Gross, S.: Cardiovascular findings in children with sickle cell anemia. Dis. Chest 52:788, 1967.

111. Burger, H. C., and Van Milaan, J. B.: Heart-vector and leads. Br. Heart J. 8:157, 1946.

112. Burger, H. C., and Van Milaan, J. B.: Heart-vector and leads. Part III. Br. Heart J. 10:229, 1949.

113. Johnston, F. D.: Lead systems: Conventional extremity and precordial lead electrocardiograms and vectorcardiography. In Electrocardiography in Infants and Children, edited by D. E. Cassels and R. F. Ziegler. Grune & Stratton, New York, 1966.

114. McFee, R., and Johnston, F. D.: Electrocardiographic leads. I. Introduction. Circulation 8:554, 1953.

115. McFee, R., and Johnston, F. D.: Electrocardiographic leads. II. Analysis. Circulation 9:255, 1954.

116. McFee, R., and Johnston, F. D.: Electrocardiographic leads. III. Synthesis. Circulation 9:868, 1954.

117. Frank, E.: An accurate clinically practical system for spatial vectorcardiography. Circulation 13:736, 1956.

118. Frank, E.: Spread of current in volume conductors of finite content. Ann. N.Y. Acad. of Sci. 65:980, 1957.

119. McFee, R., and Parungao, A.: An orthogonal lead system for clinical electrocardiography. Am. Heart J. 62:93, 1961.

120. Burgess, M. J., Green, L. S., Millar, K., Wyatt, B. S., and Abildskov, M. D.: The sequence of normal ventricular recovery. Am. Heart J. 84:660, 1972.

121. Wilson, F. N., Macleod, A. G., Barker, P. S., and Johnston, F. D.: The determination of the significance of the areas of the ventricular deflections of the electrocardiogram. Am. Heart J. 10:46, 1934.

122. Lux, R. L., Urie, P. M., Burgess, M. J., and Abildskov, J. A.: Variability of the body surface distributions of QRS, ST-T and QRS T deflection areas with varied activation sequence in dogs. Cardiovasc. Res. 14:607, 1980.

123. Urie, P. M., Burgess, M. J., Lux, R. L., Wyatt, R. F., and Abildskov, J. A.: The electrocardiographic recognition of cardiac states at high risk of ventricular arrhythmias.

124. Waller, A. D.: On the electromotive changes connected with the beat of the mammalian heart and of the human heart in particular. Philos. Trans. R. Soc. Lond. 180:169, 1889.

125. Lippmann, G.: Relations entre les pnenomenes electriques et capillaires. Ann. Chim. Phys. Ser. 5, 5:494, 1875.

126. Einthoven, W.: Die galvanometrische Registrirung des menschlichen Elektrokardiogramms, zugleich eine Berurtheilung der Anwendung des capillar Elektrometers in der Physiologie. Pfluegers Arch. Ges. Physiol. 99:472, 1903.

127. Lepeschkin, E.: Electrocardiographic instrumentation. Prog. Cardiovasc. Dis. 5:498, 1963.

128. Spach, M. D., Barr, R. C., Havstad, J. W., and Long, E. C.: Skin-electrode impedance and its effect on recording cardiac potentials. Proceedings of the Society for Pediatric Research, 36th Annual Meeting, April 1966, p. 14.

129. Ko, W. H., and Hynacek, J.: Dry electrodes and electrode amplifiers. In Biomedical Electrode Technology, edited by Miller and Harris, Academic Press, New York, 1973, pp. 169–180.

130. Dower, G. E., Moore, A. D., Ziegler, W. G., and Osborne, J. A.: On QRS amplitude and other errors produced by direct-writing electrocardiographs. Am. Heart J. 65:307, 1963.

131. Thomas, C.: Electrocardiographic measurement system response. In Pediatric Electrocardiography, edited by J. Liebman, R. Plonsey, and P. Gillette, Chap. 5. Williams & Wilkins, Baltimore, 1982.

132. Langner, P. H., Geselowitz, D. B., and Mansure, F. T.: High frequency components in the electrocardiograms of normal subjects and of patients with coronary heart disease. Am. Heart J. 62:746, 1961.

133. Geselowitz, D. B., Langner, P. H., and Mansure, F. T.: Further studies on the first derivative of the electrocardiogram, including instruments available for clinical use. Am. Heart J. 64:805, 1962.

134. Holcroft, J. W., and Liebman, J.: Notching of the QRS complex in high frequency electrocardiograms of normal children and in children with rheumatic fever. J. Electrocardiol. 3:133, 1970.

135. Berson, A. S., Lau, F. Y. K., Wojick, J. M., and Pipberger, H. V.: Distortions in infant electrocardiograms caused by high frequency

response. Am. Heart J. 93:730, 1977.

136. Riggs, T., Isenstein, B. S., and Thomas, C. W.: Spectra of normal electrocardiograms in children and adults. J. Electrocardiol. 12:377, 1979.

137. Ziegler, R. F.: Electrocardiographic Studies in Normal Infants and Children. Charles C Thomas, Springfield, Ill., 1951.

138. Wilson, F. N., Johnston, F. D., Macleod, A. G., and Barker, P. S.: Electrocardiograms that represent the potential variations of a single electrode. Am. Heart J. 9:447, 1934.

139. Wilson, F. N., Johnston, F. D., and Hill, I. G. W.: The interpretation of the galvanometric curves obtained when one electrode is distant from the heart and the other near or in contact with the ventricular surface. Part II. Observations in the mammalian heart. Am. Heart J. 10:176, 1934.

140. Langner, P. H., Jr., Okada, R. J., Moore, S. R., and Fies, H. L.: Comparison of four orthogonal systems of vectorcardiography. Circulation 17:46, 1958.

141. Watanabe, Y.: Purkinje repolarization as a possible cause of the U wave in the electrocardiogram. Circulation 51:1030, 1975.

142. Ellison, R. C., and Restiaux, N. J.: Vectorcardiography in Congenital Heart Disease. W. B. Saunders, Philadelphia, 1972.

143. Liebman, J.: Statistics related to electrocardiographic interpretation. In Pediatric Electrocardiography, edited by J. Liebman, R. Plonsey, and P. Gillette, Chap. 7. Williams & Wilkins, Baltimore, 1982.

144. Mann, H.: A method of analyzing the electrocardiogram. Arch. Intern. Med. 25:283, 1920.

145. Wilson, F. N., Johnston, F. D., and Barker, P. S.: The use of the cathode ray oscillograph in the study of the monocardiogram. J. Clin. Invest. 16:664, 1937.

146. Hellerstein, H. K.: Theory and Interpretation of the Electrocardiogram. Horn Ohio Company, Cleveland, 1954.

147. Downs, T. D., and Liebman, J.: The analysis of vectorcardiogram angular data. Fourth Annual Symposium on Biomathematics and Computing, Houston, Texas, March 24, 1966 (Presentation and Abstract).

148. Downs, T. D., Liebman, J., Agusti, R. J., and Romberg, H. C.: The statistical treatment of angular data in vectorcardiography. In Vectorcardiography 1965, edited by I. Hoffman and R. C. Taymar. North-Holland, Amsterdam, 1966.

149. Downs, T., and Liebman, J.: Statistical methods for vectorcardiographic directions. IEEE Trans. Biomed. Eng. 16:87, 1969.

150. Liebman, J., Downs, T. D., Romberg, H., and Agusti, R.: The statistical treatment of angular data in vectorcardiography. (abstr.). Am. J. Cardiol. 17:129, 1966.

151. Liebman, J.: Normal standards. In Pediatric Electrocardiography, edited by J. Liebman, R. Plonsey, and P. Gillette, Chap. 8. Williams & Wilkins, Baltimore, 1982.

152. Davignon, A., Rautaharju, P., Boiselle, E., Soumis, F., Megelas, M., and Choquette, A.: Normal ECG standards for infants and children. Pediatr. Cardiol. 1:123, 1979 and 1980.

153. Namin, E. P., and Miller, R. A.: The normal electrocardiogram and vectorcardiogram in children. In Electrocardiography in Infants and Children, edited by D. E. Cassels and R. F. Ziegler. Grune & Stratton, New York, 1966.

154. Alimurung, M. M., Lester, G. J., Nadas, A. S., and Massell, B. F.: The unipolar precordial and extremity electrocardiogram in normal infants and children. Circulation 4:420, 1951.

155. Sreenivasan, V. V., Fisher, B. J., Liebman, J., and Downs, T. D.: A longitudinal study of the standard electrocardiogram in the healthy premature infant during the first year of life. Am. J. Cardiol. 31:57, 1973.

156. Strong, W. B., Downs, T. D., Liebman, J.,

and Liebowitz, R.: The normal adolescent electrocardiogram. Am. Heart J. 83:115, 1972.

157. Liebman, J., Downs, T. D., and Priede, A.: The Frank and McFee vectorcardiogram in normal children. A detailed quantitative analysis of 10 children between the ages of two and 19 years. In Vectorcardiography 2, edited by I. Hoffman. North-Holland, Amsterdam, 1971, p. 483.

158. Kan, J. S., Liebman, J., Lee, M. H., and Whitney, A.: Quantification of the normal Frank and McFee-Parungao orthogonal electrocardiogram at ages two to ten years. Circulation 55:31, 1977.

159. Liebman, J., Lee, M. H., Rao, P. S., and Mackay, W.: Quantitation of the normal Frank and McFee-Parungao orthogonal electrocardiogram in the adolescent. Circulation 48:735, 1973.

160. Guller, B., Lau, F., Dunn, R. A., Pipberger, H. A., and Pipberger, H. V.: Computer analysis of changes in Frank vectorcardiograms of 666 normal infants in the first 72 hours of life. J. Electrocardiol. 10:19, 1977.

161. Namin, E. P., Arcilla, R. A., D'Cruz, I. A., and Gasul, B. M.: Evolution of the Frank vectorcardiogram in normal infants. Am. J. Cardiol. 13:757, 1964.

162. Namin, E. P., and D'Cruz, I. A.: The vectorcardiogram in normal children. Br. Heart J. 26:689, 1964.

163. Ferrer, P. L., and Ellison, R. C.: The Frank scalar atrial vectorcardiogram in normal children. Am. Heart J. 88:467, 1974.

164. Borun, E. R., Sapin, S. O., and Goldberg, S. J.: Scalar amplitude measurements of data recorded with cube and Frank leads from normal children. Circulation 39:859, 1969.

165. Liebman, J., Romberg, H. C., Downs, T. D., and Agusti, R.: The Frank QRS vectorcardiogram in the premature infant. In Vectorcardiography 1965, edited by I. Hoffman and R. C. Taymore. North-Holland, Amsterdam, 1966.

166. Levine, O. R., and Griffiths, S. P.: Electrocardiographic findings in healthy premature infants. Pediatrics 3:889, 1951.

167. Walsh, S. Z.: Evolution of the electrocardiogram of healthy premature infants during the first year of life. Acta. Paediatr. Scand. (Suppl.) 145:1, 1963.

168. Walsh, S. Z.: Comparative study of electrocardiograms of healthy premature and full term infants of similar weight. Am. Heart J. 68:183, 1964.

169. Costa, A. F., Faul, B. C., Ledbetter, M. K., and Oalmon, M. C.: The electrocardiogram of the premature infant. Am. Heart J. 67:4, 1964.

170. Wenger, N. K., Watkins, W. L., and Hurst, J. W.: A preliminary study of the electrocardiogram of the normal premature infant. Am. Heart J. 62:304, 1961.

171. Hubsher, J. A.: The electrocardiogram of the premature infant. Am. Heart J. 61:467, 1961.

172. Liebman, J.: The normal electrocardiogram in newborns and infants (a critical review). In Electrocardiography in Infants and Children, edited by D. E. Cassels and R. F. Ziegler. Grune & Stratton, New York, 1966, pp. 79–98.

173. Khoury, G. H., and Fowler, R. S.: Normal Frank vectorcardiogram in infancy and childhood. Br. Heart J. 29:563, 1967.

174. Tudbury, P. B., and Atkinson, D. W.: The electrocardiogram of 100 normal infants and children. J. Pediatr. 36:466, 1950.

175. Guller, B., O'Brien, P. C., Smith, R. E., Weidman, W. H., and DuShane, J. W.: Computer interpretation of Frank vectorcardiograms in normal infant: Longitudinal and cross sectional observations from birth to two years of age. J. Electrocardiol. 8:201, 1975.

176. Hänninen, P.: Vectorcardiographic studies in newborn infants. Acta Paediatr. Scand. (Suppl.) 175:3, 1967.

177. Hugenholtz, P., and Liebman, J.: The orthogonal vectorcardiogram in 100 normal children (Frank system). With some comparative data recorded by the Cube system. Circulation 26:891, 1962.

178. Ellison, R. C., and Restiaux, N. J.: Vectordiography in Congenital Heart Disease: A Method for Estimating Severity. W. B. Saunders, Philadelphia, 1972.

179. Simonson, E., Cady, L. D., and Woodbury, M.: The normal QT interval. Am. Heart J. 63:747, 1962.

180. McCammon, R. W.: Longitudinal study of electrocardiographic intervals in healthy children. Acta Paediatr. Scand. (Suppl.) 126, 1961.

181. Castellanos, A., Jr., Lemberg, L., and Castellanos, A.: The vectorcardiographic significance of upright T waves in V1 and V2 during the first month of life. J. Pediatr. 62:827, 1963.

182. Castellanos, A., Jr., Salhanick, L., Lemberg, L., and Cohen, R.: The T loop in normal children. Am. J. Cardiol. 16:336, 1965.

183. Hait, G., and Gasul, B. M.: The evolution and significance of T wave changes in the normal newborn during the first seven days of life. Am. J. Cardiol. 12:494, 1963.

184. Puech, P., Eschavissat, M., Sodi-Pallares, D., and Cisneros, F.: Normal auricular activation in the dog's heart. Am. Heart J. 47:174, 1954.

185. Puech, P.: The P wave: Correlations of surface and intraatrial electrograms. Cardiovasc. Clin. 6:43, 1974.

186. King, T. D., Barr, R. C., Herman-Giddens, G. S., Boaz, D. E., and Spach, M. S.: Isopotential body surface maps and their relationship to atrial potentials in the dog. Circ. Res. 30:393, 1972.

187. Morris, J. J., Jr., Estes, E. H., Jr., Whalen, R. E., Thompson, H. R., and McIntosh, H. D.: P wave analysis in valvular heart disease. Circulation 29:242, 1964.

188. Baneyea, J. C., and Mukherjea, S. K.: Some observations on left atrial enlargement in the electrocardiogram. Indian Heart J. 20:264, 1978.

189. Macruz, R., Perloff, J. K., and Case R. B.: A method for the electrocardiographic recognition of atrial enlargement. Circulation 17:882, 1958.

190. Ferrer, P. L., and Ellison, R. C.: Detection of atrial overload in congenital heart disease by the Frank scalar vectorcardiogram (abstr.). Circulation 68 (Suppl. IV):82, 1973.

191. Ishikawa, K., Kini, P. M., and Pipberger, H. V.: P wave analysis in 2464 orthogonal electrocardiograms from normal subjects and patients with atrial overload. Circulation 48:565, 1973.

192. Naeye, R. L.: Arterial changes during the perinatal period. Pathology 71:121, 1961.

193. Emery, J. L., and MacDonald, A. M.: The weight of the ventricles in the later weeks of intrauterine life. Br. Heart J. 22:563, 1960.

194. Liebman, J., Romberg, H. C., Downs, T. D., and Agusti, R.: The Frank QRS vectorcardiogram in the premature infant. In Vectorcardiography 1965, edited by I. Hoffman and R. C. Taymor. North-Holland, Amsterdam, 1966.

195. Emery, J. L., and Mithal, A.: Weights of cardiac ventricles at and after birth. Br. Heart J. 23:313, 1961.

196. Allenstein, B. J., and Mori, H.: Evaluation of electrocardiographic diagnosis of ventricular hypertrophy based on autopsy comparison. Circulation 21:401, 1960.

197. Griep, A. H.: Pitfalls in the electrocardiographic diagnosis of left ventricular hypertrophy: A correlative study of 200 autopsied patients. Circulation 20:30, 1959.

198. Cooksey, J. D., Dunn, M., and Massie, E.: Clinical Vectorcardiography and Electrocardiography, 2nd ed. Year Book Publishers,

Chicago, 1977.

199. Rosenfeld, I., Goodrich, C., Kassebaum, A., Winston, A. L., and Reader, G.: The electrocardiographic recognition of left ventricular hypertrophy. Am. Heart J. 63:731, 1962.

200. Scott, R. C.: The correlation between the electrocardiographic patterns of ventricular hypertrophy and the anatomic findings. Circulation 21:256, 1960.

201. Selzer, A., Naruse, D. Y., York, E., Kahn, K. E., and Matthews, H. B.: Electrocardiographic findings in concentric and eccentric left ventricular hypertrophy. Am. Heart J. 63:320, 1962.

202. Rudy, Y., and Plonsey, R.: A comparison of volume conductor and source geometry effects on body surface and epicardial potentials. Circ. Res. 46:283, 1980.

203. Rudy, Y., and Plonsey, R.: Comments on the effects of variations in the size of the heart on the magnitude of ECG potentials. J. Electrocardiol. 13:79, 1980.

204. Rudy, Y., Wood, R., Plonsey, R., and Liebman, J.: The effect of high lung conductivity on electrocardiographic potentials. Circulation 65:440, 1982.

205. Downs, T. D., Liebman, J., and Mackay, W.: Statistical methods for vectorcardiogram orientation. In Vectorcardiography 2, edited by I. Hoffman. North-Holland, Amsterdam, 1971, p. 216.

206. Liebman, J., and Nadas, A. S.: An abnormally superior vector (formerly called marked left axis deviation) (editorial). Am. J. Cardiol. 27:577, 1971.

207. Namin, E. P.: Pediatric electrocardiography and vectorcardiography. In Heart Disease in Children: Diagnosis and Treatment, edited by B. M. Gasul, R. A. Arcilla, and M. Lev. J. B. Lippincott, Philadelphia, 1966.

208. Liebman, J., and Nadas, A. S.: The vectorcardiogram in the differential diagnosis of atrial septal defect in children. Circulation 22:956, 1960.

209. Toscano-Barbazo, E., Brandenburg, R. O., and Burchell, H. B.: Electrocardiographic studies of cases with intracardiac malformations of the atrioventricular canal. Proc. Staff Meet. Mayo Clinic 31:513, 1956.

210. Liebman, J., Miller, B. L., and Gessner, I. H.: The initial QRS in children. In Vectorcardiography 2, Proceedings of the XI International Symposium on Vectorcardiography, edited by I. Hoffman. North-Holland, Amsterdam, 1971.

211. Strang, R. H., Hugenholtz, P. G., Liebman, J., and Nadas, A. S.: The vectorcardiogram in pulmonary stenosis: Correlation with the hemodynamic state with and without ventricular septal defect. Am. J. Cardiol. 12:758, 1963.

212. Mehran-Pour, M., Whitney, A., Liebman, J., and Borkat, G.: Quantification of the Frank and McFee-Parungao orthogonal electrocardiogram in valvular pulmonic stenosis. Correlations with hemodynamic measurement. J. Electrocardiol. 12:69, 1979.

213. Rosenbaum, M. B., Elizari, M. V., and Lazzara, J. O.: The hemiblocks. Oldsmar, Fla. Tampa Tracings, 1970.

214. Rosenbaum, M. B., and Elizari, M. V.: Left anterior and left posterior hemiblock. Electrocardiographic manifestations. Postgrad.

215. Liebman, J.: Interpretation of conduction abnormalities. In Pediatric Electrocardiography, edited by J. Liebman, R. Plonsey, and P. Gillette, Chap. 12. Williams & Wilkins, Baltimore, 1982.

216. Moore, E. N., Hoffman, B. F., Patterson, D. F., and Stuckey, D. H.: Electrocardiographic changes due to delayed activation of the wall of the right ventricle. Am. Heart J. 68:347, 1974.

217. Gelband, H., Waldo, A. L., Kaiser, G. A., Bowman, F. O., Malm, J. R., and Hoffman, B. F.: Etiology of right bundle branch block in patients undergoing total correction of tetralogy of Fallot. Circulation 44:1022, 1971.

218. Krongrad, E., Hefler, S. E., Bowman, F. A., Jr., Malm, J. R., and Hoffman, B. F.: Further observations on the etiology of the right bundle branch block pattern following right ventriculotomy. Circulation 50:1105, 1974.

219. Mehran-Pour, M., Borkat, G., Liebman, J., and Ankeney, J.: Resolution of surgically induced right bundle branch block. Ann. Thorac. Surg. 23:139, 1977.

220. Fedor, J. M., Walston, A., II, Wagner, G. S., and Starr, J.: The vectorcardiogram in right bundle branch block. Correlation with cardiac failure and pulmonary disease. Circulation 53:926, 1976.

221. Cannon, D. S., Wyman, M. G., and Goldreyer, B. N.: Initial ventricular activation in left sided intraventricular conduction defects. Circulation 62:621, 1980.

222. Lev, M., Unger, P. N., Rosen, K. M., and Bharati, S.: The anatomical base of the electrocardiographic abnormality left bundle branch block. Recent advances in ventricular conduction. Adv. Cardiol. 14:16, 1975.

223. Rosenbaum, M. B.: The hemiblocks. Diagnostic criteria and clinical significance. Mod. Concepts Cardiovasc. Dis. 39:141, 1970.

224. Bellet, S.: The electrocardiogram in electrolyte imbalance. Arch. Intern. Med. 96:618, 1956.

225. Surawicz, B.: Primary and Secondary T wave changes. Heart Bull. 15:31, 1966.

226. Surawicz, B.: Relationship between electrocardiogram and electrolytes. Am. Heart J. 73:814, 1967.

227. Fisch, C., Knoebel, S., Feigenbaum, H., and Greenspan, K.: Potassium and the monophasic action potential, electrocardiogram, conduction and arrhythmias. Prog. Cardiovasc. Dis. 8:387, 1966.

228. Ferencz, C.: The electrocardiogram in electrolyte disturbances and in thyroid dysfunction. In Electrocardiography in Infants and Children, edited by D. E. Cassels and R. F. Ziegler. Grune & Stratton, New York, 1966.

229. Lepeschkin, E., and Surawicz, B.: Electrocardiographic aspects of hypopotassemia. Heart Bull. 7:114, 1958.

230. Rubin, A. L., Lubash, G. D., Cohen, B. D., Brailovsky, D., Braveman, W. D., and Luckey, H. E.: Electrocardiographic changes during hemodialysis and the artificial kidney. Circulation 8:227, 1958.

231. Schwartz, W. B., Levin, H. D., and Relman, A. S.: The electrocardiogram in potassium depletion. Its relation to the total potassium deficit and the serum concentration. Am. J. Med. 16:395, 1954.

232. Weller, J. M., Lown, B., Haigue, R. V., Wyatt, N. F., Criscetrello, M., Merrill, J. P., and Levine, S. A.: Effects of acute removal of potassium from dogs: Changes in the electrocardiogram. Circulation 11:44, 1955.

233. Weaver, W. F., and Burchell, H. B.: Serum potassium and the electrocardiogram in hypokalemia. Circulation 21:505, 1960.

234. Roberts, K. E., and Magida, M. D.: Electrocardiographic alterations produced by a decrease in plasma pH, bicarbonate and sodium as compared with those produced by an increase in potassium. Circ. Res. 1:206, 1953.

235. Seta, K., Kleiger, R., Hellerstein, E. E., Lown, B., and Vitale, J. J.: Effect of potassium and magnesium deficiency on the electrocardiogram and plasma electrolytes of pure-bred beagles. Am. J. Cardiol. 17:516, 1966.

236. Hoffman, B. F., and Singer, D. H.: Effects of digitalis on electrical activity of cardiac fibers. Prog. Cardiovasc. Dis. 7:226, 1964.

237. Manning, J. W., and Wallace, R. W.: How do cerebral vascular disorders induce ECG changes? Cardiologia 52:267, 1968.

238. Burgess, M. J., Green, L. S., Miller, K., Wyatt, R., and Abildskov, J. A.: The sequences of normal ventricular recovery. Am. Heart J. 84:660, 1972.

239. Yanowitz, F., Preston, J. B., and Abildskov, J. A.: Functional distribution of right and left stellate innervation of the ventricles: Production of neurogenic electrocardiographic changes by unilateral alteration of sympathetic tone. Circ. Res. 18:416, 1966.

240. Schwartz, P. J., and Malliani, A.: Electrical alternation of the T wave: Clinical and experimental evidence of its relationship with the sympathetic nervous system and with the long Q-T syndrome. Am. Heart J. 89:45, 1975.

241. Schwartz, P. J., Periti, M., and Mallia, A.: The long Q-T syndrome. Am. Heart J. 89:378, 1975.

242. Abildskov, J. A., Burgess, M. J., Millar, K., Wyatt, R., and Baule, G.: The primary T wave: A new electrocardiographic wave form. Am. Heart J. 81:242, 1971.

243. Hansson, L., and Larsson, O.: The incidence of ECG abnormalities in acute cerebrovascular accidents. Acta Med. Scand. 195:45, 1974.

244. Ledbetter, M. K., Cannon, A. B., II, and Fonseca Costa, A. F.: The electrocardiogram in diphtheritic myocarditis. Am. Heart J. 68:599, 1964.

245. Fowler, N. O.: The electrocardiogram in pericarditis. Cardiovasc. Clin. 5:255, 1973.

246. Spodick, D. H.: Diagnostic electrocardiographic sequences in acute pericarditis: Significance of PR segment and PR vector changes. Circulation 48:575, 1973.

247. Spodick, D. H.: The electrocardiogram in acute pericarditis: Distributions of morphologic and axial changes by stages. Am. J. Cardiol. 33:470, 1974.

248. Sreenivasan, V. V., Liebman, J., Linton, D. S., and Downs, T. D.: Posterior mitral regurgitation in girls possibly due to posterior papillary muscle dysfunction. Pediatrics 42:276, 1968.

249. Parisi, A. F., Beckmann, C. H., and Lancaster, M. C.: The spectrum of ST segment elevation in the electrocardiogram of healthy adult man. J. Electrocardiol. 4:137, 1971.

4

Echocardiography

Richard A. Meyer, M.D.

Echocardiography has become indispensable in the diagnosis and management of newborns, infants, and children with and without cardiac disease. The application of M-mode technique has become well established in diagnosing anatomic abnormalities. The development of real-time two-dimensional systems has enhanced this capability. In addition, the utilization of diagnostic ultrasound has become more prevalent in the assessment of cardiac performance.

All too frequently, however, technology exceeds the clinician's ability to optimally apply equipment to clinical situations. New developments and modifications are consistently, making models obsolete almost when they are delivered, while escalating costs make purchase of new equipment nearly prohibitive. All of these factors cause confusion and uncertainty when purchasing a system.

It is the purpose of this chapter to discuss the current two-dimensional or cross-sectional instrumentation presently available and its application to selected congenital cardiac defects. In addition, the utilization of Duplex systems combining pulsed Doppler and two-dimensional echocardiography to assess cardiac flow likewise will be included. Finally, the utilization of echocardiography in assessing cardiac performance in pediatric patients will also be stressed. The scope of this chapter does not permit detailed descriptions of specific cardiac defects, but additional descriptions will be found in the chapters of this book dealing with the specific cardiac defects. Also, two books devoted entirely to pediatric echocardiography discuss the ultrasonic physics and methodology in greater depth.[26a, 57]

SAFETY OF ULTRASOUND

Since diagnostic ultrasound is accurate and pain free, it has tremendous appeal to the pediatrician as a noninvasive method. With the wide application of diagnostic ultrasound in pediatric patients, particularly in premature and full-term neonates as well as fetuses, the dictum "Do not harm" assumes even greater significance. At the present time, adverse effects resulting from the application of diagnostic ultrasound in patients have not been reported. However, one of the problems confronting investigators studying the safety of this technique is the inability to satisfactorily measure the "dose" of ultrasonic energy delivered to and absorbed by living cells. Therefore, detailed information about the ultrasonic energy levels on "thresholds" required to alter various biologic tissues is lacking.

Definitions and explanations of terminology as well as measurements of specific acoustical ouput can be found in the recent works of Eggleton[16] and Kosoff.[43] It should be pointed out, however, that in pulsed echo systems the instantaneous spatial peak intensities are several orders of magnitude higher than the average intensities since the total "on time" of the pulsed transducer is very brief. Information regarding the ultrasonic output of current diagnostic systems is important to know and directly relates to potential risks to patients. A wide range of output values was found by Carson et al. (11) and varied from 0.4 to 1700 watts/cm^2 for instantaneous spatial peak intensity in pulsed echo systems. For continuous wave obstetrical Doppler systems, the output varied from a low of 0.95 to 37 milliwatts/cm^2. At present, there appears to be no danger with the level of energy output from the current instruments; however, the margin of safety is obviously reduced when using high power outputs, and unless some benefit is to be gained, more power than absolutely necessary should be avoided.

For the purpose of risk assessment, it is probably useful to classify interaction into two categories: those related to the mechanics of wave propagation (i.e., direct effects and cavitation) and those related to the absorption of acoustical energy leading to heat generation and temperature rise. Information such as the higher susceptibility to damage of dividing cell populations, as compared to stable mature cells or differences in thermal denaturation thresholds or mechanical fragility, must all be included in the assessment of the risk of ultrasound on tissues. The evidence appears to be conclusive that with continuous wave or pulsed ultrasound there is no likelihood of damage to *organized* mammalian tissue from wave mechanics phenomenon and cavitation up to peak intensity levels of approximately 1500 watts/cm^2 at a frequency of 2 to 3 MHz.[45]

Temperature thresholds for tissue damage are time dependent and independent of the source or cause of temperature rise.[38, 45] Goss et al.[26] reported that acoustical absorption coefficients and thermal properties typical of mammalian soft tissue would require continuous wave insonation at acoustical intensity levels of 1.5 watts/cm^2 at 2.5 MHz for about 5 minutes to raise the temperature at the site of insonation to 44°C. In addition it would have to be sustained for at least 15 minutes for damage to occur. It would appear that the margin of safety for mature cells using clinical pulsed echo instrumentation and continuous wave Doppler type instrumentation would be in excess of two orders of magnitude. Fortunately, tissues do not appear to have a memory for exposure to ultrasound. Thus, unlike x-rays there is little likelihood of a cumulative effect of ultrasound once the heat generated has been dissipated.

Evidence regarding the safety of ultrasound is often contradictory, making decisions about the safety of ultrasound difficult. It is convenient to consider the large body of evidence under the following categories: epidemiological studies, laboratory studies, studies on fetuses, studies on dividing cell populations in vivo, and in vitro studies on cells in tissue culture.

To date the epidemiological studies have been reassuring. In a group of 1114 pregnant women, Hellman et al.,[30] found that neither the frequency of the ultrasonic examination nor the time of the first examination seemed to affect adversely the frequency of fetal abnormality and abortion. Bernstine[6] found the frequency of congenital malformation, abortion, and premature labor in 720 patients examined with continuous wave Doppler ultrasound to be slightly lower than those in control patients. Ziskin[101] in 1972 received no reports of any adverse effect in 17,869 pulsed echo examinations and 7,667 continuous wave Doppler examinations. Since that time there have been no untoward effects reported from the United States or Europe in several carefully designed, controlled, prospective studies. However, it may be a decade or longer before any definitive statements on the absence of any defects can be made. In studies by Smyth,[86] Warwick et al.,[95] and Mannor et al.,[53] no effects of ultrasound on the ovaries, ovulation, fertilization, implantation, abortion (or continuation of pregnancy to term) prenatal or subsequent development of the offspring, litter size, birth weight, or occurrence of abnormalities were found in the first or second generation. However, Shimizu and Shoji[84] in 1973 reported an increase in frequency of abortion and fetal malformation in pregnant mice insonated with CW ultrasound for 5 hours from a clinical diagnostic instrument on the ninth day of pregnancy. Hence, the results in mice and rats generally confirm the evidence found in clinical experience.

Caution must be exercised when interpreting and extrapolating results obtained from animal fetuses to man for two reasons, especially when animal fetuses are so much smaller than those of man. First, the relation of ultrasonic field characteristics, such as number of wavelengths in the fetus, size of the ultrasonic beam relative to the fetus, and attenuation of intensity in the tissues between the transducer and fetus, are grossly different in the two situations. Secondly, despite the care exercised in defining the ultrasonic field characteristics in water, the insertion of a small experimental animal into a field so severely distorts the field that it is impossible to know the actual intensity at each of the fetuses.

Studies involving the dividing cell population in vivo have demonstrated little correlation between a response and intensity of ultrasound used.[14, 44] In fact, the experiments of Miller et al.,[65] using very high intensities of ultrasound, failed to show any difference between the insonated cell population and the control group. Studies on the effects of ultrasound on chromosomes also have been somewhat confusing. The first reports by Macintosh and Davey[51] suggested chromosomal aberrations; however, repetition of their experiments in other laboratories failed to confirm these aberrations.[12, 41, 52, 56, 70] Presently it would seem reasonable to assume that continuous wave insonation of human lymphocytes in vitro with intensities of up to 300 milliwatts/cm^2 and durations of up to 2 hours does not cause chromosomal aberrations. Lyon and Simpson[50] carried out a study insonating the gonads of male and female mice prior to mating and found no evidence of genetic damage even with intensity levels and durations considerably higher than those used in diagnostic ultrasound. However, Liebeskind et al.[47, 48] have demonstrated chromatid exchanges in human lymphocytes and effects on DNA and growth patterns of animal cells.

In summary, it would appear at this time that diagnostic ultrasound produced by currently available equipment will not have an adverse effect on tissues in clinical practice. In August 1976, the American Institute of Ultrasound in Medicine issued a statement regarding the ultrasonic biological effects on mammalian tissues in vivo which stated in part that "in the low megahertz frequency range there have been no significant biological effects in mammalian tissues exposed to intensities below 100 milliwatts per square centimeter. Furthermore for ultrasonic exposures times less than 500 seconds and greater than 1 second such effects have not been demonstrated even at higher intensities when the product of the intensity and exposure time is less than 50 joules per centimeter square," with intensities here referring to

spatial peak temporal average as measured in a free field in water, exposure time equaling total time including off time as well as on time for a repeated pulse regimen, and a joule, the amount of heat generated by ultrasound, equaling 0.239 calories. In October 1978 the statement was modified to include the phrase "no independently confirmed."

INSTRUMENTATION

The greatest experience in pediatrics has been obtained using motion mode (M-mode) echocardiography, which continues to be the backbone of most echocardiography laboratories. It has proved extremely useful in determining the size, presence or absence of structures, and their relationship to one another. However, it provides only a single dimension view of the heart, and the recent emergence and greater acceptance of cross-sectional or two-dimensional (2-D) real-time echocardiography has tremendously enhanced the ability to visualize spatial relationships. These cross-sectional or 2-D echograms are generated using a variety of equipment: B-scan; multicrystal linear array; electronic phased array sector scanner; and mechanical sector scanner.

A stop action *B-scan* of the heart is obtained with a conventional general purpose B-scanner by rocking the transducer slowly by hand at one point on the chest through a single plane of the heart. A gated circuit which is triggered from the R wave of the patient's electrocardiogram allows the transducer to be activated during diastole or systole. A composite of multiple sequential B scans is thus built up on a storage oscilloscope and photographed with a suitable camera (Fig. 4.1). When one composite is completed and photographed, the transducer can be moved to another location and the process repeated. However, the transducer is held in a rigid transducer holder and is cumbersome to use. Because of its size and design, it lacks portability, making it impractical for bedside evaluation. Since constructing one image is quite time consuming, small infants and children find it difficult to hold still while the composite is being constructed, which is essential to preserve the plane of examination. This system does not lend itself to the evaluation of complex congenital heart disease. Furthermore, any system that depends upon stop-action recording techniques loses functional data.

The *multicrystal linear array* system employs multiple single-element crystals aligned in a row (Fig. 4.2). The crystals sequentially transmit and receive signals rapidly, either

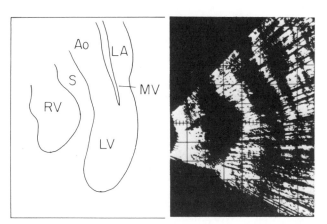

Fig. 4.1 Stop action B scan of child with an ASD taken in diastole which shows a large right ventricle (*RV*) and normal to small left atrium (*LA*). *Ao*, aorta; *LV*, left ventricle; *MV*, mitral valve; *S*, septum.

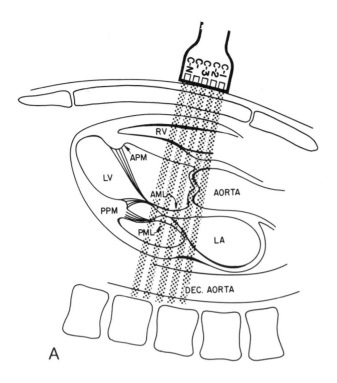

A

consuming; and, in addition, a larger ultrasonic window is provided which obviates the extremely narrow near field associated with most sector equipment. Near field resolution is better; however, the larger transducer cannot be placed between the ribs, resulting in rib artifacts, and examining from the suprasternal notch and subcostal area is not easy. Difficulty recording structures may be greater because the transducer cannot be manipulated easily since the linear array format is inflexible.

Real-time two-dimensional (2-D) echocardiograms can also be obtained with *sector scanners*. These instruments sweep a sound beam from a point source through an arc either electronically or mechanically.

In electronic scanners a properly designed array of transducer elements can be operated as a "phased array," a modality that is quite different in principle from the multicrystal systems described previously. The principal requirement is that the delays between the pulsing of successive transducer elements be small, typically less than a microsecond, compared to the 250-millisecond intervals between successive pulses used in multicrystal systems. The result is that the energy from the individual elements combines to form a single ultrasonic beam and that the direction of the beam can be controlled by varying the delay between the pulsing of individual elements. Thus, when all of the elements are pulsed at exactly the same time, the beam emanates perpendicularly to the transducer face (Fig. 4.3*A*). If the elements at the top of the transducer are pulsed later

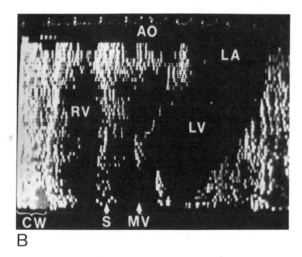

B

Fig. 4.2   (*A*) Idealized diagram of multicrystal linear array transducer and sagittal view of the heart. (*B*) One selected frame taken from the multicrystal linear array study of a patient with tricuspid atresia and VSD showing a normal-sized right ventricle (*RV*) and large left ventricle (*LV*). The aorta (*Ao*) is not overriding the septum (*S*). *AML*, anterior mitral leaflet; *APM*, anterior papillary muscle; *CW*, chest wall; *LA*, left atrium; *PML*, posterior mitral leaflet; *PPM*, posterior papillary muscle.

singly or in groups, and provide real-time two dimensional images of the heart. Echoes are displayed so that the vertical axis corresponds to crystal positions in the transducer (crystal 1 at top) and the horizontal axis corresponds to depth of tissue (with centimeter depth markers at the top of the screen). Many investigations have been performed in children with congenital heart disease by Sahn and associates.[13, 14] The advantages of this system over the stop-action B-scan are: it is in real-time, and functional data will not be lost; it can be performed at the bedside; it is less time

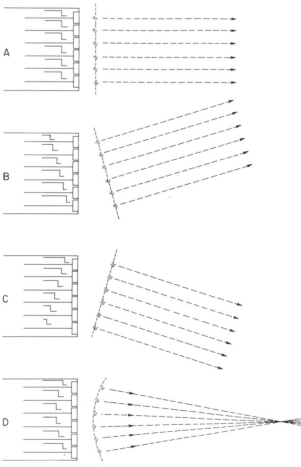

Fig. 4.3   Manner in which a phased array is used to direct beams A, B, and C and to focus beam D (see text).

than the elements at the bottom (Fig. 4.3*B*), the beam will propagate upward. If the delays are reversed, the beam will be directed downward (Fig. 4.3*C*). Finally, if the elements in the center of the transducer are delayed with respect to the edges, the beam will be focused (Fig. 4.3D). The delaying process can be operative both during transmission and (by the use of controllable delay lines) during reception.

The advantages of phased array systems are: since there are no moving parts, there is no noise, vibration, or wear; focusing can be provided in the plane of the scan, and the receiving focus can be dynamic; the sector angle can be as large as 90° and can easily be changed by instrument adjustment; simultaneous motion mode recordings can be produced; only a limited ultrasonic window is required; line density is good (100 or more per picture); and the transducer is small. The disadvantages are: the system is complex, resulting in a high cost; anterior structures are not well demonstrated; and the systems are not portable. Experience with this device in children has demonstrated its usefulness in determining spatial relationships and atrioventricular morphology.[21, 67, 72]

The *mechanical sector scanner* is the simplest real-time system and has been used extensively in the diagnosis of congenital heart disease, including transposition of the great arteries[8, 31, 32] aortic stenosis,[97, 98] coarctation of the aorta,[99] pulmonic stenosis,[96] and mitral stenosis,[33] and endocarditis.[13] In concept, this is nothing more than the mechanization of the cardiac sweep performed by the M-mode echocardiographer and is accomplished by driving a single crystal through a sector or spinning several crystals around an axle so that only one crystal is active at any given moment. These sector scans typically create a sector of 30 to 90° and are produced at a frame rate of approximately 30 frames/second (Fig. 4.4). Because only one line of information is obtained from each interrogation, and because real-time scanners operate at high scanning rates, the number of scan lines or lines containing echo data per picture is limited. With a mechanical sector scanner operating at 30 frames/second and at a pulse repetition frequency of 3000 frames/second, each individual picture or frame contains 100 lines.

The advantages of real-time mechanical sector scanners are: good line density (100 or more per picture); good resolution owing to the use of focused transducers; low cost; and only a moderate ultrasonic window is required. The disadvantages are: limited view of anterior structures owing to the use of the sectoring format in many instruments; limited sectoring angle; noise and vibration in some systems causing apprehension in patients; and impossibility of satisfactory simultaneous M-mode and 2D recordings.

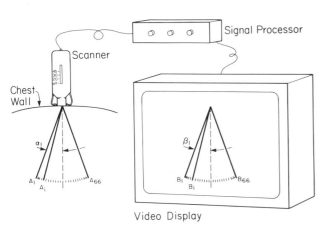

Fig. 4.4   Diagram of mechanical sector scanner.

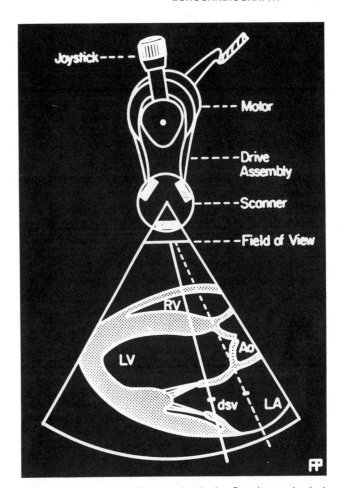

Fig. 4.5   Composite diagram of a duplex Doppler mechanical scanner. *RV*, right ventricle; *LV*, left ventricle; *LA*, left atrium.

DOPPLER

Doppler echocardiography is very complex and so it will not be possible to describe the instrumentation in detail; however, the reader is referred to an excellent review of the subject.[4] Although not new, it is only with the advent of the Duplex scanner (Fig. 4.5), which combines pulsed Doppler with two-dimensional echocardiography, that great interest has been provoked about Doppler. The pulsed Doppler system is primarily a velocity sensing system and complements the findings of echocardiography. The Doppler principle states that the frequency of a returning ultrasonic signal from a target is proportional to the velocity of that target, such as a valve leaflet, vessel wall, or the movement of the cellular components in flowing blood. This change in frequency is known as the Doppler shift, and with current instrumentation it can be displayed graphically on a monitor or paper. The Doppler shift is audible, and listening to the Doppler output provides characteristic flow signals which can be interpreted with some practice.

The graphic display of the Doppler signal uses a time interval histogram technique that is accomplished with multiple zero crossing methods to analyze the frequency of the returning sound and then plots those frequencies against time. By convention, flow toward the transducer is plotted above zero crossing line, flow away from the transducer below the base line. Blood flow within a vessel or chamber is usually laminar and produces a time interval histogram with a narrowly clustered dot pattern (Fig. 4.6). Turbulent

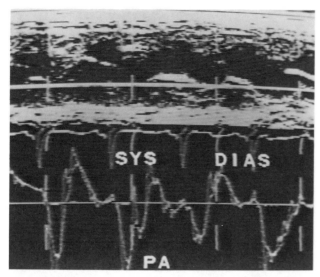

Fig. 4.6 Time interval histogram of Doppler spectral display from a normal patient showing laminar flow distal to pulmonary valve away from the transducer in systole (*SYS*) and the recoil flow toward the transducer in early diastole (*DIAS*). *PA*, pulmonary artery.

or disturbed flow, by contrast, produces a time interval histogram with a widely dispersed dot pattern, frequently referred to as spectral broadening. The presence of widely dispersed dots that are both above and below the zero crossing line illustrates marked variation in blood cell direction and velocity within the sample, with some cells moving towards and others away from the transducer.

Clinical investigations of congenital cardiac defects have been used with single crystal transducers, some of which include differentiation of ventricular septal defects from mital regurgitation,[74] noninvasive assessment of pulmonary hypertension and patent ductus arteriosus,[73] and noninvasive assessment of surgical systemic pulmonary shunts.[1] One of the major limitations of single crystal evaluations is the fact that the Doppler signal is highly sensitive to change in angulation, and attempts at recording true velocity of blood flow are difficult because of the inability to know exactly where the Doppler sample volume is in relationship to the flow vector. The "duplex" scanning system tends to minimize the angulation problem, and it also aids the investigator in positioning the Doppler sample volume precisely at a desired location.

Not only has the Duplex scanner assisted in the diagnosis of congenital cardiac disease, but also it has generated a great deal of interest in quantitation of blood flow. In order to quantitate blood flow within a vessel, certain parameters must be measured which include the cross-sectional area (A) of the vessel lumen and velocity of the blood flow. The velocity (V) can be determined by knowing the Doppler shift ($\overline{\Delta f}$) and solving the equation

$$V = \frac{c\overline{\Delta f}}{2f_0 \cos\theta},$$

where c is the velocity of sound, $\overline{\Delta f}$ is the average Doppler shift from profile or from full vessel sample gate, f_0 is the carrier frequency (3 MHz or 5 MHz), and cos θ represents the angle between the sound beam axis and the velocity vector, and constitutes one of the most difficult indices to assess. The advent of the Duplex scanner and some means of angle detection should provide the necessary vessel area

information and velocity information and, hence, provide quantitation of volume flow rate.

THE NORMAL ECHOCARDIOGRAM

M-MODE EXAMINATION

Since the echocardiographic wave forms of various structures are identical, proper interpretation of the echogram depends upon knowledge of the intracardiac anatomy as well as the relationship of structures to one another and the transducer beam position to those structures (Fig. 4.7). Normally, the ultrasonic examination begins at the left sternal border. However, if structures cannot be recorded from that position, then the transducer must be moved over the precordium in an effort to locate the desired structures.

The mitral valve, which is usually found to the left of the tricuspid valve, is in fibrous continuity with the posterior margin of the aortic root (Fig. 4.8). Hence, the mitral valve echo is continuous with and at the same depth from the chest wall as the posterior margin of the aorta. The tricuspid valve, although not in fibrous continuity with the aortic root, is related to the anterior margin of the aorta (Fig. 4.7). These important anatomic relationships enable us to identify the ventricles, whether or not M-mode or 2-D equipment is used, since the mitral valve, which is in continuity with the posterior margin of the semilunar aortic valve, always denotes the left ventricle, whereas the tricuspid valve, which is not in continuity with a semilunar valve, identifies the right ventricle. In addition it is possible to identify the left ventricle by its papillary muscles.

Normally the aorta lies to the right of and posterior to the pulmonary artery. The aortic root echo is found by scanning the mitral valve medially and superiorly along the major axis of the left ventricle (Fig. 4.8). In order to record the pulmonary artery in infants and children, it is seldom necessary to move the M-mode transducer from the aortic position but merely to direct its beam leftward and slightly superiorly (Fig. 4.7D). Echoes from the interventricular septum (Fig. 4.7) as well as from the right and left ventricle are recorded with the transducer in the mitral position. The relationship of the septum to the anterior margin of the aorta can be demonstrated by scanning the mitral valve all the way to the aorta (Fig. 4.8).

TWO-DIMENSIONAL EXAMINATION

Two-dimensional echocardiography examinations provide tomoographic images of the heart. These are obtained by directing the transducer beam along many selected cross-sectional planes through the heart that generally include: the precordial sagittal plane or long axis view of the left ventricle (Fig. 4.9); the precordial transverse plane or short axis view (Fig. 4.10 and 4.11); the apical four-chambered view (Fig. 4.12); the subxiphoid four-chambered view (Fig. 4.13); and the suprasternal notch (Fig. 4.14). Recommendations established by the American Society of Echocardiography state that the left-sided structures of a patient's heart, as we view the patient from the left hip, should appear at the right of the oscilloscope or television monitor, while the right-sided structures should appear to the left. All subsequent descriptions of the two-dimensional echograms will be according to the patient's anatomic relationships, not according to image position on the screen. Also, those structures which are closest to the transducer will appear at the top or apex of the image while those farthest away are at the bottom.

In the precordial *long axis view* of the heart, the aorta is

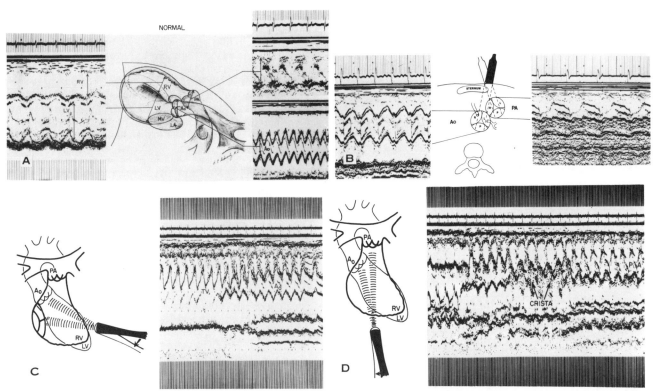

Fig. 4.7 These composite pictures demonstrate the relationships of the cardiac structures in the normal heart and the transducer positions used to record them. (*A*) Sagittal view of cardiac structures. (*B*) Transverse view of great vessels from patient's left hip. (*C*) Frontal view of relation of tricuspid valve to aorta. (*D*) Frontal view of relation of aorta to pulmonary artery. *A*$_o$, aorta; *L*, left; *LA*, left atrium; *LV*, left ventricle; *MV*, mitral valve; *P*, posterior; *PA*, pulmonary artery; *R*, right; *RV*, right ventricle; *TV*, tricuspid valve.

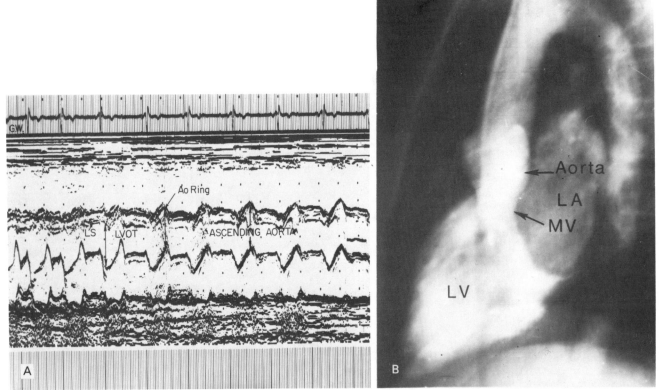

Fig. 4.8 (*A*) Echogram showing normal relation to the ventricular septum to the anterior margin of the aorta and mitral valve to the posterior margin of the aorta. *Ao*, aorta; *LS*, left septal surface; *LVOT*, left ventricular outflow tract. (*B*) Lateral left ventriculogram in patient with mitral regurgitation demonstrating mitral-aortic continuity. *LA*, left atrium; *LV*, left ventricle; *MV*, mitral valve.

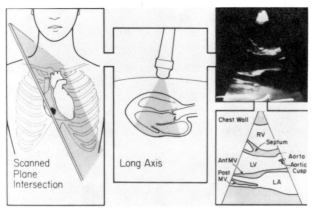

Fig. 4.9 Composite illustrating the plane of the long axis of the heart examined by mechanical sector 2D equipment.

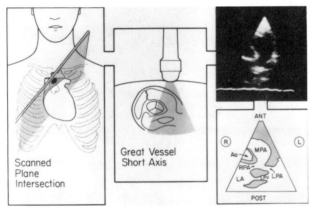

Fig. 4.10 Composite illustrating the plane of the short axis of the great arteries examined by 2D ultrasound.

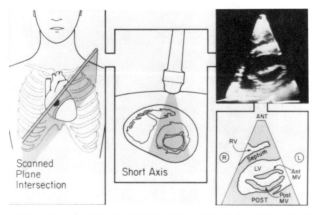

Fig. 4.11 Composite illustrating the plane of the short axis of the left ventricle examined by 2D ultrasound.

imaged to the right and the left ventricular cavity with mitral valve to the left of the screen (Fig. 4.9). Fibrous continuity of the anterior mitral valve leaflet with the posterior aortic root is clearly observed, and the left atrium is posterior to the aorta. Above the septum, varying portions of the right ventricle and right ventricular outflow tract are displayed.

Rotating the transducer 90° clockwise from long axis of the aorta provides a *short axis view* of the great vessels (Fig. 4.10). The circular aorta with its three valve cusps is displayed in the midportion of the screen, with a crescent-shaped right ventricular outflow tract above it. Angulating the transducer superiorly demonstrates the pulmonary valve just anterior and to the left of the aorta as the pulmonary trunk wraps along the left side of the aorta, subsequently dividing into the right and left pulmonary arteries below or posterior to the aorta. The left atrium resides posterior to the aorta, and with proper orientation of the transducer beam, the pulmonary veins may be seen entering the left atrium. Although the interatrial septum is seen on this view, there may be echo dropout, and the lack of echoes in the midportion of the septum is not diagnostic of an atrial septal defect.

In the *short axis view* of the left ventricle, the normal atrioventricular valves are usually differentiated by their characteristic appearances. Tilting the transducer inferiorly to the level of the mitral valve demonstrates a characteristic "fishmouth" mitral valve surrounded by the left ventricular endocardium (Fig. 4.11). Medial rotation of the transducer permits visualization of the anterior and/or tricuspid valve leaflet just to the right of the interventricular septum. The attachment of the tricuspid valve is more anterior than the mitral valve. Further angulation of the transducer inferiorly along the axis of the left ventricular cavity permits visualization of the two papillary muscles which are diagnostic of the left ventricle.

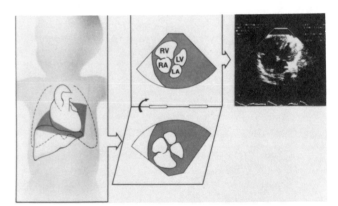

Fig. 4.12 Composite of 2D echogram from apex showing the normal 4-chambered view. *LA*, left atrium; *LV*, left ventricle; *RA*, right atrium; *RV*, right ventricle.

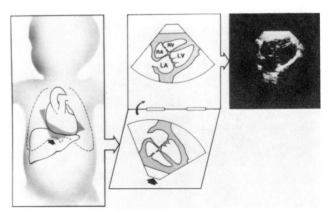

Fig. 4.13 Composite of 2D echogram from the subxiphoid position. *LA*, left atrium; *LV*, left ventricle; *RA*, right atrium; *RV*, right ventricle.

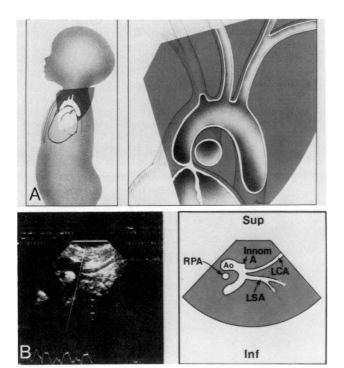

Fig. 4.14 Composite illustrating echographic plane from suprasternal notch (*A*) and echogram of aorta (*B*). *Innom A*, innominate artery; *Inf*, inferior; *LCA*, left carotid artery; *LSA*, left subclavian artery; *RPA*, right pulmonary artery; *Sup*, superior.

The transverse apical position provides a *four-chambered view* of the heart (Fig. 4.12). The transducer is placed over the apex, and the beam is directed toward the base of the heart with the plane of the beam perpendicular to the septal planes while passing through the plane of the atrioventricular valve orifices. The apex of the ventricles forms the apex of the sector and is at the top of the screen while the atria are at the bottom. The septa of the ventricles and atria, along with the mitral and tricuspid valves, form a cruciate confluence which separates these four chambers. The transducer should be oriented so that the ellipsoidal left ventricle is to the right of the screen, with the crescent-shaped right ventricle to the left. The atria are relatively circular on this view. More superior angulation of the transducer demonstrates the origin of the right ventricular outflow tract and aorta, while posterior angulation may demonstrate the entrance of the pulmonary veins. Although the entire interventricular septum is usually visualized with this approach, it and the interatrial septum may be incompletely recorded because of echo dropout.

The subxiphoid or subcostal approach usually permits more complete visualization of the interatrial septum because the beam is more perpendicular to the plane of the septum (Fig. 4.13). By rotating the transducer rightward along the horizontal plane, it is possible to visualize the inferior vena cava as it drains into the right atrium (Fig. 4.15). The orientation of the cardiac structures is such that the heart appears tilted on its left side. The liver substance is seen at the apex of the sector. Just inferior to it the right atrium can be visualized emptying into the right ventricle through the tricuspid valve. Further leftward rotation of the transducer permits the right ventricle to be visualized anterior to the left ventricle. The left atrium is recorded posterior to the right atrium and opens into the left ventricle through the mitral valve.

With the transducer in the *suprasternal notch* and the beam directed along the sagittal plane of the aortic arch, the ascending aorta can be visualized on the left side of the screen, the transverse arch at the top of the screen, and the descending aorta on the right side (Fig. 4.14). The circular right pulmonary artery can be seen just superior to and anterior to the larger left atrium.

Combining all of these views plus variations allows for a complete anatomic assessment of the heart. Specific defects must be approached with specific questions in mind so that the correct plane will be utilized to provide the desired information.

CONTRAST ECHOES

The forceful injection of dextrose-water, saline, or blood into a peripheral or central vein produces microcavitations routinely at the end of a needle or catheter. These microcavitations create multiple ultrasonic reflective interfaces that are visualized as a cloud of echoes on the oscilloscope. This technique during an echographic procedure has been used very successfully to validate structures, detect intracardiac shunts, and identify flow patterns within the heart[83, 93, 94, 100]. For example, an injection into the brachial vein of a patient can be useful to validate the right atrium, right ventricle, or pulmonary arteries. In addition there maybe "echo dropout" or failure to record the interatrial or interventricular septum. An echo contrast study can delineate the limits of the septum and confirm the spurious nature of the echo dropout (Fig. 4.16). Conversely, in a patient suspected of having a secundum atrial septal defect, the echo contrast may cross the defect from right to left atrium, verifying the presence of the defect.

THE NEWBORN

Probably the greatest contribution of pediatric echocardiography is in the newborn period. Since, in the neonate, the signs and symptoms of respiratory disease, sepsis, metabolic derangement, and abnormalities of hemoglobin may mimic those of congenital heart disease, difficulty frequently is encountered in arriving at a correct diagnosis.

HYPOPLASTIC LEFT HEART SYNDROME

The common presenting symptoms of critically ill newborns are a shock-like picture and cyanosis. Neonates with the clinical picture of shock may have the hypoplastic left heart syndrome, resulting from aortic atresia, critical aortic stenosis, aortic atresia, and mitral atresia or mitral atresia with ventricular septal defect.

Aortic Atresia

Newborns with aortic atresia have a characteristic echocardiogram that is diagnostic of this syndrome[57] (Fig. 4.17).

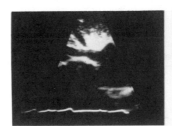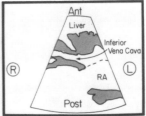

Fig. 4.15 Normal subxyphoid. Composite showing inferior vena cava draining into the right atrium (*RA*). *Ant*, anterior; *L*, left; *Post*, posterior; *R*, right.

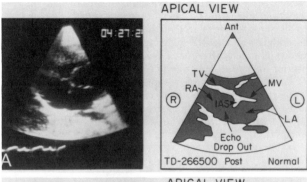

APICAL VIEW

APICAL VIEW

Fig. 4.16 Apical echograms from normal subject showing echo dropout (*A*) of portion of interatrial septum (*IAS*) and b) confirmation of intact septum using echo-contrast technique (*B*). *Ant*, anterior; *LA*, left atrium; *L*, left; *MV*, mitral valve; *Post*, posterior; *R*, right; *RA*, right atrium; *TV*, tricuspid valve.

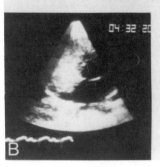
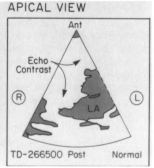

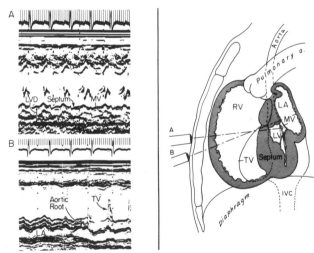

Fig. 4.17 Idealized diagram in sagittal view of patient with aortic atresia. Echogram, *A* depicts the structures recorded from transducer position *A*. Echogram *B* depicts the structures recorded as the transducer is rotated from position *A* to position *B*. *IVC*, inferior vena cava; *LA*, left atrium; *LV*, left ventricle; *MV*, mitral

The findings include: a minute to absent aortic root echo; a small posterior ventricle in the presence of a large anterior ventricle; and a mitral valve echo that is grossly distorted. The pathognomonic sign of this disease is a very tiny aortic root less than 5 mm in diameter. Identification of the aortic root is accomplished by directing the transducer beam carefully along the tricuspid valve until its anterior margin is

identified. The large pulmonary artery encroaches upon the aorta (Fig. 4.18) and may be mistaken for the aorta if a slow scan is not made. The left ventricle usually cannot be recorded, but when it is, it is usually a third or less of the normal size; on occasion, however, it may be normal or large if a ventricular septal defect (VSD) is present (Fig. 4.18). In that circumstance, the mitral valve echo appears normal, and the left ventricle is large. Since 1974, the above M-mode echocardiographic findings have provided the diagnosis of aortic atresia in 53 patients without resorting to cardiac catheterization or angiography. Also, the small aorta can be demonstrated on 2-D echo (Fig. 4.19).

Aortic Stenosis and Mitral Atresia

It is imperative to distinguish critical aortic stenosis from aortic atresia or mitral atresia with VSD since prompt surgical relief of the severe obstruction improves the circulation of these neonates. Patients with critical aortic stenosis or mitral atresia with VSD have almost normal aortic root dimensions. However, in patients with critical aortic stenosis, the left ventricular cavity is small, and the free wall and septum are quite thick. The mitral valve echo may be thick and distorted, but it is recognizable, whereas in mitral atresia with or without a VSD, the mitral valve is absent, and a left ventricle is not recordable. The left atrium in both conditions may be normal in size.

MITRAL STENOSIS

Mitral stenosis, although unusual in children, is easily diagnosed with ultrasound. The classic M-mode echographic feature is the thick, flat, square wave form of the mitral valve compared to the tricuspid valve echo. In addition, the left atrium is markedly enlarged if the obstruction is severe. Evaluation of the mitral echo is indispensable since other conditions which produce signs of pulmonary edema and inflow obstruction to the left ventricle (cor triatriatum, stenosis of pulmonary veins, supravalvular stenosis ring) may be clinically indistinguishable from mitral stenosis. A normal mitral valve echo, therefore, will focus attention on the other diagnostic possibilities, and appropriate selective angiocardiograms can be performed in order to arrive at the correct diagnosis.

COARCTATION OF THE AORTA

Frequently, neonates with coarctation of the aorta, either as an isolated defect or with associated defects, present with heart failure and/or shock. Two-dimensional echocardiography has enabled us to visualize the site of coarctation from the suprasternal notch (Fig. 4.20) and exclude any of the above diagnostic possibilities. Vigorous medical management usually results in marked improvement which leads to enhanced cardiac output. Appropriate surgical intervention can then be undertaken.

CYANOTIC HEART DISEASE

The common cardiac causes of cyanosis in the critically ill newborn include transposition of the great arteries, tricuspid atresia, pulmonary atresia, and total anomalous pulmonary venous connection.

Transposition of the Great Arteries

One characteristic feature of transposition of the great arteries (TGA) is that the anterior root echo, which in normal patients is recorded to the left of the posterior root,

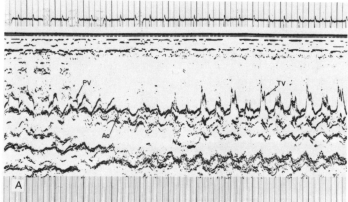

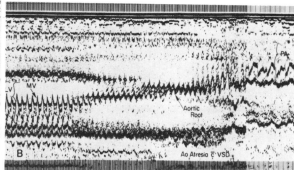

Fig. 4.18 (*A*) Echogram of patient with aortic atresia showing minute aortic root identified from tricuspid valve sweep. *Ao*, aorta; *PV*, pulmonary valve; *TV*, tricuspid valve. (*B*) Echocardiogram of patient with aortic atresia and ventricular septal defect showing large left ventricle and normal mitral valve echo. A sweep from the mitral valve to aorta demonstrates the thread-like aortic root. *LV*, left ventricle; *MV*, mitral valve; *PA*, pulmonary artery.

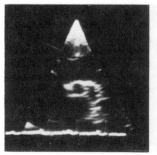

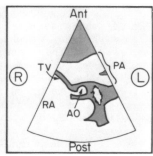

Fig. 4.19 Composite 2D echogram from a patient with aortic atresia showing tiny aortic root (*Ao*) and large pulmonary artery (*PA*) in the short axis view.

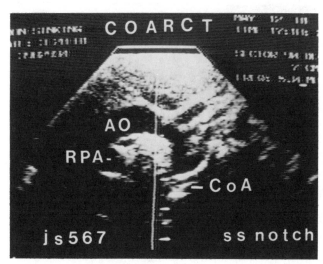

Fig. 4.20 2-D echo from suprasternal (*ss*) notch showing transverse aorta (*Ao*) and discrete coarctation (*coarct* and *CoA*). RPA, right pulmonary artery.

is now found to the right in 70% of the patients. The aorta may also reside directly anterior to the pulmonary artery (10 to 15%), or even arise to the left of the pulmonary artery (10 to 15%).

When using M-mode echocardiography, difficulty identifying the anterior aortic root from position alone may be encountered. Another helpful feature is that normally the aortic root echo is obtained by scanning the mitral valve from the apex of the left ventricle to the aortic root by directing the transducer beam across the midline of the chest over the right shoulder. In patients with TGA, the posterior pulmonary artery arises from the left ventricle more anteriorly and leftward. Therefore, the pulmonary artery is recorded to the left of sternum with the transducer beam more parallel to the sternum (Fig. 4.21). This finding is rarely present in normal patients. Two-dimensional echo has virtually eliminated the difficulty of diagnosing TGA. Since the aorta arises retrosternally in a more vertical course, the echogram of the short axis view of the great vessels demonstrates two circles (Fig. 4.22) rather than the typical crescent shaped echo of the normal pulmonary artery as it wraps around the aorta (Fig. 4.10). This 2-D echographic feature has substantially reduced the difficulties and errors arising from M-mode studies.

In addition, systolic time intervals have been helpful in identifying the pulmonary artery and aorta. The systolic time intervals of the two ventricles are altered by changes in the vascular resistance to which each ventricle is exposed. If vascular resistance is high, as in the normal aorta, the systolic time interval ratio (PEP-VET) will be high. If the vascular resistance is low, as is the case in a normal pulmonary artery, the PEP-VET ratio will be low. Thus, the PEP-VET ratios generally are reversed in patients with TGA. Although some infants may have high pulmonary vascular resistance in the newborn period, for the most part this systolic time interval information has enabled us to determine more accurately from which ventricle the aorta and pulmonary artery arises in patients with TGA.

Persistent Fetal Circulation

The syndrome of persistent fetal circulation or pulmonary hypertension of the newborn must always be considered in the differential diagnosis of the cyanotic newborn. Although the etiology of this problem appears diverse, the basic hemodynamic abnormality is severe pulmonary vasoconstriction with pulmonary hypertension and right to left shunting through the ductus arteriosus or the foramen ovale. Since cardiac catheterization poses a risk to these infants, echocardiography has played a role in the management by excluding congenital cardiac defects and obviating the need for catheterization. In persistent fetal circulation, the RPEP-

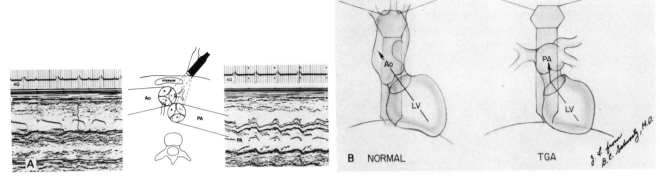

Fig. 4.21 (*A*) A composite of the great vessels in a transverse plane of a patient with transposition of the greater arteries showing the transducer position used to record the rightward and anterior aorta and leftward posterior pulmonary artery. (*B*) Idealized diagrams showing the relationships of the normal aorta to the left ventricle and pulmonary artery to the left ventricle in transposition of the great arteries. The *arrows* stress the difference in tranducer beam positions necessary to record the semilunar valves. *R*, right; *L*, left; *P*, posterior; *Ao*, aorta; *LV*, left ventricle; *PA*, pulmonary artery; *TGA*, transposition of the greater arteries.

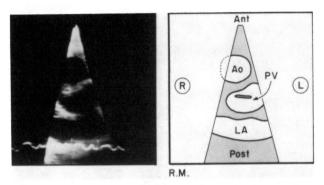

Fig. 4.22 Composite of echogram in short axis view from newborn infant with TGA showing anterior (*Ant*) rightward (*R*) position of the aorta (*Ao*). *L*, left; *LA*, left atrium; *Post*, posterior; *PV*, pulmonary valve.

RVET ratio is almost always ≥0.50, whether in the full-term infant[69] or in the premature infant with respiratory distress syndrome.[29] Furthermore, serial assessment of the right ventricular STI ratio is helpful in predicting the prognosis of these infants, since the ratio falls to normal over 24 to 48 hours in those infants in whom there is resolution of the pulmonary hypertension and cyanosis. However, there is little if any change in the right ventricular STI ratio of those who succumb.

The feature that distinguishes TGA from persistent fetal circulation is the lower left ventricular STI ratio (0.28) of the posterior great vessel in contrast to the elevated ratio (≥0.40) found in persistent fetal circulation. In addition, the right ventricular STI ratio of the aortic valve in TGA rarely exceeds 0.35 to 0.40 whereas the ratio of the pulmonic valve in persistent fetal circulation is usually 0.50 or greater. Furthermore, the pulmonary resistance can be assessed in patients with TGA using the left ventricular STI ratio in the same manner as with the right side.[27, 63]

Tricuspid Atresia and Pulmonary Atresia

Uncomplicated tricuspid atresia can readily be diagnosed by M-mode echo in the neonate. The characteristic echographic criteria are: absent tricuspid valve; a small anterior ventricular chamber with a large posterior ventricular chamber; and a large aortic root which generally does not override the septum. Absence of the tricuspid valve echo assumes

great significance since the normal valve is easily demonstrable in the normal newborn.

On 2-D echo, tricuspid atresia is suggested on the short axis view when only a single atrioventricular valve can be recorded which in the long axis is in fibrous continuity with the posterior margin of a great vessel, thus identifying it as the mitral valve. From the subcostal view, absence of the tricuspid valve is confirmed, and the size of the tricuspid ring and right ventricle can be estimated. The left ventricle may be large, and the right ventricle may be small or absent. The great vessel relationship may be determined in the short axis view. Furthermore, the relative severity of pulmonary stenosis can also be estimated.

In patients with pulmonary atresia or severe pulmonary stenosis with an intact ventricular septum, the right ventricle is usually hypoplastic but may be large. The tricuspid valve wave form is distorted and is of low amplitude. In the short axis view of the great vessels, the membrane of the pulmonary valve atresia frequently cannot be distinguished from the thick valve of severe pulmonary stenosis. With the addition of pulsed Doppler, it is possible to detect forward flow through the right ventricular outflow tract across the pulmonary valve in pulmonic stenosis but not pulmonary atresia (Fig. 4.23). In addition, it is also possible to assess the size of the right ventricle and the tricuspid ring, which would have bearing on the surgical intervention planned. From the subcostal views and suprasternal notch, it is likewise possible to assess the size of the right and left pulmonary arteries.

Total Anomalous Pulmonary Venous Connection

Total anomalous pulmonary venous return is one of the most difficult diagnoses to make using M-mode echocardiography. Often, it is confused with hypoplastic left heart syndrome because of the small left ventricular dimensions so commonly associated with the defect. With the advent of 2-D echocardiography, it is now possible to visualize the normal pulmonary veins as they drain into the left atrium. When they are absent or when there are common venous channels posterior to the left atrium, it is possible to record these findings with two-dimensional echo and Doppler and arrive at the diagnosis.[75, 80]

AORTIC OVERRIDE

Patients with tetralogy of Fallot (TOF), double outlet right ventricle (DORV), truncus arteriosus, pulmonary atre-

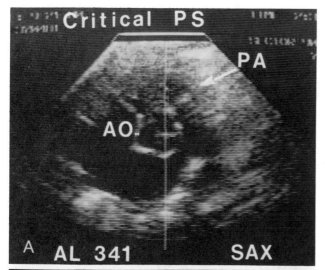

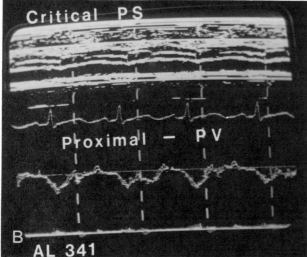

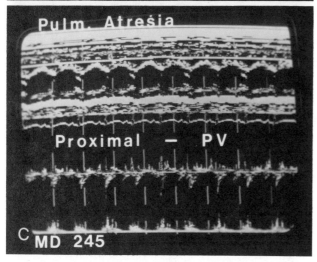

Fig. 4.23 Echograms of newborn with severe PS showing thick pulmonary valve (*A*) and forward flow by Doppler (*B*). In contrast (*C*) there is no forward flow across the pulmonary valve (*PV*) in newborn with atresia. *Ao*, aorta; *SAX*, short axis.

sia with ventricular septal defect, and an anteriorly positioned ventricular septal defect all have a common echocardiographic feature—an overriding aorta. Normally, the ven-

tricular septal echo and the anterior margin of the aortic root echo lie at the same depth from the chest wall since the membranous septum is in fibrous continuity with the anterior margin of the aorta (Fig. 4.8). Even in patients with isolated ventricular septal defect, the relationship is preserved (Fig. 4.24). Presumably, this is due to adequate development of the conal tissue of the right ventricle which serves to tether the anterior margin of the aorta in its proper position. However, in conditions with abnormal development of the conus tissue, migration of the anterior aorta occurs which permits the aorta to straddle or override the septum.

Aortic override is demonstrated on M-mode echo by rotating the transducer beam from the body of the left ventricle medially and superiorly along the mitral valve until the aortic root is recorded. If the VSD is large, septal echoes are lost and the anterior aortic margin is difficult to define. The severity of override can be estimated by measuring the aortic dimension in end-diastole (its posterior movement) and the distance from the anterior aortic margin in diastole to the left septal surfaces.[57] The ratio of the aortic to left septal surface distance to the aortic dimension represents the percentage of override of the aorta. This information may be useful to the surgeon when planning therapy since closure of the ventricular septal defect in these patients may cause varying degrees of obstruction to the left ventricular outflow tract.

False negative aortic override may occur on M-mode if the transducer is placed inferiorly along the sternum (Fig. 5.24C)[18, 58] As the transducer is rotated from the left ventricle to the anteriorly positioned aorta, an arc is inscribed. Since all radii of an arc are equal, the transducer beam does not recognize that the aorta is actually located anteriorly and fails to demonstrate aortic overriding of the septum. However, if the transducer is moved superiorly to the next interspace and another scan or sweep from the left ventricle to the aorta is made, the aortic override should be visible. Therefore, in patients who are cyanosed and/or are suspected of having one of the above diseases, this maneuver should prevent misinterpretation of false negative override.

This problem is significantly reduced and virtually absent with 2D echo. Despite transducer placement, the overriding aorta can be detected as well as the ventricular septal defect if it is large enough (usually greater than 4 to 5 mm in diameter) (Fig. 5.4.24D).

DISCONTINUITY

When aortic override is present, there is aortic-septal discontinuity. There may also be mitral-semilunar valve discontinuity. In double outlet right ventricle, this finding is produced by the subaortic conus (Fig. 4.25A) that is interposed between the mitral valve and posterior semilunar valve. Of all the M-mode echographic findings, discontinuity of the mitral and aortic valve seems to be the most difficult one to demonstrate consistently. The problem is compounded not only by technical factors,[18] but also by the fact that a subaortic conus may exist in other conditions as well.

In order to establish mitral-semilunar valve continuity, a continuous slow sweep of the mitral valve must be performed (Fig. 4.8A) that, initially, includes both the anterior and posterior leaflets and then anterior leaflet alone, which merges into the aortic cusp and posterior aortic margin. The aortic cusp echo should immediately follow the last recognizable anterior mitral leaflet echo since it is the anterior leaflet of the mitral valve that is in fibrous continuity with the bases of the posterior and left cusps of the aortic valve in the region of the membranous septum. In addition, it is

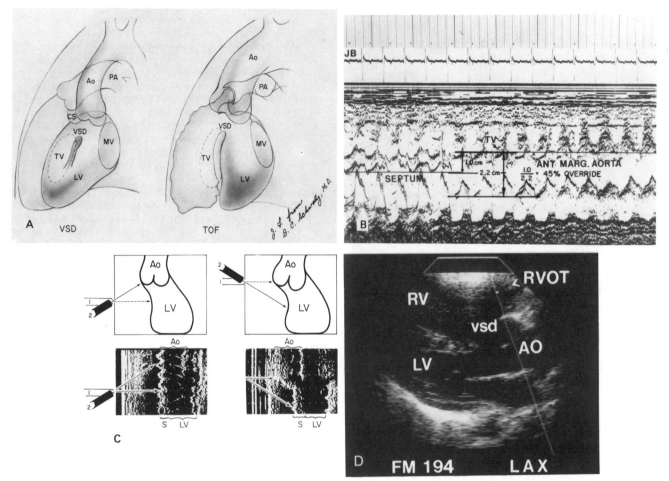

Fig. 4.24 (A) Idealized diagram in sagittal views of patient with ventricular septal defect (*VSD*) and tetralogy of Fallot (*TOF*) showing how absence of the cristasupraventricularis (*CS*) allows the aorta (*Ao*) to migrate anteriorly. The orientation of the pulmonary artery (*PA*) and relation of the mitral valve (*MV*) are shown (see text). *LV*, left ventricle; *TV*, tricuspid valve. (B) Echogram of patient with tetralogy of Fallot demonstrating aortic override and method of determining percent override. *ANT. MARG.*, anterior margin. (C) Idealized diagram and corresponding echoes show how false negative aortic overriding may occur and how to prevent it. *S*, septum (see text). (D) 2D echogram showing override and large VSD.

the depth of the end-diastolic position of the anterior leaflet of the mitral valve and posterior margin of the aorta that are compared. In our experience, we have not seen displacement in normal patients, although a normal displacement of several millimeters has been observed.[18]

If a patient has a subaortic conus, regardless of the type of defect, abrupt anterior displacement of the posterior margin of the aorta and mitral-aortic valve discontinuity (Fig. 4.25B) usually are demonstrated. However, if the aorta is severely dextroposed and farther from the mitral valve, it assumes a more retrosternal position, which means that the transducer must be angled more acutely in order to record it. Even though the posterior margin of the aorta is quite anterior, it is almost as far from the transducer as the mitral valve (Fig. 4.25C).[57] Therefore, the arc effect, which produced the false negative override of the aorta results in false negative nondisplacement of the posterior margin of the aorta. This may also occur if the transducer position is too inferior. However, if there is discontinuity of the mitral valve echo and the aortic cusp echo, and as the transducer beam is rotated from the mitral valve to the aorta, the anterior leaflet merges with the subaortic conus, not the aortic cusp (Fig. 4.25C). On rare occasions, the mitral and aortic leaflets may be in continuity which results from an unusually long anterior mitral leaflet that ascends through the ventricular

septal defect and joins the aortic valve. Under these circumstances, it would be difficult to distinguish double outlet right ventricle from tetralogy of Fallot.

The presence of a subaortic conus can be demonstrated more reliably with 2-D echo (Fig. 4.25D). Generally, the mitral valve echo appears attached to a thick immobile structure (the conus muscle) which has a semilunar valve sitting on top of it. The separation between the mitral valve and semilunar valves varies with age but is usually substantial. In addition, if the patient has double outlet right ventricle, then both great arteries should be seen arising anterior to the septum and may be recorded side by side (Fig. 4.25E).

VOLUME OVERLOAD

Right and left ventricular volume overload (Fig. 4.26) are easily detected using M-mode echo. Normal values for ventricular dimensions have been well established and can be used to assess ventricular dilatation. The conditions most commonly associated with right ventricular volume overload include secundum and primum atrial septal defects, atrioventricular canal, tricuspid, and pulmonary valve insufficiency, and partial or total anomalous pulmonary venous connection. Less common causes include left ventricular-right atrial shunts and systemic atriovenous fistula. Left

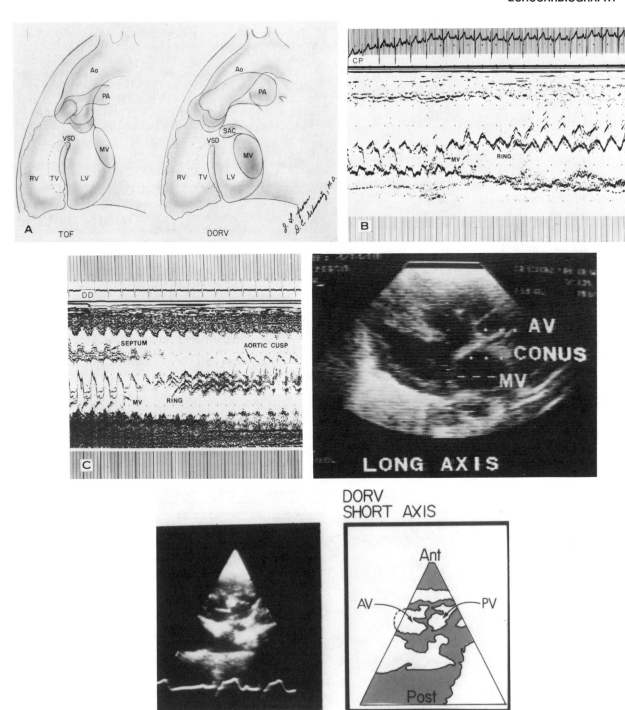

Fig. 4.25 (*A*) Idealized diagrams in sagittal view of patient with tetralogy of Fallot (*TOF*) and double outlet right ventricle (*DORV*) demonstrating the subaortic conus (*SAC*) and origin of both great vessels from the right ventricle in the patient with *DORV. Ao*, aorta; *PA*, pulmonary artery; *VSD*, ventricular septal defect; *MV*, mitral valve; *RV*, right ventricle; *LV*, left ventricle; *TV*, tricuspid valve. (*B*) Echogram of infant with double outlet right ventricle showing abrupt anterior displacement of posterior aortic margin. *MV*, mitral valve. (*C*) Echogram of patient with Taussig-Bing anomaly demonstrating nondisplacement of posterior aorta, but discontinuity of anterior mitral valve leaflet and aortic cusp. (*D*) 2D echo showing SAC and side by side position (*E*) of great vessels.

ventricular volume overload commonly is produced by aortic insufficiency, mitral insufficiency, patent ductus arteriosus, and ventricular septal defects, as well as heart failure. For the most part 2-D echocardiography does not add to the assessment of ventricular dilatation. Normal pediatric values have not yet been established; however, the important application in the future of 2-D echo may rest in the ability to

compare unusual ventricular configurations. For example, M-mode echocardiography may show a very small dimension of the left ventricle in conditions with right ventricular pressure overload and volume overload, and may suggest that the left ventricle is small, when in fact, the volume may be normal or large.

The detection of atrial volume overload by M-mode echo

has been limited primarily to the left atrium. This finding depends upon an increase in the anterior/posterior dimension of the left atrium. Evaluation of right atrial dilatation has not been as amenable to M-mode echo. However, with the advent of 2-D echo, a more accurate assessment of both may be forthcoming.

SEPTAL DEFECTS

The diagnosis of atrial or ventricular septal defects depends mainly upon indirect evidence interpreted in the clinical context of the patient. If a large right ventricle or large left ventricle and left atrium are recorded then, by deductive reasoning, the appropriate diagnosis can be made based on the associated clinical information. With 2-D echo it is possible to directly visualize an atrial septal defect or a ventricular septal defect. However, it is important to recognize that there are limitations of the technique and that attempts to diagnose an atrial septal defect from short axis or apical views of the heart rather than the subxiphoid view may be fraught with dangers since there may be significant atrial septal echo dropout (Fig. 4.16). Similarly, the ventricular septum may not be optimally examined from the apical regions but rather from the subxiphoid or long axis views of the heart (Fig. 4.24). As experience broadens, it most likely will be possible to assess the size of the defect.

ATRIOVENTRICULAR VALVES

It is possible, using M-mode echo, to detect abnormalities of the atrioventricular valves. For example, the cleft mitral valve in the ostium primum defect and atrioventricular canal is very characteristic and has been well described (Fig. 4.27). Using 2-D echo, the abnormal attachment of the cleft mitral valve in the endocardial cushion defects can be more clearly visualized and recorded (Fig. 4.28). On the short axis view of the ventricles in a patient with the complete type "C canal," a common atrioventricular valve that moves as a single valve during the cardiac cycle may be visualized stretching from the left ventricle through a large defect into the right ventricle[21, 76].

Ebstein's anomaly of the tricuspid valve can be diagnosed by recording delayed tricuspid valve closure from the M-mode echocardiogram.[64] Another helpful finding is that the tricuspid valve seems to be recorded over the entire precordium and is difficult to avoid. The displacement of the tricuspid valve, as well as its redundancy, are easily recorded on 2-D echo and, in fact, this is probably the laboratory procedure of choice in diagnosing this lesion.[67] In the apical view (Fig. 4.29A), the marked displacement of the tricuspid valve can be easily recognized, and in the short axis view (Fig. 4.29B), the obstructive nature of this large redundant valve is likewise appreciated as the valve sits in the right ventricular outflow tract. Furthermore, it is possible to accurately assess the state of the pulmonary valve, which may be stenotic in these patients.

Mitral valve prolapse is a common form of mitral valve dysfunction in children.[9] When we have suspected this clinically, we have been able to demonstrate either discrete (Fig. 4.30A) or pansystolic prolapse of the mitral valve in about 95% of our patients. Silent prolapse in our own population

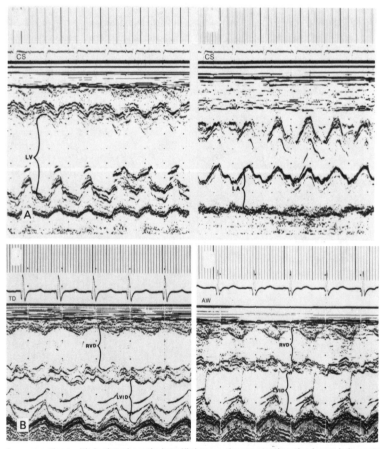

Fig. 4.26 (*A*) Echograms from a patient with isolated aortic insufficiency, demonstrating the large left ventricle (*LV*) and normal size left atrium (*LA*). (*B*) Echograms from two patients with atrial septal defect demonstrating enlarged right ventricular dimensions (*RVD*). (*Left*) Septal motion normal. (*Right*) Septal motion abnormal. *LVID*, left ventricular internal dimension.

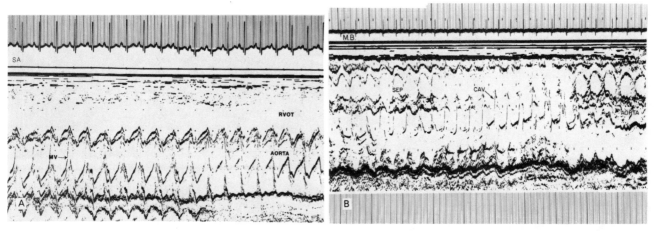

Fig. 4.27 Method for determining mitral valve prolapse. See text for discussion. *PEP*, preejection period. Echograms from a patient with ostium primum defect (*A*) and complete atrioventricular canal (*B*) showing mitral valve (*MV*) in left ventricular outflow tract in ostium primum but traversing the septal (*SEP*) echo plane in complete canal.

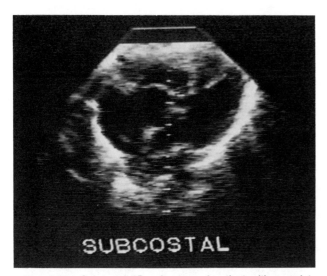

Fig. 4.28 Subcostal 2D echogram of patient with complete canal showing absence of atrial septum and part of ventricular canal with attachment of leaflets to the rim of the ventricular septum.

has occurred only twice, and those patients did not undergo cardiac catheterization. A consensus of what constitutes pathologic prolapse is lacking echographically just as it is angiographically. Therefore, in order not to overdiagnose this disease, we define prolapse as any movement of the mitral valve leaflets posterior to an imaginary line drawn parallel to the chest wall from the closure point (C point) of the mitral leaflets (Fig. 4.30*B*). The movement should occur after the onset of ventricular ejection, which can be determined from the aortic valve echo (Q to aortic cusp opening). There may be some posterior movement normally during isovolumic contraction. The prolapse may occur anytime during ventricular systole, but usually does not normalize until ventricular diastole. Using this criterion, our clinical, echographic, and angiographic correlation has been about 95%.[9] Two-dimensional echo has not increased our detection rate of mitral valve prolapse.

PATENT DUCTUS ARTERIOSUS

M-mode echocardiography has been extremely useful in assessing the effects of left to right shunting through a patent ductus arteriosus (PDA) in the premature infant, even in the

presence of severe lung disease. The left ventricle and left atrium become enlarged, and following closure of the ductus the values returned to normal.

Frequently, an echo will appear in the left atrial cavity which we think originates from the left atrial promontory and may be mistaken for the left atrial wall. A scan from the left ventricle to the left atrium should be made to identify the left atrial wall, which generally resides posterior to the left ventricular wall and is in continuity with it. This should help to prevent erroneous measurement of the left atrium.

It is possible to image and measure the PDA by 2-D echo.[79] Evidence of continuous pulmonary artery turbulence flow by pulsed Doppler[73] confirms the presence of a PDA and is helpful in some patients (Fig. 4.31). It is still not possible to quantitate the amount of shunting through the PDA, but with the advent of pulsed Doppler, it is possible to either exclude or confirm an associated ventricular septal defect (Fig. 4.32). The real value of echocardiography in the infant with a PDA is the ability to serially evaluate chamber sizes and left ventricular function. The majority of infants with a large PDA not in overt heart failure have shortening fractions greater than most normal infants (normal shortening fraction of premature infants = 33.5 ± 3.5%).[5] Following surgical or spontaneous closure of the PDA, these values return to normal. On the other hand, infants with a large PDA whose cardiac function is impaired have shortening fractions which are normal or below normal. Currently in our institution, the infant with a large PDA who has a decreased shortening fraction and enlarged chambers and who fails to respond to diuretics, digitalis, and fluid restriction undergoes surgical ligation of the duct.

VENTRICULAR OUTFLOW OBSTRUCTION

The M-mode echographic findings of valvar aortic stenosis have depended upon multiple diastolic echoes of the aortic valve, increased thickness of the septum and free wall of the left ventricle, and an eccentric diastolic closure of the aortic valve during systole. Eccentricity of the diastolic cusp echoes of the aortic valve was initially felt to be diagnostic of bicuspid aortic valve, whereas patients with tricuspid aortic valves had midluminal diastolic position of the cusp echoes. Although this finding was initially useful, it has not proven to be specific for bicuspid aortic valve since up to 17% of patients with severe tricuspid aortic stenosis will exhibit marked eccentricity. In addition, beam position will dramatically alter diastolic closure position.

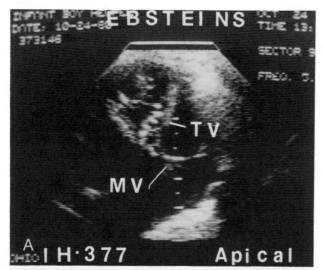

Two-dimensional evaluation from the precordial long axis view of the ascending aorta and left ventricular outflow tract has provided a means by which accurate localization of the level of obstruction in the subvalvar, valvar, or supravalvar regions can be made. In subvalvar obstructions, asymmetric hypertrophy as well as concentric left ventricular hypertrophy may be determined (premature closure of the aortic cusp and abnormal systolic anterior motion of the mitral valve can be better appreciated on M-mode). Discrete subvalvar membranes can usually be differentiated from subvalvar muscular obstruction. The degree of valve cusp separation of the domed aortic valve has permitted semiquantitation of the gradient.[97] Further narrowing of the aorta above the cusp may be recorded as an hourglass configuration, diffuse hypoplasia or a membranous diaphragm.[98, 99] Discrete coarctation or diffuse long segment narrowing of the thoracic aorta can be detected from the suprasternal notch view (Fig. 4.20).

Evaluation of pulmonary valvar stenosis has been difficult using M-mode echo; however, directing the 2-D echo beam in the long axis of the pulmonary artery facilitates detection of valvar pulmonic stenosis.[96] Normally, the pulmonary leaflet echoes move rapidly apart during systole. When fully open they lay parallel and in close apposition to the margins of the pulmonary artery, thus making the complete recording of the pulmonary valve leaflets difficult. However, in valvar pulmonic stenosis, doming and restriction of the motion of the pulmonary valve cusps permits better visualization of the leaflets (Fig. 4.29B). In addition, muscular obstruction of the right ventricular outflow tract may be visualized from the subxiphoid approach.

OTHER CONDITIONS

SINGLE VENTRICLE

In a single ventricle, the most important M-mode echocardiographic finding is the absence of the ventricular septal echo. In the majority of our patients, two atrioventricular (A V) valves were demonstrated, usually at different depths, without an intervening ventricular septal echo. On occasion, only a single AV valve is present. Another sign that helps distinguish the single ventricle from other lesions that have

Fig. 4.29 2D echograms from patient with Ebstein's anomaly showing (A) marked displacement of the tricuspid valve (TV) and (B) stenosis of the pulmonary valve (PV). Ao, aorta; MV, mitral valve; SAX, short axis.

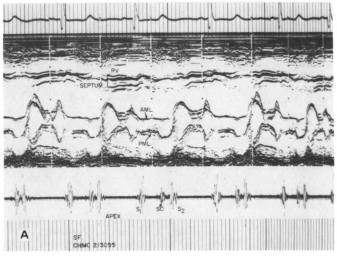

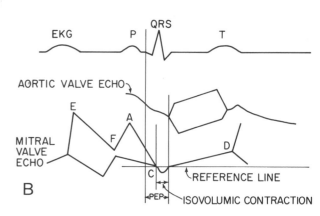

Fig. 4.30 Echograms showing prolapse of mitral leaflets. (A and B) Simultaneous echogram and phonocardiogram in patient with mitral valve prolapse showing discrete posterior mitral leaflet (PML) prolapse coincident with late systolic click (SC).

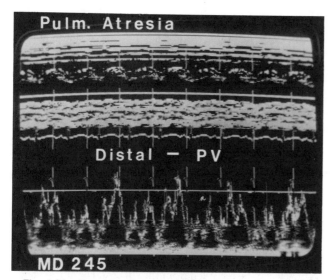

Fig. 4.31 Doppler echogram of patient with pulmonary valve (*PV*) atresia showing continuous flow from ductus arteriosus.

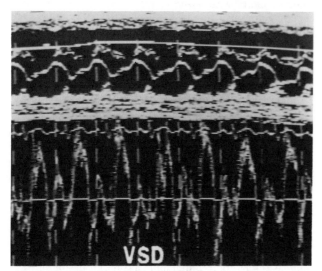

Fig. 4.32 Doppler echogram from long axis view in a patient with a *VSD* showing left to right shunt toward the transducer in systole.

a common mixing chamber is that it is difficult to record simultaneously the anterior and posterior margins of the posterior root structure arising from the ventricle. The transducer must be moved in order to record the anterior margin of the root structure. This is in contrast to either aortic atresia or tricuspid atresia. If the infundibular chamber is dilated, an echo that looks a septum may appear, but both AV valve echoes should be posterior to the "septal" echo if it is a true single ventricle.

Cross-sectional echocardiography has enhanced the ability to diagnosis a single ventricle when there is double-inlet single ventricle. Both atrioventricular valves may be recorded from the short axis parasternal view (Fig. 4.33) and the subcostal view without an intervening interventricular septal echo. These findings are highly specific and very dramatic in real-time. Very often, the interatrial septum is intact. In addition it is very easy to determine whether there is transposition of the great arteries or inversion of the infundibulum as well as to determine the status of the interatrial septum.

VENTRICULAR INVERSION

The M-mode diagnosis of this defect remains one of exclusion. The echo criteria are dependent upon recognition that there is transposition of the great arteries (TGA) and that there is discontinuity between the left atrioventricular (AV) and semilunar valves. Generally, the echographic study is very confusing, and the relationships of the cardiac structures are difficult to establish. The AV valves may be recorded with one traversing what looks like a ventricular septal echo. A first impression during the M-mode examination is that the patient has a single ventricle because the plane of the septum is often perpendicular to the sternum and parallel to the transducer beam, and the septum generally is not recorded. Analysis of the systolic time intervals of the semilunar valves suggests TGA and that the anterior systemic vessel is in the levo position. This in conjunction with the discontinuity of the left AV valve and semilunar valve should suggest the diagnosis of ventricular inversion with corrected transposition of the great arteries. Clearly, 2-D evaluation provides a much easier assessment of both the TGA and a morphologic right ventricle on the left side. Normal atrial situs can be determined by visualizing the inferior vena cava draining into the right side of the atrium (Fig. 4.15) and pulmonary veins draining into the left atrium.

CARDIAC MALPOSITION AND COMPLEX DEFECTS

Cardiac anomalies associated with cardiac malposition, polysplenia, and asplenia syndrome invariably are quite complex. However, it is possible to arrive at an accurate anatomic diagnosis with the use of echocardiography when the atrial situs is known. Atrial situs can be determined noninvasively by plain chest radiograph or barium swallow. A systematic echographic examination will generally provide the relative position of the ventricles, the relationship of the great vessels, and the presence or absence of the interventricular septum. Only a brief discussion of the method will be possible here; however, detailed descriptions of the M-

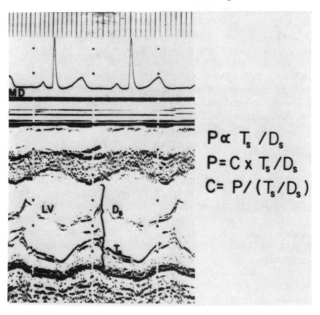

$$P \propto T_s / D_s$$
$$P = C \times T_s / D_s$$
$$C = P / (T_s / D_s)$$

Fig. 4.33 Echogram of child with aortic stenosis showing method used to measure relative wall thickness and the formula used to estimate left ventricular (*LV*) peak systolic pressure (*P*). D_s, LV dimension in systole; *C*, wall stress constant of 225; T_s, LV free wall thickness in systole.

mode technique and deductive approach to the diagnosis of these defects have been published.[59, 87]

It is helpful for two people to be present during the examination of such a patient—one performing the study and one writing down the positions of the transducer beam used to record the echoes. This is true for both M-mode and 2-D techniques. In this fashion, the relative position of various structures can be stated in left-right, superior-inferior, and anterior-posterior terms. For example, in a patient with isolated dextrocardia, the mitral valve, which is in continuity with the posterior semilunar root, may be recorded to the right of the tricuspid valve, indicating that the morphologic left ventricle is to the right. Furthermore, if the anterior great artery is the systemic artery (determined by systolic time intervals) and is to the left of the posterior great artery, then by deduction, this patient has atrioventricular discordancy and TGA. On the other hand, if a patient with isolated dextrocardia has the mitral valve echo recorded to the left, indicating that the left ventricle is to the left, and the anterior great artery echo is not systemic and is found to the right, the diagnosis of atrioventricular concordance with normally related great arteries can be made.

Thus, with echocardiography and the knowledge of atrial situs derived from a plain chest film, it is possible to define accurately important anatomic relationships in a high percentage of patients with complex cardiac defects. Clearly, 2-D echo has enhanced this capability. When catheterization is necessary, prior knowledge of pertinent anatomic relations provided by the echograms should aid in planning the study.

VENTRICULAR PERFORMANCE

Echocardiography has been used extensively to define anatomic relationships in many of the congenital cardiac defects. However, it has also emerged as an important method for assessing cardiac function in children.[34, 39, 42, 62, 81] Also, its noninvasive nature allows for serial evaluation as frequently as desired in patients who serve as their own controls. Although there are limitations to the technique, in general echo has been underutilized, and we have found serial evaluation of the shortening fraction (by M-mode), of the ejection fraction (by 2-D), and of the systolic time intervals, including isovolumic contraction time (ICT), extremely valuable in the day to day management of children. Two-dimensional echo offers greater promise for estimating volumes of chambers.

VENTRICULAR VOLUMES

Estimation of left ventricular volumes and ejection fractions using a single dimension determined by M-mode echocardiography is based upon two assumptions: the left ventricle approximates the configuration of a prolate ellipse and the left ventricle contracts symmetrically along the major axis with little shortening in the major dimension. In general, as long as the left ventricle retains its configuration, then linear regression equations can be used to reasonably estimate the ventricular volumes; however, the linear regression equations used to estimate volumes in adults[14, 43] are not satisfactory for children with smaller hearts. Conversely, the linear regression equation used to calculate the volumes in children with small hearts[32] is not satisfactory for adults. This is due in part to the fact that the major axis of the ventricle in children is not twice the minor axis but only 1½ times the minor axis and to the fact that the percent shortening of the major axis approximates 6 to 10% rather than the 20% in adults. It appears that there is a curvilinear relation-

ship between the smaller hearts of children and the larger hearts of adults. Therefore, the cubic regression equation LVD = 19.1 ± 14.6 Be + 0.62 Be (where Be is the lateral minor dimension and LVD represents left ventricular volume) was developed. This relationship provides a reasonable estimation of volumes for hearts with a minor axis dimension of 2 to 8 cm for diastole and systole. However, if the left ventricle assumes a configuration other than the prolate ellipse, then these equations and formulas are not appropriate, and there will be greater disparity between the volumes calculated by angiographic techniques and those obtained by ecocardiography. In addition, there are many potential pitfalls[6a] in using a single dimension to estimate left ventricular volumes.

The predictive accuracy of left ventricular volumes obtained by 2-D has proved encouraging.[15, 71] Part of the reason is that with 2-D echo it is now possible to obtain dimensions and planed areas from several sites along the major axis of the left ventricle. In addition, the major axis of the left ventricle can be recorded from the subcostal or apical views. From these values, five reconstruction models or algorithms have been used to estimate end-diastolic and end-systolic volumes along with ejection fractions. These algorithms include Simpson's rule, a hemisphere-cylinder, single and biplane ellipses, and area-length method. Thus far, most investigations comparing 2-D volume calculations with angiographic determinations have demonstrated Simpson's rule to be the best algorithm.

SHORTENING FRACTION

The shortening fraction of the left ventricle is one measure of its contractility and represents the ratio of the difference of the end-diastolic dimension (LVED) and end-systolic dimension (LVES) to the end-diastolic dimension expressed as $SF = \dfrac{LVED-LVES}{LVED} \times 100$. The measurement is made from the endocardial left septal surface to the endocardial surface of the posterior free wall. To minimize error and maximize reproducibility from one day to the next and from patient to patient, as well as on the same patient, a consistent recording technique must be used. Generally, a true and reliable echographic minor dimension can be obtained by scanning the left ventricle to the left atrium once a clear mitral valve echo is recorded from a perpendicular position on the chest. In addition, the dimension just inferior to the atrioventricular sulcus should be measured at the Q-wave and no later than at the R-wave of the electrocardiogram to ensure measurement prior to the isovolumic contraction period.[51] Furthermore, left ventricular filling is enhanced during expiration and decreased during inspiration; thus, we make measurement during expiration. In our laboratory the normal shortening fraction varies between 28 and 38%.

We have found the shortening fraction to be the most reliable index of left ventricular function. Single values of shortening fraction, however, are of limited use in assessing ventricular performance whereas serial evaluation provides a more reliable indication of relative change in myocardial performance. Depending upon the physiologic state, the shortening fraction will be increased or decreased. For example, in the compensated left ventricular volume overload situation (i.e., PDA,[5] VSD, MI,[54, 82] and AI), the shortening fraction is uniformly increased. In similar fashion, the shortening fraction in children is also elevated in compensated pressure overload situations such as moderate to severe aortic stenosis[39, 55] and obstructive idiopathic hypertrophic subaortic stenosis. In contrast, the shortening fraction is decreased in the poorly compensated left ventricle, regardless of etiology (i.e., pressure or volume overload, idiopathic or rheumatic congestive cardiomyopathy,[82] or adriamycin cardiotoxicity[7]). From evaluation of our data, we believe that a greater than 5% increase or decrease in the shortening fraction cannot be accounted for by differences in recording technique or by physiologic variations and probably represents a significant change in hemodynamic consequences or myocardial performance.

PEAK SYSTOLIC PRESSURE

M-mode echocardiography is useful in the estimation of left ventricular peak systolic pressure (LVPSP) in children.[3, 25, 40] Valvar aortic stenosis is characterized by concentric left ventricular hypertrophy, and the magnitude of this hypertrophy is dependent on the wall stress. The left ventricular wall thickness increases, while the left ventricular cavity size remains relatively constant, until the systolic wall stress normalizes. This relationship in a patient with normal left ventricular function can be expressed as:

$$\text{Wall stress} = \frac{\text{pressure} \times \text{cavity diameter}}{\text{wall thickness}}$$

When these measurements are obtained in children without evidence of left ventricular hypertrophy at end-systole from left ventricular echograms, the wall stress constant approximates 225. Thus:

$$\text{LVPSP} = \frac{225 \times \text{left ventricular end-systolic wall thickness}}{\text{left ventricular end-systolic cavity diameter}}$$

The LVPSP thus derived in children with aortic stenosis correlates with the LVPSP determined at cardiac catheterization (Fig. 4.33), and mild aortic insufficiency has a minimal effect on this technique. Hence, aortic valve gradients can be monitored over time at the bedside using M-mode echo and a blood pressure cuff. However, the LVPSP cannot be estimated accurately following aortic valve repair.[24]

These measurements are usually made at end-systole based on the assumption that peak stress occurs then, but Aziz et al.[3] contend that the peak stress may occur early in systole. Therefore, end-diastolic values of wall thickness and cavity diameter may also be appropriate to estimate LVPSP. The ratio

$$\frac{\bar{h} \text{ (mean of the septal and posterior wall thickness)}}{r \text{ (minor semiaxis)}}$$

also compares favorably with the LVPSP obtained during catheterization. Since these measurements at end-diastole are generally more easily and accurately made, this may be a more reliable method of estimating LVPSP.

MEAN VELOCITY OF CIRCUMFERENTIAL FIBER SHORTENING

The mean velocity of circumferential fiber shortening (mean VCF) is another parameter of left ventricular function which can be determined by M-mode echocardiography.[17, 81] It is the percentage of internal shortening of the left ventricle during systole in the minor axis per unit time and is expressed by the formula in circumferences.

$$\text{VCF} = \frac{\pi \text{ (end diastolic dimension-end systolic dimension)}}{\pi \text{ (end diastolic dimension)} \times \text{ejection time}}$$

We use left ventricular ejection time measured directly from the aortic cusp opening and closure (pulmonic in transposition). In children with heart rates of 100 beats/minute or greater, there is less than 5 milliseconds variation in left ventricular ejection time from beat to beat. Some authors

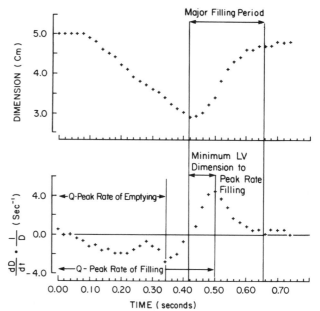

Fig. 4.34 Digitized output from M-mode echo of normal left ventricular chamber showing the various indices measured (see text).

use left ventricular wall motion or mitral valve closure to mitral valve opening to determine ejection time.

DIGITIZING

Practically speaking, the assessment of left ventricular function by M-mode echocardiography has depended upon the shortening fraction of the left ventricle and mean VCF. The application of computer-assisted analysis of the left ventricular M-mode echogram has allowed the continuous measurement of changes in the left ventricular chamber as well as septal and free wall thickness and the computation of their instantaneous rates of change throughout the cardiac cycle.[86, 93] In adults, these assessments of peak rates of change have been more sensitive as indices of early dynamic disturbance of left ventricular function than the mean or fractional change of the minor axis dimension.[86, 87]

Echograms for digitized computer analysis are recorded in the same manner as described in the section on shortening fraction to ensure optimal echoes from the left ventricular septal endocardium, posterior wall endocardium, and epicardium. The tracings should be recorded at a paper speed of at least 100 mm/second and in expanded depth so that 1 cm of tissue equals 15 to 20 mm. These precautions will minimize errors in techniques. Data points plotted from this echogram are entered into the computer, and a computer trace of this echogram is generated (Fig. 4.34).

From this computer trace, instantaneous measurements of the left ventricular dimension septal wall and free wall and their rates of change may be determined both during systole and diastole. Generally included in the left ventricular dynamic measurements during systole are: the percentage change of the left ventricular cavity dimension in systole, which is the same as the shortening fraction; the normalized peak rate of change of the cavity dimension in systole (VCF), which is the peak rate of change of the cavity dimension divided by the instantaneous or maximum cavity dimension expressed as:

$$\frac{dD}{dt} \times \frac{1}{D}$$

wherein D equals dimension and t is time in seconds; and the time interval from the onset of the QRS to the time of the minimal cavity dimension, wherein dD/dt = 0. Among the diastolic phase measurements are: the peak rate of relaxation of the cavity dimension, expressed as the peak dD/dt; the time interval from the onset of the QRS to the peak rate of increase in cavity dimension; and the duration of the rapid filling phase, which is the time interval from the minimum cavity dimension, or dD/dt = 0, to the time of sudden decrease in the rate of filling of the chamber.

These measurements are based on the assumption that the left ventricular cavity has a circular cross-section which always changes dimensions concentrically. Furthermore, it must be emphasized that the behavior of a single left ventricular dimension studied by echocardiography is not necessarily representative of the left ventricle as a whole. The full benefit of this technique in children has not been fully realized since only a limited number of studies have been performed[20, 37-39, 91] in children, but it shows promise.

SYSTOLIC TIME INTERVALS

The systolic time interval(s) (STI) of a ventricle include the preejection period (PEP) and the ventricular ejection time (VET) as well as the isovolumic contraction time (ICT). They are easily derived from echograms recorded directly from the aortic and pulmonary valve and tricuspid and mitral valves. The intervals by echo correlate well with those obtained from other direct measurements. Usually, aortic valve echograms are recorded in all pediatric patients. The pulmonary valve echograms are recorded in nearly all infants and the majority of children or young adults. If the pulmonary valve cannot be recorded in a newborn infant, the diagnosis of pulmonary valve disease is strongly considered. The mitral valve when normal is recorded virtually 100% of the time. The tricuspid may be seen but not recorded in its entirety all the time.

The derivation of STI from echograms requires high quality tracings with accurate recording of the opening and closing of the valve cusps, and an electrocardiogram where a sharp Q or S wave is easily observed (Fig. 4.35). Paper speeds of at least 75 mm/second and preferably 100 mm/second should be used to reduce timing errors. With heart rates of 100 beats/minute or greater, these errors are usually less than 5 milliseconds. Simultaneous recording of respirations using impedance plethysmography will not only serve to standardize the effects of respiratory changes but will also permit evaluation of the effects of respiratory changes on the STI. While the timing of valve cusp opening and closure are facilitated by the simultaneous recording of more than one valve cusp, frequently only a single valve cusp is recorded. In this event, the onset of ejection is the point of rapid posterior cusp movement where the thick closed valve cusp recording changes to a thin open valve cusp recording. The end of ejection occurs at the junction of the fine and thick valve cusp recording. The effect of heart rate upon PEP and VET can be minimized by deriving the ratio of PEP to VET. In addition, small changes in either measurement will produce large changes in the ratio. Hence, we have utilized this ratio in assessing various hemodynamic states. The normal mean RPEP to RVET ratio in our laboratory is 0.24 (range 0.16 to 0.30), and the mean LPEP to LVET is 0.35 (range 0.30 to 0.39).[34] Gutgesell et al.[27] found similar values.

Four factors influence the duration of PEP and VET: preload-determined by the end-diastolic volume and filling pressure of the ventricle; contractile state of the myocardium; afterload reflected by the arterial diastolic pressure; and sequence and rate of ventricular conduction. A distinct pattern of alteration of the STI evolves as the ventricular performance (i.e., contractility) diminishes: the PEP lengthens and VET shortens, producing an elevation of the STI ratio.

Changes in afterload can cause either an increase or a decrease in STI ratio. If afterload is reduced (i.e., aortic stenosis, pulmonic stenosis, aortic runoff), the PEP is shortened, and the VET is prolonged, causing a reduction in the ratio, assuming that the contractility of the ventricle is normal. If decreased cardiac performance develops as a result of chronic ventricular outflow obstruction, a gradual

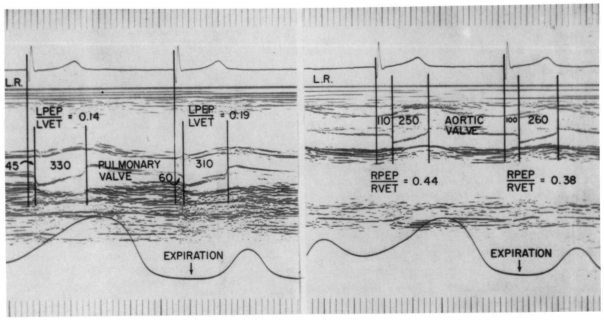

Fig. 4.35 Echogram of left and right systolic time intervals in patient with d-transposition (*dt*) of the great vessels. *LPEP*, left ventricular preejection period; *LVET*, left ventricular ejection time; *RPEP*, right ventricular preejection period; *RVET*, right ventricular ejection time.

increase in the PEP and decrease in VET will first result in normalization and ultimate elevation of the PEP/VET ratio (hence, the importance of serial assessment)!

When afterload is elevated as in pulmonary or systemic hypertension, the PEP lengthens, and the VET shortens, resulting in an increased ratio. The application of the RPEP-RVET ratio (LPEP-LVET when great arteries are transposed) has become very useful in assessing the pulmonary artery end-diastolic pressure (PAEDP) in children with large left to right shunts in whom surgery must be undertaken prior to the development of irreversible pulmonary vascular disease. Hirschfeld et al.[34] originally demonstrated and Riggs et al.[68] subsequently confirmed good correlation between the right ventricular STI and PAEDP measured at cardiac catheterization and that 95% of patients with a ratio of 0.30 or less had PAEDP less than 30 mm Hg. Silverman et al.[85] found a weaker relationship with the RPEP to RVET ratio and pressures measured in patients with large defects. However, if the patients have echoes performed in the same state as their cardiac catheterization, then the correlation between echo and pressure data is stronger. Thus, sedation of patients may be warranted when this information is vital.

It has been recommended that these children undergo repeat cardiac catheterization at intervals of 6 months to 1 year to assess pulmonary vascular resistance. We feel that these patients can be followed confidently with frequent (every 3 to 6 months) measurements of RPEP to RVET ratio. If and when the ratio begins to increase, then documentation by elective cardiac catheterization should be considered. Furthermore, the vasoreactive state of the pulmonary vascular bed may be assessed with oxygen administration. If the pulmonary hypertension is reversible, than 100% oxygen administration by mask will reduce the RPEP to RVET ratio (Fig. 4.36). If the pulmonary vascular bed is unresponsive to O_2, the RPEP to RVET ratio will remain unchanged.

Abnormalities of the ventricular conduction system can also alter the PEP to VET ratio greatly. For example, left bundle branch block selectively prolongs PEP of the left ventricle, thus elevating the LPEP to LVET ratio without affecting the RPEP to RVET ratio. Similarly, complete right bundle branch block selectively prolongs PEP of the right ventricle, thus elevating the right-sided ratio without affecting the left-sided ratio (unless there is coexisting LV disease). Thus, in the face of bundle branch block, the STI ratio alone cannot be used to assess ventricular function; but must be used in conjunction with the isovolumic contraction time.

ISOVOLUMIC CONTRACTION TIME

The isovolumic contraction time (ICT) of each ventricle represents the mechanical component of the preejection period. It is derived by measuring the interval between the atrioventricular valve closure and the semilunar valve opening of the great artery arising from the ventricle (Fig. 4.37). The LICT is the period of time from coaptation of the mitral valve to the point of initial opening of the aortic valve cusps determined echographically. Measurements derived from the isovolumic contraction phase of left ventricular systole are sensitive to changes in the inotropic state of the myocardium. Thus, LICT has potential physiologic importance as an expression of the level of myocardial contractility. In addition, it has been found to reflect the effects of preload and afterload.

Heart rate and age may influence the LICT; however, it appears from our data that the heart rate is the dominant factor. The regression equation for calculating the normal LICT (milliseconds) is: LICT = 54 − 0.23 (heart rate) with a SE of ±10.5. In patients with LV myocardial dysfunction (e.g., congestive cardiomyopathy, aberrant left coronary artery, or adriamycin cardiotoxicity), the mean LICT is prolonged.[35] As clinical improvement occurs, the LICT returns to a more normal value.

In the presence of decreased afterload (i.e., AI or PDA),[88]

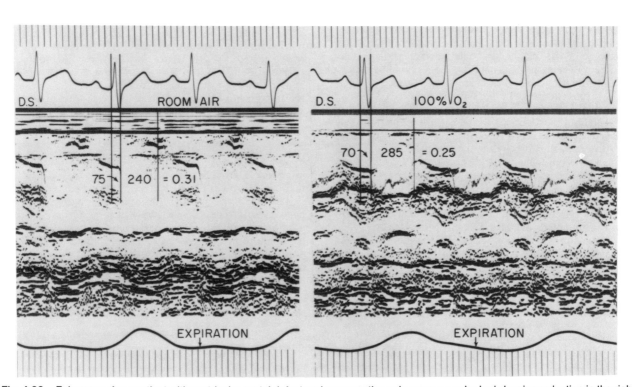

Fig. 4.36 Echograms from patient with ventricular septal defect and vasoreactive pulmonary vascular bed showing reduction in the right preejection period to right ventricular ejection time ratio following 100% oxygen administration.

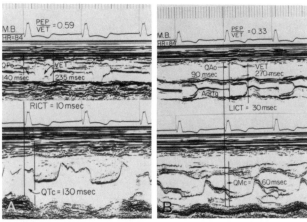

Fig. 4.37 (*A*) Echograms from normal patient showing derivation of isovolumic contraction time of the left ventricle (*LICT*) (see text). (*B*) Echograms from patient with closure of VSD and complete right bundle branch block showing application of the right isovolumic contraction time (*RICT*) to evaluate pulmonary vascular resistance (see text). PEP, preejection period; *QPo*, interval between Q wave of ECT and pulmonary valve opening; *QTc*, interval between Q wave and tricuspid valve closure; *VET*, ventricular ejection time.

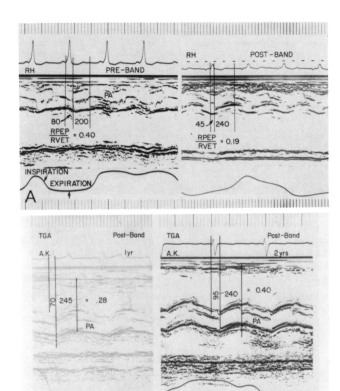

Fig. 4.38 These echograms show the reduction of the right preejection period (*RPEP*) to ventricular ejection time (*RVET*) ratios in a child. (*A*) postpulmonary artery (*PA*) banding for a large VSD and (*B*) in a child with TGA and *VSD*. (*Left*) 1 year following adequate banding. (*Right*) 2 years after banding with catheter proven pulmonary hypertension.

the LICT is shorter than normal. It is postulated that the decreased LICT in patients with PDA is related to increased systemic runoff and therefore decreased peripheral vascular resistance which allows an earlier opening of the aortic valve. Upon ligation of the PDA, the LICT returns to normal, reflecting the normalization of afterload.

In a similar manner, the RICT can be determined by measuring the interval between tricuspid closure and pulmonic opening. Studies showed that the RPEP to RVET ratio is a reliable and satisfactory method of estimating pulmonary vascular resistance. However, in patients with complete right bundle branch block (CRBBB), the RPEP is markedly prolonged, resulting in a spuriously elevated RPEP to RVET ratio, even in the face of normal pulmonary vascular resistance. Since the ICT reflects the mechanical component of the PEP and is relatively uninfluenced by conduction delays, the RICT has shown its greatest usefulness in estimating pulmonary vascular resistance in those postoperative children who are left with CRBBB following surgery for congenital heart disease.[41] It is also of value in patients without CRBBB, in whom closure of the pulmonic valve is difficult to record echocardiographically (i.e., respiratory disease), thus precluding the use of RPEP to RVET ratio to assess pulmonary vascular resistance. Also, it is not necessary to record simultaneous pulmonary and tricuspid valve echoes, as long as the R-R intervals are within 20 milliseconds for each echo.

The RICT in normal children ranges from 1 to 20 milliseconds with a mean of 10.6 ± 5.2 milliseconds.[41] Changes in heart rate and age do not alter RICT significantly. As anticipated, the RICT is correlated with right ventricular afterload, as defined by pulmonary artery end-diastolic pressure (PAEDP), and it is possible to utilize RICT to separate

patients with normal from those with elevated PAEDP. Furthermore, in patients with CRBBB, the RICT remains normal in the presence of normal PAEDP and is prolonged with elevated PAEDP. Hence, serial echocardiographic evaluation of the RICT can give an assessment of RV afterload in many children with congenital heart disease, regardless of the presence or absence of CRBBB.

POSTOPERATIVE ASSESSMENT

The regression or progression of postoperative pulmonary hypertension may be evaluated using serial systolic time intervals. If a pulmonary artery band is successful, a dramatic reduction in the RPEP-RVET ratio will occur immediately (Fig. 4.38*A*). On the other hand, progressive pulmonary hypertension may continue despite adequate pulmonary artery banding (Fig. 4.38*B*). Also, it may develop in a patient who has undergone a Mustard operation for transposition of the great arteries. Furthermore, the late development of obstructive pulmonary vascular disease may be recognized following closure of a ventricular septal defect.

REFERENCES

1. Allen, H. D., Sahn, D. J., Lange, L., and Goldberg, S. J.: Noninvasive assessment of surgical systemic to pulmonary artery, shunts by range gated pulsed Doppler echocardiography. J. Pediatr. 94:395, 1979.
2. Allen, H. D., Sahn, D. J., and Goldberg, S. J.: New serial contrast technique for assessment

of left to right shunting patent ductus arteriosus in the neonate. Am. J. Cardiol. 41:288, 1978.
3. Aziz, K. U., von Grondelle, A., Paul, M. H., and Muster, A. J.: Echocardiographic assessments of the relation between left ventricular wall and cavity dimensions and peak systolic

pressures in children with aortic stenosis. Am. J. Cardiol. 40:775, 1977.
4. Baker, D. W.: The present role of Doppler techniques in cardiac diagnosis. Prog. Cardiovasc. Dis. 21:79, 1978.
5. Baylen, B., Meyer, R. A., Korfhagen, J., Benzing, G. III, Bubb, M. E., and Kaplan, S.: Left

ventricular performance in the critically ill premature infant with patent ductus arteriosus and pulmonary disease. Circulation 55:182, 1977.

6. Bernstine, R. L.: Safety studies with ultrasonic Doppler technique. Obstet. Gynecol. 34:704–709, 1969.

6a. Bhatt, D. R., Isabel-Jones, J. B., Villoria, G. J., Nakazawa, M., Yabek, S., Marks, R. A., and Jarmakani, J. M.: Accuracy of echocardiography in assessing left ventricular dimension and volume. Circulation 57:699, 1978.

7. Biancaniello, T. M., Meyer, R. A., Wong, K. Y., Sager, C., and Kaplan, S.: Doxorubicin cardiotoxicity in children. J. Pediatr. 97:45, 1980.

8. Bierman, F. Z., and Williams, R. G.: Subxiphoid two-dimensional imaging of the atrial septum. Am. J. Cardiol. 41:354, 1978.

9. Bisset, G. S., III, Schwartz, D. C., Meyer, R. A., James F. W., and Kaplan, S.: Clinical spectrum and long term follow-up of isolated mitral valve prolapse in 119 children. Circulation 62:423, 1980.

10. Bommer, W., Miller, L., Keown, M., Mason, D. T., and DeMaria, A. N.: Real-time fast Fourier analysis of Doppler spectral information and two-dimensional echocardiography yield a noninvasive estimate of cardiac output. Circulation 62:III–199, 1980.

11. Carson, P. L., Fischella, P. R., and Oughton, T. V.: Ultrasonic power and intensities produced by diagnostic ultrasound equipment. Ultrasound Med. Biol. 3:341–350, 1978.

12. Coakley, W. T., Slade, J. S., Braeman, J. M., and Moore, J. L.: Examination of lymphocytes for chromosomal aberrations after ultrasonic irradiation. Br. J. Radiol. 45:328–332, 1972.

13. Dillon, T., Meyer, R. A., Korfhagen, J. C., Chung, K., and Kaplan, S.: Management of infective endocarditis. J. Pediatr 96:552–558, 1980.

14. Dyson, M., Franks, C., and Suckling, J.: Stimulation of healing of varicose ulcers by ultrasound. Ultrasonics 14:232–236, 1976.

15. Erton, L. W., Maughan, W. L., Shaukas, A. A., and Weiss, J. L.: Accurate volume determination in the isolated ejecting canine left ventricle by two-dimensional echocardiography. Circulation 60:320, 1979.

16. Eggleton, R. C.: Interim AIUM standard nomenclature. Reflections 4:275–292, 1978.

17. Fortuin, N. J., Hood, W. P., Sherman, E. M., and Criage, E.: Determination of left ventricular volumes of ultrasound. Circulation 44:575, 1971.

18. French, J. W., and Popp, R.: Variability of echocardiographic discontinuity in double outlet right ventricle and truncus arteriosus. Circulation 51:848, 1975.

19. Friedman, M. J., Sahn, B. J., Larson, D., Fling, A.: 2-D echo range gated Doppler (RGD) measurements of cardiac output (CO) and stroke volume (SV) in open chest dogs. Circulation 62:III–101, 1980.

20. Friedman, M. J., Sahn, D. J., Burres, H., Allen, H. D., and Goldberg, S. J.: Detection of abnormal systolic and diastolic left ventricular function in children with aortic stenosis by computerized echocardiographic analysis. Am. J. Cardiol. 41:355, 1978.

21. Fisher, D. J., Silverman, N. H., Schiller, N. B., and Hart, P. A.: Evaluation of endocardial cushion defects by phased array sector scanner. Am. J. Cardiol. 41:353, 1978.

22. Gibson, D. G.: Estimation of left ventricular size by echocardiography. Br. Heart J. 35:128, 1973.

23. Gardin, J. M., Iseri, L. T., Elkayam, U., Tobis, J., Childs, W., Burn, C. S., and Henry, W. L.: Use of Doppler echocardiography in the noninvasive assessment of left ventricular dysfunction in patients with dilated cardiomyopathy. Circulation 62:III–200, 1980.

24. Gewitz, M. H., Werner, J. C., Kleinman, C. S., Hellenbrand, W. E., and Talner, N. S.: Role of echocardiography in aortic stenosis: Pre and post-operative studies. Am. J. Cardiol. 43:67, 1979.

25. Glanz, S., Hellenbrand, W. E., Berman, M. A., and Talner, N. S.: Echographic assessment of the severity of aortic stenosis in children and adolescents. Am. J. Cardiol. 38:620, 1976.

26. Goss, S. A., Johnston, R. L., and Dunn, F.: Comprehensive compilation of empirical ultrasonic properties of mammalian tissues. J. Acoust. Soc. Am. 64:423–457, 1978.

26a. Goldberg, S. J., Allen, H. D., and Sahn, D.: Journal of Pediatric and Adolescent Echocardiography, 2nd ed. Yearbook Medical Publishers, Chicago, 1980.

27. Gutgesell, H. P., Paquet, M., Duff, D. F., and McNamara, D. G.: Evaluation of left ventricular size and function by echocardiography, results in normal children. Circulation 56: 457, 1977.

28. Gutgesell, H. P.: Echocardiographic estimation of pulmonary artery pressure in transposition of the great arteries. Circulation 57:1151, 1978.

29. Halliday, H., Hirschfeld, S., Riggs, T., and Liebman, J.: Respiratory distress syndrome: Echocardiographic assessment of cardiovascular function and pulmonary vascular resistence. Pediatrics 60:444, 1977.

30. Hellman, L. M., Duffus, G. M., Donald, I., and Sunden, B.: Safety of diagnostic ultrasound in obstetrics. Lancet 1:1133–1135, 1970.

31. Henry, W. L., Maron, B. J., Griffith, J. M., Redwood, D. R., and Epstein, S. E.: Differential diagnosis of anomalies of the great arteries by real-time two-dimensional echocardiography. Circulation 51:283, 1975.

32. Henry, W. L., Maron, B. J., and Griffith, J. M.: Cross-sectional echocardiography in the diagnosis of congenital heart disease: Identification of the relation of the ventricles and great arteries. Circulation 56:267, 1977.

33. Henry, W. L., and Kastl, D. G.: Echocardiographic evaluation of patients with mitral stenosis. Am. J. Med. 62:813, 1977.

34. Hirschfeld, S., Meyer, R. A., Schwartz, D. C., Korfhagen, J., and Kaplan, S.: Measurement of right and left ventricular systolic time intervals by echocardiography. Circulation 51:304, 1975.

35. Hirschfeld, S., Meyer, R. A., Korfhagen, J., Kaplan, S., and Liebman, J.: The isovolumic contraction time of the left ventricle: An echographic study. Circulation 54:751, 1976.

36. Hoekenga, D. E., Greene, E. R., Loeppky, J. A., Mathews, E. C., Richards, K. L., and Luft, U. C.: A comparison of noninvasive Doppler cardiographic and simultaneous Fick measurements of left ventricular stroke volume. Circulation 62:III–199, 1980.

37. Janos, G. G., Kalavathy, A., Meyer, R. A., Engel, P., and Kaplan, S.: Differentiation of constrictive pericarditis and restrictive cardiomyopathy of echocardiography. Am. J. Cardiol. 47:462, 1981.

38. Johnson, F. H., Eyring, H., and Stover, B. J.: The theory of rate processes in biology and medicine. Wiley, New York, 1974.

39. Johnson, G. L., Meyer, R. A., Schwartz, D. C., Korfhagen, J., and Kaplan, S.: Left ventricular function by echocardiography in children with fixed aortic stenosis. Am. J. Cardiol. 38:611, 1976.

40. Johnson, G. L., Meyer, R. A., Schwartz, D. C., Korfhagen, J., and Kaplan, S.: Echocardiographic evaluation of fixed left ventricular obstruction in children: Pre and postoperative assessment of ventricular systolic pressures. Circulation 56:299, 1977.

41. Johnson, G. L., Meyer, R. A., Korfhagen, J., Schwartz, D. C., and Kaplan, S.: Echocardiographic assessment of pulmonary artery pres-

sure in children with complete right bundle branch block. Am. J. Cardiol. 41:1264, 1978.

42. Kaye, H. H., Tynan, M., and Hunter, S.: Validity of echocardiographic estimates of left ventricular size and performance in infants and children. Br. Heart. J. 37:371, 1975.

43. Kossoff, G.: On the measurement and specification of acoustic output generated by pulsed ultrasonic diagnostic equipment. J. Clin. Ultrasound 6:303–309, 1978.

44. Kremkau, F. W., and Witcofski, R. L.: Mitotic reduction in rat liver exposed to ultrasound. J. Clin. Ultrasound 2:123–126, 1974.

45. Lele, P. P.: Thresholds and mechanisms of ultrasonic damage to "organized" animal tissues. In Symposium on Biological Effects Characterizations Ultrasound Sources, HEW Pub (FDA) 78-8048. Edited by D. G. Hazzard and M. L. Litz pp. 224–239, 1977.

46. Lele, P. P.: No chromosomal damage from ultrasound. N. Engl. J. Med. 287:254, 1972.

47. Liebeskind, D., Bases, R., Elequin, F., et al.: Diagnostic ultrasound: Effects on the DNA and growth patterns of animal cells. Radiology 131:177–184, 1979.

48. Liebeskind, D., Bases, R., Mendez, F., et al.: Sister chromatid exchanges in human lymphocytes after exposure to diagnostic ultrasound. Science 205:1273–1275, 1979.

49. Lorch, G., Rubenstein, S., Baker, D. W., Dooley, T., and Dodge, H.: Doppler echocardiography. Use of a graphical display system. Circulation 56:576, 1977.

50. Lyon, M. F., and Simpson, G. M.: An investigation into the possible genetic hazard of ultrasound. Br. J. Radiol. 47:712–722, 1974.

51. Macintosh, I. J. C., and Davey, D. A.: Chromosome aberrations induced by an ultrasonic fetal pulse detection. Br. Med. J. 4:92–93, 1970.

52. Macintosh, I. J. C., Brown, R. C., and Coakley, W. T.: Ultrasound and in vitro chromosome aberrations. Br. J. Radiol. 48:230–232, 1975.

53. Mannor, S. M., Serr, D. M., Tamari, I., et al.: The safety of ultrasound in fetal monitoring. Am. J. Obstet. Gynecol. 113:653–661, 1972.

54. McDonald, I.: Echocardiographic assessment of left ventricular function in mitral valve disease. Circulation 53:865, 1976.

55. McDonald, I.: Echocardiographic assessment of left ventricular function in aortic valve disease. Circulation 53:860, 1976.

56. Mermut, S., Katayama, P., Del Castillo, R., and Jones H. W.: The effect of ultrasound on human chromosomes in vitro. Obstet. Gynecol. 41:4–6, 1973.

57. Meyer, R. A.: Pediatric Echocardiography, 2nd ed. Lea & Febiger, Philadelphia, in press.

58. Meyer, R. A.: Echocardiography in congenital heart disease. Cardiovasc. Clin. 6:219, 1975.

58a. Meyer, R. A.: Echocardiography in congenital heart disease. Semin. Roetgenol. 10:277, 1975.

59. Meyer, R. A., Schwartz, D. C., Covitz, W., and Kaplan, S.: Echocardiographic assessment of cardiac malposition. Am. J. Cardiol. 33:896, 1974.

60. Meyer, R. A., Schwartz, D. C., Benzing, G., III, and Kaplan, S.: The ventricular septum in right ventricular volume overload. Am. J. Cardiol. 30:349, 1972.

61. Meyer, R. A., and Kaplan, S.: Noninvasive techniques in pediatric cardiovascular disease. Prog. Cardiovasc. Dis. 15:341, 1973.

62. Meyer, R. A., Stockert, J., and Kaplan, S.: Echographic determination of left ventricular volumes in pediatric patients. Circulation 51:297, 1975.

63. Meyer, R.: Pediatric Echocardiography. Philadelphia, Lea & Febiger, 1977, p. 200.

64. Milner, S., Meyer, R. A., Venables, A. W., and Kaplan, S.: The tricuspid valve in children: An echocardiographic and phonocardiographic study. Am. J. Cardiol. 35:157, 1975.

65. Miller, M. W., Kaufman, G. E., Castaldo, F. W., and Carstensen, E. L.: Absence of mitotic reduction in regenerating rat livers exposed to ultrasound. J. Clin. Ultrasound 4:169–172, 1976.

66. Nyborg, W. L., Gershoy, A., and Miller, D. L.: Interaction of ultrasound with simple biological systems. Ultrasonic International 1977 Conference, Conference Proceedings, pp. 19–27. IPC Science and Technology, Guilford, England, 1977.

67. Ports, T. A., Silverman, N. H., and Schiller, N. B.: Two-dimensional echocardiographic assessment of Ebstein's anomaly. Circulation 58:336, 1978.

68. Riggs, T., Hirschfeld, S., Borkat, G., Knoke, J., and Liebman, J.: Assessment of the pulmonary vascular bed echocardiographic right ventricular systolic time intervals. Circulation 57:939, 1978.

69. Riggs, T., Hirschfeld, S., Fanaroff, A., Liebman, J., Fletcher, B., Meyer, R., and Bormuth, G.: Persistence of fetal circulation syndrome: An echocardiographic study. J. Pediatr. 91:626, 1977.

70. Rott, H. D., Huber, H. J., Soldner, R., and Schwarritz, G.: Examinations of chromosomes after in vitro exposure of human lymphocytes to ultrasound. Electromedica 40:14–76, 1972.

71. Schiller, N. B., Acqiatella, H., Ports, T. A., et al.: Left ventricular volume from pained biplane two-dimensional echocardiography. Circulation 60:547, 1979.

72. Silverman, N. H., and Schiller, N. B.: Apex echocardiography: A two-dimensional technique for evaluating congenital heart disease. Circulation 57:503, 1978.

73. Stevenson, J. G., Kawabori, I., and Guntheroth, W. G.: Noninvasive detection of pulmonary hypertension in patient ductus arteriosus by pulsed Doppler echocardiography. Circulation 60:355, 1979.

74. Stevenson, J. G., Kawabori, I., and Guntheroth, W. G.: Differentiation of ventricular septal defects from mitral regurgitation by pulsed Doppler echocardiography. Circulation 56:14, 1977.

75. Stevenson, J. G., Kawabori, I., and Guntheroth, W. G.: Pulsed Doppler echocardiographic detection of total anomalous pulmonary venous return: Resolution of left atrial line. Am. J. Cardiol. 44:1155, 1979.

76. Sahn, D. J., Terry, R., and O'Rourke, R.: Multiple-crystal echocardiographic evaluation of endocardial cushion defect. Circulation 50:25, 1974.

77. Sahn, D. J., Terry, R., and O'Rourke, R.: Multiple-crystal and cross-sectional echocardiography in the diagnosis of cyanotic congenital heart disease. Circulation 50:230, 1974.

78. Sahn, D. J., Allen, H. D., McDonald, G., and Goldberg, S. J.: Real-time cross-sectional echocardiographic diagnosis of coarctation of the aorta: A prospective study of echocardiographic-angiographic correlations. Circulation 56:762, 1977.

79. Sahn, D. J., and Allen, H. D.: Real-time cross-sectional echocardiographic imaging and measurement of the patent ductus arteriosus in infants and children. Circulation 58:343, 1978.

80. Sahn, D. J., Allen, H. D., Lange, L., and Goldberg, S.: Cross-sectional echocardiographic diagnosis of the sites of total anomalous pulmonary venous drainage. Circulation 60:1317, 1979.

81. Sahn, D. J., Deely, W. J., Hagan, A. D., and Friedman, W. F.: Echocardiographic assessment of left ventricular performance in normal newborns. Circulation 49:232, 1974.

82. Schieken, R., and Kerber, R.: Echocardiographic abnormalities in active rheumatic fever. Am. J. Cardiol. 38:458, 1976.

83. Seward, J. B., Tajik, A. J., Hagler, D. J., and Ritter, D. G.: Contrast echocardiography in single or common ventricle. Circulation 55:513, 1977.

84. Shimizu, T., and Shoji, R.: An experimental safety study of mice exposed to low intensity ultrasound. Excerpta Med. Int. Congr. Ser. 277:28, 1973.

85. Silverman, N. H., Snider, A. R., and Rudolph, A. M.: Evaluation of pulmonary hypertension by M-mode echocardiography in children with ventricular septal defect. Circulation 61:1125, 1980.

86. Smyth, M. G.: Animal toxicity studies with ultrasound at diagnostic power levels. Diagnostic ultrasound, edited by C. C. Grossman. Plenum Press, New York, 1966, pp. 296–299.

87. Solinger, R., Francisco, E., and Minhas, K.: Deductive echocardiographic analysis in infants with congenital heart disease. Circulation 50:1072, 1974.

88. Stopa, A., Meyer, R. A., Korfhagen, J., and Kaplan, S.: The left isovolumic contraction time in left to right shunts. Am. J. Cardiol. 39:266, 1977.

89. St. John Sutton, M. G., Tajik, A. J., Gibson, D. G., Brown, D. J., Seward, J. B., and Guiliani, E. R.: Echocardiographic assessment of left ventricular filling and septal and posterior wall dynamics in idiopathic hypertrophic subaortic stenosis. Circulation 57:512, 1978.

90. St. John Sutton, M. G., Hagler, D. J., Tajik, A. J., Giuliani, E. R., Seward, J. B., Ritter, D. G., and Ritman, E. L.: Cardiac function in the normal newborn, additional information by computer analysis of the M-mode echocardiogram. Circulation 57:1198, 1978.

91. Sutton, M. S. J., Meyer, R., Tajik, A., and Ritman, E. L.: Computer analysis of the echocardiogram in newborns with persistent fetal circulation (PFC). Am. J. Cardiol. 43:385, 1979.

92. Tajik, A. J., Seward, J. B., Hagler, D. J., Mair, D. D., and Lie, J. T.: Two-dimensional real-time ultrasonic imaging of the heart and great vessels, technique, image orientation, structure identification, and validation. Mayo Clin. Proc. 53:271, 1978.

93. Valdes-Cruz, L. M., Pieroni, D. R., Roland, J. A., and Varghese, P. J.: Echocardiographic detection of intracardiac right-to-left shunts following peripheral vein injections. Circulation 54:558, 1976.

94. Valdes-Cruz, L. M., Pieroni, D. R., Roland, J., and Shematek, J. P. L.: Recognition of residual post-operative shunts by contrast echocardiographic techniques. Circulation 55:148, 1977.

95. Warwick, R., Pond, J. B., Woodward, B., and Connolly, C. C.: Hazards of diagnostic ultrasound—A study with mice. IEEE Trans Sonic Ultrasonics SU-17:158–164, 1970.

96. Weyman, A. E., Hurwitz, R. A., Girod, D. A., Dillon, J. C., Feigenbaum, H., and Green, D.: Cross-sectional echocardiographic visualization of the stenotic pulmonary valve. Circulation 56:769, 1977.

97. Weyman, A. E., Feigenbaum, H., Hurwitz, R. A., Girod, D. A., and Dillon, J. C.: Cross-sectional echocardiographic assessment of the severity of aortic stenosis in children. Circulation 55:773, 1977.

98. Weyman, A. E., Caldwell, R. L., Hurwitz, R. A., Girod, D. P., Dillon, J. C., Feigenbaum, H., and Green, D.: Cross-sectional echocardiographic characterization of aortic obstruction. 1. Supravalvar aortic stenosis and aortic hypoplasia. Circulation 57:491, 1978.

99. Weyman, A. E., Caldwell, R. L., Hurwitz, R. A., Girod, D. P., Dillon, J. C., Feigenbaum, H., and Green, D: Cross-sectional echocardiographic detection of aortic obstruction. Circulation 57:491, 1978.

100. Weyman, A. E., Wann, L. S., Caldwell, R. L., Hurwitz, R. A., Dillon, J. C., and Feigenbaum, H.: Negative contrast echocardiography: A new method for detecting left-to-right shunts. Circulation 59:498, 1979.

101. Ziskin, M.: Survey of patient exposure to diagnostic ultrasound. In Interaction of Ultrasound and Biological Tissue, edited by J. M. Reid, and M. R. Sikov. U. S. Food & Drug Administration, Washington, D. C., 1972.

102. Meyer, R. A.: Echocardiography in pediatric patients from cardiovascular clinics. Pediatr. Cardiovasc. Dis. 11:2, 187–225, 1981.

5

Catheterization and Angiocardiography

Jay M. Jarmakani, M.D.

INDICATIONS

The purposes of cardiac catheterization are to: delineate the cardiovascular anatomy; quantitate the shunt; quantitate the severity of valvar stenosis and/or regurgitation; determine the pulmonary vascular resistance; and determine myocardial function. Therefore, cardiac catheterization should be performed when knowledge of the above is essential for the medical and/or surgical management of the patient. Two-dimensional echocardiography (2D echo) delineates the diagnosis in many instances and eliminates the need for cardiac catheterization in some patients. In the remaining patients, 2D echo provides essential information which helps in the planning of the cardiac catheterization. The indications for cardiac catheterization in the different age groups follow.

PREMATURE INFANTS

In the premature infant the most common lesion is patent ductus arteriosus (PDA) where the clinical findings are frequently diagnostic. Contrast echocardiography confirms the diagnosis of PDA. Cardiac catheterization is not indicated unless there is evidence for an associated cardiac lesion.

INFANTS

In the infant with cyanosis of cardiac origin, cardiac catheterization is indicated. A clinical diagnosis of transposition of the great arteries (TGA), total anomalous pulmonary venous connection (TAPVC), or tricuspid atresia is an indication for emergency cardiac catheterization. Balloon septostomy in these cases can be life-saving and should not be delayed.

In noncyanotic infants with heart disease, the indications include: heart failure not responding to medical management; heart failure in the first 2 months of life responding to medical management but with a tentative diagnosis of a left to right shunt, anomalous origin of the left coronary artery, and other similar defects where the course of the lesion suggests that the patient might deteriorate further in the coming months; pulmonary disease with cardiomegaly or other evidence for vascular anomaly; cardiac defects such as ventricular septal defect (VSD), with a change in the clinical findings suggesting an increase in the pulmonary vascular resistance.

CHILDREN

In children the indications for cardiac catheterization are multiple. A change in the clinical course of a patient with a previous cardiac catheterization frequently necessitates another cardiac catheterization to evaluate: the pulmonary vascular resistance; the severity of valvar stenosis; the anatomy; and the pulmonary blood flow, since surgery may be indicated promptly.

Most children should have detailed cardiac catheterization before corrective surgery to determine the anatomy of the defect and to exclude other associated lesions. Aortic stenosis (AS) is an indication for cardiac catheterization since the severity of this lesion cannot be evaluated clinically. Finally, all children with a questionable diagnosis probably should be catheterized at 5 to 6 years of age to establish the diagnosis and to determine the operable cases, such as atrial septal defect (ASD) with moderate left to right shunt.

POSTOPERATIVE PATIENTS

Postoperatively many patients require evaluation for such lesions as: tetralogy of Fallot (TF) with a residual murmur or cardiomegaly; VSD with a residual murmur, cardiomegaly, or an increased pulmonary vascular resistance preoperatively; AS; TGA; TAPVC; and severe valvar pulmonary stenosis. In addition, any patient with unexplained deterioration in the cardiovascular status in the immediate postoperative period requires cardiac evaluation.

PATIENTS WITH DYSRHYTHMIA

Dysrhythmia is an indication for right heart catheterization to evaluate the conduction system. His bundle electrocardiogram will delineate the etiology in most cases and guide the physician in the medical management.

EQUIPMENT

The following is a brief outline of the necessary equipment for a pediatric catheterization laboratory:

1. Biplane image intensifiers are important for infants because they show the heart in two views simultaneously, and they reduce the quantity of contrast media injected.
2. Biplane film changers (6 to 12 films/second) are very helpful in many defects where a detailed knowledge of the anatomy is essential.
3. Two TV systems are necessary to view the cardiac image in the anterior-posterior and lateral views.
4. Two video systems are desirable for immediate playback of the cines.
5. A set of solid state preamplifiers are needed for pressure recordings, heart sound recording, dye and thermodilution curves, His bundle recording, and electrocardiogram monitoring. The output of these amplifiers can be fed simultaneously to an oscilloscope, and a magnetic tape system with a high-frequency recorder. The recorders should have a high-frequency response, which is essential for the recording of high-fidelity pressure, His bundle electrograms, heart sound, etc. The oscilloscope should be located in the proximity

to the TV system to observe the electrocardiogram and pressure curves during manipulation of the catheter.

6. A magnetic tape system is desirable for storing data.

7. Conventional fluid-filled pressure transducers are needed. It is desirable to have a tip pressure transducer catheter which can be used for high-fidelity recordings.

8. A defibrillator is essential and should be ready for use in seconds if needed.

9. A pacemaker unit is necessary for patients with bradycardia and can be used to convert atrial tachycardias.

10. A blood gas analyzer is essential for analysis of PO_2, PCO_2, and pH.

11. A spectrophotometric unit is needed for determination of the oxygen saturation.

12. A Van Slyke unit is desirable to quantitate the oxygen content.

13. Equipment is needed to determine oxygen consumption such as: a Douglas bag and Tissot spirometer to measure the volume of expired air or an Oxford gas analyzer.

PERSONNEL

It is desirable to have two physicians in the cardiac catheterization laboratory, especially when studying sick infants. In addition, two to three individuals should be available to assist with the procedure. They should have the following skills: a nurse familiar with the monitoring and care of infants with heart disease; a radiology technician capable of running all radiology equipment; and a person capable of running and assisting in pressure monitoring, dye dilution curves, electrophysiological studies, and blood gas analyses. In addition, these personnel should be well trained in the proper cleansing and sterilization of all equipment.

CATHETERIZATION PROCEDURE

After deciding that cardiac catheterization is indicated, the physician should discuss with the family the indications for cardiac catheterization and the benefit to the patient. In addition, he should discuss in detail all the potential complications including: dysrhythmia, arterial or ventricular puncture, arterial thrombi, etc. It is necessary to obtain written permission for cardiac catheterization from the parents or guardians, and this should include the benefit and potential complications of the procedure. It is also helpful to show the parents and the older child the cardiac catheterization laboratory and to explain briefly the sequence of the study.

PREMEDICATION

It is not recommended to sedate infants in the first 6 months of life. Infants 6 months to 1 year of age who are in severe heart failure or are severely cyanotic should be sedated in the laboratory under supervision. Older children can be sedated intramuscularly 30 minutes before catheterization with any number of different preparations which include: meperidine (Demerol, 1 mg/kg) and hydroxyzine (Vistaril, 1 mg/kg), or meperidine (1 mg/kg) and droperidol (0.03 mg/kg), or meperidine (1 mg/kg) and chlorpromazine (0.5 mg/kg), and promethazine (0.5 mg/kg). Patients with cyanotic heart disease and potential cyanotic spells should be sedated only with morphine (0.1 mg/kg subcutaneously).

PATIENT SAFETY

Patient safety in the cardiac catheterization laboratory depends on proper monitoring and support of the patient's vital signs as soon as the patient enters the laboratory. The patient should be restrained gently on the examining table to prevent motion which could lead to injury. Intravenous fluid should be started on all patients for the administration of medication and fluids. The blood pressure should be monitored frequently with a regular blood pressure unit or a Doppler unit. The patient's rectal temperature should be monitored continuously with rectal probe and thermistor. It is essential to terminate the cardiac catheterization whenever the patient's temperature approaches $39°C$, and to warm the hypothermic patient. In all small infants, the patient should be warmed with heating pads or a radiant heat.

INSERTION OF CATHETERS

The site of inserting intravascular catheters depends on the anticipated cardiovascular and visceral anomaly. In the first week of life, it is desirable to catheterize infants via the umbilical vessels. This can be achieved easily in the first 48 hours of life and is less likely after 3 days of age. The venous catheter can be maneuvered from the umbilical vein via the ductus venosus to the inferior vena cava and right atrium. The catheter should be maneuvered very gently and should not be forced, since this might rupture the veins. If it is very difficult to maneuver the catheter via the ductus venosus, it is advisable to withdraw the catheter to a position 1 to 2 cm below the ductus venosus and then inject 1 ml of contrast media to outline the path and the patency of the ductus venosus. When the ductus venosus is open it is possible to pass a balloon catheter and to perform an atrial septostomy. Using this approach, however, it is quite difficult to enter the right ventricle and the pulmonary artery. Before inserting the catheter in the umbilical vein, we usually pass the catheter through an appropriate size sheath. The sheath is kept outside the patient but can be advanced on the catheter to the right atrium when we want to change catheters. This maneuver saves time and ensures the continuous utilization of a patent ductus venosus. Extreme care should be taken to prevent air from entering the right atrium, especially in cyanotic infants. Umbilical artery catheters can also be inserted in the first 3 days of life for measurement of pressure and determination of arterial blood gases.

In the infant 1 week to 1 year of age, it is desirable to catheterize the patient via the femoral vein. The advantages of this approach include: the vessels in the leg are large, whereas the veins in the arm are quite small; the lower approach permits manuevering the catheter via the foramen ovale, whereas it is quite difficult to enter the foramen ovale from the arm; the leg approach permits performing atrial septostomy; and occasionally it is difficult to manuever the catheter from the right subclavian vein to the superior vena cava, and this can be avoided by catheterizing the femoral vein. This approach, however, cannot be used if the patient has polysplenia, since this condition is associated with interruption of the inferior vena cava.

In patients requiring retrograde arterial catheterization, the entry to the femoral artery, either percutaneous or cutdown, carries the risk of arterial thrombosis and permanent compromise of the circulation to the leg. I, therefore, prefer to perform a retrograde arterial catheterization via the right axillary artery in this age group. In children more than 1 year of age, the vein and artery should both be entered from the inguinal region. This approach is practical in all patients except those with polysplenia or severe coarctation of the aorta.

METHODS OF ENTRY

Percutaneous

The percutaneous technique can be used to enter the anticubital vein, the femoral vein, and the femoral artery. The area of entry should be cleaned thoroughly with antiseptic solution, dryed with sterilized towels, then covered with a sterile sheet with a 2 × 2 cm opening above the entry site. The patient then is covered with sterile towels, and the site of entry is infiltrated with 1% lidocaine. Using the arm approach, it is useful to apply a tourniquet proximal to the site of entry. A thin wall, short bevel needle is used to enter the vein. It is also desirable to use the needle without the stylet to avoid entering the posterior wall of the vessel. In addition, this ensures that the needle will not puncture the artery as it enters the vein. The needle should be moved in a plane medial and parallel to the artery. The needle should be directed posteriorly and slightly lateral in a 45° angle with the skin. Using this approach, it is my experience that a free flow of venous blood will come from the needle as it enters the anterior wall of the vein. The flexible end of the guide wire is then passed through the needle. This maneuver can be done with more ease if the angle of the needle with the skin is reduced to 25°. The wire should not be forced through the needle, and if there is resistance, the wire should be withdrawn and the needle should be maneuvered to obtain a free flow of blood from the needle. The skin is then cut 1 mm at the needle, and the needle is withdrawn. A dilator and sheath is passed over the wire. The dilator should be held firm at a 40° angle with the skin and rotated as it is advanced. While advancing the dilator, it is important to move the wire back and forth to ensure that the wire is free through the dilator and is not kinked. When the dilator enters the vein, the blood will flow around the wire. The sheath then should be held firm around the dilator and rotated while being advanced into the vessel. The dilator and the wire are then removed, and free bleeding should be observed before passing the catheter into the sheath. An artery can be entered percutaneously only from the inguinal region. The technique is similar to that described for the vein. It is essential that the catheter diameter is smaller than the internal diameter of the artery to allow flow around the catheter during the procedure. This eliminates leg cramps and reduces the frequency of arterial thrombosis. After the insertion of the arterial catheter the patient should be given a dose of heparin (100 units/kg, IV) in all cases when long arterial catheterization (more than 30 minutes) is anticipated. This is done to minimize arterial thrombi at the site of entry.

Direct Exposure

The vessels can be exposed by cutdown in the antecubital region, the axillary region, or the inguinal region. The inguinal region can be used in all patients except when the heart cannot be entered from the inferior vena cava, when the patient has severe coarctation of the aorta, or in the infant where retrograde arterial catheterization is necessary. In the infant, I prefer to use the axillary artery. The area of cutdown is cleansed with antiseptic solutions (pHisoHex and then Betadine), dried, and then covered by a sterile sheet, and the patient is covered with sterile towels. The region is infiltrated with 1% lidocaine.

In the inguinal region, a 2-cm long cut is made in the skin across the femoral artery 1 to 2 cm distal to the inguinal ligament. In small infants, a more distal cut is useful to utilize the superficial femoral vein and spare the deep femoral vein. When anticipating a balloon septostomy, however, the cut should be more proximal but just distal to the inguinal ligament to utilize the large vein for the entry of a balloon catheter.

In older infants and children, however, two-thirds of the cut should be medial to the femoral artery to isolate the saphenous vein. The tissues should be dissected one level at a time. The vein should be isolated for 1 to 2 cm, and two 4:0 sutures placed around the vein. The vein is then cut vertically, proximal to the distal suture to permit easy entry of the catheter. In small veins, it is desirable to do this cut at a branching site or a large segment of the vein since the cut can be enlarged by a longitudinal incision. Gentle retraction is applied to the distal end of the vein to straighten the proximal portion. A catheter guide can be used to stretch the opening in the vein to permit entry of the catheter. The distal suture is tied and the proximal sutures are retracted gently to stop the bleeding. In small infants, I introduce a dilator and a sheath over a wire into the vein. The sheath then is left in the vein during the catheterization. This speeds up the procedure and facilitates a quick change of the catheters with no additional trauma to the vein.

When it is necessary to perform a cutdown on the femoral artery, it should be well exposed for 2 to 3 cm. The artery should be surrounded by umbilical tape proximal and distal to the site of entry. Gentle snaring usually stops bleeding and prevents severe constriction which can cause arterial damage and erosion of the intima. The artery is cut perpendicularly to permit the entry of the catheter without stretching the artery. Heparin (1 to 2 ml, 100 units/ml) should be injected in the distal part of the artery.

In the auxillary region, a 2-cm incision is made perpendicular to the auxillary artery 1 to 2 cm distal to the auxillary fold. The tissue layers should be dissected one at a time. The fascia over the vessel is entered and opened proximally and distally. The basilic vein is isolated. The axillary artery lies behind two brachial nerves and lateral to the basilic vein. The artery is isolated for 2 cm and surrounded by two umbilical tapes. A disadvantage of the axillary approach can be the difficulty in advancing the catheter from the subclavian vein or artery to the superior vena cava and the ascending aorta. In addition, a descending aorta origin of the right subclavian artery is a contraindication for retrograde catheterization via the right axillary artery. The catheter should always be smaller than the lumen of the artery, and the exposed portion of the artery should be kept moist.

Arterial Closure

The arterial catheter is removed and the proximal tape is then released quickly to allow free bleeding to ensure removal of all clots around the catheter. The distal umbilical tape is loosened to permit free bleeding from the distal end of the artery; then 1 to 2 ml of diluted heparin should be injected distally to ensure the removal of clots. Two vascular clamps are then inserted around the site of the arterial cut. The opening of the artery should be flushed with diluted heparin, and the edge of the arterial wall should be well exposed. The artery is closed with 5:0 or 6:0 arterial suture on a noncutting needle. The first two sutures should be placed at the corners of the cut and are used to stretch the artery gently. Interrupted suture is placed at 1-mm intervals and should be placed about 1 mm away from the arterial edge. In each site the needle should enter all arterial layers, but in such a way that the posterior arterial wall is kept free. This can be accomplished by placing all the sutures before tying any of them. The sutures are then tied, but before tying the last suture, the distal clamp should be released to fill the artery with blood. The proximal clamp is then released after tying all sutures.

Transthoracic Puncture

In some patients with severe aortic stenosis, it is quite difficult to enter the left ventricle retrograde via the aortic valve or from the right atrium via the foramen ovale. In these cases, transthoracic ventricular puncture becomes necessary. During the procedure it is important that the patient remain quiet, and therefore general anesthesia should be used if needed. Ketamine is a short-term anesthetic and can be used safely. The lower chest and upper abdomen is cleansed with antiseptic solution and then draped. A long no. 20 spinal needle, attached to a pressure line as well as the electrocardiogram, is inserted into the skin in the subxyphoid region. The needle is directed toward the left shoulder at an angle of 45°. Advancing the needle under biplane fluoroscopy can be useful for the proper direction. When the electrocardiographic tracing shows cardiac injury, the stylet is removed and the needle is connected to a three way stopcock with a catheter for a recording of pressures. The needle is then advanced, consecutively, through the apex of the right ventricle, the ventricular septum, and into the left ventricle. The catheter is then flushed and the pressure is recorded. The procedure should be done quickly, and the needle should not be kept in the heart for more than a few minutes.

Transseptal

In patients with mitral stenosis and occasionally in patients with aortic stenosis, it is important to catheterize the left atrium. Since most of these patients have an intact atrial septum, the left atrium can be entered either retrograde via the mitral valve or transseptally. The latter procedure is performed using a catheter on a Cross and Brockenbrough transseptal needle. The needle is maneuvered into the superior vena cava and pointed to the left of the patient. It is then rotated clockwise 45° posteriorly and withdrawn gently till it is released from the superior vena cava entering the right atrium. This is usually felt, and the position of the needle should be checked by biplane fluoroscopy. The needle at this time is pointing toward the atrial septum, and with a gentle push the needle penetrates the atrial septum. The catheter is then advanced over the needle into the left atrium and the needle is pulled back.

TYPES OF CATHETERS

A number of different kinds of catheters are used in a pediatric cardiac catheterization laboratory. The following is a brief description of most of the catheters and their use.

END HOLE

A Lehman catheter is a thin-walled, flexible catheter which can be used to record the wedge pressure and pressure pullbacks across the left and right ventricular outflow tract. The disadvantage: the catheter adds (the catheter facing flow) or subtracts (the catheter is in the direction of the flow) a kinetic component to the lateral pressure in the vessels. In addition, the catheter should not be used for injection of contrast media.

SIDE HOLE AND CLOSED END (NIH)

This catheter is easy to maneuver and is very useful for pressure recording, blood sampling, and injection of contrast media. The main disadvantage of this catheter is that it cannot be passed over a wire when using the percutaneous technique.

SIDE HOLE AND END HOLE

This catheter can be passed over a wire when using the percutaneous technique and thus avoids introducing a sheath into the vessel. In addition, a thin wire can be passed through the lumen to guide the catheter into the different chambers of the heart. The catheter can also be used for injection of contrast media. The disadvantages of this catheter are that during injection of contrast media the tip might be facing the vascular or ventricular wall, and this can lead to an intramyocardial injection; furthermore, the catheter tends to recoil during injection.

END HOLE AND BALLOON (SWAN-GANZ)

This catheter has a balloon proximal to the tip which can be inflated with CO_2 to help direct the catheter into vessels in difficult cases. In addition, the balloon can be inflated in a small vessel to achieve occlusion proximal to the tip, thus permitting a recording of the wedge pressure. This catheter, however, should not be used for injection of contrast media.

SIDE HOLE AND BALLOON

This catheter has side holes and an inflatable balloon at the tip of the catheter. It is also quite useful, since it can be maneuvered easily into different cardiac chambers and vessels. The balloon at the end of the catheter prevents intramyocardial injection of contrast media.

ELECTRODE

Catheters are made which have electrodes at the tip. These can be used for intracardiac pacing or recording of His bundle.

THERMISTOR

This catheter has a thermistor on the tip which possesses a rapid response time. It can be used in conjunction with a thermodilution unit to determine cardiac output.

PRESSURE-TIP TRANSDUCER

Microtransducers of different make and design are manufactured on the tip of a regular catheter. They can be used to measure the intravascular or intraventricular pressure. The catheter used should have a side hole for baseline adjustment and calibration of the microtransducer. Such catheters have a high-frequency response and therefore can provide an accurate pressure measurement for determination of first derivative (dP/dt).

PHONOCATHETER

This catheter has a microphone mounted on the tip permitting recording of intracardiac heart sounds and murmurs.

HANDLING AND MANIPULATION OF CATHETERS

The catheter should be connected to a two core manifold with a rotating adaptor, which in turn is connected to the pressure transducer by way of a Paley manifold. The whole system should be flushed to eliminate all air bubbles. The size of the catheter should be as large as possible but should not occlude the lumen of the vein or artery. This will usually preserve the integrity of the vein or artery and eliminate erosion of the intima. It is advisable to start with an end hole catheter which permits the recording of a wedge pressure and the pull-back pressure. This catheter can then be replaced by a side hole catheter, which permits easy blood sampling and minimizes the kinetic component of the pressure. Each time a new catheter is introduced into the vessel, blood should be withdrawn through the stopcock and then flushed with heparinized 0.5 N saline and 5% glucose in water (5 units/ml) to eliminate air bubbles and clot formation. Also it should be flushed frequently during the procedure.

The catheter should be rotated and advanced gently, but it should not be rotated unless it is advanced or withdrawn. This will lead to weakening and kinking of the catheter. During sterilization and storage, the catheters should be kept straight on a piece of wood with the tip in a J shape. It is difficult to describe all of the problems in maneuvering the catheter into the correct location, but knowledge of the anatomy and a gentle curve at the end of the catheter will make the maneuvers possible. The following should be avoided: wedging the catheter in an arterial or venous branch; forcing the catheter against the vascular or ventricular chamber; and wedging the catheter in a ventricular cavity. Occasionally it is difficult to maneuver a regular catheter into the right ventricle or the pulmonary artery in patients with transposition of the great arteries. It is also quite dangerous to inject through a regular catheter in an infant with heart failure. In these cases, an end hole or side hole balloon catheter is very useful and reduces the duration of the procedure, which is extremely important in a sick infant.

MEASUREMENT OF BLOOD OXYGEN

GENERAL COMMENTS

The oxygen is carried in the blood in two forms: combined with hemoglobin (Hgb O_2), and dissolved. *Oxygen capacity* refers to the maximum amount of oxygen which combines with hemoglobin in 100 ml of blood. One gram of adult hemoglobin usually combines with 1.34 to 1.36 ml of oxygen. Thus, for a normal adult with a hemoglobin of 15 gm%, the oxygen capacity will be 1.36 multiplied by 15, or 20.4 cc oxygen/100 ml blood. This does not account for the dissolved oxygen. The amount of oxygen dissolved is affected by the partial pressure of oxygen and the temperature of the plasma. At 37°C, the amount of oxygen dissolved is 0.00003 ml of oxygen in 1 ml of blood for each mm Hg oxygen partial pressure (PO_2). Thus, the amount of oxygen dissolved in 100 ml of blood for a PO_2 of 100 mm Hg is 0.3 ml.

Oxygen content refers to the sum of oxygen combined with hemoglobin and the oxygen dissolved in the plasma. Oxygen saturation refers to the ratio of oxygen combined with hemoglobin divided by the oxygen capacity. The oxygen saturation can be calculated accurately by determining the O_2 content, the dissolved oxygen, and the oxygen capacity by the equation:

$$O_2 \text{ Saturation} = \frac{O_2 \text{ Content-Dissolved } O_2}{O_2 \text{ Capacity}}$$

Oxygen saturation can also be determined spectrophotometrically. This method is not accurate for O_2 saturation less than 47% or higher than 94%. Although oxygen content can be calculated from the partial pressure of oxygen, oxygen saturation, and hemoglobin concentration, an accurate determination of oxygen content should be determined by the Van Slyke method or some similar procedure.

RELATION OF PO₂ TO OXYGEN CONTENT

The oxygen content in the blood depends upon the PO_2, the hemoglobin concentration, and the O_2 dissociation curve for that patient. The relationship between the O_2 saturation and the PO_2 for adult hemoglobin is shown in Figure 5.1. This curve shifts to the left with alkalosis, with a decrease in PCO_2, with a decrease in temperature, or with a decrease in 2,3-diphosphoglycerate (DPG). Changes in these variables in the opposite direction will shift this curve to the right.

Fetal hemoglobin binds poorly with 2,3-DPG, and therefore the dissociation curve for fetal hemoglobin is to the left of adult hemoglobin. The patient with anemia or chronic cyanosis has an increased level of 2,3-DPG, and therefore the dissociation curve is shifted to the right. A shift to the left results in a higher saturation at a lower PO_2, and therefore the fetal hemoglobin is capable of extracting larger amounts of oxygen at the placental level. A shift to the right, on the other hand, results in a decrease in the affinity of hemoglobin for oxygen, and therefore a larger amount of oxygen is available to the tissue. The "P-50" value is a term used to show the PO_2 for a hemoglobin saturation of 50%.

INTERPRETATION OF LEVEL OF BLOOD OXYGEN

GENERAL COMMENTS

The oxygen saturation and the PO_2 of the blood are used to calculate the cardiac output, as well as the left to right or right to left shunts. In order to draw meaningful conclusions, sampling should be done in the steady state. Any of the following will affect the interpretation of the data: (a) it is crucial that the patient be quiet but not so heavily sedated as to depress respiration; (b) a restless anxious patient increases his cardiac output and thus intracardiac shunting may vary from moment to moment; (c) medications which increase cardiac output or vary pulmonary and systemic resistance should not be given before blood sampling; (d) the patient should be on room air if possible; and (e) the oxygen saturation should be obtained before injection of contrast media since the latter affects systemic and pulmonary resistance.

Accurate calculation of cardiac output using the Fick principle requires strict adherence to the following: in calculating blood flow from point *a* to point *c*, it is important that the blood at sites *a* and *c* is fully mixed, and the blood does not enter or leave the circulation between points *a* and *c*. If blood of a different saturation enters the flow at point *b* and we wish to calculate the shunt, it is very important that the blood entering at point *b* is completely mixed, and

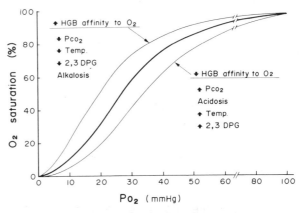

Fig. 5.1 Oxygen hemoglobin dissociation curve for adult hemoglobin (*thick line*). The *thin lines* show the effect of the different variables.

complete mixing is achieved again at point *c*. In addition, when calculating cardiac output, the oxygen consumption must be measured and not assumed, since there is too much individual variation. For calculation of cardiac output and shunts, one can use the oxygen saturation if the patient is breathing room air, but the oxygen content must be measured if the patient is breathing increased amounts of oxygen.

BLOOD OXYGEN IN THE CHAMBERS

The oxygen saturations in the superior vena cava (SVC), inferior vena cava (IVC), and coronary sinus vary considerably, and complete mixing is not achieved at the atrial level. At the junction with the heart, the inferior vena cava sample consists of hepatic flow with a low saturation and the remainder of the IVC with a higher saturation. Thus, the best site for obtaining fairly adequately mixed IVC sample is 1 cm below the IVC-right atrial junction. The coronary sinus flow can be 10% of the cardiac output, and the saturation is usually 30 to 35% less than the saturation in the SVC. The superior vena cava saturation in a normal patient is approximately 70%. A superior vena cava saturation higher than 80% suggests a high cardiac output, partial anomalous pulmonary venous connection, or a systemic arterial venous fistula. A superior vena cava saturation of less than 65% is consistent with desaturated aortic blood, low cardiac output, severe anemia, or very high metabolic rate.

The right atrial sample should be taken at the right midlateral wall with the catheter pointing to the right. This prevents sampling from the coronary sinus, the mouth of the tricuspid valve, or across an ASD. An increase in right atrial oxygen saturation of 10% in one run or 7% in two runs indicates: an ASD; partial anomalous pulmonary venous connection to the right atrium or the coronary sinus; coronary AV fistula; left ventricle right atrial communication; or VSD with tricuspid insufficiency. Occasionally, however, the increase in oxygen saturation in ASD is only partially realized at the atrial level, and a further step-up in saturation is seen at the ventricular level.

The oxygen saturation in the left atrium is normally 96% with a PO_2 of 90 to 100 mm Hg. If the patient, however, is heavily sedated or has heart failure and/or a large left to right shunt, the oxygen saturation could be as low as 88%. In addition, any major atelectasis will reduce the oxygen saturation in the left atrium. In the presence of a normal pulmonary venous oxygen saturation of 96%, a 5% step-down in oxygen saturation in the left atrium indicates a right to left interatrial shunting or a drainage of the superior vena cava into the left atrium. A step-down in the left atrium with no step-up in oxygen saturation in the right atrium is consistent with patent foramen ovale or small ASD with partial or complete obstruction to right atrial flow in patients with: valvular pulmonary atresia or very severe valvular pulmonary stenosis with intact ventricular septum, tricuspid atresia, tricuspid stenosis, or severe tricuspid insufficiency (dysplastic tricuspid valve or Ebstein's anomaly), or a systemic vein draining to the left atrium. Bidirectional shunting at the atrial level (step-down in the left atrium and step-up in the right atrium) is consistent with a large ASD and decreased right ventricular compliance, or a common atrium. When the saturation in the right atrium is equal to or higher than saturation in the left atrium, the diagnosis of TAPVC should be suspected.

The saturation in the right ventricle is approximately equal to the midright atrial saturation and usually represents complete mixing of systemic venous return. Occasionally a small step-up in the right ventricle can be seen in patients with isolated ASD. A step-up of 7% on one run or 5% on two runs is, however, consistent with VSD, rupture of sinus of valsalva to the right ventricle, or coronary AV fistula draining into the right ventricle. In the presence of a VSD a step-up in oxygen saturation can be detected in the pulmonary artery because of a direct streaming of blood from the left ventricle to the pulmonary artery via the right ventricular outflow tract. It is accepted, however, that a 5% step-up in the pulmonary artery is consistent with an aortic to pulmonary communication (PDA, aortic-pulmonary artery window, or truncus arteriosus).

The saturation from the pulmonary wedge sample is usually 96% or higher. A low saturation drawn from a wedged catheter suggests that the catheter is not wedged or the patient has atelectasis or poor ventilation in that lobe.

The oxygen saturation in the left ventricle is normally equal to the left atrial saturation in the absence of any intercardiac shunting. This is usually 96%, but in the heavily sedated patient it can be as low as 93%. A 5% step-down in left ventricular saturation is consistent with VSD with severe right ventricular outflow obstruction or pulmonary vascular resistance higher than systemic. In a patient with a common ventricle, the saturation in the right and left ventricle are approximately equal. In a patient with very large VSD and normal pulmonary vascular resistance, there is a small right to left shunt, but the step-down does not exceed 5%. The aortic saturation is usually equal to the left ventricular saturation in a normal patient. Occasionally, the saturation in the aorta and pulmonary artery are equal, and this is consistent with complete mixing at the atrial level (common atrium, TAPVC) or the ventricular level (common ventricle) or at the aortic level (truncus arteriosus). In double outlet right ventricle the saturations in the great arteries are usually different and are higher in the vessel more proximal to the ventricular septal defect. A 5% step-down in the aortic saturation is consistent with tetralogy of Fallot (TF), PDA, or aortic-pulmonary window with a high pulmonary vascular resistance. An oxygen saturation in the descending aorta equal to the saturation in the right ventricle in the presence of a relatively normal saturation in the left ventricle is consistent with severe preductal coarctation of the aorta, with the ductus supplying the descending aorta, or TGA. The diagnosis of TGA is confirmed by excluding coarctation of the aorta and an equal peak aortic and right ventricular pressure with a lower peak left ventricular pressure.

In the newborn with persistence of the fetal circulation, there is a right to left shunt at the ductal level, and the saturation in the descending aorta is reduced as compared with the ascending aorta. It is important, therefore, to obtain a right brachial blood sample to exclude this possibility before making the diagnosis of cyanotic heart disease. In some infants, the saturation in the right brachial artery might be 60 to 70%, while it is 90% in the descending aorta. This combination is consistent with TGA, severe preductal coarctation, and pulmonary to descending aortic shunt.

In the presence of an ASD or a patent foramen ovale, it is important to sample some of the pulmonary veins. In the normal patient, the saturation in the pulmonary veins is almost equal and ranges from 95 to 98% with a PO_2 of 90 to 95 mm Hg. In small infants with a large left to right shunt, both saturation and PO_2 are lower, due to the increase in blood volume in the lungs. In these cases, the left atrial saturation might be 90 to 94%. In some infants with atelectasis, the difference in saturation in the various pulmonary veins might be large, and this makes it difficult to quantitate the right to left atrial shunt or pulmonary blood flow using the Fick method because it is impossible to achieve complete mixing of pulmonary venous return before the right to left shunt.

RELATION OF INSPIRED OXYGEN AND BLOOD OXYGEN

In a normal individual breathing room air with an F_iO_2 of 20.9% and a PO_2 of 159 mm Hg (at sea level), the alveolar PO_2 is usually 95 to 100 mm Hg, and the peripheral arterial saturation is approximately 96% with a PO_2 of 90 to 95 mm Hg. In a patient with a hemoglobin concentration of 15 gm/100 ml, the oxygen content in the arterial blood is 19.6 ml/100 ml combined with hemoglobin plus 0.3 ml oxygen dissolved in the plasma. With an increase in F_iO_2 the PO_2 in the alveolar and arterial blood is increased and can reach 700 mm Hg at an F_iO_2 of 100%. This will result in a minimal increase in the oxygen combined with hemoglobin (0.8 ml/100 cc), but in a considerable increase in the dissolved oxygen (0.3 ml for each additional 100 mm Hg of PO_2). Therefore, at 100% F_iO_2, the oxygen content will be 20.4 ml of oxygen combined with hemoglobin and 2 ml of oxygen dissolved in the plasma.

In a cyanotic infant with tetralogy of Fallot and a 60% right to left shunt, or a patient with complete intracardiac mixing and a pulmonary to systemic flow ratio of 0.66, the peripheral arterial saturation will be approximately 68% with a PO_2 of 36 mm Hg. If we increase the F_iO_2 from 20 to 100%, the O_2 saturation will increase from 96 to 100% in the pulmonary venous return, and the dissolved oxygen will increase from 0.3 to 2 ml/100 ml blood. Thus, the oxygen content in the pulmonary venous blood will increase by 3 ml/100. When the above patient breathes 100% oxygen, the O_2 content in the pulmonary venous blood will be 22.5 ml/100 ml, and the aortic saturation will be 77%, or approximately 10% higher. The increase in PO_2 will be less than 10 mm Hg.

If the patient has complete mixing and a pulmonary to systemic flow (Q_p/Q_s) ratio of 3:1 then his aortic saturation on room air will be 87% with a PO_2 of 60, but it will be 100% when the patient breathes 100% oxygen, with a PO_2 of 100 to 150 mm Hg. The difference is due to the larger quantity of oxygen dissolved in a larger pulmonary blood flow (the quantity of dissolved oxygen per 100 ml of blood would remain the same, but the quantity of flow would be increased). This is a very important point since infants with cyanotic congenital heart disease and complete intracardiac mixing can have normal aortic saturation when the infant is breathing oxygen.

CARDIAC OUTPUT AND SHUNTS

FICK METHOD

According to the Fick principle, the blood flow through an organ can be quantitated if an indicator is either added to or removed from the blood during its flow through the organ. Oxygen can be used as an indicator. In a normal person, the systemic venous return is completely mixed at the pulmonary artery level, and the pulmonary venous return is completely mixed at the left ventricular level. Under steady conditions the same amount of oxygen gained in the lungs is also lost to the tissue in the systemic circulation.

Pulmonary flow (Q_p) can be calculated by the equation:

$$Q_p = \frac{\text{oxygen consumption (ml/min)}}{10 \ (PV \ O_2 - PA \ O_2)} = \text{liters/min} \qquad (1)$$

Systemic flow (Q_s) can be calculated by a similar equation:

$$Q_s = \frac{\text{oxygen consumption (ml/min)}}{10 \ (Ao \ O_2 - MVB \ O_2)} = \text{liters/min} \qquad (2)$$

where PV = pulmonary venous return, PA = pulmonary artery, Ao = aorta, MVB = systemic mixed venous blood,

and O_2 = oxygen content. In the presence of a left to right shunt, the pulmonary blood flow is equal to the systemic flow plus the amount of left to right shunt. Therefore, in order to calculate the shunt, it is important to calculate the effective pulmonary blood flow (Q_{ep}). This can be done by assuming that the left to right shunt did not exist and substituting mixed venous blood for pulmonary artery in equation 1. In this case, the effective pulmonary flow is equal to systemic flow. The quantity of the left to right shunt is equal to $Q_p - Q_{ep}$, and the percentage of shunt is equal to $100 \ (Q_p - Q_{ep})/Q_p = \%$ of Q_p.

In the presence of an isolated right to left shunt, systemic flow (Q_s) is equal to the effective systemic flow (Q_{es}) plus the right to left shunt. Q_{es} can be calculated from equation 2 assuming that aortic saturation is equal to left atrial saturation (mixed pulmonary venous return). The Q_s is calculated by using O_2 content in the ascending aorta and the mixed venous blood. Similar to that shown for the pulmonary flow, $Q_s = Q_{es} + $ right to left shunt. The right to left shunt equals $Q_s - Q_{es}$, and the percentage of right to left shunt equals $100 \ (Q_s - Q_{es})/Q_s$.

By substituting and solving the above equations the left to right shunt can be calculated by:

$$L \rightarrow R \text{ shunt} = PA \ O_2 - MVB \ O_2/PV \ O_2 - MVB \ O_2$$
$$R \rightarrow L \text{ shunt} = PV \ O_2 - Ao \ O_2/PV \ O_2 - MVB \ O_2$$

The pulmonary to systemic flow ratio can also be calculated as follows:

$$(Ao \ O_2 - MVB \ O_2)/(PV \ O_2 - PA \ O_2)$$

It should be emphasized that the O_2 content and not the saturation should be used in the above equations. It is recommended that the O_2 content be determined by the Van Slyke method, but since this procedure is quite time-consuming, the oxygen content can be determined from the oxygen capacity and the O_2 saturation in addition to the oxygen dissolved in the plasma. Neglecting the dissolved oxygen introduces only a small error in a patient breathing room air but creates a large error in a patient breathing high F_iO_2. The normal AV difference in dissolved O_2 is only 0.15 vol% for 50 mm Hg difference in PO_2. This represents a 4% error in calculating pulmonary flow in a patient with a Q_p/Q_s ratio of 1:1 and 15% error in calculating pulmonary flow in a patient with a Q_p/Q_s ratio of 4:1. In a patient breathing 100% oxygen, the error in calculation of pulmonary flow could be quite large (50 to 100% error).

In patients with atrial septal defect, others have recommended that $MVB \ O_2 = 0.33 \ SVC \ O_2 + 0.67 \ IVC \ O_2$. The retrograde flow from the right atrium to the inferior vena cava, in addition to the poor mixing in the inferior vena cava increases the O_2 saturation in the IVC and invalidates the method of averaging SVC and IVC. Therefore, only the SVC sample should be used to calculate left to right atrial shunt. In the presence of partial anomalous pulmonary venous return to the superior vena cava, calculation of the shunt is quite unreliable. In a patient with a right to left atrial shunt and different oxygen content in the pulmonary veins, it is impossible to calculate the oxygen content in the mixed pulmonary venous flow, and, therefore, pulmonary blood flow or right to left shunt at the atrial level cannot be determined. In a patient with a VSD and bidirectional shunting, the step-up or step-down in oxygen content is not fully realized at the ventricular level but is only achieved in the great arteries. Therefore, pulmonary and systemic flow or left to right and right to left shunts cannot be determined in the absence of a pulmonary artery and aortic sample, respectively. Similarly, in a patient with an aortic to pulmonary shunt or bidirectional shunt, the oxygen content distal to the site of the shunt is different in the branches of the pulmonary artery or aorta, and therefore pulmonary or systemic flow cannot be determined using the Fick principle. These are examples of some of the serious limitations in calculating cardiac output and shunt. Additional limitations in determining oxygen content include: unsteady state; sampling error; technician error; and the reproducibility of the machines used. Oxygen saturation reading can vary by 2%.

In a patient with complete intracardiac mixing and increased pulmonary blood flow, or a patient with TGA and pulmonary artery saturation higher than 85%, the difference in saturation between the pulmonary artery and the pulmonary vein could be 5 to 10%, and a combined error in determining O_2 saturation could reach 5%. Therefore, the pulmonary AV difference could be overestimated or underestimated by 100%. In a patient with TGA and bronchial collateral flow equal to 10% of systemic flow, it is quite difficult to estimate the bronchial circulation, and therefore the error in calculating pulmonary blood flow can be large. In a patient with TGA with a hemoglobin of 18 gm/100 ml, oxygen capacity is 24.5 ml. If this patient had 4% difference in O_2 saturation between the pulmonary artery and the pulmonary vein, then the AV difference is 0.98 ml oxygen/100 ml blood. If the patient had bronchial circulation with 40% difference in O_2 saturation between the aorta and the pulmonary vein (aorta = 55%, pulmonary vein = 95%), then the aortic to pulmonary venous AV difference is 9.8 ml O_2. This indicates that a bronchial circulation equal to 10% of Q_p would combine with half the O_2 extracted from the lungs. Neglecting this amount will result in 100% overestimation in pulmonary blood flow. The difference in saturation in the different pulmonary veins and the bidirectional interatrial shunting indicate that Q_p and Q_s cannot be determined by the Fick method. The error is much less in patients with tetralogy of Fallot but remains important for the same reasons.

Oxygen Consumption

Oxygen consumption can be calculated from the oxygen concentration and the volume of inspired and expired air. The volume of expired air is frequently different from the volume of inspired air. The inspired volume can be calculated from the expired air. The expired air is collected in a Douglas bag. Older patients can breathe with the nose clamped through a mouth piece connected to the bag. In infants, a plastic bell can be placed over the head. The bell is connected to a T tube and the air pump with air flow in excess of expired volume.

BP, barometric pressure
V_i, total volume of inspired air
$\dot{V}_i$ volume of inspired air per minute
V_e, total volume of expired air
$\dot{V}_e$, volume of expired air per minute
$\dot{V}O_2$, volume of oxygen consumed per minute
$\dot{V}CO_2$, volume of CO_2 expired per minute
F_iO_2, $PO_2/(BP - \text{vapor pressure})$ = Fraction of O_2 in inspired air (3)
F_iCO_2, F_iN_2, fractions of CO_2 and N_2 in inspired air and can be calculated by equation similar to equation 3
F_eO_2, F_eCO_2, F_eN_2, fraction of O_2, CO_2, and N_2, respectively, in expired air
RER, Respiratory exchange ratio = $\dot{V}CO_2/\dot{V}O_2$

This last ratio equals approximately 1 in carbohydrate metabolism and 0.7 in fat metabolism.

In order to calculate VO_2 three corrections should be made:

1. Inspired and expired air volume should be calculated at standard temperature and pressure dry (STPD), (temperature at 0°C or 273 Kelvin, and BP of 760).

2. The expired gas should be collected over 3 to 5 minutes; then the volume should be determined immediately to prevent leak or diffusion of gas, especially CO_2. The volume of a gas will vary, depending on the barometric pressure, temperature, and vapor pressure.

3. The pressure of a dry gas equals actual pressure minus vapor pressure which is fully saturated in expired air (say the BP = 720 and the vapor pressure at room temperature is 20 mm Hg). The conversion factor (STPD) to calculate gas volume at absolute temperature of 0°C or 273 Kelvin at sea level (760 mm Hg) can be calculated from the equation, $P_1 \cdot V_1/T_1 = P_2 \cdot V_2/T_2$, where P_1 = BP dry or $720 - 20 = 700$, V_1 = expired gas volume, T_1 = room temperature (25°C or $273 + 25 = 298$ Kelvin), $P_2 = 760$ mm Hg, $T_2 = 0°C$ or 273 Kelvin, V_2 = volume at STPD, and $V_2 = V_1 \times P_1/P_2 \times T_2/T_1$, after substituting $V_2 = V_1 \times 0.844$. In room air, $F_iO_2 = 0.209$; $F_iCO_2 = 0.003$, which can be neglected; $F_iN_2 = 0.790$. If $VO_2 = VCO_2$, then $F_iN_2 = F_eN_2$, but if $VO_2 > VCO_2$, then expired air is less than inspired air and $P_eN_2 > P_iN_2$, and the following equation will also be true: $V_i \times P_iN_2 = V_i \times P_eN_2$ (4) or $V_e \times F_iN_2 = V_e \times F_eN_2$ (5). V_i, which is not known, can be calculated from equation 4 or 5.

$$V_i = V_e P_e N_2/P_i N_2 \qquad (6)$$

Oxygen consumption per minute can be calculated by the equation:

$$\dot{V}O_2 = \dot{V}_i \times F_iO_2 - \dot{V}_e \times F_eO_2 \qquad (7).$$

After substituting for $\dot{V}_i$ from equation 6, $\dot{V}O_2 = \dot{V}_eF_iO_2 (P_eN_2/P_iN_2) - \dot{V}_eF_eO_2 = \dot{V}_e[F_iO_2 (P_eN_2/P_iN_2) - F_eO_2]$. To derive the partial pressure or fraction of inspired or expired air the following equations should be kept in mind: $F_iO_2 + F_iCO_2 + F_iN_2 = F_eO_2 + F_eCO_2 + F_eN_2 = 1$, and $P_iO_2 + P_iCO_2 + P_iN_2 = P_eO_2 + P_eCO_2 + P_eN_2 = BP - \text{vapor pressure}$.

INDICATOR DILUTION METHODS

The indicators used are usually liquid or gas. They must be: water soluble; nontoxic and cause no cardiorespiratory disturbances; suitable for intravenous injections in a small volume; and not metabolically degraded or excreted from the blood during the first circulation. The indicators must also be detectable and quantitated in whole blood or plasma by one of the following methods: change in light absorption at a definite wavelength; emission of light or fluorescence; emission of ionizing radiation; change in conductivity or voltage between two terminals; or change in the temperature of the circulating blood.

Dyes

Different dyes have been used for this purpose including indocyanine green, Evans blue (T-1824), methylene blue, and Coomassie blue. Evans blue was the most widely used indicator. However, it has major disadvantages; for example, it is slowly excreted, it stains the tissue and combines with albumin, and its maximal light absorption is in the red region with a wavelength of 630 to 650 μ. At this wavelength, reduced hemoglobin and oxyhemoglobin have different light absorption, and the red photocell is more sensitive to reduced hemoglobin. Therefore, any change in the ratio of reduced hemoglobin to oxyhemoglobin will affect light absorption and therefore affect dye curves obtained with Evans blue. Light absorption to reduced hemoglobin and oxyhemoglobin are equal at a wavelength of 805 μm, and at this wavelength indocyanine green has maximum absorption to light. Thus, a change in oxygen saturation does not affect the reading of a dye curve using indocyanine green. Therefore, this dye can be used in all patients irrespective of their type of heart disease. Two minor disadvantages for this dye are that the dye is unstable with time and is affected by temperature.

In performing a dye dilution curve, the dye is injected into the right or the left heart, and the blood is sampled in a peripheral artery. It is crucial that the dye and the blood are completely mixed before reaching the site of sampling. In addition, the concentration of the dye at the site of sampling must be quickly measured. This means that the intravascular catheter, stopcocks, and connecting tubes between the catheter and a cuvette should be as short as possible with a small dead space, and provide minimum resistance to flow. All tubes should be of similar diameter and fit tightly to the stopcocks to eliminate the drawing in of air. The blood should be withdrawn at a constant and fast rate; 25 ml/second is considered satisfactory.

The sampling catheter should be connected to a three way stopcock and then to a short stiff tubing which is connected to the cuvette. This line is flushed with saline. The catheter used for injection is connected to a large diameter short tubing (with 1.5-ml volume) which is connected to a three way stopcock. The dye injected (0.2 ml/kg body weight) is drawn in a small syringe (tuberculin syringe) and mounted to the stopcock. After flushing the tube, the dye is injected into the large bore tube, and withdrawal is begun through the sampling catheter until a base line is established, and the blood is passing the cuvette steadily with no air bubbles. At this point the dye is flushed quickly to the circulation using a 10-ml syringe filled with saline or the patient's blood.

A dye dilution curve can be used to determine the cardiac output and shunting. In order to determine cardiac output, the quantity of dye injected should be determined accurately, and the concentration of the dye in the blood withdrawn should be determined by calibrating the system. This can be accomplished by mixing 10 ml of blood with dye to obtain a concentration of 2.5 mg/liter and 5 mg/liter. These two syringes in addition to a third 10 ml syringe filled with blood are connected to three interconnected stopcocks and a tube to the cuvette. After flushing the cuvette with saline the blood is withdrawn first from the dye-free syringe to establish a base line or zero concentration. The stopcocks are then switched to draw blood from the syringe with a concentration of 2.5 mg/liter; then after a steady state is established the stopcocks are switched to the syringe with 5 mg/liter concentration. This permits three points for the calibration curve.

Cardiac Output. If a known amount (I) of dye is injected and the dye is completely mixed with the blood to obtain a known concentration (C), the volume (V) of the blood can be calculated by the equation: $V = I/C$ (8). The flow however is $F = V/t$ where t = time elapsed (9). After substituting equation 8 into 9, $F = I/C \times t$. The flow per second therefore can be calculated by knowing the quantity of the dye injected (*I*) and the mean concentration of dye during the sampling period (C) and the duration of the sampling period (t). The blood returning to the heart during recirculation prevents the dye concentration from reaching 0, and therefore this part of the recirculation should be excluded when calculating the mean concentration. In order to accomplish this, the downslope of the curve is extrapolated to zero using semilogarithmic paper (Fig. 5.2). The area under the curve is measured (Fig. 5.2) by planimetry. The average deflection is

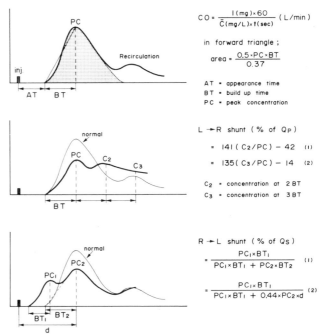

Fig. 5.2 Normal dye curves (*top panel*), left to right shunt (*middle panel*), right to left shunt (*bottom panel*).

then calculated by: area/base = mm paper. The mean concentration is the average deflection divided by the calibration mg per liter. The flow per minute (Q) is given by:

$$CO = \frac{I \text{ (mg)} \times 60}{\bar{C} \text{ (mg per liter)} \times t \text{ (sec)}} = \text{(liters/min)}$$

The above method can be used only in cases where the downslope is well identified. In a patient with a large left to right shunt or valvular insufficiency, however, the downslope cannot be established, and the area under the curve cannot be calculated. In these conditions, the forward triangle method is used to calculate cardiac output. This triangle is shown in Figure 5.2 and can be drawn by extrapolating the base line and dropping a vertical line from the point of peak concentration. It has been shown that in normal circumstances, the area of this triangle is equal to 0.37 of the total area of the dye curve excluding recirculation. Cardiac output, therefore, can be calculated by the equation:

$$Q = \frac{I \times 60}{0.5 \text{ BT} \times \text{PC}} \times 0.37$$

Left to Right Shunt. In the normal patient, the curve obtained after injecting dye into the ascending aorta is different from the curve after injecting dye into the superior vena cava. Usually the peak concentration is highest when injecting in the ascending aorta and becomes gradually less as the site of injection is moved further from the sampling site. Likewise, the peak concentration is lower and the disappearance curve is longer in patients with low cardiac output and large ventricles, valvular regurgitation, and a large left to right shunt. In the patient with left to right shunt, however, we observe a break in the downslope of the curve and a second peak (Fig. 5.2).

In the following discussion we assume that sampling is made in the femoral artery, and we change only the injection site. Injecting into the main pulmonary artery in a patient with mitral stenosis, the curve shows delay in the appearance time and lower concentration as compared with the normal curve. The difference from normal is due to the large blood volume proximal to the mitral valve and the low cardiac output. In patients with valvular insufficiency, the dye curve will be normal if we inject into a site two chambers downstream from the valve involved, i.e., injecting in the ascending aorta in a patient with mitral insufficiency or injecting in the main pulmonary artery in a patient with tricuspid insufficiency. When injecting, however, one chamber distal or proximal to that valve, the curve would have a lower peak concentration and the disappearance curve would be slow and similar to that of a very large left to right shunt, but with no break in the downslope. This is due to the large intracardiac blood volume and delayed washout of the dye.

Localization of the left to right shunt can be made by injecting into the chamber distal to the shunt and the chamber at the site of the shunt. For example, the dye curve in a patient with ASD would be normal if we injected into the left ventricle but would show a left to right shunt if we injected into the left atrium or proximal to the left atrium. This general rule can be applied to all left to right shunts. In patients with an ASD, the curves obtained by injecting into the right or left pulmonary arteries are quite different. In the right pulmonary artery curve, the concentration in the first circulation is less than in the second circulation. In contrast, the left pulmonary artery curve shows a higher concentration in the first circulation. The findings are consistent with the fact that most of the blood returning from the right lung is directly shunted across the atrial defect, while most of the blood returning from the left lung enters the left ventricle and only a small portion is shunted into the right atrium. In a patient with large ASD and PAPVC to the right atrium, the curve recorded injecting into the anomalous pulmonary vein is similar to the curve obtained after injecting into the inferior vena cava and shows a very small initial deflection (right to left shunt) and a much larger recirculation. In a patient with PAPVC and an intact atrial septum, the curves obtained after injecting into the lung with the anomalous drainage show a very long appearance time and a left to right shunt on recirculation. In contrast, the curve obtained after injecting into the lung with the normal pulmonary venous return is normal.

The quantitation of the left to right shunt is based on the concentration of the dye at the peak concentration and intervals thereafter equal to the time lapse from the appearance time to the peak concentration or build-up time (BT). It is assumed that the larger the shunt, the lower is the first peak concentration and the higher is the concentration at two build-up time (BT) and 3 BT. The ratio of the concentration after two build-up time C_{2BT} to the peak concentration PC, and the concentrations at 3 BT to the peak concentration have been correlated with the left to right shunt quantitated by the Fick method. There was a positive correlation between these ratios and the left to right shunt by the Fick method. The following equations also have been established for calculating left to right shunt from the dye curve: $L \rightarrow R$ shunt = 141 (C_{2BT}/PC) − 42 (10), $L \rightarrow R$ shunt = 135 (C_{3BT}/PC) − 14 = % of Qp (11) (Fig. 5.2).

Right to Left Shunt. The basic concept of detecting a right to left shunt is similar to that of a left to right shunt. The site of the right to left shunt can be determined by injecting into the chamber at the site of shunt and one chamber distal to the site of shunt. For example, in a patient with a right to left shunt at the atrial level, a right ventricular injection shows a normal curve, but a right atrial injection shows an early appearance (Fig. 5.2). In the presence of a right to left shunt at the ventricular level, the pulmonary artery injection shows a normal curve, but a right ventricular or a right atrial injection shows an early appearance. Occasionally, however, the right ventricular injection shows a larger right to left shunt, which indicates that the tip of the catheter is at the VSD and that most of the dye is shunted right to left before complete mixing in the right ventricle. The catheter should be positioned in the sinus of the right ventricle. In the presence of a right to left shunt at the ventricular and the atrial level, quantitating the shunt from the right atrial and right ventricular injections can be used to determine the shunt at each site. For example, in a patient with pentalogy of Fallot, the right to left shunt might show 30% of Qs in the ventricular injection and 60% in the atrial injection. Since the atrial injection reflects the sum of the atrial and ventricular shunt, the shunt at each level can be calculated.

The combination of two or more dye curves is very useful in the diagnosis of certain types of cyanotic heart disease. In a patient with truncus arteriosus, common ventricle, or tricuspid atresia, the curves obtained after injecting into the left atrium or the right atrium would be identical and show a large right to left shunt and large left to right shunt. In a patient with TAPVC, the curve obtained after injecting into the left atrium is normal, but the right atrial injection will show a right to left shunt and a large left to right shunt on recirculation. In contrast, in a patient with common atrium, the dye curve obtained after injecting into the right atrium will show bidirectional shunts. In all patients with an isolated right to left shunt at the atrial level, the dye curve is normal after injecting into the left atrium, left ventricle, right ventricle, or pulmonary artery but will show a right to left shunt with a right atrial injection. The presence of valvular insufficiency could lead to the wrong diagnosis in some cases. For example, in a patient with an isolated right to left shunt at the atrial level, the dye curve in right ventricular injection is usually abnormal (right to left shunt) when the tricuspid valve is insufficient. Likewise, in a patient with TGA, a right ventricular injection will show a normal curve but the left ventricular injection will show a delayed appearance and a large left to right shunt.

Quantitation of the right to left shunt is based on two assumptions: the area under the initial curve represents the right to left shunt; and the sum of the areas under the initial curve and the area under the normal curve represents total systemic flow. Therefore, the ratio of the area under the initial curve to the sum of the areas under the initial and the normal curves represents the degree of the right to left shunt, and this can be expressed by the equations shown in Figure 5.2.

Hydrogen

The hydrogen electrode technique is a very sensitive method for detecting a left to right or a right to left shunt. The basic principle of the method depends on the voltage change between an intracardiac platinum tip electrode and the patient's electrocardiogram lead or the cutdown site (ground lead). Initially the voltage is set at zero. Hydrogen ions (H^+) reaching the platinum tip cause an immediate change in the voltage.

For detection of a left to right shunt, the platinum tip electrode is positioned in the pulmonary artery. The patient is then given one breath of hydrogen which should be properly timed by the operator or by placing another platinum electrode in the patient's nostril. The inspired hydrogen diffuses across the alveolar capillary wall and dissolves in the capillary blood, returning to the left atrium and ventricle. In the presence of a left to right shunt, a deflection can be seen within 2 to 3 seconds after inhaling the hydrogen. A deflection after 5 seconds is due to recirculation and can be considered normal. The site of the shunt can be localized by performing consecutive curves with the catheter in the pulmonary artery, right ventricle, right atrium, and the superior vena cava. A positive curve at the ventricular level and a negative curve at the atrial level indicate a ventricular shunt or an aortic to pulmonary shunt with pulmonary valvular insufficiency. In the presence of multiple shunts, only the most proximal shunt can be determined. Thus the curve is positive in all chambers at the site of the shunt and distal to it. This method is very sensitive and will detect a 2 to 3% shunt.

The detection of a right to left shunt can be made by placing the platinum tip catheter in the left side of the heart and by injecting hydrogen dissolved in saline into the right heart. In the normal patient, the hydrogen is completely dissociated from saline during the first circulation in the lungs, and, therefore, the voltage of the platinum electrode shows no deflection. In the presence of a right to left shunt, however, the injection of hydrogen at the site of the shunt or more proximal to it results in a positive deflection.

Isotope

A radioactive isotope, iodine 125, has been used to detect and quantitate shunts. It is essential when using an isotope in the human that the isotope used have a very short half-life, is excreted quickly from the body, and can be disposed of with no hazard of contamination. Heparin labeled with radioactive iodine is used for this purpose and satisfies these conditions. The left to right shunt can be detected by placing the monitoring probe above the right lung. The injection is then made into the right pulmonary artery. The voltage change in this area above the right lung will show normal circulation, and in a normal patient the curve will be similar to the dye dilution curve after injection into the left ventricle. In a patient with a left to right shunt, there will be a break in the downslope of the curve and an early recirculation. This method is quite reliable in detecting a left to right shunt in excess of 25% of pulmonary blood flow.

Quantitation of the left to right shunt is based on the assumption that the area between the recirculation curve and the normal original curve is in proportion to the left to right shunt. The downslope of the curve is extrapolated using semilogarithmic paper to a concentration less than 1% of peak concentration. At that point, a vertical line is drawn to intersect with recorded curve. The ratio of the area between the recirculation curve and the normal curve to the normal curve is calculated; from this ratio, the actual left to right shunt can be calculated.

The right to left shunt is usually detected by positioning one probe above the head to detect circulation and the other probe above the heart. The isotope is then injected into the right side of the heart. In the normal patient, there is a delay in deflection between the heart and the head curves. In the presence of a right to left shunt, however, the deflection in the head curve takes place within 1 to 2 seconds of the heart curve. This technique is quite useful in the diagnosis of infants with cyanotic heart lesions.

Thermodilution

In this method, the indicator is a cool liquid which is usually injected into the right atrium and sampled downstream by a thermistor (in the pulmonary artery or the aorta). The cool liquid reduces the temperature of the blood flowing by the thermistor at the tip of the catheter and shows a deflection similar to that seen with a dye curve. Recirculation is not seen with thermodilution curves. The accuracy of this method depends on the following assumptions: there is minimal loss of temperature in the catheter system between the syringe and the tip of the catheter; heat exchange between the cooled blood and the cardiac chamber and vessels is minimum; there is a minimal fluctuation in

the temperature of the blood; the thermistor is very sensitive to change in temperature; and the system response is fast with a short time constant. This method is quite useful in older children for consecutive measurements of cardiac output.

The cardiac output can be calculated by the equation:

$$CO = \frac{V_i \times S_i \times C_i \times (T_b - T_i) \times 60}{\left(S_b \times C_b \int_0^\infty T_b(t)\, dt \right)} = (ml/min) \qquad (12)$$

where S_i and S_b = specific gravity of indicator and blood, respectively, in gm/cm^3; C_i and C_b, specific heat of indicator and blood, respectively, in calories/gm/degree C; V_i = volume of injectate in ml; T_b = temperature of blood in degrees C; T_i = temperature of indicator, at the point of entrance to the circulation in degrees C; $\int_0^\infty T_b (t)\, dt$ = area (A) under the thermodilution curve in sec times correction factor in degrees C.

The sum $S_i \times C_i / S_b \times C_b = 1.08$ (13). $\int_0^\infty T_b (t)\, dt$ can be written as A/rf, when A is the area of the temperature curve in mm^2, r = recording paper speed in mm/sec, f = temperature calibration factor in mm per $1°C$. After substituting in equation 12,

$$CO = \frac{1.08 \times V_i(T_b - T_i) \times 60}{A/rf} = (ml/min)$$

The thermodilution method is accurate in older children. It is important to calibrate the equipment in small children to ensure the accuracy of the determination. When using ice water it is important that the injection be made immediately after removing the syringe from the ice. The duration of injection should be less than 2 seconds. Also the catheter should be short. After completing the injection, 1 ml should be withdrawn from the catheter to avoid continuous cooling of the thermistor.

This method is quite useful in determining cardiac output in patients postoperatively, and in quantitating pulmonary blood flow in patients with TGA with intact ventricular septum by injecting in the left ventricle with the thermistor in one of the branches of the pulmonary artery.

MEASUREMENT OF PRESSURES

GENERAL COMMENTS

Intracardiac pressure can be recorded by a pressure transducer connected to an end hole catheter or side hole catheter or by a pressure-tip transducer catheter. As noted previously, it is important to use a large pore catheter to enhance the frequency response. The connecting tube between the catheter and the pressure transducer should be short, large in diameter, and stiff-walled. In addition, the catheter, stopcocks, connecting catheter, and the pressure transducer should be flushed well to eliminate all air bubbles, and the intravascular catheter should be flushed repeatedly to prevent clot formation in the catheter. The system should not have a leak. This usually results in the maximum frequency response for a given catheter and eliminates pressure damping. The frequency response for a no. 6 or 7 catheter is adequate for physiologic pressure recording. A fluid-filled catheter, however, adds a kinetic force to the actual pressure during isovolumic contraction, and it subtracts the kinetic force during isovolumic relaxation. This results in a higher ventricular pressure first derivative. In addition, the end hole catheter adds 2 to 4 mm Hg when facing the flow and it subtracts 2 to 3 mm Hg when the tip is pointed in the direction of the flow. A pressure-tip transducer catheter records the high-frequency (50 cycles/second) ventricular pressures free from the kinetic energy component, and it facilitates the accurate determination of first derivative ventricular pressure. An additional advantage of the pressure-tip transducer catheter with two transducers at the tip or one transducer and a side hole is the ability to record two pressures simultaneously from the same catheter (Fig. 5.3).

The pressure transducers should be set at the level of the midlateral chest wall. A zero base line and calibration should be obtained before recording any pressure. It is also important when using two pressure transducers to make sure that both transducers have the same gain and zero base line. It is not unusual to record a difference in the left and the right ventricular pressures in a patient with equal ventricular pressures if different transducers and amplifiers are used with poor calibration. Therefore, it is generally more reliable to obtain a pullback pressure to determine the gradient rather than using a different catheter and pressure transducer.

It is desirable to perform the recording of pressure in the following sequence: first introduce the end hole catheter into the pulmonary artery wedge position; then record the pressure pulling back from this position to the right atrium. The catheter is then replaced with a side hole catheter. This catheter is then introduced into the main pulmonary artery, and another pressure is recorded upon pullback. The pressure should be done with the patient quiet and as fast as possible to eliminate minute to minute variation in the patient's status. In addition, all pressure recordings should be done before the injection of contrast media or intravenous medications.

RIGHT HEART

The pulmonary artery wedge pressure in a normal patient reflects the pressure in the left atrium and the pulmonary veins. The mean pulmonary artery wedge pressure is approximately 2 mm Hg higher than the mean left atrial pressure and ranges from 10 to 15 mm Hg with a mean of 12. The relative position of the tip of the catheter to the heart and the pressure transducer affect the pressure reading, and therefore the wedge pressure in a posterior pulmonary segment could be 5 to 7 mm Hg higher than the wedge pressure in an anterior pulmonary segment. Neglecting this normal

difference can lead to an important error in interpretation. When it is difficult to record the wedge pressure with a Lehman catheter, the end-hole balloon catheter can be used to measure pressure in the peripheral pulmonary artery after inflating the balloon. A very low wedge pressure in the right or the left lung suggests that the patient has partial anomalous pulmonary venous connection from that lobe. A very high wedge pressure is consistent with poor wedging of the catheter, mitral stenosis or mitral insufficiency, or pulmonary venous obstruction.

The pulmonary artery pressure usually ranges from 20/10 mm Hg (mean = 13) to 35/15 mm Hg (mean = 22). The peak systolic and diastolic pressures increase with an increase in pulmonary arteriolar resistance, pulmonary venous obstruction, mitral stenosis, mitral insufficiency, or increased pulmonary blood flow. The diastolic pulmonary artery pressure is usually 1 to 3 mm Hg higher than the left atrial pressure in the normal patient. The pulmonary artery diastolic pressure can be less than 10 mm Hg in patients with severe valvar pulmonary regurgitation, or pulmonary artery banding, or pulmonary artery branch stenosis. The pulse pressure is usually less than 40% of the peak systolic pressure in patients with fixed resistance (pulmonary vascular obstructive disease or pulmonary venous obstruction). In patients with pulmonary hypertension and increase in pulmonary blood flow (hyperkinetic pulmonary hypertension), the pulse pressure exceeds 40% and can reach 60% of the peak systolic pressure. In patients with valvar pulmonary stenosis, the time to peak pressure is prolonged and shows an anacrotic notch. In patients with pulmonary artery banding or peripheral pulmonary stenosis, the pressure proximal to the stenotic area is ventriculized; both peak systolic and diastolic pressures are equal to right ventricular pressure. The difference between the two pressures, however, is in diastole. The pulmonary artery pressure in these cases has a dichrotic notch in early diastole and the lowest pressure is recorded at end diastole. In contrast, the ventricular pressure has no dicrotic notch and the lowest pressure is recorded in early diastole (Fig. 5.4).

In the presence of valvar and/or infundibular stenosis, the best pressure recording can be obtained with an end hole catheter. This facilitates the recording of the pressure in the small infundibular chamber, and it avoids the simultaneous pressure recording in two chambers. In the presence of valvar and infundibular stenosis, the transition from the pulmonary artery pressure to the infundibular pressure can be identified by observing the right ventricular pressure contour with its low peak systolic pressure. The transition from the infundibular chamber to the ventricular chamber will have no effect on the diastolic pressure but shows an increase in the peak systolic pressure.

On pullback of the catheter across a narrow segment in the peripheral pulmonary artery or in the infundibular region, it is possible to record a lower pressure than the distal pressure. The lower pressure in the narrow segment is due to two factors: (a) the actual lateral pressure in the narrow segment is usually lower than the pressure in the distal segment due to the higher velocity of flow in this segment and the conversion of lateral pressure to a kinetic energy component; (b) the kinetic energy component is subtracted from the lateral pressure when using an end hole catheter, thereby increasing the pressure difference between the narrow segment and the distal branch. In the normal patient, the gradient across the right ventricular outflow tract and the pulmonary valve is usually less than 10 mm Hg. In patients with increased pulmonary blood flow, this gradient can be higher. Although a gradient of 70 mm Hg has been described in patients with atrial septal defect, I have not

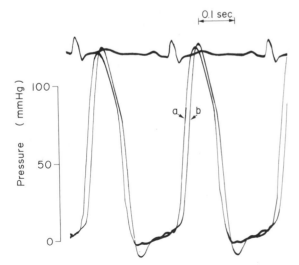

Fig. 5.3 Left ventricular pressure recorded with a tip transducer pressure catheter. *a,* The pressure recorded from the microtransducer on the tip of the catheter; *b,* the pressure recorded by the external transducer.

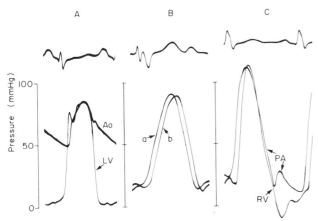

Fig. 5.4 (A) Left ventricular (LV) and aortic (Ao) pressure in a patient with tetralogy of Fallot. (B) Right ventricular pressure in a patient with isolated valvular pulmonary stenosis; a and b are similar to points a and b in Figure 5.3. (C) Simultaneous recording of right ventricular (RV) and pulmonary artery (PA) in a patient with peripheral pulmonary branch stenosis.

recorded a flow gradient in excess of 25 mm Hg in the absence of valvular or infundibular stenosis. In all patients with gradient more than 10 mm Hg, a right ventricular and pulmonary artery cineangiocardiogram should be made to rule out infundibular and valvular obstruction.

In the normal patient, the peak systolic right ventricular pressure is usually less than 35 mm Hg, and the shape of the pressure curve is rectangular. Right ventricular end-diastolic pressure averages 4 mm Hg ± 3 (SD). In the presence of a nonrestrictive VSD or very large aortic to pulmonary communication, the contour of right ventricular pressure is similar to that of the left ventricle and remains rectangular. In the presence of a restrictive VSD or an intact ventricular septum with pulmonary stenosis, the contour of right ventricular pressure is a symmetrical triangle and peaks at midsystole (Fig. 5.4B). The difference in pressure contour is quite useful in differentiating valvular pulmonary stenosis (PS) from a large VSD. During a premature ventricular contraction (PVC), the ventricular pressure is less than in a normal beat. The right ventricular pressure in the post-PVC beat is higher than in a normal beat and equal to the aortic pressure in patients with large VSD, but higher than aortic pressure in patients with isolated PS. In a patient with VSD and equal left ventricular and right ventricular pressure, the administration of tolazoline hydrochloride (Priscoline) produces a difference between left ventricle (LV) and right ventricle (RV) pressure (RV pressure < LV pressure) in patients with a restrictive VSD, but does not in patients with a large VSD.

The pullback pressure from the right ventricle to the right atrium shows no significant diastolic gradient (diastolic gradient less than 2 mm Hg in the latter half of diastole). The pressures in the right atrium, superior vena cava, and inferior vena cava are identical in the normal patient. A pressure difference between the superior or inferior vena cava and the right atrium suggests obstruction. The dominant pressure wave in the right atrium is the "a" wave, which is seen at the lateral half of the P wave on the electrocardiogram. The C wave is associated with ventricular contraction and the V wave is associated with atrial filling and peaks at the end of ventricular systole. The mean right atrial pressure ranges from 1 to 7 mm Hg (mean = 4) and the "a" wave ranges from 5 to 10 mm Hg. An increase in peak and mean right atrial pressures is observed in patients with tricuspid atresia, tricuspid stenosis, pulmonary atresia, severe pulmo-

nary stenosis with or without VSD, TAPVC, and idiopathic pulmonary hypertension. An increase in mean right atrial pressure with a dominant V wave is associated with tricuspid insufficiency, Ebstein's anomaly, and left ventricular to right atrial shunt. Equal "a" and V waves or dominant V wave with normal right atrial pressure suggests a large interatrial communication (Fig. 5.5). A prominent "a" wave occurring during ventricular systole is diagnostic of atrial ventricular block.

LEFT HEART

The pressure in the left atrium (mean, 10 to 13 mm Hg) is higher than the right atrial pressure. The V wave is dominant in the left atrium. An increase in the left atrial pressure with a prominent V wave is seen in VSD, large PDA, and mitral insufficiency. A prominent "a" wave in the left atrium is observed in patients with: decreased left ventricular compliance (coarctation of the aorta and severe aortic stenosis), left heart failure with increased left ventricular diastolic pressure, severe aortic insufficiency, and mitral stenosis. The "a" wave is dominant in patients with dominant right to left interatrial shunt, TAPVC, tricuspid atresia, and pulmonary atresia with intact ventricular septum. A mean pressure difference of more than 2 mm Hg between the left and right atrium suggests that the patient has a restrictive interatrial communication.

When recording atrial pressure, it is important to be sure that the tip of the catheter is not in the mitral or tricuspid valve region. In addition, the pressure should be recorded when the patient is quiet, and all pressure measurements should be made at end expiration. A difference in pressure contour between the left and right atrium is evidence against large interatrial communication. An equal mean pressure in the two atria, however, is not diagnostic of a large interatrial communication and can be seen in patients with increased right atrial pressure and poor interatrial communication.

A pullback pressure from the left ventricle to the left atrium usually shows no diastolic gradient. In patients with mitral stenosis, there is a diastolic gradient through all of diastole, and the gradient increases with atrial contraction.

The peak systolic left ventricular pressure ranges from 50 to 60 mm Hg in the premature infant, 65 to 80 mm Hg in the full-term infant, and averages 103 ± 10 mm Hg in normal children. The left ventricular pressure contour is rectangular in normal patients, and more triangular in patients with severe aortic stenosis. The left ventricular end-diastolic pressure (LVEDP) averages 10 ± 3 mm Hg in normal children

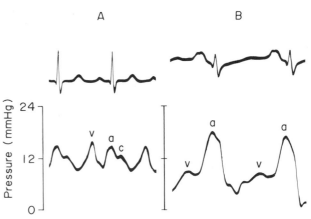

Fig. 5.5 (A) Right atrial pressure (RAP) in a patient with atrial septal defect, (B) RAP in a child with severe isolated valvar pulmonic stenosis.

and is higher than 15 mm Hg in most patients with concentric hypertrophy (aortic stenosis or coarctation of the aorta), aortic insufficiency, myopathy, and pericardial tamponade. Interestingly, left ventricular end-diastolic pressure is normal in infants in heart failure with a large left to right ventricular or ductal shunt.

In normal patients, on pullback from the left ventricle to the aorta, the pressure gradient is usually less than 5 mm Hg. The aortic pulse pressure is usually 30 to 35% of peak systolic pressure. In patients with valvular aortic stenosis, the aortic pressure has an anacrotic notch, and the time to peak pressure is usually delayed. In patients with idiopathic hypertrophic subaortic stenosis or aortic insufficiency, the anacrotic notch is not seen, and the time to peak pressure is usually normal. In these instances, however, the aortic pressure has a double peak (bisferious pulse). The pulse pressure is increased (with a low diastolic pressure) in patients with aortic insufficiency, rupture of the sinus of valsalva, large coronary arteriovenous fistula, truncus arteriosus, aortico-pulmonary window, large patent ductus arteriosus, systemic arteriovenous fistula, and surgical aortic to pulmonary shunt. The pressure in the peripheral arteries is higher than the ascending aorta due to wave reflection, and amplification of the pressure in the arteries (resonance).

In 47 children with a normal left heart studied in our laboratories, the peak systolic pressure in the femoral artery averaged 12 mm Hg (5 to 30) higher than the pressure in the ascending aorta. The average diastolic pressure in the femoral artery was 2 mm Hg less than the average diastolic pressure in the ascending aorta. The mean pressures were equal. The data suggest that mild aortic stenosis cannot be ruled out by recording the left ventricular and femoral artery pressures.

The pressure in the right arm can be higher than the pressure in the left arm in patients with supravalvular aortic stenosis (Coanda effect) or in patients with coarctation of the aorta. The pressure in the right arm is lower than the pressure in the left arm in patients with coarctation of the aorta and aberrant right subclavian artery.

CALCULATION OF VASCULAR RESISTANCE

The flow ($\dot{Q}$) in cylindrical tubes is determined by: Poiseuille's law: $\dot{Q} = P \cdot r^4/8nL$ (14), where $\dot{Q}$ = flow, P = mean pressure gradient, r = the radius of the tube, n = the viscosity of the fluid, and L = the length of the tube, conductance = $\dot{Q}/P = r^4/8nL$ (15); and resistance = $1/conductance = P/\dot{Q} = 8nL/r^4$ (16).

The calculation of resistance, described above, assumes that: the blood viscosity, the length of the vessels, and the radius of the vessels are all constant and that the pressure and flow are nonpulsatile. Since these conditions do not exist in vivo, the calculation of resistance is an approximation of the true resistance in the vascular bed. In addition, the resistance between points *a* and *b* is calculated with the assumption that: flow between these two points is nonpulsatile; the amount of fluid entering at point *a* is equal to the amount of fluid leaving at point *b*; no fluid enters or leaves the circulation between *a* and *b*, and there is no narrowing in the vessels between *a* and *b*.

Examples where the above principles are violated and the calculation of vascular resistance is inaccurate include patients with: PDA, valvar insufficiency, pulmonary AV fistula, or partial or complete obstruction in the major vessels.

The systemic vascular resistance (Rs) is calculated by the equation, Rs = (mean aortic pressure minus mean right atrial pressure)/systemic flow (liter/minute) = (mm Hg/liter/minute).

It is obvious that the size of the patient will affect the calculated Rs. For example, in an infant with a cardiac output of 1.0 liter/minute and a mean systemic pressure of 50 mm Hg the systemic vascular resistance is 50 mm Hg/liter/minute. In contrast, the resistance in an older child with similar pressure and a cardiac output of 5 liters/minute, the calculated resistance is 10 mm Hg/liter/minute. For this reason, it is important to calculate the resistance using the cardiac index. The systemic vascular resistance normalized for patient size in infants (9 to 12 mm Hg/liter/minute/m²) is usually lower than that of older children (13 to 18 mm Hg/liter/minute/m²). Occasionally, systemic vascular resistance is calculated using only mean aortic pressure and neglecting right atrial pressure. The term total systemic vascular resistance is given to this value.

The systemic vascular resistance varies with the patient's sympathetic tone, sedation, and contrast media injection. Therefore, it is important to determine the pressure and flow in the steady state before injection of contrast media.

The pulmonary vascular resistance (Rp) is calculated by the equation, Rp = (mean pulmonary artery pressure minus mean left atrial pressure)/pulmonary flow. Pulmonary vascular resistance should also be expressed in mm Hg/liter/minute/m².

In a normal individual, the pressure at the capillary level is higher than the pressure in the left atrium (waterfall phenomenon). Therefore, the mean pressure difference between the pulmonary artery and the left atrium is higher than the actual pressure difference across the pulmonary arterioles. Thus, the pulmonary vascular resistance calculated by the above equation is usually slightly higher than the actual pulmonary arteriolar resistance. This difference, however, is quite small and has no effect on the management of the patient.

In infants with PDA or VSD and large left to right shunt, the left atrial pressure is higher than normal due to the increase in pulmonary blood flow. In addition, heart failure further increases the left atrial pressure. For these reasons it is important to measure the left atrial pressure or pulmonary artery wedge pressure when calculating the pulmonary vascular resistance.

Another calculation which can lead to an erroneous conclusion is the pulmonary to systemic resistance ratio. As discussed above, systemic vascular resistance can vary during the course of cardiac catheterization, and this can exaggerate or underestimate the pulmonary vascular resistance.

The pulmonary vascular resistance is usually less than 2 mm Hg/liter/minute/m² in the normal patient and less than 3 mm Hg in the patient with hyperkinetic pulmonary hypertension. In patients with pulmonary hypertension and slightly increased pulmonary vascular resistance, it is assumed that some of the increase in resistance is due to active constriction by the smooth muscles of the pulmonary arterioles which is reversible with the administration of high F_iO_2 or α blocker (Priscoline). In the presence of a normal arterial oxygen saturation, giving oxygen has no effect on the pulmonary vascular resistance. On the other hand, Priscoline (1 mg/kg) injected slowly into the pulmonary artery produces pulmonary vasodilitation and a decrease in peripheral vascular resistance for 10 to 15 minutes after its administration. A positive response (decrease in pulmonary vascular resistance) in patients with ASD is manifested by a decrease in peak systolic pressure in the right ventricle and a decrease in peak systolic, end-diastolic, and mean pulmonary artery pressures. In patients with a large VSD, peak systolic pressure in the right ventricle and pulmonary artery remains systemic, but the diastolic and the mean pulmonary artery pressure decrease with an increase in the left to right shunt.

In the presence of a large aortic to pulmonary artery communication, the changes in the peak systolic and diastolic pressures in the great vessels are identical, but there is usually an increase in the left to right shunt.

When the patient is breathing a high F_iO_2, the calculation of the pulmonary and systemic blood flow by the Fick method should be based on O_2 content, since the dissolved oxygen in pulmonary venous blood is 2 vol%.

CALCULATION OF AORTIC AND PULMONIC VALVE AREAS

The area of a stenotic valve can be determined from the mean flow across the valve in milliliters per second and the mean pressure difference across the valve. The flow across an orifice can be determined by the equation: $F = A VC_e$ (17), where F is the flow across the orifice in milliliters per second, A = the area of the orifice in cm^2, V = velocity of flow in milliliters per second, and C_e = coefficient to compensate for orifice contraction. $V^2 = C_v^2 \, 2 \, gh$ or $V = Cv\sqrt{2 \, gh}$ (18), where g = gravity acceleration (980 cm/second), V = velocity of flow in centimeters per second, h = pressure gradient $(P_1 - P_2)$, and C_v = coefficient of velocity. Combining equations 17 and 18, we get: $A = F/(C_e \times C_v \times \sqrt{2 \, g} \times P_1 - P_2)$ (19), where $\sqrt{2 \, g} = \sqrt{1960} = 44.5$ and $A = F/(C_e \times 44.5 \sqrt{P_1 - P_2})$ (20). C for the aortic and pulmonary valve is equal to 1. F = cardiac output (milliliters per minute)/EP (seconds per minute) = (milliliters per second), where EP = systolic ejection period.

The pressure in the left ventricle and aorta or in the right ventricle and pulmonary artery can be recorded simultaneously with a double lumen catheter or a pressure-tip transducer catheter. Since these are not available in most laboratories, a pullback pressure is recorded. The systolic ejection period is defined as the period between the opening of the aortic valve (the end of isovolumic contraction) and the diacrotic notch. The mean aortic and left ventricular pressures during the ejection period are calculated by planimetry, and the difference represents the gradient across the valve (Fig. 5.6). The gradient across the pulmonic valve is calculated in a similar manner.

CALCULATION OF MITRAL VALVE AREA

The mean flow per second across the mitral valve can be calculated from the cardiac output and the diastolic filling period per minute. The diastolic filling period is the period from the end of isovolumic relaxation to the beginning of isovolumic contraction. This corresponds to the points where the left atrial pressure crosses the left ventricular pressure (Fig. 5.6). The diastolic filling period (DFP) per minute is calculated by multiplying the diastolic filling period per beat times the heart rate. The mean flow (F) across the mitral valve is calculated by the equation:

$$F = \frac{\text{Cardiac output (ml/min)}}{\text{DFP (sec/min)}} = \text{(ml/sec)}$$

The pressure in the left ventricle and left atrium or pulmonary wedge pressure are recorded simultaneously. The mean pressure gradient is calculated from the area (mm^2) between the two pressure curves and diastolic filling period per beat in millimeters by the equation, mean gradient = area (mm^2)/base (mm) × calibration.

For the mitral valve the empiric constant (C) is 0.7 when the diastolic filling period is derived from the aortic and left ventricular pressure curves, and 0.85 when the diastolic filling period is determined from the atrial and ventricular pressure (excluding isovolumic contraction and isovolumic

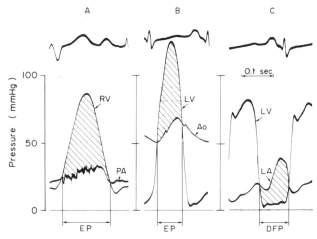

Fig. 5.6 (*A*) Right ventricular (*RV*) and pulmonary (*PA*) pressure in a patient with isolated valvular pulmonary stenosis. *EP*, ejection period. (*B*) Left ventricular (*LV*) and aortic (*Ao*) pressure in a patient with valvular aortic stenosis. (*C*) Left atrial (*LA*) and *LV* pressure in a patient with mitral stenosis. *DFP*, diastolic filling period.

relaxation periods). The constant in equation 20, therefore, will be $0.7 \times 44.5 = 31$ when using aortic pressure and $0.85 \times 44.5 = 38$ when using a ventricular and left atrial pressure to determine diastolic filling period.

CINEANGIOCARDIOGRAPHY

TYPES OF CONTRAST MEDIA

The three types of contrast media commercially available and used in pediatric cardiology (Renografin, Renovist, and Hypaque) all contain a high sodium concentration, iodine, and methylglucamine iothalamat. In older infants and children, a 70 to 80% concentration is used for injection. In small infants and premature babies a 50% concentration is used for injection.

AMOUNT OF CONTRAST MEDIA

In patients with a normal heart size, who do not have a large left to right shunt, the ventricular chambers and vessels can well be visualized by injecting 1 to 1.25 ml/kg in the atria and ventricles, 1.25 ml/kg in the pulmonary artery, and 0.75 to 1 ml/kg in the aorta. In patients with a large left to right shunt and large cardiac chambers, the amount of contrast media should be increased by 20 to 30%. The contrast media should be warmed to body temperature before it is injected and should be injected in a large bore catheter with side holes or a balloon catheter. An end hole catheter should not be used for injection of contrast media. During the injection the catheter should move freely and there should be no evidence of dysrhythmia. A test injection of 3 to 4 ml of diluted contrast (25% concentration) should be injected immediately prior to the main injection to ensure that the catheter is not wedged in the ventricle or in the coronary artery. In general, the catheter should be positioned in the ventricular sinus during ventricular injections and the length of one vertebrae above the aortic valve during aortograms.

SEQUENCE OF INJECTIONS

The sequence of cineangiocardiograms is determined by the anticipated cardiac anomaly. The most important cine for the patient should be done first (i.e., right ventricular injection in a patient with tetralogy of Fallot and pulmonary artery injection in a patient with ASD or PAPVC). It is important that the total amount of contrast media injected does not exceed 4 ml/kg of body weight, but in certain very complicated cardiac lesions it might be necessary to do an additional injection and exceed this limit.

REACTIONS TO CONTRAST MEDIA

The side effects of contrast media include: coronary vasodilitation; increase in coronary blood flow; depression in myocardial contractility; flushing of the skin and warm feeling due to peripheral vasodilitation; transient increase in blood volume; increase in acidosis in the small sick infant; and a reduction of oxygen carrying capacity by a shift in the hemoglobin dissociation curve to the right. The warm feeling experienced by the patient 1 to 2 seconds after injection can be alarming, and thus, this should be explained in advance to older patients. To avoid some of these complications, the patient should be well hydrated, and patients with heart failure should receive diuretics intravenously.

SITES OF INJECTION

It is important that the study be complete and outline all of the cardiac defects present. Occasionally when attention is focused on one defect, other associated defects are missed. This can be avoided by reviewing all the clinical data before study, and by reviewing the pressure and oxygen saturation data before beginning the injection. Each cine injection should be reviewed by video tape immediately after each injection. The complete cardiac catheterization should provide an accurate diagnosis, delineate the severity of the anatomy and the size of the cardiac chambers and the great vessels, and determine cardiac function. Axial cineangiography is very useful in most cardiac defects (see recent publications by Bargeron and co-workers). The following is a brief outline of the sites of injection for different defects:

1. In ASD or PAPVC the first injection should be made into the main pulmonary artery. A left ventricular injection will delineate an associated abnormal mitral valve, or a VSD.
2. In VSD, the first injection should be made into the pulmonary artery to delineate an associated ASD or PAPVC. In the absence of an ASD or PAPVC, this injection will show the interventricular shunt. A left ventricular injection should be done in the long axial rotated view (lateral tube) to delineate membranous and muscular defects and in the four chamber view (vertical tube) to delineate a posterior VSD or ventricular to atrial shunt.
3. In right ventricular outflow obstruction the first injection should be made into the right ventricle in the axial sitting up position (vertical tube). In TF, the size of the main pulmonary artery and branches should be delineated. In addition, the aortic arch, the size of the aortic branches, and the coronary arteries should be well visualized.
4. In mitral insufficiency, the first injection should be made into the left ventricle.
5. In aortic stenosis, the injections should be made into the left ventricle in the long axial oblique view (lateral tube) and into the ascending aorta in the AP and lateral views. When membranous subvalvular aortic obstruction is expected, a small injection should be made immediately below the aortic valve.
6. In aortic insufficiency or CA, the injection should be made into the ascending aorta approximately one vertebrae above the aortic valve.
7. In TAPVC, the first injection should be made into the main pulmonary artery. An additional injection should be made into the left atrium or the left ventricle to delineate the size of these chambers.
8. When tricuspid atresia is entertained the injection should be made into the inferior vena cava right atrial junction in the anterior-posterior and lateral views as well as the four chamber view (vertical tube).
9. With a possible diagnosis of mitral stenosis or hypoplasia of the mitral valve, a left ventricular injection should be made in the anterior-posterior and lateral views.
10. The possible diagnosis of common ventricle requires four injections into: the anatomic left ventricle in the long axial oblique view (lateral tube); the anatomic right ventricle in the four chamber view (vertical tube); and the left and right atrium in the four chamber view.
11. Double outlet right ventricle requires two ventricular injections (left and right) and a left atrial injection to delineate the aortic-mitral valve continuity.
12. In patients with valvar pulmonary atresia it is important to delineate the size of the main pulmonary artery and branches. In the absence of a large PDA one must hand-inject into a large bronchial artery and/or the pulmonary veins with an end hole catheter in the wedge position. These injections usually outline the pulmonary arteries.
13. In addition to the above injections it is important in certain defects to delineate the size and function of the right or left ventricle, and this can be accomplished by injecting into the right or left ventricle in the anterior-posterior or lateral view.

MEASUREMENT OF VENTRICULAR FUNCTION

GENERAL COMMENTS

The right and left ventricles function as a pump which is filled during diastole and empties portions of its contents during systole. The cardiac output depends on: ventricular size at end diastole (end-diastolic volume); the force of ventricular contraction; the resistance to ventricular ejection (afterload); and the heart rate. The left ventricular volume can be determined accurately from biplane cineangiocardiography by the area length method, assuming that the left ventricle is an elipsoid. Using this method the left ventricular volume can be determined for each cine frame. Thus, a ventricular volume curve can be constructed for the total cardiac cycle. The left ventricular pressure can be recorded simultaneously during cineangiocardiograms, and from left ventricular pressure and volume curves we can construct a pressure-volume loop.

In the normal patient there is no major change in left ventricular volume during isovolumic contraction and isovolumic relaxation. The left ventricular volume however, decreases during isovolumic contraction in patients with large VSD, mitral insufficiency, or left ventricular to right atrial shunt. The left ventricular volume increases during isovolumic relaxation in patients with aortic insufficiency, TF, or large VSD with equal pressure in the right and left ventricles.

The left ventricular end-diastolic volume increases in patients with poor myocardial contraction, aortic or mitral insufficiency, VSD with large left to right shunt, aortic to pulmonary communication, and systemic AV fistula with volume overload. A decrease in left ventricular size is seen in patients with hypoplasia of the left ventricle and/or hypoplasia of the mitral valve, TAPVC, large ASD, and severe aortic stenosis.

The right ventricular volume can also be determined from biplane cineangiocardiogram according to Simpson's rule method. The right ventricular end-diastolic volume increases in patients with myopathy, tricuspid or pulmonary valve insufficiency, and large left to right shunt proximal to the ventricular level.

Definition of Terms

Ventricular end-diastolic volume (EDV)
= ventricular volume at end-diastole
End-systolic volume (ESV) = ventricular volume at end-systole
Stroke volume (SV) = EDV − ESV
Ejection fraction (EF) = stroke volume/end-diastolic volume
Cardiac output = stroke volume × heart rate

CLINICAL APPLICATION

Figures 5.7 and 5.8 show normal right ventricular end-diastolic volume and output in children. The cardiac output increases linearly with body surface area in children and averages 4.5 liters/minute/m^2. In a patient, the cardiac output is dependent on: adequate filling of the ventricle ("preload"); myocardial contractility; heart rate; and the resistance to ventricular ejection (afterload). In the normal patient the left ventricular and right ventricular stroke volumes calculated from biplane cineangiocardiograms are equal to the stroke volume calculated by the Fick method or by dilution curves. In a patient with aortic or mitral insufficiency, left ventricular stroke volume derived by cine is equal to the sum of the forward stroke volume plus the regurgitant flow: left ventricular stroke volume (cine) equals forward aortic flow plus regurgitant flow. Hence, regurgitant fraction = [stroke volume (cine) minus forward flow (Fick)]/stroke volume (cine).

In a patient with VSD or PDA, the cine left ventricular stroke volume is equal to the forward flow (Q_s) plus the left to right shunt (not accounting for the diastolic interventricular shunt in VSD). Therefore, the left ventricular systolic output is an approximation of pulmonary blood flow.

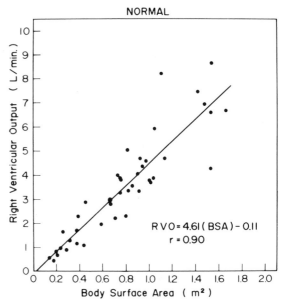

Fig. 5.8　Right ventricular cardiac output as a function of body surface area.

The right ventricular stroke volume also increases in the presence of valvar, pulmonic, or tricuspid insufficiency, and in patients with ASD or anomalous pulmonary venous connection.

The quantitation of right and left ventricular volume parameters can be used to determine the severity of valvar regurgitation or the degree of left to right shunt. For example, in the patient with mitral insufficiency, the right ventricular stroke volume and output are equal to forward systemic flow. The left ventricular stroke volume, however, is equal to the regurgitant flow and forward stroke volume. Therefore, the difference between right ventricular stroke volume and left ventricular stroke volume represents the regurgitant flow. In the presence of tricuspid insufficiency, right ventricular stroke volume is equal to left ventricular stroke volume plus the regurgitant flow.

In a patient with normal ventricular volume, the end-diastolic volume represents the initial muscle length at the beginning of contraction. In a patient with normal end-diastolic volume (normal preload) and normal ventricular pressure (normal afterload), the ventricular ejection fraction represents a crude index of ventricular contractility. An acute increase in the preload or a decrease in the afterload results in a higher ejection fraction with no change in myocardial contractility. On the other hand, an acute decrease in the preload or an increase in the afterload results in a decrease in ejection fraction with no change in myocardial contractility. The afterload represents wall tension which is equal to the sum of ventricular pressure times the radius of the ventricle.

COMPLICATIONS

One of the most common complications during cardiac catheterization is *dysrhythmia*. Paroxysmal atrial tachycardia can be terminated by moving the tip of the catheter against the right atrial wall to induce premature atrial contraction. When this maneuver is not successful a gentle thump on the chest might terminate the tachycardia. When this maneuver also is not successful, DC shock will terminate the dysrhythmia.

The second most common dysrhythmia is first or second

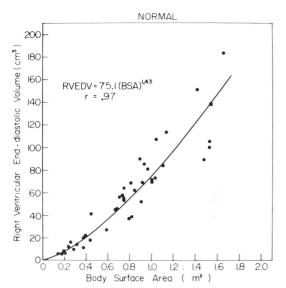

Fig. 5.7　Right ventricular end-diastolic volume as a function of body surface area.

degree heart block. This will usually occur when a large loop is formed in the right atrium or the tip of the catheter is forced against the right ventricle. When this occurs, it is important to withdraw the catheter and release the atrial loop. If this fails atropine, 0.01 mg/kg, should be given intravenously. Sinus bradycardia also can be managed by giving atropine intravenously.

Maneuvering the catheter in the ventricle occasionally causes premature ventricular contractions which can lead to ventricular tachycardia and fibrillation. This can be avoided by gently maneuvering the catheter in the ventricle and immediately withdrawing the catheter at any time ventricular tachycardia is observed. If, however, ventricular fibrillation occurs, immediate DC shock should be given to the patient.

Acidosis due to hypoventilation and heavy sedation can be managed by administering oxygen and assisted ventilation if needed. If the patient has received meperidine or morphine, the patient should be given *N*-allylnormorphine (Nalline). If the acidosis is due to low cardiac output, an effort should be made to improve cardiac output by administering an inotropic agent.

Shock and *severe hypotension* can be avoided by reducing the blood loss due to bleeding and by avoiding frequent blood sampling. In small infants who require arteriotomy, when blood loss is expected it is important to have the blood typed and cross-matched for immediate transfusion if needed. In all infants less than 5 kg, blood loss and fluid infusion should be quantitated.

Cardiac perforation by the catheter is one of the rare, but serious, complications. If this is suspected, the catheter should be left in place for withdrawal of a sample from the catheter. If the sample is blood, then it is very likely that the catheter is in a cardiac chamber or vessel and can be withdrawn. If, however, the sample is fluid-stained with blood, then the catheter is in the pericardial cavity. If the catheter has passed through the atrium or major vessels, the catheter should be left in place and the surgeon should be called to close the atrial perforation, since this is usually associated with pericardial tamponade. If the catheter has passed through the ventricle, the catheter can be withdrawn and the patient should be observed carefully for pericardial tamponade. During this period ventricular or aortic pressure should be monitored continuously and the size of the heart should be observed under fluoroscopy.

Forming a sharp curve or *knot in the catheter* is one of the serious complications. If this occurs the loop or the knot should be released and the catheter changed. This can be accomplished by pointing the tip of the catheter into a branch and then withdrawing the catheter or by introducing wire into the lumen of the catheter and moving the catheter back and forth over the wire to release the loop.

In patients with severe valvar pulmonary stenosis, passing the catheter across the pulmonic valve might reduce the pulmonary flow seriously and cause low cardiac output, bradycardia, and severe ventricular dysrhythmia. To avoid this serious complication, the catheter should not be passed across the pulmonic valve when the pressure in the right ventricle is more than systemic, and the catheter should be withdrawn from the left ventricle as soon as possible when left ventricular pressure is more than 150 mm Hg.

After completion of a retrograde arterial catheterization, the blood pressure should be measured in the limb distal to the site of entry. The artery is usually occluded when the pulse is very *weak* or the limb is cooler than the opposite limb. If either of these findings is observed, arterial embolectomy should be done immediately.

A *hypercyanotic spell* is observed frequently in cyanotic patients with reduced pulmonary blood flow when the patient is heavily sedated, has significant blood loss, or becomes hypotensive. To avoid this complication, the patient should be well hydrated, blood loss should be avoided, and the blood pressure should be kept at a normal or higher than normal level.

Electric shock is a common problem in the catheterization laboratory. This hazard can be prevented by securing all electric outlets with proper cover to keep them dry; and in all equipment connected to the patient, the current should be less than 10 μA. Equipment in the laboratory should be inspected by an electrical engineer for safety.

Patients should continue to receive intravenous fluid until they are fully awake. The site of entry should be observed for *bleeding*, and the pulse distal to the site of entry should be observed for 24 hours following the procedure.

SPECIAL PRECAUTIONS

1. All patients should receive intravenous fluid during cardiac catheterization, and cyanotic patients should be well hydrated at the time of the procedure. In small sick infants, the blood sugar should be tested and all hypoglycemic infants should receive 10% dextrose in water intravenously.

2. The temperature of all patients should be monitored by rectal thermistor connected to a monitor. Hypothermic patients should be warmed to normal temperature, and cardiac catheterization should be discontinued if the patient's temperature exceeds 38°C.

3. The patient's family should be questioned before cardiac catheterization to exclude bleeding disorders and renal dysfunction. All patients should have normal urinalysis before the procedure.

4. Digitalis should not be given on the day of the procedure since a high dose of digitalis is associated with an increased frequency of AV block.

SELECTED REFERENCES

Bargeron, L. M., Elliott, L. P., Soto, B., Bream, P. R., and Curry, G. C.: Axial cineangiography in congenital heart disease. Section I. Concept, technical and anatomic considerations. Circulation 56:1075-1083, 1977.

Bloomfield, D. A. (ed.): Dye Curves. University Park Press, Baltimore, 1974.

Burton, A. C. (ed.): Physiology and Biophysics of the Circulation. Year Book Medical Publishers, Chicago, 1965.

Elliott, L. P., Bargeron, L. M., Bream, P. R., Soto, B., and Curry, G. C.: Axial cineangiography in congenital heart disease. Section II. Specific lesions. Circulation 56:1084-1093, 1977.

Graham, T. P., Jr., Jarmakani, J. M.: Evaluation of ventricular function in infants and children. Pediatr. Clin. North Am. 18(4), 1971.

Graham, T. P., Jr., Jarmakani, J. M.: Hemodynamic investigation of congenital heart disease in infancy and childhood. Prog. Cardiovasc. Dis. 15(2), 1972.

Graham, T. P., Jr., Jarmakani, J. M., Atwood, G. F., Canent, R. V., Jr.: Right ventricular volume determinations in children. Circulation 47, January, 1973.

Grossman, W. (ed.): Cardiac Catheterization and Angiography. Lea & Febiger, Philadelphia, 1974.

Rudolph, A. (ed.): Cardiac catheterization and angiography. In Congenital Diseases of the Heart: Clinical-Psychological Considerations in Diagnosis and Management, Chap. 4. Year Book Medical Publishers, Chicago, 1974.

Wood, E. H. (ed.): Symposium on Use of Indicator-Dilution Technics in the Study of Circulation. American Heart Association, New York, 1962.

Yang, S. S. (ed.): Cardiac Catheterization Data to Hemodynamic Parameters. F. A. Davis, Philadelphia, 1972.

6

Nuclear Cardiology

Roger A. Hurwitz, M.D., and S. T. Treves, M.D.

Radionuclide angiocardiography has been successfully used for evaluation of adults with cardiovascular disease for many years; with improvements in methodology, this modality is being applied to the diagnosis and management of cardiac disorders in the pediatric population.[41] Radionuclide angiocardiography is relatively noninvasive, requiring only an intravenous injection of isotope, resulting in a reasonably small dose of radiation. The test can usually be done in 15 to 30 minutes, as an outpatient. With refinements in imaging and computer analysis, the resultant information has minimum observer intervention and is thus highly reproducible. The technique affords evaluation during intervention testing and also offers the capability to perform serial studies, providing a means to help define the course of cardiac disease in infants, children, and adolescents.

Three major radionuclide methods are used in pediatric cardiology: first pass radionuclide angiocardiography; radionuclide ventriculography gated from an accompanying electrocardiographic signal; and myocardial scintigraphy. Currently, the first two have most wide pediatric application. These radionuclide investigations can commonly provide information on anatomy, flow, intra- or extracardiac shunts, myocardial function, chamber size and output, and myocardial integrity. First-pass angiocardiography provides an anatomic delineation and time-activity curve for vascular structures during the initial transit of isotope through the circulation. This technique is used to examine the extracardiac vasculature and the shunting between the venous and systemic circulations. First pass techniques are also used to evaluate myocardial function by estimation of ejection fraction and transit times. Left ventricular function is commonly examined by gated radionuclide ventriculography (sometimes called "MUGA"). Multiple cardiac cycles are summed, with analysis of a small segment of the cycle provided by computer methods. The high count rates provided by this technique afford good statistical analysis. This technique can provide evaluation of systolic and diastolic function, as well as estimation of relative and absolute ventricular volumes. Myocardial integrity may also be determined from the cineangiographic display and regional pump performance provided by gated radionuclide ventriculography. However, the viability of myocardium is most commonly done by myocardial scintigraphy, which usually necessitates a visual interpretation to diagnose acute, chronic, or latent ischemia.

METHODOLOGY

EQUIPMENT

Basic equipment includes a gamma scintillation camera and a digital computer system, including capability for video imaging and production of hard copy. The most commonly used camera is a multipurpose Anger type. These cameras record and display images through a single large sodium iodide crystal viewed by photomultiplier tubes. A digital computer is interfaced to the camera; the computer provides static images (similar to a single frame of an angiogram) or using a closed loop format, dynamic images (a modification of cineangiographic data processing). These images may be manipulated for data analysis or storage on large magnetic discs or tape, or photographed. Also available is a multicrystal camera, which provides very high count rates. Although widely suited for first pass angiocardiography, it has little versatility.

When gamma rays are emitted from an organ, they travel in all directions. A collimator is interposed between the sodium iodide crystal and the object being imaged. This collimator literally sorts and collects photons, presenting them to the crystal through holes of certain length and thickness. This variability allows the physician to alter resolution or sensitivity. Though parallel hole collimators are customarily used in nuclear cardiology, a collimator with holes slanted at 30° has been employed to provide caudal tilt, similar to the "angled oblique" view of cardiac angiography.[22]

Computerized data acquisition and analysis is required to obtain quantitative information. The speed and immediate storage capacity of the camera-computer system may limit the type of study to be performed. Generally, static or equilibrium studies pose no problem. However, a dynamic (list or fast frame mode) first pass study to estimate ejection fraction or diastolic filling rate may only be accomplished with a newer system designed to acquire such cardiac studies.

RADIOPHARMACEUTICALS

Technetium-99m (^{99m}Tc) is the isotope most commonly used for angiography and ventricular function studies. This isotope decays with a half-life of approximately 6 hours and emits monoenergetic gamma rays of 140 keV, which is ideal for currently available gamma scintillation cameras. When given as an intravenous bolus, technetium-99m sodium pertechnetate rapidly distributes throughout the body, with accumulation in the intestine (critical, or target organ), choroid plexus, thyroid, and salivary gland (Table 6.1). Elimination is through the urine, intestine, and by physical decay. An intravascular indicator is necessary for gated equilibrium ventriculography.

Human serum albumin or autologous red blood cells can be labeled with ^{99m}Tc. The target organ in such cases is the blood, with whole body radiation slightly greater than that accumulated during first pass angiography.

When imaging the pulmonary vasculature for emboli or relative flows macroaggregated albumin can be tagged with ^{99m}Tc. This compound collects in the first capillary bed it reaches; thus, in patients with right to left shunts or in suspected pulmonary hypertension, the procedure is performed with as small an amount of particles as possible.

Different pharmaceuticals are used in myocardial scintigraphy. In the first 96 hours, infarcted myocardium may be

TABLE 6.1   RADIOPHARMACEUTICALS FOR ANGIOCARDIOGRAPHY

Radiopharmaceutical[a]	mCi/kg	Minimal Total Dose	Radiation Absorbed Dose (rad)[b]	
			Whole Body	Critical Organ
^{99m}Tc sodium pertechnetate	0.200	2.0	0.110–0.182	Intestine 1.3–2.8
^{99m}Tc human serum albumin	0.200	2.0	0.124–0.210	Blood 0.48–0.70
^{99m}Tc red blood cells	0.200	2.0	0.124–0.210	Blood 0.48–0.70
^{99m}Tc macroaggregated human serum albumin	0.030	0.2	0.013–0.030	Lung 0.20–0.40
^{99m}Tc pyrophosphate	0.050	0.2		
^{201}Tl thallous chloride	0.300	0.25	0.25–0.36	Kidney 1.1–2.4

[a] Tc, technetium-99m: physical half-life, 6 hours; Tl, thallium-201: physical half-life, 73 hours.

[b] Absorbed doses per imaging dose and in a range from 1 year old to adult.

seen by accumulation of ^{99m}Tc pyrophosphate, an infarct-avid isotope. Once the area of necrosis is established, thallium-201 is used. Essentially, this pharmaceutical accumulates in myocardium relative to flow. Unfortunately, it has a relatively long half-life of 73.3 hours; thus, the kidney becomes the critical organ.

TECHNIQUE

No patient preparation is required. Prior to ^{99m}Tc pertechnetate administration, perchlorate is given to block uptake by the thyroid gland and speed excretion of the radiopharmaceutical. Perchlorate is not necessary when equilibrium ventriculography is performed.

First pass evaluation of shunt or hemodynamic function requires a small, compact bolus. Accurate results with the first pass technique are dependent upon this bolus. A 23- or 21-gauge butterfly needle inserted into an arm vein may provide adequate access to the patient. However, an "intracatheter" inserted into an arm vein or butterfly needle inserted into the external jugular vein will help ensure a successful bolus. Since changes in intrathoracic pressure may cause fragmentation of the bolus, the injection should not be attempted while the patient is crying, sighing, or coughing. Despite these limitations, sedation is seldom needed.

To assess the adequacy of the bolus, a time-activity curve of the superior vena cava is performed before analysis. The bolus should be one of a single peak, smooth, and 3 seconds or less in duration. Currently available deconvolution programs, designed to mathematically smooth the less fragmented curves, have helped increase efficiency to more than 90%.[20]

For equilibrium studies, ^{99m}Tc is tagged to human serum albumin or red blood cells. When red blood cells are used, tagging may be done in vitro or in vivo, with certain drawbacks to each. When done properly, labeling efficiency is approximately 90% by each technique. If first pass studies are performed at the time of injection of tagged material, care must be taken to provide a small bolus with introduction into as large an intravascular catheter or needle as possible.

STRESS-INTERVENTION STUDIES

A first pass study usually may be repeated once. If planned, initial injection could be ^{99m}Tc sulfur colloid, which accumulates in the liver, resulting in little residual thoracic background activity. If ^{99m}Tc is used, a second dose would have to be somewhat larger, and background correction would be necessary. An advantage of the gated equilibrium ventriculography technique is that multiple studies may be performed from the same dose of radioactivity. Most data, especially that relating to ventricular function, has been

obtained with patients in the resting, supine position. Exercise studies, primarily in adults, have been performed in the same position, with patients lying flat and pedaling bicycle ergometers. Since the upright position has more potential for change in ventricular dimensions, greater work loads, and more compliance in the pediatric age group, investigators are beginning to study children and adolescents while seated upright on a bicycle.[9] These studies have promise for discovery of subtle, early changes in ventricular function.

APPLICATIONS

ANATOMIC DEFINITION

Most anatomic diagnoses are made by visual analysis of first pass radionuclide angiocardiograms, with examination of static images (often with frames summed to enhance the amount of activity) or by the cineangiographic mode (Fig. 6.1). Since injection is usually through a peripheral vein, patency of the more proximal venous system can be readily ascertained. An aberrant or double superior vena cava, inferior vena cava continuing into an azygous system, blockage of the inferior vena cava following previous catheter manipulation, or compression and shift by an abdominal mass are delineated by visualization of activity over the suspicious area.

We have found the radionuclide technique to be reliable in identification of blockage to one or both limbs of the intracardiac baffle following repair of transposition of the great arteries (Fig. 6.2).[23] Radionuclide data were in agreement with concurrent catheterization in 20 of 21 patients suspected of having baffle obstruction. The discrepant patient had partial superior vena cava blockage which rapidly progressed to complete obstruction. Use of radionuclides will help to identify patients requiring further invasive procedures; if the venous system is patent, the study can be used to identify and quantitate shunts and also to provide an estimate of ventricular function.

Analysis of the angiographic anatomy and quantitation of lung activity may also identify a discrepancy between size of the pulmonary arteries or vascular distribution abnormalities. This latter is very common in patients with transposition of the great arteries, who have more flow to the right lung both pre- and postoperatively. The reason for this is unknown; the unusual angle of the origin of the pulmonary artery is postulated.

First pass studies, usually employing small amounts of ^{99m}Tc labeled to aggregated human serum albumin, may also determine relative pulmonary flow after palliative shunts. Caution must be exercised, however, with interpretation of these data to quantitate the shunt, since pulmonary flow will be a resultant of intracardiac and systemic shunt contributions, unless pulmonary atresia is present.

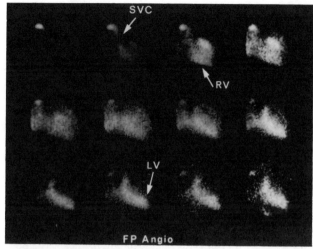

Fig. 6.1 Normal first pass angiogram, imaged in a right anterior oblique projection. *SVC*, superior vena cava; *RV*, right ventricle; *LV*, left ventricle.

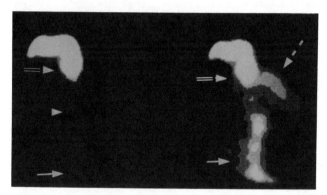

Fig. 6.2 Postoperative Mustard repair of transposition of great arteries with superior limb of baffle obstructed. *Open stem arrow*, superior vena cava; *arrowhead*, azygous vein; *arrow*, inferior vena cava; *dashed arrow*, pulmonary ventricle. Image on right follows that on left by 2 seconds.

Intracardiac anatomy may be identified by visual inspection or by use of time-activity curves. When first pass and gated equilibrium studies are used together, angiographic demonstration of vascular continuity, gross intracardiac anatomy, and time-activity patterns may help exclude major malformations. However, noninvasive sector scan echocardiography and cardiac catheterization angiography are generally superior to the radionuclide evaluation of intracardiac anatomy.

SHUNTS

Right to Left

Right to left shunts may be detected by inspection of images obtained during transit of activity through the right heart, with immediate filling of left heart chambers or aorta. To detect small amounts of shunting, time-activity curves over regions of interest separated from pulmonary vessels must be used. Abdominal aorta or carotid arteries provide suitable regions of interest.

Quantitation of the shunt has been performed in a manner similar to analysis of dye curves. A recent study using this technique showed a good correlation, with an estimation of right to left shunting by the Fick method employed during

cardiac catheterization.[31] Counting was done over the carotid arteries, with evaluation of the shunt by a modification of the forward triangle method. The radionuclide method slightly overestimated the shunt calculated at catheterization.

Left to Right

Visual inspection of the radionuclide angiocardiogram will demonstrate persistence of activity in the lungs and right heart chambers. On recirculation, the left ventricle and the aorta will be seen indistinctly, due to the shunt. This pattern is present with moderate to large shunts.

Accurate quantitation of the shunt depends upon a rapid, discrete bolus of radioactivity and the absence of major pulmonary or tricuspid insufficiency. A fragmented bolus or tricuspid or pulmonary insufficiency produces a falsely high shunt estimate. All quantitation techniques employ a time-activity curve from a region of interest in one or both lungs (Fig. 6.3).

Though visual inspection of the time-activity curve allows diagnosis of a left to right shunt, it is often not possible to accurately quantitate the shunt by curve inspection, despite the resemblance between the curve and that seen with other cardiovascular indicators. One radionuclide method uses an exponential extrapolation of count decline to an arbitrary end-point and compares the area of first transit to the area reflecting the recirculated blood.[3] The method we prefer uses a mathematical model, the gamma variate function, to separate activity due to first pulmonary transit from that caused by the shunt.[29] Use of this technique, with modifications including deconvolution, has resulted in a good correlation between estimate of Qp:Qs by radionuclide angiocardiography and cardiac catheterization.[1, 3, 29] Using our preferred technique, a Qp:Qs < 1.2 is considered normal, since the analysis of lung curves probably adds chest wall or bronchial arterial counts. Shunts >3.0 can be identified but

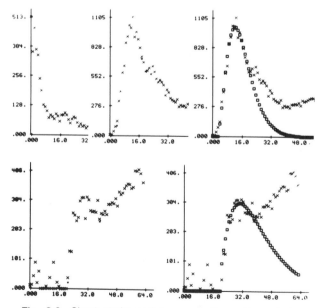

Fig. 6.3 Shunt study; activity versus time with each frame representing 0.25 seconds. *Top left* represents region over superior vena cava, demonstrating sharp, discrete bolus; *top middle* is right lung region, showing probable recirculation; *top right* has fitted curve (open squares); *bottom left* has new, subtracted curve; *bottom right* has new fitted curve (open squares). Qp:Qs, initial fitted curve divided by initial minus secondary fitted curve; Qp:Qs = 1.7. Note different activity levels requiring computer analysis.

not accurately quantitated because adequate gamma variate fit cannot be accomplished.

When a shunt is detected, the exact site is difficult to determine. These programs quantitate the total left-to-right shunt, regardless of location or number. A totally different, alternative approach to quantitation of the shunt is by use of gated equilibrium ventriculography. This technique has been used to quantitate the left-to-right shunt caused by atrial septal defects; right ventricular stroke volume is increased relative to that of the left ventricle.[7]

Analysis of shunt is probably the most commonly used radionuclide study in pediatric cardiology. Results are accurate, when compared to results from invasive estimate and are more consistent than results from most other noninvasive techniques. Radionuclide angiocardiography provides a means to accurately and serially follow hemodynamic changes and may help select those patients in whom further invasive procedures are necessary. In a group of 74 patients referred for quantitation of shunts associated with probable atrial septal defect, four invasive procedures were cancelled, surgery was done in 12 without catheterization, and 13 patients were discharged from further cardiac care after radionuclide evaluation.[24]

VENTRICULAR MEASUREMENT AND FUNCTION

General Applications

Most myocardial function data are derived from modifications of first-transit or gated equilibrium ventriculography studies. Using first pass techniques, cardiac output can be calculated using a time-activity curve obtained from a region of interest drawn over the heart and an independently calculated total blood volume.[42] This method measures forward cardiac output but has not been verified in small children or those with intracardiac shunts. In the absence of other lesions, left ventricular end-diastolic volume can be calculated.

Of greater potential value are the methods to absolutely measure diastolic and systolic left ventricular volumes, using gated equilibrium ventriculography. Techniques applying both geometric and count methods have been reported and validated in adult patients.[10, 36, 38, 39] There are certain handicaps: the radionuclide method has relatively poor resolution; the count method requires external counting of a blood sample and use of a correction factor. Though correction factors and resultant equations have been derived for adults, validation and correction factors are necessary before applying these measurements to the management of pediatric patients. Our own preliminary work suggests that less correction is necessary in smaller children, who have less thoracic attenuation.

Ventricular volume measurements may offer major improvement in the estimate of function. However, radionuclide evaluation of ventricular performance has generally focused upon systolic function. Estimation of left ventricular ejection fraction, by first pass or gated equilibrium ventriculography, has proven both reliable and valuable. Though dependent upon relative volumes, ejection fraction determination does not require an absolute measurement of volume, eliminating the mechanical and physical difficulties inherent in radionuclide volume measurement.[4, 8, 28, 30] Estimates of ejection fraction by these methods have shown good correlation with data obtained during cardiac catheterization. Radionuclide estimates of left ventricular ejection fraction may be slightly exaggerated at the extremes, being very high at high normal and low at very low normal. However, overall correlation is good, with "normal" values about 5% below those derived from cineangiography.

Additional data derived from these studies by computer intervention include regional wall motion and ejection, ejection rate, and partial (first third etc.) quantitation of these factors. To augment evaluation of myocardial performance, stress intervention studies are often necessary to assess myocardial reserve. Despite this, the systolic characteristics of the ventricle may not be sufficient for diagnosis. Thus, recent work has focused upon ventricular diastolic properties. Diastolic filling is reported to be abnormal in patients with normal ejection fraction and no prior myocardial infarction but existing coronary artery disease.[6]

Right Ventricle

The complexity of right ventricular anatomy results in imaging problems. Anatomic constraints are present in all projections when blood pool imaging is performed. Despite this, some authors describe adequate studies in adults using gated equilibrium ventriculography.[22, 27] Our own experience suggests difficulty in achieving adequate studies with gated equilibrium ventriculography due to poor separation of the right ventricle from contiguous structures. We favor use of first-transit studies, using the right anterior oblique projection and dynamic function derived from time-activity curves.

Before embarking upon a radionuclide evaluation of abnormal patients, it was necessary to define normal values for ventricular function in the pediatric group, since data were reported only for adults and adolescents.[5] We evaluated ejection fraction in 74 infants and children with normal hearts who were undergoing bone scintigraphy and found right ventricular ejection fraction to be 0.53 ± 0.06 (Fig. 6.4). Lower values tended to be present in younger patients (often with tachycardia), but there was little difference between means for different age groups. This data is comparable to that in other radionuclide studies of adults, but is slightly lower than angiographically determined ejection fractions.[5, 13]

Initial radionuclide efforts have concentrated on assessment of ventricular function in patients with chronic respiratory disease. Though right ventricular function varies widely in these patients, 38% were found to have abnormal right ventricular function, and all patients with "cor pulmonale" were identified.[5] In a smaller group of patients, our own investigations demonstrated a mean right ventricular ejection fraction for a group of children with relatively severe chronic lung disease to be 0.42, which was statistically different ($p < 0.01$) from the mean value for our normal children. Little evaluation has been performed on large groups with congenital heart disease. Sixteen asymptomatic patients were evaluated following repair of tetralogy of Fallot.[34] Although 15 had normal resting right ventricular ejection fraction, 13 demonstrated an abnormal response to exercise. Myocardial scintigraphy in this group also demonstrated increased right ventricular uptake, consistent with residual right ventricular hypertrophy.

Myocardial scintigraphy, using thallium 201, has also demonstrated right ventricular hypertrophy in patients with pulmonary hypertension. Rabinovitch and co-workers[33] found significant right ventricular uptake in patients with peak systolic pressure in the right ventricle, which was more than half that in the left ventricle. Analysis of the second half regional ejection fraction obtained by gated equilibrium ventriculography has been useful in predicting pulmonary artery systolic pressure in adults.[14] Our own preliminary work using this technique has been reasonably effective in classifying patients into those with normal or abnormal systolic pressures in the pulmonary artery.

Left Ventricle

The contours of the left ventricle allow easier differentiation from adjacent structures. Generally, borders are easier

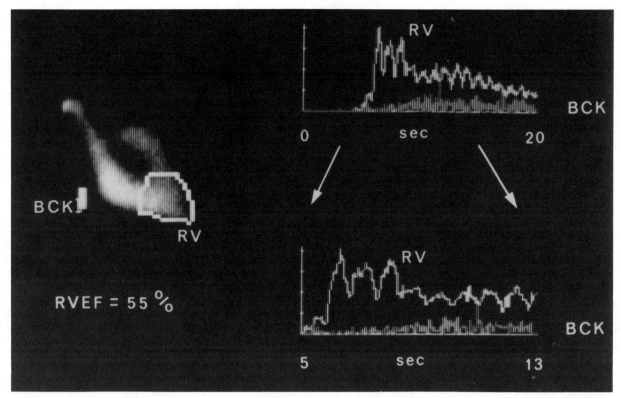

Fig. 6.4 Calculation of right ventricular ejection fraction by first pass technique. Summed right ventricular image (*RV* region) with background (*BCK*) on left. Cardiac image not necessarily diastole, but stroke volume image is outlined. Time-activity curves from background and stroke volume regions on right. Ejection fraction could be calculated from three cycles in this patient.

to define in children, who seldom have regional wall abnormalities. First pass angiocardiography is technically possible in the absence of a major left to right shunt. When imaged in the right anterior oblique projection, the ellipsoidal left ventricle allows clear delineation for a longer period and more cardiac cycles than is available for the right ventricle.

Children with normal hearts have left ventricular ejection fractions higher than those of the right ventricle.[25] Our own recently determined values were 0.68 ± 0.09 for the patients with normal hearts examined during bone scintigraphy. These values are similar to those reported in normal adults when obtained by first pass or gated equilibrium ventriculography.[4] The ejection fraction for "normal left hearts" of children undergoing cardiac catheterization for isolated right-sided lesions is also similar.[18] There have been several studies showing close correlation between left ventricular ejection fraction derived from equilibrium ventriculography and that from cineangiography.[4, 8, 22] Gated equilibrium ventriculography is relatively easy to perform, with imaging in the left anterior oblique projection providing the best septal delineation. When a slight caudal tilt is employed, the ventricle elongates and the separation from the great vessels and atrium becomes more clear.

Equilibrium ventriculography has had wide application in adults, since it lends itself to repeat study, facilitating intervention testing. Recent pediatric applications of left ventricular performance have included evaluation of the ventricle during potentially cardiotoxic cancer chemotherapy and following surgery for congenital abnormalities.[2] Since the ejection fraction can be serially followed for at least 6 hours after one dose of radioactivity, the technique has application in the postoperative intensive care unit.

Radionuclide evaluation of left ventricular ejection fraction should prove beneficial in management and selection of patients for cardiac surgery. Patients with tricuspid atresia are not considered good candidates for Fontan-type procedures when ventricular function is abnormal. Unfortunately, many of these patients have borderline or abnormal function. Recently, Harder and colleagues[21] reported nearly half of tricuspid atresia patients to have abnormal resting or dynamic exercise responses. We have studied 18 patients with tricuspid atresia with similar results. A number of these patients continue to have subnormal ventricular function following the Fontan repair. Perhaps earlier identification with radionuclide testing will result in better patient selection and follow-up.

Another group that might benefit from radionuclide examination are those relatively asymptomatic children and adolescents with aortic and/or mitral insufficiency. Assessment of ventricular volumes and ejection fraction at rest and during stress testing could determine those whose function has deteriorated. This may be especially important, since adults have been shown to develop severe heart failure in as short a period as 1 year. This occurred in 30% of patients with severe aortic insufficiency (AI) in one study.[32] Quantitation of left-sided valvar insufficiency may be effectively performed using radionuclide techniques. The left ventricular to right ventricular stroke volume ratio correlates well with results from cardiac catheterization.[26, 32, 37] We studied 28 patients with predominant AI and/or MI; stroke volume ratio correlated well with angiography in 22 of 23 patients with relatively concurrent cardiac catheterization (Fig. 6.5). A stroke ratio volume greater than 1.4 was abnormal; a stroke volume ratio more than 2.0 was associated with a significant degree of insufficiency.

MYOCARDIAL SCINTIGRAPHY

This radionuclide technique is usually employed to assess integrity of the left ventricular myocardium. As previously

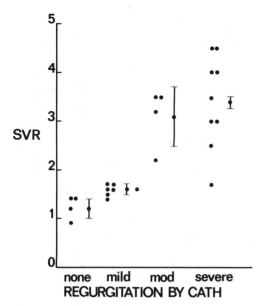

Fig. 6.5 Left ventricular to right ventricular stroke volume ratio (SVR), plotted versus aortic and/or mitral insufficiency estimated by cardiac angiography. A SVR as large as 1.4 may be found in normal patients.

stated, thallium-201 uptake in the right ventricle may be relative to its degree of hypertrophy. Lack of significant myocardial uptake has been reported in transient myocardial ischemia of the newborn; serial studies showed eventual normalization of uptake as the patients recovered.[11]

Thallium-201 imaging has been used to evaluate infants and children with anomalous coronary arteries. In one study, all seven patients with anomalous coronary arteries had scintigraphic abnormalities.[19] Unfortunately, results overlapped in eight patients with congestive cardiomyopathy; three of eight had diffusely abnormal scans, distinguishable from abnormal coronary scans, but one myopathy patient had a large scintigraphic defect. Some patients with abnormal coronary arteries have shown great improvement or even normalization after surgical therapy.[12] Our own experience is a persistent abnormality in two patients with probable early infarcts and eventual coronary ligation at the

pulmonary connection, while the patient corrected by coronary reimplant into the aorta had a scan that became normal.[16] One patient in the Toronto series showed clinical and scintigraphic improvement, but expired suddenly.[12] A possible explanation could be that subendocardial ischemia may not be detected by thallium-201 scans. For this reason, it is doubtful that these perfusion scans would be of great benefit in evaluation of patients with aortic stenosis and questionable ischemia. Scintigraphy may, however, help diagnose and manage patients with suspected myocardial compromise with Kawasaki's disease or mitral valve prolapse.[15] Myocardial imaging may also be of help in evaluation of patients with suspected myocardial injury following cardiac surgery.

CONCLUSIONS

Radionuclide angiocardiography is a reproducible and relatively noninvasive procedure that can be safely performed in pediatric patients. The first pass angiographic phase may be definitive for venous abnormalities and more obvious central abnormalities, including discrepant pulmonary flow. Quantitation of left-to-right shunting is highly reliable by the radionuclide technique. Ventricular performance, especially systolic function, is being evaluated with increasing precision. There is great potential for further intervention testing, evaluation of diastolic function, and validation of absolute ventricular volume measurements in the pediatric population.

Current investigative efforts in the nuclear field are mainly concerned with more specific evaluation of the myocardium. Positron emission computed tomography is a technique with potential value in measurement of myocardial blood flow and metabolism.[35] An obvious goal in investigation of pediatric patients would be the limitation or elimination of ionizing radiation. Nuclear magnetic resonance imaging, dependent upon atomic properties, may eventually provide information on the biochemical and structural characteristics of the myocardium without the hazard of radiation.[17] Of more current applicability is the use of ultra-short lived isotopes. First pass radionuclide angiocardiography with iridium–191m has proven effective for quantitation of shunts in infants and children.[40] In preliminary work, we have shown the feasibility of estimating ejection fraction using this isotope, which has a half-life less than 5 seconds.

REFERENCES

1. Alderson, P. O., Jost, R. G., Strauss, A. W., Boonvisut, S., and Markham, J.: Radionuclide angiocardiography: Improved diagnosis and quantification of left-to-right shunts using area ratio techniques in children. Circulation 51:1136–1143, 1975.

2. Alexander, J., Dainiak, N., Berger, H. J., Goldman, L., Johnstone, D., Reduto, L., Duffy, T., Schwartz, P., Gottschalk, A., and Zaret, B.: Serial assessment of doxorubicin cardiotoxicity in cancer patients with quantitative radionuclide angiocardiography. N. Engl. J. Med. 300:278–283, 1979.

3. Anderson, P. A., Jones, R. H., and Sabiston, D. C.: Quantitation of left-to-right cardiac shunts with radionuclide angiography. Circulation 49:512–516, 1974.

4. Ashburn, W. L., Schelbert, H. R., and Verba, J. W.: Left ventricular ejection fraction: A review of several radionuclide angiographic approaches using the scintillation camera. Prog. Cardiovasc. Dis. 20:267–284, 1978.

5. Berger, H. J., Matthay, R. A., Loke, J., Marshall, R. C., Gottschalk, A., and Zaret, B. L.: Assessment of cardiac performance with quan-

titative radionuclide angiocardiography: Right ventricular ejection fraction with reference to findings in chronic obstructive pulmonary disease. Am. J. Cardiol. 41:897–905, 1978.

6. Bonow, R. O., Bacharach, S. L., Green, M. V., Kent, K. M., and Epstein, S. E.: Impaired left ventricular diastolic filling in patients with coronary artery disease: Assessment with radionuclide angiography. Circulation 64:315–323, 1981.

7. Bough, E. W., Gandsman, E. J., Benham, I. D., Boden, W. E., North, D. L., and Shulman, R. S.: Detection and quantitation of atrial shunts in adults by gated radionuclide angiography (abstr.). Am. J. Cardiol. 45:409, 1980.

8. Burow, R. D., Strauss, H. W., Singleton, R., Pond, M., Rehn, T., Bailey, I. K., Griffith, L. L., Nickoloff, E., and Pitt, B.: Analysis of left ventricular function from multiple gated acquisition cardiac blood pool imaging: Comparison to contrast angiography. Circulation 56:4–8, 1978.

9. Covitz, W., Eubig, C., and Strong, W.: Radionuclide ejection fraction in children with heart disease (abstr.). Circulation 62(III):116, 1980.

10. Dehmer, G. L., Lewis, S. E., Hillis, L. D., Twieg, D., Falkoff, M., Parkey, W. R., and Wilerson, J. T.: Nongeometric determination of left ventricular volumes from equilibrium blood pool scans. Am. J. Cardiol. 45:293–300, 1980.

11. Finley, J. P., Howman-Giles, R. B., Gilday, D. L., Bloom, K. R., and Rowe, R. D.: Transient myocardial ischemia of the newborn infant demonstrated by thallium myocardial imaging. J. Pediatr. 94:263–270, 1979.

12. Finley, J. P., Howman-Giles, R. B., Gilday, D. L., Olley, P. M., and Rowe, R. D.: Thallium-201 myocardial imaging in anomalous left coronary artery arising from the pulmonary artery. Am. J. Cardiol. 42:675–680, 1978.

13. Fisher, E. A., Dubrow, I. W., and Hastreiter, A. R.: Right ventricular volume in congenital heart disease. Am. J. Cardiol. 36:67–75, 1975.

14. Friedman, B. J., Holman, B. L., Wynne, J., and Idoine, J.: Correlation of second half regional right ventricular ejection fraction with pulmonary artery systolic pressure (abstr.). J. Nucl. Med. 22:5, 1981.

15. Gaffney, F. A., Wohl, A. J., Blomquist, C. G.,

Parkey, R. W., and Willerson, J. T.: Thallium-201 myocardial perfusion studies in patients with the mitral valve prolapse syndrome. Am. J. Med. 64:21–26, 1978.

16. Girod, D. A., Faris, J., Hurwitz, R. A., Caldwell, R., Burt, R. W., and Siddiqui, A.: Thallium-201 assessment of myocardial perfusion in coronary anomalies in children (abstr.). Am. J. Cardiol. 43:402, 1979.

17. Goldman, M. R., Pohost, G. M., Ingwall, J. S., and Fossel, E. T.: Nuclear magnetic resonance imaging: Potential cardiac applications. Am. J. Cardiol. 46:1278–1283, 1980.

18. Graham, T. P., Jr., Jarmakani, M. M., Canent, R. V., Jr., Capp, M. P., and Spach, M. S.: Characterization of left heart volume and mass in normal children and in infants with intrinsic myocardial disease. Circulation 38:826–837, 1968.

19. Gutgesell, H. P., Pinskey, W. W., and Depwey, E. G.: Thallium-201 myocardial perfusion imaging in infants and children. Circulation 61:596–599, 1980.

20. Ham, H. R., Dobbelier, A., Viari, P., Piepsz, A., and Lenaers, A.: Radionuclide quantitation of left-to right cardiac shunts using deconvolution analysis. J. Nucl. Med. 22:688–692, 1981.

21. Harder, J. R., Gilday, D. L., deSouza, M., Freedom, R. M., Olley, P. M., and Rowe, R. D.: Radionuclide assessment of left ventricular function in patients with tricuspid atresia (abstr.). Am. J. Cardiol. 47:431, 1981.

22. Holman, B. L., Wynne, J., Zielonka, J. S., and Idoine, J. D.: A simplified technique for measuring right ventricular ejection fraction using the equilibrium radionuclide angiogram and the slant hole collimator. Radiology 138:429–435, 1981.

23. Hurwitz, R. A., Papanicolaou, N., Treves, S., Keane, J. F., and Castaneda, A.: Radionuclide angiocardiography in evaluation of patients following repair of transposition of the great arteries. Am. J. Cardiol., 49:761–765, 1982.

24. Hurwitz, R. A., Treves, S., Keane, J. F., Girod, D. A., and Caldwell, R. L.: Radionuclide angiocardiography: Current usefulness for shunt quantitation and management of patients with atrial septal defects. Am. Heart. J., 103:421–425, 1982.

25. Kurtz, D., Ahnberg, D. S., Freed, M., LaFarge, C. G., and Treves, S.: Quantitative radionuclide angiocardiography. Determination of left ventricular ejection fraction in children. Br. Heart J. 38:966–973, 1976.

26. Lam, W., Pavel, D., Bryom, E., Sheikh, A., Best, D., and Rosen, K.: Radionuclide regurgitant index: Value and limitations. Am. J. Cardiol. 47:292–298, 1981.

27. Maddahi, J., Berman, D. S., Matsouka, D. T., Waxman, A. D., Stankus, K. E., Forrester, J. S., and Swan, H. J. C.: A new technique for assessing right ventricular ejection fraction using rapid multiple-gated equilibrium cardiac blood pool scintigraphy. Circulation 60:581–589, 1979.

28. Maddox, D. E., Holman, B. L., Wynne, J., Idoine, J., Parker, J. A., Uren, R., Neill, J. M., and Cohn, P. F.: Ejection fraction image: A noninvasive index of regional left ventricular wall motion. Am. J. Cardiol. 41:1230–1238, 1978.

29. Maltz, D. L., and Treves, S.: Quantitative radionuclide angiocardiography: Determination of Qp:Qs in children. Circulation 47:1049–1056, 1973.

30. Marshall, R. C., Berger, H. J., Costin, J. C., Freedman, G. S., Woldberg, J., Cohen, L. S., Gottschalk, A., and Zaret, B. L.: Assessment of cardiac performance with quantitative radionuclide angiocardiography: Sequential left ventricular ejection fraction, normalized left ventricular ejection rate and regional wall motion. Circulation 56:820–829, 1977.

31. Peter, C. A., Armstrong, B. E., and Jones, R. H.: Radionuclide quantitation of right-to-left intracardiac shunts in children. Circulation 64:572–577, 1981.

32. Peter, C. A., Armstrong, B. E., and Jones, R. H.: Radionuclide measurements of left ventricular function: Their use in patients with aortic insufficiency. Arch. Surg. 115:1348–1352, 1980.

33. Rabinovitch, M., Fischer, K. C., and Treves, S.: Quantitative thallium-201 myocardial imaging in assessing right ventricular pressure in patients with congenital heart defects. Br. Heart J. 45:198–205, 1981.

34. Reduto, L. A., Berger, H. J., Johnstone, D. E., Hillenbrand, W., Wackers, F. J. Th., Whittemore, R., Cohen, L. S., Gottschalk, A., and Zaret, B. L.: Radionuclide assessment of right and left ventricular exercise reserve after total correction of tetralogy of Fallot. Am. J. Cardiol. 45:1013–1018, 1980.

35. Schelbert, H. R., Phelps, M. E., Hoffman, E., Huang, S., and Kuhl, D. E.: Regional myocardial blood flow, metabolism and function assessed non-invasively with positron emission tomography. Am. J. Cardiol. 46:1269–1277, 1980.

36. Slutsky, R., Karliner, J., Ricci, D., Kaiser, R., Pfisterer, M., Gordon, D., Peerson, K., and Ashburn, W.: Left ventricular volumes by gated equilibrium radionuclide angiography: A new method. Circulation 60:556–564, 1979.

37. Sorensen, S. G., O'Rourke, R. A., and Chavdhuri, T. K.: Noninvasive quantitation of valvar regurgitation by gated equilibrium radionuclide angiography. Circulation 62:1089–1098, 1980.

38. Steele, P., Kirch, D., Matthew, M., and Davies, H.: Measurement of left heart ejection fraction and end-diastolic volume by computerized, scintigraphic technique using a wedged pulmonary arterial catheter. Am. J. Cardiol. 34:179–186, 1974.

39. Strauss, H. W., Zaret, B. L., Hurley, P. J., Natarajan, T. K., and Pitt, B.: A scintiphotographic method for measuring left ventricular ejection fraction in man without cardiac catheterization. Am. J. Cardiol. 28:575–580, 1971.

40. Treves, S., Cheng, C., Samuel, A., Lambrecht, R., and Norwood, W.: Iridium-191m angiocardiography for the detection and quantitation of left-to-right shunting. J. Nucl. Med. 21:1151–1157, 1980.

41. Treves, S., Fogle, R., Lang, P.: Radionuclide angiography in congenital heart disease. Am. J. Cardiol. 46:1247–1255, 1980.

42. Weber, P. M., Dos Remedios, L. V., and Jasko, I. A.: Quantitative radioisotopic angiocardiography. J. Nucl. Med. 13:815–822, 1972.

7

Exercise Testing

Frederick W. James, M.D.

Exercise testing provides an evaluation of working performance and reveals the adaptive response to exercise at different levels of intensity. This technique identifies mechanisms which limit working performance in patients with heart disease of varying severity. Further, the change in exercise responses related to growth, severity of disease, and therapeutic interventions, i.e., medical and surgical, are appreciated when careful longitudinal studies are conducted. Relevant exercise data influence the timing of cardiac catheterization and surgical intervention, including the use of specific surgical techniques. Exercise data also help to establish the guidelines for cardiac rehabilitation after surgery and the level of involvement in physical and vocational activities. Thus, exercise testing is essential for improved clinical care and therapeutic intervention in young patients with cardiovascular or related disease.

This chapter reviews methodology and the use of clinical exercise testing in normal children and adolescents, and in those with cardiovascular disease. Highlights of specific exercise responses reflecting presence and severity of disease, and the effect of therapeutic intervention are illustrated. Additional reading in exercise-physiology, clinical and experimental exercise studies is encouraged for maximal understanding and interpretation of exercise responses.

REASONS FOR EXERCISE TESTING

The exercise procedure supplements other relevant clinical information obtained from a careful history, physical examination, and other cardiologic procedures. The reasons for performing exercise tests in young patients are: to provoke, describe and measure responses to controlled exercise

TABLE 7.1   CONTRAINDICATIONS FOR EXERCISE TESTING

Contraindications	Special Considerations
Acute inflammatory cardiac disease, e.g., pericarditis, myocarditis, acute rheumatic heart disease	Severe aortic stenosis
Uncontrolled heart failure	Severe pulmonic stenosis
Acute myocardial infarction	Serious ventricular dysrhythmia, especially associated with significant cardiac disease
Acute pulmonary disease, e.g., acute asthma, pneumonia	Coronary artery diseases, e.g., anomalous left coronary artery, homozygous hypercholesterolemia, Kawasaki's disease (acute phase)
Severe systemic hypertension: e.g., blood pressure greater than 240/120 mm Hg	Severe pulmonary vascular disease
Acute renal disease, e.g., acute glomerulonephritis	Metabolic disorders, e.g., glycogenosis Type I and V
Acute hepatitis (within 3 months after onset)	Hemorrhagic diseases
Drug overdose affecting cardiorespiratory response to exercise; e.g., digitalis toxicity, salicylism, quinidine toxicity	Orthostatic hypotension

for the purpose of detecting and determining the severity of cardiovascular disease; to identify mechanisms which explain signs and symptoms due to cardiovascular disease; to assess the effectiveness of specific medical and surgical treatment; to estimate functional capacity for reasonable participation in recreational, competitive, and vocational activities; and to estimate prognosis.

Clinical exercise testing has proven invaluable in the evaluation of children with the following cardiac problems: left ventricular outflow obstructions; chronic left or right ventricular volume overload; and cardiac rhythm and conduction disturbances. Clinical information which supports the use of this procedure in the evaluation of patients with hyperlipidemia, elevated resting blood pressure, and signs or symptoms suggestive of cardiovascular disease is rapidly developing.

METHODS

A clinical laboratory engaged in exercise testing of cardiac patients should have the capability of: measuring blood pressure and heart rate; recording multiple electrocardiographic leads; observing a continuous electrocardiographic tracing during the procedure; estimating working performance; and measuring or estimating pulmonary ventilation and gas exchange. Other measurements, such as cardiac output and systolic time intervals, are needed for further evaluation of cardiovascular performance and cardiac function.

PREPARATION

Adequate preparation of the patient and parent regarding the procedure, clothing, food intake, safety, total time for the test, and cost is strongly advised to reduce unnecessary anxiety. A brief history and physical examination by the physician and laboratory personnel before testing is advised. These requirements help to identify patients in whom the test is contraindicated or in whom the test should only be performed under special circumstances (Table 7.1).

EQUIPMENT

An exercise laboratory needs an ergometer (bicycle or treadmill); an apparatus for measuring indirectly peripheral blood pressure; a multiple channel electrocardiograph for recording electrocardiographic leads reflecting anterior and posterior, superior and inferior, and right and left wave forms from the heart; and an oscilloscope for continuous visualiza-

tion of the electrocardiogram. The recording of multiple electrocardiographic leads during exercise is superior to single lead recordings for detecting the presence and distribution of ST depression, and for evaluating cardiac dysrhythmia. This approach enhances the evaluation of congenital cardiac disease, especially cardiac malposition and other defects affecting both right and left sides of the heart. A meterologic or Douglas bag system for collecting the expiratory gas volume and an oxygen and carbon dioxide analyzer permit determination of respiratory minute volume, oxygen uptake, and carbon dioxide production. The addition of a multichannel recorder, rapid gas analyzer, and computer facilities greatly facilitates measuring pulmonary ventilation and gas exchange, systolic time intervals, and cardiac output.

Protocols

A common goal of many exercise protocols is to estimate or measure maximal oxygen uptake, an index of working performance. These continuous or intermittent protocols using a bicycle or treadmill ergometer cause an increase in working intensity over time. Most clinical laboratories use a continuous graded protocol which consists of progressive increases in work load without an intervening period of rest. The continuous graded bicycle protocol[17] described in Table 7.2 has been satisfactorily used for testing in children as young as 4 years of age and in adolescents with cardiac disease of varying severity.[18]

During a continuous graded protocol, all subjects are encouraged to perform to either a level of exhaustion, a percent of estimated maximal heart rate, or a predetermined endpoint (Table 7.3) which warrants discontinuing the study. The magnitude of the abnormal cardiovascular and electrocardiographic changes in Table 7.3 requires a medical decision to continue the exercise procedure.

Continuous graded treadmill protocols[6, 7, 19] have been successfully used in pediatric patients. Measurements of work and maximal oxygen uptake in a subject may be higher using a treadmill protocol than a bicycle protocol. On the other hand, measuring several responses to exercise (i.e., electrocardiogram, blood pressure, pulmonary ventilation and gas exchange, systolic time intervals, cardiac output, ejection fraction, and left ventricular wall motion, by scintigraphic techniques and cardiac dimensions by echographic techniques) is accomplished with greater ease using a bicycle protocol than a treadmill protocol. For most clinical evaluations of patients a bicycle or treadmill protocol which allows an assessment of multiple electrocardiographic leads, blood pressure, work and pulmonary ventilation, and gas exchange will be satisfactory.

TABLE 7.2   CONTINUOUS GRADED BICYCLE PROTOCOL WITH EXERCISE PROGRAMS I, II AND III

Exercise Level (3 min at each level)	I (BSA < 1 m^2) Work Loads (kg-m/min)	II (BSA = 1–1.19 m^2) Work Loads (kg-m/min)	III (BSA > 1.2 m^2) Work Loads (kg-m/min)	Cumulative Time (min)
1	200	200	200	3
2	300	400	500	6
3	500	600	800	9
4	600	700	1000	12
5	700	800	1200	15
6	800	900	1400	18
7	900	1000	1600	21
8	1000	1100	1800	24
9	1100	1200	2000	27
10	1200	1300	2200	30

TABLE 7.3   INDICATIONS FOR TERMINATION EXERCISE TESTS PRIOR TO REACHING PEAK VOLUNTARY CAPACITY LEVEL

The onset of a serious cardiac dysrhythmia (e.g., ventricular tachycardia, supraventricular tachycardia)

Any appearance of potential hazard to the patient:

Failure of electrocardiographic monitoring system

Symptoms such as pain, headache, dizziness, or syncope precipitated by exercise

ST depression or elevation ≥3 mm during exercise

Cardiac dysrhythmia (over 25% of beats) precipitated or aggravated by exercise

Atrioventricular block precipitated by exercise

Inappropriate rise in blood pressure with systolic pressures exceeding 230 mm Hg and diastolic pressures exceeding 120 mm Hg

Fall in systolic blood pressure below the resting level of 20 or more mm Hg during exercise

Marked signs of cutaneous vascular insufficiency (e.g., pallor)

RESPONSES OF NORMALS TO EXERCISE

The data presented in this section were recorded in normal subjects using a fixed continuous graded bicycle protocol. These data provide a reference for judging the performance of patients with heart disease. Exercise data in normal children using a continuous treadmill protocol have been provided by Riopel et al.[19] and Cumming.[6]

Caution must be taken, particularly when relying upon a single variable to reveal the severity of disease. A combination of abnormalities during exercise may produce an apparently normal response. A child with severe aortic stenosis causing a restricted cardiac output may have *normal oxygen transport* during submaximal exercise due to a marked increase in the peripheral extraction of oxygen producing an abnormally wide A-V difference. Further, a child with congenital heart block may have a *normal cardiac output* during submaximal exercise because of an abnormally large stroke volume combined with the abnormally slow ventricular rate. Due to these factors, the interplay of cardiovascular responses during exercise must be understood so that the impact of cardiovascular disease can be appreciated.

Total work, maximal power output, and total exercise time are indices of working capacity.[1, 17] Using a continuous graded bicycle protocol, these indices are positively related to body size and sex, especially in males and females having a body surface area ≥1.2 m^2. Males with body surface ≥1.2 m^2 tend to perform more work and have higher rates of work than females matched by body size. Boys and girls with body surface areas <1.2 m^2 have similar values for total work and maximal power output. These factors, sex and body size,

must be taken into account when evaluating working capacity.[1, 17]

Oxygen uptake ($\dot{V}O_2$) at submaximal levels is linearly related to working intensity. In an individual during progressive exercise, $\dot{V}O_2$ continues to rise to a level where further increases in work fail to produce incremental changes in $\dot{V}O_2$. That amount of $\dot{V}O_2$ is called the maximal oxygen uptake ($M\dot{V}O_2$) or maximal aerobic power.

$\dot{V}O_2$ and $M\dot{V}O_2$ measurements or estimates are recommended for providing a reference to evaluate other measured exercise responses. $\dot{V}O_2$ reported as a percent of measured or estimated $M\dot{V}O_2$ (%$M\dot{V}O_2$) allows meaningful interpretation of circulatory and pulmonary responses affected by the intensity of exercise, growth, level of physical training, disease, and treatment.

Carbon dioxide production ($\dot{V}CO_2$) at submaximal levels also increases with the intensity of exercise to a level where the slope changes markedly. At this level, the anaerobic threshold is reached with carbon dioxide production exceeding oxygen uptake. The respiratory rate and minute volume increase rapidly, producing audible oral breathing. The difference in serum lactate before and after maximal exercise is greater than 44 mg/dl.

Systolic blood pressure increases promptly with graded leg exercise. Generally, the greatest change from rest to maximal exercise for systolic pressure develops when working intensity exceeds approximately two-thirds of $M\dot{V}O_2$. Beyond two-thirds of $M\dot{V}O_2$, small increases in systolic pressure occur up to the level of maximal oxygen uptake. The rise in systolic pressure indicates that the increase in cardiac output is relatively greater than the decrease in systemic vascular resistance. Diastolic and mean pressures increase to a modest degree during exercise.

At peak exercise, *maximal systolic pressure* (MSP) is positively related to height, work load, and level of resting systolic pressure. The absolute level of maximal systolic pressure is higher in males with body surface area ≥1.2 m^2 than in matched females, and in those normals with body surface area <1.2 m^2.[18]

Cardiac output is linearly related to $\dot{V}O_2$ during submaximal dynamic exercise. During graded exercise, an individual's cardiac output parallels the increase in $\dot{V}O_2$ to a level where further increases in $\dot{V}O_2$ are associated with minimal or no change in cardiac output. Maximal cardiac output and the level of hemoglobin are major determinants of maximal oxygen uptake. Although the level of hemoglobin changes minimally from childhood to adolescence, maximal cardiac output increases markedly and parallels the increase in height and muscle mass. The relationship between maximal cardiac output and maximal oxygen uptake is affected by anemia,[20] cardiac disease,[8] and maldistribution of blood flow.[3]

On the *exercise electrocardiogram*, the R-R interval shortens approximately 56% from rest to peak exercise. This average change in R-R interval is due to a shortened T-P interval and Q-T interval (approximately 33%). The T wave decreases in duration by 18% in males and by 48% in females. The QRS interval varies minimally in duration during exertion. The ST segment also decreases in duration and is sometimes encroached upon by the ascending portion of the T wave. This finding potentially causes difficulty in determining ST depression at peak effort.

A base line for determining ST depression is drawn horizontally to connect the PQ or PR junctions of three to five consecutive QRS-T complexes (Fig. 7.1). Typical positions and contours of normal ST segments at rest and during exercise are illustrated in Figure 7.2. Abnormal ST depression during exercise is shown in Figure 7.3. ST depression of 1 mm or more below the base line is judged to be significant.[17, 21] The ST segment must be depressed below the base line for at least 0.06 second after the J point. The slope may

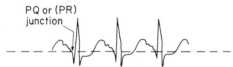

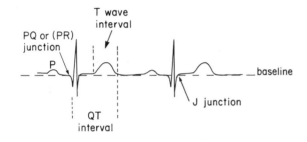

Fig. 7.1 Schematic for analyzing the exercise electrocardiogram. (*Top*) The horizontal base line connects the PQ points of consecutive QRS-T complexes at rest. (*Bottom*) The J junction and ST segment are below the base line during exercise. (Reproduced with permission from F. W. James.[16])

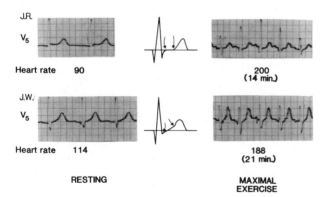

Fig. 7.2 Typical position and slope of the ST segment at rest and during exercise in normals. (*Top*) ST segment and J junction are above the base line at rest and descend to the base line at maximal exercise. (*Bottom*) At rest, the ST segment slopes upwards. Both ST segment and J junction are above the base line. During exercise, J junction is below the base line with a rapidly upward sloping ST segment. Schematic tracings illustrate normal ST segment changes during exercise. (Reproduced with permission from F. W. James.[14])

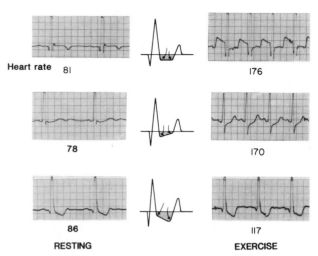

Fig. 7.3 Abnormal ST segments during exercise in children. (*Top*) Horizontal ST depression; (*Middle*) ST depression with upward ST segments; (*Bottom*) ST depression with downward sloping ST segments. Schematic tracings illustrate abnormal ST depression during exercise.

B.A.

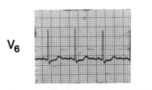

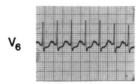

Fig. 7.4 ST depression occurring while standing and hyperventilating in an 11-year-old child without clinical evidence of cardiovascular disease.

be horizontal, upward, or downward at peak exercise (Fig. 7.3).

Exercise-induced conduction and rhythm disturbances of the heart are rare in normal children without previously documented electrocardiographic abnormalities. A recording of multiple electrocardiographic leads while standing and/or hyperventilating is advisable for the detection of ST depression (Fig. 7.4) and dysrhythmia before testing.

RESPONSES OF CARDIACS TO EXERCISE

AORTIC STENOSIS

An exercise profile consisting of ST depression of 2 mm or more, decreased total work and systolic pressure, and prolonged left ventricular ejection time in patients with aortic stenosis is characteristic of severe obstruction (resting left ventricular to aortic peak systolic gradient ≥70 mm Hg) (Figs. 7.5 to 7.8). Stroke volume during exercise also decreases with increasing severity of obstruction.[10] This abnormal profile indicating subendocardial ischemia and depressed left ventricular performance may exist in patients who are judged to have mild obstruction by routine cardiac evaluation or resting left ventricular to aortic peak systolic gradient.[21]

A substantial change in exercise response toward normal may occur in some patients as early as 3 months after adequate surgical relief of the obstruction. Complete resolution of abnormal exercise response may require many months, and the rate of improvement may also be related to the duration and severity of the obstruction before treatment.[21]

Some patients are able to maintain normal left ventricular output and oxygen transport during submaximal exercise with severe electrocardiographic signs of subendocardial ischemia. Recognition of these exercise results provides insight into the adaptation to exercise, the impact and the progression of the heart disease. A longitudinal study measuring systolic blood pressure, heart rate, working capacity, and recording the electrocardiogram provides early data on the progression of cardiac disease and the benefits of treatment (Fig. 7.9).

The common practice of doing a cardiac catheterization

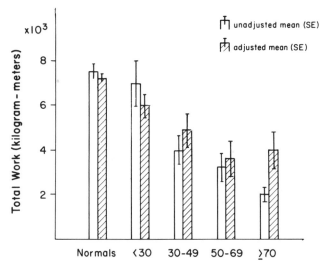

Resting LV to Ao Gradient
(mm Hg)

Fig. 7.6 Mean (±SE) total work in normals and patients with aortic stenosis. Total work is adjusted for body height (*hatched bar*). Mean total work is significantly decreased in all patient subgroups as compared to normal. The greatest depression in total work occurs in patients with resting gradient at or above 50 mm Hg.

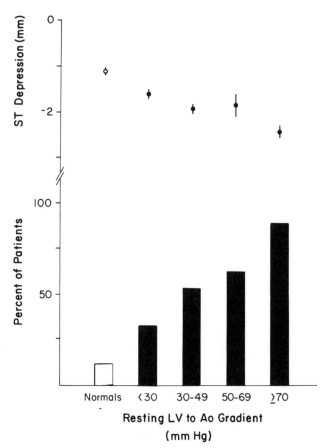

Resting LV to Ao Gradient
(mm Hg)

Fig. 7.5 Mean (±SE) ST depression during exercise in normals and patients with aortic stenosis. The frequency and magnitude of ST depression increase with increasing obstruction. The frequency of ST depression is greater in each patient subgroup than in normals.

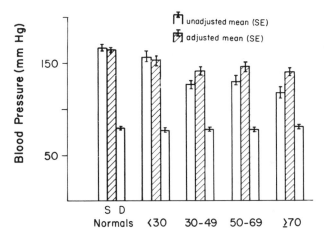

Resting LV - Ao Gradient
(mm Hg)

Fig. 7.7 Mean (±SE) blood pressure during exercise in normals and patients with aortic stenosis. Exercise systolic (*S*) pressure is adjusted for height and work-load. Mean exercise systolic pressure is significantly lower in the patient subgroups than in normals. There is no significant correlation between the peak exercise systolic pressure and resting gradient. Mean exercise diastolic (*D*) pressure is similar among normals and patients. *LV-Ao* gradient, left ventricular to aortic peak systolic gradient.

for determining the severity of aortic stenosis can be supplemented with properly performed exercise testing. Serial follow-up is recommended for patients with an abnormal exercise test. Progressive abnormal changes during longitudinal follow-up indicate increasing severity and warrant an evaluation by cardiac catheterization and possibly surgical treatment (Fig. 7.9).

Following surgical treatment for aortic stenosis, the per-

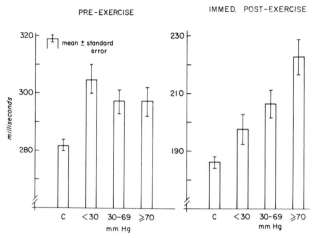

PRE-EXERCISE   IMMED. POST-EXERCISE

Fig. 7.8 Mean (± standard error) left ventricular ejection time (LVET, ordinate) before and after exercise in controls (C) and patients with aortic stenosis (abcissa). LVET is significantly prolonged at rest and after exercise in the patients. A progressive increase in LVET is seen after exercise with increasing resting gradient (mm Hg). The LVET is adjusted for heart rate, blood pressure, and body size. (Immed post-exercise, ≤1.5 minutes) (Reproduced with permission from F. W. James.[18])

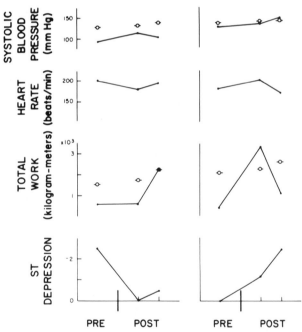

Fig 7.9 Serial exercise responses in two patients with aortic stenosis pre- and postaortic valvotomy. (*Left panel*, resting systolic gradient 100 mm Hg). Preoperatively, decreased exercise systolic pressure, total work, and ST depression are seen. Postoperatively, ST segments and total work are normal by 10 months and 29 months, respectively. Exercise systolic pressure remains depressed up to 29 months after surgery. (*Right panel*, resting systolic gradient 70 mm Hg) Preoperatively, decreased total work with normal ST segments and exercise systolic blood pressure are seen. Postoperatively (9 months), total work increases above normal with associated ST depression. At 30 months after surgery, significant ST depression and a fall in total work are seen, suggesting clinical deterioration. (Reproduced with permission from J. T. Whitmer *et al.*[21] and the American Heart Association).

sistence or the lack of resolution of exercise responses towards normal suggests significant residual obstruction, cardiovascular dysfunction, and/or an associated cardiac lesion.

TETRALOGY OF FALLOT

Cardiopulmonary responses during exercise improve markedly after corrective surgery for tetralogy of Fallot. Despite these favorable changes, impaired cardiovascular performance often persists after corrective surgery in some patients.[2, 8, 13] Maximal working capacity and heart rate are significantly lower than normal[2, 13] and are inversely related to the age at corrective surgery.[13] Cardiac output is low in relation to measured VO_2, and severe right ventricular hypertension may develop during exercise (Fig. 7.10) in patients with mild obstruction at rest.[8] These findings suggests that early surgical correction may be advisable, and physical training can potentially improve cardiopulmonary performance.

Controlled exercise testing is used also to evaluate postoperative patients for the presence of serious ventricular dysrhythmia (Fig. 7.11). In the presence of frequent or serious ventricular dysrhythmia at rest or induced by exercise following intracardiac surgery, patients should be evaluated for residual defects and considered for antiarrhythmic drug therapy. Following surgical reconstruction of the right ventricular outflow tract, residual obstruction, aggravated by exercise, may be associated with abnormal ST changes

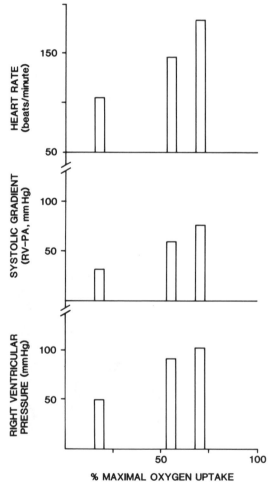

Fig 7.10 Cardiovascular responses during exercise in a patient after corrective surgery for tetralogy of Fallot. At rest (20% of maximal oxygen uptake), resting right ventricular peak systolic pressure is 50 mm Hg with an outflow tract gradient of 31 mm Hg. At two levels of exercise (55 and 70% of maximal oxygen uptake) right ventricular systolic pressure and systolic gradient increase to a peak value of 103 mm Hg and 78 mm Hg, respectively.

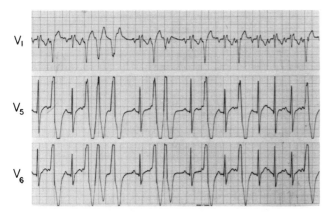

Fig 7.11 Postexercise electrocardiogram in a patient 5 years after corrective surgery for tetralogy of Fallot. "Bursts" of ventricular tachycardia are recorded immediately after exercise in the supine position.

which probably reflect right ventricular subendocardial ischemia due to the effect of exercise and right ventricular hypertension.

COARCTATION OF THE AORTA

Exercise-induced systolic hypertension and ST depression occur frequently in patients after coarctectomy.[5, 12] An increasing systolic gradient can be demonstrated between the upper and lower extremities after strenuous exercise.[5] This finding suggests an exercise-induced systolic gradient across the site of resection. During exercise, intraarterial measurements support the presence of a high systolic pressure above the site of resection producing a peak systolic gradient in some patients.[11] These intraarterial measurements fail to correlate with the size of the anastomosis or residual coarctation.

We use antihypertensive medication for those patients with systolic hypertension at rest and during exercise, and a residual gradient <30 mm Hg across the site of resection. Exercise studies are performed before and during treatment in each patient to evaluate the effectiveness of the therapy. Proper drug selection in some patients can effectively reduce the blood pressure without creating exercise intolerance. Those patients with a residual gradient ≥30 mm Hg across the site of resection should be considered for cardiac catheterization and surgical treatment.

The exercise-induced ST depression occurs in any of the precordial or inferior leads. The frequency and magnitude of ST depression in these leads are often out of proportion to the measured gradient across the site of anastomosis. The cause of the ST depression is thought to be due to ischemia; however, the reason for the ischemia is unknown. Left ventricular hypertension, residual obstruction, associated defects, and premature atherosclerosis are potential reasons justifying further clinical investigation and careful postoperative follow-up.

AORTIC INSUFFICIENCY

Exercise testing reveals a decreased working capacity, increased systolic pressure, and significant ST-depression in severe aortic insufficiency. Systolic pressure exceeding 230 mm Hg and ST depression of up to 4 mm have been recorded in some patients during exercise.[15] The level of pressure and the frequency of ST depression appear to increase in magnitude with signs of progressive enlargement of the left ventricle. The demonstration of ST depression and systolic hypertension in a patient with severe aortic insufficiency and cardiomegaly suggests myocardial ischemia and cardiovascular dysfunction. An exercise test with myocardial imaging for ejection fraction and left ventricular wall motion[4] may further asisist in the difficult problem of selecting patients for surgical treatment.

PULMONIC STENOSIS

Exercise tolerance can be depressed in patients with moderate right ventricular outflow tract obstruction. Maximal blood pressure and heart rate are generally normal. From pressure measurements during exercise at two-thirds of maximal oxygen uptake, right ventricular peak systolic pressure may exceed 190% of the resting pressure level. Right ventricular end-diastolic pressure may increase 150% above the resting level during exercise with some levels greater than 20 mm Hg.

Exercise-induced ST depression also occurs in patients with severe pulmonic stenosis. In severe obstruction, the ST segment can be depressed in leads V_2, V_3, II, III, and AVF and elevated in the leads AVF and AVL. Decreased myocardial blood flow to the right ventricular wall has been demonstrated experimentally when right ventricular peak systolic pressure exceeds 50 mm Hg.[9] Intracardiac pressure measurements as well as electrocardiographic changes and blood pressure during exercise are of potential benefit in determining the hemodynamic consequence of surgical correction of right-sided cardiac lesions.

OTHER CARDIAC LESIONS

In transposition of great arteries following Mustard operation, a depressed maximal heart rate, ST depression, and prolonged preejection period may occur. A high frequency of ST depression occurs in severe mitral insufficiency and mitral valve prolapse. After surgery for atrial septal defect, some patients have a depressed maximal heart rate, inappropriately low maximal cardiac output relative to VO_2,[8] and a decreased cardiac output which can be improved with regular physical training.

Patients with congenital complete heart block may have reasonably normal tolerance for exercise. Cardiac output particularly at submaximal exercise may be near normal at the expense of a large increase in stroke volume due to the decreased heart rate. Ventricular dysrhythmia is often provoked during exercise in these patients.

CARDIAC DYSRHYTHMIA WITH NORMAL HEART

The presence of ventricular dysrhythmia at rest does not preclude conducting an exercise test in a young patient. Patients without cardiac abnormalities and with ventricular dysrhythmia recorded before exercise or induced by exercise do not have a significant alteration in working capacity, maximal heart rate, or blood pressure response to exercise. The premature ventricular beats in these children have an equal percentage of right bundle branch block (BBB) (47%) and left BBB patterns (47%), and 6% have right and left BBB patterns. Three patterns of exercise-related ventricular dysrhythmia are recognized: ventricular dysrhythmia that is present at rest is usually suppressed or aggravated during exercise and usually reappears after exercise when the heart rate approaches control levels; ventricular dysrhythmia that is not recorded at rest may be induced by exercise; ventricular dysrhythmia which may or may not be present at rest may be induced or aggravated after exercise.

Exercise-induced ventricular dysrhythmia may resolve over time (Fig. 7.12). Further, a child with cardiac dysrhyth-

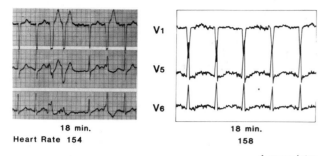

18 min.

Heart Rate 154

18 min.

158

4 years later

Fig 7.12 Serial exercise electrocardiograms in a patient with a "normal" heart and exercise induce ventricular dysrhythmia. *Left panel*, ventricular dysrhythmia with coupling is recorded. The follow-up studies revealed a decrease in the frequency of premature beats during exercise. *Right panel*, 4 years after the initial study, ventricular dysrhythmia was not recorded during the exercise procedure.

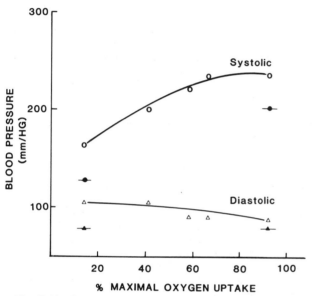

Fig. 7.13 Resting and exercise blood pressures in a patient with systemic hypertension. Systolic pressure is elevated at rest and during exercise. Diastolic pressure decreases to normal from rest to exercise. Solid circle and triangle, expected blood pressure according to height.

mia who otherwise has a normal heart and exercise test should not be restricted from recreational activities and, in many instances, athletics.

HYPERTENSION

Adolescents with a systolic pressure ≥140 mm Hg at rest will generally have excessive systolic blood pressure during exercise (Fig. 7.13). The rise in systolic pressures in hypertensive patients generally parallels the rise in normals. Occasionally, the elevated systolic pressure at rest may rise at a more rapid rate than normal during exercise or fall to a normal level during exercise. The latter has been associated with an increased cardiac output at rest.

Diastolic pressure during exercise may decrease to within normal limits as shown in Fig. 7.13. Measurements of cardiac output, blood pressure, and estimates of systemic vascular resistance can potentially contribute to the management of adolescents with borderline or essential hypertension.

ANEMIA

During submaximal exercise, patients with sickle cell anemia have low normal oxygen uptake for the level of work, increased respiratory quotient, and elevated cardiac output for the level of VO_2. This elevated cardiac output results from an increased stroke volume and heart rate. The increased cardiac output above normal is related to the hemoglobin level. Patients with hemoglobin <8 gm/dl have a 60 to 90% increase above normal for cardiac output. Blood transfusion increases oxygen transport, causing a decrease in the respiratory quotient and modest changes in cardiac output and heart rate. These changes may occur within 24 hours after transfusions therapy.

PHYSICAL ACTIVITY

An abnormal adaptive response to exercise and the level at which the abnormal response occurs are readily identified during proper exercise testing. The influence of exercise upon ventilation and respiratory gas-exchange, cardiac performance and function, myocardial perfusion, electrical stability of the heart, working performance and perceived exertion can be assessed with techniques of reasonable sensitivity and reliability. Caution must be taken when extrapolating laboratory data under controlled conditions to the field where conditions are not controlled. However, patients with cardiovascular disease whose working performance and adaptive responses to exercise are normal can probably participate in physical activities at a risk similar to that of healthy subjects. Thus, exercise data combined with other relevant clinical data provide necessary information for recommending physical activities and removing physical restrictions in specific patients.

REFERENCES

1. Adams, F. H.: Factors affecting the working capacity of children and adolescents. In Physical Activity, edited by G. L. Rarick, Chap. 4. Academic Press, New York, 1973.
2. Bjarke, B.: Oxygen uptake and cardiac output during submaximal and maximal exercise in adult subjects with totally corrected tetralogy of Fallot. In functional studies in palliated and totally corrected adult patients with tetralogy of Fallot. Scand. J. Thorac. Cardiovasc. Surg. [Suppl.] 16:9, 1974.
3. Blomqvist, C. G.: Exercise physiology: Clinical aspects. Cardiovasc. Clin. 9(3):1, 1978.
4. Borer, J. S., Bacharach, S. L., Green, M. V., Kent, K. M., Henry, W. L., Rosing, D. R., Seides, S. F., Johnston, G. S., and Epstein, S. E.: Exercise induced left ventricular dysfunction in symptomatic and asymptomatic patients with aortic regurgitation: Assessment

with radionuclide cineangiography. Am. J. Cardiol. 42:351, 1978.
5. Connor, T. M.: Evaluation of persistent coarctation of aorta after surgery with blood pressure measurement and exercise testing. Am. J. Cardiol. 43:74, 1979.
6. Cumming, G. R., Everatt, D., and Hastman, L.: Bruce treadmill test in children: Normal values in a clinical population. Am. J. Cardiol. 41:69, 1978.
7. Cumming, G. R.: Maximal exercise capacity of children with heart defects. Am. J. Cardiol. 42:613, 1978.
8. Epstein, S. E., Beiser, G. D., Goldstein, R. E., Rosing, D. R., Redwood, D. R., and Morrow, A. G.: Hemodynamic abnormalities in response to mild and intense upright exercise following operative correction of an atrial septal defect or tetralogy of Fallot. Circulation

47:1065, 1973.
9. Fixler, D. E., Archie, J. P., Ullyot, D. J., Buckberg, G. D., and Hoffman, J. I. E.: Effects of acute right ventricular systolic hypertension on regional myocardial blood flow in anesthetized dogs. Am. Heart J. 85:491, 1973.
10. Godfrey, S.: Exercise Testing in Children. W. B. Saunders, Philadelphia, 1974, Chap. 3.
11. Hanson, E., Eriksson, B. Q., and Sorhenson, S. E.: Intra-arterial blood pressures at rest and during exercise after surgery for coarctation of the aorta. Eur. J. Cardiol. 11:245, 1980.
12. James, F. W., and Kaplan, S.: Systolic hypertension during submaximal exercise after correction of coarctation of the aorta. Circulation 50(Suppl II):II-34, 1974.
13. James, F. W., Kaplan, S., Schwartz, D. C., Chou, T. C., Sandker, M. J., and Naylor, V.: Response to exercise in patients after total

surgical correction of tetralogy of Fallot. Circulation 54:671, 1976.

14. James, F. W.: Exercise testing in children and young adults: an overview. In Exercise and the Heart Cardiovascular Clinics, edited by N. K. Wenger. F. A. Davis, Philadelphia, 1978.

15. James, F. W., Donner, R., and Kaplan, S.: Exercise responses in children with progressive aortic regurgitation. Am. J. Cardiol. 41:389, 1978.

16. James, F. W.: Exercise ECG test in children. In Exercise Electrocardiography: Practical Approach, edited by E. K. Chung. Williams & Wilkins, Baltimore, 1979.

17. James, F. W., Kaplan, S., Glueck, C. J., Tsay, J-Y., Sandker, M. J., and Sarwar, C. J.: Responses of normal children and young adults to controlled bicycle exercise. Circulation 61:902, 1980.

18. James, F. W.: Exercise testing in normal individuals and patients with cardiovascular disease. In Pediatric Cardiovascular Disease, edited by M. A. Engle. F. A. Davis, Philadelphia, 1981.

19. Riopel, D. A., Taylor, A. B., and Hohn, A. R.: Blood pressure, heart rate, electrocardiographic changes in healthy children during treadmill exercise. Am. J. Cardiol. 44:697, 1979.

20. Sproule, B. J., Mitchell, J. H., and Miller, W. F.: Cardiopulmonary physiological responses to heavy exercise in patients with anemia. J. Clin. Invest. 39:378, 1960.

21. Whitmer, J. T., James, F. W., Kaplan, S., Schwartz, D. C., and Knight, M. J. S.: Exercise testing in children before and after surgical treatment of aortic stenosis. Circulation 63:254, 1981.

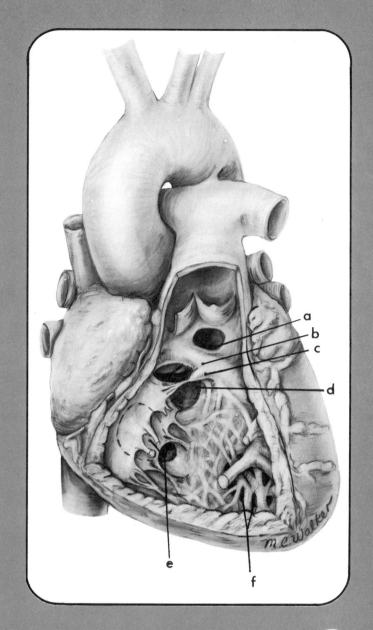

Part 2

CONGENITAL DEFECTS

8

Atrial Septal Defects and Atrioventricular Canal

Robert H. Feldt, M.D., William D. Edwards, M.D., Francisco J. Puga, M.D.,
James B. Seward, M.D., and William H. Weidman, M.D.

Secundum-type atrial septal defects are common and usually not associated with other intracardiac abnormalities. Abnormalities in the development of the atrioventricular canal result in one or more defects involving the atrioventricular septum and the atrioventricular valves. Several types of defects make up the complex of atrioventricular canal defects: partial atrioventricular canal, complete atrioventricular canal, common atrium, and isolated ventricular septal defect of the atrioventricular canal type. All the defects have some features in common; however, important differences exist in the clinical course, natural history, and treatment which make differential diagnosis necessary.

SECUNDUM ATRIAL SEPTAL DEFECT

Secundum-type atrial septal defect (ASD) is one of the most common congenital cardiac defects (7%), and the ratio of affected females to males is 2:1.[17] In most cases, the cause is unknown; however, there are reports of several families in which more than one member had an ASD, and in some of these families, the defect was probably transmitted as a result of a genetic abnormality.[8, 35] Holt and Oram[24] described families in which several members had ASD in association with bony abnormalities of the upper extremities and usually nonapposition of the thumb; this association is now well established.

PATHOLOGY

The embryonic atrium is partially divided by two septa, so that flow from the right atrium to the left atrium occurs throughout intrauterine life. The sequence of atrial septation is well illustrated by Netter[40] and described by Van Mierop.[66]

Septum primum is an incomplete partition in which the anteroinferior free edge lies above the atrioventricular canal and becomes lined by tissue derived from the superior and inferior endocardial cushions. The resultant ostium primum is subsequently sealed by endocardial cushion tissue, but not before fenestrations in the septum primum coalesce to form ostium secundum. To the right of the septum primum, anterosuperior infolding of the atrial roof results in the formation of septum secundum, a thick-walled muscular structure that expands posterioinferiorly to form an incomplete partition overlying ostium secundum. This posteroinferior deficiency in septum secundum is the fossa ovalis.

Postnatally, left atrial pressure exceeds right atrial pressure, and the valve of the fossa ovalis (septum primum) is forced against the lumbus (septum secundum), thereby effecting functional closure of the foramen (valvular-competent patent foramen ovale). In 30 to 35% of adult hearts,[61] this communication remains potentially patent. Rarely, premature closure of the foramen ovale may occur during intrauterine life.[30]

In some persons, the valve of the fossa ovalis may be redundant and may result in aneurysms of the fossa ovalis valve.[57] Atrial septal defects commonly involve the fossa ovalis and are due to deficiency of the valve or the limbus of the fossa ovalis, fenestrations of the fossa ovalis valve, or combinations of these. Since the ostium secundum is generally enlarged, such defects are commonly called secundum (or ostium secundum) atrial septal defects (Fig. 8.1).

Most secundum atrial septal defects are isolated anomalies. However, when the defect coexists with another malformation, the latter is generally the more significant lesion. An important group of associated lesions relate to abnormalities of the mitral valve. Mitral stenosis (Lutembacher's syndrome) is usually the result of rheumatic fever and is now uncommon. Mitral valve prolapse with or without mitral regurgitation is more commonly seen.[26]

PHYSIOLOGY

With the exception of the very small defects, the size of the defect has less effect on the flow of blood from the left to the right atrium than it does on the relative filling resistances in the right and left ventricles. The direction in which blood flows through the defect is primarily related to the difference in pressures in the right and left atria throughout the cardiac cycle. The pressures in the atria are determined mainly by the relative compliances of their respective ventricles. During the early months of life, the wall thicknesses of the right and left ventricles are similar, and the comparable filling characteristics may result in only minimal shunting. With increasing age, the maturation of the pulmonary vascular bed results in decreases both in pulmonary vascular resistance and in right ventricular wall thickness, and thus can result in an increase in the left-to-right shunt.

Most commonly, the dominant shunt is left to right because the left atrial pressure exceeds the right during the major part of the cardiac cycle. A small right-to-left shunt of blood returning via the inferior vena cava is usually present and occurs at the onset of ventricular contraction or during early ventricular diastole. Further, phasic changes during respiration also influence the amount of left-to-right shunting.[32] Superior vena caval blood return is directed toward the tricuspid valve and participates less in the right-to-left shunt. The nearness of the right pulmonary vein orifices to the ASD results in preferential shunting of blood from the right lung, compared with that from the left lung.[60]

Despite the large increase in pulmonary blood flow (often three to four times normal), pulmonary artery pressure almost always is normal until early adult life.[70] Systemic

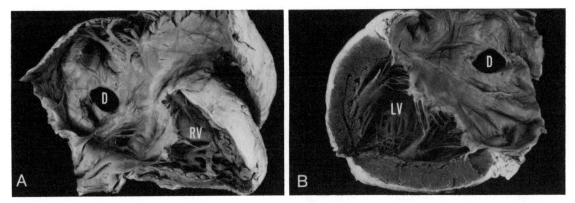

Fig. 8.1 Secundum atrial septal defect (*D*) viewed from right atrium (*A*) and left atrium (*B*). *LV*, left ventricle; *RV*, right ventricle. The right atrium and right ventricle are greatly dilated, and the left ventricle is of normal size.

blood flow is usually normal despite the large left-to-right shunt. Although the pulmonary arteries may have medial hypertrophy and intimal proliferation, pulmonary vascular changes greater than grade 2 (Heath and Edwards' classification) are rare.

The development of irreversible pulmonary hypertension in the setting of an isolated atrial septal defect is uncommon and in some cases represents the coincidental occurrence of such a defect with primary plexogenic pulmonary arteriopathy.[67]

A pressure gradient across the pulmonary valve often occurs as a result of the great increase in blood flow from the dilated right ventricle across the normal pulmonary valve into the dilated pulmonary artery. This peak systolic pressure gradient is often as high as 40 mm Hg.[70]

Secundum ASD only rarely causes myocardial dysfunction in children, but studies on adult patients have shown decreased left ventricular stroke work.[31] The effects of long-standing right ventricular volume overload in the adult remain uncertain, although recent echocardiographic studies have suggested that certain parameters of left ventricular function remain normal well into adult life.[53]

MANIFESTATIONS

Clinical Features

Although symptoms have been noted in infancy,[74] most infants with this defect are asymptomatic, and frequently their condition goes undetected until they are of school age. In our experience, only 13 of 170 patients (8%) seen during a 20-year period had their condition detected and diagnosed when they were less than 2 years of age. Eight of the 13 had heart failure.[59]

Most patients with a moderate left-to-right shunt, that is, a ratio of pulmonary blood flow to systemic blood flow (Qp/Qs) of 1.5 to 3.0, and normal pulmonary artery pressure are asymptomatic, and those with symptoms usually complain only of mild fatigue and dyspnea. The frequency of fatigue and dyspnea increases in patients who have larger left-to-right shunts (Qp/Qs >3), and cardiac failure occasionally occurs. Many patients with moderately large left-to-right shunts have no appreciable symptoms.

Palpation of the chest reveals a systolic impulse along the lower left sternal border, resulting from systolic contraction of a dilated right ventricle. The first cardiac sound may be accentuated. The second sound is moderately split (duration 0.04 second or more), partly as a result of the delayed emptying of the dilated right ventricle; respiration affects

the splitting minimally. The pulmonary valve closure is usually slightly increased in intensity, even in the absence of pulmonary hypertension.

The increased flow of blood across the pulmonary valve produces an ejection-type systolic murmur, maximal over the upper left sternal border and transmitted into the upper lung fields. The increased volume of blood shunted from the left to the right atrium across the tricuspid valve results in a middiastolic murmur, maximal along the lower left sternal border. The latter murmur may be heard at the apex. Jugular venous pulses are normal in the absence of heart failure and tricuspid valve insufficiency.

The clinical diagnosis of ASD is usually easy in children. However, it is not possible clinically to differentiate ASD from partial anomalous pulmonary venous connection. Patients can be sent to surgery without further study,[39] provided all features are completely typical and the surgeon is prepared for the possibility of partial anomalous pulmonary venous connection. The diagnosis may be more difficult in older patients. The murmurs are frequently variable and are suggestive of rheumatic heart disease because of the rather high frequency of mitral insufficiency and tricuspid insufficiency in older patients with ASD.

Phonocardiographic Features

Splitting of the first heart sound is commonly apparent on precordial phonocardiography. The second sound is almost always moderately split with accentuation of the pulmnary component, and the degree of splitting frequently remains relatively constant throughout the respiratory cycle. The ejection murmur is always located at the pulmonary valve, and the middiastolic murmur is localized to the inflow tract of the right ventricle.[3]

Electrocardiographic Features

The mean QRS axis in the frontal plane ranges from +95 to +170° in most cases and is associated with a clockwise loop directed inferiorly to the right in the frontal projection (Fig. 8.2). In 6% of the cases, the QRS loop is counterclockwise in the frontal plane.

There is always some variant of RSR' in lead V_1, and in about half the cases, there are changes in P waves, suggestive of atrial enlargement.[14]

Radiologic Features

The heart is usually enlarged, with a cardiothoracic ratio greater than 0.50. The aortic arch is small, and there is distinct enlargement of the main pulmonary artery and its

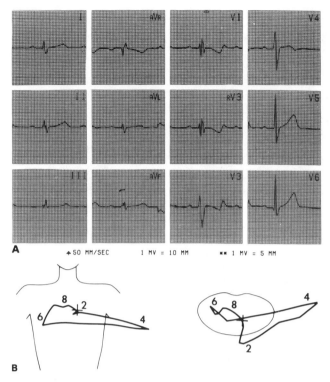

Fig. 8.2 Electrocardiogram (*A*) and vectorcardiogram (*B*) of 6-year-old with secundum ASD. Both are compatible with right ventricular volume overload.

major branches. Pulmonary vascular markings are increased, but it is often difficult to quantitate the left-to-right shunt from a roentgenographic assessment of peripheral vascularity (Fig. 8.3). Some patients with large left-to-right shunts have normal heart size on the roentgenogram.

Echocardiographic Features

Volume overload of the right side of the heart, secondary to left-to-right shunting at the atrial level, is characterized by increased right atrial and right ventricular dimensions and paradoxical ventricular septal motion[13, 47] (Fig. 8.4). These abnormal, but indirect, M-mode echocardiographic features of right ventricular volume overload are present in more than 98% of patients.[47]

The primary advantage of the 2D echocardiographic technique is the ability to visualize the atrial septal defect directly.[33, 62] Patients with a large secundum ASD usually have a convincing absence of midseptal echoes (Fig. 8.5*A*). However, false echo dropout in the area of the thin valve of the fossa ovalis is commonly encountered when the apical four-chamber view is used,[62] which makes this particular projection less diagnostic. When feasible, the subcostal transducer position is preferred for direct visualization of an ASD (Fig. 8.5*B*). From the subcostal position, the ultrasonic beam is more perpendicular to the atrial septum and false dropout is minimized.

Contrast echocardiography has been very helpful in enhancing the recognition of the secundum ASD.[56] A high percentage of patients with an uncomplicated ASD will have a small right-to-left shunt, which can be detected by peripheral venous contrast echocardiography.[56] However, when the shunt is predominantly left to right, appreciation of a "negative contrast" effect (that is, visualization of a bolus of undyed blood distorting a bolus of dye-enhanced blood)[71] can be confidently visualized in a high percentage of patients (Fig. 8.6).

By utilizing multiple transducer positions for direct visualization and contrast echocardiography for appreciation of right-to-left and left-to-right shunts, nearly all instances of secundum ASD can be confidently diagnosed by noninvasive echocardiography.

CARDIAC CATHETERIZATION

The presence of a secundum ASD is suspected when oxygen saturation is greater in right atrial blood than in blood from the superior and inferior venae cavae. An increase of 10% in oxygen saturation in one series of blood samples or an increase of 5% in two series usually indicates an interatrial communication. A ventricular septal defect with insufficiency of the tricuspid valve, a left ventricular-right atrial shunt, or partial and complete atrioventricular canal can produce similar findings. Anomalous connection of some or

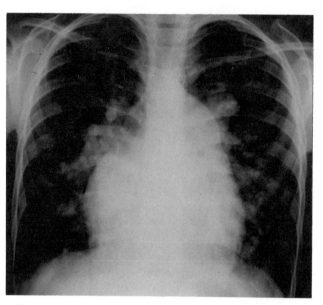

Fig. 8.3 Roentgenogram of 7-year-old with secundum ASD, showing cardiomegaly, prominent main pulmonary artery, and prominent pulmonary vascular markings.

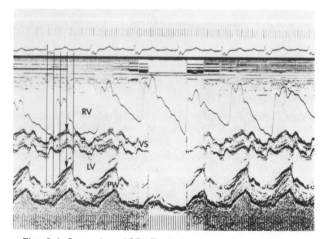

Fig. 8.4 Secundum ASD. Typical echocardiographic features include increased right ventricular (*RV*) dimension and paradoxical motion of ventricular septum (*VS*). (Paradoxical septal motion is defined as systolic anterior motion of the left, right, or both septal echoes). Both posterior wall (*PW*) and *VS* move anteriorly with each systole. (Vertical lines assist in appreciating paradoxical septal motion.) *LV*, left ventricle. Carotid tracing is shown in right ventricular cavity.

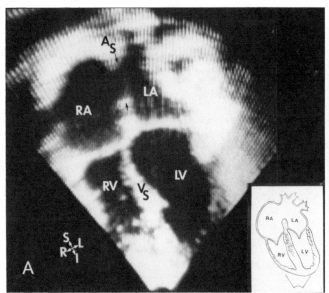
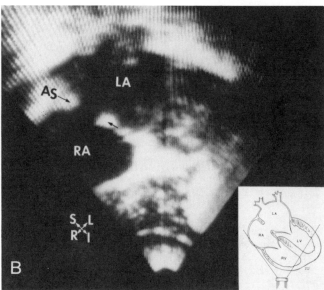

Fig. 8.5 Secundum ASD: 2D echocardiography. (*A*) Apical four-chamber view in patient with large secundum ASD. There is prominent echo dropout in midportion of atrial septum (*AS*) (*small arrows*). However, because echo beam is parallel to atrial septum, the potential for false dropout of echoes in area of fossa ovalis makes this view less diagnostic. *RA*, right atrium; *LA*, left atrium; *RV*, right ventricle; *LV*, left ventricle; *VS*, ventricular septum; *L*, left; *I*, inferior; *R*, right; *S*, superior. (Reproduced with permission from J. B. Seward et al.[55]). (*B*) Subcostal four-chamber view in same patient, showing prominent echo dropout in midarterial septum, consistent with secundum ASD.

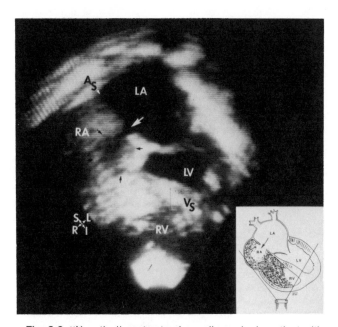

Fig. 8.6 "Negative" contrast echocardiography in patient with secundum ASD. After peripheral venous injection of echo contrast material a cloud of echoes fills the right atrium (*RA*) and right ventricle (*RV*). In midportion of atrial septum (*AS*), a "negative" contrast effect is visualized (*arrows*) as a darker (undyed) bolus of blood entering the contrast-enhanced blood of right atrium. This observation is diagnostic of left-to-right shunt at atrial level. *LA*, left atrium; *LV*, left ventricle; *VS*, ventricular septum; *L*, left; *R*, right; *I*, inferior; *S*, superior. (Reproduced with permission from J. B. Seward et al.[55])

all of the pulmonary veins to the right atrium or defects of the atrioventricular canal also can result in increased oxygen saturation of blood in the right atrium. Anomalous pulmonary venous connection to the cavae or systemic arteriovenous fistula also will produce a saturation step-up in the

right atrium and may be mistaken for a shunt at the atrial level. Recognition of these less common shunts is facilitated by attention to the level of saturation change (cavae versus atrium), dye dilution, and angiographic techniques.

Generally, the right ventricular pressure is not elevated, although peak systolic gradients across a normal pulmonic valve of as high as 40 mm Hg have been reported. Pulmonary artery pressure is usually normal, as is the calculated pulmonary arterial resistance (less than 4 units/m²). Studies of adult patients have documented an increased frequency of pulmonary hypertension and elevated pulmonary arterial resistance. Elevated pulmonary arterial resistance, which reflects the degree of pulmonary vascular obstruction, is usually mild to moderate, and severe pulmonary vascular obstructive disease (pulmonary arterial resistance greater than 10 units/m²) has been reported only rarely.[54]

Angiocardiographic volume studies[19] have shown significant elevations in right ventricular end-diastolic volume and right ventricular stroke index and normal values for right ventricular ejection fraction. Other studies have suggested decreases in left ventricular stroke work.[31]

DIFFERENTIAL DIAGNOSIS

Secundum-type ASD is distinguished from partial atrioventricular canal by the absence of the murmur of mitral insufficiency and by the typical clockwise QRS loop in the frontal plane.

Infrequently, secundum ASD defect is associated with mitral insufficiency and mitral valve prolapse with or without mitral insufficiency. Anatomically, the mitral defect does not resemble the deformity in partial atrioventricular canal.

Ventricular septal defects with shunting of blood from the left ventricle into the right atrium are also part of the differential diagnosis of atrial septal defect.

Current methods of echocardiography have a crucial role in separating secundum atrial septal defect from all the defects mentioned above. The echo features are frequently so typical as to be diagnostic and eliminate the need for cardiac catheterization.

CLINICAL COURSE

Secundum-type ASD is compatible with a long life. There are reports of patients living into the 7th and 8th decades.[11] Some patients 50 years old or older have had symptoms for less than 10 years.[64]

Although this condition does not usually manifest itself in infancy cardiac failure may rarely develop in an infant with an uncomplicated ASD. Spontaneous closure of an ASD encountered in infancy also has been documented.[37]

Patients with ASD frequently remain active and tolerate the defect for many years, in part because the architecture of the right ventricle is conducive to ejection of a large stroke volume. Few patients have been studied more than once by cardiac catheterization. In one series of eight such patients, none had a change in the calculated pulmonary vascular resistance.[76]

If pulmonary vascular obstruction develops, with increased pulmonary artery pressure, the left-to-right shunt diminishes, pulmonary blood flow decreases, and murmurs across the tricuspid and pulmonary valves are diminished. Splitting of the second sound diminishes, and intensity of the pulmonary valve closure sound increases. A pulmonary ejection "click" may develop. If a right-to-left shunt develops, cyanosis is noted.

Pulmonary hypertension rarely develops during the childhood years, but some patients less than 8 years of age who have an ASD have had significant pulmonary hypertension. In a collaborative study of 298 patients[76] whose ages ranged from less than 1 year to 96 years, only 7 had significant pulmonary hypertension, that is, a ratio of pulmonary artery systolic pressure to systemic artery systolic pressure (Pp/Ps) equal to or greater than 0.5, in the presence of a large pulmonary blood flow. The youngest patient was 8 months old, and three patients were less than 12 years old. Eighteen patients had pulmonary vascular obstructive disease; six of these were between 3 and 12 years of age. Occasionally, particularly after pregnancy or recurrent respiratory infections, pulmonary vascular disease develops early in adult life, and its course is usually progressive.[54]

Cardiac failure increases in frequency among patients who are in the 2nd and 3rd decades of life.[22] Endocarditis is an extremely rare complication. Death is uncommon through the 3rd decade. Thereafter, heart failure, coronary artery disease, and atrial fibrillation are the usual precipitating causes of death.

There is uncertainty regarding the natural history and proper management of patients with small ASD. Serial catheterization studies of such patients have failed to document deterioration over average follow-up of about 10 years.[1] It remains to be seen whether deterioration or sequelae of a possible right-to-left shunt will occur over longer periods.

OTHER ATRIAL SEPTAL DEFECTS

The sinus venosus atrial septal defect accounts for 5 to 10% of atrial septal defects and is located posterior to the fossa ovalis. Most commonly, the defect is rimmed by atrial septal tissue only anterioinferiorly, while its posterior aspect is the right atrial free wall and its superior border is often absent, owing to an overriding superior vena cava. Infrequently, the defect may be directly posterior to the fossa ovalis or posteroinferior, whereby the inferior vena cava may join both atria.

The sinus venosus defect is commonly associated with anomalous connection of the right pulmonary veins to either the right atrium or the superior vena cava near the caval-atrial junction. Pulmonary veins from the right upper lobe or, less commonly, the entire right lung connect anomalously, while the remaining veins joint the left atrium normally.

Two-dimensional echocardiography permits direct examination of the atrial septum, and by the use of multiple tomography projections, in particular the subcostal approach, the sinus venosus atrial septal defect can be visualized.[38]

The coronary sinus atrial septal defect, a rare anomaly, lies inferior and slightly anterior to the fossa ovalis, at the anticipated site of the coronary sinus ostium.[48] It is usually part of a developmental complex that includes absence of the coronary sinus and a persistent left superior vena cava that joins the roof of the left atrium. This anomaly may be associated with complete atrioventricular canal, particularly in the asplenia syndrome, and the atrial septal defects of both malformations then merge.

When isolated, coronary sinus and sinus venosus defects have the same clinical manifestations as secundum atrial septal defects. Defects of the sinus venosus type are more likely to show right-to-left shunting on indicator dye-dilution curves from injections into the superior vena cava and none from injections into the inferior vena cava. These features may lead to the diagnosis during cardiac catheterization.

TREATMENT

Elective surgical repair of significant ASDs is the treatment of choice. The age at which repair is done depends on the experience of the surgeon; however, there is no obvious advantage in delaying surgery after the patient reaches 4 or 5 years of age. While the risk of surgical morbidity and mortality increases in the adult years, surgical repair frequently results in an excellent result in the symptomatic patient.[52]

For experienced cardiac surgeons, elective repair of ASD is simple and safe. The usual approach is through a median sternotomy, although a right anterolateral thoracotomy below the breast can be used and provides a better cosmetic result. Usually, closure can be accomplished by direct approximation of the edges of the defect, which are everted toward the right atrium; occasionally, with very large defects, a patch of pericardium or Teflon can be used to achieve closure.

For high sinus venosus atrial septal defects associated with partial anomalous pulmonary venous connection to the superior vena cava, repair requires construction of a tunnel that directs anomalous pulmonary venous flow through the ASD into the left atrium.

Complications of surgery in children are rare. Factors that seem to influence surgical mortality and moribidity are the presence of pulmonary hypertension, preoperative heart failure or left ventricular dysfunction characterized by elevated left atrial pressures, and pulmonary congestion and edema occasionally seen during the postoperative period.[5, 75]

Postoperative dysrhythmias are common.[29] Most frequently observed rhythm disturbances are supraventricular in origin, although transitory atrioventricular conduction defects also can be seen. These rhythm changes are usually transitory and can be managed pharmacologically. Postoperative atrial dysrhythmias are particularly frequent in patients undergoing repair of a sinus venosus defect,[28] possibly due to the proximity of the sinus node.

ATRIOVENTRICULAR CANAL DEFECTS

The embryologic development of the atrioventricular canal involves septation of the common atrioventricular

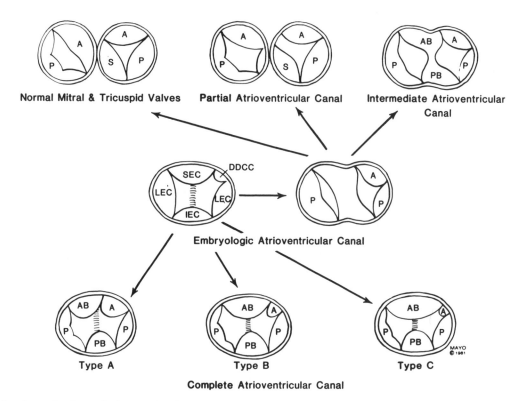

Fig. 8.7 Embryology of atrioventricular canal and spectrum of atrioventricular canal defects. *Center panel* (embryologic atrioventricular canal), superior (*SEC*) and inferior (*IEC*) endocardial cushions fuse, thereby forming two orifices. Lateral endocardial cushion (*LEC*) on left forms posterior (*P*) mitral leaflet, *LEC* on right forms posterior tricuspid leaflet, and *LEC* on the right and dextrodorsal conus cushion (*DDCC*) form anterior tricuspid leaflet (*A*). *Top panel*, fused superior and inferior endocardial cushions form anterior mitral and septal (*S*) tricuspid leaflets in normal heart. In partial form of atrioventricular canal, anterior mitral leaflet is cleft, and medial triscuspid commissure is widened. In intermediate form, anterior (*AB*) and posterior (*PB*) bridging leaflets are fused in midline. *Bottom panel*, complete forms of atrioventricular canal. With progression from type A to type C, anterior bridging leaflet becomes larger, anterior tricuspid leaflet becomes smaller, and medial triscuspid papillary muscle migrates from ventricular septum to moderator band to anterior tricuspid papillary muscle. Anterior bridging leaflet is attached by chordae tendineae to ventricular septal summit in type A but not in type B or C (so-called free-floating leaflet).

orifice into mitral and tricuspid valves and closure of the atrial septum (ostium primum) above and the ventricular septum below. This is accomplished by proliferation of the endocardial cushions and the dextrodorsal conus swelling[40, 66] (Fig. 8.7).

Growth of the superior and inferior endocardial cushions toward one another results in an H-shaped atrioventricular orifice. Two lateral cushions later form, and eventually a portion of the dextrodorsal conus swelling interposes between the superior and right lateral endocardial cushions. Fusion of the superior and inferior cushions completely separates the orifices of the mitral and tricuspid valves. The development of leaflets and tensor apparatus involves cushion tissue and excavation and undermining of the subjacent ventricular myocardium, with later attenuation of the muscular component.

The anterior mitral leaflet forms first, in part from the superior cushion and half of the inferior cushion. Then, the posterior mitral and anterior tricuspid leaflets develop, the former associated with the left lateral cushion and the latter with both the right lateral endocardial cushion and the dextrodorsal conus swelling. The posterior leaflet forms in part from the right lateral cushion, and the septal leaflet originates in part from the inferior endocardial cushion (with no contribution from the superior cushion).

Tissue from the superior and inferior endocardial cushions subdivides the atrioventricular orifice and proliferates along the atrial septal rim of the ostium primum; with the development of the atrioventricular septum, basal septation of the atria is achieved. The secondary interventricular foramen is eventually closed by proliferation of the inferior endocardial cushion.

Faulty development of the endocardial cushions and of the atrioventricular septum is believed to be responsible for the broad range of atrioventricular canal defects. The anterior leafleft of the mitral valve is almost always deformed, and occasionally, the septal leaflet of the tricuspid valve is involved. The severity of the defect in the anterior leaflet of the mitral valve may vary from a small notch to a complete cleft of the entire leaflet with loss of tissue.

Three types of complete atrioventricular canal have been identified by differences in the anterior bridging leaflet of the common atrioventricular valve[50] (Figs. 8.7 and 8.8). In the most frequent type (Fig. 8.8*A*), the anterior bridging leaflet has chordal insertions into the right crest of the ventricular septum. There is a limited interventricular communication between the chordae and the anterior and posterior bridging leaflets. In the second type (Fig. 8.8*B*), the anterior bridging leaflet has chordal insertions into one papillary muscle in the right ventricle; the ventricular septal defect is large. In these two types, there are usually no other intracardiac defects.

When other major defects, such as pulmonary stenosis, transposition of the great arteries, double-outlet right ventricle, or splenic anomalies, coexist with complete atrioventricular canal, the anterior bridging leaflet has chordal insertions into the anterior tricuspid papillary muscle (Fig. 8.8*C*). The ventricular septal defect is large.

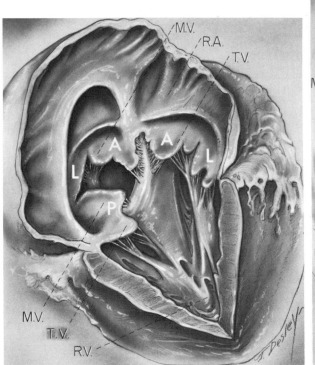

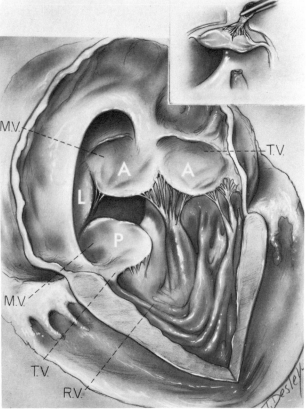

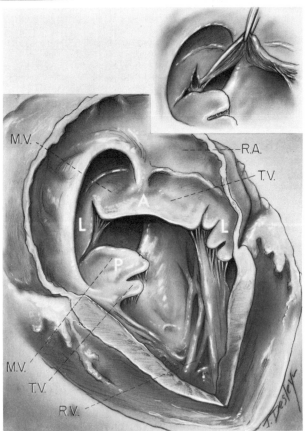

Fig. 8.8 Illustrations of various types of complete atrioventricular canal. (*A*) The most frequent form (type A) originally classified according to anterior bridging leaflet (*A*) being divided and attached to septum. Current interpretation has only the left-sided portion of anterior leaflet as the anterior briding leaflet, and the right-sided portion is the true anterior tricuspid leaflet. *P* is posterior bridging leaflet, and *L* represents the two lateral leaflets that correspond to posterior mitral and tricuspid leaflets. *MV* and *TV* indicate mitral and tricuspid portions of leaflets, and *RA* and *RV* indicate right atrium and right ventricular. (*B*) The least frequent form of complete atrioventricular canal (type B) originally classified because of the common anterior leaflet was believed to be divided but attached by chordae only in the right ventricle. Current

Infrequently, defects in atrioventricular septal formation may result in a ventricular septal defect in the position seen in complete atrioventricular canal but unassociated with other abnormalities of the atrioventricular valves or defects in the atrial septum.

PARTIAL ATRIOVENTRICULAR CANAL

This defect is one-fourth as frequent as the secundum-type atrial septal defect and also differs in that the sex frequency is approximately equal. The left-to-right shunt usually is large and produces volume overloading of the right ventricle. In addition, there are various degrees of mitral insufficiency, resulting in volume overload of the left ventricle.

Partial atrioventricular canal defect is associated with four abnormalities that may occur alone or in combination: primum atrial septal defect; paratricuspid inlet ventricular septal defect (ventricular septal defect of the atrioventricular canal type); cleft anterior mitral leaflet; and widened medial tricuspid commissure (so-called cleft septal tricuspid leaflet).

The most frequent form of partial atrioventricular canal consists of a primum atrial septal defect and a cleft anterior mitral leaflet, the latter of which is usually associated with mitral insufficiency. The atrial septal defect lies anteroinferior to the fossa ovalis and is bordered by a crescentic rim of atrial septal tissue, posterosuperiorly, and by mitral-tricuspid valvular continuity, anterioinferiorly (Fig. 8.9). The defect results from deficiency of atrial septum at the site of the embryonic ostium primum and from deficiency of the atrioventricular septum, whereby the ventricular septal summit attains a scooped-out appearance.

Manifestations

Clinical Features. The lesion is frequently discovered in infancy because of the prominence of cardiac murmurs. Symptoms, including heart failure, may occur in infancy and most commonly occur when the defect is associated with severe mitral insufficiency or other significant cardiac defects. Symptoms of dyspnea, fatigue, and recurrent respiratory infections can occur early in life. Growth failure is more common than in secundum ASD. Partial atrioventricular canal is less likely to go undetected into adult life than is secundum atrial septal defect. The severity of symptoms frequently depends on the severity of insufficiency of the atrioventricular valves.[42]

The left anterior chest wall is often prominent. The heart is overactive and, if mitral insufficiency is significant, there is often an apical systolic thrill. The right and left ventricular impulses can be palpated over the left sternal border and at the apex, respectively. On auscultation, the first sound is normal and the second sound is split during both inspiration and expiration. The degree of accentuation of the pulmonary valve closure depends on the pulmonary artery pressure, and the pulmonary second sound is increased in patients who have pulmonary hypertension. An ejection systolic murmur, which is transmitted into the upper lung fields, is heard over the upper left sternal border. A holosystolic murmur of mitral insufficiency usually can be heard at the apex, with transmission into the lower left part of the thorax. There is often a low-pitched middiastolic murmur heard either at the left lower sternal border or at the apex.

Electrovectorcardiographic Features. Changes in the P waves, indicating atrial enlargement, are present in about 60% of patients. Electrophysiologic studies[68] have shown a prolongation of the internodal conduction time, which may account for the first-degree heart block that commonly occurs.[43]

The mean QRS axis in the frontal plane ranges from -30 to $-170°$, with most axes directed between -30 and $-90°$. The initial QRS vector forces are usually directed inferiorly to the right, and the QRS loop moves counterclockwise, superiorly and to the left (Fig. 8.10). The frontal plane loop usually lies above the isoelectric line; less often, it is a figure-of-eight loop lying along the horizontal isoelectric line.[43] Anatomic and electrophysiologic studies have shown that this abnormal vectorcardiographic pattern is associated with a specific anomaly of the conduction system.[10, 18]

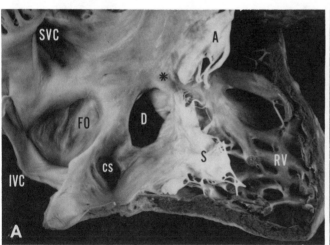
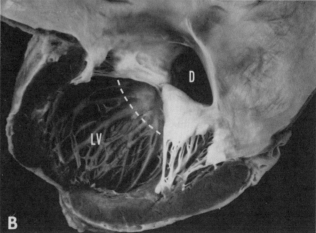

Fig. 8.9 Partial atrioventricular canal (primum atrial septal defect, *D*) and cleft anterior mitral leaflet viewed from right atrium (*A*) and left atrium (*B*). Commissure (*) between septal (*S*) and anterior (*A*) tricuspid leaflets is widened. *Dashed line* indicates anticipated extent of normal anterior mitral leaflet. *FO*, foramen ovale; *CS*; coronary sinus ostium; IVC, inferior vena cava; SVC, superior vena cava; LV, left ventricle.

interpretation has the anterior briding leaflet larger and overhanging the ventricular septum. (*C*) The form of complete atrioventricular canal that is most often associated with other major cardiac anomalies (type C) (originally classified that the common anterior leaflet was undivided and unattached). Currently, it is believed that the anterior bridging leaflet is very large and the anterior tricuspid leaflet (unlabeled but between *A* and *L* on tricuspid side) is very hypoplastic. (Reproduced with permission from G. C. Rastelli *et al.*[50])

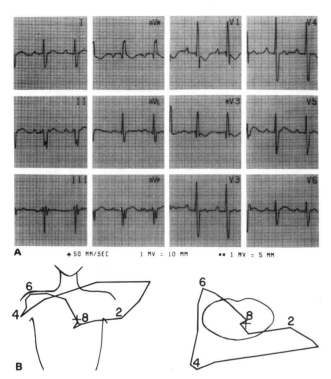

Figure 8.10 Electrocardiogram (*A*) and vectorcardiogram (*B*) of 4-month-old with partial atrioventricular canal defect, severe mitral insufficiency, and pulmonary hypertension. Findings are compatible with right ventricular overload. Mean frontal plane QRS axis is −70°.

Usually, a delay in right ventricular depolarization, indicating right ventricular volume overload, is present. Patients with mitral insufficiency may have additional evidence of left ventricular hypertrophy.[14]

Radiologic Features. The heart is usually large on a plain roentgenogram of the chest, with an average cardiothoracic ratio of 0.60. Assessment of left ventricular enlargement is difficult because of displacement by the enlarged right ventricle. Because the mitral insufficiency jet is often directed into the right atrium, left atrial enlargement may not be apparent.

Echocardiographic Features. The M-mode echocardiographic features include inferior displacement of the mitral valve echo, narrowing of the left ventricular outflow tract, and multiple systolic and diastolic echoes of the mitral valve.[73] A unifying feature of the atrioventricular canal defect (partial or complete) is seen on apex-to-base scans of the ventricular septum, which show apparent movement of the mitral valve through the plane of the left ventricular septum (Fig. 8.11). However, as opposed to complete atrioventricular canal, large dropout of ventricular septal echoes is not present in partial atrioventricular canal.[20] This feature is best appreciated on 2D echocardiography.[21]

In atrioventricular canal defect, the atrioventricular valves are displaced toward their morphologic ventricle, with the septal portion of each atrioventricular valve inserting at the same level to the crest of the ventricular septum. The lower atrial septum is normally a relatively thick structure, and false dropout is rare. In atrioventricular canal defect, this portion of the atrial septum is conspicuously absent and accounts for the diagnostic 2D echocardiographic picture. There is no visible ventricular septal defect below the insertion of the atrioventricular valves of partial canal (Fig. 8.12).

The characteristic cleft anterior leaflet of the mitral valve

is visible by utilizing short-axis parasternal echo projections (Fig. 8.13). Normally, the mitral valve has a "fishmouth" appearance, whereas patients with cleft mitral valve have a break in the anterior leaflet, producing a "horseshoe" appearance during diastole.

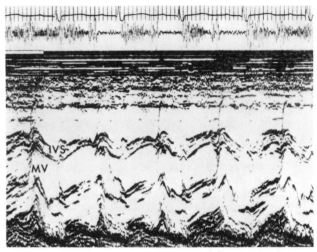

Fig. 8.11 Partial atrioventricular canal. Characteristic M-mode echocardiographic feature of atrioventricular canal is apparent movement of atrioventricular valve through plane of ventricular septum (this results from inferior displacement of both atrioventricular valves and insertion at same level to crest of ventricular septum). Additional features include multiple mitral valve (*MV*) echoes, paradoxical ventricular septal motion, and abutment of the mitral and septal echoes (narrowed left ventricular outflow tract). *IVS,* interventricular septum.

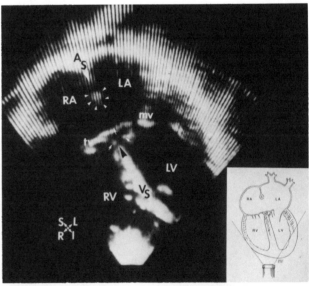

Fig. 8.12 Partial atrioventricular canal. An apical four-chamber view demonstrates diagnostic 2D echocardiographic features of (1) insertion of both septal portions of atrioventricular valves (*mv* and *tv*) to crest of ventricular septum (*VS, black arrowhead*) (normally, tricuspid valve inserts lower than mitral valve); (2) absence of echoes in inferior atrial septum (*AS*) (see *inset*); and (3) multiple atrioventricular valve echoes. *Small arrowheads* highlight the bulbous-appearing AS above primum atrial septal defect. *Small arrows* point to multiple chordae inserting onto crest of VS. *RA,* right atrium; *LA,* left atrium; *LV,* left ventricle; *L,* left; *RV,* right ventricle; *R,* right; *S,* superior; *I,* inferior. (Reproduced with permission from J. B. Seward et al.[55])

Cardiac Catheterization and Angiocardiography

A large left-to-right shunt can be demonstrated at the atrial level by a significant higher oxygen saturation of the blood from the right atrium, compared with blood returning through the inferior and superior venae cavae. Because of the anatomic position of the atrial septal defect, blood samples taken from the inflow portion of the right ventricle may have increased oxygen saturation. The calculated left-to-right shunt usually exceeds 50%. Most patients have a small right-to-left shunt that is measurable by indicator dye-dilu-

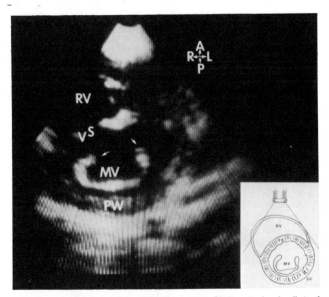

Fig. 8.13 Partial atrioventricular canal. Cleft anterior leaflet of mitral valve (*MV*) is best visualized from parasternal short-axis scans of left ventricle. Normally, anterior leaflet completes the circle, producing a "fishmouth" appearance in the normal state and a "horseshoe" appearance (*small arrows*) when cleft. *RV*, right ventricle; *VS*, ventricular septum; *PW*, posterior wall; *A*, anterior; *L*, left; *P*, posterior; *R*, right.

tion curves. Right ventricular pressure in most patient is less than 60% of systemic pressure. Significant elevation of calculated pulmonary vascular resistance is unusual.[44] Detectable tricuspid insufficiency is also unusual. The left ventricular angiocardiogram demonstrates a "gooseneck" deformation of the outflow tract of the left ventricle, resulting from an abnormality in the mitral valve and its attachments[2, 50] (Fig. 8.14).

Course

These patients usually have more severe symptoms than do patients with secundum ASD, and the symptoms occur at an earlier age. The increased severity of symptoms is related to associated defects or significant mitral insufficiency that may occur in infancy. Heart failure is more common than in secundum ASD, with a frequency approaching 20%. Heart failure occurs most frequently in childhood, but it may not occur until the 4th or 5th decade.[72] Endocarditis is a rare complication.

Dysrhythmia has been found in 20% of patients in one series, and this frequently has led to clinical deterioration.[58] Atrial fibrillation, nodal bradycardia, paraoxysmal ventricular tachycardia, and complete heart block have occurred. As with secundum ASD, pulmonary vascular obstructive disease occurs only rarely and infrequently is the cause of death.[58] Pulmonary venous hypertension, owing to mitral insufficiency, may also develop.

Differential Diagnosis

Those lesions occasionally confused with the most common variety of partial atrioventricular canal include: secundum atrial septal defect with or without mitral regurgitation; common atrium; complete atrioventricular canal; and anomalous pulmonary venous connection.

Electrocardiographic and vectorcardiographic findings usually exclude secundum ASD and anomalous pulmonary venous connection. The crucial role of echocardiography in separating these lesions cannot be overemphasized.

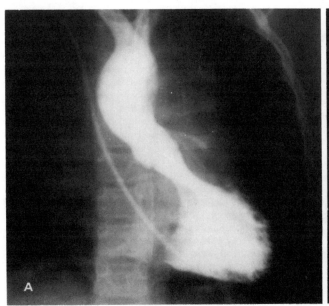
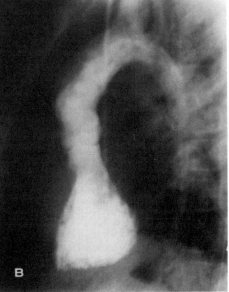

Fig. 8.14 Frontal (*A*) and lateral (*B*) views of left ventriculogram of patient with partial atrioventricular canal. Frontal view shows elongation and narrowing of left ventricular outflow tract. Right side of ventricular silhouette is scalloped and indented, and this correlates with abnormal attachment of mitral valve. Lateral view shows intact ventricular septum on edge and confirms absence of interventricular shunting as expected in this form of defect.

Treatment

Surgical techniques applicable to this anomaly are well standardized, safe, and reproducible.[69] The edges of apposition of the mitral cleft should be approximated with a few fine, interrupted, nonabsorbable sutures, and an adequately shaped patch of pericardium or Teflon should be used to close the primum atrial septal defect.

Results of surgical repair of partial atrioventricular canal defect have been excellent. A surgical risk of less than 5% is to be expected, with increased mortality and moribidity usually associated with long-standing symptoms or pulmonary hypertension (or both). Seven to ten percent of the patients require mitral valve replacement during the late postoperative period, because of residual mitral insufficiency. Losay *et al.*[34] have found that 25% of patients with significant preoperative mitral insufficiency require mitral valve replacement at the initial or subsequent operations. Complete heart block has been reported, but with improvement in surgical technique, such block should be a rare complication.

COMMON ATRIUM

Common atrium is characterized by virtual absence of the atrial septum, with the lowermost boundary of the defect formed by either atrioventricular valve tissue or the ventricular septum. This anomaly is always associated with atrioventricular canal defect.[65] At one end of the spectrum are patients with coexistent secundum and primum atrial septal defects and an intervening band of atrial septal muscle. At the other extreme are patients with absence of the entire septum, except for a small muscular cord. The latter group usually represents patients with complex congenital heart disease associated with splenic anomalies, in whom combined secundum, primum, and coronary sinus atrial septal defects merge. In this setting, transposition of the great arteries, double-outlet right ventricle, univentricular heart, anomalous pulmonary venous connection, and iosmerism of the atrial free walls are common.

Manifestations

Clinical Features. Most patients fatigue easily and are short of breath. If elevation of the pulmonary vascular resistance develops, the symptoms are more severe and resemble those associated with complete atrioventricular canal. In general, symptoms are more likely to develop earlier in life in these patients than in patients with partial atrioventricular canal. The symptoms are usually more severe, and occasionally, infants may be critically ill with heart failure and may fail to thrive.

Cyanosis varies from constant and obvious to very mild and present only with exertion. The heart is overactive, with a right ventricular impulse. The second sound is often constantly split during respiration, with the loudness of the pulmonary valve closure dependent on the severity of pulmonary hypertension. An ejection systolic murmur transmitted into the lungs is present over the upper left sternal border. A separate holosystolic murmur of mitral insufficiency is heard at the apex, with transmission into the axilla. In the absnece of pulmonary vascular disease, a middiastolic murmur over the lower left sternal border as a result of an increase in right atrial to right ventricular blood flow is commonly detected. Patients with common atrium and additional cardiac lesions and asplenia have Howell-Jolly bodies in the red blood cells of a peripheral blood smear.

Electrovectorcardiographic Features. The electrocardiogram is similar to that in other forms of atrioventricular canal defect. Abnormal frontal plane P axes have been reported in most cases.[25] The mean QRS axis in the frontal plane lies above the isoelectric line. All electrocardiograms show right ventricular hypertrophy, which increases if pulmonary vascular obstructive disease occurs. The frontal and horizontal QRS loops are identical with those seen in partial atrioventricular canal.[43]

Radiologic Features. The heart is enlarged, the main pulmonary artery is prominent, and the pulmonary vascular markings are increased. These features are indistinguishable from those seen in other forms of partial atrioventricular canal or in complete atrioventricular canal.

Echocardiographic Features. M-mode echocardiographic features are nonspecific and are usually similar to those of partial or complete atrioventricular canal.[20, 73] Because 2D echocardiography permits direct visualization of the atrial septum, common atrium can be diagnosed noninvasively. In addition to the absence of atrial septal echoes, features of the atrioventricular canal defect are invariably present (that is, inferiorly displaced atrioventricular valves with insertion at the same level to the crest of the ventricular septum).

Cardiac Catheterization and Angiocardiography

The hemodynamic diagnosis of common atrium depends on the demonstration of almost complete mixing of systemic venous and pulmonary venous blood. The oxygen saturations of pulmonary artery and systemic artery blood are nearly identical.[15] Pulmonary blood flow exceeds systemic flow, except in patients with severe pulmonary vascular obstructive disease. Indicator dye-dilution curves may be helpful in making the diagnosis of complete mixing. Right ventricular pressure is elevated more often than in secundum atrial septal defect or partial atrioventricular canal. Only infrequently, however, is the pulmonary vascular resistance significantly elevated.[44]

Angiocardiography shows a large globule-shaped single atrial structure.[25] Selective left ventricular angiocardiograms show the typical "gooseneck" deformity seen in partial and complete atrioventricular canal.[50]

Differential Diagnosis

Patients with complete atrioventricular canal complicated by severe pulmonary vascular obstructive disease may present features similar to those of common atrium. Clinically, the former can be suspected if there is a large increase in the pulmonary second sound and no diastolic murmur is heard over the lower sternum. Cardiac catheterization is indicated if severe pulmonary vascular obstructive disease is suspected. Total anomalous pulmonary venous connection may resemble common atrium. The electrocardiogram is extremely helpful in that, in total anomalous pulmonary venous connection, it has the characteristics of that seen in secundum ASD—the frontal plane QRS axis is directed toward the right, and the loop in the frontal projection is clockwise.

The echocardiographic features of common atrium are virtually pathognomonic, so that this examination should be employed if the diagnosis is suspected. An echocardiographic study should exclude other lesions in the differential diagnosis.

Treatment

Common atrium requires surgical repair, which should be employed early in life because there are usually symptoms and because these patients are at risk for development of pulmonary vascular obstructive disease. Most reports suggest that good results are achieved.[15]

COMPLETE ATRIOVENTRICULAR CANAL

This defect is uncommon, and the sex frequency is equal. It is more often associated with Down's Syndrome than are other forms of atrioventricular canal.[6, 63]

Complete atrioventricular canal is characterized by a large combined atrioventricular septal defect, by a single atrioventricular valve that takes origin from both atria, and by pronounced deficiency of the inlet ventricular septum and atrioventricular septum resulting in a scooped-out appearance.[65] The atrial portion of the defect is a large primum atrial septal defect. The ventricular portion, resulting from deficiency of the inlet septum, extends to the level of the membranous septum, which is usually deficient or absent. The length of the left ventricle from crux to apex is foreshortened, and the length from apex to aortic valve is increased.[9, 45] The left ventricular outflow tract is long and narrow and has been referred to angiographically as the "gooseneck" deformity. The distance from crux to aortic valve is also usually increased.

The common atrioventricular valve usually has five major leaflets and commissures. The interventricular communication lies between the two bridging leaflets and, in most cases, beneath these two leaflets. The posterior bridging leaflet overhangs the ventricular septum and usually has extensive chordal attachments to it, sometimes obliterating this potential interventricular communication. The anatomic relationship between the anterior bridging leaflet and the underlying ventricular septum is variable and forms the basis for subclassification as described by Rastelli et al.[50] and recently reevaluated by Piccoli et al.[46] (Fig. 8.8).

In type A (Fig. 8.8A), the anterior bridging leaflet is committed almost entirely to the left ventricle, and its commissure with the anterior tricuspid leaflet lies along the right anterosuperior rim of the ventricular septum. Beneath this commissure is either a distinct medial papillary muscle or, more commonly, multiple direct chordal insertions into the septum. Rastelli et al.[50] considered the anterior bridging and anterior triscuspid leaflets to represent a divided and attached common anterior leaflet.

In the rare type B (Fig. 8.8B), the anterior bridging leaflet is larger and overhangs the ventricular septum somewhat more than in type A. The medial papillary muscle attaches apically on the trabecula septomarginalis or on the moderator band. Since chordal anchors are not present between the anterior bridging leaflet and the underlying ventricular septum, free interventricular communication exists. Rastelli et al.[50] considered the anterior bridging and anterior tricuspid leaflets to represent a divided but unattached common anterior leaflet.

In type C (Fig. 8.8C), the anterior bridging leaflet is larger and overhangs the ventricular septum more than in type A or B. The medial papillary muscle attaches to the anterior tricuspid papillary muscle, and the anterior tricuspid leaflet is generally very small. The anterior bridging leaflet is not attached to the ventricular septum (so-called free-floating leaflet), and free interventricular communication is possible. Rastelli et al.[50] considered this leaflet to represent an undivided, unattached common anterior leaflet.

The intermediate form of atrioventricular canal usually resembles the complete form, except for fusion of the anterior and posterior bridging leaflets atop the ventricular septum. Surgically, the bridging leaflets often have insufficient tissue from which to reconstruct a competent anterior mitral leaflet.[7]

Manifestations

Clinical Features. Symptoms invariably occur early in infancy as a result of the large increase in pulmonary blood flow associated with pulmonary hypertension and complicated by insufficiency of the common atrioventricular valve. Severe cardiac failure, repeated respiratory infections, and failure to thrive are frequent complications. The patients are usually small and undernourished.[42]

In the absence of severe pulmonary vascular obstructive disease, there is no clinical evidence of systemic arterial oxygen desaturation. The heart is overactive, the first sound may be accentuated, and the second sound is usually split in inspiration only, with accentuation of the pulmonary valve closure. A loud, holosystolic murmur can be heard along the lower left sternal border and at the cardiac apex, resulting from mitral insufficiency. A separate ejection systolic murmur can be heard over the upper left sternal border as a result of the increased flow of blood from a dilated right ventricle across the normal pulmonary valve into the dilated pulmonary artery. A middiastolic murmur can be heard along the lower left sternal border and frequently at the apex as a result of increased blood flow across the common atrioventricular valve. However, the physical findings may be indistinguishable from those of the uncomplicated VSD or partial atrioventricular canal.

Electrovectorcardiographic Features. The electrocardiographic pattern is diagnostic. Prolonged PR interval is common. The mean electric axis of the QRS lies above the isoelectric line, and the vector loop in the frontal plane is directed counterclockwise.[43] All patients have right ventricular hypertrophy. The horizonal loop is directed clockwise; it lies anteriorly and to the right before passing into the right posterior quadrant (Fig. 8.15). Because a clockwise QRS loop

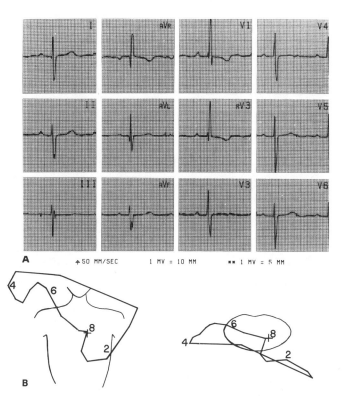

Fig. 8.15 Electrocardiogram (A) and vectorcardiogram (B) of 4-year-old with complete atrioventricular canal defect showing right ventricular hypertrophy. Mean frontal plane QRS axis is −100°, typical of this defect.

is common in the horizontal plane, many patients do not have visible Q or tall R waves in the left chest leads. Many patients also have left ventricular hypertrophy, but because of the unusual ventricular depolarization, left ventricular hypertrophy may not be evident on the electrocardiogram.

Radiologic Features. The heart is always enlarged. Enlargement of the right atrium is suggested by an increased convexity of the right border, and the increase in size of the left atrial appendage may give a characteristic flattening of the left heart border. The pulmonary artery is prominent, and the pulmonary vascular markings are increased (fig. 8.16).

Echocardiographic Features. The characteristic M-mode observation common to both complete and partial atrioventricular canal defects is the apparent movement of the anterior leaflet of the mitral valve through the plane of the ventricular septum. The differential feature from partial atrioventriicular canal is the large dropout of septal echoes separating the two components (tricuspid and mitral) of the inferiorly displaced common atrioventricular valve[22, 73] (Fig. 8.17).

Two-dimensional echocardiography is the more informative examination for the diagnosis and classification of complete atrioventricular canal.[55, 73] In contradistinction to the partial form, complete atrioventricular canal is characterized by the visualization of a posteriorly positioned inflow (atrioventricular canal) ventricular septal defect. Both atrioventricular valves are displaced inferiorly. The morphologic subgroups (Rastelli types A, B, and C) also can be recognized by characteristic chordal insertions and anatomy of the anterior portion of the common atrioventricular valve (Fig. 8.18).

Cardiac Catheterization and Angiocardiography

Right heart catheterization reveals increased oxygen saturation at both the right atrial and right ventricular levels. Pulmonary artery systolic pressure is invariably at or near systemic level,[44] in contrast to partial atrioventricular canal in which the pulmonary artery systolic pressure is usually

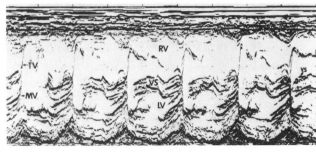

Fig. 8.17 Complete atrioventricular canal. M-mode echocardiographic features consistent with atrioventricular canal demonstrate the atrioventricular valve [tricuspid (*TV*) and mitral (*MV*) components] and apparent diastolic movement through plane of ventricular septum (*VS*). Complete atrioventricular canal is distinguished from partial atrioventricular canal (with use of M-mode echocardiography) by larger dropout of ventricular septal (*VS*) echoes separating mitral (*MV*) and tricuspid (*TV*) components of common atrioventricular valve. With inferior scanning, the apparent single atrioventricular valve can be separated into more distinct tricuspid and mitral components separated by ventricular septal echo. *LV*, left ventricle; *RV*, right ventricle.

60% or less than systemic pressure. The pulmonary blood flow is increased as a result of left-to-right shunting at both atrial and ventricular sites, and the severity of shunting depends on the relationship of pulmonary to systemic vascular resistances. The hemodynamic abnormality in complete atrioventricular canal may be complicated by severe insufficiency of the common atrioventricular valve, allowing blood to shunt freely between all four chambers.

As with other forms of atrioventricular canal, selective angiocardiograms from the left ventricle invariably reveal the typical "gooseneck" deformity[49, 50] (Fig. 8.19).

Course

If complete atrioventricular canal is not complicated by other major defects, death often occurs before 15 years of age (median age, 2 years). If other major defects are present, death occurs earlier (median age, 4 months). The mean age at the time of death has been reported to be usually less than 1 year.

The chief causes of death in infancy are either heart failure or pneumonia. Progressive pulmonary vascular disease is common and may progress more rapidly than in patients with ventricular septal defect. Several pulmonary vascular disease (calculated pulmonary resistance, more than 10 units/m^2) has occurred in children who are less than 2 years of age.[44]

The differential diagnosis of complete atrioventricular canal includes partial atrioventricular canal, large secundum atrial septal defect, common atrium, anomalous pulmonary venous connection, and ventricular septal defect. While electrocardiographic and vectorcardiographic features are helpful in differentiating these lesions, the echocardiographic findings are now so clearly documented as to be an extremely reliable diagnostic tool.

Treatment

Surgical repair for complete atrioventricular canal is indicated whenever unmanageable symptoms are encountered or, on an elective basis, prior to 2 years of age. After that age, significant pulmonary vascular obstructive disease is likely to occur. Until recently, the surgical management of the symptomatic infant with complete atrioventricular canal

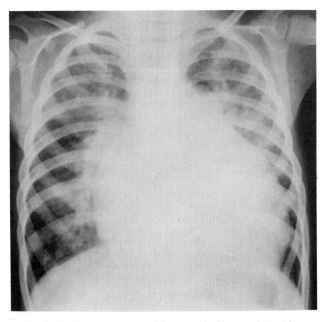

Fig. 8.16 Roentgenogram of 3-year-old with complete atrioventricular canal showing pronounced cardiomegaly, prominence of the main pulmonary artery, and large increase in pulmonary vascular markings.

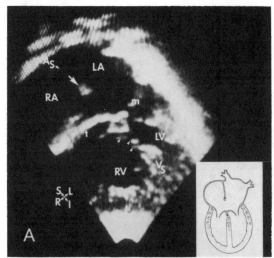

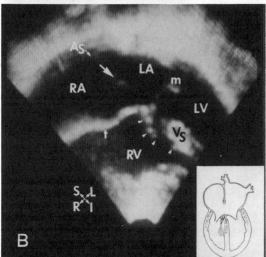

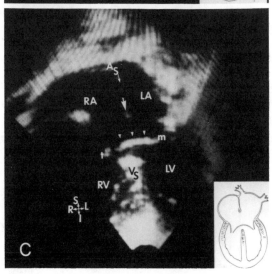

was controversial. Some advocated pulmonary artery banding in the symptomatic infant, followed by complete repair at a later age.[16] Alternatively, it is believed best to correct the defects completely, even in infants less than 6 months of age, because the surgical risk of banding and later complete repair is higher.[27] Pulmonary artery banding tends to be an ineffective method of palliation in those infants with moderate to severe atrioventricular valve insufficiency.

Surgical repair of complete atrioventricular canal requires a careful assessment of the intracardiac anatomy. Repair is started by splitting the anterior briding leaflet into mitral and tricuspid components (for types B and C). The mitral components of the anterior and posterior common leaflets are then approximated with a few fine interrupted sutures. A single patch, usually of Teflon, is used to close both the ventricular and atrial components of the septal defect. The patch is attached with interrupted sutures to the right aspect of the ventricular septum away from the crest which contains the conduction bundle. The mitral and tricuspid septal leaflets are then attached to the septal patch at a level corresponding to that of the atrioventricular anulus, allowing for the deficiency in the inlet septum. The atrial portion of the patch is then sutured to the rim of the ostium primum defect, thus completing the repair. After completion of the repair and restoration of the circulation, the function of the reconstructed mitral valve can be evaluated by obtaining double sampling indicator dye-dilution curves.

At the Mayo Clinic, surgical mortality has been 17% (38% for infants less than 6 months of age and 6% for older patients). In a group of 58 patients, 48 of whom were followed from 1 to 9 years, there were two late deaths and three instances of late mitral valve replacement. Two-thirds of surviving patients are considered to be in Class I (NYHA classification). Surgical mortality rates of from 10 to 35% have been reported from other centers.[12, 23, 36] Berger and co-workers[4] reported a 5-year survival rate of 91% for patients leaving the hospital after repair. Ideal age for operation was 14 months. Coexistent anomalies, such as tetralogy of Fallot or double-outlet right ventricle, may significantly alter the operative results.

As with other forms of congenital heart disease, preexisting pulmonary vascular disease at operation influences the ultimate result of surgery. While not many patients who have had successful repair of complete atrioventricular canal defect have had a postoperative cardiac catheterization, preliminary data suggest that pulmonary resistance remains low postoperatively in those who had preoperative pulmonary resistance less than 5 units/m^2. Those with preoperative resistance between 5 and 13 units/m^2 tended to have persistent or further elevations of pulmonary resistance postoperatively.

Reconstruction of the left atrioventricular valve is strongly preferred over valve replacement at the time of the initial surgical procedure. The long-term fate of the reconstructed mitral valve remains unknown, although most patients who have undergone operation have seemed to tolerate the mild to moderate mitral insufficiency commonly seen. Endocarditis prophylaxis should be rigorously given to these patients.

Fig. 8.18 Complete atrioventricular canal. Rastelli subtypes as visualized by 2D echocardiography. General features include primum atrial septal defect (absence of echoes in lower atrial septum) and inflow ventricular septal defect below the atrioventricular valve. Rastelli subtypes of complete atrioventricular canal are distinguished by different chordal insertions and support of anterior (bridging) leaflet of atrioventricular valve. (*A*) Type A, chordae (*arrowheads*) to crest of ventricular septum (*VS*). (*B*) Type B, chordae (*arrowheads*) insert into right ventricle. (*C*) Type C, unattached common anterior leaflet (*arrowheads*) visualized as plate of echoes over crest of *VS*; note mitral (*m*) and tricuspid (*t*) components of common atrioventricular valve of complete atrioventricular canal. Large *white arrow* points to bulbous portion of atrial septum (*AS*) above primum atrial septal defect. *LA*, left atrium; *LV*, left ventricle; *RV*, right ventricle; *RA* right atrium; *L*, left; *R*, right; *S*, superior, *I*, inferior.

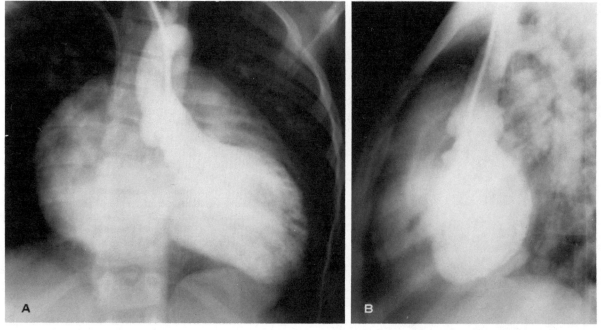

Fig. 8.19 Frontal (*A*) and lateral (*B*) views of left ventriculogram taken in early systole of patient with complete atrioventricular canal (type A). Note elongated and narrowed left ventricular outflow tract and regurgitant jet directed primarily into right atrium, which is commonly seen in this defect. Lateral view shows filling of structures anterior to left ventricle, representing interventricular shunt and left ventricular right atrial shunt.

VENTRICULAR SEPTAL DEFECT OF THE ATRIOVENTRICULAR CANAL TYPE

Ventricular septal defects in the inlet portion of the ventricular septum have been described as similar to the ventricular septal component of complete atrioventricular canal.[41] Defects of the atrioventricular valves may or may not be present, and associated straddling of the tricuspid valve has been described.[51] The defect involves the atrioventricular septum and thereby resembles that of a primum atrial septal defect; however, owing to the attachment of the atrioventricular valves to the posterior aspect of the defect,

the communication becomes interventricular rather than interatrial.

Defects also categorized under this heading include abnormally shaped paramembranous defects. Because of this confusion, ventricular septal defects of the atrioventricular canal type should be classified as one form of defect of the inlet muscular ventricular septum.

The history, physical examination, roentgenographic features, hemodynamics, and echocardiographic features are similar to those seen in the usual ventricular septal defect. In some cases, the electrocardiogram shows features similar to those in patients with other forms of atrioventricular canal.

References

1. Andersen, M., Lyngborg, K., Møller, I., and Wennevold, A.: The natural history of small atrial septal defects: Long-term follow-up with serial heart catheterizations. Am. Heart J. 92:302, 1976.

2. Baron, M. G., Wolf, B. S., Steinfeld, L., and Van Mierop, L. H. S.: Endocardial cushion defects: Specific diagnosis by angiocardiography. Am. J. Cardiol. 13:162, 1964.

3. Barritt, D. W., Davies, D. H., and Jacob, G.: Heart sounds and pressures in atrial septal defect. Br. Heart J. 27:90, 1965.

4. Berger, T. J., Blackstone, E. H., Kirklin, J. W., Bargeron, L. M., Jr., Hazelrig, J. B., and Turner, M. E., Jr.: Survival and probability of cure without and with operation in complete atrioventricular canal. Ann. Thorac. Surg. 27:104, 1979.

5. Beyer, J.: Atrial septal defect: Acute left heart failure after surgical closure. Ann. Thorac. Surg. 25:36, 1978.

6. Bharati, S., and Lev, M.: The spectrum of common atrioventricular orifice (canal). Am. Heart J. 86:553, 1973.

7. Bharati, S., Lev, M., McAllister, H. A., Jr., and Kirklin, J. W.: Surgical anatomy of the atrioventricular valve in the intermediate type of common atrioventricular orifice. J. Thorac. Cardiovasc. Surg. 79:884, 1980.

8. Bizarro, R. O., Callahan, J. A., Feldt, R. H., Kurland, L. T., Gordon, H., and Brandenburg, R. O.: Familial atrial septal defect with prolonged atrioventricular conduction: A syndrome showing the autosomal dominant pattern of inheritance. Circulation 41:677, 1970.

9. Blieden, L. C., Randall, P. A., Castaneda, A. R., Lucas, R. V., Jr., and Edwards, J. E.: The "goose neck" of the endocardial cushion defect: Anatomic basis. Chest 65:13, 1974.

10. Boineau, J. P., Moore, E. N., and Patterson, D. F.: Relationship between the ECG, ventricular activation, and the ventricular conduction system in ostium primum ASD. Circulation 48:556, 1973.

11. Colmers, R. A.: Atrial septal defects in elderly patients: Report of three patients aged 68, 72 and 78. Am. J. Cardiol. 1:768, 1958.

12. Cooper, D. K. C., de Leval, M. R., and Stark,

J.: Results of surgical correction of persistent complete atrioventricular canal. J. Thorac. Cardiovasc. Surg. 27:111, 1979.

13. Diamond, M. A., Dillon J. C., Haine, C. L., Chang, S., and Feigenbaum, H.: Echocardiographic features of atrial septal defect. Circulation 43:129, 1971.

14. DuShane, J. W.: The electrocardiogram in infants and children with low pressure left-to-right shunts. In Electrocardiography in Infants and Children, edited by D. E. Cassels and R. F. Ziegler. Grune & Stratton, New York, 1966, p. 131.

15. Ellis, F. H., Jr., Kirklin, J. W., Swan, H. J. C., DuShane, J. W., and Edwards, J. E.: Diagnosis and surgical treatment of common atrium (cor triloculare-biventriculare). Surgery 45:160, 1959.

16. Epstein, M. L., Moller, J. H., Amplatz, K., and Nicoloff, D. M.: Pulmonary artery banding in infants with complete atrioventricular canal. J. Thorac. Cardiovasc. Surg. 78:28, 1979.

17. Feldt, R. H., Avasthey, P., Yoshimasu, F. Kurland, L. T., and Titus, J. L.: Incidence of

congenital heart disease in children born to residents of Olmsted County, Minnesota, 1950–1969, Mayo Clin. Proc. 46:794, 1971.

18. Feldt, R. H., DuShane, J. W., and Titus, J. L.: The atrioventricular conduction system in persistent common atrioventricular canal defect: Correlations with electrocardiogram. Circulation 42:437, 1970.

19. Graham, T. P., Jr., Jarmakani, J. M., Atwood, G. F., and Canent, R. V., Jr.: Right ventricular volume determinations in children: Normal values and observations with volume or pressure overload. Circulation 47:144, 1973.

20. Hagler, D. J.: Echocardiographic findings in atrioventricular canal defect. In Atrioventricular Canal Defects, edited by R. H. Feldt, D. C. McGoon, P. A. Ongley, G. C. Rastelli, J. L. Titus, and L. H. S. Van Mierop. W. B. Saunders, Philadelphia, 1976, p. 87.

21. Hagler, D. J., Tajik, A. J., Seward, J. B., Mair, D. D., and Ritter, D. G.: Real-time wide-angle sector echocardiography: Atrioventricular canal defects. Circulation 59:140, 1979.

22. Hairston, P., Parker E. F., Arrants, J. E., Bradham, R. R., and Lee, W. H., Jr. The adult atrial septal defect: Results of surgical repair. Ann. Surg. 179:799, 1974.

23. Hardesty, R. L., Zuberbuhler, R., and Bahnson, H. T.: Surgical treatment of atrioventricular canal defect. Arch. Surg. 110:1391, 1975.

24. Holt, M., and Oram, S.: Familial heart disease with skeletal malformations. Br. Heart J. 22:236, 1960.

25. Hung, J.-S., Feldt, R. H, Kincaid, O. W., and Ritter, D. G.: Electrocardiographic and angiocardiographic features of common atrium (abstr.). Circulation 42(Suppl. 3):167, 1970.

26. Hynes, K. M., Frye, R. L., Brandenburg, R. O., McGoon, D. C., Titus, J. L., and Giuliani, E. R.: Atrial septal defect (secundum) associated with mitral regurgitation. Am. J. Cardiol. 34:333, 1974.

27. Kirklin, J. W., and Blackstone, E. H.: Management of the infant with complete atrioventricular canal. J. Thorac. Cardiovasc. Surg. 78:32, 1979.

28. Kyger, E. R., III, Frazier, O. H., Cooley, D. A., Gillette, P. C., Reul, G. J., Jr., Sandiford, F. M., and Wukasch, D. C.: Sinous venosus atrial septal defect: Early and late results following closure in 109 patients. Ann. Thorac. Surg. 25:44, 1978.

29. Lancelin, B., Crépieux, A., Diebold, B., Abbou, B., Goujon, J., Apoil, E., Pauly-Laubry, C., and Maurice, P.: Les troubles du rythme après fermeture des communications inter-auriculaires: A propos de 300 cas. Arch. Mal. Coeur 70:1283, 1977.

30. Lev, M., Arcilla, R., Rimoldi, H. J. A., Licata, R. H., and Gasul, B. M.: Premature narrowing or closure of the foramen ovale. Am. Heart J. 65:638, 1963.

31. Levin, A. R., Liebson, P. R., Ehlers, K. H., and Diamant, B.: Assessment of left ventricular function in secundum atrial septal defect: Evaluation by determination of volume, pressure, and external systolic time indices. Pediatr. Res. 9:894, 1975.

32. Levin, A. R., Spach, M. S., Boineau, J. P., Canent, R. V., Jr., Capp, M. P., and Jewett, P. H.: Atrial pressure-flow dynamics in atrial septal defects (secundum type). Circulation 37:476, 1968.

33. Lieppe, W., Scallion, R., Behar, V. S., and Kisslo, J. A.: Two-dimensional echocardio-

graphic findings in atrial septal defect. Circulation 56:447, 1977.

34. Losay, J., Rosenthal, A., Castaneda, A. R., Bernhard, W. H., and Nadas, A. S.: Repair of atrial septal defect primum: Results, course, and prognosis. J. Thorac. Cardiovasc. Surg. 75:248, 1978.

35. Lynch, H. T., Bachenberg, K., Harris, R. E., and Becker, W.: Hereditary atrial septal defect: Update of a large kindred. Am. J. Dis. Child. 132:600, 1978.

36. Midgley, F. M., Galioto, F. M., Shapiro, S. R., Perry, L. W., and Scott, L. P.: Experience with repair of complete atrioventricular canal. Ann. Thorac. Surg. 30:151, 1980.

37. Mody, M. R. Serial hemodynamic observations in secundum atrial septal defect with special reference to spontaneous closure. Am. J. Cardiol. 32:978, 1973.

38. Nasser, F. N., Tajik, A. J., Seward, J. B., and Hagler, D. J.: Diagnosis of sinus venosus atrial septal defect by two-dimensional echocardiography. Mayo Clin. Proc. 56:568, 1981.

39. Neal, W. A., Moller, J. H., Varco, R. L., and Anderson, R. C.: Operative repair of atrial septal defect without cardiac catheterization. J. Pediatr. 86:189, 1975.

40. Netter, F. H.: The Ciba Collection of Medical Illustrations, edited by F. F. Yonkman, Vol. 5. Ciba Pharmaceutical Company, Summit, N.J., 1969, p. 119.

41. Neufeld, H. N., Titus, J. L., DuShane, J. W., Burchell, H. B., and Edwards, J. E.: Isolated ventricular septal defect of the persistent common atrioventricular canal type. Circulation 23:685, 1961.

42. Ongley, P. A., Pongpanich, B., and Feldt, R. H.: The clinical profile of the atrioventricular canal defects. In Atrioventricular Canal Defects, edited by R. H. Feldt, D. C. McGoon, P. A. Ongley, G. C. Rastelli, J. L. Titus, and L. H. S. Van Mierop. W. B. Saunders, Philadelphia, 1976, p. 44.

43. Ongley, P. A., Pongpanich, B., Spangler, J. G., and Feldt, R. H.: The electrocardiogram in atrioventricular canal. In Atrioventricular Canal Defects, edited by R. H. Feldt, D. C. McGoon, P. A. Ongley, G. C. Rastelli, J. L. Titus, and L. H. S. Van Mierop. W. B. Saunders, Philadelphia, 1976, p. 51.

44. Park, J. M., Ritter, D. G., and Mair, D. D.: Cardiac catheterization findings in persistent common atrioventricular canal. In Atrioventricular Canal Defects, edited by R. H. Feldt, D. C. McGoon, P. A. Ongley, G. C. Rastelli, J. L. Titus, and L. H. S. Van Mierop. W. B. Saunders, Philadelphia, 1976, p. 76.

45. Piccoli, G. P., Gerlis, L. M., Wilkinson, J. L., Lozsadi, K., Macartney, F. J., and Anderson, R. H.: Morphology and classification of atrioventricular defects. Br. Heart J. 42:621, 1979.

46. Piccoli, G. P., Wilkinson, J. L., Macartney, F. J., Gerlis, L. M., and Anderson, R. H.: Morphology and classification of complete atrioventricular defect. Br. Heart J. 42:633, 1979.

47. Radtke, W. E., Tajik, A. J., Gau, G. T., Schattenberg, T. T., Giuliani, E. R., and Tancredi, R. G.: Atrial septal defect: Echocardiographic observations; studies in 120 patients. Ann. Intern. Med. 84:246, 1976.

48. Raghib, G., Ruttenberg, H. D., Anderson, R. C., Amplatz, K., Adams, P., Jr., and Edwards, J. E.: Termination of left superior vena cava in left atrium, atrial septal defect, and absence of coronary sinus: A developmental complex.

Circulation 31:906, 1965.

49. Rastelli, G. C., Kincaid, O. W., and Ritter, D. G.: Angiocardiography of persistent common atrioventricular canal. In Atrioventricular Canal Defects, edited by R. H. Feldt, D. C. McGoon, P. A. Ongley, G. C. Rastelli, J. L. Titus, and L. H. S. Van Mierop. W. B. Saunders, Philadelphia, 1976, p. 110.

50. Rastelli, G. C., Kirklin, J. W., and Titus, J. L.: Anatomic observations on complete form of persistent common atrioventricular canal with special reference to atrioventricular valves. Mayo Clin. Proc. 41:296, 1966.

51. Rastelli, G. C., Ongley, P. A., and Titus, J. L.: Ventricular septal defect of atrioventricular canal type with straddling right atrioventricular valve and mitral valve deformity. Circulation 37:816, 1968.

52. St. John Sutton, M. G., Tajik, A. J., and McGoon, D. C.: Atrial septal defect in patients aged 60 years or older: Operative results and long-term postoperative follow-up. Circulation 64:402, 1981.

53. St. John Sutton, M. G., Tajik, A. J., Mercier, L.-A., Seward, J. B., Giuliani, E. R., and Ritman, E. L.: Assessment of left ventricular function in secundum atrial septal defect by computer analysis of the M-mode echocardiogram. Circulation 60:1082, 1979.

54. Saksena, F. B., and Aldridge, H. E.: Atrial septal defect in the older patient: A clinical and hemodynamic study in patients operated on after age 35. Circulation 42:1009, 1970.

55. Seward, J. B., Tajik, A. J., and Hagler, D. J.: Two-dimensional echocardiographic features of atrioventricular canal defect. In Pediatric Echocardiography—Cross Sectional, M-Mode and Doppler, edited by N.-R. Lundström. Elsevier/North Holland Biomedical Press, Amsterdam, 1980, p. 197.

56. Seward, J. B., Tajik, A. J., Hagler, D. J., and Ritter, D. G.: Peripheral venous contrast echocardiography. Am. J. Cardiol. 39:202, 1977.

57. Silver, M. D., and Dorsey, J. S.: Aneurysms of the septum primum in adults. Arch. Pathol. Lab. Med. 102:62, 1978.

58. Somerville, J.: Ostium primum defect: Factors causing deterioration in the natural history. Br. Heart J. 27:413, 1965.

59. Spangler, J. G., Feldt, R. H., and Danielson, G. K.: Secundum atrial septal defect encountered in infancy. J. Thorac. Cardiovasc. Surg. 71:398, 1976.

60. Swan, H. J. C., Hetzel, P. S., Burchell, H. B., and Wood, E. H.: Relative contribution of blood from each lung to the left-to-right shunt in atrial septal defect: demonstration by indicator-dilution techniques. Circulation 14:200, 1956.

61. Sweeney, L. J., and Rosenquist, G. C.: The normal anatomy of the atrial septum in the human heart. Am. Heart J. 98:194, 1979.

62. Tajik, A. J., Seward, J. B., Hagler, D. J., Mair, D. D., and Lie, J. T.: Two-dimensional real-time ultrasonic imaging of the heart and great vessels: Technique, image orientation, structure identification, and validation. Mayo Clin. Proc. 53:271, 1978.

63. Tenckhoff, L., and Stamm, S. J.: An analysis of 35 cases of the complete form of persistent common atrioventricular canal. Circulation 48:416, 1973.

64. Tikoff, G., Schmidt, A. M., Kuida, H., and Hecht, H. H.: Heart failure in atrial septal defect. Am. J. Med. 39:533, 1965.

65. Titus, J. L., and Rastelli, G. C.: Anatomical features of persistent common atrioventricular canal. In Atrioventricular Canal Defects, edited by R. H. Feldt, D. C. McGoon, P. A. Ongley, G. C. Rastelli, J. L. Titus, and L. H. S. Van Mierop. W. B. Saunders, Philadelphia, 1976, p. 13.

66. Van Mierop, L. H. S.: Embryology of the atrioventricular canal region and pathogenesis of endocardial cushion defects. In Atrioventricular Canal Defects, edited by R. H. Feldt, D. C. McGoon, P. A. Ongley, G. C. Rastelli, J. L. Titus, and L. H. S. Van Mierop. W. B. Saunders, Philadelphia, 1976, p. 1.

67. Wagenvoort, C. A., and Wagenvoort, N.: Pathology of Pulmonary Hypertension. John Wiley & Sons, New York, 1977, pp. 56–94, 138.

68. Waldo, A. L., Kaiser, G. A., Bowman, F. O., Jr., and Malm, J. R.: Etiology of prolongation of the P-R interval in patients with an endocardial cushion defect: Further observations on internodal conduction and the polarity of the retrograde P wave. Circulation 48:19, 1973.

69. Ward, R. E., Anderson, R. M., Goldberg, S. J., Allen, H. D., and Sahn, D.: Septum primum defect repair. Ann. Thorac. Surg. 24:291, 1977.

70. Weidman, W. H., Swan, H. J. C., DuShane, J. W., and Wood, E. H.: A hemodynamic study of atrial septal defect and associated anomalies involving the atrial septum. J. Lab. Clin. Med. 50:165, 1957.

71. Weyman, A. E., Wann, L. S., Caldwell, R. L., Hurwitz, R. A., Dillon, J. C., and Feigenbaum, H.: Negative contrast echocardiography: A new method for detecting left-to-right shunts. Circulation 59:498, 1979.

72. Weyn, A. S., Bartle, S. H., Nolan, T. B., and Dammann, J. F., Jr.: Atrial septal defect—primum type. Circulation 32 (Suppl. 3):13, 1965.

73. Williams, R. G., and Rudd, M.: Echocardiographic features of endocardial cushion defects. Circulation 49:418, 1974.

74. Wyler, F., and Rutishauser, M.: Symptomatic atrial septal defect in the neonate and infant. Helv. Paediatr. Acta 30:399, 1976.

75. Young, D.: Later results of closure of secundum atrial septal defect in children. Am. J. Cardiol. 31:14, 1973.

76. Zaver, A. G., and Nadas, A. S.: Atrial septal defect—secundum type. Circulation 32(Suppl. 3):24, 1965.

9

Ventricular Septal Defect

Thomas P. Graham, Jr., M.D., Harvey W. Bender, M.D., and Madison S. Spach, M.D.

Ventricular septal defects (VSD) have served as excellent models for study of the interrelationships of anatomic and physiologic variables in lesions which allow communication between the systemic and pulmonary circulations. In view of the vagaries presented clinically by many patients, the clinician cannot be satisfied with simple detection of the defect. Clinical assessment must be made of the size of the defect, the magnitude of hemodynamic overload, and the status of the pulmonary vascular resistance. The effect on the patient depends primarily on the size of the defect and, in large communications, on the resistance to blood flow through the lungs. This chapter presents a discussion of isolated VSD with classification of the lesion into four anatomic-physiologic groups[16, 32, 56]: small defect with low pulmonary vascular resistance; moderate defect with variable pulmonary vascular resistance; large defect with mild to moderate elevation of pulmonary vascular resistance; and large defect with marked elevation of pulmonary vascular resistance.

Roger[53] in 1879 first defined the clinical signs of an underlying VSD. The term Roger's defect (maladie de Roger) is used to indicate small VSDs. In 1897, Eisenmenger described the postmortem findings in a cyanotic patient who died at age 32 with a large VSD and overriding aorta. The patient had a history of cyanosis and dyspnea since infancy, with these symptoms worsening with effort. Physical findings included murmurs of both tricuspid and pulmonary insufficiency. Autopsy showed right ventricular hypertrophy and dilatation, a dilated tricuspid valve ring, a large VSD with overriding of the aorta, atherosclerosis of the pulmonary arteries, and hemorrhagic pulmonary infarction secondary to pulmonary thrombosis.[66] Abbott,[1] who noted that Dalrymple first described this entity in 1847, coined the term Eisenmenger's complex. This eponym is now commonly applied to the condition of a VSD, with marked elevation of pulmonary vascular resistance and a predominant right to left shunt. The term Eisenmenger's syndrome commonly is used to indicate any defect allowing free communication between the pulmonary and systemic circuits with a predominant right to left shunt secondary to marked elevation of primary vascular resistance.

Variation of the position of defects in the ventricular septum and their relationship to the conduction system have been emphasized by a number of investigators over the past decade.[6, 23, 43, 45, 62] The combined anatomic-physiologic studies of Dammann and Ferencz[15] and Edwards[22] have provided information leading to a better understanding of the importance of changes in pulmonary vascular resistance in determining the net shunt across large defects. Finally, advances in the surgical correction of ventricular septal defects at an early age[2, 3, 5, 7, 39, 50] have brought into focus the necessity of an understanding of the underlying pathophysiological state by those who share in the care of patients with this lesion.

PREVALENCE

The experience at our institutions has been quite similar to that reported by Nadas and Fyler[47] and Keith et al.[36] in that approximately 20% of congenital heart patients have a ventricular septal defect as a solitary lesion. Most centers now report VSD as the most commonly encountered lesion if one excludes a bicuspid aortic valve from consideration. The incidence of VSD in all live births is approximately 1.5 to 2.5 per 1,000.[32, 36, 47, 48] The lower prevalence found by groups caring for adults with congenital heart disease is probably in large part due to spontaneous closure of a significant number of defects. VSD is found slightly more frequently in females as compared to males with the experience of Hoffman and Rudolph[32] representative of most series (56% female, 44% males). VSD is the most common lesion in the majority of the described chromosomal syndromes including the 13-trisomy, 18-trisomy, and 21-trisomy groups, as well as in rarer syndromes associated with the 4-group, 5-group, and the C-mosaic group.[48] In the majority of patients with VSD (>95%), the defect is unassociated with a chromosomal abnormality, and the cause is unknown. A multifactorial etiology has been assumed in which interaction between hereditary predisposition and environmental influences results in the defect.[48]

PATHOLOGY

The pathologic anatomy is depicted schematically in Figure 9.1. For a detailed review of the surgical implications of the variances in position, the reports of Becu *et al.*[6] Edwards,[23] Lincoln *et al.*,[43] and Titus *et al.*[62] should be consulted. From the right ventricular aspect the defect can be related to the crista supraventricularis (Fig. 9.1, *b*) and its septal band, the pulmonary valve, the papillary muscle of the conus (Fig. 9.1, *c*), the septal leaflet of the tricuspid valve, and the atrioventricular fibrous ring. The most common defect, the membranous or infracristal defect, lies in the outflow tract of the left ventricle immediately beneath the aortic valve. When viewed from the right heart, the defect is beneath the crista supraventricularis and posterior to the papillary muscle of the conus, (Fig. 9.1, *g*). This is the location for approximately 80% of defects seen at surgery or at autopsy.[6, 23, 43, 45] The term membranous ventricular septal defect is somewhat inaccurate, because these defects involve varying amounts of muscular tissue adjacent to the membranous septum. With the membranous defect, there can be a variable degree of malalignment between the infundibular septum and the anterior ventricular septum such that the aortic valve appears to override the defect.[43] In addition, when the septal commissure of the tricuspid valve is deficient

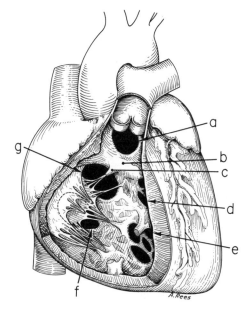

Fig. 9.1 Anatomical position of ventricular septal defects (VSD). The positions of the most commonly encountered VSDs are shown as viewed from the right septal surface with the right ventricular free wall removed. The positions of these defects are illustrated in relation to the morphology of the right ventricle. (*a*) Defect located in the outflow tract of the right ventricle between the crista supraventricularis and pulmonary valve, the supracristal VSD. (*b*) The crista supraventricularis. (*c*) Papillary muscle of the conus. (*d* and *e*) Muscular ventricular septal defects. (*f*) Area outlining location of isolated ventricular defect of the atrioventricular canal variety. (*g*) Defect located just inferior to the crista supraventricularis, the so-called "membranous" or infracristal defect (most common location).

at its attachment to the atrioventricular membranous septum, a left ventricular to right atrial shunt can occur.[43]

Embryologically, closure of the interventricular foramen is primarily dependent upon three factors: continued growth of connective tissue situated on the crest of the muscular septum; downward growth of ridges dividing the conus and truncus arteriosus; and projections into the atrioventricular canal from the right-sided cushions. Thus, with multiple factors involved in the closure of the region encompassing the membranous septum (interventricular foramen), it is not unexpected that the most common defect occurs at this site.

Defects positioned in the outflow tract of the right ventricle beneath the pulmonary valve are usually called supracristal, infundibular, conal, or subpulmonary (Fig. 9.1, *a*). Supracristal defects constitute approximately 5 to 7% of defects seen at surgery or autopsy,[6, 23, 43, 45] except in Japan or other Far Eastern countries where the percentage is much higher, approximately 29%.[61]

Isolated defects which are posterior and inferior to the membranous defect and lie beneath the septal cusp of the tricuspid valve and inferior to the papillary muscle of the conus previously have been called atrioventricular canal defects (Fig. 9.1, *f*). We agree with other authors that this is a misnomer because most of these defects have no abnormalities of the mitral or tricuspid valves, and the common atrioventricular bundle does not pass beneath the defect, as would be anticipated for a true atrioventricular canal defect.[43] We have termed these posterior defects. Such posterior defects have been reported in 8% of 50 patients undergoing elective repair.[43]

Defects in the muscular septum are frequently multiple and comprise 5 to 20% of defects found at surgery or autopsy.[6, 23, 38, 43, 45, 65] There have been two recent attempts to classify muscular defects by location.[38, 65] In surgical reports, apical defects are the most common. These defects are frequently difficult to visualize from the right ventricle because they are usually multiple with bordering and overlying trabeculae and tortuous channels (Fig. 9.1, *e*). The left ventricular view usually shows fewer overlying trabeculae, and multiple defects from the right ventricular side frequently coalesce to form a single defect on the left side.

Another type of muscular defect which has been described is a central defect (Fig. 9.1, *d*). This defect is posterior to the trabecula septomarginalis (septal band of the crista) and in the midportion of the ventricular septum. Commonly, it is partially hidden by overlying trabeculae when viewed from the right ventricle and can give the impression of multiple defects. From the left ventricular view, this usually appears as a single, rounded-off defect well away from the apex and the anterior and posterior left ventricular walls.

Small defects near the septal-free wall margins have been termed marginal defects. These defects are usually multiple, small, tortuous, and distributed all along the ventricular septal-free wall margins. They are seldom large enough to warrant surgical closure.

Posterior muscular defects also have been defined. These defects are usually slit-like with the long axis nearly parallel to the long axis of the septum. When viewed from the right ventricle, the defect may reach the posterior ventricular wall and may be partially hidden by the septal leaflet of the tricuspid valve. It is inferior to the membranous or infracristal defect and slightly anterior to the posterior ("AV canal type") defect.

All of these muscular defects may occur in combination with other muscular or nonmuscular defects. The so-called "swiss cheese" type of multiple muscular defects is a rare anomaly in which there are virtually as many defects as there is remaining septum.

Of considerable importance is the relationship of the atrioventricular conduction pathways and the position of the defect. With a membranous defect, the bundle of His lies in a subendocardial position as it courses the posterior-inferior margin of the defect. Therefore, this part of the defect is watched closely by surgeons to avoid damage to the bundle of His which can produce complete heart block. In posterior ("AV canal type") defects, the bundle of His passes anterosuperiorly to the defect.[45] In muscular ventricular septal defects and supracristal defects there is little danger of heart block since the conduction tissue is generally far removed.

Right bundle branch block (RBBB) occurs frequently after surgery for VSD. Recent studies have indicated that the pattern of RBBB can be due to the ventriculotomy[25, 40, 49] or it can be due to damage to the right bundle itself which can course along the posterior-inferior margin of infracristal defects.[49] Okoroma et al.[49] in a retrospective analysis found a 60% prevalence of an RBBB pattern in 26 patients having muscular defects closed using a transverse ventriculotomy and a 44% prevalence of an RBBB pattern in 38 patients having infracristal defects closed through an atrial approach. Krongrad et al.[40] demonstrated the appearance of an RBBB pattern at the time of ventriculotomy in 12 of 15 patients (80%) having a vertical ventriculotomy incision. These investigators found that the total QRS prolongation occurred with a specific 1 cm incision of a stepwise ventriculotomy during a sequence of stepwise incisions. Their results suggest that the ventriculotomy-induced RBBB pattern is unlikely to be due to disruption of a continuous Purkinje network but more likely is due to disruption of a distal branch or branches of the right bundle.[40]

PHYSIOLOGY

The primary anatomic variable which determines the physiologic state of the patient is the size of the defect. In small or medium-sized defects, this component presents a limiting barrier to the magnitude of the left to right shunt; however, in large defects which approximate the size of the aortic orifice there is essentially no resistance to flow across the opening itself, and the relative resistance offered by the systemic and pulmonary circulations regulates the magnitude of flow across the defect. Thus the initial conditions of defect size and circulatory resistances determine the magnitude of systemic and pulmonary flow, the pressures in the two circulations, and the work characteristics of the atria and ventricles.

The physiologic parameters of shunt flow, intracardiac pressure, and ventricular volume can be estimated indirectly by clinical examination and determined more quantitatively by cardiac catheterization and cineangiocardiography. The pulmonary artery pressure can be measured accurately, and estimations can be made of total pulmonary blood flow. The pulmonary resistance can be calculated by dividing the flow by the pressure difference across the pulmonary circuit, although this variable cannot be measured directly. These calculations are useful in estimating the resistance to the flow of blood through the lungs, although they are based on an approximation that assumes the pulmonary circulation to be a rigid system of tubes. Obviously, there are inherent errors in the absolute values obtained, since the pulmonary bed is a distensible one of varying compliance. As pointed out by Burton,[11] pulmonary resistance is a dynamic phenomenon and is directly related to the transmural pressure distending the vessels and the force of perfusion. Thus for a given vascular tone, pulmonary resistance will vary with the force of perfusion.

EFFECT OF PULMONARY VASCULAR RESISTANCE ON CARDIOVASCULAR STRUCTURE AND FUNCTION

Rudolph[55] and Dammann and Ferencz[15] have emphasized the role of pulmonary vascular resistance in determining the magnitude of the left to right shunt in the neonatal and subsequent growth periods. Following birth, the small muscular pulmonary arteries normally change from the fetal state with a small lumen and a thick medial muscle layer to thin-walled structures with increased lumen size. The rate of decline in pulmonary vascular resistance which accompanies these changes is such that the right ventricular pressure is approximately at adult levels within 7 to 10 days. In the presence of large defects, the rate of this maturational process appears to be delayed, and the increased pulmonary vascular resistance acts as a protective mechanism against massive shunting of blood through the lungs. Considerable evidence indicates that elevation of left atrial pressure (pulmonary venous pressure) may play an important role in maintaining this phase of peripheral pulmonary vascular constriction.[55]

Dammann et al.[15] pointed out that when pulmonary vessels are stretched to the limit of their surrounding fibrous jacket, the pressure-flow curve becomes linear. Thereafter, further increase in flow is associated with elevation of pressure to the point that the vessels are stretched to their limit and probably are injured. Such events can produce inflammatory arteritis. On the other hand, less severe, more chronic injury eventually can result in a thickened adventitia, an increase in medial hypertrophy, and an intimal injury. Although the progressive changes of pulmonary hypertension are well documented, the basic mechanisms involved in this end stage of markedly sclerotic and damaged vessels remain to be clarified.

During the first few months of life, in patients with large defects, a gradual decline of pulmonary vascular resistance usually occurs, and it results in augmentation of the left to right shunt. Owing to the large pulmonary flow which develops during this interval, the large blood volume handled by the left atrium may result in elevated left atrial pressure and pulmonary venous hypertension. The increased return to the left heart results in an enlarged left atrium and left ventricle as well as an increase in the left ventricular muscle mass.[35] With a markedly increased volume overload of the left ventricle, the stress may produce left ventricular failure; this is particularly likely to occur in infants between the ages of 1 to 3 months. Compensatory mechanisms which allow the infant to adapt to this large volume load include the Frank-Starling effect, increased sympathetic cardiac stimulation, and myocardial hypertrophy. The rapidity of the development of myocardial hypertrophy is probably one of the major factors in the ability of an infant to compensate adequately for a VSD with a large left to right shunt.

Usually, pulmonary and aortic peak systolic pressures equilibrate in the presence of moderate elevation of pulmonary vascular resistance with a large left to right shunt. The pulmonary vascular response with time in this setting is variable.[16, 51, 55, 64] In some patients, little change occurs in pulmonary vascular resistance, and the magnitude of the left to right shunts remains stable. However, in some patients the dilatation and stretch of the pulmonary vessels and the increased vasoconstrictive tone is followed by hypertrophy of the media, continued pulmonary hypertension, and gradual development of intimal sclerotic changes. Although this complication is emphasized in the literature, with rare exceptions these changes are limited to large defects where there is a common ejectile force from both ventricles. If an increase in pulmonary vascular resistance occurs, there is a resultant diminution of pulmonary blood flow, alleviation of the increased volume overload of the left heart, and a gradual decrease in the size of the left atrium and left ventricle as well as a decrease in the left ventricular muscle mass. Finally, if pulmonary vascular resistance exceeds that of the systemic circulation, the pressures in the two circuits remain equal but the direction of flow across the defect becomes predominantly right to left. Although this sequence of events is probably the usual one in those patients who develop the Eisenmenger reaction, there are some patients who appear to persist throughout infancy with elevation of pulmonary vascular resistance, balanced shunting, and probably normal or near normal left ventricular size and muscle mass. These patients frequently do not show any evidence of left ventricular decompensation either in infancy or childhood. Right ventricular decompensation eventually occurs, but this complication is usually delayed to late adolescence or early adulthood.

The abnormal workload of the right ventricle depends upon the interaction of pulmonary resistance and the magnitude of left to right shunt. In small defects, the right ventricular peak systolic pressure remains normal, and its workload and wall thickness also remain normal. In moderate-sized defects, the interaction of magnitude of the left to right shunt and pulmonary resistance is such that mild to moderate elevation of pulmonary artery pressure occurs with proportional extrasystolic work being required of this chamber. Mild to moderate right ventricular hypertrophy accompanies this elevated systolic pressure. In the presence of large defects with a common systolic ejectile thrust, considerable extra work is required of the right ventricle to overcome increased resistance during ejection. The right ventricle then hypertrophies to a greater extent with considerable increase in muscle mass. With moderate to large left to right shunts, the right ventricle also enlarges secondary to the degree of diastolic shunting from left ventricle to right ventricle. We have found in patients with considerable elevation of left ventricular volumes secondary to large defects that right ventricular volumes are also increased, but to a lesser degree.[27] Since normally the major shunting occurs during ventricular systole and is ejected into the outflow tract of the right ventricle, the right ventricle does not enlarge to the same extent as the left ventricle.

CLASSIFICATION OF PHYSIOLOGIC STATES

Small Defect with Low Pulmonary Vascular Resistance

Small ventricular septal defects can be defined as defects whose size imposes a high resistance to flow with a resultant large pressure difference between the two ventricles during ventricular systole, a small left to right shunt, normal right heart pressures, and essentially normal work characteristics of the ventricles. The magnitude of the left to right shunt in this situation is directly related to the size of the defect, and there is little or no tendency for an increase in pulmonary vascular resistance. The pressure gradient across the defect favors the left ventricle throughout the cardiac cycle and can result in a continuous left to right shunt.[42] Some small defects have diastolic shunting from left to right ventricle with blood flow across the defect directly into the body of the right ventricle during diastole with accentuation following atrial contraction. The onset of ventricular systole is characterized by an earlier rise in left ventricular pressure as compared to that of the right and augmentation of the shunt during isovolumic contraction. The major gradient and left to right shunt occurs during ventricular ejection with the direction of flow across the infracristal or supracristal defect being diverted into the outflow tract of the right ventricle and pulmonary artery. Following closure of the semilunar valves, isovolumic relaxation may be associated with a continuing left to right shunt with the flow now being directed into the body of the right ventricle. In some patients the left to right shunt stops transiently at the end of isovolumic relaxation during a brief interval of early diastole when left ventricular pressure occasionally falls below that of the right. None of these patients have right to left shunting across the defect at this time; presumably, the failure to reverse flow here is related to inertial effects with deceleration of blood flow in the left to right direction. Phonocardiographic studies in this group indicate that the holosystolic murmur is associated with the large pressure gradient across the defect lasting throughout ventricular systole. The absence of a murmur during diastole, although flow continues across the defect, is most likely related to the lack of turbulence due to the small quantity of blood being shunted at this time.

Moderate Defect with Variable Pulmonary Vascular Resistance

Moderate-sized defects are large enough to permit a moderate to large shunt, yet small enough to offer some resistance to flow, and therefore result in a lower peak systolic pressure in the right ventricle than in the left ventricle. There is considerable variation in the size of the defect in this group; however, these patients generally have a defect that is less than 1 cm^2 per m^2 of body surface area.[56] Defects in this group are associated with a systolic pressure difference of 15 mm Hg or more between the two ventricles during ventricular ejection. It is unusual for this group to have marked elevation of pulmonary vascular resistance; most have moderate to large left to right shunts with volume overload of the left atrium and left ventricle and left ventricular hypertrophy (Fig. 9.2A). Right ventricular systolic work and muscle mass vary according to the elevation in right ventricular pressure.

The intracardiac pressure flow events throughout the cardiac cycle occur in the same fashion as described for small defects until right ventricular systolic pressures reach a level of 70 to 80 mm Hg or from 70 to 85% of systemic pressure. Patients with right ventricular pressures at this level have a left to right gradient of 15 to 30 mm Hg throughout ventricular ejection. Left ventricular pressure rises more rapidly with the onset of systole than does right ventricular pressure, and this gradient is maintained throughout systole into the initial portion of isovolumic relaxation. The left ventricular pressure, however, falls more rapidly than that of the right with the development of a transient right to left gradient during relaxation. This is associated with a small right to left shunt across the defect into the outflow portion of the left ventricle. With the commencement of diastole, the pressure relationships across the defect favor the left ventricle, and flow again occurs from left ventricle to right ventricle. In this group, the small volume of blood which is shunted from the right ventricle into the left ventricle during isovolumic relaxation is returned to the right ventricle and thus does not enter the systemic circulation. Thus these patients have no direct shunting of blood from the right ventricle into the aorta since right ventricular pressure during systole remains below that of the aorta. Phonocardiographic studies in this group indicate, as in smaller defects, that the murmur is holosystolic and can be related to the left to right pressure gradient continuing through the entire period of ventricular ejection.

In many infants during the first year of life, very large left

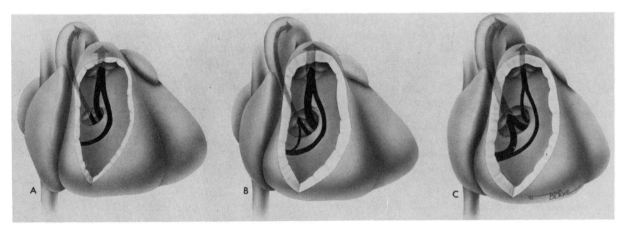

Fig. 9.2   Influence of size of defect and pulmonary vascular resistance upon net shunts. Anatomic-physiologic categories of ventricular septal defects are illustrated. The anterior aspect of the heart is viewed with the right ventricular free wall removed. (A) With moderate-sized defects, the pulmonary vascular resistance remains normal to slightly elevated. As indicated by the *arrows*, the net shunt is purely left to right, and there is increased pulmonary blood flow with augmented volume overload on the left heart. (B) In large ventricular septal defects with mild to moderate elevation of pulmonary vascular resistance, there is a large left to right shunt with marked increase in pulmonary blood flow, and equal pressure in both ventricles. Right ventricular hypertrophy results, and there is frequently a small right to left shunt into the systemic circulation. There is increased volume overload of the left ventricle, and the right ventricle is usually mildly to moderately dilated as well as moderately hypertrophied. (C) With large ventricular defects and marked elevation of pulmonary vascular resistance, the total volume of blood handled by the heart approaches normal. Here the resistance to flow of blood to the lungs is markedly increased so that the major flow across the defect occurs in a right to left direction into the systemic circulation (Eisenmenger's complex). Pulmonary blood flow approaches normal with resultant normal volume load on the left ventricle; the predominant abnormal workload is placed on the right ventricle.

to right shunts may be present with right ventricular pressures which are normal or only mildly to moderately elevated. In these patients the size of the defect is restrictive to flow, but the total amount of flow across the defect is relatively large for a small infant. In these patients, if the defect remains the same size and continues to be restrictive to flow, the absolute amount of shunting will become less significant as the child becomes larger.

Figure 9.3B illustrates the pressure-volume characteristics of the left ventricle in a patient with a medium-sized defect and normal right heart pressures.[33] Pulmonary flow was more than twice systemic flow and resulted in a large increase in the pressure-volume work. For comparison the pressure-volume loop labeled A is that of a postoperative patient who had normal hemodynamics and normal pressure-volume work.

Large Defects with Mild to Moderate Elevations of Pulmonary Vascular Resistance

Defects can be considered large when they are greater than 1 cm^2 per m^2 of body surface area, and approximate the size of the aortic orifice. Because of the nonrestrictive character of the defect, the pulmonary circulation is subjected to the common ejectile force of both ventricles during most of the period of ventricular ejection. Large left to right shunts ensue with systemic pressures in both ventricles and frequently a small systemic right to left shunt (Fig. 9.2B).

The interventricular pressure relationships and their influence on flow across large defects are illustrated in Figure 9.4. As in the smaller defects, the period of diastole shows fluctuations in the pressure gradient which favor the left ventricle and are associated with flow across the defect into the body of the right ventricle. This flow from left ventricle to right ventricle is accentuated with atrial contraction. Diastolic shunting can be readily seen in lateral cineangiocardiograms with filming rates of 60 per second. With the onset of systole, left ventricular pressure rises before that of the right with augmentation of flow across the defect immediately preceding opening of the aortic valve. The period of early ventricular ejection is characterized by maintenance

of a left ventricular gradient with left to right shunting across the defect into the outflow tract of the right ventricle. During the latter period of ventricular ejection, right ventricular pressure exceeds that of the left and obliterates the left to right shunt at this point. Some patients develop a direct right to left shunt into the aorta during this interval when left ventricular pressure has dropped considerably below that of the pulmonary artery and aorta. As the cycle continues into the relaxation period, the more rapid and earlier fall in left ventricular pressure accentuates the right to left gradient. This results in a right to left shunt into the left ventricle. This blood appears to mix in the upper portion of the left ventricular chamber (Fig. 9.4) and remains there despite some diastolic left to right shunting, and a small portion may be ejected from this chamber into the aorta with the subsequent beat. This right to left shunting from right ventricle to left ventricle can be readily appreciated in lateral cineangiocardiograms with rapid filming rates.

Figure 9.5 presents the relationships of the interventricular pressures and the direction of flow across the defect throughout the cardiac cycle in this group of patients. During diastole there is a left to right shunt into the body of the right ventricle (A), with augmentation of the left to right gradient and shunt during early systole (B). Phonocardiography in this group of patients demonstrates that the systolic murmur is most prominent during early ventricular ejection (C) when most of the left to right shunt occurs. This murmur stops or shows marked diminution during the latter third of systole when right ventricular pressure has exceeded that of the left and has resulted in a cessation of left to right flow (D). During relaxation (E), the right to left shunt across the defect is associated with an increasing left ventricular volume at the time when all valves are closed.

The work characteristics of the left ventricle in this situation are illustrated in Figure 9.3C. Note the large area of the pressure-volume loop, the decreasing volume during early systole, and the increasing volume during early relaxation due to the right to left shunt into the left ventricle.

Jarmakani and coworkers[35] have determined left ventricular (LV) and left atrial (LA) volumes and muscle mass in

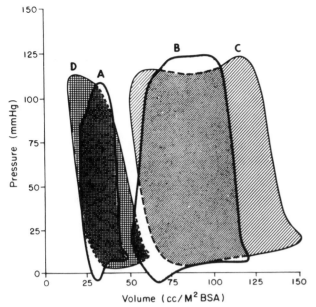

Fig. 9.3 Pressure-volume characteristics of the left ventricle with varying hemodynamic states of ventricular septal defects.[33] The pressure-volume loops shown were derived from simultaneously recorded pressure and biplane cineangiocardiographic volume data. Each volume determination was correlated with instantaneous pressure. The area of each loop represents the net systolic pressure-volume work done by the left ventricle during one cardiac cycle. The above data were obtained from patients 6 to 9 years old. In addition to indicating the net work of the left ventricle, the shape of each loop demonstrates characteristic changes ini volume during various portions of the cardiac cycle. (A) Normal ventricular septum. This loop was derived in a patient 3 years after surgical repair of his defect with the patient's preoperative loop shown in B. The net work represented is 28 g·m. Note that during isovolumic contraction, there is a rapid fall in volume during ventricular ejection; during isovolumic relaxation, the volume remains stable and then increases during diastole. (B) Moderate-sized defect with large left to right shunt and normal right ventricular pressure. The left to right shunt in this patient comprised 60% of total pulmonary blood flow. Note the marked increase in area of the loop; the work per stroke represented here is 93 g·m. The change in slope of the curve during periods of "isovolumic" contraction and relaxation shows a decrease in volume (left to right flow across the defect) during these intervals. (C) Large defect with moderate elevation of pulmonary vascular resistance. In this patient the right and left ventricular systolic pressures were equal, and there was a large left to right shunt which comprised 70% of pulmonary blood flow. Note the markedly increased area of the pressure-volume loop with stroke work of 124 g·m. The configuration of the pressure-volume loop in this situation with a systemic systolic pressure in the right ventricle shows a decreasing volume during "isovolumic" contraction due to the left to right shunt. The period of "isovolumic" relaxation is characterized by an increasing volume due to the right to left shunt across the defect at this time (see Figs. 9.4 and 9.5). (D) Large defect with marked elevation of pulmonary vascular resistance. This child demonstrated equal peak systolic ventricular pressures and net shunts across the defect which were equal with essentially normal pulmonary blood flow. Note that the area of pressure-volume loop approximates normal with stroke work of 43 g·m. The decreasing left ventricular volume during "isovolumic" contraction results from a left to right shunt across the defect. The "isovolumic" right to left shunt produces an increase in left ventricular volume during "isovolumic" relaxation, as also is present in loop C.

58 patients with isolated ventricular septal defect. LV end diastolic volume and mass and LA maximal volumes in patients who had left to right shunts of 35% or more were increased, and these variables showed a linear increase with

increasing left to right shunt. The total left ventricular systolic output as quantitated from cineangiocardiography provides an estimate of total pulmonary blood flow in VSD patients, although it does not account for diastolic left to right shunting, which can be sizeable.

Right ventricular end-diastolic volume also is increased in patients who have large left to right shunts with the increase being proportional to but less than the corresponding increase in left ventricular end-diastolic volume.[27] This increase in right ventricular size can be accounted for by the significant diastolic and "isovolumic" shunting from left to right ventricle which occurs in patients with large defects.

Large Defects with Marked Elevation of Pulmonary Vascular Resistance.

Left ventricular pressure-volume work is normal in this situation. The shunt across the defect is predominantly right to left (Fig. 9.2C), although the timing and direction of flow occur in the same manner as described above (Fig. 9.5). Diastole and early systole are associated with left to right shunting. The period of early ventricular ejection, however,

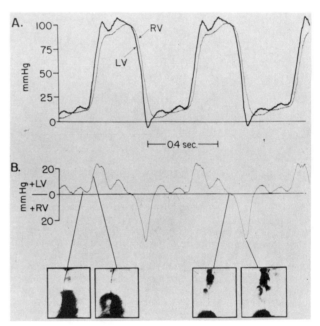

Fig. 9.4 Intraventricular pressure relationships and their influence on flow across large defects.[42] These data were recorded from the patient with pressure-volume loop C in Figure 9.3. Right and left ventricular pressures were recorded simultaneously. (A) Simultaneous right and left ventricular pressures. (B) Continuous pressure difference across the defect throughout the cardiac cycle with cineangiocardiographic pictures (below) demonstrating the effect of pressure difference across the defect on flow. Note that during diastole the pressure gradient is predominantly in favor of the left ventricle. During this interval, diastolic shunting from left ventricle to right ventricle can frequently be visualized with augmentation of the shunt occurring with atrial contraction. With the onset of "isovolumic" contraction there is an augmentation of the pressure gradient with the cine frames, indicating an augmented left to right shunt during this interval prior to opening of the aortic valve. Although the right ventricle has a "systemic" pressure, during early ejection the instantaneous left ventricular pressure is greater than that of the right. During the later part of ventricular ejection, right ventricular pressure exceeds that of the left. The period of "isovolumic" relaxation is characterized by a more rapid fall in left ventricular pressure with a prominent right to left gradient which results in right to left flow across the defect into the left ventricle as shown in the time-related cine frames following ejection of contrast media into the right ventricle (lower right).

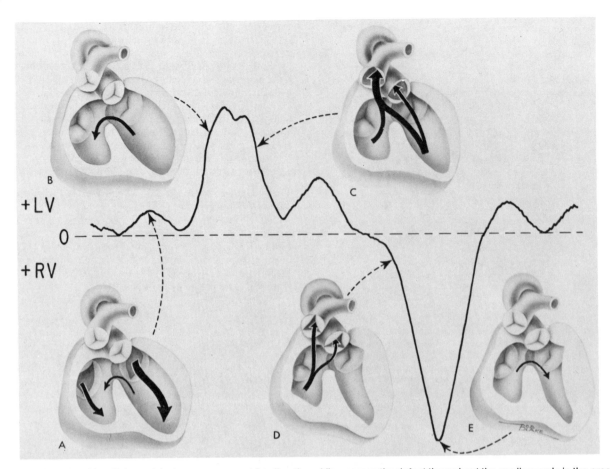

Fig. 9.5 Relationship of interventricular pressures and the direction of flow across the defect throughout the cardiac cycle in the presence of large ventricular septal defects.[42] The continuous pressure difference curve (see Fig. 9.4) across the defect is shown with a schematic representation of the state of the ventricles and valves during various portions of the cardiac cycle. The flow pattern indicated by the *solid lines* represents the direction of flow through the heart found in patients with large defects, hyperkinetic pulmonary hypertension, and large left to right shunt. (*A*) During diastole, a larger volume of flow occurs across the mitral as compared to the tricuspid valve with spillover of blood across the defect from the left ventricle into the body of the right ventricle. (*B*) During "isovolumic" contraction, when all valves are closed, there is accentuation of the predominant left ventricular pressure gradient with augmentation of flow across the defect into the right ventricle. (*C*) Early ventricular ejection is characterized by the right ventricle ejecting blood into the pulmonary artery and the left ventricle ejecting blood into aorta, as well as the large amount of blood across the defect. The shunted blood is directed through the outflow tract of the right ventricle into the pulmonary artery. (*D*) The terminal period of ventricular ejection is characterized by the right ventricular pressure exceeding that of the left; this cuts off left to right flow and can produce a small shunt from the right ventricle into the aorta. (*E*) "Isovolumic" relaxation is characterized by a predominant right ventricular pressure gradient with flow occurring across the defect into the left ventricle at a time when all valves are closed.

is associated with a very small left to right shunt across the defect. In late systole, significant right to left flow occurs from right ventricle into aorta with continuation of this right to left shunt during the early relaxation period. Similar findings have been shown in patients with tetralogy of Fallot.[41]

The left ventricular pressure-volume loop in this situation approximates normal (Fig. 9.3D), indicating that the magnitude of work per stroke is normal. However, the shape of the loop shows considerable fluctuation in left ventricular volume since it decreases during early systole and increases during the relaxation period. The small total stroke volume indicated by the loop is consistent with the minor left to right shunt during systole. The murmur generated by the flow across the defect during early ejection is minimal or absent, and there is no murmur associated with the period of right to left shunting. The explanation for this physical finding probably is the interrelationship of the size of the defect and the instantaneous flow (velocity) characteristics which fail to produce significant turbulence to generate an audible murmur.

MANIFESTATIONS

CLINICAL FEATURES

History

The dynamic nature of the physiologic changes which occur after birth emphasizes that the clinical state of the patient depends primarily upon the size of the defect, the state of pulmonary vascular resistance, and the variation of these two parameters with age.[16, 32] Most commonly, the murmur is detected at 2 to 6 weeks of age when the infant returns for the initial checkup after discharge from the hospital. However, the murmur occasionally can be heard during the first days of life, especially in the presence of small or moderate-sized defects associated with a normal fall in pulmonary vascular resistance. With small defects, the clinical course is benign. When the child is seen for cardiac evaluation, the clinical setting is usually one of a healthy infant. Small ventricular septal defects continue with a benign course throughout infancy and childhood. The only danger to these patients is endocarditis, which is rare before the age of 2 years.

From 1 to 12 months, severe symptoms are due primarily to left ventricular failure secondary to a large left to right shunt. The initial symptoms consist of tachypnea with increased respiratory effort, excessive sweating due to increased sympathetic tone, and fatigue when feeding. Since feeding is the most strenuous activity that the infant undergoes in the early months, the feeding history becomes important. The story is usually that of an infant who tires with feeding with these symptoms beginning usually during the first month and progressing in severity as pulmonary vascular resistance falls. There is a slightly earlier onset of symptomatology for prematures as compared to full-term infants.[32] It is not unusual for symptoms of failure to be preceded by respiratory infection. This complication makes it difficult to clarify the degree to which the respiratory distress is due to heart failure versus the infection.

The cardiovascular basis for the respiratory symptoms in the absence of infection probably is related to pulmonary edema of mild to moderate degree with elevated pulmonary venous pressure, and decreased lung compliance. It has been shown in dogs that a decrease in lung compliance does not occur with increased pulmonary flow or increased pulmonary arterial pressure alone, but occurs with an increase in left atrial pressure.[9] It is well known, of course, that many patients with isolated ASDs, large left to right shunts, and normal or only slightly elevated left atrial pressures have normal lung compliance and usually no symptoms of dyspnea.[17] In adults with mitral stenosis, lung compliance generally is normal until pulmonary wedge pressure exceeds 15 mm Hg.[19] In infants with a large left to right shunt secondary to a VSD, dyspnea can occur with mean left atrial pressures slightly lower than 15 mm Hg and is undoubtedly related to some degree of pulmonary edema.

Some infants with large defects have very little decrease in pulmonary vascular resistance in the first few months of life with the development of only mild to moderate left to right shunting. These infants do well without passing through the phase of high output cardiac failure. Their mild clinical course disguises the underlying physiologic abnormality, because this group can develop pulmonary vascular obstructive disease with ultimate reversal of shunting.

The clinical course following the development of left ventricular failure is variable. In some infants with large defects, pulmonary resistance continues to fall with augmentation of the left to right shunt and accentuation of heart failure. However, the majority of infants improve under medical therapy. Hypertrophy of the left ventricle which enables this chamber to handle large flows probably accounts for some of this improvement. A number of patients show evidence of gradual decrease in the magnitude of the left to right shunt between 6 and 24 months. With such a history, it is of paramount importance to assess accurately the cause of increased resistance to left to right flow; this can result from: progression of pulmonary vascular resistance; decrease in the relative size of the defect; and the development of hypertrophy of the outflow tract of the right ventricle with resultant functional and/or anatomic obstruction in this area.

With large left to right shunts, these infants appear thin, and are underweight. In those who have gradual diminution of the shunt, symptoms and growth improve. If large shunts stabilize, the infant continues with retarded growth, tachypnea, and excessive sweating. Hoffman and Rudolph[32] have reported that a decrease in the size of the defect as related to body surface area occurs in more than half of patients with large VSDs. The frequency of spontaneous closure of large defects is approximately 5 to 10%. Spontaneous closure of small defects occurs in well over 60%, and it usually does so during infancy.

When the patient is first seen after 2 years of age, the clinical setting is somewhat different from that of the infant in the first year of life. Although a few have heart failure after 18 months, the majority of patients are stable except for frequent respiratory infections. Since this group has survived the danger period of high output failure in infancy, they present the problem of estimating the size of the defect, and in those with moderate to large defects, evaluation of the status of the pulmonary vascular resistance. Evaluation of the history during the period of 9 months to 3 years can be difficult, because the clinical improvement may be due to progression of pulmonary hypertension. This group presents a challenge in designing proper therapy. Our experience has been similar to that of others,[16, 32, 37] in that patients with large defects, high pulmonary artery pressure, and large left to right shunts with heart failure in infancy are at risk during this interval to develop further elevation of pulmonary vascular resistance. In the past, considerable emphasis has been placed on the possible progression of pulmonary hypertension, which by history may be inapparent in children between the ages of 5 and 16 years. Overwhelming evidence indicates that this problem occurs, with rare exceptions, in only one group of patients—those with a large defect. If the defect is small or moderate in size, it is unlikely that the pulmonary vascular bed will progress from a state of low resistance to high resistance during this age period. The history alone may be of little help because there are usually only mild symptoms of a subjective nature, for example, shortness of breath and decreased exercise tolerance. One must rely on other diagnostic modalities for evaluating these patients.

A history of cyanosis not documented by physical examination is most difficult to evaluate. In particular, cyanosis during the early weeks of life is often transient and frequently presents only with superimposed stress. Persistent cyanosis from birth suggests a more complicated lesion than isolated ventricular septal defect. However, the occurrence of cyanosis after infancy suggests reversal of the shunt because of progressive pulmonary vascular disease or the development of significant infundibular pulmonary stenosis.

In patients with the Eisenmenger complex, Wood[66] found that the majority had a history of cyanosis since infancy. It was his impression that the syndrome was commonly established at birth or developed during the first 2 years of life. He found that usually neither cyanosis nor breathlessness progressed markedly during childhood or adolescence, but that deterioration occurred as young adults. Squatting was found in 15% of his patients, and hemoptysis occurred in 33% of patients but never before 24 years of age. It occurred in 100% of patients by 40 years of age and was a contributing cause of death in 29%. He felt that it could herald a downhill course, but this is not an invariable course of events.

Physical Examination

An accurate evaluation of the physical examination, electrocardiogram, and cardiac roentgenograms usually allows one to classify each patient's status into one of the four anatomic-physiologic groups, since interaction of the underlying physiologic variables results in a rather specific profile. Although the purpose of evaluation of these patients is to classify the situation into one of the four categories, it should be emphasized that these categories are used merely as guidelines. At times it is difficult to clarify borderline situations, for example, to determine if a patient with a large defect has mild or moderate elevation of pulmonary vascular resistance. In severely ill infants, clinical evaluation often leaves much to be desired, and one frequently has to resort to echocardiography and cardiac catheterization for clarification of the diagnosis and physiological consequences.

Small Defects

In accord with the very mild hemodynamic changes associated with small defects, these children appear quite healthy. By palpation, the precordial activity is normal. A thrill can be palpable along the lower left sternal border at the third or fourth intercostal space. This thrill is associated with a grade IV/VI holosystolic murmur which can appear plateau, crescendo, or crescendo-decrescendo (Fig. 9.6A). It frequently envelops and can bury the aortic component of the second sound and extends slightly past it. Unlike most cases of mitral insufficiency, the murmur of VSD has, in addition to its high frequency components, those which are of lower frequency, and these give it a characteristic harsh quality. Because of the high frequency components of the murmur, it is accentuated when auscultation is carried out with the diaphragm. In some patients the murmur can extend up along the left parasternal region, owing to ejection across the outflow tract of the right ventricle. The murmur also can radiate to the right of the sternum. In patients with a supracristal defect, the murmur and thrill usually are maximal at the second left intercostal space, and there frequently is a thrill in the suprasternal notch.

It should be emphasized that the holosystolic quality of the murmur correlates with a continuous pressure gradient across the defect and provides indirect evidence that the right ventricular systolic pressure is significantly less than the left. However, patients with muscular defects may have short murmurs which cut off in midsystole, presumably because of closure of the defect due to systolic contraction of septal musculature (Fig. 9.6B). These patients are usually differentiated from patients with an innocent murmur by the fact that the murmur is well localized to the left sternal border and is heard best with the diaphragm rather than the bell because of its high frequency components. This type of murmur is most common in infancy and has a high likelihood of disappearance during the first year of life because of the frequent occurrence of spontaneous closure of such defects.

The heart sounds in small ventricular septal defect are usually normal. Some patients, however, have wide splitting of the second sound. Occasionally, a prominent third sound is heard over the apical region. Knowledge of the location of the right ventricular area[57] projected onto the chest wall (Fig. 9.7) is helpful in differentiating the murmurs of isolated pulmonic stenosis or mitral insufficiency from that of VSD. If there is associated pulmonic stenosis or mitral insufficiency in a patient with VSD, these lesions may be suspected when the systolic murmur is transmitted into areas not indicated by the right ventricular projection. It should be remembered, however, that the supracristal VSD can project high onto the left sternal border as indicated above.

Moderate-sized Defects

In the presence of large shunts, children may appear with normal height and decreased weight. Precordial activity is accentuated, and extends over both the right and left ventricular areas, as indicated in Figure 9.7. The hyperdynamic precordium becomes more prominent as left ventricular volume increases owing to increased pulmonary blood flow. In patients with large shunts for 4 to 6 months or longer, the left anterior thorax bulges outward.

The murmur with moderate-sized defects is usually associated with a thrill, is holosystolic, and is harsh in nature (Fig. 9.6C, 1 and 2). Its duration and character suggest a significant pressure gradient across the defect. As in small defects, this murmur is most prominent over the right ventricular area along the lower left sternal border. A prominent third sound with a short early middiastolic rumble (Fig. 9.6C, 1) is frequently audible at the apex when pulmonary blood flow is approximately twice that of systemic or greater. The first sound in the apical region is frequently accentuated in these patients who have increased left ventricular end diastolic volume and workload as illustrated in Figure 9.3B. The second sound is frequently widely split, and usually there is a slight variation with respiration. The intensity of the pulmonary component is usually normal or only slightly increased.

Large Defects with Moderate Elevation of Pulmonary Vascular Resistance

In infants, this group of defects presents a diagnostic problem in differentiation from other lesions. These patients show tachypnea with increased respiratory effort, increased sweating, particularly about the forehead, and markedly increased precordial activity. Jugular venous pulsations are difficult to evaluate in the infant but may be prominent with accentuation of a and v waves. The anterior-posterior diameter of the chest frequently is increased.[17] By palpation, an abnormal left ventricular tap in the apical region usually is present and becomes more marked as the volume load of the left ventricle increases. Also, there is a right ventricular lift which is diffusely felt over the entire right ventricular area. In infants it may be difficult to differentiate the right and left ventricular components of the precordial activity, and diffusely increased activity over the precordium may be the principle finding. Frequently, the thrust of the main pulmonary artery against the chest wall can be palpated during systole as well as closure of the pulmonary valve.

The murmur from the defect is located over the right ventricular area, usually is decrescendo in nature, and disappears during the latter third of systole before closure of the aortic valve (Fig. 9.6D). These characteristics differ from those in patients maintaining a significant systolic pressure gradient across the defect throughout ventricular ejection. The pulmonary component of the second sound is usually loud, and splitting is narrow but detectable in most patients. Some patients have a murmur which extends into the upper left parasternal region. This murmur may be generated by ejection of blood into the pulmonary artery or may be due to mild infundibular pulmonary stenosis. A few patients may exhibit an early faint diastolic decrescendo murmur in this region as a result of mild pulmonary insufficiency. The presence of an early diastolic decrescendo murmur, however, should alert one to the possibility of associated aortic insufficiency. There is usually a prominent third sound and a diastolic rumble in the left ventricular apical area.

Large Defects and Marked Elevation of Pulmonary Vascular Resistance

These patients are those with marked pulmonary hypertension secondary to elevated pulmonary resistance. Since the right ventricle is capable of handling for a number of years the increased systolic work required in the presence of a ventricular septal defect, these patients frequently appear well compensated in childhood. Those patients with moderate to large right to left shunts will be cyanotic even at rest. This is rare in infants, is occasionally seen by the age of 2 to 3 years, but is more frequently seen in the adolescent and young adult.

Since the workload of the left ventricle approximates normal (Fig. 9.3D), a hyperdynamic chest motion is not present as it is in the other groups. Palpation reveals a

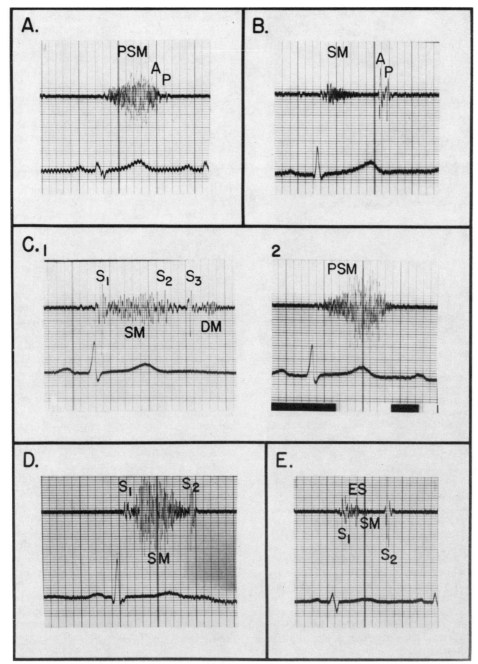

Fig. 9.6 Phonocardiographic findings in ventricular septal defects with varying physiologic states. (*A*) Small defect with normal right ventricular pressure and minimal left to right shunt. The prominent murmur is harsh in quality and pansystolic (*PSM*). Note the prominent splitting of S_2, as commonly occurs in small defects. (*B*) Small defect with nonholosystolic murmur in the presence of normal right ventricular systolic pressure. This illustrates the occasional occurrence of an early systolic murmur from a ventricular defect where the murmur ends well before the second sound because of functional closure of the defect during ventricular contraction. (*C*) Moderate-sized defect with mild elevation of right ventricular systolic pressure and prominent left to right shunt. (*1*) Phonocardiogram obtained at the apex illustrates the prominent S_3 and diastolic rumble (*DM*) (*2*) This tracing was recorded in the third inner space adjacent to the sternum. Note that the murmur is most prominent in this area; also demonstrated are the harsh quality and holosystolic nature of the bruit. (*D*) Large defect with "equal" ventricular systolic pressures and large left to right shunt. This tracing was obtained from the left parasternal region in the third interspace. Notice the decrescendo nature of the murmur, which shows marked diminution or termination before S_2. (*E*) Large defect with marked elevation of pulmonary vascular resistance and equal bidirectional shunting. This shows a predominant ejection sound (*ES*), a short ejection murmur (*SM*), and a single or closely split S_2 with a loud pulmonary component.

prominent right ventricular lift which is usually maximal in the xiphoid region. There may be a very short or no systolic murmur from the VSD (Fig. 9.6*E*). These patients may have a short pulmonary ejection murmur along the upper left parasternal region. In the presence of a loud, harsh holosystolic murmur in a patient known to be physiologically in this group, one should suspect associated tricuspid insufficiency, since the murmur from flow across the defect should be minimal in intensity and duration and usually not audible. Many patients have an early diastolic murmur of pulmonary insufficiency.[66] The second sound is quite loud, with a palpable and markedly accentuated pulmonary component

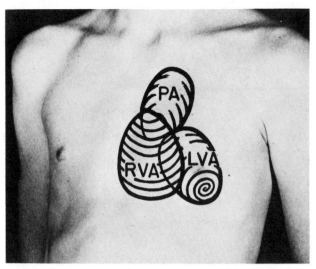

Fig. 9.7 Projection of cardiac structure areas into the chest wall. These regions correspond to surface locations where impulses, thrills, sounds, and murmurs are transmitted maximally by events in the right ventricle, left ventricle, and pulmonary artery. The murmur of a ventricular septal defect occurs predominantly in the right ventricular area (RVA). Auscultation in the pulmonary artery (PA) area provides information in evaluating the second sound and in differentiating the murmur of associated pulmonary stenosis from that of an isolated infracristal ventricular septal defect. The supracristal defect murmur usually occurs maximally over the pulmonary artery area. Analysis of events over the left ventricular area (LVA) is helpful in evaluating the size and function of the left ventricle. With increasing left ventricular volume overload, precordial motion is accentuated in this area. The areas may shift on the body surface depending upon the underlying hemodynamic state in patients with ventricular defects. As the cardiac dimensions are altered, their positions as related to the torso become altered; for example, with a marked volume overload of the left ventricle, the LVA shifts leftward into the axillary region. With normal left ventricular activity in the presence of marked right ventricular hypertrophy, the RVA may extend over a larger area of the left precordium.

along the upper left sternal border. It is usually single or closely split, although Wood[66] found it to be single in only 55% of his patients. The pulmonary artery impulse also usually can be easily palpable. There is no diastolic rumble at the apex as in patients with increased volume loading of the left ventricle. However, a third sound can be present which is usually right ventricular in origin and is present along the left sternal border.

ELECTROVECTORCARDIOGRAPHIC FEATURES

The electrocardiogram is valuable in providing indirect information concerning the work characteristics of the heart in patients with VSD. For accurate appraisal of the electrocardiogram in these patients, not only must one keep in mind the work characteristics of both ventricles, as they are determined by the previously discussed varying physiologic states, but several additional variables which influence the projection of electrical events within the heart onto the body surface. Particularly important are: increasing volume overload of the left ventricle while the right ventricle primarily is affected with a systolic overload; alterations in ventricular thickness which produce changes in the sequence of ventricular excitation; and overall cardiac enlargement which causes an abnormal geometric relationship between the heart and points on the body surface.

In small VSD, the electrocardiogram is usually normal. However, a few patients with small defects demonstrate a

rsr' in Lead V1. In addition, left axis deviation can be seen in the absence of an AV canal position of the defect.

In moderate-sized defects, there may be no right ventricular hypertrophy; however, mild or moderate elevation of right ventricular pressure can result in right ventricular hypertrophy, which is evident in Lead V4R or 1 as a rsR' pattern with the R' increasing in amplitude with increasing right ventricular pressure. Since most of these patients have moderately large left to right shunts with volume overload of the left ventricle, left ventricular hypertrophy is the rule.

In isolated VSD, the familiar electrocardiogram of the enlarged left ventricle with an increased mass and dilated chamber includes prominent Q, R, and T waves in limb leads II, III, aVF, and V6. These changes are illustrated in Figure 9.8A. Note the prominent Q wave (greater than 0.4 mv), tall R, and symmetrical, peaked T wave in lead V6.

In infants with a similar hemodynamic pattern, the electrocardiographic features frequently are not as distinctive as in older children. In this age group, the presence of a counterclockwise QRS loop in the frontal plane can be helpful as an index of left ventricular hypertrophy. Some infants with large defects early in their course may show only increased biphasic voltages over the midprecordium (greater than 4.5 mv). Patients with large VSD and equal ventricular pressures demonstrate right ventricular hypertrophy. The main clinical implication of discerning the work characteristics of the heart is to detect those patients who show abnormal volume overloading of the left ventricle, indicating the presence of a significant left to right shunt in the face of right ventricular hypertrophy. DuShane et al.[21] have described the features of the elecrocardiogram in these patients. In patients with large pulmonary blood flow, left atrial hypertrophy is evidenced by biphasic P waves which are usually most prominent in Leads I, aVR, and V6. In addition, lead V1 frequently shows a biphasic P wave with a prominent negative deflection. Evidence of left atrial enlargement provides indirect evidence of left ventricular overload (in the absence of mitral valve disease). Figures 9.8B and C represent typical electrocardiograms of patients with large defects with increased pulmonary flow and combined ventricular hypertrophy. Note the prominent Q, tall R, and peaked T waves in Lead V6 in the presence of right ventricular hypertrophy. In the presence of combined ventricular hypertrophy, the right ventricular hypertrophy pattern in Lead V1 usually consists of a QRS complex of the rsR' pattern or one with a prominent negative deflection on the upstroke of the R wave (rR').

In patients with large defects and marked elevation of pulmonary resistance, in whom there is essentially normal volume work by the left ventricle, evidence of left ventricular and left atrial hypertrophy is usually absent (Fig. 9.8D). Here right ventricular hypertrophy produces a QRS pattern in Lead V1 with slurring of the upstroke of the R wave, a delay in the onset of the intrinsicoid deflection, and absent or minor S waves. In addition, the P waves do not suggest left atrial enlargement and the T waves are frequently more peaked in the midprecordial leads (V2 to V4) rather than V5 and V6.

Isolated posterior defects of the "AV canal type" frequently produce the characteristic changes seen in the usual complete AV canal defects with superior orientation of the electrical forces and counterclockwise rotation of the QRS loop in the frontal plane. In these defects, the conduction system abnormality is largely responsible for "programming" the sequence of ventricular excitation such that the wave fronts spread from the diaphragmatic surface of the left ventricle in a cephalad direction.[58]

The vectorcardiogram also is useful in establishing the general hemodynamic status of the heart in isolated ventric-

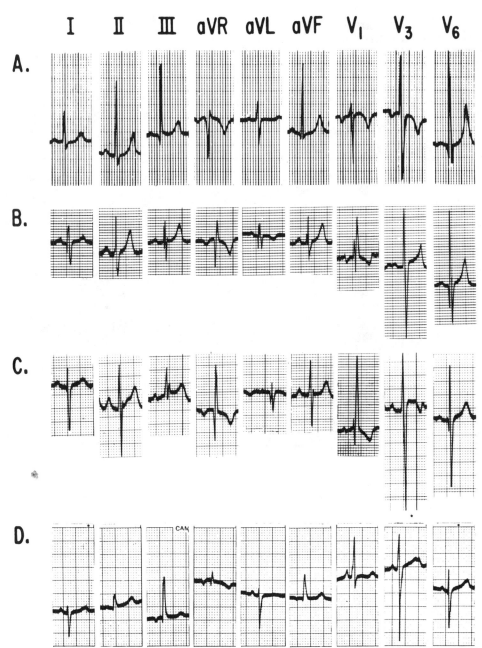

Fig. 9.8 Electrocardiographic findings in varying hemodynamic states in ventricular septal defects. These tracings were obtained in children whose ages varied from 4 to 12 years. (*A*) Moderate-sized defect with normal pulmonary resistance and large left to right shunt. Note the absence of right ventricular hypertrophy. Left ventricular volume overload is evidenced by the prominent R wave in lead II and by the prominent Q and R waves in lead V6. Note the tall, symmetrically peaked T waves in leads II and V6. (*B*) Large defect and hyperkinetic pulmonary hypertension with large left to right shunt. This tracing demonstrates combined ventricular hypertrophy. Left ventricular overload is evidenced by the large Q and tall R in lead V6. Note also the prominently peaked T waves in leads II and V6. Right ventricular hypertrophy with the rsR′ in lead V1 indicates associated right ventricular overload. (*C*) Large defect with hyperkinetic pulmonary hypertension with more right ventricular hypertrophy than shown in *B*. Note the rsR′ in lead V1 with the prominent R′ as well as the large S wave in lead V6. Left ventricular overload in the presence of this degree of right ventricular hypertrophy is indicated by the prominent Q and moderately tall R wave in lead V6. (*D*) Large defect with marked elevation of pulmonary vascular resistance. This tracing demonstrates right ventricular hypertrophy in the absence of left ventricular overload. Lead V1 usually demonstrates a slurred upstroke of the R wave and the absence of an rsR′. Note in lead V6 the lack of prominent Q and T waves.

ular septal defects. Figure 9.9 demonstrates three characteristic Frank vectorcardiograms, illustrating changes in patients with moderate and large defects. In moderate-sized defects (Fig. 9.9*A*) with left ventricular overload and essentially normal right ventricular pressures, the frontal plane usually demonstrates a thin loop which is elongated and points downward to the left. The rotation in the horizontal plane remains normal with the major orientation of the loop leftward and slightly anterior. In large defects, with right ventricular hypertrophy and left ventricular volume overload, combined ventricular hypertrophy (Fig. 9.9*B*) is more prominently seen in the horizontal plane with diagonal orientation of the loop, which is rather thin, with the first half of the loop oriented anteriorly and to the left and the terminal part of the loop to the right and posteriorly. The horizontal loop usually rotates in a clockwise direction or in

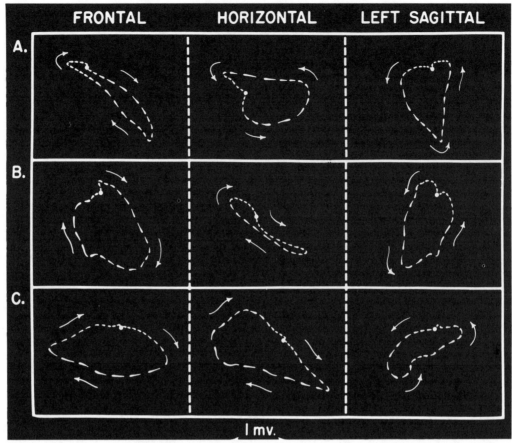

Fig. 9.9 Vectorcardiographic findings in varying hemodynamic states in ventricular septal defects. These are Frank vectorcardiograms from 8 to 10 year old children. (*A*) Moderate-sized defect with left ventricular overload and normal right ventricular pressure. The frontal plane demonstrates a thin QRS loop which is elongated in an inferior and leftward direction. In the horizontal plane, the rotation maintains a normal counterclockwise direction with a major portion of the loop oriented leftward and slightly anteriorly. (*B*) Large defect with hyperkinetic pulmonary hypertension. Biventricular hypertrophy is evidenced here in the horizontal plane by the rather thin loop which is oriented diagonally. The first half of the loop is directed anteriorly and to the left with the terminal part being oriented to the right and posteriorly. The rotation is abnormal in a clockwise direction. (*C*) Large defect with marked elevation of pulmonary resistance. This demonstrates pure right ventricular hypertrophy with the initial portion of the QRS loop directed leftward and anteriorly, clockwise rotation of the loop in the horizontal plane, and the major portion of the loop oriented anteriorly and rightward.

a figure-of-eight manner. Finally, in large defects with markedly elevated pulmonary resistance and normal left ventricular workload, pure right ventricular hypertrophy is seen with the initial portion of the loop directed leftward and anteriorly, clockwise rotation in the horizontal plane, with the major portion of the loop oriented anteriorly and rightward (Fig. 9.9C). The initial forces in this group tend to be oriented anteriorly and leftward. The rotation of the horizontal loop is clockwise.

RADIOLOGIC FEATURES

With small defects, the chest x-ray usually shows normal heart size and normal pulmonary vascularity.

Patients with moderate-sized defects show cardiac enlargement of varying severity and increased pulmonary vascular markings. This condition is illustrated in Figure 9.10A. Note the downward elongation and lateral position of the left ventricular apex. Pulmonary vascular resistance is normal to slightly increased. This results in the pulmonary vascular markings being increased in both the central and peripheral portions of the lung fields. Barium swallow with lateral and right oblique chest films can be helpful in assessing left atrial enlargement but is seldom indicated. Left atrial enlargement is quite frequent in medium-sized and large

defects with moderate elevation of pulmonary vascular resistance; in both these conditions, the shunt is large. However, in small defects and in large communications with very high pulmonary vascular resistance, the left atrium is usually normal in size.

In patients with large defects, moderately elevated pulmonary resistance, and large left to right shunts, the x-ray findings are those of generalized cardiac enlargement, increased pulmonary vascular markings, prominence of the main pulmonary artery, and right ventricular hypertrophy (Fig. 10B and 9.10D). Because all these patients have "equal" right and left ventricular systolic pressures, the right ventricle hypertrophies to accommodate its systolic workload and enlarges to a moderate degree. This hypertrophy and enlargement frequently results in the left ventricular apex being displaced posteriorly. This group of patients has a low position of the diaphragms, which gives the chest an emphysematous-like appearance.[17] Large defects with marked elevation of pulmonary vascular resistance have essentially normal size hearts (Fig. 9.10C). Right ventricular hypertrophy with the cardiac apex rotated slightly upward and to the left and posteriorly is characteristic and is associated with marked prominence of the main pulmonary artery and its adjacent vessels with decreased pulmonary vascularity in the outer third of the lung fields. In patients who develop

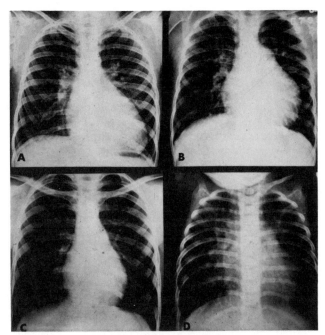

Fig. 9.10 Chest roentgenograms in patients with ventricular septal defects and varying hemodynamic states. (A) 7-year-old child with a moderate-sized defect with low pulmonary vascular resistance and a large left to right shunt. Left ventricular overload is evidenced by the prominent projection of the cardiac apex downward and to the left. The pulmonary vascularity is accentuated both in the hilar and peripheral regions of the lung. (B) 5-year-old child with a large defect, moderate elevation of pulmonary vascular resistance, and a large left to right shunt. Elevated pressures in the pulmonary artery and right ventricle are suggested by a combination of prominence of the main pulmonary artery segment and rounding of the left heart border. Left ventricular overload due to the large left to right shunt is indicated by the generalized cardiac enlargement. The pulmonary vascular markings are accentuated. A barium esophagram revealed left atrial enlargement. (C) 8-year-old child with a large defect, markedly elevated pulmonary resistance, small left to right shunt, and moderate right to left shunt. This film is typical of Eisenmenger's reaction. The normal cardiac size is related to normal pulmonary blood flow with the resultant normal left heart dimensions. The pulmonary vessels are prominent in the hilar region with no accentuation peripherally. (D) 9-month-old infant with a large defect, hyperkinetic pulmonary hypertension, and large left to right shunt. This child had heart failure and growth retardation. Note the cardiac enlargement, marked increase in pulmonary vascularity, and suggestive left atrial enlargement.

marked elevation of pulmonary vascular resistance after initially having a large shunt, the left ventricle and left atrium may remain somewhat enlarged for a period of time, as the dilatation and hypertrophy slowly regress or remain unchanged while the child grows.

ECHOCARDIOGRAPHIC FEATURES

M-mode echocardiography is extremely useful in detecting abnormalities of the atrioventricular and semilunar valves, great vessel abnormalities, and the presence or absence of a ventricular septum. In addition, the technique is useful in providing an index of left to right shunt by measurement of left atrial and left ventricular dimensions. Left ventricular shortening fraction and systolic time intervals can aid in assessment of ventricular function when afterload is not increased. M-mode measurements also can be useful in providing indirect assessment of pulmonary vascular resistance. Patients who show a decrease in the ratio of the right

ventricular pre-ejection period to ejection time while breathing 100% O$_2$ in general can be expected to have a reactive pulmonary vascular bed.[31]

Two-dimensional echocardiography is extremely useful in visualization of defects using both subcostal or precordial views. Defects which are approximately 3 mm or greater in diameter can be detected by experienced echocardiographers.[8, 12, 13] In addition, valvular and great vessel abnormalities can be readily defined with 2D studies.

CARDIAC CATHETERIZATION

The purposes of the cardiac catheterization are primarily to: document the presence of the defect or defects; evaluate the magnitude of shunting across the defect; estimate pulmonary vascular resistance; estimate the workload of the two ventricles; document or rule out the presence of associated defects; and provide the surgeon with a clear anatomic picture of the location of the defect or defects in those patients in whom operation is required. Just as the clinical syndromes differ, the indications and the objectives of the catheterization procedure vary from patient to patient. The extent to which catheterization is used depends upon the experience of the physician; the indications for the procedure should be based on the procurement of information not apparent or available by other clinical means. Since conventional diagnostic techniques are sufficiently accurate to appraise the anatomic and physiologic state of the patient with a small defect, it is not necessary to catheterize children whose evaluations indicate that they have small defects.

Cardiac catheterization yields the maximum amount of useful information in two groups of patients: infants with suspected VSD with evidence of a large left to right shunt and/or heart failure and patients with evidence suggesting increased pulmonary vascular resistance with moderate or small left to right shunts. In most symptomatic infants with suspected VSD, catheterization is necessary since these children may have associated defects which will alter the management. We usually recommend catheterization for: all infants with heart failure or with evidence of a large left to right shunt without definite heart failure and for patients with moderate or large left to right shunts for whom surgery is contemplated. Improvements in echocardiographic imaging now allow accurate diagnosis in many patients with isolated defects and can delay or obviate the need for catheterization in selected patients.

We first perform a right heart catheterization with measurement of the pressures and oxygen saturations in the pulmonary circuit, right heart, and femoral artery for estimating pulmonary and systemic blood flows. Thereafter, indicator dilution curves (either arterial dye or radioisotope)[59] are recorded to further document the presence and magnitude of the intracardiac shunt in any situation in which oxygen-derived shunt data are not consistent with the clinical estimation of shunting or the estimated pulmonary vascular resistance is elevated. Simultaneous pulmonary artery and aortic or peripheral arterial pressures are obtained for estimation of pulmonary and systemic vascular resistances. Frequently, in infancy the left heart can be catheterized through a patent foramen ovale. In this situation a rapid pullback from left ventricle to left atrium to right atrium and then rapid manipulation of the catheter into right ventricle provides a means for assessment of the relative pressures in right and left ventricle to aid in determining the size of the ventricular defect. In addition, the pullback from left atrium to right atrium provides a method to gauge the size of the atrial defect. In the presence of only a dilated foramen ovale there is usually a mean pressure gradient from left atrium to right atrium of ≤ 5 mm Hg.

If a patent ductus arteriosus is not traversed in patients with pulmonary hypertension, left heart catheterization is performed for retrograde aortography. Calculations of left ventricular (LV) end-diastolic volume, LV ejection fraction, LV systolic output, LV muscle mass, and left atrial maximal volume can be performed relatively easily, and comparisons can be made with normal values.[18, 29] These data can be valuable in providing further information regarding pulmonary flow[35] and cardiac function. On the levogram phase of a right heart injection, one can detect the presence or absence of a left to right shunt at the atrial level and anomalies of pulmonary venous return.

In patients in whom surgery is indicated, we feel left ventricular cineangiocardiography is mandatory to document the location and number of ventricular septal defects. This information is extremely valuable to the surgeon in planning the operation and in being able to locate all of the defects quickly after the intracardiac part of the operation has begun. Dr. L. M. Bargeron of the University of Alabama has developed a long axis, oblique view which has proven extremely useful in visualizing the ventricular septum, in accurately delineating the size and number of defects, and in evaluating the left ventricular outflow tract.[4, 24] With this method the patient is first turned across the table so that the long axis of the left ventricle lies along the long axis of the catheterization table. With the catheterization performed from the patient's right groin, the patient's legs are pulled toward the operator until the long axis of the left ventricle lies along the long axis of the table as viewed on fluoroscopy. The patient's right shoulder then is elevated from 30 to 45°. Small test injections are performed to be sure that the long axis of the left ventricle is adequately visualized on the lateral screen and the ventricular septum is perpendicular to the lateral image intensifier. With the newer

angiographic systems, this long axis view can be obtained by angling the image intensifiers without moving the patient.

Figure 9.11 demonstrates clearly the presence of multiple ventricular septal defects in two patients evaluated by Dr. Bargeron using this technique. This method also is useful in ruling out the absence of a ventricular septum, although we have found that echocardiography is usually diagnostic and serves as a valuable adjunct to cineangiocardiography.

If the long axis view does not clearly delineate the defect(s), left ventricular injection with the 4-chamber or hepatoclavicular view should be performed. This view more clearly displays the posterior ventricular septum, and also is useful for demonstrating a left ventricular to right atrial communication.[24]

The patient with a tricuspid valve overriding the ventricular septum can present a difficult diagnostic challenge. These patients usually have hypoplasia of the right ventricle and a large ventricular septal defect of the atrioventricular canal type. Echocardiography can be diagnostic. Right atrial angiocardiography in the 4-chamber view also is useful in demonstrating contrast which appears to pass directly from right atrium into left ventricle. In addition, volume calculations of the right ventricle will demonstrate hypoplasia of this chamber.

In patients with a diastolic murmur suggesting semilunar valvular insufficiency, an aortogram is required for detection and estimation of the degree of aortic insufficiency. In addition, information regarding coronary artery distribution is useful in situations in which a ventriculotomy is to be performed in order to rule out the presence of left anterior descending coronary arising from the right coronary or a single main coronary artery with the anterior descending branch crossing the outflow tract of the right ventricle. These abnormalities are very rare, however, in isolated ventricular defects.

It is to be emphasized that clinical assessment of the

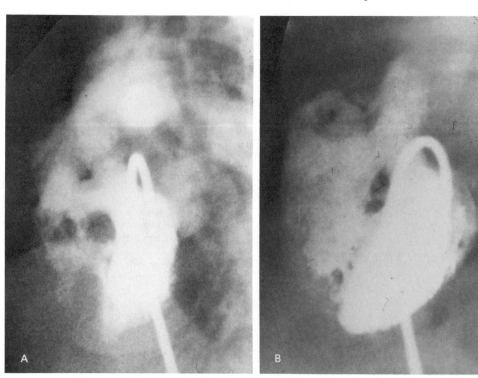

Fig. 9.11   Left ventricular cineangiocardiography in ventricular septal defect (VSD). Tilted oblique view of ventricular septum and left ventricular outflow tract demonstrates clearly multiple VSDs in two different patients. This technique was developed by Dr. L. M. Bargeron of the University of Alabama, who kindly furnished these figures.

physiologic state of the patient is just as important as evaluating the physiologic data obtained. Although usually such data fit with the predictions made clinically, occasionally catheterization studies indicate the magnitude of the left to right shunt and pulmonary resistance values to be at variance with that predicted. There remains controversy as to the best method for evaluating pulmonary vascular resistance. In patients whose systemic vascular resistance is normal, the pulmonary resistance to systemic resistance (Rp/Rs) ratio generally provides the pertinent information. In situations in which the systemic resistance may be variable, the evaluation of pulmonary arteriolar resistance, in terms of the pressure drop across the pulmonary bed divided by the pulmonary blood flow, is a more useful means for estimation of a patient's pulmonary resistance. However, since catheterization represents evaluation of the physiologic status over a very brief interval, the physician must not be lulled into complete dependence upon such technical data for the final answer. Left atrial and left ventricular volume studies provide further indices of pulmonary blood flow. These volumes are invariably increased in patients with left to right shunts greater than 35%, and the increase is proportional to the degree of left to right shunting.[35]

Finally, in those patients in whom pulmonary resistance appears to be elevated to an extent that surgery might be precluded, the inhalation of 100% oxygen and the injection of tolazoline into the pulmonary artery with repeated measurements of flow and pressures are indicated to determine whether or not the pulmonary vascular resistance can be reduced. In patients in whom pulmonary vascular resistance appears to be increased at the time of cardiac catheterization but whose subsequent course and clinical data suggest a sizeable left to right shunt, then a repeat cardiac catheterization is indicated to re-evaluate the patient's status regarding operability. It is essential in these patients to rule out associated defects which could cause pulmonary venous hypertension such as cor triatriatum or mitral stenosis.

DIFFERENTIAL DIAGNOSIS

In isolated VSD, the most common differential diagnostic problems arise in infants with large left to right shunts and in older children who have marked elevation of pulmonary vascular resistance. Cardiac catheterization is particularly helpful in the infant group to prove the presence of a ventricular defect or defects plus the presence or absence of associated defects.

Endocardial cushion defects usually can be suspected from the electrocardiogram and vectorcardiogram; however, a few isolated VSDs may present with left axis deviation and a counterclockwise loop in the frontal plane. If this presents a diagnostic problem, left ventricular angiocardiography in the anterior-posterior view will demonstrate the characteristic gooseneck deformity in the endocardial cushion defect.

Double outlet right ventricle also can present with a large left to right shunt. These patients usually have a counterclockwise loop in the frontal plane. Biplane cineangiocardiography usually will demonstrate the subaortic conus, and in the lateral view the separation of aortic and mitral valves leads one to this diagnosis. Echocardiography can be useful in this situation in showing posterior discontinuity between aortic root and mitral valve.

By auscultation, pure infundibular pulmonary stenosis can sound very similar to a ventricular septal defect, particularly if there has been spontaneous closure or diminution in the size of a VSD with persistence of the pulmonary stenosis. When the stenosis is severe, with greater than systemic systolic pressures in the right ventricle, the marked right ventricular hypertrophy evidenced in the electrocardiogram and prolongation of the murmur past aortic closure provide useful diagnostic clues to the diagnosis of infundibular pulmonary stenosis. It is common for these patients to have a VSD, even though it may be small. Left ventricular cineangiocardiography is useful to demonstrate a VSD, as it is important to close the defect at the time that the stenosis is relieved.

Occasionally, mild or moderate subaortic stenosis may be confused with a small VSD because of the overlap in the areas where the murmur is projected in these two conditions. The murmur in subaortic stenosis, however, usually radiates well to the upper right sternal border as well as toward the apex. In patients in whom the murmur suggests either a small VSD or subaortic stenosis, the presence of significant left ventricular hypertrophy on the electrocardiogram suggests subaortic stenosis.

Truncus arteriosus with increased pulmonary blood flow without cyanosis may be mistaken for VSD; however, accentuation of the arterial pulse pressure makes one suspicious of a large aortic-pulmonary flow. In addition, the chest film usually shows a concavity at the site of the main pulmonary artery in truncus arteriosus as well as rather high takeoffs for the right and left pulmonary artery. Retrograde aortography is essential in ruling out truncus arteriosus, aortico-pulmonary window, and patent ductus arteriosus in situations where these lesions are suspected.

In the presence of a known VSD, associated lesions may present diagnostic problems. Associated aortic insufficiency[20] is indicated by a high-pitched, early diastolic decrescendo murmur in the second or third left interspace. It is unusual to detect the associated murmur of aortic insufficiency before 2 years of age. Once the aortic insufficiency becomes apparent, it may progress in severity, particularly in adolescence. Endocardial fibroelastosis involving the left ventricle can occur in the presence of a VSD, although this is a rare combination. Biplane cineangiocardiographic studies to determine the contraction characteristics of the left ventricle are helpful in evaluating the functional status of the left ventricular muscle. In isolated VSD, the ejection fraction of the left ventricle generally is 0.60 or greater whereas with associated myocardial disease the ejection fraction is usually less than 0.45.

In patients with corrected transposition of the great arteries with ventricular septal defect and in those patients with common ventricle without pulmonic stenosis, the clinical picture may simulate isolated VSD. The electrocardiogram is useful for differentiating these patients, because Q waves in lead V1 or V4R occur commonly in the former two conditions and rarely in isolated VSD. Vectorcardiographic analysis shows an orientation of the initial forces far leftward in corrected transposition, whereas in VSD, these forces are anteriorly positioned more in the midline or to the right. In addition, the echocardiogram has been found helpful in identifying these patients.

Patients with L-transposition of the great arteries and large ventricular septal defect can present with heart failure with minimal cyanosis. These patients are usually differentiated by the marked right ventricular hypertrophy on the electrocardiogram and by echocardiography.

TREATMENT

Optimal therapy rests upon accurate diagnosis of the defect and evaluation of the physiologic parameters. Of importance in the overall management of the patient is attention to details in communication with the parents. They should be informed of the implications of repeated evaluations and the clinical courses which can ensue. In the presence of a small defect, follow-up should emphasize the continuing benign nature of the lesion and provide reassurance to the family that the child should be managed normally. In these patients it is important to emphasize that prophylactic antibiotics should be given to protect from endocarditis at times of probable bacteremia. These instances include any dental procedure which involves moderate dental manipulation, other oropharyngeal surgery, gastrointestinal surgery, and genitourinary manipulation or surgery.

Parents frequently are interested in the risk of congenital heart disease in future children. The recurrence risk in ventricular septal defect is 4.4% if there is only one affected first-degree relative.[48] The risk is approximately doubled with two affected first-degree relatives and is considerably higher in the rare families with multiple affected relatives.[48]

TREATMENT DURING INFANCY

In most infants with heart failure, we perform cardiac catheterization. With the onset of heart failure, a trial of medical therapy is indicated because the majority can be managed adequately without resorting to early surgical intervention.

Initial therapy is with digoxin in a dose of 0.05 mg/kg p.o. or 0.04 mg/kg i.m. or i.v. as the usual digitalizing dose. Maintenance digoxin doses range from 0.010 to 0.020 mg/kg/day p.o. in two divided doses. Furosemide is used in a dose of 1 mg/kg intramuscularly or intravenously in the child with severe symptomatology; it can be repeated daily for several days if needed, but electrolytes and blood urea nitrogen should be checked between doses. In patients who require chronic diuretic management we prefer to use aldactazide, a drug which combines hydrochlorthiazide and aldactone, in a dose of 1 to 2 mg/kg/day of each drug. An alternative regimen which can be helpful in difficult patients is furosemide 2 to 5 mg/kg/day combined with aldactodone. With this combination potassium loss is seldom a problem, and potassium supplementation usually is not needed. Potassium supplementation is difficult to achieve in most infants because of the bad taste.

Systemic afterload reduction with hydralazine or prazosin orally is attractive on a theoretical basis, but controlled clinical trials have not been performed to prove their effectiveness. A selective systemic vasodilator with little or no pulmonary vasodilator activity might prove useful in selected patients with chronic failure who respond poorly to the usual therapy.

The question as to how long one should pursue medical management in the presence of continued symptomatology and poor growth is a difficult one and the answer varies with the patient and with the physician. There is the possibility that the shunt may diminish in size as a result of a decrease in the size of the defect or as a result of a patient's overall growth with the defect remaining unchanged in size. On the other hand, infants with large left to right shunts who develop pulmonary infections have a significant mortality on medical management alone. Our present policy is to begin each infant with medical management including digoxin and diuretics if needed and to resort to early correction when such management appears to be a failure. Factors of importance in this evaluation include growth failure, life threatening or repeated pulmonary infections, elevated pulmonary artery pressure, and inability of a family to cope with long-term medical therapy.

Neither age nor patient size should be prohibitive factors in considering a patient for surgical correction. Pulmonary artery banding[26] does not offer an advantage in terms of morbidity or mortality over primary closure of an isolated defect at any age or patient size. However, one can make a case for banding in the critically ill infant with multiple ventricular defects. The status of closure and overall results in a number of institutions indicate that repair should be accomplished with a mortality rate of approximately 5% or less.[2, 3, 5, 7, 39, 50]

Medical Management in Children after Infancy

The majority of patients with ventricular septal defect remain rather stable following infancy. Emphasis is needed to ensure that the child is handled as normally as possible within the limits of his or her condition. Heart failure rarely supervenes past infancy; should it occur, endocarditis should be suspected as well as associated lesions such as aortic insufficiency. Patients who have large left to right shunts require vigorous treatment for intercurrent pulmonary infections. However, it is not our policy to utilize continuous antibiotic prophylaxis.

Patients who have significant elevation of pulmonary artery pressure at their initial catheterization have a repeat catheterization performed at 6 to 9 months of age in order to clarify the physiologic state. Those who continue to show pulmonary arterial hypertension with a predominant left to right shunt then have correction performed at approximately 9 to 12 months of age.

The small group of patients who have developed severe pulmonary vascular obstructive disease with predominant right to left shunts by the time of referral are subjected to cardiac catheterization for confirmation of the diagnosis and clarification of the physiologic state. This group is considered inoperable with presently available techniques. Here the physician must resort to continuous support of the family with judicious advice concerning regulation of activities and avoidance of stressful pursuits. Red cell volume reduction with reduction in blood viscosity can decrease systemic resistance, increase systemic blood flow, and improve oxygen transport in patients whose polycythemia is excessive.[54] This procedure must be done judiciously with careful replacement of red cell volume with a plasma expander. Such patients usually feel better with a decrease in number and severity of headaches, although the benefit usually lasts only for several weeks to several months. Although it is difficult to predict the length of survival, most survive comfortably, function rather well, and live into their 20s and 30s. Wood[66] found the average age of death of patients with the Eisenmenger complex was 33 years. In his group, 29% died of hemoptysis, 17% of heart failure, 14% died suddenly, presumably from dysrhythmias, 26% died during attempted operative repair, and the remainder died with endocarditis, cerebral abscess, cerebral thrombosis, or pregnancy (<5% in each group).

SURGICAL MANAGEMENT

Small Ventricular Septal Defects

Since the long-term prognosis is excellent in these patients, surgery is not indicated. At present, the risk of surgery is greater than that of the natural course of the disease.

Moderate-Sized Defects with Large Left to Right Shunts

In patients who have evidence of normal or mild elevation of pulmonary artery pressure with large shunts, we recommend cardiac catheterization in the first year of life. If the data confirm the impression, then operation is not recommended at this time. These patients are followed medically. If subsequent information indicates that the pulmonary artery pressure may be increasing, then catheterization is repeated. However, if all data indicate continued normal or only mild elevation of pulmonary artery pressure, then catheterization is not repeated until approximately a year before the child is to enter school. If the patient again shows a large left to right shunt of greater than twice the systemic flow, surgery usually is recommended. Occasionally, infants will present with voluminous left to right shunts with low pulmonary resistance and considerable growth retardation. These infants are usually catheterized in the first 6 months of life. Recatheterization is then performed at approximately 1 year of age, and if the shunt has not diminished and considerable growth retardation continues then surgical correction is performed.

Large Ventricular Septal Defects with Hyperkinetic Pulmonary Hypertension

This group presents a particular challenge in recommending optimal therapy if the left to right shunt is only moderate in magnitude. Our criteria for surgery are similar to those suggested by others.[2, 3, 5, 39, 50] With pulmonary to systemic flow ratios greater than 1.5 and with pulmonary to systemic vascular resistance ratios of 0.5 or less, surgery usually is recommended. It should be emphasized again that criteria vary from institution to institution with the indication for surgery being dictated by local experience. Although physiologic data obtained at cardiac catheterization are quite useful, clinical and laboratory information including electrocardiograms, chest film, echocardiography, and volume determinations are also quite valuable in assessing shunt size and vascular resistance. A large left atrium and left ventricle are helpful confirmatory signs of increased pulmonary blood flow in borderline situations.

In the infant with hyperkinetic pulmonary hypertension and a large left to right shunt, catheterization is performed in infancy. If the infant continues to show growth failure and repeated pulmonary infections, surgery is recommended. Generally, catheterization is performed again prior to operation in order to be certain the defect has not decreased in size and the pulmonary artery pressure has not come down to a near normal range which would indicate that further medical therapy might be indicated.

The larger patient (approximately $\geq$7 kg) generally will have the operation performed using cardiopulmonary bypass, whereas deep hypothermia and circulatory arrest are used for small infants.

Many defects can be repaired using a right atrial approach with the avoidance of a ventriculotomy. Although the ventriculotomy scar is to be avoided when possible, there are no data at present indicating a difference in early or late postoperative morbidity or mortality with closure using a ventriculotomy versus an atriotomy.

Multiple muscular defects can present a difficult operative problem. Left ventricular angiocardiography should provide as precise a localization of these defects as possible. An atrial approach is attempted first, but all defects may not be accessible for closure from the right side. In this situation, an apical left ventriculotomy can be used with a single patch utilized to close these defects in most patients.

Defects Associated with Aortic Insufficiency

This group presents a difficult problem in management in that the aortic insufficiency (AI) frequently becomes the major consideration. The frequency of this complication is approximately 5%.[46] The best opportunity to repair the aortic valved and prevent progressive AI undoubtedly is early in the course of this complication. As soon as significant

AI is present, then repair should be undertaken. The problem of defining significant AI remains. We use the following criteria: widened aortic pulse pressure of greater than 50 mm Hg; filling of the body of the left ventricle (LV) following aortic root contrast injections; failure of clearing of contrast from the LV with one systole following aortic root injection; and increased LV end-diastolic volume in the absence of a left to right shunt of $\leq$35%.

Van Praagh and McNamara[63] presented anatomic data on patients with ventricular septal defect and aortic insufficiency, and noted several important features. Patients with supracristal defects have herniation of the right coronary leaflet through the VSD; this leaflet may cause a mild to moderate right ventricular outflow gradient, and the aortic comissures usually are normal. Patients with infracristal VSDs have herniation of the right and/or the noncoronary cusp, have frequent abnormalities of aortic commissures (usually the right-noncoronary), and frequently have associated infundibular pulmonary stenosis.

Primary defect closure without aortic valve surgery is indicated in patients with left to right shunts $\leq$35%, and mild AI. Closure of the defect may prevent progression of the valvular lesion. In patients with more significant AI, Spencer et al.[60] have demonstrated that valvuloplasty can be performed with a low mortality (1 of 20 patients). Followup evaluation from 6 months to 12 years postoperatively indicated no AI or only mild residual AI in all but one patient who showed moderate AI. Approximately half of the patients had infracristal and half supracristal VSDs,[60] as has been noted by others.[63] Utilizing the technique described by Spencer et al.,[60] our results have been satisfactory in approximately 50% of such patients. In these patients, the ventricular septal defect is easily closed, but the difficult portion of the procedure is the repair of the aortic valve. Utilizing hypothermic protection of the arrested heart, the aorta is opened and the valve is inspected from above. The corpora Arantii are identified, and the free edge of the aortic valve leaflets is carefully measured. The redundant portion of the aortic leaflet is then plicated at the commissure utilizing teflon felt to reinforce these sutures. Suturing of abnormal commissures also may be necessary particularly in the group with infracristal defects.[60] These patients must be followed for an extended period in order to assess the long-term function of these plicated valves. Aortic valve replacement is reserved for patients with severe aortic AI and left ventricular volume overload, who usually are symptomatic.

COURSE AND PROGNOSIS

SMALL VENTRICULAR SEPTAL DEFECTS

Patients with small defects have an excellent prognosis, and there are no data that suggest a decreased life expectancy in these patients in the absence of complications from endocarditis. A large number of these defects close spontaneously, this number approaches 75 to 80% with the majority closing in the first 2 years of life. Many will show an aneurysm of the ventricular septum after spontaneous closure has occurred. An early systolic click can be heard in many of these patients due to systolic expansion followed by rapid deceleration of the aneurysm. There are no data at present to indicate that such aneurysms are associated with morbidity or mortality. These patients usually are followed indefinitely in order to detect spontaneous closure of the defect, to emphasize the importance of prophylactic antibiotics for endocarditis, and to observe for the occasional patient who develops aortic insufficiency. In some of these, catheterization will show that the prolapsed aortic leaflet partially closes the moderate-sized ventricular septal defect and limits the left to right shunt.

MODERATE-SIZED DEFECTS

Patients with moderate-sized defects may develop large left to right shunts in infancy, and their main danger is that of heart failure between 1 and 6 months of age. Usually, this group can be managed medically without surgical intervention during infancy. If catheterization demonstrates that the right ventricular pressure is normal or only mildly elevated, most of these patients will have decreasing shunts over the first year of life. Many will never require operative intervention. These patients as well as those with large defects can develop significant infundibular pulmonary stenosis which can progress in severity and require surgical intervention.

Approximately 15 to 20% of these patients continue to have large left to right shunts following infancy. If the clinical signs indicate that the shunt remains large by 4 to 5 years of age, then repeat catheterization is performed at this time, and operation usually recommended if the pulmonary flow exceeds twice the systemic flow.

LARGE DEFECTS

The patients with large defects are the most difficult to handle because of the dangers of mortality in the first year of life due to heart failure and associated pulmonary infections as well as the problem of development of elevated pulmonary vascular resistance. Those patients who respond poorly to medical therapy and continue to show signs of a large left to right shunt with growth failure and pulmonary infection are operated upon in the first year of life.

The problem of when to operate in order to prevent pulmonary vascular obstructive disease in children with large ventricular septal defects and pulmonary hypertension also remains a difficult one. DuShane and coworkers[20] showed that the development of pulmonary vascular disease did not occur in patients operated under 2 years of age but occurred in 28% of 50 patients whose operation was performed after 2 years of age. In addition, there was a progressively higher frequency of increased postoperative pulmonary resistance in the older patients. These data indicate the pulmonary vascular obstructive changes can occur as early as 2 years of age.

There are at present limited data on long term evaluation following operative correction of patients with moderate or large left to right shunts. Most patients have excellent results following operation with normal growth and development and normal activity. Jarmakani et al.[34] reported pre- and postoperative LV volume data in patients with large VSD repaired at an average age of 5 years. The patients were restudied an average of 1.6 years following operation and were found to have no significant residual shunts. These patients, however, had LV end-diastolic volume of 118% of normal, LV wall mass 134% of normal, and mildly depressed LV ejection fraction (LVEF) of 86% of normal.

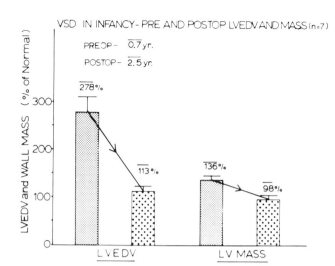

Fig. 9.12 Pre- and postoperative left ventricular end-diastolic volume and wall mass for seven infants who were operated upon at an average age of 12 mo. (Reproduced with permission from T. P. Graham, Jr. et al.[28]).

Maron and coworkers[44] reported abnormal responses to intense upright exercise in 5 of 11 asymptomatic patients studied 3 to 15 years following successful VSD surgery at an average age of 15 years. All five patients with an abnormal exercise response were operated upon after 10 years of age, and the magnitude of the abnormal response was directly related to the age of operation.

We have been interested in the possibility that infants requiring operation for VSD early in life might show a better postoperative LV performance.[14, 28] Figure 9.12 shows pre- and postoperative values for LVEDV and LV mass for seven infants who required VSD closure at an average age of 12 months.[28] Preoperative Qp/Qs averaged 3.1:1, right ventricular pressure (RVP) averaged 96 mm Hg, and RVP/LVP was 1.0 in all patients. Recatheterization at an average of 1.5 years following operation showed that LVEDV had decreased from 278 to 113% of normal and LV mass from 136 to 98% of normal.

These data indicate that "early" closure of large VSDs in the first year of life is associated with a better result in terms of left ventricular function and regression of hypertrophy than operation later in childhood. In evaluating "early" ($\leq$12 months) versus "late" operative results, multiple factors must be considered including mortality, postoperative rhythm or conduction disturbances, pulmonary vascular resistance, ventricular function, and psychological impact. In patients with large defects, there are no data to indicate a difference in mortality in older patients versus infants for surgical groups with a broad experience in infant cardiac surgery. Thus repair in infancy is preferable in those symptomatic patients with large defects in whom a significant diminution in defect size during the first 18 months of life is unlikely.

REFERENCES

1. Abbott, M. E.: Congenital heart disease. Nelson's Loose-Leaf Medicine, Vol. 5. Thomas Nelson & Sons, New York, 1932, p. 207.
2. Agosti, J., and Subramanian, S.: Corrective treatment of isolated ventricular septal defect in infancy. J. Pediatr. Surg. 10:785–793, 1975.
3. Arciniegas, E., Farooki, Z. Q., Hakimi, M., Perry, B. L., and Green, E. W.: Surgical closure of ventricular septal defect during the first twelve months of life. J. Thorac. Cardiovasc. Surg. 80:921–928, 1980.

4. Bargeron, L. M., Jr., Elliott, L. P., Soto, B., Bream, P. R., and Curry, G. C.: Axial cineangiography in congenital heart disease. Section I. Concept, technical and anatomic consideration. Circulation 56:1075–1083, 1977.
5. Barratt-Boyes, B. G., Neutze, J. M., Clarkson, P. M., Shardey, G. C., and Brandt, P. W. T.: Repair of Ventricular Septal Defect in the first two years of life using profound hypothermia—Circulatory arrest techniques. Ann. Surg. 184:376–390, 1976.

6. Becu, L. M. Fontana, R. S., DuShane, J. W., Kirklin, J. W., Burchell, H. B., and Edwards, J. E.: Anatomic and physiologic studies in ventricular septal defect. Circulation 14:349, 1956.
7. Bender, H. W., Jr., Fisher, R. D., Walker, W. E., and Graham, T. P., Jr.: Reparative cardiac surgery in infants and small children: Five years experience with profound hypothermia and circulatory arrest. Ann. Surg. 190:437–443, 1979.

8. Bierman, F. Z., Fellows, K., and Williams, R. G. Prospective identification of ventricular septal defects using subxiphoid two-dimensional echocardiography. Circulation 62:807, 1980.

9. Borst, H. G., Berglund, E., Whittenberger, J. L., Mead, J., McGregor, M., and Collier, C.: The effect of pulmonary vascular pressure on the mechanical properties of the lungs of anesthetized dogs. J. Clin. Invest. 36:1708, 1957.

10. Brotmacher, L., and Campbell, M.: The natural history of ventricular septal defect. Br. Heart J. 20:97, 1958.

11. Burton, A. C.: The relation between pressure and flow in the pulmonary bed. In Pulmonary Circulation, edited by W. R. Adams and I. Veith. Grune & Stratton, New York, 1959.

12. Canale, J. M., Sahn, D. J., Allen, H. D., Goldberg, S. J., Valdez-Cruz, L. M., and Ovitt, T. W.: Factors affecting real-time, cross-sectional echocardiographic imaging of perimembranous ventricular septal defects. Circulation 63:689–697, 1981.

13. Cheatham, J. P., Latson, L. A., and Gutgesell, H. P. Ventricular septal defect in infancy: Detection with two dimensional echocardiography. Am. J. Cardiol. 47:85, 1981.

14. Cordell, D., Graham, T. P., Jr., Atwood, G. F., Boerth, R. C., Boucek, R. J., and Bender, H. W.: Left heart volume characteristics following ventricular septal defect closure in infancy. Circulation 54:294–298, 1976.

15. Dammann, J. F., Jr., and Ferencz, C.: The significance of the pulmonary vascular bed in congenital heart disease. III. Defects between the ventricles or great vessels in which both increased pressure and blood flow may act upon the lungs and in which there is a common ejectile force. Am. Heart J. 52:210, 1956.

16. Dammann, J. F., Jr., Thompson, W. M., Jr., Sosa, O., and Christlieh, I.: Anatomy, physiology and natural history of simple ventricular septal defects. Am. J. Cardiol. 5:136, 1960.

17. Davies, H., Williams, J., and Wood, P.: Lung stiffness in states of abnormal pulmonary blood flow and pressure. Br. Heart J. 24:129, 1962.

18. Dodge, H. T., Sandler, H., Ballew, D. W., and Lord, J. D., Jr.: The use of biplane angiocardiography for the measurement of left ventricular volume in man. Am. Heart J. 60:762, 1960.

19. Donald, K. E.: Disturbances in pulmonary function in mitral stenosis and left heart failure. Prog. Cardiovasc. Dis. 1:298, 1958.

20. DuShane, J. W., Krongrad, E., Ritter, D. G., and McGoon, D. C.: The fate of raised pulmonary vascular resistance after surgery in ventricular septal defect. In The Child with Congenital Heart Disease after Surgery, edited by R. D. Rowe and B. S. L. Kidd. Futura, Mount Kisco, N.Y., 1976.

21. DuShane, J. W., Weidman, W. H., Braundenburg, R. O., and Kirklin, J. W.: The electrocardiogram in children with ventricular septal defect and severe pulmonary hypertension. Circulation 22:49, 1960.

22. Edwards, J. E.: Functional pathology of the pulmonary vascular tree in congenital cardiac disease. The Lewis A. Conner Memorial Lecture. Circulation 15:164, 1957.

23. Edwards, J. E.: Malformations of the ventricular septal complex. In Pathology of the Heart, 3rd ed., edited by S. E. Gould. Charles C Thomas, Springfield, Ill., 1968, pp. 280–294.

24. Elliott, L. P., Bargeron, L. M., Jr., Bream, P. R., Soto, B., and Curry, G. C.: Axial cineangiography in congenital heart disease. Section II. Specific lesions. Circulation 56:1084–1093, 1977.

25. Gelband, H., Waldo, A. L., Kaiser, G. A., Bowman, F. O., Jr., Malm, J. R., and Hoffman, B.: Etiology of right bundle branch block in patients undergoing total correction of tetralogy of Fallot. Circulation 44:1022, 1971.

26. Goldblatt, A., Bernhard, W. F., Nadas, A. S., and Gross, R. E.: Pulmonary artery banding: Indications and results in infants and children. Circulation 32:172, 1965.

27. Graham, T. P., Jr., Atwood, G. F., Boucek, R. J., Jr., Cordell, D., and Boerth, R. C. Right ventricular volume characteristics in ventricular septal defect. Circulation 54:800–804, 1976.

28. Graham, T. P., Jr., Cordell, G. D., and Bender, H. A., Jr.: Ventricular function following surgery. In The Child with Congenital Heart Disease after Surgery, edited by R. D. Rowe and B. S. L. Kidd. Futura, Mount Kisco, N.Y., 1976.

29. Graham, T. P., Jr., Jarmakani, J. M., Canent, R. V., Jr., and Morrow, M. N.: Left heart volume estimations in infancy and childhood: Reevaluation of methodology and normal values. Circulation 43:895, 1971.

30. Halloran, K. H., Talner, N. S., and Browne, M. J.: A study on ventricular septal defect associated with aortic insufficiency. Am. Heart J. 69:320, 1965.

31. Hirschfield, S., Meyer, R., Schwartz, D. C., Korfhagen, J., and Kaplan, S.: The echocardiographic assessment of pulmonary artery pressure and pulmonary vascular resistance. Circulation 52:642, 1975.

32. Hoffman, J. I. E., and Rudolph, A. M.: The natural history of ventricular septal defects in infancy. Am. J. Cardiol. 16:634, 1965.

33. Jarmakani, M. M., Edwards, S. B., Spach, M. S., Canent, R. V., Jr., Capp, M. P., Hagan, M. J., Barr, R. C., and Jain, V.: Left ventricular pressure-volume characteristics in congenital heart disease. Circulation 37:879, 1968.

34. Jarmakani, J. M., Graham, T. P., Jr., Canent, R. V., Jr., and Capp, M. P.: The effect of corrective surgery on left heart volume and mass in children with ventricular septal defect. Am. J. Cardiol. 27:254, 1971.

35. Jarmakani, M. M., Graham, T. P., Jr., Canent, R. V., Jr., Spach, M. S., and Capp, M. P.: Effect of site of shunt on left heart volume characteristics with ventricular septal defect and patent ductus arteriosus. Circulation 40:411, 1969.

36. Keith, J. D., Rowe, R. D., and Vlad, P.: Heart Disease in Infancy and Childhood. The Macmillan Company, New York, 1967, p. 3.

37. Kidd, L., Rose, V., Collins, G., and Keith, J.: Ventricular septal defect in infancy. Am. Heart J. 69:4, 1965.

38. Kirklin, J. K., Castaneda, A. R., Keane, J. F., Fellows, K. E., and Norwood, W. I. Surgical management of multiple ventricular septal defects. J. Thorac. Cardiovasc. Surg. 80:485–493, 1980.

39. Kirklin, J. W.: Current status of corrective surgery for ventricular septal defects. In The Child with Congenital Heart Disease after Surgery, edited by R. D. Rowe and B. S. K. Kidd. Futura, Mount Kisco, N.Y., 1976.

40. Krongrad, E., Hefler, S. E., Bowman, F. O., Jr., Malm, J. R., and Hoffman, B. F.: Further observations on the etiology of the right bundle branch block pattern following right ventriculotomy. Circulation 50:1105, 1974.

41. Levin, A. E., Boineau, J. P., Spach, M. S., Canent, R. V., Jr., Capp, M. P., and Anderson, P. A. W.: Ventricular pressure-flow dynamics in tetralogy of Fallot. Circulation 34:4, 1966.

42. Levin, A. E., Spach, M. S., Canent, R. V., Jr., Boineau, J. P., Capp, M. P., Jain, V., and Barr, R. C.: Ventricular pressure-flow dynamics in ventricular septal defect. Circulation 35:430, 1967.

43. Lincoln, C., Jamieson, S., Shinebourne, E., and Anderson, R. H.: Transatrial repair of ventricular septal defects with reference to their anatomic classification. J. Thorac. Cardiovasc. Surg. 74:183, 1977.

44. Maron, B. J., Redwood, D. R., Hirshfield, J. W., Jr., Goldstein, R. E., Morrow, A. G., and Epstein, S. E.: Postoperative assessment of patients with ventricular septal defect and pulmonary hypertension: Response to intense upright exercise. Circlation 48:864, 1973.

45. Milo, S., Ho, S. Y., Wilkinson, J. L., and Anderson, R. H.: Surgical anatomy and atrioventricular conduction tissues of hearts with isolated ventricular septal defects. J. Thorac. Cardiovasc. Surg. 79:244–255, 1980.

46. Nadas, A. S., Thilenius, O. G., LaFarge, C. G., and Hauck, A. J.: Ventricular septal defect with aortic regurgitation: Medical and pathologic aspects. Circulation 29:862, 1964.

47. Nadas, A. S., and Fyler, D. C.: Pediatric Cardiology, 3rd ed. W. B. Saunders, Philadelphia, 1972, p. 348.

48. Nora, J. J., and Fraser, F. L. C.: Medical Genetics. Lea and Febiger, Philadelphia, 1974, pp. 334–338.

49. Okoroma, E. O., Guller, B., Maloney, J. D., and Weidman, W. H.: Etiology of right bundle branch block pattern after surgical closure of ventricular septal defects. Am. Heart J. 90:14, 1975.

50. Rein, J. G., Freed, M. D., Norwood, W. I., and Castaneda, A. R.: Early and late results of closure of ventricular septal defect in infancy. Ann. Thoracic. Surg. 24:19–26, 1976.

51. Ritter, D. G., Feldt, R. H., Weidman, W. H., and DuShane, J. W.: Ventricular septal defect. Circulation 32 (Suppl. 3):42, 1965.

52. Rizzoli, G., Blackstone, E. H., Kirklin, J. W., Pacifico, A. D., and Bargeron, L. M.: Incremental risk factors in hospital mortality rate after repair of ventricular septal defect. J. Thorac. Cardiovasc. Surg. 80:494–505, 1980.

53. Roger, H.: Recherches cliniques sur la communication congenitale des deux coeurs, par inocclusion du septum interventriculaire. Bull. Acad. Med. Paris 8:1074, 1879.

54. Rosenthal, A., Nathan, D. G., Margy, A., and Nadas, A. S.: Acute hemodynamic effect of red cell volume reduction in polycythemia of cyanotic congenital heart disease. Circulation 42:297, 1970.

55. Rudolph, A. M.: The effects of postnatal circulatory adjustments in congenital heart disease. E. Mead Johnson Award Address, October, 1964. Pediatrics 36:763, 1965.

56. Savard, M., Swan, H. J. C., Kirklin, J. W., and Wood, E. H.: Hemodynamic alterations associated with ventricular septal defect. In Symposium on Congenital Heart Disease, edited by A. D. Bass and G. K. Moe. American Association for the Advancement of Science, Washington, D.C., 1960, p. 141.

57. Shah, P. M., Slodki, S. J., and Luisada, A. A.: A review of the classic areas of auscultation of the heart: A physiologic approach. Am. J. Med. 36:293, 1964.

58. Spach, M. S., Boineau, J. P., Long, E. C., Gabor, J. P., and Gallie, T. M.: Genesis of the vectorcardiogram (electrocardiogram) in endocardial cushion defects. In Vectorcardiography 1965, edited by I. Hoffman and R. C. Taymor. North-Holland, Amsterdam, 1966.

59. Spach, M. S., Canent, R. V., Jr., Boineau, J. P., White, A. W., Jr., Sanders, A. P., and Baylin, G. J.: Radioisotope-dilution curves as an adjunct to cardiac catheterization. Am. J. Cardiol. 16:165, 1965.

60. Spencer, F. C., Doyle, E. F., Danilowicz, D. A., Bahnson, H. T., and Weldon, C.S.: Long-term evaluation of aortic valvuloplasty for aortic insufficiency and venticular septal defect. J. Thorac. Cardiovasc. Surg. 65:15, 1973.

61. Tatsuno, K., Ando, M., Takao, A., Hatsune, K., and Konno, S.: Diagnostic importance of aortography in conal ventricular-septal defect. Am. Heart J. 89:171–177, 1975.

62. Titus, J. L., Daugherty, G. W., and Edwards, J. E.: Anatomy of the atrioventricular conduction system in ventricular septal defect. Circulation 28:72, 1963.

63. Van Praagh, R., and McNamara, J. J.: Anatomic types of ventricular septal with aortic

insufficiency. Am. Heart J. 75:604, 1968.
64. Weidman, W. H., DuShane, J. W., and Kirklin, J. W.: Observations concerning progressive pulmonary vascular obstruction in children with ventricular septal defects. Am. Heart J.

65:148, 1963.
65. Wennik, A. C. G., Oppenheimer-Dekker, A., and Moulaert, A. J.: Muscular ventricular septal defects: A reappraisal of the anatomy. Am. J. Cardiol. 43:259–264, 1979.

66. Wood, O.: The Eisenmenger syndrome or pulmonary hypertension with reversed central shunt. Br. Med. J. 2:701, 755, 1958.

10

Left Ventricular-Right Atrial Communication

Thomas A. Riemenschneider, M.D.

An unusual group of defects of the ventricular septum permits communication between left ventricle and right atrium.[29] Although these defects are being encountered with increasing frequency, the diagnosis is often not suspected on the basis of clinical findings. Frequently the diagnosis is made at the time of catheterization or occasionally not until the defect has been visualized at the time of operation.

Thurnman[35] in 1838 reported the first case of a left ventricular-right atrial shunt in which a ventricular septal defect was associated with a cleft in the septal leaflet of the tricuspid valve. Merkel[24] and Preicz[28] reported different malformations of the tricuspid valve associated with a ventricular septal defect. In 1949, Perry et al.[27] proposed a classification for left ventricle-right atrial communications based on the type of defect of the tricuspid valve. The first successful surgical repair of this defect was reported by Kirby et al.[14] in 1954. Braunwald and Morrow[4] reported the first angiographic demonstration of a left ventricular-right atrial communication by injection of contrast material into the left ventricle. The prevalence of this group of defects has been estimated as slightly less than 1% of all congenital cardiac defects[18] with a slight predominance of females over males.[29]

PATHOLOGY

Left ventricular-right atrial communications may be divided into two main groups, depending upon whether the defect is located above or below the tricuspid valve. Rarely, lesions may be encountered in which both supravalvular and infravalvular areas are involved (Table 10.1, group III).[3, 33] Defects below the valve are always associated with a malformation of the septal leaflet.

The membranous ventricular septum is divided by the insertion of the septal leaflet of the tricuspid valve into atrioventricular and interventricular portions.[12] The position of the tricuspid valve, below the mitral valve in the sagittal plane, places the atrioventricular portion of the septum in a location common to both the left ventricle and the right atrium (Fig. 10.1).[8] Supravalvular defects (type I) are located in the atrioventricular membranous septum above the septal tricuspid leaflet and anterior to the coronary sinus (Fig. 10.2). Occasionally the inferior margin of the defect extends into the attachment of the tricuspid leaflet.[33] These defects are caused by failure of fusion of the dextrodorsal conus ridge with the right tubercle of the ventral endocardial cushion.

Infravalvular defects are located below the insertion of the tricuspid valve (type II) and may be classified as anterior, central, or communis (canal) according to position: anterior,

in the membranous septum immediately below the anterior half of the septal leaflet; central, in both the membranous septum and the adjoining muscular septum beneath the septal leaflet; and communis, in the position of an isolated ventricular septal defect of the endocardial cushion type.

TABLE 10.1   CLASSIFICATION AND PREVALENCE OF LEFT VENTRICULAR-RIGHT ATRIAL COMMUNICATIONS

I. Supravalvular		32%
II. Infravalvular-tricuspid		62%
A. Septal defect		
1. Anterior		70%
2. Central		16%
3. Communis		14%
B. Tricuspid defect		
1. Perforation		42%
2. Malformation		28%
3. Cleft		12%
4. Widened commissure		18%
III. Combined		6%

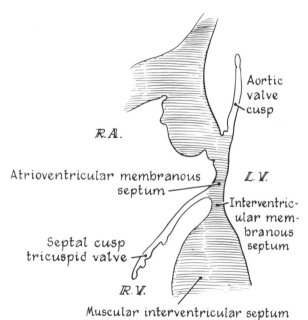

Fig. 10.1 Atrioventricular septum. Note location which is superior to septal tricuspid insertion and common to both the left ventricle and right atrium. *R.A.*, right atrium; *R.V.*, right ventricle; *L.V.*, left ventricle.

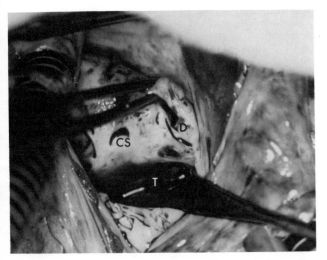

Fig. 10.2 Supravalvular defect on the atrioventricular septum photographed during cardiopulmonary bypass. The right atrium has been opened and a retractor is positioned in the tricuspid valve opening.[7] An elongated defect (10 × 2 mm) (*D*) can be visualized above the septal leaflet (*T*) and anterior to the coronary sinus (*CS*). The surgeon is grasping the thickened edge of the defect with his forceps. *T*, tricuspid valve opening.

Failure of fusion of the tubercles with the conus ridges and the crest of the muscular interventricular septum results in a membranous septal defect, while failure of the right tubercles of the endocardial cushions to meet and fuse causes a malformation of the septal leaflet of the tricuspid valve[15, 26] Abnormalities of the septal leaflet of the tricuspid valve are of four types: perforation; malformation; cleft, or widened commissure either anterior or posterior to the septal leaflet.[29] The valvular defect may freely override the septal defect or may be partially or totally fused to it.

Defects of the communis type tend to be large and in most cases are associated with a cleft septal leaflet or a widened commissural space. They differ from the usual endocardial cushion defect in that the mitral valve and interatrial septum are intact, there is no deformity of the outflow tract of the left ventricle, and the communication is mainly from the left ventricle to the right atrium. Acquired left ventricular-right atrial communications have also been reported to occur as a consequence of: endocarditis[1, 5]; chest trauma[7, 13]; and mitral valve replacement.[21, 31]

Associated malformations have been documented in one-third of reported cases. The commonest associated lesion is atrial septal defect. Less frequently left ventricular-right atrial communications have been associated with: subaortic stenosis; persistent left superior vena cava; transposition of the great arteries; bicuspid aortic valve; ventricular septal defect; pulmonic stenosis; patent ductus arteriosus; cleft mitral valve; tetralogy of Fallot; coarctation of the aorta; and aneurysm of the membranous septum.[29]

The marked difference in pressure during systole between the left ventricle and right atrium, which is present at birth, results in a large volume overload of the right ventricle, enlargement of the main pulmonary artery, and increased blood flow through the lungs. Increased pulmonary venous return leads to a volume overload of the left chambers of the heart, causing increased left ventricular work. Frequently the heart is unable to maintain an adequate output and failure supervenes. Because a portion of the left ventricular volume is shunted to the right atrium, the aortic knob is not enlarged and often appears hypoplastic relative to the prominent main pulmonary artery.

MANIFESTATIONS

Clinical Features

A heart murmur is common in the newborn period and is often present on the first day of life. Poor weight gain, frequent respiratory infections, dyspnea, and fatiguability are encumbered especially in the first year of life. Approximately one of four patients develops heart failure, most frequently during the first month of life.

Physical examination reveals a loud harsh holosystolic murmur and a thrill located at the lower left sternal border. Especially in the supravalvular type of left ventricular-right atrial communication there may be radiation of the murmur to the right upper sternal border. A middiastolic murmur is heard less frequently, usually at the apex and occasionally along the left sternal border. The pulmonary component of the second sound is widely split with inspiration but narrows with expiration.[19]

Electrovectorcardiographic Features

Tall peaked P waves, together with a prolonged PR interval in leads II, V3R, or V_1, reflect the severity of right atrial enlargement (Fig. 10.3). Right ventricular conduction delay

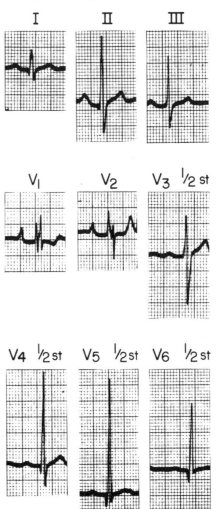

Fig. 10.3 Electrocardiogram in an 18-year-old with left ventricular-right atrial communication. Note prolonged PR interval in lead II and peaked P waves in V_1. Right ventricular conduction delay and evidence of left ventricular hypertrophy are also present.

is often noted in V3R and V_1. Left ventricular hypertrophy is commonly present and in those cases with larger shunts may be associated with right ventricular hypertrophy. Evidence of pure right ventricular hypertrophy is seen infrequently. Shakibi et al.[32] have reported that vectorcardiographic analysis of the frontal QRS loop will reveal a leftward and more superiorly oriented axis, situated midway between the normal QRS and that position usually occupied by an endocardial cushion defect. Left axis deviation with combined ventricular hypertrophy is noted in the communis type defect. Vectorcardiography of the communis type defect reveals a superiorly oriented counterclockwise frontal loop and biventricular enlargement.

Radiologic Features

Cardiomegaly, right atrial enlargement out of proportion to the remainder of the cardiac silhouette, and increased pulmonary vascularity are striking findings.[16] The combination of a prominent right atrium with combined ventricular enlargement, prominent pulmonary artery, and relatively hypoplastic aortic arch combine to produce a ball-like, or globular, configuration in the frontal plane which is strongly suggestive of a left ventricular-right atrial defect.[9, 10]

Echocardiographic Features

Nanda and associates[25] have reported echocardiographic findings of "high frequency, low amplitude oscillations of the systolic segment" of the tricuspid valve in patients with infravalvular defects (Fig. 10.4). In one patient this finding disappeared following repair of the defect. Systolic flutter could not be demonstrated in patients with atrial or ventric-

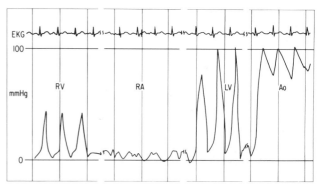

Fig. 10.5 Pressure tracing obtained during cardiac catheterization of a 15-year-old with supravalvular type of left ventricular-right atrial communication (see Fig. 10.2). The catheter could be repeatedly passed across the aortic valve, into the left ventricle, through the defect into the right atrium and across the tricuspid valve into the right ventricle. The continuous pullback tracing demonstrates typical pressures for each of these chambers. *RA*, right atrium; *RV*, right ventricle; *LV*, left ventricle; *Ao*, ascending aorta.

ular defects or a fistula from aorta to right atrium. They speculate that the flutter is due to passage of a jet of blood from left ventricle to right atrium through the defect in the tricuspid valve. Systolic flutter was not present in one patient with a supravalvular defect described by Nanda's group. They suggest that the presence of systolic flutter will help differentiate the infravalvular type of left ventricular-right atrial communication. Based on this report we have correctly predicted a supravalvular type of left ventricular-right atrial communication (Fig. 10.2) in a 15-year-old in whom echocardiography demonstrated no evidence of systolic tricuspid flutter.

CARDIAC CATHETERIZATION

An increase in oxygen saturation at the level of the right atrium is the hallmark of this defect and in about one-third of the cases is associated with a smaller increase in the right ventricle. The strong systolic jet of blood across the defect may at times be responsible for an increase in oxygen saturation in the lower portion of the superior vena cava at its junction with the right atrium. The presence of an intact interatrial septum is suggested by inability to pass the catheter into the left atrium and by inequality of left and right atrial pressures when the catheter enters the left atrium through the foramen ovale. Available data indicate that the pulmonary to systemic flow ratio averages 2.6:1 but may be as high as 5.3:1.

Right atrial pressure is usually normal. Although severe pulmonary hypertension is uncommon, 50% of patients demonstrate moderate elevation of pulmonary artery pressure. Retrograde arterial catheterization may result in passage of the catheter across the defect from left ventricle into right atrium (Fig. 10.5).

ANGIOCARDIOGRAPHY

The most important diagnostic aid is angiocardiography. Selective injection of dye into the left ventricle reveals the passage of contrast medium across the ventricular septum with immediate opacification of the dilated right atrium, a finding which is diagnostic of left ventricular-right atrial shunt (Fig. 10.6). If the defect is infravalvular, contrast material may fill the right atrium and right ventricle simultaneously. The outflow tract of the left ventricle is noted to

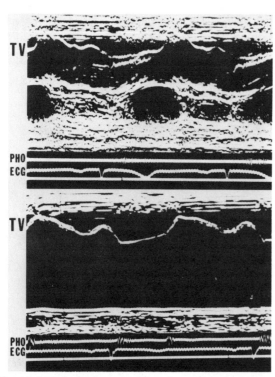

Fig. 10.4 Echocardiogram of the tricuspid valve in congenital left ventricular-right atrial communication. In the *upper panel* the tricuspid valve echocardiogram shows a low amplitude, high frequency systolic flutter and an undulating movement in diastole. The postoperative echocardiogram, in the *lower panel*, shows absence of systolic flutter. *TV*, tricuspid valve; *PHO*, phonocardiogram; *ECG*, electrocardiogram. (Courtesy of Dr. Navin C. Nanda.[25])

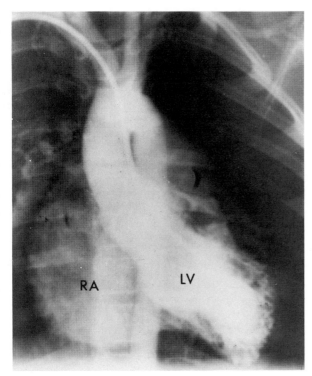

Fig. 10.6 Left ventricular angiocardiogram in a 4-year-old with left ventricular-right atrial communication. Note opacification of the dilated right atrium (*RA*) with the major portion of contrast still in the left ventricle (*LV*).

be normal in appearance, thus excluding an endocardial cushion defect. Since the mitral valve is almost always intact, the left atrium is not visualized.

DIFFERENTIAL DIAGNOSIS

On the basis of physical findings, the major lesion to be differentiated is ventricular septal defect. Although the murmur and thrill may be similar in characteristics and location, the diagnosis of left ventricular-right atrial communication is suggested by close splitting of the second sound, radiation of the murmur to the right upper sternal border, a middiastolic murmur at the left lower sternal border, and evidence on x-ray and electrocardiogram of right atrial and right ventricular enlargement.

Variable splitting of the pulmonic sound with expiratory narrowing usually excludes a secundum atrial septal defect or combined atrial and ventricular septal defect. The rare occurrence of mitral insufficiency (2% of recorded cases) is helpful in differentiation from the endocardial cushion defects. Inability to pass the catheter across the atrial septum is unusual in atrial septal defect and endocardial cushion defect. The angiocardiogram, which demonstrates immediate opacification of the right atrium from the left ventricle with no evidence of mitral insufficiency or outflow tract obstruction, excludes other malformations.

COURSE AND TREATMENT

Symptoms are more severe and the prevalence of heart failure is greatest in the first months of life. Thereafter, gradual improvement occurs in most patients. The course may be complicated by endocarditis (6% of recorded cases)[2, 6, 23, 27, 36], or atrial dysrhythmias (5% of recorded cases).[17, 20] There have been no reports of spontaneous closure of left ventricular-right atrial communications, although a marked decrease in size of the defect has been noted in two cases at the time of repeat cardiac catheterization.[22] Furthermore, the presence of an aneurysm of the membranous septum has been documented in association with a left ventricular-right atrial communication, raising the possibility that aneurysmal formation may represent a stage in spontaneous closure of this defect.[30] Nevertheless, the high frequency of endocarditis and the usually large shunt through the defect suggest that in most cases surgical intervention is indicated.

Cardiopulmonary bypass is necessary for adequate exploration and repair of the defect. At operation, an enlarged right atrium is noted. When the defect is supravalvular, a palpable thrill is present at the lower right atrium, while infravalvular defects are associated with a palpable thrill at the atrioventricular groove.[34] The atrium should be opened widely to visualize the defect and to examine the entire interatrial septum for associated defects. The supravalvular type of defect is easily closed by direct suture. Infravalvular defects may be associated with varying degrees of fibrosis and fusion of the septal leaflet of the tricuspid valve over the ventricular septal defect.[11] The tricuspid leaflet must be resected to visualize the septal defect in its entirety. Following mobilization of the septal leaflet, fibrous tissue should be resected, the defect closed with a patch, and the septal leaflet reconstructed. Occasionally a prosthetic tricuspid valve will be required.[34] The surgeon must be aware of the intimate association of these defects with the conduction system of the heart, as well as the close relationship of the superior margin of the defect to the right and posterior cusps of the aortic valve.

Postoperative complications occurred in 17% of the cases reported. The most common complications after surgery were heart failure (6%), complete heart block (4%), and cardiac dysrhythmias (3%).

REFERENCES

1. Aberg, T., Johansson, L., Michelsson, M., and Rhedin, B.: Left ventricular-right atrial shunt of septic origin. J. Thorac. Cardiovasc. Surg. 61:212, 1971.
2. Barclay, R. S., Reid, J. M., Coleman, E. N., Stevenson, J. G., Welsh, T. M., and McSwann, N.: Communication between the left ventricle and right atrium. Thorax 22:473, 1967.
3. Bouchard, F., Wolff, R., and Kalmanson, D.: Communication between the left ventricle and the right atrium: Diagnosis catheterization and intracardiac phonocatheterization. Arch. Mal. Coeur. 54:1319, 1961.
4. Braunwald, E., and Morrow, A. G.: Left ventricular-right atrial communication: Diagnosis

by clinical, hemodynamic and angiographic methods. Am. J. Med. 28:913, 1960.
5. Cantor, S., Sanderson, R., and Cohn, K.: Left ventricular-right atrial shunt due to bacterial endocarditis. Chest 60:552, 1971.
6. Deverall, P. B., Taylor, J. F. N., Aberdeen, E., and Waterston, D. J.: Left ventricular-right atrial communication. Ann. Thorac. Surg. 8:498, 1969.
7. Dunseth, W. and Ferguson, T. B.: Acquired cardiac septal defect due to thoracic trauma. J. Trauma 5:142, 1965.
8. Edwards, J. E.: The pathology of ventricular septal defect. Semin. Roentgenol. 1:2, 1966.
9. Elliott, L. P.: Other forms of left to right shunt.

Semin. Roentgenol. 1:120, 1966.
10. Elliott, L. P., Gedgaudas, R., Levy, M. J., and Edwards, J. E.: The roentgenologic findings in left ventricular-right atrial communication. Am. J. Roentgenol. 93:304, 1965.
11. Gerbode, F., Hultgren, H., Melrose, D., and Osborn, J.: Syndrome of left ventricular-right atrial shunt: Successful surgical repair of defect in five cases with observation of bradycardia on closure. Ann. Surg. 148:433, 1958.
12. Gould, S. E.: Pathology of the Heart, 2nd ed. Charles C Thomas, Springfield, Ill., 1960, p. 45.
13. Kanber, G. J., Fort, M. L., Trege, A., Meadows, W. R., and Sharp, J. T.: Left ventricular-right

atrial communication with aortic insufficiency of probable traumatic origin. Am. J. Cardiol. 20:879, 1967.

14. Kirby, C. K., Johnson, J. J., and Zinsser, H. F.: Successful closure of a left ventricular-right atrial shunt. Ann. Surg. 145:392, 1957.

15. Kramer, T. C.: The partitioning of the truncus and conus and the formation of the membranous portion of the interventricular septum in the human heart. Am. J. Anat. 71:343, 1942.

16. Kramer, R. A., and Abrams, H. L.: Radiologic aspects of operable heart disease. VII. Left ventricular-right atrial shunts. Radiology 78:171, 1962.

17. Latham, J.: Communication between the left ventricle and the right auricle. Apropos of a case operated successfully. Cardiologia (Basel) 42:287, 1963.

18. Laurichesse, J., Ferrane, J., Renais, J., Scebat, L., and Legegre, J.: Communication between the left ventricle and the right auricle. Arch. Mal. Coeur. 57:703, 1964.

19. Letham, A., and Segal, B.: Auscultatory and phonocardiographic signs of ventricular septal defect with left to right shunt. Circulation 25:318, 1962.

20. Levy, M., and Lillehei, C. W.: Left ventricular-right atrial canal: Ten cases treated surgically. Am. J. Cardiol. 10:623, 1962.

21. Marten, J. L., and Hildner, F. J.: Left ventricular-right atrial communication following

valve replacement. J. Thorac. Cardiovasc. Surg. 58:558, 1969.

22. McCue, C.: Personal communication, 1980.

23. Mellins, R. B., Cheng, G., Ellis, K., Jameson, A. G., Malm, J. R., and Blumenthal, S.: Ventricular septal defect with shunt from left ventricle to right atrium: Bacterial endocarditis as a complication. Br. Heart J. 26:584, 1964.

24. Merkel, G: Zur casuistik der fotalen herzenkrankungen. Virchows Arch. Pathol. Anat. Physiol. 48:488, 1869.

25. Nanda, N. C., Gramiak, R., and Manning, J. A.: Echocardiography of the tricuspid valve in congenital left ventricular-right atrial communication. Circulation 51:268, 1975.

26. Patten, B. M.: Human Embryology, 2nd ed. McGraw-Hill, New York, 1953, p. 656.

27. Perry, E. L., Burchell, H. B., and Edwards, J. E.: Cardiac clinics: Congenital communication between the left ventricle and the right atrium: Coexisting ventricular septal defect and double tricuspid orifice. Mayo Clin. Proc. 24:198, 1949.

28. Preicz, H.: Beitrage zur lehre von den angeborenen herzanomalien. Beitr. Pathol. Anat. 7:234, 1890.

29. Riemenschneider, T. A., and Moss, A. J.: Left ventricular-right atrial communication. Am. J. Cardiol. 19:710, 1967.

30. Russell, E., Spindola-Franco, H., and Eisenberg, R.: Left ventricular-right atrial commu-

nication with aneurysm of the membranous interventricular septum. Br. J. Radiol. 54:463, 1978.

31. Seabra-Gomes, R., Ross, D. N., and Gonzalez-Lavin, L.: Iatrogenic left ventricular-right atrial fistula following mitral valve replacement. Thorax 28:235, 1973.

32. Shakibi, J. G., Aryanpur, I., Paydar, M., Yazdanyar, A., and Siassi, B.: The vectorcardiogram as an aid to diagnosis in left ventricular-right atrial communication. J. Electrocardiol. 10:337, 1977.

33. Taguchi, K., Ogawa, A., and Seo, Y.: Clinical problems associated with the anatomy and surgery of atrioventricular septal defects with left ventricular-right atrial shunt. Basic anatomical study on a new A-V canal classification. Jpn. J. Thorac. Surg. 16:536, 1963.

34. Taguchi, K., Matsuura, Y., Yoshizaki, E., and Tamura, M.: Surgery of atrioventricular septal defects with left ventricular-right atrial shunt: Report of 23 cases. J. Thorac. Cardiovasc. Surg. 56:265, 1968.

35. Thurnman, J.: On aneurysms of the heart. Med. Chir. Trans. R. Med. Chir. Soc. Lond. 21:187, 1838.

36. Yacoub, M. H., Mansur, A., Towers, M., and Westbury, H.: Bacterial endocarditis complicating left ventricle to right atrium communication. Br. J. Dis. Chest 66:8082, 1972.

11

Patent Ductus Arteriosus

Michael A. Heymann, M.D.

ANATOMY

The ductus arteriosus, a large channel found normally in all mammalian fetuses, develops from the distal portion of the left sixth aortic arch and connects the main pulmonary trunk with the descending aorta about 5 to 10 mm distal to the origin of the left subclavian artery in a full-term infant. If there is a right aortic arch the ductus arteriosus may be on the right, joining the right pulmonary artery and the right aortic arch just distal to the right subclavian artery, but more commonly it is on the left joining the left pulmonary artery and the proximal portion of the left subclavian artery.[42] Rarely the ductus arteriosus may be bilateral. It varies in length but in the fetus close to term it has a diameter of approximately 10 mm which is similar to that of the descending aorta.[32, 61]

The microscopic structure of the ductus arteriosus is quite different from that of the adjacent pulmonary trunk or aorta. Although the wall thicknesses of the ductus arteriosus and the adjacent great arteries are similar, the media of the latter are composed mainly of circumferentially arranged layers of elastic fibers, whereas the media of the ductus arteriosus consists largely of dense layers of smooth muscle arranged spirally in both leftward and rightward directions. The intimal layer of the ductus arteriosus is thicker than that of the adjoining arteries and contains an increased amount of mucoid substance. There are also small thin-walled vessels in its subendothelial region.[20, 29]

PHYSIOLOGY

ROLE IN THE FETUS

By about the sixth week of gestation, the ductus arteriosus is sufficiently developed to carry the major proportion of the right ventricular output. The relative sizes of the great arteries and the ductus arteriosus reflect the proportions of cardiac output (combined ventricular output) carried by them.[32, 61] Based on studies performed on fetal lambs, the right ventricle ejects about two-thirds of the combined ventricular output and since flow to the lungs accounts for only about 6 to 8%, the ductus arteriosus carries between 55 and 60% of the combined ventricular output.[33] The ductus arteriosus therefore permits flow to be diverted away from the high resistance pulmonary circulation to the descending aorta and particularly to the low resistance placental circulation. A large pulmonary blood flow during fetal life would represent wasted circulation and the ductus arteriosus therefore reduces the total work load of the fetal ventricles.[33]

Whether or not the ductus arteriosus plays an active physiologic role during fetal life is unknown. It had been considered a relatively passive structure until recent evidence suggested that active relaxation may be produced and maintained by prostaglandins E_2 and I_2 (see below).[10, 11, 13, 34]

NORMAL POSTNATAL CLOSURE

Postnatal closure of the ductus arteriosus is effected in two stages. Initially contraction of the medial smooth muscle in the wall of the ductus arteriosus produces shortening, increased wall thickness, and protrusion into the lumen of the thickened intima (intimal cushions), resulting in functional closure.[29] This generally occurs within 10 to 15 hours after birth in full-term human infants,[52, 59] but the timing varies in different species.[2, 18] The second stage of closure is usually completed by about 2 to 3 weeks in human infants and is produced by infolding of the endothelium, disruption and proliferation of the subintimal layers, and small hemorrhages and necrosis in the subintimal region. As a result, there is connective tissue formation with fibrosis and permanent sealing of the lumen to produce the ligamentum arteriosum.[20]

The exact mechanisms responsible for the initial postnatal closure of the ductus arteriosus are not yet fully understood. During fetal life, the PO_2 to which the ductus arteriosus is normally exposed is between 18 and 28 torr.[33] An increase in PO_2, as occurs with the initiation of ventilation after birth, has been shown to produce constriction of the ductus arteriosus in mature fetal animals.[10, 11, 19, 21, 33, 41, 48, 54] Of great importance is the relationship of this response to increasing PO_2 and gestational age. In fetal lambs of about 0.6 gestation (term, 150 days), the ductus arteriosus is not constricted by increased oxygen even at extremely high concentrations. As shown diagrammatically in Figure 11.1, with advancing gestation the amount of constriction in response to increasing PO_2 is greater and the level of PO_2 required to initiate a response falls.[48]

Other factors, such as the release of vasoactive substances (e.g., acetylcholine, bradykinin, or endogenous catecholamines), may contribute to postnatal closure of the ductus arteriosus under physiological conditions.[33, 48, 54] Of greater importance is the role of prostaglandins in the physiology of the ductus arteriosus. Exogenous prostaglandins E₁ (PGE_1), E₂ (PGE_2), and prostacyclin (PGI_2) dilate isolated ductus arteriosus strips or rings obtained from close-to-term fetal lambs.[10-13] Inhibitors of prostaglandin synthesis either in vitro or when administered in vivo to pregnant animals near term produce constriction of the ductus arteriosus,[10, 11, 34] suggesting that prostaglandins play an active role in maintaining the ductus arteriosus in a dilated state during normal fetal life. The exact sites of production of these prostaglandins in vivo are unclear. PGE_2 and PGI_2 are formed intramurally in the ductus arteriosus and exert their action locally on muscle cells.[10, 11, 13] Endogenous PGI_2 production is about

10-fold that of PGE_2; however, PGE_2 is three orders of magnitude more potent than PGI_2 as a relaxer of the ductus arteriosus.[10, 11] Prostaglandins are detectable only in very low concentrations in adult plasma and most are not thought to act as circulating hormones because of their rapid catabolism in the lungs.[11] The fetus, however, has high circulating concentrations of prostaglandins, particularly PGE_2, probably due to low fetal pulmonary blood flow and therefore decreased prostaglandin catabolism in the lungs, as well as to the fact that the placenta produces prostaglandins.[10, 11, 13]

At birth, the placental source is removed, and the marked increase in pulmonary blood flow allows effective removal of circulating PGE_2. Thus, patency or closure of the ductus arteriosus represents a balance between the constricting effects of oxygen, and perhaps certain vasoconstrictive substances, and the relaxing effects of several prostaglandins.

As with the effects of oxygen, the effects of prostaglandins as well as of inhibitors of their synthesis vary at different gestational ages.[10, 11] Indomethacin constricts rings of ductus arteriosus from immature fetal lambs more than it does rings from close-to-term lambs. Both PGE_2 and PGI_2 relax the ductus arteriosus from immature lambs more than that from mature animals, reflecting a significantly greater sensitivity to PGE_2 and PGI_2 of the immature ductus arteriosus.

PERSISTENT PATENCY

PHYSIOLOGIC CONSIDERATIONS OF A LEFT TO RIGHT SHUNT

General

As with all left to right shunts there are three major interrelated factors that control the magnitude of shunting if there is a patent ductus arteriosus (PDA). These are: the diameter of the ductus arteriosus, which governs the resistance offered to flow; the pressure difference between the aorta and the pulmonary artery; and the systemic and pulmonary vascular resistances.

Normally, after birth, the systemic vascular resistance is high, whereas the pulmonary vascular resistance falls when ventilation begins. As a result systemic arterial blood pressure becomes higher than that in the pulmonary artery. With a small PDA a high resistance to flow is offered across the ductus arteriosus, so that the left to right shunt will be small despite the large pressure difference. However, with a large communication, pressures will tend to become equal, and the magnitude of shunting will then be determined by the relationship of the systemic and pulmonary vascular resistances. For this reason left to right shunting through a PDA has been defined as dependent shunting.[57, 58] Since systemic vascular resistance is generally high and does not change significantly after birth, changes in pulmonary vascular resistance will be the major determinant in regulating the left to right shunting through a PDA. This is particularly important in the first 2 months after birth when the pulmonary vascular resistance is normally decreasing.

The physiologic features associated with left to right shunting through a PDA will depend on the magnitude of the left to right shunt and the ability of the infant to handle the extra volume load.[62, 64] Left ventricular output, which normally is high in the immediate newborn period,[46] is even further increased by the volume shunted left to right through the PDA. The resultant increase of pulmonary venous return to the left atrium and left ventricle will increase ventricular diastolic volume and thereby increase left ventricular stroke volume by evoking the Frank-Starling mechanism. Left ventricular dilatation will result in an increased left ventricular

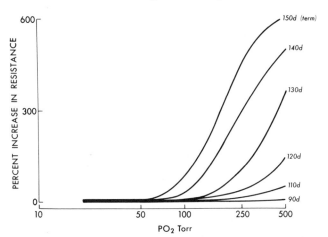

Fig. 11.1 Diagrammatic representation of the relationship between increasing PO_2 and the resistance across the isolated perfused ductus arteriosus of fetal lambs of different gestational ages.[48] With advancing gestation the level of PO_2 required to initiate constriction falls and the amount of constriction increases.

end-diastolic pressure with secondary increase in left atrial pressure. This may lead to overt left heart failure with left atrial dilatation and pulmonary edema. Right ventricular failure may occur if there is a large PDA with pulmonary hypertension or pulmonary edema and an elevated left atrial pressure, in which case pulmonary vascular resistance may be increased. The net result of both these situations is an increased pressure load for the right ventricle. Left to right shunting through a stretched, incompetent foramen ovale secondary to left atrial dilatation is a fairly common association.[62]

Several compensatory physiologic mechanisms are involved in an attempt to improve myocardial performance and thereby maintain a normal systemic output. In addition to the Frank-Starling mechanism the sympathetic adrenal system is stimulated as is the development of myocardial hypertrophy. Increased sympathetic stimulation leads to direct stimulation of nerve fibers within the myocardium, with local norepinephrine release as well as an increase in circulating catecholamines released from the adrenal glands. As a result, both the force of contraction and heart rate are increased. These mechanisms are responsible for the rapid heart rate and the sweating seen often in infants with heart failure. If the increased volume load persists, hypertrophy of the ventricular myocardium will develop.

These compensatory mechanisms are generally well developed in older children or adults; however, they are not as well developed in newborn infants and are even less so in prematurely born infants. It is most important, therefore, to consider the state of maturity, that is, the gestational age at the time of birth, of an infant who has a PDA with left to right shunting. It has become apparent recently that many physiologic functions present in older children reach full maturation at different rates and periods of gestation. For example, sympathetic innervation of the left ventricular myocardium may only be completed at term,[25, 43] so that in an infant born prematurely it is likely that sympathetic stimulation of the left ventricular myocardium would be incomplete or even absent. Likewise the myocardium in an immature animal responds less to stretch (Frank-Starling mechanism) than does that in a more mature animal.[23] The structure of the immature fetal myocardium too is quite different from that at term in that there are far fewer contractile elements.[23] Premature infants often have lower than normal serum Ca^+ concentrations, and this too may affect myocardial performance.[73] It is probably for one or all of these reasons that premature infants with left to right shunts through a PDA develop left ventricular failure considerably earlier than their full-term counterparts and, in addition, with a considerably smaller volume load. The altered myocardial structure may be partly responsible for the poor response to digitalis of immature infants with left ventricular failure.

Of considerable importance as well is the maintenance of myocardial perfusion. Since coronary blood flow to the left ventricle occurs mainly during diastole and depends on the systemic arterial-intramyocardial diastolic pressure differences as well as the duration of diastole, alterations in either can affect coronary blood flow.[38] A reduction in aortic diastolic pressure occurs in a large PDA, and with a significant shunt left ventricular end-diastolic pressure may be increased and cause an increase in subendocardial intramyocardial pressure. The development of tachycardia will reduce the diastolic period. All three factors which determine adequate myocardial perfusion are therefore jeopardized in the presence of a large PDA.

Delivery of oxygen to the myocardium depends not only on the coronary blood flow but also the oxygen content of arterial blood and the ability of arterial blood to deliver oxygen at the tissue sites. A low hemoglobin caused by physiologic anemia in the newborn period, particularly in premature infants, or by repeated blood sampling as occurs with intensive neonatal care, will jeopardize oxygen delivery to the myocardium as well as to other organs. A further important factor, particularly in premature infants, is the amount of fetal hemoglobin present. Since fetal hemoglobin has a low affinity for the organic phosphates such as 2,3-diphosphoglycerate the facilitation of oxygen delivery to peripheral tissues is reduced. This effect is greater with higher amounts of fetal hemoglobin.[16]

Effects on the Pulmonary Circulation and Lungs

A small communication has little or no effect on the pulmonary arterial circulation. However, with a large communication systemic and pulmonary arterial pressures will equalize, and because of the high flow and high pressure the small pulmonary arteries will not undergo their normal postnatal maturational changes. The medial smooth muscle does not regress as rapidly as normal nor to the same extent so that the pulmonary vascular resistance will fall more slowly and less completely than usual.[37]

Initially the increase in pulmonary vascular resistance is associated with only an increased amount of medial smooth muscle. However, true pulmonary vascular disease may subsequently occur, manifested by intimal damage with cellular proliferation, hyalinization, and finally thrombosis and fibrosis of the small pulmonary arteries. As more small pulmonary arteries become involved in this process, the left to right shunt diminishes, and eventually a right to left shunt will occur. In severe pulmonary vascular obstructive disease arteriovenous malformations may form with resultant hemoptysis.

Pulmonary edema occurs commonly in premature infants with only a moderate shunt and without severe heart failure. Capillary permeability in newborn animals is greater than in adults, and it is possible that this is even more pronounced in prematures. A small elevation in pulmonary venous pressure could therefore produce significant pulmonary edema.

DELAYED CLOSURE IN TERM INFANTS

Although functional closure of the ductus arteriosus is generally completely effected within the first day after birth, it may be delayed for several days. Since pulmonary vascular resistance will have fallen normally, flow will occur from the aorta into the pulmonary artery throughout this period of functional patency. On careful auscultation, therefore, a murmur may be heard in the first few hours of life in many infants[6, 7, 52] or animals.[2, 18] Two particular murmurs have been described in human infants; a crescendo systolic murmur and a continuous murmur with a crescendo systolic and diminuendo diastolic component. Neither murmur is very loud (grade 1 to 2/6), and both may be accentuated or possibly only heard during inspiration; the murmurs are best heard in the second to third left intercostal space and do not radiate widely. Since pulmonary arterial pressure is normal, the pulmonic component of the second sound is of normal intensity, and the second sound is often well split.[6] As the ductus arteriosus constricts, the diastolic component becomes inaudible and leaves only a crescendo systolic murmur that usually disappears by the third to fifth day of life. The electrocardiogram and chest roentgenogram in these infants are normal. The echocardiogram is also likely to be within normal limits, since a significant left to right shunt is not present and left atrial size is not significantly increased. Hemodynamic studies have been performed in some of these infants and have demonstrated small left to right shunts with essentially normal arterial pressures.[52]

During the initial period of constriction any condition that lowers arterial blood PO_2 or perhaps increases circulating blood PGE_2 concentrations may delay normal closure. Likewise before true anatomic closure occurs, the functionally closed ductus arteriosus may be dilated by a reduced arterial blood PO_2,[51] or increased PGE_2 concentration. This may occur in asphyxial states and in the presence of any one of many different pulmonary diseases (e.g., meconium aspiration). A nonpulmonary cause of arterial hypoxemia, living at high altitude, has been shown to produce delayed closure of the ductus arteriosus. The incidence of PDA is about 30 times greater at high altitude (4,500 to 5,000 m) than at sea level.[1] With pulmonary disease with hypoxemia and possibly acidemia, there is an increase in pulmonary vascular resistance that will affect the magnitude of left to right shunting through the dilating ductus arteriosus. With severe pulmonary disease or persistent pulmonary hypertension of the newborn, no shunt or even a right to left shunt through the PDA may occur. This will lead to a lower PO_2 in the lower extremities than in the upper. This difference in PO_2 may persist for many days, and with pulmonary disease the ductus arteriosus may remain patent for several weeks.

The initial constriction of the ductus arteriosus is most prominent at its pulmonary arterial end and extends progressively toward the aorta, thus accounting for the typical cone shape of the small PDA in which the diameter at the aortic end is considerably larger than at the pulmonary end. Even after the pulmonary arterial end has completely closed, the dilated aortic end of the ductus arteriosus may be apparent for many weeks. This ductus ampulla, or ductus "bump", may be evident on the chest roentgenogram (Fig. 11.2A) for several weeks.[4] Persistence of the ductus ampulla (Fig. 11.2B) for many months or even years has been well demonstrated by angiograms in older children.

PERSISTENT PATENCY IN PREMATURE INFANTS

Delayed closure of the ductus arteriosus in preterm infants is well recognized.[3, 5, 9, 15, 28, 40, 44, 53, 56, 59, 68, 71] With the advent of techniques for maintenance of ventilation in premature infants the survival, particularly of small premature infants, has improved dramatically.[30] Since the constrictor response of the ductus arteriosus to oxygen and the dilator effect of PGE_2 are closely related to gestational age,[10, 11, 48] it is not surprising that there is an extremely high incidence of PDA in small preterm infants, particularly those with pulmonary disease. No accurate statistics are available; however, in our institution approximately 45% of infants under 1750 gm birth weight have clinical evidence of PDA, and infants under 1200 gm birth weight have a prevalence closer to 80%. Based on the number of deliveries at our institution this makes the incidence of PDA 8 per 1000 of *all* live births.

Manifestations

The clinical features depend on the magnitude of left to right shunt through the PDA and the ability of the infant to initiate compensatory mechanisms to handle the extra volume load. Since many premature infants have respiratory distress syndrome, the stage of development of this disease will determine the pulmonary vascular resistance and therefore the shunt. As mentioned previously, the maturity of the infant and the development of the myocardium will determine the ability to handle the shunt.

Three fairly distinct patterns of clinical presentation are recognized in these infants.

Patent Ductus Arteriosus with No Lung Disease. In the first group there is little or no underlying pulmonary disease (usually infants whose birth weight exceeds 1500 gm). However, smaller infants are encountered, and in many instances their mothers have received steroid therapy prior to delivery. A systolic murmur is first heard 3 to 5 days after birth, and as the left to right shunt increases this murmur becomes louder and more prolonged, extending to and often beyond the second heart sound into early diastole. The murmur is generally best heard at the left sternal border in the second and third intercostal spaces. The classical continuous machinery murmur, described for older children with PDA, is not usual in premature infants in whom the murmur generally has a high frequency "rocky" quality. The pulmonic component of the second sound may become moderately accentuated. In the most mature infants in this group a middiastolic flow rumble due to increased diastolic flow across the normal mitral valve may be heard at the apex. If the shunt becomes large enough a third heart sound due to rapid ventricular filling during diastole may be heard at the apex. The precordium becomes increasingly more hyperactive, the pulse pressure widens, and the peripheral pulses become more prominent and bounding as the left to right shunt increases.

If the shunt becomes sufficiently large, clinical evidence of left ventricular failure may appear. This includes tachycardia, tachypnea, and rales on auscultation of the lung fields. Associated with the development of pulmonary edema

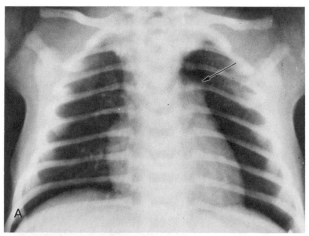
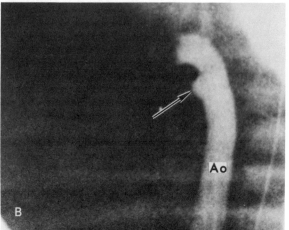

Fig. 11.2 (A) Posterior-anterior chest roentgenogram of a 2-day-old infant demonstrating the typical ductus "bump" (B) Angiogram in the lateral position of a 5-day-old infant demonstrating the ampulla of the ductus arteriosus.

there may be an increase in arterial blood PCO_2. If left ventricular failure progresses a significant number of these infants develop episodes of apnea often associated with severe bradycardia. Enlargement of the liver is usually fairly late.

The electrocardiogram is generally not helpful early in the disease, but if a moderately large shunt persists for several weeks left ventricular and left atrial hypertrophy may become evident. The chest roentgenogram may show enlargement of both the left atrium and ventricle if there is a moderately large shunt, but it is common for heart size to be normal. The pulmonary vascularity is often increased. Dilatation of the ascending aorta is not usually seen in premature infants, but may occur with a protracted moderately severe shunt.

The echocardiogram has become very useful in assessing the magnitude of shunting.[5, 65, 69] It also can be used to exclude congenital cardiac lesions with similar clinical findings and left ventricular failure due to poor intrinsic myocardial function.[65] Since left atrial diameter varies with the size of the infant, we have related left atrial diameter to the aortic diameter and calculated the left atrial (LA) diameter to the aortic root (Ao) diameter ratio (Fig. 11.3). The normal LA to Ao ratio in infants is between 0.8 and 1.0. A ratio greater than 1.2 indicates left atrial enlargement which, in the absence of left ventricular failure due to some other cause (such as aortic stenosis or volume overload), indicates a significant left to right shunt. In the premature infant this is most likely to be through a PDA. Real time (two-dimensional) echocardiography has proven even more useful in the management of these infants. Left atrial and left ventricular size and left ventricular activity can be assessed more accurately. The dynamics of both left ventricular and descending aortic wall motion also can give an indication of the magnitude of shunt. Direct visualization of the ductus arteriosus (Fig. 11.4), although not always possible, confirms the diagnosis. Contrast echocardiography can detect the left to right shunt and also give some idea about blood flow in the thoracic descending aorta. Doppler techniques have recently been applied to the evaluation of flow patterns in infants with PDA. Flow from the aorta into the pulmonary artery

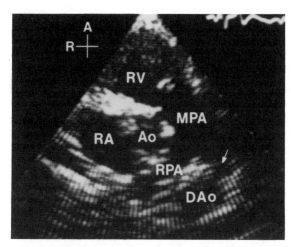

Fig. 11.4 Real time echocardiogram in short axis view demonstrating a patent ductus arteriosus (indicated by *arrow*). *A*, anterior; *R*, right; RV, right ventricle; MPA, main pulmonary artery; RA, right atrium; Ao, ascending aorta; RPA, right pulmonary artery; DAo, descending aorta.

can be detected, and velocity profiles of flow in the descending aorta in infants with PDA have been characterized.[26, 67]

Cardiac catheterization and angiography in these infants generally reveals moderate elevation of pulmonary arterial pressures and left to right shunting through the ductus arteriosus.[15]

The majority of infants in this group do not develop severe left ventricular failure, and those that do are generally easily managed with conventional medical therapy of cardiac failure, fluid intake restriction, and maintenance of hematocrit above 45%. Very rarely intractable cardiac failure develops, and surgical closure may be required. If left alone the ductus arteriosus in the vast majority of these infants closes spontaneously, generally within 2 to 3 months after birth.

Patent Ductus Arteriosus in Infants Recovering from Lung Disease. The second and most common group of infants develops left to right shunting while recovering from severe or moderately severe respiratory distress syndrome. These infants usually weigh between 1000 and 1500 gm at birth. The idiopathic respiratory distress syndrome is generally evident within a few hours after birth and, if this follows the usual course, starts to improve after 3 to 4 days. As this improvement continues, early clinical evidence of a left to right shunt through a PDA occurs. In addition, at about this age, fluid administration generally is increased in order to deliver adequate calories; this could aggravate the deleterious effects of the left to right shunt on left ventricular function. It is probable that the ductus arteriosus has been patent since birth and that the pulmonary disease with a resultant increase in pulmonary vascular resistance has prevented a large left to right shunt. As the pulmonary disease improves, oxygenation increases and the ductus arteriosus should constrict. However, the majority of these infants are quite immature so that a good constrictor response to oxygen is not likely to occur. Many of these infants are still maintained on mechanical ventilators or continuous positive airway pressure (CPAP) so that careful clinical assessment is required in order to establish the presence of a shunt through the ductus arteriosus. In many instances the murmurs are not audible until the infant is briefly detached from the ventilator or CPAP system. Since recovery from the respiratory distress syndrome is often not continuously progressive but is interspersed by periods of deteriorating lung function, left to right shunting and therefore the murmur

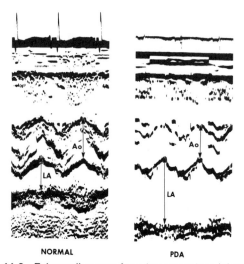

Fig. 11.3 Echocardiograms from two premature infants, one without clinical evidence of a PDA and the other with a large left to right shunt through a PDA which was subsequently ligated. *LA*, left atrial diameter; *Ao*, aortic root diameter; *PDA*, with patent ductus arteriosus.

may be intermittent for several days. It is common for the murmur to disappear and reappear several times within short periods of time. Initially a systolic murmur alone will be heard; however, as the shunt increases the murmur will extend into diastole. The murmur is similar in distribution and quality to that in the first group of premature infants with PDA. Because the second group of infants is generally more immature than the first, left ventricular failure occurs in them when clinically there seems to be a smaller amount of left to right shunting. A third sound is often heard, but a middiastolic flow rumble is very uncommon. The pulmonic component of the second sound is generally already accentuated due to the pulmonary disease but may become louder as the shunt increases. Increasing precordial activity is a good indication of the magnitude of shunting in these infants, and increased heart rate, pulse pressure, and bounding pulses with a rapid upstroke are often detectable early. Since the majority of these infants have the indwelling umbilical arterial catheters, careful monitoring of the umbilical arterial blood pressure often will show a widening pulse pressure and fall in diastolic pressure as left to right shunting develops.

Rales as an index of pulmonary edema and left ventricular failure are unreliable since they may be suppressed by the positive pressure ventilatory assistance used in these infants. However, in those that have recovered sufficiently from their respiratory distress syndrome to have been extubated, rales may be heard in the lung fields. Apneic episodes are also common in this group of infants and may or may not be associated with short periods of bradycardia.

A deterioration in the ventilatory status of an infant recovering from respiratory distress syndrome is often a good indication that there is a significant left to right shunt through a PDA. However, other causes, such as recurring lung disease and pneumothorax or sepsis, should be actively excluded. Deterioration of the ventilatory status is manifested by the requirement for an increasing concentration of inspired oxygen, alterations in ventilator rate or pressure settings, increased requirements of CPAP, and assisted ventilation and increasing arterial blood PCO_2. The electrocardiogram often shows increased right ventricular forces due to the underlying pulmonary disease but is generally of little help. A chest roentgenogram will show the parenchymal changes of respiratory distress syndrome, and increased pulmonary vascularity may therefore be extremely difficult to assess. Cardiomegaly is variable, particularly if the infant is being artificially ventilated; however, increasing cardiomegaly may indicate an increasing shunt.

Since many of the changes described may be due to deterioration of underlying pulmonary disease it is important to be able to assess the contribution to the clinical picture of left ventricular failure. For this purpose, the echocardiogram is often very helpful. An increasing LA to Ao ratio will be produced by increasing left to right shunting, whereas a ratio that remains constant and within normal limits will indicate noncardiac causes of deterioration. Changes in the variables assessed by real time echocardiography similarly will help determine the role of shunting through the PDA.

Patent Ductus Arteriosus Associated with Lung Disease. The third group consists of infants who have severe respiratory distress syndrome from birth. They either show little improvement of the pulmonary disease when clinical deterioration or clinical evidence of a left to right shunt through the PDA occurs or they fail to show any improvement in respiratory status at an age when they should start to recover from the primary pulmonary disease. They too are extremely sensitive to small increases in Na^+ and fluid administration. The majority of infants in this group weigh

under 1000 gm at birth. They require ventilatory assistance by mechanical respirators or CPAP. Deterioration generally is manifested by the need for increasing pressures or rates on the ventilators, the necessity to increase CPAP or to institute mechanical ventilation in an infant who has previously been maintained on CPAP, and by increasing oxygen requirements. Failure to improve is manifested by the inability to wean the infant from ventilatory support. An increase in arterial blood PCO_2 is common. Murmurs may be difficult to hear, and in some of these infants the ductus arteriosus may be so widely patent that a murmur is not produced.[71] Changes in the ventilatory status may be due to progression of the primary pulmonary disease, and it is often even more difficult to separate left ventricular failure from increasing pulmonary problems than in the previous group. Increasing precordial activity, bounding pulses, and a widening arterial pulse pressure suggest the development of left to right shunting. When present, the murmur is usually only systolic, the pulmonic component of the second sound is accentuated, and a gallop rhythm is usually heard. The electrocardiogram and chest x-ray are usually not particularly helpful but, as outlined above, the echocardiogram is often very useful.

Management

Confirmation of Diagnosis. Infants with birth weights under 1500 gm who have clinical evidence of significant left to right shunting are statistically more likely to have a PDA.[45] However, more severe forms of congenital heart disease should be considered. Clinical evaluation combined with a chest roentgenogram and electrocardiogram often cannot differentiate a PDA from such lesions as truncus arteriosus or aortopulmonary fenestration unless an additional anomaly, for example, a right aortic arch, is present. The echocardiogram may be valuable in distinguishing truncus arteriosus from PDA, since distinctly separate aortic and pulmonic valves will exclude the former.

If medical management is unsuccessful and surgical closure is considered, cardiac catheterization and angiocardiography are recommended in some institutions. The value of angiocardiography in assessing the magnitude of left to right shunt has recently been superceded by echocardiograms. However, confirmation of the anatomic lesion can be done only by angiocardiography. In most instances complete catheterization is not required, and retrograde aortography suffices. Since a large proportion of infants with suspected PDA have an umbilical arterial catheter in place, it is generally a simple procedure to replace this catheter with a new one and advance it into the thoracic aorta. Angiography gives only a rough estimate of the magnitude of shunting and can only distinguish a small from a large shunt. Recently, single film aortography performed in the intensive care nursery by injecting contrast material into the umbilical arterial catheter has been suggested[71] as an alternative confirmatory test.

Our current practice in infants in whom the clinical and echocardiographic evidence is strongly in favor of a PDA with left to right shunting is medical management without retrograde aortography to confirm the diagnosis. If any doubt or question as to the diagnosis occurs, retrograde aortography should always be performed.

Relationship to Necrotizing Enterocolitis. One of the major factors involved in the development of necrotizing enterocolitis is bowel ischemia. It has become apparent recently that a PDA with significant left to right shunting and left ventricular failure may be one of the major contributing conditions in the production of bowel ischemia. Decreased systemic blood flow and moderate hypotension are common in premature infants with left ventricular failure due to a PDA and may predispose to the development of necrotizing enterocolitis. We therefore carefully monitor abdominal girth and residual gastric volumes prior to feeding and perform hematests on all stools and gastric aspirates in all premature infants with a PDA. When signs of necrotizing enterocolitis develop in an infant with significant left to right shunting through a PDA, it has been our experience that early surgical closure of the ductus arteriosus has significantly reduced the mortality. Therefore, if persistent abdominal distention, increasing residuals before feedings, blood in the stools or gastric aspirate, decreasing bowel sounds, and particularly intramural air occur in association with a significant left to right shunt through a PDA, surgical closure is considered.

Treatment. An important consideration in treating a premature infant with a PDA is maintenance of an adequate hematocrit and hemoglobin. A reduction in hemoglobin requires an increased cardiac output to maintain peripheral oxygenation and with a left to right shunt and an already compromised myocardium, anemia may further impair cardiac function. In addition, since myocardial oxygen delivery is dependent on blood oxygen content, a low hemoglobin may be associated with myocardial ischemia. Since arterial blood gas sampling is common, the hematocrit often falls and care must be taken to maintain this above 45%. Since peripheral tissue oxygen delivery is retarded by fetal hemoglobin, exchange transfusion replacing fetal hemoglobin with adult hemoglobin may help to facilitate peripheral oxygenation.[16] Since the majority of premature infants require repeated blood sampling and blood transfusions, this is, in fact, generally accomplished. Maintenance of electrolyte, glucose, and nutritional requirements must be carefully attended to. Caloric intake is often a major problem, and intravenous hyperalimentation may be required. Since volume overload may precipitate left ventricular failure, Na$^+$ and fluid administration are generally restricted to low maintenance amounts. Previously, left ventricular failure was treated by digitalization and the use of diuretics, particularly furosemide. More recently it has become evident that in very small preterm infants digitalis is relatively ineffective, and in view of potential toxic reactions, digitalis now is rarely used. All the above are aimed at supportive treatment of the results of a left to right shunt with myocardial failure. Recently treatment has been aimed at removing the shunt and its effects by closing the ductus arteriosus. The timing of such a maneuver and the method to be employed are still not generally agreed upon and currently are under investigation.

Surgical closure before 10 days of age results in a reduced duration of ventilatory support and hospital stay and a lower morbidity.[14] The use of oral or intravenous (lyophilized) indomethacin to constrict the ductus arteriosus has led to successful nonsurgical closure in a large proportion of treated infants[24, 36, 74]; the effects of indomethacin apparently are best when it is administered before 10 days of age and in less mature infants.[47] Originally indomethacin was administered only to infants in whom standard medical management had failed and surgery was contemplated.[24, 36] Dose schedules vary but generally 0.2 mg/kg is given by nasogastric tube or intravenously. A maximum of three doses, 12 to 24 hours apart, can be given if there is little or no initial response. Indomethacin should not be administered to infants with renal dysfunction (serum creatinine > 1.6 mg/dl or BUN > 20 mg/dl), overt bleeding, shock, necrotizing enterocolitis, or any suspicion thereof, or if there is electrocardiographic evidence of myocardial ischemia. The side effects, oliguria

and hyponatremia, do not always occur, and when they do they are transient; no obvious long-term adverse effects have been experienced.[49] Indomethacin, when used correctly, has a high success rate and relatively few and minor side effects. Therefore, administration to infants with PDA before they show obvious major hemodynamic complications has been suggested and is currently under investigation. As with early surgical ligation, it is probable that this approach will reduce morbidity associated with a PDA. If after 48 to 72 hours of adequate medical management left ventricular failure is still uncontrolled, surgical closure is performed. Despite the small risk of recanalization, ligation rather than division of the ductus arteriosus is recommended, since the tissues in premature infants are very friable. Surgery can now be performed with minimal morbidity and mortality.[17]

PERSISTENT PATENCY IN TERM INFANTS

The incidence of isolated patent ductus arteriosus in full-term infants is about 1 in 2000 live births,[8, 50] accounting for about 5 to 10% of all types of congenital heart disease. Unlike the ductus arteriosus in premature infants in whom failure of closure is due to developmental retardation, the ductus arteriosus in full-term infants is abnormal and failure to constrict is probably related to a significant structural abnormality.

Exposure to rubella during the first trimester of pregnancy is associated with a high frequency of multiple congenital abnormalities, and the cardiovascular system is involved in about 60% of these infants. Rubella virus interferes with the normal formation of arterial elastic tissue, and in particular derivatives of the sixth aortic arch are involved. Patency of the ductus arteriosus is generally present, often associated with peripheral pulmonic stenosis and systemic arterial stenosis, especially of the renal arteries.

Patency of the ductus arteriosus may occur in more than one member of a family, suggesting possible genetic factors in certain instances; it has been produced by genetic inbreeding in certain species of animals, particularly poodles.[41]

Manifestations

In mature infants and older children the factors determining the clinical features are the same as in premature infants, namely: the size of the communication; the relationship between pulmonary and systemic vascular resistances; and the ability of the myocardium to handle the extra volume load.

Small Ductus Arteriosus. With a small communication, pulmonary vascular resistance and therefore pulmonary arterial pressure fall normally after birth. However, since the resistance to flow across the ductus arteriosus is high only a small left to right shunt develops. Pulmonary blood flow is only minimally increased, and left ventricular failure does not occur. Therefore, few patients are symptomatic, and attention is often brought to this condition only by the murmur detected at a routine physical examination.

Physical growth is normal except in those children in whom maternal rubella has been present. The peripheral pulses may be full and the arterial pulse pressure is slightly increased unless the shunt is very small. Precordial activity is generally normal with no increased apical impulse. Auscultation reveals normal first and second heart sounds, and the only significant abnormal finding may be the presence of a murmur. In early infancy before pulmonary vascular resistance has fallen completely there may be a short period in which no murmur is heard. A short systolic murmur may then be heard which may progress on to the typical continuous murmur heard in older children. It is best heard in the second left intercostal space and is often accentuated when the patient is recumbent or during inspiration. Administration of a vasopressor agent such as phenylephrine will raise systemic vascular resistance and increase left to right shunt, and the murmur will become longer and louder. The important features of the characteristic continuous murmur first described by Gibson[27] are the late systolic accentuation and continuation through the second sound into diastole. The murmur generally starts shortly after the first sound, peaks at the second heart sound, and fades away, ending in the last third of diastole.

The electrocardiogram and chest roentgenogram are usually normal in these children; however, slight prominence of the main and peripheral pulmonary arteries may be seen on the roentgenogram (Fig. 11.5A).

Moderate Ductus Arteriosus. In infants a moderately large left to right shunt may produce symptomatology related to left ventricular failure. Poor feeding, irritability, and tachypnea may be present, and there is often slow weight gain. The symptoms generally increase until about the second to third month of age. If the left ventricular failure does

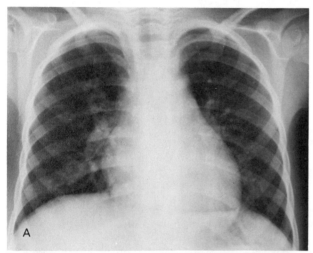

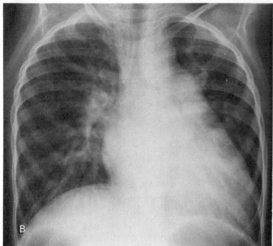

Fig. 11.5 Posterior-anterior chest roentgenograms in two children each with a patent ductus arteriosus. (A) A 4-year-old child with a small left to right shunt. Slight cardiomegaly and prominence of the pulmonary vascularity are present. (B) A 4-year-old child with a very large left to right shunt. A double density and elevation of the left main stem bronchus are present due to left atrial enlargement. The left ventricle, main and peripheral pulmonary arteries, and ascending aorta are prominent. Pulmonary venous congestion is also present.

not produce severe disease at this stage, compensatory myocardial hypertrophy will occur, and in many instances these infants improve considerably. Some in fact are only detected on a subsequent routine physical examination, but close questioning will reveal the previous abnormal history. General physical development is slightly retarded, and easy fatigability may be present in the older child. The pulse rate is often increased and the peripheral pulses are full and bounding. The systemic arterial pressure is widened with a low diastolic pressure. The precordium is hyperdynamic and left ventricular enlargement produces a thrusting apical impulse. A systolic thrill may be palpable at the upper left sternal border. Both the first and second sound may be difficult to hear, as it is often masked by a loud murmur. A third heart sound is often heard at the apex. The progression from a systolic murmur to a continuous murmur is considerably more rapid in these infants than it is in those with a small shunt. The continuous murmur is more intense, has more extensive radiation, and is generally well heard posteriorly. It has a much harsher quality with low frequency components and, due to the large flow and great turbulence, there are eddy sounds that vary from beat to beat and give the murmur a "machinery" quality.

If heart failure occurs the murmur may lose its continuous nature and occupy only systole. A middiastolic low frequency rumbling murmur is generally heard at the apex. Early pulmonic or aortic ejection sounds may occur. The increased left ventricular stroke may produce a functional systolic pressure difference across the aortic valve and this may be manifested, although rarely, by a soft ejection systolic murmur. In early infancy left ventricular failure with increased left atrial size and pressure often induces a left to right shunt through a stretched and incompetent foramen ovale.[62] Depending on the magnitude of left to right atrial shunting, right ventricular hyperactivity may become evident, and the right ventricular outflow murmur typical of atrial left to right shunting may be heard. In addition, a middiastolic flow rumble due to the increased flow across the tricuspid valve may be audible at the lower left sternal border.

The electrocardiogram may be relatively normal during infancy, but left ventricular hypertrophy is usual in older infants and children. The mean frontal plane axis is generally normal. Left ventricular hypertrophy is manifested by a deep Q wave and a tall R wave in leads II, III, AVF and the left precordial leads V_5 and V_6. The T waves in these leads are generally upright and also show increased amplitude. A pattern compatible with left bundle branch block has also been described in some children. A widened P wave indicating left atrial enlargement may also be present. If there is a left to right atrial shunt as well as moderate pulmonary hypertension, right ventricular hypertrophy may develop and produce an increased amplitude of the R waves in the right precordial leads. Right atrial enlargement may increase the height of the P wave.

The chest roentgenogram shows an enlarged heart with prominence of the left ventricle and the typical signs of left atrial enlargement (Fig. 11.5B). The main pulmonary artery segment is prominent, and the pulmonary vascular markings in the peripheral lung fields are increased (Fig. 11.5B). The ascending aorta is often very prominent and may be associated with unfolding of the aortic arch. The echocardiogram will demonstrate an increased left atrial diameter, and an estimate of left to right shunt may be made from the LA to Ao ratio. With a significant left to right atrial shunt, paradoxical interventricular septal movement may be apparent.

Large Ductus Arteriosus. Infants with a large patent ductus arteriosus are invariably symptomatic. They are irritable, feed poorly, fail to gain weight normally, tire easily—

particularly while feeding—and sweat excessively. They have increased respiratory effort and respiratory rates, also aggravated by feeding, and are prone to develop recurrent upper respiratory infections and pneumonia. These symptoms indicative of severe left ventricular failure with pulmonary edema may occur early in infancy.

Many of the typical physical signs may be absent when there is severe left ventricular failure. However, tachycardia and tachypnea are present, and if there is pulmonary edema, rales will be heard throughout the lung fields. The respiratory signs may be suggestive of bronchopneumonia. The peripheral pulses are bounding with a rapid upstroke and a wide pulse pressure unless there is severe left ventricular failure when the pulse volume decreases. The precordium is markedly hyperdynamic, and clinical evidence of cardiac enlargement is present. The left ventricular apical impulse is thrusting and, if right ventricular enlargement occurs, may be accompanied by a left parasternal impulse. A systolic thrill is often palpable. The first and second heart sounds are accentuated and a third sound is usually heard at the apex. Occasionally no murmur is heard, especially when there is severe failure. When left ventricular failure is controlled, a moderately loud systolic murmur is best heard in the pulmonary area or occasionally in the third or fourth intercostal spaces. The murmur peaks late in systole, and the prolongation into diastole is variable; the murmur generally ends within the first third of diastole. Nonspecific ejection type systolic murmurs have also been described. The typical continuous murmur heard with a small or moderate-sized PDA may be heard but is less usual. A prominent middiastolic mitral flow rumble is generally audible at the apex.

The electrocardiogram shows more prominent left ventricular enlargement with deep Q and taller R waves than in the previous group. The T waves may be diphasic or even inverted. Right ventricular hypertrophy may be evident with upright T waves in the right precordial leads and increased R wave amplitude in the right precordial leads. Left atrial enlargement as demonstrated by a widened P wave will also be seen. The chest roentgenogram shows striking enlargement of the heart with predominant left atrial and left ventricular enlargement. The main pulmonary artery segment is usually markedly enlarged and the peripheral pulmonary vascular markings are markedly accentuated. Evidence of left ventricular failure with increased pulmonary venous markings and interstitial fluid may also be seen. With an enlarged left atrium or pulmonary arteries, lobar collapse or emphysema due to bronchial compression may occur.

Infants with large left to right shunts through a PDA may not survive the resultant cardiac failure without treatment. However, a certain proportion is capable of compensating adequately and survives the initial period. A moderate or large left to right shunt either undetected in infancy or treated but allowed to persist will eventually lead to the development of obstructive pulmonary vascular disease. As pulmonary vascular resistance increases, pulmonary hypertension increases until systemic levels are reached. The left to right shunting decreases, and this leads to improvement in the infant's symptomatology and signs generally between 8 and 15 months after birth. Feeding problems, poor weight gain, and the increased sweating previously present disappear, and there are far fewer episodes of respiratory infection. The murmur becomes shorter and the diastolic component may be completely lost. The middiastolic rumble decreases and disappears, and the first heart sound becomes softer. The second heart sound remains markedly accentuated, but the third heart sound disappears. Precordial hyperactivity diminishes, and the pulses become less bounding. The chest roentgenogram will show decreasing pulmonary vascularity,

and a decrease in heart size may also be noted. The period of time over which these changes occur is variable and may take several years.

As the increased pulmonary vascular resistance progresses to irreversible pulmonary vascular disease, the symptoms and clinical features change even further. The murmur continues to shorten until it eventually disappears. The second sound becomes single and progressively louder, an ejection systolic click occurs, and a faint blowing early diastolic regurgitant murmur due to pulmonary incompetence may be heard at the upper left sternal edge. Left ventricular hyperactivity disappears, and the right ventricular parasternal impulse increases. The electrocardiogram shows increasing right ventricular hypertrophy with dominant R waves in the right precordial leads. Peaked P waves indicative of right atrial enlargement may also occur. The chest roentgenogram shows increasing right ventricular enlargement with decreasing left ventricular size, a large main pulmonary artery, and progressive decrease in peripheral vascular markings.

Cyanosis, often more pronounced in the lower than in the upper limbs, begins to appear; initially it occurs only with exertion but eventually becomes continuous, as persistent right to left shunting across the ductus arteriosus occurs. The final picture, if allowed to progress, is one of irreversible pulmonary vascular disease with marked right to left shunting. The precordial activity is now dominantly right ventricular, and the pulses are either of normal or small volume. The second heart sound is generally palpable in the pulmonic area, and a diastolic thrill may also be felt. The first heart sound is slightly accentuated and the pulmonic component of the second heart sound is markedly accentuated. A harsher and longer early diastolic blowing murmur caused by pulmonic incompetence is heard at the left sternal border. A blowing systolic murmur due to secondary tricuspid insufficiency may be heard at the lower left sternal border. The electrocardiogram shows right axis deviation in the frontal plane with marked right ventricular hypertrophy and eventually T wave inversion in older patients. The chest roentgenogram shows moderate cardiomegaly with predominant enlargement of the right ventricle and a markedly enlarged main pulmonary artery with prominence of the central vessels but no peripheral plethora. Right atrial enlargement may be evident.

CARDIAC CATHETERIZATION

Based on careful clinical evaluation, principally the characteristic continuous murmur, together with the electrocardiogram, chest roentgenogram and echocardiogram, the clinical diagnosis of PDA is almost always possible. Whether or not the majority of these children require cardiac catheterization is still a matter of discussion. However, confirmation of the suspected clinical diagnosis is occasionally dependent on catheterization. In children with pulmonary hypertension the exact site of communication needs to be determined since it may be impossible to differentiate between a PDA or ventricular septal defect with pulmonary vascular disease. In addition, the reactivity of the small pulmonary arteries as shown by the response to pulmonary vasodilators needs to be evaluated. If there is a large PDA with considerable shunting, the possibility of an additional intracardiac lesion should be excluded, and this must be done by catheterization as it may be impossible clinically. Although aortopulmonary fenestration is clinically different in most instances, this lesion should be considered and excluded by catheterization. Patients with truncus arteriosus too may present with clinical findings indistinguishable from PDA. In a small or moderate-sized patent ductus arteriosus demonstration of the anatomy may be beneficial to the surgeon. Although the anatomy is usually consistent, abnormal orientation and attachment of the ductus arteriosus has been encountered.

The risks and complications associated with percutaneous cardiac catheterization are well established and are very low but certainly need to be taken into consideration in making the final decision. Obviously, if any question arises as to the diagnosis, cardiac catheterization is mandatory.

Right heart catheterization alone is usually sufficient to confirm the diagnosis. However, if an additional lesion such as ventricular septal defect is suspected, retrograde catheterization may be required if the interatrial septum is intact and the left ventricle cannot be entered prograde. The venous catheter can usually be passed from the main pulmonary artery through the ductus arteriosus into the descending aorta, and in infants it is often very difficult to manipulate the catheter into the branch pulmonary arteries. In rare instances the catheter passes proximally into the aortic arch and one of the major arterial branches. In this situation catheter position alone will not confirm the diagnosis of PDA, as aortopulmonary fenestration can result in a similar catheter position. If the venous catheter cannot be passed through the ductus arteriosus, retrograde aortic catheterization is indicated in order to define the anatomy.

An increase of pulmonary arterial blood oxygen content of greater than 0.5 ml/dl or a saturation increase of greater than 4 to 5% from that in right ventricular blood indicates a significant left to right shunt at the pulmonary arterial level. Occasionally an increase in oxygen saturation is noted in blood just below the pulmonic valve due to pulmonary regurgitation. It is often difficult to measure pulmonary blood flow accurately from the blood oxygen data, and therefore the true magnitude of left to right shunting usually cannot be calculated. Preferential streaming of oxygenated blood from the PDA into one or another of the major pulmonary arteries is common, and therefore a sample from either one does not reflect mixed pulmonary arterial blood oxygen saturation.[62] In the presence of left ventricular failure with pulmonary edema, pulmonary venous blood oxygen saturation may be reduced. If the foramen ovale is incompetent a left to right atrial shunt may be detected by an increase in oxygen saturation in right atrial blood. A large increase in oxygen saturation at the right atrial level may mask a smaller rise of saturation in the pulmonary artery, even though the rise represents a significant shunt at the pulmonary arterial level. With significant pulmonary hypertension and right to left shunting through the PDA, oxygen saturation of blood in the descending aorta will be reduced as compared with that obtained in the ascending aorta. Bidirectional shunting may be present until pulmonary vascular disease is extremely severe when right to left shunting alone occurs.

A small left to right shunt may not be detected by blood oxygen saturation data alone. An increase in oxygen saturation in pulmonary arterial blood is not diagnostic of a PDA but may be present in lesions such as aortopulmonary fenestration or a high ventricular septal defect (supracristal) in which streaming may direct the highly saturated blood into the pulmonary artery.

With a small communication, pulmonary arterial blood pressures are normal, but systemic arterial pulse pressure may be slightly widened. With a moderate sized defect, pulmonary arterial systolic, diastolic, and mean blood pressures may be slightly elevated. Systemic arterial diastolic blood pressure falls, whereas systemic arterial pulse pressure increases. Both left and right atrial mean pressures will be moderately elevated in the presence of a moderate shunt. With a large shunt, pulmonary and systemic arterial pressures are equal, left atrial mean pressure may be increased

to about 10 mm Hg, and a prominent "V" wave is seen. Left ventricular end-diastolic pressure may be elevated, and with a large flow a diastolic pressure gradient between the left atrium and left ventricle is demonstrated. A small systolic pressure difference between the left ventricle and aorta is also encountered occasionally when there is a large shunt. Since calculation of pulmonary blood flow in PDA is often inaccurate, the calculation of pulmonary vascular resistance is also inaccurate.[62]

Inhalation of hydrogen with placement of the platinum electrode in the pulmonary artery will be able to detect even a small left to right shunt at that level. Withdrawal of the electrode into the right ventricle will not detect the shunt and thus indicates the level of the left to right shunting.

ANGIOCARDIOGRAPHY

Although angiocardiography cannot accurately measure the magnitude of left to right shunting, it probably still gives the most valuable information obtained during catheterization. Good demonstration of the anatomy can be obtained by injecting the contrast medium into a catheter passed through the PDA into the aorta from the pulmonary artery (Fig. 11.6). However, if this technique is unsatisfactory, retrograde aortography will delineate the anatomy. As shown in Figure 11.6, the aortic end of the PDA is usually widely dilated, and the ductus narrows down at the pulmonary arterial end. This is the usual picture in the majority of children, but occasionally a long ductus arteriosus of similar diameter throughout is seen. In most instances the lateral

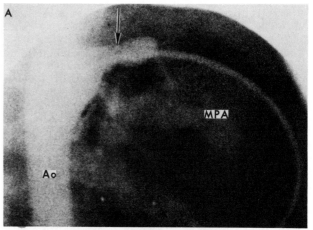
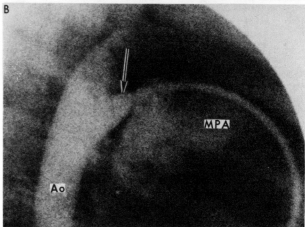

Fig. 11.6 Angiograms in the lateral position in two children each with a patent ductus arteriosus. The variable anatomy in this lesion is demonstrated, *Ao*, aorta; *MPA*, main pulmonary artery.

projection or occasionally the left anterior oblique projection demonstrates the anatomy most clearly. It is important to remember that in infants in whom severe heart failure is present a PDA is often associated with a ventricular septal defect or interatrial communication, and selective aortography is essential in these infants to exclude a PDA.

RADIONUCLIDE ANGIOGRAPHY

The course of an intravenously injected radionuclide (usually technetium-99m pertechnetate) can be traced with a scintillation camera as it courses through the heart and great vessels.[70] With good technical resolution, anatomical definition of the heart and great vessels is possible. A left to right shunt with a pulmonary systemic flow ratio of greater than 1.4 is easily detected by reappearance of the radionuclide in the right heart or lungs.[72] The magnitude of left to right shunting can be calculated from dilution curves obtained with the scintillation camera. Localization of the level of shunting can be determined, but with a shunt at the pulmonary arterial level a PDA cannot be differentiated from an aortopulmonary window. However, the anatomy of a truncus arteriosus has been defined by this technique.[70] Although relatively new, this noninvasive technique may become useful.

DIFFERENTIAL DIAGNOSIS

Venous Hum. The continuous bruit produced by flow through the large veins in the neck is often confused with the continuous murmur of a PDA. The venous hum varies in intensity with head and neck position as well as the phase of respiration and is usually obliterated by firm pressure over the neck, by turning the head to one side or by lying flat.

Total Anomalous Pulmonary Venous Connection. Unobstructed total anomalous pulmonary venous connection to the innominate vein occasionally produces a continuous murmur very much like a venous hum. The other features of this lesion serve to differentiate it from a PDA.

Ruptured Sinus of Valsalva. Rupture of one of the sinuses of Valsalva into either the right atrium or right ventricle is accompanied by a continuous murmur. However, onset of symptoms and signs in this condition is generally abrupt and often follows trauma to the chest. The murmur is usually heard lower in the precordium.

Arteriovenous Communications. Arteriovenous fistulae involving one of the coronary arteries, an intercostal artery, or an internal mammary artery may be associated with continuous murmurs similar to those occurring in PDA. The murmurs are generally more superficial and sound extracardiac in origin. Origin of one of the pulmonary arteries from the aorta (hemitruncus arteriosus) may also produce a continuous murmur, as may lobar sequestration in which an anomalous artery arising from the aorta supplies one or more pulmonary lobes. Pulmonary arteriovenous fistulae may produce a continuous murmur but when large enough to do so are usually associated with cyanosis and classical x-ray findings.

Anomalous Origin of the Left Coronary Artery from the Pulmonary Artery. In this lesion, retrograde flow occurs from the right coronary artery and then the pulmonary artery. If this retrograde flow is sufficiently large a continuous murmur may be heard, but this is rare. The clinical presentation and electrocardiogram are diagnostic of this condition.

Absent Pulmonary Valve. This lesion is invariably associated with massive dilatation of the pulmonary arteries and almost always is associated with a ventricular septal defect. The murmur has been described as "sawing wood" in character and is not really continuous but has more of a to and fro character. The massively dilated pulmonary artery evident on chest roentgenogram generally allows for accurate differentiation.

Aortic Insufficiency Associated with a Ventricular Septal Defect. Prolapse of one aortic sinus complicates ventricular septal defects, particularly supracristal defects. The murmur is not strictly continuous and there is generally separation between the systolic murmur produced by the ventricular septal defect and the blowing regurgitant diastolic murmur produced by the incompetence. However, accurate clinical differentiation may be difficult.

Peripheral Pulmonic Stenosis. Although commonly associated with a PDA, peripheral pulmonic stenosis may occur as an isolated defect and give rise to a soft continuous murmur heard best in the infraclavicular areas and conducted to the axillae. Stenosis may occur in only one pulmonary artery producing a unilateral murmur. This lesion may be difficult to distinguish clinically from a PDA.

Truncus Arteriosus. Truncus arteriosus may not be accompanied by cyanosis in early infancy, and with a low pulmonary vascular resistance and increased pulmonary blood flow there may be a continuous murmur. Absence of the pulmonary artery segment on the posterior-anterior chest roentgenogram suggests this diagnosis; furthermore, the relatively common occurrence of right aortic arch with truncus arteriosus excludes the diagnosis of isolated PDA.

Aortopulmonary Fenestration. This defect may be extremely difficult to differentiate from a PDA. The murmur is generally heard best lower down the left sternal border and is often mistaken for the murmur of a high ventricular septal defect.

Pulmonary Atresia. When pulmonary atresia is accompanied by markedly enlarged bronchial arteries supplying pulmonary blood flow, a continuous murmur may be heard. However, cyanosis is present, and the peripheral pulses are not bounding as in PDA. The chest roentgenogram also shows absence of the pulmonary artery segment.

COMPLICATIONS

Endarteritis. Bacterial endarteritis has become extremely uncommon, although it was once a serious complication of PDA. Since the advent of surgical correction of many congenital heart defects, the prevalence of endocarditis, particularly in defects associated with left to right shunts, has declined dramatically. In a recent survey of major congenital heart defects, PDA had the lowest frequency which was attributed to early surgical closure.[39]

Aneurysm Formation. Marked dilatation of a PDA or of the ampulla of the closed ductus arteriosus has been described. The massive dilatation that occurs may be diagnosed as a mediastinal mass. It has also been found as an incidental finding at autopsy.

TREATMENT

Since surgical repair of an uncomplicated PDA is accompanied by minimal risk in all but the smallest preterm infants, closure should be recommended soon after the diagnosis is made. Indomethacin is ineffective in all but preterm infants and therefore should not be used in this situation. The criteria for operative intervention in premature infants were discussed earlier. In older infants or children the complications resulting from isolated PDA including failure to grow, recurrent respiratory infections, cardiac failure and enlargement, lobar emphysema or collapse, bacterial endarteritis, and the eventual development of irreversible pulmonary vascular disease are all indications for early surgical correction. If intractable cardiac failure is present, intravenous infusion of epinephrine, isoproterenol, or dopamine may be beneficial[63] prior to immediate surgical closure.

A technique has been described for occluding the isolated PDA using a transfemoral catheter.[55, 66] A wire is manipulated from the femoral artery through the PDA and out through a femoral vein. An Ivalon foam plastic plug is then advanced over the wire from the arterial side into the PDA. Since in older children the ductus arteriosus is generally conical in shape, the plug is well wedged into the ductus arteriosus. This technique has been quite successful in specifically selected cases but has not yet been performed in very young children.

The usual surgical approach to closure of the PDA involves division or transsection of the ductus rather than simple suture ligation since recanalization has been reported following single suture ligation. In an extremely large PDA suture ligation is dangerous in view of the potential for tearing and hemorrhage.

The decision to recommend surgical closure in children with moderately increased pulmonary vascular resistance is not quite as simple. If a good response to a pulmonary vasodilator such as tolazoline has occurred, surgical closure is advised. However, if the response is poor or equivocal the decision is considerably more difficult. Some children respond extremely well and show significant improvement after closure, whereas others show a progressive increase in pulmonary vascular resistance after closure. Fortunately, the latter are encountered only rarely. The only contraindication to surgical closure of an isolated PDA is severe pulmonary hypertension with irreversible pulmonary vascular disease. If the PDA is closed in these children they are incapable of maintaining an adequate systemic output in response to stress, and rapid deterioration and death generally occur.

ROLE OF THE DUCTUS ARTERIOSUS IN CONGENITAL CARDIAC MALFORMATIONS

In right ventricular outflow obstruction lesions such as pulmonary atresia, the normal flow patterns in fetal life are altered, and development of the ductus arteriosus is probably abnormal.[61] The diameter and orientation of the ductus arteriosus are typical in this situation and can be diagnostic at the time of aortography (Fig. 11.7). Since maintenance of a PDA is generally essential for maintenance of pulmonary blood flow, the constrictor response to an increase in PO_2 is undesirable. Despite the hypoxemia in these infants, the ductus arteriosus closes, and recently attempts have been made at pharmacologic prevention of this closure prior to the creation of a surgical aortopulmonary communication. Prostaglandin E_1 has been administered in a larger number of cases and has produced dilatation of the ductus arteriosus with a significant increase in systemic arterial PO_2.[22, 35] Systemic oxygenation is markedly improved, acidemia reversed, and the infants can generally be stabilized for several hours

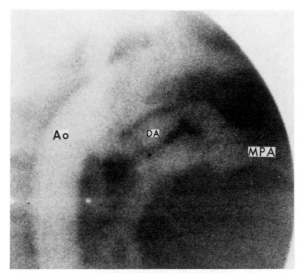

Fig. 11.7 Angiogram in the lateral position in a newborn infant with pulmonary atresia. The typical anatomy associated with right ventricular outflow obstruction is demonstrated. The aorta is widely dilated and the aortic isthmus is wider than the descending aorta. The typical narrow tortuous ductus arteriosus with an acute rather than the normal obtuse inferior angle with the aorta is present. This orientation is consistent with aortic to pulmonary arterial blood flow in fetal life. *Ao*, aorta; *DA*, ductus arteriosus; *MPA*, main pulmonary artery.

prior to palliative surgery. Maintenance of patency for a more prolonged period has been produced by infiltrating the wall of the ductus arteriosus with formalin at the time of thoracotomy.[60] This procedure too may be only temporary, and subsequent correction or the creation of an aortopulmonary shunt may be required.

Maintenance of systemic blood flow in lesions such as aortic atresia or interrupted aortic arch also may be dependent on patency of the ductus arteriosus. PGE_1 has proven extremely valuable in improving lower body perfusion in many infants with aortic arch interruption. Acidemia is often reversed and renal function markedly improved so that the infants can be stabilized and returned to reasonable electrolyte balance before corrective surgery is undertaken.[22, 31]

It has recently been shown that the ductus arteriosus plays an important role in the presentation of infants with juxtaductal aortic coarctation. Localized coarctation generally is produced by a well-circumscribed posterior shelf protruding into the aortic lumen at a point opposite the insertion of the ductus arteriosus.[61] If the ductus arteriosus remains patent or if there is a well-formed ductus ampulla even when the ductus arteriosus is closed, obstruction by the juxtaductal coarctation may not occur. However, as the ductus arteriosus closes and the ampulla retracts, progressive interference with flow occurs, and the clinical symptoms and signs will develop. The sudden occurrence of acute left ventricular failure in infants with juxtaductal coarctation of the aorta may be produced by rapid constriction of the ductus arteriosus in the postnatal period. PGE_1 has been of great benefit in the management of these infants as well.[22, 31]

REFERENCES

1. Alzamora-Castro, V., Battilana, G., Abugattas, R., and Sialer, S.: Patent ductus arteriosus and high altitude. Am. J. Cardiol. 5:761, 1960.
2. Amoroso, E. C., Dawes, G. S., and Mott, J. C.: Patency of the ductus arteriosus in the newborn calf and foal. Br. Heart J. 20:92, 1958.
3. Auld, P. A. M.: Delayed closure of the ductus arteriosus. J. Pediatr. 69:61, 1966.
4. Baden, M., and Kirks, D. R.: Transient dilatation of the ductus arteriosus—the "ductus bump". J. Pediatr. 84:858, 1974.
5. Baylen, B. G., Meyer, R. A., Kaplan, S., Rin-

genburg, W. E., and Korfhagen, J.: The critically ill premature infant with patent ductus arteriosus and pulmonary disease: An echocardiographic assessment. J. Pediatr. 86:423, 1975.
6. Braudo, M., and Rowe, R. D.: Auscultation of

the heart. Early neonatal period. Am. J. Dis. Child. 101:575, 1961.

7. Burnard, E. D.: A murmur that may arise from the ductus arteriosus in the human baby. Proc. R. Soc. Med. 52:77, 1959.

8. Carlgren, L-E.: The incidence of congenital heart disease in children born in Gothenburg 1941–1950. Br. Heart J. 21:40, 1959.

9. Clarkson, P. M., and Orgil, A. A.: Continuous murmurs in infants of low birth weight. J. Pediatr. 84:208, 1974.

10. Clyman, R. I.: Ontogeny of the ductus arteriosus response to prostaglandins and inhibitors of their synthesis. Semin. Perinatol. 4:115, 1980.

11. Clyman, R. I., and Heymann, M. A.: Pharmacology of the ductus arteriosus. Pediatr. Clin. North Am. 28:77, 1981.

12. Coceani, F., and Olley, P. M.: The response of the ductus arteriosus to prostaglandins. Can. J. Physiol. Pharmacol. 51:220, 1973.

13. Coceani, F., and Olley, P. M.: Role of prostaglandins, prostacyclin, and thromboxanes in the control of prenatal patency and postnatal closure of the ductus arteriosus. Semin. Perinatol. 4:109, 1980.

14. Cotton, R. B., Stahlman, M. T., Bender, H. W., Graham, T. P., Catterton, W. Z., and Kovar, I.: Randomized trial of early closure of symptomatic patent ductus arteriosus in small preterm infants. J. Pediatr. 93:647, 1978.

15. Danilowicz, D., Rudolph, A. M., and Hoffman, J. I. E.: Delayed closure of the ductus arteriosus in premature infants. Pediatrics 37:74, 1966.

16. Delivoria-Papadopoulos, M., Roncevic, N. P., and Oski, F. A.: Postnatal changes in oxygen transport of term, premature, and sick infants: The role of red cell 2,3-diphosphoglycerate and adult hemoglobin. Pediatr. Res. 5:235, 1971.

17. Edmunds, L. H., Jr., Gregory, G. A., Heymann, M. A., Kitterman, J. A., Rudolph, A. M., and Tooley, W. H.: Surgical closure of the ductus arteriosus in premature infants. Circulation 48:856, 1973.

18. Evans, J. R., Rowe, R. D., Downie, H. G., and Rowsell, H. C.: Murmurs arising from the ductus arteriosus in normal newborn swine. Circ. Res. 12:85, 1963.

19. Fay, F. S.: Guinea pig ductus arteriosus. I. Cellular and metabolic basis for oxygen sensitivity. Am. J. Physiol. 221:470, 1971.

20. Fay, F. S., and Cooke, P. H.: Guinea pig ductus arteriosus. II. Irreversible closure after birth. Am. J. Physiol. 222:841, 1972.

21. Fay, F. S., and Jobsis, F. F.: Guinea pig ductus arteriosus. III. Light absorption changes during response to O_2. Am. J. Physiol., 223:588, 1972.

22. Freed, M. D., Heymann, M. A., Lewis, A. B., Reischer, S., and Kensey, R. C.: PGE_1 in infants with ductus arteriosus dependent cyanotic cogenital heart disease. The U.S. experience. Circulation, 64:899, 1981.

23. Friedman, W. F.: The intrinsic physiologic properties of the developing heart. In Neonatal Heart Disease, edited by E. M. Sonnenblick. Grune & Stratton, New York, 1973, p. 21.

24. Friedman, W. F., Kurlinski, J., Jacob, J., DiSessa, T. G., Gluck, L., Merritt, T. A., and Feldman, B. H.: The inhibition of prostaglandin and prostacyclin synthesis in the clinical management of patent ductus arteriosus. Sem. Perinatol. 4:125, 1980.

25. Friedman, W. F., Pool, P. E., Jacobowitz, D., Seagren, S. C., and Braunwald, E.: Sympathetic innervation of the developing rabbit heart. Circ. Res. 23:25, 1968.

26. Gentile, R., Stevenson, G., Dooley, T., Franklin, D., Kawabori, I., and Pearlman, A.: Pulsed Doppler echocardiographic determination of time of ductal closure in normal newborn infants. J. Pediatr. 98:443, 1981.

27. Gibson, G. A.: Persistence of the arterial duct and its diagnosis. Edinburgh Med. J. 8:1, 1900.

28. Girling, D. J., and Hallidie-Smith, K. A.: Persistent ductus arteriosus in ill and premature babies. Arch. Dis. Child. 46:177, 1971.

29. Gittenberger-De Groot, A. C., Van Ertbruggen, I., Moulaert, A. J. M. G., and Harinck, E.: The ductus arteriosus in the preterm infant: Histologic and clinical observations. J. Pediatr. 96:88, 1980.

30. Gregory, G. A., Kitterman, J. A., Phibbs, R. H., Tooley, W. H., and Hamilton, W. K.: Treatment of the idiopathic respiratory-distress syndrome with continuous positive airway pressure. N. Engl. J. Med. 284:1333, 1971.

31. Heymann, M. A., Berman, W., Rudolph, A. M., and Whitman, V.: Dilatation of the ductus arteriosus by prostaglandin E1 in aortic arch abnormalities. Circulation 59:179, 1979.

32. Heymann, M. A., and Rudolph, A. M.: The effects of congenital heart disease on the fetal and neonatal circulation. Prog. Cardiovasc. Dis. 15:115, 1972.

33. Heymann, M. A., and Rudolph, A. M.: Control of the ductus arteriosus. Physiol. Rev. 55:62, 1975.

34. Heymann, M. A., and Rudolph, A. M.: Effects of acetylsalicylic acid on the ductus arteriosus and circulation in fetal lambs in utero. Circ. Res. 38:418, 1976.

35. Heymann, M. A., and Rudolph, A. M.: Ductus arteriosus dilatation by prostaglandin E1 in infants with pulmonary atresia. Pediatrics 59:325, 1977.

36. Heymann, M. A., Rudolph, A. M., and Silverman, N. H.: Closure of the ductus arteriosus in premature infants by inhibition of prostaglandin synthesis. N. Engl. J. Med. 295:530, 1976.

37. Hoffman, J. I. E.: Abnormal pulmonary circulation. In Pediatric Pulmonary Physiology and Disease, edited by E. M. Scarpelli, P. A. M. Auld, and H. S. Goldman, Lea & Febiger, Philadelphia, 1975.

38. Hoffman, J. I. E., and Buckberg, G. D.: Regional myocardial ischemia—causes, prediction and prevention. Vasc. Surg. 8:115, 1974.

39. Johnson, D. H., Rosenthal, A., and Nadas, A. S.: A forty-year review of bacterial endocarditis in infancy and childhood. Circulation 51:581, 1975.

40. Kitterman, J. A., Edmunds, L. H., Jr., Gregory, G. A., Heymann, M. A., Tooley, W. H., and Rudolph, A. M.: Patent ductus arteriosus in premature infants: Incidence, relation to pulmonary disease and management. N. Engl. J. Med. 287:473, 1972.

41. Knight, D. H., Patterson, D. F., and Melbin, J.: Constriction of the fetal ductus arteriosus induced by oxygen, acetylcholine and norepinephrine in normal dogs and those genetically predisposed to persistent patency. Circulation 47:127, 1973.

42. Knight, L., and Edwards, J. E.: Right aortic arch: Types and associated cardiac anomalies. Circulation 50:1047, 1974.

43. Lebowitz, E. A., Novick, J. S., and Rudolph, A. M.: Development of myocardial sympathetic innervation in the fetal lamb. Pediatr. Res. 6:887, 1972.

44. Lees, M. H.: Commentary: Patent ductus arteriosus in premature infants—a diagnostic and therapeutic dilemma. J. Pediatr. 86:132, 1975.

45. Levin, D. L., Stanger, P., Kitterman, J. A., and Heymann, M. A.: Congenital heart disease in low birth weight infants. Circulation 52:500, 1975.

46. Lister, G., Walter, T. K., Versmold, H. T., Dallman, P. R., and Rudolph, A. M.: Oxygen delivery in lambs: Cardiovascular and hematologic development. Am. J. Physiol. 237:H668, 1979.

47. McCarthy, J. S., Zies, L. G., and Gelband, H.: Age-dependent closure of the patent ductus arteriosus by indomethacin. Pediatrics 62:706, 1978.

48. McMurphy, D. M., Heymann, M. A., Rudolph, A. M., and Melmon, K. L.: Developmental change in constriction of the ductus arteriosus: Response to oxygen and vasoactive substances in the isolated ductus arteriosus of the fetal lamb. Pediatr. Res. 6:231, 1972.

49. Merritt, T. A., White, C. L., Jacob, J., Kurlinski, J., Martin, J., DiSessa, T. G., Edwards, D., Friedman, W. F., and Gluck, L.: Patent ductus arteriosus treated with ligation or indomethacin: A follow-up study. J. Pediatr. 95:588, 1979.

50. Mitchell, S. C., Korones, S. B., and Berendes, H. W.: Congenital heart disease in 56,109 births: Incidence and natural history. Circulation 43:323, 1971.

51. Moss, A. J., Emmanouilides, G. C. Adams, F. H., and Chuang, K.: Response of ductus arteriosus and pulmonary and systemic arterial pressure to changes in oxygen environment in newborn infants. Pediatrics 33:937, 1964.

52. Moss, A. J., Emmanouilides, G. C., and Duffie, E. R., Jr.: Closure of the ductus arteriosus in the newborn infant. Pediatrics 32:25, 1963.

53. Neal, W. A., Bessinger, F. B., Jr., Hunt, C. E., and Lucas, R. V.: Patent ductus arteriosus complicating respiratory distress syndrome. J. Pediatr. 86:127, 1975.

54. Oberhansli-Weiss, I., Heymann, M. A., Rudolph, A. M., and Melmon, K. L.: The pattern and mechanisms of response to oxygen by the ductus arteriosus and umbilical artery. Pediatr. Res. 6:693, 1972.

55. Porstmann, W., Wierny, L., Warnke, H., Gerstberger, G., and Romaniuk, P. A.: Catheter closure of patent ductus arteriosus: 62 cases treated without thoracotomy. Radiol. Clin. North Am. 9:203, 1971.

56. Powell, M. L.: Patent ductus arteriosus in premature infants. Med. J. Aust. 2:58, 1963.

57. Rudolph, A. M.: Congenital Diseases of the Heart. Year Book Medical Publishers, Chicago, 1974.

58. Rudolph, A. M.: The changes in the circulation after birth: Their importance in congenital heart disease. Circulation 41:343, 1970.

59. Rudolph, A. M., Drorbaugh, J. E., Auld, P. A. M., Rudolph, A. J., Nadas, A. S., Smith, C. A., and Hubbell, J. P.: Studies on the circulation in the neonatal period. The circulation in the respiratory distress syndrome. Pediatrics 27:551, 1961.

60. Rudolph, A. M., Heymann, M. A., Fishman, N., and Lakier, J. B.: Formalin infiltration of the ductus arteriosus: A method for palliation of infants with selected congenital cardiac lesions. N. Engl. J. Med. 292:1263, 1975.

61. Rudolph, A. M., Heymann, M. A., and Spitznas, U.: Hemodynamic considerations in the development of narrowing of the aorta. Am. J. Cardiol. 30:514, 1972.

62. Rudolph, A. M., Mayer, F. E., Nadas, A. S., and Gross, R. E.: Patent ductus arteriosus. A clinical andhemodynamic study of patients in the first year of life. Pediatrics 22:892, 1958.

63. Rudolph, A. M., Mesel, E., and Levy, J. M.: Epinephrine in the treatment of cardiac failure due to shunts. Circulation 28:3, 1963.

64. Rudolph, A. M., Scarpelli, E. M., Golinki, R. J., and Gootman, N.: Hemodynamic basis for clinical manifestations of patent ductus arteriosus. Am. Heart J. 68:447, 1964.

65. Sahn, D. J., Allen, H. D., Goldberg, S. J., Solinger, R., and Meyer, R. A.: Pediatric echocardiography: A review of its clinical utility. J. Pediatr. 87:335, 1975.

66. Sato, K., Fujino, M., Kozuka, T., Naito, Y., Kitamura, S., Nakano, S., Ohyama, C., and Kawashima, Y.: Transfemoral plug closure of patent ductus arteriosus: Experience in 61 consecutive cases treated without thoracotomy. Circulation 51:337, 1975.

67. Serwer, G. A., Armstrong, B. E., and Anderson,

P. A. W.: Noninvasive detection of retrograde descending aortic flow in infants using continuous wave Doppler ultrasonography. J. Pediatr. 97:394, 1980.

68. Siassi, B., Emmanouilides, G. C., Cleveland, R. J., and Hirose, F.: Patent ductus arteriosus complicating prolonged assisted ventilation in respiratory distress syndrome. J. Pediatr. 74:11, 1969.

69. Silverman, N. H., Lewis, A. B., Heymann, M. A., and Rudolph, A. M.: Echocardiographic assessment of ductus arteriosus shunt in premature infants. Circulation 50:821, 1974.

70. Strauss, H. W., Wagner, H. N., Jr., Wesselhoeft, H., and Hurley, P. J.: Radionuclide angiocardiography in pediatrics. In Pediatric Nuclear Medicine, edited by A. E. James, H. N. Wagner, and R. E. Cooke. W. B. Saunders, Philadelphia, 1974.

71. Thibeault, D. W., Emmanouilides, G. C., Nelson, R. J., Lachman, R. S., Rosengart, R. M. and Oh, W.: Patent ductus arteriosus complicating the respiratory distress syndrome in preterm infants. J. Pediatr. 86:120, 1975.

72. Treves, S., Maltz, D. L., and Adelstein, S. J.: Intracardiac shunts. In Pediatric Nuclear Medicine, edited by A. E. James, H. N. Wagner, and R. E. Cooke. W. B. Saunders, Philadelphia, 1974.

73. Tsang, R. C., Light, I. J., Sutherland, J. M., and Kleinman, L.: Possible pathogenetic factors in neonatal hypocalcemia of prematurity. J. Pediatr. 82:423, 1973.

74. Yeh, T. F., Luken, J. A., Thalji, A., Raval, D., Carr, I. and Pildes, R. S.: Intravenous indomethacin therapy in premature infants with persistent ductus arteriosus—a double-blind controlled study. J. Pediatr. 98:137, 1981.

12

Aortic Stenosis

William F. Friedman, M.D., and Lee N. Benson, M.D.

Each of the specific congenital cardiovascular malformations that causes obstruction to the ejection of blood from the left ventricle will be discussed separately. These malformations include valvar aortic stenosis, the discrete form of subaortic stenosis, narrowing of the supravalvar ascending aorta, and some forms of idiopathic hypertrophic subaortic stenosis (see Chapter 48).

VALVAR AORTIC STENOSIS

Valvar aortic stenosis (AS) has been considered to occur in approximately 3 to 6% of patients with congenital cardiovascular defects. It is not widely appreciated that the congenital bicuspid aortic valve may actually be the most common congenital malformation of the heart.[50, 105] This anomaly is often undetected in early life, and since bicuspid valves may become stenotic with time, it may become of clinical significance only in adult life. At that time a congenitally deformed valve may be indistinguishable from one in which the stenosis has been acquired, and for this reason the true prevalence of the congenital malformation may be grossly underestimated.[106] Valvar aortic stenosis occurs far more often in males than in females, with the sex ratio approximating 4:1. The prevalence of associated cardiovascular anomalies may be as high as 20%.[16] Patent ductus arteriosus and coarctation of the aorta occur most frequently with valvar AS, and all three of these lesions may coexist. There is also a high prevalence of a bicuspid, but not necessarily stenotic, aortic valve in association with coarctation of the aorta.[116] Less commonly, ventricular septal defect or isolated pulmonic stenosis are associated with valvar aortic stenosis.

PATHOLOGY

Thickening and increased rigidity of the valve tissue and varying degrees of commissural fusion comprise the basic malformation (Fig. 12.1). Most often the aortic valve is bicuspid with a single, fused commissure and an eccentrically placed orifice; a third incomplete or rudimentary commissure may sometimes be apparent. Less commonly, the stenotic aortic valve is unicuspid and dome-shaped with no or one lateral attachment to the aorta at the level of the orifice. Rarely, the valve has three fused cusps with a stenotic, central office. The aortic valve ring may be relatively underdeveloped in infants and young children with severe valvar

AS, a lesion which represents a segment of the spectrum extending to the hypoplastic left heart syndrome and the aortic hypoplasia and atresia. The dynamics of blood flow associated with a congenitally deformed aortic valve commonly lead to thickening of the cusps and ultimately to calcification in later life. Secondary calcification of the valve is extremely rare in childhood. When the obstruction is hemodynamically significant, concentric hypertrophy of the left ventricular wall and dilatation of the ascending aorta occur.

PHYSIOLOGY

The essential hemodynamic abnormality produced by the obstruction to left ventricular outflow is the pressure gradient between the left ventricle and aorta during the systolic ejection period. This gradient rarely exceeds 200 mm Hg. Since blood flow across stenotic heart valves is turbulent, the transvalvar pressure gradient is not a simple linear function of the flow, but rather is directly proportional to the square of the flow rates across the valve.[58] Thus, a doubling of blood flow across a stenotic aortic valve is associated with approximately a quadrupling of the pressure gradient. In addition, the ejection gradient varies with changes in the contractile state of the left ventricle and peripheral vascular resistance in the absence of changes in cardiac output. The gradient may increase under the influence of positive inotropic stimuli or decrease when distal systemic resistance is increased. Accurate determination of the severity of valvar stenosis by measurement of the transvalvar pressure gradient alone is not possible. Because the gradient is determined primarily by the flow, as well as by the size of the orifice, it is clear that to assess the hemodynamic severity of obstruction, it is necessary to measure both the transvalvar flow rate and pressure gradient simultaneously. When valvar insufficiency exists, the flow across the valve is the sum of the effective cardiac output and of the regurgitant flow. Because most clinical techniques for measuring blood flow record only the effective cardiac output, the valvar flow may be underestimated, and the severity of the stenotic lesion may be falsely exaggerated if allowance is not made for the associated insufficiency. In addition, since alterations in heart rate modify the fraction of the cardiac cycle during which blood flows across cardiac valves, changes in rate alter the velocity of transvalvar blood flow

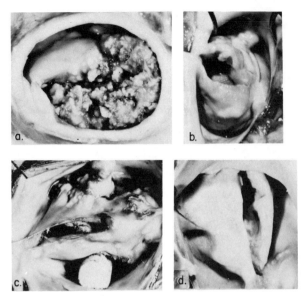

Fig. 12.1 Aortic valve, as seen from above, is shown in four patients who died of congenital valvar aortic stenosis. *a* and *b*, dome-shaped, unicuspid, unicommissural valves. The patient whose valve is shown in *a* had a peak systolic gradient of 90 mm Hg; in *b*, the gradient was 125 mm Hg. The bicuspid valves shown in *c* and *d* were responsible for gradients of 70 mm Hg and 90 mm Hg, respectively.

at any given level of cardiac output; an increase in heart rate shortens diastole relatively more than systole and therefore increases the total time available for flow across the aortic valve. A peak systolic pressure gradient exceeding 75 mm Hg, in association with a normal cardiac output, or an effective aortic orifice less than 0.5 cm²/m² of body surface area, is considered to reflect critical obstruction to left ventricular outflow.[46, 47] The effective systolic orifice area of the aortic valve is calculated using the Gorlin formula[58]: area (cm²) = [blood flow (ml per sec)]/[√mean gradient (mm Hg) × K (44.5)]. The mean systolic gradient is determined by planimetry after adjusting left ventricular and systemic arterial pressure tracings for pulse delay. The normal outflow orifice approximates 2.0 cm²/m² body surface area; areas of 0.5 to 0.8 cm²/m² signify moderate obstruction; and when the area is larger than 0.8 cm²/m² the obstruction is considered to be mild.

The mean left atrial pressure is usually normal, unless severe obstruction is present. While the V wave is the tallest wave in the left atrial pressure pulse of normal subjects, the A wave predominates in AS because of usually forceful left atrial contraction, diminished ventricular compliance, or a combination of these factors.[16] A vigorous atrial contraction tends to elevate the left ventricular end-diastolic pressure without elevating the mean left atrial pressure to the same extent. The augmentation of left ventricular filling by left atrial contraction in aortic stenosis prevents the pulmonary venous pressure from rising to levels which would produce pulmonary congestion, while maintaining the left ventricular end-diastolic pressure at the level necessary for effective left ventricular contraction.

Most children with AS have a left ventricular end-diastolic pressure in the upper normal range. When this pressure is elevated, it indicates either that left ventricular function is impaired and/or that left ventricular hypertrophy is sufficiently severe to have reduced the compliance of this chamber. The left ventricular pressure pulse exhibits a rounded or peaked, (instead of flat-topped) summit as the contraction of the ventricle becomes progressively more isometric with

more severe obstruction to left ventricular outflow. (Fig. 12.2) Mechanical pulsus alternans occur rarely in younger patients with aortic stenosis, even when the obstruction is severe.[27] The ascending limb of the central aortic pressure pulse rises steeply during early ejection but is soon interrupted by an anacrotic notch, following which the pressure rises more slowly. With increasing degrees of stenosis the initial steep rise becomes progressively shorter, and the anacrotic shoulder occupies a lower level on the pressure pulse.[55]

The resting cardiac output and stroke volume are generally within normal limits. During exercise, most children with critical stenosis show an elevation of the cardiac output with an associated increase in the transvalvar pressure gradient.[28] When left ventricular failure occurs, the cardiac output decreases, and the left ventricular end-diastolic, left atrial, and pulmonary vascular pressures increase.

The blood supply to the myocardium may be compromised in patients with aortic stenosis despite wide patency of the coronary arteries.[18, 87] Oxygen supply to the myocardium is determined by coronary blood flow and arterial oxygen content. Since intramyocardial compressive forces are greatest in the subendocardium, it may be expected that flow to that region of left ventricle would be entirely diastolic in the presence of the elevated left ventricular systolic pressure. In patients with AS, coronary vasodilatation may give an inadequate response to an increase at rest or with exercise in the demands of the myocardium for oxygen. Once subendocardial vessels are maximally dilated, the coronary artery driving pressure and the duration of diastole are the principal determinants of the magnitude of subendocardial flow. Diastole is shortened, especially at high heart rates, when systolic ejection lengthens across the stenotic orifice. Moreover, coronary driving pressure is reduced if left ventricular end-diastolic pressure is high or if aortic diastolic pressure is low, e.g., with heart failure or aortic insufficiency. In critical aortic stenosis, the redistribution of flow away from the subendocardium and the resulting ischemia of that portion of ventricular muscle may be estimated by relating the diastolic pressure time index (DPTI), the area between the aortic and left ventricular pressures in diastole, to the systolic pressure time index (SPTI), a measure of myocardial oxygen demands.[65, 66] Inadequate subendocardial oxygen de-

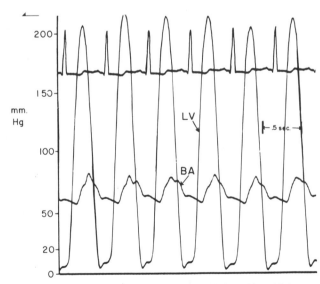

Fig. 12.2 Simultaneous left ventricular (*LV*) and brachial artery (*BA*) pressure tracings, in valvar aortic stenosis. The systolic pressure gradient was 129 mm Hg.

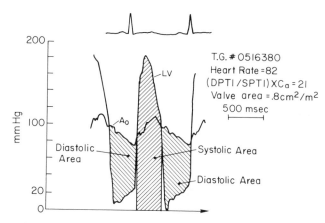

Fig. 12.3 Redrawn aortic (A_o) and left ventricular (LV) pressure curves used for calculation of the subendocardial flow index. The systolic pressure time index ($SPTI$) is the area under the LV curve during aortic ejection. The diastolic pressure time index ($DPTI$) is the area under the A_o curve during the period when A_o pressure is greater than LV, minus the LV end-diastolic pressure. The ratio $DPTI \times$ arterial oxygen content (Ca)/$SPTI$ is proportional to myocardial oxygen consumption.

livery has been shown to exist when the ratio DPTI × arterial oxygen content/SPTI falls below 10 (Fig. 12.3).

MANIFESTATIONS

Clinical Features

Aortic stenosis may be responsible for severe obstruction to left ventricular outflow without the clinical symptoms of diminished cardiac reserve that are so frequent in other forms of congenital heart disease. Conversely, in an occasional patient with mild obstruction, the clinical findings may be striking. Most children with AS are asymptomatic and grow and develop normally. Initial attention is usually called to these children only when murmur is detected on a routine examination. When symptoms occur, those most commonly noted are: fatigability, exertional dyspnea, angina pectoris, and syncope.[16] Less frequently described are: abdominal pain, profuse sweating, and epistaxis. The obstruction is at least moderately severe if there is a history of fatigability and exertional dyspnea. Exertional syncope occurs usually only in patients with critical stenosis and is related to inability of the left ventricle to increase its output and to maintain cerebral flow during exercise.[16] The disparity between the oxygen supply to the left ventricle and myocardial oxygen requirements is responsible for anginal pain.

Endocarditis occurs in approximately 4% of patients with valvar aortic stenosis; no correlation appears to exist with severity of obstruction. Sudden death is another potential threat, occurring in various series in from 1 to 19% of patients.[46, 51, 74] The children who have died in this manner had severe obstruction, and most had been symptomatic before death[31, 69]; frequently, a temporal relation exists to strenuous physical activity.[86] The precise cause of death in these patients is poorly understood, but ventricular dysrhythmias, perhaps initiated by acute myocardial ischemia, is probably the most common inciting event. Speculation exists that an abrupt rise in intracavitary pressure excites a reflex hypotensive syncope that promotes acute ischemia and ventricular fibrillation.

When the degree of AS is significant, a left ventricular lift is usually palpable. If the systolic pressure gradient across the aortic valve exceeds approximately 25 mm Hg, a precordial systolic thrill is often palpated over the base of the heart with transmission to the jugular notch and along the carotid arteries. Ordinarily the obstruction is mild if neither a left ventricular lift nor a thrill is present. The increased force of left atrial contraction in the presence of left ventricular hypertrophy results in a palpable presystolic expansion. The latter sign is almost always associated with a severe degree of obstruction and an elevated left ventricular end-diastolic pressure.

A systolic aortic ejection sound may be heard at the cardiac apex when the valve is mobile and can be differentiated from a pulmonic ejection sound and from the tricuspid valve closure sound by its prominence at the apex, its failure to change in intensity during respiration, and its temporal relation to the onset of the carotid upstroke (Fig. 12.4).[15] The aortic ejection sound is more often heard in patients with mild or moderate stenosis than in those with severe stenosis. In most instances the opening of the aortic valves is responsible for the ejection sound. Disappearance of the ejection sound suggest that progression of stenosis has occurred. The abnormal behavior of the second heart sound in many patients with severe aortic stenosis can be attributed to prolongation of left ventricular emptying which accompanies a greatly increased resistance to left ventricular ejection. Delayed closure of the aortic valve leads to a single or a closely split second heart sound.[16] With more severe degrees of obstruction (transvalvar systolic pressure gradients exceeding 75 mm Hg), there is little or no widening of the interval between the aortic and pulmonic components during inspiration. Less often, the aortic closure sound actually precedes the pulmonic sound during expiration; i.e., paradoxical splitting is present.

An early diastolic filling sound (third heart sound) is a common finding in normal children and is detected even more frequently in children with aortic stenosis. In the absence of PR-interval prolongation, the presence of a fourth (atrial) heart sound reflects increased vigor of atrial systole during active ventricular filling. This is especially true in older children and adolescents, in whom a physiologic fourth heart sound is infrequently heard. In patients with aortic stenosis the presence of a fourth heart sound is generally associated with severe obstruction, insofar as hypertrophy of the left ventricle increases the resistance to passive filling of the latter chamber.[16, 20]

The systolic murmur which is characteristic of valvar aortic stenosis starts after the completion of left ventricular isometric contraction or with the ejection sound, and is rhomboid shaped, loud, harsh, and best heard at the base of the heart (Fig. 12.4). The murmur, like the thrill, radiates to the jugular notch and carotid vessels as well as to the apex. The configuration, but not the duration of the murmur, may be helpful in assessing the severity of stenosis, since the murmur tends to reach its peak during the last 60% of ventricular systole when the gradient exceeds 75 mm Hg, although the converse is not always true.[16, 46, 55] In approximately one-fourth of the patients with valvar aortic stenosis, an early diastolic murmur of aortic insufficiency is present. Since the regurgitation is usually not hemodynamically significant, the diastolic murmur is faint, and the arterial pulse pressure is normal. However, erosion of the valve leaflets by endocarditis may produce aortic insufficiency severe enough to be the predominant lesion.

Indirect Pulse Tracings

The external jugular venous pulse frequently reveals an increased amplitude of the atrial contraction (A) wave, even in the absence of pulmonary hypertension.[15, 16] Indirect carotid arterial pulse tracings may be of particular diagnostic help and show a prominent anacrotic notch or shoulder,

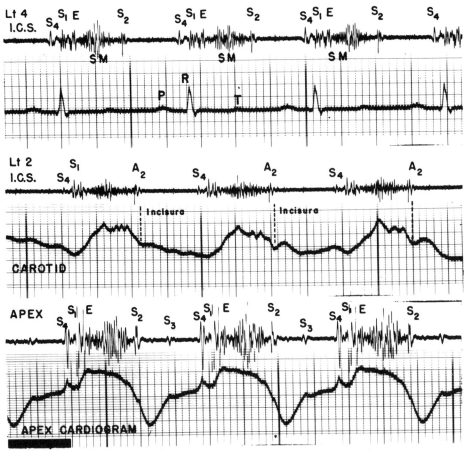

Fig. 12.4 Phonocardiogram, indirect arterial carotid pulse tracing, and apex cardiogram in a patient with valvar aortic stenosis. The carotid pulse tracing exhibits a prolonged upstroke with a systolic plateau. The apex cardiogram shows a presystolic pulsation and a sustained systolic plateau. S_1, S_2, S_3, and S_4 refer to the first, second, third, and fourth heart sounds. *SM*, systolic murmur; *E*, ejection sound. (Reproduced with permission from E. Braunwald et al.[16])

followed by a rounded or delayed peak, often with superimposed systolic vibrations ("carotid shudder") and a delayed incisura (Fig. 12.4). Additional alterations in the systemic arterial pressure pulse include: a decreased rate of rise of intraarterial pressure; a narrow pulse pressure; and a prolongation of the ejection period (time interval from the onset of the anacrotic rise to the incisura) and the upstroke time (time interval from the onset of the anacrotic rise to the peak) (Fig. 12.5) While the various pulse characteristics are helpful in identifying the presence of aortic stenosis, attempts to assess its severity by pulse analysis have not always been successful.[15, 64]

Electrovectorcardiographic Features

Although the electrocardiographic findings may vary with the severity of obstruction,[51, 70] a normal or near normal electrocardiogram does not exclude severe stenosis.[16, 101, 104] The lack of a good correlation between the electrocardiogram and the transvalvar pressure gradient emphasize the potential hazard of overreliance on the electrocardiogram in patient management.[45] In patients under 10 years of age the electrocardiogram appears to be a more reliable guide in indicating the severity of the stenosis than in older patients (Fig. 12.6).[16] The findings in the younger age group that tend to accompany severe obstruction are T wave vectors in the frontal plane to the left of −40°, widening of the angle between the mean QRS and T forces in the frontal plane in excess of 100°, an S wave in V1 greater than 16 mm, and an R wave in V5 exceeding 20 mm. It is important to recognize,

however, that some patients in whom these voltages are exceeded do not have severe stenosis. The most reliable index of the severity of obstruction in patients not receiving digitalis is the left ventricular "strain pattern," which consists of the findings of left ventricular hypertrophy combined with ST segment depressions and T wave inversion in the left precordial leads (Fig. 12.7). This pattern generally indicates that severe aortic stenosis is present. In a collaborative study, a formula was proposed for predicting the severity of AS; the formula utilized the intensity of the cardiac murmur and the magnitude of the R and Q waves in lead V6. Mild stenosis (gradient less than 50 mm Hg) was predicted accurately in 80% of patients; however, the formula also predicted the presence of mild stenosis in 20% of patients with measured gradients in excess of 80 mm Hg (117, 118).

The vectocardiogram best demonstrates the major influences of the left ventricular wall in the later phases of the QRS loop, and left ventricular hypertrophy is reflected in the abnormal displacement of the mean spatial QRS vector in a posterior, superior, and leftward direction, with maximal QRS forces exceeding 1.4 mv and QRS-T angle exceeding 60° (Fig. 12.7).[51] Infrequently, depolarization of the posterobasal left ventricle and/or the superior aspect of the interventricular septum results in large terminal rightward vectors. The right bundle branch block patterns observed in this settng[88] are the result of left rather than right ventricular hypertrophy. Correlations that have been reported between the vectorcardiographic alterations and the severity of obstruction in patients with aortic stenosis have not been

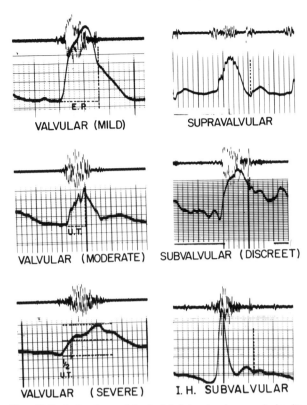

VALVULAR (MILD)

SUPRAVALVULAR

VALVULAR (MODERATE)

SUBVALVULAR (DISCREET)

VALVULAR (SEVERE)

I. H. SUBVALVULAR

Fig. 12.5 Indirect carotid arterial pulse tracings and simultaneous phonocardiograms in patients with various forms of obstruction to left ventricular outflow. *E.P.*, ejection period; *U.T.*, upstroke time. The indirect carotid pulse normally rises rapidly to a single rounded peak and then declines to the incisura. The contour of the pulse in idiopathic hypertrophic (*I.H.*) subaortic stenosis (*lower right*) differs from the others and exhibits a rapid rise, a midsystolic dip, and a secondary systolic rise. (Reproduced with permission from E. Braunwald *et al.*: Circulation (Suppl. 4):29–30, 1964.)

verified in other studies.[46, 70] Occasionally, the vectorcardiogram may indicate the presence of severe aortic stenosis when the electrocardiogram does not.

Exercise Testing

Treadmill or bicycle exercise is employed frequently in the evaluation of children with aortic stenosis.[2, 22, 61, 68, 70, 73, 122] Several laboratories have reported that exercise-induced ST depression ≥ 1 mm indicates a transvalvar pressure difference in excess of 50 mm Hg. Reports exist, however, of patients with significant ST depression and left ventricle to aortic pressure differences less than 30 mm Hg.[73] A relationship appears to exist between symptoms evoked during exercise, such as dyspnea, chest pain, dizziness, or palpitations, and work capacity and blood pressure, and changes in the electrocardiogram during exercise.

During monitored exercise, a fall or a lack of rise in systolic blood pressure suggests the presence of severe obstruction[103]; an inverse relationship appears to exist between severity of obstruction and total expended work or exercise time.[73]

Hemodynamic studies at rest and with exercise in children with valvar AS suggest that even severe aortic stenosis is usually associated with relatively normal cardiac function during exercise.[98] In contrast to adult studies, relatively few children show a reduction in stroke volume with increasing left ventricular end-diastolic pressure, suggesting ventricular dysfunction. Interpretation must be cautious in patients with aortic insufficiency, since true forward stroke volume is underestimated by the Fick technique.

Radiologic Features

The overall heart size is normal or the degree of enlargement is minimal in most patients. Concentric left ventricular hypertrophy accompanies moderate or severe obstruction and is manifested by rounding of the cardiac apex in the frontal projection and posterior displacement in the lateral view (Fig. 12.8). Striking left ventricular enlargement may exist in the presence of severe obstruction, although the roentgenographic size of the left ventricle does not correlate closely with the size of the aortic orifice, the left ventricular systolic pressure, or the peak transvalvar pressure gradient. Left atrial enlargement strongly suggests that a severe degree of stenosis exists.[16]

Severe obstruction may also produce pulmonary congestion and enlargement of the pulmonary artery, right ventricle, and right atrium. Poststenotic dilatation of the ascending aorta is a common finding in patients with a valvar AS. Roentgenographic evidence of calcification of the valve does not usually occur in the pediatric age group but is a relatively common finding in adults with congenital AS.

Echocardiographic Features

The single crystal ultrasound findings that may suggest the diagnosis of aortic valve stenosis include diminished systolic valve echo excursions toward the aortic wall, multiple diastolic echoes, eccentric diastolic closure lines, and an increased dimension of the aortic root (Fig. 12.9).[34, 59, 94, 124] The aortic eccentricity index (one-half the internal diameter of the aortic root divided by the shortest distance to the aortic wall in diastole) has been used to identify the presence of a bicuspid aortic valve. The index for normal values is usually 1.0 to 1.2; in bicuspid valves this value ranges from 1.5 to 4.5. Real time cross-sectional echocardiography reveals impaired mobility of cusp tissue, an alteration in the phasic movement of the aortic valve with reduced lateral and increased superior excursions of valve echoes, and an increase in the internal aortic root dimension beyond the level of the valve annulus (Fig. 12.10).[121, 124] A correlation has been shown by cross-sectional echo methods between the peak systolic pressure gradient and the rate of maximal aortic cusp separation/aortic root diameter, although refinements in the technique are required.[119] Moreover, the validity of cusp separation measurements has been questioned.[23]

An increase in left ventricular wall thickness by echocardiography implies severe obstruction, and estimates of left ventricular pressure have been derived from measurements of posterior left ventricular wall thickness in end-systole divided by end-systolic diameter × 225 (Fig. 12.11).[5] The difference between the echo-derived left ventricular pressure and the cuff-measured arterial blood pressure provides an estimate of the transvalvar aortic gradient (Fig. 12.12).[12, 56, 60, 75, 108] It would also appear that end-diastolic dimensions may be accurate for predicting left ventricular peak systolic pressure by echocardiography. Using measurements of left ventricular end-diastolic posterior and septal wall thickness and left ventricular minor axis, a regression equation has been developed in which left ventricular systolic pressure (mm Hg) equals 6 + 298 (H/R) ± 13.4; H equals mean of posterior and septal end-diastolic wall thickness at the equator, and R equals the end-diastolic minor semiaxis (half the end-diastolic minor axis).[1] The presence of aortic insufficiency may reduce the predictive accuracy of both of these determinations.

Pulse Doppler echocardiography allows inspection of the pattern of flow velocity within the circulation.[76] The technique detects the altered and disturbed turbulence of flow in patients with aortic stenosis; current investigations seek to

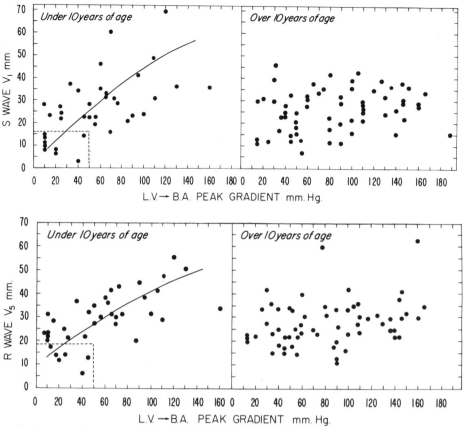

Fig. 12.6 Relationship between depth of the S wave in Lead V1 (*top*) and height of the R wave in lead V5 and the systolic pressure gradients in patients with aortic stenosis. An S wave in V1 less than 11 mm and an R wave in V5 less than 18 mm always denoted a systolic gradient less than 50 mm Hg in children below the age of 10 years. *L.V.*, left ventricle; *B.A.*, brachial artery. (Reproduced with permission from E. Braunwald et al.[16])

quantify the severity of obstruction with pulse Doppler ultrasound.[63, 126]

CARDIAC CATHETERIZATION

Cardiac catheterization is more important for establishing the site and severity, rather than the presence, of obstruction to left ventricular outflow, since the malformation is usually readily diagnosed by clinically examination.[45] Catheterization is indicated in any child with a clinical diagnosis of AS in whom the clinical examination, roentgenogram, or resting or exercise electrocardiogram suggests the possibility of severe obstruction.[45, 46] Even in the absence of such findings, catheterization should be prformed if symptoms exist which might be related to AS.

Precise assessment of the site and severity of obstruction is best obtained by combined right and left heart catheterization. Right heart catheterization is helpful in detecting or excluding associated malformations such as patent ductus arteriosus, ventricular septal defect, or pulmonic stenosis. If a coexistent left to right shunt is excluded and pulmonary hypertension is present, the obstruction to left ventricular outflow is generally severe, and prompt surgical treatment should be considered.

There are a number of techniques that may be employed to catheterize the left side of the heart. Whenever possible we prefer the retrograde approach by percutaneous puncture. Cardiac output is measured by the indicator-dilution, thermodilution, or Fick technique. Retrograde left heart catheterization allows withdrawal pressure recordings across

the site of stenosis, and left ventricular angiocardiography can be carried out permitting an evaluation of the size of the left ventricular cavity, the thickness of the wall, the degree of deformity and mobility of the aortic valve leaflets, the competency of the mitral valve, the patency of the coronary arteries, and the diameter of the aortic root and ascending aorta. If aortic insufficiency is thought to be present, cineangiocardiography is performed with injection of contrast material into the aortic root. The severity can be assessed qualitatively by cineaortography and quantitatively by left ventriculography with calculation of regurgitant volume by subtraction of net forward flow (calculated by the Fick method) from angiographically determined total forward flow.[80] The typical angiocardiographic features of valvar stenosis are thickening of the aortic cusps and of the left ventricular cavity, poststenotic dilatation of the ascending aorta, and, occasionally, a jet of contrast material entering the ascending aorta through a central or eccentric, narrowed valve orifice (Fig. 12.13a).[113] The leaflets of the bicuspid valve are domed in systole, and a central jet corresponds to the orifice of the stenotic valve. In contrast, the stenotic orifice of the unicommissural valve can be visualized by the systolic jet in contact with the posterior wall of the aorta with leaflet tissue and valve motion seen only anteriorly.[113] If retrograde left heart catheterization is unsuccessful, the left ventricle may be entred by the transseptal method or by direct percutaneous puncture.[16, 55] When combined with the indicator-dilution method, the latter technique permits simultaneous determination of the transvalvar flow rate and pressure gradient but does not allow precise localization of the site of obstruction.

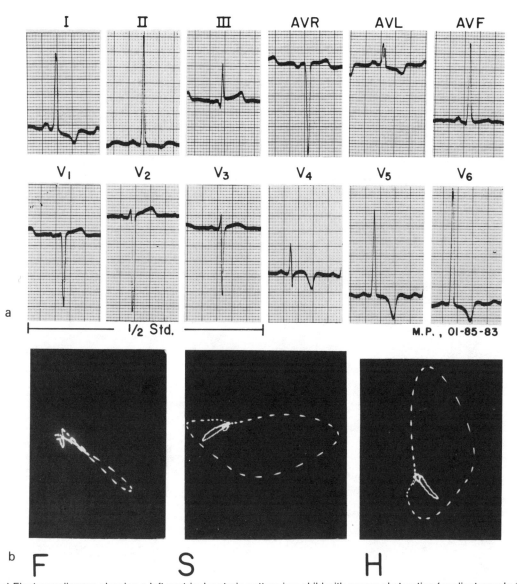

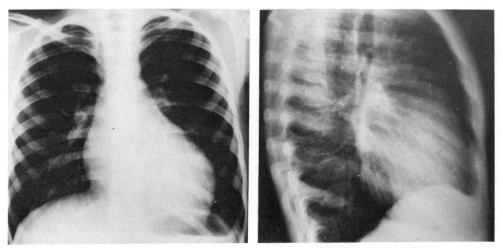

Fig. 12.7 (*a*) Electrocardiogram showing a left ventricular strain pattern in a child with severe obstruction (gradient equals 110 mm Hg.) (*b*) Vectorcardiogram (VCG) by the Frank system in a boy with a 150 mm Hg peak systolic gradient. There is posterior displacement of the QRS loop, increased maximum spatial voltage, and reduced 0.01- and 0.02-sec vectors, and an abnormal QRS-T angle. *F*, *S*, and *H* refer to the frontal, sagittal, and horizontal vector loops, respectively.

Fig. 12.8 Roentgenograms of a 13-year-old boy with severe valvar aortic stenosis (systolic gradient equals 116 mm Hg). The heart is moderately enlarged, and left ventricular hypertrophy is evident.

NATURAL HISTORY

Progression in the stenosis differs in various studies. It is clear that congenital AS is frequently a progresive disorder, even early in life, in a significant fraction of patients presenting initially with mild obstruction.[25, 33, 44] Thus, clinical deterioration may be anticipated because of an intensification of the severity of obstruction, rather than the development of significant aortic insufficiency. The intensification of obstruction is usually the result of the increase in cardiac output that occurs with body growth. Occasionally, a decrease has been noted in the area of the orifice as an added factor in the progression of obstruction. The onset of symptoms or changes in the phonocardiogram or graphic pulse

tracings, chest roentgenograms, electrocardiograms, or vectorcardiograms do not appear to be reliable markers of progressive obstruction in any individual patient.[44] Accordingly, we recommend repeat hemodynamic evaluation at approximately 5- to 10-year intervals in asymptomatic children with mild to moderate AS (Fig. 12.14).[49, 50]

TREATMENT

Since the malformed aortic valve is a potential site of bacterial infection, careful prophylaxis should be followed in all patients, regardless of the severity of obstruction. Avoidance of strenuous physical activity is advised if severe stenosis is present. Participation in competitive sports should probably also be restricted in patients with milder degrees of obstruction. Digitalis should be administered to patients with symptoms of diminished cardiac reserve and should also be considered in patients with left ventricular hypertrophy, even if they are not in heart failure.[45, 49]

The most critical decision concerns the advisability of

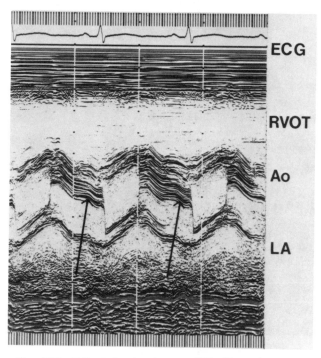

Fig. 12.9 Echocardiogram from a child with aortic stenosis showing multiple diastolic closure lines in the aortic lumen (*Ao*) (*arrows*). Although cusp separation appears normal, a 50 mm Hg peak systolic gradient was measured at cardiac catheterization. *LA*, left atrium; *RVOT*, right ventricular outflow tract. (Courtesy of Thomas DiSessa, M.D.)

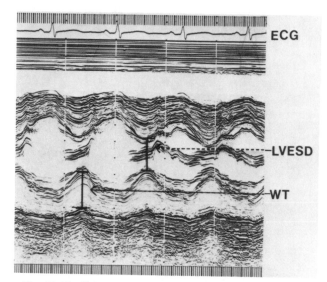

Fig. 12.11 Echocardiogram of the left ventricle below the level of the mitral valve, at the level of the chordae tenineae, demonstrating the proper technique for determining the left ventricular peak systolic pressure in patients with aortic stenosis. Estimated left ventricular peak systolic pressure (*LVPSP*) equals 225 × LV wall thickness (*WT*)/LV end-systolic dimension (*LVESD*). (Courtesy Thomas DiSessa, M.D.)

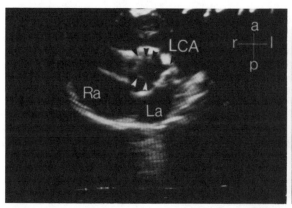
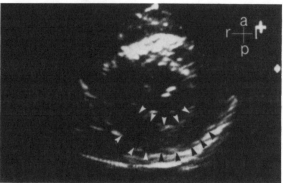

Fig. 12.10 Short axis 2D view through the base of the heart (*left panel*) reveals an eccentric, thickened bicuspid aortic valve (*arrows*). In the same patient, a short axis view of the left ventricle (*right panel*) reveals a thickened left ventricular wall (*arrows*). *a*, anterior; *Ra*, right atrium; *La*, left atrium; *LCA*, left coronary artery. (Courtesy Thomas DiSessa, M.D.)

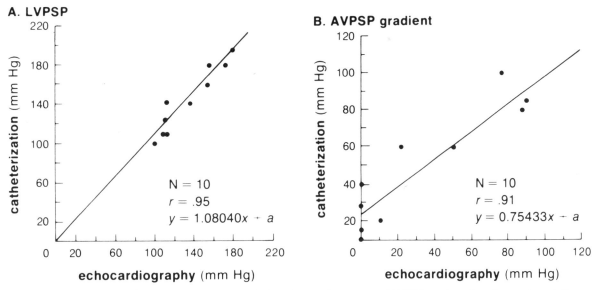

A. LVPSP

B. AVPSP gradient

A. catheterization (mm Hg) vs echocardiography (mm Hg)

N = 10
r = .95
$y = 1.08040x + a$

B. catheterization (mm Hg) vs echocardiography (mm Hg)

N = 10
r = .91
$y = 0.75433x + a$

Fig. 12.12 Reliability of echocardiography in estimating LV peak systolic pressure (*LVPSP*) and aortic valve peak systolic pressure gradient (*AVPSP*) in children compared with pressures obtained at cardiac catheterization. (Reproduced with permission from A. D. Hagan et al.[60])

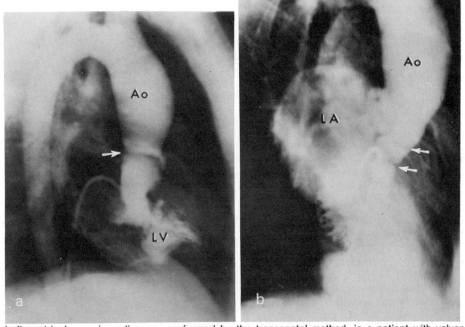

Fig. 12.13 (*a*) Left ventricular angiocardiogram, performed by the transseptal method, in a patient with valvar aortic stenosis. *Ao*, poststenotic dilatation of the aorta; *LV*, left ventricle. The *arrow* denotes the thickened valve cusps. (*b*) Selective angiocardiogram in a patient with discrete subvalvar stenosis (denoted by *bottom arrow*). There is associated mitral insufficiency, as is evident in the reflux of dye into an enlarged left atrium (*LA*) The aortic valve (*top arrow*) is normal, and the right coronary artery is visualized.

surgical treatment. Among the factors influencing the indications, techniques, and results of operation are the patient's age, the nature of the valvar deformity, and the experience of the surgical team. The decision to advise operation depends more often on the presence of severe obstruction than on the symptoms described by the patient.[16, 46] Operation is recommended for any child with critical stenosis, i.e., a peak systolic pressure gradient exceeding 75 mm Hg, measured in the basal state, or a calculated effective orifice less than 0.5 cm^2/m^2 of body surface area. In the presence of symptoms

or a left ventricular strain pattern on the electrocardiogram, or an abnormal exercise-electrocardiogram, operation may be recommended with less rigid regard to the hemodynamic assessment of the severity of stenosis.[46] Once the presence of severe stenosis has been established, the potential hazard of sudden death dictates that surgical treatment not be postponed unnecessarily. Operation is carried out under direct vision after institution of cardiopulmonary bypass, and the fused commissures are opened. When this is done precisely and judiciously, the commissural incision enlarges the valve

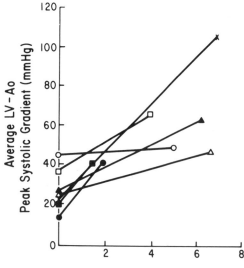

REFERENCE	NUMBER OF PATIENTS	AVERAGE AGE (yrs.)	
		1st CATH	2nd CATH
■ HOHN, et. al. (67)	4	6,10,10,45	N.A.
● BENTIVOGLIO, et. al. (6)	1	27	29
□ EL-SAID, et. al. (33)	18	7	11
○ HURWITZ (71)	19	9	14
▲ FRIEDMAN, et. al. (44)	9	6.8	13.1
△ COHEN, et. al. (25)	15	8.5	15.1
X BANDY and VOGEL (3)	1	5	12

Fig. 12.14 Composite of serial hemodynamic studies in the literature showing the relationship between time and left ventricular (*LV*)-aortic (*Ao*) pressure gradients in patients with aortic stenosis. (Reproduced with permission from W. F. Friedman *et al.*[48])

orifice and does not result in significant aortic insufficiency.[35] When operation is performed by an experienced surgeon, a mortality rate less than 2%[107] can be expected. The small size of the aorta in very young children creates technical problems for the surgeon, and for this reason operative results are enhanced if the patient's weight exceeds 10 kg.

Long term follow-up studies indicate that aortic valvotomy is a safe and effective means of treatment with excellent relief of symptoms (Fig. 12.15).[26, 46, 107, 110] Occasionally, aortic insufficiency may be progressive and require prosthetic valve replacement. Moreover, following commissurotomy the valve leaflets remain somewhat deformed, and it is possible that further degenerative changes, including calcification, will lead to significant stenosis in later years.[48] Since the valves are not rendered normal, antibiotic prophylaxis is indicated in the postoperative patient, even if the systolic pressure gradient has been abolished.[54]

VALVAR AORTIC STENOSIS IN INFANCY

This malformation may create unique problems in infants and therefore deserves special comment.[17, 19, 79, 90] Although isolated valvar aortic stenosis seldom causes symptoms in infancy, occasionally the lesion is responsible for profound and intractable heart failure. In spite of apparently normal coronary arteries, infarction of left ventricular papillary muscles may occur in some infants, resulting in an acquired form of mitral insufficiency, which intensifies the heart failure state. Moreover, endocardial fibroelastosis may result from reduced subendocardial oxygen delivery, and myocardial

degeneration may be prominent.[17] The symptomatic infant is irritable, pale, and hypotensive and presents with tachycardia, cardiomegaly, and pulmonary congestion, manifested by dyspnea, tachypnea, subcostal retractions, and diffuse rales. Cyanosis secondary to pulmonary venous unsaturation may be observed. The systolic murmur is often atypical, best heard at the apex or along the lower left sternal border, and may be confused with that caused by a ventricular septal defect. In some infants with heart failure, the murmur may be absent or extremely soft, but it becomes louder when myocardial contractility is improved with medical measures. Often the response to medical management of the infant with heart failure is poor.[79]

The electrocardiographic findings may not be characteristic; left ventricular hypertrophy and/or strain as well as right atrial enlargement and right ventricular hypertrophy may be detected shortly after birth. The electrocardiographic signs of right heart involvement result from volume loading of the right ventricle due to left-to-right shunting across the foramen ovale and from pulmonary hypertension secondary to elevated left ventricular diastolic and left atrial pressures. Survival past the neonatal period does not preclude subsequent difficulties, and deterioration may recur with the onset of anemia.

The seriously ill newborn with AS must be considered to be a medical emergency.[37, 85] Cardiac catheterization and angiocardiography may be indicated in the first 24 hours of life. Hemodynamic findings frequently include left to right shunting at the atrial level, an elevated left atrial and left ventricular end-diastolic pressure, and a small pressure drop

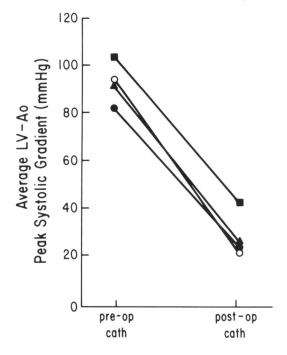

REFERENCE	NUMBER OF PATIENTS	CATH INTERVAL (yrs.)	
■ JACK and KELLY (72)	15	5.8	
▲ CONKLE, et. al. (26)	32	0.5	1
● FISHER, et. al. (35)	18 bicuspid	1.5	
○ FRIEDMAN, et. al. (48)	7 tricuspid		

Fig. 12.15 A composite of hemodynamic studies before and after aortic valvotomy in three series. *LV*, left ventricular; *Ao*, aortic. (Reproduced with permission from W. F. Friedman *et al.*[48]).

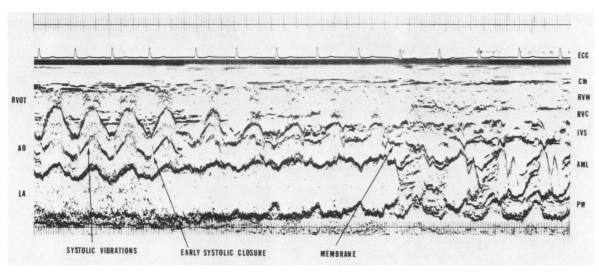

Fig. 12.16   M-mode scan of the long axis of the left ventricle in discrete subvalvar aortic stenosis. Noted are systolic vibrations and early systolic closure of the aortic valve (*Ao*). An extralinear echo in the left ventricular outflow (membrane) probably represents the subvalvular membranous stenosis. (Courtesy of Thomas DiSessa, M.D.)

across the aortic valve as a result of a markedly reduced cardiac output. Right to left shunting across a patent ductus arteriosus is encountered occasionally. The lesion may be distinguished from the hypoplastic left heart syndrome echocardiographically and angiographically by the presence of normal or enlarged left ventricular cavity and normal or dilated ascending aorta. Establishment of the diagnosis and prompt valvotomy are justified since prolonged periods of stabilization are uncommon with medical therapy. Poor myocardial performance resulting from endocardial fibroelastosis, subendocardial ischemia, and reduced left ventricular compliance, and inadequate relief of obstruction with or without aortic insufficiency are some of the factors accounting for high operative mortality and morbidity.[17, 85] Open repair under direct vision is the preferred type of operation.

DISCRETE SUBAORTIC STENOSIS

This malformation accounts for 8 to 10% of all cases of congenital aortic stenosis and occurs more frequently in males than in females by a ratio of 2:1.[95] The lesion consists of a membraneous diaphragm or fibrous ring encircling the left ventricular outflow tract just beneath the base of the aortic valve (Fig. 12.13*b*).

Differentiation between valvar and subvalvar aortic stenosis is extremely difficult from clinical findings alone.[16, 55] A systolic ejection sound is rarely heard, and the diastolic murmur of aortic insufficiency is more common than it is in valvar aortic stenosis. Dilatation of the ascending aorta is common, but valvar calcification is not observed.

Echocardiography may be useful in the distinction of valvar and subvalvar stenosis. The finding by single crystal methods of a fine, high intensity echo in the left ventricular outflow tract can suggest the presence of a subaortic diaphragm.[100] Multiple, thick echoes from a level near the annular attachment of the anterior mitral leaflet and below the sinuses of Valsalva have been observed with fibromuscular subaortic obstruction. Also noted are preclosure of the aortic valve, with associated high frequency systolic vibrations (Fig. 12.16)[29]; the ratio of the dimension of the narrowed subaortic area to the aortic root has been employed to estimate the severity of obstruction.[7, 84] Cross-sectional echo

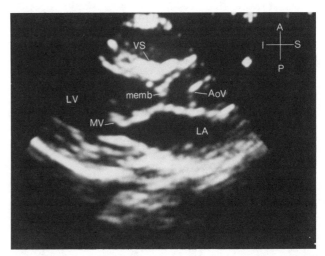

Fig. 12.17   Two-dimensional long axis view in discrete membranous subaortic stenosis. A discrete membrane (*memb*) is imaged in the left ventricular (*LV*) outflow tract, beneath and parallel to the aortic valve (*AoV*), extending from the ventricular septum (*VS*) to the anterior leaflet of the mitral valve (*MV*). *LA*, left atrium. (Courtesy of Josephine Isabel-Jones, M.D.)

studies reveal persistent, prominent echoes in the subaortic left ventricle in both systole and diastole (Fig. 12.17).[30, 120, 123, 124] Echocardiography also has the potential for identifying hypertrophic subaortic stenosis when it coexists with fixed subaortic stenosis and for distinguishing between the two forms of obstruction (vide infra).

Definitive differentiation between valvar and subvalvar obstruction is best accomplished by recording the pressure as a catheter is withdrawn across the outflow tract and valve (Fig. 12.18)[13, 14, 24] or by localizing the site of obstruction with selective axial left ventricular angiocardiography (Fig. 12.13*b*).[82]

Mild degrees of aortic valvar insufficiency are often observed in patients with discrete subaortic stenosis and are probably caused by thickening of the valve and impaired mobility of the cusps.[91] Because of the likelihood of both progressive obstructive and aortic insufficiency, the presence of even mild to moderate subaortic stenosis warrants consideration of elective operation[95, 114] The risks of operation in patients with discrete subaortic stenosis and valvar aortic stenosis are essentially the same.[78] Surgery consists of excising the membrane or fibrous ridge and may be expected to improve the hemodynamics and frequently may be curative.[21, 62, 102] In a small number of patients, secondary muscular hypertrophy of the outflow tract and a pressure gradient may persist following the operative relief of valvar or discrete subvalvar aortic stenosis.[16] Ultimately, this form of outflow obstruction may resolve (Fig. 12.19).

UNCOMMON FORMS OF SUBAORTIC STENOSIS

Occasionally, valvar and subvalvar aortic stenosis coexist in the same patient, producing a tunnel-like narrowing of the left ventricular outflow tract.[89] Associated findings are often a small ascending aorta, hypoplasia of the aortic valve ring, and thickened valve leaflets. The subvalvar fibrous process usually extends onto the aortic valve cusps and almost always makes contact with the ventricular aspect of the anterior mitral leaflet at its base. The presence of "tunnel stenosis" may be suspected angiographically from the appearance of the outflow tract and the aortic root. Operative treatment is complicated by the frequent necessity for prosthetic replacement of the aortic valve as well as for enlarging

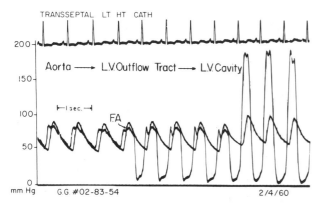

Fig. 12.18 Pressure recorded as the catheter was withdrawn from the aorta into the left ventricle in a patient with discrete subaortic stenosis. The increase in pressure from the subvalvar chamber to the main cavity of the left ventricle (*L.V.*) localizes the obstruction to the outflow tract of the ventricle. *F.A.*, femoral artery. (Reproduced with permission from Braunwald *et al.*[48])

the aortic annulus, proximal aorta, and left ventricular outflow tract. Experience is accumulating in interposing a valve containing prosthetic conduit from the apex of the left ventricle to the descending aorta.[96, 97, 115] Alternative operations to the left ventricular apical-aortic conduit incorporate aortoventriculoplasty methods for widening the aortic valve ring, as well as the subaortic outflow tract.[10, 83]

Several lesions other than a discrete membrane or ridge may produce subaortic stenosis. Among these are abnormal adherence of the anterior leaflet of the mitral valve to the left septal surface and the presence in the left ventricular outflow tract of accessory endocardial cushion tissue.[9, 39, 109] In some patients with atrioventricular canal, the part of the ventricular septum that contributes to the wall of the left ventricular outflow tract is deficient, and the ventricular aspect of the anterior leaflet of the common atrioventricular valve is adherent to the posterior edge of the deficient septum, resulting in a narrow left ventricular outflow tract. Malalignment of the conal ventricular septum, resulting in an inferior ventricular septal defect, produces a leftward superior deviation and insertion of the conal septum obstructing left ventricular outflow.[38, 92] In patients with single ventricle and an outflow chamber, the bulboventricular foramen serves as a potential site of aortic outflow obstruction. Additional rarer causes of subaortic stenosis include redundant dysplastic left atrioventricular valve tissue in patients with corrected transposition of the great arteries, and patients with anomalous muscle bundles of the left ventricular outflow tract.[39, 93]

A muscular type of subaortic stenosis may result from a convergence of all the mitral chordae into one of two fused papillary muscles producing the "parachute" deformity of the mitral valve that is often seen in association with supravalvular stenosis of the left atrium and coarctation of the aorta.[112] In some of these patients discrete membranous subvalvar aortic obstruction has also been noted.

In patients with common ventricle and ventricular septal defect, muscular subaortic stenosis has been shown to develop after surgical banding of the pulmonary artery.[37, 40]

SUPRAVALVAR AORTIC STENOSIS

Supravalvar aortic stenosis is a congenital narrowing of the ascending aorta that may be localized or diffuse, originating at the superior margin of the sinuses of Valsalva just above the level of the coronary arteries.

The clinical picture of supravalvar aortic stenosis may

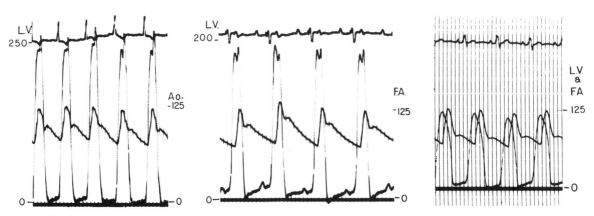

Fig. 12.19 Simultaneous pressure tracings recorded in the left ventricle and aorta prior to operation in a patient with discrete congenital subaortic stenosis (*left*); pressures recorded 3 weeks after operation (*center*) and 19 months postoperatively (*right*). The discrete obstruction was completely relieved at operation, and hypertrophic subaortic stenosis was responsible for the residual obstruction noted in the center tracing. Subsequently the latter resolved. (Reproduced with permission from E. Braunwald *et al.*: Circulation 29 and 30 (Suppl. 4): 1964.)

differ in major respects from that observed in the other forms of obstruction to left ventricular outflow. Chief among these differences is the association of supravalvar aortic stenosis with idiopathic infantile hypercalcemia,[11] a disease probably related to deranged vitamin D metabolism.[8, 41–43, 53] The designations supravalvar aortic stenosis syndrome or Williams syndrome[125] have been applied to the distinctive picture produced by coexistence of the cardiac and multiple system disorder. Other manifestations of this syndrome include mental retardation, "elfin facies," narrowing of peripheral systemic and pulmonary arteries, inguinal hernia, strabismus, and abnormalities of dental development. Occasionally, there is moderate thickening of the aortic cusps, and valvar pulmonary stenosis may occur in association with the narrowing of peripheral pulmonary arteries. Rarely, patients have mitral valve abnormalities.

Hypervitaminosis D in the pregnant rabbit has resulted in craniofacial abnormalities and malformations resembling supravalvar aortic stenosis in the offspring.[41–43] Skin fibroblast cultures from patients with William's syndrome show enhanced metachromasia upon addition of vitamin D_3 and calcium.[4] In humans, chromosome studies have revealed normal karyotypes, with the exception of one patient who demonstrated a 46/47 mosaic pattern with an extra chromosome resembling the 19 to 20 group. Most commonly, supravalvar aortic stenosis is a feature of the distinctive syndrome described above. However, the aortic anomaly and peripheral pulmonary arterial stenosis are also seen in familial and sporadic forms unassociated with the other features of the syndrome. Genetic studies suggest that when the anomaly is familial, it is transmitted as an autosomal dominant with variable expression.[77] Some family members may have supravalvar pulmonic stenosis either as an isolated lesion or in combination with the supravalvar aortic anomaly. It is helpful to classify patients according to their clinical presentation into (1) nonfamilial, sporadic cases: normal facies and intelligence; (2) familial: normal facies and intelligence; and (3) nonfamilial syndrome with abnormal facial appearance and mental retardation. In contrast to the other forms of aortic stenosis, there appears to be no sex predilection in any of these 3 categories.

PATHOLOGY

Supravalvar aortic stenosis may be separated into three categories, although some patients may have findings of more than one type.[99] Most common is the hourglass type, in which a constricting annular ridge at the superior margin of the sinuses of Valsalva is produced by extreme thickening and disorganization of the aortic media (Fig. 12.20). Although the lumen of the aorta is reduced, the constriction may not be evident on gross inspection of the external surface of the vessel. It has been suggested that this lesion results from a developmental exaggeration of the normal transverse supravalvar aortic plica. The membranous type is produced by a fibrous or fibromuscular semicircular diaphragm with a small central opening stretched across the lumen of the aorta. The hypoplastic type is characterized by uniform hypoplasia of the ascending aorta.

In supravalvar stenosis, the coronary arteries are subjected to the elevated pressure that exists within the left ventricle, because they arise proximal to the site of outflow obstruction. These vessels are often dilated and tortuous.[106] Commonly, their lumina are narrowed by a thickened medial layer, and premature coronary arteriosclerosis has been observed. In addition, if the free edges of some or all of the aortic cusps are adherent to the site of supravalvar stenosis, there may be interference with coronary arterial inflow. The

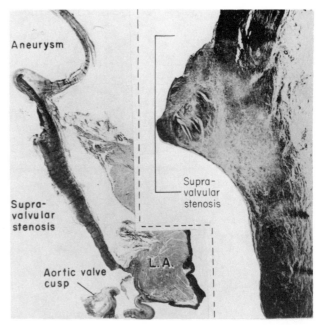

Fig. 12.20 Photomicrographs of aortic roots of two patients with supravalvar aortic stenosis. Section on the *left* includes aortic valve, ascending aorta, and the wall of an aortic aneurysm. Note that the medial layer of the aortic wall is markedly thickened, distal to the superior margin of the sinus of Valsalva. The section on the *right* shows the most common pathologic finding. The medial layer is thickened markedly, creating a triangular infolding or hillock whose apex points to the lumen. Also observed are foci of necrosis and calcification. Characteristically, the elastic fibers are broken, and there is an irregular increase in smooth muscle cells. (*Right panel* reproduced with permission from M. Peron: Archives of Pathology 71:453, 1961.)

formation of thoracic aortic aneurysms has been described in several patients.

MANIFESTATIONS

Clinical Features

Patients with the supravalvar aortic stenosis syndrome are often mentally retarded and bear a marked facial resemblance to one another. The typical appearance is similar to the "elfin facies" observed in the severe form of idiopathic infantile hypercalcemia and is characterized by a high prominent forehead, epicanthal folds, underdeveloped bridge of the nose and mandible, overhanging upper lip, strabismus, and anomalies of dentition (Fig. 12.21). Recognition of this distinctive appearance, even in infancy, should lead promptly to suspicion of underlying multiple system disease. Also, a positive family history in a patient with a normal appearance and signs suggesting left ventricular outflow obstruction should alert the physician to a diagnosis of either supravalvar aortic stenosis or idiopathic hypertrophic subaortic stenosis. Patients with supravalvar aortic stenosis appear to be subject to the same risks of unexpected sudden death and endocarditis as those with valvar aortic stenosis.

With a few exceptions, the physical findings resemble those observed in patients with valvar aortic stenosis. Among these exceptions are the frequent accentuation of the sound of aortic valve closure due to the elevated pressure in the aorta proximal to the stenosis, the infrequency of an ejection sound, and the more prominent transmission of a thrill and murmur into the jugular notch and along the carotid vessels. The narrowing of the peripheral pulmonary arteries that

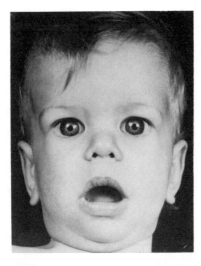
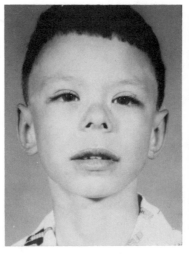
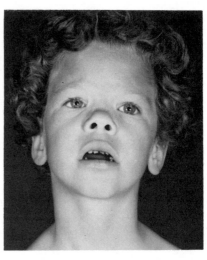

Fig. 12.21 Characteristic facial appearance in patients with supravalvar aortic stenosis and mental retardation. Note the high, prominent forehead, epicanthal folds, underdeveloped bridge of the nose, and mandible and overhanging upper lip. Strabismus is noted in the middle panel. (*Left panel*, reproduced with permission from Garcia, *et al.*[52])

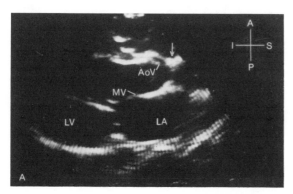
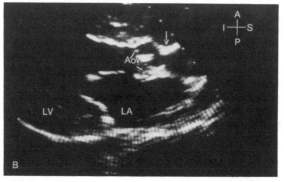

Fig. 12.22 A two-dimensional long axis parasternal view of the left ventricle (*LV*) during systole (*panel A*) and diastole (*panel B*). Note the narrowed supravalvar region (*arrow*) and normal aortic valve mobility (*AoV*). *MV*, mitral valve; *LA*, left atrium. (Courtesy Thomas DiSessa, M.D.)

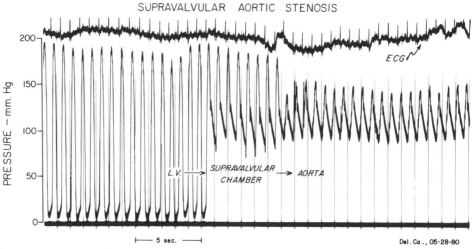

Fig. 12.23 Continuous pressure recording as a catheter was withdrawn from the left ventricle (*L.V.*) through the supravalvar chamber and into the aortic arch of a patient with supravalvar aortic stenosis. *ECG*, electrocardiogram. (Reproduced with permission from R. L. Kahler *et al.*[77])

frequently coexists in these patients may produce a continuous murmur that may help distinguish this anomaly from valvar AS. This distinction is reinforced by the disparity between the arterial presssures in the upper extremities in supravalvar aortic stenosis; the systolic pressure in the right arm tends to be the higher of the two and may even exceed that in the femoral arteries. The disparity in pulses may relate to the tendency of a jet stream to adhere to a vessel wall (Coanda effect) and selective streaming of blood into the innominate artery.[36, 57]

Electrocardiographic, Echocardiographic, and Radiologic Features

When obstruction is severe, the electrocardiogram generally reveals left ventricular hypertrophy. However, biventricular, or even right ventricular, hypertrophy may be observed if significant narrowing of peripheral pulmonary arteries coexists. In a number of patients without significant right-sided lesions the vectorcardiogram has shown displacement of the maximum transverse QRS loop rightward and posteriorly and a tendency for initial forces to be directed leftward, perhaps reflecting posterobasal left ventricular hypertrophy or a manifestation of left posterior hemiblock.[53] Single crystal echocardiography has been of limited help in localizing obstruction to the supravalvar aorta. However, the level of narrowing of the outflow tract may be observed clearly by 2D echocardiography (Fig. 12.22). Roentgenographically, in contrast to valvar and discrete subvalvar aortic stenosis, poststenotic dilatation of the ascending aorta is rarely seen. Most often the sinuses of Valsalva are dilated and the ascending aorta and the aorta arch are of normal size or appear small.

CARDIAC CATHETERIZATION

Retrograde aortic catheterization is the most valuable technique for localizing the site of obstruction to the supravalvar area and to assess the degree of hemodynamic abnormality. The diagnosis is confirmed by the demonstration of a pressure gradient just above the aortic valve (Fig. 12.23) and a constriction at this level by aortography (Fig. 12.24 a). The angiogram may also permit visualization of narrowed segments of the aorta distal to the obstruction. At right heart catheterization, the presence of stenosis of peripheral pulmonary arteries may be detected by continually recording pressure as the catheter is withdrawn from a peripheral pulmonary artery to the body of the right ventricle and by right ventricular angiocardiography (Fig. 12.24 b).

TREATMENT

For several reasons, supravalvar aortic stenosis may be less amenable to operative treatment than either valvar or discrete subvalvar stenosis.[45] The lumen of the aorta at the supravalvar level may be widened by the insertion of an oval- or diamond-shaped fabric prosthesis in those patients with a normal ascending aorta. If the aorta is hypoplastic, this procedure merely displaces the pressure gradient distally, without abolishing the obstruction. Under these circumstances, treatment may necessitate replacement or widening of the entire hypoplastic aorta with an appropriate prosthesis. Stricter criteria should be employed for the selection of patients with supravalvar obstruction for operation, since surgery is usually more difficult and often less effective than in other forms of aortic stenosis. Operation may be recommended when relatively little hypoplasia of the ascending aorta and arch exists and when the obstruction is discrete and severe, i.e., with a systolic gradient exceeding 75 mm Hg.

DIFFERENTIAL DIAGNOSIS

Clinical differentiation of the various types of aortic stenosis from other types of heart disease usually is not difficult because of the physical findings. However, differential diagnosis presents special problems with infants. The critically ill infant with valvar AS in heart failure may be in such

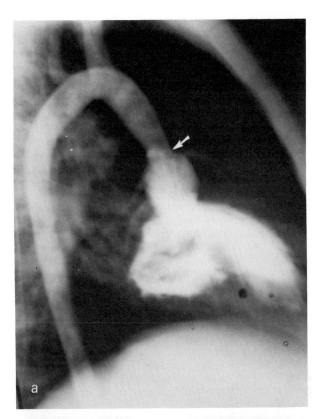

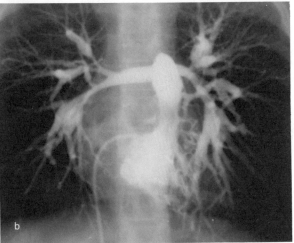

Fig. 12.24 (a) Aortogram in a patient with supravalvar aortic stenosis, showing dilated sinuses of Valsalva and an aortic constriction just above the sinuses (arrow). (b) Angiocardiogram with right ventricular injection showing multiple sites of stenosis of the peripheral pulmonary arteries in a patient with supravalvar aortic stenosis. (Reproduced with permission from R. L. Kahler et al.[77])

profound shock that he is difficult to distinguish from the patient with severe coarctation of the aorta. An electrocardiogram showing pure left ventricular hypertrophy with strain during the first weeks of life points to the former diagnosis. A patent ductus arteriosus in infancy may present with a harsh systolic murmur and electrocardiographic evidence of left axis deviation and left ventricular hypertrophy; the peripheral pulses are bounding rather than diminished, and the roentgenogram reveals increased pulmonary vascularity and a prominent pulmonary artery segment. Also to be distinguished from valvar AS in infancy are the hypoplastic left heart syndrome and endocardial fibroelastosis. Helpful points of differentiation are the absence on the electrocardiogram of left ventricular hypertrophy and characteristic echocardiographic findings in the former, and a somewhat later onset of symptoms and cardiac enlargement in the latter. Occasionally, in infants the location of the murmur of AS at the lower sternal border and apex and its harsh quality may lead to the suspicion of a ventricular septal defect. However, the electrocardiographic pattern of combined ventricular hypertrophy and the roentgenographic appearance of pulmonary arterial hypervascularity in infants with ventricular septal defect usually lead to a correct diagnosis.

In the older patient the common malformations to consider in the differential diagnosis include pulmonic stenosis, peripheral pulmonary arterial stenosis, and rheumatic aortic stenosis. Mild pulmonic stenosis with intact ventricular septum may resemble mild AS, because an ejection systolic murmur at the base of the heart and a normal electrocardiogram and chest roentgenogram may be found in both conditions. However, the nature of the cardiac impulse and the relative intensity of the second heart sound on either side of the upper sternal border are helpful in distinguishing one from the other. When the pulmonic stenosis is more severe, a lift is palpable along the left lower parasternal area, indicative of right ventricular enlargement, instead of the forceful and localized apical thrust indicative of left ventricular enlargement. Also, pulmonic stenosis is often accompanied by poststenotic dilatation of the pulmonary trunk on chest roentgenograms, and the electrocardiogram demonstrates right instead of left ventricular hypertrophy.

Peripheral pulmonary arterial stenosis may give rise to an ejection systolic murmur heard best at the base of the heart. Usually, however, there is no thrill, the murmur is not loud, and although widely transmitted to the precordium and back, it does not radiate to the neck vessels. If the obstruction is severe, right ventricular hypertrophy may be observed on the electrocardiogram and roentgenogram.

The most important point in the differentiation of congenital from rheumatic aortic stenosis is the age of the child when the murmur is first heard. Rheumatic aortic stenosis is not seen in early childhood and is extremely rare during the first decade of life. Usually, there is a history of acute rheumatic fever and evidence of involvement of the mitral valve. In addition, rheumatic aortic stenosis is often accompanied by aortic insufficiency. Calcification of the aortic valve may be observed in both congenital and rheumatic aortic valvular stenosis after the age of 20 years.

PROGNOSIS

The prognosis in the various forms of AS varies with the severity of obstruction. Mild stenosis may be compatible with a normal life. However, even when the obstruction is mild, the hazard of endocarditis remains, and there is a tendency for sclerosis and calcification of the aortic valve to develop in later life so that a note of caution regarding the prognosis is necessary. Although sudden death usually occurs in patients with signs of severe obstruction, demise may occur unexpectedly, even in patients who are relatively asymptomatic.

The worst prognosis is encountered in infants in heart failure. With the exception of infants, death in children is rarely due to heart failure; ventricular dysrhythmias are probably the most common cause of a fatal outcome.

Since the various forms of AS are susceptible to early recognition and definition, intelligent selection of patients for surgical treatment is important. In the majority, effective relief of obstruction to left ventricular outflow can be accomplished. However, residual AS or aortic insufficiency may occur following surgery. Moreover, the residual deformity of the valve after a valvotomy still places the patient at risk of endocarditis. Thus, it is possible that many of these patients may ultimately require replacement of the aortic valve.

REFERENCES

1. Aziz, K. U., van Grondelli, A., Paul, M. M., and Muster, A. J.: Echocardiographic assessment of the relationship between left ventricular wall and cavity dimensions and peak systolic pressure in children with aortic stenosis. Am. J. Cardiol. 40:775, 1977.
2. Bache, R. J., Wang, Y., and Jorgensen, C. R.: Haemodynamic effects of exercise in isolated valvular aortic stenosis. Circulation 44:1003, 1971.
3. Bandy, G. E., and Vogel, J. H. K.: Progressive congenital valvular aortic stenosis. Chest 60:189, 1971.
4. Becroft, D. M., and Chamber, D.: Supravalvular aortic stenosis-infantile hypercalcemia syndrome: In vitro hypersensitivity to Vitamin D_2 and calcium. J. Med. Genet. 13:223, 1976.
5. Bennet, D. H., Evans, D. W., and Raj, M. V. J.: Echocardiographic left ventricular dimensions in pressure and volume overload: Their use in assessing aortic stenosis. Br. Heart. J. 37:371, 1975.
6. Bentivoglio, L. G., Sagarminaga, J., Uricchio, J., and Goldberg, H.: Congenital bicuspid aortic valve: A clinical and hemodynamic study. Br. Heart J. 22:321, 1960.
7. Berry, T. E., Aziz, K. U., and Paul, M. H.: Echocardiographic assessment of discrete subaortic stenosis in childhood. Am. J. Cardiol. 43:951, 1979.
8. Beuren, A.: Supravalvular aortic stenosis: A complex syndrome with and without mental retardation. Birth Defects 8, 5:45, 1972.
9. Bjork, V. O., Hultquist, G., and Lodin, H.: Subaortic stenosis produced by an abnormally placed anterior mitral leaflet. J. Thorac. Cardiovasc. Surg. 41:659, 1961.
10. Bjornstad, P. G., Rastan, H., Keutel, J., Beuren, A. J., and Koncz, J.: Aortoventriculoplasty for tunnel subaortic stenosis and other obstructions of the left ventricular outflow tract. Circulation 60:59, 1979.
11. Black, J. A., and Bonham-Carter, R. E.: Association between aortic stenosis and facies of severe infantile hypercalcemia. Lancet 11:745, 1963.
12. Blackwood, R. A., Bloom, K. R., and Williams, C. M.: Aortic stenosis in children: Experience with echocardiographic prediction of severity. Circulation 57:263, 1978.
13. Block, P. C., Powell, W. J., Jr., Dinsmore, R., and Goldblatt, A.: Coexistent fixed congenital and idiopathic hypertrophic subaortic stenosis. Am. J. Cardiol. 31:523–526, 1973.
14. Bloom, K. R., Meyer, R. A., Bove, K. E., and Kaplan, S.: The association of fixed and dynamic left ventricular outflow obstruction. Am. Heart J. 89:586, 1975.
15. Bonner, A. J., Jr., Sacks, H. N., and Tavel, M. E.: Assessing the severity of aortic stenosis by phonocardiography and external carotid pulse recordings. Circulation 48:247, 1973.
16. Braunwald, E., Goldblatt, A., Aygen, M. M., Rockoff, S. D., and Morrow, A. G.: Congenital aortic stenosis. I. Clinical and hemodynamic findings in 100 patients. Circulation 27:426, 1963.
17. Broderick, T. W., Higgins, C. B., Guthaner, D. F., Friedman, W. F., Stevenson, J. G., and Frinch, J. W.: Critical aortic stenosis in neonates. Radiology 129:393, 1978.
18. Buckberg, G., Eber, L., Herman, N., and Gorlin, R.: Ischemia in aortic stenosis: Hemodynamic prediction. Am. J. Cardiol. 35:778, 1975.
19. Burnell, R. M., Ghadiale, P. E., Joseph, M. C., and Paneth, M.: Management of critical valvular outflow obstruction in neonates. Thorac. 25:116, 1970.
20. Caulfield, W. H., deLeon, A. C., Jr., Perloff, J. K., and Steelman, R. B.: The clinical significance of the fourth heart sound in aortic stenosis. Am. J. Cardiol. 28:179, 1971.
21. Champsaur, G., Trussler, G. A., and Mustard, W. T.: Congenital discrete subvalvar aortic stenosis: Surgical experience and long-term follow-up in twenty pediatric patients. Br. Heart J. 35:443, 1973.
22. Chandramouli, B., Ehruka, D. A., and Lauer, R. M.: Exercise-induced electrocardiographic changes in children with congenital aortic stenosis. J. Pediatr. 87:725, 1975.
23. Chang, S., Clements, S., and Chang, J.: Aortic stenosis: Echocardiographic cusp separation and surgical description of the aortic valve in 22 patients. Am. J. Cardiol. 39:499, 1977.
24. Chung, K. J., Manning, J. A., and Gramiak, R.: Echocardiography in coexisting hypertrophic subaortic stenosis and fixed left ventricular outflow obstruction. Circulation 49:673, 1974.
25. Cohen, L. S., Friedman, W. F., and Braunwald, E.: Natural history of mild congenital aortic stenosis elucidated by serial hemody-

namic studies. Am. J. Cardiol. 30:1, 1972.

26. Conkle, D. M., Jones, M., and Morrow, A. G.: Treatment of congenital aortic stenosis: An evaluation of the late results of aortic valvotomy. Arch. Surg. 107:649, 1973.

27. Cooper, T., Braunwald, E., and Morrow, A. G.: Pulsus alternans in aortic stenosis: Hemodynamic observations in 50 patients studied by left heart catheterization. Circulation 18:64, 1958.

28. Cueto, L., and Moller, J. H.: Hemodynamics of exercise in children with isolated aortic valvular disease. Br. Heart J. 35:93, 1973.

29. Davis, R. M., Feigenbaum, M., Chang, S., Konecke, L. L., and Dillon, J. C.: Echocardiographic manifestations of discrete subaortic stenosis. Am. J. Cardiol. 33:277, 1974.

30. DiSessa, T. G., Hagan, A. D., Isabel-Jones, J. B., Ti, C. C., Mercier, J. C., and Friedman, W. F.: Two-dimensional echocardiographic evaluations of discrete subaortic stenosis from the apical long axis view. Am. Heart J. 6:774, 1981.

31. Doyle, E. F., Arumughan, P., Lara, E., Rutkowski, M. R., and Killy, B.: Sudden death in young patients with congenital aortic stenosis. Pediatrics 53:481, 1974.

32. Edmunds, L. M., Wagner, H. R., and Heymann, M. A.: Aortic valvulotomy in neonates. Circulation 61:421, 1980.

33. El-Said, G., Galioto, F. M., Jr., Mullins, C. E., and McNamara, D. G.: Natural hemodynamic history of congenital aortic stenosis in childhood. Am. J. Cardiol. 30:6, 1972.

34. Feizi, D., Symons, C., and Yacoub, M.: Echocardiography of the aortic valve. I. Studies of normal aortic valve, aortic stenosis, aortic regurgitation and mixed aortic valve disease. Br. Heart J. 36:341, 1974.

35. Fisher, R. D., Mason, D. T., and Morrow, A. G.: Results of operative treatment in congenital aortic stenosis. J. Thorac. Cardiovasc. Surg. 59:218, 1970.

36. French, J. W., and Guntheroth, W. G.: An explanation of asymmetric upper extremity blood pressure in supravalvular aortic stenosis: The Coanda effect. Circulation 42:31, 1970.

37. Freed, M., Rosenthal, A., and Plauth, W. H., Jr.: Development of subaortic stenosis after pulmonary artery banding (abstr.). Circulation 47 and 48 (Suppl. III):7, 1973.

38. Freedom, R. M., Culham, J. A. G., and Rowe, R. D.: Angiocardiography of subaortic obstruction in infancy. Am. J. Roentgenol. 129:813, 1977.

39. Freedom, R. M., Dische, M. R., and Rowe, R. D.: Pathologic anatomy of subaortic stenosis and atresia in the first year of life. Am. J. Cardiol. 39:1035, 1977.

40. Freedom, R. M., Sondheimer, H., Dische, R., and Rowe, R. D.: Development of subaortic stenosis after pulmonary arterial banding for common ventricle. Am. J. Cardiol. 39:78, 1977.

41. Friedman, W. F., and Roberts, W. C.: Vitamin D and the supravalvar aortic stenosis syndrome: The transplacental effects of vitamin D on the aorta of the rabbit. Circulation 34:77, 1966.

42. Friedman, W. F.: Vitamin D embryopathy. Adv. Teratol. 3:85, 1968.

43. Friedman, W. F., and Mills, L. F.: The relationship between vitamin D and the craniofacial and dental anomalies of the supravalvular aortic stenosis syndrome. Pediatrics 43:12, 1969.

44. Friedman, W. F., Modlinger, J., and Morgan, J.: Serial hemodynamic observations in asymptomatic children with valvar aortic stenosis. Circulation 43:91, 1971.

45. Friedman, W. F., and Pappelbaum, S. J.: Indications for hemodynamic evaluation and surgery in congenital aortic stenosis. Pediatr. Clin. North Am. 18:1207, 1971.

46. Friedman, W. F.: Congenital aortic valve disease: Natural history, indications and results of surgery. In New Aspects in Congenital, Valvular and Coronary Artery Disease, edited by D. Morse. Futura, Mt. Kisco, N.Y., 1975, p. 43.

47. Friedman, W. F.: Indications for and result of surgery in congenital aortic stenosis. Adv. Cardiol. 17:1976, p. 2.

48. Friedman, W. F., Novak, V., and Johnson, A. D.: Congenital aortic stenosis in adults. Cardiovasc. Clin. 9(3):235, 1979.

49. Friedman, W. F.: Congestive heart failure. In Current Pediatric Therapy, 9th Ed. W. B. Saunders, Philadelphia, 1980, p. 128.

50. Friedman, W. F.: Congenital heart disease in infancy and childhood. In Heart Disease, edited by E. Braunwald. W. B. Saunders, Philadelphia, 1980, p. 967.

51. Gamboa, R., Hugenholtz, P. G., and Nadas, A. S.: Comparison of electrocardiograms and vectorcardiograms in congenital aortic stenosis. Br. Heart J. 27:344, 1965.

52. Garcia, R. E., Friedman, W. F., Kaback, M. M., and Rowe, R. D.: Idiopathic hypercalcemia and supravalvular aortic stenosis: Documentation of a new syndrome. N. Engl. J. Med. 271:117, 1964.

53. Gaum, W. E., Chou, T. C., and Kaplan, S.: The vectorcardiogram and electrocardiogram in supravalvular aortic stenosis and coarctation of the aorta. Am. Heart J. 84:620, 1972.

54. Gerson, W. M., and Hayes, C. J.: Bacterial endocarditis in patients with pulmonary stenosis, aortic stenosis or ventricular septal defect. Circulation 55–56 (Suppl I):I-83, 1977.

55. Glancy, D. L., and Epstein, S. E.: Differential diagnosis of type and severity of obstruction to left ventricular outflow. Prog. Cardiovasc. Dis. 14:153, 1971.

56. Glanz, S., Hellenbrand, W. E., Berman, M. A., and Talner, N. S.: Echocardiographic assessment of the severity of aortic stenosis in children and adolescents. Am. J. Cardiol. 38:620, 1976.

57. Goldstein, R. E., and Epstein, S. E.: Mechanism of elevated innominate artery pressures in supravalvular aortic stenosis. Circulation 42:23, 1970.

58. Gorlin, R., and Gorlin, S. G.: Hydraulic formula for calculation of area of stenotic mitral valve, other cardiac valves, and central circulatory shunts. Am. Heart J. 41:1, 1951.

59. Gramiak, R., and Shah, P.: Echocardiography in the normal and diseased aortic valve. Radiology 96:1, 1970.

60. Hagan, A. D., DiSessa, T. G., Samtag, L., Friedman, W. F., and Vieweg, W. V. R.: Reliability of echocardiography in diagnosing and quantitating valvular aortic stenosis. J. Cardiovasc. Med. 5:391, 1980.

61. Halloran, K. H.: A telemetered exercise electrocardiogram in congenital aortic stenosis. Pediatrics 47:31, 1971.

62. Hardisty, R. L., Griffith, B. P., Mathews, R. A., Siewers, R. D., Neches, W. M., Park, S. C., and Bahnson, H. T.: Discrete subvalvular aortic stenosis. An evaluation of operative therapy. J. Thorac. Cardiovasc. Surg. 74:352, 1977.

63. Hattle, L., Angelsen, E. A., and Tromsdal, A.: Non-invasive assessment of aortic stenosis by Doppler ultrasound. Br. Heart J. 43:284, 1980.

64. Hawker, R. E., Seara, C. A., and Krovetz, L. J.: Distalward modification of the arterial pulse wave in children with clinical aortic stenosis. Circulation 50:181, 1974.

65. Hoffman, J. I. E., and Buckberg, G. D.: The myocardial supply:demand ratio—A critical review. Am. J. Cardiol. 41:327, 1978.

66. Hoffman, J. I. E.: Determinants and prediction of transmural myocardial perfusion. Circulation 58:381, 1978.

67. Hohn, A. R., Van Praagh, S., Moore, A. A. D., Vlad, P., and Lambert, E. C.: Aortic stenosis. Circulation 31 and 32 (Suppl. III):4, 1965.

68. Hossack, K. F., and Neilson, G. M.: Exercise testing in congenital aortic stenosis. Aust. N.Z. J. Med. 9:164, 1979.

69. Hossack, K. F., Neutze, J. M., Lowe, J. B., and Barratt-Boyes, B. G.: Congenital valvular aortic stenosis. Natural history and assessment for operation. Br. Heart J. 43:561, 1980.

70. Hugenholtz, P. G., Lees, M. M., and Nadas, A. S.: The scalar electrocardiogram, vectorcardiogram, and exercise electrocardiogram in the assessment of congenital aortic stenosis. Circulation 26:79, 1962.

71. Hurwitz, R. A.: Valvar aortic stenosis in childhood: Clinical and hemodynamic history. J. Pediatr. 82:228, 1973.

72. Jack, W. D., and Kelly, D. T.: Long-term follow-up of valvulotomy for congenital aortic stenosis. Am. J. Cardiol. 38:231, 1976.

73. James, F. W.: Exercise testing in normal individuals and patients with cardiovascular disease. Cardiovasc. Clin. 11(2):227, 1981.

74. Johnson, A. M.: Aortic stenosis, sudden death, and the left ventricular baroreceptors. Br. Heart J. 33:1, 1971.

75. Johnson, G. L., Mayer, R. A., Schwartz, D. C., Korfhager, J., and Kaplan, S.: Left ventricular function by echocardiography in children with fixed aortic stenosis. Am. J. Cardiol. 38:611, 1976.

76. Johnson, S. L., Baker, D. W., Lute, R. A., and Dodge, H. T.: Doppler echocardiography. The localization of cardiac murmurs. Circulation 48:810, 1973.

77. Kahler, R. L., Braunwald, E., Plauth, W. H., Jr., and Morrow, A. G.: Familial congenital heart disease. Am. J. Med. 40:384, 1966.

78. Katz, N. M., Buckley, M. J., and Liberthown, R. R.: Discrete membranous subaortic stenosis. Report of 31 patients, review of the literature, and delineation of management. Circulation 56:1034, 1977.

79. Keane, J. F., Berhard, W. F., and Nadas, A. S.: Aortic stenosis surgery in infancy. Circulation 52:1138, 1975.

80. Kennedy, J. W., Twiss, R. D., Blackmon, J. R., and Dodge, H. T.: Quantitative angiocardiography. III. Relationships of left ventricular pressure, volume, and mass in aortic valve disease. Circulation 38:838, 1968.

81. Kelly, D. T., Wulfsberg, E., and Rowe, R. D.: Discrete subaortic stenosis. Circulation 46:309, 1972.

82. Kelly, M. J., Higgins, C. B., and Kirkpatrick, S. E.: Axial left ventriculography in discrete subaortic stenosis. Radiology 135:77, 1980.

83. Konno, S., Imai, Y., Iida, Y., Nakajima, M., and Tatsuno, K.: A new method for prosthetic valve replacement in congenital aortic stenosis associated with hypoplasia of the aortic valve ring. J. Thorac. Cardiovasc. Surg. 70:909, 1975.

84. Kruger, S. K., French, J. W., Forker, A. P., Caudell, C. C., and Popp, R. L.: Echocardiography in discrete subaortic stenosis. Circulation 59:506, 1979.

85. Lakier, J. B., Lewis, A. B., Heymann, M. A., Stanger, P., Hoffman, J. I. E., and Rudolph, A. M.: Isolated aortic stenosis of the neonate: Natural history and hemodynamic considerations. Circulation 50:801, 1974.

86. Lambert, E. C., Menon, V. A., Wagner, H. R., and Vlad, P.: Sudden unexpected death from cardiovascular disease in children. Am. J. Cardiol. 34:89, 1974.

87. Lewis, A. L., Heymann, M. A., Stanger, P., Hoffman, J. I. E., and Rudolph, A. M.: Evaluation of subendocardial ischemia in valvar aortic stenosis in children. Circulation 49:978, 1974.

88. Liebman, J., and Plonsey, R.: Electrocardiography. In Heart Disease in Infancy and Childhood, edited by A. J. Moss, F. H. Adams, and G. C. Emmanouilides. Williams & Wilkins,

Baltimore, 1977, p. 85.

89. Maron, B. J., Redwood, O. R., Roberts, W. C., Henry, W. L., Morrow, A. G., and Epstein, S. F.: Tunnel subaortic stenosis left ventricular outflow tract obstruction produced by fibromuscular tubular narrowing. Circulation 54:404, 1976.

90. Moller, J. H., Nakib, A., Eliot, R. S., and Edwards, J. E.: Symptomatic congenital aortic stenosis in the first year of life. J. Pediatr. 69:728, 1966.

91. Morrow, A. G., Fort, L., III, Roberts, W. C., and Braunwald, E.: Discrete subaortic stenosis complicated by aortic-valvular regurgitation. Clinical, hemodynamic, and pathologic studies and the results of operative treatment. Circulation 31:163, 1965.

92. Moulaert, A. J., Bruins, C. C., and Oppenheimer-Dekker, A.: Anomalies of the aortic arch and ventricular septal defects. Circulation 53:1011, 1976.

93. Moulaert, A. J., and Oppenheimer-Dekker, A.: Anteriolateral muscle bundle of the left ventricle, bulboventricular flange and subaortic stenosis. Am. J. Cardiol. 37:78, 1976.

94. Nanda, N. C., Gramiak, R., Shah, P. M., Stewart, S., and DeWeese, J. A.: Echocardiography in the diagnosis of idiopathic hypertrophic subaortic stenosis coexisting with aortic valve disease. Circulation 50:752, 1974.

95. Newfeld, E. A., Muster, A. J., Paul, M. M., Idriss, F. S., and Richie, W. L.: Discrete subvalvular aortic stenosis in childhood. Am. J. Cardiol. 38:53, 1976.

96. Nihill, M. R., Cooley, D. A., Norman, J. C., Hallman, G. L., and McNamara, D. G.: Hemodynamic observations in patients with left ventricle to aorta conduit. Am. J. Cardiol. 45:573, 1980.

97. Norman, J. C., Nihill, M. R., and Cooley, D. A.: Valved apicoaortic composite conduits for left ventricular outflow tract obstructions. Am. J. Cardiol. 45:1265, 1980.

98. Orsmond, G. S., Bessinger, F. B., and Moller, J. A.: Rest and exercise hemodynamics in children before and after aortic valvotomy. Am. Heart J. 99:76, 1980.

99. Peterson, T. A., Todd, D. B., and Edwards, J. E.: Supravalvular aortic stenosis. J. Thorac. Cardiovasc. Surg. 50:73, 1965.

100. Popp, R. L., Silverman, J. F., French, J. W., Stinson, E. B., and Harrison, D. C.: Echocardiographic findings in discrete subvalvular aortic stenosis. Circulation 49:226, 1974.

101. Reeve, R., Kawamata, K., and Selzer, A.: Reliability of vectorcardiography in assessing the severity of congenital aortic stenosis. Circulation 34:92, 1966.

102. Reis, R. L., Peterson, L. M., Mason, D. T., Simon, A. L., and Morrow, A. G.: Congenital fixed subvalvular aortic stenosis. An anatomical classification and correlations with operative results. Circulation 43 and 44 (Suppl. I and II): 1971.

103. Riopel, D. A., Taylor, A. B., and Hohn, A. R.: Blood pressure response to treadmill exercise in children with aortic stenosis (abstr.). American Academy of Pediatrics, 46th Annual Meeting, New York, 1977.

104. Reynolds, J. L., Nadas, A. S., Rudolph, A. M., and Gross, R. E.: Critical congenital aortic stenosis with minimal electrocardiographic changes. N. Engl. J. Med. 262:276, 1960.

105. Roberts, W. C.: Anatomically isolated aortic valvular disease: The case against its being of rheumatic etiology. Am. J. Cardiol. 49:151, 1970.

106. Roberts, W. C.: Valvular, subvalvular, and supravalvular aortic stenosis: Morphologic features. Cardiovasc. Clin. 5:97, 1973.

107. Sandor, G. G. S., Olley, P. M., Trusler, G. A., Williams, W. G., Row, R. D., and Morch, J. E.: Long-term follow-up of patients after valvotomy for congenital valvular aortic stenosis in children. J. Thorac. Cardiovasc. Surg. 80:171, 1980.

108. Schwartz, A., Vignola, P. A., Walker, H. J., King, M. E., and Golblatt, A.: Echocardiographic estimation of aortic valve gradient in aortic stenosis. Ann. Intern. Med. 89:329, 1978.

109. Sellers, R. D., Lillehei, C. W., and Edwards, J. E.: Subaortic stenosis caused by anomalies of the atrioventricular valves. J. Thorac. Cardiovasc. Surg. 48:289, 1964.

110. Shackelton, J., Edwards, F. R., Bickford, B. J., and Jones, R. S.: Long-term follow-up of congenital aortic stenosis after surgery. Br. Heart J. 34:47, 1972.

111. Sharlatzadeh, A. N., Kenj, M., and Girod, D.: Discrete subaortic stenosis. A report of 20 cases. J. Thorac. Cardiovasc. Surg. 63:258, 1972.

112. Shone, J. D., Sellers, R. D., Anderson, R. C., Adams, P., Jr., Lillehei, C. W., and Edwards, J. E.: The developmental complex of "parachute mitral valve," supravalvular ring of left atrium, subaortic stenosis, and coarctation of aorta. Am. J. Cardiol. 11:714, 1963.

113. Simon, A. L., and Reis, R. L.: The angiographic features of bicuspid and unicommissural aortic stenosis. Am. J. Cardiol. 28:353, 1971.

114. Sommerville, J., Stone, S., and Ross, O.: Fate of patients with fixed subaortic stenosis after surgical removal. Br. Heart J. 43:629, 1980.

115. Stansel, H. C., Tabry, I. I., Hellenbrand, W. E., Talner, N. S., and Kelley, M. J.: Apical-aortic shunts in children. Am. J. Surg. 135:547, 1978.

116. Tawes, R. L., Jr., Berry, C. L., and Aberdeen, E.: Congenital bicuspid aortic valve associated with coarctation of the aorta in children. Br. Heart J. 31:127, 1969.

117. Wagner, M. R., Weidman, W. M., Ellison, R. C., and Miettinen, D. S.: Congenital valvular aortic stenosis. Clinical detections of small pressure gradient. Am. J. Cardiol. 37:757, 1976.

118. Wagner, M. R., Weidman, W. M., Ellison, R. C., and Miettinen, O. S.: Indirect assessment of severity of aortic stenosis. Circulation 55 and 56 (Suppl. 1):20, 1977.

119. Weyman, A. J., Feigenbaum, H., Dillon, J. C., and Chang, S.: Cross-sectional echocardiography in assessing the severity of valvular aortic stenosis. Circulation 52:828, 1975.

120. Weyman, A. J., Feigenbaum, H., Hurwitz, R. A., Girod, D. A., Dillon, J. C., and Chang, S.: Cross-sectional echocardiography evaluating patients with discrete subaortic stenosis. Am. J. Cardiol. 37:358, 1976.

121. Weyman, A. J., Feigenbaum, H., Hurwitz, R. A., Girod, D. A., Dillon, J. C., and Chang, S.: Localization of left ventricular outflow tract obstruction by cross-sectional echocardiography. Am. J. Cardiol. 60:33, 1976.

122. Whitmer, J. T., James, F. W., Kaplan, S., Schwartz, D. C., and Knight, M. J. S.: Exercise testing in children before and after surgical treatment of aortic stenosis. Circulation 63:254, 1981.

123. Wilcox, W. D., Seward, J. B., Haglan, D. J., Mau, D. O., and Tajik, A. J.: Discrete subaortic stenosis: Two-dimensional echocardiographic features with angiographic and surgical correlation. Mayo Clin. Proc. 55:425, 1980.

124. Williams, D. E., Sahn, D. J., and Friedman, W. F.: Cross-sectional echocardiographic localization of the sites of the left ventricular outflow tract obstruction. Am. J. Cardiol. 37:250, 1976.

125. Williams, J. C. P., Barrett-Boyes, B. G., and Lowe, J. B.: Supravalvular aortic stenosis. Circulation 24:1311, 1961.

126. Young, J. B., Quinones, M. A., Waggoner, A. D., and Miller, R. R.: Diagnosis and quantification of aortic stenosis with pulsed doppler echocardiography. Am. J. Cardiol. 45:987, 1980.

13

Coarctation of the Aorta

Welton M. Gersony, M.D.

Coarctation of the aorta (CA) occurs as a constriction of the aorta, either discrete or of significant length, which is almost invariably located at the junction of the ductus arteriosus and the aortic arch just distal the left subclavian artery. Intracardiac lesions are often present with coarctation (CA) which may or may not affect the diagnostic features and clinical course of the disease. The basic lesion was described 200 years ago, and the precise physical findings which were outlined by Wernicke[15] in 1875 remain applicable today. Surgical treatment for CA has been available for over 35 years.[9, 20] Success depends upon the anatomy of the aortic arch, associated anomalies, the age of the patient, and other hemodynamic features.

Classification of coarctation of the aorta is based upon the presence or absence of severe isthmic narrowing as opposed to discrete obstruction and major associated lesions. Anatomically, CA is in a juxtaductal position, but it is very important to ascertain whether lower trunk blood flow is supplied predominantly by the left ventricular output via the ascending aorta (adult type), or by right heart blood flow into the pulmonary artery and across the patent ductus arteriosus (PDA) to the descending aorta (infantile type). The latter physiological state is most often encountered with long segment isthmic narrowing and severe intracardiac abnormalities. "Infantile coarctation" is not a specific descriptive term, since numerous infants are recognized to have "adult" type of discrete coarctation with left-to-right shunt across a juxtaposed ductus arteriosus.

Isolated coarctation of the aorta is the fifth or sixth most common of the congenital cardiovascular defects.[30] Among infants, CA ranked 4th in the New England Regional Study of congenital heart defects, accounting for 7.5% of all the infants under 1 year of age with cardiac malformations.[17] This may represent an underestimation since it has become apparent that newborn infants may not display a difference in blood pressure between the upper and lower extremities in the first few days of life.[53] The evolution of CA appears to be an active process in some babies, resulting in an increasing degree of obstruction and blood pressure gradient with time. Furthermore, even among older children and adolescents, CA is often overlooked by primary physicians who may not recognize the findings which characterize this disorder.[61]

Isolated CA in older patients is more common in males. The male to female ratio is 1.74 to 1,[5] whereas CA in infancy is associated with only a slight male predominance.[17] There appears to be no evidence for a Mendelian pattern of inheritance in the majority of patients.[5] The frequency of associated congenital cardiac defects is high; these include: PDA, ventricular septal defect (VSD), aortic stenosis (AS) and insufficiency (AI), and mitral valve abnormalities. Bicuspid aortic valve is the most frequently encountered associated malformation, occurring in as many as 85% of the cases in some series.[10, 65] Cerebral aneurysms appear to be an associated anomaly in a few patients with CA, predisposing these individuals to cerebrovascular accidents in the presence of severe hypertension. Seven percent of patients in one large series has noncardiac malformations, the most common of which were hypospadius, club foot, and ocular defects.[5] Coarctation of the aorta is the most common cardiovascular abnormality found with Turner's syndrome.

The prognosis for patients with CA is predicated on the anatomic features, early recognition, and surgical technique. Successful repair of this lesion in the presence of associated cardiac lesions has been accomplished in the first weeks of life, but most patients with isolated CA are operated upon beyond the first year.

PATHOLOGY

Coarctation of the aorta occurs in the form of a preductal segmental tubular hypoplasia or as a more discrete juxtaductal obstruction. Often, both components are present. A hemodynamic theory as to the genesis of CA best explains the various types of anatomic and physiological abnormalities which are observed, ranging from interruption of the aortic arch, to severe isthmal narrowing and finally to discrete coarctation (Fig. 13.1).[29, 56] It is postulated that CA is initiated in the presence of a cardiac abnormality which results in decreased antegrade aortic blood flow and proportionately increased flow through the pulmonary artery and PDA. A contraductal shelf-like structure[41] bifurcates ductal blood flow retrograde into the left subclavian and antegrade to the descending aorta. Antegrade aortic flow supplies the innominate, left carotid, and vertebral arteries, but very little blood reaches the aortic isthmus proximal to the left subclavian artery. This results in isthmic tubular hypoplasia. In cases of hypoplasia of the left heart, the ascending aorta is hypoplastic. If the genesis for decreased ascending aortic flow is based on less severe abnormalities, such as a bicuspid

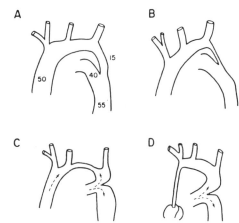

Fig. 13.1   (A) Normal fetal flow pattern. Numbers represent the approximate percentage of total cardiac output. Note that only 15% of cardiac output flows across the aortic isthmus distal to the left subclavian artery. (B) Isthmic hypoplasia with no contraductal shelf. (C) Bifurcation complex with development of contraductal shelf. Left subclavian supplied via the ductus arteriosus. Tubular hypoplasia is present in the segment between the left carotid and subclavian artery where ductal and aortic flow meet. (D) Aortic valve atresia, hypoplasia of the ascending aorta, and bifurcation complex. Ductal flow profuses great vessels. (Reproduced with permission from A. I. Schaffer, and K. Ellis.[56])

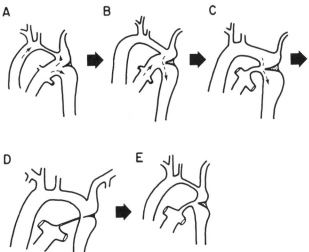

Fig. 13.2   Metamorphosis of coarctation. (A) Fetal prototype. No flow obstruction. (B) Late gestation. Aortic ventricle increases output and dilates hypoplastic segment. Antegrade aortic bypass shelf via ductal orifice. (C) Neonate. Ductal constriction initiates obstruction by removing bypass and increasing antegrade arch flow. (D) Mature juxtaductal stenosis. Bypass completely obliterated; intimal hypoplasia on edge of shelf aggravates stenosis. Collaterals develop. (E) Infantile type fetal prototype persists. Intracardiac left heart obstruction precludes an increase in antegrade aortic before or after birth. Both isthmal hypoplasia and contraductal shelf are present. Lower body flow often depends on patency of the ductus. (Reproduced with permission from A. I. Schaffer and K. Ellis.[56])

aortic valve or a malalignment type of VSD, only isthmal narrowing occurs. Occasionally, severely hypoplastic segments of the aortic isthmus may become completely atretic, resulting in an interrupted arch with the left subclavian artery arising either proximal or distal to the interruption. The nature of the CA lesion depends on the ultimate flow across the aortic isthmus proximal to the left carotid artery (Fig. 13.2). If the segment remains patent but narrow, then the "infantile" type of CA occurs (Fig. 13.3), usually with

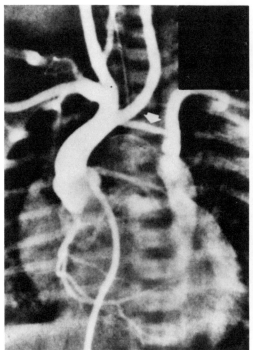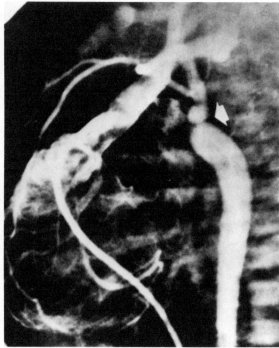

Fig. 13.3   Infantile coaractation showing bifurcation complex and segmental hypoplasia between left carotid and subclavian arteries (*arrows*).

right to left ductal flow to the descending aorta and almost invariably with an associated VSD. If antegrade aortic flow becomes normal after birth, isthmal narrowing will not be prominent. However, the exaggeration of the contraductal shelf[11] associated with bifurcating ductal flow results in potential obstruction of aortic blood flow. When the ductus is closed either spontaneously or surgically, a discrete "adult" CA is produced.[53, 63]

The hemodynamic theory nicely accounts for numerous features of the coarctation syndrome: e.g., isthmal narrowing, persistent contraductal shelf, and an increased frequency of lesions which can decrease antegrade aortic blood flow in utero. The role of ectopic ductal tissue within the aorta in the pathogenesis of coarctation of the aorta has been debated for over a century,[6] and, indeed, ductal tissue has been identified within the infant aorta.[27, 50, 67] However, ectopic ductal tissue does not explain tubular hypoplasia of the isthmus nor the obvious role of the juxtaductal shelf in determining the pathologic features of CA. In addition, CA is often associated with a large PDA after birth.

The relationship between aortic arch anomalies and VSD is well established.[42] The site and size of the VSD, as well as the presence of muscular bands which may divert blood flow away from the ascending aorta, have been postulated to be important in the pathogenesis of CA. There is a so called malalignment VSD located above the level of the papillary muscle of the conus which involves the inferior part of the conus septum. This results in the extension of the conus along the posterior edge of the defect where it can obstruct the anterior portion of the left ventricular outflow tract. In this situation, the aortic orifice is narrowed and displaced posteriorly. The resultant decreased antegrade aortic blood flow increases the likelihood that anomalies of the aortic arch will occur. On the other hand, when the VSD lies below the conus septum, either there will be no malalignment or the anterior displacement of the conus septum and parietal muscle band will cause right ventricular outflow obstruction

and aortic overriding (tetralogy of Fallot). In such cases, CA is virtually never identified.[56]

Coarctation of the aorta is frequently associated with biscuspid aortic valve,[12, 65] mitral valve anomalies,[51] and an increased frequency of other aortic arch abnormalities.[56] It has been recently postulated[40] that when spontaneous closure of central muscular VSDs occur, associated abnormalities of the aortic and mitral valve apparatus may remain. This type of VSD may explain the coarctation syndrome in some patients who have associated mitral or aortic valve lesions, but are without a clinical VSD at the time of evaluation.

The external appearance of the aorta at the site of the coarctation reveals an hour glass deformity of the outer contour. This may or may not be associated with a longer segment of isthmal narrowing which can be recognized externally. The aorta distal to the coarctation is usually dilated. Microscopic examination of the area of coarctation reveals thickening of the aortic media projecting into the aortic lumen as a shelf-like deformity. In older patients, the aortic intima is also thickened.

A localized area of intimal thickening and distortion of the media is often recognized distal to the contraductal shelf. This appears to be caused by the jet of blood across the coarctation which erodes the intimal area over a small patch of distal aorta. If there is a marked disruption of elastic tissue, a saccular aneurysm can develop later in life. Intimal dissection can also occur. In addition, this is the site where bacterial aortitis may become established.

COARCTATION OF THE AORTA IN INFANCY

The frequency of associated anomalies among symptomatic infants with coarctation of the aorta is high.[23, 30, 43] Two-thirds of the babies have associated PDA. Thirty to thirty-five percent have VSD, and it is in this group that urgent surgery during infancy is most often required. Only fifteen to twenty percent of babies who present with heart failure in the first few months of life with CA have an isolated abnormality; most patients without major intracardiac malformations are recognized later in life. Although the presence of a bicuspid aortic valve is common at all age levels, the rare patient with severe associated aortic stenosis is likely to present in early infancy.[64] Mitral valve abnormalities are common, but severe mitral dysfunction occurs in only 10% of the symptomatic infants.[30] In addition, CA occurs as part of the transposition complex, being especially common with transposition of the great arteries (TGA) and double outlet right ventricle (Taussig-Bing abnormality). In addition to the valvular abnormalities and other congenital heart lesions, a number of infants present with CA and cardiomyopathy.[23] Coarctation syndrome also includes variations of left heart hypoplasia with small ventricular chambers and endocardial fibroelastosis.

CA with associated anomalies is the second leading cause of heart failure in the newborn with heart disease. As a general principle, the more severe the associated lesions, the earlier the infant will be recognized to have heart failure. The mortality rate for patients with complex coarctation syndromes is highest in the first 2 months of life.[30]

MANIFESTATIONS

Clinical Features

The symptomatic baby with coarctation of the aorta with or without associated anomalies most often presents with heart failure and failure to thrive. In the most severe cases, the patient is in low cardiac output. Physical examination reveals an irritable debilitated infant who is dyspneic and tachypneic. The baby usually weighs no more than a few ounces above birth weight and has a weak cry and ashen color. Cardiac examination reveals a heaving left ventricular precordium, and a nonspecific systolic murmur along the left mid and upper sternal border, which often is heard over the back. A harsh pansystolic murmur may be audible at the left lower sternal border when a VSD is present, but the continuous murmur of a PDA is rarely noted. Likewise, a rough right upper sternal border bruit of AS is usually not identified. In the most severely ill patients, virtually no murmurs are audible. The liver is enlarged and pulmonary rales may be heard at the lung bases. There may be puffiness about the face and extremities. In patients with a normal cardiac output, the brachial and radial pulses are easily palpable, but the femoral and pedal pulses are weak or absent. However, in a number of patients, there may be no differences in the character of the lower and upper extremity pulses; both are weakly palpable or virtually absent. Blood pressures should be measured by the flush or[18] Doppler ultrasound technique[24] in both arms and one leg. Hypertension is usually noted in the upper limbs and diminished blood pressure is present in the lower extremities. The differences are found in the systolic and/or mean pressures, whereas the diastolic pressures tend to be similar. Systolic gradients will range between 20 and 140 mm Hg. Variations in upper extremity pressure occur on the basis of the position of the subclavian arteries relative to the coarctation. Right arm pressure will be the most consistently elevated, but in the rare instance of an aberrant right subclavian artery arising distal to the coarctation, the observed right arm blood pressure will be low.

In a number of instances, almost no blood pressure gradient or pulse differences will be found on physical examination. There are two explanations for this observation. (1)

The baby with a long segment isthmus coarctation and the right ventricle will perfuse the lower body via the PDA at virtually systemic pressure. A relatively low blood pressure is recorded both in the arms and in the legs, reflecting heart failure. In these cases, a large VSD and pulmonary artery hypertension can be expected. If there is some degree of obstruction at the ductal level, the pressure in the lower extremities may be slightly less than the upper, but these differences are not likely to be striking. (2) When the left ventricle is supplying lower extremity blood flow across the coarctation with or without a left to right shunt at the level of the PDA or VSD, a major gradient should be present between the arms and the legs. However, in the presence of severe heart failure, the lower cardiac output provided by the left ventricle will result in diminished blood flow and, therefore, a smaller gradient across the coarctation.

It is extremely important that palpation of the pulses and careful blood pressure determination by the flush or Doppler method be repeated following vigorous medical anticongestive measures. Often, as the baby's condition improves with treatment, the gradients will become prominent, and unless the physical examination is repeated, CA may be overlooked. It is impressive indeed when a baby in whom all the pulses were weak and no gradient was measured between the upper and lower extremities is reexamined, and vigorous brachial and radial pulses, weak or absent femoral and pedal pulses, and a 40 or 50 mm Hg difference between the upper and lower extremity blood pressures become evident.

Electrocardiographic Features

In an infant with CA in the first few months of life, the electrocardiogram reveals right ventricular hypertrophy, often with a strain pattern. This is noted regardless of the hemodynamic blood flow patterns across the ductus arteriosus. In the presence of CA in prenatal life, the right ventricle is subject to the same afterload as the left ventricle, since the right ventricle contributes blood flow into the aorta via the ductus arteriosus just proximal to or at the site of coarctation. When lower body blood flow is provided by the right ventricle in the neonate with "preductal" coarctation, the explanation for continued right ventricular hypertrophy is obvious; the right ventricle is providing systemic pressure. However, even when a discrete coarctation remains after birth, right ventricular hypertrophy remains dominant. As a patient with isolated CA is followed into the second year of life, a left ventricular hypertrophy pattern gradually emerges. If marked left ventricular enlargement and strain is recognized in the first few weeks of life, associated lesions of the left heart should be suspected.

Echocardiographic Features

The echocardiogram is most useful in determining the associated abnormalities including the status of the aortic and mitral valves and the presence or absence of a VSD. Discrete CA as well as narrowing of the aortic isthmus also may be demonstrated by 2D echocardiography (Fig. 13.4).[55] Doppler studies in conjunction with ultrasound are extremely useful in identifying CA in the infant age group.

Radiologic Features

Chest x-rays show the heart to be generally enlarged with prominent pulmonary vascularity consistent with heart failure. However, a characteristic inverted E sign may be noted on the frontal view with a barium study. These findings will be most evident in patients with short segment coarctation,

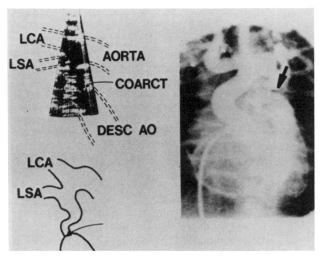

Fig. 13.4 Angiocardiogram (*right*) and echocardiographic still frame from an infant with a long segment tortuous coarctation are shown, along with a line drawing of the anatomy (*below*). The angiocardiogram is an AP projection while the echo view and line drawing are the equivalent of right lateral projections. The position of the coarctation (*coarct*) is shown by curved arrows on the echo still frame and the line drawing. (Reproduced with permission D. J. Sahn *et al.*[55])

but a number of infants will have isthmic narrowing terminating in a discrete obstruction which also can be identified in this manner. Since detailed diagnostic studies are required in order to plan medical and surgical management of these infants, it is rarely advisable to obtain a barium swallow, especially in critically ill babies.

CARDIAC CATHETERIZATION

The purpose of hemodynamic studies is not only to demonstrate the coarctation of the aorta, but also to determine the presence and severity of associated defects which are so often present in the infant group. It is important to obtain detailed information in order to assess the relative importance of the CA as it affects the overall hemodynamic state. Decisions as to the type and timing of surgical intervention are made on the basis of this study, which must be comprehensive and complete.

A large gradient across the coarcted area with hypertension in the proximal aorta suggests that the left ventricle is providing impetus for blood flow to the lower body and also indicates that cardiac output is not unduly decreased. A small or absent gradient suggests either a low cardiac output state or the physiology of preductal coarctation. The latter implies isthmal narrowing, and in all probability lower body blood flow is being provided by the right ventricle. Masking of severe CA by marked collateral blood flow is rarely a factor in the infant. If the ascending aorta is not entered with the catheter, then the systolic blood pressure gradient between the left ventricle and the distal aorta or a lower extremity defines the hemodynamic severity of the CA. It must be remembered, however, that a gradient across the aortic valve will also produce differential pressures between these catheter locations.

ANGIOCARDIOGRAPHY

Left ventricular angiography is helpful in demonstrating the important features of CA in infancy. If the PDA and pulmonary artery fill from an aortic root or left ventricular

contrast injection and the descending aorta is visualized, this suggests a physiological "postductal" coarctation. On the other hand, if the descending aorta is filled primarily from the pulmonary artery, this indicates a "preductal" type of physiological arrangement, with lower body blood flow being supplied by the right heart. Left ventricular angiography (Fig. 13.5) is also helpful in demonstrating the anatomy of the coarctation area. The presence or absence of a VSD is documented. The anatomic features of the mitral and aortic valves can be visualized; the presence and degree of severity of mitral insufficiency and/or AS is determined. In addition, angiography can be utilized to determine left ventricular performance and chamber size. In patients with VSD, selected angled view of left ventricular angiograms should be utilized to determine the location of a VSD and rule out the possibility of multiple communications.

The aim of cardiac catheterization in the infant with multiple abnormalities is essentially to determine whether elimination of the CA will be of sufficient hemodynamic benefit to warrant delay in surgical repair of other potentially correctable lesions. For example, it is important to determine by left and right ventricular pressures, systolic pressure differences, and angiography whether a VSD appears to be large and/or complicated. Left to right shunts at the atrial level are commonly found among infants with severe CA and left ventricular failure. In most instances, this is due to a dilated foramen ovale secondary to elevated left ventricular end-diastolic pressure and subsequent left atrial hypertension. However, cases of true atrial septal defects of both the secundum and primum types have been documented, and occasionally occur even in the presence of a VSD.[23]

TREATMENT

The treatment of coarctation of the aorta during infancy has become more surgically oriented in recent years. This is due to improving techniques in anesthesia, operative proce-

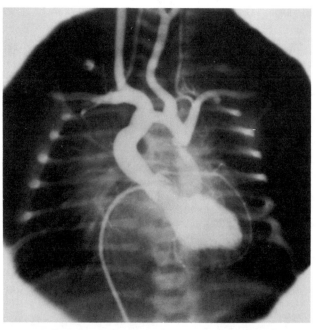

Fig. 13.5 Left ventricular angiogram. Coarctation of the aorta is demonstrated along with valvular aortic stenosis. The absence of a ventricular defect is documented, and there is no mitral insufficiency.

dure, and postoperative care. Critically ill infants with CA no longer are managed medically in the presence of heart failure and failure to thrive. The high operative mortality of past decades is no longer a stimulus for prolonged medical management in the face of a poor clinical course. The risk-benefit ratio has shifted in recent years towards surgical treatment not only because of lower operative mortality, initially, but also because reoperation is less often necessary.

The specific surgical approaches to complex coarctation syndromes in infancy are dictated by the associated lesions. However, one important generalization appears to be appropriate. In the majority of instances, it is the CA which results in the major hemodynamic burden and is ultimately most responsible for cardiac decompensation during infancy.

A number of factors account for this. The neonatal left ventricle does not respond well to severe afterload soon after birth; in patients with elevated left ventricular and proximal aortic pressures, left to right shunts across a VSD and/or PDA are exaggerated; and a physiologic preductal CA results in a right ventricle which must supply blood to the lower body while also pumping a large volume of blood to the lungs at systemic pressure. Some degree of pulmonary vasoconstriction is invariably present as well. Thus, CA primarily causes an increased afterload requirement for the left and right ventricles and indirectly results in a greater preload burden for the left and/or right ventricle in the presence of intracardiac or great artery communications.

Experience with combined CA and VSD has indicated that repair of the CA is the procedure that is associated with major benefit to the infant.[44, 62] Repairing the VSD alone would only be advantageous when the CA is trivial and, in most instances, this is not the case. A number of approaches to CA and VSD in infancy have been utilized. A standard management plan has been to repair the CA, and if pulmonary artery pressure remains elevated at the completion of the anastomosis, a pulmonary artery banding is carried out.[35, 45, 59, 64] Closing the VSD directly along with repair of the CA utilizing open heart surgical technique via a median sternotomy has been advocated,[52] but in most instances such an aggressive approach is not warranted. In recent years some institutions, including our own, have advocated repair of the CA withing banding, even in the presence of an isolated membranous VSD.[44, 62] This is done regardless of whether or not the VSD appears to be large. Afterwards, if the patient cannot be managed medically because of a large left to right shunt, a direct repair of the membranous VSD is carried out within days or weeks. In the experience of those who utilize this approach, this is rarely necessary, in that the patient improves dramatically after relief of the coarctation. In over 50% of the infants in our series,[62] the VSD became smaller or closed; pulmonary artery hypertension was no longer present, and a second operation was not needed. In most of the other cases, elective surgery for the VSD was carried out later in childhood. Banding of the pulmonary artery at initial operation is reserved for infants with multiple defects or large apical muscular communications, and for patients with single ventricle or other complex lesions. In these situations, surgical procedures for elimination of interventricular left to right shunts would not be feasible in early infancy, and a long-term palliated status is preferable.

Babies with CA and AS rarely have severe aortic valve obstruction; therefore, coarctation surgery alone is sufficient to carry such patients into later childhood. Rarely, however, a combined procedure is necessary. Similarly, mitral valve abnormalities, including stenosis and/or insufficiency, do not generally require surgical intervention during infancy.[16, 31, 68] With rare exceptions, these patients do well with repair of the coarctation alone. Over the years, mitral function often will improve; the apparent early severe insufficiency having been exaggerated prior to coarctation repair in the presence of hypertension, heart failure, and left ventricular dilatation. In a few instances, however, mitral valvuloplasty and even replacement have been required.

It is important to emphasize that the apparent presence of primary myocardial or endocardial disease, even with endocardial fibroelastosis, should not be a contraindication for coarctation repair in severely ill babies. Afterload reduction, by elimination of aortic obstruction caused by the coarctation, improves cardiac dynamics. Furthermore, a number of such patients will show markedly improved left ventricular function and with time will prove not to have the structural endocardial or myocardial disease which had been suspected.

SURGICAL PROCEDURES

The purposes of surgical management of coarctation of the aorta in infants are twofold: to relieve obstruction, and to avoid restenosis. Several types of procedures have been advocated. These include: end to end anastomosis,[25, 35] patch aortoplasty,[14, 54, 69] and the subclavian flap procedure.[47, 66] In addition, conduit insertion between the ascending and descending aorta have also been utilized for severe long segment obstruction.[46] Although the long-term results regarding the frequency of recoarctation are not available for the aortoplasty and subclavian flap procedures, it is to be expected that there will be a lower frequency of residual gradient utilizing these techniques which involve longitudinal incisions, than after resection and end to end anastomosis (Fig. 13.6A). On a theoretical basis, scarring in the region of the incision would be less likely to cause the napkin-ring type of constriction which has occurred later in childhood after the end to end anastomosis. The newer approaches seem especially useful in cases with tubular hypoplasia of the aortic isthmus with discrete coarctation at the site of the ductus arteriosus.

In the patch aortoplasty technique (Fig. 13.6B), the aorta is opened longitudinally and any existing membrane is excised. The aortotomy is extended from the inferior portion of the left subclavian artery to the largest portion of the

A. Resection with end-to-end repair

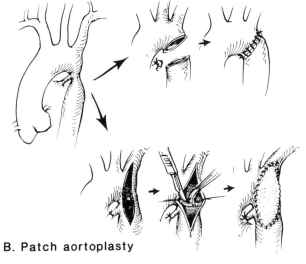

B. Patch aortoplasty

Fig. 13.6 Surgical techniques for repair of coarctation of the aorta. (Reproduced with permission from P. S. Hesslein.[25])

descending aorta. After excision of a fibrous shelf, an elliptical woven Dacron patch is inserted to expand the diameter of the lumen. The subclavian flap procedure (Fig. 13.7), which may be more desirable in that no exogenous material is utilized, consists of dividing the distal subclavian artery and inserting a flap of the proximal portion of this vessel between the two sides of the longitudinally split aorta throughout the coarcted segment. Regardless of the type of operative procedure for repair of the CA, the ductus arteriosus is always ligated and divided.

Operative mortality and morbidity depend on the circumstances under which surgery is carried out (e.g., age and condition of the patient, emergency status, experience of the surgeon, etc.) as well as the presence and severity of associated lesions. Recent mortality figures range from 8 to 32%,[3, 21, 36] and residual obstruction and/or recoarctation has been described in 16 to 33% of survivors of end to end anastomosis procedures with or without isthmus resection.[8, 13, 22, 35] Data regarding the newer operative techniques suggest that residual coarctation is less common.[7, 47] However, comparing resection versus patch aortoplasty it also has been reported that postoperative hypertension is virtually the same and that a residual gradient is related more to early age at operation rather than technique of repair.[25]

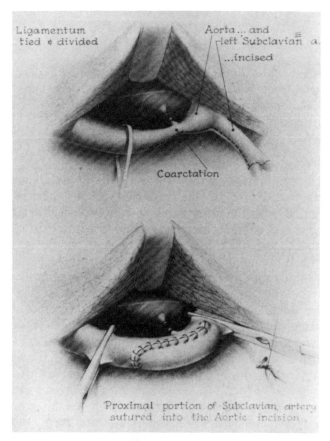

Fig. 13.7 Surgical repair of coarctation utilizing left subclavian artery flap. Drawing depicts the operative technique employed. The dotted line (*upper drawing*) indicates the location of transection of the left subclavian artery and longitudinal incision on the subclavian artery and aorta. The flap considerably enlarges the cross-sectional area of the aorta (*lower drawing*). (Reproduced with permission from W. S. Pierce *et al.*[47])

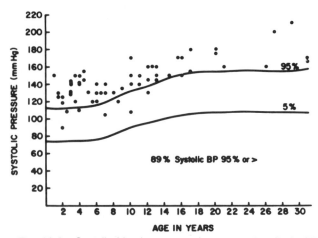

Fig. 13.8 Systolic blood pressures in upper extremity in 65 patients over 1 year of age with isolated coarctation of the aorta. (Reproduced with permission from M. A. Strafford *et al.*[61])

COARCTATION OF THE AORTA IN OLDER CHILDREN

Clinical Features

Coarctation of the aorta recognized after infancy rarely is associated with symptomatology. An occasional child will complain about weakness and/or pain in the legs after exercise, but the majority will have no complaints. The physical examination is characteristic. The pathognomonic features include differential blood pressure between the upper and lower extremities with systolic hypertension present in one arm (almost always the right) or both upper extremities. Absent or decreased femoral and pedal pulses are characteristic.

In a recent review of physical findings in 65 patients with CA over 1 year of age,[61] all had differential blood pressures between the upper and lower extremities, and 89% had systolic hypertension in the upper extremity greater than the 95th percentile for age (Fig. 13.8). Mean upper extremity blood pressure in the 65 patients was 145 ± 12 mm Hg; lower extremity blood pressure was 70 ± 10 mm Hg. Although absent femoral and pedal pulses are the hallmark of the disease, in only 40% of patients were the femoral pulses completely absent. Weakly palpable femoral pulses with a pulse lag were evident in 44%; the pulses were characterized as normal in 16%. Palpable pedal pulses were noted in 23% of the patients.

A short systolic murmur is often heard along the left sternal border at the third and fourth intercostal space. The murmur is well transmitted to the back and neck. The interscapular systolic murmur over the region of the CA is quite characteristic. Often, the typical murmur of mild AS can be heard in the third right intercostal space, and an apical systolic ejection click is also common. The latter findings suggest that an aortic valve deformity is present in addition to CA, but it is rare that a major degree of obstruction across the aortic valve is present. Among patients with well developed collateral blood flow, systolic or continuous murmurs may be heard over the left and right chest laterally and posteriorly.

Electrocardiographic Features

Among asymptomatic patients with isolated CA, either a normal electrocardiogram or the pattern of left ventricular hypertrophy can be expected. Occasionally, a left ventricular strain pattern over the left precordial leads is recognized. This could occur in the presence of severe hypertension or suggest the presence of myocardial disease and/or left heart valvular lesions.

Radiologic Features

Marked cardiac enlargement is rarely noted in the chest x-ray. However, there are a number of other findings which should alert the physician to the presence of CA. In a recent study, 48 patients with CA had a retrospective review of the preoperative chest films.[39] In only four was the chest x-ray interpreted as normal. Rib notching (Fig. 13.9) was present in 11, all over 5 years of age. The aorta was abnormal in 43 patients. Findings included arch abnormalities, localized inverted "3" signs (Fig. 13.10), and prominence of the descending aorta. A barium swallow may be helpful for the demonstration of aortic abnormalities, but an adequately penetrated chest radiograph is often sufficient. It has been suggested that it is more difficult to diagnose CA by chest x-ray in younger patients.[33] However, in this series, the percentage of individuals with coarctation who showed radiologic signs in the 1 to 5-year age group was similar to the older patients.

CARDIAC CATHETERIZATION

The findings at cardiac catheterization among older children have been well documented. Cardiologists vary in their decision as to whether cardiac catherization should be carried out prior to surgical intervention. It can be argued that the physical findings and radiologic features are pathonomonic for this condition, and that in a patient with characteristic findings, hemodynamic studies and angiography are unnecessary. If there are clinical or laboratory indications that an associated lesion is present, the CA is nevertheless repaired initially through a left thoracotomy, leaving the intracardiac defect to be reevaluated at a later time. Even a

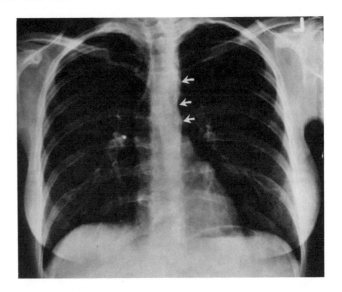

Fig. 13.10 Localized poststenotic dilatation: "3" sign (*arrows*). Obvious rib notching. (Reproduced with permission from E. C. Martin *et al.*[39])

hitherto unsuspected associated defect can be documented by cardiac catheterization and angiography after repair of the CA. Since complicating intracardiac defects are rare in the older child with CA, subsequent studies will not often be necessary; therefore, the majority of patients might never require catheterization.

Retrograde aortography in patients with CA can be associated with complications. Attempts at manipulation across a severe coarctation has resulted in perforation of collateral vessels. Since the pressure gradient across the coarctation will depend on blood flow as well as the degree of narrowing, and this is altered by the number and size of collateral vessels, obtaining a pullback pressure tracing across the coarctation is not necessarily an accurate measure of severity. In any event, the gradient can be determined by blood pressure measurements at the bedside.

On occasion, delineation of severe long segment coarctation is helpful to the surgeon prior to operation, so that a bypass procedure can be planned in advance. However, cardiac catheterization may be most helpful in the mildest cases of CA, and among patients in whom radiographic signs cannot be demonstrated on plain films or barium swallow. If only a small gradient exists between the upper and lower extremity systolic blood pressure, and if there are no clinical or laboratory findings suggestive of increased intercostal collateral blood flow, clamping of the distal coarcted segment at surgery may be inadvisable. Thus, in this situation, the nature of the obstruction and collateral flow might best be demonstrated by angiography prior to intervention. Aortography, while providing an excellent demonstration of the site of coarctation, still should not be used as the final indicator of the severity of hemodynamic obstruction, since the angle from which the coarcted segment of aorta is viewed may result in a less than accurate assessment of the size of the lumen at the site of constriction. In marginal situations, the physician must evaluate the clinical, hemodynamic, and angiographic data together in order to best assess severity and advisability of surgical intervention.

Angiography also demonstrates the condition known as pseudocoarctation of the aorta.[60] In this situation the aorta appears to be kinked or buckled, and a small ridge is noted distal to the left subclavian, similar to that seen in obstruc-

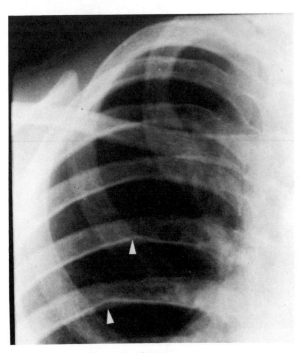

Fig. 13.9 Detail from a chest roentgenogram with light technique showing rib notching (white arrowheads).

tive cases (Fig. 13.11). However, in pseudocoarctation there is no systolic hypertension or difference between upper and lower extremity blood pressures. Collateral circulation is not increased. Such cases are usually recognized in adults on the basis of the appearance of an aneurysm of the aortic arch. Rupture has been reported rarely.

When the typical physical findings and radiographic data suggestive of CA are not present or when neurofibromatosis is suspected, an aortogram must be carried out in order to rule out abdominal coarctation.[48, 49] The renal and mesenteric arteries may also be involved (Fig. 13.12).[2, 49] Abdominal or low thoracic long segment coarctation has also been noted as an acquired lesion in patients with an inflammatory type of aortitis similar to Takayashu's disease.[19]

TREATMENT

The poor prognosis of untreated coarctation of the aorta is well known. Twenty percent of patients die between the first and second decade of life and 80% expire before the age of 50.[4] It is agreed that CA should be repaired during childhood.

The timing of surgical intervention has been influenced by concerns about the growth of the anastomotic site. In the early years, recommendations were made to repair this lesion at the age of 10 or 11 years, an age when the cross-sectional area of the aorta is similar to that seen in the adult. However, experimental data and clinical experience have indicated that surgery can be done at a much younger age without recurrent coarctation.[22]

Recent reports appear to have added to the importance of repairing CA early in life. A study of patients 20 years following repair[38] carried out during adolescence or young adulthood revealed late cardiovascular complications in the

majority of cases. Another report described less postoperative hypertension in patients operated upon at under 5 years of age than in the older age group.[34] Such data suggest that repair early in childhood may be important in preventing late hypertension. There is also a decreased frequency of endocarditis and cerebral hemorrhage due to associated cerebral aneurysms if the coarctation is eliminated early in life.

Improvements in surgical technique have made safe, early operative intervention feasible for the patient with asymptomatic isolated CA with little possibility of recurrence. Furthermore, patients in whom surgical correction has been delayed into late adolescence or adulthood, appear to have a greater risk of premature death and debilitation from cardiovascular disease.

Of course, consideration of optimal timing of surgical intervention is not possible unless the child with CA is identified and referred to a medical center by the primary physician at an early age. Thus, a greater emphasis on early detection seems warranted. However, our experience suggests that early diagnosis is not common.[61] Among 65 consecutive patients in whom uncomplicated CA was diagnosed after 1 year of age, the median age of diagnosis was 10 years. Only 14% of the cases had the specific diagnosis of CA made at the time of referral. The remaining referrals were made after an incidental notation of hypertension or a cardiac murmur, either at a routine physical examination or under special circumstances. Cardiac murmurs which appeared to the primary physician to be of significance resulted in referral at a median age of 6 years and hypertension at 18 years. Almost half of the patients referred because of elevated blood pressure had additional delays in referral even after hypertension was recognized, since the difference in upper and lower extremity blood pressures were not recognized. It

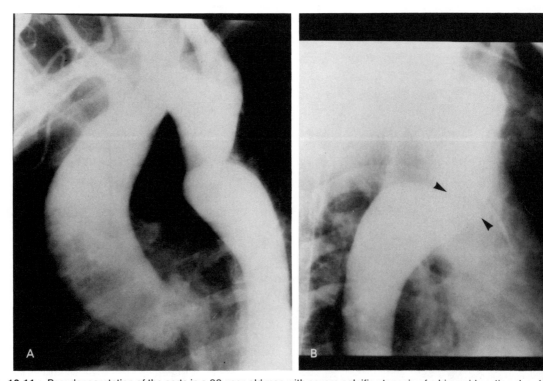

Fig. 13.11   Pseudocoarctation of the aorta in a 22-year-old man with severe calcific stenosis of a bicuspid aortic valve. (*A*) An aortogram, right posterior oblique view, shows poststenotic dilatation of the ascending aorta and kinking of the arch beyond the left subclavian. (*B*) A biplane roentgenogram, left posterior oblique view, confirms the absence of significant constriction of the aortic lumen as well as infolding and kinking of the posterior lateral wall.

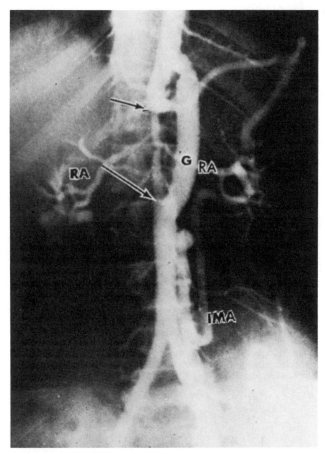

Fig. 13.12 Abdominal aortogram demonstrating a coarctation of the abdominal aorta just below the celiac axis. A patent graft (*G*) provides a bypass around the coarctation (between arrows). Dilated splenic and inferior mesenteric (*IMA*) arteries provide collateral circulation. The superior mesenteric artery does not opacify. The renal arteries (*RA*) appear hypoplastic. (Reproduced with permission from T. A. Riemenschneider et al.[49])

is important to emphasize that primary physicians must be educated that as part of routine pediatric care, blood pressure in lower as well as upper extremities should be measured.

At the present time, we advise elective surgical correction of CA between the ages of 2 and 4 years and earlier in the presence of sever hypertension and symptoms of heart failure or cardiomegaly. Utilizing this approach, it is possible that the late cardiovascular complications in adolescence and young adulthood can be avoided. Even in the rare instance when a second procedure might be required, this is preferable to long-standing hypertension, chronic left ventricular hypertrophy, and eventual myocardial dysfunction. It is distressing that less than one-third of patients with isolated CA are identified prior to 5 years of age.

SURGICAL TECHNIQUE AND POSTOPERATIVE COURSE

Primary anastomosis is the surgical treatment of choice for the majority of patients with CA. For those few patients in which the length of the coarctation is too great to allow primary repair, a Dacron graft may be utilized. A few patients will be expected to have a PDA, but in most instances it is the ligamentum arteriosus which is divided.

A rare complication which is of great concern is that inadequate spinal artery pressure during clamping of the distal aorta at the time of repair may lead to spinal cord ischemia and paresis.[57] This has been described both in patients with severe and mild CA and limited collateral blood flow. Surgery can be avoided in many patients with trivial gradients both at rest and during exercise and with no hypertension, but among those in whom operation is deemed advisable, every effort must be made to avoid this complication. This can be accomplished by utilizing patch grafts with partial aortic occlusion, or by the use of temporary or permanent Dacron conduits to bypass the coarcted segment. Extracorporeal circulation may be required under these circumstances.

A recent study indicates that patients with unusually severe upper body hypertension during the operation and low descending aortic pressure distal to the clamp are most prone to spinal cord ischemia.[1] It is postulated that arterial hypertension in the cerebral circulation results in high cerebral spinal fluid pressure throughout the length of the spinal column. Resultant high venous pressure may obstruct flow of low pressure arterial blood into areas of the spinal cord supplied from arteries below the coarctation. Cerebral spinal fluid monitoring was utilized by these authors, so that the potential for this complication could be recognized. The use of agents such as nitroprusside during surgery, which rapidly lower arterial blood pressure, may temporarily exaggerate cerebral spinal fluid pressure elevation and thus lead to the physiologic events which could predispose a patient to paresis.

Rebound hypertension immediately following surgery is common, especially among patients with moderate to severe upper extremity hypertension prior to operation.[26] Perhaps because such elevations of pressure tend to be treated more vigorously in recent years, the syndrome of severe constriction of mesenteric arteries associated with gangrene of the intestines no longer appears to be encountered. However, a mild form of mesenteric arteritis is frequently recognized in patients who manifest hypertension and abdominal pain 1 to 5 days after surgery for CA. Prolonged restriction of oral feedings after surgery may be helpful as a preventive measure. Severe postoperative hypertension should be treated. Intramuscular reserpine administered on one or two occasions may result in dramatic improvement.[26] A short course of hydralazine is also effective. It is rare that a patient will require chronic antihypertensive therapy following discharge from the hospital.

After successful repair of coarctation of the aorta, an unrestricted life should be recommended. Routine antibiotic prophylaxis for the prevention of endocarditis should be continued. Associated lesions, such as mitral and aortic valve deformities and small intracardiac shunts, should be observed, but intervention is rarely necessary during childhood or young adult years. Late recoarctation in patients repaired after 1 year of age is unusual.[28, 58]

Whether there is a resurgence of hypertension during adolescence or young adult life, in patients who had been documented to be normotensive for many years, is questionable. Such cases have been reported,[34, 38] but whether the frequency of hypertension in these patients is greater than would be expected in the general population is unknown. The postoperative patients with CA tend to be observed more carefully and have blood pressure determinations more often, so that the possibility of recognition of hypertension is greater in this population. Even if late hypertension may occasionally occur, there can be no doubt that the surgical relief of coarctation early in life has favorably altered the prognosis for patients with this anomaly.

REFERENCES

1. Berendes, J., Bredée, J., and Schipperheyn, J.: Paraparesis after surgical correction of aortic coarctation (abstr.). Circulation, vol. 64, Supp. IV., Oct., 1981.
2. Bjork, V. O., and Intont, F.: Coarctation of the abdominal aorta with right renal artery stenosis. Ann. Surg. 160:54, 1964.
3. Berman, L. B., Neches, W. H., Patnode, R. E., Fricker, F. J. Matthews, R. A., Park, S. C.: Coactation of the aorta in children: Late results after surgery. Am. J. Dis. Child. 134:464, 1980.
4. Campbell, M.: Natural history of coarctation of the aorta. Br. Heart J. 32:63, 1970.
5. Campbell, M., and Polani, P. E.: The etiology of coarctation of the aorta. Lancet 1:463, 1961.
6. Cassels, D. E.: The Ductus Arteriosus. Charles C Thomas, Springfield, Ill., 1973, a) p. 161; b) p. 180.
7. Connor, T. M., and Baker, W. P.: A comparison of coarctation resection and patch angioplasty using postexercise blood pressure measurements. Circulation 64, No. 3, 1981.
8. Connors, J. P., Hartmann, A. F., Jr., and Weldon, C. S.: Considerations in the surgical management of infantile coarctation of aorta. Am. J. Cardiol. 36:489, 1975.
9. Crafoord, C., and Nylin, G.: Congenital coarctation of the aorta and its surgical treatment. J. Thorac. Surg. 14:347, 1945.
10. Edwards, J. E.: Coarctation of the aorta. In Pathology of the Heart, 2nd ed., edited by S. E. Gould, Charles C Thomas, Springfield, Ill., 1960.
11. Edwards, J. E.: Malformations of the thoracic aorta. In Pathology of the Heart and Blood Vessels, 3rd ed., edited by S. E. Gould. Springfield, Ill., Charles C Thomas, 1968, p. 422.
12. Edwards, J. E., Carey, L., Newfield, H. N., and Lester, R. G.: Congenital Heart Disease. W. B. Saunders, Philadelphia, 1965, pp. 25, 217, 680, 684, 695.
13. Eshaghpour, E., and Olley, P. M.: Recoarctation of the aorta following coarctectomy in the first year of life: A follow-up study. J. Pediatr. 80:809, 1972.
14. Fleming, W. H., Sarafian, L. B., Clark, E. B., Dooley, K. J., Hofschire, P. J., Hopeman, A. R., Ruckman, R. N., and Mooring, P. K.: Critical aortic coarctation: Patch aortoplasty in infants less than age 3 months. Am. J. Cardiol. 44:687–690, 1979.
15. Flexner, J.: Coarctation of the aorta (adult type): Clinical and experimental studies. Am. Heart J. 11:572, 1936.
16. Freed, M. D., Keane, J. F., Van Praagh, R., Castaneda, A.R., Bernhardt, W. F., and Nadas, A. S.: Coarctation of the aorta with congenital mitral regurgitation. Circulation 48:1175–1184, 1974.
17. Fyler, D. C., Buckley, L. P., Hellenbrand, W. E., and Cohn, H. E.: Report of the New England Regional Infant Cardiac Program, Supplement to Pediatrics, Vol. 65, No. 2, Feb. 1980.
18. Goldring, D., and Wohltman, H.: Flush method for blood pressure determinations in newborn infants. J. Pediatr. 40:285, 1952.
19. Gonzalez-Corna, J. L., Villavicencio, L., Molina, B., and Bessudo, L.: Non-specific obliterative aortitis in children. Ann. Thorac. Surg. 4:193, 1967.
20. Gross, R. E., and Hufnagel, C. A.: Coarctation of the aorta: Experimental studies regarding its surgical correction. N. Engl. J. Med. 233:287, 1945.
21. Hallman, G. L., Yashar, J. J., Bloodwell, R. D., and Cooley, D. A.: Surgical correction of coarctation of the aorta in the first year of life. Ann. Thorac. Surg. 4:106, 1967.
22. Hartmann, A. F., Jr., Goldring, D., Hernandez, A., Behrer, M. R., Schad, N., Ferguson, T.,

and Burford, T.: Recurrent coarctation of the aorta after successful repair in infancy. Am. J. Cardiol. 25:405, 1970.
23. Hartmann, A. F., Goldring, D., Strauss, A. W., Hernandez, A., McKnight, R. C., and Weldon, C. S.: Coarctation of the aorta. In Heart Disease in Infants, Children, and Adolescents, 2nd ed., edited by A. J. Moss, F. H. Adams, and G. C. Emmanouilides. Williams & Wilkins, Baltimore, 1977, p. 199.
24. Hernandez, A., Goldring, D., and Hartmann, A. F., Jr.: Measurement of blood pressure in infants and children by the Doppler ultrasonic technique. Pediatrics 48:788, 1971.
25. Hesslein, P. S., McNamara, D. G., Morriss, M. J., Hallman, G. L., and Cooley, D. A.: Comparison of resection versus patch aortoplasty for repair of coarctation in infants and children. Circulation Vol. 64, July, 1981.
26. Ho, E. C. K., and Moss, A. J.: The syndrome of mesenteric arteritis following surgical repair of aortic coarctation. Pediatrics 49:40, 1972.
27. Ho, S. Y., and Anderson, R. H.: Coarctation, tubular hypoplasia and the ductus arteriosus. Br. Heart J. 41:268–274, 1979.
28. Hubbell, M. M., O'Brien, R. G., Krovetz, L. J., Mauck, H. P., and Tompkins, D. G.: Status of patients 5 or more years after correction of coarctation of the aorta over age 1 year. Circulation 60 (1):74–80, 1979.
29. Hutchins, G. M.: Coarctation of the aorta explained as a branch point of the ductus arteriosus. Am. J. Pathol. 63:203–214, 1971.
30. Keith, J. D., Rowe, R. D., and Vlad, P.: Coarctation of the aorta. In Heart Disease in Infancy and Childhood, 3rd ed. Macmillan, New York, 1978, p. 226.
31. Khoury, G., Hawes, C. R., and Grow, J. B.: Coarctation of the aorta with obstructive anomalies of the mitral valve and left ventricle. J. Pediatr. Vol. 75, No. 4, Oct. 1969.
32. Kirklin, J. W., Burchell, H. B., Pugh, D. G., Purke, E. C., and Mills, S. D.: Surgical treatment of coarctation of the aorta in a ten-week-old infant: Report of a case. Circulation 6:411, 1952.
33. Lester, R. G., Margulis, A. R., and Nice, C. M.: Roentgenographic evaluation of coarctation of the aorta in infants. J.A.M.A. 163:1022–1026, 1957.
34. Liberthson, R. R., Pennington, D. G., Jacobs, M. L., and Daggett, W. M.: Coarctation of the aorta: Review of 234 patients and clarification of management problems. Am. J. Cardiol., 43:835–840, 1979.
35. Litwin, S. B., Bernhard, W. F., Rosenthal, A., and Gross, R. E.: Surgical resection of coarctation of the aorta in infancy. J. Pediatr. Surg. 6:307, 1971.
36. Macmanus, O., Starr, A., Lambert, L. E., and Grunkemeler, G.: Correction of aortic coarctation in neonates: Mortality and late results. Ann. Thorac. Surg. 24:544–549, 1977.
37. Malm, J. R., Blumenthal, S., Jameson, A. G., and Humphreys, G. H., II: Observations on coarctation of the aorta in infants. Arch. Surg. 86:110, 1963.
38. Maron, B. J., Humphries, J. O., Rowe, R. D., and Mellits, E. D.: Prognosis of surgically corrected coarctation of the aorta: A 20-yr. postoperative appraisal. Circulation 47:119–126, 1973.
39. Martin, E. C., Strattford, M. A., and Gersony, W. M.: Initial detection of coarctation of the aorta: An opportunity for the radiologist. Am. J. Roentgenol. 137:1015–1017, 1981.
40. Moene, R. J., Oppenheimer-Dekker, A., and Wenink, A. C.: Relation between aortic arch hypoplasia of variable severity and central muscular ventricular septal defects: Emphasis on associated left ventricular abnormalities. Am. J. Cardiol. 48:111–116, 1981.

41. Moffat, D. B.: Pre- and postnatal changes in the left subclavian artery and their possible relationship to coarctation of the aorta. Acta Anat. 43:346–357, 1960.
42. Moulaert, A. J., Bruins, C. C., and Oppenheimer-Dekker, A.: Anomalies of the aortic arch and ventricular septal defect. Circulation 53:1011–1015, 1976.
43. Nadas, A. S., and Fyler, D. C.: Pediatric Cardiology, 3rd ed. W. B. Saunders, Philadelphia, 1972, p. 460.
44. Neches, W. H., Park, S. C., Lenox, C. C., Zuberbuhler, J. R., Siewers, R. D., and Hardesty, R. L.: Coarctation of the aorta with ventricular septal defect. Circulation 55:189–194, 1977.
45. Pelletier, C., Davignon, A., Ethier, M. F., and Stanley, P.: Coarctation of the aorta in infancy. J. Thorac. Cardiovasc. Surg. 57:171, 1969.
46. Pennington, D. G., Liberthson, R. R., Jacobs, M., Scully, H., Goldblatt, A., and Daggett, W. M.: Critical review of experience with surgical repair of coarctation of the aorta. J. Thorac. Cardiovasc. Surg. 77:217, 1979.
47. Pierce, W. S., Waldhausen, J. A., Berman, W., and Whitman, V.: Late results of the subclavian flap procedure in infants with coarctation of the thoracic aorta. Circulation, Suppl. 1, Vol. 58, No. 3, Sept. 1978.
48. Pyorala, K., Heinonen, O., Koselo, P., and Heikel, P. E.: Coarctation of the abdominal aorta. Review of twenty-seven cases. Am. J. Cardiol. 6:650, 1960.
49. Riemenschneider, T. A., Emmanouilides, G. C., Hirose, F., and Linde, L. M.: Coarctation of the abdominal aorta in children: Report of three cases and review of the literature. Pediatrics 44(5), 1969.
50. Rosenberg, H. S.: Coarctation of the aorta: Morphology and pathogenetic considerations. Perspect. Pediatr. Pathol. 1:339–368, 1973.
51. Rosenquist, G. C.: Congenital mitral valve disease associated with coarctation of the aorta. Circulation 49:985–993, 1974.
52. Rowe, R. D., and Vlad, P.: Diagnostic problems in the newborn: Origins of mortality in congenital cardiac malformation. In Heart Disease in Infancy, edited by B. G. Barratt-Boyes, J. M. Neutze, and E. A. Harris, Longman, New York, 1973, p. 3.
53. Rudolph, A. M., Heyman, M. A., and Spitznas, U.: Hemodynamic considerations in the development of narrowing of the aorta. Am. J. Cardiol. 30:514–525, 1972.
54. Sade, R. M., Taylor, A. B., and Chariker, E. P.: Aortoplasty compared with resection for coarctation of the aorta in young children. Ann. Thorac. Surg. 28:346, 1979.
55. Sahn, D. J., Allen, H. D., McDonald, G., and Goldberg, S. J.: Real-time cross-sectional echocardiographic diagnosis of coarctation of the aorta. Circulation 56 (5):762–769, 1977.
56. Schaffer, A. I., and Ellis, K.: Hemodynamic genesis of aortic coarctation and other arch anomalies. In Advances in Heart Disease. Grune & Stratton, New York, to be published.
57. Schuster, S. R., and Gross, R. E.: Surgery for coarctation of the aorta: A review of 500 cases. J. Cardiovasc. Surg. 43:54, 1962.
58. Simon, A. B., and Zloto, A. E.: Coarctation of the aorta. Longitudinal assessment of operated patients. Circulation 50:456, 1974.
59. Sinha, S. N., Kardatzke, M. L., Cole, R. B., Muster, A. J., Wessel, H. U., and Paul, M. H.: Coarctation of the aorta in infancy. Circulation 40:385, 1969.
60. Smyth, P. T., and Edwards, J. E.: Pseudocoarctation, kinking or buckling of the aorta. Circulation 46:1027, 1972.
61. Strattford, M. A., Griffiths, S. P., and Gersony, W. M.: Coarctation of the aorta: A study in delayed detection. Pediatrics 69:159–163, 1982.

62. Strattford, M. A., Hayes, C. J., Griffiths, S. P., Hordof, A. J., Edie, R. N., Bowman, F. O., Malm, J. R., and Gersony, W. M.: Management of the infarct with coarctation of the aorta and ventricular septal defect (abstr.) Am. J. Cardiol. 45:450, 1980.

63. Talner, N. S., and Berman, M. A.: Postnatal development of obstruction in coarctation of the aorta: Role of the ductus arteriosus. Pediatrics 56:562–569, 1975.

64. Tawes, R. L., Aberdeen, E., Waterston, D. J.,

and Bonham-Carter, R. E.: Coarctation of the aorta in infants and children. Circulation 39–40 (Suppl. I):173–184, 1969.

65. Tawes, R. L., Berr, C. L., and Aberdeen, E.: Congenital bicuspid aortic valves associated with coarctation of the aorta in children. Br. Heart J. 31:127–128, 1969.

66. Waldhausen, J. A., and Nahrwold, D. L.: Repair of coarctation of the aorta with a subclavian flap. J. Thorac. Cardiovasc. Surg. 51:532, 1966.

67. Wielenga, G., and Dankmeijer, J.: Coarctation of the aorta. J. Pathol. Bacteriol. 95:265–274, 1968.

68. Wood, W. C., Wood, J. C., Lower, R. R., Bosher, L. H., and McCue, C. M.: Associated coarctation of the aorta and mitral valve disease. J. Pediatr. Vol. 87, No. 2, Aug. 1975.

69. Vosschulte, K.: Isthmusplastik zur behandlung der aortem isthmusstenose. Thoraxchirugie 4:443, 1957.

14

Anomalies of the Aortic Arch Complex

Norman J. Sissman, M.D.

Anomalies of the aortic arch complex have been known since the 18th century. In 1939, Wolman[123] described the syndrome produced by a double aortic arch. Gross described the first surgical correction of the same entity in 1945. Since then the experiences of diagnosticians, surgeons, radiologists, and pathologists have accumulated. Numerous reviews on the subject have appeared; that of Stewart et al.[107] is the most extensive and contains a full bibliography. Others emphasize various aspects.[15, 45, 58, 79, 100]

The incidence of anomalies of this type is not known, as many are asymptomatic. On the basis of published cases, it is clear that the number of children presenting because of difficulties due to a lesion in this group of anomalies is small. There is no predilection of these anomalies for either sex. The association with other cardiac defects will be discussed as they are described individually.

EMBRYOLOGY AND ETIOLOGY

Congdon[22] made many of the basic observations on morphologic development of the aortic arches in the human. Barry[7] provided a clear summary and analysis of these data; others[45, 100, 107] have used this information as a basis for classification of anomalies and also as reasonable background for conclusions about their pathogenesis. Barry's semidiagrammatic illustrations of the developmental changes leading to the mature aorta and its branches are reproduced in Figure 14.1.

Stewart et al.[107] have introduced a schema, the "hypothetic double aortic arch," to conceptualize the developmental origin of almost all anomalies of the aortic arch complex. If one assumes that these defects result either from regression and atrophy of embryonic vascular structures which normally remain patent, or from the maintenance of patency in structures which normally regress, one can reconstruct a sequence of events leading to any set of defects. Figure 14.2, reproduced from Stewart et al., retains the method of shading used by Barry (Fig. 14.1) to identify embryonic vessels or segments of vessels. Theoretic explanations of the pathogenesis of defects of the aortic arch complex are derived from this schema by postulating changes in the normal sequence of embryonic events at the six sites indicated in the figure by *arrows*.

Anomalies of the aortic arch complex have been produced

experimentally by many methods.[49, 51, 93, 106, 120–122] However, none has been implicated directly in the occurrence of aortic arch anomalies in the human.

Undoubtedly the theory of multifactorial inheritance, applied by Nora[81] to other types of congenital heart disease will be used also to elucidate the etiologies of aortic arch anomalies. Although the nature of the genetic background and the relevant environmental factors has yet to be identified, recent observations[50, 61, 66, 71, 92, 99] have suggested that the size and continuity of the aortic arch and its branches are related to blood flow through them during intrauterine life.

CLASSIFICATION

Anomalies of the aortic arch complex form a diverse group in their anatomic and clinical manifestations. Various classifications have been published.[45, 79, 100, 107]

Table 14.1 lists the anomalies considered in this chapter. This list is clinically oriented and, because of the important role that radiology has in diagnosis of these diseases, the classification emphasizes aspects of the anomalies that can be appreciated from study of various types of x-ray examinations of the thorax.

I. ANOMALIES OF POSITION, COURSE, AND COMPOSITION OF THE AORTA

A. DOUBLE AORTIC ARCH

Pathology

A double aortic arch is characterized by the presence of both left and right aortic arches which arise from a branching of the ascending aorta, pass on both sides of the trachea and esophagus, and unite posteriorly to form a single descending aorta which may, in its upper portion, lie to the right or left of the vertebral column, more commonly the latter. According to the hypothetic double aortic arch schema, this anomaly occurs as a result of a failure of regression of the embryonic right eighth dorsal aortic segment. All cases reported to date have had a left-sided ductus arteriosus. The luminal size of the two arches in relation to each other varies considerably. They may be equal in size, or one may be smaller;

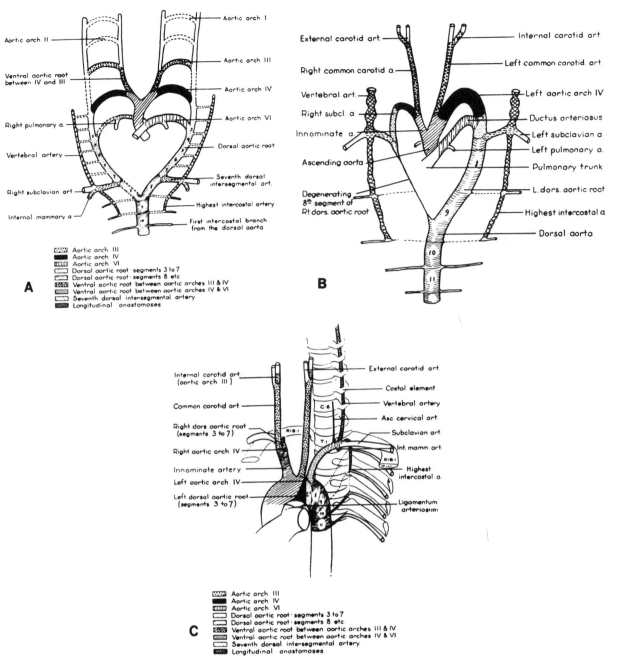

Fig. 14.1 Diagrams of how components of the aortic arch system change size and configuration during embryonic development and contribute to the normal adult structures. The scheme of identification is the same in all three drawings. The components which do not normally persist in the adult are indicated by *dashed lines.* The Arabic numbers indicate the segments of each dorsal aortic root and the dorsal aortas. (*A*) Embryonic arch complex in the human embryo. (*B*) Aortic arch complex in a human embryo of 15-mm crown-rump length. (*C*) Adult aortic arch complex. (Reproduced with permission from A. Barry.[7])

indeed, one of them may be represented by only an atretic strand. Figure 14.3 illustrates in a diagrammatic manner the features of a double aortic arch. Among the 14 cases reported by Stewart *et al.*[107] three patients had other anomalies. Higashino and Ruttenberg[48] reviewed 16 cases of double aortic arch associated with intracardiac defects; 15 of the 16 were cyanotic and included tetralogy of Fallot and transposition of the great arteries. Several cases with coarctation in one of the aortic branches[89, 107] have been reported.

Manifestations

Clinical Features. The majority of patients manifest symptoms early in infancy which are severe enough to be

life-threatening. The symptoms and signs are those of a vascular ring. As with all vascular rings, there are no alterations of normal cardiac physiology and no changes in the electrocardiogram or other tests of cardiac function.

Radiologic Features. Details of the radiologic manifestations have been described.[58, 79, 107] Conventional films of the chest may show emphysematous changes in the lungs common to patients with partial respiratory obstruction. The mediastinum may be widened and the presence of a right aortic arch alone, or with a left arch in addition, may be recognized. Narrowing of the trachea by components of the arches from the left and/or the right side may be seen in the posteroanterior view and from the anterior aspect of the trachea in the lateral projection. Barium swallow shows the following features:[58, 79] (a) There is compression of the esophagus from its posterior aspect by a rounded mass (the junction of two arches with the upper descending aorta). (b) The esophagus is indented by the two arches from both the left and right sides in the posteroanterior projection. The lateral indentations may be of equal or unequal size and may be at the same or different cephalocaudal levels. (c) There may be a similar indentation of the esophagus from its anterior aspect which is transmitted to the esophagus by deviation of the trachea caused by the ring. Figure 14.4 illustrates some of these characteristics in a 6-year-old boy with a double aortic arch proven at surgery. Cross-sectional echocardiography and computed tomography of the thorax may aid in diagnosis.

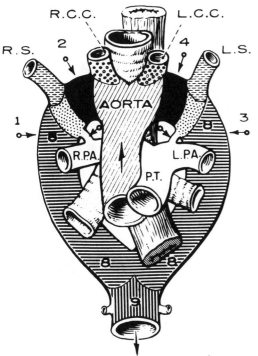

Fig. 14.2 Diagram of Edwards' hypothetic double aortic arch and bilateral ducti arteriosi. The ascending and descending aorta are each depicted in midline positions. The scheme of identification is the same as in Fig. 14.1. *Arrows* point to the four key locations where regression is thought to occur. *Arrow 1* indicates the eighth segment of the right dorsal aorta; *arrow 2*, the right fourth arch; *arrows 3 and 4*, the corresponding two positions on the left; and the *unnumbered arrows*, the ducti arteriosi. *P.T.*, pulmonary trunk; *R.P.A.*, right pulmonary artery; *L.P.A.*, left pulmonary artery; *R.S.*, right subclavian artery; *L.S.*, left subclavian artery; *R.C.C.*, right common carotid; *L.C.C.*, left common carotid. (Reproduced with permission from J. R. Stewart *et al.*[107])

TABLE 14.1   ANOMALIES OF THE AORTIC ARCH COMPLEX

I. Anomalies of position, course or composition of the aorta
  A. Double aortic arch
  B. Double lumen aortic arch
  C. With left aortic arch and left upper descending aorta
    1. Aberrant right subclavian artery
    2. Aberrant brachiocephalic arteries other than the right subclavian
      a. Aberrant brachiocephalic arteries without compression of the trachea
      b. Aberrant innominate or left common carotid arteries causing compression of the trachea
    3. Ductus arteriosus sling
    4. Subclavian steal
  D. Circumflex retroesophageal aortic arch
  E. Right aortic arch
    1. Without retroesophageal component
    2. With retroesophageal component
II. Abnormalities of length, size, or continuity of the aorta
  A. Cervical aorta
  B. Pseudocoarctation of the aorta
  C. Hypoplasia of the aorta
  D. Complete interruption of the aortic arch
III. Anomalies of the pulmonary arterial system
  A. Anomalous left pulmonary artery ("vascular sling")
  B. Unilateral absence of a pulmonary artery
  C. Origin of one pulmonary artery from the ascending aorta

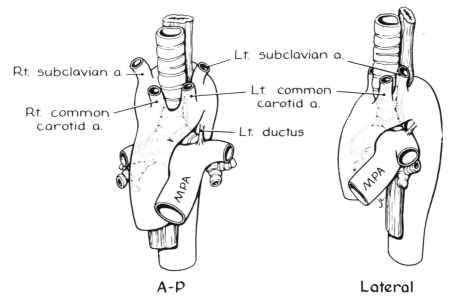

A-P   Lateral

Fig. 14.3 Anatomy of a double aortic arch. In this illustration both arches are of equal size. Note that each carotid and subclavian artery (*a.*) arises separately and that the trachea and esophagus are impinged upon the anterior (*A*), posterior (*P*), and right (*Rt.*) and left (*Lt.*) sides. *MPA*, main pulmonary artery. (Reproduced with permission from J. R. Stewart *et al.*[107])

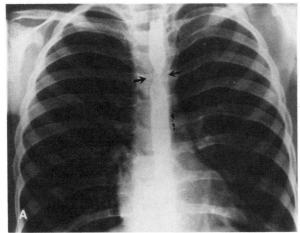

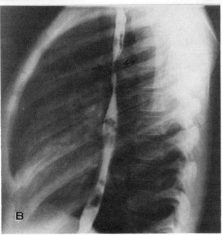

Fig. 14.4 X-ray in a 6-year-old with a double aortic arch. *Arrows* point to the indentations on the barium-filled esophagus made from the anterior, posterior, and left and right aspects. The upper descending aorta is on the left. The aortic knobs appear to be the same diameter on both sides. The heart and the lung fields are normal. (*A*) Posteroanterior projection. (*B*) Left lateral projection.

Bronchoscopy and bronchography rarely add enough information to justify their risks but occasionally are necessary to appreciate the nature of associated respiratory tract abnormalities. Aortography will delineate the anomaly, although nonpatent components of the ring will not be visualized.

Treatment

Surgery is indicated only when symptoms are severe enough to interfere with the patient's health or are life-threatening. Because the symptoms are occasionally episodic, a decision regarding surgery may be difficult. Medical treatment consists in allowing the patient to assume the most comfortable body position, careful feeding with soft foods, treatment of infection if present, and reassessment at frequent intervals. When surgery is done, the left anterolateral approach is favored because the majority have a left arch as the smaller of the two or else have a smaller right arch which joins the left upper descending aorta in such a manner that it can be satisfactorily ligated from the left side. Operative mortality in recent series[28, 44, 84, 116, 124] is about 5%.

B. DOUBLE LUMEN AORTIC ARCH

In 1969 Van Praagh and Van Praagh[118] reported a pathologic heart specimen in which the arch of the aorta, between the origins of the innominate artery and the left subclavian artery, had two separate lumina. Comparison of the appearance of this heart with certain mammalian embryo reconstructions suggested strongly that the double lumen resulted from persistence of a fifth arterial arch. Izukawa et al.[52] described two additional cases, one diagnosed during life by arteriography. All three hearts had other intracardiac defects that probably masked any physical signs arising from the double lumen arch.

Although this anomaly should have no untoward physiologic effects, awareness of its existence may aid in the diagnosis of future cases by aortography or autopsy.

C. ANOMALIES WITH LEFT AORTIC ARCH AND LEFT UPPER DESCENDING AORTA

Aberrant Right Subclavian Artery

Pathology. In this lesion the right subclavian artery arises as the fourth branch of the aorta distal to the origin of the left subclavian artery, then courses to the right arm at an obliquely upward angle posterior to the esophagus. Figure 14.5 illustrates the usual anatomy. According to the hypothetical double aortic arch schema of Edwards (Fig. 14.2), this anomaly occurs as a result of abnormal regression of the fourth aortic arch (*arrow 2*) and persistence of patency of the right eighth dorsal aortic segment. The anomaly exists frequently in cases of tetralogy of Fallot,[112] and is important in this circumstance because of the difficulty of using this vessel to perform a Blalock-Taussig anastomosis. An aberrant right subclavian artery occurs also in association with an otherwise uncomplicated coarctation of the aorta.[107]

Manifestations. *Clinical Features.* Dysphagia has long been attributed to pressure on the esophagus by this vessel and has been called dysphagia lusoria. Modern authors[8, 42, 72] refute previous clinical conclusions and deny that major symptoms are caused by this anomaly, although Smith *et al.*[102] recently recorded a case of a teenager with pain on swallowing attributed to an aberrant right subclavian artery and relieved by reconstructive vascular surgery. When the vessel is present with a coarctation of the aorta, the blood pressure in the right arm is elevated or depressed depending on the site of origin of the artery in relation to the coarctation.

Radiologic Features. The diagnosis is made by barium swallow.[58, 79, 107] In the posteroanterior projection, the vessel

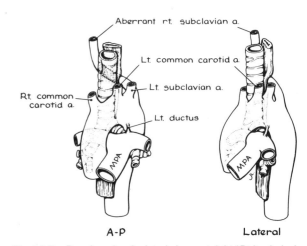

Fig. 14.5 Drawing of an isolated aberrant right (*Rt.*) subclavian artery (*a.*). Note that the aberrant vessel passes posteriorly to the esophagus at an angle upward toward the right shoulder. *Lt.*, left; *MPA*, main pulmonary artery; *A-P*, anterior-posterior. (Reproduced with permission from J. R. Stewart *et al.*[107])

causes a linear defect in the barium-filled esophagus at an angle approximately 70° from the horizontal, beginning on the left of the esophagus at about the level of the third to fourth thoracic vertebra and emerging on the right about the level of the second or third vertebra. In the lateral view the indentation is from the posterior aspect; it is more shallow than indentations produced by the aorta when it is retroesophageal, and may extend over a longer segment of the esophagus because of its oblique course. Figure 14.6 illustrates the radiologic characteristics. There is almost never a need for further radiologic diagnostic procedures, unless the anomaly is part of a more complex combination of cardiac defects.

Treatment. Almost always no treatment is needed for an aberrant right subclavian artery. When surgery is indicated for severe symptoms attributed to pressure from the anom-

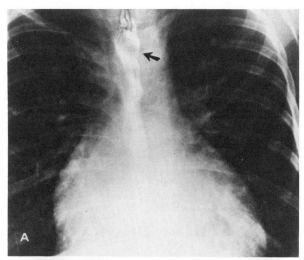

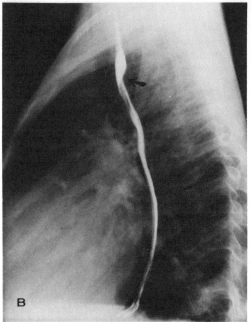

Fig. 14.6 X-rays in an 8-year-old with an aberrant right subclavian artery. Note the indentation, indicated by the *arrows*, on the esophagus from its posterior aspect, making an angle in the posteroanterior projection (*A*) upward toward the right arm at the level of the third thoracic vertebra. In the lateral view (*B*), the indentation is long and shallow. The patient had an associated ventricular septal defect with a moderate left to right shunt.

alous subclavian artery, reconstruction of the artery (rather than simple ligation) is recommended[102] to prevent possible development of claudication or a subclavian-vertebral steal syndrome.

Aberrant Brachiocephalic Arteries Other Than the Right Subclavian

Pathology. Abnormal sites of origin and courses of brachiocephalic vessels other than the right subclavian artery are common. These have been reviewed by Bosniak,[16] the most common are origin of the left common carotid artery from the innominate and independent origin of the left vertebral artery from the aortic arch. Gross[41] and Gross and Neuhauser[42] first described patients in whom tracheal compression was caused by what they believed to be abnormal origins and courses of the innominate or left common carotid arteries, which may be drawn taut against the anterior wall of the trachea as they course to their destinations. Since then there has been controversy[30, 63, 76] regarding the frequency of symptoms caused by anomalous arteries of this type, the significance of radiologic characteristics,[78] and methods of diagnosis and management. Fearon and Shortreed[31] and Mustard et al.[76] found many infants with symptoms of tracheal compression by an anomalous innominate artery requiring surgical relief. Others[11, 30] caution against overdiagnosis. Ericsson and Soderlund[30] and Maurseth[63] emphasize the association of symptomatic compression of the trachea by aberrant innominate or left common carotid arteries with esophageal atresia and tracheoesophageal fistula.

Manifestations. *Clinical Features.* Symptoms, when they occur, begin early in infancy. They are stridor, cough, dyspnea and, at times, cyanosis on exertion and recurrent periods of apnea. Apneic spells have an especially grave prognosis. Berdon et al.[11] emphasize the importance of differentiating this "reflex apnea" from other causes of apnea, such as central nervous system disease. Both Berdon et al.[11] and Swischuk[111] stress the role of "physiologic crowding" of the superior mediastinum in producing anterior indentation of the trachea on x-ray, and the contribution of tracheal abnormalities to symptoms of stridor, dyspnea, and cough. These conditions can be expected to improve as the patient grows.

Radiologic Features. In older asymptomatic patients, aberrant brachiocephalic arteries are usually detected as incidental features of arteriograms performed for other reasons. Symptomatic infants may show a round anterior indentation of the lower trachea in the lateral chest film, the significance of which has been questioned.[111] Indications for bronchoscopy, tracheography, and aortography have been debated[11, 31]; only the last has been advocated by most authorities, and then only to confirm a probable diagnosis.

Treatment. If respiratory difficulty can be demonstrated to be caused by these anomalous vessels and is severe enough to require surgical intervention, freeing up the offending vessels and suturing them to the bony structures of the anterior thoracic wall may relieve pressure on the trachea.

Ductus Arteriosus Sling

Binet et al.[13] reported a case of a 7-week-old infant with a history of dyspnea, wheezing during feeding, and an episode of asphyxia. The clinical presentation resembled an anomalous left pulmonary artery, but at surgery a normal left pulmonary artery was found and a 4-mm diameter vessel ran from the right pulmonary artery between the trachea and esophagus to join the aorta opposite the origin of an anomalous right subclavian artery. The anomalous vessel was diagnosed as aberrant ductus arteriosus "sling"; its surgical division relieved the infant of her symptoms.

Subclavian Steal

When normal flow of blood into a subclavian artery is blocked proximal to the origin of the vertebral artery, reversal of direction of blood flow in the vertebral artery may result, draining blood from the brain via the vertebral. This has been given the picturesque name of subclavian steal. The designation, subclavian steal syndrome, is reserved for cases in which symptoms of cerebral ischemia occur.[10] Although the majority of cases have occurred in adults, a few of congenital etiology or following surgery for congenital heart disease have been reported in children.

Pathology. Patel and Toole[85] reviewed 125 cases, mostly in adults with atherosclerotic narrowing of the lumen of the subclavian artery. Becker et al.[10] analyzed 20 cases of congenital origin; 13 had right aortic arch with left-sided steal. Congenital lesions included stenosis, atresia or isolation of subclavian arteries, or aortic obstruction proximal to subclavian artery origins. In some cases[98, 110] the runoff was into the pulmonary arterial system through a patent ductus arteriosus which was in continuity with the isolated subclavian artery. Folger and Shah[35] found 12 cases with radiologic characteristics of the steal following Blalock-Taussig anastomoses; seven had symptoms. Cerebral symptoms usually do not occur unless additional factors, such as arterial desaturation or disease of extra- or intracerebral vessels, are present.

Manifestations. *Clinical Features.* Cerebral symptoms are motor or sensory with vertigo, dizziness, blurred vision, headaches, diplopia, and syncope. They may be brought on or exacerbated by exercise, particularly of the arm supplied by the diseased subclavian artery. In addition, there may be intermittent pain, numbness, and fatigue in this limb. Physical examination shows decreased blood pressure and diminished delayed pulses in the affected arm. There may be systolic or continuous murmurs accompanied by a thrill over the location of the involved subclavian artery. The neurological examination is usually normal, although there may be motor or sensory long tract signs.

Radiologic Features. The radiologic aspects have been reviewed by Patel and Toole[85] and Steinberg and Halpern.[105] No unique changes are seen on conventional x-rays of the chest and neck. The diagnosis is established by injection of contrast material into the aortic arch or the carotid or vertebral arteries on the unaffected side. The affected subclavian artery does not fill from the aorta. In later phases of the study, after the contrast material has been cleared from the normal carotid-vertebral system, retrograde filling of the opposite vertebral artery with subsequent visualization of the affected subclavian artery will establish the diagnosis of subclavian steal.

Treatment. No treatment is indicated if the patient is asymptomatic. If the symptoms are mild, restraint of arm exercise may bring relief. If this is not successful or if the symptoms are more severe, surgery may be indicated. Raising the pressure in the distal portion of the affected subclavian artery by creating a shunt is the preferred operation.[46]

D. CIRCUMFLEX RETROESOPHAGEAL AORTIC ARCH

Patients have been reported[12, 25, 75, 97] with a left aortic arch which, in its terminal portion, turns medially, crosses the midline behind the esophagus, and descends to the right of the thoracic spine. The converse situation, in which a right aortic arch crosses the midline and descends to the left of the spine is also an established anomaly. Both lesions have been designated by D'Cruz et al.[25] as circumflex retroesophageal aortic arch.

Pathology

Patients with a left aortic arch and a right descending aorta may have an aberrant right subclavian artery or may have normal branches arising from the aorta. The ductus arteriosus (usually a ligamentum) may be either right or left-sided.

Eight of the nine patients in one series[25] with a right aortic arch and left-sided descending aorta also had intracardiac lesions, mostly tetralogy of Fallot and truncus arteriosus. It is common in cases with circumflex retroesophageal aortic arch for the arch to be elongated and extend to a higher than usual level in the thorax.

Manifestations

Clinical Features. When the ductus arteriosus (or ligamentum) is on the side opposite the aortic arch, a vascular ring is formed. Symptoms are of variable severity, depending on the tightness of the ring. Aside from those produced by an associated intracardiac defect, there are no specific findings.

Radiologic Features. On conventional x-rays of the chest, the laterality of the aortic arch and its elongation may be identified in the mediastinum. On the barium swallow the aorta, as it crosses behind the esophagus, will produce a large rounded horizontal impression from the posterior aspect at or just below the level of the aortic knob as illustrated in Figure 14.8. A similar indentation may be seen in cases of right aortic arch with a retroesophageal component and in some cases of double aortic arch. Aortography will establish the diagnosis, although, in cases with a vascular ring, the ligamentum arteriosus will not be identified because of its nonpatency.

Treatment

When a vascular ring is present, surgical intervention is indicated only when symptoms are severe enough to be disabling or life threatening. Division of the ligamentum arteriosus should loosen the ring sufficiently to relieve symptomatology.

E. RIGHT AORTIC ARCH

When the ascending aorta and the aortic arch pass anterior to the right main stem bronchus and then posteriorly in an arch to the right of the trachea and esophagus, a right aortic arch is present. Analysts of this entity have classified it into various subgroups[25, 32, 58, 59, 100, 108] but, from a clinical point of view, there are two main types of right aortic arch: one without a retroesophageal component (mirror image branching) and one with a retroesophageal component that is not a circumflex aortic arch.

Right Aortic Arch without a Retroesophageal Component

Pathology. Most commonly, the branches of this type of right aortic arch are in a mirror image relationship to normal. That is, the first branch is a left innominate artery after which the right common carotid and right subclavian arteries arise separately. The majority of patients with this type of right aortic arch have a left ductus or ligamentum arteriosus connecting the left subclavian artery with the left pulmonary artery, but some have a right ductus arteriosus from the arch of the aorta to the right pulmonary artery; those with bilateral ducti arteriosi have associated congenital intracardiac defects over 90% of which are tetralogy of Fallot or truncus arteriosus. In Edwards' hypothetic double aortic arch schema (Fig. 14.2), this anomaly results from abnormal regression at the site of *arrow 3* and persistence or regression of one or both ducti arteriosi.

Manifestations. *Clinical Features.* This anatomic arrangement does not produce symptoms, physical signs, or electrocardiographic abnormalities.

Radiologic Features. A right aortic arch without a retroesophageal component has the same radiologic features as a normal aortic arch but with reversed laterality (Fig. 14.7). Absence of the left-sided aortic knob may be the feature which first leads to suspicion of a right arch. The presence of an associated intracardiac defect of the conotruncal type influences the radiologic picture. Mirror-image right aortic arch may be confused radiologically with a double aortic arch in which the right arch is large and the left small. Aortography will delineate the anatomy of the arch.

Right Aortic Arch with a Retroesophageal Component

Pathology. In this group, a portion of the right aortic arch extends to the left behind the esophagus. The extension is usually in the form of a diverticulum, from which an aberrant left subclavian arises associated with a left-sided ductus or ligamentum arteriosum. Some authors include a

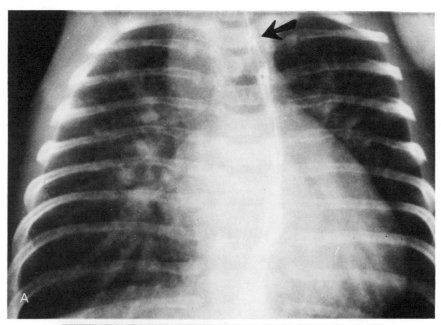

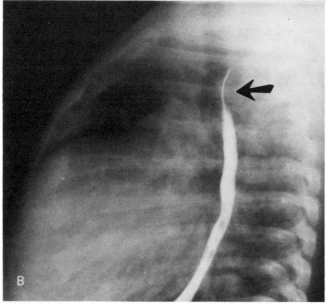

Fig. 14.7 X-rays showing the features of a right aortic arch without a retroesophageal component. The patient was a 2-month-old with a truncus arteriosus. Note the knob of the enlarged trunk in the right upper mediastinum and the right upper descending aorta. The left upper mediastinum shows an absence of the left aortic knob. The arrows point to an indentation made on the barium-filled esophagus by an aberrant left retroesophageal subclavian artery. (*A*) Posteroanterior projection. (*B*) Left lateral projection.

right-sided circumflex aortic arch under this classification category. Cases of right aortic arch with a retroesophageal component may have symptoms of a vascular ring, the ring being composed of the ascending aorta anteriorly, the arch of the aorta on the right, the diverticulum and left subclavian artery posterior to esophagus, and the ductus or ligamentum arteriosus on the left. This type of right aortic arch is usually not associated with intracardiac defects in contrast to the mirror image type. One review[108] revealed 88% of cases without intracardiac defects.

Manifestations. *Clinical Features.* Symptoms of a vascular ring are of variable severity and age of onset. Physical examination reveals only signs associated with the ring.

Radiologic Features. The features on conventional films of the chest are the same as those of mirror image right aortic arch except for the lesser frequency of manifestations of associated intracardiac defects. Barium swallow shows an indentation in the barium-filled esophagus from its posterior aspect which varies in size (depending on the nature of the retroesophageal component) from that of a large round diverticulum to a more slender angulated aberrant left subclavian artery. The differential diagnosis radiologically is that of a double aortic arch with a large right arch, but in this anomaly no left arch can be seen, and thus there is no indentation of the esophagus from the left and right as there may be in a double aortic arch. Aortography will show the configuration of patent components of the anomaly.

Treatment. No treatment is indicated unless the symptoms of a vascular ring are severe enough to be disabling. When they are, division of the ductus arteriosus and/or ligation and division of the left subclavian artery together with freeing up of the adjacent structures will provide loosening of the ring and relief of symptoms.

II. ABNORMALITIES OF LENGTH, SIZE, OR CONTINUITY OF THE AORTA

A. CERVICAL AORTIC ARCH

Patients with such elongation of the aorta that the apex of the arch is in a cervical position, and with additional specific abnormalities of the brachiocephalic arteries and descending thoracic aorta, have been described.[64, 70, 74]

Pathology

Mullins *et al.*[74] list three features they consider essential to the definition of the "complex" of the cervical aortic arch: cervical position of the apex of the aortic arch; separate origin of the carotid contralateral to the arch with anomalous origin, from the descending aorta, of the subclavian artery contralateral to the arch; and retroesophageal descending thoracic aorta crossing contralateral to the side of the aortic arch. The anomaly appears to occur equally frequently with left- and right-sided arches. Although rare, intracardiac defects may also be present.[70] Narrowing of the arch with obstruction[114] and aneurysm of the descending aorta[73] have also been reported.

Two embryologic explanations for the anomaly have been postulated: persistence of the embryonic third aortic arch rather than the fourth as a component of the adult arch and failure of the normal postbranchial elongation of the neck and arm vessels when the heart descends into the thorax. The high frequency of associated right aortic arch and abnormalities of the brachiocephalic vessels favor the first explanation.

Manifestations

Clinical Features. Patients ranged in age from 3 months to 44 years when they were first seen. Several presented symptoms of vascular ring with both respiratory and swallowing difficulties. All showed abnormal physical findings. A thrill and systolic murmur was detected radiating from the apex of the arch in the supraclavicular area or thorax. A pulsating aneurysmal mass can be observed in the supraclavicular area. Compression of the mass causes pathognomonic diminution of the volume of the femoral pulses.[74] Abnormalities of the peripheral pulses may be present depending on the nature of associated defects of the aortic arch or brachiocephalic arteries.

Radiologic Features. On conventional films of the chest, the arch of the aorta may be seen, in the posteroanterior view, to extend to a higher level than normal.[101] The upper mediastinum on the side of the arch is widened, and the arch may produce a well-defined opacity in the apex of the affected hemithorax. The upper descending aorta may be identified as abnormal if it is right-sided. With barium swallow the esophagus is deviated by a large rounded posterior impression, as in patients with circumflex retroesophageal aortas. The exact nature of the anomaly is confirmed by aortography. Figure 14.8 demonstrates the x-ray findings on barium swallow in a young girl.

Treatment

No treatment is necessary in asymptomatic patients. Surgery has been performed for symptoms of a vascular ring, to relieve a subclavian steal, to remove or bypass aortic obstruction when it is present, or to repair associated intracardiac defects. One adult with an aneurysm of the descending aorta has been reported.[73] It is important to identify the true nature of the aneurysmal neck mass to avoid misdirected surgery such as reported by Beaven and Fatti[9] where the aortic arch was ligated in the mistaken impression that it was an aneurysm of the right common carotid artery.

B. PSEUDOCOARCTATION OF THE AORTA

In pseudocoarctation of the aorta, the distal portion of the aortic arch and the proximal portion of the upper descending aorta are abnormally elongated, tortuous, and kinked. The anomaly is believed to be congenital in origin. Reviews have been published.[38, 55] Smyth and Edwards[103] make a convincing argument that this entity is simply a mild subclinical form of coarctation of the aorta.

Pathology

The distal segment of the aortic arch and the proximal upper descending aorta are abnormally elongated and fixed anteriorly in their midportion at the site of the ligamentum arteriosum. This results in an aortic configuration which has the form of a reversed "E" or number "3," when viewed from the left side. There is an association with other congenital heart defects, particularly lesions of the aortic valve.[55, 104] Some adults are reported to have developed thinning and weakness leading to aneurysms distal to the kink.[38, 87]

Manifestations

Clinical Features. Usually no symptoms are produced by this anomaly. On physical examination the majority of patients have a late systolic murmur of ejection character, loudest at the base of the heart and transmitted well to the posterior thorax. Blood pressures are normal, an important distinguishing point from coarctation of the aorta, but there may be "delayed" pulses in the legs.[27, 40] There are no alterations of cardiac function and no electrocardiographic abnormalities.

The main condition from which kinking of the aorta must be distinguished is true coarctation of the aorta.[1] In pseu-

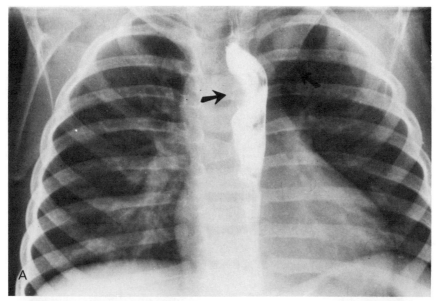

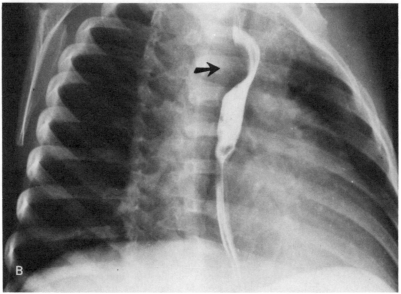

Fig. 14.8 Barium-swallow x-rays to illustrate the characteristics of a retroesophageal aorta. The patient is a 4-year-old. The ascending aorta is left-sided and the elongated portion of the arch widens the mediastinum on the left and extends into the apex of the left lung. The upper descending aorta begins its descent on the left, crosses to the right behind the esophagus at the level of the fourth rib, and then descends on the right side of the vertebral column. At the point where it crosses the midline, the aorta indents the esophagus from its right and posterior aspects with a large rounded shadow which is typical of the deformity made also by a right aortic arch with a retroesophageal component. (*A*) Posteroanterior projection. (*B*) Right anterior oblique projection.

docoarctation, there is no blood pressure elevation in the arms, no dilated collateral circulation, no dilation of the ascending aorta, and no pressure gradient across the area of kinking. Aneurysmal dilatation of the aorta may develop; at least one patient[38] died of rupture of such an aneurysm.

Radiologic Features. On plain x-rays of the chest, the knob of the aortic arch is abnormally elongated. Below the area of insertion of the ligamentum arteriosum (the "kink") the tortuous aorta presents as an opaque rounded upwardly convex shadow, due to the efferent limb of the kink being seen "head-on," as it were. In the lateral and left anterior oblique views, the actual configuration of the abnormal segment of aorta in the shape of a figure "3" may be discerned. The distal segment of the anomaly may cause an indentation in the barium-filled esophagus similar to that produced by the poststenotic segment of the aorta in a true coarctation. No evidence of collateral circulation is seen

radiologically. Aortography will define the lesion more completely.

Treatment

No treatment is indicated for pseudocoarctation. However, long-term follow-up is indicated to detect increasing dilatation and aneurysm formation. If this develops, surgical resection should be carried out[38]; Prian *et al.*[87] recommended partial bypass during resection to avoid untoward results from clamping an aorta around which no collateral circulation has developed.

C. HYPOPLASIA OF THE AORTA

Pyörälä *et al.*[88] reported a child with hypoplasia of the entire aorta and reviewed the literature of similar cases. Neufeld *et al.*[78] described another case, as did Eklöf *et al.*[29]

These patients had normal aortic valves and aortic valve ring size, and normal sized left ventricular chambers; thus, this condition can be considered different and separate from the more common hypoplastic left heart syndrome. Nine of the 15 cases of supravalvular aortic stenosis and hypercalcemia reported by Antia et al.[3] also had aortic hypoplasia. Laurie[61] attributed sudden death in young adults (in 14 of 500 consecutive autopsies) to aortic hypoplasia and consequent myocardial ischemic fibrosis; this has not been observed by others.

Pathology

The degree of narrowing of the aortic lumen and length of involved aorta vary (Arvidsson[6] measured the diameters of ascending and descending aortas from angiocardiograms performed on children. He devised a formula for the calculation of the expected cross-sectional area of the aorta of any normal child whose body surface area is known). Although the etiology of this condition is unknown, aortic hypoplasia is a major component of the syndrome of hypercalcemia and supravalvular aortic stenosis.

Manifestations

Clinical Features. Symptoms, when present, are similar to those in patients with aortic stenosis. Mental retardation and facial features associated with the syndrome of hypercalcemia and supravalvular aortic stenosis may be present. Systemic hypercalcemia and supravalvular aortic stenosis may be present. Systemic hypertension has been described.[88] Physical signs are those of aortic stenosis, except that no systolic click is present. Hypertension of varying degree in the left ventricle is reflected in the physical findings and in electrocardiographic signs of left ventricular hypertrophy.

Radiologic Features. The appearance of patients with this anomaly also is similar in many ways to that of patients with aortic stenosis, but there is no poststenotic dilatation of the ascending aorta. The arch of the aorta may appear smaller than normal. Left heart catheterization and aortography will identify the lesion. Comparison of the size of the aorta with Arvidsson's calculated standards will quantitate roughly the degree of hypoplasia.

Treatment

If the hypoplasia is limited to favorably located relatively short segments of the aorta, it may be possible to replace these segments with prosthetic vessels. Without surgery patients should be treated medically, as are patients with inoperable aortic stenosis.

D. COMPLETE INTERRUPTION OF THE AORTIC ARCH

Complete interruption of the aortic arch differs clinically in many important respects from classic coarctation of the aorta. The entity has been described in detail.[26, 69, 90, 117]

Pathology

In this anomaly, a segment of the aortic arch is absent or atretic, and the continuity of the aorta is interrupted. Celoria and Patton[20] divided patients into three groups according to the site of interruption: type A, interruption distal to the left subclavian artery; type B, interruption between the left carotid and left subclavian arteries; and type C, interruption proximal to the origin of the left carotid artery. In types A and B, subgroups have been designated A2 and B2 when the right subclavian artery arises anomalously from the distal aortic segment. Most series report Type B to be the most common; Type C is rare.[80, 117] Almost all cases have a patent

ductus arteriosus. The first edition of this chapter described an infant with complete interruption of the aortic arch in whom the ductus was not patent; Dische et al.[26] reviewed eight other similar cases. Almost all cases of complete interruption of the aortic arch have associated intracardiac anomalies in addition to patency of the ductus.[80, 117] Ventricular septal defects are almost always present, usually with pulmonary hypertension; other associated lesions are: muscular subaortic stenoses; bicuspid aortic valves; truncus arteriosus; and aortic-pulmonary window.[68] The main pulmonary artery is often dilated. The two most common types of complete interruption of the aortic arch are, according to the hypothetic double aortic arch schema of Edwards (Fig. 14.2), the result of abnormal complete regression and atrophy of embryonic vessels at the site of *arrows 3* or *4*. Van Praagh et al.[117] and others[71] speculate that this regression may be initiated by reduced antegrade blood flow in the ascending aorta, during embryogenesis, secondary to preexisting intracardiac defects.

Manifestations

Clinical Features. Symptoms appear early and are severe (the few patients with solitary interruption of the aortic arch have had symptoms resembling those of a postductal coarctation).[26] Symptoms are initially those of a large left to right shunt. Physical signs are variable, depending on the nature and severity of the intracardiac defect, the degree of increased pulmonary vascular resistance, the size of the ductus arteriosus, and the severity of myocardial failure. Inevitably, however, right to left ductal flow becomes restricted, and signs of hypoperfusion of the legs, acidosis, and oliguria develop. The electrocardiogram shows features of either left or combined ventricular hypertrophy. Cardiac catheterization will define the physiologic situation. On retrograde arterial catheterization from the femoral artery, the catheter may traverse the patent ductus arteriosus into the pulmonary artery.

Radiologic Features. The characteristics are essentially those of a large left to right shunt usually at the ventricular level. Jaffe[54] emphasized plain film findings that should alert one to the possibility of aortic arch interruption: midline trachea, hypoplastic ascending aorta, absence of the aortic knob, unusual patterns of rib notching. These radiologic features, however, are usually seen only in the minority of patients who survive infancy without surgery; in the more common case presenting in early infancy with severe heart failure these findings are frequently not observed.[80] Angiography will outline the arterial anatomy as well as associated defects; large volume left ventricular injections with axial views are most informative.[80] Aortography, especially via the right arm, may be helpful; if tortuosity of the right subclavian artery prevents successful catheterization, retrograde injection of contrast into the right radial artery will usually be satisfactory.[80] Cross-sectional echocardiography may contribute also to accurate diagnosis. Figure 14.9 shows posteroanterior and left lateral projections from a retrograde cineaortogram performed on a 5-week-old with type A interrupted aortic arch.

Treatment

Until recently no satisfactory treatment has been available, and early death has been the rule. Now, administration of prostoglandin E₁ has been shown to dilate the ductus arteriosus, and thus to improve flow to the lower half of the body and to ameliorate the metabolic acidosis that is such a prominent aspect of the clinical picture.[36, 47, 125] Usually

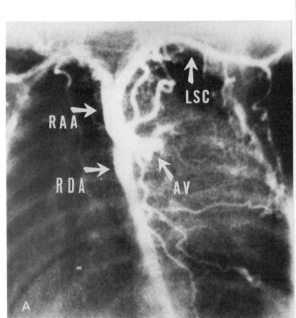
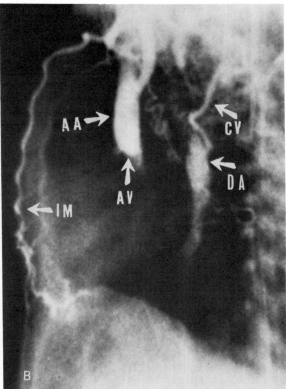

Fig. 14.9 Frames from a cineaortogram of a 5-week-old boy with complete interruption of the aortic arch, type A. Injection was made retrogradely into the left brachial artery. In the lateral view, note the gap representing the absent segment of the aortic arch beginning just distal to the origin of the left subclavian artery. The descending aorta is to the right of the vertebral column and is filled by retrograde flow through internal mammary, intercostal, and other large collateral arteries. This collateral circulation appears artifactually to be greater on the left because of the introduction of the contrast material into the left brachial artery. Differences in magnification of the intrathoracic structures in the two projections are the result of a different tube-patient length. (*A*) Posteroanterior projection. (*B*) Left lateral projection. *AA*, ascending aorta; *AV*, aortic valve; *CV*, collateral vessels; *DA*, descending aorta; *IM*, internal mammary artery; *LSC*, left subclavian artery; *RAA*, right ascending aorta; *RDA*, right descending aorta.

0.05 mg/kg/minute is administered intravenously and may be continued for as long as necessary before surgery is performed. A multicenter study[36] reported that prostoglandin infusions were useful in about three-fourths of infants with interruption of the aortic arch: femoral pulses improved, acidemia became less severe, and urine flow increased. In comparison with its effect on patients with cyanotic heart disease, beneficial effects of prostaglandin in acyanotic infants were less dependent on an age of less than 96 hours but took longer to become fully developed (up to 90 minutes of infusion). Complications of the drug were usually minor and reversible;[62] respiratory depression was the most serious problem, but most often was seen in infants weighing less than 2 kg. Structural changes that weaken the ductal wall, previously reported,[39] were not observed in any of the 492 infants in the multicenter study.[36]

Newer surgical techniques also have improved the prognosis for this group of patients.[82, 109, 125] Sturm *et al.*[109] have reviewed methods of restoring aortic continuity; the insertion across the aortic interruption of an expanded polytetrafluorethylene graft is currently the preferred technique. How best to approach the associated defects is still evolving; whether one should attempt to correct all defects or to stage the repair and band the pulmonary artery at the time of aortic repair depends partly on the nature of the associated defects and the condition of the patient during surgery. Norwood and Stellin[82] successfully treated one patient with an associated valvular aortic atresia with an aortic graft, banding of the pulmonary artery, and the insertion of a left

ventricular apex-aortic valved conduit. In a recent series of eight patients,[125] five of six receiving prostoglandin E_1 responded well, and all seven in whom aortic grafts were inserted had satisfactory immediate postoperative courses. However, four of the seven died (within a year) of complications of their associated defects and second attempts to correct these surgically.

III. ANOMALIES OF THE PULMONARY ARTERIAL SYSTEM

Three anomalies of the pulmonary arterial system will be considered: anomalous left pulmonary artery ("vascular sling"); unilateral absence of a pulmonary artery; and origin of one pulmonary artery from the ascending aorta. These three anomalies probably have a common embryologic etiology, that is, regression of the proximal segment of the sixth aortic arch or failure of this segment of the arch to establish normal connections with the more peripheral vessels of the developing lung buds.

A. ANOMALOUS LEFT PULMONARY ARTERY ("VASCULAR SLING")

Pathology

In all described cases[43, 58, 94, 113] the anomalous pulmonary artery is the left one, and the anatomy has been essentially the same. The left pulmonary artery arises from an elongated main pulmonary artery, courses initially to the right, then turns dorsally and to the left, encircling the right stem bronchus just distal to the carina, passing to the left between the trachea and the esophagus, and emerging from the left border of the mediastinum to enter the left lung, where it branches normally. There is constriction of either the right main stem bronchus or the posterior wall of the trachea, or both. Contro et al.[23] called this anomaly "vascular sling." There is a high frequency of other anomalies, both of the cardiovascular system and elsewhere,[43, 58, 60, 94, 113] most commonly patent ductus arteriosus, atrial septal defect, and persistent left superior vena cava, and those of the respiratory system, such as ring tracheal cartilage and congenital stenosis of the trachea and main bronchus.[21]

Manifestations

Clinical Features. Symptoms usually begin within the first weeks of life and are severe, resulting in death within a few months, unless surgical intervention is successful. Patients have stridor, dyspnea, intermittent cyanosis, apneic spells, and repeated respiratory infections. A few patients develop symptoms later in childhood, and occasionally the anomaly is discovered accidentally on chest x-rays.[43] Because of ball-valve obstruction of the right stem bronchus, there may be emphysematous changes in the right lung and shift of the trachea to the left.

Radiologic Features. Hyperexpansion of the right lung together with a shift of the trachea to the left secondary to ball-valve obstruction of the right main stem bronchus may be seen. Atelectasis is sometimes present. In the lateral view there may be indentation of the trachea from its posterior aspect. "Caudal migration" of the hilum of the left lung and forward deflection of the right main bronchus have been described.[18] The indentation of the barium-filled esophagus is uniquely from its anterior aspect and sometimes from the right as well. It is a round vessel shadow, usually at a lower level than the indentations made by other vascular rings. Figure 14.10 illustrates these findings. Although bronchography and bronchoscopy may be difficult and even dangerous in these ill infants, they are sometimes indicated to assess the extent and nature of associated respiratory tract abnormalities.[43, 94] Cardiac catheterization and angiocardiography will usually establish the diagnosis and define associated intracardiac defects. Figure 14.11 shows an angiocardiographic frame of the patient whose plain films are shown in Fig. 14.10.

Treatment

The prognosis is poor without treatment in severely ill infants. Thus prompt surgical alleviation is indicated. The surgical procedure[23, 53, 94] consists of detachment of the left pulmonary artery at its origin and anastomosis of its proximal end to the main pulmonary artery after the anomalous vessel is brought anterior to the trachea. The operation is difficult. Reviews[43, 58, 94, 113] indicate a postoperative mortality rate of about 50%. Symptoms may not be completely relieved in survivors, and occlusion of the repositioned left pulmonary artery is common. Thus, older patients and those with non-life-threatening symptoms may do better with conservative management. Complete delineation of associated cardiac and respiratory tract anomalies will help in deciding whether repositioning of the sling alone, or together with intracardiac and tracheobronchial procedures, is indicated.

B. UNILATERAL ABSENCE OF A PULMONARY ARTERY

There are two groups of patients with unilateral absence of one pulmonary artery: those associated with intracardiac defects, and those with isolated ones. Reviews of the subject have been published.[2, 33, 34, 86]

Pathology

There is no branch of the pulmonary artery to the affected side. Usually in the hilum of the affected lung, a vessel can be identified which branches into the periphery of the lung in a fashion similar to the branching of a normal pulmonary artery, although it is smaller than normal. Blood flow through this vessel comes either through a ductus arteriosus or through bronchial collaterals.[86] The affected pulmonary artery is almost always on the side opposite that of the aortic arch. In about 20% of isolated cases, there is pulmonary hypertension in the "unaffected" lung. When an intracardiac defect with a left to right shunt coexists, more than 85% of patients develop pulmonary hypertension.[86] Older patients have extensive bronchial collateral circulation.

Manifestations

Clinical Features. Patients with this anomaly may be divided into two categories. The majority have no symptoms and may not come to the attention of physicians until their teens or later. This group may have repeated pulmonary infections associated with coexisting bronchiectasis or malformations of the bronchial tree, and, later in life, may manifest hemoptysis from the affected lung. Physical examination is normal, except for the possible presence of an ejection type murmur originating from the pulmonary outflow area. The electrocardiogram is normal. In the smaller second group of patients, pulmonary hypertension, with its associated symptoms, physical signs, and electrocardiographic manifestations, dominates the clinical picture when there is no pulmonic stenosis. Definitive diagnosis is made by cardiac catheterization and angiocardiography. Information about the type and extent of collateral circulation to the affected lung can be obtained by aortography. Pulmonary function studies will be consistent with the presence of a ventilated but underperfused lung.

Radiologic Features. Conventional x-rays of the chest may show diminished "lacey" pulmonary vascular markings on the affected side. In the lung field normally connected with the main pulmonary artery and the right ventricle, the pulmonary vascular markings will be increased because it is receiving the entire cardiac output. There may be signs of pulmonary hypertension on the "unaffected" side. The lung with diminished pulmonary flow is usually smaller in volume than normal[95] and may show evidence of associated malformations of the tracheobronchial tree. Tomography and lung scans may aid in the diagnosis.

Treatment

Most patients are asymptomatic and need no treatment. When pulmonary infections occur, they should be treated. If there is severe unilateral bronchiectasis or other bronchial pathology with disabling pulmonary infections or atelectasis, or if there is major hemoptysis, pneumonectomy should be considered. Pool et al.[86] emphasize the importance of correcting an intracardiac left to right shunt as early as possible to prevent the development of pulmonary vascular disease.

C. ORIGIN OF ONE PULMONARY ARTERY FROM THE ASCENDING AORTA

Pathology

This entity has been reviewed.[19, 56, 83] The anomalous pulmonary artery usually arises from the side of the aorta, but

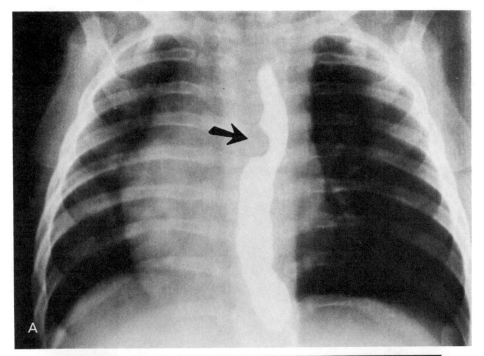

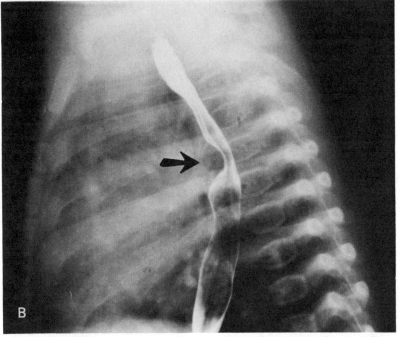

Fig. 14.10   X-rays of a 3-month-old with an anomalous left pulmonary artery, a vascular sling. The heart is shifted to the right because of mesocardia. The left pulmonary artery makes a relatively small, rounded indentation on the barium-filled esophagus from the right and *anterior* aspects, and the trachea is pushed anteriorly from behind. Angiocardiographic opacification of the pulmonary arterial tree is illustrated in Fig. 14.11. (*A*) Posteroanterior projection. (*B*) Left lateral projection.

it may arise from its posterior aspect. The site of origin may be anywhere from 1 cm above the aortic valve to just proximal to the arch. The size of the orifice of the anomalous pulmonary artery varies from small to normal. In 85% of cases, the anomalous pulmonary artery is the right one.[56] The majority of patients have associated patent ductus arteriosi; a few have a ventricular septal defect or tetralogy of Fallot.[17, 91] Pulmonary vascular obstruction has not been found in patients under 6 months of age; in older patients abnormalities were present in the "systemic" lung in the

majority, and, in two patients, changes were found in both lungs.[56]

Two embryologic mechanisms have been hypothesized to explain this anomaly. For unknown reasons, the proximal portion of a sixth aortic arch fails to develop, regresses abnormally after development, or fails to establish a patent connection with the vascular plexus of the affected lung bud. Flow to the lung is maintained through the distal segment of the sixth aortic arch (the ductus arteriosus), and this constitutes the connection of the right pulmonary artery

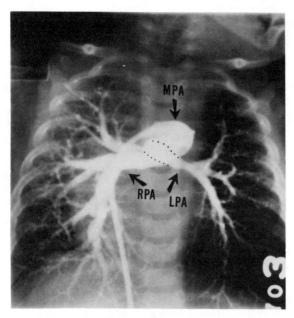

Fig. 14.11 Angiocardiographic opacification in a posteroanterior projection of the pulmonary arterial tree of the same patient whose x-rays are shown in Fig. 14.10. The catheter tip is in the main pulmonary artery, where the injection was made. The pulmonary valve lies in an almost completely sagittal plane in front of the right border of the vertebral column. The anomalous left pulmonary artery, outlined by the *dotted lines*, arises from the posterior aspect of the main pulmonary artery and then courses to the left lung hilum between the trachea and the esophagus. The left pulmonary artery appears smaller in diameter and less well opacified than the right. *LPA*, left pulmonary artery; *MPA*, main pulmonary artery; *RPA*, right pulmonary artery.

with the aorta. Cucci *et al.*[24] have proposed another explanation: because the sixth aortic arch arises from the dorsal aspect of the truncus arteriosus, a rotation of about 45° of the angle of the truncal ridges could result in origin of the right pulmonary artery from the portion of the truncus which becomes the aorta.

Manifestations

Clinical Features. The manifestations of this anomaly are the results of a left to right shunt from the aorta into the anomalous pulmonary artery and the development of pulmonary hypertension in one or both pulmonary arteries. Patients are uniformly symptomatic within the first few months of life. When no treatment is given, most die before 6 months of age. The symptoms are those of respiratory distress, poor weight gain, and heart failure. If the volume of the left to right shunt through the anomalous pulmonary artery is large there may be signs of an aortic runoff, that is, bounding pulses and increased systemic pulse pressure. There may be a continuous murmur from flow through the anomalous vessel. The electrocardiogram usually shows combined ventricular hypertrophy. Cardiac catheterization and angiocardiography will establish the diagnosis and reveal the physiologic status.

Radiologic Features. X-rays will show enlargement usually of both ventricles and the left atrium. The aorta may or may not be enlarged. Close inspection of the pulmonary vascular markings might suggest that the origin of blood flow into the two lungs was from different sources. Since the entire output of the right ventricle must perfuse the "normal" lung there is almost invariably an increase in the pulmonary vascular markings in that lung field. The size and

number of the pulmonary vessels in the anomalous lung field depend on the volume of blood flow through that lung which in turn is related to the size of the right pulmonary artery and the right-sided pulmonary vascular resistance. A lung scan with venous injection of radionuclides reveals uptake only in the normally vascularized lung. Left ventricular angiocardiography or aortography will outline the anomalous pulmonary artery (Fig. 14.12).

Treatment

Early diagnosis and surgical correction is imperative not only to relieve symptoms and signs of failure but hopefully to forestall the development of pulmonary vascular disease. The procedure of choice is anastomosis of the aberrant pulmonary artery to the main pulmonary artery, either directly or with a graft, and correction of associated defects. This has been done successfully in 12 of 18 reported attempts.[56] Prognosis after surgery is good.

GENERAL CONSIDERATIONS

The clinical manifestations of anomalies of the aortic arch complex vary greatly because of the multiplicity of the anatomic forms of the lesions and the varying degrees of severity of the individual entities. Some patients may be entirely asymptomatic and have their abnormalities discovered on a routine chest x-ray; at the other extreme, severe respiratory difficulty may begin shortly after birth and lead to early death unless treated successfully.

The physical examination of patients with vascular rings reveals the objective manifestations of the symptoms. The first step in the differential diagnosis is to determine whether the clinical picture results from a vascular ring or from some other acquired or congenital disease of the respiratory or upper gastrointestinal tracts. It should be noted that vascular rings are a rare cause of infantile respiratory distress or dysphagia.[4]

Every patient with respiratory symptoms or dysphagia or both should have conventional x-rays of the chest and a

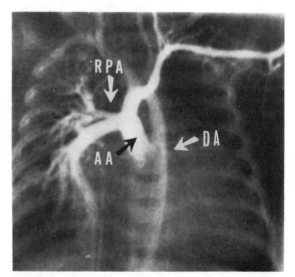

Fig. 14.12 Frame from a retrograde cineaortogram in posteroanterior projection of a 6-week-old boy with origin of the right pulmonary artery (*RPA*) from the ascending aorta (*AA*). Injection was made into the left brachial artery. A large normally branching right pulmonary artery is seen arising from the ascending aorta; in the lateral view, not illustrated, it arose from the posterior aspect of the aorta. The aorta and its branches are otherwise normal. *DA*, descending aorta.

barium swallow examination. These two simple and safe procedures will almost invariably lead to at least a suspicion of a vascular ring. In analysis of chest x-rays and esophagrams, the following questions should be asked: On which side of the mediastinum is the aortic arch? Is the aortic arch of normal or abnormal length, size, and configuration? On which side of the vertebral column is the upper descending aorta? What are the characteristics of the indentations and deviations made on the trachea and on the barium-filled esophagus? What additional intracardiac lesions, if any, can be diagnosed from the cardiac series?

Bronchoscopy and tracheobronchography may be difficult and even risky when patients are small and acutely ill, but they may be necessary to assess associated malformations of the lower respiratory tract. Cross-sectional echocardiography has accurately diagnosed coarctation of the aorta[96, 119] and can be of value in other aortic arch anomalies as well. Computed tomography has visualized thoracic vascular structures accurately.[65] Lung scanning with radionuclides[37] can provide valuable information about the source and volume of blood flow to the lungs. Cardiac catheterization is necessary for complete evaluation, particularly interruption of the aortic arch and anomalies of the pulmonary arteries.

Selective angiocardiography and aortography will, in most cases, provide a clear delineation of anomalous arteries. However, many diagnoses can be made firmly without the added risk of contrast studies. In addition, it should be kept in mind that important components of vascular rings may be nonpatent and thus not visualized by angiocardiography. Tonkin et al.[115] argue that axial cineangiography, combined with barium esophagography, provides such complete anatomic information as to warrant its use in all cases of suspected vascular rings.

The mere presence of an anomaly of the aortic arch complex does not dictate surgical correction. When symptoms of a vascular ring are mild and do not interfere with general growth and development, medical treatment, including appropriate feeding instructions, positioning for sleep, explanation and reassurance to parents, and periodic reevaluation, may suffice. Symptoms may lessen and disappear with increasing age. However, when symptoms are progressively more severe, interfere with adequate growth and development, or in themselves threaten life, prompt surgical correction is indicated.

REFERENCES

1. Acevedo, R. E., Thilenius, O. G. Moulder, P. V., and Cassels, D. E.: Kinking of the aorta (pseudocoarctation) with coarctation. Am. J. Cardiol. 21:442, 1968.
2. Anderson, R. C., Char, F., and Adams, P., Jr.: Proximal interruption of a pulmonary arch (absence of one pulmonary artery): Case report and a new embryologic interpretation. Dis. Chest 34:73, 1958.
3. Antia, A. V., Wiltse, H. E., Rowe, R. D., Pitt, E. L., Levin, S., Ottesen, O. E., and Cooke, R. E.: Pathogenesis of the supravalvular aortic stenosis syndrome. J. Pediatr. 71:431, 1967.
4. Apley, J.: The infant with stridor. Arch. Dis. Child. 28:423, 1953.
5. Arciniegas, E., Hakimi, M., Hertzler, J. H., Farooki, Q., and Green, E. W.: Surgical management of congenital vascular rings. J. Thorac. Cardiovasc. Surg. 77:721, 1979.
6. Arvidsson, H.: Angiocardiographic measurements in congenital heart disease in infancy and childhood. I. The size of the ascending and descending aorta. Acta Radiol. [Diagn.] (Stockh.) 1:981, 1963.
7. Barry, A.: The aortic derivatives in the human adult. Anat. Rec. 111:221, 1951.
8. Beabout, J. W., Stewart, J. R., and Kincaid, O. W.: Aberrant right subclavian artery. Dispute of commonly accepted concepts. Am. J. Roentgenol. Radium. Ther. Nucl. Med. 92:855, 1964.
9. Beaven, T. E. D., and Fatti, L.: Ligature of aortic arch in the neck. Br. J. Surg. 136:414, 1946.
10. Becker, A. E., Becker, M. J., and Edwards, J. E.: Congenital anatomic potentials for subclavian steal. Chest 60:4, 1971.
11. Berdon, W. E., Baker, D. H., Bordiuk, J., and Mellins, R.: Innominate artery compression of the trachea in infants with stridor and apnea. Radiol. 92:272, 1969.
12. Berman, W., Jr., Yabek, S. M., Dillon, T., Neal, J. F., Akl, B., and Burstein, J.: Vascular ring due to left aortic arch and right descending aorta. Circulation 63:458, 1981.
13. Binet, J. P., Conso, J. F., Losay, J., Narcy, Ph., Raynaud, E. J., Beaufils, Fr., Dor. C., and Bruniaux, J.: Ductus arteriosus sling: Report of a newly recognized anomaly and its surgical correction. Thorax 33:72, 1978.
14. Binet, J. P., and Langlois, J. P.: Aortic arch anomalies in children and infants. J. Thorac. Cardiovasc. Surg. 73:248, 1977.

15. Blake, H. A., and Manion, W. C.: Thoracic arterial arch anomalies. Circulation 26:251, 1962.
16. Bosniak, M. A.: An analysis of some anatomic-roentgenologic aspects of the brachiocephalic vessels. Am. J. Roentgenol. 91:1222, 1964.
17. Calder, A. L., Brandt, P. W. T., Barratt-Boyes, B. G., and Neutze, J. M.: Variant of tetralogy of Fallot with absent pulmonary valve leaflets and origin of one pulmonary artery from the ascending aorta. Am. J. Cardiol. 46:106, 1980.
18. Capitanio, M. A., Ramos, R., and Kirkpatrick, J. A.: Pulmonary sling: Roentgen observations. Am. J. Roentgenol. Radium Ther. Nucl. Med. 112:28, 1971.
19. Caudill, D. R., Helmsworth, J. A., Daoud, G., and Kaplan, S.: Anomalous origin of the left pulmonary artery from ascending aorta. J. Thorac. Cardiovasc. Surg. 57:493, 1969.
20. Celoria, G. C., and Patton, R. B.: Congenital absence of the aortic arch. Am. Heart J. 58:407, 1959.
21. Cohen, S., and Landing, B.: Tracheostenosis and bronchial abnormalities associated with pulmonary artery sling. Ann. Otol. Rhinol. Laryngol. 85:582, 1976.
22. Congdon, E. D.: Transformation of the aortic-arch system during the development of the human embryo. Carnegie Institute of Washington Publication 277. Contrib. Embryol. 14(68): 47, 1922.
23. Contro, S., Miller, R., White, H., and Potts, W. J.: Bronchial obstruction due to pulmonary artery anomalies. I. Vascular sling. Circulation 17:418, 1958.
24. Cucci, C. E., Doyle, E. F., and Lewis, E. W., Jr.: Absence of a primary division of the pulmonary trunk. An ontogenic theory. Circulation 29:124, 1964.
25. D'Cruz, I. A., Cantez, T., Namin, E. P., Licata, R., and Hastreiter, A.: Right sided aorta, Part II. Right aortic arch, right descending aorta, and associated anomalies. Br. Heart J. 28:725, 1966.
26. Dische, M. R., Tsai, M., and Baltaxe, H. A.: Solitary interruption of the arch of the aorta. Am. J. Cardiol. 35:271, 1975.
27. Dungan, W. T., Char, F., Gerald, B. E., and Campbell, G. S.: Pseudocoarctation of the aorta in childhood. Am. J. Dis. Child. 119:401, 1970.

28. Eklöf, O., Ekstrom, G., Erikkson, B. O., Michaelsson, M., Stephensen, O., Soderlund, S., Thoren, C., and Wallgren, G.: Arterial anomalies causing compression of the trachea and/or oesophagus. Acta Paediatr. Scand. 60:81, 1971.
29. Eklöf, O., Ilah, D. O., and Zetterqvist, P.: Aortic hypoplasia. Acta Paediatr. Scand. 53:377, 1964.
30. Ericsson, N. O., and Soderlund, S.: Compression of the trachea by an anomalous innominate artery. J. Pediatr. Surg. 4:424, 1969.
31. Fearon, B., and Shortreed, R.: Tracheobronchial compression by congenital cardiovascular anomalies in children. Syndrome of apnea. Ann. Otol. Rhinol. Laryngol. 72:949, 1963.
32. Felson, B., and Palayew, M. J.: The two types of right aortic arch. Radiology 81:745, 1963.
33. Ferencz, C.: Congenital abnormalities of pulmonary vessels and their relation to malformations of the lung. Pediatrics 28:993, 1961.
34. Finney, J. O., and Finckum, R. N.: Congenital unilateral absence of the left pulmonary artery with right aortic arch and normal conus. South. Med. J. 65:1079, 1972.
35. Folger, G. M., Jr., and Shah, K. D.: Subclavian steal in patients with Blalock-Taussig anastomosis. Circulation 31:241, 1965.
36. Freed, M. D., Heymann, M. A., Lewis, A. B., Roehl, S. L., and Kensey, R. C.: Prostoglandin E₁ in infants with ductus arteriosus-dependent congenital heart disease. Circulation 64:899, 1981.
37. Gates, G. F., Orme, H. W., and Dore, E. K.: The hyperperfused lung. Detection in congenital heart disease. J.A.M.A. 233:782, 1975.
38. Gay, W. W., Jr., and Young, W. G., Jr.: Pseudocoarctation of the aorta: A reappriasal. Circulation 38 (Suppl. 6):80, 1968.
39. Gittenberger-de Groot, A. C., Moulaert, A. J., Harink, E., and Becker, A. E.: Histopathology of the ductus arteriosus after prostoglandin E₁ administration in ductus dependent cardiac anomalies. Br. Heart J. 40:215, 1978.
40. Griffin, J. F., Congenital kinking of the aorta (pseudocoarctation). N. Engl. J. Med. 271:726, 1964.
41. Gross, R. E. The Surgery of Infancy and Childhood. W. B. Saunders, Philadelphia, 1953.
42. Gross, R. E., and Neuhauser, E. B. D.: Compression of the trachea or esophagus by vas-

cular anomalies: Surgical therapy in 40 cases. Pediatrics 7:69, 1951.

43. Gubiner, C. H., Mullins, C. E., and Mc-Namara, D. G.: Pulmonary artery sling. Am. J. Cardiol. 45:311, 1980.

44. Hallman, G. L., and Cooley, D. A.: Congenital aortic vascular ring. Surgical considerations. Arch. Surg. 88:666, 1964.

45. Harley, H. R. S.: The development of anomalies of the aortic arch and its branches. With the report of a case of right cervical aortic arch and intrathoracic vascular ring. Br. J. Surg. 46:561, 1959.

46. Herring, M.: The subclavian steal syndrome: A review. Am. Surg. 43:220, 1977.

47. Heymann, M. A., Berman, W., Jr., Rudolph, A. M., and Whitman, V.: Dilatation of the ductus arteriosus by prostaglandin E₁ in aortic arch abnormalities. Circulation 59:169, 1979.

48. Higashino, S. M., and Ruttenberg, H. D.: Double aortic arch associated with complete transposition of the great vessels. Br. Heart J. 30:579, 1968.

49. Hodach, R. J., Gilbert, E. F., and Fallon, J. F.: Aortic arch anomalies associated with the administration of epinephrine in chick embryos. Teratology 9:203, 1974.

50. Hutchins, G. M.: Coarctation of the aorta explained as a branch-point of the ductus arteriosus. Am. J. Pathol. 63:203, 1971.

51. Ingalls, T. H., Curley, F. J., and Prindle, R. A.: Experimental production of congenital anomalies. N. Engl. J. Med. 247:758, 1952.

52. Izukawa, T., Scott, M. E., Durrani, F., and Moes, C. A. F.: Persistent left fifth aortic arch in man. Br. Heart J. 35:1190, 1973.

53. Jacobson, J. H., II, Morgan, B. C., Andersen, D. H., and Humphreys, G. H., II: Aberrant left pulmonary artery: A correctable cause of respiratory obstruction. J. Thorac. Cardiovasc. Surg. 39:602, 1960.

54. Jaffe, R. B.: Complete interruption of the aortic arch. 1. Characteristic radiographic findings in 21 patients. Circulation 52:714, 1975.

55. Kavanaugh-Gray, D., and Chiu, P.: Kinking of the aorta (pseudocoarctation): report of six cases. Can. Med. Assoc. J. 103:717, 1970.

56. Keane, J. F., Maltz, D., Bernhard, W. F., Corwin, R. D., and Nadas, A. S.: Anomalous origin of one pulmonary artery from the ascending aorta. Circulation 50:588, 1974.

57. Keith, J. D., Rowe, R. D., and Vlad, P.: Heart Disease in Infancy and Childhood. Macmillan, New York, 1958.

58. Klinkhamer, A. C.: Esophagography in Anomalies of the Aortic Arch System. Williams & Wilkins, Baltimore, 1969.

59. Knight, L., and Edwards, J. E.: Right aortic arch. Circulation 50:1047, 1974.

60. Landing, B. H.: Syndromes of congenital heart disease with tracheobronchial anomalies. Am. J. Roentgenol. Radium Ther. Nucl. Med. 123:686, 1975.

61. Laurie, W.: Aortic hypoplasia as a possible cause of sudden death. Med. J. Aust. 2:710, 1968.

62. Lewis, A. B., Freed, M. D., Heymann, M. A., Roehl, S. L., and Kensey, R. C.: Side effects of therapy with prostaglandin E₁ in infants with critical congenital heart disease. Circulation 64:893, 1981.

63. Maurseth, K.: Tracheal stenosis caused by compression from the innominate artery. Ann. Radiol. 9:287, 1966.

64. McCue, C. M., Mavck, P., Jr., Tinglestad, J. B., and Kellett, G. N.: Cervical aortic arch. Am. J. Dis. Child. 125:738, 1973.

65. McLoughlin, M. J., Weisbrod, G., Wise, D. J., and Young, H. P. H.: Computed tomography in congenital anomalies of the aortic arch and great vessels. Radiology 138:399, 1981.

66. Meurs-van Woezik, H. V., and Klein, H. W.: Calibres of aorta and pulmonary artery in hypoplastic left and right heart syndromes: Effects of abnormal bloodflow? Virchows Arch. [Pathol. Anat.] 364:357, 1974.

67. Moene, R. J., Oppenheimer-Dekker, A., and Wenink, A. C. G.: Relation between aortic arch hypoplasia of variable severity and central muscular ventricular septal defects: Emphasis on associated left ventricular abnormalities. Am. J. Cardiol. 48:111, 1981.

68. Moes, C. A. F., and Freedom, R. M.: Aortic arch interruption with truncus arteriosus or aorticopulmonary septal defect. Am. J. Radiol. 135:1011, 1980.

69. Moller, J. H., and Edwards, J. E.: Interruption of the aortic arch: Anatomic patterns and associated cardiac malformations. Am. J. Roentgenol. Radium Ther. Nucl. Med. 95:557, 1965.

70. Moncada, R., Shannon, M., Miller, R., White, H., Friedman, J., and Shuford, W. H.: The cervical aortic arch. Am. J. Roentgenol. 125:591, 1975.

71. Moore, G. W., and Hutchins, G. M.: Association of interrupted aortic arch with malformations producing reduced blood flow to the fourth aortic arch. Am. J. Cardiol. 42:467, 1978.

72. Moore, T. C.: Esophageal obstruction due to anomalous right subclavian artery. J. Indiana State Med. Assoc., 52:1117, 1959.

73. Morris, T., and Ruttley, M.: Left cervical aortic arch associated with aortic aneurysm. Br. Heart J. 40:87, 1978.

74. Mullins, C. E., Gillette, P. C., and McNamara, D. G.: The complex of cervical aortic arch. Pediatr. 51:210, 1973.

75. Murthy, R., Mattioli, L., Diehl, A. M., and Holder, T. M.: Vascular ring due to left aortic arch, right descending aorta and right patent ductus arteriosus. J. Pediatr. Surg. 5:550, 1970.

76. Mustard, W. T., Bayliss, C. E., Fearon, B., Petton, D., and Trusler, G. A.: Tracheal compression by the innominate artery in children. Ann. Thorac. Surg. 8:312, 1969.

77. Mustard, W. T., Trimble, A. W., and Trusler, G. A.: Mediastinal vascular anomalies causing tracheal and esophageal compression and obstruction in childhood. Can. Med. Assoc. J. 87:1301, 1962.

78. Neufeld, H. N., Wagenvoort, C. A., Ongley, P. A., and Edwards, J. E.: Hypoplasia of ascending aorta. Am. J. Cardiol. 10:746, 1962.

79. Neuhauser, E. B. D.: The roentgen diagnosis of double aortic arch and other anomalies of the great vessels. Am. J. Roentgenol. 56:1, 1946.

80. Neye-Bock, S., and Fellows, K. E.: Aortic arch interruption in infancy: Radio- and angiographic features. Am. J. Radiol. 135:1005, 1980.

81. Nora, J. J.: Multifactorial inheritance hypothesis for the etiology of congenital heart disease. The genetic environmental interaction. Circulation 38:604, 1968.

82. Norwood, W. I., and Stellin, G. J.: Aortic atresia with interruped arch. Reparative operation. J. Thorac. Cardiovasc. Surg. 81:239, 1981.

83. Odell, J. E., and Smith, J. C., II: Right pulmonary artery arising from ascending aorta. Am. J. Dis. Child. 105:53, 1963.

84. Park, C. D., Waldhausen, J. A., Friedman, S., Aberdeen, E., and Johnson, J.: Tracheal compression by the great arteries in the mediastinum. Arch. Surg. 103:626, 1971.

85. Patel, A., and Toole, J. F.: Subclavian steal syndrome: Reversal of cephalic blood flow. Medicine (Baltimore) 44:289, 1965.

86. Pool, P. E., Vogel, J. H. K., and Blount, Jr., S. G.: Congenital unilateral absence of a pulmonary artery. Am. J. Cardiol. 10:706, 1962.

87. Prian, G. W., Kinard, S. A., Read, C. T., and Diethrich, E. B.: Pseudocoarctation. Vasc. Surg. 6:198, 1972.

88. Pyörälä, K., Keikel, P. E., and Halonen, P. I.: Hypoplasia of the aorta. Am. Heart. J. 57:289, 1959.

89. Raju, S., Ratliff, J., Timmis, H., Watson, D., and Suzuki. A.: "Internal coarctation" associated with double aortic arch. J. Thorac. Cardiovasc. Surg. 66:192, 1973.

90. Roberts, W. C., Morrow, A. G., and Braunwald, E.: Complete interruption of the aortic arch. Circulation 26:39, 1962.

91. Robin, E., Silberberg, B., Ganguly, S. N., and Magnisalis, K.: Aortic origin of the left pulmonary artery. Variant of tetralogy of Fallot. Am. J. Cardiol. 35:324, 1975.

92. Rudolph, A. M., Heymann, M. A., and Spitznas, U.: Hemodynamic considerations in the development of narrowing of the aorta. Am. J. Cardiol. 30:514, 1972.

93. Ryeter, Z.: Experimental morphology of the aortic arches and heart loop in chick embroys. Adv. Morphog. 2:333, 1962.

94. Sade, R. M., Rosenthal, A., Fellows, K., and Castaneda, A. R.: Pulmonary artery sling. J. Thorac. Cardiovasc. Surg. 69:333, 1975.

95. Sage, M. R., and Brown, J. H.: Congenital unilateral absence of a pulmonary artery. Australas. Radiol. 16:228, 1972.

96. Sahn, D. J., Allen, H. D., McDonald, G., and Goldberg, S. J.: Real-time cross-sectional echocardiographic diagnosis of coarctation of the aorta. A prospective study of echocardiographic-angiographic correlations. Circulation 56:762, 1977.

97. Schlamowitz, S. T., DiGiorgi, S., and Gensini, G. G.: Left aortic arch and right descending aorta. Am. J. Cardiol. 10:132, 1962.

98. Shaher, R. M., Patterson, P., Stranahan, A., Older, T., Farina, M., and Bishop, M.: Congenital pulmonary and subclavian arteries steal syndrome. Am. Heart J. 84:103, 1972.

99. Shinebourne, G. A., and Elseed, A. M.: Relation between fetal flow patterns, coarctation of the aorta, and pulmonary blood flow. Br. Heart J. 36:492, 1974.

100. Shuford, W. H., and Sybers, G.: The Aortic Arch and its Malformations: with Emphasis on its Angiocardiographic Features. Charles C Thomas, Springfield, Ill., 1973.

101. Shuford, W. H., Sybers, R. G., Milledge, R. D., and Brinsfield, D.: The cervical aortic arch. Am. J. Roentgenol. Radium Ther. Nucl. Med. 116:519, 1972.

102. Smith, J. M., III, Reul, G. J., Jr., Wukasch, D. C., and Cooley, D. A.: Retroesophageal subclavian arteries: Surgical management of symptomatic children. Cardiovasc. Dis., Bulletin of the Texas Heart Institute, 6:331, 1979.

103. Smyth, P. T., and Edwards, J. E.: Pseudocoarctation, kinking or buckling of the aorta. Circulation 46:1027, 1972.

104. Steinberg, I.: Anomalies (pseudocoarctation) of the arch of the aorta. Am. J. Roentgenol. 88:73, 1962.

105. Steinberg, I., and Halpern, M.: Roentgen manifestations of the subclavian steal syndrome. J. Roentgenol. 90:528, 1963.

106. Stephan, F.: Contribution experimentle a l'etude du development du systeme circulatoire chez l'embryon de poulet. Bull. Biol. Fr. Belg. 86:217, 1952.

107. Stewart, J. R., Kincaid, O. W., and Edwards, J. E.: An Atlas of Vascular Rings and Related Malformations of the Aortic Arch System. Charles C Thomas, Springfield, Ill., 1964.

108. Stewart, J. R., Kincaid, O. W., and Titus, J. L.: Right aortic arch: Plain film diagnosis and significance. Am. J. Roentgenol. Radium Ther. Nucl. Med. 97:377, 1966.

109. Sturm, J. T., vanHaeckeren, D. W., and Borkat, G.: Surgical treatment of interrupted aortic arch in infancy with expanded polytetrafluoroethylene grafts. J. Thorac. Cardiovasc.

Surg. 81:245, 1981.
110. Sunderland, C. O., Lees, M. H., Bonchek, L. I., Kidd, H. J., and Rosenberg, J. A.: Congenital pulmonary artery-subclavian steal. J. Pediatr. 81:927, 1972.
111. Swischuk, L. E.: Anterior tracheal indentation in infancy and early childhood.: Normal or abnormal? Am. J. Roentgenol., Radium Ther. Nucl. Med. 112:12, 1971.
112. Taussig, H. B.: Congenital Malformations of the Heart, 2nd ed., Vol. II. The Commonwealth Fund, Harvard University Press, Cambridge, Mass., 1960.
113. Tesler, V. F., Balsara, R. H., and Niguidula, F. N.: Aberrant left pulmonary artery (vascular sling): Report of five cases. Chest 66:402, 1974.
114. Tiraboschi, R., Crupi, G., Locatelli, G., Ho, S. Y., and Parenzan, L.: Cervical aortic arch with aortic obstruction: Report of two cases. Thorax 35:26, 1980.
115. Tonkin, I. L., Elliott, L. P., and Bargeron, Jr.,

L. M.: Comcomitant axial cineangiography and barium esophagography in the evaluation of vascular rings. Radiology 135:69, 1980.
116. Tucker, B. L., Meyer, B. W., Lindesmith, G. G. Stiles, Q. R., and Jones, J. C.: Congenital aortic vascular ring. Arch. Surg. 99:521, 1969.
117. Van Praagh, R., Bemhard, W. F., Rosenthal, A., Parisi, L., and Fyler, D.: Interrupted aortic arch: Surgical treatment. Am. J. Cardiol. 27:200, 1971.
118. Van Praagh, R., and Van Praagh, S.: Persistent fifth arterial arch in man. Am. J. Cardiol. 24:279, 1969.
119. Weyman, A. E., Caldwell, R. L., Hurwitz, R. A., Girod, D. A., Dillon, J. C., Feigenbaum, H., and Green, D.: Cross-sectional echocardiographic detection of aortic obstruction. 2. Coarctation of the aorta. Circulation 57:498, 1978.
120. Wilson, J. G: Teratogenic activity of several azo dyes chemically related to trypan blue. Anat. Rec. 123:313, 1955.

121. Wilson, J. G., and Karr, J. W.: Effects of irradiation on embryonic development. Am. J. Anat. 88:1, 1951.
122. Wilson, J. G., and Warkany, J.: Aortic arch and cardiac anomalies in the offspring of vitamin A deficient rats. Am. J. Anat. 85:113, 1949.
123. Wolman, I. J.: Syndrome of constricting double aortic arch in infancy: Report of case. J. Pediatr. 14:527, 1939.
124. Wychulis, A. R., Kincaid, O. W., Weidman, W. H., and Danielson, G. K.: Congenital vascular ring: Surgical considerations and results of operation. Mayo Clin. Proc. 46:182, 1971.
125. Zahka, K. G., Roland, M. A., Cutilletta, A. F., Gardner, T. J., Donahoo, J. S., and Kidd, L.: Management of aortic arch interruption with prostaglandin E$_1$ infusion and microporous expanded polytetrafluoroethylene grafts. Am. J. Cardiol. 46:1001, 1980.

15

Tetralogy of Fallot

Warren G. Guntheroth, M.D., Isamu Kawabori, M.D., and David Baum, M.D.

Tetralogy of Fallot (TF) identifies a type of cyanotic congenital heart disease with pressure in the right ventricle equal to the aortic pressure due to a large ventricular septal defect and obstruction to right ventricular outflow. In addition, the terms pink, or acyanotic, tetralogy (etc) are frequently used to describe patients with a VSD and a milder degree of pulmonic obstruction in which there is no appreciable right to left shunting.

The first anatomic description of a case of TF was by Stensen in 1671[62], over 200 years before Fallot published his series of cases. Sandifort[56] described some of the clinical manifestations of the disorder in 1777. Shortly thereafter, Hunter[22] described the characteristic "paroxysms of difficulty in breathing." Fallot's series of articles in 1888[13] won the inevitable eponym for him by describing four anatomic findings: pulmonary stenosis (or atresia), dextroposition of the aortic origin, VSD, and hypertrophy of the right ventricle. However, the diagnosis of TF during life was not made with any consistency until Taussig's work in the 1930s and 1940s.[65]

As with other forms of congenital defects, the prevalence of TF varies from clinic to clinic, depending on the age distribution in the clinic. Certainly a large majority of cyanotic patients over 1 year of age have tetralogy. The overall prevalence is on the order of 10% of all forms of congenital heart disease. The distribution between males and females is approximately equal, although some series report a 60:40 ratio for males.[24, 51] There is no apparent correlation between the appearance of tetralogy and maternal rubella or any specific genetic disorder, although there is a higher than expected prevalence of older maternal age at the time of conception of affected children.[51]

PATHOLOGY

The spectrum of pathology is as broad as the spectrum of physiologic disturbance; the degree of obstruction to pul-

monic flow is the factor crucial to both. The obstruction may be mild enough to permit net left to right shunting through the ventricular septal defect, or it may be as severe as atresia. The site of the obstruction is also variable and may involve one or more of the following locations: the infundibulum of the right ventricle, the pulmonic valve, the annulus of the pulmonic valve, and the branches of the pulmonary artery. Rowe et al.[24] summarizes the consensus that "all patients with tetralogy have narrowing of the infundibulum to some degree."[24] Although a majority of patients have some abnormality of the pulmonary valve, approximately one-third of tetralogies will have infundibular stenosis as the only substantial obstruction.

Kjellberg and colleagues[28] and Grant and associates[14] point out that the relationship between infundibular stenosis and a ventricular septal defect reflects disturbed development of the bulbar (outflow) muscular components. Van Praagh et al.[69] describe the condition as a "monology," attributable to underdevelopment of the infundibulum, in what seems to us an oversimplified explanation. In particular, Kjellberg's anatomic scheme better explains the varying nature and severity of infundibular stenosis, based upon two arms of the crista supraventricularis, with the important advantage that the types may be recognized clinically on the basis of selective angiocardiography[28] and surgical experience.[27]

Normally, the crista supraventricularis is barely raised above the surface of the right ventricle (Fig. 15.1A). The parietal band normally courses anteriorly, somewhat inferiorly, and to the subject's right, toward the free wall of the right ventricle. The septal band descends more sharply along the septal surface, anteriorly and toward the patient's left; near its termination it blends with fibers of the moderator band, which traverse the apical part of the ventricular cavity to the low, free wall of the right ventricle. The outflow tract above the crista contracts with the other muscular components of the right ventricle, but there is normally no obstruction of any part of the outflow tract, even during systole.

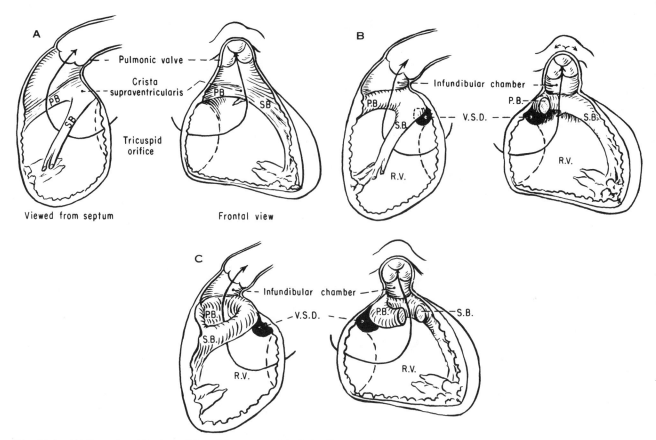

Fig. 15.1 (*A*) Normal architecture of the crista supraventricularis. The superior margin is relatively indistinct; the lower margin separates the inflow from the outflow tracts of the right ventricle. Note that even with hypertrophy of the crista and its parietal band (*PB*) and septal band (*SB*), no localized obstruction to outflow would occur (see Fig. 15.10*C*). (*B*) In addition to the ventricular septal defect (*V.S.D.*) and generalized hypertrophy of the right ventricle, the parietal band (*P.B.*) is abnormally positioned, running superiorly, anteriorly, and toward the septum. An infundibular chamber is separated from the body of the right ventricle by the hypertrophied crista and the abnormal parietal band. *R.V.*, right ventricle. (*C*) In the most severe forms of infundibular stenosis, both the parietal and septal bands are abnormally positioned, running superiorly and anteriorly; with hypertrophy of the musculature, a severe obstruction to flow develops. The infundibular chamber, the pulmonary valve annulus, and the pulmonary trunk may be hypoplastic, or atretic.

With generalized hypertrophy of the right ventricle, but with normally positioned crista supraventricularis, as in isolated valvular pulmonic stenosis, the entire outflow tract may be markedly narrowed in a tubular fashion, but the outflow tract opens fully during diastole. In the presence of a VSD, however, components of the crista may be abnormally placed and hypertrophied, infringing on the outflow tract even in diastole. Most commonly, the parietal band of the crista is displaced superiorly and is directed more toward the septum (toward the patient's left), and with right ventricular hypertrophy an obstruction to ejection occurs (Fig. 15.1*B*). There is ordinarily a normally developed outflow tract distal (in a flow sense) to the crista which results in the so-called third ventricle, or infundibular chamber. Much less commonly, only the septal band of the crista will be directed more superiorly, and, with hypertrophy, the outflow tract will be compromised.[28]

In the most severe forms of tetralogy all the bulbar elements are involved. Both the septal and parietal bands course in an abnormally superior direction, and the parietal band is directed toward the patient's left. With hypertrophy of all bulbar elements, the outflow channel may be hypoplastic (Fig. 15.1*C*), or atretic.

All forms of infundibular stenosis may obstruct progressively with increasing hypertrophy, although the progression will be most striking in the group with an abnormally di-

rected parietal band, which may progress from a clinical picture of a left to right shunt in infancy to that of a right to left shunt at the age 3 or 4. The infundibulum in this group will be well developed, and this finding can not readily be reconciled with Van Praagh's proposal that underdevelopment of the infundibulum is the primary anomaly in all forms of tetralogy.[69]

A recent report recommended abandoning the terminology for the crista, because of conflicting uses of the term, particularly the septal band;[2] although their criticism is valid, their newer terminology based on anatomy rather than embryology is inadequate to describe the variations in obstructive muscle bundles. An earlier anatomic study, however, seems to confirm older theories of morphogenesis, namely unequal truncal partition.[5] In addition, they found evidence of abnormal conal rotation, to the subject's left and anteriorly.

Valvular abnormalities occur in the great majority of tetralogies. The valve is frequently bicuspid or may have fused leaflets, and the annulus may be hypoplastic. The literature does not adequately distinguish stenosis due to inadequate opening of the leaflets from stenosis due to a small annulus, although the distinction has surgical significance. Inadequate circumference of the annulus prevents complete relief of the obstruction unless the annulus is cut through and a wedge is added, a procedure which inevitably will create some degree of insufficiency of the pulmonary valve.

Atresia of the pulmonic valve or infundibulum occurs in approximately 25% of autopsy series,[24] although in an operative series, the frequency of atresia was only 7%.[42] The atretic valve may appear to be reasonably intact but fused and hypoplastic, although more commonly there is relatively thick muscle between the outflow tract and the pulmonary trunk. The pulmonary trunk may vary from a faint cord to a normal-sized trunk and branches. In the former instance it is difficult to decide whether the case should be classified as a severe tetralogy (pseudotruncus arteriosus) or as a true truncus arteriosus with absent pulmonary arteries (type IV). If there is a common pulmonary artery or main pulmonary artery branches, TF should be diagnosed; if the major arteries supplying the lungs are tortuous and unjoined, suggesting bronchial arteries, truncus may be inferred.

The pulmonary valve leaflets may be hypoplastic enough to produce pulmonary insufficiency. This is not a particularly common disorder, but when it occurs it is apt to be in association with TF. The main pulmonary artery is then frequently aneurysmally dilated.

Unilateral absence of a pulmonary artery is found in a small number of patients with TF.[47] Most commonly, the left pulmonary artery is absent, and the right pulmonary artery may be unusually dilated. In some of these patients, the pulmonary valve leaflets are hypoplastic or absent. Circulation to the abnormal lung is accomplished by bronchial arteries and other collateral vessels, and the scant venous return from that lung is to the left atrium.

The VSD in TF is usually large and is located directly under the right cusp of the aortic valve. It is separated from the pulmonary valve by the crista supraventricularis, and thus is upstream of the obstruction. The common bundle of the atrioventricular conduction system runs along its inferior margin, on the left side of the summit of the ventricular septum.

Atrial septal defect occurs in approximately 15% of patients with tetralogy of Fallot.[24] When it is present, the clinical entity is sometimes called pentalogy of Fallot or, pentad. Endocardial cushion defects may also occur with the other features of TF.

Overriding aorta was initially regarded as an inherent feature of TF but it is no longer considered a sine qua non. Overriding is produced by an anterior extension of the aortic root, relative to the ventricular septum. In the milder forms of tetralogy, the development of the conal region is not seriously distorted, and there is no appreciable overriding of the aorta, although the usual relationship of the septal defect to the aortic root permits easy visualization of the aortic cusps from the right ventricle. In the more severe forms there is as much as 75% overriding, and the distinction between TF and partial transposition of the great arteries depends upon continuity between the anterior leaflet of the mitral valve and elements of the aortic[68] valve.

The presence and degree of overriding is actually easier to determine from radiographic contrast techniques than from autopsy specimens, considering the customary technique of creating a "filet" of the organ by cutting through the valves. Fig. 15.2 is based on the classification suggested by Kjellberg and coauthors[28] from lateral angiocardiographic views of the heart. In the normal position with no overriding (left, upper), the ascending aorta arches anteriorly, so that a line projected from the first part of the ascending aorta would be directed posteriorly into the left ventricle. The plane of the ventricular septum runs obliquely anteriorly and toward the left, causing some overlap of the outlines of the two ventricles

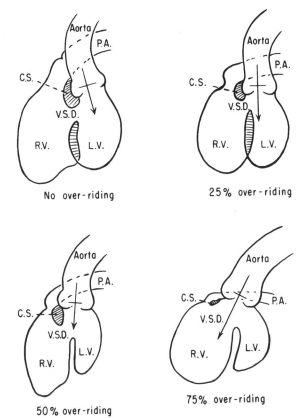

Fig. 15.2 Classification of overriding aorta, drawn from lateral projections of angiocardiograms, after Kjellberg et al.[28] P.A., pulmonary artery; C.S., crista supraventricularis; V.S.D., ventricular septal defect; R.V., right ventricle; L.V., left ventricle. A line is extended from the axis of the first part of the ascending aorta. In patients with no overriding, the aorta curves posteriorly toward the left ventricle. With marked (75%) overriding, the aorta faces anteriorly, into the right ventricle, the left ventricle is small, and the septum runs directly laterally and is convex posteriorly.

when they are filled with contrast material; the septum bulges anteriorly into the right ventricle, as it does in the normal subject. In tetralogies with 25% overriding, the line projected from the ascending aorta is truly vertical, and approximately 25% of the aortic orifice faces the right ventricle. The ventricular septum is not appreciably different in orientation from the normal. With 50% overriding, the aorta straddles the septum, the plane of which is directed laterally toward the midaxilla. In extreme cases, with 75% overriding, the septum frequently is convex toward the *left* ventricle and inclines posteriorly as it courses superiorly. In these severe deformities, the ascending aorta is large in all its dimensions.[57]

Shaner et al. denied that the large aorta in patients with TF reflected abnormal truncal septation and Grant[14] agreed that the increased size is secondary to increased aortic flow, presumably secondary to collateral flow to the lung.[14] This explanation is inadequately supported by clinical correlations: patients with a moderately large ductus arteriosus have much larger flows through their ascending aorta and have a less prominent aorta than do some patients with quite modest collateral circulation to the lung. Quantifying bronchial arterial flow requires special techniques[6]; the few studies reported have found the bronchial flow considerably less than 50% of the normal cardiac output, and the average cardiac output is 3.59 liters per min per m², close to normal. Second, other forms of cyanotic congenital heart disease with inadequate pulmonary blood flow but with normal position of the great vessels, particularly tricuspid atresia, do not have a prominent aorta although their collateral circulation is comparable to patients with tetralogy.

Collateral circulation to the lung in TF is invariably increased in comparison to that of the normal bronchial arteries. Ordinarily, this collateral circulation is modest, and is simply responsive to the decrease in flow in the pulmonary arteries.[16] In some instances, the collateral circulation is unaccountably large[33] and can cause serious problems during cardiopulmonary bypass, unless identified and ligated.[40]

The total pulmonary flow will, by definition, constitute the pulmonary venous return. This volume will eventually determine the size of the left ventricle, and in severely cyanotic patients, in whom the aortic flow arises largely from the right ventricle, the left ventricle will be smaller than normal for age. This is in contrast to autopsy findings in ASD, where the left ventricle appears small relative to the very large right ventricle but is normal for age. In ASD, all of the aortic flow comes from the left ventricle, and cardiac output will be normal except in heart failure.

Right aortic arch, with the aortic knob and the descending aorta on the right, occurs in approximately 25% of patients with TF. When this condition is present, the left subclavian artery arises in the right hemithorax directly from the distal aorta. In subjects without heart disease, or with heart disease other than tetralogy, who have a right aortic arch, the left subclavian invariably originates from an aortic diverticulum,[70] and usually crosses anterior to the esophagus. In rare instances of right aortic arch, a double arch may be found, with an incomplete arch to the left, supplying the left carotid, subclavian, and vertebral arteries, terminating in a ductus arteriosus.[16]

The coronary arteries in TF may have surgically important variations from the normal origin and course.[10, 34] The anterior descending artery may originate from the right coronary artery in association with marked overriding of the aorta. More treacherous to the surgeon is a single, right coronary artery which gives off a left branch, coursing anterior to the pulmonary trunk. Similarly, a left coronary artery originating normally may then course anteriorly between the aorta and pulmonary artery and then laterally in front of the pulmonary trunk. In the latter two circumstances, the anomalous coronary artery may run deep, under the myocardium of the right ventricular outflow tract. Accidental interruption of these vessels is catastrophic when hypoplasia of the pulmonary annulus requires an incision paralleling the outflow tract. In almost all patients with TF, the infundibular branch of the right coronary artery is enlarged and may present a problem with respect to the right ventriculotomy.

PHYSIOLOGY

There are certain consequences of the combination of a large VSD and obstruction to pulmonary blood flow. The right and left ventricles will be at essentially identical pressures during systole, and the left ventricular pressure is controlled by the carotid baroreceptors; thus, the right ventricular pressure is limited to systemic pressure levels. This explains the rarity of heart failure in TF in childhood; since the heart is doing no extra volume work, the heart size is never more than mildly enlarged. Any deficiency in volume of the pulmonary venous return can be made up by a right to left shunt through the ventricular septal defect. The magnitude of the right-to-left shunt and the pulmonary blood flow will be determined by the relatively fixed obstruction of valvular or infundibular stenosis, the relatively fixed right ventricular pressure, and the variable systemic vascular resistance. In the normal cardiovascular system, the pulmonary vascular resistance is less than 1/10 of the systemic. In TF, the total (outflow and vascular) resistance to flow across the pulmonic circuit exceeds the systemic resistance and in severe cases, the pulmonic resistance may be three or four times the systemic resistance; consequently, the pulmonary blood flow may be one-third or one-fourth of the systemic blood flow. This limitation of pulmonary blood flow has unfortunate consequences because this reduces the amount of oxygen which can be picked up in the lungs, and can result in hypoxia. Whereas mild cyanosis (hypoxemia) produces relatively mild disorders, hypoxia can have serious metabolic and physiologic consequences.

Compensation for hypoxia may occur in two principal ways: the development of collateral circulation to the lungs and polycythemia. The former usually requires several years, whereas polycythemia may occur in early infancy when the usual phyisologic drop in hematocrit fails to occur. In most neonates with tetralogy, hypoxemia is not a problem, and even cyanosis may not be apparent in the first few months of life. The explanation for the relatively benign course in early infancy is not certain. Taussig[65] has postulated that this is due to patency of the ductus arteriosus, which subsequently closes, precipitating cyanosis and hypoxia. The increasing level of general activity, with associated increased oxygen consumption, is the most likely explanation. The newborn infant is asleep most of the time. After the first 2 months, the amount of sleep decreases and more organized activity increases, and, with it, the total oxygen demands increase in the face of a limited ability to pick up oxygen from the lungs.

The development of polycythemia is an important compensation to hypoxemia. Normal hematocrit or hemoglobin levels in a cyanotic child usually indicate a relative iron deficiency. Iron therapy can produce striking improvement in these children by improving the oxygen-carrying capacity of the blood, even though the apparent cyanosis may be exaggerated by more reduced hemoglobin. At the other extreme, viscosity may increase rapidly after the 60 to 65% level of hematocrit.[55] There is no proof that secondary polycythemia *causes* thromboses, although there is certainly an association between the two phenomena; it is possible that a common factor for both may be hypoxia. Reducing the hematocrit by phlebotomy may increase the hypoxia, and usually causes a transient state of hypercoagulability. Therefore, phlebotomy is probably not of value unless heart failure is present, in which case reduction of viscosity may be of appreciable benefit. Polycythemia has an apparent role in bleeding tendencies in the immediate postoperative period. Improvement is reported by preoperative exchange of blood with plasma[38] but excessive reduction in oxygen-carrying capacity prior to surgical correction carries a substantial risk.

Paroxysmal hyperpnea is a somewhat alarming complication. These episodes are also called paroxysmal dyspnea,[65] anoxic spells,[46, 72] hypoxic spells, blue spells,[24] and syncopal attacks.[72] These paroxysms are characterized by increasing rate and depth of respiration, with increasing cyanosis progressing to limpness, syncope and, occasionally, ending in convulsions, cerebral vascular accidents, and death. The prevalence of spells in TF varies from 20% in older patients[71, 72] to 70% in autopsied cases[24]; in surgical patients the prevalence is 35%.[24, 42] The onset of symptoms may be as early as the 1st month of life but may occur as late as at 12 years of age, with a peak frequency between 2 and 3 months.

In severely cyanotic patients, the attacks may occur at any time of the day, but in patients with only occasional episodes, the paroxysms commonly occur in the morning after a full night of sleep.[42, 46] Crying, defecation, and feeding are the most frequent precipitating events.[65] These stiuations, have in common increased oxygen demands, and cause increased arterial PCO_2 and lowered pH and PO_2, all of which might stimulate hyperpnea and initiate an attack. Curiosuly, the attacks are not restricted to patients with severe cyanosis; we have observed typical paroxysms in patients with normal arterial saturations (during catheterization and therefore, under sedation). Conversely, some patients with severe desaturation do not develop spells. On the average, hyperpneic spells are more often seen in younger patients who are cyanotic at rest. The arterial oxygen saturation *during* a spell is uniformly low.

Hyperpnea is the crucial event in maintaining these spells regardless of initiating events. Whereas in normal subjects hyperpnea increases arterial PO_2, in patients with TF, hypernea lowers the PO_2.[67] In the normal individual, hyperpnea causes an increase in cardiac output from both ventricles, presumably through a reduction in the intrathoracic pressure, which would cause an improved pressure gradient favoring systemic venous return and an increase in the effective filling pressure of the right ventricle.[19] In tetralogy, however, the increase in systemic flow is unmatched on the pulmonary side, since the greatest resistance to flow is the relatively fixed obstruction at the infundibulum and pulmonary valve. Since the systemic blood flow is made up of pulmonary venous return plus the right to left shunt through the ventricular septal defect, the net result of hyperpnea is an increased shunt, resulting in an increase in arterial PCO_2, and a decrease in PO_2 and pH. These three changes in arterial composition tend to further stimulate respiration, and a vicious cycle is begun.[17] Hyperpnea not only increases the right to left shunt but increases the oxygen consumption through the increased work of breathing, which adds to the problem of an infant already dependent on anaerobic metabolism. As hypoxia develops, systemic vascular resistance decreases,[29] further increasing right to left shunting.

The mechanism whereby a paroxysm of hyperpnea is initiated is less clear but probably involves variations in arterial composition and respiratory center sensitivity. During prolonged sleep, the diminished oxygen requirements of a patient are adequately met through the limited pulmonary blood flow, and arterial PO_2, PCO_2, and pH are restored toward normal. The child awakes in reasonable metabolic balance, with a fully responsive respiratory drive. On most days spells do not occur, probably due to a gradual shift in the blood gases and a gradual reduction in respiratory drive. If, prior to the adjustment, a relatively sudden increase in activity or a Valsalva-like maneuver (crying or bowel movement) occurs, the resulting increase in right to left shunt with attendant increase in PCO_2 and decrease in PO_2 and pH may initiate hyperpnea.

Other theories of etiology of blue spells are compatible with the cycle proposed by us. Wood[72] suggested that the spells are due to obstructive spasm of the right ventricular infundibulum which, others speculate, is the result of a release of endogenous catecholamines in the myocardium.[21] Increased infundibular obstruction would further decrease the pulmonary blood flow and could initiate the cycle by decreasing pulmonary venous return. However, this mechanism does not explain paroxysmal hyperpnea in patients with pulmonary atersia, in whom infundibular spasm is irrelevant.

It is unfortunate that Wood used "spasm" in reference to infundibular obstruction. A basic characteristic of cardiac muscle which distinguishes it from skeletal muscle and smooth muscle is the absence of spasm, or tetanus. On the other hand, increased resistance to flow through the infundibulum has been shown in a variety of conditions having in common decreased filling of the right ventricle. Tachycardia from pacing or from spontaneous tachyrythmia has been shown to cause a marked drop in arterial saturation, with no change in systemic pressure or resistance but a marked decrease in pulmonary flow.[25, 60] This right to left shunting would stimulate hyperpnea. Whether increased inotropism can exaggerate infundibular obstruction has not been demonstrated. A sudden decrease of systemic vascular resistance[20] could theoretically increase right to left shunting and initiate hyperpnea.

Metabolic acidosis, secondary to profound hypoxia is clearly a stimulant to the respiratory center, and prolonged attacks of paroxysmal hyperpnea have been successfully terminated with intravenous sodium bicarbonate.[54] Rudolph,[53] however, proposed a mechanism different from hyperpnea: inadequate venous return secondary to supine posture and inactivity. He cautioned against restraint and sedation; yet, two of the effective treatments of these spells are morphine[65] and general anesthesia,[72] and we found that sleep in tetralogy improved the arterial oxygen saturation.[17]

The natural history suggests that spells involve ventilatory drive. The spells diminish in frequency and severity 2 or 3 years from onset, regardless of surgery. Similar adaptation to hypoxemia occurs in normal subjects living at altitude. Both high altitude natives and patients with tetralogy after surgical repair retain a permanent insensitivity of respiratory response to hypoxemia in adult life.[59]

Squatting is a characteristic posture of children with tetralogy of Fallot when resting after exertion.[65] Increased venous return has been suggested as the mechanism which improves recovery.[20, 35] Although squatting undoubtedly prevents pooling in the legs after exercise, squatting cannot be expected to produce a sustained increase in venous return. Brotmacher[8] suggested that the improvement is actually associated with a decrease in venous return from the legs or, more directly, a decrease in flow to the legs. Because the venous return from the large muscle groups in the legs has an extremely low saturation after exercise, and since pulmonary venous return is relatively fixed, the right to left shunt would cause a marked decrease in arterial oxygen saturation, high PCO_2, and increased lactate. We have studied squatting and the knee-chest position in seven patients and have shown that these positions cause a sustained decrease in flow in the inferior vena cava. Arterial oxygen saturation improved, and arterial lactate decreased as a result of the decreased venous return from the leg muscles. The squatting also produced an increase in resistance to arterial flow in the legs, thereby reducing the venous washout from the muscles.[18]

Exercise limitation is a predictable consequence of a relatively fixed obstruction to pulmonary blood flow. Although cardiac output can increase as in the normal, pulmonary blood flow cannot increase proportionally. This results in an increasing right to left shunt, progressive dyspnea, and hypoxemia.

MANIFESTATIONS

Clinical Features

The complaints of patients reflect their dominant handicap: hypoxia. The age at onset of symptoms varies markedly from children in whom heart disease is unsuspected to infants cyanotic from birth who may die in the first 2 or 3 months of life. The degree of obstruction to pulmonic flow is the governing factor. Infants who develop cyanosis during the 1st month of life invariably have severe pulmonic stenosis or atresia and will frequently develop paroxysmal hyperpnea, polycythemia, marked dyspnea on exertion, exercise intolerance, and irritability. Curiously, if these patients survive, they frequently improve after the 1st year or two of life, possibly due to the development of collateral blood vessels. Headaches are a later complaint related to hypoxia, but the apparent delay in their appearance is probably dependent on the development of speech. Squatting may be obvious even in infancy: many severely cyanotic infants prefer to lie in a knee-chest position. In preschool children, squatting is most obvious. Older children may not take advantage of the position as they become more socially aware.

Physical examination reveals that most children are underdeveloped and undernourished.[3] The degree of cyanosis varies from a deep purple to undetectable desaturation. Clubbing usually is not well developed for the first few months, but older children may present full-blown osteoarthropathy with paddle-shaped phalanges. In the earlier or milder cases, there is a subtle fullness or convexity only in the nailbed, progressing to a convexity of the entire nail.

The blood pressure is usually normal, although after several years of marked cyanosis and polycythemia, systemic hypertension may develop. Polycythemia also is thought to cause the distended appearance of retinal veins in severe TF.

The liver is rarely enlarged, corresponding to the rarity of heart failure. Similarly, distension of neck veins and edema are rare in childhood, although in older children and adults chronic hypoxia may culminate in heart failure. Splenomegaly suggests bacterial endocarditis or some process unrelated to the cardiovascular pathophysiology.

The cardiac impulse usually is maximal at the lower left sternal border, although in patients with a significant left to right shunt, there may be a prominent apical impulse as well. There may be a systolic thrill palpable, depending on the loudness of the murmur.

The second sound in the pulmonic area may be normally loud, or even louder than normal, but will not be split. This audible component of the second sound is produced by closure of the aortic valve; the pulmonic component is rarely audible, although it is possible to record it with the phonocardiogram (Fig. 15.3). One clue to the aortic origin of the audible component is the increase in intensity of that component at the third and fourth left interspaces, compared to that of the second interspace.

The systolic murmur is varied in intensity and character. The murmur is produced by flow across the obstruction at the right ventricular infundibulum or, less often, across the pulmonic valve. Since the pressures in the two ventricles are essentially equal, there is little chance that the murmur is produced by flow across the septal defect. Also, since the right ventricle has two outlets, peak ejection is not as delayed as in isolated pulmonic stenosis, and the systolic murmur tends to have a peak intensity relatively early in systole and is of more uniform intensity throughout systole than in isolated pulmonic stenosis. The murmur is usually most intense at the third left interspace. Absence of a systolic murmur may indicate pulmonary atresia, but severe degrees of infundibular stenosis may be associated with little or no murmur. Polycythemia, decreased systemic vascular resistance, and increased infundibular obstruction may be responsible for lessened murmurs.

A crescendo-decrescendo murmur at the base, peaking at the second sound, may indicate a patent ductus arteriosus,

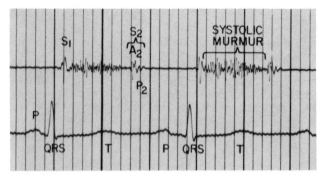

Fig. 15.3 Phonocardiogram in the second left interspace from a patient with tetralogy of Fallot. The pulmonic component (P_2) of the second sound (S_2) was recorded, but its intensity was so low that it was inaudible; thus, the audible second sound in the pulmonic area was actually produced by the aortic closure (A_2). The systolic murmur ended before A_2.

although this is rare, except in pulmonary atresia. More often, particularly in children over 1 year of age, such a murmur indicates the presence of collateral circulation through bronchial arteries. In this instance, the murmur is apt to be more intense over the paravertebral area. In the rare cases of absent or hypoplastic pulmonic valve, an ejection murmur is followed by a decrescendo diastolic murmur, described as to-and-fro.

Routine laboratory results are exceptionally valuable in following the course of the disease in patients with cyanotic congenital heart disease. If the child is receiving a normal iron intake, the hematocrit or hemoglobin serves as an indicator of the average level of hypoxia. A child who appears normally saturated at rest but who has polycythemia for his age very probably develops cyanosis with exertion. A rapidly rising hematocrit or hemoglobin is a reliable clue to the need for surgical assistance. Hypochromic or microcytic erythrocytes on a blood smear indicate a relative iron deficiency.[55] In marked polycythemia, the platelets may appear diminished both on smear or by platelet count.

Electrovectorcardiographic Features

The electrocardiogram ordinarily shows right ventricular hypertrophy (Fig. 15.4). Right bundle branch block is uncommon if this term is reserved for QRS complexes of duration greater than normal for age,[50] although rsR or slurred R patterns are frequent. Tall, peaked P waves (P pulmonale) are relatively uncommon in children but more common in older patients. Strain pattern consisting of wide QRS-T angle and ST-segment shift is unusual, compared to its incidence in isolated pulmonic stenosis.

In acyanotic tetralogy, the electrocardiogram may reveal combined hypertrophy and occasionally a startlingly normal record.[15] In patients with large collateral flow, left ventricular dominance may be observed.[33]

The vectorcardiogram demonstrates major forces to the right and anterior, and usually inferior. The loops are ordinarily clockwise in the frontal and horizontal planes, and in the more marked degrees of right ventricular hypertrophy, clockwise in the sagittal plane (Fig. 15.4). There is no unusual terminal slowing.

Radiologic Features

Characteristically, the heart is not enlarged in its overall dimensions. The configuration of the silhouette indicates the relative dominance of the right ventricle by the anterior extension of the cardiac mass and cocking up of the apex. In

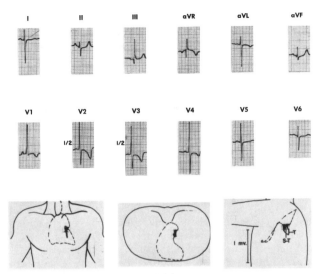

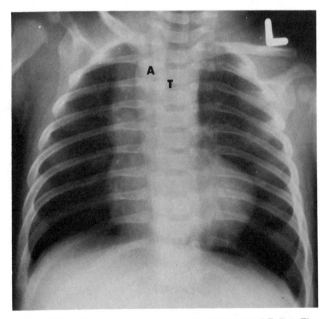

Fig. 15.4 Electrocardiogram and Frank vectorcardiogram from a 7-year-old with tetralogy of Fallot. The electrocardiogram is full standard except for V2 and V3, which are half-standard. The vector loops slightly exceed 1 mV in their largest dimension. There is obvious evidence for right ventricular hypertrophy, with the major forces deviated to the right and anterior. (Reproduced with permission from W. G. Guntheroth.[15])

Fig. 15.5 Radiogram of a child with tetralogy of Fallot. The heart is not enlarged and exhibits the characteristic boot shape. The aorta (A) descends to the right of the patient's trachea (T). The pulmonary vascular markings are diminished.

the majority of patients with deficient conal development, the region of the normal main pulmonary artery is deficient. The cocked-up apex (Fig. 15.5) and deficient conus produce the characteristic boot shape, or coeur en sabot. In the less common instances of predominantly valvular pulmonic stenosis, the pulmonary artery may be normally developed or may even show poststenotic dilatation. The pulmonary vascular markings are typically diminished, particularly beyond the mesial third of the lung fields. In pink tetralogy, the lung fields may appear normal or even somewhat engorged. Similarly, the collateral circulation may occasionally be so generous as to cause the appearance of increased

vascularity. However, the usual radiologic appearance of collateral vessels in severe forms of tetralogy is a uniformly fine, reticular pattern, which lacks the progressive diminution of vessel caliber toward the periphery.

The aortic arch is on the right in one fourth of the patients, which may be recognized on the plain films by displacement of the trachea to the left of the midline. On barium swallow, the esophagus is also shifted to the left, whereas with the normal left arch, the esophagus and trachea are displaced to the right of the midline. As a natural consequence of a right aortic arch, the left subclavian artery must course from right to left. In tetralogy, the left subclavian arises directly from the aorta and produces a shallow, oblique impression on the barium-filled esophagus.[70] (In subjects without heart disease and right aortic arch, or with nontetralogy heart defects, the left subclavian invariably originates from an aortic diverticulum, producing a larger, more transverse indentation on the esophagus.) The ascending aorta may be abnormally prominent in some on the plain radiogram (Fig. 15.5).

Echocardiographic Features

Although many details of anatomy and function are provided by M-mode, 2D, and Doppler echocardiography, we continue to base surgical decisions on cardiac catheterization and angiocardiography. Nevertheless, ultrasonic studies provide vital information in the neonate and frequently aid the interpretation of other anatomic and physiologic details (Figs. 15.6 and 15.7).

We have found that the Doppler technique, with either M-Mode or 2D echo, aids in identification of the great vessels, and their relative position, of particular importance in the cyanotic neonate (Fig. 15.8).[63]

CARDIAC CATHETERIZATION

The right atrial pressure is usually normal, although somewhat high "a" waves may be found. The right ventricular systolic pressure is essentially the same as that of the left ventricle and aorta. The contour of the right ventricular pressure pulse is similar to the normal left ventricular pulse, with a rapid upstroke and an overshoot and plateau, in contrast to isolated, severe pulmonic stenosis, in which the upstroke is more delayed, creating a triangular pulse contour. The pulmonary artery pressure is usually less than normal

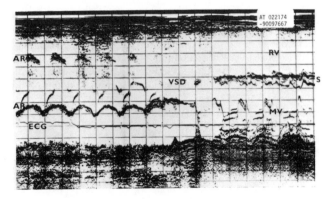

Fig. 15.6 Echocardiogram from a child with tetralogy of Fallot, demonstrating characteristic features of an increased depth of the right ventricular cavity (RV), and overriding aorta, judged from the straddling of the septum (S) by the aortic root (AR), seen on the left. The ventricular septal defect (VSD) is indicated by absence of reflections. The record shows reasonably good evidence of continuity of the mitral anterior leaflet (MV) with the posterior aortic root. (Recording supplied by Dr. Steve Johnson.)

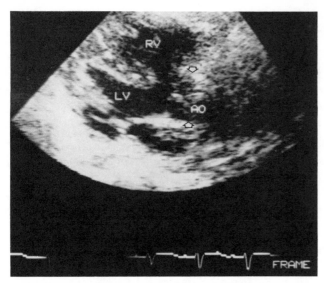

Fig. 15.7 Two-dimensional evaluation in tetralogy of Fallot. The aorta (*AO*), left ventricle (*LV*), and right ventricle (*RV*) are imaged in long axis from standard left parasternal approach in diastole. The large aortic root (bracketed by *arrows*) overrides the ventricular septum, with posterior wall of the aortic root relating normally to the anterior leaflet of the mitral valve, but the anterior aortic root overrides well into the right ventricular cavity, giving rise to dropout of the ventricular septal echo. The pulmonary trunk is not visualized in this sector. (Courtesy of Dr. J. Geoffrey Stevenson.)

in TF; in isolated pulmonic stenosis, the mean pulmonary artery pressure is normal in the absence of failure. On gradual withdrawal of the catheter from the pulmonary artery, a third kind of pressure chamber may be encountered, with diastolic pressure approximating zero but with a systolic pressure considerably below that of the body of the right ventricle (Fig. 15.9). The systolic pressure in this infundibular chamber may be equal to or greater than that of the pulmonary artery, depending upon whether valvular stenosis is present in addition to the infundibular obstruction. The reliability of these measured gradients depends on the type of catheter used. An angiocardiographic catheter with holes distributed over a centimeter of length may produce a false "intermediate pressure chamber" by mechanically averaging from above and below a value. Generally, one can safely deduce the total severity of obstruction from the overall pressure drop between the body of the right ventricle and the pulmonary arteries, and the relative contribution of anatomic sites to the obstruction from the angiographic studies. (In severe obstruction, the catheter will occupy a substantial part of the cross-sectional area and may critically reduce the already marginal pulmonary flow and initiate a severe hyperpneic paroxysm.) Of additional diagnostic significance is catheter entry of the aorta from the right ventricle. This occurrence does not necessarily indicate overriding aorta but constitutes irrefutable evidence of a ventricular septal defect in the absence of transposition of the aorta.

Oxygen saturations of blood in the right heart are not particularly helpful. A measurable increase in saturation at the right ventricular level is common but not large, except in the pink tetralogy. If the left atrium is entered, desaturation at that site suggests an atrial septal defect; however, normal saturation in the left atrium does not rule out pentalogy of Fallot.

Oxygen consumption is decreased in the usual patient. Cardiac output is minimally increased over the normal, and pulmonary flow is, of course, reduced.[6] The usual calculation of pulmonary blood flow based on oxygen saturation in the

pulmonary artery will underestimate the true pulmonary blood flow, since bronchial artery flow may be substantial, and by virtue of precapillary anastomoses, participates in gas exchange.[16]

Dye dilution techniques can help to localize the occurrence and site of right to left shunts. However, selective angiocardiograms yield the same information and anatomic information as well.

ANGIOCARDIOGRAPHY

Angiocardiography is mandatory prior to complete surgical repair and almost as important when considering a palliative procedure. Angiocardiograms, either with full size filming or cines, are essential in two planes, preferably as simultaneously filmed biplane studies. The contrast material should be injected selectively into the right ventricle with a power injector, although in infants under 5 kg a hand injection may be satisfactory. Additional sites of injection may be advisable, depending upon the adequacy of visualization of the left heart by the forward flow of contrast material.

Right ventricular architecture has been discussed in the pathology section. It is usually possible to identify the components of the crista supraventricularis in relation to infundibular stenosis (Fig. 15.10). In evaluating the lumen of the outflow tract, "spasm" of the outflow tract during contrast injection is frequently due to extrasystoles induced by mechanical stimulus of the catheter. In addition to infundibular architecture, stenosis of the pulmonary valve and annulus may be determined as well as stenosis of peripheral branches of the pulmonary arteries. The caliber of the annulus, the main pulmonary artery, and branches of the pulmonary arteries is of crucial importance relative to choice of operative approach. As discussed in the section on pathology, overriding of the aorta is best judged from the lateral projection of the angiocardiogram. This is so, in part, because of the tendency of the interventricular septum to run in a true, lateral direction in TF, whereas in the normal, the septum projects obliquely toward the left and anteriorly. Although streaming may produce misleading results, it is frequently possible to estimate the size of the VSD from the angiocardiogram. If the aorta is unusually large and overriding, the pulmonary trunk is generally small, a major factor limiting early complete repair. The left ventricular size may be obvious from spillover immediately after right ventricular injection, or after the contrast material returns from the pulmonary veins. Small left atrial and ventricular volumes indicate somewhat greater risk of complete repair, and some centers considers this to be an indication for a shunt operation, with the expectation that the resulting increase in pulmonary venous return will gradually improve the capacity of the left heart.

Coronary artery anomalies may be of lethal consequence if a major branch is interrupted; consequently, it is our practice to perform an aortic root injection of contrast material to demonstrate the number and distribution of the coronary arteries. This injection will also demonstrate the extent and origin of collateral vessels to the lung. If the bronchial flow is substantial, surgical considerations may require selective injection.[40] When the main branches of the pulmonary arteries are not identifiable by antegrade flow from right-sided injections of contrast material, they may be demonstrated by retrograde injection from an end-hole catheter gently wedged into the corresponding pulmonary vein.[58]

We routinely obtain a radiogram of the abdomen approximately 10 minutes after angiocardiograms. Considering the frequent coexistence of congenital anomalies and the risk of endocarditis, this small effort provides important information on the genitourinary tract.

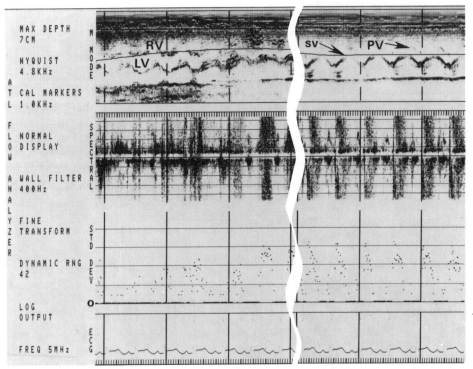

Fig. 15.8 Duplex Doppler-echocardiographic flow record, fast Fourier transform format. At the top of the figure, an M-mode echocardiographic tracing demonstrates the relationshiop of the Doppler sample volume (SV, the location from which Doppler flow information is evaluated) to known structures: right ventricle (RV), left ventricle (LV), and pulmonic valve (PV). The spectral Doppler flow record depicts the flow characteristics at the position of the Doppler sample volume. The standard deviation of Doppler shift is an index of the degree of spectral broadening, or "turbulence." An electrocardiogram is present for timing. From a standard precordial approach, the right ventricle and left ventricle are recorded on the *left*, and the Doppler sample volume and imaging plane are swept to the right ventricular outflow tract and pulmonic valve. On the *left*, the Doppler sample volume is in the left ventricle. The spectral flow record demonstrates a smooth wave form, indicative of normal left ventricular flow; the standard deviation is low for this portion of the record. As the sample volume is moved into the ventricular septal echo in the region of the ventricular septal defect (Fig. 15.6), there is broadening of the spectral record and an increase in standard deviation, indicating the presence of a flow disturbance, the ventricular septal defect. Near the *middle* of the figure, the Doppler sample volume is in the right ventricular outflow tract, and a greater degree of spectral broadening is present, with greater standard deviation, suggesting an additional flow disturbance from subpulmonic stenosis. As the sweep is completed and with the sample volume positioned distal to the pulmonic valve in the main pulmonary artery at the right of the figure, there is further spectral broadening, suggesting additional obstruction at the pulmonic valve. In this patient, the majority of spectral broadening appears to be subvalvar. (Courtesy of Dr. J. Geoffrey Stevenson.)

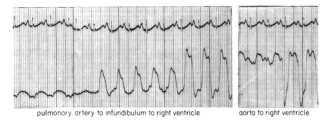

pulmonary artery to infundibulum to right ventricle   aorta to right ventricle

Fig. 15.9 Pressure records obtained at catheterization in an 18-month-old. On the *left*, the catheter was withdrawn gradually from the pulmonary artery into the right ventricular infundibulum and then into the body of the right ventricle. The record on the right was obtained by withdrawing the catheter from the ascending aorta into the body of the right ventricle. Pressure in the right ventricle was 100 mm Hg, in the infundibulum it was 60, and in the pulmonary artery it was 10. (Reproduced with permission from B. C. Morgan et al.[43])

DIFFERENTIAL DIAGNOSIS

The diagnosis of tetralogy of Fallot must be differentiated from varied forms of congenital heart disease, considering the functional spectrum: intensely blue, hypoxic infants with ischemic lungs at one extreme, to young adults with no detectable cyanosis and slightly plethoric lung fields. Most of the discussion here will deal with the customary image of TF: cyanosis, ischemic lungs, and right ventricular hypertrophy. With the last criterion, it is possible to exclude conditions which may closely resemble TF on physical examination or ordinary radiograms, particularly tricuspid atresia. Tricuspid atresia, with right ventricular hypoplasia, will exhibit left ventricular dominance or hypertrophy on electrocardiogram. A true truncus arteriosus with hypoplastic pulmonary arteries may show combined or left ventricular hypertrophy but may be impossible to distinguish from severe forms of TF, even on angiocardiography. Fortunately, taxonomy is less urgent than therapeutic considerations, and if the pulmonary arteries are markedly hypoplastic, even palliative surgery may be ineffective. Occasionally, left ventricular hypertrophy is found in patients with moderately severe pulmonic stenosis in whom collateral circulation has developed to an unusual extent,[33] or in whom an unusually large ductus arteriosus is patent. In these instances the pulmonary vascular markings are apt to be normal or increased in appearance.

Ebstein's anomaly may be distinguished by radiography as well as the electrocardiogram. The heart is considerably

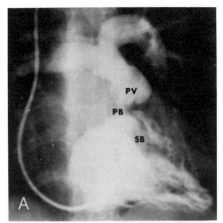

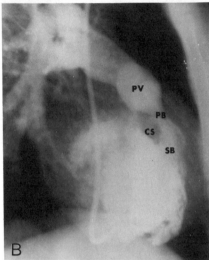

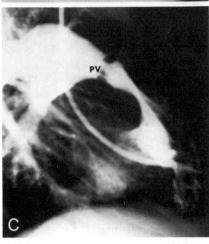

Fig. 15.10 (*A*) Frontal projection of selective right ventricular angiocardiogram. There is stenosis of both the pulmonic valve (*PV*) and infundibulum. The infundibular stenosis is of the type drawn in Fig. 15.1*B*, with a hypertrophied but normally positioned septal band (*SB*) and a parietal band (*PB*) which is abnormally directed toward the patient's left, crossing the outflow tract of the right ventricle. (*B*) Lateral projection simultaneous with *A*. The valvular pulmonic stenosis is more obvious in *B*. The central body of the crista supraventricularis (*CS*) is clear. There is some contrast material behind the crista which has crossed the ventricular septal defect and is immediately under the aortic valve. (*C*) For contrast, this lateral angiocardiogram is from a patient with valvular pulmonic stenosis and an intact ventricular septum. There is diffuse narrowing of the infundibulum, but the crista supraventricularis and its bands are normally positioned.

enlarged in the typical Ebstein's, particularly the right atrium, whereas the heart volume in TF is not significantly increased. The bizarrely slurred, wide QRS complexes associated with giant P waves are almost pathognomonic of Ebstein's, and this type of electrocardiogram pattern is not compatible with tetralogy. Doppler echocardiography will demonstrate abnormal tricuspid anatomy and tricuspid regurgitation of a major degree.

The patients with cyanosis, diminished pulmonary vascular markings, and right ventricular hypertrophy include at least two other entities that may be difficult to differentiate from TF. Eisenmenger's syndrome, or ventricular septal defect with pulmonary vascular obstruction, should be relatively easy to distinguish; the peripheral vascular markings are diminished but the central vessels are quite prominent. Although poststenotic dilatation may occur in the tetralogies with some valvular stenosis, it rarely produces central pulmonary vessels as prominent as those found in Eisenmenger's. Auscultation should provide the essential difference through the loud—even—palpable—pulmonic closure in pulmonary vascular obstruction. However, the second sound in the pulmonic area in TF may be single and relatively loud, representing aortic closure, which may be confirmed by hearing the same sound louder at the lower left sternal border.

Transposition of the great arteries with ventricular septal defect and pulmonic stenosis may be relatively difficult to differentiate in infancy. Echocardiography may help by demonstrating the relative positions of the great vessels. A single ventricle with pulmonic stenosis usually may be differentiated by 2-dimensional echocardiography from the ordinary form of TF with a ventricular septal defect of more moderate size. The degree of septation is sometimes in doubt after right ventricular injection of contrast. In these instances, a left ventricular injection of contrast material may be helpful.

Isolated pulmonic stenosis, with an intact aortic root and a right to left shunt through a patent foramen ovale may require catheterization and angiocardiography for differentiation, although we believe we can successfully separate the two by pulsed Doppler echocardiography. If the stenosis is severe, the patient with an intact aortic root may develop right heart dilatation, hepatomegaly, and other signs of heart failure, clearly separating this condition from tetralogy. For the moderately severe pulmonic stenosis, with right ventricular pressures close to systemic levels, the differentiation is particularly difficult. Exercise performed while brachial artery and right ventricular pressures are recorded simultaneously frequently will increase the right ventricular pressure in intact ventricular septum whereas the systemic pressure will change relatively little; this is a consequence of the increase in stroke volume in both ventricles, against a relatively fixed resistance to right ventricular outflow and a decreasing vascular resistance on the left. For similar reasons, isoproterenol should increase right ventricular systolic pressure to a greater extent than the left in isolated pulmonic stenosis, whereas in TF the two pressures should remain essentially identical. In tetralogy, contrast material injected from either the right atrium or right ventricle will opacify the aorta early, whereas the aorta will not opacify with right ventricular injections when the aortic root is intact. If a ventricular septal defect exists, selective angiocardiograms with injection into the right ventricle will almost invariably demonstrate the ventricular septal defect, even when there is no appreciable arterial desaturation; this shunt may be enhanced by extrasystoles due to the mechanical stimulation by the catheter. Finally, although a left aortic arch does not favor either diagnosis, a right aortic arch is strongly in favor of tetralogy and against pulmonic stenosis with intact aortic root.

TREATMENT AND COURSE

Management of patients with tetralogy of Fallot should be compatible with the philosophy for any other form of congenital heart disease—the most normal activity possible for the individual. Restrictions, if any, should be imposed by the disorder, not by parents or physicians.

Certain precautions are necessary in the management of these patients. With hypoxia, the requirement for increased oxygen-carrying capacity requires increased iron for hemoglobin. Whereas the normal infant has stores of iron adequate for the first few months of life, the diet of the infant with cyanotic congenital heart disease should contain more iron than that available from human or cow's milk. Most cereals, egg yolk, and meat are convenient sources, but supplemental iron may be indicated.

The patient should be protected against endocarditis, primarily by scrupulous dental hygiene, and in the event of dental extraction or tonsillectomy, by prophylaxis with penicillin or a suitable substitute in the case of allergy to penicillin.[1] Considering that the offending organism is frequently streptococcus viridans, and considering its natural habitat, the mouth, these precautions seem reasonable. However, one should not use penicillin promiscuously, with every fever, abrasion, or ordinary surgical procedure. Although experimental evidence from animals suggests that large injections of penicillin and streptomycin are superior in protection,[12] a strong case may still be made for the less traumatic approach of oral penicillin, since it makes frequent dental care more acceptable. There is no doubt that good daily dental hygiene will provide more protection than one day antibiotic coverage for extractions, since chewing alone in the presence of caries and gingival disease will cause bacteremia.

Dehydration should be prevented in any child, but it is a more urgent problem in patients with marked polycythemia, since the available plasma volume is diminished. However, there is no reason for panic with a brief episode of vomiting or diarrhea in a patient with a hematocrit in the 40 to 50% range. Intravenous fluids are not without hazard of paradoxical embolism if the needle is unplugged by forceful flushing. It is wise to post a conspicuous sign on the crib of any cyanotic child receiving parenteral fluids, stating that a clotted needle should not be forcibly unplugged.

Anemia, or hypovolemia, following a bleeding episode, may present an urgent therapeutic problem by creating an acute reduction in oxygen-carrying capacity, requiring transfusion. Lesser degrees of anemia, including the "relative" anemia of a normal hemoglobin or hematocrit in the presence of cyanosis, may cause an appreciable worsening of symptoms, with lessened exercise tolerance, greater dyspnea, and increased frequency of paroxysmal hyperpnea. The response to iron therapy, orally or by injection, is very gratifying, sometimes as dramatic as though a surgical shunt had been performed. This clinical improvement is an adequate basis for considering polycythemia as physiologic, at reasonable levels. Although viscosity rises with an increase in hematocrit, the viscosity does not rise sharply until levels of 60 to 70% have been reached.[55] Accordingly, unless heart failure is present, there is no evidence that venesection is necessary. Cerebral vascular accidents in patients with cyanosis and polycythemia is more likely due to the hypoxemia which stimulated the polycythemia rather than to the polycythemia *per se.*[37] These "strokes" are best treated conservatively, with oxygen therapy; more vigorous measures, such as low-molecular-weight dextran and hypothermia, are of unproved value. It is also important to rule out a brain abscess.

Brain abscesses are a grave but infrequent complication in any patient with right to left shunting. Patients with tetralogy of Fallot seem somewhat more susceptible than patients with other forms of cyanotic congenital heart disease, but this may reflect their relatively greater longevity and cumulative exposure. Such patients may have headache, vomiting, marked lethargy, personality changes, convulsions, and focal neurological signs. Papilledema is common. They may or may not have fever and other signs of infection, and curiously almost never have bacterial endocarditis. Blood cultures are commonly negative, but when they are positive, streptococcus viridans is the most frequent offender. Spinal taps should be done only after consultation with a neurosurgeon, in deference to the possibility of cerebral herniation. When obtained, the spinal fluid will usually have increased protein, but the sugar will ordinarily be normal, and no organisms will grow on culture. The electroencephalogram and computerized tomography may help localize the abscess; technetium scans have been particularly useful in localizing even the early nidus of infection, prior to abscess formation. The most common location is in the right parietooccipital region. Treatment consists of antibiotics and surgical drainage of an actual abscess. The mortality is high, and an aggressive neurosurgical approach is justified. With early diagnosis, and vigorous antibiotic therapy, it is sometimes possible to stop the infective process short of actual necrosis and abscess.

Paroxysmal hyperpnea may respond dramatically to morphine in relatively large doses, 0.2 mg per kg of body weight.[65] The effect is probably due to the depressing effects of morphine on the respiratory center. We have disproved the assertion that morphine inhibits the positive inotropic effects of catecholamines.[64] An additional therapeuitc step that can be instituted by the mother or medical personnel is to place the child in a knee-chest, or fetal, posture. Rudolph[53] advocates the head-down position to assist the systemic venous return, which he suspects is the primary problem in spells. This position, however, has serious disadvantages to respiratory mechanics and causes systemic vasodilatation through a false signal to the carotid baroreceptors.[44] Any situation producing systemic vasodilatation is deleterious, and pure alpha-adrenergic drugs such as phenylephrine may be useful in aborting attacks. Oxygen should be administered, although the results are not dramatic. If the attack has gone on for a considerable length of time and the patient has not responded to the measures listed, it is quite probable that metabolic acidosis has developed from prolonged anaerobic metabolism.[54] Treatment with intravenous sodium bicarbonate may help interrupt the attack. Glucose supplementation is wise, since hypoglycemia may result from accelerated utilization and depleted glycogen stores endangering the available substrate for the brain. Occasionally, general anesthesia will be necessary to interrupt the attack,[72] probably by a general suppression of central nervous system activity, and by depression of respiration. Propranolol has proved to be of great value for both acute and longer term management of patients with paroxysms.[21, 52] Suppression usually is obtained with 1 mg/kg four times daily. The favorable response to beta blockade has been attributed to negative inotropic effects on the infundibular myocardium. However, patients with pulmonary atresia also respond to propranolol; the favorable response logically would require noncardiac mechanisms. Hypoxia in acute experiments in animals causes hyperpnea and a decrease in systemic vascular resistance. Beta-adrenergic blockade prevents this decrease in peripheral resistance,[25] which would diminish right to left shunting in a tetralogy. Propranolol can slow tachyrhythmias,[25, 60] which would improve right ventricular filling and thereby lessen infundibular obstruction. In our study on five normal adult volunteers, the ventilatory response to hypoxemia was blocked by propranolol in four. This suggests that beta blockade may prevent the vicious cycle of hypoxemia and hyperpnea.

The management of the ductus-dependent patient with pulmonary atresia by intravenous prostaglandin E_1 will be discussed in the chapter on pulmonary atresia.

Palliative operations for patients with TF have not been vitiated by the development of complete repair with cardiopulmonary bypass, although the shunting operations should be regarded as preliminary to more complete correction. The simpler type of operation with its relatively slight mortality may provide an infant or child with several years of existence at a near normal level, by relieving hypoxia secondary to inadequate pulmonary blood flow. Although surgical shunts are mechanically inefficient, they overcome the crucial disability of inadequate pulmonary blood flow. Critically small pulmonary arteries may enlarge following surgery and by improving pulmonary venous return, the shunts have the additional virtue of improving the capacity of the left atrium and ventricle in anticipation of total correction. Also, by reducing the hypoxic stimulus for polycythemia with its attendant hemorrhagic tendency, the postoperative course after complete repair should be safer in those patients who have had a prior shunt operation.

Of the systemic-pulmonic arterial shunt procedures, the Blalock-Taussig operation is preferred if the vessels are of adequate size. The shunt is of moderate size, rarely large enough to cause heart failure or pulmonary hypertension, and at the time for complete repair can be simply ligated at its insertion. The Pott's procedure, anastomosis of the descending aorta to the left pulmonary artery, has been abandoned because of the difficulty of takedown at the time of complete repair. It has been replaced by the Waterston shunt, between the ascending aorta and the right pulmonary artery. The effect of the Waterston shunt is difficult to predict from the physical size of the anastomosis, and too large a flow may cause heart failure and even pulmonary vascular disease in time. Kinking and aneurysm formation may obstruct continuity between the right and left pulmonary arteries. For these reasons, the Waterston procedure is recommended only in those infants in whom a satisfactory Blalock-Taussig anastomosis cannot be established.

Following Lillehei's pioneering work,[32] surgical repair of tetralogy of Fallot has been performed either primarily or after earlier palliation. The ventricular septal defect is closed by a Dacron patch, and the infundibular stenosis is relieved by excision of the obstructing muscle bundles and, when necessary, by pulmonary valvulotomy. If relief of the obstruction remains incomplete, an outflow patch of pericardium or Dacron may be incorporated into the ventriculotomy closure, enlarging the ventricular exit. In those cases where the pulmonary annulus and main pulmonary artery are small, the outflow tract gusset may be extended across the valve ring into the pulmonary artery, exchanging obstruction for pulmonic insufficiency. In large series utilizing this general approach, the operative mortality is 5 to 10%.[4, 11, 49]

In symptomatic infants with TF, early definitive repair has been advocated and performed with low operative mortality.[7, 45, 66] Hypoplasia of the pulmonary arteries is a relative contraindication for early intervention, or a pulmonary annulus small enough to require surgical disruption.[26] In these infants, shunt operations in the first year of life allow a period of further growth without the risks of increasing polycythemia and other complications of hypoxemia. Ebert et al.[66] have developed an alternative of enlarging the right ventricular outflow tract, without closing the ventricular septal defect; after a relatively brief interval, based on the growth of the pulmonary arteries, the ventricular septal defect is closed. Obviously, conduits or replacement valves, with no growth potential, should be used with the knowledge that reoperation will be required.

Medical problems in postoperative care occur, no matter the age or operative technique. Bleeding problems postoperatively are particularly common in older patients and in those with very high hematocrits preoperatively.[31] Generally, the most successful treatment is fresh, whole blood, but the possibility of bleeding from a major vessel should be entertained. A challenging problem can occur if poor cardiac output occurs early in the postoperative period. Urinary output diminishes, and capillary filling is delayed. Blood should be given in aliquots, and the central venous pressure (CVP) monitored. In most cases of TF, the CVP will be high, and a high value should not deter administration of enough fluid to restore good capillary perfusion. Adequate perfusion may require an abnormally large circulating volume, which may cause capillary leakage in both the pulmonary and peripheral circulation. This "third spacing" is common to other conditions, such as "shock lung," and poses a therapeutic dilemma. We believe that the extra volume is mandatory to avoid metabolic acidosis, and that pulmonary function should be compensated by continuous positive airway pressure. Additional therapeutic measures are digitalization and a dopamine infusion. Dopamine produces hemodynamic responses similar to isoproterenol[1] but without tachycardia and also produces a greater increase in renal flow.[39]

Heart block is now an uncommon but serious problem of postoperative management. Pacing is mandatory in the immediate postoperative period, but most infants and children can be "weaned" by gradual reduction in the pacemaker frequency, after the first week. Although the cumulative mortality of acquired heart block is worrisome, the inference that "prophylactic" pacing abolishes the risk of mortality is not consistent with available statistics. The average mortality for 70 children with chronic pacemakers from Toronto and Boston was 27%, according to a report presented at the International Symposium in Toronto in 1975. These youngsters averaged one operation per year for various failures of wires and batteries, threshold increase, and infection. Thus, when weighing the indication for pacemaker therapy, it appears that mortality may not be altered; the choice may logically be based on morbidity. We continue to regard heart failure and syncope as the major indications for chronic pacing in children.

Right bundle branch block (RBBB) is found commonly after right ventriculotomy and causes no known problems. Kulbertus et al.[30] reported that bifascicular block (RBBB plus left anterior fascicular block) greatly increased the chance of complete A-V block and sudden death. This was not confirmed in a larger follow-up,[61] and sudden death was attributed to exercise-induced ventricular tachycardia.[23] However, in a series of 395 postop patients, dysrhythmias were not exercise induced, and the patients with bifascicular block had a relatively benign course.[71]

Heart failure occurs transiently in many patients postoperatively, particularly in those with outflow-tract patches; heart failure thereafter usually indicates a more permanent problem such as a reopened septal defect. However, some degree of cardiomegaly persists in many postop tetralogies. In the absence of residual shunts, pulmonary valvular insufficiency probably accounts for the right ventricular enlargement, and this appears to be reasonably well tolerated if moderate, and if there is no substantial tricuspid insufficiency.[48]

In general terms, the early course of the patient with TF

is a good basis for prognosis. The infant with cyanosis in the 1st month of life rarely survives the 1st year without surgical assistance, whereas the mildest forms, the pink tetralogies may survive to 40 years of age without operation.[36] The course for the usual patient is one of gradual worsening of cyanosis. Except for complications, the course does not change rapidly after infancy, but a gradual decline almost invariably occurs after puberty. After a shunt operation, there is no doubt that the symptoms are less and the chances for survival are improved, although not to the extent that

definitive repair should be postponed indefinitely. The development of fibrotic and calcified bands in the infundibulum, bleeding tendencies, and a general decline in vigor argue against indefinite procrastination of definitive surgery. Although an occasional patient survives to a fairly advanced age, this should not obscure the fact that very few survive the first 20 years of life without surgery.[24] On the other hand, this limited prognosis does not justify attempts at surgical correction of this complicated abnormality by inadequately experienced teams.

REFERENCES

1. American Heart Association: Prevention of bacterial endocarditis. Circulation 56:139A, 1977.
2. Anderson, R. H., Becker, A. E., and Van Mierop, L. H. S.: What should we call the "crista". Brit. Heart J. 39:856, 1977.
3. Baum, D., and Stern, M. P.: Adipose hypocellularity in cyanotic congenital heart disease. Circulation 55:916, 1977.
4. Beach, P. M., Bowman, F. O., Kaiser, G. A., and Malm, J. R.: Total correction of tetralogy of Fallot in adolescents and adults. Circulation (Suppl. 1) 44:1, 1971.
5. Becker, A. E., Conner, M., and Anderson, R. H.: Tetralogy of Fallot: A morphometric and geometric study. Am. J. Cardiol. 35:402, 1975.
6. Bing, R. J., Vandam, L. D., and Gray, F. D.: Physiological studies in congenital heart disease. II. Results of preoperative studies in patients with tetralogy of Fallot. Bull. Hopkins Hosp. 80:121, 1947.
7. Bonchek, L. I., Starr, A., Sunderland, C. O., and Menashe, V. D.: Natural history of tetralogy of Fallot in infancy. Circulation 48:392, 1973.
8. Brotmacher, L.: Hemodynamic effects of squatting during repose. Brit. Heart J. 19:559, 1957.
9. Clay, R. C., Elliott, S. R., II, and Scott, H. W., Jr.: Changes in blood volume following operation for pulmonic stenosis: Studies with Evans blue and radioactive phosphorous. Bull. Hopkins Hosp. 89:337, 1951.
10. Dabizzi, R. P., Caprioli, G., Aiazzi, L., Castelli, C., Baldrighi, G., Parenzan, L., and Baldrighi, V.: Distribution and anomalies of coronary arteries in tetralogy of Fallot. Circulation 61:95, 1980.
11. Daily, P. O., Stinson, E. B., Griepp, R. B., and Shumway, N. E.: Tetralogy of Fallot: Choice of surgical procedure. J. Thorac. Cardiovasc. Surg. 75:358, 1978.
12. Durack, D. T.: Current practice in prevention of bacterial endocarditis. Brit. Heart J. 37:478, 1975.
13. Fallot, A.: Contribution a l'anatomie pathologique de la maladie bleue (cyanose cardiaque). Marseille Med. 25:77, 138, 207, 270, 341, 403, 1888.
14. Grant, R. P., Downey, F. M., and MacMahon, H.: The architecture of right ventricular outflow tract in the normal human heart and in the presence of ventricular septal defect. Circulation 24:223, 1961.
15. Guntheroth, W. G.: Pediatric Electrocardiography. W. B. Saunders, Philadelphia, 1965, p. 95.
16. Guntheroth, W. G., Arcasoy, M. M., Phillips, L. A., and Figley, M. M.: Demonstration of collateral circulation to the lungs with angiocardiographic studies in congenital heart disease. Am. Heart J. 64:293, 1962.
17. Guntheroth, W. G., Morgan, B. C., and Mullins, G. L.: Physiologic studies of paroxysmal

hyperpnea in cyanotic congenital heart disease. Circulation 31:70, 1965.
18. Guntheroth, W. G., Morgan, B. C., Mullins, G. L., and Baum, D.: Venous return with knee-chest position and squatting in tetralogy of Fallot. Am. Heart. J. 75:313, 1968.
19. Guyton, A. C.: Cardiac Output and Its Regulation. W. B. Saunders, Philadelphia, 1963, p. 135.
20. Hamilton, W. F., Winslow, J. A., and Hamilton, W. F., Jr.: Notes on a case of congenital heart disease with cyanotic episodes. J. Clin. Invest. 29:20, 1950.
21. Honey, M., Chamberlain, D. A., and Howard, J.: The effect of beta-sympathetic blockade on arterial oxygen saturation in Fallot's tetralogy. Circulation 30:401, 1964.
22. Hunter, W.: Three cases of malformation of the heart. Medical Observations and Inquiries by a Society of Physicians in London 6:291, 1784.
23. James, F. W., Kaplan, S., and Chou, Te-C.: Unexpected cardiac arrest in patients after surgical correction of tetralogy of Fallot. Circulation 52:691, 1975.
24. Keith, J. D., Rowe, R. D., and Vlad, P.: Heart Disease in Infancy and Childhood, 3rd Ed. MacMillan, New York, 1978.
25. King, S. B., and Franch, R. H.: Production of increased right-to-left shunting by rapid heart rates in patients with tetralogy of Fallot. Circulation 44:265, 1971.
26. Kirklin, J. W., Blackstone, E. H., Pacifico, A. D., Brown, R. N., and Bargeron, L. M., Jr.: Routine primary repair vs. two-stage repair of tetralogy of Fallot. Circulation 60:373, 1979.
27. Kirklin, J. W., and Karp, R. B.: The Tetralogy of Fallot from a Surgical Viewpoint. W. B. Saunders, Philadelphia, 1970.
28. Kjellberg, S. R., Mannheimer, E., Rudhe, U., and Jonsson, B.: Diagnosis of Congenital Heart Disease, 2nd ed. Year Book Medical Publishers, Chicago, 1959.
29. Kontos, H. A., and Lower, R. R.: Role of beta-adrenergic receptors in the circulatory response to hypoxia. Am. J. Physiol. 217:756, 1969.
30. Kulbertus, H. E., Coyne, J. J., and Hallidie-Smith, K. A.: Conduction disturbances before and after surgical closure of ventricular septal defect. Am. Heart J. 77:123, 1969.
31. Leachman, R. D., Hallman, G. L., and Cooley, D. A.: Relationship between polycythemia and surgical mortality in patients undergoing total correction for tetralogy of Fallot. Circulation 32:65, 1965.
32. Lillehei, C. S., Cohen, M., Warden, H. E., Read, R. C., Aust, J. B., DeWall, R. A., and Varco, R. L.: Direct vision intracardiac surgical correction of the tetralogy of Fallot, pentalogy of Fallot, and pulmonary atresia defects. Report of first ten cases. Ann. Surg. 142:418, 1955.
33. Lintermans, J. P., Guntheroth, W. G., and

Figley, M. M.: Extensive accessory pulmonary arteries in the presence of relatively normal primary pulmonary arteries. Am. Heart J. 71:527, 1966.
34. Longenecker, C. G., Reemtsma, K., and Creech, O., Jr.: Anomalous coronary artery distribution associated with tetralogy of Fallot: A hazard in open cardiac repair. J. Thorac. Cardiovasc. Surg. 42:258, 1961.
35. Lurie, P. R.: Postural effects in tetralogy of Fallot. Am. J. Med. 15:297, 1953.
36. Marquis, R. M.: Longevity and the early history of the tetralogy of Fallot. Br. Med. J. 1:819, 1956.
37. Martelle, R. R., and Linde, L. M.: Cerebrovascular accidents with tetralogy of Fallot. Am. J. Dis. Child. 101:206, 1961.
38. Maurer, H. M., MacCue, C. M., Robertson, L. W., and Haggins, J. C.: Correction of platelet dysfunction and bleeding in cyanotic congenital heart disease by simple red cell volume reduction. Am. J. Cardiol. 35:831, 1975.
39. McDonald, R. H., Goldberg, L. I., McNay, J. L., and Tuttle, E. P.: Effects of dopamine in man, augmentation of sodium excretion, glomerular filtration rate, and renal plasma flow. J. Clin. Invest. 43:1116, 1964.
40. McGoon, D. C., Baird, D. K., and Davis, G. D.: Surgical management of large bronchial collateral arteries with pulmonary stenosis or atresia. Circulation 52:109, 1975.
41. Miller, R. A., Lev, M., and Paul, M. H.: Congenital absence of the pulmonary valve: The clinical syndrome of tetralogy of Fallot with pulmonary regurgitation. Circulation 26:266, 1962.
42. Morgan, B. C., Guntheroth, W. G., Bloom, R. S., and Fyler, D. C.: A clinical profile of paroxysmal hyperpnea in cyanotic congenital heart disease. Circulation 31:66, 1965.
43. Morgan, B. C., Guntheroth, W. G., Figley, M. M., Dillard, D. H., and Merendino, K. A.: Operable congenital heart disease. Pediatr. Clin. North Am. 13:105, 1966.
44. Morgan, B. C., Guntheroth, W. G., and McGough, G. A.: Effect of position on leg volume: Case against the Trendelenburg position. J.A.M.A. 187:1024, 1964.
45. Murphy, J. D., Freed, M. D., Keane, J. F., Norwood, W. I., Castaneda, A. R., and Nadas, A. S.: Hemodynamic results after intracardiac repair of tetralogy of Fallot by deep hypothermia and cardiopulmonary bypass. Circulation 62:I168, 1980.
46. Nadas, A. S.: Pediatric Cardiology, 3rd ed. W. B. Saunders, Philadelphia, 1972, p. 557.
47. Nadas, A. S., Rosenbaum, H. D., Wittenborg, M. H., and Rudolph, A. M.: Tetralogy of Fallot with unilateral pulmonary atresia: A clinically diagnosable and surgically significant variant. Circulation 8:328, 1953.
48. Nottin, R., Blondeau, Ph., D'Allaines, C., Carpentier, A., Bouchard, F., and Dubost, Ch.: A study of long-term hemodynamic results fol-

lowing complete repair of tetralogy of Fallot. Thorac. Cardiovasc. Surgeon 27:211, 1979.

49. Pacifico, A. D., Kirklin, J. W., and Blackstone, E. H.: Surgical management of pulmonary stenosis in tetralogy of Fallot. J. Thorac. Cardiovasc. Surg. 74:382, 1977.

50. Park, M. K., and Guntheroth, W. G.: How to Read Pediatric ECGs. Year Book Publishers, Chicago, 1981.

51. Polani, P. E., and Campbell, M.: An aetiological study of congenital heart disease. Ann. Hum. Genet. 19:209, 1955.

52. Ponce, F. E., Williams, L. C., Webb, H. M., Riopel, D. A., and Hohn, A. R.: Propranolol palliation of tetralogy of Fallot: Experience with long-term drug treatment in pediatric patients. Pediatrics 52:100, 1973.

53. Rudolph, A. M.: Right ventricular obstruction with ventricular septal defect (Fallot's tetralogy). In Paediatric Cardiology, edited by H. Watson, C. V. Mosby, St. Louis, 1968, p. 556 ff.

54. Rudolph, A. M., and Danilowicz, D.: Treatment of severe spell syndrome in congenital heart disease. Pediatrics 32:141, 1963.

55. Rudolph, A. M., Nadas, A. S., and Borges, W. H.: Hematologic adjustments to cyanotic congenital heart disease. Pediatrics 11:454, 1953.

56. Sandifort, E.: Observations, quoted by L. R. Bennet. Bull. Hist. Med. 20:539, 1946.

57. Shaner, R. F.: Malformations of the truncus arteriosus in pig embryos. Anat. Rec. 118:539, 1954.

58. Singh, S. P., Rigby, M. L., and Astley, R.: Demonstration of pulmonary arteries by contrast injection into pulmonary vein. Br. Heart J. 40:55, 1978.

59. Sorenson, S. C., and Severinghaus, J. W.: Respiratory insensitivity to acute hypoxia persisting after correction of tetralogy of Fallot. J. Appl. Physiol. 25:21, 1968.

60. Steeg, C. N., and Hordof, A.: The hemodynamic effects of supraventricular tachycardia in ventricular septal defect with pulmonary outflow tract obstruction. Am. Heart J. 90:245, 1975.

61. Steeg, C. N., Krongrad, E., Davachi, F., Bowman, F. O., Jr., Malm, J. R., and Gersony, W. M.: Post-operative left anterior hemiblock and right bundle branch block following repair of tetralogy of Fallot. Circulation 51:1026, 1975.

62. Stensen, N.: Quoted by H. I. Goldstein. Bull. Hist. Med. 22:526, 1948.

63. Stevenson, J. G., Kawabori, I., and Guntheroth, W. G.: Pulsed Doppler echocardiographic evaluation of the cyanotic newborn: Identification of the pulmonary artery in transposition of the great arteries. Am. J. Cardiol. 46:849, 1980.

64. Tanz, R. D., and Guntheroth, W. G.: The response of mammalian cardiac muscle to certain sympathomimetics in the presence of morphine. Proc. Soc. Exp. Biol. Med. 122:754, 1966.

65. Taussig, H. B.: Congenital Malformations of the Heart, 2nd ed., vol. 2. Harvard University Press, Cambridge, Mass., 1960, p. 3.

66. Tucker, W. Y., Turley, K., Ullyot, D. J., and Ebert, P. A.: Management of symptomatic tetralogy of Fallot in the first year of life. J. Thorac. Cardiovasc. Surg. 78:494, 1979.

67. Van Lingen, B., and Whidborne, J.: Oximetry in congenital heart disease with special reference to the effects of voluntary hyperventilation. Circulation 6:740, 1952.

68. Van Praagh, R., and Van Praagh, S.: The anatomy of common aortico-pulmonary trunk (truncus arteriosus communis) and its embryological implications: A study of 57 neocropsy cases. Am. J. Cardiol. 16:406, 1965.

69. Van Praagh, R., Van Praagh, S., Nebesar, R. A., Muster, A. J., Sinha, S. N., and Paul, M. H.: Tetralogy of Fallot: Underdevelopment of the pulmonary infundibulum and its sequelae. Am. J. Cardiol. 26:25, 1970.

70. Velasquez, G., Nath, P. H., Castaneda-Zuniga, W. R., Amplatz, K., and Formanck, A.: Aberrant left subclavian artery in tetralogy of Fallot. Am. J. Cardiol. 45:811, 1980.

71. Wessel, H. U., Bastanier, C. K., Paul, M. H., Berry, T. E., Cole, R. B., and Muster, A. J.: Prognostic significance of arrhythmia in tetralogy of Fallot after intracardiac repair. Am. J. Cardiol. 46:843, 1980.

72. Wood, P.: Attacks of deeper cyanosis and loss of consciousness (syncope) in Fallot's tetralogy. B. Heart J. 20:282, 1958.

16

Congenital Absence of the Pulmonary Valve

George C. Emmanouilides, M.D., and Barry G. Baylen, M.D.

Congenital absence of the pulmonary valve is a relatively rare cardiac malformation. In the majority of cases this lesion is associated with a ventricular septal defect (VSD), obstructive pulmonary valve annulus, and massive dilatation of the pulmonary arteries. This combination of lesions is better known as tetralogy of Fallot with absent pulmonary valve. Isolated congenital absence of the pulmonary valve (with intact ventricular septum) has been described also but less frequently.

Since the first description of this lesion by Chevers[6] in 1847, there have been at least 250 cases reported in the literature, including 12 cases of absent pulmonary valve with intact ventricular septum.[4, 13, 15, 18, 32, 37, 40, 41] Absence of the pulmonary valve has also been described in association with patent ductus arteriosus,[21, 26, 43] atrial septal defect,[7, 52] double outlet right ventricle,[1, 11, 26] endocardial cushion defect, Marfan's syndrome,[8] VSD without valve ring stenosis,[5, 14, 47] tricuspid atresia,[17] transposition of the great arteries,[39] Uhl's anomaly,[22] and anomalous origin of right or left pulmonary artery from the ascending aorta.[4, 51]

In the majority of cases, there is absence of mature valvular tissue, which leads to pulmonary valvular insufficiency. An irregular and occasionally smooth, slight rim of primitive connective tissue is usually present at the expected area of the valve (Fig. 16.1). In some instances, incomplete or defective but mature valvular tissue may be present, and in these cases the prognosis is relatively good. Although survival beyond infancy is not infrequent, a number of infants with the severe form of this syndrome die early with signs of severe respiratory distress and intractable cardiac failure.[15] The pulmonary problems are due to tracheobronchial compression caused by the massively dilated pulmonary arteries and usually determine the prognosis.[15, 39]

PATHOLOGY

The heart is usually very large owing to the dilated right ventricle and prominent infundibulum. The pulmonary trunk and its main branches are dilated (Fig. 16.1). At times the pulmonary artery is massively dilated, reaching aneurysmal proportions. At the expected area of the pulmonary valve, there is usually a ring of nodular, gelatinous tissue which most likely represents primitive valvular tissue. The pulmonary valve annulus is usually constricted and hypoplastic and is often associated with a narrow, long, tortuous infundibulum. In cases with VSD and infundibular stenosis, the internal arrangement of the heart is that of tetralogy of Fallot. The VSD is large and is located in the membranous septum beneath the aortic valve. The aorta is dilated, and frequently a right aortic arch is present.

The rudimentary pulmonary valvular tissue consists of a large avascular mass of pale-staining, highly cellular, primi-

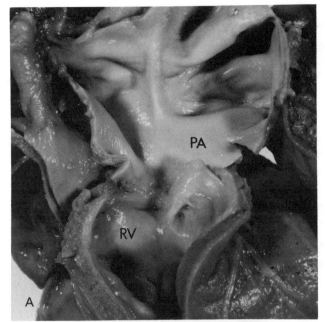

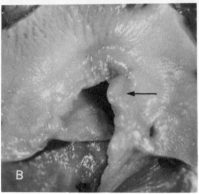

Fig. 16.1 (*A*) Photograph of the opened right ventricle (*RV*) and pulmonary artery (*PA*) of a 3-month-old infant with the syndrome of tetralogy of Fallot with absent pulmonary valve. Note the relatively dilated but thickened infundibulum, rudimentary valve tissue at the level of the pulmonary valve annulus, and the massive dilatation of the pulmonary artery and the major branches. (Reproduced with permission from G. C. Emmanouilides *et al.*[15] and the Dun-Donnelley Publishing Corporation.) (*B*) Cephalad view of the pulmonary valve annulus of a 30-day-old infant with the syndrome of tetralogy of Fallot and absent pulmonary valve. Note that instead of normal valve leaflets, only small nodules of gelatinous tissue are present (*arrow*).

tive connective tissue which projects into the lumen. It has been suggested that the wall of dilated pulmonary artery is abnormal.[29, 44] Histologic findings similar to those seen in Marfan's syndrome (cystic medial necrosis) have been described only in a few cases, but no abnormalities of the wall architecture were found in the majority of instances.[32, 34, 35] The coexistence of Marfan's syndrome and absent pulmonary valve has been reported in one case in which a ventricular septal defect and aneurysm of the left sinus of Valsalva were also present.[8] It appears that there is a relationship between the orientation of the infundibulum and pulmonary arterial dilatation. When the infundibulum is oriented towards the right, the right pulmonary artery becomes aneurysmal, whereas a vertical or leftward oriented infundibulum is associated with bilateral or left pulmonary artery dilatation.[24] The valvular ring stenosis plays an important role in

the pathogenesis of dilatation of the pulmonary arteries (poststenotic dilatation).[15, 24]

Recently the association of "agenesis" of the ductus arteriosus with this syndrome has been described in four severely affected infants with massive dilatation of the pulmonary arteries.[15] It has been suggested that the massive in utero dilatation of the pulmonary arteries in these infants may be pathogenetically related with the agenesis of the ductus arteriosus. This is supported by the fact that, in cases of absence of the pulmonary valve with intact ventricular septum, where a normally located ductus arteriosus is present in utero, aneurysmal dilatation of the pulmonary arteries is not present.[29, 34, 42] It appears that the ductus arteriosus in utero, because of the low placental vascular resistance, promotes forward flow in spite of the presence of pulmonary valvular insufficiency.[24]

Recently, Rabinovitch and associates[39] in a detailed postmortem study of three severely affected infants using special morphometric techniques have shown that, in addition to the massively dilated central pulmonary arteries compressing the main stem bronchi, there was a rather bizarre pulmonary arterial branching pattern (Figs. 16.2 and 16.3). The normally branching single segmental arteries were replaced by tufts of vessels which entwined and compressed the intrapulmonary smaller bronchi along their root from hilar to periphery. Moreover, in one case the number of bronchial generations was definitely decreased, and in another one the alveolar multiplication was severely impaired. These findings may explain why, in certain patients with the severe form of the syndrome, surgical relief of compression of the main stem bronchus alone will not alleviate or reverse their severe respiratory obstructive disease.[39]

MANIFESTATIONS

Clinical Features

The diagnosis of absent pulmonary valve often can be suspected by the clinical features.[3, 11, 24, 29, 42] Immediately after birth the majority of the severely affected infants with

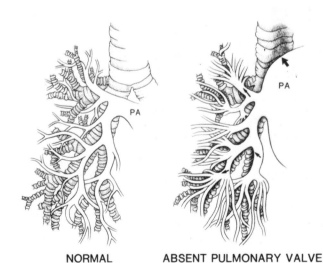

NORMAL   ABSENT PULMONARY VALVE

Fig. 16.2 Diagrammatic representation of normal pulmonary artery (*PA*) branching and the abnormal pattern seen in cases of absent pulmonary valve syndrome—tufts of vessels emerging at segmental artery level that entwine the bronchi. *Arrows* denote large right pulmonary artery compressing right main stem bronchus. (Reproduced with permission from M. Rabinovitch *et al.*[39])

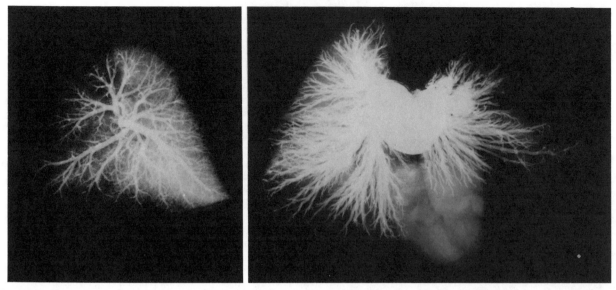

Fig. 16.3 Postmortem arteriograms from a 14-day-old normal infant (*left*) and from a 4-day-old patient with absent pulmonary valve syndrome associated with a ventricular septal defect and *d*-transposition of the great arteries (*right*), showing tufts of vessels in both lungs. (Note the hypoplasia of the left lung.) (Reproduced with permission from M. Rabinovitch *et al.*[39])

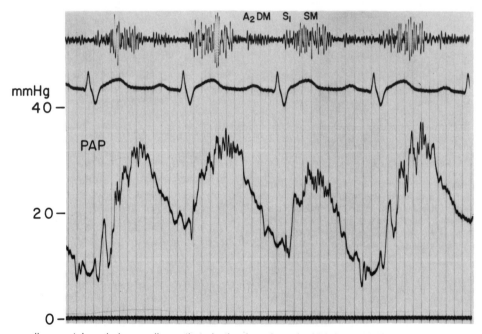

Fig. 16.4 Phonocardiogram taken during cardiac catheterization in a 6-week-old infant with the syndrome of tetralogy of Fallot and absent pulmonary valve. Note the prominent ejection systolic murmur, the single second sound (aortic closure), and the decrescendo diastolic murmur of pulmonary valvular insufficiency ("to and fro" murmur). There was a 60 mm Hg pressure gradient across the stenotic pulmonary valve annulus. At autopsy only minimal primitive dysplastic tissue was present at the area of pulmonary valve ring (see Fig. 16.1*A*). A_2, aortic closure; *DM*, diastolic murmur; *PAP*, pulmonary artery pressure, S_1, first heart sound; *SM*, systolic murmur.

this syndrome develop varying degrees of respiratory distress. Cyanosis is not always present except early in the neonatal period. The respiratory distress is due to the partial bronchial obstruction caused by external compression from the massively dilated pulmonary arteries. The respiratory difficulty at times is relieved when the infant is placed in the prone position. Cardiac decompensation and death occur early in many instances.[15, 24] In isolated pulmonary valvular insufficiency, there are typically no associated symptoms, although symptoms of right ventricular failure during middle age have been reported in a few cases.

Physical examination reveals a characteristic rough sys-

tolic and diastolic ("to and fro") murmur[16] (Fig. 16.4). In cases with VSD there is moderate cyanosis, rapid respiratory rate, abdominal breathing, and overexpansion of the thorax accompanied with intercostal retractions. Inspiratory and expiratory wheezes are frequently present. A systolic and sometimes a diastolic thrill is palpable maximally at the left sternal border. The "to and fro" murmur is heard best at the upper left sternal border and is widely transmitted over the precordium. The murmur consists of a rough ejection systolic component due to valve ring stenosis and a rough decrescendo diastolic component. Between the two murmurs there is a short pause when a single second sound is heard.

The single second sound is heard loudest at the lower left sternal border and apex; it is due to the closure of the aortic valve. The discontinuity of the characteristic "to and fro" murmur distinguishes it from the typical continuous murmur of a patent ductus arteriosus.[16] In isolated pulmonary valvular insufficiency, a moderately loud, rough "to and fro" murmur is also heard at the upper left sternal border accompanied with a systolic thrill. Because of the obstructive nature of the respiratory distress, hepatomegaly is difficult to evaluate. However, massive liver enlargement may be present in some infants with profound heart failure.

In patients with minimal or no symptoms, the second sound may be split, suggesting that some functional valvular tissue is present. In such cases a bicuspid pulmonary valve is found at autopsy. In those patients who survive the first year of life, the respiratory symptoms improve spontaneously, and the cyanosis disappears. The loss of cyanosis is due to the reversal of the initial right to left shunt, as a result of the decrease in pulmonary vascular resistance which normally occurs during the neonatal period. Thus, most of the patients beyond the neonatal period have predominantly left to right shunts. With the reduction of pulmonary vascular resistance, the pulmonary regurgitation will also diminish and thus decrease the diastolic right ventricular overload and lessen the diastolic right to left shunting at the ventricular level. A small amount of diastolic right to left shunting may persist even in the presence of a moderate left to right ventricular systolic shunt.

Electrovectorcardiographic Features

Evidence of right ventricular hypertrophy is always present in cases of tetralogy of Fallot and absent pulmonary valve. Biventricular hypertrophy may be present in cases with VSD and bidirectional or left to right shunt. In isolated pulmonary insufficiency, usually mild degrees of right ven-

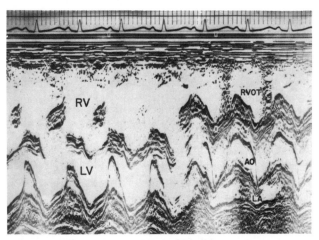

Fig. 16.6 M-mode echocardiogram recorded in a 3-day-old infant with tetralogy of Fallot and absent pulmonary valve. Note septal aortic discontinuity and aortic override. Small left atrial and ventricular dimensions suggest reduced pulmonary blood flow. A markedly enlarged right ventricle with volume overload pattern and abnormal septal motion were recorded at a lower level. *Ao*, aorta; *LA*, left atrium; *RV*, right ventricle; *LV*, left ventricle; *RVOT*, right ventricular outflow tract.

tricular hypertrophy may be suggested by an rsR' pattern in the right precordial leads.

Radiologic Features

A moderately enlarged heart with massively dilated right, main, and left pulmonary arteries is seen in routine chest roentgenograms (Fig. 16.5). However, in the presence of a right aortic arch and overinflation of the lung with displacement of the heart to the left, the aneurysmally dilated pulmonary arteries may not be as obvious.[2, 15, 35, 50] The dilated pulmonary artery may be medially placed and hidden within the mediastinal silhouette. The hilar densities may resemble a tumor mass but can be easily identified by fluoroscopy, which demonstrates pulsation synchronous with the heart beat. A prominent bulge in the left upper cardiac border due to the dilated outflow tract of the right ventricle may also be present. A possible explanation for the prominent infundibulum and occasional medial or rightward displacement of the pulmonary trunk is the leftward rotation of the heart.[42] Thus, the infundibulum forms the upper left border of the heart, then curves to the right and terminates medially. This displaces the pulmonary trunk toward the midline or to the right of the spine. The peripheral pulmonary vascular markings are usually normal, although they may be increased in older infants and children with dominant left to right shunts. Frequently, however, unilateral obstructive emphysema and segmental pulmonary atelectasis may be present with the heart shifted to the opposite hemithorax.[15, 24, 34, 35]

In isolated congenital pulmonary valvular insufficiency, the chest roentgenograms may be normal or show prominent main and left pulmonary arteries. Fluoroscopy may reveal increased pulmonary arterial pulsations and occasionally a hilar dance. However, the dilatation of the pulmonary arteries usually does not reach the aneurysmal proportions seen in tetralogy of Fallot with absent pulmonary valve.

Echocardiographic Features

Both M-mode and 2D echocardiography may be useful in demonstrating varying degrees of dilatation of the right

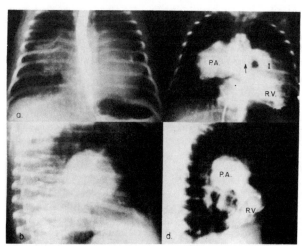

Fig. 16.5 Roentgenographic features of a 2½-month-old infant with the syndrome of tetralogy of Fallot with absent pulmonary valve. (a and b) Frontal and lateral views, respectively, of thoracic roentgenograms. Cardiomegaly with marked prominence of the upper left cardiac border. This prominence represents an enlarged, levorotated infundibulum. The large, rounded hilar density extending into the right hemithorax seen in the frontal view is also apparent in the lateral view as well and represents an aneurysmal dilatation of the pulmonary artery (*P.A.*) (c and d) Selective angiocardiograms from the right ventricle (*R.V.*) The right ventricle is enlarged. The infundibular tract (*I*) and the huge pulmonary artery (*P.A.*) are opacified. The location of the pulmonary annulus is marked with an *arrow*. The aorta opacifies from the right ventricle, indicating the presence of a VSD with right to left shunt. (Reproduced with permission from H. D. Ruttenberg et al.[42])

ventricle and right ventricular outflow tract. The pulmonary valve cannot be easily visualized. However, in older children an abnormal linear echo thought to be derived from the rudimentary pulmonary valve tissue is recorded anteriorly to the dense echo from the subpulmonary muscle mass.[31] Overriding of the aorta with an enlarged right ventricle and paradoxical motion of the intraventricular septum (ventricular volume overload) are the echocardiographic characteristics of this anomaly. Two dimensional echocardiography, in addition, may demonstrate the aneurysmal dilatation of the pulmonary trunk and its main branches (Fig. 16.6).

CARDIAC CATHETERIZATION

In cases with VSD and outflow obstruction during the newborn period and early infancy, the right ventricular pressure usually is at systemic levels and there is predominantly a right to left shunt at the ventricular level. In the absence of significant outflow obstruction, as the pulmonary vascular resistance falls, the right ventricular pressure falls and the shunt becomes predominantly left to right. A systolic pressure gradient virtually always is present between the right ventricle and the pulmonary artery. The magnitude of the gradient depends upon the degree of constriction of the pulmonary valve annulus. The diastolic pressure in the pulmonary artery usually is equal to that of the right ventricle. This is due to the pulmonary insufficiency which is reflected in the contour of the pulmonary arterial pressure showing a wide pulse pressure and absence of the incisural notch. Many times it is difficult to obtain an accurate pulmonary arterial pressure because of artifacts caused by turbulence in the pulmonary artery and the severe respiratory distress present in the very young infant. A properly damped catheter system and a relatively steady state are necessary for adequate pulmonary arterial pressure recordings. In severely affected cyanotic infants with respiratory distress, sedation is definitely contraindicated during the cardiac catheterization because of the danger of respiratory arrest.

In isolated valvular insufficiency, catheterization reveals normal peak right ventricular and pulmonary systolic pressures. There is usually a small systolic gradient across the pulmonary valve which is the result of the high velocity of blood flow via the normal annulus due to the increased right ventricular stroke volume consequent to regurgitation.

ANGIOCARDIOGRAPHY

Right ventricular angiocardiograms demonstrate the location and severity of constriction of the pulmonary valve annulus, the orientation of the infundibulum, and the dilatation of the pulmonary arteries (Figs. 16.5 and 16.7). Valve leaflets cannot be identified, but a discrete ridge of tissue may be present at the level of the stenotic valvular ring (Fig. 16.5). The infundibulum is usually dilated and seldom is found to be mildly stenotic. The right ventricle is dilated, and a right to left shunt may be seen when there is significant outflow obstruction, as seen in tetralogy of Fallot. A prolonged emptying of the right ventricular cavity due to pulmonary insufficiency is usually seen. Injection of contrast material in the pulmonary artery will demonstrate the presence of pulmonary valvular insufficiency, as well as the extent of the aneurysmal dilatation (Fig. 16.7). Atresia of the left pulmonary artery also has been reported in a few instances.[24, 30] In rare instances, an anomalous origin of a right or left pulmonary artery from the ascending aorta may be present.

Recently, analyses of ventricular volume data in a number

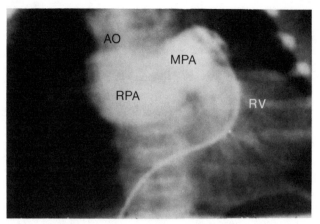

Fig. 16.7 Photograph of a cine frame of a pulmonary artery injection obtained in an infant 24 hours old, with the syndrome of tetralogy of Fallot and absent pulmonary valve. Note the marked aneurysmal dilatation of the main (*MPA*) and right (*RPA*) pulmonary arteries. The dilatation of the left pulmonary artery is less obvious, and the pulmonary valve ring stenosis is not visible in this view. There is some regurgitation of contrast material in the right ventricular outflow tract. The massively dilated right pulmonary artery was not seen in the chest roentgenogram partly because of superimposition of the right aortic arch (*AO*). *RV*, right ventricle. (Reproduced with permission from G. C. Emmanouilides et al.[15])

of infants with the syndrome of tetralogy of Fallot and absent pulmonary valve suggest the presence of marked differences in right ventricular end-diastolic volume (RVEDV) between the very sick infants and the children surviving this syndrome, i.e., the sick infants have very large RVEDV in contrast to surviving older children who have normal or near normal RVEDV.[19] Moreover, the relative size of the dilated right pulmonary artery correlates with the morbidity and mortality of these infants; the very sick newborn infants have relatively larger right pulmonary arteries than the older infants and children.[19] In addition, abnormalities of the branching of the hilar pulmonary arteries can be easily diagnosed on the conventional cineangiogram.[39]

TREATMENT

The prognosis of infants with this syndrome is related to the extent of tracheobronchial obstruction secondary to the dilatation of the pulmonary arteries. Pulmonary complications, such as obstructive emphysema and atelectasis, especially during the course of minor respiratory infections are usually the cause of death. There are a number of infants reported with mild or moderate respiratory obstructive symptoms who improved spontaneously by their first birthday. This improvement may be accounted for by several factors: maturational changes in the structure of the tracheobronchial tree, whereby the weak cartilaginous, muscular, and elastic support of the newborn trachea and bronchi becomes strengthened and renders the walls of these airway passages firmer and more resistant to outside compressive forces; growth changes which make the lumina of these structures larger, and thus the same outside force produces less obstruction; and the altered hemodynamics postnatally with reduction of pulmonary vascular resistance, and/or the relative increase in valvular ring stenosis, resulting in decrease in pulmonary arterial pressure and thus less distension of the dilated pulmonary arteries.[24, 46]

The majority of infants with the severe form of this syndrome die early in infancy mainly from severe respiratory distress and hypoxemia. A variety of surgical procedures, such as aneurysmorrhaphy,[34] aneurysmectomy with suspension of the pulmonary artery to the retrosternal fascia,[3] and transection of the dilated pulmonary arterial segment, together with an anastomosis either to the superior vena cava or to the main pulmonary artery, have been suggested for the relief of the respiratory obstruction.[27, 48] However, the results are far from satisfactory.

Definitive correction of the lesion with or without replacement of the pulmonary valve has been performed in older patients with good results.[4, 9, 10, 12, 20, 45, 49] It appears that valve insertion at the pulmonary annulus leads to a better hemodynamic result, as suggested by postoperative exercise performance and improvement of right ventricular function.[20] At least 14 patients have been reported as having total correction with insertion of a prosthetic valve with apparently excellent results.[4, 10, 12, 20] However, in some centers, pulmonary valve replacement is recommended only when there is pulmonary hypertension.[36, 45] In spite of the recent strides in infant surgery, definitive correction of this lesion in the severely symptomatic infant has not been as successful.[20, 36] Only occasional infants survive such a procedure.[4, 12] It appears that the severity of the pulmonary manifestations of the syndrome is the main determinant of successful surgery and ultimate survival of these infants. It has been suggested that the angiographic detection of abnormalities of the branching pattern of the segmental pulmonary arteries may become useful in assessing preoperatively these infants.[39] It is possible that these vascular changes may be of such severity that they preclude survival, with or without surgical intervention.[39]

REFERENCES

1. Baker, W. P., Kelminson, L. L., Turner, W. M., and Blount, S. G.: Absence of pulmonic valve associated with double outlet right ventricle. Circulation 36:452, 1967.
2. Borg, S. A., Young, L. W., and Roghair, G. C.: Congenital avalvular pulmonary artery and infantile lobar emphysema. A diagnostic correlation. Am. J. Roentgenol. Radium Ther. Nucl. Med. 125:412, 1975.
3. Bove, E. L., Shaher, R. M., Alley, R. M., and McKneally, M.: Tetralogy of Fallot with absent pulmonary valve and aneurysm of the pulmonary artery: Report of two cases presenting as obstructive lung disease. J. Pediatr. 81:339, 1972.
4. Calder, A. L., Brandt, P. W., Barratt-Boyes, B. G., and Neutze, J. M.: Variant of tetralogy of Fallot with absent pulmonary valve leaflets and origin of one pulmonary artery from the ascending aorta. Am. J. Cardiol. 46:106, 1980.
5. Campeau, L., Gilbert, G., and Aerichide, N.: Absence of the pulmonary valve: Report of two cases associated with other congenital lesions. Am. J. Cardiol. 8:113, 1961.
6. Chevers, N.: *Recherches sur les maladies de l'artere pulmonaire.* Arch. Gen. Med. 15:488, 1847.
7. Chiemmongkoltip, P., Replogle, R. L., and Arcilla, R. A.: Congenital absence of the pulmonary valve with atrial septal defect surgically corrected with aortic homograft. Chest 62:200, 1972.
8. Childers, R. W., and McRea, P. C.: Absence of the pulmonary valve. Circulation 29:598, 1964.
9. Cornell, G., Colocathis, B., and Subramanian, S.: Heterograft valve implant in tetralogy of Fallot with absent pulmonary valve. Ann. Thorac. Surg. 22:51, 1971.
10. Daenen, W., de Leval, M., Stalpaert, G., Vander Hauwaert, L., and Stark, J.: Surgical management of tetralogy of Fallot with absent pulmonary valve. Eur. J. Cardiol. 8:99, 1978.
11. D'Cruz, J. A., Lendrum, B. L., and Novak, G.: Congenital absence of the pulmonary valve. Am. Heart J. 68:728, 1964.
12. Dunnigan, A., Oldham, H. N., and Benson, D. W.: Absent pulmonary valve syndrome in infancy: Surgery reconsidered. Am. J. Cardiol. 48:117, 1981.
13. Durnin, R. E., Willner, R., Virmani, S., Lawrency, T. Y., and Fyler, D. C.: Pulmonary regurgitation with ventricular septal defect and pulmonic stenosis: Tetralogy of Fallot variant. Am. J. Roentgenol. Radium Ther. Nucl. Med. 106:42, 1969.
14. Elliot, L. P., Shanklin, D. R., and Schiebler, G. L.: Congenital insufficiency of the pulmonary valve with a ventricular septal defect. Dis. Chest 42:534, 1962.
15. Emmanouilides, G. C., Thanopoulos, B., Siassi, B., and Fishbein, M.: "Agenesis" of ductus arteriosus associated with syndrome of tetralogy of Fallot and absent pulmonary valve. Am.

J. Cardiol. 37:403, 1976.
16. Fontana, M. E., and Wooley, C. F.: The murmur of pulmonic regurgitation in tetralogy of Fallot with absent pulmonary valve. Circulation 57:986, 1978.
17. Freedom, R. M., Patel, R. G., Bloom, K. R., Duckworth, J. W., Silver, M. M., Dische, R., and Rowe, R. D.: Congenital absence of the pulmonary valve associated with imperforate membrane type of tricuspid atresia, right ventricular tensor apparatus and intact ventricular septum: A curious developmental complex. Eur. J. Cardiol. 10:171, 1979.
18. Harris, B. C., Shaver, J. Q., Kroetz, F. W., and Leonard, J. J.: Congenital pulmonary valvular insufficiency complicating tetralogy of Fallot. Am. J. Cardiol. 23:864, 1969.
19. Hiraishi, S., Bargeron, L. M., Emmanouilides, G. C., Friedman, W. F., and Jarmakani, J. M.: Right and left ventricular volume characteristics in infants and children with absent pulmonary valve (abstr.) Am. J. Cardiol. 1982.
20. Ilbawi, M. N., Idriss, F. S., Muster, A. J., Wessel, H. U., Paul, M. H., and DeLeon, S. Y.: Tetralogy of Fallot with absent pulmonary valve: Should valve insertion be part of the intracardiac repair?: J. Thorac. Cardiovasc. Surg. 81:906, 1981.
21. Ito, T., Engle, M. A., and Holswade, G. R.: Congenital insufficiency of the pulmonic valve: A rare cause of neonatal heart failure. Pediatrics 28:712, 1961.
22. Kaul, U., Arora, R., and Rani, S.: Uhl's anomaly with rudimentary pulmonary valve leaflets: A clinical, hemodynamic, angiographic and pathologic study. Am. Heart J. 100:673, 1980.
23. Knight, L., and Edwards, J. E.: Right aortic arch. Types of associated cardiac anomalies. Circulation 50:1047, 1974.
24. Lakier, J. B., Stanger, P., Heymann, M. A., Hoffman, J. I. E., and Rudolph, A. M.: Tetralogy of Fallot with absent pulmonary valve: Natural history and hemodynamic considerations. Circulation 50:167, 1974.
25. Layton, C. A., McDonald, A., McDonald, L., Towers, M., Weaver, J., and Yacoub, M.: The syndrome of absent pulmonary valve: Total correction with aortic valvular homografts. J. Thorac. Cardiovasc. Surg. 63:800, 1972.
26. Lendrum, B. L., and Shaffer, A. B.: Isolated congenital pulmonic valvular regurgitation. Am. Heart J. 57:298, 1959.
27. Litwin, S. B., Rosenthal, A., and Fellows, K.: Surgical management of young infants with tetralogy of Fallot, absence of pulmonary valve and respiratory distress. J. Thorac. Cardiovasc. Surg. 65:552, 1973.
28. MacCartney, F. J., and Miller, G. A. H.: Congenital absence of the pulmonary valve. Br. Heart J. 32:483, 1970.
29. Miller, R. A., Lev, M., and Paul, M. H.: Congenital absence of the pulmonary valve. The

clinical syndrome of tetralogy of Fallot with pulmonary regurgitation. Circulation 26:266, 1962.
30. Nadas, A. S., Rosenbaum, H. D., Wittenborg, M. H., and Rudolph, A. M.: Tetralogy of Fallot with unilateral pulmonary atresia. A clinically diagnosable and surgically significant variant. Circulation 8:328, 1953.
31. Nagai, Y., Komatsu, Y., Nakamura, K., Sato, Y., and Takao, A.: Echocardiographic findings of congenital absence of the pulmonary valve with tetralogy of Fallot. Chest 75:481, 1979.
32. Nagao, G. I., Daoud, G. I., McAdams, A. J., Schwartz, D. C., and Kaplan, S.: Cardiovascular anomalies associated with tetralogy of Fallot. Am. J. Cardiol. 20:206, 1967.
33. Onesti, S. J., and Harned, H. S.: Absence of the pulmonary valve associated with tetralogy of Fallot. Am. J. Cardiol. 20:206, 1967.
34. Osman, M. Q., Meng, C. C. L., and Girdany, B. R.: Congenital absence of the pulmonary valve: Report of eight cases with review of the literature. Am. J. Roentgenol. Radium Ther. Nucl. Med. 106:58, 1969.
35. Pernot, C., Hoeffel, J. C., Henry, M., Worms, A. M., Stehlin, M. D., and Louis, J. P.: Radiological patterns of congenital absence of the pulmonary valve in infants. Radiology 102:619, 1972.
36. Pinsky, W. W., Nihill, M. R., Mullins, C. E., Harrison, G., and McNamara, D. G.: The absent pulmonary valve syndrome. Circulation 57:159, 1978.
37. Pouget, J. M., Kelly, C. E., and Pilz, C. G.: Congenital absence of pulmonic valve: Report of case in 73-year old man. Am. J. Cardiol. 19:732, 1969.
38. Price, B. O.: Isolated incompetence of the pulmonary valve. Circulation 23:596, 1961.
39. Rabinovitch, M., Grady, S., Saver, U., Buhlmeyer, K., Castaneda, A. R., and Reid, L.: Intrapulmonary abnormalities in patients with absent pulmonary valve syndrome. Am. J. Cardiol. 50:804, 1982.
40. Rose, J. S., Levin, D. C., Coldstein, S., and Laster, W.: Congenital absence of the pulmonary valve associated with congenital aplasia of the thymus (DiGeorge's syndrome). Am. J. Roentgenol. Radium Ther. Nucl. Med. 122:97, 1974.
41. Rowe, R. D., Vlad, P., and Keith, J. D.: Atypical tetralogy of Fallot: A noncyanotic form with increased lung vascularity. Circulation 12:230, 1955.
42. Ruttenberg, H. D., Carey, L. S., Adams, P. A., Jr., and Edwards, J. E.: Absence of the pulmonary valve in the tetralogy of Fallot. Am. J. Roentgenol. Radium Ther. Nucl. Med. 91:500, 1964.
43. Smith, R. D., DuShane, J. W., and Edwards, J. E.: Congenital insufficiency of the pulmonary valve including a case of fetal cardiac

failure. Circulation 20:554, 1959.
44. Soulié, P., Vernant, P., Sterba, S., Bouchard, F., Albou, E., Lanfranchi, J., and Letac, B.: *Insufficience pulmonaire congenital et communication interventriculaire.* Arch. Mal. Coeur 60:172, 1967.
45. Stafford, E. G., Mair, D. D., McGoon, D. C., and Danielson, G. K.: Tetralogy of Fallot with absent pulmonary valve: Surgical considerations and results. Circulation 47-48(Suppl. III):24, 1973.
46. Stanger, P., Lucas, R. V., and Edwards, J. E.: Anatomic factors causing respiratory distress in acyanotic congenital cardiac disease: Special reference to bronchial obstruction. Pedi-

atrics 43:760, 1969.
47. Venables, A. W.: Absence of the pulmonary valve with ventricular septal defect. Br. Heart J. 24:293, 1962.
48. Waldhausen, J. A., Friedman, S., Nicodemus, H., Miller, W., Rashkind, W., and Johnson, J.: Absence of the pulmonary valve in patients with tetralogy of Fallot: Surgical management. J. Thorac. Cardiovasc. Surg. 57:669, 1969.
49. Weldon, C., Rowe, R. D., and Gott, V. L.: Clinical experience with the use of aortic valve homografts for reconstruction of the pulmonary artery, pulmonary valve, and outflow portion of the right ventricle. Circulation 37 (Suppl. II):51, 1968.

50. Wolfe, R. R., Smothermon, M. M., Miles, V. N., Wessenberg, R., and Nora, J. J.: Atypical radiographic findings in neonates with absent pulmonary valve and tetralogy of Fallot. Chest 72:245, 1977.
51. Zach, M., Beitzke, A., Singer, H., Hofler, H., and Schellman, B.: The syndrome of absent pulmonary valve and ventricular septal defect. Anatomical features and embryologic considerations. Basic Res. Cardiol. 74:54, 1979.
52. Zajtchuk, R., Gonzales-Lavin, L., and Replogle, R. L.: Pulmonary artery aneurysm associated with atrial septal defect and absent pulmonary valve. J. Thorac. Cardiovasc. Surg. 65:699, 1973.

17

Pulmonary Stenosis

George C. Emmanouilides, M.D., and Barry G. Baylen, M.D.

Obstructive lesions involving the right ventricle and pulmonary arterial tree, isolated or in association with other congenital cardiac defects, occur in 25 to 30% of all individuals with congenital heart disease. These lesions may involve the right ventricular cavity or outflow tract, the pulmonary valve, and the pulmonary trunk or the pulmonary arterial branches. In approximately half of the instances, there is an intact ventricular septum. When the ventricular septum is intact, a common physiologic derangement characterizes the lesions, i.e., increased impedance to the right ventricular output which is proportional to the degree of obstruction. The site and degree of obstruction are very important in understanding the clinical manifestations, the natural history, and the prognosis of these lesions.

In this chapter the following pathologic entities are discussed: pulmonary valvular stenosis, primary infundibular stenosis, the "two-chambered" right ventricle due to anomalous muscle bundles, and the supravalvular pulmonary arterial stenoses, all with intact ventricular septum. In addition, a brief discussion of the cardiovascular malformations associated with the rubella syndrome is included. Pulmonary atresia with intact ventricular septum is discussed elsewhere (Chapter 18).

PULMONARY VALVULAR STENOSIS WITH INTACT VENTRICULAR SEPTUM

The most frequent lesion, producing obstruction to right ventricular output, is pulmonary valvular stenosis. Narrowing of the infundibulum, owing to secondary hypertrophy of its septal and parietal muscle bands, is frequently present, especially in more severe forms of obstruction (Fig. 17.1). A patent foramen ovale or, less frequently, an atrial septal defect (ASD) may also be present in many instances. A number of terms have been used in referring to this lesion such as isolated, pure, simple, or uncomplicated pulmonary stenosis; pulmonary stenosis with normal aortic root; and pulmonary stenosis with intact ventricular septum.[1, 65, 99, 177, 193] The latter term is used in this chapter.

Pulmonary stenosis (PS) was first described by Morgagni,[132] and subsequently an account of its pathology was

given by Meckel.[120] The clinical description of the cyanotic form of this entity and its separation from tetralogy was first attempted by Fallot;[54] he introduced the term "trilogy," which is still used by French authors. Although earlier studies based on postmortem material have suggested that this lesion was rare, with the introduction of cardiac catheterization in the diagnosis of congenital heart disease, numerous reports have appeared indicating that the frequency of this cardiac malformation is relatively high.[2, 65, 99, 139, 177, 193] A rather conservative estimate of the prevalence of PS with intact ventricular septum may be 8 to 10% of all congenital cardiac defects.[1, 65, 99, 193] Familial occurrence of PS has been reported, and its probability of recurrence in siblings has been estimated to be 2.9%.[143] Varying degrees of obstruction may produce entirely different pictures, and thus terms such as mild, moderate, and severe pulmonary stenosis have been introduced, descriptive primarily of the functional significance of the lesion.[49, 52, 65, 99, 105]

PATHOLOGY

In pulmonary valvular stenosis with intact ventricular septum, the basic problem resides in the pulmonary valve. In its classical, severe form, the pulmonary valve takes the shape of a conical fibrous funnel, which projects superiorly into the pulmonary trunk and is formed by the fusion of the valve leaflets (Fig. 17.1). The fused leaflets can be recognized from the pulmonary arterial side as three equidistant raphes radiating to the pulmonary arterial wall. In some instances, four raphes may be present, and in one series a bicuspid valve was found in 20% of autopsied cases of PS. The shape of the valve apparatus and its opening is influenced by the degree of thickness and rigidity of the fused cusps.[19] The valve may be short, thick, and rigid. In older children and adults, small warty vegetations or calcifications around the valve opening also may be present. In extremely severe cases, the opening of the valve may be 1 to 2 mm in diameter. In moderate stenosis only a partial, peripheral fusion of the cusps occurs, leaving the central portion of each leaflet relatively free, producing a larger valve orifice than in severe stenosis.

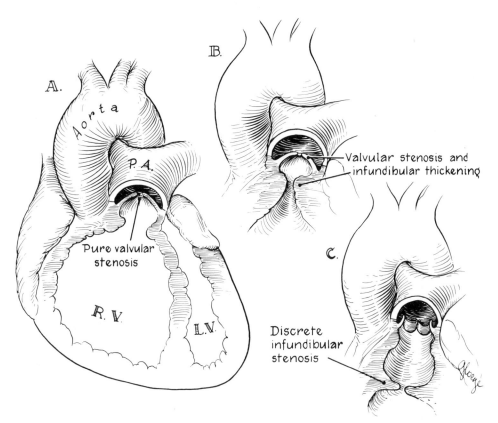

Fig. 17.1 Diagrammatic portrayal of pulmonary valvular stenosis with intact ventricular septum (*A*.), valvular stenosis with secondary infundibular thickening (*B*.), and primary infundibular stenosis with discrete narrowing in the proximal portion of the infundibulum (*C*.). *P.A.*, pulmonary artery; *R.V.*, right ventricle; *L.V.*, left ventricle.

Recently, a distinctive type of familial pulmonary valvular stenosis called "pulmonary valvular dysplasia" has been described.[92, 101, 108] It is characterized by stenosis of the valve without fusion of its cusps. The obstruction is due to markedly thickened, immobile cusps which consist of disorganized myxomatous tissue. The annulus of the valve may also be narrowed with this type of obstruction.[101] Dysplastic pulmonary valves also may be present in some apparently nonfamilial cases of PS and in the majority of patients with Noonan's syndrome, even those with mild stenosis.[99, 142]

Secondary changes due to valvular obstruction occur in the right ventricle and pulmonary arteries. The right ventricle may show severe hypertrophy with the chamber appearing smaller than normal. This hypertrophy is particularly noticeable in the infundibular region, producing narrowing of the outlet of the right ventricle (Fig. 17.1). The endocardium of the infundibulum may be opaque, and the tricuspid valve is often thickened with fibrous tissue along the line of closure and at the points of attachment of the chordae tendineae. These tricuspid valve changes are believed to be the result of a reaction to the excessive physical stresses placed upon the valve apparatus, which may also cause tricuspid insufficiency. The right atrium may be dilated, and its wall may be thickened. In the majority of cases, a patent foramen ovale and, less commonly, an ASD may be present.

A distinct pathologic entity, consisting of hypoplastic right ventricle, hypoplastic tricuspid valve, pulmonic stenosis, and ASD also has been described.[38, 61, 99, 121, 177, 203] The right ventricle in these cases contains very dense fine trabeculae filling its apical portion and outflow tract. These anatomical characteristics suggest that a failure of absorption of the normally present embryonic ventricular spongy mesenchymatous tissue has occurred during development.[99]

Small myocardial infarcts involving subendocardial areas of the ventricular wall and papillary muscles of the right ventricle were found in a number of patients dying with severe PS and massive right ventricular hypertrophy.[60] These changes have been attributed to subendocardial ischemia and may occur more frequently than clinically suspected, especially in infants with critical PS.

The pulmonary arterial trunk is usually dilated, except in cases of valve dysplasia, and a "jet" lesion may be found in its wall. The dilatation begins from the pulmonary valve ring, which may be, in some cases, smaller than normal. This dilatation may extend occasionally into the left pulmonary artery. The mechanism by which dilatation occurs is probably related to the high velocity of blood ejected through the small valvular opening.[87, 159] The kinetic energy of the blood flow is converted to lateral pressure, and the stream is deflected laterally or even completely reversed, so that "eddies" of alternating high and low pressure are produced. These cause repeated impacts, and over a long time the elastic wall undergoes structural fatigue and distension.[87, 151] The degree of poststenotic dilatation is not always proportional to the severity of the stenosis. Very mild cases of valvular PS are frequently associated with pronounced dilatation of the main pulmonary artery. It has been postulated also that the poststenotic dilatation may be the result of a separate and distinct malformation of the pulmonary artery itself. Poststenotic dilatation of the pulmonary artery may not always be present in newborns with severe pulmonary valve stenosis but may develop within a few months after birth. In addition, dilatation of the main pulmonary artery is always absent in patients with isolated infundibular stenosis and in those with pulmonary valvular stenosis associated with bilateral pulmonary arterial stenoses, where the pulmonary arterial trunk is usually smaller than its distal branches.

The aorta arises normally from the left ventricle, and there is always a left aortic arch. Right aortic arch is extremely rare and, when present, infundibular stenosis should be suspected with an associated spontaneously closing or closed ventricular septal defect.[173] Prominent bronchial arteries may be present only in older patients with severe PS. Hypoplasia of the lung is also described in association with congenital pulmonary valvular stenosis.[41, 104] The left ventricular cavity may be normal or increased in size. In cases of severe PS and large atrial right to left shunt, and especially in those cases associated with hypoplasia of the right ventricle, the left ventricular wall may show moderate to marked hypertrophy.[78]

Histologic evidence for a rather widespread cardiovascular disease has been reported recently by Becu et al.[12] Varying degrees of myocardial dysplasia and necrosis, coronary arterial occlusive lesions, and abnormal aortic wall histology were found at autopsy in a number of unoperated and operated patients with severe pulmonary valve stenosis. In those who survived surgery, hypertrophic cardiomyopathy was commonly present. The majority of the affected patients were infants, and only in one infant were the features of Noonan's syndrome present. Because of the presence of a thick, poorly mobile cusp tissue (valvular dysplasia) and some other congenital stigmata, it is possible that some of these cases may represent variants of Noonan's syndrome.[12, 99, 142] Pulmonary valvular stenosis also has been found in association with "prune belly" syndrome.[109]

The most likely pathogenetic mechanism of the obstruction is a maldevelopment of the distal part of the bulbus cordis from which the valves develop.[98] However, it is difficult to understand how a developmental abnormality of the bulbus cordis may lead to fusion of the apparently well-formed cusps of the pulmonary valve in a heart in which the development of the ventricular septum has been completed.[131] Since closure of the ventricular septum depends upon the development of the more proximal connections of the bulbus cordis, Brock[19] postulated that it is possible to have a malformed valve with the rest of the structures developed from the bulbus cordis showing only slight abnormality. That pulmonary valvular stenosis or atresia may be the result of fetal endocarditis also has been postulated for a long time.[147] The association of pulmonary valvular or supravalvular stenosis with multiple somatic abnormalities, such as peculiar facies, short stature, webbed neck, mental retardation, etc., without gross chromosomal abnormalities suggests that genetic factors may play an important role in the pathogenesis of the obstruction.[100, 108, 142, 143, 149]

PHYSIOLOGY

The principal functional derangement in PS is obstruction to ejection of blood from the right ventricle. This leads to an increase in right ventricular pressure which is proportional to the degree of obstruction. In fetal life, as the stenosis develops, an increase in right ventricular muscle mass occurs. This is accomplished by hyperplasia and hypertrophy of the right ventricular muscle fibers which are proportional to the severity of the stenosis. In mild or moderate degrees of PS, the hypertrophied right ventricle is able to maintain normal output with minimal or no effects upon the fetal pattern of circulation. However, in severe forms of PS, the right ventricular output may fall, and the pattern of the circulation in the fetus may resemble that of pulmonary atresia although the right ventricular chamber is definitely larger.[166]

The fetal or neonatal myocardial response to major after-

loads is apparently different from that of the adult. It has been demonstrated in animals that the myocardium of either ventricle responds to obstruction primarily by hypertrophy of the muscle fibers with minimal or no hyperplasia. Since there is no simultaneous increase in capillaries, the diffusion distance between the capillary and the most distant portion of the hypertrophied myocardial cell increases. In contrast, in the newborn animal, marked hyperplasia of the muscle cells associated with an increase in the number of capillaries takes place, and thus the relationship between cells and capillaries remains normal. This developmental property of the fetal and neonatal myocardium is very important because it provides the fast-growing individual the capacity to generate high ventricular pressures that maintain normal blood flow across the obstruction.[166]

Since the ventricular septum is intact, the pressure generated in the right ventricle may exceed that of the left ventricle. Thus the right ventricle may perform more pressure work than the left ventricle, a distinct hemodynamic difference from other types of obstruction, i.e., tetralogy of Fallot. Emptying of the right ventricle is modified by the increased resistance of the pulmonary orifice. The pressure rise during ventricular contraction occurs more or less continuously toward a peak, which is succeeded by a pressure fall with the same continuous course (Fig. 17.2). The more severe the PS, the closer to the end of systole is the peak. As a consequence of this high pressure work, marked right ventricular hypertrophy develops. This tends to maintain a normal stroke volume. If stenosis is severe and remains fixed as the individual grows or as increased demands are placed upon the heart, the right ventricle eventually dilates, and heart failure may ensue. In experimental animals, right-sided failure occurred only when the diameter of the pulmonary artery was reduced to less than one-third of its original size.[36] With right ventricular failure pulmonary flow decreases, but oxygenation of the body at rest may continue to be sufficient, owing to the increased oxygen extraction by the tissues (wide arteriovenous difference in oxygen content). With exercise this compensatory mechanism becomes insufficient, and peripheral cyanosis may result. The cyanosis is usually due to a right to left shunt through the foramen ovale or through an ASD. The right to left atrial shunt depends upon the presence of greater diastolic pressure in the right ventricle caused by the marked muscular hypertrophy (decreased compliance). Diminution of the right ventricular cavity and decreased compliance also explain the central cyanosis usually seen in the syndrome of pulmonary stenosis and hypoplastic right ventricle.[203] In rare cases of severe PS, the presence of right ventricular endocardial fibrosis (most likely the result of chronic subendocardial ischemia) is the basis of low compliance and increase in end-diastolic pressure. The right atrial pressure may be modified in severe PS with a high peaked "a" wave, produced by the forceful atrial systole in response to the increased filling resistance of the ventricle.

MANIFESTATIONS

Clinical Features

In general, the clinical manifestations are quite distinctive, so a diagnosis can be made without special laboratory procedures. The majority of patients are asymptomatic, and they are discovered during routine examination. When symptoms are present, they may vary, depending upon the degree of obstruction and the level of myocardial compensation, from mild exertional dyspnea and mild cyanosis to signs and symptoms of heart failure.

Patients with mild PS are asymptomatic. Those with

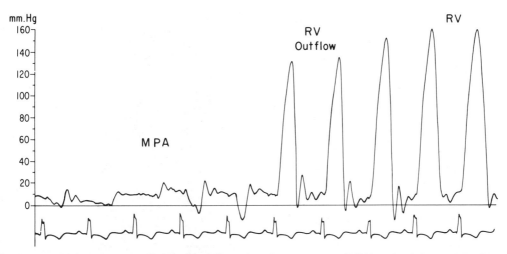

Fig. 17.2 Continuous withdrawal pressure tracing from the main pulmonary artery (*MPA*) to the right ventricle (*RV*). As the catheter approaches the pulmonary valve, the amplitude of the pressure wave during systole decreases and becomes negative, owing to a Venturi effect. The sudden increase in systolic gradient as the catheter passes the valve confirms the presence of severe valvular stenosis. Note the difference between the pressure pulse waves recorded in the right ventricular outflow area and main right ventricular cavity, shown in Figure 17.9.

moderate PS are usually asymptomatic during the first 2 to 3 years of life but later may develop *dyspnea* and *fatigability* with exertion. Children with severe PS may have dyspnea and fatigability even with moderate exercise. Occasionally, in some of the latter patients, strenuous exercise may provoke syncope and even sudden death. Precordial pain is common in such patients, and even epigastric pain on effort has been described. Episodes of fainting and chest pain are related to inability to increase the critically low cardiac output with exercise with a concomitant decrease in myocardial perfusion and the development of dysrhythmias. These are signs of poor prognosis and an indication for immediate surgical relief of the stenosis. Patients with severe PS may develop signs and symptoms of right ventricular failure in infancy or early childhood. Some of these infants may rapidly develop cardiomegaly with signs of tricuspid insufficiency and in order to survive require emergency surgical treatment.[112] It appears that the hypertrophied right ventricle is unable to maintain the necessary cardiac output for survival and growth of these infants because of the very narrow and fixed pulmonary valve orifice.

Growth and development in children with PS are usually normal. Even those infants with severe PS who develop heart failure early in life are remarkably well developed and nourished. The presumably characteristic moon face is a common finding in chubby-looking, healthy children, and it is not as helpful a diagnostic feature.[4, 204]

Cyanosis, a relatively common finding in severe PS, is absent with mild PS and infrequently seen with moderate PS. It is usually due to a venoarterial shunt at the atrial level. However, mild peripheral cyanosis may be present in patients with severe PS and intact atrial septum. In the majority of cases, cyanosis, when present, is minimal because of the small size of the interatrial communication allowing a small venoarterial shunt. However, in the presence of a large ASD, due to a larger venoarterial shunt, the cyanosis may be more pronounced, and polycythemia and clubbing may also be present.

Mixing of the right and left atrial blood takes place when a large ASD is present, even in the absence of very high right ventricular pressures. This is particularly true in infants with PS and hypoplastic right ventricle, or in cases of hypoplasia of the right ventricle without apparent PS.[61, 82, 100, 183, 203] Here the venous inflow, because of the high filling resistance of the right ventricle, is forced to enter the left side of the heart, causing marked cyanosis. Thus, cyanosis as an isolated criterion of severity of stenosis is not always reliable, i.e., patients with severe obstruction and intact atrial septum or a very small communication between the atria may have no or minimal cyanosis, whereas patients with more cyanosis may have less severe degrees of obstruction.

Squatting is extremely rare in isolated PS. If there is history of squatting in a moderately cyanotic child, the diagnosis of PS with intact ventricular septum should be accepted with caution.

Prominent venous pulsations ("a" waves) in the neck usually indicate the presence of severe stenosis. These presystolic pulsations may be felt on palpation of the liver without evidence of cardiac failure. However, in the presence of heart failure, previously noted prominent "a" waves may be overshadowed by prominent systolic "v" waves. In many instances, despite large "a" waves recorded during cardiac catheterization, venous pulsations in the neck are not detectable.[99] This is particularly true in infants and young children.[65]

Cardiomegaly may be detected only in severe PS, particularly when cardiac decompensation is present. Right ventricular overactivity, manifest as a mild lower left parasternal lift or marked heave, is invariably present with moderate or severe PS. With right ventricular dilatation and failure, a diffuse apical impulse may be palpated at the fifth or sixth left intercostal space near the anterior axillary line.

A *systolic thrill* is almost invariably felt at the second and third intercostal space along the left sternal border. It may also be felt at the suprasternal notch and the lower left sternal border if the corresponding murmur is very loud. Occasionally it may be absent in very young infants with mild PS, and especially in those with severe PS and heart failure.

The striking feature of valvular PS on auscultation is *a loud, ejection type systolic murmur* with maximum intensity at the upper left sternal border. This murmur is well conducted to the rest of the precordium, the neck, and the back. Phonocardiographically, the murmur has a crescendo-decrescendo configuration with its peak in mid or late systole, and it is usually of medium or high frequency.[17, 189] In mild stenosis, the murmur is much shorter, and its peak never passes midsystole. In severe PS, the crescendo part of the murmur is more prolonged, and the aortic component of the second sound is usually obscured by the murmur (Fig. 17.3). This is in contrast to the systolic murmur of tetralogy of Fallot, where the more severe the stenosis, the shorter the murmur becomes, and its peak appears earlier. The mechanism responsible for this behavior of the murmur in these two conditions is the prolongation of mechanical systole of the right ventricle, which is proportional to the degree of obstruction in PS with intact ventricular septum, as long as there is good myocardial compensation. In newborn or young infants with critical PS and heart failure, the systolic murmur in the upper left sternal border may be faint and unimpressive and is not accompanied with a thrill. The absent pulmonary closure sound, the associated cardiomegaly, and the presence of a louder tricuspid regurgitation holosystolic murmur in the lower left sternal border are highly suggestive signs for the diagnosis of severe PS in these infants.[112, 163, 177]

The *first heart sound* is not remarkable. An early *ejection sound* ("click") is heard in the upper sternal border and may be transmitted down to the lower sternal border.[89] This sound may be mistaken for the second component of a split first heart sound (Fig. 17.4). It can be easily distinguished, though, by its sharp high-pitched quality, the location, and the fact that it usually becomes louder during expiration. Its mechanism of production is most likely related to the sudden opening of the thickened but relatively flexible stenotic valve rather than the sudden expansion of the aterial wall as previously has been postulated.[57, 89] The presence of a "click" usually denotes mild or moderate valvular stenosis, although exceptions to this rule occur. This sound typically occurs 0.08 second after the Q wave in the electrocardiogram. When

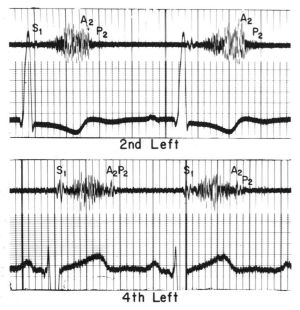

Fig. 17.3 Phonocardiograms of an 8 year old with severe pulmonary valvular stenosis and marked infundibular hypertrophy. (*Upper*) Before operation (right ventricle (RV) pressure, 170/0-10). Note the prolonged crescendo part of the murmur and the delay in its peak. The second sound is widely split with the aortic component (*A₂*) completely masked by the murmur and the pulmonary component (*P₂*) barely demonstrable. (*Lower*) One year after operation (RV pressure, 70/0-5). Moderate degree of obstruction was still present due to residual infundibular hypertrophy. Note the earlier appearance of the peak of the murmur and the aortic component of the second sound clearly identifiable.

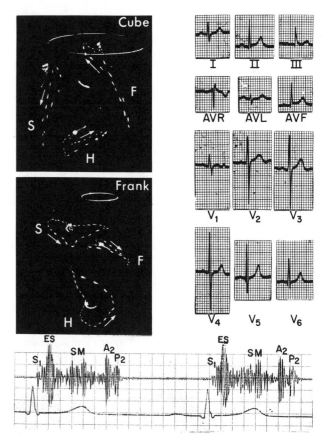

Fig. 17.4 Electrocardiogram, vectorcardiogram, and phonocardiogram of 6 year old with mild pulmonary valvular stenosis (right ventricle pressure, 44/0-2). Note the difference between the two vectorcardiographic systems. The inscription of the QRS loop in the horizontal plane is clockwise with the cube system but counterclockwise with the corrected system of Frank. The electrocardiogram suggests mild right ventricular hypertrophy. The phonocardiogram demonstrates the systolic ejection sound (click) (*ES*), the crescendo decrescendo systolic murmur (*SM*), and the variable splitting of the second sound with the pulmonary component (*P₂*) of less intensity than the aortic component (*A₂*).

the "click" occurs earlier, it signifies more severe stenosis and may become indistinguishable from the first heart sound. The second sound is usually split, and the degree of splitting is proportional to the degree of obstruction. The pulmonary component of the second sound may be normal or decreased in intensity or may be inaudible.[189]

Occasionally, in mild stenosis with marked dilatation of the pulmonary trunk, the pulmonary closure sound may be louder than normal. There appears to be a correlation between the severity of the stenosis and the intensity of the pulmonary component of the second sound, the intensity being inversely proportional to the severity of obstruction. These subtle changes in the intensity of the pulmonary closure sound can be readily detected by phonocardiography. The width of the splitting of the second sound varies from 0.04 to 0.10 second or more. In mild to moderate PS, the second sound shows normal variation of splitting with respiration, i.e., widening with inspiration and narrowing of the splitting with expiration. In severe PS it is difficult to assess the respiratory variation of the splitting, and when the obstruction is extremely severe, the second sound is not audible at the upper left sternal border because the aortic component is completely masked by the murmur. In such patients the aortic closure sound is heard as a single second heart sound of normal intensity in the lower precordium and apex. A fourth heart sound is heard quite often at the lower precordium in patients with severe PS. It is associated with large "a" waves in the right atrium and has the same significance as the "giant" presystolic venous "a" waves in the neck. A presystolic murmur occasionally may be heard as an extension of the fourth heart sound, owing probably to some degree of tricuspid stenosis.[139] When a third heart sound is heard, the presence of an associated ASD or an anomalous pulmonary vein emptying into the right atrium should be suspected. Early diastolic regurgitant murmurs are rare and occur after distortion of the pulmonary valvular ring or cusps by secondary complications such as progressive poststenotic dilatation of the pulmonary trunk, endocarditis, or surgical valvulotomy.

Electrovectorcardiographic Features

The electrocardiogram and vectorcardiogram are probably the most useful of all laboratory diagnostic aids in assessing severity of obstruction to right ventricular output, irrespective of the location of the obstruction. With very few exceptions, a reasonable estimate of the severity of the obstruction can be made by a properly obtained electro- or vectorcardiogram.[9, 48, 59, 63, 122]

In *mild PS*, the electrocardiogram may be normal in 30 to 40% of the cases. The only abnormality may be a slight rightward QRS mean frontal axis. The amplitude of the R wave, with the exception of the newborn period, never exceeds 15 mm and is usually less than 10 mm. Frequently, an abnormality of the intraventricular conduction is seen manifested as rsR' or rR' in the right precordial leads. The R/S ratio in the same leads is greater than 1.0, and the T waves are normal. These abnormalities are reflected in the vectorcardiogram, which may show a figure-of-eight QRS loop in the horizontal plane. The loop maintains its normal counterclockwise direction with the initial forces directed briefly to the right and anteriorly and then to the left and slightly posteriorly, passing anteriorly to the E point and forming a figure-of-eight pattern. The frontal loop is not unusual while the sagittal QRS loop is directed inferiorly and slightly anteriorly. The T loop has normal orientation (Fig. 17.4).

In *moderate PS* a normal electrocardiogram may be seen in approximately 10% of the cases. The mean frontal QRS axis is usually right (90 to 130°), and the anterior forces in the horizontal plane are more prominent. An rR' or RS complex with a ratio of more than 4:1 in the right precordial leads with a magnitude of the R wave less than 20 mm is usually recorded. The T waves may be upright or negative. The vectorcardiogram shows anterior and rightward orientation of the QRS loop, more than in mild stenosis. With the cube system a clockwise rotation in the horizontal plane is usually present, even in patients in whom left ventricular pressure still exceeds that of the right ventricle. The Frank system may show a counterclockwise directed loop suggestive of relative left ventricular dominance.[63]

In *severe PS*, the electrocardiogram is usually abnormal, although occasionally cases with normal tracings have been observed. The mean frontal QRS axis may range from 110 to 150° or more. A dominant R wave may be seen in AVR. In the right precordial leads a qR, Rs, or a pure R is usually present. The magnitude of the R waves is usually more than 20 mm, and the T waves may be negative or upright. The R/S ratio in the left precordial leads is equal to or less than 1.0. With extremely severe obstruction, a qR pattern with a tall R wave is present in V1, but there is no abrupt transition in the pattern of the QRS complex in the midprecordium (Fig. 17.5). Instead there is gradual decline of the R/S ratio

such that in V6 or V7, small R and deep S waves are present. Sometimes the very tall R waves may extend up to V6, and only in V7 or V8 may equiphasic QRS complexes be encountered. The T waves may remain discordant from V4R to V4 or V5. The P waves are abnormally tall and peaked in lead II and in the right precordial leads, indicating right atrial hypertrophy.

The vectorcardiogram shows a clockwise rotation of the QRS loop in the horizontal plane with the initial forces directed to the left and anteriorly, followed by a broad limb that is directed to the right and anteriorly.[63] The direction of the initial vector to the left and anteriorly is an indication of severe right ventricular hypertrophy and accounts for the abscence of Q waves in the left precordial leads. In very severe cases of PS the T loops are discordant, i.e., the mean T vector in every plane is exactly opposite the mean QRS vector of the same plane (Fig. 17.5).

In patients between 2 and 20 years old with severe PS, there is a good correlation between the height of the R wave in lead V4R or V1 (when there is a pure R) and the right ventricular systolic pressure at rest. The height of the R wave in millimeters multiplied by a factor 5 gives a number which approximates the right ventricular pressure in mm Hg.[166]

In infants and some older children with severe PS with hypoplastic right ventricle, the mean QRS frontal axis may be more leftward than expected (30 to 70°) with clear evidence of left ventricular hypertrophy associated with right atrial dilatation.[99] Moreover, in spite of the presence of right ventricular hypertension, the anterior forces are not as prominent.[203] Rarely, left axis deviation or superiorly oriented frontal vector loop may be present with PS.[48] In these cases, a conduction abnormality of the left bundle may be present, isolated, or in association with endocardial cushion defect or Noonan's syndrome with cardiomyopathy. In these instances, despite the superior counterclockwise orientation of the frontal vector loop, the relationship between the maximum rightward spatial vector in the vectorcardiogram and the right ventricular pressure was found to be practically the same as that observed in patients with inferiorly oriented clockwise frontal vector loop.[48]

Radiologic Features

In the majority of cases of PS with intact ventricular septum, a characteristic cardiac contour is present.[24, 99, 177] The most striking feature is a prominent main pulmonary artery segment caused by poststenotic dilatation of the pulmonary trunk and sometimes the left pulmonary artery as well (Fig. 17.6). This finding is present in 80 to 90% of the cases but may be absent in infants and small children.[65] In cases of pulmonary valve dysplasia or rubella syndrome with valvular or supravalvular stenosis, the pulmonary artery segment in the roentgenogram may not be prominent.[50] In certain instances, in spite of angiocardiographic evidence of a dilated main pulmonary trunk, the dilatation is not seen in the posteroanterior roentgenogram. A right anterior oblique view of the heart in these cases may demonstrate the pulmonary arterial bulge.

In approximately 50% of the cases, some prominence of the right atrial segment of the cardiac contour may be seen. The apex of the heart is usually rounded and is pointed downward. In the lateral view, right ventricular hypertrophy is identified by an increased contiguity of the anterior border of the heart to the thoracic wall. However, in many instances, because of an enlarged right atrial appendage, identification of the anterior border of the ventricle is difficult. Right ventricular enlargement may be suspected in the left anterior oblique position by a marked anterior bulge of the cardiac

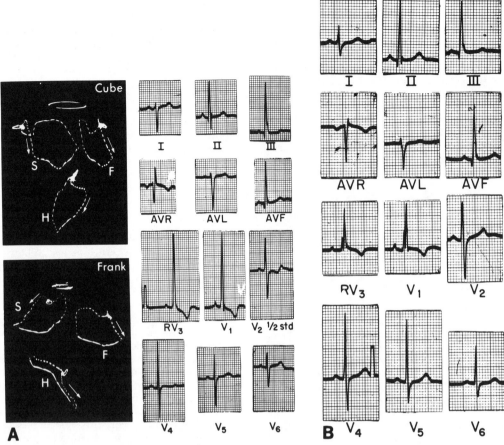

Fig. 17.5 Electrocardiogram and vectorcardiogram of a 12 year old with severe pulmonary valvular stenosis (right ventricle pressure, 170/5-15). (*A*) Before operation. Note tall qR complexes in *III* and *AVF*, tall R and inverted T in right pecordial leads, and deep S in V_5 and V_6. The vectorcardiogram in both recording systems (cube and Frank) shows large voltage with abnormal inscription and orientation of the QRS loops anteriorly and to the right. The T loops are discordant (have opposite direction) to the QRS loops in the horizontal plane in both recording systems. (*B*) Postoperative electrocardiogram 1 year later. Note the change in QRS frontal axis and the R in right precordial lead (rR′). The RS ratio in V_5 and V_6 is inverted now.

shadow. When marked right ventricular enlargement is present, this may be reflected in the spinal overlapping of the left ventricle, which is merely displaced posteriorly by the large right ventricle. The left atrium, left ventricle, and aorta are of normal size. With rare exceptions, a left aortic arch is present. The *pulmonary vascularity* is usually normal, except in patients with right ventricular failure or venoarterial shunt at the atrial level in whom a reduction of pulmonary vascular markings is seen due to reduction of pulmonary flow. The lack of objective criteria in evaluating vascular markings led to the erroneous impression that PS is associated with reduction in pulmonary vascular markings. In some severe cases without signs of heart failure, slender right hilar vessels and diminished vascular markings in the mid- and outer lung fields may be seen. However, if cardiomegaly is present, these findings may be explained on the basis of low normal pulmonary flow.

In cases of mild and moderate PS, the heart size is usually normal. In severe PS, the cardiac size may be only slightly enlarged as long as right ventricular compensation exists. When cardiac failure develops, moderate or marked cardiomegaly may be seen. This increase in cardiac size is due mainly to right ventricular and right atrial dilatation. The chamber dilatation may obscure a previously bulging main

pulmonary artery and thus change the typical contour of PS described earlier.

Echocardiographic Features

Evaluation of the anatomy and function of the pulmonary valve has been less satisfactory than that of the other cardiac valves. This limitation is partially due to its anterior (near field) location.[71, 198]

M-Mode. The most commonly observed abnormality is the abnormal presystolic cusp motion, the "A" dip, in addition to reduced valve opening[198] (Fig. 17.7). However, these findings are highly variable and may be seen with other conditions associated with right ventricular dysfunction such as Uhl's anomaly. Fluttering and preclosure of the pulmonary valve may be observed in the presence of infundibular PS but also with VSD and PDA. In patients with major PS, septal and right ventricular wall hypertrophy is seen. Moreover, serial assessment of right ventricular cavity dimensions can be easily made. The right ventricular cavity is usually normal.

2-D. The 2-D echo may show an unusually prominent pulmonary valve with restricted systolic motion. The latter finding has been likened to the angiographic finding of "doming" of the valve (Fig. 17.8). Poststenotic dilatation of

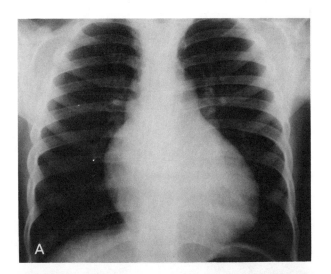

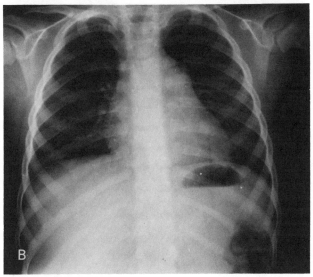

Fig. 17.6 Roentgenograms of two children with pulmonary valvular stenosis and intact ventricular septum. (*A*) Eight year old with severe stenosis (RV pressure, 170/0-10) with prominent right cardiac border and rounded apex pointing downward. Pulmonary vascularity is normal. The main pulmonary artery segment is not particularly prominent. (*B*) One year old with moderate degree of stenosis (RV pressure, 80/0-6). Note prominent main pulmonary artery segment and borderline cardiomegaly with slightly prominent right cardiac border and apex.

the pulmonary trunk and its main branches may be visualized.[200] The ventricular cavity and tricuspid valve also can be easily assessed. Contrast echocardiography may detect the presence of right to left intraatrial shunt by injecting in a peripheral vein.

CARDIAC CATHETERIZATION

Although the diagnosis of PS can be easily made without cardiac catheterization, and even its severity can be estimated from the physical signs, chest roentgenogram, electrocardiogram, and vectorcardiogram, physiologic studies, and angiocardiography are indicated in cases which require surgical treatment. It is not only of interest to know the level of right ventricular pressure proximal to the obstruction, but information about the location of the obstruction and pres-

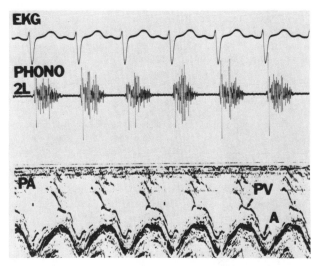

Fig. 17.7 M-mode echocardiogram and phonocardiogram recorded from a child with moderate valvular pulmonic stenosis (gradient 50 mm Hg). Note the early ejection click, which varies in intensity with respiration, followed by a high frequency ejection murmur peaking in midsystole. The echocardiogram shows "thickening" of the pulmonic valve cusps and a prominent presystolic A-dip. *PV* pulmonary valve; *PA*, pulmonary artery.

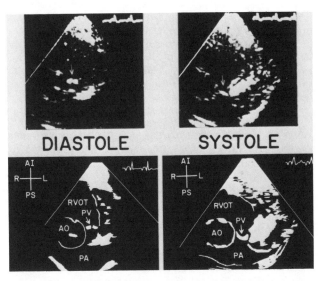

Fig. 17.8 Single frame 2-D echocardiograms (*above*) and corresponding diagrams (*below*) from a 1-month-old infant with severe valvular pulmonic stenosis. Short axis orientation through a plane of the aortic root (*AO*) and right ventricular outflow tract (*RVOT*). Thickened pulmonary valve (*PV*) leaflets (*arrow*) seen in diastole persist within the small pulmonary annulus in systole. Poststenotic dilatation of the pulmonary artery (*PA*) is present. *R*, right; *L*, left; *AI*, anteroinferior; *PS*, posterosuperior.

ence or absence of other cardiac defects is of help to the surgeon.[2, 21, 99]

In the usual case of PS with intact ventricular septum, blood oxygen data do not show a left to right shunt. In cases with severe obstruction and an associated interatrial communication, a right to left shunt can be detected by comparing the oxygen saturation of samples obtained from a pulmonary vein and left atrium. The systemic arterial saturation should be equal to or slightly higher than that of the left atrium.

The most important information obtained by cardiac catheterization is the demonstration of the stenosis and evaluation of its severity, as manifest by elevation of right ventricular pressure and a major pressure gradient across the site of obstruction. Carefully obtained withdrawal pressure tracings from the pulmonary artery to the right ventricle provide useful information concerning the site of stenosis and its severity.

Resting peak systolic pressures in the right ventricle over 30 to 35 mm Hg as well as pressure gradients across the stenotic area of more than 10 to 15 mm Hg are considered abnormal. In mild degrees of PS the pulmonary arterial pressures are normal. In severe forms of PS, there is a marked reduction of mean pulmonary arterial pressure and obliteration of the usual pulsatile configuration of the pressure tracing. A negative systolic pressure, owing to a Venturi effect, is frequently recorded in the most severe cases immediately distal to the site of obstruction (Fig. 17.2). As the catheter passes the stenotic valve, a sudden change in the pressure tracing from low pressure pulmonary arterial to high pressure right ventricular pressure curve is seen. In cases of obstruction distal to the valve, this abrupt change of pressure may occur more peripherally at the origin of the main pulmonary branches or at the pulmonary trunk.

Associated infundibular stenosis may sometimes be suspected from the withdrawal pressure tracing. The typical pressure tracing of isolated primary infundibular stenosis consists of a low pressure pulmonary arterial curve followed by a ventricular curve of low systolic pressure (equal to the peak pulmonary arterial pressure) and finally a right ventricular tracing of considerably higher peak systolic pressure. In some cases of combined valvular and discrete infundibular stenosis, two pressure gradients may be encountered, one at the valvular and one at the infundibular level. In severe valvular stenosis with a diffuse infundibular narrowing, a characteristic infundibular pressure pulse pattern is seen.[194]

Because of the high velocity of the blood ejected through the narrowed lumen of the infundibulum, the pressure in the area of the infundibulum is decreased (Venturi effect). During early systole both main ventricular and infundibular pressure tracings show the same initial rise, but as the blood begins to flow at high velocity through the outflow tract, the pressure there begins to fall, whereas in the body of the right ventricle the pressure remains high throughout systole. During the remaining portion of systole, the contraction of the hypertrophied infundibular muscle causes further reduction in the lumen of the outflow tract, thereby increasing the velocity of the blood flowing through it and consequently decreasing the pressure which falls away rapidly toward zero (Fig. 17.9).

The end-diastolic pressure in the right ventricle may be normal or elevated with severe obstruction or right ventricular failure. Tall right atrial "a" waves are usually present in severe PS, particularly when the atrial septum is intact or only a small foramen ovale is present. These atrial contraction waves result in partial doming reflected well in the echocardiogram of the pulmonary valve (Fig. 17.7).[198]

The pulmonary valve area can be calculated using Gorlin's[70] formula and normally is about 2.0 cm^2/m^2 of body surface area. In mild to moderate PS, the valve area may range from 1.0 to 2.0 cm^2/m^2 whereas in severe stenosis the pulmonary valve area may be as small as 0.25 cm^2/m^2. However, in the presence of an associated infundibular narrowing, the calculation of valve area using this formula is not valid.[166] The formula measures flow across an orifice rather than across an elongated tube or more than one site of obstruction.

The resting cardiac output is usually normal, even in cases

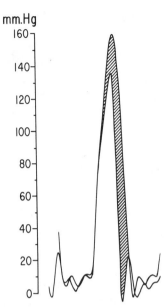

Fig. 17.9 Illustration of the difference between the systolic pressure tracings recorded in the outflow tract and main right ventricular cavity. The tracings of Figure 17.2 have been superimposed using the scalar electrocardiogram to ensure correct timing. Note the difference in peak systolic pressure and the descending portions of the two curves. These differences are due to viscous resistance to flow through the narrow contracting infundibulum and suggest the presence of secondary hypertrophic infundibular stenosis.

of severe PS, but with exercise or infusion of isoproterenol, an increase in systolic gradient across the obstruction is usually observed.[134, 141, 181] This increase in pressure gradient is due primarily to an increase in the rate of contraction of the right ventricle and consequently the increase in velocity of the blood ejected across the obstruction.[151] The stroke volume does not increase and in patients with severe obstruction remains normal or decreases slightly.[88, 91, 95, 106, 174] The increase in cardiac output with exercise is accomplished by an increase in heart rate. In extreme obstruction, a marked increase in heart rate may be detrimental, leading to a reduction of cardiac output by shortening the diastolic filling time. In these patients, the expected rise in right ventricular systolic pressure with exercise is not seen and, instead, a drop in pressure may be noted. Occasionally, in young infants with critical obstruction, during cardiac catheterization if marked tachycardia develops, a relatively low right ventricular systolic pressure may be recorded. The latter may be mistaken as evidence of less severe stenosis. In severe PS both the shortening of the diastolic filling time by the prolongation of systole and the increase in diastolic filling resistance by the hypertrophied muscle limit considerably the diastolic reserve capacity of the right ventricle. The greater or the stiffer the hypertrophied muscle mass, the greater the impedance to filling and the greater the handicap during tachycardia. The markedly hypertrophic right ventricle is capable of generating a great ejective force but, being bulky, stiff, and slow to dilate, has a markedly increased diastolic filling resistance. It apparently functions well when adequate diastolic filling is ensured by slow heart rate, but its performance is diminished during tachycardia.

Although cardiac output determination during cardiac catheterization is essential in evaluating the severity of PS as reflected in the pressure gradient across the pulmonary valve, the data collected and analyzed by the Joint Study of the Natural History of Congenital Heart Disease suggests that the most important correlation between peak systolic pressure difference across the pulmonary valve and possible hemodynamic factors influencing the pressure gradient is the heart rate.[49, 145] When the pressure gradient is adjusted for heart rate, the inclusion of the cardiac output in the calculations does not improve the correlation. However, it has been demonstrated that acute increase of the right ventricular output induced by closure of the patent foramen ovale or ASD using a balloon catheter during cardiac catheterization in cases of pulmonary stenosis with moderate venoarterial shunt accentuates the pressure gradient across the pulmonary valve.[28]

The classification of mild, moderate, and severe pulmonary stenosis is based upon correlations made between clinical and hemodynamic observations. When the resting right ventricular systolic pressure is less than 50 mm Hg, the stenosis is characterized as mild. In moderate PS, the pressure in the right ventricle approaches or equals that of the left ventricle. A right ventricular pressure higher than the systemic pressure is usually evidence of severe PS. Resting right ventricular pressures as high as 250 to 300 mm Hg have been recorded in some instances of extreme obstruction. One precaution must be considered during catheterization in cases of severe stenosis, especially in young cyanotic infants: the danger of critically obstructing the markedly stenotic valve opening by the catheter.

Indicator dilution curves may be helpful in detecting left to right shunts at the atrial or ventricular level. When the indicator is injected into the right chamber of the heart a venoarterial shunt can be easily detected by the early appearance time.

ANGIOCARDIOGRAPHY

Angiocardiography is very useful in the diagnosis of PS by providing information about the location and severity of the stenosis. The use of biplane cineangiocardiographic equipment with image intensification has improved considerably the yield of information usually obtained by simple or roll film biplane angiocardiography. It offers a more dynamic view of ventricular performance simultaneously in both anteroposterior and lateral views. A selective injection of contrast medium into the right ventricle provides the most useful information.

The right ventricular cavity is usually normal in size and has prominent trabeculations. The ventricular wall in severe stenosis is thickened. The size and configuration of the infundibulum during systole and diastole are well outlined. The thickness and the size of the orifice of the pulmonary valve are seen fairly well as the jet of the ejected "opacified" blood enters the dilated main pulmonary artery (Fig. 17.10).

The typical stenotic valve is slightly thickened, domes during systole, and returns to a normal configuration during diastole. The annulus is usually normal but may be moderately hypoplastic in young children with severe PS. Poststenotic dilatation of the main pulmonary trunk and sometimes of the left pulmonary artery is usually seen. However, there is no correlation between the degree of dilatation and severity of stenosis. In rare instances of PS due to a *dysplastic valve*, the leaflets are not anatomically fused but because of their thickness are relatively immobile.[92] The main pulmonary trunk is moderately hypoplastic in these cases, and it further limits the mobility of the valve. Thus, the angiographic picture of the thickened valve changes very little during the cardiac cycle. The sinuses of Valsalva are very narrow and remain so during diastole. The thickened valve edges when seen in profile appear like vertically oriented filling defects. The annulus is always small.[92] Varying degrees

of diffuse narrowing of the outflow tract of the right ventricle, due to muscular hypertrophy, may be seen in patients with severe PS. A further narrowing, usually involving the mid-portion of the infundibulum, can be seen during mid- to late systole, but it disappears during diastole. In some instances of extremely severe PS, the systolic narrowing of the infundibulum appears to produce almost complete obliteration of the lumen. In the frontal projection, the boundaries of the narrowing consist of the parietal band of the crista supraventricularis on the right and the septal band of the crista on the left. In the lateral view, the markedly hypertrophied crista bulges anteriorly, and the anterior bulge is made by the parietal band.

In mild cases of PS, there is no infundibular abnormality. The valve leaflets may be thickened and, depending on the degree of stenosis, their range of motion during the cardiac cycle may be somewhat limited. Selective left ventricular angiocardiograms show a normal size left ventricle and aorta. In certain cases of severe PS, the hypertrophied ventricular septum may bulge into the left ventricular cavity.

Ventricular volume studies in patients with PS and intact ventricular septum have shown that right and left ventricular function is usually normal.[140] However, in those cases associated with a major venoarterial intraatrial shunt, varying degrees of depressed ventricular function have been observed.[140] Thus, ventricular volume studies may be useful in assessing myocardial function in the latter group of patients.

DIFFERENTIAL DIAGNOSIS

The diagnosis of PS with intact ventricular septum usually is not difficult because of its relatively distinct features. Mild PS should be differentiated from conditions such as idiopathic dilatation of the pulmonary arterial trunk, ASD, pulmonary artery stenosis, straight back syndrome, mitral valve prolapse, aortic stenosis, and innocent murmurs. Moderate or severe PS without cyanosis must be differentiated from VSD with PS and left to right shunt. When cyanosis is present, tetralogy of Fallot should be excluded. In addition, during the neonatal period, other lesions such as transposition of the great arteries or pulmonary atresia with intact ventricular septum have to be differentiated. Complicated lesions, with the main defect being pulmonary stenosis, must also be differentiated from cases of pure stenosis.

Idiopathic dilatation of the main pulmonary arterial trunk is sometimes very difficult to distinguish from mild PS, although such differentiation is rather academic since both conditions have a benign prognosis and require no treatment. An early systolic ejection click at the upper left sternal border, split second sound, and dilatation of the pulmonary artery segment with normal heart size and normal pulmonary vascularity in the chest roentgenogram, all features of idiopathic dilatation of the pulmonary artery, may be easily confused with signs of mild PS. An early ejection systolic murmur, usually not as harsh as in PS and unaccompanied by a thrill, may also be present. The electrocardiogram and vectorcardiogram are always normal. Evidence of right ventricular hypertrophy in the electrocardiogram suggests the diagnosis of PS.

Atrial septal defect with left to right shunt should be differentiated from mild PS. The murmur in ASD, although heard best at the left base, is not as loud and harsh as the one of PS and usually is not accompanied with a thrill. The splitting of the second sound is usually fixed and not as wide as in PS. There is usually a mid-diastolic murmur at the lower left sternal border in ASD with large left to right shunt. The precordium is more active in ASD, and there is

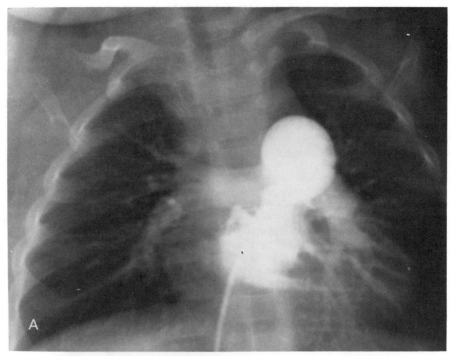

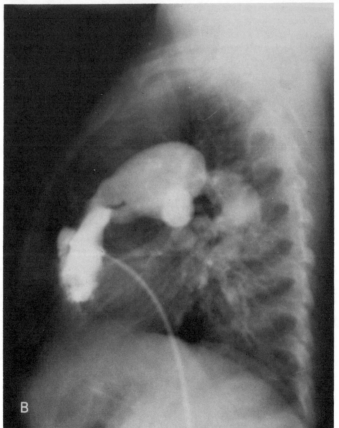

Fig. 17.10 Selective right ventricular angiocardiogram of 1 year old with pulmonary valvular stenosis (right ventricle pressure, 80/0-8). (A) Anteroposterior view showing marked dilatation of the pulmonary trunk. (B) Lateral view showing thickened pulmonary valve, marked poststenotic dilatation of the pulmonary trunk, and mild encroachment of the crista supraventricularis in the right ventricular outflow tract. The origin of the left pulmonary artery appears to be somewhat narrowed.

always right ventricular overactivity. In ASD there is always an increase in pulmonary vascular markings in the chest roentgenogram, whereas right atrial and right ventricular enlargement may be present in both conditions. The electro-

cardiogram and vectorcardiogram may not be as helpful, but echocardiography is useful in differentiating the two conditions.

Pulmonary arterial stenosis is commonly associated with

varying degrees of valvular stenosis; thus, the physical signs may be similar to those of "pure" valvular stenosis. However, bilateral pulmonary artery stenosis can be easily suspected by the wide transmission of the systolic murmur to the axillae and back. Family history of siblings with pulmonary stenosis, history of maternal rubella, or the presence of intrahepatic cholestasis may all be helpful in suspecting the diagnosis of pulmonary arterial stenosis.[14, 40, 116, 155, 157]

Straight back syndrome, associated with varying degrees of pectus excavatum deformity, should be differentiated from mild pulmonary stenosis because frequently it manifests with a short ejection systolic murmur in the pulmonary area and a split second sound of normal intensity.[40, 153] It is usually not associated with an ejection click. In some instances the electrocardiogram may show a rSR′ pattern in the right precordial leads, suggesting right ventricular hypertrophy. The pathogenesis of the murmur and the ECG conduction abnormality may be related to pectus deformity, compressing the right ventricle against the spine. The pectus excavatum deformity and the narrow chest seen and confirmed by a lateral roentgenogram should be helpful in the differentiation from mild to moderate PS.

Mitral valve prolapse occasionally may manifest with a click and systolic murmur heard best at the mid and upper left sternal border and should be differentiated from mild PS. This unusual transmission of the click and the murmur has been attributed either to the prolapse of the more medial portion of the valve or to the direction of the regurgitant flow towards the left atrial appendage. The typical changes in auscultatory findings with various positions and the echocardiogram are most helpful in differentiating this condition from pulmonary valvular stenosis (see Chapter 32).

Aortic valvular stenosis, especially in young infants, may be difficult to distinguish from PS. This is because the location of the murmur is frequently at the left sternal border, and the electrocardiogram may show signs of right ventricular hypertrophy rather than left ventricular overloading. In addition, the ejection sound (click) when present may be widely transmitted, and its changes with respiration may not be as pronounced as they are in older children and adults because of the frequent and shallow breathing of the young infants. Echocardiography is quite useful in the differentiation of these two conditions.

Innocent murmurs can be easily differentiated from murmurs due to PS. Although their location may be similar, innocent murmurs are shorter in duration and are not accompanied by a thrill. The quality of the murmurs is different also, the innocent murmur being more vibratory or musical. The second sound is normally split, and there is no ejection sound present with innocent murmurs.

Ventricular septal defect associated with PS and left to right shunt is usually characterized by a very loud holosystolic murmur with midsystolic accentuation heard best at the left sternal border, high or low. There is usually a palpable thrill and biventricular or right ventricular heave with mild to moderate cardiomegaly. There is no ejection click, and the second sound is split with the pulmonary component diminished or sometimes inaudible. The chest roentgenogram may be diagnostic if left atrial or left ventricular dilatation are present together with increase in pulmonary vascular markings. The electrocardiogram and vectorcardiogram show evidence of combined ventricular hypertrophy or only right ventricular hypertrophy in cases where more severe obstruction to right ventricular output is present. Echocardiography may be very useful in the diagnosis by demonstrating the relative size of the cardiac chambers, the presence of a VSD, the size of the infundibulum, and the status of the pulmonary valve.

Severe pulmonary valvular stenosis with intact ventricular septum and cyanosis due to venoarterial shunt at the atrial level frequently resembles *tetralogy of Fallot*, and differentiation may be at times difficult. In both conditions, besides the cyanosis, a loud, ejection type systolic murmur and right ventricular hypertrophy are present. Cyanosis is usually more prominent in tetralogy of Fallot and correlates well with symptoms whereas this is not true with isolated PS. The murmur in PS is usually long and obliterates the aortic component of the second sound, in contrast to the murmur in tetralogy of Fallot, which ends before the single second sound. The chest roentgenogram shows a decrease in pulmonary vascularity but normal heart size in tetralogy of Fallot, in contrast to isolated PS, in which normal vascularity and mild to moderate cardiomegaly may be present. A right aortic arch, seen in approximately 25 to 30% of cases of tetralogy of Fallot, very seldom occurs in cases of isolated PS. In addition, poststenotic dilatation of the pulmonary arterial trunk, a very common finding in pulmonary valvular stenosis, is not seen in tetralogy of Fallot. The electrocardiogram and vectorcardiograms are similar in both conditions. However, in cases of severe PS, more pronounced degrees of right ventricular hypertrophy with discordant T waves in the right precordial leads are seen. Although echocardiography is extremely valuable in differentiating noninvasively these two conditions, selective angiocardiography is the procedure of choice for final confirmation of the diagnosis.

Pulmonary valvular stenosis can be easily differentiated from *primary* or *secondary pulmonary hypertension* due to peripheral pulmonary vascular obstruction. The absence of the typical stenosis murmur and the loudness of the pulmonary closure sound suggest pulmonary hypertension. Not infrequently, a murmur of pulmonary valvular insufficiency may be heard at the left sternal border in patients with pulmonary hypertension.

Pulmonary atresia with intact ventricular septum in newborn and very young infants must be differentiated from severe pulmonary valvular stenosis. Both conditions may manifest with signs of right ventricular failure, cyanosis, and decreased pulmonary vascular markings. In the commonest type of pulmonary atresia, the right ventricle is usually hypoplastic, and there is no significant cardiomegaly. The electrocardiogram shows left ventricular dominance with normal or right QRS frontal axis. In the less common type, in which the right ventricle is dilated and there is tricuspid regurgitation, the clinical findings may be very similar to those of severe PS. Only selective angiocardiography will differentiate the two lesions by demonstrating either atresia or extreme narrowing of the pulmonary valve. In both conditions, emergency surgery is mandatory for survival.

Ebstein's anomaly of the tricuspid valve may sometimes simulate very severe PS with cardiomegaly and heart failure. Cyanosis and decreased pulmonary vascularity may also be present. The typical physical and electrocardiographic findings, however, in the two conditions make their differential diagnosis not difficult.

Corrected transposition of the great arteries, where the aorta forms the left upper portion of the cardiac border and simulates a pulmonary arterial bulge, sometimes may create a problem in differential diagnosis. Echocardiography is extremely useful in suspecting the diagnosis, but cardiac catheterization and angiocardiography are usually needed for final confirmation.

Pulmonary valvular stenosis and endocardial fibrosis of the right ventricle have been described in association with *malignant carcinoid disease* of the bowel with liver metastases. It has been suggested that the cardiac findings are sequelae of the hemodynamic effects of increased secretion of serotonin. This rare disease is more commonly seen in adults and older children, and it is associated with abdominal pain, diarrhea, flushing, and facial telangiectases.

PULMONARY STENOSIS WITH SMALL VENTRICULAR SEPTAL DEFECT

Clinically these patients are indistinguishable from those with isolated PS. It appears that infundibular stenosis is seen relatively more frequently than valvular stenosis, and in these cases, the embryologic basis for the development of the lesions may be similar to that of tetralogy of Fallot. However, hemodynamically this combination of lesions does not behave like tetralogy of Fallot. The right ventricular pressure may exceed considerably that of the left ventricle when stenosis is severe, because the VSD is very small (restrictive).[86, 195] The typical triangular right ventricular pressure contour seen in isolated PS is retained in these cases. In addition, the increase in systolic pressure of the postextrasystolic beat in these patients differentiates them from patients with tetralogy of Fallot. In order to demonstrate the small VSD, selective angiocardiography from the right ventricle is necessary.

PULMONARY STENOSIS WITH INTERATRIAL LEFT TO RIGHT SHUNT

Mild PS may sometimes be associated with an ASD and a left to right shunt.[6, 158] In such instances, the amount of blood shunted is inversely proportional to the degree of obstruction. The cardiac findings cannot be distinguished from those of PS without left to right shunt. The presence of an inflow mid-diastolic murmur over the lower left sternal border may suggest associated ASD with left to right shunt. The roentgenologic examination is quite helpful in these cases, demonstrating mild to moderate cardiomegaly, increased pulmonary vascularity, and a prominent pulmonary artery segment. The simple or contrast 2-D echocardiogram may visualize the ASD.

PULMONARY STENOSIS WITH PATENT DUCTUS ARTERIOSUS

This combination is relatively rare, in contrast to supravalvular pulmonary artery stenosis, which is frequently associated with PDA in patients with rubella syndrome.[50] The clinical and roentgenographic features of PDA may dominate the picture, and only the additional presence of a loud, ejection systolic murmur with a thrill in the upper left sternal border and an ejection click with a prominent right ventricular heave may suggest the presence of an associated pulmonary valvular stenosis. The electrocardiogram may show biventricular hypertrophy. Echocardiography may be useful in demonstrating the associated PS.

ENDOCARDIAL CUSHION DEFECTS WITH PULMONARY STENOSIS

Clinically, this combination of lesions behaves like tetralogy of Fallot, but it can be distinguished by the electrocardiographic and vectorcardiographic findings of superiorly oriented mean QRS frontal axis with counterclockwise inscription of the QRS loop.[168] A prominent right border of the heart, suggesting right atrial enlargement and moderate to marked cardiomegaly, may be seen more frequently in this lesion than in isolated PS. The echocardiogram could easily detect the abnormalities of the atrioventricular valves and the septal defects.

PULMONARY VALVULAR OR SUBVALVULAR STENOSIS WITH AORTIC STENOSIS

This combination of lesions is relatively rare.[133, 139, 171] The clinical findings are those of aortic and pulmonary stenosis combined with decreased or absent second sound, moderate cardiomegaly, and normal pulmonary vascularity. Echocardiography may be helpful in the diagnosis of the associated aortic valvular stenosis. The electrocardiogram and vectorcardiogram may show evidence of biventricular hypertrophy with right or left predominance, depending upon the dominant lesion. Definite diagnosis, however, is established only by right and left heart catheterization and angiocardiography.

NOONAN'S SYNDROME

In this syndrome, approximately 50% of affected individuals have congenital malformations of the heart.[142, 143, 184] Pulmonary stenosis is the commonest lesion and is usually due to dysplasia of the pulmonary valve. Hypertrophic cardiomyopathy affecting the left ventricle associated with or without PS has been described in up to 25% of the cases.[144] The signs and severity of PS may not be as typical as those with pure PS. The ejection click is frequently absent, and the electrocardiogram may show left axis deviation. The duration and loudness of the cardiac murmur may not always be indicative of severity of the stenosis, i.e., a short and relatively soft murmur may be associated with severe PS proven at cardiac catheterization. The characteristic facial appearance and the phenotypic stigmata of the syndrome should alert the examiner to the possible association with these cardiac abnormalities.[142] Echocardiography will easily detect the thickened pulmonary valve and the associated cardiomyopathy.[144] These patients require thorough investigation by cardiac catheterization and angiocardiography. The syndrome is apparently transmitted as a dominant trait.[143]

PULMONARY STENOSIS OR OBSTRUCTION DUE TO ACQUIRED CAUSES

Intracardiac neoplasms or extrinsic lesions compressing the cardiac structures, although rare, have been described.[170] These lesions may involve the right ventricular wall, the pulmonary valve, pericardium, or mediastinum and may be malignant or benign. The obstruction may be progressive or stationary and occurs in all age groups. It may be associated with symptoms and is suggested by a loud, ejection systolic murmur at the upper left sternal border without severe right ventricular hypertrophy in the electrocardiogram. Echocardiography may prove to be most helpful in the diagnosis of these acquired right ventricular obstructions. Angiocardiography usually establishes the diagnosis, although the exact nature of the lesion cannot be suspected before surgery and histologic examination.

TREATMENT

The treatment of pulmonary valvular stenosis with intact ventricular septum is primarily surgical. Medical treatment is necessary in cases with heart failure before surgical intervention. Prophylaxis against endocarditis is also indicated in all cases of PS.

Direct relief of the PS is usually accomplished surgically, employing closed or open techniques.[20, 30, 43, 137, 146] Transventricular closed valvulotomy, employing expendable valvulotomes, was used extensively in the early stages of cardiac surgery with relatively good results. Subsequently, the open transarterial technique with or without hypothermia and inflow occlusion was introduced with excellent results. With the introduction of cardiopulmonary bypass, almost all pulmonary valvulotomies are performed now under direct vision. The valve is usually approached from an incision in the pulmonary arterial trunk. In rare instances with significant infundibular obstruction, resection of infundibular muscle can be also accomplished through the pulmonary valve. Right ventriculotomy is used only when the infundibular obstruction cannot be relieved transarterially or when a VSD is present. Exploration of the right atrium and repair of an ASD or a patent foramen ovale is also performed at the same time.

However, in extremely ill infants, the closed or open valvulotomy, using inflow occlusion, is used as an emergency procedure. As techniques of bypass surgery have improved, very young infants can be safely operated now with very low mortality. The results of surgery are generally excellent.[30, 51, 154, 175] Occasionally, in cases of severe stenosis, a persistent systolic gradient between the right ventricle and the pulmonary artery equal to or greater than that observed preoperatively is measured immediately postoperatively. This may be an indication for reestablishing the cardiopulmonary bypass and proceeding with further infundibular resection. In rare instances, fatal right ventricular failure ensues (suicidal right ventricle) after an apparently successful valvotomy, because of postoperative clampdown of the infundibular area.[20] Recently, it has been suggested that after adequate surgical relief of the pulmonary valve stenosis, there is no need to explore and proceed with infundibular resection in cases where immediately postoperatively the right ventricular pressure was found to be at systemic levels.[129] Continuous postoperative right ventricular pressure monitoring invariably demonstrated a reduction of right ventricular pressure up to 50% within the first 24 hours.[129] Propanolol given immediately after valvotomy has been recommended in order to distinguish postoperative right ventricular hypertension due to hypertrophy from that caused by residual fixed infundibular or pulmonary annulus obstruction.[135] A fall in right ventricular pressure denotes dynamic rather than discrete obstruction. The functional infundibular stenosis present in most cases of severe PS resolves itself with time, a fact that has been well documented.[151, 94]

Only 10 of 294 patients operated on for pulmonary valvular stenosis had pressure gradients more than 50 mm Hg at cardiac catheterization 4 to 8 years after surgery, and only one of these had an open transarterial valvotomy using cardiopulmonary bypass (U.S. Joint Study of Congenital Heart Defects).[145] These observations support the recommendation for surgical intervention in children with resting gradients in excess of 50 mm Hg.

When pulmonary stenosis is due to a *dysplastic valve*, narrowing of the valve annulus is also present.[92, 101] In these cases, simple valvulotomy does not relieve the pressure gradient. Removal of the thickened valve tissue plus a widening of the annulus and proximal main pulmonary artery by insertion of a patch are needed in order to relieve the obstruction.[182, 192] This procedure invariably results in pulmonary valvular insufficiency, which is better tolerated than persistent obstruction. The late effects of pulmonary valvular insufficiency created at surgery by removal of the cusps and/or placement of an outflow patch are not known. Diastolic overloading of the right ventricle may appear late in life, especially following chronic vascular obstructive or emphysematous lung disease.

Successful pulmonary valvuloplasty results in abolition of the pressure gradient across the pulmonary valve. However, small pressure gradients may persist for longer periods.[51, 56, 174] In general, there is prompt symptomatic improvement. The systolic murmur becomes shorter in duration, and there is regression of the widely split second sound with the pulmonary component becoming more audible. A gradual improvement in the electrocardiogram and vectorcardiogram is observed. These changes usually appear later than the clinical improvement and apparently reflect the slow involution of the ventricular hypertrophy following reduction in the right ventricular work.

The indications for pulmonary valvotomy may be summarized as follows.

Symptomatic infants or older children should be operated as soon as possible. Medical management, digitalization, and other anticongestive measures may be helpful in the older child but usually are not successful in young infants with signs of heart failure and may waste invaluable time. Diagnostic studies such as cardiac catheterization in these infants should be performed only if the cardiologist feels that the baby can tolerate the procedure or the delay of the operation. One of the few emergencies in pediatric cardiology where substantial help can be offered is the infant with severe PS in failure. Closed or open valvotomy with or without the use of cardiopulmonary bypass is the procedure of choice.[125, 126]

The older symptomatic child with classical signs of PS should be operated upon. With few exceptions, cardiac catheterization and angiocardiography should be performed prior to surgery, in order to determine the severity and location of the obstruction.

Asymptomatic patients with severe pulmonary stenosis and intact ventricular septum should be operated upon on an elective basis, usually before school age. Surgical relief of the stenosis may be carried out even earlier if the stenosis is extremely severe by physiologic criteria. Such patients have right ventricular systolic pressures at rest well above systemic levels (greater than 130 mm Hg) as well as elevated diastolic pressures. Patients with resting right ventricular systolic pressure equal to or near systemic values should be operated on an elective basis. To some pediatric cardiologists, a right ventricular pressure of 70 mm Hg constitutes an indication for pulmonary valvotomy, but it is obvious that this arbitrary figure may be misleading, if one does not take into consideration cardiac output, age, symptoms, and other variables.

Asymptomatic patients with moderate pulmonary stenosis should be followed at regular intervals (once or twice a year) to evaluate the progression of the lesion. Some of these patients may never need surgical correction. Cardiac catheterization is indicated to evaluate the degree of obstruction and the response to exercise if progressive right ventricular hypertrophy is seen in the electrocardiogram. Some patients may need repeat cardiac catheterization studies, especially if symptoms appear which cannot be explained on the basis of clinical evaluation.[130]

Patients with mild pulmonary valvular stenosis do not need operation or evaluation by cardiac catheterization or angiocardiography. However, prophylaxis against endocarditis is recommended in these individuals, despite their hemodynamically insignificant lesion. They should not be restricted in their physical activities and should be treated like normal children.

ASSESSMENT OF SEVERITY, COURSE, AND PROGNOSIS

The course and prognosis of patients with PS and intact ventricular septum is determined primarily by the severity of obstruction. Symptoms are notoriously unreliable in reflecting hemodynamic severity. Chest roentgenograms may not be as informative until cardiac dilatation occurs, and even the electrocardiogram may prove to be insensitive, particularly in adults.[52, 138]

The most reliable assessment of severity of pulmonary stenosis is usually made by pressure measurements obtained during cardiac catheterization. The diagnosis of mild PS is made when right ventricular pressure at rest does not exceed 60 mm Hg or the pressure gradient across the pulmonary valve is less than 40 mm Hg. Severe PS is present when right ventricular pressure at rest is higher than 100 mm Hg or the pressure gradient across the valve is more than 80 mm Hg. Moderate PS is considered when right ventricular pressure or pressure gradients fall between the above mentioned values.[49, 145]

Whereas the physical signs and electrocardiographic findings in general may differentiate those patients with mild or severe stenosis, accurate clinical assessment of those with moderate stenosis cannot always be certain. Attempts have been made to correlate hemodynamic measurements with clinical, phonocardiographic, and electrovectocardiographic variables in order to predict the degree of valvular obstruction. Unfortunately, no one variable alone can reliably predict the severity of stenosis. Therefore, multivariate analysis has been employed recently for this purpose[49]

Prediction equations have been developed using universally available data obtained during the U.S. Joint Study of Congenital Heart Defects. The most important variables were found to be the auscultatory findings and the electrocardiogram.[49, 145]

An estimate of the pressure gradient across the pulmonary valve can be given by the following equation:

Pressure gradient RV − PA mm Hg
$$= 10.5 \text{ (ISM)} + 2.6 \text{ } (S_1) + S_2 \text{ Score} + \text{T score}$$

where the following data show that: ISM = intensity of systolic murmur graded 1–6; S_1 = S wave in lead I in mm where 1 mm = 0.1 mv; S_2 score = −10 if P_2 is normal, +2 if P_2 is audible but diminished, and +15 if P_2 is inaudible; T score: T score = +15 if T wave in V1 = diphasic when R wave in V1 is greater than 10 mm; otherwise the T score is 0. Using this equation, if the estimated gradient is under 35 mm Hg, cardiac catheterization shows a gradient no more than 65 mm Hg. If the estimated gradient is between 35 and 50 mm Hg, a small number of cases show a higher actual gradient. However, if the estimation is greater than 50 mm Hg, cardiac catheterization should probably be performed.

Most cardiologists agree that mild pulmonary valvular stenosis has a benign course and does not require treatment. There was not a single death among 214 patients with mild pulmonary stenosis during a follow-up of 4 to 8 years.[105] However, there is still controversy regarding the course and prognosis of asymptomatic patients with moderate PS.[138, 201] In a group of 21 adult asymptomatic patients with PS, with an average follow-up period of 15 years, no cardiac symptoms or other complications have developed.[94] Based upon these observations, recommendations have been made that, at least in older children and adult asymptomatic patients, surgery is not indicated even when the PS is severe (i.e., right ventricular pressure more than 100 mm Hg).[94] However, only two patients, ages 35 and 42, in these series had severe PS, and no repeat evaluation by cardiac catheterization was made 12 and 18 years later.[138]

Experience from most centers as well as data from the Natural History Study suggest that infants and children with moderate and severe valvular stenosis may develop progressively increasing degrees of outflow obstruction.[105, 145] This is particularly true during the periods of rapid growth, i.e., infancy and adolescence. Approximately 50% of patients with moderate or severe PS (right ventricular pressures between 90 and 120 mm Hg) are asymptomatic, whereas one-third of those with the most severe stenosis (right ventricular pressure greater than 120 mm Hg) were symptomatic. It appears that the development of symptoms during the first 2 years of life is always associated with severe obstruction.[197]

Progressive changes in the electrocardiogram suggestive of increasing stenosis are noted frequently at all ages and with all degrees of severity. This is more striking in young infants in whom the electrocardiogram may be normal or show borderline right ventricular hypertrophy during the first year of life but progresses to definite hypertrophy or to a strain pattern in later childhood. Hypertrophy of the right ventricular outflow tract is a major factor in the development of this progression.

Serial catheterization data in children with PS, especially in the absence of cardiac output measurements, are difficult to evaluate.[105, 130, 179] However, the data indicate that only a few patients with mild or moderate PS show progressive increase or obstruction as indicated by an increase in right ventricular pressure. In the majority of patients there is no change in right ventricular pressure, and in some instances there is a reduction in the pressure gradient across the pulmonary valve.[51, 111] The latter suggests that as the child grows, the stenotic pulmonary orifice increases in size. Serial catheterization data in cases of severe PS are also lacking, since the majority of these patients undergo surgical correction. However, clinical and electrocardiographic data suggest that a progression in the severity of obstruction is more commonly seen in this group of patients. Increasing severity of obstruction may be relative and can be explained by the disproportionate physical growth of the child.[32, 128, 145] This is particularly true in fast-growing premature infants with moderate to severe PS.

After growth has ceased, the only likely cause of further narrowing of the valve would be fibrosis or bland vegetations on the cusps. Progressive infundibular narrowing due to myocardial hypertrophy is another factor in the natural course of severe pulmonary valvular stenosis and may explain the rapid deterioration of some of these patients.[93] Development of myocardial fibrosis, especially in the older individual, has been described as another factor responsible for the deteriorating course in such patients.[119] Regardless of the magnitude of right ventricular pressure, a history of heart failure was associated with a relatively poor surgical prognosis.

Studies also indicate that most patients with moderate or severe PS may have a normal or low normal cardiac output at rest but a subnormal response to exercise.[89, 91, 95, 106, 174] A similar response to exercise was also observed in some patients postoperatively. The importance of the myocardial factor in response to exercise and the similarities of the response of these patients to that of patients with myocardial fibrosis has been emphasized by several authors.[119, 174] In contrast, studies on the cardiac performance of patients with mild PS indicate that they have normal cardiac output and normal response to exercise[91, 106, 174] From available data, prediction of the course of moderate stenosis cannot be made.

Endocarditis should be listed among the complications of pulmonary valvular stenosis. Surgical correction of the lesion does not prevent the development of this complication, and these patients should receive the recommended prophylaxis against endocarditis. Sudden death at any age and anoxic spells in very sick cyanotic infants have also been observed.[61]

PRIMARY INFUNDIBULAR STENOSIS

Primary infundibular stenosis with intact ventricular septum is a relatively rare malformation. It was first described by Elliotson.[47] The prevalence of this entity varies from 2 to 10% of all cases of obstructive lesions to the right ventricular outflow. However, infundibular stenosis associated with ventricular septal defect (tetralogy of Fallot) or secondary to pulmonary valvular or supravalvular stenosis is more commonly seen.[15] Combined subvalvular aortic and pulmonic stenosis due to muscular hypertrophy of the ventricular septum have also been reported.

PATHOLOGY

There are two types of primary infundibular stenosis: the more common type in which a fibrous band, at the junction of the main cavity of the right ventricle and the infundibulum, produces a stenosis of the proximal portion of the infundibulum and divides the cavity into two chambers; and the type in which the infundibulum appears shrunken with a thick muscular wall forming a narrowed outlet to the right ventricle. In the second type the narrowed area may be short or long, immediately below the pulmonary valve or lower in the outflow tract (Fig. 17.1).

The right ventricular outflow tract, developmentally, is derived from the bulbus cordis. Infundibular stenosis is probably caused by an arrest of involution of the bulbus cordis, which normally is incorporated by the end of the second month of intrauterine life with the ventricular sinus and forms the infundibulum or outflow tract.[98]

PHYSIOLOGY

The main physiologic derangement of primary infundibular stenosis is the same as that of pulmonary valvular stenosis with intact ventricular septum, i.e., obstruction of ejection of blood from the right ventricle. The principal difference between the two lesions is the location of obstruction. If the obstruction is discrete immediately below the pulmonary valve, the hemodynamic consequences are practically identical to those of valvular stenosis and depend mainly upon the degree of obstruction. Diffuse muscular obstruction, however, primary or secondary to severe valvular stenosis, is usually dynamic in nature and may vary in severity.[94] Such obstruction invariably becomes more severe during isoproterenol infusion or exercise by further constriction of the hypertrophied infundibulum. Patients with discrete infundibular stenosis do not show a change in the calculated stenotic area during isoproterenol infusion.[70] The increase in pressure gradient across the stenotic area during isoproterenol infusion in the latter patients is proportional to the flow across the obstruction.

MANIFESTATIONS

Clinical Features

The manifestations of primary infundibular stenosis are indistinguishable from those of pulmonary valve stenosis with intact ventricular septum. The symptoms and signs depend primarily upon the degree of obstruction. Cyanosis of moderate degree may be present when severe infundibular stenosis is associated with a patent foramen ovale which allows a right to left shunt. Dyspnea on exertion, fatigue, and signs of right ventricular failure may be seen with severe degrees of obstruction. Patients with mild or moderate stenosis are usually asymptomatic. The physical findings are dominated by a loud, harsh, ejection type systolic murmur associated with a thrill, which is heard best at the third and second left intercostal space at the sternal border. The murmur is widely transmitted over the precordium and back, and is usually heard better at the fourth than at the first intercostal space. The first sound is usually normal, and the second sound is widely split with the pulmonary component markedly diminished. The location of maximum intensity of the murmur depends upon the site of obstruction. When the obstruction is immediately below the valve, the site of maximum intensity of the murmur is identical to that of valvular stenosis. If the obstruction is located low in the outflow tract, the murmur may be louder at the lower left sternal border. Usually, there is no ejection click.

The duration of the murmur depends upon the severity of the obstruction. The aortic closure sound may be obscured by the murmur in cases of severe obstruction, as it is with severe valvular stenosis.[34, 189, 202] It is very difficult clinically to distinguish primary infundibular from valvular PS.

Electrovectorcardiographic Features

The electrocardiogram and vectorcardiogram are indistinguishable from those of valvular stenosis with the same degree of obstruction (Fig. 17.11). Since the musculature of the infundibular chamber is not as hypertrophied in this type of stenosis, large forces may not be seen in the electrocardiogram and vectorcardiogram. It appears that progressive electrocardiographic changes indicating increasing severity of right ventricular hypertrophy are more frequently seen in cases of primary infundibular stenosis than valvular stenosis.[105]

Radiologic Features

The roentgenographic features of infundibular stenosis are similar to those of valvular stenosis, with the exception of the absence of poststenotic dilation of the pulmonary trunk. Occasionally, if a large infundibular chamber is present, a bulge in the area of the main pulmonary artery segment may be attributed erroneously to pulmonary arterial dilatation. Cardiomegaly, decreased pulmonary vascularity, and specific chamber enlargement may be seen, depending upon the severity of the lesion.

Echocardiographic Features

Echocardiography appears to be useful in the noninvasive differentiation between valvular and infundibular stenosis.[199] The M-mode echo may show a fluttering of the pulmonary valve, which lies within the turbulent stream of blood distal to the obstruction. In severe infundibular stenosis, no presystolic opening of the pulmonary valve ("A" wave) is recorded, suggesting that the small pressure changes produced by atrial systole fail to reach the valve leaflets.

2-D echocardiography is also very helpful in the diagnosis. The size of the right ventricular outflow tract, the ventricular septum, the pulmonary valve, and the site of obstruction can be delineated. In addition, the fluttering of the pulmonary valve can be well visualized.

CARDIAC CATHETERIZATION

Cardiac catheterization, in most instances, may establish the diagnosis of infundibular stenosis by demonstrating the typical withdrawal pressure gradient described earlier. This

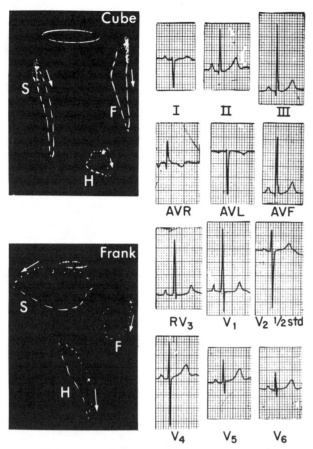

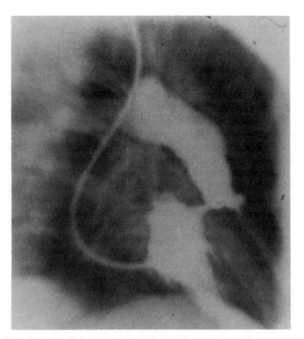

Fig. 17.12   Selective cineangiocardiogram from the right ventricle in the same 9 year old as in Figure 17.11 with primary discrete infundibular stenosis (right anterior oblique view). Note the markedly narrowed proximal end of the infundibulum. The encroachment of the septal and parietal bands of the crista supraventricularis at the side of the constriction is evident. The narrowed lumen of the ostium infundibuli did not change in caliber during systole and diastole. The right ventricle is divided into an inflow and outflow chamber. The pulmonary valve and trunk are normal.

Fig. 17.11   Electrocardiogram and vectorcardiogram of 9 year old with severe primary infundibular stenosis of the proximal discrete type (right ventricle pressure, 146/0-6; infundibular chamber, 20/0-3; main pulmonary artery, 20/6). Note tall qR complexes in III and AVF, and tall R and upright T waves in right precordial leads. The vectorcardiogram shows abnormal inscription and orientation of the QRS loops anteriorly and to the right.

tracing is usually obtained in cases with a relatively large infundibular chamber and is characterized by absence of a systolic gradient across the pulmonary valve and the presence of pressure gradient between the outflow area and the main right ventricular cavity. When the stenosis is immediately below the pulmonary valve, the pressure tracing obtained is indistinguishable from that seen in pulmonary valvular stenosis. Simultaneous recording of the intracardiac electrocardiogram may be helpful in localizing the site of obstruction. Without angiocardiography, on the basis of intraventricular pressure gradient alone, it is difficult to make the diagnosis of primary infundibular stenosis, since obstruction due to an anomalous muscle bundle gives similar intraventricular pressure gradients.

ANGIOCARDIOGRAPHY

Selective angiocardiography from the right ventricle is the best procedure for demonstration of primary infundibular stenosis. The location, the extent, and the severity of the stenosis are well visualized in either the biplane angiocardiogram or the lateral or oblique cineangiocardiogram (Fig. 17.12). In the usual type of stenosis with an infundibular chamber, the constricted area is further narrowed down during systole and becomes less narrow during diastole. The distal chamber appears to be normal in size or somewhat dilated during the cardiac cycle. When the narrowing in-

volves a major portion of the outflow tract, no definite infundibular chamber is seen and no great changes in size of this chamber during systole and diastole are noted. In all types of primary infundibular stenosis, there is always narrowing but it is more pronounced during systole. The pulmonary valve is usually normal, and there is no poststenotic dilatation of the main pulmonary trunk.

DIFFERENTIAL DIAGNOSIS

The lesions from which primary infundibular stenosis must be differentiated are the same as described in the section on pulmonary valvular stenosis. However, isolated infundibular stenosis must be differentiated from an isolated VSD, especially when the murmur of stenosis is maximally heard at the lower left sternal border. The murmur of the VSD is usually holosystolic and well localized, except in cases of supracristal VSD where the murmur is conducted towards the upper left sternal border. A middiastolic rumble at the apex, with a left ventricular heave, is commonly found when a large left to right shunt is present. In these cases, the electrocardiogram and vectorcardiogram, together with the chest roentgenogram, are most helpful in the differential diagnosis. Less combined ventricular hypertrophy with evidence of left atrial hypertrophy and increased pulmonary vascularity are usually present with VSD. A small VSD with a small shunt is usually characterized by a normal electrocardiogram in contrast to the infundibular stenosis, in which right ventricular hypertrophy is present. A widely split second sound with a pulmonary component decreased in intensity may differentiate the infundibular stenosis from a VSD. Echocardiography may be useful in suspecting the diagnosis, but cardiac catherization and angiocardiography are necessary for differentiation between valvular discrete infundibular stenosis and right ventricular obstruction due to anomalous muscle bundles (two-chamber right ventricle).

TREATMENT

The treatment of primary infundibular stenosis is surgical. The principles described for the treatment of valvular PS can be applied here as well. Surgical resection of the fibrotic narrowed area, with resection of the hypertrophied muscle if necessary, can be easily accomplished using cardiopulmonary bypass. In rare instances, if the infundibulum is hypoplastic and there is narrowing of the valvular ring, widening of the outflow tract using a pericardial or suitable plastic patch may be necessary.[173, 175, 202] The course of patients with primary infundibular stenosis is usually similar to that of valvular stenosis. No actual distinction has been made between the two lesions regarding their natural history. However, there is some indication that primary infundibular stenosis may progress in severity relatively faster than valvular PS.[105] Antibiotic prophylaxis against endocarditis is recommended.

RIGHT VENTRICULAR OBSTRUCTION DUE TO ANOMALOUS MUSCLE BUNDLES

This congenital cardiac malformation, also known as "double chamber right ventricle," is characterized by aberrant hypertrophied muscular bands that divide the right ventricular cavity into a proximal high pressure chamber and a low pressure chamber located distal to the hypertrophied muscle bands.[26, 62, 79, 84, 107, 110, 115, 164, 190]

PATHOLOGY

Anatomically, the aberrant hypertrophied muscle bundles constitute a muscle mass, pyramidal in shape, which runs between the ventricular septum from an area immediately inferior to the septal leaflet of the tricuspid valve to the anterior wall of the right ventricle. Usually, there are two bundles: the ventral bundle (superficial when viewed through a ventriculotomy) which attaches to the wall of the right ventricle adjacent to the septum, and the dorsal bundle, which is larger and has its attachment at the base of the anterior papillary muscle. The right ventricular cavity is divided into a proximal chamber, which consists of the proximal portion of the sinus of the right ventricle, and the infundibulum. In tetralogy of Fallot and isolated infundibular stenosis, the obstruction involves the infundibular area, so there is a clear anatomic distinction between these entities and obstruction caused by anomalous muscle bundles. The hypertrophied muscle bundles in the infundibulum, in the case of tetralogy, protrude from the walls into the cavity of the infundibulum but do not cross the cavity from one wall to another. In contrast, the anomalous muscle bundles cross the cavity of the right ventricle and lie proximal to the infundibular area. Their usual site of occurrence is the distal or apical part of the inflow or sinus portion of the right ventricle. The orientation of these muscle bundles is different from that of the moderator band. The septal attachment of the moderator band is usually at the apical third of the ventricular septum, in contrast to the anomalous muscle bundles which have their septal attachments basally, near the tricuspid ring. Although both types of muscle bundles, moderator and aberrant, attach to the anterior wall of the right ventricle, the moderator band lies toward the septal side of the cavity and does not ordinarily obstruct the cavity. In contrast, the anomalous muscle bundles cross the main channel of the right ventricle and, being placed in the main

stream of blood from tricuspid to pulmonary valve, may cause obstruction.

The origin of these muscle bundles is unknown. They may be due to a localized aberrant overgrowth of the trabeculated myocardium very early in the development of the embryonic heart. The bundles themselves might be pathogenetic in the formation of the VSD and pulmonic stenosis.

It has been suggested that the right ventricular subdivision and obstruction in this malformation represent an arrested incorporation of the primitive bulbus cordis into the right ventricular body.[98] An improper expansion of the bulboventricular junction may result in incomplete fusion of the bulbar and endocardial cushion elements that normally close the superior portion of the ventricular septum, which may explain the frequent association of a VSD with this malformation. It has also been postulated that the obstruction in the "double chamber right ventricle" is due to an elevated origin of an hypertrophied moderator band from the septal band.[164] In the most severe form, this band originates near the crista supraventricularis, resulting in an orientation quite unlike that of normal moderator band and producing a major intrachamber pressure gradient. According to this view, this muscular tissue appears to be "anomalous" only in representing developmental retardation of a normal right ventricular structure.[164] An associated discrete subaortic stenosis is also reported in some instances, supporting the concept of inadequate bulbar incorporation as an etiologic mechanism.[11]

PHYSIOLOGY

The aberrant muscle bundles may not be obstructive at all, especially early in infancy, or they may cause varying degrees of obstruction within the ventricular cavity. For blood to pass from the right ventricular inflow to the outflow area, it must course either above the muscle bundles, between the latter and the tricuspid valve, or it must pass through the narrow channel between the bundles and the septal wall (Fig. 17.13). During ventricular contraction, the diameter of these channels is markedly reduced, and sometimes the lumen of the one adjacent to the septum may be completely obliterated. The main *hemodynamic* consequence to the obstruction is an elevation of pressure within the proximal inflow portion of the right ventricle. Exercise or isoproterenol infusion usually results in a marked increase of systolic pressure in the proximal chamber.

MANIFESTATIONS

Clinically, patients with obstruction due to hypertrophic aberrant muscle bundles and intact ventricular septum closely resemble those with isolated pulmonary valvular or infundibular stenosis. When a VSD is present, the features may be dominated by those of VSD. Since some of these patients may have associated pulmonary vascular stenosis, their clinical differentiation becomes very difficult.

A loud, crescendo-decrescendo, long systolic murmur, indistinguishable from that of isolated valvular or infundibular stenosis, is heard at the left sternal border. This murmur, although louder at the second and third left intercostal spaces, can also be heard well at the lower left sternal border and is usually associated with a thrill. The pulmonary valve closure sound may not be as delayed or as soft as would be expected from the length of the murmur if the obstruction were at infundibular or valvular level.

In general, the *electrocardiogram, vectorcardiogram,* and *chest roentgenogram* fail to differentiate this type from other types of obstruction to right ventricular outflow. How-

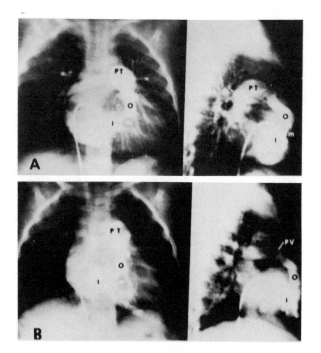

Fig. 17.13 Right ventriculograms of a 3½ year old with pulmonary valvular stenosis, intact ventricular septum, and anomalous muscle bundle in the right ventricle causing obstruction to pulmonary outflow. (*A, left*) Anteroposterior view during diastole. A filling defect is seen in the midportion of the right ventricle (*m*). The routes of flow of opaque material are seen to be between the crista supraventricularis (*c*) and the muscle mass, and also between the mass and the apex of the right ventricle. (*A, right*) Lateral view at the same time as *A, left*. Stenotic pulmonary valve (*PV*) is illustrated. (*B, left*) Anteroposterior view during systole. The filling defect has remained unchanged. The channel between the mass and the crista supraventricularis is the only evident communication between inflow and outflow portions of the right ventricle. (*B, right*) Lateral view during systole. The small diameter of the communication between inflow and outflow portions of the right ventricle is apparent. (Reproduced with permission from R. V. Lucas, Jr., *et al.*[110] and the American Heart Association.)

ever, it has been suggested that the electrocardiogram and vectorcardiogram in some instances may show evidence of diminished terminal right ventricular forces similar to those seen in isolated infundibular stenosis.

In a recent report involving 30 patients with "double chamber right ventricle," an upright T-wave in lead V3R was the only finding suggestive of right ventricular hypertrophy in 40% of the cases.[107] This finding should alert the cardiologist to the possibility of the presence of anomalous muscle bundles prior to cardiac catheterization in cases of isolated VSD.[107]

Echocardiography may be very useful in suspecting the diagnosis of anomalous right ventricular muscle bundles.[33] Abnormal tissue densities in the right ventricle and pulmonary valve flutter may be detected. In addition, the 2-D echo may visualize intraventricular tissue "masses." Similar tissue densities also may be seen in infundibular stenosis or right ventricular tumors, but when such echo findings are seen in patients with an apparently small VSD, they should lead to suspicion that the VSD is complicated.[33] In one patient followed for 19 years with the clinical diagnosis of a small VSD, the echocardiogram was responsible for a change in diagnosis and referral for cardiac catheterization, which demonstrated severe intraventricular obstruction. Thus, it has been recommended that echocardiography should be

done in children and adults who have been followed for many years with the clinical diagnosis of a small VSD.[33]

CARDIAC CATHETERIZATION

Cardiac catheterization may suggest the presence of an obstruction within the ventricular cavity by the demonstration of a pressure gradient between the distal and proximal portion of the body of the right ventricle. When associated pulmonary valvular stenosis is present, an additional pressure gradient may be detected between the infundibulum and the pulmonary artery. In cases of isolated anomalous muscle bundle obstruction, the systolic pressure in the ventricular cavity beyond the obstruction is equal to that in the pulmonary artery.

ANGIOCARDIOGRAPHY

Angiocardiography is the best tool for accurate diagnosis of this lesion. Biplane selective angiocardiography should always be performed when evidence of an intraventricular pressure gradient is found during cardiac catheterization. In the anterior view, filling defects within the right ventricle between the outflow and inflow areas are usually seen (Fig. 17.13). These filling defects are seen well below the crista supraventricularis. In the lateral view, the right ventricular filling defects may extend from just below the crista to the anterior wall near the apex. Usually, the filling defects are constant and do not change with systole and diastole. However, they may be seen best only during systole. In addition, one or several channels or routes of blood flow may traverse the obstruction. Marked changes in the configuration of the right ventricular cavity during systole and diastole are seen.

TREATMENT

The *treatment* of this type of obstruction is surgical. Advance knowledge of the presence of anomalous muscle bundles causing obstruction to the right ventricular outflow is most helpful to the surgeon. In the past, there have been several instances in which an associated VSD or pulmonary valvular stenosis have been corrected but, because of inability to recognize the obstructing abnormal muscular bands, the patients did not survive. Certain features of this condition seen at surgery should alert the surgeon to suspect the existence of obstructing anomalous muscle bundles within the body of the right ventricle.[190] Thus, during ventricular contraction, the presence of a "dimple" in the ordinarily smooth, ballooned right ventricular surface strongly suggests the presence of a muscular band. The dimpling is more prominent when associated pulmonary valvular stenosis is present. This deformity is usually found near the anterior interventricular groove about midway between the base and the apex of the heart and corresponds to the parietal attachment of the ventral limb of the anomalous bundle.[190] On opening the right ventricle through a transverse or longitudinal cardiotomy, the obstructing muscle masses become immediately apparent and may completely or partially obscure the view of the tricuspid valve. Transection of the origin of the bundles from the septum and parietal attachment of the superficial bundle is performed first. This permits reflection of the muscle mass so that the relationship of the insertion of the larger of the bundles at the base of the anterior papillary muscle can be visualized and injury to the latter structure and the tricuspid valve is avoided[190] A search for a small, closing VSD should be always carried out because of the frequent association between these two lesions.

The *course* and *prognosis* of patients with this type of

right ventricular obstruction is not known. Progressive obstruction has been observed in patients in whom there was an associated VSD.[79] Spontaneous closure of an associated VSD may occur, resulting in an isolated right ventricular obstruction due to anomalous muscle bundles.[33, 194] It is possible that some of the cases of anomalous muscle bundle obstruction and intact ventricular septum, in the absence of pulmonary valvular stenosis, may have been cases associated with VSD which have closed spontaneously. All patients who have been surgically corrected showed definite subjective improvement postoperatively.

PULMONARY ARTERIAL STENOSIS WITH INTACT VENTRICULAR SEPTUM

Stenosis of the pulmonary artery, isolated or in association with other congenital cardiac defects, is common. Its overall frequency has been reported to be 2 to 3% of all patients with congenital heart disese.[58, 136] It may be single, involving the main pulmonary trunk or either of its branches, or multiple, involving both main and several smaller peripheral arterial branches.[39, 50, 66] Pulmonary artery stenosis is referred to frequently as supravalvular or postvalvular pulmonary stenosis or coarctation of the pulmonary artery.

Isolated pulmonary artery stenosis was first reported by Mangars[114] and then Schwalbe[167] described a case with absent right pulmonary artery and stenosis on the left. However, with the application of cardiac catheterization and particularly angiocardiography, reports involving small or large series of patients with this lesion have appeared with increasing frequency.[3, 7, 10, 14, 16, 37, 46, 50, 75, 83, 96, 117, 156, 157] In approximately two-thirds of the cases, other associated cardiac defects are present. Pulmonary valvular stenosis and VSD are the most frequent cardiac lesions associated with pulmonary artery stenosis.[7, 65] PDA and ASD are also frequent, perhaps more so in cases associated with the rubella syndrome.[50, 81, 162] Tetralogy of Fallot with hypoplasia or pulmonary branch atresia or pulmonary artery stenosis also has been frequently seen.[65, 117] Pulmonary arterial stenosis may also be associated with transposition of the great arteries and mitral atresia. Supravalvular aortic stenosis in association with multiple pulmonary arterial stenoses, mental retardation, and peculiar facies was described as a separate syndrome.[14, 157, 187] Pulmonary arterial stenoses also have been reported in association with Noonan's syndrome,[142] Alagille's syndrome[5] (arteriohepatic dysplasia), cutis laxa,[83] and Ehlers-Danlos syndrome.[99] Isolated pulmonary artery stenosis, single or multiple, with intact ventricular septum, however, is not rare, and its frequency is, by far, greater than that of isolated infundibular stenosis.

PATHOLOGY

The pulmonary artery and its branches developmentally have their origin from three separate vascular components. The proximal portion of the main pulmonary trunk adjacent to and immediately above the semilunar valve is probably derived from the bulbus cordis. The remainder of the trunk arises from the common truncus arteriosus. The proximal segments of the right and left pulmonary arteries are formed from the sixth branchial arches on either side. While the dorsal portion of the right sixth arch disappears completely, the one on the left persists as the ductus arteriosus and later as the ligamentum arteriosum. The peripheral portions of the pulmonary arterial branches are derived from the "postbranchial pulmonary vascular plexus," which lies in close relation to the growing lung buds.[90] The pathogenesis of pulmonary arterial stenosis is not known. It appears that

multiple factors and many types of pathologic changes may produce the same end result, i.e., narrowing of the lumen of the pulmonary arteries. The high frequency of associated intracardiac anomalies suggests that the pathogenesis of these lesions is developmental in origin. Any teratogenic insult upon the components of the developing pulmonary arteries may arrest their development, leading to atresia or hypoplasia or stenosis, involving different levels of the pulmonary arterial tree. At least one teratogenic agent, the rubella virus, has been implicated in the pathogenesis of these lesions.[23, 50, 117, 162] In the stenosis associated with the rubella syndrome, it appears that interference with the normal formation of elastic tissue may be the principal mechanism of the lesion.[23]

Peripheral stenoses of the pulmonary arteries in association with supravalvular aortic stenosis, mental retardation, and peculiar facies have been also described as a characteristic syndrome, probably associated with infantile hypercalcemia.[14, 96] However, genetic factors in the etiology of these lesions cannot be excluded. In several instances, pulmonary artery stenosis was observed in siblings or mother and child, or in families with history of congenital heart disease.[66, 117, 157]

Recently, a hereditary syndrome consisting of intrahepatic cholestasis, varying degrees of peripheral pulmonary artery stenoses, or diffuse hypoplasia of the pulmonary artery and its branches has been reported by several groups (Alagille's syndrome, or arteriohepatic dysplasia).[5, 42, 72, 155, 160] Thus, isolated pulmonary arterial stenosis may be associated with a number of familial and hereditary or environmental factors, and its frequency has been underestimated.[55]

In general, the stenosis may be single or multiple and may involve the main pulmonary trunk, its main branches, or the secondary and smaller branches at their bifurcations, unilaterally or bilaterally. Very rarely, the pulmonary trunk stenosis may be due to a membranous or ring-like constriction immediately distal to the valve. The narrowed segment of the vessel usually consists of fibrous intimal thickening with varying degrees of medial thickening, resulting in a very thick wall. The distal portion of the vessel often is dilated and appears as a vein-like structure. However, in cases of rubella syndrome, the pulmonary arterial trunk may be diffusely hypoplastic without apparent histologic abnormality. The stenosis frequently involves the origin of the main pulmonary arterial branches (at the bifurcation) where considerable intimal thickening may be present as well as microscopic changes in the elastic tissue. In these cases, dilatation of the pulmonary arterial branches distal to the stenosis is usually present. The narrowing may be localized or segmental, may involve longer segments of the main arterial branches, or may take the form of generalized hypoplasia. Frequently, a combination of these types of lesions may be encountered in the same individual.

A useful classification of pulmonary arterial stenosis has been proposed by Gay et al.[66] The stenoses have been classified in four types (Fig. 17.14): stenosis involving the main pulmonary trunk or the right and left main branch; stenosis involving the bifurcation of the pulmonary artery extending into both branches; multiple peripheral stenoses; and a combination of main and peripheral stenoses. In approximately two-thirds of the cases, the stenosis involves the main pulmonary trunk, its bifurcation, or its main branches. When the stenosis is localized, dilatation of the vessel distal to the narrowing is usually present. With elongated constrictions, only minimal poststenotic dilatation, if any, is seen, and no dilatation at all is noted in the hypoplastic form. The pulmonary trunk usually is not dilated, even with severe stenosis involving its distal portion or the bifurcation and both branches (prestenotic dilatation). Only

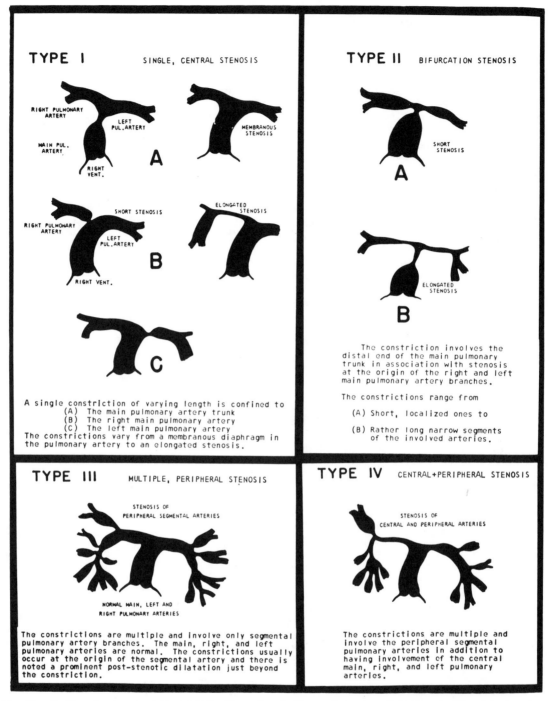

Fig. 17.14 Classification of pulmonary artery stenosis. (Reproduced with permission from B. B. Gay *et al.*[66] and the American Journal of Roentgenology.)

occasionally, mild degrees of prestenotic dilatation are seen but never to the extent seen in obstructive pulmonary hypertension.[37]

Depending upon the degree of obstruction, right ventricular hypertrophy may or may not be present. Marked hypertrophy of the right ventricle may develop with severe degrees of obstruction. A patent foramen ovale or an ASD may also be present in patients with pulmonary artery stenosis and intact ventricular septum.

PHYSIOLOGY

The physiologic derangement in these lesions of the pulmonary arterial tree is similar to that of isolated pulmonary

valvular or infundibular stenosis, the only difference being the location of the obstruction. Thus, depending upon the degree of obstruction, mild to marked elevation of the right ventricular and pulmonary arterial (proximal to stenosis) systolic pressure are present. In the majority of cases, the obstruction is central, i.e., involving the proximal vascular tree. This results in a limited volume capacity of the pulmonary trunk proximal to the obstruction. The right ventricular stroke volume cannot be easily accommodated by the small thick-walled compartment of the pulmonary artery in these cases, as it can when the pulmonary arterial compartment is considerably larger, i.e., in individuals with primary pulmonary hypertension. When the obstruction is severe, right ventricular ejection time is prolonged, and the pulmonary trunk (proximal to the obstruction) behaves as an extension of the right ventricular outflow tract. The narrow orifice of the stenotic area of the vessel, not the true valvular orifice, determines the duration and forcefulness of ventricular contraction. The pulmonary arterial pressure proximal to the obstruction is of the same magnitude as that of the right ventricle, and the pulmonary valve remains open as long as there is systolic pressure gradient between the distal pulmonary artery and the right ventricle. This explains the delay in pulmonary valve closure seen in this condition despite the very high systolic pressure in the pulmonary trunk. The pressure tracing proximal to the stenosis resembles that of the right ventricle with high systolic and low diastolic pressure. In cases of severe multiple peripheral stenoses involving many small arterial branches bilaterally, closure of the pulmonary valve occurs earlier and approximates closure of the aortic valve.[148] In the presence of associated valvular stenosis, the hemodynamics are essentially the same, the only difference being that in these cases the valvular obstruction is the determinant of ventricular function. With unilateral pulmonary artery stenosis, in the absence of increased pulmonary flow, the right ventricular pressure is normal. The capacitance of the unobstructed artery and its tributaries is adequate to accommodate the right ventricular stroke volume, and thus hypertension does not occur. However, with exercise or with large left to right shunts, the volume of the unobstructed pulmonary vascular tree may reach its limits, and pulmonary hypertension may ensue.

Bilateral pulmonary artery stenosis may be regarded as beneficial to the patient when associated cardiac lesions with left to right shunt are present. The stenosis reduces the flow to the lungs and thus tends to prevent volume overloading of the heart.

MANIFESTATIONS

Clinical Features

Patients with mild or moderate bilateral pulmonary stenosis, as well as those with unilateral stenosis, are usually asymptomatic. *Dyspnea* on exertion, easy fatigability, and signs of heart failure may be seen in cases with severe obstruction involving the main or both branches of the pulmonary artery or involving multiple small peripheral branches. Right ventricular overactivity with or without cardiomegaly and signs of heart failure, when present, are usually indistinguishable from those seen in pulmonary valvular stenosis of similar severity. However, subtle differences in auscultatory findings may sometimes differentiate the two conditions. The *first sound* is usually normal and *is not followed by an ejection click*. The *second sound* is usually split, and the pulmonary component is normal or only slightly increased in intensity, a distinct difference from valvular stenosis. The width of the splitting depends upon the severity of stenosis, as in valvular stenosis, and there is some respiratory variation of the splitting, except in cases with very severe degrees of obstruction. There is an *ejection systolic murmur* of varying intensity at the upper sternal border, and it is well transmitted to the axilla and back but not to the neck. In patients with multiple peripheral pulmonary arterial stenoses, the second sound in the pulmonary area may be so loud that pulmonary hypertension is suspected. However, in multiple peripheral pulmonary stenoses, soft blowing systolic or continuous murmurs may be heard over both lung fields, and in the back, a distinct difference from pulmonary hypertension when no murmurs or a very short, early systolic murmur may be heard at the left upper sternal border. A continuous murmur occasionally may be present in cases with main or distal branch stenosis, especially when increased pulmonary flow is present.[37, 46, 65, 139, 150]

In the phonocardiogram, the murmur of pulmonary artery stenosis usually begins well after the first sound, has a crescendo-decrescendo configuration, covers the aortic closure sound, and may partially cover the pulmonary closure sound.[150] These features are more pronounced when the record is obtained from the right upper sternal border or axilla. When associated lesions are present, it is very difficult to suspect pulmonary artery stenosis on the basis of clinical findings. The murmurs of mild pulmonary artery stenosis may be erroneously considered innocent or functional.[50] When a PDA with a continuous murmur is present, coexisting pulmonary artery stenosis is suspected by the presence of a loud systolic murmur over the right subclavicular and axillary areas.[50] Since pulmonary valvular stenosis is a commonly associated lesion, transmission of the murmur to the left axilla is not as helpful as suspecting associated pulmonary artery stenosis, especially when the latter lesion is mild.

Electrovectorcardiographic Features

The electrocardiogram and vectorcardiogram are indistinguishable from those of pulmonary valvular stenosis. Normal tracings are usually recorded from patients with mild degree of stenosis. Varying degrees of right ventricular hypertrophy are seen in cases with more severe obstruction.

A relatively high frequency of left axis deviation with counterclockwise direction of the frontal QRS vector was noted in a group of infants with the rubella syndrome and pulmonary artery stenosis and was attributed to myocardial damage from the rubella virus.[76] Similarly, left axis deviation and counterclockwise QRS frontal vector was also seen in a number of infants with the supravalvular pulmonic stenosis syndrome[157] and Noonan's syndrome.[142]

Radiologic Features

In patients with mild and moderate stenosis, the chest roentgenogram shows normal heart size and normal vascularity, as in pulmonary valvular stenosis. However, unlike the latter lesion, the main pulmonary artery segment is not prominent. The pulmonary vascular markings may be normal bilaterally, even in cases of unilateral pulmonary artery stenosis. Only when severe unilateral stenosis is present and there is increased pulmonary flow is there a detectable difference in the degree of vascularity between the two lung fields. When the stenosis is bilateral and severe, varying degrees of right atrial and ventricular enlargement may be seen. When cardiac failure is present, more cardiac enlargement and a definite decrease in pulmonary vascularity are noted.

Echocardiographic Features

Hypertrophy of the right ventricular wall reflecting the degree of obstruction can be detected by the echocardiogram. Since the diastolic pressure in the proximal artery is low, the systolic time intervals of the right ventricle will be consistent with the low overall pulmonary vascular resistance. These echo findings will be similar to those seen in patients with pulmonary arterial banding.[64]

The 2-D echo will show the main pulmonary artery and its branches, as well as the right ventricular cavity and the pulmonary valve. Proximal stenoses up to the bifurcation and the origin of the main pulmonary branches may be visualized, but more distal stenoses are impossible to assess.[163] The presence of other associated lesions such as large ASD and VSD and aortic and pulmonary valve stenosis can be easily detected.

CARDIAC CATHETERIZATION

Cardiac catheterization is usually the first step in confirming the clinical diagnosis of pulmonary artery stenosis. Carefully obtained withdrawal pressure tracings from the more distal branches toward the main pulmonary arterial branches, pulmonary trunk, and right ventricle usually will demonstrate systolic pressure gradients across the narrowed segments of the vessels (Fig. 17.15).

Small pressure gradients, however, may sometimes be artifactual, being produced by the discrepancy between the size of the vessel and the size of the catheter.[31] In very young infants, and especially preterm infants, mild to moderate pressure gradients between the main pulmonary arterial branches and the pulmonary trunk may be recorded normally and may disappear with growth of the infant. These normal pressure gradients are due most likely to disparity between the size of the lumen of the main pulmonary trunk and that of the main pulmonary branches.[31, 45] In general, systolic pressure gradients more than 10 mm Hg may be considered abnormal in the absence of increased pulmonary flow due to associated shunting lesions and in individuals beyond the first few months of life. With unilateral stenosis, a pressure gradient is usually present across the constricted segment of the vessel with the proximal pulmonary artery pressure being within normal limits. However, with exercise or in the presence of associated left to right shunt, accentuation of the pressure gradient may be observed with a concomitant increase in the proximal arterial pressure.

In cases of stenosis of the pulmonary arterial trunk and its bifurcation, or in bilateral main branch stenosis, the pressure distal to the stenosis is usually low, and the tracing shows a slow pressure rise and fall with a broad systolic peak. However, the pressure tracing proximal to the obstruction shows certain characteristics which may be helpful in suspecting the diagnosis, especially if only one or none of the main branches could be entered. The pressure tracing proximal to the obstruction has a contour identical to that of the right ventricle as far as height and time are concerned up to the dicrotic notch. The dicrotic notch is usually quite low and is followed by a low diastolic pressure which is similar to that distal to the obstruction. This wide pressure pulse recorded

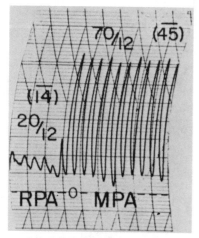

Fig. 17.15 Pressure record during withdrawal of catheter from right pulmonary artery (*RPA*) to maintain pulmonary artery (*MPA*), in a 21 month old with bilateral pulmonary artery stenosis and small patent ductus arteriosus. There is abrupt increase in pressure as the stenotic area is traversed. Note the low diastolic pressure in the main pulmonary artery. (Reproduced with permission from Emmanouilides *et al.*[50] and the American Heart Association.)

in the proximal pulmonary artery becomes more pronounced with increasing severity of obstruction. The descending limb of the curve becomes steeper and the dicrotic notch deeper with very low diastolic pressure, with the overall configuration of the tracing resembling that of the right ventricle.[3, 50] In many instances, because of this similarity of right ventricular and pulmonary trunk tracings, and because the branches of the pulmonary artery cannot be entered, pressures obtained from the pulmonary trunk may be falsely interpreted as representing ventricular tracings. Thus, in the past, it was common that such cases, in the absence of an angiocardiogram, were diagnosed as pulmonary valvular stenosis. Intracardiac electrocardiography and phonocardiography may also be helpful in the diagnosis in such instances.

The characteristic contour of the pressure tracing proximal to the stenosis is attributed to the altered function of the pulmonary trunk.[3] The wall of the pulmonary trunk is usually very thick and fibrotic, with reduced elasticity. The prestenotic portion of the pulmonary trunk becomes an extension of the right ventricular outflow tract, and since the right ventricular function is determined by the degree of obstruction at the bifurcation or at the main pulmonary arterial branches, the pressure in the pulmonary trunk reflects pressure changes of the ventricle rather than those of the distal pulmonary circulation. As long as the pulmonary artery pressure distal to the obstruction is lower than the right ventricular pressure, the pulmonary valve remains open. Closure of the valve occurs during the early phase of isometric relaxation of the ventricle, which results in a sudden increase in the volume capacity of the pulmonary trunk with a corresponding fall in pressure and formation of the dicrotic notch. The slow descent of the diastolic pressure seen in the tracing reflects the relatively slow rate of diastolic runoff of blood from the main pulmonary trunk to the distal branches. This slow diastolic runoff is a consequence of the obstruction and the impaired elastic recoil of the thick fibrotic wall of the pulmonary trunk.

When stenosis is severe, the diastolic descent is nonexistent and the tracing becomes plateau-shaped. As the obstruction sites are located more peripherally, the characteristic pressure tracing in the pulmonary trunk becomes less obvious and, when the obstruction involves multiple small peripheral branches, it is almost indistinguishable from that of primary pulmonary hypertension.

Right to left shunt at the atrial level through a patent foramen ovale is often present in severe cases with right ventricular pressures higher than systemic. Frequently, there is an associated valvular stenosis.[50, 117] Evaluation of the severity of either lesion can be easily made by careful withdrawal pressure tracings. This is crucial, especially to the cardiac surgeon, and has important therapeutic implications. If the pressure in the main pulmonary trunk is moderately elevated, this suggests that pulmonary artery stenosis is the dominant lesion. In contrast, when the dominant lesion is pulmonary valvular stenosis, elevation of the right ventricular pressure with normal or only slightly increased pulmonary trunk pressure is noted. However, it is difficult sometimes to predict the severity of peripheral stenoses in such cases because of the masking effect of the valvular upon the supravalvular obstruction. Angiocardiography is the procedure of choice in appraising the severity of supravalvular stenoses in such a combination of lesions.

ANGIOCARDIOGRAPHY

Selective angiocardiography is the most valuable single tool in the diagnosis of pulmonary artery stenosis.[7, 50, 66, 117] The exact location, extent, and distribution of these lesions can be easily visualized with this procedure. Usually, a selective biplane angiocardiogram from the right ventricle will give all the necessary information. The right pulmonary artery stenosis and the multiple peripheral stenoses are best seen in the anteroposterior view, while stenosis involving the pulmonary trunk or the origin of the left main branch can be recognized in the lateral view (Fig. 17.16). Half axial selected oblique views are currently used for better delineation of the lesions.[8] The main pulmonary trunk is usually normal or hypoplastic. In rare instances, prestenotic dilatation may be present in stenoses involving distal branches. In severe unilateral obstruction, a delayed filling of the respective pulmonary veins may be noted. Angiocardiography must be performed in all patients in whom major pulmonary artery stenosis is suspected during cardiac catheterization, especially when the main pulmonary branches could not be entered. In addition, it is recommended that aortographic studies should always be performed in order to exclude the presence of frequently associated systemic arterial lesions.

DIFFERENTIAL DIAGNOSIS

Isolated pulmonary artery stenosis may be clinically suspected by the presence of the characteristic systolic murmur which is widely transmitted to the axillae and the back, the absence of a pulmonary ejection click, the widely split second sound with normal respiratory variation, and a normal or slightly increased in intensity pulmonary component. The

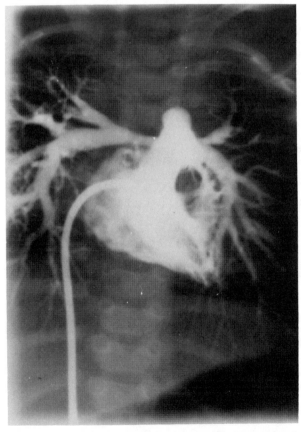

Fig. 17.16 Right ventricular angiocardiogram of an 8 months old with severe main trunk and bilateral pulmonary artery stenosis (right ventricle pressure, 120/0-10, pulmonary trunk pressure, 100/12). Anteroposterior view showing small pulmonary trunk and severe proximal stenosis of the right pulmonary artery. The corresponding lateral view showed hypoplasia of the pulmonary trunk and stenosis of the bifurcation.

electrocardiogram, vectorcardiogram and echocardiogram are helpful in assessing the severity of the obstruction. The entities discussed in the differential diagnosis of pulmonary valve stenosis also must be differentiated from isolated pulmonary artery stenosis. Since pulmonary artery stenosis is commonly associated with other intracardiac and extracardiac malformations, the features of the predominant lesion will determine the clinical picture in these complicated cases. A history of maternal rubella, familial congenital heart disease, or prolonged neonatal jaundice, and the finding of facies or features suggesting Noonan's syndrome or the idiopathic hypercalcemia syndrome, should make one suspicious that pulmonary arterial stenosis could be the underlying cause of the systolic murmur.

A rather common murmur which simulates that of mild pulmonary artery stenosis is that heard in many preterm infants with less than 2200 gm birth weight. This widely transmitted, short, high-pitched systolic murmur persists for 2 to 3 months and eventually disappears.[45] It is most likely produced by either relative pulmonary branch stenosis due to hypoplasia of the pulmonary arterial branches or an unusual alignment of the main pulmonary artery with its branches.

TREATMENT

Mild to moderate isolated unilateral or bilateral stenosis does not require surgical correction. However, well-localized main pulmonary artery or trunk stenosis of severe degree should be surgically relieved. The operation is performed with the use of cardiopulmonary bypass, but the results are not uniformly encouraging.[50, 118, 178] In pulmonary trunk stenosis, the narrowed area of the vessel is opened, and a pericardial or plastic elliptoid patch is used to widen the lumen of the vessel. When the narrowing involves the bifurcation and origin of both main arteries and is well localized, a similar plastic procedure may be carried out. However, it is important for the success of any corrective procedure, first, to rule out associated multiple peripheral stenoses and, second, to establish by angiocardiography the well-localized, centrally located obstruction. With the introduction of the newer soft plastic grafts, severely stenotic lesions may be successfully bypassed, especially in older children. The indications for operation, except for the above limitations, are similar to those of pulmonary valvular or infundibular stenosis with intact ventricular septum.

Routine prophylaxis against endocarditis in these patients is also recommended. The natural history of these lesions is not well documented. The prognosis is related to the severity of obstruction and should be more or less similar to that of valvular stenosis. Although in multiple peripheral pulmonary arterial stenoses of severe degree, the prognosis is probably similar to that of primary pulmonary hypertension, localized stenosis of the trunk and main branches is not always as easily amenable to surgical correction as is pulmonary valvular or infundibular stenosis. Thus, for the same degree of obstruction, patients with valvular stenosis have a better prognosis because they can be corrected more easily and with less risk. Progressive increase in the degree of obstruction of pulmonary artery stenosis may occur. Whether this is the result of a discrepancy between the rate of growth of the normal portion of the vessel and the stenotic segments, or a reflection of increased cardiac output, is not known. On the other hand, in many cases, pressure gradients recorded early in life disappear with growth.[80, 191] Poststenotic aneurysmal dilatation of the small elastic arteries may be complicated by arteritis, thrombosis, or pulmonary hemorrhage.[65, 139] Death early in infancy or later, in cases of severe pulmonary artery stenosis, has also been reported.[113] Severe pulmonary artery stenosis in late adult life is apparently very rare. It is conceivable that either these cases are missed and are considered cases of valvular stenosis or the patients die early in life. The most likely explanation for this is that the obstruction becomes less with growth.

CONGENITAL RUBELLA SYNDROME

The teratogenic effects of rubella infection acquired early in pregnancy have been well documented since the first report of Gregg in 1941.[73] Congenital heart disease with congenital cataracts and deafness have been the most frequent abnormalities associated with a history of maternal rubella during the first trimester of pregnancy.[74] However, knowledge of the pathogenesis of congenital rubella has been considerably expanded following the successful cultivation of the rubella virus in tissue cultures in 1962 and observations made during the rubella epidemic in the United States in 1964.[165] Since then, the natural history of rubella infection has been studied extensively, and new information regarding the pathogenetic, clinical, epidemiologic, and preventive aspects of congenital rubella has been acquired.[77] Thus, the clinical profile of the rubella syndrome has been expanded to include manifestations which were not recognized prior to the epidemic in 1964 (Table 17.1).

It is well established now that rubella virus infection acquired in utero persists throughout pregnancy and is present at birth. Virus can be recovered from fetal tissues obtained by therapeutic abortions performed weeks or months after maternal rubella infection. At birth, virus can be cultured from pharyngeal secretions, urine, cerebrospinal fluid, and other tissues. Infants with congenital rubella infection may continue to shed virus for months after birth, but with advancing age the shedding of virus decreases. Virus has been recovered from affected organs for as long as 10 years. These infants with congenital rubella have serum rubella neutralizing antibody titers comparable to those observed in their mothers, and levels of antibody appear to persist for many years. Persistent asymptomatic congenital rubella infection may occur in infants who appear normal during early months of life but later on may develop subtle psychomotor disturbances. It has been also shown that these infants are contagious and must be isolated to prevent spread of infection to susceptible women in the early stages of pregnancy. The introduction of a live attenuated rubella virus vaccine appears to have effectively reduced the frequency of congenital rubella.[127] However, there are some questions about its effectiveness in eliminating rubella infection in the population.[196]

CARDIOVASCULAR LESIONS

The spectrum of cardiovascular lesions related to the rubella syndrome has been widened in recent years (Table 17.2). Early reports indicated that the most frequent anomaly was PDA.[22] The implication of maternal rubella as a possible cause of stenosis of the pulmonary arteries was first made by Arvidsson and associates.[7] In 1963, Rowe[161] reported frequent association of varying degrees of pulmonary artery stenosis in offspring of mothers who had contracted rubella during an epidemic in New Zealand. His observations were subsequently confirmed.[50, 81, 113, 186] Localized stenosis or diffuse hypoplasia of the pulmonary trunk with or without narrowing of its bifurcation, isolated pulmonary branch stenosis, bilateral or unilateral, as well as multiple peripheral stenoses, have all been described in association with the rubella syndrome. These lesions may be isolated or associated with PDA, pulmonary valve stenosis, or ASD. However, the frequency of isolated pulmonary artery stenoses in the rubella syndrome may be as high as that of PDA. In the majority of cases, the stenoses may be mild or moderate and may escape clinical detection. Ventricular septal defect, valvular or supravalvular aortic stenosis, tetralogy of Fallot, coarctation of the aorta, tricuspid atresia, and transposition of the great vessels also have been reported in association with the rubella syndrome.[162, 163]

Generalized systemic arterial lesions have been described.[23, 53, 113] These lesions may involve large and medium size vessels, such as the aorta and coronary, cerebral, mesenteric, and renal arteries.[185] Diffuse hypoplasia of the abdominal aorta has been described in severely affected infants with the rubella syndrome.[172] Focal intimate thickening consisting of loose fibroblastic tissue and fragmentation of the elastic fibers in the vacuolated media are the principal histologic features described in the lesions of the aorta and large arteries.[23, 180] In the small arteries, the lesions consist of extensive focal intimate thickening, localized to areas of deficient elastic tissue in the wall, and almost invariably involving the internal elastic lumina. The wall of the pulmonary trunk may show varying degrees of thickness and fibrosis. The main cause of stenosis in the case of the right and left pulmonary arteries may be generalized hypoplasia without intimal thickening.[176] The ductus arteriosus shows a decrease in both smooth muscle and elastic tissue. All lesions described may be progressive.

Myocardial injury, suggested by the electrocardiographic

TABLE 17.1 MANIFESTATIONS OF CONGENITAL RUBELLA

Common	Uncommon or Rare
History of maternal rubella	Glaucoma
Low birth weight	Cloudy cornea
Cataracts	Interstitial pneumonitis
Microphthalmia	Myocarditis
Retinopathy	Hepatitis
Congenital heart disease	Generalized adenopathy
Deafness	Encephalitis
Thrombocytopenic purpura	Renal artery stenosis with hypertension
Hepatosplenomegaly	Dermatoglyphic "abnormalities"
Bone lesions	Hemolytic or hypoplastic anemia
Large anterior fontanelle	Obstructive jaundice
Psychomotor retardation	Spastic quadraparesis
	Inguinal hernia

TABLE 17.2 CARDIOVASCULAR MALFORMATIONS ASSOCIATED WITH CONGENITAL RUBELLA

Pulmonary arterial stenoses[a]
Patent ductus arteriosus[a]
Pulmonary valvular stenosis
Systemic arterial stenoses
Hypoplasia of the abdominal aorta
Ventricular septal defect
Atrial septal defect
Tetralogy of Fallot
Coarctation of the aorta
Aortic valvular or supravalvular stenosis
Transposition of the great arteries
Tricuspid atresia
Multiple valvular sclerosis

[a] Commonest.

examination, has been observed in several infants. Marked swelling of muscle fibers and loss of cross-striation with small pyknotic and larger vacuolated nuclei and minimal evidence of inflammatory response have been described in infants with the rubella syndrome dying from heart failure.[102]

Cardiovascular disease in the rubella syndrome is probably the result of focal damage to vessels in both pulmonary and systemic circulations, but the pathogenesis is obscure. Impaired formation of the elastic tissue, due to interference with the fibroblastic or myoblastic activity by the rubella virus, is probably responsible for the development of the vascular lesions. Rubella virus inhibits mitosis and increases the number of chromosomal breaks in human embryonic cells grown in tissue culture. The growth retardation and the hypoplasia of various organs and arterial vessels is most likely the result of interference with fetal and postnatal cell multiplication by the rubella virus.[77]

The clinical picture of neonates and young infants with cardiovascular involvement in rubella syndrome depends upon the severity of the lesions and the associated abnormalities of other organs and systems. Signs of heart failure may appear early in life, and in the majority of these infants a PDA or other associated cardiac lesions is present.[113] Newborns with lower birth weights may develop heart failure earlier than those with larger birth weights. The diagnosis of heart failure in these infants may be difficult because of the presence of hepatosplenomegaly and tachypnea due to noncardiac causes. A low grade interstitial pneumonitis with tachypnea, cough, and cyanosis may be present during the early weeks of life and should be excluded before the diagnosis of heart failure is made. However, the two conditions may coexist.

The prognosis of infants with cardiovascular malformations due to rubella virus depends upon the nature of the lesion and its severity. In the majority of cases, pulmonary arterial stenoses of mild to moderate degree do not progress and may disappear with growth. However, severe obstructions usually remain severe or get worse. Since the virus affects many other organs and systems, it is difficult sometimes to dissociate effects of noncardiac lesions from those of cardiovascular lesions. Slow growth and development, mental retardation, or other sequelae of the rubella syndrome may modify the effects of the cardiovascular lesions upon the overall health of the individual.[123] For example, surgical correction of a hemodynamically significant cardiac lesion, i.e., a PDA with large left to right shunt, in an infant with the rubella syndrome may not necessarily result in improvement of the rate of growth as it would in another infant with the same cardiac lesion but without the stigmata of congenital rubella.

REFERENCES

1. Abrahams, D. G., and Wood, P.: Pulmonary stenosis with normal aortic root. Br. Heart J. 13:519, 1951.
2. Adams, F. H., Veasy, L. G., Jorgens, J., Diehl, A., LaBree, J. W., Shapiro, M. J., and Dwan, P. F.: Congenital valvular pulmonary stenosis with or without an interatrial communication: Physiologic studies as diagnostic aids. J. Pediatr. 38:431, 1951.
3. Agustsson, M. H., Arcilla, R. A., Gasul, B. M., Bicoff, J. P., Nassif, S. I., and Lendrum, B. L.: The diagnosis of bilateral stenosis of the primary pulmonary branches based on characteristic pulmonary trunk pressure curves: A hemodynamic and angiocardiographic study. Circulation 26:421, 1962.
4. Ainsworth, H., Hunt, J., and Joseph, M.: Numerical evaluation of facial pattern in children with isolated pulmonary stenosis. Arch. Dis. Child. 54:662, 1979.
5. Alagille, D., Odievre, M., Gautier, M., and Dommergues, J. P.: Hepatic ductular hypoplasia associated with characteristic facies, vertebral malformations, retarded physical, mental and sexual development, and cardiac murmur. J. Pediatr. 86:63, 1975.
6. Arnett, E. N., Aisner, S. C., Lewis, K. B., Tecklenberg, P., Brawley, R. K., and Roberts, W. C.: Pulmonary valve stenosis, atrial septal defect and left to right interatrial shunting with intact ventricular septum: A distinct hemodynamic-morphologic syndrome. Chest 78:759, 1980.
7. Arvidsson, H., Carlsson, E., Hartmann, A., Jr., Tsifutis, A., and Crawford, C.: Supravalvular stenoses of the pulmonary arteries. Report of eleven cases. Acta Radiol. 56:466, 1961.
8. Bargeron, L. M. J., Elliot, L. P., Soto, P. R., Bream, P. R., and Curry, G. C.: Axial cineangiography in congenital heart disease. Circulation 56:1048, 1977.
9. Bassingthwaighte, J. B., Parkin, T. W., DuShane, J. W., Wood, E. H., and Burchell, H. B.: The electrocardiographic and hemodynamic findings in pulmonary stenosis with intact ventricular septum. Circulation 28:893, 1963.
10. Baum, D., Khoury, G. H., Ongley, P. A., Swan, H. J. C., and Kincaid, O. W.: Congenital stenosis of the pulmonary artery branches. Circulation 29:680, 1964.
11. Baumstark, A., Fellows, K. E., and Rosenthal, A.: Combined double chambered right ventricle and discrete subaortic stenosis. Circulation 57:299, 1978.
12. Becu, L., Somerville, J., and Gallo, A.: "Isolated" pulmonary valve stenosis as part of more widespread cardiovascular disease. Br. Heart J. 38:472, 1976.
13. Berman, W., Jr., Gross, R., Marawala, Z., and Carlsson, E.: The measurement of pulmonic valve area by angiocardiographic and hemodynamic methods. Cardiovasc. Radiol. 1:77, 1978.
14. Beuren, A. J., Schulze, C., Eberle, P., Harmjanz, D., and Apitz, J.: The syndrome of supravalvular aortic stenosis, peripheral pulmonary stenosis, mental retardation and similar facial appearance. Am. J. Cardiol. 13:471, 1964.
15. Blount, S. G., Jr., Vigoda, P. S., and Swan H.: Isolated infundibular stenosis. Am. Heart J. 57:684, 1959.
16. Bourassa, M. G., and Campeau, L.: Combined supravalvular aortic and pulmonic stenosis. Circulation 28:572, 1963.
17. Bousvaros, G., and Palmer, W.: Phonocardiographic features of the systolic murmur in pulmonary artery stenosis. Br. Heart J. 27:374, 1965.
18. Bouvrain, Y., Bourthoumieux, A., and Nezry, R.: Souffles systoliques a irradiations axillaires et retrecissement des branches de l'artére pulmonaire. Arch. Mal. Coeur 54:999, 1961.
19. Brock, R. C.: *The Anatomy of Congenital Pulmonic Stenosis.* Paul B. Hoeber, New York, 1957.
20. Brock, R. C.: The surgical treatment of pulmonic stenosis. Br. Heart J. 23:337, 1961.
21. Campbell, M.: Relationship of pressure and valve area in pulmonary stenosis. Br. Heart J. 22:101, 1960.
22. Campbell, M.: Place of maternal rubella in the etiology of congenital heart disease. Br. Med. J. 1:691, 1961.
23. Campbell, P. E.: Vascular abnormalities following maternal rubella. Br. Heart J. 27:134, 1965.
24. Castaneda-Zuniga, W. R., Formanek, A., and Amplatz, K.: Radiologic diagnosis of different types of pulmonary stenoses. Cardiovasc. Radiol. 1:45, 1978.
25. Chesler, E., Mitha, A. S., Matisonn, R. E., and Rogers, M. N.: Subpulmonic stenosis as a result of noncalcific constrictive pericarditis. Chest 69:425, 1976.
26. Coates, J. R., McCleanthan, J. E., and Scott, L. P.: The double chambered right ventricle. A diagnostic and operative pitfall. Am. J. Cardiol. 14:561, 1964.
27. Cohn, L. H., Senders, J. H., Jr., and Collins, J. J., Jr.: Surgical treatment of congenital unilateral pulmonary arterial stenosis with contralateral pulmonary hypertension. Am. J. Cardiol. 38:857, 1977.
28. Cotter, L., Pusey, C. D., and Miller, G. A.: Extreme right ventricular hypoplasia after relief of severe pulmonary stenosis. Use of balloon catheter occlusion of atrial septal defect in assessing right ventricular function. Br. Heart J. 44:469, 1980.
29. Dalby, A. J., and Forman, R.: Acquired pulmonary stenosis. S. Afr. Med. J. 55:218, 1979.
30. Danielson, G. C., Exarhos, N. D., Weidman, W. H., and McGoon, D. C.: Pulmonic stenosis with intact ventricular septum. J. Thorac. Cardiovasc. Surg. 61:228, 1971.
31. Danilowicz, D. A., Rudolph, A. M., Hoffman, J. I. E., and Heymann, M.: Physiologic pressure differences between main and branch pulmonary arteries in infants. Circulation 45:410, 1972.
32. Danilowicz, D., Hoffman, J. I., and Rudolph, A. M.: Serial studies of pulmonary stenosis in infancy and childhood. Br. Heart J. 37:808, 1975.
33. Danilowicz, D., and Ishmael, R.: Anomalous right ventricular muscle bundle: Clinical pitfalls and extracardiac anomalies. Clin. Cardiol. 4:146, 1981.
34. Daoud, G., Kaplan, S., Benzing, G., III, and Gallaher, M. E.: Auscultatory findings of pure infundibular stenosis. Am. J. Dis. Child. 108:73, 1964.
35. Danneimer, I. P., and Venter, C. P.: Haeman-

giosarcoma of the pulmonary valve presenting as a pulmonary stenosis. A case apart. S. Afr. Med. J. 54:873, 1978.

36. Davis, J. E., Hyatt, R. E., and Howell, D. S.: Right-sided congestive heart failure in dogs produced by controlled progressive constriction of the pulmonary artery. Circ. Res. 3:252, 1955.

37. D'Cruz, I. E., Agustsson, M. H., Bicoff, J. P., Weinberg, M., Jr., and Arcilla, R. A.: Stenotic lesions of the pulmonary arteries: Clinical and hemodynamic findings in 84 cases. Am. J. Cardiol. 13:441, 1964.

38. DeCastro, C. M., Nelson, W. P., Jones, R. C., Hall, R. J., Hopeman, A. R., and Jahnke, E. J.: Pulmonary stenosis: Cyanosis, interatrial communication and inadequate right ventricular distensibility following pulmonary valvotomy. Am. J. Cardiol. 26:540, 1970.

39. Delaney, T. B., and Nadas, A. S.: Peripheral pulmonic stenosis. Am. J. Cardiol. 13:451, 1964.

40. DeLeon, A. C., Jr., Perloff, J. K., Twigg, H., and Majd, M.: The straight back syndrome: Clinical cardiovascular manifestations. Circulation 32:193, 1965.

41. DeTroyer, A., Yernault, J. C., and Englert, M.: Lung hypoplasia in congenital pulmonary valve stenosis. Circulation 56:647, 1977.

42. Devloo-Blancquaert, A., Van Den Bosaert-Van Hegesvelde, A. M., Van Aken Craen, R., Essermont-Wirtsen, M., Kunnen, M., and Hooft, C.: Supravalvular pulmonic and aortic stenoses and intrahepatic bile duct hypoplasia. Acta Paediatr. Belg. 33:95, 1980.

43. Dilley, R. B., Longmire, W. P., and Maloney, J. V.: An elevation of the clinical results in the surgical treatment of isolated valvular pulmonic stenosis by the closed transventricular, hypothermic, and cardiopulmonary bypass techniques. J. Thorac. Cardiovasc. Surg. 45:789, 1958.

44. Driscoll, S. G.: Histopathology of gestational rubella. Am. J. Dis. Child. 118:49, 1969.

45. Dunkle, L. M., and Rowe, R. D.: Transient murmurs simulating pulmonary artery stenosis in premature infants. Am. J. Dis. Child. 124:666, 1972.

46. Eldredge, W. J., Tingelstad, J. B., Robertson, L. W., Mauck, H. P., and McCue, C. M.: Observations on the natural history of pulmonary artery coarctations. Circulation 45:404, 1972.

47. Elliotson, J.: *The Recent Improvements in the Art of Distinguishing the Various Diseases of the Heart.* Longmans & Company, London, 1830.

48. Ellison, R. C., and Restiaeux, N. J.: *Vectorcardiogram in Congenital Heart Disease. A Method of Estimating Severity.* W. B. Saunders, Philadelphia, 1972, p. 60.

49. Ellison, R. C., Freedom, R. M., Keane, J. F., Nugent, E. W., Rowe, R. D., and Miettinen, O. S.: Indirect assessment of severity in pulmonic stenosis. Circulation 56 (Suppl. 1):114, 1977.

50. Emmanouilides, G. C., Linde, L. M., and Crittenden, I. H.: Pulmonary artery stenosis associated with ductus arteriosus following maternal rubella. Circulation 29:514, 1964.

51. Engle, M. A., Holswade, G. R., Goldberg, H. D., Lukas, D. S., and Glenn, F.: Regression after open valvotomy of infundibular stenosis accompanying severe valvular pulmonic stenosis. Circulation 17:862, 1958.

52. Engle, M. A., Ito, T., and Goldberg, H. P.: The fate of the patient with pulmonic stenosis. Circulation 39:544, 1964.

53. Esterly, J. R., and Oppenheimer, E. H.: Pathological lesions due to congenital rubella. Arch. Pathol. 87:380, 1969.

54. Fallot, A.: *Contribution a l'anatomie pathologique que la maladie bleue (cyanose cardiaque).* Marsielle med. 25:77, 1888.

55. Feigl, A., Feigl, D., Yahini, J. H., Deutsch, V., and Neufeld, H. N.: Supravalvular aortic and peripheral pulmonary arterial stenoses. A report of eight cases in two generations. Isr. J. Med. Sci. 16:496, 1980.

56. Finnegan, P., Ihenacho, H. N. C., Singh, S. P., and Abrams, L. D.: Haemodynamic studies at rest and during exercise in pulmonary stenosis after surgery. Br. Heart J. 36:913, 1974.

57. Flanagan, W. H., and Shah, P. M.: Echocardiographic correlate of presystolic pulmonary ejection sound in congenital valvular pulmonic stenosis. Am. Heart J. 94:633, 1977.

58. Fouron, J. C., Favreau-Ethier, M., Marion, P., and Davignon, A.: Les stenoses pulmonaires peripheriques congenitales: Presentation de 16 observations et revue de la literature. Can. Med. Assoc. J. 96:1084, 1967.

59. Fowler, R. S., Newnham, L., Jones, M., Lamont, G., and O'Beirne, H.: A simple method for ECG and VCG assessment of the severity of pulmonary valve stenosis. Eur. J. Cardiol. 5:453, 1977.

60. Franciosi, R. A., and Blanc, W. A.: Myocardial infarcts in infants and children. I. A necropsy study in congenital heart disease. J. Pediatr. 73:309, 1968.

61. Freed, M. D., Rosenthal, A., Bernhard, W. F., Litwin, S. B., and Nadas, A. S.: Critical pulmonary stenosis with diminutive right ventricle in neonates. Circulation 48:875, 1973.

62. Gale, G. E., Heimann, K. W., and Barlow, J. B.: Double-chambered right ventricle: A report of five cases. Br. Heart J. 31:291, 1969.

63. Gamboa, R., Hugenholtz, P. C., and Nadas, A. S.: Corrected (Frank), uncorrected (cube), and standard electrocardiographic lead systems in recording augmented right ventricular forces in right ventricular hypertension. Br. Heart J. 28:62, 1966.

64. Garcia, E. J., Riggs, T., Hirschfeld, S., and Liebman, J.: Echocardiographic assessment of the adequacy of pulmonary arterial banding. Am. J. Cardiol. 44:487, 1979.

65. Gasul, B. M., Arcilla, R. A., and Lev, M.: Heart Disease in Children. J. P. Lippincott, Philadelphia, 1966.

66. Gay, B. B., Franch, R. H., Shuford, W. H., and Rogers, J. V.: Roentgenologic features of simple and multiple coarctations of the pulmonary artery and branches. Am. J. Roentgenol. 90:599, 1963.

67. Goitein, K. J., Neches, W. H., Park, S. C., Matthews, R. A., Lenox, C. C., and Zuberbuhler, J. R.: Electrocardiogram in double chamber right ventricle. Am. J. Cardiol. 45:604, 1980.

68. Goldberg, S. J., Areias, J. C., Spitaels, S. E., and Villeneuve, V. H.: Echo Doppler detection of pulmonary stenosis by time-interval histogram analysis. J.C.U. 7:183, 1979.

69. Gomez-Engler, H. E., Grunkemeier, G. L., and Starr, A.: Critical pulmonary valve stenosis with intact ventricular septum. Thorac. Cardiovasc. Surg. 27:160, 1979.

70. Gorlin, R., and Gorlin, S. G.: Hydraulic formula for calculation of the area of the stenotic mitral valve, other cardiac valves, and central circulatory shunts. Am. Heart J. 41:1, 1951.

71. Gramiak, R., Nanda, N. C., and Shah, P. M.: Echocardiographic detection of the pulmonary valve. Radiology 102:153, 1972.

72. Greenwood, R. D., Rosenthal, A., Crocker, A. C., and Nadas, A. S.: Syndrome of intra-hepatic biliary dysgenesia and cardiovascular malformations. Pediatrics 58:243, 1976.

73. Gregg, N. M.: Congenital cataract following German measles in the mother. Trans. Ophthalmol. Soc. Aust. 3:35, 1941.

74. Gregg, N. M.: Rubella during pregnancy of the mother with its sequelae of congenital defects in the child. Med. J. Aust. 1:313, 1945.

75. Gyllensward, A., Lodin, H., Lundberg, A., and

Moller, T.: Congenital multiple peripheral stenoses of the pulmonary artery. Pediatrics 19:399, 1957.

76. Halloran, K. H., Sanyal, S. K., and Gardner, T. H.: Superiorly oriented electrocardiographic axis in infants with the rubella syndrome. Am. Heart J. 72:600, 1966.

77. Hanshaw, J. B., and Dudgeon, J. A.: Viral Diseases of the Fetus and Newborn, In Major Problems in Clinical Pediatrics, Vol. 17, W. B. Saunders, Philadelphia, 1978.

78. Harrink, E., Becker, A. E., Gittenberger-DeGroot, A., Oppenheimer-Dekker, A., and Verspille, A.: The left ventricle in congenital isolated pulmonary valve stenosis. A morphological study. Br. Heart J. 39:429, 1977.

79. Hartmann, A. F., Jr., Tsifutis, A. A., Arvidsson, H., and Goldring, D.: The two-chambered right ventricle: Report of nine cases. Circulation 26:279, 1962.

80. Hartmann, A. F., Jr., Elliot, L. P., and Goldring, D.: The course of peripheral pulmonary artery stenosis in children. J. Pediatr. 73:212, 1968.

81. Hastreiter, A. R., Joorabchi, B., Pujatti, G., Van der Horst, R. L., Patersil, G., and Sever, J. L.: Cardiovascular lesions associated with congenital rubella. J. Pediatr. 71:59, 1967.

82. Haworth, S. G., Shinebourne, E. A., and Miller, G. A. H.: Right-to-left interatrial shunting with normal right ventricular pressure: A puzzling hemodynamic picture associated with some rare congenital malformations of the right ventricle and tricuspid valve. Br. Heart J. 37:386, 1975.

83. Hayden, J. G., Taler, N. S., and Klaus, S. M.: Cutis laxa associated with pulmonary artery stenosis. J. Pediatr. 72:506, 1968.

84. Hindle, W. V., Engle, M. A., and Hagstrom, J. W. C.: Anomalous right ventricular muscles: A clinicopathologic study. Am. J. Cardiol. 21:487, 1968.

85. Hoeffel, J. C., Ravault, M. C., Worms, A. M., and Pernot, C.: Atypical pulmonary stenosis: Radiological features. Am. Heart J. 98:315, 1979.

86. Hoffman, J. I. E., Rudolph, A. M., Nadas, A. S., and Gross, R. E.: Pulmonic stenosis, ventricular septal defect, and right ventricular pressure above systemic level. Circulation 22:405, 1960.

87. Holman, E.: On circumscribed dilatation of an artery immediately distal to a partially occluding band. Post-stenotic dilatation. Surgery 36:3, 1954.

88. Howitt, G.: Haemodynamic effects of exercise in pulmonary stenosis. Br. Heart J. 28:152, 1966.

89. Hultgren, H. N., Reeve, R., Cohn, K., and McLeod, R.: The ejection click of valvular pulmonic stenosis. Circulation 40:631, 1969.

90. Huntington, G. S.: The morphology of the pulmonary artery in the mammalian. Anat. Rec. 17:165, 1919.

91. Ikkos, D., Jonsson, B., and Linderholm, H.: Effect of exercise in pulmonary stenosis with intact ventricular septum. Br. Heart J. 28:316, 1966.

92. Jeffery, R. F., Moller, J. H., and Amplatz, K.: The dysplastic pulmonary valve: A new roentgenographic entity. Am. J. Roentgenol. Ther. Radium Nucl. Med. 114:322, 1972.

93. Johnson, A. M.: Hypertrophic infundibular stenosis complicating simple pulmonary valve stenosis. Br. Heart J. 21:429, 1959.

94. Jonson, L. W., Grossman, W., Dalen, J. E., and Dexter, L.: Pulmonic stenosis in the adult. Long-term follow-up results. N. Engl. J. Med. 387:1159, 1972.

95. Jonsson, B., and Lee, S. J. K.: Hemodynamic effects of exercise in isolated pulmonary stenosis before and after surgery. Br. Heart J. 30:60, 1968.

96. Jue, K. L., Noren, G. R., and Anderson, R.

C.: The syndrome of idiopathic hypercalcemia in infancy with associated heart disease. J. Pediatr. 47:1130, 1965.

97. Kaplan, S., and Adolph, R. J.: Pulmonic valve stenosis in adults. Cardiovasc. Clin. 10:327, 1979.

98. Keith, A.: The Hunterian Lectures on Malformations of the Heart. Lancet 2:359, 1909.

99. Keith, J. D., Rowe, R. D., and Vlad, P.: Heart Disease in Infancy and Childhood, 3rd ed. Macmillan, New York, 1978.

100. Klinge, T., and Laursen, H. B.: Familial pulmonary stenosis with underdeveloped or normal right ventricle. Br. Heart J. 37:60, 1974.

101. Koretzky, E. D., Moller, J. H., Korns, M. E., Schwartz, C. J., and Edwards, J. E.: Congenital pulmonary stenosis resulting from dysplasia of the valve. Circulation 60:43, 1969.

102. Korones, S. B., Ainger, L. E., Monif, G. R., Roane, J., Sever, J. L., and Fuste, F.: Congenital rubella syndrome: New clinical aspects with recovery of virus from affected infants. J. Pediatr. 67:166, 1965.

103. Krugman, S., and Katz, S. L.: Rubella immunization: A five-year progress report. N. Engl. J. Med. 290:1375, 1974.

104. Levin, D. L., Heymann, M. A., and Rudolph, A. M.: Morphological development of the pulmonary vascular bed in experimental pulmonic stenosis. Circulation 59:179, 1979.

105. Levine, R. O., and Blumenthal, S.: Pulmonic stenosis in five congenital cardiac defects. Circulation 31 and 32 (Suppl. III):33, 1965.

106. Lewis, J. M., Montero, A. G., Kinard, S. A., Jr., Dennis, E. W., and Alexander, J. K.: Hemodynamic response to exercise in isolated pulmonic stenosis. Circulation 29:854, 1964.

107. Li, M. D., Coles, J. C., and McDonald, A. C.: Anomalous muscle bundle of the right ventricle. Its recognition and surgical treatment. Br. Heart J. 40:1040, 1978.

108. Linde, L. M., Turner, S. W., and Sparkes, R. S.: Pulmonary valvular dysplasia: A cardiofacial syndrome. Br. Heart J. 35:301, 1973.

109. Lockhart, J. L., Reeve, H. R., Bredael, J. J., and Krueger, R. P.: Siblings with prune belly syndrome and associated pulmonic stenosis, mental retardation and deafness. Urology 14:140, 1979.

110. Lucas, R. V., Jr., Marshall, R. J., Morgan, D. Z., and Warden, H. E.: Anomalous muscle bundle of the right ventricle with intact ventricular septum: A newly recognized cause of right ventricular obstruction. Circulation 28:759, 1963.

111. Lueker, R. D., Vogel, J. H. K., and Blount, S. G., Jr.: Regression of valvular pulmonary stenosis. Br. Heart J. 32:779, 1970.

112. Luke, M. J.: Valvular pulmonic stenosis in infancy. J. Pediatr. 68:90, 1966.

113. Lynfield, J., Vichitbandha, P., Yao, A. C., Rodriguez-Torres, R., Karlson, K. E., and Kauffman, S.: Neonatal heart failure following rubella in utero. Am. J. Cardiol. 17:130, 1966.

114. Mangars. Rec. Period. Soc. Med. Paris, T.X., 1802, p. 74. Cited by E. Schwalbe in ref. 167, p. 427.

115. Maron, B. J., Ferrans, V. J., and White, R. J.: Unusual evolution of acquired infundibular stenosis in patients with ventricular septal defect. Clinical and morphologic observations. Circulation 48:1092, 1973.

116. McCarron, W. E., and Perloff, J. K.: Familial congenital valvular pulmonary stenosis. Am. Heart J. 88:397, 1974.

117. McCue, C. M., Robertson, L. W., Lester, R. G., and Mauck, H. P., Jr.: Pulmonary artery coarctations: A report of 20 cases with review of 319 cases from the literature. J. Pediatr. 67:222, 1965.

118. McGoon, D. C., and Kincaid, O. W.: Stenosis of branches of the pulmonary artery: Surgical repair. Med. Clin. North Am. 48:1083, 1964.

119. McIntosh, H. D., and Cohen, A. L.: Pulmonary stenosis: The importance of the myocardial factor in determining the clinical course and surgical results. Am. Heart J. 65:715, 1963.

120. Meckel, J. R. Handbuch der menschlichen Anatomie, Vol. 3, p. 59. Buchhandlung des Hallischen Waisenhauses, Berlin, 1817.

121. Mehl, S. J., Kaltman, A. J., Kronzon, J., Dworkin, L., Adams, P., and Spencer, F. C.: Combined tricuspid and pulmonic stenosis. Clinical, echocardiographic, hemodynamic, surgical and pathological features. J. Thorac. Cardiov. Surg. 74:55, 1977.

122. Mehra-Pour, M., Whitney, A., Liebman, J., and Borkat, G.: Quantification of the Frank and MacFee-Parungao orthogonal electrocardiogram in valvular pulmonic stenosis. Correlation with hemodynamic measurements. J. Electrocardiol. 12:69, 1979.

123. Michael, R. H., and Kenny, F. M.: Postnatal growth retardation in congenital rubella. Pediatrics 43:251, 1969.

124. Miettinen, O. S., and Rees, J. K. II. Methodology. Report from the Joint Study on the Natural History of Congenital Heart Disease. Circulation 56: (Suppl. 1) 1, 1977.

125. Miller, G. A. H., Restifo, M., Shinebourne, E. A., Paneth, M., Joseph, M. C., Lennox, S. C., and Kerr, I. H.: Pulmonary atresia with intact ventricular septum and critical pulmonary stenosis presenting in the first month of life. Investigation and surgical results. Br. Heart J. 35:9, 1973.

126. Mistrot, J., Neal, W., Lyons, G., Moller, J., Lucas, R., Castaneda, A., Varco, R., and Nicoloff, D.: Pulmonary valvotomy under inflow stasis for isolated pulmonary stenosis. Ann. Thorac. Surg. 21:30, 1976.

127. Modlin, J. F., Brandling-Bennett, A. D., Witte, J. J., Campbell, C. C., and Meyers, J. D.: A review of five years experience with rubella vaccine in the United States. Pediatrics 55:20, 1975.

128. Mody, M. R.: The natural history of uncomplicated valvular pulmonic stenosis. Am. Heart J. 90:317, 1975.

129. Mohr, R., Milo, S., Smolinsky, A., and Goor, D.: Right ventricular pressure drop 24 hours after open heart surgery for isolated pulmonary valve stenosis: The phenomenon and its surgical implication (abstr.). Circulation 64 (Suppl. IV):127, 1981.

130. Moller, J. H., and Adams, P., Jr.: The natural history of pulmonary valvular stenosis: Serial cardiac catheterizations in 21 children. Am. J. Cardiol. 16:654, 1965.

131. More, G. W., Hutchins, G. M., Brito, J. C., and Kang, H.: Congenital malformations of the semilunar valves. Hum. Pathol. 11:367, 1980.

132. Morgagni, J. B.: De sedibus et causis morborum (The seats and causes of diseases). Epist. 17:435, 1761. Translation by Benjamin Alexander, 1769.

133. Moss, A. J., Adams, F. H., Latta, H., O'Loughlin, B. J., and Longmire, W. P., Jr.: Congenital stenosis of the aortic and pulmonary valvular areas of the heart: Indications for early surgical relief. J. Dis. Child. 95:46, 1958.

134. Moss, A. J., and Quivers, W. W.: Use of isoproterenol in the evaluation of aortic and pulmonic stenosis. Am. J. Cardiol. 11:734, 1963.

135. Moulaert, A. J., Buis-Liem, T. N., Geldoff, W. C., and Rohmer, J.: The postvalvulotomy propranolol test to determine reversibility of the residual gradient in pulmonary stenosis. J. Thorac. Cardiovasc. Surg. 71:865, 1976.

136. Mudd, C. M., Walter, K. F., and Wilman, V. L.: Pulmonary artery stenosis: Diagnostic and therapeutic consideration. Am. J. Med. Sci. 249:125, 1965.

137. Mustard, W. T., Jain, S. C., and Trusler, G. A.: Pulmonary stenosis in the first year of life. Br. Heart J. 30:255, 1968.

138. Nadas, A.: Pulmonic stenosis. Indications for surgery in children and adults. Editorial. N. Engl. J. Med. 287:1196, 1972.

139. Nadas, A. S., and Fyler, D. C.: Pediatric Cardiology, 3rd. ed. W. B. Saunders, Philadelphia, 1972, p. 551.

140. Nakazawa, M., Marks, R. A., Isabel-Jones, J., and Jarmakani, J. M.: Right and left ventricular volume characteristics in children with pulmonary stenosis and intact ventricular septum. Circulation 53:884, 1976.

141. Neal, W. A., Lucas, R. V., Roa, S., and Moller, J. H.: Comparison of the hemodynamic effects of exercise and isoproterenol infusion in patients with pulmonary valve stenosis. Circulation 49:948, 1974.

142. Noonan, J. A.: Hypertelorism with Turner phenotype: A new syndrome with associated congenital heart disease. Am. J. Dis. Child. 116:373, 1968.

143. Nora, J. J., Torres, F. G., Sinha, A. K., and McNamara, D. G.: Characteristic cardiovascular anomalies of XO Turner's syndrome. XX and XY phenotype and XO/XX Turner mosaic. Am. J. Cardiol. 25:639, 1970.

144. Nora, J. J., Lortscher, R. H., and Spangler, R. D.: Echocardiographic studies of left ventricular disease in Ullrich-Noonan syndrome. Am. J. Dis. Child. 129:1417, 1975.

145. Nugent, E. W., Freedom, R. M., Nora, J. J., Ellison, R. C., Rowe, R. D., and Nadas, A. S.: Clinical course in pulmonic stenosis. Circulation 56 (Suppl. 1):15, 1977.

146. Oakley, C. M., Braimbridge, M. V., Bentall, H. H., and Cleland, W. P.: Reversed interatrial shunt following complete relief of pulmonary valve stenosis. Br. Heart J. 26:662, 1964.

147. Oka, M., and Angrist, G. M.: Mechanism of cardiac valvular fusion and stenosis. Am. Heart J. 74:37, 1967.

148. Orell, S. R., Karnell, J., and Wahlgren, F.: Malformation and multiple stenosis of the pulmonary arteries with pulmonary hypertension. Acta Radiol. 54:449, 1960.

149. Patterson, D. F., Haskins, M. E., Schnarr, W. R.: Hereditary dysplasia of the pulmonary valve in beagle dogs. Pathologic and genetic studies. Am. J. Cardiol. 47:631, 1981.

150. Perloff, J. K., and Lebauer, E. J.: Auscultatory and phonocardiographic manifestations of isolated stenosis of the pulmonary artery and its branches. Br. Heart J. 31:314, 1969.

151. Rao, P. S., Awa, S., and Linde, L. M.: Role of kinetic energy in pulmonary valve pressure gradients. Circulation 48:65, 1973.

152. Rao, P. S., Liebmann, J., and Brokat, G.: Right ventricular growth in a case of pulmonic stenosis with intact ventricular septum and hypoplastic right ventricle. Circulation 53:389, 1976.

153. Rawlings, N. S.: The "straightback" syndrome. A new cause of pseudo-heart disease. Am. J. Cardiol. 5:333, 1960.

154. Reid, J. M., Coleman, E. N., Stevenson, J. G., Inall, J. A., and Doig, W. B.: Long-term results of surgical treatment for pulmonary valve stenosis. Arch. Dis. Child. 51:79, 1976.

155. Riely, C. A., Labrecque, D. R., Ghent, C., Horwich, A., and Klatskin, G.: A father and son with cholestasis and peripheral pulmonic stenosis. J. Pediatr. 92:406, 1978.

156. Rios, J. C., Walsh, B. J., Massumi, R. A., Sims, A. J., and Ewy, G. A.: Congenital pulmonary branch stenosis. Am. J. Cardiol. 24:318, 1969.

157. Roberts, N., and Moes, C. A. F.: Supravalvular pulmonary stenosis. J. Pediatr. 82:838, 1973.

158. Roberts, W. C., Shemin, R. J., and Kent, K.

M.: Frequency and direction of interatrial shunting in valvular pulmonic stenosis with intact ventricular septum and without left ventricular inflow and outflow obstruction. An analysis of 127 cases treated by valvulotomy. Am Heart J. 99:142, 1980.

159. Rodbard, S., Ikeda, K., and Montes, M.: Mechanisms of poststenotic dilatation. Circulation 28:791, 1963.

160. Rosenfield, M. S., Kelley, M. J., Jensen, P. S., et al.: Radiology of arteriohepatic dysplasia. A.J.R. 135:1217, 1980.

161. Rowe, R. D.: Maternal rubella and pulmonary stenoses: Report of eleven cases. Pediatrics 32:180, 1963.

162. Rowe, R. D.: Cardiovascular disease in the rubella syndrome. Cardiovasc. Clin. 4:5, 1973.

163. Rowe, R. D., Freedom, R. M., Mehrizi, A., and Bloom, K. R.: The Neonate with Congenital Heart Disease, 2nd ed. W. B. Saunders, Philadelphia, 1981.

164. Rowland, T. W., Rosenthal, A., and Castaneda, A. R.: Double-chambered right ventricle. Experience with 17 cases. Am. Heart J. 89:455, 1974.

165. Rubella Symposium. Am. J. Dis. Child. 110:345, 1965.

166. Rudolph, A. M.: Congenital Diseases of the Heart. Yearbook Medical Publishers, Chicago, 1974.

167. Schwalbe, E.: Morphologie der Missbildungen. Pt. 3, p. 426. Cited by D'Cruz[37].

168. Scott, L. P., Hauck, A. J., and Nadas, A. S.: Endocardial cushion defect with pulmonic stenosis. Circulation 25:653, 1962.

169. Semb, B. K., Tjönneland, S., Stake, G., and Aabyholm, G.: "Balloon valvulotomy" of congenital pulmonary valve stenosis with tricuspid valve insufficiency. Cardiovasc. Radiol. 2:239, 1979.

170. Seymour, J., Emanuel, R., and Pattinson, N.: Acquired pulmonary stenosis. Br. Heart J. 30:776, 1968.

171. Shemin, R. J., Kent, K. M., and Roberts, W. C.: Syndrome of valvular pulmonary stenosis and valvular aortic stenosis with atrial septal defect. Br. Heart J. 42:442, 1979.

172. Siassi, B., Klyman, G., and Emmanouilides, G. C.: Hypoplasia of the abdominal aorta associated with the rubella syndrome. Am. Dis. Child. 20:476, 1970.

173. Slade, P. R.: Isolated infundibular stenosis. J. Thorac. Cardiov. Surg. 45:775, 1963.

174. Stone, F. M., Bessinger, F. B., Jr., Lucas, R. V., Jr., and Moller, J. H.: Pre- and post-operative rest and exercise hemodynamics in children with pulmonary stenosis. Circulation 49:1102, 1974.

175. Swan, H., Hederman, W. P., Vigoda, P. S., and Blount, S. G., Jr.: The surgical treatment of isolated infundibular stenosis. J. Thorac. Cardiovasc. Surg. 38:319, 1959.

176. Tang, J. S., Kauffman, S. L., and Lynfield, J.: Hypoplasia of the pulmonary arteries in infants with congenital rubella. Am. J. Cardiol. 27:491, 1971.

177. Taussig, H. B.: Congenital Malformations of the Heart, 2nd ed., vol. 2. The Commonwealth Fund, Harvard University Press, Cambridge, 1960.

178. Thrower, W. B., Abelmann, W. H., and Harken, D. E.: Surgical correction of coarctation of the main pulmonary artery. Circulation 21:672, 1960.

179. Tinker, J., Howitt, G., Markman, P., and Wade, E. G.: The natural history of isolated pulmonary stenosis. Br. Heart J. 27:151, 1965.

180. Tondury, G., and Smith, D. W.: Fetal rubella pathology. J. Pediatr. 48:867, 1966.

181. Trucone, N. J., Steeg, C. N., Dell, R., and Gersony, W. M.: Comparison of the cardiocirculatory effects of exercise and isoproterenol in children with pulmonary and aortic valve stenosis. Circulation 56:79, 1977.

182. Vancini, M., Roberts, K. D., Silove, E. D., and Singh, S. P.: Surgical treatment of congenital pulmonary stenosis due to dysplastic leaflets and small valve anulus. J. Thorac. Cardiovasc. Surg. 79:464, 1980.

183. Van Der Havwaert, L. G., and Michaelsson, M.: Isolated right ventricular hypoplasia. Circulation 45:466, 1971.

184. Van Der Havwaert, L. G., Fryns, J. P., Dumoulin, M., and Logghe, N.: Cardiovascular malformations in Turner's and Noonan's Syndrome. Br. Heart J. 40:500, 1978.

185. Vargheese, P. J., Izukawa, T., and Rowe, R. D.: Supravalvular aortic stenosis as part of rubella syndrome with discussion of pathogenesis. Arch. Dis. Child. 45:63, 1970.

186. Venables, A. W.: The syndrome of pulmonary stenosis complicating maternal rubella. Br. Heart J. 27:49, 1965.

187. Vernant, P., Corone, P., Rossignol, A. M., Bielman, C.: Etude de 120 observations de syndrome de Williams et Beuren. Arch. Mal. Coeur 73:661, 1980.

188. Viewez, W. V., Brodhead, C. L., Neil, D. J., and Folkerth, T. L.: Hodgkin's disease of the anterior mediastinum presenting as pulmonic stenosis. South. Med. J. 69:1094, 1976.

189. Vogelpoel, L., and Schrire, V.: Auscultatory and phonocardiographic assessment of pulmonary stenosis with intact ventricular septum. Circulation 22:55, 1960.

190. Warden, H. E., Lucas, R. V., and Varco, R.

L.: Right ventricular obstruction resulting from anomalous muscle bundles. J. Thorac. Cardiovasc. Surg. 41:53, 1966.

191. Wasserman, M. P., Vargheese, P. J., and Rowe, R. D.: The evolution of pulmonary arterial stenosis associated with congenital rubella. Am. Heart J. 76:638, 1968.

192. Watkins, L. J., Donahoo, J. S., Harrington, D., Haller, J. A., Jr., and Neill, C. A.: Surgical management of congenital pulmonary valve dysplasia. Ann. Thorac. Surg. 24:498, 1977.

193. Watson, H.: Paediatric Cardiology. C. V. Mosby, St. Louis, 1968.

194. Watson, H., and Lowe, K. G.: Ventricular pressure flow relationships in isolated valvular stenosis. Br. Heart J. 24:431, 1962.

195. Watson, H., McArthur, P., Somerville, J., and Ross, D.: Spontaneous evolution of ventricular septal defect into isolated pulmonary stenosis. Lancet 2:1225, 1969.

196. Weinstein, L., and Chang, T. W.: Prevention of rubella: Commentary. Pediatrics 55:5, 1975.

197. Wennevold, A., and Jacobsen, J. R.: Natural history of valvular pulmonary stenosis in children below the age of two years. Long-term follow-up with serial heart catheterizations. Eur. J. Cardiol. 8:371, 1978.

198. Weyman, A. E., Dillon, J. C., Feigenbaum, H., and Chang S.: Echocardiographic patterns of pulmonary valve motion in valvular pulmonic stenosis. Am. J. Cardiol. 34:644, 1974.

199. Weyman, A. E., Dillon, J. C., Feigenbaum, H., and Chang, S.: Echocardiographic differentiation of infundibular from valvular pulmonary stenosis. Am. J. Cardiol. 36:21, 1975.

200. Weyman, A. E., Hurwitz, R. A., Girod, D. A., Dillon, J. C., Feigenbaum, H., and Greene, D.: Cross-sectional echocardiographic visualization of the stenotic pulmonary valve. Circulation 56:769, 1977.

201. White, P. D., Hurst, J. W., and Fennell, R. H.: Survival to the age of seventy-five years with congenital pulmonary stenosis and patent foramen ovale. Circulation 2:558, 1950.

202. Williams, G. R., Richardson, W. R., Cayler, G. C., and Campbell, G. C.: Infundibular pulmonic stenosis with intact ventricular septum. Am. Surgeon 27:307, 1961.

203. Williams, J. C. P., Barratt-Boyes, B. G., and Lowe, J. B.: Underdeveloped right ventricle and pulmonary stenosis. Am. J. Cardiol. 11:458, 1963.

204. Wood, P.: Congenital pulmonary stenosis with left ventricular enlargement associated with atrial septal defect. Br. Heart J. 4:11, 1942.

18

Pulmonary Atresia with Intact Ventricular Septum

George C. Emmanouilides, M.D., Barry G. Baylen, M.D., and Ronald J. Nelson, M.D.

Pulmonary atresia with intact ventricular septum is a relatively rare cardiac malformation. It was first recognized in 1783, and it consists of complete atresia of the pulmonary valve associated with intact ventricular septum and varying degrees of hypoplasia of the right ventricle. Its frequency approximates 1% of all congenital cardiac anomalies.[4,35,55] There is no apparent sex predilection; however, males are slightly favored over females.[38]

PATHOLOGY

The mechanisms responsible for the development of this lesion are not known. Since pulmonary atresia can be considered an extreme form of pulmonic stenosis resulting in complete obstruction to the pulmonary outflow tract, its pathogenesis must be similar to that of pulmonic stenosis.

It has been postulated that pulmonary stenosis or atresia may be the result of fetal endocarditis caused by viral or other organisms.[56] The association between the rubella virus and pulmonary artery stenoses due to vasculitis is well established. It seems logical to assume that the insulting agent producing pulmonary atresia must be present much earlier than that which results in pulmonic stenosis.

In more than 80% of patients, the atresia involves the pulmonary valve (Fig. 18.1).[55] The pulmonary cusps are fused and form a diaphragm-like membrane with two or three discernible raphae. In the remaining 20% of patients there is combined infundibular and valvular atresia.[21,44,55] In the majority of instances, the pulmonary valve ring and main pulmonary trunk are hypoplastic (Fig. 18.2). The extreme narrowing or atresia of the infundibulum is due to hypertrophy of the right and left posterior muscle bundles attached to the pulmonary valve cusps.[1] In some instances there is only infundibular atresia, with the pulmonary valve being hypoplastic but not atretic. Occasionally, no valve structure is present, and the atresia involves the pulmonary trunk which becomes a cord-like structure up to the bifurcation.

There is a great variation in the size of the right ventricle, and a rather simple classification based on the right ventricular size has been proposed.[11,24,38] The two types described, one with a diminutive and the other with a large right ventricle, represent the two extremes of a spectrum.[11,50,67] There are, however, a number of intermediate forms of this lesion with normal or only slightly hypoplastic right ventricle. The right ventricle was found to be markedly hypoplastic in 50% of the cases reported by Van Praagh *et al.*,[67] whereas 10% had normal and 26% moderately hypoplastic ventricles. Thus, each case must be assessed individually, since there is obviously a continuum from the massively enlarged to the diminutive right ventricle.

In those cases with hypoplastic right ventricle, the ventricular cavity may be very small and the walls thickened. The endocardium is white, thickened, and has the appearance of fibroelastosis. The tricuspid valve is usually proportional to the size of the ventricle. The cusps may be hypoplastic, with short and thickened cordae tendineae resulting in varying degrees of tricuspid stenosis.[8,19,24,67,71] In cases with normal or dilated ventricles, secondary endocardial fibroelastosis is less commonly seen. The tricuspid valve is usually competent in those cases with normal right ventricular size and incompetent in those with dilated ventricles (Fig. 18.2). Ebstein's anomaly of the tricuspid valve is also associated with this malformation, resulting in massive cardiomegaly.[3,38,50,67] Very rarely, congenital absence of the tricuspid leaflets is seen.[33] In addition, in some instances, a very thin-walled right ventricle (Uhl's anomaly) also is described in association with pulmonary atresia and intact ventricular septum.[10,13]

A recent quantitative and morphologic study of the pulmonary arteries in a relatively large number of patients revealed marked hypoplasia of the right and left pulmonary arteries (0 to 3 mm) in 6 and 18%, respectively.[67] In 10% of the cases marked hypoplasia of the main pulmonary trunk was found.[67]

The right atrium is always dilated and reaches aneurysmal proportions when tricuspid insufficiency is present. There is always a patent foramen ovale or a true atrial septal defect (ASD). In the presence of a large foramen ovale, the left atrium, left ventricle, and aorta are slightly enlarged. The aortic arch is invariably left-sided. The aortic isthmus at birth does not show the usual reduction in diameter as compared with the ascending or descending aorta.[56] The ductus arteriosus (PDA) which provides the pulmonary flow may vary in size but usually is very small (Fig. 18.2). The medial wall of the muscular pulmonary arteries is apparently thinner than normal.[30,68]

In some instances, with hypoplastic or normal size right ventricle but competent tricuspid valve, there are communications between the right ventricular cavity and coronary circulation.[14,29,34,38,55,62,70] These represent ectatic sinusoidal channels which arise from the right ventricular trabeculae and connect with the coronary arteries (Fig. 18.3). These sinusoidal channels are kept open presumably by the high right ventricular pressure and allow egress of blood during systole from the completely obstructed right ventricle towards the systemic circulation, via the coronary arterial system (right-sided "circular" shunt).[21]

Patients with pulmonary atresia and intact ventricular septum have almost invariably visceroatrial situs solitus, a normal ventricular relationship, and a normal great vessel relationship. There is only one documented case of a pulmonary atresia with intact ventricular septum associated with corrected transposition of the great arteries.[63] A coexisting aortic stenosis has been reported rarely.[47]

PHYSIOLOGY

In the fetus, pulmonary atresia with intact ventricular septum is compatible with survival as long as an interatrial communication is present (Fig. 18.1). In spite of the complete

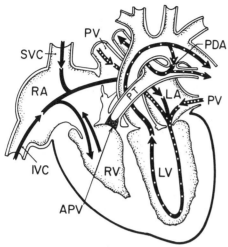

Fig. 18.1 Diagrammatic portrayal of the heart and the circulatory pathways in pulmonary atresia with intact ventricular septum. Note that the blood from the systemic veins enters the left atrium (*LA*) through a patent foramen ovale or an atrial septal defect; there it mixes with the blood coming from the pulmonary veins. The pulmonary flow is provided exclusively by the ductus arteriosus and/or the bronchial arteries. *APV*, atretic pulmonary valve; *IVC*, inferior vena cava; *LV*, left ventricle; *PDA*, patent ductus arteriosus; *PT*, pulmonary trunk; *RA*, right atrium; *RV*, right ventricle; *SVC*, superior vena cava.

obstruction to the right ventricular output and the resultant bypass of the pulmonary circulation, the fetus seems to tolerate this lesion well. The venous return from the superior and inferior vena cava bypasses the right ventricle, and through the foramen ovale or an ASD reaches the systemic circulation via the left chambers of the heart. The right ventricular output does not contribute to the effective cardiac output, except in cases where large sinusoidal communications exist with the coronary arteries.[21,27,50,62] The right ventricular output is proportional to the degree of tricuspid insufficiency or the size and extent of the sinusoidal communications with coronary arteries.

The circulatory pattern in pulmonary atresia resembles that of tricuspid atresia. The left ventricle provides the total fetal cardiac output which may be somewhat lower than that of the combined ventricular output in the normal fetus. The aorta and its isthmus are dilated since they receive the total cardiac output. The blood supply to the lungs, besides the bronchial circulation, is provided by the flow through the PDA from the aorta. The size of the PDA most likely determines the magnitude of pulmonary flow in utero and consequently the size of the pulmonary vascular tree. It appears that the smaller the PDA, the more hypoplastic are the pulmonary arteries. It has been postulated that in pulmonary atresia, in utero, the blood reaching the lungs has slightly higher PO_2 than that in normal circulation.[56] This may alter the development of the pulmonary circulation by producing less constriction of the pulmonary arterioles and thus less development of the medial layer of smooth muscle. Thus, the postnatal reduction of pulmonary vascular resistance may occur more rapidly in these patients.

The PDA is small and elongated, suggesting that the reduced flow through it may in turn influence its development. The size and patency of the PDA are of paramount

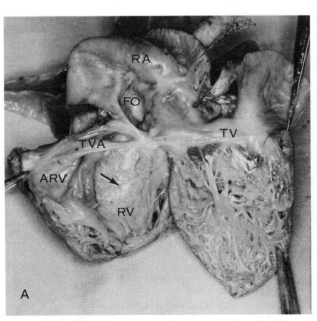

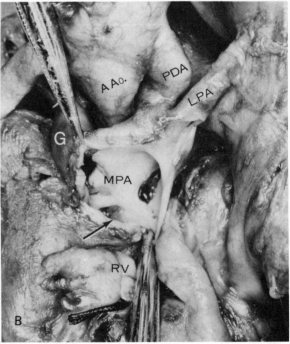

Fig. 18.2 (*A*) Photograph of the opened right ventricle (*RV*) and right atrium (*RA*) of a 4-day-old with pulmonary atresia and intact ventricular septum (type II). The right atrium and right ventricle are massively dilated, and there was Ebstein's anomaly of the tricuspid valve (*TV*). The posterior leaflet of the tricuspid valve is rudimentary and displaced inferiorly (*arrow*). *ARV*, atrialized right ventricular wall; *FO*, foramen ovale; *TVA*, tricuspid valve annulus. (*B*) Photograph of the opened right ventricle (*RV*) and main pulmonary artery (*MPA*) of the same patient. The pulmonary valve is atretic (*arrow*). The hypoplastic pulmonary artery was receiving blood from a patent ductus arteriosus (*PDA*) which is elongated and partially constricted at the pulmonary arterial junction. This patient underwent ascending aorta-main pulmonary artery anastomosis at 3 days of age using a 4 mm in diameter microporous expanded polytetrafluoroethylene arterial prosthesis (*G*).[26] *AAo.*, ascending aorta; *LPA*, left pulmonary artery.

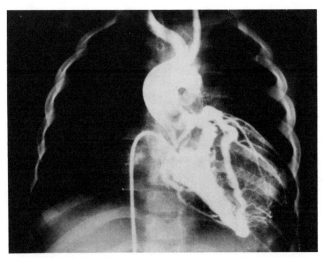

Fig. 18.3 Right ventriculogram. The right ventricular cavity is of near normal size. The pulmonary valve is atretic. Note the large sinusoidal communication between the right ventricle and the tortuous left anterior descending coronary artery. The aorta is filled via the large sinusoids from the right ventricle. Note also the minimal tricuspid regurgitation present. (Reproduced with permission from M. Quero Jimenez et al.[50])

importance for the postnatal survival of these infants. Immediately after birth there is a reduction of blood flow across the interatrial communication because of the elimination of the placental flow. The interatrial communication for a few weeks or months appears to be adequate. There is an obligatory complete admixture of systemic and pulmonary venous return in the left atrium, and as long as there is low pulmonary flow there is no impedance to flow from the right atrium (Fig. 18.1). However, as pulmonary flow increases, left atrial pressure may increase and thus impede the flow from the right atrium. Under these circumstances, in order to maintain the flow of systemic venous return to the left atrium, a higher right atrial pressure must be generated.

The degree of postnatal hypoxemia in these patients depends upon the magnitude of the pulmonary flow which, in turn, depends on the size of the PDA. Since the ductus arteriosus is relatively hypoplastic in the majority of these patients and it appears to constrict with the increase in arterial PO_2, it soon becomes inadequate to maintain pulmonary blood flow. A profound hypoxemia and tissue hypoxia may result. As hypoxia ensues, some relaxation of the ductal tissue may occur, permitting more blood to enter the pulmonary circulation. Thus, a fine balance between pulmonary flow, ductus constriction, and systemic hypoxemia may exist in these patients.

MANIFESTATIONS

Clinical Features

Infants with pulmonary atresia and intact ventricular septum may appear normal immediately after birth. However, they soon become cyanotic and tachypneic. The degree of cyanosis depends upon the magnitude of pulmonary blood flow. As the cyanosis becomes more severe, metabolic acidosis due to hypoxemia may develop, and the respirations become deep and labored. Cyanosis is invariably present in both groups of patients, those with hypoplastic and those with normal or dilated right ventricles. Signs of heart failure such as hepatomegaly, peripheral edema, and apical gallop, may be present at the first examination. These signs are

seen more frequently in patients with a large right ventricle and tricuspid insufficiency.[8, 19, 59]

Heart murmurs may not be present initially in infants with competent tricuspid valve and hypoplastic right ventricle. Soft systolic or continuous murmurs may be heard subsequently, due to flow across the PDA. Short, nonspecific systolic murmurs may also be heard at the upper or lower left sternal border, thought to be either ductal or tricuspid in origin. In patients with a large right ventricle and tricuspid insufficiency, holosystolic murmurs and thrills are usually present and the second sound is single. Diastolic sounds or murmur may also be heard in cases with large right ventricle and tricuspid insufficiency due to malformation of the tricuspid valve (Fig. 18.4).

Electrocardiographic Features

The electrocardiographic findings are not typical and vary according to the size and thickness of the right ventricle.[25, 34, 55] The PR interval is usually normal, and there is always evidence of right atrial enlargement, especially after the first few weeks of life. Occasionally left atrial enlargement is present manifested as notched broad P waves in leads II or terminal inversion in the right precordial leads.

The QRS mean frontal axis may be normal or rightward. It is rare that the QRS axis is less than zero. Normal or, rarely, left QRS frontal axis is present in cases with marked hypoplasia of the right ventricle. In these cases, the anterior forces are not as prominent as are those with larger right ventricles. However, the main feature of the electrocardiogram is the relative dominance of the left ventricular forces. Infants with large right ventricles usually may show evidence of right ventricular hypertrophy with or without associated left ventricular hypertrophy (Fig. 18.4). A qR pattern in the right precordial leads is present in these cases and occasionally is seen in cases with hypoplastic but markedly thickened right ventricle with secondary endocardial fibroelastosis. The left ventricular dominance is characteristic of tricuspid atresia as well. However, the presence of normal or rightward QRS axis in pulmonary atresia with intact ventricular septum may distinguish this lesion electrocardiographically from tricuspid atresia. Equivocal or normal electrocardiographic tracings may also be seen occasionally.

As the infants grow, progressive changes in the electrocardiogram may occur. The degree of right axis deviation, right atrial dilatation, and right ventricular hypertrophy appear to increase. In addition, neonates with normal tracings or tracings showing left ventricular hypertrophy may acquire signs of right ventricular loading in subsequent recordings.

Radiologic Features

In half of the cases the chest roentgenograms, if taken the first 2 or 3 days of life, may appear normal. However, moderate or marked cardiomegaly may be present at birth, especially in those instances with massive tricuspid insufficiency and signs of right ventricular failure.[14, 34, 35, 55] This massive cardiomegaly occurs in utero as a consequence of tricuspid insufficiency and right ventricular and atrial dilatation (Fig. 18.5). The only two other conditions that present with such cardiomegaly at birth are severe forms of Ebstein's anomaly or isolated tricuspid insufficiency with or without congenital thinning of the right ventricular wall (Uhl's anomaly).[10] A mediastinal teratoma may occasionally present with such a roentgenographic picture.[14] The pulmonary vascular markings are usually reduced. The right atrium is prominent as well as the left ventricle. There is almost always a left aortic arch present. The presence of right aortic arch associated with pulmonary atresia should lead to the suspicion

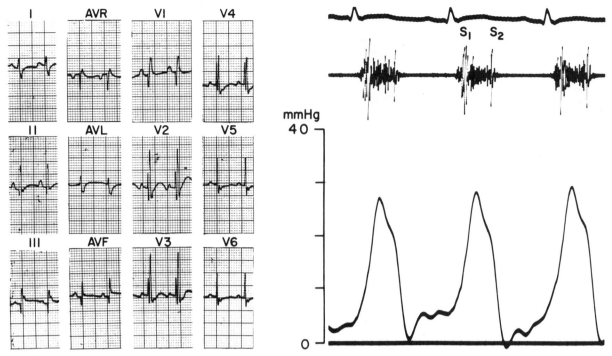

Fig. 18.4 Electrocardiogram, phonocardiogram, and right ventricular pressures in the same infant as in Figure 18.2, obtained at 2 days of age. Note the QRS frontal axis (100°) and the rsR' in *V1* and rsr's' in *V2, V3, V5*, findings compatible with Ebstein's anomaly. The holosystolic murmur was recorded at the left lower sternal border and is due to tricuspid insufficiency. The second sound is single (S_2). The right ventricular pressure is not elevated as it is usually in cases of pulmonary atresia with intact ventricular septum and competent tricuspid valve.

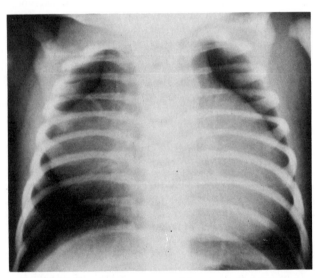

Fig. 18.5 Chest roentgenogram of the same infant as in Figures 18.2 and 18.4, showing massive cardiomegaly and decreased pulmonary vascular markings. The cardiomegaly is due to massively dilated right atrium and right ventricle. This picture may also be seen in newborns with severe Ebstein's anomaly without pulmonary atresia, as well as in severe cases of isolated congenital tricuspid insufficiency.

of tetralogy of Fallot with pulmonary atresia or more complex cardiac malformations associated with visceral heterotaxia.[55]

Echocardiographic Features

The M-mode echocardiogram is useful in defining the size of the right ventricle and the thickness of its wall. The degree of hypoplasia or dilatation of the right ventricle can be easily determined. The atretic pulmonary valve membrane, if of adequate size, can be recorded on the M-mode and can resemble an opening valve with a deep "a" wave.[39, 64]

Two-dimensional (2D) echocardiography usually will demonstrate the atretic pulmonary valve together with other characteristics of the right ventricular cavity and tricuspid valve. The hypoplastic main pulmonary artery and its branches also may be visualized. The echocardiographic evaluation of the tricuspid valve is very important in determining the degree of right ventricular hypoplasia. In certain instances of tricuspid atresia, the M-mode echocardiogram may falsely suggest the presence of a patent tricuspid valve by tracking the moving atrioventricular diaphragm. This can be easily clarified by the 2D echocardiogram which will usually detect the diaphragm or demonstrate the open, although stenotic, tricuspid valve.[24, 45, 55] The atrial septum also can be visualized, and an estimate of the size of the foramen ovale or ASD can frequently be made. When a restrictive interatrial communication is present, varying degrees of bulging of the atrial septum can be identified by 2D echocardiography.[58]

CARDIAC CATHETERIZATION

When pulmonary atresia is suspected in a cyanotic neonate, cardiac catheterization and angiocardiography are indicated for establishing the diagnosis. Accurate diagnosis is very important, not only for its prognostic value but for its implications regarding surgical treatment. After stabilization of the infant's condition following his transfer to the cardiac center, cardiac catheterization should be performed on an emergency basis. This is because the infant's survival depends on the patency of the ductus arteriosus, and deterioration of his condition may rapidly take place within a few hours.

In the newborn infant, an umbilical arterial catheter should be placed in the aorta for monitoring blood gases, pH, and blood glucose. If the PO_2 is markedly decreased and there is acidosis and/or hypoglycemia, alkali and glucose should be administered during the preparation for cardiac catheterization. The use of continuous infusion of prostaglandin E_2 for the maintenance of patency of the ductus arteriosus has changed considerably the approach in managing these very cyanotic, sometimes moribund infants. Within a few minutes a dramatic improvement in the oxygenation of the infant can be accomplished, and subsequent cardiac catheterization and angiocardiographic studies can be performed with less risk and greater safety.[7, 20, 31, 46]

Cardiac catheterization can be accomplished via the umbilical vessels during the first week of life and should be tried first.[40] The previously placed umbilical arterial catheter can be easily exchanged by a new one, and an aortogram can be obtained in order to delineate the size of the PDA and the pulmonary arteries. Right heart catheterization can be accomplished also using the umbilical vein by traversing the ductus venosus. However, the ductus venosus is not always patent. In order to establish its patency, a test injection of 0.5 to 1.0 ml of contrast material in the portal sinus is performed, and if the structure is closed, we proceed with a cutdown or percutaneous technique using the right femoral vein. The catheter is easily passed from the right atrium to the left atrium and left ventricle in a similar manner as it does in cases of tricuspid atresia. The right ventricle, when extremely hypoplastic, is difficult to enter. Inability to enter the right ventricle from the right atrium is usually a sign of tricuspid atresia. When the catheter enters the right ventricle, a selective angiocardiogram is usually obtained.

The mean right atrial pressure is usually elevated, and there are prominent "a" waves. In contrast, the left atrial "v" waves are not prominent because of the reduced pulmonary venous return. The "a" and "v" waves in the left atrium are equal, and the mean pressure is always 2 to 3 mm Hg less than that of the right atrium. The right ventricular systolic pressure is markedly elevated above systemic levels and may reach 120 to 150 mm Hg. The left ventricular pressure is usually normal. The contour of the right ventricular pressure tracing is triangular, characteristic of right ventricular outflow obstruction. The right ventricular end-diastolic pressure may also be elevated to levels up to 10 to 15 mm Hg. In cases with a dilated right ventricle and tricuspid insufficiency or associated Ebstein's anomaly, the right ventricular pressure may be only moderately elevated (Fig. 18.4). The pulmonary artery can be entered only through the PDA from the aorta. However, this procedure is not recommended because of the danger of completely obstructing the narrow PDA and inducing severe hypoxemia and acidosis. The pulmonary arterial pressure when measured is always lower than that of the systemic pressure. The presence of a continuous murmur is evidence of lower pulmonary artery pressure.

The systemic venous saturation is decreased and may be as low as 30%, with the PO_2 as low as 15 mm Hg. The right atrial and ventricular oxygen saturations are similar to those of the inferior and superior vena cava. The degree of systemic arterial undersaturation depends upon the magnitude of the pulmonary flow. Due to the streaming of the blood shunted from the right atrium and incomplete mixing, the left atrial oxygen saturation may be lower than that of the left ventricle. The pulmonary venous saturation is usually normal and, if the infant receives 100% oxygen, the systemic arterial PO_2 may be as low as 20 to 25 mm Hg and as high as 35 to 40 mm Hg. If oxygenation of the tissues is adequate, arterial pH is normal, but with severe degrees of hypoxemia it may

decrease to as low as 7.0. However, with the use of prostaglandin E_2, these severe degrees of hypoxemia and acidosis can be easily avoided.

ANGIOCARDIOGRAPHY

Selective angiocardiography is essential in establishing the diagnosis and providing detailed information regarding the size of the right ventricle and of the pulmonary arteries. This can be accomplished by a right and left ventricular injection. If, however, the pulmonary arteries cannot be well delineated by a left ventricular injection, an aortogram should be performed with the retrograde arterial catheter tip near the entrance of the PDA (Fig. 18.6).

The size of the right ventricle may be variable, and the tricuspid valve may be hypoplastic or incompetent (Fig. 18.7). Usually a hypoplastic outflow tract is present which ends blindly at the level of the atretic pulmonary valve (Fig. 18.7). The pulmonary valve ring is usually narrow, and no contrast material enters the pulmonary artery. A simultaneous opacification of the pulmonary artery via the PDA using a retrograde arterial catheter and the right ventricle by a venous catheter has been used successfully to evaluate patients with pulmonary atresia and intact ventricular septum.[22] This double catheter technique allows precise localization of the atresia, whether valvular, infundibular, or both, and at the same time provides information about the size of the pulmonary trunk if present and its main branches. In a few instances the right ventricular infundibulum is atretic also, so there is a considerable distance between the right ventricular cavity and pulmonary artery, a very important finding regarding the surgical management of the infant.

In many patients, usually in those with a relatively competent tricuspid valve, large coronary sinusoids are filled

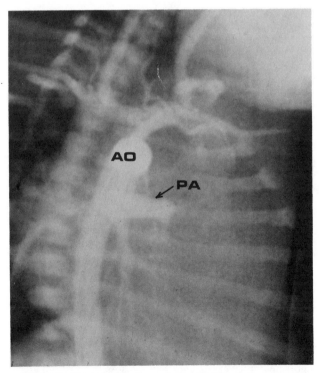

Fig. 18.6 Frame from a cineaortogram obtained via a retrograde umbilical arterial catheter in the same infant as in Figures 18.2, 18.4, and 18.5. The patient is in right anterior oblique position. Note the hypoplastic pulmonary artery (*PA*) filling from the aorta (*AO*) via a patent ductus arteriosus (visualized well in the left anterior oblique position). The pulmonary valve is atretic.

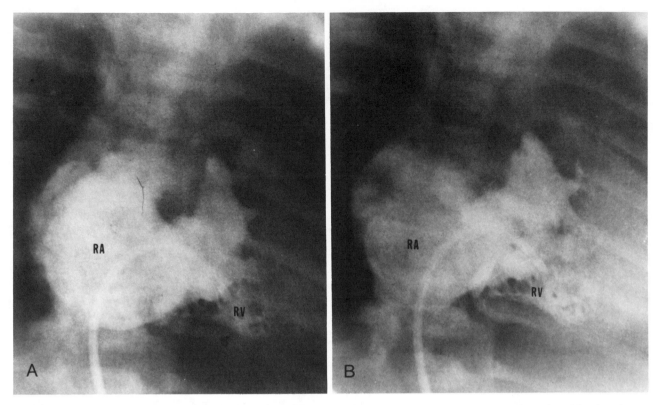

Fig. 18.7 Anteroposterior view. Systolic (*A*) and diastolic (*B*) cine frames from a right ventriculogram of a 3-day-old with pulmonary atresia and intact ventricular septum. Note the atretic right ventricular outflow tract, the massive tricuspid insufficiency, the near normal sized right ventricle, and the huge right atrium. The hypoplastic pulmonary artery (not shown here) opacified from the aorta via a small ductus arteriosus. *RA*, right atrium; *RV*, right ventricle.

during systole from the right ventricle communicating with the coronary arteries. These right ventricular coronary artery anastomoses may become quite large and empty, in part, into the ascending aorta or coronary sinus (Fig. 18.3). In cases of enormous dilatation of the right atrium and right ventricle, the contrast medium may be so diluted that the anatomy of the right ventricle and pulmonary valve may be obscured. In such cases, in order to demonstrate the presence of pulmonary atresia, it may be necessary to inject selectively into the infundibulum of the right ventricle. Venous or selective right atrial angiocardiography alone is not recommended because the small right ventricle may be bypassed by the contrast material which readily enters the left atrium and left ventricle. These findings may lead to an incorrect diagnosis of tricuspid atresia.

DIFFERENTIAL DIAGNOSIS

The diagnosis of pulmonary atresia with intact ventricular septum may be suspected in infants who develop cyanosis immediately after birth and have the following associated findings: reduced pulmonary vascular markings in the chest roentgenogram; left ventricular dominance in the electrocardiogram with normal or right QRS axis and/or associated right ventricular hypertrophy; a systolic murmur may or may not be present.

There are several complex cyanotic cardiac lesions which may show left ventricular dominance in the electrocardiogram. These include tricuspid atresia with or without transposition of the great arteries, persistent truncus arteriosus, severe pulmonic stenosis with intact ventricular septum, common ventricle and simple D-transposition of the great

arteries. Some of these entities may be differentiated by the presence of increased pulmonary flow and prominent pulmonary arteries. Both M-mode and 2D echocardiography are found to be very useful in differentiating many of the simple and complex forms of cyanotic congenital heart disease from pulmonary atresia and intact ventricular septum. However, for definitive diagnosis, cardiac catheterization and angiocardiography are necessary.

TREATMENT

The majority of these infants need immediate and special attention because of their severe progressive hypoxemia. Oxygen administration, anticongestive measures, and correction of acid-base disturbances may be helpful on a temporary basis. The survival of these infants depends entirely on our ability to help them increase their pulmonary flow, either medically or surgically.

Immediate improvement in oxygenation may be accomplished by the use of E-type prostaglandins.[7, 20, 31, 46] This biologically active peptide apparently results in ductal smooth muscle relaxation, thus maintaining continuous patency of the ductus arteriosus and securing increased pulmonary flow. This medical manipulation of the ductus arteriosus usually allows these very ill infants to improve and to stabilize so surgical intervention may be deferred for several hours or days. The drug can be administered parenterally either via the umbilical artery or peripheral vein. Recently an oral preparation of prostaglandin E_2 has been used in a small number of newborns with ductus-dependent pulmonary flow with considerable success and without major complications.[61]

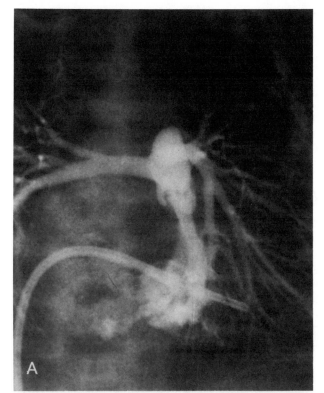

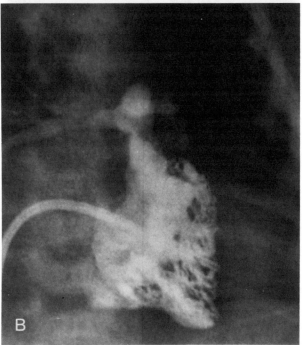

Fig. 18.8 Anteroposterior view. Systolic (*A*) and diastolic (*B*) cine frames from a right ventriculogram obtained 4 weeks after closed pulmonary valvotomy of the patient shown in Figure 18.7. Note the almost normal sized right ventricle, the enlargement of the right ventricular outflow tract, and the pulmonary valve annulus. Only small tricuspid insufficiency is present. The pulmonary arteries are only moderately hypoplastic, and the pulmonary valve appears to be thickened. The right ventricular pressure from preoperative systemic levels dropped to $^{30}/_{5}$ mm Hg postoperatively. At 1 year of age, the infant was asymptomatic, acyanotic, with normal electrocardiogram and chest roentgenogram.

The surgical therapy of these infants aims at increasing the pulmonary flow. This can be accomplished either by pulmonary valvotomy, creation of an aortopulmonary shunt, or both.[2, 4, 12, 16–18, 26, 27, 36, 37, 41, 43, 45, 48, 52, 54, 65, 66, 69] A successful pulmonary valvotomy by relieving the obstruction may result in gradual enlargement and growth of the right ventricle.[4, 16, 28, 36, 41, 48, 51]

During cardiac catheterization, it is essential to arrive at a conclusion about the type of surgical procedure needed to alleviate the patient's condition. In the presence of an extremely hypoplastic right ventricle and markedly hypoplastic or atretic infundibulum, the creation of a systemic arterial shunt is recommended.[36, 57, 66] In these cases, it is advisable that a balloon atrial septostomy be performed at the end of cardiac catheterization. This is done in order to ensure a wide patency of the formen ovale and prevent partial closure of the valve of the foramen by the increased pulmonary venous return resulting from the anastomotic procedure.[51]

Pulmonary valvotomy alone is recommended when the right ventricular cavity is of normal or near normal size in spite of the presence of tricuspid insufficiency. The valvotomy can be performed by using closed or open techniques, depending upon the anatomy and the preference of the surgeon.[4, 16, 52] If the anatomy is ideal, i.e., the pulmonary valve annulus is not very hypoplastic and pulmonary arteries are not markedly hypoplastic, an excellent surgical result can be achieved (Figs. 18.7 and 18.8). The use of prostaglandin E₂ postoperatively for several days may obviate the need for an additional aortopulmonary shunting procedure. By pharmacologically maintaining the patency of the ductus arteriosus for a few days, an adaptation of the right ventricle occurs so its forward flow progressively increases to a point where there is no need for the additional (ductus arteriosus or surgical shunt) derived pulmonary flow.

However, between the two extremes, there is a large number of infants in whom valvotomy alone is not as successful, and there is a need for a systemic to pulmonary artery surgical shunt.[3, 18, 63] The systemic to pulmonary artery shunts used include: the Blalock-Taussig shunt, the Potts anastomosis, and the Waterston-Cooley shunt. The selection of the particular procedure depends upon the age of the patient and the size of the pulmonary artery. Recently, direct ascending aorta to main pulmonary artery or subclavian to right or left pulmonary artery anastomosis, using a polytetrafluroethylene prosthetic graft, has been performed with excellent results.[12, 26, 37] It appears that such a technique may replace the Blalock-Taussig shunt and avoid the sacrifice of the subclavian artery.[12] Occasionally, as an alternative to shunt procedures, formalin infiltration of the adventitia of the ductus arteriosus was used in order to maintain patency of the ductus.[57] This palliative approach at present is seldom recommended.

With accurate preoperative anatomic evaluation of each case and the appropriate surgical procedure, in conjunction with the pre-, intra-, and postoperative use of the E-type prostaglandins, a number of these infants may survive and some may reach normal hemodynamics.[16, 36, 45, 48, 52, 66, 69]

PROGNOSIS

Without surgical palliation or correction, the prognosis for these infants is dismal. Although some may survive for a few months, survival beyond a year of age is exceptional.[5, 53] With aggressive surgical intervention, in spite of a relatively high immediate surgical mortality, a number of these patients may be helped because of the potential of further growth of the right ventricle and the pulmonary arterial tree. Future improvements in the surgical techniques and in the intra- and postoperative management may result in further increases in survival of these infants.

Infants with the smallest, hypoplastic, thick right ventricles do not show adequate growth of their ventricle, even after successful pulmonary valvotomy. It is possible that some of these infants who survived palliative systemic pulmonary shunts and have adequate size pulmonary arteries may become candidates for a right ventricular bypass operation (Fontan procedure). Infants with very large, dilated, thin walled, right ventricles and massive tricuspid insufficiency have the worst prognosis and seldom survive a few days to a few weeks of life with or without palliative surgery.

However, in those infants with normal or moderately hypoplastic right ventricles who survive surgery, the prognosis depends to a great extent upon the growth potential of the right ventricle. These patients should be recatheterized within a few months in order to assess the size of the right ventricle and its outflow tract, the status of the tricuspid valve, and the sinusoidal-coronary artery communications, as well as the ASD and the pulmonary arteries. If there still is an obstruction in the outflow tract, its relief by reconstruction is recommended. By relieving the existing right ventricular hypertension, it is possible that right ventricular growth can be promoted, and obliteration of the sinusoidal-coronary artery communications can ensue.[36, 45, 48]

REFERENCES

1. Arom, K. V., and Edwards, J. E.: Relationship between right ventricular muscle bundles and pulmonary valve. Significance in pulmonary atresia with intact ventricular septum. Circulation 54 (Suppl. 3):79, 1976.
2. Aziz, K. U., Olley, P. M., Rowe, R. D., Trusler, G. A., and Mustard, W. T.: Survival after systemic to pulmonary arterial shunts in infants less than 30 days old with obstructive lesions of the right heart chambers. Am. J. Cardiol. 36:479, 1975.
3. Benton, J. W., Jr., Elliott, L. P., Adams, P., Jr., Anderson, R. C., Hong, C. V., and Lester, R. G.: Pulmonary atresia and stenosis with intact ventricular septum. Am. J. Dis. Child. 104:161, 1962.
4. Bowman, F. O., Malm, J. R., Hayer, C. J., Gersony, W. M., and Ellis, K.: Pulmonary atresia with intact ventricular septum. J. Thorac. Cardiovasc. Surg. 37:124, 1976.
5. Buckley, L. P., Dooley, K. J., and Fyler, D. C.: Pulmonary atresia and intact ventricular septum in New England (abstr.). Am. J. Cardiol. 37:124, 1976.
6. Campbell, M.: Results of surgical treatment for pulmonary atresia. Br. Heart J. 22:527, 1960.
7. Cocceani, F., and Olley, P.: The response of the ductus arteriosus to prostaglandins. Can. J. Physiol. Pharmacol. 51:980, 1973.
8. Cole, R. B., Muster, A. J., Lev, M., and Paul, M. H.: Pulmonary atresia with intact ventricular septum. Am. J. Cardiol. 21:23, 1968.
9. Costa, A.: Atresia congenita dell'ostio della pulmonare, con setto interventriculare chiuso e dotto de Bottalo persistente in uomo de 20 anni. Clin. Med. Ital. 61:567, 1930.
10. Cote, M., Davignon, A., and Fouron, J. C.: Congenital hypoplasia of right ventricular myocardium (Uhl's anomaly) associated with pulmonary atresia in a newborn. Am. J. Cardiol. 31:658, 1973.
11. Davignon, A. L., Greenwold, W. E., DuShane, J. W., and Edwards, J. E.: Congenital pulmonary atresia with intact ventricular septum. Clinico-pathologic correlation of two anatomic types. Am. Heart J. 62:591, 1961.
12. de Leval, M. R., McKay, R., Jones, M., Stark, J., and Macartney, F. J.: Modified Blalock-Taussig shunt. Use of subclavian artery orifice as flow regulator in prosthetic systemic-pulmonary artery shunts. J. Thorac. Cardiovasc. Surg. 81:112, 1981.
13. Descalzo, A., Canadas, M., Cintado, C., Castillo, J. Q., Garcia, E., and Ariza, S.: Uhl's anomaly associated with pulmonary atresia. Hum. Pathol. 11(Suppl.):375, 1980.
14. Desilets, D. T., Marcano, B. A., Emmanouilides, G. C., and Gypes, M. T.: Severe pulmonary valve stenosis and atresia. Radiol. Clin. North Am. 6:367, 1968.
15. Dhanavaravibul, S., Nora, J. J., and McNamara, D. G.: Pulmonary valvular atresia with intact ventricular septum: Problems in diagnosis and results of treatment. J. Pediatr. 77:1010, 1970.
16. Dobell, A. R., and Grignon, A.: Early and late results of pulmonary atresia. Ann. Thorac. Surg. 24:264, 1977.
17. Donahoo, J. S., Gardner, T. J., Zahka, K., and Kidd, B. S.: Systemic-pulmonary shunts in neonates and infants using microporous expanded polytetrafluoroethylene: Immediate and late results. Ann. Thorac. Surg. 30:146, 1980.
18. Edmunds, L. H. Jr., Fishman, N. H., Heymann, M. A., and Rudolph, A. M.: Anastomosis between aorta and right pulmonary artery (Waterston) in neonates. N. Engl. J. Med. 284:464, 1971.
19. Elliott, L. P., Adams, P., Jr., and Edwards, J. E.: Pulmonary atresia with intact ventricular septum. Br. Heart J. 25:489, 1963.
20. Elliott, R. B., Starling, M. B., and Neutze, J. M.: Medical manipulation of the ductus arteriosus. Lancet 1:140, 1975.
21. Freedom, R. M., and Harrington, D. D.: Contributions of intramyocardial sinusoids in pulmonary atresia and intact ventricular septum to a right-sided circular shunt. Br. Heart J. 36:1061, 1974.
22. Freedom, R. M., White, R. I., Jr., Ho, C. S., Gingell, R. L., Hawker, R. E., and Rowe, R. D.: Evaluation of patients with pulmonary atresia and intact ventricular septum by double catheter technique. Am. J. Cardiol. 33:892, 1974.
23. Freedom, R. M., Culham, G., Moes, F., Olley, P. M., and Rowe, R. D.: Differentiation of functional and structural pulmonary atresia: Role of aortography. Am. J. Cardiol. 41:914, 1978.
24. Freedom, R. M., Dische, M. R., and Rowe, R. D.: The tricuspid valve in pulmonary atresia and intact ventricular septum: A morphological study of 60 cases. Arch. Pathol. Lab. Med. 102:28, 1978.
25. Gamboa, R., Gersony, W. M., and Nadas, A. S.: The electrocardiogram in tricuspid atresia and pulmonary atresia with intact ventricular septum. Circulation 34:24, 1966.
26. Gazzaniga, A. E., Lamberti, J. J., Stewers, R. D., Sperling, D. R., Dietrick, W. R., Arcilla, R. A., and Replogle, R. L.: Microporous expanded polytetrafluoroethylene arterial prosthesis for construction of aorto-pulmonary shunts. J. Thorac. Cardiovasc. Surg. 72:357, 1976.
27. Gersony, W. M., Bernhard, W. F., Nadas, A. S., and Gross, R. E.: Diagnosis and surgical treatment of infants with critical pulmonary outflow obstruction. Circulation 34:765, 1967.
28. Graham, T. P., Jr., Bender, H. W., Atwood, G. F., Page, D. L., and Sell, C. G. R.: Increase in right ventricular volume following valvulotomy for pulmonary atresia or stenosis with intact ventricular septum. Circulation 49 and 50(Suppl. II):69, 1974.
29. Grant, R. G.: Unusual anomaly of coronary vessels in malformed heart of child. Heart 13:396, 1926.
30. Haworth, S. G., Sauer, U., and Buhlmeyer, K.: Effect of prostaglandin E₁ on pulmonary circulation in pulmonary atresia. A quantitative morphometric study. Br. Heart J. 43:306, 1980.
31. Heymann, M. A., and Rudolph, A. M.: Ductus arteriosus dilatation by prostaglandin E in infants with pulmonary atresia. Pediatrics 59:325, 1977.
32. Hunter, J. M.: Observations and Enquiries 6:291, 1783. Cited by Peacock (49).
33. Kanjuh, V. I., Stevenson, J. E., Amplatz, K., and Edwards, J. E.: Congenitally unguarded tricuspid orifice with coexistent pulmonary atresia. Circulation 30:911, 1964.
34. Keith, J. D., Rowe, R. D., and Vlad, P.: Heart Disease in Infancy and Childhood, 3rd ed. Macmillan, New York, 1978.
35. Kiefer, S. A., and Lewis, S. C.: Radiological aspects of pulmonary atresia with intact ventricular septum. Br. Heart J. 25:655, 1963.
36. Laks, H., Hellenbrand, W., Stansel, H. C., Pennell, R., Kleinman, C., Lister, G., Kopf, G., and Talner, N.: Improved results in the treatment of pulmonary atresia with intact ventricular septum (abstr.). Circulation 64 (Suppl. 4):IV 30, 1981.
37. Lamberti, J. J., Campbell, C., Replogle, R. L., Anagnostopoulos, C., Lin, C. Y., Chiemmonskoltip, P., and Arcilla, R.: The prosthetic (Teflon) central aorto-pulmonary shunt for cyanotic infants less than three weeks old: Results and long term follow-up. Ann. Thorac. Surg. 28:568, 1979.
38. Lauer, R. M., Fink, H., Petry, E. L., Dunn, M. I., and Diehl, A. M.: Angiographic demonstration of intramyocardial sinusoids in pulmonary atresia with intact ventricular septum. N. Engl. J. Med. 271:68, 1964.
39. Lewis, B. S., Amitai, N., Simcha, A., Merin, G., and Gotsman, M. S.: Echocardiographic diagnosis of pulmonary atresia with intact ventricular septum. Am. Heart J. 97:92, 1979.
40. Linde, L. M., Higashino, S. M., Berman, G., Sapin, S. O., and Emmanouilides, G. C.: Umbilical vessel cardiac catheterization and angiocardiography. Circulation 34:984, 1966.
41. Luckstead, E. G., Mattioli, L., Grossly, I. K., et al.: Two-stage palliative surgical approach for pulmonary atresia with intact septum (Type I). Am. J. Cardiol. 29:490, 1972.
42. Mangiardi, J. L., Sullivan, J. J., Bifulco, E., and Lukash, L.: Congenital tricuspid stenosis with pulmonary atresia. Am. J. Cardiol. 11:726, 1963.
43. Moller, J. H., Girod, D., Amplatz, K., and Varco, R.: Pulmonary valvotomy in pulmonary atresia with hypoplastic right ventricle. Surgery 58:630, 1970.
44. Morgan, B. C., Stacy, G. S., and Dillard, D. H.: Pulmonary valvular and infundibular atresia with intact ventricular septum. Am. J. Cardiol. 16:746, 1965.

45. Moulton, A. L., Bowman, F. O., Jr., Edie, R. N., Hayes, C. J., Ellis, K., Gersony, W. M., and Malm, J. R.: Pulmonary atresia with intact ventricular septum. Sixteen-year experience. J. Thorac. Cardiovasc. Surg. 78:327, 1979.
46. Neutze, J. M., Starling, M. B., Elliott, R. B., and Barratt-Boyes, B. G.: Palliation of cyanotic congenital heart disease in infancy with E-type prostaglandins. Circulation 55:238, 1977.
47. Patel, R. G., Freedom, R. M., Bloon, K. R., and Rowe, R. D.: Truncal or aortic valve stenosis in functionally single arterial trunk. A clinical, hemodynamic and pathologic study of six cases. Am. J. Cardiol. 42:800, 1978.
48. Patel, R. G., Freedom, R. M., Moes, C. A. F., Bloom, K. R., Olley, P. M., Williams, W. G., Trusler, G. A., and Rowe, R. D.: Right ventricular volume determinations in 18 patients with pulmonary atresia and intact ventricular septum: Analysis of factors influencing right ventricular growth. Circulation 61:428, 1980.
49. Peacock, T. B.: Malformation of the heart: Atresia of the orifice of the pulmonary artery. Trans. Pathol. Soc. Lond. 20:61, 1869.
50. Quero-Jimenez, M., Herraiz, S. I., Moreno, G. F., Vasquez, M. E., Tomas, F. I., Gonzalez, D. C., and Alvarez, D. F.: Atresia pulmonar con tabique interventricular integro. Estudio de 28 casos. Arch. Inst. Cardiol. Mex. 46:182, 1976.
51. Rao, P. S., Liebmann, J., and Brokat, G.: Right ventricular growth in a case of pulmonic stenosis with intact ventricular septum and hypoplastic right ventricle. Circulation 53:389, 1976.
52. Rigby, M. L., Silove, E. D., Astley, R., and Abrams, L. D.: Pulmonary atresia with intact ventricular septum. Open heart surgical correction at 32 hours. Br. Heart J. 39:573, 1977.
53. Robicsek, F., Bostoen, H., and Sanger, P. W.: Atresia of the pulmonary valve with normal pulmonary artery and intact ventricular sep-

tum in a 21 year old woman. Angiology 17:896, 1966.
54. Rook, G. C., and Gootman, N.: Pulmonary atresia with intact interventricular septum: Operative treatment with survival. Am. Heart J. 81:476, 1971.
55. Rowe, R. D., Freedom, R. M., Mehrizi, A., and Bloom, K. B.: The Neonate with Congenital Heart Disease, 3rd ed. W. B. Saunders, Philadelphia, 1981.
56. Rudolph, A. M.: Congenital Diseases of the Heart. Yearbook Medical Publishers, Chicago, 1974.
57. Rudolph, A. M., Heyman, M. A., Fishman, N., and Lakier, J. B.: Formalin infiltration of the ductus arteriosus: A method for palliation of infants with selected congenital cardiac lesions. N. Engl. J. Med. 272:1263, 1975.
58. Sahn, D. J., Allen, H. D., Anderson, R., and Goldberg, S. J.: Echocardiographic diagnosis of atrial septal aneurysm in an infant with hypoplastic right heart syndrome. Chest 73:227, 1978.
59. Schrire, V., Sutin, G. J., and Barnard, C. N.: Organic and functional pulmonary atresia with intact ventricular septum. Am. J. Cardiol. 8:100, 1961.
60. Shams, A., Fowler, R. S., Trusler, G. A., Keith, J. D., and Mustard, W. T.: Pulmonary atresia with intact ventricular septum: Report of 40 cases. Pediatrics 47:370, 1971.
61. Silove, E. D., Coe, J. Y., Shiu, M. F., Brunt, J. D., Page, A. J., Singh, S. P., and Mitchell, M. D.: Oral prostaglandin E₂ in ductus-dependent pulmonary circulation. Circulation 63:682, 1981.
62. Sissman, N. J., and Abrams, H. L.: Bidirectional shunting in a coronary artery-right ventricular fistula associated with pulmonary atresia and intact ventricular septum. Circulation 32:582, 1965.
63. Steeg, C. N., Ellis, K., Bransilver, B., and Ger-

sony, W. M.: Pulmonary atresia with intact ventricular septum complicating corrected transposition of the great arteries. Am. Heart J. 82:382, 1971.
64. Takahashi, O., Eshashpour, E., and Kotler, M. N.: Tricuspid and pulmonic valve echos in tricuspid and pulmonary atresia. Chest 76:487, 1979.
65. Trusler, G. A., and Fowler, R. S.: Surgical management of pulmonary atresia with intact ventricular septum and hypoplastic right ventricle. J. Thorac. Cardiovasc. Surg. 59:740, 1970.
66. Trusler, G. A., Yamamoto, N., Williams, W. G., Izukawa, T., and Rowe, R. D.: Surgical treatment of pulmonary atresia with intact ventricular septum. Br. Heart J. 38:147, 1976.
67. Van Praagh, R., Ando, M., Van Praagh, S., Senno, A., Hougen, T. J., Novak, G., and Hastreiter, A. R.: Pulmonary atresia: Anatomic considerations. In The Child with Congenital Heart Disease after Surgery, edited by B. S. Kidd and R. D. Rowe. Mt. Kisco, New York, Futura Publishing Co., 1976, p. 103.
68. Wagenvoort, C. A., and Edwards, J. E.: The pulmonary arterial tree in pulmonary atresia. Arch. Pathol. 71:646, 1961.
69. Weisz, D., Gootman, N., Silbert, D., Voleti, C., and Wisoff, B. G.: Pulmonary atresia with intact ventricular septum. Results of surgery. N.Y. State J. Med. 77:2068, 1977.
70. Williams, R. R., Kent, G. B., Jr., and Edwards, J. E.: Anomalous cardiac blood vessel communicating with the right ventricle: Observations in a case of pulmonary atresia with an intact ventricular septum. Arch. Pathol. 42:480, 1951.
71. Zuberbuhler, J. R., and Anderson, R. H.: Morphological variations in pulmonary atresia with intact ventricular septum. Br. Heart J. 41:281, 1979.

19

Tricuspid Atresia

Amnon Rosenthal, M.D., and Macdonald Dick, II, M.D.

In tricuspid atresia there is complete agenesis of the tricuspid valve with no direct communication between the right atrium and right ventricle. An interatrial defect, hypoplasia of the right ventricle, and a communication between the systemic and pulmonary circulation, usually via a ventricular septal defect (VSD), are invariably present. The malformation, first described by Kuhne,[32] in 1906 is uncommon. It comprises 2.7% (61/2251) of infants with cardiac disease registered with the New England Regional Infant Cardiac Program between 7/1/68 and 6/30/74.[50] This represents an incidence of 0.056 per 1000 live births in the New England area.

A prevalence of 1.1 to 2.4%[9, 23, 30, 43] is reported in clinical series, and 3%[30, 43] is reported in autopsy reports of patients with congenital heart disease. Tricuspid atresia is slightly more common in males (55%).[9] Extracardiac anomalies are present in 20% of patients and most often involve the gastrointestinal or musculoskeletal system.[50] Tricuspid atresia may be associated with the cat's-eye syndrome,[18] Christmas disease,[35] Down syndrome, and asplenia.[50] Intrauterine

growth retardation is present in 4%[51] and prematurity (maternal gestation less than 36 weeks) in 6%.[50] Etiology is unknown. Polyhydramnios and maternal toxemia are said to be common,[53] and tricuspid atresia has been reported after thalidomide ingestion.[37]

PATHOLOGY

The development of the tricuspid valve is intimately related to right ventricular sinus development. Van Praagh[64] observed that in tricuspid atresia, the tricuspid dimple is directly above the posterior part of the muscular ventricular septum. He postulates, therefore, that tricuspid atresia results from malalignment between the ventricular loop and the atria. Since normal development of the right ventricle may be one of the factors resulting in a swing of the ventricular apex to the appropriate direction, underdevelopment of this chamber may cause malalignment between the ventricular loop and the atrioventricular canal, such that the ventricular septum blocks the tricuspid orifice.[1]

During fetal life in tricuspid atresia, if the ventricular septum is intact, the lungs are supplied via the ductus arteriosus and bronchial vessels, and the ductus arteriosus is small because it supplies flow only to the lung. The ascending aorta and isthmus are large since they carry nearly the entire cardiac output. If however, a VSD is present, the diameter of the ductus and ascending aorta depend on the size and flow through the defect. In infants who also have transposition and a VSD, the ductus arteriosus (PDA) is likely to be normal in size since blood is ejected directly from the left ventricle to the pulmonary artery and flows through the PDA into the descending aorta. Under these circumstances, however, a small VSD results in a ductus which may be larger than normal, and the diminished flow to the ascending aorta produces tubular hypoplasia of the arch.

In tricuspid atresia, the right ventricular cavity is composed largely of conus and incompletely formed sinus portion. In the presence of a large VSD, the right ventricular sinus may be better developed, and the pulmonary arteries are large. If the ventricular septum is intact at birth, the right ventricle is only a remnant or may be absent, and the pulmonary valve and trunk are atretic. The atretic tricuspid valve is usually muscular, represented by a dimple in the floor of the right atrium (Fig. 19.1). Less frequently, the atresia is fibrous (17%).[65] Membranous or fibrous atresia may be associated with Ebstein's anomaly,[49] atrioventricular canal, or the classical form of tricuspid atresia.[64] The interatrial communication necessary for survival is usually a patent foramen ovale (80%), a secundum atrial septal defect (ASD), or, rarely, a primum associated with a complete endocardial cushion defect.[1, 9] The VSD is usually in the basal or muscular portion of the ventricular septum, but multiple defects have been observed.[30] Obstruction to pulmonary blood flow may be due to a restrictive small VSD, a long narrow tract in a tiny right ventricle, directly in the subpulmonary area or, rarely, to valvar pulmonary stenosis. In patients with D-transposition of the great arteries, the obstruction is usually subpulmonary or pulmonary, whereas in those with normally related great arteries, it is often at the VSD. When pulmonary atresia or intact ventricular septum is present, a PDA or large collateral aortopulmonary vessels are mandatory for survival.

Tricuspid atresia is uniformly associated with other cardiac anomalies. These may produce decreased, normal, or increased pulmonary blood flow and thus affect the physiology and clinical manifestations and dictate the type of treatment. To categorize these, a number of classifications have been devised.[3, 9, 13, 30, 32, 65] None are entirely satisfactory because of the variability in type and severity of associated defects. The most useful classification is that proposed by Kuhne[32] and later modified by Edwards and Burchell[13] Keith et al.,[30] and Tandon and Edwards.[61] A simplified version is outlined in Table 19.1 There are two main types: one with normally related great arteries (type I) and the other with D-transposition of the great arteries (type II). Each type is further subdivided into several categories, depending upon the presence of pulmonary stenosis (PS) or atresia and the absence or size of the VSD. Patients with L-transposition or malposition of the great arteries and a D or L loop are designated as type III. These latter patients may also have varying degrees of pulmonary obstruction, subaortic stenosis, or coarctation of the aorta, and they account for 3 to 7% of tricuspid atresia patients.[9, 30, 50]

Additional cardiovascular malformations are present in 30% of all patients but are less common in patients with normally related great arteries (18%) than in those with transposition of the great arteries (63%).[10] The most commonly associated vascular abnormalities are: persistent left superior vena cava (16%), coarctation of the aorta (8%), and patent ductus arteriosus (3%).[10] Coarctation of the aorta (CA), hypoplasia of the aortic arch, and patent ductus arteriosus (PDA) are a frequent complex of lesions present in patients with tricuspid atresia, transposition of the great arteries, and large pulmonary blood flow (Type IIc).[23] (Fig. 19.2) Juxtaposition of the atrial appendages occurs in approximately 10 to 40% of patients with tricuspid atresia and D-transposition.[9, 50] Right aortic arch is reported in 3% of patients[10, 62] but is more frequent in those with dextrocardia[66] and transposition.[10]

MANIFESTATIONS

Clinical Features

Cyanosis or murmurs occur in more than 50% of patients with tricuspid atresia in the 1st day of life.[9] Of the infants registered in the New England Regional Infant Cardiac Program, 57% were hospitalized by 1 week of age, 78% by 1 month, and all but one within 6 months of age.[50] In general, the clinical picture in tricuspid atresia and diminished or normal pulmonary blood flow is one of cyanosis and its sequelae, whereas in those with excessive pulmonary blood flow, it is heart failure. The latter is a less common form of presentation, not often recognized until a few months of age, and is characteristic of infants with D-transposition.

Central cyanosis is the most frequent presenting symptom. It results from the obligatory right to left shunt via an ASD, and its intensity is largely dependent on pulmonary blood flow. It is most severe in infants with intact ventricular septum or PS and least severe in those with a large VSD and heart failure (types Ic and IIc). Hypoxemia, when severe, is associated with acidemia, and leads to hyperventilation by stimulation of arterial and cerebral chemoreceptors. Cyanosis may be minimal or absent in patients with transposition of the great arteries and large pulmonary blood flow. In older patients, chronic severe hypoxemia results in secondary polycythemia and its consequences.[52] Exertional dyspnea and fatigue on effort are common, and squatting may be present.

Hypoxic spells occur in 16 to 45% of infants with tricuspid

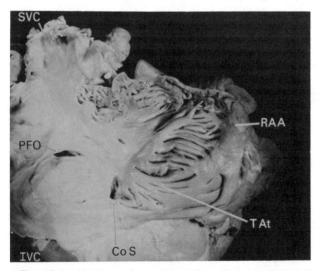

Fig. 19.1 Heart specimen viewed through an opened right atrium showing muscular atresia of the tricuspid orifice (*TAt*). The right atrial appendage (*RAA*) is large, and the patent foramen ovale (*PFO*) is smaller than in most infants with tricuspid atresia. *CoS*, coronary sinus; *IVC*, inferior vena cava; *SVC*, superior vena cava.

TABLE 19.1   TRICUSPID ATRESIA: TYPES AND FREQUENCY[a]

Patient Type	Clinical CHMC[9, b] No. (%)	Pathology[30] Specimens No. (%)	Combined Clinical and Necropsy[10c] No. (%)
I. Normally related great arteries	71 (70)	99 (69)	478 (73)
a. Intact ventricular septum with pulmonary atresia		13	
b. Small ventricular septal defect and pulmonary stenosis		73	
c. Large ventricular septal defect without pulmonary stenosis		13	
II. D-Transposition of the great arteries	23 (23)	40 (28)	156 (24)
a. Ventricular septal defect with pulmonary atresia		3	
b. Ventricular septal defect with pulmonary stenosis		11	
c. Ventricular septal defect without pulmonary stenosis		26	
III. L-Transposition of the great arteries	7 (7)	4 (3)	19 (3)
Total	101	143	653

[a] All cases confirmed by cardiac catheterization, angiography, surgery, and/or autopsy.

[b] CHMC, Children's Hospital Medical Center, Boston.

[c] Collected from five clinical and three necropsy series.

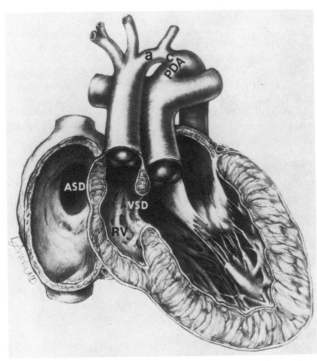

Figure 19.2   Heart specimen illustrating a common variant of tricuspid atresia type IIc: D-transposition of the great arteries associated with coarctation of the aorta (c), hypoplasia of the aortic arch (a), patent ductus arteriosus (PDA), small ventricular septal defect (VSD) and hypoplasia of the right ventricle (RV). Note the adequate atrial septal defect (ASD).

atresia, usually in those infants under 6 months of age with diminished pulmonary blood flow.[9, 46] Their appearance may be related to spontaneous diminution or closure of the VSD,[21, 48] severe or progressive infundibular[12, 21] or valvar PS, or constriction of the PDA. The physiology is similar to hypoxic spells in infants with tetralogy of Fallot and is an ominous sign indicating critically low pulmonary flow and an urgent need for surgery. Death is reported in 4% of infants.

Heart failure due to increased pulmonary flow is common in infants with tricuspid atresia and D-transposition of the great arteries (type IIc) but may occur in infants with normally related great arteries and a large VSD or a PDA (type Ic). In patients with PS, a surgically created systemic

to pulmonary artery anastomosis with a large stoma (Pott or Waterston) often leads to the development of heart failure. Cyanosis may be absent or mild, but hypoxemia can be demonstrated. Dyspnea, fatigue during feeding, frequent respiratory infections, and excessive perspirations are common. Weight maturation is delayed. Tachypnea, tachycardia, hepatomegaly and, less frequently, pulmonary rales are present. Severe right-sided failure with giant "a" waves in the jugular venous pulse suggests a restrictive atrial communication. Death usually occurs within 3 years after the onset of severe failure.[9]

Infants with severe cyanosis and iron deficiency anemia and older children with polycythemia are prone to develop cerebrovascular accidents.[47] The episodes may follow an acute febrile illness, a hypoxic spell, or cardiac catheterization. They may occur in 2% of patients. In older children, hemiplegia may result from a brain abscess, emboli associated with endocarditis, or complication of a systemic to pulmonary artery shunt.

Brain abscess occurs in 1.3 to 5% of patients with tricuspid atresia and is a serious, potentially lethal complication.[10, 15] The rate of development of brain abscess has been estimated at one per 273 patient years. Because of an obligatory right to left intracardiac shunt, the phagocytic filtering action of the pulmonary capillary bed is by passed and transient bacteremia may colonize the brain previously damaged by hypoxemia or hypoperfusion and thus may produce an abscess. A brain abscess should always be suspected in any cyanotic patient over 2 years of age with headaches, focal neurologic signs, or seizures. It represents an emergency situation. A combination of radionuclide brain scan, electroencephalogram and computerized axial tomography, when supplemented by a thorough history and physical examination, will nearly always lead to the correct diagnosis and localization of the lesion. Treatment is with antibiotics and surgical aspiration. Mortality among all cyanotic patients with brain abscess in the last decade has been 38%, with nearly half of the survivors having residual neurologic impairment related to the abscess.[15]

Endocarditis occurs in 17 to 25% of patients surviving shunt surgery for tricuspid atresia.[9, 62] The rate of development of endocarditis has been estimated at one per 72 patient years.

Patients with D-transposition of the great arteries, pulmonary hypertension, and large pulmonary flow are candidates for the development of pulmonary vascular obstructive disease within the first year of life. Pulmonary hypertension and the development of vascular obstructive disease is very unusual in patients with normally related great arteries in the absence of a large systemic to pulmonary artery shunt.[9] Patients with a Potts anastomosis develop obstructive disease, possibly due to growth in the orifice size with time. Patients with a Waterston shunt could be expected to have a similar course whereas those with Blalock-Taussig anastomosis rarely develop vascular obstructive disease. Symptoms are indistinguishable from those observed in other patients with Eisenmenger's syndrome.

Life-threatening dysrhythmias are encountered in 7% of patients.[9] Atrial dysrhythmias, particularly atrial fibrillation, tend to develop in older patients with long-standing shunt-anastomoses and chronic left ventricular volume overload. The onset of dysrhythmia in such patients aggravates pre-existing heart failure. Atrial tachycardia or flutter during cardiac catheterization in patients with diminished pulmonary blood flow will tend to potentiate the hypoxemia, produce acidemia, and lead to hypotension.

Examination of infants with tricuspid atresia and diminished pulmonary blood flow discloses marked cyanosis, hyperventilation, and a relatively quiet cardiac impulse at the lower left sternal border. In older infants and children, there is delayed growth, clubbing, and a left precordial prominence. Delayed height and weight maturation occur in 40 to 70% of all patients with tricuspid atresia.[10, 40] There is a prominent "a" wave in the jugular venous pulse which may be accompanied by a palpable presystolic pulse wave over the precordium when the foramen ovale is restrictive. Cardiac impulse is hyperactive at the apex. A thrill is uncommon. The first heart sound is single and accentuated. The second heart sound is single in patients with pulmonary atresia, severe PS, or transposition of the great arteries. In some patients with pulmonary stenosis, the second sound may be widely split and P2 diminished. A prominent S4 may be present if the foramen ovale is restrictive. A systolic ejection click is often audible at the left parasternal border. A regurgitant or ejection systolic murmur, generated by the VSD and/or PS, is heard along the left sternal border. Diminution in intensity of the murmur suggests the development of severe PS,[12] pulmonary atresia, or closure of the VSD. When pulmonary blood flow is large, S1 is prominent, and a third heart sound or mid-diastolic rumble is audible. In patients with a systemic to pulmonary artery shunt and normal pulmonary artery pressure, there is a continuous murmur.

Electrovectorcardiographic Features

The electrocardiogram features are: superior and leftward QRS axis in the frontal plane, right atrial hypertrophy, absent or markedly diminished right ventricular forces, and increased left ventricular forces. Right ventricular and anterior (R in V2) forces may be more evident when the right ventricle is better developed (Fig. 19.3).[58] A tall R wave and deep Q in lead V6 suggest increased pulmonary flow, and a small r with shallow q is seen in those with diminished pulmonary flow (Fig. 19.4).[8] The QRS axis in the frontal plane in 87% of type I patients (normally related great arteries) is between 0 and −90° and in the remainder is at 0

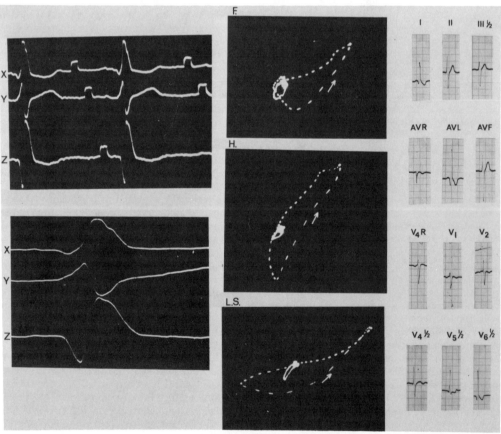

Fig. 19.3 The Frank and standard electrocardiogram and vectorcardiogram in a 3-year-old with tricuspid atresia, D-transposition of the great arteries, large ventricular septal defect, and pulmonary vascular obstructive disease. The frontal loop (*F*) is counterclockwise, leftward, and predominantly superior. The counterclockwise horizontal loop (*H*) and dominant left ventricular forces suggest systemic pressure in the left ventricle with hypoplasia of the right ventricle. The standard electrocardiogram shows a superior QRS axis of −40°, left ventricular hypertrophy, diminished right ventricular forces, and ST-T wave changes.

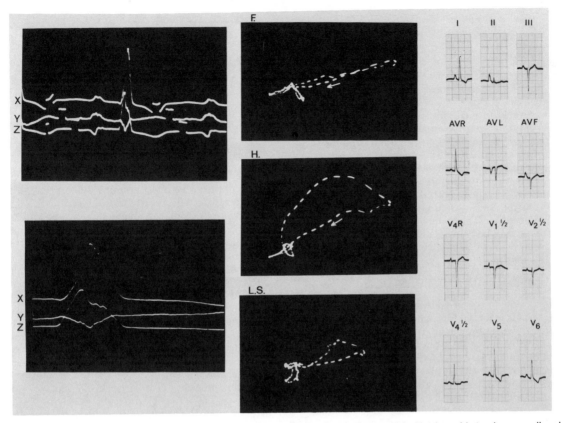

Fig. 19.4 The Frank and standard electrocardiogram and vectorcardiogram of an 8-year-old with tricuspid atresia, normally related great arteries, and diminished pulmonary blood flow. The frontal loop (F) is superior, leftward, and has a figure of eight configuration (frontal plane elevation, 352°). The horizontal plane configuration is unusual, being clockwise and posterior. The maximal spatial vector to the left is 3.26 mV (normal 1.1 to 2.1 mV), elevation 352° and azimuth 338°. Note the virtual absence of rightward and anterior electromotive forces. The standard electrocardiogram shows P tricuspidale (taller than the R wave), a superior QRS axis of −15°, left ventricular hypertrophy, absence of right ventricular forces, and ST-T wave changes.

to +90°, with very rare exception. QRS axis in type II patients is evenly distributed between the left superior (0 to −90°) and the left inferior (0 to 90°) quadrant.[9] A rightward axis is exceedingly rare.[9, 58] Of six patients with a rightward axis (superior or inferior), four had L-transposition of the great arteries, one had D-transposition of the great arteries, and one had normally related great arteries.[9] The abnormal superior QRS axis [51] is present in the majority of patients with tricuspid atresia.[9, 22, 45] It may be secondary to early origin to the left bundle from the common bundle which leads to an abnormal sequence of depolarization with a superior and counterclockwise loop in the frontal plane.[25, 26] Right atrial hypertrophy is present in 70 to 80%.[9, 45] It may be accompanied by left atrial hypertrophy in 30% of patients, particularly those with increased pulmonary flow.[23] Occasionally, the P wave configuration has a spike and dome pattern. There is no relationship between P wave amplitude and mean interatrial gradient or size of the ASD.[9] Prolongation of the PR interval occurs in less than 15% of patients.[58] Ischemic ST depression and T wave changes are common, especially in patients with increased pulmonary flow and left ventricular volume overload.

In patients with tricuspid atresia, the frontal plane loop is usually leftward, counterclockwise, and superior, but in some patients, particularly those with transposition, it may be leftward and inferior. The horizontal loop is oriented to the left and more posterior than normal. Rotation is counterclockwise (Fig. 19.3) and less frequently is clockwise (Fig. 19.4) or figure of eight. There is usually a marked decrease of early anterior and leftward forces resembling the vector-

cardiogram of an anterolateral myocardial infarction or left bundle branch block.[14] A more anterior displacement of the horizontal loop and the presence of a terminal rightward force are indicative of a larger right ventricular cavity and VSD. Terminal slowing of the QRS complex is common, but initial delay may also be seen. There is left ventricular dominance with an increase in left maximal spatial vector and reduced rightward forces.[14] There is no relationship between left maximal spatial vector and pulmonary blood flow or the presence or absence of transposition of the great arteries. Wide loops in all planes suggest increased pulmonary flow,[8] and narrow loops suggest reduced pulmonary flow.

Echocardiographic Features

Adequate echocardiographic scanning in normal infants should always show some portion of the tricuspid valve. In older children, this may not be possible. In infants, the absence of tricuspid valve echos in association with reduced right ventricular dimension may be taken as strong presumptive evidence of tricuspid atresia. In patients with tricuspid atresia, the two semilunar valves are usually identified (unless pulmonary atresia is present) and a tricuspid valve echo cannot be found. There is normal mitral semilunar continuity when the great arteries are normally related. Left ventricular dimension is occasionally normal but usually increased. The presence of a large VSD is suggested by the "dropping out" of septal echos during part of the scanning. The 2D echocardiogram is particularly useful in assessing the relationship of the great arteries, size of interatrial communication, and size of the VSD. The echocardiogram features may resemble those of a single ventricle.

Radiologic Features

The roentgenographic findings in patients with diminished pulmonary flow (Table 19.1) are: a normal to mildly increased cardiac silhouette, concavity in the region of the main pulmonary artery, and diminished pulmonary vascular markings. By contrast, those with increased pulmonary flow have gross cardiac enlargement and plethoric pulmonary vasculature often accompanied by pulmonary congestion. A transition from increased to decreased pulmonary vasculature on serial chest roentgenograms suggests diminution in pulmonary blood flow. This is often attributable to spontaneous closure of the VSD, which occurs in 38% of patients with tricuspid atresia.[48] The right heart border, formed by the right atrium, may be convex and prominent. A straight and flattened border may be due to left-sided juxtaposition of the atrial appendage.

CARDIAC CATHETERIZATION

A presumptive diagnosis based on the clinical picture and noninvasive tests is essential for an adequate cardiac catheterization study and its proper interpretation. Introduction of the venous catheter via the groin is preferable to antecubital or axillary approach since it facilitates manipulation of the catheter to the left heart chambers. The right ventricular cavity cannot be entered by the catheter directly from the right atrium because the tricuspid valve is atretic. Similar difficulties may be encountered in infants with pulmonary atresia or stenosis and an intact ventricular septum when the right ventricle and tricuspid orifice are very small. In very cyanotic neonates, the catheter frequently cannot and should not be advanced beyond the left atrium and left ventricle. Great caution must be exercised in these infants with pulmonary obstruction and reduced pulmonary flow to avoid a hypoxic spell. The right ventricle and pulmonary arteries are, therefore, rarely entered. In older infants and children, a balloon tip catheter can frequently be guided through the foramen ovale into the left atrium and left ventricle and via a VSD into the right ventricle and occasionally into the pulmonary artery. An arterial retrograde catheter may be manipulated into the pulmonary artery and sometimes into the right ventricle if a large aortopulmonary shunt is present (Fig. 19.5, C and D) or directly through the aortic valve into the right ventricle in patients with transposition of the great arteries (Fig. 19.5B).

In tricuspid atresia, the entire systemic venous blood is directed to the left atrium, where it mixes with pulmonary venous blood. Complete mixing is achieved at the left atrial level and, consequently, left and right ventricular, pulmonary artery, and systemic arterial saturations are nearly identical. When the great arteries are normally related, mixed venous blood from the left ventricle is pumped directly to the aorta and indirectly to the pulmonary artery through a VSD and a hypoplastic right ventricle or via a PDA or aorticopulmonary collaterals if the ventricular septum is intact. In complete transposition, the pulmonary artery fills directly from the left ventricle and the aorta indirectly through a VSD and the hypoplastic right ventricle. Systemic arterial hypoxemia is always present. The degree of hypoxemia is dependent on the pulmonary to systemic flow ratio. If hypoxemia is severe, metabolic acidosis is present. Arterial PCO_2 is usually normal. Pulmonary, systemic, and effective pulmonary flow can be calculated if oxygen consumption is measured. Pulmonary arterial saturation may be assumed to equal systemic arterial saturation since there is complete admixture of blood in the left atrium. The anatomic right to left shunt is the flow across the foramen ovale. The physiologic shunt is the difference between the systemic and effective pulmonary flow. The anatomic left to right shunt is the entire pulmonary flow since it is derived from the VSD, PDA, or aortopulmonary collaterals. The physiologic shunt is the difference between the pulmonary and effective pulmonary flow.

In the presence of a superior vena cava to right pulmonary artery anastomosis (Glenn shunt),[24] neither a mixed systemic venous nor pulmonary arterial saturation can be determined, and systemic or pulmonary blood flow cannot be calculated by the Fick principle. In infants with D-transposition, coarctation of the aorta, and a systemic PDA, systemic blood flow can be calculated because there is complete mixing in the left atrium and differential cyanosis is absent.

The right atrial pressure is usually elevated and is equal to or greater than left atrial pressure. If left atrial or ventricular filling pressure rises or the foramen ovale is restrictive, the right atrial pressure will rise further to maintain systemic output. An increase in left atrial volume and pressure predisposes to closure of the flap of the foramen ovale. A large "a" wave is often present on the pressure tracing, especially when the right atrium contracts against the increased resistance of a small foramen ovale. A mean interatrial gradient equal to or greater than 3 mm Hg across the atrial septum is demonstrated in only 6% of patients at initial cardiac catheterization.[9]

In the presence of a large VSD, the right ventricular pressure is equal to left ventricular pressure. The pulmonary artery pressure is usually normal when the great arteries are normally related because of the frequent association of a restrictive VSD or PS (type Ib). Pulmonary artery hypertension may be present initially (type Ic), but pulmonary flow frequently diminishes with time due to diminution in the size of the VSD or to the development of PS. In patients with complete transposition and no pulmonary stenosis (type IIc), pulmonary artery hypertension persists, and vascular obstructive disease invariably develops.

Indicator dye dilution studies are not sufficiently specific to be of diagnostic value. Injection of dye into the right atrium and sampling in the systemic artery demonstrates an early appearance time.

ANGIOCARDIOGRAPHY

The diagnosis of tricuspid atresia is best established by angiography. The right atrial angiogram shows a large dilated right atrium with contrast material refluxing to the inferior vena cava and hepatic veins and simultaneously spilling via the foramen ovale into the left atrium and producing the so-called "waterfall" or "onionskin" appearance. This is best visualized in the left anterior oblique or lateral projection. The right ventricle inflow does not opacify from the right atrium, and the negative shadow or right ventricular "window"[6] thus created (in the anterior projection) by the absence of the right ventricular sinus is characteristic but not pathognomonic of tricuspid atresia (Fig. 19.5A). An inferiorly malpositioned right atrial appendage, total anomalous pulmonary venous return to the coronary sinus, and other right-sided obstructive lesions with a large right to left shunt at the atria may occasionally mimic this appearance. A selective left ventricular angiogram (preferably in the anterior and lateral projection) is essential for identification of the hypoplastic right ventricle, delineation of the ventricular defect and type of pulmonary obstruction, and assessment of the pulmonary arteries. The right ventricle appears as a sliver or appendage medial and directly

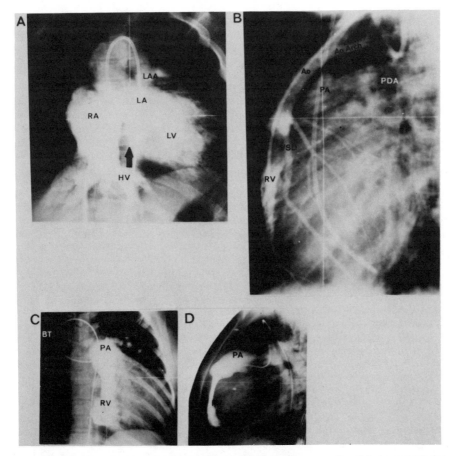

Fig. 19.5 (*A*) Right atrial angiocardiogram in an 8-year-old with tricuspid atresia, normally related great arteries, ventricular and atrial septal defects, and severe pulmonary stenosis. Hypoxic spells at 5 months of age required a Waterston anastomosis. Note the clear or "window" area (*arrow*) which the right ventricle should fill. Contrast material injected into the right atrium (*RA*) flows via an atrial defect into the left atrium (*LA*) and through the mitral valve into the large left ventricle (*LV*). The hepatic veins (*HV*) and left atrial appendage (*LAA*) also fill. A second catheter is in the ascending aorta. (*B*) Right ventricular angiogram in a 4-year-old with tricuspid atresia and transposition of the great arteries. The hypoplastic right ventricle (*RV*) was entered in a retrograde manner via the small ascending aorta (*Ao*). The aortic arch (*Ao Arch*) is very hypoplastic; a patent ductus arteriosus (*PDA*) and ventricular septal defect (*VSD*) are present. The pulmonary artery (*PA*) is large, and pulmonary hypertension is present. (*C* and *D*) Selective anterior (*C*) and lateral (*D*) films from a right ventricular angiocardiogram of a 21-year-old with tricuspid atresia and normally related great arteries (type Ib). The arterial catheter was advanced in a retrograde fashion to the aortic arch, via a right Blalock-Taussig anastomosis into the pulmonary artery (*PA*) and then through the pulmonary valve into a hypoplastic right ventricle (*RV*). The pulmonary valve and infundibulum are of adequate size, and there is no ventricular septal defect. Spontaneous closure of the interventricular defect (proven at a later postmortem examination) had resulted in gradual diminution of pulmonary blood flow requiring a Blalock-Taussig anastomosis at 14 months of age.

anterior to the left ventricle (Fig. 19.6*A*). The left ventricular cavity may be normal in infants but is usually very dilated in older children with or without a large aortopulmonary shunt. When the VSD is large and pulmonary flow has increased, the right ventricular sinus is often better developed than in children with a small defect and/or severe PS and diminished pulmonary flow (Fig. 18.5*B*). In patients with transposition of the great arteries, a very small right ventricle may be associated with hypoplasia of the aortic arch, PDA, and coarctation of the aorta (Figs. 19.2 and 19.5*B*).[27] A restrictive VSD in patients with L-malposition will result in subaortic stenosis with a systolic pressure gradient between the left ventricle and ascending aorta. Selective left ventricular angiography will distinguish these patients with tricuspid atresia from those with double inlet (or atrioventricular canal), single left ventricle, and right ventricular outflow chamber.

In patients with diminished pulmonary flow, left ventricular end-diastolic volume is somewhat increased and the ejection fraction is slightly diminished, whereas in patients with increased pulmonary blood flow, the left ventricular

end-diastolic volume is further increased but the ejection fraction may be normal. The largest left ventricular end-diastolic volume and poorest ejection fraction occur in patients with increased pulmonary blood flow due to a large systemic to pulmonary artery anastomosis present over a decade.[33] Patients with tricuspid atresia develop left ventricular dysfunction and failure as a consequence of long-standing left ventricular volume overload. The left ventricle receives both systemic and pulmonary venous blood from the left atrium and is the sole pump supplying the systemic and pulmonary circulations. The development and severity of heart failure are dependent on the magnitude of pulmonary flow and the duration of volume overload.

DIFFERENTIAL DIAGNOSIS

The characteristic findings in most infants with tricuspid atresia are: cyanosis from or soon after birth; leftward and superior QRS axis with left ventricular hypertrophy on the electrocardiogram; and reduced pulmonary blood flow on chest x-ray. By contrast, most other cyanotic infants have

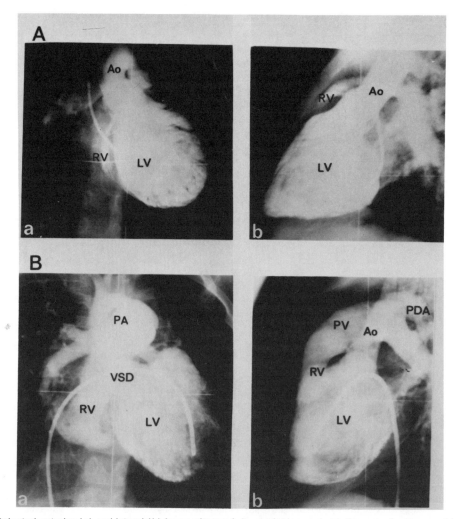

Fig. 19.6 (*A*) Selected anterior (*a*) and lateral (*b*) frames from a left ventricular angiocardiogram of a 5-year-old with tricuspid atresia, normally related great arteries, small ventricular septal defect, pulmonary stenosis (type Ib), and a Waterston shunt. The left ventricle (*LV*) is dilated, right ventricle (*RV*) markedly hypoplastic, and pulmonary anulus somewhat small. The pulmonary arteries fill from the right ventricle via a ventricular septal defect and through the ascending aorta to right pulmonary artery shunt. *Ao*, aorta. (*B*) Selected anterior (*a*) and lateral (*b*) films from a left ventricular angiocardiogram of a 6-year-old girl with tricuspid atresia, large ventricular septal defect (*VSD*), and a patent ductus arteriosus (*PDA*) (type Ic). The right ventricle (*RV*) here is not as hypoplastic; the pulmonary valve (*PV*) anulus and pulmonary artery (*PA*) are large, and pulmonary artery hypertension is present.

right ventricular hypertrophy on the electrocardiogram. Neonates, who present in a similar manner, however, include those with pulmonary atresia and an intact ventricular septum; critical pulmonary stenosis with a diminutive right ventricle; tricuspid stenosis with a VSD; single ventricle with PS; D-transposition with PS or atresia and hypoplastic right ventricle; Ebstein's anomaly; or patients with overriding tricuspid valve. Infants with tetralogy of Fallot and those with transposition and an intact ventricular septum usually can be distinguished by the electrocardiogram, which shows right axis deviation and right ventricular hypertrophy. Infants with severe PS or pulmonary atresia and intact ventricular septum often have cardiomegaly and are in heart failure, and the QRS is not usually superior. Those with Ebstein's anomaly nearly always have cardiomegaly. The 2D echocardiogram is most helpful. Careful scanning in those with tricuspid atresia reveals a normal pulmonary valve (except in types Ia and IIa), hypoplastic right ventricle, and the absence of any portion of the tricuspid valve. Overriding of the tricuspid valve can also be diagnosed from the echocardiogram.[34]

Patients presenting with heart failure and mild or no

cyanosis should be distinguished from those with an isolated large VSD; double inlet single left ventricle with right ventricular outflow chamber; double outlet right ventricle with pulmonary stenosis; transposition of the great arteries, VSD, and normal tricuspid valve; complex coarctation; and atrioventricular canal or truncus arteriosus. The presence of right ventricular hypertrophy on the electrocardiogram or vectorcardiogram virtually excludes tricuspid atresia. The echocardiogram may be diagnostic, but a definitive diagnosis should be established by cardiac catheterization and angiography.

TREATMENT

Treatment of patients with tricuspid atresia is surgical. Palliative surgery, for all types of tricuspid atresia, is designed to improve blood flow when it is diminished, reduce pulmonary blood flow when it is excessive, and eliminate major interarterial obstruction when present. Associated cardiovascular lesions may also require repair.

Neonates with severe hypoxemia, whose pulmonary blood flow is dependent in part or completely on patency of the ductus arteriosus, will benefit from infusion of prostaglandin E_1-(0.05 to 0.1 μg/kg/minute). Dilatation of the PDA will increase pulmonary flow, improve systemic blood oxygenation, and stabilize the infant in preparation for surgical palliation. Prostaglandin E_1 is most effective in neonates under 4 days of age and in those with the lowest PaO_2 (<40 mm Hg).[17] Infants receiving prostaglandin infusion should be closely monitored for side effects and complications, which include cutaneous vasodilatation, hypotension, apnea, hyperthermia, and seizures.[39] The acutely ill and hypoxemic infant requires oxygen and intravenous sodium bicarbonate to correct metabolic acidosis. Supportive medical therapy includes the administration of iron or blood transfusion in infants with anemia and decongestive measures in those with heart failure.

All patients should be advised of precautions against endocarditis and brain abscess. Vocational and recreational guidance and counseling is required in older patients.

In patients with diminished pulmonary blood flow, palliative surgery is done to increase pulmonary flow and improve systemic oxygen saturation. Indications for surgery in a cyanotic infant are one or more documented hypoxic spells and significant or progressive hypoxemia. Palliative surgery in infants under 1 month of age is best achieved by a central aortopulmonary shunt utilizing prosthetic material (e.g., Gore-Tex tube), an ascending aorta to right pulmonary artery anastomosis (Waterston) and, less often, a subclavian to pulmonary artery anastomosis (Blalock-Taussig). Between 1 month and 1 year of age, the procedure of choice is a Blalock-Taussig shunt, and after age 1, a Blalock-Taussig shunt or right main pulmonary artery to superior vena cava anastomosis (Glenn).[24] The latter is an end-to-side anastomosis with complete or partial ligation of the superior vena cava just above the right atrial junction (Fig. 19.7, A and B).[24] The disadvantages of the Waterston shunt include kinking of the right pulmonary artery, excessive pulmonary flow because of inability to regulate the size of the orifice, the tendency of the anastomosis to increase further in size with age, development of heart failure and left ventricular dysfunction, pulmonary artery hypertension and, later on, pulmonary vascular obstructive disease. Blalock-Taussig anastomosis, on the other hand, provides a more appropriate pulmonary flow without the complications of intractable failure, pulmonary hypertension, or vascular obstructive disease. It is, however, technically difficult to obtain a satisfactory Blalock-Taussig shunt in very young infants. One would prefer, therefore, if possible to delay the shunt procedure until the infant is older. Unfortunately, this is often not feasible. The Glenn procedure is the most physiologic shunt because it avoids an increased volume load on the left ventricle and delivers approximately one-third of total systemic venous blood directly to the pulmonary artery at a low

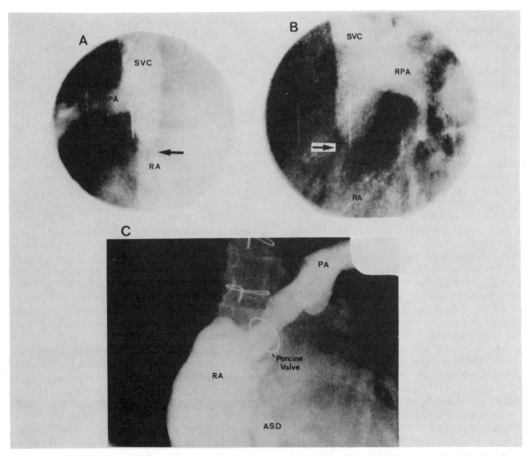

Fig. 19.7 Angiograms from a 20-year-old with tricuspid atresia, normally related great arteries, and diminished pulmonary blood flow (Table 19.1). Injection of contrast material in the superior vena cava (*SVC*) at age 15 years reveals both in the anterior (*A*) and lateral (*B*) view that a previously created anastomosis between end of the right pulmonary artery (*RPA*) and side of the superior vena cava (*SVC*) (Glenn) is functioning. A small communication between the superior vena cava and right atrium (*RA*) persists despite ligation of the superior vena cava (*arrow*) (*C*). Following a Fontan procedure at age 19 years, a right atrial angiocardiogram shows contrast material flowing through a prosthetic conduit containing a porcine valve xenograft (mounted on a metal ring) into the pulmonary artery (*PA*). Incomplete closure of the atrial septal defect (*ASD*) resulted in a small residual right to left shunt.

pressure. Furthermore, it may serve as a first stage for subsequent surgery employing a right atrial to pulmonary artery conduit. However, the Glenn shunt is an unsatisfactory operation in infants under 6 months of age because the pulmonary arteries are too small. In the neonate, the pulmonary vascular resistance may also be elevated, and perfusion from a low pressure systemic venous vessel may not be possible. Pulmonary infection or atelectasis will also raise vascular resistance and have a similar effect. Other disadvantages of the Glenn shunt include: thrombosis and occlusion resulting in a superior vena cava syndrome; gradual decrease in perfusion to the ipsilateral lung through the development of venous collaterals, hemoconcentration, peripheral vascular occlusion, and competition with aortopulmonary collateral circulation; differential distribution of pulmonary flow with decreased perfusion to the contralateral lung; and the development of stenosis or atresia of the right ventricular outflow tract. Five years after an initially satisfactory anastomosis, the systemic arterial saturation usually declines because of the aforementioned factors. The presence of a persistent left superior vena cava with a communicating innominate vein must be excluded prior to performing a Glenn shunt; otherwise, it may create a "steal syndrome," draining right superior vena cava blood via the innominate vein into the coronary sinus and right atrium.[24, 25] There is limited experience to date with a new palliative procedure described by Annecchino et al.[2] in infants and children with diminished pulmonary blood flow (Type Ib). The operation involves reconstruction of the right ventricular outflow tract and/or enlargement of the VSD.

Balloon atrial septostomy is seldom necessary except when a considerable interatrial pressure gradient ($\geq$ 3 mm Hg) is demonstrated at cardiac catheterization because of an obstructive foramen ovale.[10, 36, 55, 57] In older infants and children, if an obstruction to systemic venous return through the foramen ovale is demonstrated, a shunt procedure should be accompanied by creation of an atrial septal defect. An obstructive foramen is suggested by unremitting right heart failure, giant "a" waves in the jugular venous pulse, presystolic hepatic venous pulse,[36] and a very prominent fourth heart sound. At cardiac catheterization, there is a high mean right atrial pressure and "a" wave, large interatrial pressure gradient, and a small atrial communication on right atrial cinengiogram. Aneurysm of the fossa ovale can, on rare occasions, also lead to obstruction at the atrial level by inserting into the mitral orifice.[19]

Infants with transposition, increased pulmonary flow, pulmonary artery hypertension and heart failure require pulmonary artery banding within the first 6 months of life for control of the failure and prevention of pulmonary vascular obstructive disease. It is rare for infants with normally related great arteries or L-transposition and increased pulmonary flow to require banding.[63] On careful observation through the first year of life, most of these infants will gradually exhibit diminishing pulmonary flow through decrease in the size of the VSD[21] and/or the development of PS.[12] Successful palliation by banding of the pulmonary arteries and creation of an aorticopulmonary window (proximal to the pulmonary artery band) has been performed in a patient with transposition when a VSD has become restrictive.[44]

The overall mortality for both medically and surgically treated infants with tricuspid atresia in the New England Regional Infant Cardiac Program is shown in Table 19.2. All but one of the surgically managed infants had closed heart procedures (e.g., aortopulmonary shunt, pulmonary artery banding). At our institution the palliative procedure for relief

TABLE 19.2. CRUDE FIRST YEAR MORTALITY OF MEDICAL AND SURGICAL TREATMENT OF INFANTS WITH TRICUSPID ATRESIA (1969 to 1976)[50]

	Total (No.)	Dead (No.)	Mortality (%)
Medical treatment	21	10	48
Surgical treatment	55	22	40
Total	76	32	42

of hypoxemia with the best early survival and greatest durability has been the Blalock-Taussig anastomosis. Operative mortality for the Blalock-Taussig shunt was 23% between 1950 and 1980 and improved from 39 to 13% in the last decade.[10] In general, the surgical mortality is inversely related to age[9, 50, 62] and to weight of the patient.[9]

The surgical experience with a physiologic procedure[16, 31] for patients with tricuspid atresia has been very promising.[4, 5, 20, 59, 60] A right atrial to main pulmonary artery direct anastomosis or conduit (with or without a valve) channels the systemic venous return directly into the lung. ASD is closed and main pulmonary artery is ligated just above the pulmonary valve (Fig. 18.7C). A previously existing Glenn anastomosis is not disturbed, but a systemic to pulmonary artery arterial shunt must be closed to reduce pulmonary pressure and avoid excessive pulmonary flow. In a modification of the above procedure, a right atrial to right ventricular conduit with or without a valve is used[4, 5] (Fig. 19.8 A and B). The patient's right ventricle, if not extremely hypoplastic, is thus able to generate some forward pressure and the pulmonary valve and trunk are utilized. Here it is imperative that the VSD be closed and the patient have a nonobstructive right ventricular outflow tract and an adequate-sized pulmonary valve annulus and main pulmonary artery.

The Fontan and Bandet[16] or Kreutzer et al.[31] procedure is, at present, performed in older symptomatic patients with decreased pulmonary blood flow. Candidates most suitable for the procedure are children between the ages of 4 and 15[7, 20] with: normal pulmonary vascular resistance and a mean pulmonary artery pressure less than 20 mm Hg; adequate-sized main and branch pulmonary arteries (a pulmonary artery-aortic diameter ratio of 0.75 or more)[7]; normal sinus rhythm; and normal left heart with good left ventricular function. The left ventricular end-diastolic pressure should be below 12 mm Hg. In the absence of pulmonary vascular obstructive disease, successful surgery probably depends most upon an adequate gradient between the right and left atrium. With normal or low left atrial pressure, only a small rise in right atrial pressure is necessary to produce an adequate pulmonary and systemic flow. The operation is contraindicated in patients with pulmonary vascular obstructive disease or left ventricular dysfunction. Such patients develop severe right-sided failure and low cardiac output following surgery. Dysrhythmias such as nodal tachycardia may also result in an increase in left atrial pressure, increased right atrial pressure, and right-sided failure. Although the absence of sinus rhythm is not invariably associated with clinical deterioration,[4] atrial systole does provide the major pulsatile support to pulmonary blood flow.[56] Transient superior vena cava syndrome and right heart failure with edema, ascites, and hepatomegaly are not uncommon in the immediate postoperative period.[4, 42] Complete closure of the ASD is required to avoid a residual right to left shunt (Fig. 19.7C). With improved patient selection and operative techniques, the operative mortality has gradually declined

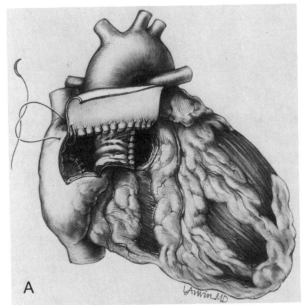

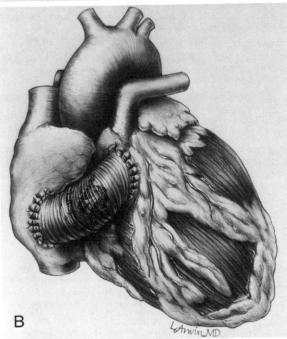

strated resting systemic venous hypertension with a mean right atrial pressure of approximately 12 to 16 mm Hg,[5, 35, 60] relatively low resting cardiac output,[35, 60] and normal left ventricular end-diastolic pressure.[54] Systemic venous pressure may increase significantly with even minor degrees of obstruction to right atrial emptying. Such obstruction may be caused by small or stenotic pulmonary arteries, by persistent mild valvar pulmonary stenosis in instances in which the pulmonary valve has been incorporated in the repair, by stenosis or calcification of the procine valve, thrombosis of the conduit, or by obstruction at any of the suture lines.[4] Some of the long-term, residua and sequelae after the Fontan procedure or one of its modifications are shown in Table 19.3.

The overall survival of patients with tricuspid atresia is shown in Figure 19.9. With appropriate management, more than 50% of patients survive to the second decade of life. This compares to less than 10% without surgical therapy.[9] Infants with diminished pulmonary flow and those with severe heart failure are unlikely to survive beyond infancy without surgery. After a large atrition in infancy, there seems to be a period of clinical stability up to approximately the age of 15, after which mortality increases, predominantly owing to heart failure but also as a result of pulmonary

TABLE 19.3   LONG-TERM RESIDUA AND SEQUELAE AFTER THE FONTAN PROCEDURE OR ITS MODIFICATIONS[5, 45, 60]

Right-sided obstruction to flow
   Narrow anastomosis of either end of conduit
   Residual pulmonary valve stenosis when right ventricle is used
   Porcine valve or homograft calcification
   Thrombosis of conduit
   Fibrosis of Dacron tube
Intracardiac and extracardiac shunts
   Right to left through
      interatrial leak
      intrapulmonary shunts
   Left to right through
      residual ventricular septal defect
      incomplete aortopulmonary shunt or pulmonary artery ligation
      extensive aortopulmonary collaterals
Atrial or ventricular dysrhythmias
Complete heart block
Systemic venous hypertension
   Liver dysfunction
   Varicose veins

Fig. 19.8 Modification of the Fontan procedure utilizing a right atrial to right ventricular valveless pericardial conduit (*A*) or a prosthetic conduit containing a porcine valve (*B*). In the former procedure (*A*) an incision is made in the right ventricular infundibulum, and a flap of the right atrial appendage is folded back and sutured to the right edge of the ventriculotomy to form the floor of the conduit. A patch of pericardium is then sutured over the flap to form the roof of the conduit. Both modifications utilize the right ventricular chamber and incorporate the pulmonary valve into the repair.

from 14% (11/80 patients)[4, 5, 20, 54, 60] to less than 7%.[20, 54] Marked symptomatic improvement has been observed in most patients surviving surgery. The procedure leads to normal systemic arterial oxygen saturation, maintenance of normal left ventricular volume load, and reduction of the risk of systemic embolization and brain abscess. Long-term postoperative cardiac catheterization studies have demon-

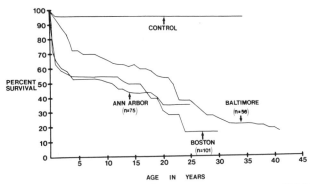

Fig. 19.9 Survival curves of patients with tricuspid atresia[9, 10, 62] compared with a control population. (Reproduced with permission from M. Dick and A. Rosenthal.[10])

vascular obstructive disease, dysrhythmias and other complications associated with large right to left shunt. Exceptional patients, with normal or only slightly increased pulmonary flow, may survive beyond the third decade.[28]

REFERENCES

1. Ando, M., Satomi, G., and Takao, A.: Atresia of triscupid or mitral orifice: Anatomic spectrum and morphogenetic hypothesis. In Etiology and Morphogenesis of Congenital Heart Disease, edited by R. Van Praagh and A. Takao. Futura Publishing Co., Mount Kisco, N.Y., 1980.
2. Annecchino, F. P., Chauve, A., Quaegebeur, J., and Fontan, F.: Palliative reconstruction of right outflow tract in tricuspid atresia. A report of 5 cases. Ann. Thorac. Surg. 29:317, 1980.
3. Astley, R., Oldham, J. S., and Parsons, G.: Congenital tricuspid atresia. Br. Heart. J. 15:287, 1953.
4. Behrendt, D. M., and Rosenthal, A.: Cardiovascular status after repair by Fontan procedure. Ann. Thorac. Surg. 29:322, 1980.
5. Bowman, F. O., Jr., Malm, J. R., Hayes, C. J. et al.: Physiologic approach to surgery for tricuspid atresia. Circulation (Suppl.) 58: 1–83, 1978.
6. Campbell, M., and Hills, T. H.: Angiocardiography in cyanotic congenital heart disease. Br. Heart J. 12:65, 1950.
7. Choussat, A., Fontan, F., Besse, P. et al.: Selection criteria for Fontan's Procedure. In: Pediatric Cardiology 1977, edited by R. H. Anderson, and E. A. Shinebourne, Edinburgh, Churchill Livingstone, p. 1978, p. 559.
8. Davachi, F., Lucas, R. V., and Moller, J. H.: The electrocardiogram and vectorcardiogram in tricuspid atresia. Correlation with pathologic anatomy. Am. J. Cardiol. 25:18, 1970.
9. Dick, M., Fyler, D. C., and Nadas, A. S.: Tricuspid atresia: The clinical course in 101 patients. Am. J. Cardiol. 36, 1975.
10. Dick, M., and Rosenthal, A.: The clinical profile of tricuspid atresia. In Tricuspid Atresia, edited by P. S. Rao. 1982. Futura Publishing Co., Mt. Kisco, N.Y., in press, 1982.
11. Diehl, A. M., Lauer, R. M., and Shankar, K. R.: Tricuspid atresia. In Heart Disease in Infants, Children and Adolescents, edited by A. J. Moss and F. H. Adams. Williams & Wilkins, Baltimore, 1968.
12. Dolara, A., Fazzini, P. F., Marchi, F., et al.: Changing clinical features in tricuspid atresia without transposition of the great arteries. Report of two cases. Acta Cardiol. (Brux) 24:275, 1969.
13. Edwards, J. E., and Burchell, H. B.: Congenital tricuspid atresia: A classification. Med. Clin. North Am. 33:1177, 1949.
14. Ellison, R. C., and Restieaux, N. J.: Vectorcardiography in congenital heart disease. W. B. Saunders, Philadelphia, 1972.
15. Fischbein, C. A., Rosenthal, A., Fischer, E. G., Nadas, A. S., and Welch, K.: Risk factors for brain abscess in patients with congenital heart disease. Am. J. Cardiol. 34:97, 1974.
16. Fontan, F., and Bandet, E.: Surgical repair of tricuspid atresia. Thorax 26:240, 1971.
17. Freed, M. D., Heymann, M. A., Lewis, A. B., et al.: Prostaglandin E₁ in infants with ductus arteriosus-dependent congenital heart disease. Circulation 64:899, 1981.
18. Freedom, R. M., and Gerald, P. S.: Congenital cardiovascular disease and the "Cat-eye" syndrome. Am. J. Dis. Child. 126:16, 1973.
19. Freedom, R. M., and Rowe, R. D.: Aneurysm of the atrial septum in tricuspid atresia diagnosed during life and therapy. Am. J. Cardiol. 38:265, 1976.
20. Gale, A. W., Danielson, G. K., McGoon, D. C. et al.: Fontan procedure for tricuspid atresia. Circulation 62:91, 1980.

21. Gallaher, M. E., and Fyler, D. C.: Observations in changing hemodynamics in tricuspid atresia without associated transposition of the great arteries. Circulation 35:381, 1967.
22. Gamboa, R., Gersony, W. M., and Nadas, A. S.: The electrocardiogram in tricuspid atresia and pulmonary atresia with intact ventricular septum. Circulation 34:24, 1966.
23. Gasul, B. M., Arcilla, R. A., and Lev, M.: Heart Disease in Children. J. B. Lippincott, Philadelphia, 1966.
24. Glenn, W. W. L., Ordway, N. K., Talner, N. S., and Call, B. P., Jr.: Circulatory bypass of the right side of the heart. VI. Shunt between superior vena cava and distal right pulmonary artery: Report of clinical application in thirty-eight cases. Circulation 31:172, 1965.
25. Guller, B., DuShane, J. W., and Titus, J. L.: The arterioventricular conduction system in two cases of tricuspid atresia. Circulation 40:217, 1969.
26. Guller, B., Titus, J. L., and DuShane, J. W.: Electrocardiographic diagnosis of malformations associated with tricuspid atresia: Correlation with morphologic features. Am. Heart J. 78:180, 1969.
27. Gypes, M. T., Marcano, B. A., and Desilets, D. T.: Tricuspid atresia, transposition and coarctation of the aorta. Radiology 97:633, 1970.
28. Jordan, C., and Sanders, C. A.: Tricuspid atresia with prolonged survival: A report of two cases. Am. J. Cardiol. 18:112, 1966.
29. Keane, J. F., Williams, R., Treves, S., and Rosenthal, A.: Assessment of the postoperative patient by noninvasive techniques. Prog. Cardiovasc. Dis. 18:57, 1975.
30. Keith, J. D., Rowe, R. D., and Vlad, P.: Heart disease in infancy and childhood. Macmillan, New York, 1958.
31. Kreutzer, G., Gulindez, E., Bono, H., et al.: An operation for correction of tricuspid atresia. J. Thorac Cardiovasc. Surg. 66:613, 1973.
32. Kuhne, M.: Über zwei Fälle Kongenitaler Atresia des ostium venosum dextrum. Jahresb. Kinderheilk. 63:225, 1906.
33. LaCorte, M. A., Dick, M., Scheer, G., LaFarge, C. G., and Fyler, D. C.: Left ventricular function in tricuspid atresia. Angiographic analysis in 28 patients. Circulation 52:996, 1975.
34. LaCorte, M. A., Fellows, K. E., and Williams, R. G.: Overriding atrioventricular valve: Echocardiographic and angiographic features. Am. J. Cardiol., in press, 1982.
35. Lawson, R., Rullman, D., Brodeur, M., et al.: Tricuspid atresia with Christmas disease-hemophilia B. J. Thorac. Cardiovasc. Surg. 69:585, 1975.
36. Lenox, C. C., and Zuberbuhler, J. R.: Balloon septostomy in tricuspid atresia after infancy. Am. J. Cardiol. 25:723, 1970.
37. Lenz, W., and Pliess, G.: The pathology of thalidomide embryopathy and associated defects of the heart. In Memorias del IV Congreso Mundial de Cardiologia. Congenitos Hemodinamica I-A:150, 1963 (Mexico).
38. Levy, R. J., Rosenthal, A., Fyler, D. C., et al.: Birthweight of infants with congenital heart disease. Am. J. Dis. Child. 132:249, 1978.
39. Lewis, A. B., Freed, M. D., Heymann, M. A., et al.: Side effects of therapy with prostaglandin E₁ in infants with critical congenital heart disease. Circulation 64:893, 1981.
40. Malhuish, B. P., and Van Praagh, R.: Juxtaposition of the atrial appendages. A sign of congenital heart disease. Br. Heart J. 30:269, 1968.
41. Mehrizi, A., and Drash, A.: Growth disturbance in congenital heart disease: J. Pediatr. 61:418, 1962.
42. Miller, R. A., Pahlajani, D., Serratto, M., et al.: Clinical studies after Fontan's operation for tricuspid atresia. Am. J. Cardiol. 33:157, 1974.
43. Nadas, A. S., and Fyler, D. C.: Pediatric Cardiology, 3rd ed. W. B. Saunders, Philadelphia, 1972.
44. Neches, W. H., Park, S. C., Lenox, C. C., Zuberbuhler, J. R., and Bahnson, H. T.: Tricuspid atresia with transposition of the great arteries and closing ventricular septal defect. J. Thorac. Cardiovasc. Surg. 65:538, 1973.
45. O'Neill, C. A.: Left axis deviation in tricuspid atresia and single ventricle. Circulation 12:612, 1955.
46. Patel, R., Fox, K., Taylor, J. F. H., and Graham, G. R.: Tricuspid atresia: Clinical course in 62 patients. Br. Heart. J. 40:1408, 1978.
47. Phornphutkul, C., Rosenthal, A., Nadas A. S., and Berenberg, W.: Cerebrovascular accidents in infants and children with cyanotic congenital heart disease. Am. J. Cardiol. 32:329, 1973.
48. Rao, P. S.: Natural history of the ventricular septal defect in tricuspid atresia and its surgical implications. Br. Heart J. 39:276, 1977.
49. Rao, P. S., Jue, K. L., Isabel-James, J., and Ruttenberg, H. D.: Ebsteins malformation of the tricuspid valve with atresia. Am. J. Cardiol. 32:1004, 1973.
50. Report of the New England regional infant cardiac program. Pediatrics: 65(No. 2, Suppl.):388, 392–403, 1980.
51. Rihl, J., Terplan, K., and Weiss, F.: Über einen Fall von Agenesie der Tricuspidalklappe. Med. Klin. 25:1543, 1929.
52. Rosenthal, A.: Extracardiac abnormalities in cyanotic congenital heart disease. Hosp. Med. 10:46, 1974.
53. Rowe, R. D., and Mehrizi, A.: The neonate with congenital heart disease. W. B. Saunders, Philadelphia, 1968.
54. Sanders, S. P., Wright, J. F., Keane, J. F., et al.: Fontan operation for tricuspid atresia. Circulation 62(Suppl. III):210, 1980.
55. Sato, T., Onoki, H., Kano, I., et al.: Balloon atrial septostomy in an infant with tricuspid atresia. Tohoku J. Exp. Med. 101:281, 1970.
56. Sharrett, G. P., Johnson, A. M. and Monro, J. L.: Persistence and effects of sinus rhythm after Fontan procedure for tricuspid atresia. Br. Heart J. 42:74, 1979.
57. Singh, S. P., Astley, R., and Parsons, C. G.: Hemodynamic effects of balloon septostomy in tricuspid atresia. Br. Med. J. 1:225, 1968.
58. Somlyo, A. P., and Halloran, K. H.: Tricuspid atresia: An electrocardiographic study. Am. Heart J. 63:171, 1962.
59. Stadford, V., Armstrong, R. G., and Cline, R. E. L.: Right atrial-pulmonary artery allograft for correction of tricuspid atresia. J. Thorac. Cardiovasc. Surg. 66:105, 1973.
60. Stanton, R. E., Lurie, P. R., Lindensmith, G. G., et al.: The Fontan procedure for tricuspid atresia. Circulation. 64(Suppl. II):140, 1981.
61. Tandon, R., and Edwards, J. E.: Tricuspid atresia: A re-evaluation and classification. J. Thorac. Cardiovasc. Surg. 67:530, 1974.
62. Taussig, H. B., Keinonerr, R., Momberger, N., et al.: Long term observations in the Blalock-Taussig operation. IV. Tricuspid atresia. Johns Hopkins Med. J. 132:135, 1973.
63. Tingelstad, B., Lower, R. R., Howell, T. R., et al.: Pulmonary artery banding in tricuspid atresia without transposition of the great arteries. Am. J. Dis. Child. 121:434, 1971.

64. Van Praagh, R.: Anatomic types of tricuspid atresia: Autopsy study of 46 cases. Personal communication, 1975.
65. Van Praagh, R., Ando, M., and Dungan, W. T.: Anatomic types of tricuspid atresia: Clinical and developmental implication. Circulation 44:II–115, 1971.
66. Wittenborg, M. H., Neuhauser, H. B. D., and Sprunt, W. H.: Roentgenographic findings in congenital tricuspid atresia with hypoplasia of the right ventricle. Am. J. Roentgenol. Radium Ther. Nucl. Med. 66:712, 1951.

20

Ebstein's Anomaly

Lodewyk H. S. Van Mierop, M.D., Gerold L. Schiebler, M.D., and Benjamin E. Victorica, M.D.

Congenital anomalies which produce stenosis or incompetence of the tricuspid valve are uncommon. The most common is Ebstein's anomaly of the tricuspid valve; congenital isolated incompetence or stenosis due to other types of valvar dysplasia are rare.

In 1866, Ebstein described in great detail an autopsy which he had performed on a 19-year-old laborer.[33] The man had a history of dyspnea, cyanosis, and palpitations since early youth. The complaints which precipitated his admission were swelling of the legs, fever, and cough. At postmortem examination, a curious anomaly of the tricuspid valve was found (Fig. 20.1). The valve was markedly redundant and had an abnormal origin from the right ventricular wall below the tricuspid valve anulus. Only the anterior cusp of the tricuspid valve originated from its normal position. Ebstein also discussed what he conceived to be the possible pathophysiology of the lesion and correlated this with the clinical findings.[102] Following Ebstein's publication, reports of similar cases were published.[37, 52, 114, 127] It was not until 1949 that the presence of the anomaly, now known by its eponym, was diagnosed during life[117] and shortly thereafter by others.[99, 109] This was followed by reports which established Ebstein's anomaly as a clinical entity.[34, 45, 60, 74, 100, 119] Hernandez, et al.[54] were able to make the diagnosis by simultaneously recording intracavitary pressures and electrocardiograms, an approach suggested earlier.[107, 108]

The prevalence of Ebstein's anomaly among patients with congenital heart disease is about 0.5%.[58, 94] A much lower percentage (0.03%) was reported by Simcha and Bonham–Carter.[106] Over 500 cases have been reported from all parts of the globe. The sexes are equally affected, and familial occurrence of Ebstein's anomaly has been reported.[31, 46, 69, 123]

Ebstein's anomaly has no particular association with any syndromic entity, although associations have been reported with Bonnevie–Ullrich,[15] Marfan, and Down syndromes.[13] A remarkably high frequency of Ebstein's anomaly has been reported among infants born to mothers who received lithium during pregnancy[87, 124]

PATHOLOGY AND PATHOGENESIS

The pathology of Ebstein's anomaly of the tricuspid valve is extremely variable.[4, 34, 42, 66, 120, 129] The two characteristic features are redundancy of valve tissue and adherence of a variable portion of the medial (septal) and posterior cusps to the right ventricular wall, resulting in an origin of the free portion of the valve cusp from the right ventricular wall some distance away from the atrioventricular junction. The redundancy is marked and obvious if a relatively large portion of the valve cusps is free. If most valve tissue is adherent to the right ventricular wall, the redundancy may be less apparent. Redundancy involves all cusps, although the anterior cusp is always less affected. The free portion of the valve usually has a crumpled and nodular appearance. The area of adherence may be small, in which case the true origin of the cusp at the atrioventricular anulus is close to the apparent or "false" origin, or it may extend all the way down to the ring formed by the parietal band, the crista supraventricularis, the septal band, the moderator band, and the anterior papillary muscle. The portion of the right ventricle between the atrioventricular junction and the downward displaced or false origin of the valve forms a common chamber with the right atrium and is said to be "atrialized," since, in a functional sense, it has become part of the right atrium.

The degree of impairment of right ventricular function depends largely on the extent to which the right ventricular inflow portion is atrialized and how intimately the valve tissue is adherent to the right ventricular wall (Figs. 20.2 to 20.4). In some cases the wall of the atrialized portion of the right ventricle is almost normally formed, and the redundant valve tissue is superficially adherent to the trabeculae carneae, so that on cross-section the right ventricle appears to consist of an outer muscular and an inner fibrous layer with trabeculae in between. At the other extreme are found cases where adherence is so intimate that the involved right ventricular wall is reduced to a paper-thin fibrous sac and has lost much of its ability to contract. The nonatrialized portion of the right ventricular wall is usually of normal thickness.

Occasionally the membrane formed by the redundant valve tissue is imperforate; usually one or more openings are present. One of these is constant, being located close to the crista supraventricularis, and is homologous to the normal tricuspid valve orifice. It is generally of moderate or small size, causing some degree of stenosis and often incompetency. Other openings, if present, are generally found near the anterior and other papillary muscles and merely represent abortive attempts at formation of chordae tendineae. Occasionally a very large single opening is found. In such cases almost all the cusp tissue, particularly that of the medial cusp, is adherent to the ventricular wall.

Embryologically the tricuspid valve cusps are primarily derived from the interior of the embryonic right ventricular myocardium by a process of undermining of the right ventricular wall, the same process which is responsible for the formation of trabeculae carneae (Fig. 20.5A). The inner layer of ventricular myocardium is freed from the remainder of

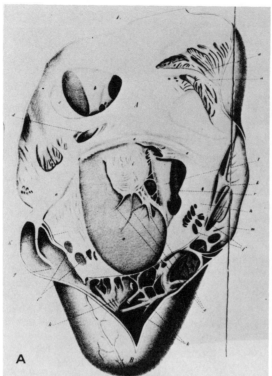
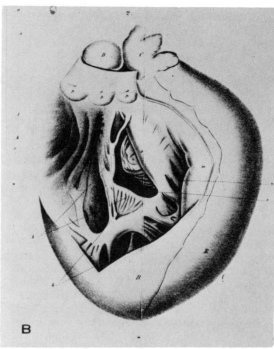

Fig. 20.1 Figures from Ebstein's original article. The same letters refer to both figures. (*A*) The right atrium and right ventricle opened by an incision from the right side of the superior vena cava. (*B*) The right ventricular outflow tract. The incision went from the apex of the right ventricle (about 1 cm to the right of the longitudinal sulcus) along the anterior wall of the right ventricle into the pulmonary trunk. *A*, right atrium; *a*, pectinate muscles; *b*, valve which does not quite close the foramen ovale; *c*, Eustachian valve; *d*, coronary sinus ostium; *B*, right ventricle; *e*, right anulus fibrosis; *h*, anterior, and *h₁*, the posterior portion of the membrane arising from *e* through which there are many small openings labeled *f*; *i*, rudimentary septal leaflet of the tricuspid valve with its chordae tendineae *g* inserted on the endocardium of the ventricular septum; *r*, tricuspid valve ostium; *k*, chordae tendineae and papillary muscles attached between the outer wall of the membrane *h* and *h₁* and the wall of the right ventricle; *l*, papillary muscles to which the anterior part of the membrane *h* is inserted with a superior and inferior limb; *m*, anterior wall of the right ventricle; *q*, posterior wall of the right ventricle; *n*, right ventricular outflow; *o*, ventricular septum; *p*, pulmonary trunk and valve with normal valve leaflets; *C*, left atrial appendage; *D*, ascending thoracic aorta; *E*, left ventricle.

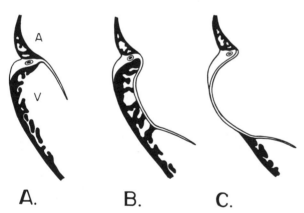

Fig. 20.2 Section through the right atrioventricular junction. *A.*, normal heart (*A*, right atrium; *V*, right ventricle); *B.*, mild degree of Ebstein's anomaly; *C.*, severe Ebstein's anomaly. Note in *B.* and *C.* the apparent displacement of the tricuspid valve.

the right ventricular wall and forms a muscular skirt. The atrial side of the skirt near the atrioventricular orifice is partially covered by endocardial cushion tissue. Perforations appear in the apical portion of the skirt which enlarge until only papillary muscles and chordae tendineae remain. Although initially muscular, the chordae and the cusps later become fibrous. The anterior cusp is formed very early in development and already is "free" in a 16-mm embryo. The

posterior and medial cusps develop much later, the latter not being fully formed even in a 3-month-old fetus.

Ebstein's anomaly of the tricuspid valve could be explained pathogenetically by an abnormality in the process of undermining which remains incomplete and never reaches the anulus (Fig. 20.5*B*). The development of large perforations which normally result in the formation of chordae and papillary muscles, does not take place at all or remains abortive—hence the redundancy of the valve. The normal origin of most of the anterior cusp is probably related to its early liberation.

Associated anomalies are common. An interatrial communication, either a patent foramen ovale or an atrial septal defect at the fossa ovalis, is present in over half of the cases. An ostium primum type of atrial septal defect has been reported in a few instances.[52, 123] If interatrial communications are excluded, the frequency of associated anomalies still remains high. Most common are pulmonary stenosis or atresia and VSD, either alone or in combination with other lesions.[23, 29, 39, 41, 58, 74, 78, 81, 100] Much less common are patent ductus arteriosus, tetralogy of Fallot, right aortic arch,[189] coarctation of the aorta, transposition of the great arteries,[65] and prolapse of the mitral valve.[92]

PHYSIOLOGY

The physiology of Ebstein's anomaly almost defies categorization, since the pathology varies so enormously. The

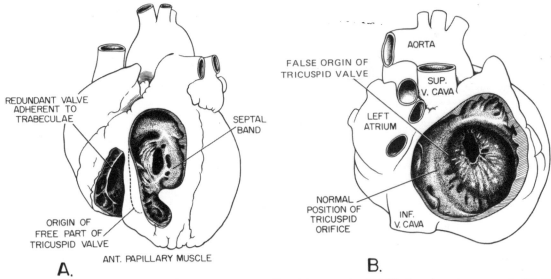

Fig. 20.3 Pathologic specimen of an adult with milder form of Ebstein's anomaly. (*A*.) Windows have been cut into the right ventricle proximal and distal to the false origin of the tricuspid valve. Note that the redundant valve tissue is rather superficially adherent to the trabeculae carneae, so that on cross-section, the right ventricle appears to consist of an outer muscular and an inner fibrous layer with trabeculae in between. (*B*.) Right atrial view of same case—showing an enlarged right atrium. Note redundant tricuspid valve tissue and the downward displacement of the valve.

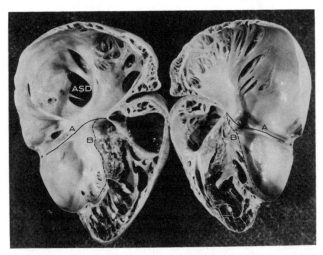

Fig. 20.4 Specimen of the severe form of Ebstein's anomaly in an infant. Section through right atrium and ventricle parallel to the septum. *A*, Position of tricuspid anulus; *B*, false origin of tricuspid valve. The wall of the "atrialized" right ventricle (between *A* and *B*) is reduced to a paper-thin sac. Note position of right coronary artery, transected at *A*. *ASD*, Atrial septal defect.

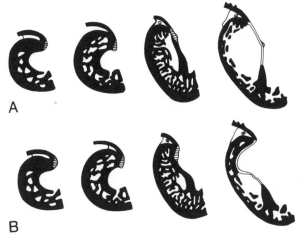

Fig. 20.5 Concept of the pathogenesis of Ebstein's anomaly. (*A*) Normal development of atrioventricular valve cusp. (*B*) Ebstein's anomaly. (Reproduced with permission from L. H. S. Van Mierop and I. H. Gessner: *Progress in Cardiovascular Diseases* 15:67, 1972.)

anomaly may be of such a mild degree that the valve mechanism functions normally. Such cases are more likely to survive well into adult life. Ebstein's anomaly has been reported as an incidental finding at autopsy.[51]

Cyanosis is caused primarily by a right to left shunt at the atrial level. This bypass of the right ventricle may be caused by a number of factors which keep the mean right atrial pressure above the mean left atrial pressure, thus causing the shunt. Elevation of right atrial pressure may be secondary to stenosis or occasionally atresia of the anomalous tricuspid valve ostium, to insufficiency, or both. Stenosis and insufficiency probably coexist in most cases.

During atrial systole a portion of the blood in the right atrium is propelled into the atrialized ventricle, which dilates to accommodate this blood. During ventricular systole the blood contained in the atrialized ventricle is forced back into the true atrium. This "ping-pong" effect is particularly pronounced in those cases in which the atrialized right ventricle has a relatively well-developed muscular wall.

Any element of tricuspid insufficiency in the newborn period is enhanced by the normally present right ventricular hypertension. As the pulmonary artery and right ventricular systolic pressures fall postnatally, the magnitude of the tricuspid insufficiency, the mean right atrial pressure, the right to left shunt, and the peripheral arterial desaturation decrease. Thus, the intense cyanosis seen in the neonate becomes less apparent or disappears. When episodes of recurrent cyanosis occur, paroxysmal tachycardia should be suspected. Tachycardia enhances tricuspid insufficiency, putting in reverse the above sequence and producing or increasing the right to left shunt.[18] The shortened diastolic filling period of the distal, nonatrialized right ventricle further impedes right ventricular filling and raises right atrial pressure. With prolonged tachycardia myocardial failure may ensue.

Although cyanosis may disappear early in life, it almost invariably recurs. Presumably with time there is diminished efficiency of the anomalous valve and associated myocardial structures. Tricuspid insufficiency dilates the right ventricular outflow tract and all proximal right heart structures, including the tricuspid valve orifice. This initiates a vicious cycle whereby insufficiency begets more insufficiency. The resultant increased right atrial pressure causes a greater right to left shunt and more cyanosis. Although a right to left atrial shunt is the usual finding in Ebstein's anomaly of the tricuspid valve, bidirectional or left to right shunts may occur in some cases, e.g., if an atrial septal defect is present in cases with the mild form of the anomaly.

If the foramen ovale is anatomically closed the patient usually remains acyanotic. The absence of an interatrial communication, however, often causes a pronounced increase in right atrial pressure, increasing the height of the *a* wave. The increased atrial pressure may exceed the right ventricular and the pulmonary artery diastolic pressure. Thus, the right atrium can open the pulmonary valve in late diastole and perfuse the pulmonary bed. Both the right ventricular and pulmonary artery systolic pressure complex may then be preceded by an *a* wave complex.

MANIFESTATIONS

Clinical Features

Since the pathology and the accompanying physiology are so variable, Ebstein's malformation presents on the stage as an actor with many masks.

The occurrence of Ebstein's anomaly cannot be correlated to prenatal event, birth order, or maternal age.[100] The occurrences of cyanosis, heart failure, presence of a murmur, or growth retardation are too nonspecific to be helpful. The only feature that suggests the diagnosis of Ebstein's anomaly is bouts of rapid heart action, particularly if they occur in a cyanotic child.

The malformation may be so pronounced as to cause intrauterine or neonatal death.[58, 74, 109] Symptoms are common in newborns, and in one large series, one-half the infants had symptoms during the first months of life.[100] Cyanosis, cardiac murmur, and severe heart failure are the obvious manifestations.[37, 94, 100, 126] Cyanosis tends to diminish or disappear with time. Eventually, however, cyanosis recurs, usually between the ages of 5 and 10 years.[37]

In some cases the valve is so redundant that it produces right ventricular outflow obstruction, thus mimicking severe pulmonic valve stenosis or atresia with intact ventricular septum.[83] After infancy, if symptoms occur, their onset is often vague and insidious. Most common are dyspnea on exertion, profound weakness or fatigue, and cyanosis.[100] The individual is often more limited by fatigue than by dyspnea.[43, 115] The degree of cyanosis may have little relationship to the individual's ability to perform physical work.

Episodes of paroxysmal tachycardia occur in about 25% of individuals with Ebstein's anomaly,[65, 100, 119] (Some authors report a lower[106] or higher[13] frequency.) Neurologic symptoms are frequent, particularly syncope associated with exertion, emotion, or a paroxysm of superventricular tachycardia. Other neurologic symptoms are dizzy spells, transient visual loss, and manifestations of thromboembolism. Cardiac failure in older children and adults usually presents only in the terminal stage of this disease, although it may occur

during a bout of supraventricular tachycardia. Exertion, emotion, or paroxysms of atrial tachycardia may precipitate precordial or epigastric anginal pain.[100, 119] Less frequent manifestations are squatting, severe headaches, protracted cough, particularly after exertion or emotion, and marked photophobia.[100]

Most individuals are of normal height and weight.[100] Individuals with an Ebstein's anomaly may also have an unusual facial coloration which has been described as "florid,"[17, 59] "flushed,"[18] a "violaceous hue,"[10, 18] and "red-cheeked."[17, 44] Only rarely is the pulsation of tricuspid insufficiency noted in the distended neck veins or liver. More often, the neck veins are either normal or, in the presence of systemic venous hypertension, simply distended. Hepatomegaly and splenomegaly may be present owing to heart failure.

The arterial blood pressure and peripheral arterial pulses are usually normal. Occasionally, we and others have observed systemic hypertension.[20] The mechanism of this is not clear. In some cases, renal disease is present.[32, 44]

The chest contour may be normal, particularly in acyanotic patients. Bilateral or left chest prominence is usually noted in individuals with cardiomegaly or cyanosis. The cardiac impulse is usually normal and well localized in acyanotic individuals, whereas in cyanotic patients, the impulse is usually diminished and diffuse. A systolic thrill may be present, often best felt to the left of the lower sternal border or laterally.

The heart rate and rhythm are usually normal. Tachycardia, premature ventricular contractions, and atrial fibrillation may be present. In many children who have either a stable, mild form of the anomaly or who are still in the early stages of a more progressive form, the auscultation may not be very revealing. Some individuals have no murmur, regardless of the severity of the anomaly.

The systolic murmur present in the majority of individuals is probably secondary to tricuspid insufficiency or right ventricular outflow obstruction. It may vary in intensity from a grade 1/6 to a 5/6 murmur and is usually maximal along the lower left sternal border in the third and fourth intercostal spaces. At times, it may be maximal over the apex. Frequently, the murmur is a short, low intensity decrescendo bruit. At other times the murmur, although remaining basically a decrescendo murmur, occupies one-half or two-thirds of systole. Finally, it may be a crescendo-decrescendo murmur that occupies the entirety of systole, obscuring portions of the first and second heart sounds. The first sound, which is either normal or slightly diminished in intensity, is usually comprised of two main components. The second constituent of the first sound is greater in intensity than the first. This second component, maximal in the fourth left intercostal space near the sternal border, often has a metallic, clicking quality resembling an ejection sound. It is usually delayed in relation to the first component.

The second sound with its two main components, the aortic and pulmonic, may be normal in the asymptomatic, acyanotic child. When a right bundle branch block pattern is present, the aortic-pulmonary interval is longer and moves normally with the phases of respiration. In deeply cyanotic individuals with decreased pulmonary flow, the pulmonic component often is diminished or inaudible.

The third sound is often more prominent than normal; and this is a prime clue that more pathology exists than might be suspected. Whether this sound is caused by increased filling of the right ventricle or represents the opening snap or other vibrations of the abnormal tricuspid valve remains unsettled. At times, the third sound may initiate, or be encompassed by, a short, middiastolic murmur, which has a superficial high-pitched quality that has been called "scratchy."[125] It is not unlike that which is heard in many cases of atrial septal defect, where it is thought to represent relative tricuspid stenosis. Recognition of this diastolic murmur is difficult, particularly when the murmur is intermittent or its intensity is poorly correlated with the phases of respiration.

A loud fourth sound may also be present, which in time may be replaced by a prominent late diastolic murmur. With prolongation of the PR interval, however, this murmur may begin earlier, and it blends with the previously described middiastolic murmur. Thus, one may hear a systolic murmur that partially obliterates S1 and S2, a silent hiatus, and a prominent mid- and late diastolic murmur. The hiatus may be so short that the systolic and diastolic murmurs appear to blend and form a continuous murmur.[81, 115]

Murmurs of tricuspid origin may increase with inspiration, but in our experience not as frequently as had been described. The continuous sounding murmur may resemble a pericardial friction rub. In turn, prominent systolic, diastolic, and atrial components of a pericardial rub, not infrequently heard in Ebstein's anomaly, may occupy enough of the cardiac cycle to suggest a continuous murmur.[100] Such a pericarditis[73, 95, 100] has been attributed to chronic severe elevation of systemic venous and coronary sinus pressure which leads to the extravasation of blood products into the pericardial space.

On rare occasions a midsystolic click is noted,[41] but when present, this sound is usually obscured by the coexistent systolic murmur. When the murmurs are soft, the metallic, clicking components of the widely split first and second sounds produce combinations of sounds that comprise a triple, quadruple, or quintuple rhythm. It is characteristic of Ebstein's anomaly that the tonal qualities of the heart sounds themselves are often unusual.

Electrocardiographic Features

The electrocardiographic patterns in Ebstein's anomaly are of inordinate value. On rare occasions the electrocardiogram may be normal.[115] All cases observed by us, however, have had abnormal tracings, as did the 67 patients reported upon by Giuliani et al.[43] The electrocardiographic abnormalities usually fall into two categories: those with a right bundle branch block (RBBB) pattern (Fig. 20.6) and those with Wolff-Parkinson-White syndrome (Fig. 20.7). With RBBB there is generally right axis deviation, and in some cases the terminal, slurred portion of the QRS loop is directed rightward and superiorly, causing an S1, S2, S3 pattern. The axis may be normal or show left-axis. Usually a normal sinus rhythm is present, but supraventricular tachycardia, atrioventricular nodal rhythm, atrial flutter, atrial fibrillation, nodal or ventricular premature beats, and other dysrhythmias may occur. Dysrhythmias other than supraventricular tachycardia occur more commonly in the adult.

Characteristically the PR interval is prolonged, which is frequently associated with an increased duration of the P wave. The P waves most often indicate right atrial enlargement or show nonspecific abnormalities. In cases with a giant right atrium, the P wave becomes wide and notched, resembling that seen in biatrial enlargement. Right atrial enlargement produces abnormally tall P waves seen in precordial leads V2 and V3.[100] Individuals who have an increase in both the height and the duration of the P waves usually have symptoms and may die within a short time.[100] Conversely, those who have normal P waves are asymptomatic.

Although the QRS complexes may be normal initially,[81, 100] eventually the QRS duration is increased. This increase is

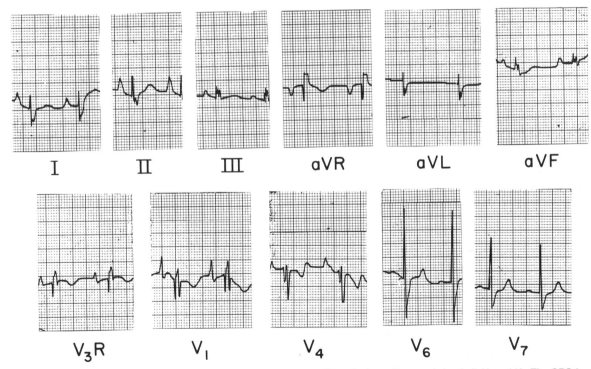

Fig. 20.6 Electrocardiogram of an 11-year-old with Ebstein's anomaly. Note the large P waves in leads *II*, *V₃* and *V₁*. The QRS forces are relatively posterior, suggesting left ventricular hypertrophy or decreased right ventricular forces, with marked delay of the terminal rightward, slightly anterior and superior QRS forces giving a right bundle branch block pattern. Note the low voltage and splintered QRS complexes, the low voltage of the R complex in the right precordial leads, and the first degree A-V block with a PR interval of 0.20 second.

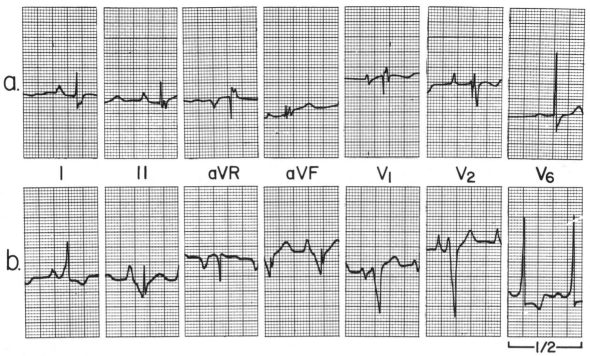

Fig. 20.7 Electrocardiogram of a 12-year-old with Ebstein's anomaly and intermittent Wolff-Parkinson-White syndrome. (*a.*) Right bundle branch block (RBBB) pattern. (*b.*) Wolff-Parkinson-White (W-P-W) pattern. There is coexistent first degree heart block. (Reproduced with permission from B. L. Miller and B. E. Victorica: *Vectorcardiography 2*, edited by I. Hoffman, pp. 597–609. North-Holland Publishing Company, Amsterdam, 1971).

secondary to a prolongation of the terminal QRS depolarization, which produces variable degrees of right bundle branch block. Thus, the QRS complex frequently becomes notched, slurred, or splintered. The R and S waves in the standards leads tend to be small, with a total height of less than 7 mm. This is particularly true in adults, or in children with a severe form of the disease. Serial tracings show a progressive decrease in QRS voltage and a progressive increase in notching and slurring.

On rare occasions, a right ventricular hypertrophy pattern is seen.[20, 63] Rarely, the R and R' wave in V_1 exceeds 9 mm.[41, 58, 100] If it does, one should consider another lesion. With a splintered, notched QRS complex, the right ventricular activation time may be greater than 0.04 sec. Serial tracings generally show progression of right ventricular activation from normal to abnormal.

A qR pattern in the right precordial leads, followed by a diphasic or negative T waves in leads V_1 to V_4, was thought to suggest Ebstein's anomaly.[107] The pattern is almost never seen in children.[100] In over half of the cases, there is no Q wave in lead V_6, although this wave then appears in leads V_7 or V_8.[100]

Left ventricular hypertrophy is not seen. Thus, we may see a child who has congenital heart disease, but who has neither right nor left ventricular hypertrophy. This is a valuable clue in distinguishing Ebstein's malformation from other clinical entities.

The QT interval is usually normal, although with marked prolongation of the QRS duration it increases *pari passu*. ST-segment and T-wave changes are variable, most profound in late stages of the disease, and accentuated by digitalis therapy. The second and less frequent pattern noted in the electrocardiogram is the Wolff-Parkinson-White (W-P-W) conduction anomaly (Fig. 20.7). The W-P-W syndrome is reported in about 5% of the cases. In contrast, this syndrome occurred in about 25% of two large groups of cases,[100]

and is present in 4 of the 18 children in the University of Florida series. Sodi-Pallares *et al.*[107] first drew attention to this association and interpreted the electrocardiogram of Yater and Shapiro's patient as showing the W-P-W pattern. Although the W-P-W pattern can occur with many other types of congenital heart disease, 30% of all cases having coexistent congenital heart disease and the W-P-W electrocardiographic pattern have Ebstein's anomaly of the tricuspid valve.[99] Considering that the Ebstein anomaly comprises less than 1% of all cases of congenital heart disease, this frequency is highly significant. Since the W-P-W syndrome may be transient or intermittent, the frequency of the W-P-W syndrome in Ebstein's anomaly is minimal. The associated W-P-W pattern is always type B, resembling left bundle branch block, with predominant S waves in the right precordial leads. Thus a patient having congenital heart disease and a type B W-P-W syndrome on the electrocardiogram should be suspected of having Ebstein's anomaly. The presence of the W-P-W pattern increases the individual's propensity to supraventricular paroxysmal tachycardia.[41, 100]

Vectorcardiographic Features

The vectorcardiogram from several series of cases of Ebstein's anomaly has been reported.[14, 16, 22, 70] The P loops are usually increased in size and have the contour of right atrial enlargement. The mean P vector is directed leftward, inferior and anterior, so that its maximal voltage is noted in leads II, V_2, and V_3. The P loop is usually equal to or greater in size than the accompanying T loop (Fig. 20.8).

The inscription of the QRSsÊ loop in the frontal plane is usually clockwise, with the mean QRS vecotr directed rightward and inferior. There is marked slowing of the terminal portion, usually in the right superior and anterior quadrant, producing a right bundle branch block pattern. At times, the mean QRS vector in the frontal plane is normal. Rarely, the QRSsÊ loop is counterclockwise in the frontal plane[41] with

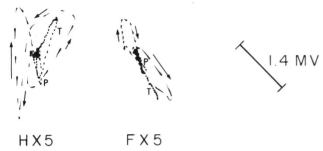

HX5   FX5

Fig. 20.8 Vectorcardiogram (Grishman cube system) of a 6-year-old boy with Ebstein's anomaly.

prolongation of the rightward and superior QRS forces producing left axis deviation.

In the horizontal plane, the QRSsÊ loop's initial and middle forces are inscribed in a normal counterclockwise direction. The initial rightward and anterior QRS forces are usually diminished or not present, producing a small or absent q wave in lead V_6. An absent or diminished, slurred Q loop or, in the absence of a Q loop, an initially slurred R loop has been ascribed in some cases to ventricular septal fibrosis.[14] The anterior QRS forces are usually diminished, so that the area encompassed by the loop is preponderantly leftward and posterior. Terminally, the QRSsÊ loop swings rightward, either anterior or posterior to the E point. This terminal portion shows marked slowing, the hallmark of right bundle branch block. The pattern and location of this terminal delay in the QRS loop is variable. These QRSsÊ loop features in combination with large P loops are characteristic of Ebstein's anomaly. The T loop may be normal and concordant with the initial and middle forces of the QRSsÊ loop, but discordant with its terminal portion. In the later stages of the disease process with digitalization and/or myocardial disease, an ST-vector change and profound T-loop changes usually occur.

The presence of the W-P-W pattern on the vectorcardiogram is indicated by an abnormal degree of slowing of the initial portion of the QRSsÊ loop (Fig. 20.9). This initial delay is the expression of the delta wave of the electrocardiogram and is the distinctive feature of the W-P-W syndrome. These initial slowed QRSsÊ forces are usually directed leftward, posterior, and superior. In the type B variety of W-P-W syndrome, which mimics left bundle branch block, the remainder of the QRSsÊ loop is predominantly leftward, posterior, and superior. The P loops are unaffected by this syndrome. It does, however, alter ventricular repolarization, causing attendant ST-vector and T-loop changes.[91]

Phonocardiographic Features

The phonocardiogram in Ebstein's malformation has been described by several groups.[74, 86, 100, 119] Such studies have clarified our auscultatory findings and have confirmed their variability. The phonocardiogram shows the following features: the Q-S_1 interval is increased to 0.05 second or more. The first sound complex is normal or diminished in intensity with the second component of the first sound usually more intense than the first component. The systolic murmur, varied in intensity, is either decrescendo or crescendo-decrescendo and of moderate frequency and intensity. It is maximal along the lower left sternal border or laterally over the left precordium. In childhood the components of the second heart sound are usually normal, but the aortic-pulmonary interval is increased in the presence of right bundle branch block. In the cyanotic individual with a low cardiac output, the pulmonic component may not be detectable. The aortic

component is of maximal intensity along the lower left sternal border or the apex. The early diastolic sound may be an opening snap of the tricuspid valve or a third heart sound. The latter frequently initiates or is encompassed by a low frequncy middiastolic murmur. A prominent fourth sound may be replaced by a presystolic murmur. With first-degree atrioventricular block, the mid- and late diastolic murmurs may be superimposed.[100] On rare occasions, the phonocardiogram records a pericardial friction rub.

Echocardiographic Features

M-mode echocardiography has been used as a noninvasive method for the diagnosis of Ebstein's anomaly.[26, 64, 71, 112] It is possible in this anomaly to obtain an echo from the downward displaced tricuspid valve further to the left on the precordium than in patients in whom the valve is in the normal position. The pattern of movement of the echo from the anterior tricuspid valve cusp is abnormal. The reason for this is believed to be either a reduced compliance of the functioning, distal portion of the right ventricle or possibly a mechanical factor related to the abnormal large anterior cusp.

The most significant and possibly pathognomonic finding is a closure of the tricuspid valve, which is considerably later (0.06 second or more) than that of the mitral valve (Fig. 20.10). This late closure, at first believed to be due to the presence of right bundle branch block, has been shown to be due to some other, possibly mechanical factor,[71] since it is not present in patients with any other anatomic or electrocardiographic abnormality. It is also reported to be present in patients who have Ebstein's anomaly associated with Wolff-Parkinson-White syndrome.[112] Some of these M-mode features, however, are nondiagnostic, since they are also seen in other forms of right ventricular volume overload.[48] Two-dimensional echocardiography is a valuable addition to the diagnosis of Ebstein's anomaly. This method not only permits the detection of the displaced septal tricuspid valve leaflet (Fig. 20.11), but can also estimate the morphologic severity of the anomaly.[88]

Radiologic Features

Profound variability is present. Rarely the chest roentgenograms are normal.[2, 115] In infancy, cardiac size varies from slight to massive enlargement,[100] and pulmonary vascular markings are diminished.

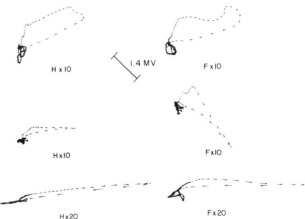

H x 10   1.4 MV   F x 10

H x 10   F x 10

H x 20   F x 20

Fig. 20.9 Vectocardiogram (Grishman cube system) of three cases of Ebstein's anomaly associated with Wolff-Parkinson-White syndrome. (Reproduced with permission from B. L. Miller and B. E. Victorica: *Vectorcardiography 2*, edited by I. Hoffman, pp. 597–609. North-Holland Publishing Company, Amsterdam, 1971).

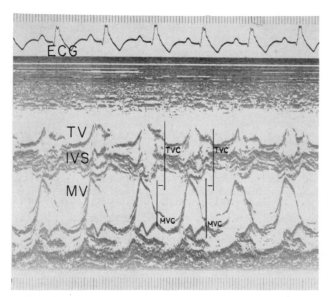

Fig. 20.10 Echocardiogram in Ebstein's anomaly. Interval between closure of mitral and tricuspid valves is 0.09 second.

In older children and adults, the chest roentgenograms generally can be grouped into a number of types (Fig. 20.12);

1. The overall heart size is normal, only slightly enlarged, with normal pulmonary vascular markings. The cardiac contour is unusual, however, in that there is a marked convexity of the heart shadow to the right of the sternum, indicating right atrial enlargement. The apex is elevated, suggesting right ventricular enlargement. The aortic knob is normal in size, but the pulmonary artery segment is hidden from view. Often a straight line can be drawn from the aortic knob to the apex of the heart.

2. The left heart border slopes downward as seen in left ventricular enlargement. This in association with normal pulmonary vascularity may suggest aortic stenosis.

3. Massive right atrial enlargement causes shelving of the right heart border and alters the position of the remaining cardiac structures. A similar shelving on the left side is produced by the dilated and displaced right ventricular outflow tract. This accounts for the box-shaped or funnel-shaped cardiac silhouette seen in the more severe forms of Ebstein's anomaly.

4. In some cases the cardiac silhouette is nonspecific or resembles that seen in other cardiac malformations.

Certain roentgenographic features are commonly seen in any of the above groups:

1. The pulmonary segment is normal or small.
2. Left atrial enlargement is never seen.
3. The aortic knob may be normal or small. Ebstein's anomaly is the only cyanotic congenital malformation of the heart in which *both* the pulmonary artery and aorta may be smaller than normal.
4. Pulmonary vascular markings may be either normal or decreased. If the pulmonary vascularity appears normal, the individual is usually acyanotic. In cyanotic patients, the vascularity is usually decreased.
5. Even in the presence of heart failure, the pulmonary venous markings are not increased and evidence of pleural effusion is not seen.

In some patients, the x-ray appearance in Ebstein's anomaly remains stable. We have followed several individuals for over 10 years in whom the cardiac silhouette has showed little or no change. In our experience[2, 100] the cardiac pulsa-

tions in children with Ebstein's anomaly as noted at fluoroscopy have not been distinctive. Occasionally calcification may be seen in the abnormal tricuspid valve.[117]

CARDIAC CATHETERIZATION

Much has been written about the dangers of cardiac catheterization in individuals with Ebstein's malformation.[17, 74] A number of deaths occurred in the early days of cardiac catheterization, and this led some investigators[125] to advise against carrying out the procedure if Ebstein's anomaly was suspected. The heart is unusually irritable, a circumstance which should not be surprising considering the high frequency of naturally occurring dysrhythmias. Dysrhythmias during cardiac catheterization have been reported to be about 20 to 30%. In an international cooperative study of 505 cases of Ebstein's anomaly in whom 363 catheterizations were carried out,[123] 13 deaths were reported for a frequency of 3.6%. An additional six cases developed cardiac arrest during the procedure but survived. With increased experience, improved techniques, better monitoring equipment, safer contrast materials, and improved defibrillators, the high fatality rate has decreased, and at present the indications for cardiac catheterization in patient with Ebstein's anomaly are no different from those in patients with other cardiac anomalies.

Cardiac catheterization, to be diagnostic, must demonstrate that a portion of the right ventricle functions as right atrium because of the abnormal distal location of the tricus-

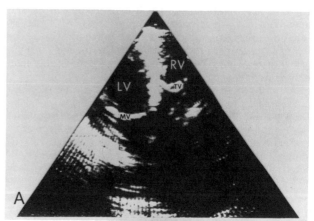

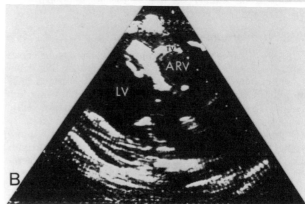

Fig. 20.11 Two-dimensional echocardiogram (apical-four chamber view) of a 5-year-old with Ebstein's anomaly. In systole (*A*), note the displaced origin of the septal tricuspid leaflet (*TV*). In diastole (*B*), the sail-like redundant leaflet forms a concavity toward the atrialized right ventricle (*ARV*).

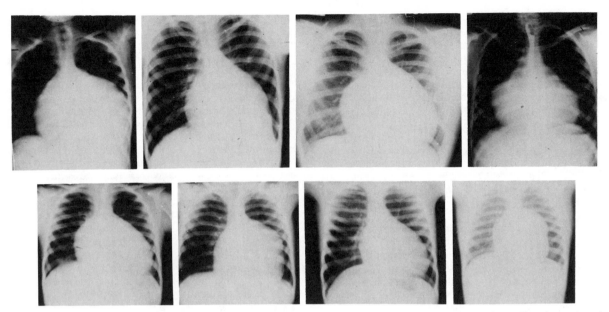

Fig. 20.12   Anteroposterior chest radiograph of eight patients with Ebstein's anomaly, showing variability in cardiac size and contour.

pid valve. *All* other information obtained by cardiac catheterization may be seen in other clinical entities.

Specific information regarding "atrialization" of a portion of the right ventricle may be obtained by utilizing the intracavitary electrocardiogram.[54, 121, 122, 128] Its value was established by Hernandez *et al.*[54] In three cases they showed, by simultaneously recording an intracavitary electrocardiogram and right heart pressures, three different combinations of these parameters. With the catheter in the distal portion of the right ventricle, right ventricular pressure and muscle potentials were recorded. On pullback from the right ventricle, right *ventricular* muscle potentials continued to be recorded over a certain distance, while the pressure dropped to atrial levels. Finally, on withdrawal of the catheter to the right atrium, the electrocardiogram changed from a ventricular to an atrial pattern, while the pressure remained the same. Such a sequence of events is diagnostic of Ebstein's anomaly. Unfortunately, if in a case of suspected Ebstein's anomaly the above events do not occur, the diagnosis is not excluded.[80] For, on withdrawal of the catheter from the distal right ventricle into the atrium, the catheter may slide along the normally attached portion of the anterior leaflet, and thus the simultaneously recorded intracavitary electrocardiogram and pressure recordings are normal. This is more likely to occur if catheterization is carried out from the saphenous vein, because the catheter will usually enter the distal right ventricle along the superior border of the tricuspid anulus, e.g., the point where the anterior leaflet has normal attachments. If there is only a very mild degree of Ebstein's deformity, then during the pullback tracing the catheter may not stay long enough in this small atrialized right ventricle to allow detection of a distinct zone of ventricular muscle potential with right atrial pressure. Indeed, in mild forms of Ebstein's anomaly with minimal valve displacement, all presently available techniques may be inconclusive.

Hernandez and his group[54] also pointed out the value of stimulating the myocardium of these three aforementioned areas of the right heart with a catheter. In the functional right ventricle and in the "atrialized ventricle" one would produce a ventricular ectopic beat, whereas in the right atrium myocardial stimulation would evoke a premature atrial complex.

The large cavity formed by the right atrium and the atrialized right ventricle can be outlined by a large loop formed by the catheter. In most cases, the maneuver requires no special effort. Usually a right to left atrial shunt is present. At times, a concomitant left to right shunt is present which may be predominant and suggest an isolated atrial septal defect.

The hemodynamic findings depend on whether there is tricuspid stenosis, tricuspid insufficiency, or both. In the presence of predominant tricuspid stenosis, the right atrial pressure tracing will show a prominent "a" wave, and a diastolic pressure difference would be recorded across the tricuspid valve. Predominant tricuspid insufficiency would cause large "ac" and "v" waves of equal magnitude or a dominant "v" wave. At times, in the atrial pressure pulse an abnormal systolic wave, the "s" wave, may be interposed between the "ac" and "v" waves.

The change in pressure on withdrawal of the catheter from the right ventricle may indicate leftward displacement of the tricuspid valve. This finding is only diagnostic when the displacement is pronounced, since an enlarged right atrium may lead to lesser degrees of tricuspid valve displacement.

The right ventricular chamber can usually be entered, although at times this presents difficulties. The pulmonary artery is more difficult to enter, because of the unusual position and deformity of the tricuspid valve. This difficulty may be increased when a portion of the leaflet obstructs the right ventricular outflow tract. The frequency of dysrhythmias caused by catheter probing in the area of the outflow tract may be such that the operator settles for a less than ideal right heart catheterization.

The right ventricular pressure is usually normal in Ebstein's anomaly, although cases have been reported in which the right ventricular systolic pressure has been as high as 45 mm Hg.[60, 100, 110] The right ventricular pressure tracing may have a normal contour, although in the presence of right bundle branch block, the ascending limb may have a slower rise than normal. Right ventricular end-diastolic pressure may be elevated due to an increase in atrial systolic pressure as manifested by a tall "a" wave. This same atrial impulse may be transmitted to the pulmonary artery, where it appears as a prominent presystolic pulsation. Thus, on rare occasions, the right atrial, right ventricular, and the pulmonary artery pressure contours resemble each other. At times, when the catheter in the distal right ventricle is pulled back to the atrialized right ventricle, and then to the right atrium, one may record a different pressure contour in each of these three areas.[41] Both systemic and pulmonary blood flow may be diminished, particularly in cyanotic individuaals.[81, 100]

ANGIOCARDIOGRAPHY

Soloff and colleagues[109] were the first to diagnose Ebstein's anomaly by angiocardiography. This may show an enlarged right atrium which extends leftward beyond its usual boundary. A notch might be apparent at the site of the anomalous origin of the tricuspid valve. The right ventricle and pulmonary artery generally are smaller than normal (Fig. 20.13).

When a large right to left atrial shunt is present, there is immediate opacifaction of the left atrium, the left ventricle, and the aorta. Such cases may simulate tricuspid atresia. Usually, however, the right to left shunt and slow propagation of contrast medium through the right heart cause all cardiac chambers to be opacified simultaneously. This may make it difficult to identify anatomical structures.

Selective right ventricualr angiocardiography[36] is a superior means of showing the position of the displaced tricuspid valve, the size of the right ventricle, the thickness of the wall of the sinus and outflow portions of the right ventricle, and the site and size of the pulmonary valve ring and pulmonary artery. In the lateral view, the abnormal origin of the tricuspid valve is seen to be located far anteriorly. A crude estimation may also be made of the amount of tricuspid insufficiency.

Since the right coronary artery indicates the location of the tricuspid valve anulus, a discrepancy in position between the opacified right coronary artery and the anomalous origin of the tricuspid valve indicates the size of the atrialized right ventricle and is diagnostic of Ebstein's anomaly.[36]

Opacification of the right heart produces a trilobed appearance. These three "lobes," consisting of the enlarged right atrium, the atrialized ventricle, and the distal right ventricle, are separated inferiorly by two notches. The proximal notch is caused by the tricuspid anulus, whereas the distal notch is produced by the origin of the displaced tricuspid valve (Fig. 20.13).

Cineangiocardiography[38] also demonstrates the absence of the opening and closing movements of the normal tricuspid valve apparatus and the function of the atrialized right

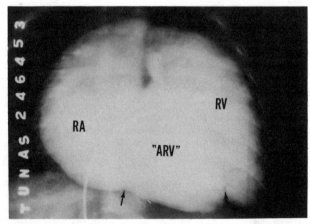

Fig. 20.13 Angiocardiogram showing trilobed appearance of heart. *RA*, right atrium; *RV*, right ventricle; "*ARV*", atrialized portion of right ventricle. *Arrows* indicate position of tricuspid valve anulus and "displaced" valve origin.

ventricle. The volume variation of the right ventricular infundibulum has been commented upon.[35]

DIFFERENTIAL DIAGNOSIS

Patients with the more severe forms of Ebstein's anomaly present no problem in diagnosis. Difficulties may arise in individuals who have mild forms of the malformation with little or no cardiomegaly, or in whom associated anomalies cloud the picture.

Complex forms of tetralogy of Fallot may present with a large heart, particularly when associated with endocardial cushion defect and atrioventricular valve incompetence. However, the incompetence usually involves the left atrioventricular valve component rather than the right. Occasionally tetralogy of Fallot also may be associated with type B Wolff-Parkinson-White syndrome. Nonetheless, the clinical, radiographic, and electrocardiographic findings are quite different.

Pulmonary atresia with intact ventricular septum associated with pronounced tricuspid valve insufficiency may simulate Ebstein's anomaly in many respects, and the differentiation may be difficult, particularly since the patients are almost always newborns, the same age group in which Ebstein's anomaly is frequently associated with pulmonary atresia. In pulmonary atresia with intact septum, however, the electrocardiogram generally shows a left dominant pattern without evidence of right ventricular conduction delay.

The rare form of congenital tricuspid insufficiency due to dysplasia of the tricuspid valve[11] but without downward displacement of the valve and the very rare Uhl's anomaly[118] of the right ventricle may closely resemble Ebstein's anomaly. It may be nearly impossible to differentiate them with certainty during life, even if angiocardiography and intracavitary electrocardiographic studies are done.

Large pericardial effusions or cardiomyopathy may produce radiographic findings similar to those seen in Ebstein's anomaly, but the history, the clinical, and the electrocardiographic findings will generally help one to arrive at the correct diagnosis. The same is true in patients with malignant carcinoid syndrome or rheumatic heart disease. In nearly all conditions which in some way mimic Ebstein's anomaly, particularly when associated with cyanosis and diminished pulmonary vascular markings, the electrocardiogram will show either right or left ventricular dominance. In Ebstein's anomaly, the tracing almost always shows *neither* right nor left ventricular hypertrophy. Even in those few cases in which right ventricular hypertrophy is present electrocardiographically, the R waves in the right precordial leads rarely exceed 9 mm and are not often associated with marked ST and T-wave changes. In the newborn period, type B Wolff-Parkinson-White syndrome associated with Ebstein's anomaly may be misinterpreted as left ventricular hypertrophy and result in an erroneous diagnosis of tricuspid atresia or pulmonary atresia with intact ventricular septum.[94]

TREATMENT

Individuals with Ebstein's anomaly should be encouraged to enter lines of activity that are rewarding but that do not require prolonged strenuous exertion. Furthermore, they should be cautioned not to engage in athletic competition under conditions from which they cannot withdraw gracefully when symptoms develop. Older children and adults usually learn to live within certain limits.

Other aspects of therapy include general medical care, antibiotics for infections and measures designed to combat heart failure when this supervenes. Individuals with heart failure who live at high altitudes should be encouraged to move to sea level.[81] Dysrhythmias can be treated with anti-dysrhythmic drugs or cardioversion.

Palliative surgical procedures have little to offer. A systemic artery-pulmonary artery shunting procedure appears to be contraindicated in Ebstein's anomaly. A superior vena cava-right pulmonary artery shunt (Glenn procedure) gives at best mediocre long-term results.

Hunter and Lillehei[55] advocated ligation and marsupialization of the thin atrialized portion of the right ventricle, realignment of the tricuspid cusps to the right atrioventricular anulus, and annuloplasty to narrow the circumference of the dilated tricuspid ostium and closure of the patent foramen ovale. Hardy and associates[49, 50] successfully employed a modification of the Hunter-Lillehei technique. Barnard and Schrire[7] were the first to excise the malformed valve and replace it with a prosthesis attached to the true anulus. Valve replacement with either a mechanical or "biological" prosthesis quickly became the most commonly used surgical approach[25, 57, 62, 68, 116] and continues to find ardent advocates[6, 19, 79, 84]. Others, however, are less satisfied and recommend a return to some type of plastic repair.[27, 75]

Data contained in an international cooperative study of 505 cases of Ebstein's anomaly indicate that very careful selection of cases remains of the utmost importance.[123]

COURSE AND PROGNOSIS

Most authors report a mean age of death of about 20 years.[37, 39, 41, 119] Others quote a somewhat younger[65] or older[72] age. About one-third of the patients die before the age of 10 years, most in infancy. There are many reports, however, of survival beyond the sixth decade,[1, 51, 72, 85, 113] and it is quite possible that a number of asymptomatic individuals with the mild form of the anomaly are missed.

The presence of associated anomalies, massive tricuspid insufficiency, heart failure, and dysrhythmias carries a poor prognosis. The latter probably accounts for the majority of cases of sudden death, a not uncommon outcome in Ebstein's anomaly, particularly in older children and adults. Not surprisingly, the larger the heart and the more pronounced the cyanosis, the poorer the prognosis. The main complications of Ebstein's anomaly are cerebral abscess and paradoxical embolism. Endocarditis is extremely rare.

Information on the natural history of Ebstein's anomaly, based on an experience of 67 patients was recently provided by Giuliani et al.[43] Mortality in this series was found to be affected primarily by four factors: functional class III or IV; cardiomegaly; cyanosis or hypoxia; and diagnosis in infancy.

TRICUSPID VALVE INSUFFICIENCY

Congenital tricuspid valve insufficiency as an isolated anomaly is rare.[3, 90, 94] In most instances it is associated with severe stenosis or atresia of the right ventricular outflow tract, either at the infundibular or valvar level, or both. In some of these, the insufficiency is functional and not due to a tricuspid valve anomaly. In others, some or all of the valve cusps are dysplastic and tethered to the right ventricular myocardium by anomalous, short chordae tendineae.

The features of tricuspid valve dysplasia have been well described.[11] These authors emphasized the great variation in the severity of the dysplasia from slight nodular thickening of the cusps of an otherwise normal valve apparatus to irregularly thickened, redundant cusps with abnormal chordae tendineae and papillary cases; there may be agenesis of part or even all[11, 56, 105] of the tricuspid valve and in others the valve is merely represented by a ridge of nodular thickening. Only two of the 10 cases of tricuspid valve dysplasia

without downward displacement of the valve described[11] had no right ventricular outflow obstruction. All but one were less than 1 year of age at death. Tricuspid valve dysplasia undoubtedly represents a spectrum which includes Ebstein's anomaly, and the pathogenesis of all the various forms is probably similar.

The manifestations of severe congenital tricuspid insufficiency in neonates and infants are remarkably similar.[8, 9, 61, 90] They include extreme cardiomegaly, heart failure, cyanosis, a precordial thrill and harsh pansystolic murmur, and decreased second sound, and the electrocardiogram demonstrates right axis deviation and a right bundle branch block pattern. In some cases, there may be evidence of left atrial enlargement as well. Chest x-rays confirm the presence of a massively enlarged heart, and the vascular pattern of the lungs is diminished.

Cardiac catheterization demonstrates the presence of tricuspid insufficiency and enormous enlargement of the right-sided cardiac chambers. The right ventricular pressure may be normal or elevated. This may explain the failure of the opacification of the pulmonary arteries on angiocardiography in some infants who do not have right ventricular outflow tract obstruction. Apparently the free regurgitation across the tricuspid valve makes it impossible for the right ventricle to generate enough pressure to open the pulmonary valve in the presence of the neonatal, high pulmonary vascular resistance. The prognosis of congenital tricuspid insufficiency is poor, probably in part because of the high frequency of associated severe pulmonary stenosis or atresia. Surgical treatment has little to offer these infants, and the mortality in cases in which it was attempted approached 100%. Patients with milder forms of tricuspid valve dysplasia have a much better prognosis and may be asymptomatic for many years.[9]

A transient form of tricuspid insufficiency in the newborn is a recognized entity.[40, 101] The picture resembles that seen in congenital tricuspid insufficiency due to malformed tricuspid valve, but with vigorous medical treatment the infant's condition improves. Eventually the cardiovascular status becomes normal. Schiebler et al.[101] suggested that a sudden closure of the ductus arteriosus and the foramen ovale immediately after birth, forcing the right heart to pump the entire systemic venous return through the pulmonary vascular bed which still has a high vascular resistance, could lead to an overload of the right ventricle and secondary tricuspid insufficiency. With reduction of the pulmonary vascular resistance, the right ventricular pressure drops and the tricuspid insufficiency disappears. On the other hand, transient congenital tricuspid insufficiency seen in babies might be due to late development of the medial cusp of the tricuspid valve.[104] Freymann and Kallfelz[40] felt the second explanation to be more plausible, in part because in the case described by them the foramen ovale was still patent at 4 days of age and the infant's recovery appeared later than could be anticipated by the theory proposed by Schiebler et al.[101]

All 14 term infants with the syndrome reported by Bucciarelli et al.[21] had experienced significant perinatal stress. The two babies that died had histologic evidence of right ventricular anterior papillary muscle necrosis. This, and the commonly seen ECG evidence of myocardial ischemia led the authors to propose that the syndrome was due to a reversible form of papillary muscle dysfunction.

TRICUSPID STENOSIS

Congenital tricuspid stenosis is usually associated with other anomalies, most commonly severe pulmonic stenosis or atresia, with secondary hypoplasia of the right ventricle.

The tricuspid anulus in this complex is small, but the valve apparatus, although dimunitive in size, is usually normally formed. The narrow tricuspid ostium in these cases, therefore, should more properly be referred to as being hypoplastic rather than stenotic, even though in some cases a certain degree of commissural fusion coexists. Tricuspid valve hypoplasia has also been described in association with ventricular septal defect, tetralogy of Fallot, double outlet right ventricle, single ventricle, and mitral stenosis.[24, 41, 92, 97] In all of these, the clinical manifestations will be determined by the associated anomalies.

Isolated tricuspid stenosis is rare, and many cases reported in adults are almost certainly acquired, probably secondary to rheumatic valvulitis. Gueron et al.[44] commented upon the strong predominance of females in this group.

Isolated congenital tricuspid stenosis is extremely rare.[12, 67, 77] In some cases there is associated moderate or severe hypoplasia of the right ventricle.[28, 30, 76, 96, 98, 111] Curiously this combination has a strong tendency to occur in families,[28, 76, 96] a circumstance for which there is no explanation. In the few cases in which chromosome studies were done, they were normal.[28]

The clinical manifestations of isolated congenital tricuspid stenosis resemble those seen in tricuspid atresia, and the two anomalies may be difficult to distinguish, even with angiocardiography. Cyanosis is present in both, and in both the electrocardiogram may demonstrate left axis deviation, right atrial hypertrophy, and left ventricular hypertrophy with absent or reduced right ventricle electrical activity. It is important, however, to make the distinction, since in some cases of tricuspid stenosis corrective surgery may be possible.[5, 30, 77, 98]

REFERENCES

1. Adams, J. C. L., and Hudson, R.: A case of Ebstein's anomaly surviving to the age of 79. Br. Heart J. 18:129, 1956.
2. Amplatz, K., Lester, R. G., Schiebler, G. L., Adams, P., Jr., and Anderson, R. C.: The roentgenologic features of Ebstein's anomaly of the tricuspid valve. Am. J. Roentgenol. 81:788, 1959.
3. Amtia, A. U., and Osunkoya, B. O.: Congenital tricuspid incompetence. Br. Heart J. 31:664, 1969.
4. Anderson, K. R., Zuberbuhler, J. R., Anderson, R. H., Becker, A. E., and Lie, J. S.: Morphologic spectrum of Ebstein's anomaly of the heart. Mayo Clin. Proc. 54:174, 1979.
5. Barbero-Marcial, M., Nuno-Conceição, N., Verginelli, G., Ebaid, M., Snitcowsky, R., and Zerbini, E. J.: Congenital tricuspid stenosis treated by a palliative open operation: Report of a case. J. Thorac. Cardiovasc. Surg. 69:562, 1975.
6. Barbero-Marcial, M., Verginelli, G., Awad, M., Ferreira, S., Ebaid, M., and Zerbini, E. J.: Surgical treatment of Ebstein's anomaly. J. Thorac. Cardiovasc. Surg. 78:416, 1979.
7. Barnard, C. N., and Schrire, V.: Surgical correction of Ebstein's malformation with prosthetic tricuspid valve. Surgery 54:302, 1963.
8. Barr, P. A., Celermajer, J. M., Bowdler, J. S., and Cartmill, T. B.: Severe congenital tricuspid incompetence in the neonate. Circulation 49:962, 1974.
9. Barritt, D. W., and Urich, H.: Congenital tricuspid incompetence. Br. Heart J. 18:133, 1956.
10. Bayer, V. O., Rippert, R., Wolter, H. H., and Loogen, F.: Klinische und physiologische Befunde beim Ebstein-Syndrome: Bericht über 3 Fälle. Z. Kreislaufforsch. 43:98, 1954.
11. Becker, A. E., Becker, M. J., and Edwards, J. E.: Pathologic spectrum of dysplasia of the tricuspid valve. Arch. Pathol. 91:167, 1971.
12. Bharati, S., McAllister, H. A., Tatooles, C. J., Miller, R. A., Weinberg, H. and Buckeleres, H. G.: Anatomic variations in underdeveloped right ventricle related to tricuspid atresia and stenosis. J. Thorac. Cardiovasc. Surg. 72:383, 1976.
13. Bialostozky, D., Horwitz, S., and Espino-Vela, J.: Ebstein's malformation of the tricuspid valve. Am. J Cardiol. 29:826, 1972.
14. Bialostozky, D., Medrano, G. A., Munoz, L., and Contreras, R.: Vectorcardiographic study and anatomic observations in 21 cases of Ebstein's malformation of the tricuspid valve. Am. J. Cardiol. 30:354, 1972.
15. Bieber, G.: Sindrome de Bonnevie-Ullrich associata a cardiopatia congenita (Sindrome de Ebstein). Riv. Clin. Pediatr. 65:148, 1960.
16. Bilger, R., So, C. S., Emmrich, J., Steim, H.,

and Reindell, H.: Über das Elektrokardiogramm und Vektorkardiogramm des Ebstein-Syndroms. Arch. Kreislaufforsch. 35:238, 1961.
17. Blacket, R. B., Sinclair-Smith, B. C., Palmer, A. J., Halliday, J. H., and Maddox, J. K.: Ebstein's disease: A report of five cases. Australas. Ann. Med. 1:26, 1952.
18. Blount, S. G., Jr., McCord, M. C., and Gelb, I. J.: Ebstein's anomaly. Circulation 15:210, 1957.
19. Bove, E. L., and Kirsh, M. M.: Valve replacement for Ebstein's anomaly of the tricuspid valve. J. Thorac. Cardiovasc. Surg. 78:229, 1979.
20. Brown, J. W., Heath, D., and Whitaker, W.: Ebstein's disease. Am. J. Med. 20:322, 1956.
21. Bucciarelli, R. L., Nelson, E. M., Egan, E. A., Eitzman, D. V., and Gessner, I. H.: Transient tricuspid insufficiency of the newborn: A form of myocardial dysfunction in stressed newborns. Pediatrics 59:330, 1977.
22. Cabrera, E., Gaxiola, A., Ferrer, G., and Costa Rocha, J.: El vectocardiograma en la enfermedad de Ebstein. Arch. Inst. Cardiol. Mex. 32:702, 1962.
23. Caddell, J. L., and Browne, M. J.: Right ventricular hypertension and pulmonary stenosis in Ebstein's anomaly of the heart. Am. J. Cardiol. 11:100, 1963.
24. Calleja, H. B., Hosier, D. M., and Kissane, R. W.: Congenital tricuspid stenosis. The diagnostic value of cineangiocardiography and hepatic pulse tracing. Am. J. Cardiol. 6:821, 1960.
25. Cartwright, R. S., Smeloff, E. A., Cayler, G. G., Fong, W. Y., Huntley, A. C., Blake, J. R., and McFall, R. A.: Total correction of Ebstein's anomaly by means of tricuspid replacement. J. Thorac. Cardiovasc. Surg. 47:755, 1964.
26. Crews, T. L., Pridie, R., Benham, R., and Leathem, A.: Auscultatory and phonocardiographic findings in Ebstein's anomaly: Correlation of first heart sound with ultrasonic records of tricuspid valve movement. Circulation 42 (Suppl III):113, 1970.
27. Danielson, S. K., Maloney, J. D., and DeVloo, R. A. E.: Surgical repair of Ebstein's anomaly. Mayo Clin. Proc. 54:185, 1979.
28. Davachi, F., McLean, R. H., Moller, J. H., and Edwards, J. E.: Hypoplasia of the right ventricle and tricuspid valve in siblings. J. Pediatr. 71:869, 1967.
29. DeLeon, A. C., Jr., Perloff, J. K., and Blanco, P.: Congenital pulmonic stenosis complicating Ebstein's anomaly of the tricuspid valve. Am. J. Cardiol. 14:695, 1964.
30. Dimich, I., Goldfinger, P., Steinfeld, L., and Lukban, S. B.: Congenital tricuspid stenosis:

Case treated by heterograft replacement of tricuspid valve. Am. J. Cardiol. 31:89, 1073.
31. Donegan, C. K., Moore, M., Wiley, T., Hernandez, F. A., Krovetz, L. J., Green, J. R., Jr., and Schiebler, G. L.: Familial Ebstein's anomaly of the tricuspid valve. Am. Heart J. 75:375, 1968.
32. Drummond, K. N., Vernier, R. L., Worthen, H. G., and Good, R. A.: The associated occurrence of the nephrotic syndrome and congenital heart disease. Pediatrics 31:103, 1963.
33. Ebstein, W.: Über einen sehr seltenen Fall von Insufficienz der Valvula tricuspidalis, bedingt durch eine angeborene hochgradige Missbildung derselben. Arch. Anat. Physiol. 238, 1866.
34. Edwards, J. E.: Pathologic features of Ebstein's malformation of the tricuspid valve. Mayo Clin. Proc. 28:89, 1953.
35. Elliott, L. P., and Hartmann, A. F., Jr.: The right ventricular infundibulum in Ebstein's anomaly of the tricuspid valve. Radiology 89:694, 1967.
36. Ellis, K., Griffiths, S. P., Burris, J. O., Ramsay, G. C., and Fleming, R. J.: Ebstein's anomaly of the tricuspid valve: Angiocardiographic considerations. Am. J. Roentgenol. 92:1338, 1964.
37. Engle, M. A., Payne, T. P. B., Bruins, C., and Taussig, H. B.: Ebstein's anomaly of the tricuspid valve: Report of three cases and analysis of clinical syndrome. Circulation 1:1246, 1950.
38. Fabian, C. E., Mundt, W. P., and Abrams, H. L.: Ebstein's anomaly: The direct demonstration of contractile synchrony between the two parts of the right ventricle. Invest. Radiol. 1:63, 1966.
39. Fontana, R. S., and Edwards, J. E.: Congenital Cardiac Disease: A Review of 357 Cases Studied Pathologically. W. B. Saunders, Philadelphia, 1962.
40. Freymann, R., and Kallfelz, H. C.: Transient tricuspid incompetence in a newborn. Eur. J. Cardiol. 2:467, 1975.
41. Gasul, B. M., Arcilla, R. A., and Lev, M.: Heart Disease in Children. Diagnosis and Treatment. J. B. Lippincott, Philadelphia, 1966.
42. Genton, E., and Blount, S. G., Jr.: The spectrum of Ebstein's anomaly. Am. Heart J. 73:395, 1967.
43. Giuliani, E. R., Fuster, V., Brandenburg, R. O., and Mair, D. D.: Ebstein's anomaly. The clinical features and natural history of Ebstein's anomaly of the tricuspid valve. Mayo Clin. Proc. 54:163, 1979.
44. Goni, L. F., Brodsky, B. M., Saavedra, V. J., Romero, T., and Martinez, C.: Ebstein's disease. Arch. Inst. Cardiol. Mex. 34:576, 1964.

45. Gøtzsche, H., and Falholt, W.: Ebstein's anomaly of the ticuspid valve: A review of the literature and report of 6 new cases. Am. Heart J. 47:587, 1954.

46. Gueron, M., Hirsch, M., Stern, J., Cohen, W., and Levy, M. J.: Familial Ebstein's anomaly with emphasis on the surgical treatment. Am. J. Cardiol. 18:105, 1966.

47. Gueron, M., Hirsch, M., Borman, J., and Appelbaum, A.: Isolated tricuspid valvular stenosis: The pathology and merits of surgical treatment. J. Thorac. Cardiovasc. Surg. 63:760, 1972.

48. Gussenhoven, W. J., Spitaels, S. E. C., Bom, N., and Becker, A. E.: Echocardiographic criteria for Ebstein's anomaly of tricuspid valve. Br. Heart J. 43:31, 1980.

49. Hardy, K. L., May, E. A., Webster, C. A., and Kimball, K. C.: Ebstein's anomaly: A functional concept and successful definitive repair. J. Thorac. Cardiovasc. Surg. 48:927, 1964.

50. Hardy, K. L., and Rose, B. B.: Ebstein's anomaly: Further experience with definitive repair. J. Thorac. Cardiovasc. Surg. 58:553, 1969.

51. Harris, R. H. D.: Ebstein's anomaly: Discovered in a 75-year-old subject in the dissecting laboratory. Can. Med. Assoc. J. 83:653, 1960.

52. Heigel, A.: Über eine besondere Form von Entwicklungsstörung der trikuspidal Klappe. Virchows Arch. [Pathol. Anat.] 214:301, 1913.

53. Henderson, C. B., Jackson, F., and Swan, W. G. A.: Ebstein's anomaly diagnosed during life. Br. Heart J. 15:360, 1953.

54. Hernandez, F. A., Rochkind, R., and Cooper, H. R.: The intracavitary electrocardiogram in the diagnosis of Ebstein's anomaly. Am. J. Cardiol. 1:181, 1958.

55. Hunter, S. W., and Lillehei, C. W.: Ebstein's malformation of the tricuspid valve: Study of a case together with suggestion of a new form of surgical therapy. Dis. Chest. 33:297, 1958.

56. Kanjuh, V. I., Stevenson, J. E., Amplatz, K., and Edwards, J. F.: Congenitally unguarded tricuspid orifice with coexistent pulmonary atresia. Circulation 30:911, 1964.

57. Kay, J. H., Tsuji, H. K., Redington, J. V., Yamada, T., Kagawa, Y., and Kawashima, J.: The surgical treatment of Ebstein's malformation with right ventricular aneurysmorrhapy and replacement of the tricuspid valve with a disc valve. Dis. Chest. 51:537, 1967.

58. Keith, J. D., Rowe, R. D., and Vlad, P.: Heart Disease in Infancy and Childhood. Macmillan, New York, 1958, p. 314.

59. Kerwin, A. J.: Ebstein's anomaly: Report of a case diagnosed during life. Br. Heart J. 17:109, 1955.

60. Kezdi, P., and Wennemark, J.: Ebstein's malformation: Clinical findings and hemodynamic alterations. Am. J. Cardiol. 2:200, 1958.

61. Kincaid, O. W., Swan, H. J. C., Ongley, P. A., and Titus, J. L.: Congenital tricuspid insufficiency: Report of two cases. Mayo Clin. Proc. 37:640, 1962.

62. Kitamura, S., Johnson, J. L., Redington, J. V., Mendez, A., Zubiate, P., and Kay, J. H.: Surgery for Ebstein's anomaly. Ann. Thorac. Surg. 11:320, 1971.

63. Kjellberg, S. R., Mannheimer, E., Rudhe, U., and Jonsson, B.: Diagnosis of Congenital Heart Disease, 2nd ed. Year Book Medical Publishers, Chicago, 1959, p. 678.

64. Kotler, N. N., and Tabatznik, B.: Recognition of Ebstein's anomaly by ultrasound technique. Circulation 44 (Suppl. II):34, 1971.

65. Kumar, A. E., Fyler, D. C., Miettinen, O. S., and Nadas, A.: Ebstein's anomaly. Clinical profile and natural history. Am. J. Cardiol. 28:84, 1971.

66. Lev, M., Liberthson, R. R., Joseph, R. H., Seten, C. E., Kunske, R. D., Eckner, F. A. O., and Miller, R. A.: The pathologic anatomy of

67. Lewis, T.: Congenital tricuspid stenosis. Clin. Sci. 5:261, 1945.

68. Lillehei, C. W., and Gannon, P. G.: Ebstein's malformation of the tricuspid valve. Method of surgical correction utilizing a ball-valve prosthesis and delayed closure of atrial septal defect. Circulation 32(Suppl.I):9, 1965.

69. Lo, K. S., Loventhal, J. P., and Walton, J. A.: Familial Ebstein's anomaly. Cardiology 64:246, 1979.

70. Lowe, K. G., Emslie-Smith, D., Robertson, P. G. C., and Watson, H.: The scalar, vector and intracardiac electrocardiogram in Ebstein's anomaly. Br. Heart J. 30:617, 1968.

71. Lundström, N-R: Echocardiography in the diagnosis of Ebstein's anomaly of the tricuspid valve. Circulation 47:597, 1973.

72. Makous, N., and Vander Veer, J. B.: Ebstein's anomaly and life expectancy. Report of a survival to over age 79. Am. J. Cardiol. 18:100, 1966.

73. Masanti, J. G., Navarret, E., Perretta, A., Perez Acebo, J. E., Malenchini, M., and Belensky, A.: Anomalia de Ebstein de la valvula tricuspide asociada a derrame pericardico. Rev. Assoc. Med. Argent. 78:659, 1964.

74. Mayer, F. E., Nadas, A. S., and Ongley, P. A.: Ebstein's anomaly: Presentation of ten cases. Circulation 16:1057, 1957.

75. McFaul, R. C., Davis, Z., Giuliani, E. R., Ritter, D. G., and Danielson, G. K.: Ebstein's malformation. Surgical experience at the Mayo Clinic. J. Thorac. Cardiovasc. Surg. 72:940, 1976.

76. Medd, W. E., Neufeld, H. N., Weidman, W. H., and Edwards, J. E.: Isolated hypoplasia of the right ventricle and tricuspid valve in siblings. Br. Heart J. 23:25, 1961.

77. Medd, W. E., and Kinmonth, J. B.: Congenital tricuspid stenosis: A case treated by open operation. Br. Med. J. 1:598, 1962.

78. Mehrizi, A., Folder, G. M., Jr., and Puri, P.: Ebstein malformation of the tricuspid valve associated with ventricular septal defect. Bull. Hopkins Hosp. 116:89, 1965.

79. Melo, J., Saylam, A., Knight, R., and Starr, A.: Long-term results after surgical correction of Ebstein's anomaly. J. Thorac. Cardiovasc. Surg. 78:233, 1979.

80. Moles, S. S., Jacoby, W. J., Jr., and McIntosh, H. D.: Ebstein's malformation: Discordant intracavitary electrocardiographic and pressure relationship. Am. J. Cardiol. 14:720, 1964.

81. Nadas, A. S.: Pediatric Cardiology, 2nd ed. W. B. Saunders, Philadelphia, 1963.

82. Neufeld, H. N.: Personal communication, 1966.

83. Newfeld, E. A., Cole, R. B., and Paul, M. H.: Ebstein's malformation of the tricuspid valve in the neonate. Functional and anatomic outflow obstruction. Am. J. Cardiol. 19:727, 1967.

84. Ng, R., Somerville, J., and Ross, D.: Ebstein's anomaly: Late results of surgical correction. Eur. J. Cardiol. 9:39, 1979.

85. Oldenberg, F. A., and Nichol, A. D.: Ebstein's anomaly in the adult. Ann. Intern. Med. 52:710, 1960.

86. Ongley, P. A., Sprague, H. B., Rappaport, M. B., and Nadas, A. S.: Heart Sounds and Murmurs. Grune & Stratton, New York, 1960, p. 309.

87. Park, J. M., Sridaromont, S., Ledbetter, E. O., and Terry, W. M.: Ebstein's anomaly of the tricuspid valve associated with prenatal exposure to lithium carbonate. Am. J. Dis. Child. 134:704, 1980.

88. Ports, T. A., Silverman, N. H., and Schiller, N. B.: Two-dimensional echocardiographic assessment of Ebstein's anomaly. Circulation 58:336, 1978.

89. Rebolledo, J. E.: Ebstein's anomaly with right aortic arch. J. Pediatr. 71:66, 1967.

Ebstein's disease. Arch. Pathol. 90:334, 1970.

90. Reisman, M., Hipona, F. A., Bloor, C. N., and Talner, N. S.: Congenital tricuspid incompetence. J. Pediatr. 66:869, 1965.

91. Reynolds, G.: Ebstein's disease: A case diagnosed clinically. Guys Hosp. Rep. 99:276, 1950.

92. Riker, W. L., Potts, W. J., Grana, L., Miller, R. A., and Lev, M.: Tricuspid stenosis or atresia complexes: A surgical and pathologic analysis. J. Thorac. Cardiovasc. Surg. 45:423, 1963.

93. Roberts, W. C., Glancy, D. L., Seningen, R. P., Maron, B. J., and Epstein, S. E.: Prolapse of the mitral valve associated with Ebstein's anomaly of the tricuspid valve. Am. J. Cardiol. 38:377, 1976.

94. Rowe, R. D., and Mehrizi, A.: The Neonate with Congenital Heart Disease. W. B. Saunders, Philadelphia, 1968, p. 308.

95. Sabatini, R., and Zizine, C.: Un cas de maladie d'Ebstein associée à une pericardite. Pediatrie 16:730, 1961.

96. Sackner, M. A., Robinson, M. J., Jamison, W. L., and Lewis, D. H.: Isolated right ventricular hypoplasia with atrial septal defect or patent foramen ovale. Circulation 24:1388, 1961.

97. Salazar, E., Benavides, P., Contreras, R., and Espino-Vela, J.: Congenital mitral and tricuspid stenoses. Am. J. Cardiol. 16:758, 1965.

98. Sapirstein, W., and Baker, C. B.: Isolated tricuspid valve stenosis. Report of a surgically treated case. N. Engl. J. Med. 269:236, 1963.

99. Schiebler, G. L., Adams, P., Jr., and Anderson, R. C.: The Wolff-Parkinson-White syndrome in infants and children. A review and a report of 28 cases. Pediatrics 24:585, 1959.

100. Schiebler, G. L., Adams, P., Jr., Anderson, R. C., Amplatz, K., and Lester, R. G.: Clinical study of twenty-three cases of Ebstein's anomaly of the tricuspid valve. Circulation 19:165, 1959.

101. Schiebler, G. L., Van Mierop, L. H. S., and Krovetz, L. J.: Diseases of the tricuspid valve. In Heart Disease in Infants, Children and Adolescents, edited by A. J. Moss, and F. H. Adams. Williams & Wilkins, Baltimore, 1968, pp. 492–516.

102. Schiebler, G. L., Gravenstein, J. S., and Van Mierop, L. H. S.: Ebstein's anomaly of the tricuspid valve. Translation of original description with comments. Am. J. Cardiol. 22:867, 1968.

103. Seward, J. B., Tajik, A. J., Feist, D. J., and Smith, H. C.: Ebstein's anomaly in an 85 year old man. Mayo Clin. Proc. 54:193, 1979.

104. Shakibi, J. G., and Diehl, A. M.: Postnatal development of the heart and prevalence of congenital heart disease in normal Swiss albino mice: An explanation for transient neonatal tricuspid insufficiency. Circulation 44(Suppl.II):116, 1971.

105. Sherman, F. E.: An Atlas of Congenital Heart Disease. Lea & Febiger, Philadelphia, 1963, pp. 226, 227, 249.

106. Simcha, A., and Bonham-Carter, R. E.: Ebstein's anomaly: Clinical study of 32 patients in childhood. Br. Heart J. 33:46, 1971.

107. Sodi-Pallares, D., Acevedo, J. S., Cisneros, F., Marsico, F., and Alvarado, A.: Wolff-Parkinson-White syndrome in Ebstein's disease: Possibility of diagnosing this anomaly by means of intracavitary leads. Presented at Second World Congress of Cardiology, Washington, D.C., 1954.

108. Sodi-Pallares, D., and Calder, R. M.: New Bases of Electrocardiography. C. V. Mosby, St. Louis, 1956, p. 270.

109. Soloff, L. A., Stauffer, H. M., and Zatuchni, J.: Ebstein's disease. Report of the first case diagnosed during life. Am. J. Med. Sci. 222:554, 1951.

110. Sumner, R. G., Jacoby, W. J., Jr., and Tucker, D. H.: Ebstein's anomaly associated with car-

diomyopathy and pulmonary hypertension. Circulation 30:578, 1964.

111. Svane, S.: Congenital tricuspid stenosis: Report on six autopsied cases. Scand. J. Thorac. Cardiovasc. Surg. 5:232, 1971.

112. Tajik, A. J., Gau, G. T., Giuliani, E. R., Ritter, D. G., and Schattenberg, T. T.: Echocardiogram in Ebstein's anomaly with Wolff-Parkinson-White pre-excitation syndrome, Type B. Circulation 47:813, 1973.

113. Talner, N.: Personal communication, 1966.

114. Taussig, H. B.: Congenital Malformations of the Heart. The Commonwealth Fund, New York, 1947.

115. Taussig, H. B.: Congenital Malformations of the Heart, 2nd ed., Vol. 2. The Commonwealth Fund, Harvard University Press, Cambridge, Mass., 1960.

116. Timmis, J. J., Hardy, J. D., and Watson, D. G.: The surgical management of Ebstein's anomaly: The combined use of tricuspid valve replacement, atrioventricular plication and atrioplasty. J. Thorac. Cardiovasc. Surg. 53:385, 1967.

117. Tourniaire, A., Deyrieux, F., and Tartulier, M.: Maladie d'Ebstein: Essai de diagnostic clinique. Arch. Mal Coeur 42:1211, 1949.

118. Uhl, H. S. M.: A previously undescribed congenital malformation of the heart: Almost total absence of the myocardium of the right ventricle. Bull. Hopkins Hosp. 91:197, 1952.

119. Vacca, J. B., Bussmann, D. W., and Mudd, J. G.: Ebstein's anomaly: Complete review of 108 cases. Am. J. Cardiol. 2:210, 1958.

120. Van Mierop, L. H. S.: In The CIBA Collection of Medical Illustrations, edited by F. H. Netter, Vol. 5, The Heart. CIBA Pharmaceutical Products, Summit, N.J., 1969, pp. 143–144.

121. Watson, H.: Electrode catheters and the diagnosis of Ebstein's anomaly of the tricuspid valve. Br. Heart J. 28:161, 1966.

122. Watson, H., and Lowe, K. G.: Intracavitary potentials in type B ventricular pre-excitation. Br. Heart J. 29:505, 1967.

123. Watson, H.: Natural history of Ebstein's anomaly of tricuspid valve in childhood and adolescence. Br. Heart J. 36:417, 1974.

124. Weinstein, M. R., and Goldfield, M. D.: Cardiovascular malformations with lithium use during pregnancy. Am. J. Psychol. 132:529, 1975.

125. Wood, P.: Diseases of the Heart and Circulation, 2nd ed. Eyre and Spottiswoode, London, 1956, pp. 188, 356.

126. Yamauchi, T., and Cayler, G. G.: Ebstein's anomaly in the neonate: A clinical study of three cases observed from birth through infancy. Am. J. Dis. Child. 107:165, 1964.

127. Yater, W. M., and Shapiro, M. J.: Congenital displacement of the tricuspid valve (Ebstein's disease): Review and report of a case with electrocardiographic abnormalities and detailed histologic study of the conduction system. Ann. Intern. Med. 11:1043, 1937.

128. Yim, B. J. B., and Yu, P. N.: Value of an electrode catheter in diagnosis of Ebstein's disease. Circulation 17:543, 1958.

129. Zuberbuhler, J. R., Allwork, S. P., and Anderson, R. H.: The spectrum of Ebstein's anomaly of the tricuspid valve. J. Thorac. Cardiovasc. Surg. 77:202, 1979.

21

Transposition of the Great Arteries

Milton H. Paul, M.D.

The most common abnormal anatomic relationship between the great arteries and the ventricles is complete transposition of the great arteries. Transposition of the great arteries literally means that the aorta and pulmonary artery are placed across (*trans* = across, *ponere* = to place), rather misplaced across the ventricular septum so that each great artery arises completely above the wrong ventricle: aorta from the right ventricle and pulmonary artery from the left ventricle. The most common clinical representation of the transposition abnormality is understood to represent complete, physiologically uncorrected, transposition of the great arteries (TGA). Functionally, this type of transposition is characterized by poorly oxygenated systemic venous blood being misdirected to the systemic circulation and highly oxygenated pulmonary venous blood similarly misdirected to the pulmonary circulation.

In recent years intensive morphologic studies have been motivated by the realistic urgency of expanding corrective surgery, and many complex arterioventricular relationships have now been accurately characterized and described. Although it is essential to consider TGA within the framework of a comprehensive classification of abnormal arterioventricular relationships, this presentation concerns itself primarily with the most common clinical form, i.e., complete, physiologically uncorrected, transposition of the great arteries.

TGA is a lethal and common malformation. Without treatment about 30% of these infants die in the 1st week of life, 50% within the first month, 70% within 6 months, and 90% within the first year[113, 154] (Fig. 21.1). In contrast to the grim hopelessness of only a few years ago, modern aggressive medical and surgical interventions can provide such infants with considerable hope for an adolescent and adult life. The diagnosis must be considered in any neonate with cyanosis, respiratory distress, or cardiac failure, and such an infant should be treated promptly in a cardiac center which has the experience and facilities for neonatal intensive care, diagnostic intervention, and surgical treatment.

The earliest recorded anatomic observations on TGA were by Baillie (1797). Farre (1814) first used this term to indicate that the great vessels were misplaced across the ventricular septum. Early extensive studies in morphology, pathogenesis, and classifications were by von Rokitansky, Spitzer, Pernkopf and Wintinger, and Harris and Farber; these have been reviewed and extended by Van Praagh[220, 221] and others (see Chapter 28).

The recognition of TGA during life resulted from the clinical and roentgenographic observations of Fanconi (1932) and Taussig (1938). The surgical innovations by Blalock and Hanlon, Albert, Senning, Mustard, Rastelli, and Jatene, and the revolutionary palliative procedure of balloon atrial septostomy by Rashkind and Miller have stimulated an avalanche of clinical and experimental work which has transformed the earlier grim prognosis associated with this malformation to one of hope and continuing challenge.

TGA is one of the most common forms of serious heart disease in newborns and infants, and this diagnosis currently represents about 10% of all infants with heart disease of sufficient severity to have cardiac catheterization, cardiac surgery, or fatal outcome as registered in an infant cardiac registry program within the first year of life.[59] As the result of a decade of widespread success with palliative and corrective procedures, the clinical prevalence of TGA is increasing rapidly in childhood and adolescence.

The incidence varies from 19.3 to 33.8 per 100,000 live births[113] with a strong (60 to 70%) male preponderance.[59] Epidemiologic and genetic surveys have suggested some other associations, e.g., increased prevalence in infants of diabetic mothers[179] or prenatal exposure to sex-hormone

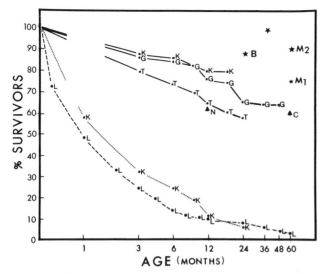

Fig. 21.1 Survival of infants with TGA. Interrupted lines indicate series before the era of balloon atrial septostomy (1966) and intraatrial repair (1964). Solid lines indicate series after these procedures were introduced. L, 742 cases of TGA, 669 of whom died in the years 1957 to 1964; K, 245 cases of TGA seen before 1966. T, 80 infants with TGA treated with balloon atrial septostomy and other indicated nonatrial surgical palliative procedures, 1966 to 1970. G, 47 infants with TGA and intact ventricular septum treated with balloon atrial septostomy, palliative surgical procedures of all forms and late (usually 1 to 2 years of age) intraatrial repair, 1967 to 1972. K (solid line), 39 infants with TGA treated as in series G, 1969 to 1970. N, 52 infants with TGA treated with balloon atrial septostomy and/or surgical atrial septectomy with survival to 1 year of age, 1968 to 1971. C, 120 consecutive infants with TGA with balloon atrial septostomy and treated as in series G, 1966 to 1973, at Children's Memorial Hospital, Chicago. The above intervention survival rates from 1966 to 1973 do not reflect current improved palliative and early corrective management programs as do; B, 58 consecutive infants treated, 1978 to 1980, with balloon atrial septostomy and Mustard or Senning intraatrial repair at a relatively earlier age. M_1, 5-year actuarial survival rate (75%) following Mustard operation performed from 1963 to 1973 on 105 patients with isolated TGA and M_2, 5-year actuarial survival rate (93%) following Mustard operation on 100 patients from 1973 to 1979. References: L[113] (1969); K[97] (1976); T[212] (1972); G[70] (1975); N[59] (1973); C (1976) (M. H. Paul, unpublished data); B[128] (1981); M_1, M_2[209] (1980).

therapy,[133, 147] but these have not been confirmed.[241] Analysis of pairs of siblings with congenital heart malformations of different types has recorded an excess of pairs for TGA with tetralogy of Fallot.[55] The occurrence of TGA is not related to parental age per se,[58, 113] but when birth order is considered a twofold increased frequency was noted when the mother had three or more previous children. Extracardiac congenital anomalies are infrequent (9%) in infants with TGA compared to incidences with truncus arteriosus (48%), ventricular septal defect (33%), or tetralogy of Fallot (31%).[59]

PATHOLOGY

The term *transposition of the great arteries* refers to a specific type of malposition of the great arteries[219] (see Chapter 28) and specifically indicates that both great arteries are completely misplaced across the ventricular septum so as to arise from morphologically inappropriate ventricles; hence, these are discordant ventriculoarterial alignments, i.e., right ventricle to aorta and left ventricle to pulmonary artery. The common clinical type, i.e., with situs solitus of

the viscera and atria, and concordant atrioventricular (right atrium to right ventricle and left atrium to left ventricle) and discordant ventriculoarterial alignments, is often termed complete transposition of the great arteries.[189]

The modifying term *complete* in complete transposition has, by common usage, come to indicate that the transposed great arteries are *physiologically uncorrected*; systemic venous blood flows predominantly to the aorta and pulmonary venous blood to the pulmonary artery. Thus, the term *complete* in this usage is contrasted to the term *corrected* as in corrected transposition, i.e., *physiologically corrected*; systemic venous blood flows to the pulmonary artery, and pulmonary venous blood to the aorta. It should, however, be recognized that both the typical physiologically uncorrected and physiologically corrected transposition are *complete transpositions*, i.e., both great arteries completely misplaced across the ventricular septum and arising from morphologically inappropriate ventricles.

Using the segmental situs terminology and abbreviations[217] favored by Van Praagh (see Chapter 28), the clinical material in this chapter almost exclusively concerns TGA {S,D,D}; transposition of the great arteries (TGA) with situs solitus of the viscera and atria (S), D-loop (solitus) ventricles (D), and D-position (solitus) of the semilunar valves (D); where solitus indicates usual or normal, and D indicates dextro or right. D-position (solitus) of the semilunar valves indicates that the aortic valve is to the right relative to the pulmonary valve. If the transposed aortic valve happens to be directly anterior to the transposed pulmonary valve this may be expressed as TGA {S,D,A}; if the transposed aortic valve is somewhat to the left of the transposed pulmonary valve, then it is TGA {S,D,L}. A rare type of transposition has been described[218, 234] in which the aorta is posteriorly positioned but nevertheless arises from the anterior morphological right ventricle.

TGA {S,L,L} is the segmental description of the usual *corrected transposition* heart with discordant atrioventricular and ventriculoarterial alignments with situs solitus (S), L-loop (inversus) ventricles, and L-position (inversus) of the semilunar valves.

An additional modifying term, *simple*, has sometimes been applied[109] to exclude from consideration hearts with complete transposition having certain complex associated malformations such as: tricuspid atresia, mitral atresia, common AV orifice, and univentricular hearts with or without small outlet chamber. This chapter is concerned exclusively with this simple type of complete transposition and includes transposition with intact ventricular septum, ventricular septal defect (VSD), patent ductus arteriosus (PDA), straddling tricuspid orifice-valve, or left ventricular outflow tract obstruction, a group comprising in all about 80% of complete transposition malformations (Table 21.1). Surgical papers, however, often use the term simple or isolated transposition of the great arteries to designate a subgroup of TGA patients with intact ventricular septum but *without* any other significant associated lesion, hence excluding: large VSD, large PDA, and significant left ventricular outflow tract obstruction.[209]

Abnormal development—growth and absorption— of the distal infundibulum (conus) is considered to be a major factor in the morphogenesis of abnormally aligned great arteries.[66, 221] The normal infundibulum is *subpulmonary*, *left-sided*, and *anterior* and prevents fibrous continuity between the pulmonary and tricuspid valve structures. This normal subpulmonary infundibulum is the solitus (or noninverted) infundibulum. In typical TGA (Fig. 21.2 and Chapter 28, Figs. 28.7 and 28.8), the infundibulum is *subaortic*, *right-sided*, and *anterior*, and it prevents aortic-tricuspid

TABLE 21.1   TRANSPOSITION^a OF THE GREAT ARTERIES WITH D-VENTRICULAR LOOP: 200 AUTOPSIED CASES

Simple	No.	Complex	No.
1. TGA {S,D,D} with IVS $\frac{\bar{s}\ PS\ (89)}{\bar{c}\ PS\ (5)}$	94	7. TGA {S,D,D} with TAtr	6
2. TGA {S,D,D} with VSD	38	8. TGA {S,D,D} with overriding TV	5
3. TGA {S,D,D} with VSD $\frac{\bar{c}\ PS\ (17)}{\bar{c}\ PAtr\ (4)}$	21	9. TGA {S,D,D} with DISV$_L$	6
4. TGA {S,D,D} with VSD $\bar{c}$ Coa Pre	10	10. TGA {S,D,D} with DICV	1
5. TGA {S,D,L}	6	11. TGA {S,D,Drb} with MAtr	6
6. TGA {I,D,D} with VSD $\bar{c}$ PAtr	1	12. TGA {A,D,D} with Asplenia (5) Polysplenia (1)	6
	170		30

^{a} The types of transposition complexes with D-ventricular loop. Modified from autopsy study by Van Praagh *et al.*[220] The Children's Medical Center, Boston. Of 243 cases of transposition of the great arteries (TGA), 200 (82%) had D- and 43 (18%) L-ventricular loop. IVS, intact ventricular septum; PS, pulmonary stenosis; VSD, ventricular septal defect; PAtr, pulmonary atresia; Coa Pre, preductal coarctation of aorta; TAtr, tricuspid atresia; TV, tricuspid valve; DISV$_l$, double inlet single (left) ventricle with infundibular outlet chamber; DICV, double inlet common ventricle; MAtr, mitral atresia; S, solitus; D, dextro; L, levo; I, inversus; A, ambiguous.

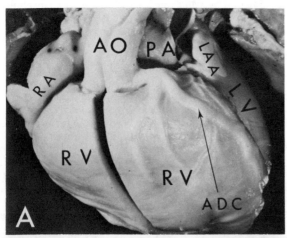

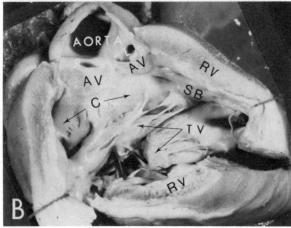

Fig. 21.2   Morphology in typical complete transposition of the great arteries. (*A*) Right ventricle anterior surface with aorta (*AO*) arising anterior and to right of pulmonary artery (*PA*) and anterior descending coronary (*ADC*) arising, as in the normal, from left coronary artery. *RA*, right atrium; *LAA*, left atrial appendage; *LV*, left ventricle. (*B*) Right ventricle interior with prominent subaortic conus (*C*). *AV*, aortic valve; *TV*, tricuspid valve; *R,L*, right and left coronary artery orifices.

fibrous continuity. The absence (absorption) of left-sided infundibulum permits fibrous continuity between the pulmonary and mitral valve structures. The right-sided subaortic infundibulum of TGA has been viewed as representing infundibular inversion (Chapter 28). Furthermore, the situs

of the infundibulum is inverted, whereas the situs of the great arteries and the ventricles is noninverted (solitus). Experimental genetic studies concerned with a dominant gene that controls visceral situs[106] seem relevant to the development and etiology of the common form of transposition, TGA {S,D,D}, which appears to result from isolated infundibular inversion (the atria, ventricles, and great arteries being noninverted).

The clinically relevant pathologic details of ventricular septal defects and left ventricular outflow-tract obstructions are considered under Angiography and Corrective Surgery.

PHYSIOLOGY

The dominant physiologic abnormalities in TGA are a deficiency of oxygen supply to the tissues and an excessive right and left ventricular workload. The systemic and pulmonary circulations function in parallel rather than the series arrangement in the normal infant; hence, the greatest portion of the output of each ventricle is recirculated to that ventricle. (Fig. 21.3*A*). Only a relatively small proportion of blood is exchanged by intercirculatory shunts between the two circulations to eventually reach the appropriate vascular bed. The systemic arterial oxygen saturation is thus dependent upon one or more of the following anatomic paths for this exchange: intracardiac (patent foramen ovale, ASD, VSD) and extracardiac (PDA, bronchopulmonary collateral circulation).

The net volume of blood passing left to right from the pulmonary circulation (left atrium, left ventricle, pulmonary arteries) to the systemic circulation (right atrium, right ventricle, aorta) represents the *anatomic left to right shunt* and is, in fact, the *effective systemic blood flow* (i.e., oxygenated pulmonary venous return perfusing the systemic capillary bed). (Fig. 21.3*B*). Conversely, the net volume of blood passing right to left from the systemic circulation to the pulmonary circulation represents the *anatomic right to left shunt* and is, in fact, the *effective pulmonary blood flow* (systemic venous return perfusing the pulmonary capillary bed). The effective pulmonary blood flow, effective systemic blood flow, net anatomic right to left, and net anatomic left to right shunts are each equal to each other, and this quantity is the *intercirculatory mixing volume*. The net volume exchanged between systemic and pulmonary circulations must be equal over a given short interval of time, since any major differences will result in a depletion of the blood volume of one circulation at the expense of overloading the other. The volumes of anatomic right to left and left to right shunted blood that participate in functional gas ex-

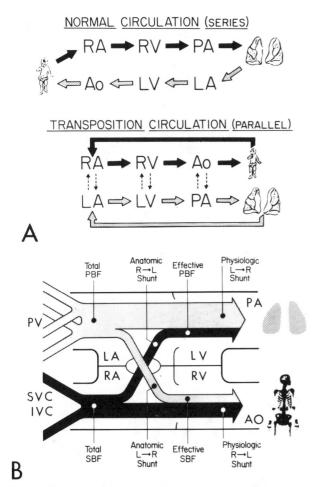

NORMAL CIRCULATION (SERIES)

TRANSPOSITION CIRCULATION (PARALLEL)

A

B

Fig. 21.3 The circulation pathways in complete transposition. (*A*) Systemic and pulmonary circulation pathways: in series, with normally related great arteries; in parallel, with TGA. *Solid arrows*, relatively unoxygenated blood; *stippled arrows*, oxygenated blood; *dashed arrows*, intercirculatory shunts. (*B*) Circulation schema demonstrating flows and shunts in infants with TGA and intact ventricular septum; *PV*, pulmonary veins; *SVC, IVC*, superior and inferior vena cava; *LA, RA*, left and right atrium; *LV, RV*, left and right ventricle; *PA*, pulmonary artery; *AO*, aorta; *PBF* and *SBF*, pulmonary and systemic blood flow; *R→L, L→R*, right to left and left to right.

by subpulmonary or pulmonary stenosis or increased pulmonary vascular resistance, the arterial oxygen saturation will be lowered in spite of adequate-sized anatomic shunting sites.[8, 118, 119, 120, 180, 187]

The physiologic mechanisms that quantitatively control the equalization of interchange between the two circulations remain speculative. Angiography has in general confirmed the anticipated shunting patterns. These appear to be determined by local pressure gradients which in turn are influenced by respiratory cycle phase, local pathology, the compliance of the cardiac chambers, and the volume of blood flow and the vascular resistance in each of the circulations. With intact ventricular septum, the interatrial shunt is from right atrium to left atrium during ventricular diastole, since left ventricular resistance to filling is less than right ventricular. The shunt is from left atrium to right atrium in ventricular systole, since the left atrium is less distensible than the right, and the net pressure in the left atrium is higher during ventricular systole.[29, 100] Flow patterns are less well substantiated in the presence of large VSD.[164] When the defect is quite large, peak systolic pressures in the ventricles are equal; during ventricular systole some right ventricular output flows preferentially to the lower resistance pulmonary circulation. During ventricular diastole, increased pulmonary venous return to the left heart favors shunting of oxygenated blood to the right ventricle. The relationship of right to left atrial and ventricular compliances and pulmonary to systemic vascular resistances are clearly operative. Other important hydraulic aspects are the location of the VSD, the influence of left ventricular outflow tract obstructions, and other infrequent abnormalities, such as straddling of the right atrioventricular valve across the VSD. Infants with a large VSD but without pulmonary stenosis or increased pulmonary vascular resistance may have torrential pulmonary blood flow with marked left ventricular volume overload and usually high arterial oxygen saturation, unless severe heart failure with pulmonary edema intervenes.

If a large PDA persists in the neonate, bidirectional shunting can be demonstrated by angiography; however, as the pulmonary vascular resistance and pulmonary artery pressures fall only systemic to pulmonary ductal shunting persists.[230]

A major role has been postulated for the bronchopulmonary collateral circulation in TGA.[6, 103, 173] Bronchopulmonary anastomotic channels have been visualized by angiography in over 30% of infants with TGA under 2 years of age, and balloon occlusion studies have demonstrated that these bronchopulmonary anastomotic channels functionally and freely communicate with the pulmonary vascular bed proximal to the pulmonary capillary bed.[6] In addition to representing a potential intercirculatory (right to left) mixing pathway, these bronchopulmonary communications may play a role in the accelerated and more widespread pulmonary vascular disease process observed in TGA patients.

Application of the Fick principle for calculating pulmonary and systemic blood flow in infants with TGA can have major sources of error. Oxygen consumption is usually reduced in the severely hypoxemic infant, and assumed values are unreliable.[96] Systemic and pulmonary arteriovenous oxygen differences may be quite small; consequently, minor errors in oxygen saturation measurement introduce large errors in calculations of flow. The bronchopulmonary collateral circulation which enters the pulmonary vascular circuit far distal to the usual catheter sampling sites may represent a significant portion of the pulmonary capillary flow, and since the true mixed pulmonary artery saturation present at the precapillary level cannot be sampled a relatively high pulmonary blood-flow calculation will result. A modest bronchopulmonary contribution (20%) to the pulmonary precap-

change at the pulmonary and systemic capillary levels are relatively small in comparison to the large portions of blood recirculating within each circulation. Thus, the *physiologic left to right shunt* represents the volume of the pulmonary venous blood recirculating through the lungs without having passed through the body, and the *physiologic right to left shunt* is the volume of systemic venous blood reentering the systemic circulation without having passed through the lungs.

The extent of intercirculatory mixing in TGA depends on the number, size, and position of the anatomic communications, and on the total blood flow through the pulmonary circuit. In the neonate with an intact ventricular septum and a closed or closing ductus arteriosus, severe hypoxemia secondary to inadequate mixing at the foramen ovale level is usually present. When the interatrial or interventricular shunting sites are of adequate size, the level of arterial oxygen saturation is influenced primarily by the pulmonary to systemic blood-flow ratio, with a high pulmonary blood flow resulting in relatively high arterial oxygen saturation, as long as the left ventricle can maintain the high output state satisfactorily. If the pulmonary blood flow is decreased illary blood flow can result in 30% overestimation of pulmonary blood flow; hence, calculated pulmonary vascular resistance should be viewed as minimum values.[6, 103]

The pulmonary blood flow in TGA is often less when derived from angiographic stroke volume measurements than from Fick measurements. With intact ventricular septum, the pulmonary blood flow by angiography is within the range for normal infants in the first few months of life, but averages approximately twice the normal flow in older infants and children, possibly because of progressive changes in pulmonary vascular resistance and ventricular compliance which occur with age.[67, 95]

The *determinants of the magnitude of pulmonary blood flow* in TGA remain obscure. A major fall in pulmonary artery pressure and vascular resistance occurs during the first few weeks of life in TGA with intact ventricular septum, and therefore the early maturation of the pulmonary circulation has been considered similar to that of the normal infant.[213] Left ventricular compliance progressively increases during this time, as manifest by decreasing left ventricular muscle mass.[12, 109] The outputs of the two ventricles are determined presumably by their respective preloads, compliances, and afterloads, but must constantly be autoregulated to meet the special requirements of the transposition circuit, i.e., that the net flow from pulmonary to systemic circuit equal the net flow from systemic to pulmonary circuit.

In the palliated TGA neonate with intact ventricular septum and large interatrial communication, the hemodynamic pattern should resemble that found in infants with isolated large atrial septal defects, i.e., as the pulmonary vascular resistance falls the pulmonary ventricle circulates an increased blood volume at low pressure.[180, 192] This increased level of pulmonary blood flow should result in improved intercirculatory mixing and systemic arterial oxygen saturation, assuming an adequate-sized and favorably placed anatomic shunt. Some newborn infants, however, with quite large anatomic interatrial communications from balloon septostomy or even surgical septectomy, do not manifest much improved systemic arterial oxygen saturation, or respond only gradually. These response patterns may result from: an inadequately increased pulmonary blood flow associated with delayed fall in pulmonary vascular resistance; unfavorable patterns of intercirculatory streaming; unfavorable ventricular compliance relationships; or, rarely, dynamic left ventricular outflow tract stenosis.[8]

If the pulmonary blood flow decreases in an older infant or child with TGA as a consequence of increasing left ventricular outflow tract stenosis or pulmonary vascular resistance, the intercirculatory mixing and systemic arterial oxygen saturation will also decrease. The resultant systemic hypoxemia will further lower peripheral systemic resistance, increase the systemic blood flow and the physiologic right to left shunt, and thus further increase systemic hypoxemia.[119]

We have observed a prevalent but clinically silent maldistribution pattern of pulmonary blood flow in TGA patients.[137] Pulmonary angiograms, radionuclide lung images, and chest roentgenograms indicate that approximately half the patients with complete TGA have a significantly greater proportion of blood flow distributed to the right lung than normal (Fig. 21.4). The perfusion disparity between the lungs is not present in newborns with TGA, is progressive but variable in its extent, and may in time result rarely in complete cessation of effective perfusion of the left lung. The maldistribution is dependent upon a common anatomic feature found in transposition, both TGA {S,D,D,} and TGA {S,L,L}, i.e., abnormal rightward inclination of the main pulmonary artery which results in a straightening of the flow direction from left ventricle to main pulmonary artery to

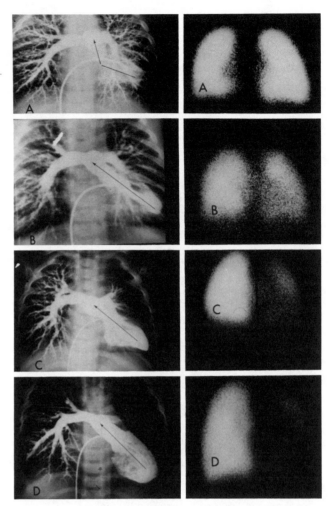

Fig. 21.4 Abnormal distribution of pulmonary blood flow favoring the right lung in TGA observed prior to corrective cardiac surgery.[137] Pulmonary and radionuclide angiograms from four patients. (*A*) Normal right-left distribution; (*B*) slight; (*C*) moderate; (*D*) marked preferential rightward distribution.

right pulmonary artery. Under these circumstances the momentum of blood flow in the main pulmonary artery carries the blood preferentially into the right pulmonary artery. The momentum effect, inoperative in the neonatal period, is enhanced progressively by increased blood flow velocity, resulting from the development of mild fibromuscular or dynamic left ventricular outflow tract stenosis and the increased left ventricular stroke output which commonly appear after the first months of life.

In the neonate with intact ventricular septum, the systemic arterial PO_2 may be as low as 15 to 25 mm Hg, with resultant anaerobic glycolysis and severe metabolic acidemia. The newborn infant may not manifest acidemia in the first day or two of life, perhaps because of favorable blood-tissue dissociation characteristics or tissue resistance factors. Inevitably, unless intracardiac mixing is improved by palliative or corrective intervention, severe hypoxemia results in advanced acidemia, hypoglycemia, hypothermia, and eventual death.

Arterial blood gases are quite helpful for discriminating cyanotic infants with TGA from those with lung disease. The contrast between systemic arterial and pulmonary venous blood gases while breathing air is striking in TGA with poor mixing. The pulmonary venous blood reflects chemoreceptor stimulated hyperventilation; the PO_2 levels may be increased to as high as 110 mm Hg, and the PCO_2 levels reduced to 15 to 25 mm Hg. In contrast, systemic arterial PO_2 levels are rarely higher than 35 mm Hg, and the PCO_2 is usually normal or only slightly elevated (<45 mm Hg) because of the limited anatomic left to right shunt. The response of systemic arterial PO_2 to 100% oxygen administration is primarily related to the extent of intercirculatory mixing. When systemic arterial PO_2 values are less than 30 mm Hg in air and remain below 35 mm Hg in high oxygen atmosphere, poor intracardiac mixing is present.[130]

TGA physiology and anatomy appear compatible with normal *fetal* survival and relatively normal gestational development; indeed the average birth weight and size of these infants are greater than normal. The course of fetal circulation is modified since the right heart ejects blood directly into the ascending aorta, in contrast to the sequence in the normal fetus where the right ventricle ejects into the descending aorta via the PDA. In the fetus with TGA, the superior vena caval blood will be directed through the tricuspid valve to the right ventricle and ascending aorta and provide blood of slightly lower PO_2 to the coronary and cerebral circulations than in the normal fetus. The blood entering the pulmonary circulation, derived mainly from the inferior vena caval return which has shunted across the patent foramen ovale, may be expected to have a PO_2 somewhat higher than that found in normal fetuses. The effects of a slightly lower than normal PO_2 on the fetal central nervous system and a slightly higher than normal PO_2 on the fetal pulmonary circulation remain undefined.

Ventricular Function

Right and left ventricular function has been assessed most extensively in the atrial-palliated and the intraatrial physiologically corrected patient, although there are important initial data for the anatomically corrected patient.[105] Ventricular function has been expressed in terms of volume,[17, 68, 73, 74, 91, 95, 105, 145] pressure-velocity,[64, 68] or systolic-time interval indices.[2, 54, 81, 82] As a generalization, right ventricular function is depressed both before and after intraatrial repair procedures. Preoperative myocardial hypoxemia or some intrinsic anatomic-geometric factors have been considered possible causes for the dysfunction. Prerepair findings indicate right ventricular dysfunction with increased right ventricular end-diastolic volume (RVEDV) and decreased right ventricular ejection fraction (RVEF); left ventricular end-diastolic volume (LVEDV) may be normal in the neonate or young infant and increased in the older infant, and left ventricular ejection fraction (LVEF) is usually normal or increased.

Observations after the Mustard or Senning procedure indicate that right ventricular function remains or is further decreased from normal (mean RVEF 0.42 to 0.47).[68, 74, 91]

Echocardiographic estimates[54, 145] of right ventricular function are to some extent in agreement with volume measurements, suggesting that right ventricular function is depressed and apparently poorly adapted to maintain systemic ventricular function.

These objective findings of depressed right ventricular function appear somewhat in contrast to clinical and subjective opinions on many postoperative patients who appear to have achieved remarkably normal levels of physical activity, growth, and development. Furthermore, there is no evidence from the limited data available that intraatrial repair, even in early infancy (1 to 2 months of age) promotes late normal right ventricular function.[17, 74] A comparative study of the systemic ventricular response to afterload stress (methoxamine infusion) 1 year after intracardiac repair in infants

with tetralogy of Fallot, VSD, and TGA (intraatrial repair) identified systemic (RV) dysfunction only in TGA patients (mean age at surgery, 0.7 ± 0.1 months), which was not evident in the systemic (LV) ventricle of the age-matched infants with repaired tetralogy of Fallot or large VSD.[25]

In contrast to the prevalent abnormal right ventricular function findings after physiological correction, preoperative normal left ventricular function is relatively well preserved. These ventricular function studies, together with the frequency of dysrhythmias, have supported continuing efforts for achieving anatomic surgical correction, i.e., left ventricle as systemic ventricle. Ventricular function studies 1 to 1½ years after two-stage anatomic correction show normal left (systemic) and right (pulmonary) ventricular function as judged by normal end-diastolic pressure and ejection fraction, and indicate normalization of abnormal precorrection right ventricular function (Fig. 21.5).[105]

Pulmonary Vascular Disease

The early development and widespread presence of *pulmonary vascular obstruction* in patients with TGA is now broadly documented by autopsy findings, biopsy studies, and hemodynamic data.[36, 141, 225, 240] Compared to other forms of congenital heart disease, TGA has an apparent accelerated rate of development and an increased frequency of this complication. Histologic evidence for advanced pulmonary vascular disease *grade 3 or greater* using Heath-Edwards

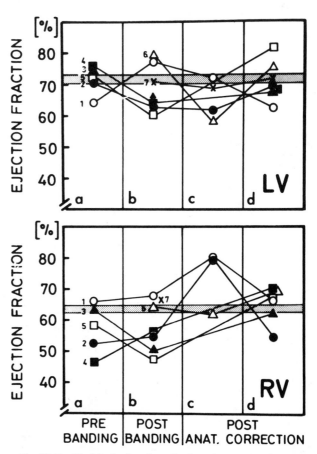

Fig. 21.5 Ventricular function after two-stage anatomic correction for TGA with intact ventricular septum. Ejection fraction of the left (*LV*) and right (*RV*) ventricle: (*a*) pre- and (*b*) postpulmonary artery banding; (*c*) early (mean 43 days); and (*d*) late (mean 671 days) after anatomic correction. (Reproduced with permission from P. E. Lange *et al.*[105]

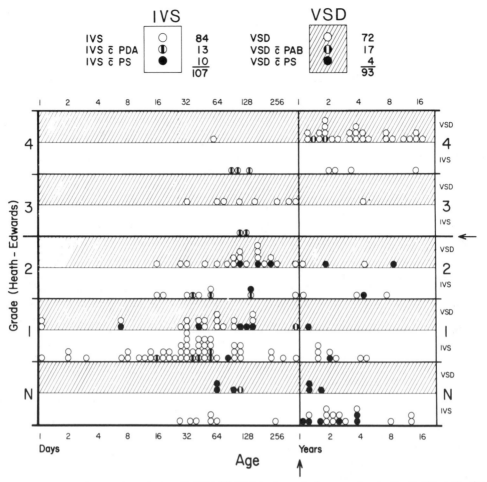

Fig. 21.6 Pulmonary vascular disease in patients with TGA.[141] Histologic analysis according to Heath-Edwards classification of lung specimens from 200 patients; 107 with intact ventricular septum (*IVS*) or small ventricular septal defect (*VSD*) and 93 with large VSD. *N*, normal vascular histology; *PDA*, patent ductus arteriosus; *PAB*, pulmonary artery banding; *PS*, pulmonary stenosis; age, plotted with geometric progression in days and years; *vertical arrow* indicates 1 year of age; *horizontal arrow* indicates separation between grades 1 to 2 pathology and grades 3 to 4 pathology. Grade 3, occlusive intimal fibrosis, and grade 4, plexiform lesions and vascular dilatation, represent advanced pulmonary vascular disease.

(H-E) classification[78] is almost the rule in infants over 1 year of age with large VSD and pulmonary-artery pressures at or near systemic level. In our clinic,[141] 25 of 28 children older than 1 year with persistent large VSD had *grade 4, H-E*, histologic changes present (Fig. 21.6). Major subpulmonary or pulmonary stenosis (i.e., peak systolic pulmonary artery pressure less than 50% of peak systolic left ventricular pressure) usually prevents the early occurrence of advanced pulmonary vascular disease in patients with large VSD and increased pulmonary blood flow. Even in infants and children with TGA and intact ventricular septum, extensive abnormal histologic changes have been noted, although the process seems somewhat slower and much less prevalent than with large VSD.[143] Markedly advanced pulmonary vascular disease (*grade 4*, H-E, or mean pulmonary artery pressure >45 mm Hg) was found in eight of 135 children with TGA and intact ventricular septum. Microthrombi, in addition to the classical vascular pathology, were identified in the pulmonary vessels of 23% of the lung specimens, and these may represent an etiologic factor. The persistence of a large PDA in infants with intact ventricular septum has been implicated as a cause for increased pulmonary vascular disease,[141, 230] as has prolonged hypoxemia or polycythemia.[225]

A summary of four comprehensive histologic studies[36]

indicates that patients with TGA and large VSD have a frequency of pulmonary vascular changes *grade 3* or greater in 20% before 2 months of age, 25% from 3 to 12 months, and 78% after 12 months of age. The comparable findings for patients with intact ventricular septum were 1% before 2 months, 17% from 3 to 12 months, and 34% after 12 months of age.

The implications of these findings are clear in regard to the timing of palliative or corrective surgery. Infants with intact ventricular septum, after satisfactory palliation with balloon atrial septostomy (or surgical septectomy), should not have corrective surgery unduly delayed beyond 8 to 12 months of age and when feasible, repair probably should be performed earlier. Infants with large VSD and pulmonary hypertension should either have palliative pulmonary artery banding within the first 2 or 3 months of age or, when feasible have early intracardiac repair with closure of the defect. A persistent large PDA should be treated surgically in the neonatal period.

Rarely, the occurrence or progression of pulmonary vascular obstruction has been noted even after successful intraatrial correction in infants with preoperative documentation of minimal pulmonary hypertension.[19, 140, 175]

The pathogenesis of the more accelerated and widespread pulmonary vascular disease in TGA is undoubtedly multifactorial. Although the pulmonary vascular bed may be functionally normal at birth, histologic studies indicate that shortly thereafter an accelerated pathologic process occurs. Recent, more sophisticated pulmonary vascular morphometry has shown that in addition to the marked increases in pulmonary vascular muscularity and intimal hyperplasia with vessel obstruction, there is a reduction in the number of intraacinar pulmonary arteries in patients with elevated pulmonary vascular resistance.[162] Hypoxemia, both systemic (chemoreceptor reflexes) and pulmonary (local effects), can induce pulmonary arteriolar vasoconstriction.[6, 180] Intense systemic hypoxemia is commonly present, and local pulmonary hypoxemia can result from increased bronchial arterial vessels and bronchopulmonary anastomoses carrying hypoxemic systemic blood to the precapillary pulmonary arterioles. Thus, increased pulmonary vascular flow, pressure, and vasoconstrictive factors, possibly in association with abnormal platelet and red cell factors, can result in increased pulmonary vessel shear stress, endothelial damage, microthrombi, and the early induction and rapid progression of vascular disease.[6, 83]

The quantitative assessment of pulmonary vascular resistance at catheterization in TGA can be beset with problems. Failure to enter the pulmonary artery precludes a meaningful estimate of resistance because of a reasonably high frequency of subpulmonary stenosis. Application of the Fick principle tends to overestimate pulmonary blood flow and hence underestimate pulmonary vascular resistance. Oxygen comsumption measurements should be made whenever possible because of the wide variance in predictive tables and the additional influence of the hypoxemic state.[96] Increased blood viscosity, particularly in older infants and children, is an important but as yet inadequately defined component of the measured pulmonary vascular resistance.[144] A limited comparison of Fick-estimated pulmonary vascular resistance with histologic grading suggests that patients with advanced pathology (grade 4, H-E) will usually have pulmonary vascular resistances greater than 7 to 8 units and mean pulmonary artery pressures greater than 55 mm Hg.[141]

MANIFESTATIONS

Clinical Features

Cyanosis, hypoxemic deterioriation, or heart failure with early death summarizes the usual clinical course in the untreated infant with complete transposition of the great arteries. The clinical manifestations and course are predominantly influenced by the extent of intercirculatory mixing. This in turn depends on several anatomic and functional factors that can be integrated into a useful clinical classification (Table 21.2). The infant with an isolated very small

TABLE 21.2 TRANSPOSITION OF THE GREAT ARTERIES (TGA): PHYSIOLOGIC-CLINICAL CLASSIFICATION[a]

I. TGA (IVS or small VSD), with increased PBF and small ICS
II. TGA (VSD large), with increased PBF and large ICS
III. TGA (VSD and PVO), with restricted PBF
IV. TGA (VSD and LVOTS), with restricted PBF

[a] IVS, intact ventricular septum; VSD, ventricular septal defect; PBF, pulmonary blood flow; ICS, intercirculatory shunting; PVO, pulmonary vascular obstruction; LVOTS, left ventricular outflowtract stenosis.

VSD as judged by angiographic and hemodynamic observations should be classified with the intact ventricular septum group in regard to most clinical features.

Prominent *cyanosis* is an early and almost universal finding in the neonate with TGA who has inadequate intercirculatory mixing (group I) or relatively decreased pulmonary blood flow (group IV). The cyanosis may be initially mild but is rapidly progressive. Mild cyanosis, in infants with intact ventricular septum, is likely to be associated with a persistent, large PDA (14% of intact ventricular septum group),[230] but only rarely is mild cyanosis the result of a large, naturally occurring secundum ASD. Cyanosis was recognized by the nursery staff or physician within the first hour of life in 56% and during the first day of life in 92% of neonates with TGA and intact ventricular septum.[111] In infants with a large interventricular shunt, the cyanosis is usually mild (group II).

Early diagnosis and prompt therapy for the neonate with intact ventricular septum is particularly critical. Undue emphasis has been placed in the past on diagnostic features, such as significant systolic murmur, heart failure, cardiomegaly, and cardiopulmonary distress; these observations have been derived from infant populations that were heterogeneous in age and associated defects. It must be recognized that beyond cyanosis, the clinical examination is often unrewarding in regard to positive physical findings.[111]

Differential cyanosis, i.e., cyanosis of the upper body greater than that of the lower body, is rare and indicates the presence of a large PDA with reversed pulmonary to systemic blood flow. In the neonate with intact ventricular septum and uncomplicated large PDA, this pattern may be transiently observed. In the older infant or child, this pattern may suggest an aortic arch anomaly, such as preductal coarctation of the aorta or interruption of the aortic arch, or severe pulmonary vascular obstructive disease with PDA.

Clubbing of the digits is usually observed only in infants with prominent cyanosis surviving beyond 5 or 6 months of age. Squatting, a distinctive clinical finding in severely cyanotic children with tetralogy of Fallot, is not observed in the TGA patient with increased pulmonary blood flow. Hypoxic "spells" in an infant with TGA and increased pulmonary blood are a consequence of inadequate intracardiac shunting and the resultant hypoxemia and metabolic acidosis. These spells are characterized by extreme irritability, persistent labored breathing, and intense cyanosis but without the characteristic unconscious spells seen with severe tetralogy of Fallot. In a few infants with intact ventricular septum, increased dynamic left ventricular outflow stenosis, recognized by echocardiography, appears to be the mechanism responsible for these acute clinical symptoms.[8]

On *physical examination* the neonate, if seen early, will appear healthy and well developed except for cyanosis. Two pictures emerge centering around either hypoxemia or heart failure; one extreme is the severely cyanotic, hypoxemic infant, and the other is the mildly or moderately cyanotic infant with prominent heart failure.

Most infants with intact ventricular septum or small VSD become severely hypoxemic and critically ill in the first few days or weeks of life, but a high index of suspicion is necessary for early diagnosis, since even the chest roentgenogram and electrocardiogram may be normal in appearance at this time.[111] With a large VSD, cyanosis may be minimal and heart failure may not become evident until after the first few weeks of life.

Sixty-two percent of a consecutive series of 50 infants less than 2 weeks old with TGA and intact ventricular septum referred to our center were judged to be well developed and in good general condition.[111] All were cyanotic (82% moderate or severe, 18% mild). Mild tachpynea and dyspnea were present in half of the infants. The peripheral pulses were normal or slightly prominent. The liver edge was palpable below the right costal margin in most infants. Gross hepatomegaly was not noted in the group with isolated intact ventricular septum, but was present at times in the infant with large VSD or PDA.

Auscultation indicated that early systolic ejection sounds were rare; the first heart sound was normal or loud. The second heart sound was split in one-third of the infants with the pulmonary component of normal intensity. In the other two-thirds the second heart sound was considered to be single or very narrowly split with increased intensity. Others have found splitting to be present in about half of such patients.[60, 233] A third heart sound was sometimes heard. No systolic murmur was heard in 42% of the neonates, and those heard were soft, grade 2/6 or less. These systolic murmurs were ejection in quality, maximum at the mid- and upper left sternal border, and probably represent a functional left ventricular outflow-tract murmur. Middiastolic ventricular inflow murmurs were rarely heard in infants with intact ventricular septum.

A *large PDA* can modify the clinical findings in the neonate with intact ventricular septum.[230] Characteristically these infants present quite early with more prominent tachypnea and relatively slight cyanosis. However, signs indicative of a large PDA, such as a continuous murmur, bounding pulses, and a prominent middiastolic rumble, are present in less than half of this group. In most infants with TGA, the PDA closes during the first days or week of life without any apparent clinical repercussions. The frequency of PDA reported in autopsy series is relatively high because of the predominant early age of death when the ductus is still normally anatomically patent. Autopsy analysis restricted to infants greater than 12 weeks of age at death indicated a 23% frequency of open ductus with intact ventricular septum.[30] Angiographic analysis of a consecutive series of 81 neonates with TGA and intact ventricular septum[230] demonstrated 39 with PDA at the time of the initial balloon atrial septostomy procedure; 21 were considered quite small and did not influence the clinical course. Of the 18 infants with an initially large and functionally significant PDA, six experienced a relatively abrupt spontaneous closure or narrowing with sudden clinical deterioration by 1 month of age, six had occult spontaneous PDA closure probably over the course of several months, and there were six infants who were followed with a moderately large PDA beyond 3 months of age (Fig. 21.25).

The neonate with a *large ventricular septal defect* may not manifest any heart disease initially, although mild cyanosis, most evident during crying, is often noted in the nursery. Characteristically signs of left heart failure develop within 2 to 6 weeks. Tachypnea and tachycardia become prominent; cyanosis, although evident with stress and crying, may remain quite mild and be overlooked. Heart murmurs also may not be present initially, but a prominant grade 3 to 4/6 pansystolic murmur, third heart sound with middiastolic rumble, gallop rhythm, and narrowly split second heart sound with loud pulmonary component usually emerge in these infants. Spontaneous closure of a VSD or diminution in size occurs in 10 to 15% of infants, and the best predictor for closure is an initial small defect.[158] Aortic isthmus narrowing with pre- or juxtaductal coarctation, sometimes with reduced femoral pulses, is an uncommon but particularly malignant associated malformation with a large VSD, more usually present with double outlet right ventricle (Taussig-Bing type).

Neonates with TGA, VSD, and *severe pulmonary stenosis or atresia* have diminished pulmonary blood flow. They represent a relatively small proportion (5 to 8%) of the neonatal transposition population. Clinical findings are similar to those in the infant with tetralogy of Fallot with severe pulmonary stenosis or atresia, and the cyanosis is extreme from birth.

A *left ventricular outflow tract fibromuscular ridge* (subpulmonary stenosis) may develop in the infant with intact ventricular septum after the neonatal period. It is usually associated with a modest peak systolic left ventricular outflow tract pressure difference (20 to 30 mm Hg) and distinctive angiographic and echocardiographic findings. Characteristically, a somewhat long ejection systolic murmur becomes progressively more evident after the first few months of age. The murmur is best heard at the mid left sternal border and sometimes is transmitted prominently toward the right sternal and clavicular area. Additionally, a dynamic type of left ventricular outflow tract narrowing occurs in some infants characterized best on cineangiography or echocardiography by exaggerated posterior systolic bulging of the interventricular septum with mitral valve opposition.[7, 156] The clinical implications of these modest degrees of subpulmonary stenosis with intact ventricular septum remain poorly defined. The rare occurrence of severe progressive anatomic subpulmonary stenosis constitutes a major problem for surgical management,[125] as does the infrequent occurrence of severe dynamic left ventricular outflow tract obstruction.[8]

Subaortic outflow tract stenosis is extremely rare, despite the very prominent subaortic conus present in TGA. It has been reported following palliative pulmonary artery banding for TGA with VSD[177] and observed only once in our clinic in an unoperated infant (Fig. 21.20C). Clinical diagnosis would be difficult except for 2D echocardiography.

Progressively advancing *pulmonary vascular disease* may not be evident early from physical findings. A secondary increase in cyanosis with increasing hematocrit in infants who have had successful palliative procedures should always raise the suspicion of a decrease in pulmonary blood flow caused by progression either in pulmonary vascular disease or in left ventricular outflow tract stenosis. With advanced pulmonary vascular obstructive disease an early systolic ejection sound is commonly heard. There may be no murmurs present or only a faint short ejection systolic murmur. Eventually, in later childhood or adolescence, a high-pitched, blowing early decrescendo diastolic murmur of pulmonary insufficiency and a blowing apical murmur of mitral insufficiency result from gross dilation of the left heart.

Hematologic abnormalities, including polycythemia, thrombocytopenia, and impaired blood-coagulation mechanisms,[229, 231] may be responsible for serious pre- and perioperative complications. These abnormalities seem related to both duration and severity of the cyanosis. Despite intense cyanosis, advanced polycythemia or thrombocytopenia are rarely present in the infant under 6 to 9 months of age, but are commonly observed in the poorly palliated or uncorrected older infant or child.[153] Even with normal platelet counts, older cyanotic infants and children have been found to have diminished platelet survival times and to be in a state of compensated thrombocytolysis with relative and absolute megathrombocytosis.[65, 229] In some instances this increased peripheral destruction of platelets and increased thrombopoiesis might be caused by a chronic, disseminated intravascular coagulopathy. Palliative or corrective surgery resulting in increased systemic arterial oxygen saturation has normalized thrombocytopenic platelet counts and corrected coagulopathies. Similarly, erythrophoresis (acute red cell volume reduction with plasma or albumin replacement) has been employed to improve temporarily coagulation abnormalities in cyanotic congenital heart disease prior to surgery.[232]

Prolonged polycythemia may be associated with a number of other adverse effects. Thrombotic lesions have been noted in the lungs, kidney, and central nervous system to an extent greater than in noncyanotic patients.[140, 148, 225] Subtle functional abnormalities in other systems may be related to prolonged intense hypoxemia, e.g., decreased respiratory center sensitivity to hypoxia and hypercarbia persisting even following successful correction in children and adults with cyanotic heart disease.[194] Polycythemia and the associated increased circulating oxygen content is advantageous until the hematocrit reaches about 65%; beyond this level the hydraulic stresses of high blood viscosity may outweigh the advantages of the increased circulating oxyhemoglobin. *Hypochromic microcytic anemia* is also an unfavorable state. It can be recognized by observing high erythrocyte counts with relatively normal hemoglobin and hematocrit levels and should be corrected with short courses of oral iron therapy.

Spontaneous *cerebrovascular accidents*, particularly in infants under 2 years of age, are an infrequent but tragic complication in the inadequately palliated and uncorrected infant (Table 21.3). The most common presentation is sudden onset of hemiparesis. The recent decrease in frequency is probably related to programs achieving more satisfactory early palliation and earlier corrective surgery. Polycythemia and the increased blood viscosity associated with severe cyanosis have been regarded as responsible for cerebral, mesenteric, renal, and pulmonary thromboses; however, hypochromic, microcytic anemia in conjunction with severe hypoxemia has also been implicated as a mechanism for cerebrovascular accidents.[155]

Brain abcesses have been infrequent and occur almost always in patients over 2 years of age, in contrast to cerebrovascular accidents which occur most commonly in infants less than 2 years of age.[51] Symptoms, such as persistent headache, or, less frequently, slowly developing neurologic abnormalities, distinguish this complication from acute cerebrovascular accident.

Preschool-age children with prolonged uncorrected cyanotic heart disease as a group have been observed to have slightly lower intelligence quotient scores and to perform less well with perceptual motor tasks than children with asymptomatic acyanotic heart disease.[61] Palliative and corrective surgery have been demonstrated to have beneficial effects on weight and linear growth; however, the long-term effects of intense, prolonged early cyanosis are not yet fully evaluated.[178]

Electrocardiographic Features

Dysrhythmias are rarely noted prior to palliative or corrective surgery but are of considerable importance following intraatrial corrective surgery. The most usual electrocardiographic findings are right axis deviation with right or combined ventricular hypertrophy; these findings, however, vary considerably, depending upon age, anatomic, and physiologic factors.[28, 187] The electrocardiogram in the first days of life may appear entirely normal (Fig. 21.7A). About half the infants with intact ventricular septum have a normal neonatal right ventricular hypertrophy pattern on the 1st day of life.[187] In our neonatal series even by the time of referral to a center, 22% were still considered to have a normal neonatal electrocardiogram.[111] Within days, however, abnormal right ventricular hypertrophy appears in almost all infants. Initially, this may be identified solely by the persistence, beyond 3 to 5 days of age, of a positive T wave in the right precordial leads. Right axis deviation predominates when the septum is intact; in contrast, one-third of the infants with large VSD have normal QRS axis deviation. Left or normal axis deviation occurs rarely in simple TGA but has been noted when associated with AV canal type defect, or VSD with hypoplastic right ventricle with or without straddling tricuspid valve.[47, 102, 171]

Right ventricular hypertrophy is present in about 80% of the patients with intact ventricular septum or small VSD, and combined ventricular hypertrophy is present in about 60 to 80% of patients with large VSD (Fig. 21.7B and C). These electrocardiographic patterns are modified by left ventricular outflow tract stenosis or increased pulmonary vascular resistance. A Q wave in V6 is usually present (70%) in TGA with large VSD, but is infrequent (15%) when the ventricular septum is intact.[187] Isolated left ventricular hypertrophy is rarely encountered and suggests TGA with VSD with hypoplasia of the right ventricle associated with straddling of the tricuspid valve (Fig. 21.7D).[102, 171]

The vectorcardiogram has been considered useful for assessing left ventricular pressure and hypertrophy in TGA, since the scalar electrocardiogram does not consistently reflect these left heart parameters in the presence of dominant right ventricular voltages.[117, 170] A clockwise horizontal plane loop indicates a dominant right ventricular mass, usually with left ventricular peak systolic pressures less than two-thirds of systemic pressures, suggesting that the patient does

TABLE 21.3 BALLOON ATRIAL SEPTOSTOMY[a]

Reference	Study Interval	No. Patients	Death (Hospital) Early	Death (Medical) Late	CVA[b]	Mortality, *Nonsurgical*, after BAS[c]	
						No.	%
202	1966–1971	52	3	4	3	7/52	13
53	1966–1972	93	6	6	5	12/93	13
97	1969–1975	85	8	3	—	11/85	13
70	1967–1972	62	6	5	2	11/62	18
165	1965–1972	64	8	10	6	18/64	28
20	1966–1972	86	5	23	5	28/86	33
128	1974–1980	125	6	7	—	13/125	10

[a] Frequency of early and late *nonsurgical* mortality and cerebral vascular accidents following balloon atrial septostomy (522 infants).

[b] CVA, cerebral vascular accident; —, not recorded.

[c] BAS, balloon atrial septostomy.

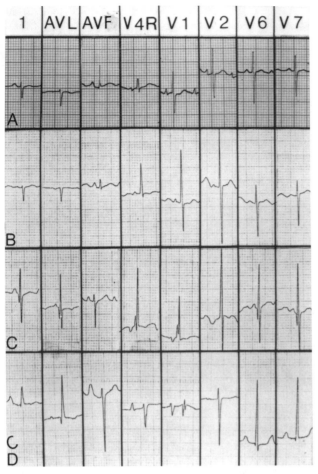

Fig. 21.7 Electrocardiogram, transposition of the great arteries. (*A*) Infant 1 day old with intact ventricular septum. No abnormal ventricular hypertrophy for age. Positive T wave in V4R, V1 as well as in V6, V7. (*B*) Infant 8 days old with intact ventricular septum. Abnormal right ventricular hypertrophy. (*C*) Infant 5 months old with VSD of AV canal type. Left axis deviation and combined ventricular hypertrophy. (*D*) Child 18 months old with straddling or overriding tricuspid valve and large ventricular septal defect of AV canal type. Left axis deviation and left ventricular hypertrophy.

not have a large VSD, severe left ventricular outflow tract stenosis, or markedly increased pulmonary vascular resistance. In contrast, a counterclockwise horizontal plane loop indicates influence from the left ventricular muscle mass and is usually associated with left ventricular peak systolic pressures at least two-thirds right ventricular pressure. In individual patients, changes in the horizontal loop configuration usually reflect changes in left ventricular pressure, but exceptions have been noted. Although serial electrocardiograms and vectorcardiograms may be helpful, pulmonary vascular disease has been shown to progress before electrovectorcardiographic changes are present.[170]

Radiologic Features

Roentgenographic findings are of major diagnostic assistance (Fig. 21.8). Sometimes the chest x-ray can establish the diagnosis at a glance; however, in the neonate particularly, the findings may be normal. A diagnostic triad of observations include: oval or egg-shaped cardiac silhouette with narrow superior mediastinum; modest cardiomegaly; and increased pulmonary vascular markings.

In the first few days and weeks of life, the chest x-ray may appear normal, particularly in the infant with intact ventricular septum. The heart is usually slightly enlarged, but one-third of the neonates have no cardiac enlargement. Pulmonary vascular markings are considered normal in from one-third to one-half the neonates seen, and the typical oval-shaped silhouette is not present in one-third to one-half of these infants.[111] In another series, the diagnostic triad was observed in only 10% of newborn infants.[38] The vascular pedicle or superior mediastinal silhouette is narrow because of the usual anteroposterior relationships of the great arteries and the hypoplasia of thymus tissue associated with cyanosis and stress.[146] Following effective palliation with atrial septostomy or septectomy or intracardiac repair in the infant, there is often prominent widening of the previously narrow mediastinal silhouette due to reappearance of thymic tissue.[146]

The left cardiac border extends in a smooth convex line towards the cardiac apex which is displaced to the left and inferiorly. Absence of the main pulmonary artery segment which normally produces a slightly convex bulge on the left cardiac border below the aortic knob is the usual finding. The right cardiac border is represented by a slightly enlarged right atrium and is full and rounded. An uncommon, but important anatomic variation, left-sided juxtaposition of the atrial appendages can rarely be recognized from any distinctive cardiac configuration.[215] Right aortic arch is relatively uncommon: 4% in patients with intact ventricular septum and 11% in patients with associated VSD.[69, 124]

After the first few weeks of life, cardiac enlargement becomes evident, and the pulmonary vascular markings appear increased in almost every infant with TGA without prominent left ventricular outflow tract stenosis. In some neonates, however, even following adequate balloon atrial septostomy the pulmonary vascular markings do not appear increased initially, and these infants often have persistent low systemic arterial oxygen saturation. Such observations support the hypothesis that functionally the pulmonary vascular bed may remain relatively vasoconstricted, and the resultant inadequate increase in pulmonary blood flow minimizes the functional effectiveness of an adequate balloon atrial septostomy.[77] In some infants during the months following balloon atrial septostomy, clinical deterioration may occur characterized by increasing cyanosis with progressive diminution in pulmonary vascularity secondary to a progressive form of left ventricular outflow tract obstruction. Recognition and assessment by echocardiography and angiography is important for this subset of infants who need early surgical intervention.[8, 206]

The pulmonary vascular markings in infancy appear particularly prominent when a large VSD is present with low pulmonary vascular resistance. If advanced pulmonary vascular obstruction is present (in older infants and children), the hilar vessels are enlarged, but the peripheral pulmonary vessels appear small and constricted; the left cardiac border is often grossly distorted by a dilated pulmonary artery trunk and left pulmonary artery. Pulmonary vascular markings remain increased in the face of moderate left ventricular outflow tract stenosis, and only severe obstruction or atresia is associated with diminished pulmonary vascular markings.

Echocardiographic Features

Two-dimensional echocardiography is extremely useful in the anatomic and functional assessment of patients with TGA; success depends largely on the skill of the operator in acquiring a complete examination and correctly synthesizing the information from numerous recorded image planes. Al-

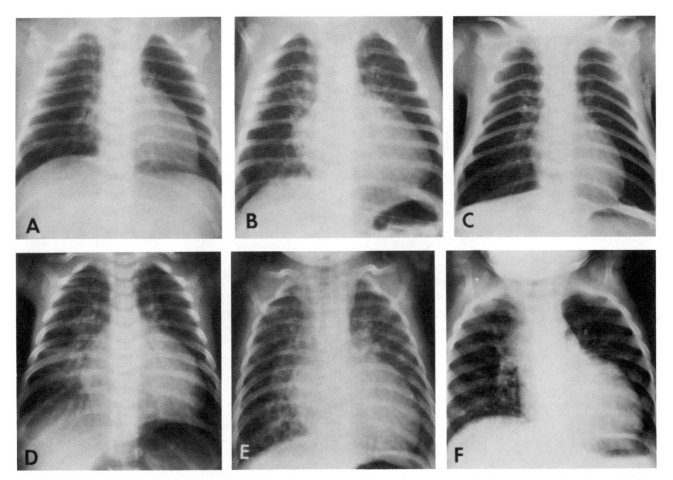

Fig. 21.8 Frontal chest roentgenograms, complete transposition of the great arteries. (*A, B, C*) Three infants 1 day of age with intact ventricular septum and no significant PDA. Note variations in cardiac size, shape, and pulmonary vasculature. (*D, E*) Two infants 10 weeks of age with large VSD. Note cardiomegaly and increased pulmonary vasculature. Only infant in *E* has a reasonably classic oval-shaped cardiac silhouette. (*F*) Infant 19 months of age with intact ventricular septum and severe pulmonary vascular obstruction; pressures were pulmonary artery, 85/45, and aorta, 80/50 mm Hg; pulmonary vascular resistance, 10 units. At 7 days of age, pressures were left ventricle, 35/5 and right ventricle, 85/7 mm Hg with quite small VSD and closed PDA.

though M-mode echocardiography can establish the diagnosis, the elements of diagnosis require much care to avoid error.[72] Sometimes both great vessels may be recorded simultaneously (so-called parallel great vessel recording) with the transducer angled toward the right shoulder from the 3rd or 4th intercostal space. Since parallel great vessels have been recorded in normal neonates, this finding is not diagnostic without further identification of the great vessel connections by semilunar valve analysis. Recognition of an anterior vessel as the aorta and the posterior vessel as the pulmonary artery, even if imaged as single structures, may be established by analysis of the opening and closing times of the respective semilunar valves; the pulmonary valve (posterior) opens earlier and closes later than the aortic valve (anterior).[81] Semilunar valve-closure intervals, however, may not be helpful in identifying the respective great vessels when there is marked pulmonary artery hypertension, since the valve closures may be simultaneous because of equivalent afterloads. Confusion may arise in analysis of the M-mode echocardiogram in 5% to 10% of patients with TGA where the aortic root is anterior but slightly to the left of the posterior pulmonary artery, since the transducer notes a left-sided anterior great vessel in a position similar to the pulmonary artery in hearts with normally related great vessels. In these situations the opening and closing times of

the semilunar valves again may be helpful in deciding the identification of the great vessels.

M-mode echocardiography has been useful in distinguishing the nature of left ventricular outflow tract obstruction as either a dynamic obstruction caused by exaggerated posterior systolic ventricular septal motion with systolic anterior movement of the mitral valve or a fixed obstruction caused by a subpulmonic fibromuscular ridge (Fig. 21.9*A* and *B*).[7, 8] M-mode echocardiography also provides a means of assessing pulmonary artery pressures and left ventricular and right ventricular function by utilizing the systolic time intervals derived from the semilunar valve recordings.[26, 54, 81, 82] M-mode echocardiography can detect an overriding or straddling tricuspid valve in TGA with VSD[102] and the interatrial baffle after the Mustard operation,[5] but 2D sector scanning is much more revealing.

Real-time wide angle 2D echocardiography provides an accurate means of establishing the anatomic diagnosis of TGA, as well as revealing major associated lesions. Imaging from the subxiphoid-subcostal positions provides a flexible acoustical window that allows for wide angulation and rotation of the transducer beam to optimize simultaneous visualization of the great arteries (ascending aorta and main pulmonary artery with its primary branches) and their respective ventricular alignments (Fig. 21.10*A*).[23] Additional

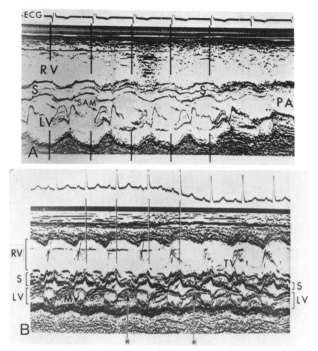

Fig. 21.9   M-mode left ventricular echocardiograms showing (A) prominent systolic anterior movement (SAM) of the anterior mitral valve leaflet (arrows) with slight narrowing of subpulmonary outflow tract (*) in infant with TGA and intact ventricular septum with 16 mm Hg peak systolic pressure difference between left ventricle (LV) and pulmonary artery (PA). (B) Severe dynamic left ventricular outflow tract obstruction in 3-month-old infant with TGA and intact ventricular septum with severe cyanotic spell and peak systolic left ventricular pressures varying from 65 to 100 mm Hg during cardiac catheterization; RV, 110 mm Hg. Note the marked early systolic bulging (small arrows) of the interventricular septum (S) and the prominent SAM (*) resulting in cavity obstruction. TV, tricuspid valve; MV, mitral valve.

imaging from the apex (four-chamber view) is useful in establishing the posterior vessel-pulmonary artery identity from its branching morphology (Fig. 21.10B). Spatial orientation of the great arteries can be appreciated from short-axis scans at the base of the heart.[123]

2D, high resolution, echocardiographic imaging of the interatrial septum after balloon atrial septostomy can assess if a satisfactory tear has been made in the septum primum flap of the fossa ovalis to provide for interatrial shunting (Fig. 21.11).[22] After interatrial corrective surgery, 2D imaging is useful for examining the structure of the surgically revised atria, and assessing if superior or inferior vena caval segment narrowing exists or if there is baffle narrowing of the pulmonary venous blood flow pathway (Fig. 21.12). Infrequent but surgically important atrioventricular valve abnormalities, such as straddling tricuspid valve, anomalous mitral valve attachments,[128] and displaced accessory tricuspid valve tissue aneurysms (Fig. 21.21B) can be detected with careful 2D imaging.

CARDIAC CATHETERIZATION

Cardiac catheterization assumes an emergency priority, particularly for the neonate with poor intercirculatory mixing, in view of the need for early diagnosis and treatment. Successful management includes prompt initiation of supportive medical therapy, such as oxygen, acid-base therapy, antibiotics and, in patients with large intercirculatory shunts, digoxin and diuretics.

The suspected diagnosis is confirmed by cardiac catheterization and angiography; in the neonate palliation should always be attempted at the same time by balloon catheter atrial septostomy. Meaningful information can be safely obtained if optimum cardiac catheterization techniques are judiciously employed.[180] Diagnostic studies and balloon catheter atrial septostomy can be successfully accomplished by direct cutdown on the femoral vein or its branches,[132, 167] percutaneous femoral vein entry,[85] or umbilical vein cathe-

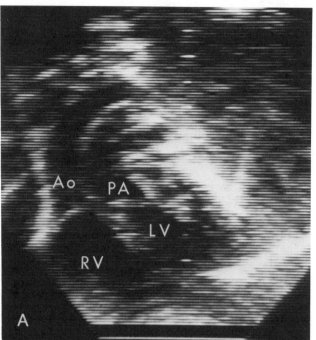

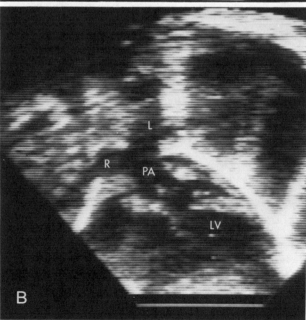

Fig. 21.10   2D echocardiogram in TGA. (A) Imaging from subcostal position establishes transposition demonstrating right-sided (anterior) aorta alignment with right-sided (anterior) morphologically right ventricle. (B) Imaging from apex displays bifurcation (branch pulmonary arteries, R and L) of the left-sided posterior great artery establishing it as the pulmonary artery. Ao, aorta; PA, pulmonary artery; RV, right ventricle; LV, left ventricle; R, right branch; L, left branch.

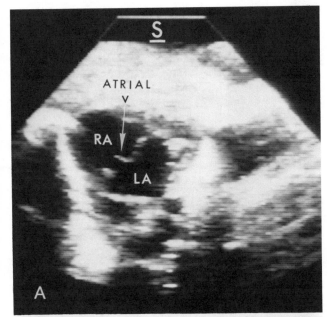

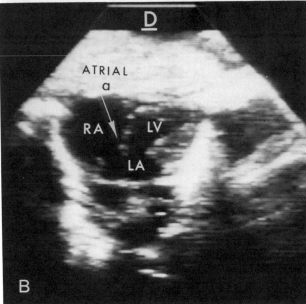

Fig. 21.11 2D echocardiographic imaging of interatrial septum immediately following catheter balloon atrial septostomy procedure which produced secundum-type defect bordered by the flail remnants of the torn septum primum. Images (A) during atrial v wave (ventricular systole-S) with left to right interatrial shunting, and (B) during atrial a wave (late ventricular diastole-D) with right to left interatrial shunting.

terization.[142] The hazards of catheterization in the newborn and young infant are minimized by: having the procedure performed by a staff skilled and experienced with infant cardiac catheterization; maintaining optimum body temperature with external thermal regulating devices; avoiding respiratory depression by not using sedation; providing a humidified high oxygen environment during the preparatory and angiocardiographic phases of the study; avoiding intracardiac trauma from rough cardiac manipulation or unnecessarily large or stiff catheters; restricting angiographic media dosage to the minimum; treating metabolic acidosis promptly; replacing excessive blood losses promptly; insti-

tuting endotracheal intubation and assisted ventilation if cardiorespiratory depression is advanced due to hypoxemic acidosis or massive left heart failure; and proceeding with therapeutic balloon atrial septostomy promptly once the diagnosis is established by 2D echocardiography or by single left ventricular angiogram rather than attempting extensive hemodynamic and angiographic investigations.

For some infants additional observations on the following items can assume major importance in planning appropriate palliative or corrective surgery; pulmonary artery pressure, pulmonary blood flow and pulmonary vascular resistance, morphological details of pulmonary or subpulmonary stenosis, VSD site and size, great vessel alignment in relation to the VSD and infundibular musculature, atrioventricular valve abnormalities, and presence of PDA or coarctation of the aorta.

Entrance into the pulmonary artery in the neonate may

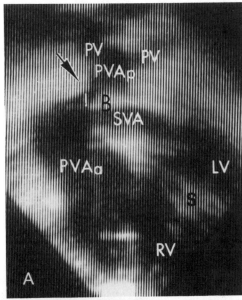

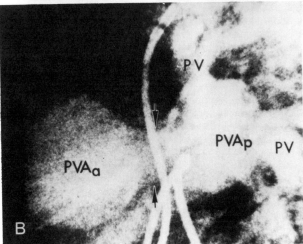

Fig. 21.12 Pulmonary venous atrium stenosis after Mustard operation for transposition of the great arteries. (A) 2D echocardiogram and (B) cineangiogram demonstrating moderately severe narrowing of the isthmus (I) between the posterior (PVAp) and anterior (PVAa) segments of the new pulmonary venous atrium. The narrowed isthmus is adjacent to the interatrial baffle. PV, pulmonary vein; B, baffle; SVA, systemic venous atrium; S, septum; RV, right ventricle.

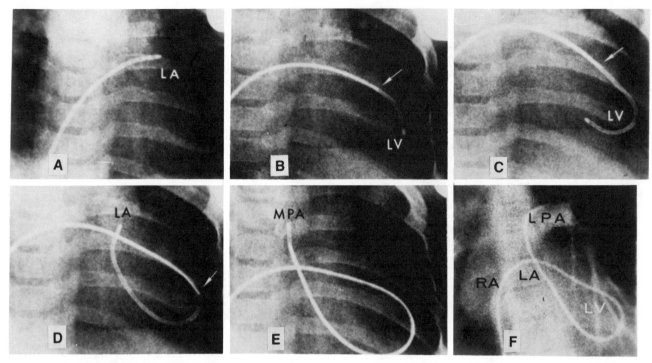

Fig. 21.13 Cineangiogram frames, frontal illustrating J-maneuver for entering pulmonary artery in transposition patients using standard angiography catheter and spring guide wire (see text for details). *Arrow* indicates tip of guide wire; *LA*, left atrium; *LV*, left ventricle; *LPA*, left pulmonary artery; *MPA*, main pulmonary artery; *RA*, right atrium.

be difficult, time-consuming, and traumatic. Aside from the importance of these measurements for later comparisons, such measurements are usually not essential for management at this stage, since the peak systolic pulmonary arterial and left ventricular pressures are almost always equal in neonates except when there is severe subpulmonary stenosis or pulmonary atresia which can be easily recognized by angiography.

Several techniques have been proposed for catheterizing the pulmonary artery in TGA. The use of a balloon-guided catheter[93] or the skilled manipulation of a standard 5F or 6F angiographic catheter in the "J" maneuver[131, 116] are the most commonly employed methods and, in the absence of severe left ventricular outflow tract obstruction, are almost always successful in entering the pulmonary artery after the neonatal period. The balloon-guided catheter technique requires that the special catheter be directed across the interatrial communication to the left atrium where the balloon is inflated. The catheter usually advances rapidly to the left ventricle, either to form a curve with the tip directed to the outflow tract or to become wedged in the apex. If the latter occurs, the catheter tip is best withdrawn to the mitral level and then advanced and withdrawn slowly with lesser degrees of balloon inflation until the catheter tip is carried into the left ventricular outflow tract where it can be then advanced rapidly into the pulmonary artery. It has been found helpful to stress the terminal portion of the balloon-guided catheter initially by stretching the shaft slightly at a point 1 to 2 cm behind the balloon tip to facilitate the essential "J" bending in the ventricle.

A standard, closed end, multiple sidehole angiographic catheter (5F or 6F) can also be successfully employed (Fig. 21.13). The catheter tip is advanced first toward the left ventricular apex, and at this point a spring guidewire is passed within 2 to 3 cm of the tip. The catheter is then pressed gently against the left ventricular wall, causing the tip of the catheter to "J" flex, with the tip of the wire acting

as a fulcrum. In order to obtain a satisfactory "J" loop in the left ventricle, it may on occasion be necessary first to form a large catheter loop within the left atrium by advancing the catheter with its tip arrested in the region of the right pulmonary veins and then advance the entire loop into the ventricle. Once there is a well-formed loop in the left ventricle it can be rotated and manipulated into the outflow tract. Several maneuvers are then helpful to enter the pulmonary artery: rotation of the catheter often flips the tip through the pulmonary valve, and repeated withdrawal or advancing of the "J"-looped catheter a few centimeters will eventually maneuver the tip into the main pulmonary artery if it has been flipping back into the mitral orifice.

In patients with major conal or conoventricular type VSD, it is often possible to manipulate the catheter directly from the right ventricle through the VSD into the pulmonary artery. If the pulmonary artery is not entered, pulmonary vein wedge pressures should be obtained and if they are normal, it is unlikely that the pulmonary artery pressure is elevated.

Catheterization findings are consistent with the detailed discussions under *Physiology* and with the classification schema (Table 21.2). In the newborn with markedly inadequate intercirculatory mixing (group I), the oxygen saturation in the vena cava may be as low as 20%, although usually it is about 40%. There is usually only a small increase of 5 to 10% in the right atrium and right ventricle; the systemic arterial saturation is quite similar to that in the right ventricle. Pulmonary venous saturation is generally normal, and there may be 4 to 8% decrease in the left atrium or left ventricle. If a large PDA is present with bidirectional shunting in the neonate, the pulmonary artery oxygen saturation may be lower than that in the left ventricle. Right and left atrial pressures may be normal or low, but usually they are slightly elevated; the right atrial A wave and the left atrial V wave are the dominant components, and the left atrial mean and V wave pressures are usually somewhat higher than the right atrial. Right ventricular and aortic systolic pressures are usually normal for age, but the aortic pulse pressure may be increased reflecting hypoxemic systemic vasodilation. If the ductus is closed or small, the peak systolic pulmonary pressures after the first week or two of life are usually lowered to about one-third the systemic levels. In older infants left ventricular and pulmonary artery pressures vary widely and reflect the status of the left ventricular outflow tract and the pulmonary vascular resistance.

In the infant with a large intercirculatory communication (group II, VSD), the vena cavae saturations are modestly reduced, and there is usually an increase in oxygen saturation at the atrial level of 5 to 10% due to interatrial shunting. A large increase in oxygen saturation is observed in the right ventricle to levels of 70 to 85%, and similar levels are noted in the aorta. A systemic arterial oxygen saturation greater than 85% with room air breathing, however, suggests that a single or common ventricle is present.[120] The pulmonary venous oxygen saturation may be reduced slightly because of left heart failure and pulmonary perfusion-ventilation abnormalities. Similar saturations are noted in the left atrium and left ventricle; but the pulmonary artery saturation may be somewhat lower than that in the left ventricle due to right to left shunting through the VSD. Saturation in the pulmonary artery is almost always higher than in the aorta; however, with extensive intracardiac mixing the saturations may be quite similar. Left atrial pressures may be quite elevated, up to 20 mm Hg or more, with quite prominent V waves. With a large defect, the left and right ventricular systolic and end-diastolic pressures and pulmonary and aortic systolic pressures may be essentially identical; the pulmonary arterial end-diastolic and mean pressures, however, are commonly lower than the systemic levels, reflecting the lower pulmonary vascular resistance.

When there is left ventricular outflow tract stenosis associated with a large VSD (group IV), the findings depend on the severity of the pulmonary outflow tract obstruction. In the neonate, when severe, and when the ductus arteriosus is small or closed, the systemic arterial oxygen saturation may be quite low (30% to 50%) and the findings are similar to those in tetralogy of Fallot with severe pulmonary stenosis or pulmonary atresia.

In infants after a few months of age and children with *intact ventricular septum*, it is common to find a modest peak systolic pressure difference ranging from 20 to 40 mm Hg across the left ventricular outflow tract at a subpulmonary site together with increased pulmonary blood flow. Such pressure differences are quite rare in the neonate but become increasingly evident after the first few months of life. In our late postoperative (intraatrial correction) hemodynamic survey, 13 of 42 of the children had such findings. They usually reflect a relatively mild degree of anatomic fibromuscular ridge or dynamic interventricular septal bulge obstruction that can be detected by cineangiography and echocardiography as well as by pressure measurement.

Balloon Atrial Septostomy

In the newborn infant less than 48 to 72 hours of age, the umbilical vein can be used successfully for balloon atrial septostomy[142] as well as for diagnostic catheterization. More commonly, however, surgical[132] or percutaneous needle[203] access to the femoral vein is employed. Using a skin incision parallel and just below the level of the inguinal crease, one should achieve adequate exposure of the saphenous bulb and its tributaries, which include the long saphenous vein, the proximal and distal femoral vein, and any deep perforating vessels to control any accidental bleeding. An adequate-

sized balloon septostomy catheter can usually be inserted into the saphenous bulb close to the saphenofemoral junction or, alternatively, into the femoral vein just distal to this junction so that the bulb and its tributaries remain undisturbed. Repair of the vessel after removal of the catheter is always attempted, since, even if there is some degree of narrowing, the continuing flow into the femoral vein facilitates patency for future percutaneous catheterizations.

There are currently available double-lumen (5F, 5.5F, 6.5F) as well as single-lumen (4F, 5F) balloon atrial septostomy catheters (Fig. 21.14). The catheter should be advanced across the foramen ovale into the left atrium or a pulmonary vein and the position of the tip *established with certainty* in the left atrium prior to proceeding. Location of the catheter tip is most readily established by visually confirming the posterior position of the tip in the lateral or left anterior oblique view or entry of the catheter into a pulmonary vein. Double-lumen catheters permit observations of pressure curves, removal of blood samples, and angiography to confirm the location. Once the position is verified, the balloon is inflated with diluted angiographic contrast medium to at least 12 to 15 mm diameter and then rapidly withdrawn across the atrial septum with an abrupt, short tug. The balloon and interatrial septum are displaced toward the inferior vena cava, and the septum primum flap of the fossa ovalis is ruptured as the balloon is carried in a single movement from the left atrium to the right atrial inferior vena caval junction. The catheter should then immediately be advanced and the balloon pushed cephalad out of the inferior vena caval orifice into the right atrium toward the superior vena cava to verify crossing the septum and to avoid obstruction to inferior vena caval return while the balloon is being deflated. This same procedure should be repeated several times with increasing balloon volumes so that withdrawal of the balloon, inflated tensely to a diameter of at least 15 mm, is achieved without much resistance being perceived at the atrial septum level. Slow or gentle withdrawal of the balloon from left to right atrium is considered by some to be counterproductive by dilating the foramen ovale without actually tearing the septum primum flap.

Complications of the procedure are rare when the above precautions are observed, but the operator must be knowledgeable and skilled to avoid chamber perforation or atrioventricular valve or pulmonary vein damage.[163] Other injuries that have been reported include damage to the inferior vena cava,[46] which probably can be minimized by utilizing an adequately inflated balloon so that it is not pulled deep into the inferior vena cava. Intracardiac rupture of the balloon occurs infrequently, but it is important to avoid introducing air bubbles during inflation with the contrast medium so as to prevent air embolization. Rubber fragmentation and embolization[224] from a ruptured balloon has been virtually abolished by new materials and fabrication techniques. Deflation failure of the balloon in the right atrium after septostomy, a rare complication in the past,[84] should be obviated by the new fabrication techniques.

Should levoposition of the right atrial appendage (juxtaposition of atrial appendages) be present, the catheter tip, still in the right atrial appendage, may falsely appear to conform to conventional criteria for left atrial positioning.[42, 176, 215] With this anomaly the right atrial appendage is more posterior than normal and occupies the left upper heart border in the anteroposterior view. The operator should suspect levoposition of the right atrial appendage if the catheter tip cannot be directed into a pulmonary vein or pass posteriorly quite as much as usual. Selective right atrial angiograms will verify the diagnosis.

In the neonate, satisfactory rupture of the septum primum

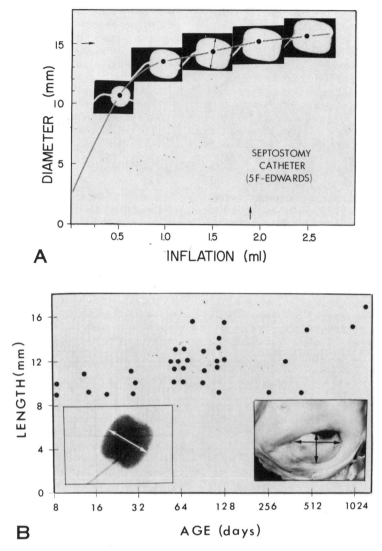

Fig. 21.14 Balloon atrial septostomy. (*A*) Relationship between volume of inflation and diameter of distended catheter balloon for 5F septostomy catheter. *Arrows* indicate that for this particular configuration 1.8 ml inflation reproducibly results in 15 mm diameter. (*B*) Fossa ovalis autopsy measurements. Maximum length without compensation for fixation shrinkage in 34 patients with complete transposition. Age, in days, plotted with geometric progression. (Reproduced with permission from E. A. Fisher and M. H. Paul.[53])

flap covering the fossa ovalis is nearly always effected by proper balloon atrial septostomy technic. In older infants with TGA and large VSD, a thick interatrial flap may preclude successful balloon catheter rupture. If necessary, resort can be had to a cardiac catheter enclosing an extendable blade which has proven a safe and effective procedure for enlarging interatrial communications.[150]

ANGIOCARDIOGRAPHY

An accurate anatomic diagnosis and assessment of associated malformations are essential for successful surgical therapy; 2D echocardiography and angiographic studies provide this information. Selective cardiac chamber and great vessel angiographic injections should be performed to identify: the spatial relationships and connection relationships of the cardiac chambers and outflow vessels[13, 219]; the conus morphology, semilunar atrioventricular valve, and atrioventricular valve-ventricular septal defect relationships[102]; and the associated cardiac malformations, e.g., ventricular septal defect, left ventricular outflow tract obstructions, patent

ductus arteriosus, straddling tricuspid valve components, or coarctation of the aorta.

In the lateral angiocardiogram in TGA with intact ventricular septum, the aorta usually forms a wide, open arch with the ascending portion proceeding far ventrally. The aortic valve cusp level is higher (4th to 5th thoracic vertebral level) than in the normal heart (7th thoracic vertebral level) and reflects the well-developed subaortic conus characteristic of TGA. Deviation from the above occurs particularly when a large VSD with atypical conal morphology (bilateral conus or deficient conus) is present, or with the rare form of posterior transposition.[218, 234]

The ascending aorta in the usual TGA with situs solitus is typically anterior and to the right of the pulmonary artery in an oblique relationship; the large main pulmonary artery arises slightly to the left and definitely posterior to the aorta. These usual relationships are present angiographically in over 90% of infants with complete physiologically uncorrected transposition of the great arteries, categorized symbolically as TGA {S,D,D}. Variations and some ambiguity may arise when angiographically the transposed aortic valve

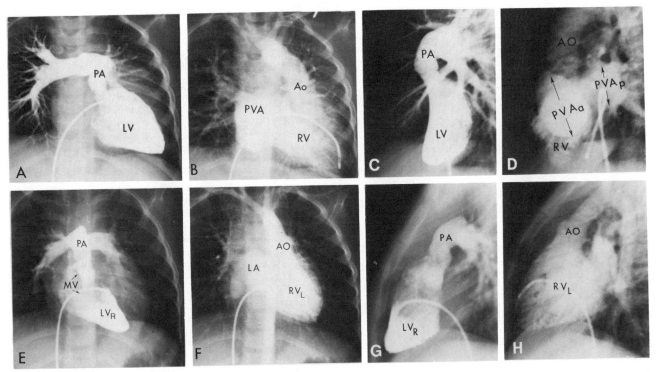

Fig. 21.15 Angiocardiograms (A to D) illustrating variant leftward position of aortic valve in 4-year-old child with complete *physiologically uncorrected* transposition; TGA {S,D,L} following intraatrial (Mustard) repair. (A) Frontal view, selective injection into left-sided morphologically left ventricle (LV). (B) Frontal view, after pulmonary circulation and opacification of new pulmonary venous atrium (PVA), right-sided, morphologically right ventricle (RV) and L-(left) positioned aortic (Ao) valve. (C) Lateral view of A. (D) Lateral view of B. PVAa, anterior segment; PVAp, posterior segment of pulmonary venous atrium. Angiocardiograms (E to H) illustrating leftward position of aortic valve in 4-year-old child with complete *physiologically corrected* transposition; TGA {S,L,L}. (E) Frontal view, selective injection into right-sided morphologically left ventricle (LV$_R$). (F) Frontal view, after pulmonary circulation and opacification of left atrium (LA) and left-sided morphologically right ventricle (RV$_L$) and L-(left) positioned aortic (AO) valve. (G) Lateral view of E. (H) Lateral view of F.

appears to lie directly anterior to the transposed pulmonary valve, and more particularly when the transposed aortic valve lies anterior and slightly to the left of the transposed pulmonary valve (6 to 14%).[57, 182, 187] The segmental findings in the latter instance, TGA {S,D,L} are: situs solitus of viscera and atria (S), ventricular D-loop (D), and an apparent L-position of the semilunar valves (L) (Fig. 21.15A to D). This configuration is to be differentiated, particularly in the anteroposterior angiographic view, from the usual physiologically corrected transposition of the great arteries, TGA {S,L,L} (Fig. 21.15E to H). In viewing the anteroposterior angiocardiogram one must consider that a minor rotation of the subject from the flat anteroposterior position during angiography can project the ascending aorta either to the left or the right of the thoracic spine and pulmonary artery, since the proximal portion of the ascending aorta is in an anterior substernal location.

Identification and localization of the conal musculature and semilunar-atrioventricular valve relationships can be helpful in analyzing the more complex variations (see Chapter 28).[41, 75] The tricuspid valve is best visualized using selective right ventricular injection in the frontal or anterior oblique views by noting intraatrial bulging of the leaflets during ventricular systole and during diastole by the negative silhouette of the orifice as nonopacified blood enters the ventricle. Continuity of the anterior leaflet of the mitral valve with the pulmonary valve is best visualized in the latter or left anterior oblique views in diastole when the anterior leaflet is noted to form the posterior wall of the left ventricular outflow tract. In the frontal view the line of attachment of the posterior mitral valve leaflets can best be

seen in diastole. Straddling or overriding tricuspid valve with VSD[102] must be suspected whenever hypoplasia of the right ventricle is observed; lesser degrees of straddling or anomalous chordal attachments, however, have been noted. The diagnosis can best be established by right or left ventricular selective injection made near the VSD, which facilitates biventrical opacification and visualization of the tricuspid valve orifice in diastole (Fig. 21.16). The straddling tricuspid orifice and valve leaflets are noted to project further than normal to the left and posterior of the septum and into the left ventricle just beneath the posteriorly arising pulmonary artery.

The site and size of a VSD can be visualized by angiography, particularly when an appropriate left anterior oblique rather than lateral view is employed (Fig. 21.17). In many instances the VSD is an uncomplicated anatomic component of the surgical repair, but when there are various types of atypical conus (bilateral, deficient, or displaced), or straddling atrioventricular orifices, valve leaflets or their attachments, foreknowledge of the precise size and location of the VSD and its relationship to the semilunar and atrioventricular valves can be helpful.[205]

The various forms of left ventricular outflow tract stenosis can be best discriminated by selective axial left ventricular cineangiographic views.[14, 188, 193, 206] Small peak systolic pressure differences (<20 mm Hg) between left ventricle and main pulmonary artery have been attributed to a "functional" stenosis similar to that observed in patients with secundum ASD with high pulmonary blood flow. However, in TGA with intact ventricular septum such systolic pressure differences are commonly associated with a recog-

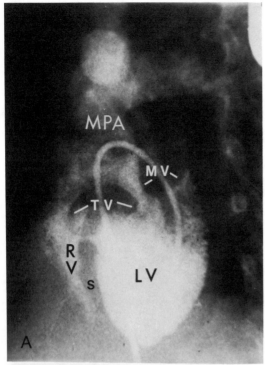

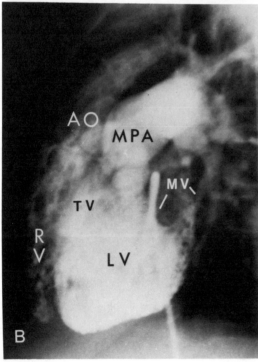

Fig. 21.16 Angiocardiogram in TGA with VSD, straddling tricuspid valve, and hypoplastic right ventricle. (A, B) Left ventricular injection shows tricuspid valve (TV) straddling the interventricular septum (S); note hypoplastic right ventricle (RV). LV, left ventricle; MV, mitral valve; MPA, main pulmonary artery; AO, aorta.

nizable septal bulge abnormality. Minor degrees of abnormal protrusion of the upper muscular ventricular septum into the left ventricular outflow tract in systole are subtle but can be appreciated angiographically in the lateral and left anterior oblique views. In the anteroposterior view the localized bulging septum may produce a small radiolucent filling defect in the outflow tract. Furthermore, echocardiography

has clearly identified a dynamic form of left ventricular outflow obstruction caused by septal motion and systolic anterior movement of the mitral valve (Fig. 21.9). Occasionally, the entire ventricular septum encroaches convexly and posteriorly during systole, and the left ventricle appears small and flattened (Fig. 21.18). A more obvious angiographic subpulmonic ridge-like obstruction is associated with somewhat larger left ventricular outflow tract pressure gradients and reflects a subvalvar fibrous muscular ridge obstruction, often with an underlying abnormal septal bulge.[52, 206] This fibromuscular ridge or discrete obstructing ring is probably an impact lesion and angiographically appears as a prominent irregular curvilinear radiolucent line during systole in the region of the mitral valve. The ridge is often most prominent medially and may demarcate sharply a small subpulmonic vestibule (Fig. 21.19). Isolated pulmonary valve stenosis is infrequent as a major lesion but thickened valve cusps may be observed. The fibromuscular tunnel type of stenosis can best be recognized in the left anterior oblique view as an extensive, narrow, fixed restrictive passage extending from above the VSD for some length toward the pulmonary valve. This form is commonly associated with a VSD of the conal septal malalignment type, with posterior and leftward displacement of some components of the conal septum and hence crowding of the left ventricular outflow tract (Fig. 21.20A).[220] Subpulmonic obstruction resulting from aneurysms of the membranous ventricular septum or redundant displaced tricuspid valve tissue displaced into the left ventricular outflow tract may be recognized by careful angiographic assessment (Fig. 21.21A).[172, 223] Persistent subpulmonic obstruction can also be caused by anomalous septal attachments of straddling mitral valve tissue, particularly in the left-sided type of Taussig-Bing double outlet right ventricle complex,[109] a malformation which can be mistaken for TGA without careful echocardiographic and angiographic assessment.[138]

DIFFERENTIAL DIAGNOSIS

The initial diagnosis of TGA can be treacherous in the newborn period because of the frequent absence of an overtly abnormal auscultation, chest roentgenogram, or electrocardiogram. Indeed, these negative findings in a comfortable well-developed cyanotic newborn should suggest this diagnostic possibility. Once disease is suspected several *noncardiac clinical entities* in particular must be considered in the differential diagnosis, including idiopathic respiratory distress syndrome, persistent fetal circulation syndrome, and neonatal polycythemic syndrome. The immediate clinical course and its integration with umbilical arterial blood gas data, blood hematocrit, and chest x-ray findings sometimes can resolve these diagnoses. Anatomic confirmation as to normal or abnormal cardiac morphology is essential and can readily be achieved with 2D echocardiography. In regards to *cardiac malformations*, it is appropriate to consider malformations with the early onset of cyanosis, such as pulmonary atresia with VSD or severe tetralogy of Fallot, tricuspid atresia with diminished (or increased) pulmonary blood flow, total anomalous pulmonary venous connection, pulmonary atresia or stenosis, truncus arteriosus, Ebstein's anomaly of the tricuspid valve, and hypoplastic left heart syndrome.

TREATMENT

Palliative Therapy

In the past the keystone to improved survival and ultimate corrective surgery has been the successful application of

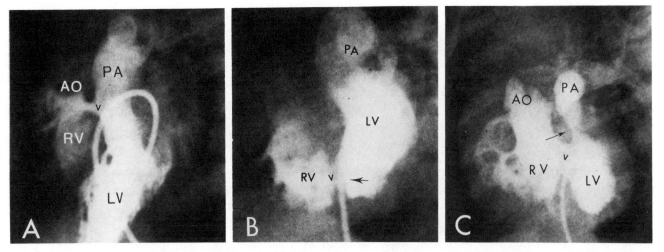

Fig. 21.17 Angiocardiograms of VSD in TGA, left anterior oblique view. (A) Small supracristal defect (v) in 6-week-old infant. (B) Apical muscular defect in 2-year-old infant with pulmonary vascular obstruction. Pressures were pulmonary artery (PA), 75/40 mm Hg, and aorta (AO), 80/50 mm Hg; pulmonary vascular resistance, 7 units. (C) Large defect (v) of conal septal malalignment type with severe subpulmonary obstruction (arrow) in 5-year-old child with previous subclavian-pulmonary shunt. RV, right ventricle; LV, left ventricle.

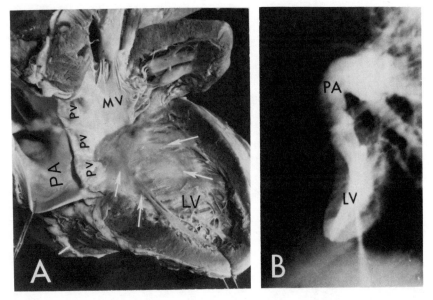

Fig. 21.18 Septal bulge in TGA. (A) Autopsy specimen from 2-year-old child showing moderately prominent convex bulging (arrows) of interventricular septum toward left ventricular (LV) cavity. Surprisingly, cardiac catheterization studies in this child indicated a peak systolic left ventricular outflow tract pressure gradient of 58 mm Hg. Note mitral valve (MV) to pulmonary vlave (PV) fibrous continuity and absence of any discrete fibromuscular ridge at the septal impact site of the mitral valve (cf. Fig. 21.19E and F). (B) Superimposed systolic and diastolic angiographic frames from 4-year-old child 2 years after intraatrial repair illustrating abnormally prominent posterior septal bulging into the left ventricular cavity during systole. No localized fibromuscular ridge stenosis was visualized. Pressures were LV apex, 60/8; LV outflow, 24/8; and pulmonary artery (PA), 24/18 mm Hg.

several palliative procedures: balloon atrial septostomy, surgical septectomy, partial venous correction,[10] pulmonary artery banding, and systemic-pulmonary shunts. To achieve maximum survival rates, a dedicated team of pediatric cardiologists, anesthesiologists, and cardiovascular surgeons available day and night, and an infant intensive care unit with specialized nursing expertise are necessary.

Accumulated experiences over the past decade clearly establish the value of *balloon atrial septostomy* for the initial management of the *severely hypoxic* neonate with TGA; survival during the 1st month of life has improved from 20% before septostomy was introduced to 90 to 95% presently (Fig. 21.1).[71, 107, 128, 152, 166] Furthermore, by improving oxygenation and acid-base balance, successful balloon

atrial septostomy decreases the operative risk for any early surgical cardiac procedure. Accordingly, balloon septostomy should be attempted in all neonates as the first step in any management program.

Several clinics have reported earlier experiences (Table 21.3) with reliance on balloon atrial septostomy alone for *prolonged* palliation. When corrective surgery was electively delayed beyond the first year of life, a significant interval morbidity and mortality occurred from complications, including cerebrovascular accidents, progressive pulmonary vascular disease, and intravascular thrombosis. A multicenter study reported 25% accumulated mortality by 1 year of age for infants with TGA and intact ventricular septum palliated only by balloon atrial septostomy (1972 to 1974).[59]

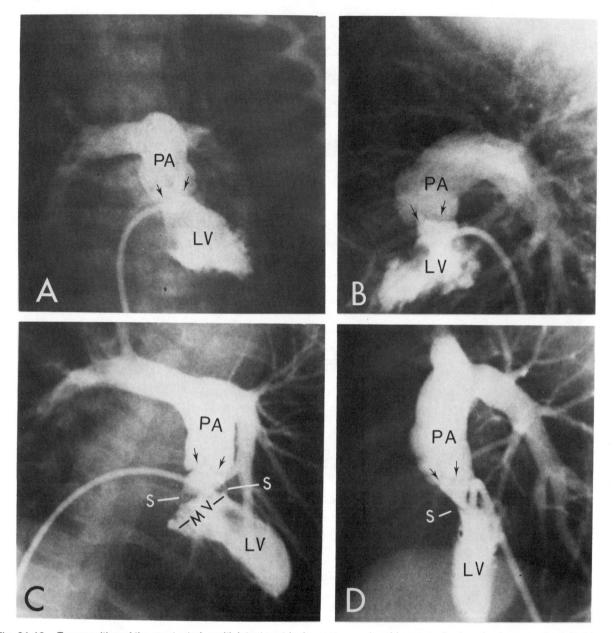

Fig. 21.19 Transposition of the great arteries with intact ventricular septum and rapid progression in subpulmonary stenosis. (A and B) Frontal and lateral angiograms at 2 days of age. Pressures were right ventricle, 70/7 and left ventricle (LV), 35/5 mm Hg, and there was no systolic murmur. (C and D) Same patient at 4 months of age. A systolic murmur was first noted at 2 months of age and progressed to grade 3/6 with marked increase in cyanosis, and pressures were now RV, 80/6; LV, 80/6; and pulmonary artery (PA), 14/10 mm Hg.

A large single series (1966 to 1978) report indicates 86% survival to 6 months after balloon atrial septostomy and any indicated intervening palliative surgery.[107] Accordingly, many have adopted a policy of early elective definitive intraatrial repair in the second 6 months of life for infants with intact ventricular septum or small VSD who have satisfactory initial improvement with balloon atrial septostomy.

There is not complete agreement on criteria for satisfactory post balloon atrial septostomy improvement.[76, 79] Some accept an increase in systemic arterial saturation of 10% or more, together with a reduction in the interatrial mean pressure gradient to less than 2 mm of Hg, plus clinical improvement as evidence for good results[71, 139]; others define good palliation as systemic arterial saturation of at least 70% with an interatrial pressure difference that is minimal[158], and

a third group defines good results in terms of survival, absence of cerebrovascular accident, and maintenance of systemic arterial oxygen saturation at 60% or greater for more than 6 months (Table 21.4, Fig. 21.22).[202]

Excluding poor technical performance, a number of anatomic and physiologic factors may be responsible for unsatisfactory improvement. The fossa ovalis may be relatively small or the valve of the foramen ovale may be quite thick (Fig. 21.23).[101, 127] Repeat balloon atrial septostomy is rarely effective,[11] and only in a few selected cases is catheter blade atrial septostomy indicated.[150] Two-dimensional echocardiographic imaging of the interatrial septum can establish the anatomic results of the balloon septostomy.[22] It has been suggested that adequately palliated infants have an interatrial defect of at least 10 to 12 mm in diameter created by the septostomy maneuver, but more commonly defects up

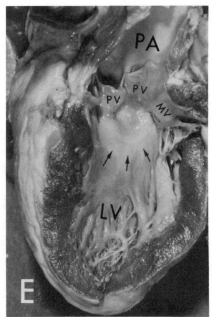

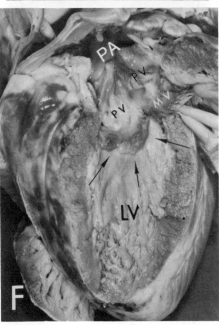

Fig. 21.19 (*E* and *F*) Autopsy specimens illustrating left ventricular outflow tract with fibromuscular ridge pathology (*arrows*). Note relationship of mitral valve (*MV*) impact region to site of ridge. (*E*) Pathologic specimen, early fibromuscular ridge in 2-month-old infant. (*F*) Pathologic specimen, moderately severe fibromuscular ridge obstruction in 2-year-old child with peak systolic pressure gradient of 64 mm Hg across left ventricular outflow tract. *PV*, pulmonary valve; *S*, subpulmonary stenosis.

to 15 mm diameter are observed.[11, 33] Despite the presence of adequate-sized anatomic communications, inadequate intercirculatory mixing and disappointing clinical improvement have been noted. In these cases it can be postulated that a delayed fall in the pulmonary vascular resistance with consequent low pulmonary blood flow and left atrial volumes result in inadequate functional interatrial mixing.[77]

In this regard it has recently been shown that neonates with TGA and intact ventricular septum with an unsatisfactory arterial oxygen saturation response to balloon atrial

septostomy often respond to infusions of prostaglandin E_1 (0.10 μg/kg/minute or less) with a substantial increase in arterial oxygenation. In 21 infants the mean PaO_2 before infusion of 23 mm Hg increased to 32 mm Hg during the infusion.[18, 56, 104] Although the beneficial effect undoubtedly depends on an adequate intraatrial communication, infusions probably should be started as soon as feasible prior to emergency balloon atrial septostomy in those neonates who are severely hypoxemic and acidotic in an early effort to raise pulmonary venous return and increase intraatrial shunting. Dilation of the ductus provides increased pulmonary blood flow as a consequence of an obligatory ductal (systemic to pulmonary) shunt with consequent *increase* in pulmonary venous return, left atrial pressures, intraatrial (pulmonary to systemic) shunting, and systemic arterial oxygen saturation. After balloon atrial septostomy, these beneficial effects can be useful as a temporary palliative support measure for a few hours or days to await a natural decrease in pulmonary vascular resistance and to avoid an early Blalock-Hanlon or intraatrial baffle procedure in the newborn. Frequently, however, stopping the prostaglandin infusion is followed promptly by a return to severe hypoxemia, and in these patients early corrective surgery may be urgently indicated. A role for a bridging therapeutic interval of pulmonary vasodilator therapy has been proposed for this and other circumstances; intravenous tolazoline hydrochloride (Priscoline) infusion has been reported to be effective by increasing systemic arterial oxygen saturation after an inadequate physiological response to an anatomically successful balloon atrial septostomy.[136]

In the early weeks following balloon atrial septostomy, a few infants manifest deterioration characterized by increasing cyanosis and hypercyanotic spells. This can be ascribed to a more extensive form of dynamic left ventricular outflow tract obstruction characterized by prominent posterior systolic bulging of the ventricular septum coupled with mitral valve opposition.[8, 206] In addition, a subpulmonary fibrous ridge-like obstruction appears to develop at this site, further compromising pulmonary blood flow. Echocardiography and left ventricular axial cineangiography can identify the details of this complication, and in some infants progressive diminution in the pulmonary vascular markings on the plain chest radiograph provides a late index of suspicion.[206]

Surgical creation of an atrial septal defect by the Blalock-Hanlon operation[24] or one of its modifications[45] has been a widely applied palliative surgical procedure for TGA (Fig. 21.24). An interatrial septal defect is created by excising the posterior aspect of the interatrial septum in a relatively simple closed heart procedure than can be performed rapidly on even the smallest infant.

Atrial septectomy provides systemic arterial oxygen-saturation levels higher than balloon atrial septostomy alone; mean systemic arterial oxygen saturation levels range as high as 79%, and these increases are well maintained for long periods of time (Table 21.4).[16, 33, 43, 115, 208] Closure or marked narrowing of an atrial septal defect after surgical septectomy and requiring a secondary septectomy has been observed rarely.[115] Some early series of atrial septectomy had a 30% operative mortality, but current operative mortality for the Blalock-Hanlon procedure is about 5 to 10%.[33, 71, 115] The critical interval of the Blalock-Hanlon operation occurs while the clamps across both the atria and the right pulmonary veins in the region of the intraatrial sulcus are in place during resection of the dorsal portion of the atrial septum. It is important that the infant enter this phase of the operation with optimal circulatory and acid-base balance parameters. Postoperative atrial dysrhythmias have been transient and rarely of clinical significance.[129]

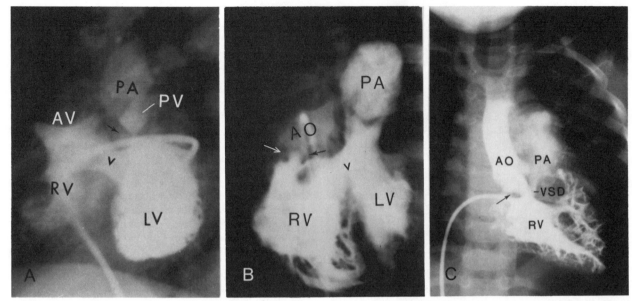

Fig. 21.20 Angiocardiograms illustrating subpulmonary and subaortic conal musculature obstructing outflow tracts in transposition. (*A*) Left anterior oblique view showing large conoventricular malalignment type of defect (*v*) with posterior and leftward displacement of conal musculature (*arrow*), severely narrowing the pulmonary outflow tract. *PA*, pulmonary artery; *PV*, pulmonary valve; *LV*, left ventricle; *RV*, right ventricle. (*B*) Left anterior oblique view showing prominent obstructing subaortic conus (*arrows*) in 23-month-old infant with pulmonary artery banding at 5 months of age for large VSD. Pressures were RV, 105/11; aorta (*AO*), 85/55; LV, 105/12; PA, 12/9 mm Hg. (*C*) Frontal view showing prominent obstructing subaortic conal musculature (*arrow*) in 21-month-old infant. Pressures were: RV, 105/6; AO, 60/40; LV, 35/6; PA, 16/9 mm Hg. In this rare occurrence of subaortic stenosis with TGA, there was no previous surgery, and no right ventricular outflow tract pressure gradient was present at the initial neonatal catheterization.

Advocates for early additional palliation with elective surgical atrial septectomy after neonatal emergency balloon atrial septostomy were concerned with the frequency of cerebrovascular accidents, repeated hospitalization, and persistent severe cyanosis in infants palliated only with balloon atrial septostomy who were awaiting corrective surgery at 12 or more months of age. One large center reporting an experience with intracardiac repair (Mustard) in 205 patients observed that despite the use of balloon atrial septostomy since 1966 there was no decrease in their practice of atrial septectomy (55% of infants) between those having repair before 1973 and those operated on between 1973 to 1979. In contrast, other large centers have curtailed palliation with atrial septectomy and advocate that corrective surgery be performed early for an infant or neonate with intact ventricular septum, if clinical improvement from the balloon atrial septostomy is inadequate or serious deterioration occurs subsequently. One series of 80 consecutive Mustard procedures from 1970 to 1980 reported only one palliative surgical septectomy.[157] The long-term results of early intraatrial correction at less than 2 to 3 months of age has not yet been adequately evaluated—but earlier intraatrial corrective surgery is becoming a more usual practice.[94, 157, 210]

Transposition associated with large VSD without left ventricular outflow tract stenosis is complicated by two major problems: heart failure and pulmonary vascular disease. *Surgical constriction of the pulmonary artery* can provide effective palliation for both these complications in infants.[141, 197] In view of the inevitability of early pulmonary vascular obstructive changes in this group, *palliative* or *corrective* surgical intervention, preferably before 3 or 4 months of age, seems mandatory.[36, 141] Atrial septectomy may be indicated at the same time as the pulmonary artery banding if an initial balloon atrial septostomy is unsuccessful. Operative mortality for banding has ranged from 10 to 58%.[44] The pulmonary artery in infants with TGA should be banded more loosely than in infants with normally related great arteries, since the former need a somewhat higher pulmonary blood flow for optimum intercirculatory mixing.[207] Hemodynamically major muscular subaortic stenosis has been reported as an infrequent late consequence of pulmonary artery banding, perhaps analagous to the muscular subpulmonary obstruction observed following pulmonary artery banding in children with normally related great arteries.[177]

Infants with TGA and VSD with severe pulmonary stenosis or pulmonary atresia have been successfully palliated with *systemic-pulmonary* (or rarely caval-pulmonary) *anastomosis*. Statistics are quite limited; in infants older than a month of age early surgical mortality can be 10 to 15%, but in the neonatal period the surgical risk has been reported higher.[4]

The infant with intact ventricular septum and a PDA appears to be at great risk for complications and early death. In one atrial septostomy series, 16 of 17 infants with large PDA expired, despite various nonsurgical and surgical palliative interventions.[165] Similarly, disastrous results were reported from a series of 144 infants with TGA and various associated lesions undergoing balloon atrial septostomy (1966 to 1978), where 18 of 24 infants with large PDA failed to survive.[107] Urgent closure of a large PDA is usually mandatory because of rapidly progressive left heart failure. Atrial septostomy or septectomy, although providing an adequate anatomic interatrial communication, may not provide effective interatrial mixing after abrupt spontaneous or surgical closure of the PDA. There is usually a marked decrease in systemic arterial saturation and clinical deterioration, perhaps the result of a pulmonary vascular bed that, preconditioned to the early high pulmonary artery blood pressures and flow, does not permit adequate pulmonary venous return after the ligation of the PDA to provide satisfactory interatrial mixing (Fig. 21.25). Of additional concern is the observation that a PDA appears to be asso-

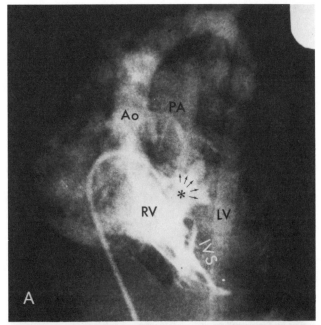

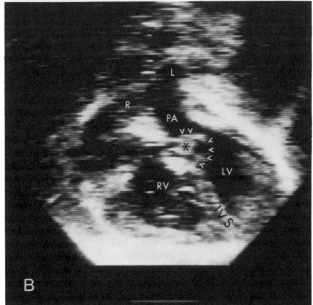

Fig. 21.21 (*A*) Cineangiogram, four-chamber view, and (*B*) 2D echocardiogram, subxiphoid imaging position, in 18-month-old infant with TGA with VSD and outpouching (*) of accessory tricuspid valve leaflet tissue causing subpulmonic obstruction. Pressures were: LV, 60/9 mm Hg; LV outflow tract, 22/9 mm Hg; and PA, 22/10 mm Hg. *RV* and *LV*, right and left ventricles; *PA*, pulmonary artery; *Ao*, aorta; *IVS*, intact ventricular septum.

ciated with a high frequency of late pulmonary vascular disease. The following management program seems indicated: balloon atrial septostomy initially as with all infants with TGA. If the PDA remains large and left and right heart failure are evident, the ductus should be surgically closed promptly and corrective intraatrial surgery done concurrently; if the ductus remains patent but there is no heart failure, continuing close observation is essential, since abrupt cyanotic deterioration can occur with spontaneous ductal closure and necessitate urgent operative intervention; if the ductus remains patent and the clinical status satisfactory,

early corrective surgery with closure of the ductus should be undertaken, probably no later than at 4 to 6 months of age because of the apparent increased risk of pulmonary vascular disease.

Corrective Surgery

Intraatrial Physiological Correction. Physiological correction of TGA became a reality with the venous procedure described by Mustard[134] for the intraatrial redirection of venous return based upon the concepts of Albert[1] and Senning.[186] In the Mustard operation, after resection of most of the atrial septum, a baffle is fashioned from pericardium or synthetic material to direct the pulmonary venous return to the tricuspid orifice and right ventricle and to direct the systemic venous return to the mitral orifice and left ventricle

TABLE 21.4 RESULTS OF PALLIATIVE PROCEDURES SYSTEMIC ARTERIAL OXYGEN SATURATION (%)[a]

Reference	165	212	53	115	43	80
Patients (no.)	(20)	(75)	(30)	(66)	(38)	(33)
Procedure	BAS	BAS	BAS	SAS	SAS	SAS
TGA (IVS)						
Preprocedure	41	43 ± 12	31 ± 11	45	55[b]	47[b]
Postprocedure	64	62 ± 12	57 ± 12			
Late follow-up		58 ± 9	55 ± 10	78	75[b]	73[b]
TGA (VSD)						
Preprocedure	53	56 ± 12	56 ± 11	64		
Postprocedure	74	67 ± 12	70 ± 11			
Late follow-up		59 ± 11	75 ± 12	81		

[a] BAS, balloon catheter atrial septostomy; SAS, surgical atrial septectomy.

[b] Data combined for intact ventricular septum (IVS) and ventricular septal defect (VSD) group; TGA, transposition of the great arteries.

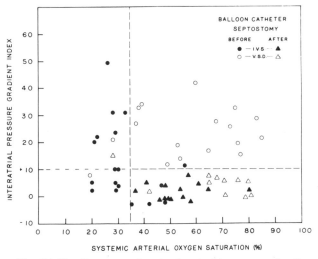

Fig. 21.22 Response of systemic arterial oxygen saturation and interatrial pressure gradient index to balloon atrial septostomy. Interatrial pressure gradient index greater than 10 indicates left atrial hypertension (mean and V wave) relative to right atrial pressures. Note: some infants with intact ventricular septum (*IVS*) have high preseptostomy left atrial pressures; almost all large interatrial pressure gradients are abolished by septostomy; and infants with VSD have relatively higher preseptostomy systemic arterial oxygen saturations and more modest postseptostomy increases in saturation compared to infants with intact ventricular septum.

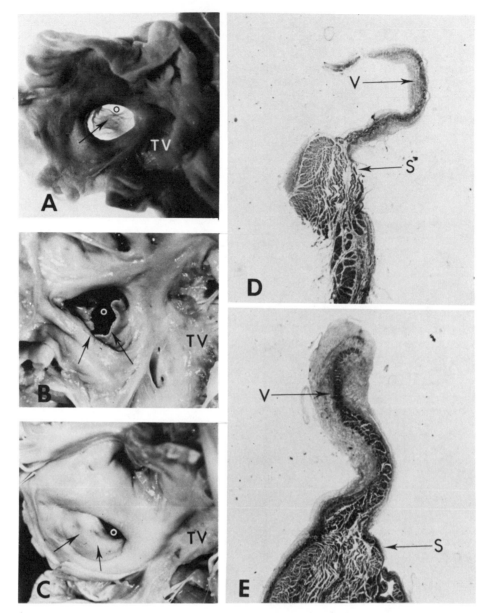

Fig. 21.23 Fossa ovalis morphology and balloon atrial septostomy. (*A*) Normal premature infant (32 weeks) with trans-illuminated fossa ovalis showing right atrial view of thin septum primum valve and elliptical patent foramen ovale (*o*). (*B*) Full-term infant with TGA and intact ventricular septum who expired 6 hours after anatomically effective balloon atrial septostomy, with long linear tear in the shunt limiting septum primum valve. (*C*) Two-month-old infant with TGA and large VSD with markedly thickened septum primum valve which resisted repeated attempts of balloon catheter withdrawal. (*D*) Usual histologic appearance of thin valve noted in most neonates with TGA, particularly with intact ventricular septum. (*E*) Thick, fibromuscular valve encountered in some older infants (2 to 3 months) particularly with large VSD. *S*, atrial septum fossa ovalis margin; *TV*, tricuspid valve; *V*, septum primum valve tissue.

(Figs. 21.26 to 21.28). In terms of connections, the surgery imposes a discordant atrioventricular connection upon the existing discordant arterioventricular connection, thus resulting in a physiological correction. Using techniques of cardiopulmonary bypass or profound hypothermia with circulatory arrest, this operation has been successfully applied to neonates, infants, and children.[3, 40, 71, 151, 198, 200, 202, 209, 211] Many clinics have achieved a remarkably low operative risk, particularly for infants with simple transposition and intact ventricular septum 6 months of age or older.[94, 157, 202, 211] One large series concerns 249 cases with intact ventricular septum and without other major lesions.[200] Hospital mortality in infants operated during the first year of life was 6%; between 6 and 12 months of life, 2%, and in older children, 10%. A

more recent large series reports a hospital mortality of 11 in the first 105 patients operated on from 1963 to 1973 and only 2 in the subsequent 100 patients operated on from 1973 to 1979.[209]

The *optimum timing for intraatrial corrective surgery* is still debated, but the advantages of early, definitive repair versus delayed, two stage correction for various anatomic and physiologic subgroups have been stressed.[200, 211] There is a strong trend in congenital cardiac surgery toward primary correction of any lesion at the earliest age when feasible *with good results*.[15, 99] Certainly, for the young infant with simple TGA, there have been reports of low (<5%) operative mortality during an interval spanning the first few weeks and months of life.[3, 211] Particular care must be observed in this

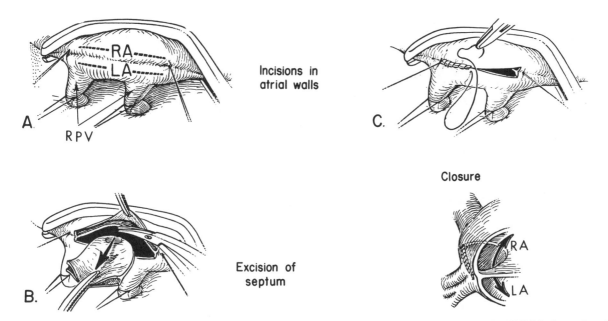

Fig. 21.24   Blalock-Hanlon operation. (*A*) Clamp placed across both atria (*RA*, *LA*) and right pulmonary veins (*RPV*) in the region of the interatrial sulcus. (*B*) Excision of posterior portion of atrial septum. (*C*) Closure of atrial incision with resultant surgically created atrial septal defect. (Modified from D. A. Cooley and G. L. Hallman: Surgical Treatment of Congenital Heart Disease. Lea & Febiger, Philadelphia, 1966.)

age group in the placement and tailoring of the intraatrial baffle and in the enlargement of the pulmonary venous atrium to avoid obstruction to systemic or pulmonary venous return. Some clinics presently follow a two-stage corrective program if the clinical status is unsatisfactory after balloon atrial septostomy, promptly resorting to surgical atrial septectomy when indicated with a view toward intraatrial correction at about 1 year of age. However, the advocates of early correction consider this program to have several disadvantages: septectomy in itself carries a mortality and morbidity ranging from 5 to 25%; delay in corrective surgery with the attendant prolonged interval of moderate hypoxemia may favor the development of pulmonary vascular disease, central nervous system complications, depressed myocardial performance, or other more subtle systemic pathology; and multiple operations may have adverse effects on family affairs as compared to a single, early initial corrective operation.

Several other ingenious intraatrial operative procedures are now being used, and advantages are claimed over the Mustard operation relative to surgical technique and electrophysiological and hemodynamic results.[186, 190, 228] In particular, Senning[185, 186] described a technique which rerouted the systemic and pulmonary venous return without resort to avascular pericardium or other patch material by arranging flaps of the interatrial septum and right atrial free wall to form the new venous channels. This procedure, using viable atrial tissue has the theoretical advantage of optimizing the potential for atrial chamber growth and contractility. Initially, the results with this technic were not uniformly satisfactory, and little was heard about it after the introduction of the widely successful Mustard procedure. Recently, the Senning procedure has been revived[160] and has been applied to infants with low hospital mortality (2 of 68 infants with IVS).[37, 149, 160] These proponents state that the Senning procedure is easier to perform and that caval and pulmonary venous obstruction is more readily avoided, particularly in the small infants, although some are advocating pericardial patch augmentation.[37] More objective late follow-up data including electrophysiological and hemodynamic studies[17]

will be needed before the superiority of one or another intraatrial surgical technique can be established.

Surgical correction of *transposition with a large ventricular septal defect* becomes more complicated and the operative mortality is higher. Problems encountered with closure of the defects are related anatomically to their size and position and the adjacent conal septal morphology and atrioventricular valve, and physiologically, to the frequent coexisting increased pulmonary vascular resistance and pulmonary vascular disease.

The more usual conoventricular and atrioventricular canal type defects can be exposed and closed readily through the tricuspid orifice, avoiding an incision in the systemic ventricle.[87] Some defects of the atrioventricular canal type and the conal septum malalignment type have components of the tricuspid valve tension apparatus which may be intimately related to the defect, and valve function can be at risk.[204] In the latter type of defect, the conal septum (parietal band) can be markedly malaligned relative to the plane of the ventricular septum and directed leftward posteriorly, often encroaching upon the pulmonary outflow tract and causing obstruction (Fig. 21.20*A*).[220] The type of surgical repair selected can be much influenced by the relationship of the VSD to the aorta. When a defect is unusually large, with absence of the basilar portion of the ventricular septum both posteriorly and anteriorly, a direct intraventricular repair may be achieved by appropriate placement of an intraventricular prosthesis.[98] More commonly, when the defect is supracristal in position the pulmonary valve is adjacent to or overriding the defect, the defect is closed by a patch so that the left ventricle drains to the pulmonary artery, and physiological correction is achieved by the usual intraatrial baffle procedure.

Operative results with early pulmonary artery banding before 2 to 3 months of age and later second stage intraatrial correction have been disappointing until recently, with the reported combined mortality of pulmonary artery banding and late correction being 25% or greater.[3, 196] Anatomic correction (great artery switch) has recently been applied to this subgroup of palliated patients at 1 to 2 years of age with

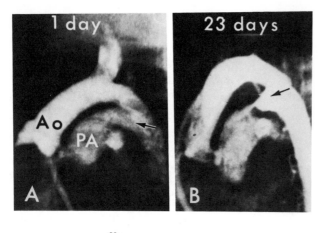

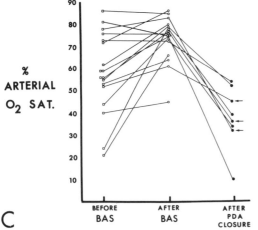

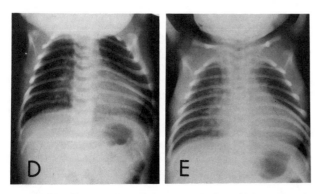

Fig. 21.25 Transposition of the great arteries with intric-ular septum and PDA. Cineangiograms showing (A) Large PDA diagnosed at 1 day of age—arterial oxygen saturation was 74%; (B) Subsequent severe narrowing was noted at 23 days of age when arterial oxygen saturation was 34%. Ao, aorta; PA, pulmonary artery. (C) Changes in systemic arterial oxygen saturation in 18 infants with TGA, intact ventricular septum, and large PDA. Measurements made before and after balloon atrial septostomy (BAS) and following spontaneous or surgical closure of the ductus. Frontal chest roentgenograms showing (D) moderately enlarged heart with increased pulmonary vascular markings in 5-day-old infant with arterial oxygen saturation of 76%. (E) Rapid clinical deterioration by 9 days of age with severe left heart failure requiring emergency surgery for closure of PDA. PDA, patent ductus arteriosus.

a surgical risk of 10 to 15%. At present, several clinics are aggressively applying primary corrective surgery for the management of the very young infant with large VSD with improved surgical outcome: intraatrial repair with patch

closure of the VSD by 3 to 4 months of age[37, 210]; or anatomic correction of the great arteries with closure of the VSD by 3 to 6 months of age. Recent improvements are related to more complete understanding and attention to the early progression of pulmonary vascular disease, increased care of the tricuspid valve apparatus, and improved myocardial preservation and extracorporeal support during the surgery.

Palliative Mustard Operation

Elevated pulmonary vascular resistance markedly increases the risk of corrective surgery with closure of the VSD. Advanced pulmonary vascular disease characterized by calculated pulmonary vascular resistances greater than 10 units or grade 4 (H-E) histologic changes are considered a contraindication to closure of the VSD.[122] Extensive grade 4 (H-E) pathology has been observed even in patients with lower pulmonary vascular resistance levels of 6 to 8 units.[141] Intraatrial baffle repair without closure of the VSD (palliative Mustard operation) has been accomplished with low surgical risk and substantial hemodynamic and clinical benefit.[27, 114, 122] Mean systemic arterial oxygen saturations have been increased in two series from preoperative levels of 68 to 74% to postoperative levels of 87 to 90%. This procedure should be reserved for patients in whom peripheral unsaturation is a major cause of symptomatology, since there is no favorable postoperative change in the pulmonary artery pressures or calculated pulmonary vascular resistances. The inevitability of advanced pulmonary vascular disease previously prevalent in older infants and children with TGA and large VSD is presently markedly reduced by the management policy during the past decade of early pulmonary artery banding, and by the more recent success with early (2 to 4 months of age) corrective surgery with closure of the VSD.

The concept of the palliative Mustard operation also can be successfully applied to patients with pulmonary vascular disease with intact ventricular septum by creating concurrently a ventricular septal defect in the apical segment of the muscular septum: in one child there was an increase of systemic arterial oxygen saturation from 46% preoperatively to 93% postoperatively.[201]

Left Ventricular Outflow Tract Stenosis

Adequate surgical relief of *severe* left ventricular outflow tract stenosis may be difficult and depends on the anatomic type and severity of the obstruction, as well as the state of the ventricular septum. With *intact ventricular septum*, transpulmonary resection of the obstruction at the time of intraatrial repair is sometimes performed if a major obstruction is caused by a short, discrete fibromuscular subvalvar shelf.[88] However, because access is often limited and extensive resection carries excessive risk, residual pressure gradients are common. If the obstruction is severe and extensive or a large residual gradient is not well tolerated, a left ventricular to pulmonary artery conduit has been suggested and successfully employed.[89, 125]

With a VSD, a moderate subpulmonary obstruction, by reducing pulmonary blood flow and pressure, may function to prevent heart failure and limit the risk of early pulmonary vascular disease. As long as intercirculatory mixing and systemic arterial oxygen saturation is satisfactory and the peak systolic pulmonary artery pressure is less than about 50% of systemic pressures, intracardiac surgery can be delayed with careful follow-up until the optimum age for physiological or anatomic corrective surgery.

With a VSD and *severe* left ventricular outflow obstruc-

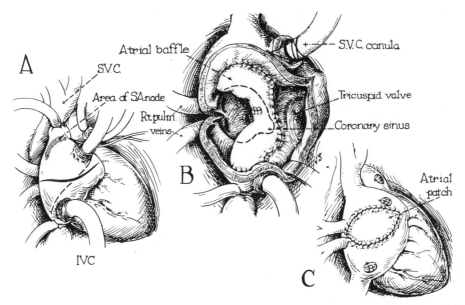

Fig. 21.26 Intraatrial correction (Mustard operation). (*A*) Superior vena caval drainage catheter placed to avoid *Area of SA node*. (*B*) After excision of the atrial septum, a pericardial baffle of suitable geometry is sutured in place to form a new systemic venous atrium which extends from the superior (*SVC*) and inferior (*IVC*) vena cava to the mitral valve and effectively separates and redirects the two circulations. Redundant baffle pericardium can be further trimmed to prevent pulmonary venous obstruction. (*C*) The pulmonary venous atrium can be expanded by insertion of a patch in the initial atrial incision. *Rt. pulm.*, right pulmonary.

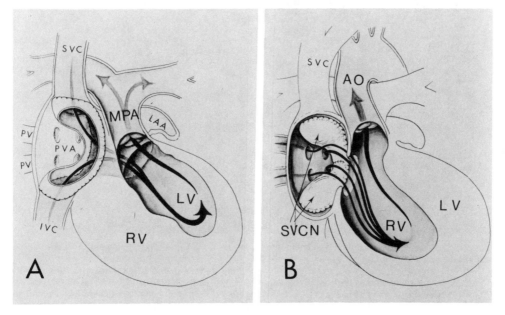

Fig. 21.27 Circulation pathways of the systemic (*A*) and pulmonary (*B*) venous return after intraatrial repair (Mustard operation). *SVC, IVC*, superior and inferior vena cava; *SVCN*, systemic venous baffle conduit; *PV*, pulmonary veins; *PVA*, pulmonary venous atrium; *RV, LV*, right and left ventricle; *AO*, aorta; *MPA*, main pulmonary artery; *LAA*, left atrial appendage.

tion, there is inadequate pulmonary blood flow and marked hypoxia, and a palliative systemic to pulmonary arterial shunt (Waterston, Blalock or Gore-tex tube shunt) is usually urgently required. Second stage intracardiac correction can be carried out at 2 to 4 years of age usually with the Rastelli operation[126, 131, 168, 169] and infrequently with direct excision of the outflow obstruction, closure of the VSD, and intraatrial repair.

The Rastelli operation when feasible has been considered the operation of choice for TGA with VSD and extensive muscular or fibromuscular left ventricular outflow tract ob-

struction (tunnel stenosis) since it achieves complete bypass of the left ventricular outflow tract obstruction and an anatomical as well as physiological correction of the transposition physiology. In this procedure (Fig. 21.29) the proximal main pulmonary artery is divided from the left ventricle, and the cardiac end is oversewn; the left ventricular output is diverted to the aorta by creating a conduit within the right ventricle which carries blood ejected through the VSD into the aorta; and the right ventricle is connected to the distal end of the divided pulmonary artery by means of an external prosthetic conduit. The VSD must be adequate in diameter

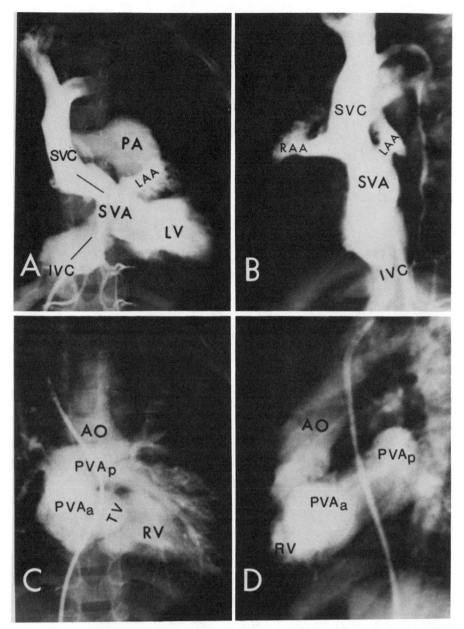

Fig. 21.28 Angiocardiograms showing systemic and pulmonary venous atrial morphology following intraatrial baffle repair (Mustard) operation. (A) Frontal and (B) lateral views of the systemic veins (SVC and IVC, superior and inferior vena cava), systemic venous atrium (SVA), left ventricle (LV), and pulmonary artery (PA). Note the very adequate conduit diameters and absence of constriction in the superior and inferior limbs of the systemic venous atrium. LAA and RAA, left and right atrial appendages. (C) Frontal and (D) lateral views of the new pulmonary venous atrium (PVA). This chamber consists of a posterior segment (PVAp) receiving the pulmonary veins and an anterior segment (PVAa) that formerly was a portion of the original right atrium. The PVAa empties via the tricuspid valve (TV) into the right ventricle (RV) and aorta (AO).

to permit a completely unobstructed outflow from the left ventricle. Enlargement of the defect by anterior excision is often necessary.

Intracardiac repair at an early age with either the Rastelli operation or direct excision of the obstruction and intraatrial repair had, until recently, a high mortality in patients less than 4 to 5 years of age.[32, 126, 159] More recently, quite satisfactory operative survival and good results have been obtained with the Rastelli operation in children 2 years or older.[126, 131] Unfavorable anatomic variants precluding normal placement of the VSD patch are characterized by having anomalous tricuspid valve connections crossing the VSD because of abnormal chordae or papillary muscle attachments.[131]

Left ventricular outflow tract obstruction by an aneurysm or pouch of the membranous septum, almost always with a VSD, is uncommon but can be readily diagnosed by angiography and 2D echocardiography. Unlike extensive conal septum obstructions, these can usually be excised with closure of the VSD in infancy with low surgical risk.[223] Anatomic correction can also be applied to this subgroup if the left ventricular outflow obstruction is of a correctable form.

Arterial Anatomic Correction

Although intraatrial repair, with physiological correction, has achieved widespread success, pursuit of an anatomic curative operation has continued. This has been stimulated

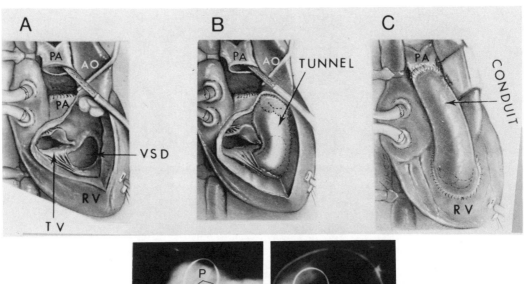

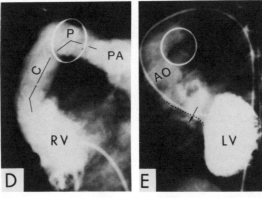

Fig. 21.29   Rastelli operation for transposition of the great arteries with VSD and extensive left ventricular outflow tract obstruction. (*A, B,* and *C*) Details of surgical procedure (modified, from Rastelli, G. C., McGoon, D. C., and Wallace, R. B., J. Thorac. Cardiovasc. Surg. 58:545, 1969; with permission of C. V. Mosby Co.) (*A*) Interior of right ventricle (*RV*), demonstrating relationship of ventricular septal defect (*VSD*), tricuspid valve (*TV*), and aortic valve. (*B*) Left ventricle is connected to aorta (*AO*) by tunnel patch extending between VSD and aorta. (*C*) Completed repair with RV connected to the distal end of pulmonary artery (*PA*) by valve-bearing prosthetic conduit or aortic homograft. (*D, E*) Lateral angiograms with selective left ventricle (*LV*) and RV injections after Rastelli operation in 5-year-old child. (*E*) Note small (left to right) leak across tunnel patch (*arrow*), and (*D*) valve-bearing prosthetic conduit (*C*) between RV and PA.

by infrequent late obstructive and dysrhythmic complications with the baffle operation, the spectre of right ventricular dysfunction and tricuspid valve insufficiency, and some dissatisfaction with current results in infants with large VSD. Since 1954, there have been a number of ingenious procedures used for anatomic correction of TGA by direct contraposition of the transposed vessels,[39, 86, 135] but clinical success was not achieved until 1975.[92] Initial major technical tasks concerned transfer of the coronary ostia, which are closely related to the aortic valve, and the reconstruction of the right ventricular outflow tract and pulmonary trunk.

The anatomic challenge has been met with the application of novel surgical techniques.[21, 92, 108, 156, 238, 239, 240] In general the great arteries are transected in a manner that allows direct reanastomosis of the distal aortic segment to the proximal pulmonary artery segment. Transfer of the coronary arteries to the pulmonary root is facilitated by their excision from the aortic sinuses with a generous cuff of adjacent aortic wall. The proximal aortic segment has usually been connected to the distal pulmonary artery with an intervening tubular conduit (Fig. 21.30),[235] but a direct end-to-end anastomosis technique (Fig. 21.31)[92] for pulmonary outflow reconstruction is also feasible.

A critical functional consideration concerns the adequacy of the left ventricle, which preoperatively faces the pulmonary circulation and postoperatively must suddenly cope with the systemic resistance. Adequate systemic left ventricular function poses little problem for TGA patients with

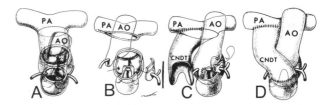

Fig. 21.30   Anatomic (arterial) correction of transposition of the great arteries according to Williams *et al.*[235] (*A*) The great arteries are divided sufficiently long to permit direct anastomosis of the distal aorta (*AO*) to the proximal pulmonary artery (*PA*). (*B*) Coronary arteries are excised from the aortic sinuses with generous margin of adjacent aortic wall. (*C*) Coronary artery sections are sutured into adjacent pulmonary valve sinuses. (*D*) Tubular conduit (*CNDT*) is used to connect the proximal aorta to the distal pulmonary artery. (Modified from W. G. Williams *et al.*[235])

additional lesions that maintain a high peak systolic pressure after birth in the left ventricle, e.g., large VSD with or without pulmonary artery banding or a major but easily resectable left ventricular outflow tract stenosis, but any abnormality in the pulmonary valve itself is a contraindication to anatomic correction. However, in patients with intact ventricular septum, where the left ventricular mass diminishes rapidly after birth, anatomic correction theoretically must be accomplished shortly after birth, or in older infants who have had systemic pressures maintained in the left

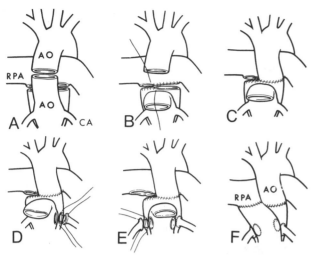

Fig. 21.31 Anatomical (arterial) correction of transposition of the great arteries according to Jatene *et al.*[92] illustrating technical modifications which limit need for conduit reconstruction of pulmonary outflow. After transection of the great arteries (*A*), the relationships and size of the connecting segments of the two vessels are mutually adjusted by reconstructive suture placement (*B*) to achieve optimum final alignments (*C, F*). The coronary arteries are excised (*D, E*) with a cuff of surrounding tissue from the aorta (*AO*) and reimplanted into the new systemic outflow vessel. (Modified from A. D. Jatene *et al.*[92])

ventricle. A "conditioning" method has been devised for this subgroup to redevelop the left ventricular myocardium by pressure loading the ventricle with an early first stage pulmonary artery banding operation by 2 months of age followed after a 3- to 6-month interval by a second stage anatomic corrective procedure.[237] Early experiences also include some atrial palliated infants who had pulmonary artery banding beyond 1 year of age with successful augmentation of left ventricular muscle mass. There is a 10% early surgical mortality from the first stage banding and 15% from the anatomic correction; improved surgical survival is reported as experience accumulates.[239] One to 2½ years after anatomic correction, left and right ventricular function as judged by ejection fraction and end-diastolic pressures at rest is normal (Fig. 21.5).[105, 239] Reduction in right ventricular afterload results in an increase of ejection fraction to normal, suggesting that the abnormal right ventricular function commonly observed in TGA may be reversible after anatomic correction. The coronary and aortic anastomoses appear to grow satisfactorily; dysrhythmias are infrequent; slight aortic insufficiency and right ventricular outflow obstruction have been observed. Although the long-term results of anatomic correction are not known, the evidence suggests it eventually will have a major role in the management of patients with physiologically uncorrected transposition of the great arteries.

Complications of Intraatrial Repair

Persistent abnormalities and new complications following intraatrial repair have represented a major although decreasing problem.[35, 121, 200, 209] These include: residual interatrial shunts, caval and pulmonary venous obstruction, tricuspid valve insufficiency, right ventricular dysfunction, and dysrhythmias. Most of these data concern the Mustard procedure which has had to date much wider application and longer follow-up than the Senning procedure. All recent series of either intraatrial technic report a

much reduced frequency of caval obstruction and dysrhythmias.[17, 149, 156, 209, 210]

Residual *intraatrial baffle shunts* occur most commonly at the superior right atrial-baffle suture line and favor systemic to pulmonary venous shunting (Fig. 21.32*A*)[199] In the absence of major coexistent systemic venous obstruction there is usually little or no arterial unsaturation, and reoperation for this problem is rarely needed.

Subclinical narrowing at the superior vena caval entrance and mild pulmonary venous atrial (posterior segment) hypertension are commonly detected at cardiac catheterization; however, gross obstruction to either the systemic venous or pulmonary venous return is an infrequent but serious complication (Fig. 21.32*B*). The young infant has been considered at greater risk for venous obstruction because of the limited anatomic spaces involved. Improper suture lines, contraction of patch materials, scar tissue, adhesions involving the baffle or the atrial wall, and too large or improper geometry of the baffle have been implicated as causes of obstruction.

The anatomically unobstructed pathway from superior vena cava to systemic venous atrium generally has a pressure difference of less than 4 mm Hg.[199] Several clinics have observed a higher frequency of late caval narrowing when using Dacron baffle material and strongly favor pericardial tissue,[175, 199] but others who have used thin knitted Dacron baffles have not found gross caval obstruction.[161, 216]

Pulmonary venous obstruction, which may be evident early after surgery or become prominent a few weeks or months later, is a serious complication and may have a fatal outcome when severe. Proper geometry and insertion of the patch material to avoid encroachment on the interatrial pathways plus enlargement of the pulmonary venous atrium with a patch graft have markedly reduced this complication.[199, 209] Prompt suspicion should be aroused by a postoperative chest x-ray with pulmonary congestion and pulmonary edema. The diagnosis is confirmed at catheterization by observing a significant mean pressure difference between the posterior and anterior segments of the pulmonary venous atrium. The systemic venous return "conduit," even when not obstructing pulmonary venous return significantly, can be shown to segment the pulmonary venous atrium into two identifiable chambers: a posterior-superior segment and an anterior-inferior segment (Figs. 21.28*D* and 21.12*B*). Attempts should be made during postoperative catheterization to enter the pulmonary veins or posterior pulmonary venous atrial segment using retrograde arterial manipulation of the catheter to traverse in succession the femoral artery, aorta, right ventricle, and tricuspid valve, and then enter both the anterior and posterior pulmonary venous atrial segments. If the posterior segment cannot be entered, the status of the pulmonary venous chambers can be assessed by comparing simultaneously recorded pulmonary artery wedge pressure and right ventricular end-diastolic pressure. Noninvasive anatomic assessments of caval narrowing and of pulmonary venous obstruction by the baffle can be obtained from 2D echocardiography.[9]

Tricuspid valve insufficiency has been recognized postoperatively, and some deaths have been attributed to this.[214] Most clinics, however, report tricuspid insufficiency to be uncommon postoperatively, particularly in patients with intact ventricular septum.[35, 121, 161, 209] Manipulation and damage of the tricuspid valve or its support apparatus during VSD repair, or prolonged right ventricular dysfunction are considered possible mechanisms leading to tricuspid insufficiency.

The *depressed right ventricular function* that has been

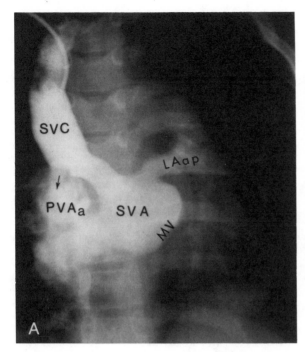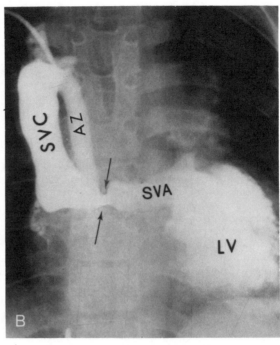

Fig. 21.32 Angiograms illustrating baffle complications after intraatrial repair. (*A*) Right to left shunt (*arrow* indicates leak) at superior vena cava (*SVC*)-baffle conduit junction with early opacification of anterior segment of pulmonary venous atrium (*PVAa*). *SVA*, systemic venous atrium; *LV*, left ventricle; *MV*, mitral valve. (*B*) Severe constriction (*arrows*) at SVC-baffle junction with horizontal displacement of upper limb of SVA and limited decompression via azygous vein (*AZ*) with mean pressure in SVC, 15 mm Hg; and in SVA, 4 mm Hg.

uniformly reported in resting volume-function studies is in sharp contrast to the remarkable clinical performance of many postoperative children during play.[64, 67, 91, 227] Nevertheless, objective radionuclide angiographic assessment during exercise has unmasked right ventricular dysfunction not evident at rest in most postoperative (intraatrial repair) patients examined. Additional studies are necessary to ascertain whether the observed depressed right ventricular function can be prevented by performing intraatrial repair in the neonatal period. It is likely, however, that geometric factors (right ventricle unsuitable as systemic ventricle) rather than early hypoxemic myocardial damage are the mechanism behind the observed early and late right ventricular dysfunction, and this consideration probably favors the eventual application of anatomic correction surgery.

Postoperative dysrhythmias, early or late in onset and transient or permanent, have been commonly encountered during long-term follow-up studies on intraatrial baffle surgery with the frequency ranging from 4 to 75%, a disparity in part due to the differences in the definition of a dysrhythmia. Consequently, numerous modifications in surgical technique have been suggested. Several of these have resulted in a higher frequency of persistent postoperative normal sinus rhythm and a lower frequency of dysrhythmias, particularly after introduction of techniques that have minimized sinoatrial node or sinoatrial nodal artery damage.[34, 49, 210, 216]

The types of dysrhythmia can be classified as: passive—such as changes in P wave morphology, bradycardia with depression or failure of initiation, or propagation of sinoatrial impulses, and sino-atrial block; active—such as atrial and ventricular premature beats, supraventricular or ventricular tachycardia, and atrial flutter or fibrillation; and AV conduction abnormalities—first to third degree atrioventricular block, and atrioventricular dissociation by default.

Holter monitoring provides essential sensitivity in detecting and evaluating dysrhythmias.[181, 195, 216] In fact, almost every patient has some type of dysrhythmia postoperatively with prolonged monitoring,[195] but many of these rhythms are seen in normals and preoperative patients, so that the frequency of acquired dysrhythmia must be assessed with control data. The mechanisms for these dysrhythmias after the Mustard or Senning operation are evident in that all parts of the cardiac conduction system are vulnerable to trauma in these operations. With TGA with intact ventricular septum, the damage is usually confined to the sinus node or sinus node artery and atrium; but with associated VSD or subpulmonary stenosis, the distal conduction system is in jeopardy during patch closure or resection of the obstruction. Controversy has centered around the presence or absence of specific internodal tracks, and if these exist, whether their disruption is a cause of dysrhythmia.[90] Animal experiments[184] show that a small amount of atrial tissue in continuity from SA to AV node is required to maintain sinus rhythm or provide a stable input into the AV node from other atrial pacemaker sites; otherwise junctional rhythm results. Atrial activation mapping[236] during various steps of the Mustard procedure has confirmed that the main atrial muscle bands, the sulcus terminalis and the interatrial band (Bachman's bundle), are able to conduct up to three times faster than the right atrial appendage musculature, and that they provide an anterior and posterior input into the atrioventricular node. Wide excision of the interatrial septum, coronary sinus cutback, and an atriotomy which transects the crista are associated with retrograde activation patterns. Observations such as these and others have led to changes in surgical (Mustard) technique including: direct cannulation of the superior vena cava or cannulation via the right atrial appendage rather than at the superior vena cava-atrial junction; avoiding transverse atriotomy and coronary sinus cutback; careful avoidance of the sinus node artery; careful placement of the baffle suture line away from the sinus and atrioventricular nodes; and preservation of the anterior muscle track input into the atrioventricular node by preservation of ridge of septum.

Several late follow-up studies in a large number of patients, ranging over a period of 1 to 8 years, indicate active or passive dysrhythmias occurring at some time in 40 to 50% of the patients.[48, 49] Recent frequencies for adequate follow-up periods may be as low as 10%.[34, 216]

Following intraatrial repair, in the past the most common postoperative electrocardiographic change noted was a decrease in the mean amplitude of the P wave without any change in QRS axis.[48] These changes suggest that tracings sometimes regarded as "sinus" rhythm postoperatively do not have a sinus origin or normal atrial conduction sequence and strongly implicate sinoatrial node damage. Sinus or atrial pacemaker slowing and slow junctional rhythms are also observed but may not become evident for 6 to 12 months following surgery. The bradycardia often progresses, usually stabilizing several years after surgery.

A type of postintraatrial repair dysrhythmia, categorized as a tachycardia-bradycardia, has occurred in about 5% of long-term survivors. The patient manifests at times marked bradycardia, sinoatrial arrest or block with atrioventricular junctional escape, and slow junctional rhythms, as well as episodes of tachyarrhythmia, such as flutter or ectopic atrial tachycardia. In most patients no treatment is necessary for the bradycardia; however, even in asymptomatic individuals, Holter tape monitoring has revealed episodes of sinus arrest and severe bradycardia, particularly during sleep, sometimes with intermittent bursts of supraventricular tachyarrhythmia. Symptomatic patients are candidates for an electrical pacemaker (atrial) insertion to provide safe pharmacologic therapy of the tachyarrhythmia when drugs other than digitalis are necessary, since the damaged intrinsic cardiac pacemaker function may be severely further depressed with therapy. Resort to electrical pacemaker therapy is generally recommended: for heart rates sustained below 40 without symptoms; for bradycardia with clear hypocirculatory associated symptoms; for safe pharmacologic therapy in the brady-tachycardia syndrome; and for sustained surgical complete atrioventricular block.

Electrophysiologic studies have examined the mechanisms of dysrhythmia in the postoperative period.[50, 62, 63, 181] All studies have confirmed that damage to the sinus node, either direct or via sinus node artery damage is one of the major mechanisms for dysrhythmia. Sinus node damage is manifest as a prolonged sinus escape time or a junctional escape after overdrive atrial pacing, or as a prolonged sinoatrial conduction time. These studies also suggest that atrial muscle damage is a mechanism for the observed dysrhythmias, based on the finding of prolonged atrial tissue refractory periods and localized areas of delayed conduction which may provide the determinants for reentry mechanisms. Reentry tachycardias have been induced by rapid atrial pacing or extrastimulus testing, with the tachycardias originating from the sinoatrial area or from within atrial muscle.

Sudden, unexplained death, probably dysrhythmic, has been reported with a frequency of 2 to 9%.[112, 183, 195, 216] One survey of patients with unexplained sudden death[183] found that 37% showed only normal sinus rhythm; 29% revealed junctional rhythm; and in 34%, there were recorded episodes of supraventricular tachycardia, atrioventricular dissociation, bradycardia-tachycardia syndrome, or complete heart block. Bifascicular block and ventricular premature beats have also been observed. Many of these patients with sudden unexplained death had a documented satisfactory hemodynamic result and were asymptomatic, despite dysrhythmias.

The remarkable change in prognosis for the neonate with TGA over the past two decades reflects many major advances in medicine and surgery. Nevertheless, today, both the unoperated infant and the physiologically or anatomically "corrected" infant with TGA provoke continuing inquiry into important unresolved problems including: morphogenesis and physiology of TGA; accelerated pulmonary vascular disease; acquired left ventricular outflow tract stenosis; late postoperative dysrhythmias; and adequacy of ventricular function at rest and exercise.

REFERENCES

1. Albert, H. M.: Surgical correction of transposition of the great arteries. Surg. Forum 5:75, 1954.

2. Alpert, B. S., Bloom, K. R., Olley, P. M., Trusler, G. A., Williams, C. M., and Rowe, R. D.: Echocardiographic evaluation of right ventricular function in complete transposition of the great arteries: Angiographic correlates. Am. J. Cardiol. 44:270, 1979.

3. Arciniegas, E., Farooki, Z. Q., Hakimi, M., Perry, B. L., and Green, E. W.: Results of the Mustard operation for dextro-transposition of the great arteries. J. Thorac. Cardiovasc. Surg. 81:580, 1981.

4. Aziz, K. U., Olley, P. M., Rowe, R. D., Trusler, G. A., and Mustard, W. T.: Survival after systemic to pulmonary arterial shunts in infants less than 30 days old with obstructive lesions of the right heart chambers. Am. J. Cardiol. 36:479, 1975.

5. Aziz, K. U., Paul, M. H., and Muster, A. J.: Echocardiographic localization of interatrial baffle in D-transposition of the great arteries following Mustard operation. Am. J. Cardiol. 38:67, 1976.

6. Aziz, K. U., Paul, M. H., and Rowe, R. D.: Bronchopulmonary circulation in D-transposition of the great arteries: Possible role in genesis of accelerated pulmonary vascular disease. Am. J. Cardiol. 39:432, 1977.

7. Aziz, K. U., Paul, M. H., and Muster, A. J.: Echocardiographic assessment of left ventricular outflow tract in D-transposition of the great arteries. Am. J. Cardiol. 41:543, 1978.

8. Aziz, K. U., Paul, M. H., Idriss, F. S., Wilson, A. D., and Muster, A. J.: Clinical manifestations of dynamic left ventricular outflow tract stenosis with D-transposition of the great arteries with intact ventricular septum. Am. J. Cardiol. 44:290, 1979.

9. Aziz, K. U., Paul, M. H., Bharati, S., Cole, R. B., Muster, A. J., Lev, M., and Idriss, F. S.: Two dimensional echocardiographic evaluation of Mustard operation for D-transposition of the great arteries. Am. J. Cardiol. 47:654, 1981.

10. Baffes, T. G.: A method for surgical correction of transposition of the great vessels. Surg. Gynecol. Obstet. 102:227, 1956.

11. Baker, F., Baker, L., Zoltun, R., and Zuberbuhler, J. R.: Effectiveness of the Rashkind procedure in transposition of the great arteries in infants. Circulation 53–54 (Suppl. I):I–6, 1971.

12. Bano-Rodrigo, A., Quero-Jimenez, M., Moreno-Granado, F., and Gamallo-Arnat, C.: Wall thickness of ventricular chambers in transposition of the great arteries. J. Thorac. Cardiovasc. Surg. 79:592, 1980.

13. Barcia, A., Kincaid, O. W., Davis, G. D., Kirklin, J. W., and Ongley, P. A.: Transposition of the great arteries: An angiographic study. Am. J. Roentgenol. 100:249, 1967.

14. Bargeron, L. M., Jr., Elliott, L. P., Soto, B., Bream, P. R., and Curry, G. C.: Axial cineangiography in congenital heart disease. Circulation 56:1075, 1977.

15. Barratt-Boyes, B. G.: Profound hypothermia. In Heart Disease in Infancy, edited by B. G. Barratt-Boyes, J. M. Neutze, and E. A. Harris. Williams & Wilkins, Baltimore, 1973.

16. Behrendt, D. M., Kirsh, M. M., Orringer, M. B., Perry, B., Sigmann, J., Stern, A., and Sloan, H.: The Blalock-Hanlon procedure: A new look at an old operation. Ann. Thorac. Surg. 20:424, 1975.

17. Bender, H. W., Jr., Graham, T. P., Jr., Boucek, R. J., Jr., Walker, W. E., and Boerth, R. G.: Comparative operative results of the Senning and Mustard procedures for transposition of the great arteries. Circulation 62 (Suppl. I):I-197, 1980.

18. Benson, L. N., Olley, P. M., Patel, R. G., Coceani, P., and Rowe, R. D.: Role of prostaglandin E1 infusion in the management of transposition of the great arteries and an intact ventricular septum. Am. J. Cardiol. 44:691, 1979.

19. Berman, W., Jr., Whitman, V., Pierce, W. S., and Waldhausen, J. A.: The development of pulmonary vascular obstructive disease after successful Mustard operation in early infancy. Circulation 58:181, 1978.

20. Beuren, A. J., Keutel, J., Gandjour, A., Vesselinova, T., Stoermer, J., and Hayek, H.: Balloon atrial septostomy: Results in 91 infants. Dtsch. Med. Wochenschr. 97:148, 1972.

21. Bex, J. P., Lecompte, Y., Baillot, F., and Hazan, E.: Anatomical correction of transposition of the great arteries. Ann. Thorac. Surg. 29:86, 1980.

22. Bierman, F. Z., and Williams, R. G.: Subxi-

phoid two-dimensional imaging of the interatrial septum in infants and neonates with congenital heart disease. Circulation 60:80, 1979.

23. Bierman, F. Z., and Williams R. G.: Prospective diagnosis of D-transposition of the great arteries in neonates by subxiphoid two-dimensional echocardiography. Circulation 60:1496, 1979.

24. Blalock, A., and Hanlon, C. R.: The surgical treatment of complete transposition of the aorta and the pulmonary artery. Surg. Gynecol. Obstet. 90:1, 1950.

25. Borow, K. M., Keane, J. F., Castaneda, A. R., and Freed, M. D.: Systemic ventricular function in patients with tetralogy of Fallot, ventricular septal defect and transposition of the great arteries repaired during infancy. Circulation 64:878, 1981.

26. Bourlon, F., Fouron, J.-C., Battle-Diaz, J., Ducharme, G., and Davignon, A.: Relation between isovolumic relaxation period of left ventricle and pulmonary artery pressure in D-transposition of the great arteries. Br. Heart J. 43:226, 1980.

27. Byrne, J., Clarke, D., Taylor, J. F. N., Macartney, F., de Leval, M., and Stark, J.: Treatment of patients with transposition of the great arteries and pulmonary vascular obstructive disease. Br. Heart J. 40:221, 1978.

28. Calleja, H. B., Hosier, D. M., and Grajo, M. Z.: The electrocardiogram in complete transposition of the great vessels. Am. Heart J. 69:31, 1965.

29. Carr, I.: Timing of bidirectional atrial shunts in transposition of the great arteries and atrial septal defect. Circulation 44 (Suppl. II):II-70, 1971.

30. Cassels, D. E., Bharati, S., and Lev, M.: The natural history of the ductus arteriosus in association with other congenital heart defects. Perspect. Bio. Med. 4:541, 1975.

31. Celermajer, J. M., Venables, A. W., and Bowdler, J. D.: Catheterization of pulmonary artery in transposition of the great arteries. Circulation 41:1053, 1970.

32. Chiarello, L., Agoti, J., Vlad, P., and Subramanian, S.: Management of left ventricular outflow tract obstruction in complex transposition: A critical review of our experience. Circulation 51–52 (Suppl. II):II-169, 1975.

33. Clarkson, P. M., Barratt-Boyes, B. G., Neutze, J. M., and Lowe, J. B.: Results over a ten-year period of palliation followed by corrective surgery for complete transposition of the great arteries. Circulation 45:1251, 1972.

34. Clarkson, P. M., Barratt-Boyes, B. G., and Neutze, J. M.: Late dysrhythmias and disturbances of conduction following Mustard operation for complete transposition of the great arteries. Circulation 53:519, 1976.

35. Clarkson, P. M., Neutze, J. M., Barratt-Boyes, B. G., and Brandt, P. W. T.: Late postoperative hemodynamic results and cineangiographic findings after Mustard atrial baffle repair for transposition of the great arteries. Circulation 53:525, 1976.

36. Clarkson, P. M., Neutze, J. M., Wardhill, J. C., and Barratt-Boyes, B. G.: The pulmonary vascular bed in patients with complete transposition of the great arteries. Circulation 53:539, 1976.

37. Coto, E. O., Norwood, W. I., Lang, P., and Castaneda, A. R.: Modified Senning operation for treatment of transposition of the great arteries. J. Thorac. Cardiovasc. Surg. 78:721, 1979.

38. Counahan, R., Simon, G., and Joseph, M.: The plain chest radiograph in D-transposition of the great arteries in the first month of life. Pediatr. Radiol. 1:217, 1973.

39. Danielson, G. K., Tabry, I. F., Mair, D. D., and Fulton, R. E.: Great vessel switch operation without coronary relocation for trans-

position of the great arteries. Mayo Clin. Proc. 53:675, 1978.

40. DeBoer, A., Miller, R., and Otto, R.: Correction of transposition of the great vessels with previous Baffes procedure. J. Pediatr. Surg. 10:925, 1975.

41. Deutsch, V., Shem-Tov, A., Yahini, J. G., and Neufeld, H. N.: Cardioangiographic evaluation of the relationship between atrioventricular and semilunar valves: Its diagnostic importance in congenital heart disease. Am. J. Roentgenol. 110:474, 1970.

42. Deutsch, V., Shem-Tov, A., Yahini, J. G., and Neufeld, H. N.: Juxtaposition of atrial appendages: Angiocardiographic observations. Am. J. Cardiol. 34:240, 1974.

43. Deverall, P. B., Tynan, M. J., Carr, I., Panagopoulos, P., Aberdeen, E., and Bonham-Carter, R. E.: Palliative surgery in children with transposition of the great arteries. J. Thorac. Cardiovasc. Surg. 58:721, 1969.

44. Dooley, K. J., Parisi-Buckley, L., Fyler, D. C., and Nadas, A. S.: Results of pulmonary arterial banding in infancy. Am. J. Cardiol. 36:484, 1976.

45. Edwards, W. S., and Bargeron, L. M., Jr.: More effective palliation of transposition of the great arteries. J. Thorac. Cardiovasc. Surg. 49:790, 1965.

46. Ehmke, D. A., Durnin, R. E., and Lauer, R. M.: Intra-abdominal hemorrhage complicating a balloon atrial septostomy for transposition of the great arteries. Pediatrics 45:289, 1970.

47. Elliott, L. P., Anderson, R. C., Tuna, N., Adams, P., Jr., and Neufeld, H. N.: Complete transposition of the great vessels. II. An electrocardiographic analysis. Circulation 27:1118, 1963.

48. El-Said, G., Rosenberg, H. S., Mullin, C. E., Hallman, G. L., Cooley, D. A., and McNamara, D. G.: Dysrhythmias after Mustard's operation for transposition of the great arteries. Am. J. Cardiol. 30:526, 1972.

49. El-Said, G., Gillette, P. C., Cooley, D. A., Mullins, C. E., and McNamara, D. G.: Protection of the sinus node in Mustard's operation. Circulation 53:788, 1976.

50. El-Said, G. M., Gillette, P. C., Mullins, C. E., Nihill, M. R., and McNamara, D. G.: Significance of pacemaker recovery time after the Mustard operation for transposition of the great arteries. Am. J. Cardiol. 38:448, 1976.

51. Fischbein, C. A., Rosenthal, A., Fischer, E. G., Nadas, A. S., and Welch, K.: Risk factors for brain abscess in patients with congenital heart disease. Am. J. Cardiol. 34:97, 1974.

52. Fisher, E. A., Muster, A. J., Lev, M., and Paul, M. H.: Angiocardiographic and anatomic findings in transposition of the great arteries with left ventricular outflow tract gradients. Am. J. Cardiol. 25:95, 1970.

53. Fisher, E., and Paul, M. H.: Transposition of the great arteries: Recognition and management. Cardiovasc. Clin. 2:211, 1970.

54. Fouron, J.-C., Vallot, F., Bourlon, F., Lombaert, M., Ducharme, G., and Davignon, A.: Isovolumic contraction time of right ventricle in D-transposition of great arteries. Br. Heart J. 44:204, 1980.

55. Fraser, F. C., and Hunter, A. D. W.: Etiologic relations among categories of congenital heart malformations. Am. J. Cardiol. 36:793, 1975.

56. Freed, M. D., Heymann, M. A., Lewis, A. B., Roehl, S. L., and Kensey, R. C.: Prostaglandin E1 in infants with ductus arteriosus-dependent congenital heart disease. Circulation 64:899, 1981.

57. Freedom, R. M., Harrington, D. P., and White, R. I., Jr.: The differential diagnosis of levo-transposed or malposed aorta: An angiocardiographic study. Circulation 50:1040, 1974.

58. Fuhrmann, W.: A family study in transposi-

tion of the great vessels and in tricuspid atresia. Humangenetik 6:148, 1968.

59. Fyler, D. C.: Report of the New England Regional Infant Cardiac Program. Pediatrics 65 (Suppl.):377, 1980.

60. Fyler, D. C., Gallaher, M. E., and Nadas, A. S.: Auscultation in the evaluation of children with heart disease. Cardiovasc. Dis. 10:363, 1968.

61. Fyler, D. C., Silbert, A. R., and Rothman, K. J.: Five year follow up of infant cardiacs: Intelligence quotient. In The Child with Congenital Heart Disease after Surgery, edited by B. S. L. Kidd, and R. D. Rowe. Futura Publishing Co., Mount Kisco, N.Y., 1976.

62. Gillette, P. C., El-Said, G., Sivarajan, N., Mullins, C. E., Williams, R. L., and McNamara, D. G.: Electrophysiological abnormalities after Mustard's operation for transposition of the great arteries. Br. Heart J. 36:186, 1974.

63. Gillette, P. C., Kugler, J. D., Garson, A., Jr., Gutgesell, H. P., Duff, D. F., and McNamara, D.: Mechanisms of cardiac arrhythmias after the Mustard operation for transposition of the great arteries. Am. J. Cardiol. 45:1225, 1980.

64. Godman, M. J., Friedli, B., Pasternac, A., Kidd, B. S. L., Trusler, G. A., and Mustard, W. T.: Hemodynamic studies in children four to ten years after the Mustard operation for transposition of the great arteries. Circulation 53:532, 1976.

65. Goldschmidt, B., Sarkadi, B., Gardos, G., and Matlary, A.: Platelet production and survival in cyanotic congenital heart disease. Scand. J. Haematol. 13:110, 1974.

66. Goor, D. A., and Edwards, J. E.: The spectrum of transposition of the great arteries: With special reference to developmental anatomy of the conus. Circulation 48:406, 1973.

67. Graham, T. P., Jr., Jarmakani, J. M., Canent, R. V., Jr., and Jewett, P. H.: Quantification of left heart volume and systolic output in transposition of the great arteries. Circulation 44:899, 1971.

68. Graham, T. P., Jr., Atwood, G. F., Boucek, R. J., Jr., Boerth, R. C., and Bender, H. W., Jr.: Abnormalities of right ventricular function following Mustard's operation for transposition of the great arteries. Circulation 52:678, 1975.

69. Guerin, R., Soto, B., Karp, R. B., Kirklin, J. W., and Barcia, A.: Transposition of the great arteries. Determination of the position of the great arteries in conventional chest roentgenograms. Am. J. Roentgenol. Radium Ther. Nucl. Med. 110:747, 1970.

70. Gutgesell, H. P., and McNamara, D. G.: Transposition of the great arteries: Results of treatment with early palliation and late intracardiac repair. Circulation 51:32, 1975.

71. Gutgesell, H. P., Garson, A., and McNamara, D. G.: Prognosis for the newborn with transposition of the great arteries. Am. J. Cardiol. 44:96, 1979.

72. Hagler, D. J.: The utilization of echocardiography in the differential diagnosis of cyanosis in the neonate. Mayo Clin. Proc. 51:143, 1976.

73. Hagler, D. J., Ritter, D. G., Mair, D. D., Davis, G. D., and McGoon, D. C.: Clinical, angiographic, and hemodynamic assessment of late results after Mustard operation. Circulation 57:1214, 1978.

74. Hagler, D. J., Ritter, D. G., Mair, D. D., Tajik, A. J., Seward, J. B., Fulton, R. E., and Ritman, E. L.: Right and left ventricular function after the Mustard procedure in transposition of the great arteries. Am. J. Cardiol. 44:276, 1979.

75. Hallerman, F. J., Kincaid, O. W., Ritter, D. G., and Titus, J. L.: Mitral-semilunar valve relationships in the angiography of cardiac malformations. Radiology 94:63, 1970.

76. Hawker, R. E., Krovetz, L. J., and Rowe, R.

D.: An analysis of prognostic factors in the outcome of balloon atrial septostomy for the transposition of the great arteries. Johns Hopkins Med. J. 134:95, 1974.

77. Hawker, R. E., Freedom, R. M., Rowe, R. D., and Krovetz, L. J.: Persistence of the fetal pattern of circulation in transposition of the great arteries. Johns Hopkins Med. J. 134:107, 1974.

78. Heath, D., and Edwards, J. E.: The pathology of hypertensive pulmonary vascular disease: A description of six grades of structural changes in the pulmonary arteries with special reference to congenital cardiac septal defects. Circulation 18:533, 1958.

79. Henry, C. G., Goldring, D., Hartman, A. F., Weldon, C. S., and Strauss, A. W.: Treatment of D-transposition of the great arteries: Management of hypoxemia after balloon atrial septostomy. Am. J. Cardiol. 47:299, 1981.

80. Hermann, V., Laks, H., Kaiser, G. C., Barner, H. B., and Willman, V. L.: The Blalock-Hanlon procedure for simple transposition of the great arteries. Arch. Surg. 110:1387, 1975.

81. Hirschfeld, S. S., Meyer, R. A., and Kaplan, S.: Measurement of right and left ventricular systolic time intervals by echocardiography. Circulation 51:304, 1975.

82. Hirschfeld, S. S., Meyer, R. A., Schwartz, D. C., Korfhagen, J., and Kaplan, S.: The echocardiographic assessment of pulmonary artery pressure and pulmonary vascular resistance. Circulation 52:642, 1975.

83. Hoffman, J. I. E., Rudolph, A. M., and Heymann, M. A.: Pulmonary vascular disease with congenital heart lesions: Pathologic features and causes. Circulation 64:873, 1981.

84. Hohn, A. R., and Webb, H. M.: Balloon deflation failure: A hazard of "medical" atrial septostomy. Am. Heart J. 83:389, 1972.

85. Hurwitz, R., and Girod, D. A.: Percutaneous balloon atrial septostomy in infants with transposition of the great arteries. Am. Heart J. 91:618, 1976.

86. Idriss, F. S., Goldstein, I. R., Grana, L., French, D., and Potts, W. J.: A new technique for complete transposition of the great vessels. Circulation 24:5, 1961.

87. Idriss, F. S., Aubert, J., Paul, M. H., Nikaidoh, H., Lev, M., and Newfeld, E. A.: Transposition of the great vessels with ventricular septal defect. Surgical and anatomic considerations. J. Thorac. Cardiovasc. Surg. 68:732, 1974.

88. Idriss, F. S., DeLeon, S. Y., Nikaidoh, H., Muster, A. J., Paul, M. H., Newfeld, E. A., and Albers, W.: Resection of left ventricular outflow obstruction in D-transposition of the great arteries. J. Thorac. Cardiovasc. Surg. 74:343, 1977.

89. Imamura, E. S., Morikawa, T., Tatsuno, K., Konno, S., Arai, T., and Sakakibara, S.: Surgical considerations of ventricular septal defect associated with complete transposition of the great arteries and pulmonary stenosis. Circulation 44:914, 1971.

90. Isaacson, R., Titus, J. L., Merideth, J., Feldt, R. H., and McGoon, D. C.: Apparent interruption of atrial conduction pathways after surgical repair of transposition of great arteries. Am. J. Cardiol. 30:533, 1972.

91. Jarmakani, J. M., and Canent, R. V., Jr.: Preoperative and postoperative right ventricular function in children with transposition of the great vessels. Circulation 50 (Suppl. II):II-39, 1974.

92. Jatene, A. D., Fontes, V. F., Souza, L. C. B., Paulista, P. P., Abdulmassih, N., and Sousa, J. E. M. R.: Anatomic correction of transposition of the great arteries. J. Thorac. Cardiovasc. Surg. 83:20, 1982.

93. Jones, S. M., and Miller, G. A. H.: Catheterization of the pulmonary artery in transposition of the great arteries using a Swan-Ganz flow directed catheter. Br. Heart J. 35:298, 1973.

94. Kawabori, I., Guntheroth, W. G., Morgan, B. C., Mohri, H., and Dillard, D. H.: Surgical correction in infancy to reduce mortality in transposition of the great arteries. Pediatrics 60:83, 1977.

95. Keane, J. F., Ellison, R. C., Rudd, M., and Nadas, A. S.: Pulmonary blood flow and left ventricular volume in transposition of the great arteries and intact ventricular septum. Br. Heart J. 35:521, 1973.

96. Kennaird, D. L.: Oxygen consumption and evaporative water loss in infants with congenital heart disease. Arch. Dis. Child. 51:34, 1976.

97. Kidd, B. S. L.: The fate of children with transposition of the great arteries following balloon atrial septostomy. In The Child with Congenital Heart Disease after Surgery, edited by B. S. L. Kidd, and R. D. Rowe. Futura Publishing Co., Mount Kisco, N.Y., 1976.

98. Kinsley, R. H., Ritter, D. G., and McGoon, D. C.: The surgical repair of positional anomalies of the conotruncus. J. Thorac. Cardiovasc. Surg. 67:395, 1974.

99. Kirklin, J. W., Pacifico, A. D., Hannah, H., III, and Allarde, R. R.: Primary definitive intracardiac operations in infants: Intraoperative support techniques. In Advances in Cardiovascular Surgery, edited by J. W. Kirklin. Grune & Stratton, New York, 1973.

100. Kjellberg, S. R., Mannheimer, E., and Rudhe, U.: Diagnosis of Congenital Heart Disease, 3rd ed. Year Book Publishers, Chicago, 1959.

101. Korns, M. E., Garabedian, H. A., and Lauer, R. M.: Anatomic limitation of balloon atrial septostomy. Hum. Pathol. 3:345, 1972.

102. LaCorte, M. E., Fellows, K. E., and Williams, R. G.: Overriding tricuspid valve: Echocardiographic and angiographic features. Am. J. Cardiol. 37:911, 1976.

103. Lakier, J. B., Stanger, P., Heymann, M. A., Hoffman, J. I. E., and Rudolph, A. M.: Early onset of pulmonary vascular obstruction in patients with aortopulmonary transposition and intact ventricular septum. Circulation 51:875, 1975.

104. Lang, P. L., Freed, M. D., Bierman, F. Z., Norwood, W. I., and Nadas, A. S.: Use of prostaglandin E1 infusion in the management of transposition of the great arteries. Am. J. Cardiol. 44:76, 1979.

105. Lange, P. E., Onnasch, D. G. W., Stephan, E., Wessel, A., Radley-Smith, R., Yacoub, M. H., Regensberger, D., Bernard, A., and Heintzen, P. H.: Two stage anatomic correction of complete transposition of the great arteries: Ventricular volumes and muscle mass. Herz 6:336, 1981.

106. Layton, W. M., and Manasek, F.: Cardiac looping of early iv/iv mouse embryo. In Etiology and Morphogenesis of Congenital Heart Disease, edited by R. Van Praagh and A. Takao. Futura Publishing Co., Mount Kisco, N.Y., 1980, p. 109.

107. Leanage, R., Agnetti, A., Graham, G., Taylor, J., and Macartney, F. J.: Factors influencing survival after balloon atrial septostomy for complete transposition of great arteries. Br. Heart J. 45:559, 1981.

108. Lecompte, Y., Zannini, L., Hazan, E., Jarreau, M. M., Bex, J. P., Tu, T. R., and Neveau, J. Y.: Anatomic correction of transposition of the great arteries: New technique without use of a prosthetic conduit. J. Thorac. Cardiovasc. Surg. 82:629, 1981.

109. Lev, M., Rimoldi, H. J., Paiva, R., and Arcilla, R. A.: The quantitative anatomy of simple complete transposition. Am. J. Cardiol. 23:409, 1969.

110. Lev, M., Bharati, S., Meng, C. C. L., Liberthson, R. R., Paul, M. H., and Idriss, F.: A concept of doublet outlet right ventricle. J. Thorac. Cardiovasc. Surg. 64:271, 1972.

111. Levin, D. L., Paul, M. H., Muster, A. J., Newfeld, E. A., and Waldman, J. D.: The clinical diagnosis of D-transposition of the great vessels in the neonate. Arch. Intern. Med. 137:1421, 1977.

112. Lewis, A. B., Lindesmith, G. G., Takahaski, M., Stanton, R. E., Tucker, B. L., Stiles, Q. R., and Myer, B. W.: Cardiac rhythm following the Mustard procedure for transposition of the great vessels. J. Thorac. Cardiovasc. Surg. 73:919, 1977.

113. Liebman, J., Cullum, L., and Belloc, N.: Natural history of transposition of the great arteries: Anatomy and birth and death characteristics. Circulation 40:237, 1969.

114. Lindesmith, G. G., Stanton, R. E., Lurie, P. R., Takahashi, M., Tucker, B. L., Stiles, Q. R., and Meyer, B. W.: An assessment of Mustard's operation as a palliative procedure for transposition of the great vessels. Ann. Thorac. Surg. 19:514, 1975.

115. Litwin, S. B., Plauth, W. H., Jr., Jones, J. E., and Bernard, W. F.: Appraisal of surgical atrial septectomy for transposition of the great arteries. Circulation 43–44(Suppl. I):I-7, 1971.

116. Macartney, F. J., Scott, O., Deverall, P., and Hepburn, F.: New preformed catheter for entry into pulmonary artery in complete transposition of the great arteries. Br. Heart J. 37:525, 1975.

117. Mair, D. D., Macartney, F. J., Weidman, W. H., Ritter, D. G., Ongley, P. A., and Smith, R. E.: The vectorcardiogram in complete transposition of the great arteries: Correlation with anatomic and hemodynamic findings and calculated left ventricular mass. J. Electrocardiol. 3:217, 1970.

118. Mair, D. D., Ritter, D. G., Ongley, P. A., and Helmholz, H. F., Jr.: Hemodynamics and evaluation for surgery of patients with complete transposition of the great arteries and ventricular septal defect. Am. J. Cardiol. 28:632, 1971.

119. Mair, D. D., and Ritter, D. G.: Factors influencing intercirculatory mixing in patients with complete transposition of the great arteries. Am. J. Cardiol. 30:653, 1972.

120. Mair, D. D., and Ritter, D. G.: Factors influencing systemic arterial oxygen saturation in complete transposition of the great arteries. Am. J. Cardiol. 31:742, 1973.

121. Mair, D. D., Danielson, G. K., Wallace, R. B., and McGoon, D. C.: Long term follow up of Mustard operation survivors. Circulation 49–50(Suppl. II):II-46, 1974.

122. Mair, D. D., Ritter, D. G., Danielson, G. K., Wallace, R. B., and McGoon, D. C.: The palliative Mustard operation: Rationale and results. Am. J. Cardiol. 37:762, 1976.

123. Maron, B. J., Henry, W. L., Griffith, J. M., Freedom, R. M., Kelley, D. T., and Epstein, S. F.: Identification of congenital malformations of the great arteries in infants by real-time two-dimensional echocardiography. Circulation 52:671, 1975.

124. Mathew, R., Rosenthal, A., and Fellows, K.: The significance of right aortic arch in D-transposition of the great arteries. Am. Heart J. 87:317, 1974.

125. McGoon, D. C.: Left ventricular and biventricular extracardiac conduits. J. Thorac. Cardiovasc. Surg. 72:7, 1976.

126. McGoon, D. C., Wallace, R. B., and Danielson, G. K.: The Rastelli operation: Its indications and results. J. Thorac. Cardiovasc. Surg. 65:65, 1973.

127. Meng, C. C. L., Wells, C. R., Valdes-Dapena, M., Arey, J. B., Black, I. F. F., and O'Riordan, A.: The anatomy of the foramen ovale in relation to balloon atrial septostomy. Pediatr. Res. 7:304, 1973.

128. Mocellin, R., Henglein, D., Brodherr, S.,

Schober, J. G., Schumacher, G., Schreiber, R., Sebening, F., and Buhlmeyer, K.: (Prognosis of newborns with transposition of the great arteries after balloon-atrioseptostomy and after surgical atrial inversion.) Herz 6:235, 1981.

129. Moene, R. J., Roos, J. P., and Eygelaar, A.: Cardiac arrhythmias following the creation of an atrial septal defect in patients with transposition of the great arteries. Thorax 28:147, 1973.

130. Motsch, K., Munster, W., Ruth, P., and Portsmann, W.: (The oxygen tension in the capillary blood of infants with complete transposition of the great vessels before and after balloon atrial septostomy). Dtsch. Gesundheitsw. 26:2306, 1971.

131. Moulton, A. L., de Leval, M. R., Macartney, F. J., Taylor, J. F. N., and Stark, J.: Rastelli procedure for transposition of the great arteries, ventricular septal defect, and left ventricular outflow tract obstruction. Early and late results in 41 patients (1971 to 1978). Br. Heart J. 45:20, 1981.

132. Mullins, C. E., Neches, W. H., and McNamara, D. G.: The infant with transposition of the great arteries. I. Cardiac catheterization protocol. Am. Heart J. 84:597, 1972.

133. Mulvihill, J. J., Mulvihill, C. G., and Neill, C. A.: Congenital heart defects and prenatal sex hormones. Lancet 1:1168, 1974.

134. Mustard, W. T.: Successful two-stage correction of transposition of the great vessels. Surgery 55:469, 1964.

135. Mustard, W. T., Chute, A. L., Keith, J. D., Sirek, A., Rowe, R. D., and Vlad, P.: A surgical approach to transposition of the great vessels with extracorporeal circuit. Surgery 36:39, 1954.

136. Muster, A. J.: Diagnosis and treatment of pulmonary vasoconstriction following palliative procedures in congenital heart disease. Chest 76:247, 1979.

137. Muster, A. J., Paul, M. H., van Grondelle, A., and Conway, J. J.: Asymmetrical distribution of pulmonary blood flow between the right and left lungs in D-transposition of the great arteries. Am. J. Cardiol. 38:352, 1976.

138. Muster, A. J., Bharati, S., Aziz, K. U., Idriss, F. S., Paul, M. H., Lev, M., Carr, I., Deboer, A., and Anagnostopoulos, C.: Taussig-Bing anomaly with straddling mitral valve. J. Thorac. Cardiovasc. Surg. 77:832, 1979.

139. Neches, W. H., Mullins, C. E., and McNamara, D. G.: The infant with transposition of the great arteries. II. Results of balloon atrial septostomy. Am. Heart J. 84:603, 1972.

140. Newfeld, E. A.: Pulmonary thrombosis and vascular disease after Mustard operation for transposition of the great arteries. Am. J. Cardiol. 37:115, 1976.

141. Newfeld, E. A., Paul, M. H., Muster, A. J., and Idriss, F. S.: Pulmonary vascular disease in complete transposition of the great arteries: A study of 200 patients. Am. J. Cardiol. 34:75, 1974.

142. Newfeld, E. A., Purcell, C., Paul, M. H., Cole, R. B., and Muster, A. J.: Transumbilical balloon atrial septostomy in 16 infants with transposition of the great arteries. Pediatrics 54:495, 1974.

143. Newfeld, E. A., Paul, M. H., Muster, A. J., and Idriss, F. S.: Pulmonary vascular disease in transposition of the great vessels and intact ventricular septum. Circulation 59:525, 1979.

144. Nihill, M. R., McNamara, D. G., and Vick, R. L.: The effects of increased blood viscosity on pulmonary vascular resistance. Am. Heart J. 92:65, 1976.

145. Ninomiya, K., Duncan, W. J., Cook, D. H., Olley, P. M., and Rowe, R. D.: Right ventricular ejection fraction and volumes after Mustard repair: Correlation of two dimensional echocardiograms and cineangiograms. Am. J.

Cardiol. 48:317, 1981.

146. Nogrady, M. B., and Dunbar, J. S.: Complete transposition of the great vessels: Re-evaluation of the so called "typical configuration" on plain films of the chest. J. Can. Assoc. Radiol. 20:124, 1969.

147. Nora, J. J., and Nora, A. H.: Birth defects and oral contraceptives. Lancet 1:941, 1973.

148. Oppenheimer, E. H.: Arterial thrombosis (paradoxical embolism) in association with transposition of the great vessels. Johns Hopkins Med. J. 124:202, 1969.

149. Parenzan, L., Locatelli, G., Alfieri, O., Villani, M., and Invernizzi, G.: The Senning operation for transposition of the great arteries. J. Thorac. Cardiovasc. Surg. 76:305, 1978.

150. Park, S. C., Neches, W. H., Zuberbuhler, J. R., Lenox, C. C., Mathews, R. A., Fricker, F. J., and Zoltun, R. A.: Clinical use of blade atrial septostomy. Circulation 58:600, 1978.

151. Parr, G. V., Blackstone, E. H., Kirklin, J. W., Pacifico, A. D., and Lauridsen, P.: Cardiac performance early after interatrial transposition of venous return in infants and small children. Circulation 49–50 (Suppl. II):II-8, 1974.

152. Parsons, C. G., Astely, R., Burrows, F. G. O., and Singh, S. P.: Transposition of great arteries. A study of 65 infants followed for 1 to 4 years after balloon septostomy. Br. Heart J. 33:725, 1971.

153. Paul, M. H., Currimhoy, Z., Miller, R. A., and Schulman, J.: Thrombocytopenia in cyanotic congenital heart disease. Circulation 24:1013, 1961.

154. Paul, M. H., Muster, A. J., Cole, R. B., and Baffes, T. G.: Palliative management for transposition of the great arteries, 1957–1967. Ann. Thorac. Surg. 6:321, 1968.

155. Phornphutkul, C., Rosenthal, A., and Nadas, A. S.: Cerebrovascular accidents in infants and children with cyanotic congenital heart disease. Am. J. Cardiol. 32:329, 1973.

156. Piccoli, G. P., and Hamilton, D. I.: Interposition of a modified aortic homograft conduit as main pulmonary trunk in anatomic correction of transposition of the great arteries. J. Thorac. Cardiovasc. Surg. 82:429, 1981.

157. Piccoli, G. P., Wilkinson, J. L., Arnold, R., Musumeci, F., and Hamilton, D. I.: Appraisal of the Mustard procedure for the physiological correction of "simple" transposition of the great arteries: Eighty consecutive cases, 1970–1980. J. Thorac. Cardiovasc. Surg. 82:436, 1981.

158. Plauth, W. H., Jr., Nadas, A. S., Bernhard, W. F., and Cross, R. E.: Transposition of the great arteries: Clinical and physiological observations on 74 patients treated by palliative surgery. Circulation 37:316, 1968.

159. Porter, C. J., Gillette, P. C., McNamara, D. G., and Cooley, D. C.: Transposition of the great arteries, ventricular septal defect and pulmonary stenosis: Early and late results of repair by Mustard procedure. Am. J. Cardiol. 37:162, 1976.

160. Quaegebeur, J. M., Rohmer, J., Brom, A. G., and Tinkelenberg, J.: Revival of the Senning operation in the treatment of transposition of the great arteries. Thorax 32:517, 1977.

161. Quaegebeur, J. M., and Brom, A. G.: The trousers-shaped baffle for use in the Mustard operation. Ann. Thorac. Surg. 25:240, 1978.

162. Rabinovitch, M., Haworth, S. G., Castaneda, A. R., Nadas, A. S., and Reid, L. M.: Lung biopsy in congenital heart disease: A morphometric approach to pulmonary vascular disease. Circulation 58:1107, 1978.

163. Rashkind, W. J.: The complications of balloon atrioseptostomy. J. Pediatrics 76:649, 1970.

164. Rashkind, W. J.: Shunting at the ventricular level in transposition of the great vessels. Circulation 44 (Suppl. II):II-71, 1971.

165. Rashkind, W. J.: Balloon atrioseptostomy. Adv. Cardiol. 11:2, 1974.

166. Rashkind, W. J.: Transposition of the great arteries: Before the Mustard operation. Ten year's experience with balloon atrioseptostomy. In The Child with Congenital Heart Disease after Surgery, edited by B. S. L. Kidd, and R. D. Rowe. Futura Publishing Co., Mount Kisco, N.Y., 1976.

167. Rashkind, W. J., and Miller, W. W.: Creation of an atrial septal defect without thoracotomy. J.A.M.A. 196:991, 1966.

168. Rastelli, G. C.: A new approach to "anatomic" repair of transposition of the great arteries. Mayo Clin. Proc. 44:1, 1969.

169. Rastelli, G. C., McGoon, D. C., and Wallace, R. B.: Anatomic correction of transposition of the great arteries with ventricular septal defect and subpulmonary stenosis. J. Thorac. Cardiovasc. Surg. 58:545, 1969.

170. Restieaux, N. J., Ellison, R. C., Albers, W. H., and Nadas, A. S.: The Frank electrocardiogram in complete transposition of the great arteries: Its use in assessments of left ventricular pressure. Am. Heart J. 83:219, 1972.

171. Riemenschneider, T. A., Vincent, W. R., Ruttenberg, H. D., and Desilets, D. T.: Transposition of the great vessels with hypoplasia of the right ventricle. Circulation 38:386, 1968.

172. Riemenschneider, T. A., Goldberg, S. J., Ruttenberg, H. D., and Gyepes, M. T.: Subpulmonic obstruction in complete D-transposition produced by redundant tricuspid tissue. Circulation 39:603, 1969.

173. Robertson, B.: The intrapulmonary arterial pattern in normal infancy and in transposition of the great arteries. Acta Paediatr. Scand. [Suppl.] 184:7, 1968.

174. Rodriguez-Fernandez, H. L., Kelly, D. T., Collado, A., Haller, J. A., Jr., Krovetz, L. J., and Rowe, R. D.: Hemodynamic data and angiographic findings after Mustard repair for complete transposition of the great arteries. Circulation 46:799, 1972.

175. Rosengart, R., Fishbein, M., and Emmanouilides, G. C.: Progressive pulmonary vascular disease after surgical correction (Mustard procedure) of transposition of the great arteries with intact ventricular septum. Am. J. Cardiol. 35:107, 1975.

176. Rosenquist, G. C., Stark, J., and Taylor, J. F. N.: Anatomical relationships in transposition of the great arteries: Juxtaposition of the atrial appendages. Ann. Thorac. Surg. 18:456, 1974.

177. Rosenthal, A., Freed, M. D., Fyler, D. C., and Levin, S.B.: Observations on the development of subaortic stenosis following pulmonary artery banding. Chest 65:420, 1974.

178. Rosenthal, A., and Castaneda, A.: Growth and development after cardiovascular surgery in infants and children. Prog. Cardiovasc. Dis. 18:27, 1975.

179. Rowland, T. W., Hubbell, J. P., Jr., and Nadas, A. S.: Congenital heart disease in infants of diabetic mothers. J. Pediatr. 83:815, 1973.

180. Rudolph, A. M.: Congenital Diseases of the Heart. Year Book Publishers, Chicago, 1974.

181. Saalouke, M. G., Rios, J., Perry, L. W., Shapiro, S. R., and Scott, L. P.: Electrophysiologic studies after Mustard's operation for D-transposition of the great vessels. Am. J. Cardiol. 41:1104, 1978.

182. Schneeweiss, A., Bliedeu, L. C., Shem-Tov, A., Fiegel, A., and Neufeld, H. N.: Wide vascular pedicle on thoracic roentgenogram in complete transposition of the great arteries. Clin. Cardiol. 5:75, 1982.

183. Scott, L. P., Saalouke, M. G., Shapiro, S. R., Rios, J. C., and Perry, L. W.: Sudden unexpected death following Mustard's procedure for D-transposition of the great arteries. Circulation 54 (Suppl. II):II-89, 1976.

184. Sealy, W. C., and Seaber, A. V.: Cardiac rhythm following exclusion of the sinoatrial node and most of the right atrium from the remainder of the heart. J. Thorac. Cardiovasc. Surg. 77:436, 1979.

185. Senning, A.: Surgical correction of transposition of the great vessels. Surgery 45:966, 1959.

186. Senning, A.: Correction of the transposition of the great arteries. Ann. Surg. 182:287, 1975.

187. Shaher, R. M.: Complete Transposition of the Great Arteries. Academic Press, New York, 1973.

188. Shaher, R. M., Moes, C. A. F., and Khoury, G.: Radiologic and angiographic findings in complete transposition of the great vessels with left ventricular outflow tract obstruction. Radiology 88:1092, 1967.

189. Shinebourne, E. A., Macartney, F. J., and Anderson, R. H.: Sequential chamber localization: Logical approach to diagnosis in congenital heart disease. Br. Heart J. 38:327, 1976.

190. Shumacker, H. B., Jr.: A new operation for transposition of the great vessels. Surgery 50:773, 1961.

191. Shumway, N. E., Griepp, R. B., and Stinson, E. B.: Surgical management of transposition of the great arteries. Am. J. Surgery 130:233, 1975.

192. Silove, E. D., Tynan, M. J., and Simcha, A. J.: Thermal dilution measurement of pulmonary and systemic blood flow in secundum atrial septal defect, and transposition of great arteries with intact ventricular septum. Br. Heart J. 34:1142, 1972.

193. Silove, E. D., and Taylor, J. F.: Angiographic and anatomical features of subvalvar left ventricular outflow obstruction in transposition of the great arteries. The possible role of the anterior mitral valve leaflet. Pediatr. Radiol. 1:87, 1973.

194. Sorenson, S. C., and Severinghaus, J. W.: Respiratory insensitivity to acute hypoxia persisting after correction of tetralogy of Fallot. J. Appl. Physiol. 25:221, 1968.

195. Southall, D. P., Keeton, B. R., Leanage, R., Lam, L., Joseph, M. C., Anderson, R. H., Lincoln, C. R., and Shinebourne, E. A.: Cardiac rhythm and conduction before and after Mustard's operation for complete transposition of the great arteries. Br. Heart J. 43:21, 1980.

196. Stark, J.: Primary definitive intracardiac operations in infants. Transposition of the great arteries. In Advances in Cardiovascular Surgery, edited by J. W. Kirklin. Grune & Stratton, New York, 1973.

197. Stark, J., Tynan, M., Tatooles, C. J., Aberdeen, E., and Waterston, D. J.: Banding of the pulmonary artery for transposition of the great arteries and ventricular septal defect. Circulation 41–42 (Suppl. II):II-116, 1970.

198. Stark, J., de Leval, M., Waterston, D. J., Graham, G. R., and Bonham-Carter, R. E.: Corrective surgery of transposition of the great arteries in the first year of life. Results in 63 infants. J. Thorac. Cardiovasc. Surg. 67:673, 1974.

199. Stark, J., Silove, E. D., Taylor, J. F. N., and Graham, G. R.: Obstruction of systemic venous return following the Mustard operation for transposition of the great arteries. J. Thorac. Cardiovasc. Surg. 68:742, 1974.

200. Stark, J., Singh, A., de Leval, M., and Taylor, J. F. N.: Early vs. late Mustard operation for "simple" transposition of the great arteries. In The Child with Congenital Heart Disease after Surgery, edited by B. S. L. Kidd, and R. D. Rowe. Futura Publishing Co., Mount Kisco, N.Y., 1976.

201. Stark, J., de Leval, M., and Taylor, J. F. N.: Mustard operation and creation of ventricular septal defect in a child with transposition of the great arteries, intact ventricular sep-

202. Subramanian, S., and Wagner, H.: Correction of transposition of the great arteries in infants under surface-induced deep hypothermia. Ann. Thorac. Surg. 16:391, 1973.

203. Sunderland, C. O., Nichols, G. M., Henken, D. P., Linstone, F., Menashe, V. D., and Lees, M. H.: Percutaneous cardiac catheterization and atrial balloon septostomy in pediatrics. J. Pediatrics 89:584, 1976.

204. Tabry, C. F., McGoon, D. C., Danielson, G. K., Wallace, R. B., Tajik, A. J., and Seward, J. B.: Surgical management of straddling atrioventricular valve. J. Thorac. Cardiovasc. Surg. 77:191, 1979.

205. Thiene, G., Razzolini, R., and Dalla-Volta, S.: Aorto-pulmonary relationship, arterioventricular alignment, and ventricular septal defects in complete transposition of the great arteries. Eur. J. Cardiol. 4:13, 1976.

206. Tonkin, I. L., Sansa, M., Elliott, L. P., and Bargeron, L. M., Jr.: Recognition of developing left ventricular outflow tract obstruction in complete transposition of the great arteries. Radiology 134:53, 1980.

207. Trusler, G. A., and Mustard, W. T.: A method of banding the pulmonary artery for large isolated ventricular septal defect with and without transposition of the great arteries. Ann. Thorac. Surg. 13:351, 1972.

208. Trusler, G. A., and Kamat, P. V.: Late results of palliative procedures in transposition of the great arteries. In The Child with Congenital Heart Disease after Surgery, edited by B. S. L. Kidd, and R. D. Rowe. Futura Publishing Co., Mount Kisco, N.Y., 1976.

209. Trusler, G. A., Williams, W. G., Izukawa, T., and Olley, P. M.: Current results with the Mustard operation in isolated transposition of the great arteries. J. Thorac. Cardiovasc. Surg. 80:381, 1980.

210. Turley, K., and Ebert, P. A.: Total correction of transposition of the great arteries. Conduction disturbances in infants younger than three months of age. J. Thorac. Cardiovasc. Surg. 76:312, 1978.

211. Turley, K., Tucker, W. Y., and Ebert, P. A.: The changing role of palliative procedures in the treatment of infants with congenital heart disease. J. Thorac. Cardiovasc. Surg. 79:194, 1980.

212. Tynan, M.: Haemodynamic effects of balloon atrial septostomy in infants with transposition of the great arteries. Br. Heart J. 34:791, 1972.

213. Tynan, M.: Transposition of the great arteries: Changes in the circulation after birth. Circulation 46:809, 1972.

214. Tynan, M., Aberdeen, E., and Stark, J.: Tricuspid incompetence after the Mustard operation for transposition of the great arteries. Circulation 45 (Suppl. I):I-111, 1972.

215. Tyrrell, M. J., and Moes, C. A. F.: Congenital levoposition of the right atrial appendage: Its relevance to balloon septostomy. Am. J. Dis. Child. 121:508, 1971.

216. Ullal, R. R., Anderson, R. H., and Lincoln, C.: Mustard's operation modified to avoid dysrhythmias and pulmonary and systemic venous obstruction. J. Thorac. Cardiovasc. Surg. 78:431, 1979.

217. Van Praagh, R.: The segmental approach to diagnosis in congenital heart disease. Birth Defects 8:4, 1972.

218. Van Praagh, R., Perez-Trevino, C., Loperz-Cuellar, M., Baker, F. W., Zuberbuhler, J. F., Zuero, M., Perez, V. M., Moreno, F., and Van Praagh, S.: Transposition of the great arteries with posterior aorta, anterior pulmonary artery, subpulmonary conus and fibrous continuity between aortic and atrioventricular valves. Am. J. Cardiol. 28:621, 1971.

219. Van Praagh, R., Durhin, R. E., Jockin, H.,

Wagner, H. R., Korns, M., Garabedian, H., Ando, M., and Calder, A. L.: Anatomically corrected malposition of the great arteries (S,D,L). Circulation 51:20, 1975.

220. Van Praagh, R., Weinberg, P. M., Calder, A. L., Buckley, L. F. P., and Van Praagh, S.: The transposition complexes: How many are there? In Second Henry Ford Hospital International Symposium on Cardiac Surgery, edited by J. C. Davila. Appleton-Century-Crofts, New York, 1977, pp. 207–213.

221. Van Praagh, R., Layton, W. M., and Van Praagh, S.: The morphogenesis of normal and abnormal relationships between the great arteries and the ventricles: Pathologic and experimental data. In Etiology and Morphogenesis of Congenital Heart Disease, edited by R. Van Praagh and A. Takao. Futura Publishing Co., Mount Kisco, N.Y., 1980, pp. 271–316.

222. Van Praagh, R., Weinberg, P. M., Matsuoka, R., and Van Praagh, S.: Malpositions of the heart and the segmental approach to diagnosis. In Heart Disease in Infants, Children and Adolescents, edited by F. H. Adams and G. C. Emmanouilides, 3rd ed., Ch. 21. Williams & Wilkins, Baltimore, 1982.

223. Vidne, B. A., Subramanian, S., and Wagner, H. R.: Aneurysm of the membranous ventricular septum in transposition of the great arteries. Circulation 53:157, 1976.

224. Vogel, J. H. K.: Balloon embolization during atrial septostomy. Circulation 42:155, 1970.

225. Wagenvoort, C. A., Nauta, J., van der Schaar, P. J., Weeda, H. W. H., and Wagenvoort, N.: The pulmonary vasculature in complete transposition of the great vessels judged from lung biopsies. Circulation 38:746, 1968.

226. Wagenvoort, C. A.: Grading of pulmonary vascular lesions—a reappraisal. Histopathology 5:595, 1981.

227. Wagner, H. R., and Teske, D. W.: Transposition of the great arteries: Problems of ventricular function before and after Mustard procedure. In The Child with Congenital Heart Disease after Surgery, edited by B. S. L. Kidd and R. D. Rowe. Futura Publishing Co., Mount Kisco, N.Y., 1976.

228. Waldhausen, J. A., Pierce, W. S., Berman, W., Jr., and Whitman, V.: Modified Shumacker repair of transposition of the great arteries. Circulation 60 (Suppl. I):I-110, 1979.

229. Waldman, J. D., Czapek, E. E., Paul, M. H., Schwartz, A. D., Levin, D. L., and Schindler, S.: Shortened platelet survival in cyanotic heart disease. J. Pediatr. 87:77, 1975.

230. Waldman, J. D., Paul, M. H., Newfeld, E. A., Muster, A. J., and Idriss, F. S.: Transposition of the great arteries with intact ventricular septum and patent ductus arteriosus. Am. J. Cardiol. 39:232, 1977.

231. Wedemyer, A. L., Castaneda, A. R., Edson, J. R., and Krivit, W.: Serial coagulation studies in patients undergoing Mustard procedure. Ann. Thorac. Surg. 15:120, 1973.

232. Wedemyer, A. L., and Lewis, J. H.: Improvement in hemostasis following phlebotomy in cyanotic patients with heart disease. J. Pediatr. 83:46, 1973.

233. Wells, B.: The sounds and murmurs in transpositions of the great vessels. Br. Heart J. 25:748, 1963.

234. Wilkinson, J. L., Arnold, R., Anderson, R. H., and Acerete, F.: "Posterior" transposition reconsidered. Br. Heart J. 37:757, 1975.

235. Williams, W. G., Freedom, R. M., Culham, G., Duncan, W. J., Olley, P. M., Rowe, R. D., and Trusler, G. A.: Early experience with arterial repair of transposition. Ann. Thorac. Surg. 32:8, 1981.

236. Wittig, J. H., de Leval, M. R., and Stark, J.: Intraoperative mapping of atrial activation before, during and after the Mustard operation. J. Thorac. Cardiovasc. Surg. 73:1, 1977.

237. Yacoub, M. H.: The case for anatomic correction of transposition of the great arteries. J. Thorac. Cardiovasc. Surg. 78:3, 1979.
238. Yacoub, M. H., Radley-Smith, R., and Hilton, C. J.: Anatomical correction of complete transposition of the great arteries and ventricular septal defect in infancy. Br. Med. J. 1:1112, 1976.
239. Yacoub, M., Bernhard, A., Lange, P., Radley-Smith, R., Keck, E., Stephan, E., and Heintzen, P.: Clinical and hemodynamic results of the two-stage anatomic correction of simple transposition of the great arteries. Circulation 62(Suppl. I):I–190, 1980.
240. Yamaki, S., and Tezuka, F.: Quantitative analysis of pulmonary vascular disease in complete transposition of the great arteries. Circulation 54:805, 1976.
241. Yasuda, M., and Miller, J. R.: Prenatal exposure to oral contraceptives and transposition of the great vessels in man. Teratology 12:239, 1975.

22

Corrected Transposition (L-Transposition) of the Great Arteries and Splenic Syndromes

Herbert D. Ruttenberg, M.D.

CORRECTED TRANSPOSITION OF THE GREAT ARTERIES

Congenitally corrected transposition of the great arteries (hereafter referred to as corrected transposition) is an unusual cardiac malformation because the normal hemodynamic pathways are not altered by the malformation: transposition of the great arteries with inversion of the ventricles and atrioventricular (AV) valves. With this arrangement, systemic venous blood enters an anatomic left ventricle and is ejected into a posterior pulmonary trunk. Pulmonary venous blood returns into an anatomic right ventricle and is ejected into an anterior aorta. Thus, in the rare case when no additional cardiac anomaly is present, a hemodynamically normal heart exists.

The first accurate anatomic description was reported by Rokitansky.[44] He observed that transposition of the great vessels was "corrected by the position of the ventricular septum." Since that time, "corrected transposition of the great vessels" has become the most popular term used to describe this condition. Spitzer[51] proposed the term "inverted transposition." More recently, Lev and Rowlatt[32] suggested the term "mixed levocardia with corrected transposition." Mixed levocardia, however, may be a misleading term since corrected transposition commonly occurs with dextrocardia. With the advent of cardiac surgery and the development of surgical techniques for correction of complete transposition, Schiebler and coworkers[50] proposed the term "congenital corrected transposition of the great vessels." This term implies that the condition was present at birth and would not, therefore, be confused with surgically corrected transposition of the great arteries.

Van Praagh[55] proposed defining malpositions of the heart and great arteries in embryologic terms which separately label the great arteries, ventricular loop, and the visceral situs. Thus, in the case of situs solitus, corrected transposition would be defined as L-transposition with L-loop and visceral-atrial situs solitus. Other currently used terms are "L-transposition of the great arteries with ventricular inversion" and "AV discordance with ventricular-great artery discordance."[1] In this chapter the traditional term "corrected transposition" will be used because it is preferred by the author for simplicity and to avoid confusion with regard to situs. It should be noted that isolated ventricular inversion (without L-transposition)[6] and ventricular inversion with D-transposition can occur, and L-malposition may be present with inverted (D-loop) of the ventricles.[6] These anomalies are rare.

Since Anderson and associates[3] first described the clinical manifestations of corrected transposition in 1957, more than 300 cases have been reported. Although corrected transposition is potentially a hemodynamically normal heart, it is usually associated with one or a combination of intracardiac malformations. For this reason, the clinical manifestations and treatment of patients with corrected transposition will depend largely on the associated defects.

EMBRYOLOGY

Most authors agree that the embryological defect in corrected transposition is an abnormal rotation of the bulboventricular loop. De la Cruz and associates[11] proposed that corrected transposition in visceral-atrial situs solitus develops when the primitive heart tube, or bulboventricular loop, loops to the left (L-loop) instead of the right (D-loop). In addition, there is a lack of spiral rotation of the truncoconal septum. Grant[25] proposed that corrected transposition, as well as ventricular inversion, dextroversion, or levoversion, are disturbances of "polarity" in conotruncal development. He postulated that abnormalities in the timing or distribution of differential growth could produce cardiac abnormalities wherein the position of the cardiac chambers and great arteries were abnormal with respect to the body axes, but the components themselves might be normally developed and lead to normal hemodynamics. His theory differs from previous ones in that he proposes that the primary defect is the formation of the L-loop in situs solitus or a D-loop in situs inversus and that the lack of coiling of the truncal septum is a secondary development.

PATHOLOGY

In this section, an attempt will be made to define corrected transposition with commonly accepted anatomic terms: inversion of the AV valves and ventricles, with transposition of the great arteries. There must be two ventricles present so that each AV valve empties into its respective ventricle. When one AV valve is atretic, the potential valve orifice should be so located that it would have opened into its ventricle had it not been atretic. The above definition, therefore, excludes cases of common ventricle with inversion of the infundibulum, a condition in which the arrangement of the great arteries (L-transposition) is similar to that of corrected transposition (see Chapter 25), but in which both AV valves empty into a common ventricular chamber. This condition has also been called "corrected transposition with rudimentary ventricle,"[1] "single ventricle with congenitally corrected transposition,"[39] and "double inlet left ventricle."[12] The distinction between corrected transposition and common ventricle with infundibular inversion and transposition is important since these conditions are very similar in their clinical manifestations, but have a different prognosis in relation to surgical correction. Some of the early reports and a recent report[20] of corrected transposition include cases of common ventricle.

Most cases of corrected transposition are associated with a situs solitus position of the heart and abdominal viscera, while a few occur with situs inversus. The terms solitus and inversus, as used here, indicate the basic positions (situs) of the abdominal organs and chambers of the heart. In situs solitus, the arterial atrium, anatomic left ventricle, and stomach are located on the left side of the body, while the venae cavae and venous atrium are to the right of the arterial chamber. Situs inversus implies a mirror image arrangement so that the left-right relationships are reversed. The location of the arterial atrium and the stomach on the same side is a constant relationship which is present in virtually all cases of congenital cardiac disease, with the exception of cases of asplenia or polysplenia. In corrected transposition, the inverted nature of the ventricles is an exception to the definition of the basic situs of the organs of the body so that a more specific term is required. Thus, the term visceral-atrial situs solitus in corrected transposition is preferred. This term implies that the atria, venae cavae, and abdominal viscera are in their usual location. Conversely, visceral-atrial situs inversus is the term applied when corrected transposition is associated with a mirror image position of the abdominal organs, venae cavae, and atria.

When corrected transposition occurs with visceral-atrial situs solitus, systemic venous blood passes from the right atrium through the inverted (mitral) AV valve into the inverted right-sided pulmonary ventricle. The pulmonary ventricle is defined as inverted since it has the anatomic characteristics of a left ventricle. It is smooth-walled, lacks a crista supraventricularis, and has a posterior outflow tract (Fig. 22.1a). As in the normal left ventricle, the septal leaflet of the bicuspid AV valve forms the posterolateral wall of the outflow tract and is in fibrous continuity with the semilunar valve (in this case, the pulmonary valve) (Fig. 22.2). The pulmonary trunk, in this arrangement, is located posteriorly near the midline, and its valve lies in the same transverse plane as the aortic valve in a normal heart. Systemic venous blood is ejected into the posterior pulmonary trunk, passes through the lungs, and is returned to a normal left atrium. The pathway of the blood is then through a tricuspid (inverted) AV valve into the inverted left-sided systemic ventricle which has the architecture of a right ventricle (Fig. 22.1b). It is coarsely trabeculated and possesses a crista supraventricularis and infundibular chamber which separate elements of the atrioventricular valve from the semilunar (aortic) valve. The infundibulum is located at the left anterior basilar aspect of the heart so that the aortic valve is superior to the pulmonic valve. The aorta takes origin from the infundibulum, which places it anterior and to the left of the pulmonary trunk (Fig. 22.2); the ascending portion of the aorta forms the left upper border of the heart. The coronary arterial pattern is also inverted. The right coronary artery arises above the right aortic sinus and gives off the anterior descending branch. The left coronary artery arises above the left sinus, continues around posteriorly, and gives off a conal branch and the posterior descending artery. The anterior sinus is noncoronary.

Recent classifications of arterial transposition have added the term "L-malposition" in two situations where the aorta arises to the left of the pulmonary trunk: both arteries arise from the same ventricle, and a left-sided aorta arises from an anatomic left ventricle while the medial pulmonary trunk arises from the anatomic right ventricle.[6]

Since corrected transposition often occurs with various forms of dextrocardia, it is appropriate to define the dextrocardias as used in this chapter. (The reader is referred to Chapter 28 for a more complete discussion of cardiac malpositions. In this chapter, the dextrocardias are classified in a different manner).

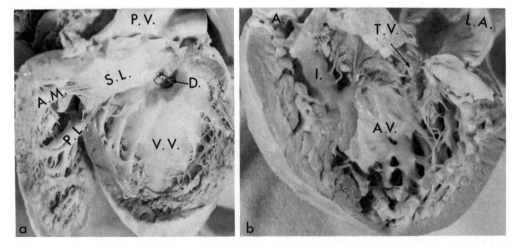

Fig. 22.1 Pathology of corrected transposition with visceral-atrial situs solitus. (a) Inverted right-sided venous ventricle (V.V.), right lateral view, demonstrating characteristics of anatomic left ventricle: smooth-walled chamber, fibrous continuity between septal leaflet (S.L.) of mitral valve and semilunar valve (P.V., pulmonary valve), and posterior outflow tract. Inverted nature of atrioventricular valve is demonstrated. P.L., posterior-lateral; A.M., anterior-medial papillary muscles; D, ventricular septal defect, surgically closed. (b) Inverted left-sided arterial ventricle (A.V.), left lateral view, demonstrating characteristics of anatomic right ventricle: coarsely tuberculated chamber, separation of aortic valve (A.) from the inverted atrioventricular valve (T.V., tricuspid valve) by anterior infundibular chamber (I.). L.A., left atrium.

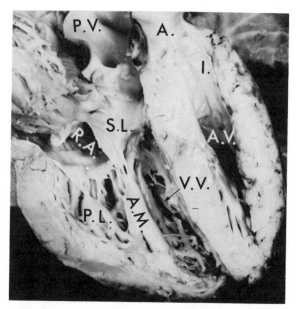

Fig. 22.2 Pathology of corrected transposition in visceral-atrial situs solitus. Anterior view demonstrating side by side relation between the inverted right-sided venous ventricle (*V.V.*) and inverted left-sided arterial ventricle (*A.V.*). The septal leaflet (S.L.) of the inverted (mitral) venous atrioventricular valve forms part of the pulmonary outflow tract, which is located posterior and medial to the ascending aorta. The pulmonary valve (*P.V.*) is located inferior to the aortic valve (*A.*) which takes origin from the infundibular chamber (*I.*) at the left anterobasal portion of the heart. *A.M.*, anterior-medial papillary muscles; *P.L.*, posterior-lateral papillary muscles; *R.A.*, right atrium.

Dextrocardia is the nonspecific or generic term applied to cardiac position in which the apex points toward the right hemithorax. The three main forms of dextrocardia are mirror image dextrocardia, dextroversion, and extrinsic dextrocardia. We will concern ourselves with the first two forms since these are commonly associated with corrected transposition. Extrinsic dextrocardia implies that the heart is displaced to the right either by an extrinsic mass or by hypoplasia of the right lung. Mirror-image dextrocardia virtually always occurs with visceral-atrial situs inversus. In this case, the relationship of the cardiac chambers and great arteries is the mirror image of the arrangement found in the usual or situs solitus heart. Dextroversion, as described by Grant,[24] involves a twisting or version of the ventricles to the right (as in the turning of a page), while the atria remain in the situs solitus position. In other words, dextroversion is the term applied to a dextrocardia associated with visceral-atrial situs solitus. This cardiac malposition may occur with or without corrected transposition. Various degrees of dextroversion occur. In mild dextroversion ("mesoversion"), the heart appears midline (Fig. 22.5B) while the right-sided ventricle forms the apex of the heart to the right (Fig. 22.7). In its severest form, the ventricles are rotated 180° to the right so that the left-sided arterial ventricle lies anterior and may form the right border of the heart. As dextroversion occurs in the situs solitus heart, "levoversion" may occur in visceral-atrial situs inversus. Levoversion, then, is a twisting of the ventricles to the left in visceral-atrial situs inversus (*i.e.*, levoversion is the mirror image of dextroversion).

Fontana and Edwards[17] reported corrected transposition to occur in 1.4% of 357 specimens of congenital cardiac disease. The prevalence in general population may be slightly higher since undoubtedly there are people with corrected transposition whose condition remains undetected.

ASSOCIATED MALFORMATIONS

The most commonly associated cardiac abnormalities are ventricular septal defect (VSD), pulmonary stenosis, malpositions of the cardiac apex (dextroversion, mirror image dextrocardia, and levoversion) and rhythm disturbances. The frequency of VSD has been reported as high as 80% in one large series in which pulmonary stenosis was an accompanying lesion in 80% of these.[14] The VSD is usually large and located in the membranous septum near the pulmonary valve beneath the crista supraventricularis (Fig. 22.1), which separates the defect from the aortic valve. Supracristal,[40] muscular, and multiple defects are far less common.

Pulmonary outflow tract obstruction is also common and has been reported to occur in 70%.[14] It is usually either valvular or subvalvular. Subpulmonary stenosis may be produced by either a fibrous ring, or an accumulation of fibrous or myxomatous tissue,[34] or a fibromuscular tunnel.[5]

The frequency of systemic AV valvular insufficiency has been reported in one-third of cases.[50] At necropsy, most cases have an Ebstein-like malformation of the tricuspid (systemic) valve. In contrast to Ebstein's anomaly of the pulmonary tricuspid valve, the circumference of the valve and the systemic ventricle are not enlarged, the anterior leaflet is frequently cleft, and the malformed valve may interfere with the ventricular outflow tract.[2] Other cases of incompetent systemic AV valve are thickened deficient leaflets, annular dilatation, abnormal papillary muscle, and anomalous insertion of the chordae tendineae.[1, 29]

Other cardiac lesions which are frequently associated with corrected transposition are ASD and PDA. These usually accompany pulmonary stenosis, VSD, or atrial AV valvular insufficiency in various combinations. Less common lesions are coarctation of the aorta, aortic insufficiency, aortic valvular stenosis, mitral atresia, and tricuspid atresia.

MANIFESTATIONS

Clinical Features

The symptoms of patients with corrected transposition are related to the associated lesions. It is well documented that patients with corrected transposition and no associated malformation live normal lives. In such cases, the possibility exists, however, that symptoms may result from arrhythmias.

The majority of patients with corrected transposition present with severe cardiac symptoms during the first months of life. In 33 cases,[50] 75% had symptoms during the 1st month of life. The associated lesions in practically all were large VSD, with or without pulmonary arterial obstruction. They present with corresponding symptoms: heart failure with large left to right shunts; or, cyanosis and apneic spells with pulmonary arterial obstruction and right to left shunts. In the latter cases, squatting may occur in the older age group.

Typically, the findings on physical examination are manifestations of the associated lesions. However, one finding which is peculiar to the malformation may suggest corrected transposition to the astute observer; this is a loud, single second sound, frequently palpable, and maximal at the mid-left sternal border. This sound represents aortic valvular closure and is loud because of the proximity of the aortic valve to the chest wall. The pulmonary component of the second sound is seldom heard since the valve is posterior. In corrected transposition with no associated malformation, the finding of a loud aortic closure is frequently accompanied by a soft ejection murmur at the midsternal border. This murmur may result from turbulence associated with rapid ejection of blood into the pulmonary artery by the anatomic left ventricle. Bradycardia, as a result of heart block, is another finding which should alert the physician to this malformation. The murmur of arterial AV valvular insufficiency is usually pansystolic, is loudest at the lower left sternal border, and may be confused with the murmur of a ventricular septal defect. When a VSD coexists with "mitral" insufficiency, it may be difficult to identify separately the lesion on the basis of physical examination. When pulmonary stenosis is present, either as an isolated lesion or with a ventricular septal defect, a harsh systolic ejection murmur is heard maximal at the mid or lower left sternal border.

Electrovectorcardiographic Features

The electrocardiographic and vectorcardiographic features in this condition are manifestations of the abnormal direction of initial ventricular depolarization. Anderson *et al.*[3] first described the reversal of the precordial Q wave pattern, and suggested that this pattern may reflect a mirror image arrangement of the ventricular conduction system. The AV node, bundle of His, and the bundle branches are, in fact, mirror image in distribution.[33] This hypothesis is supported by the findings in six cases with normal hemodynamic states.[16, 23, 46, 47] In these cases the electrocardiographic and vectorcardiographic features were: reversal of the Q wave pattern in the precordial leads; large Q wave in lead III; left axis deviation; and clockwise rotation of the QRS loop in the frontal plane (Fig. 22.3).

The majority of cases with corrected transposition have associated cardiac malformations which influence to varying degrees the ventricular depolarization. Malposition of the cardiac apex has the most profound influence. For this reason, the findings in cases with cardiac malposition will be discussed separately.

In corrected transposition without cardiac malposition, the initial QRS vectors are directed to the left, anteriorly and superiorly, in over 90% of the cases (Figs. 22.3b and 22.4c and d).

The direction of the initial QRS vectors is manifested in the vectorcardiogram by a straight, leftward efferent limb of the QRS loop in the horizontal plane (absence of the Q loop) and in the electrocardiogram by Q waves in V4R and V1 and in lead III, with absence of the Q waves in lead V6 (Fig. 22.4b). In about 30% of these cases, the Q wave in lead III is abnormally large, simulating an infarction pattern (Figs. 20.2a and 22.4d).

Despite the fact that many patients with corrected transposition have ventricular septal defects, the Q loop of the vectorcardiogram is absent, and there is no Q wave in lead V6. The ventricular hypertrophy patterns, however, as

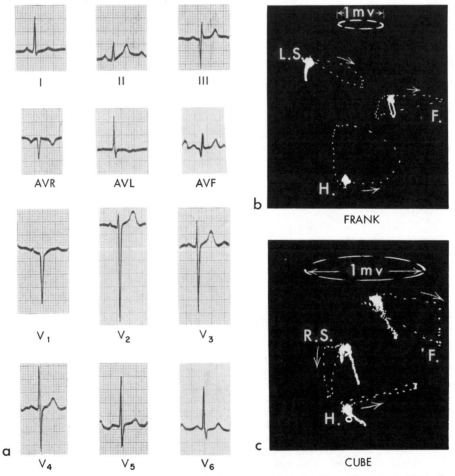

Fig. 22.3 Electrocardiographic and vectorcardiographic features in corrected transposition with no associated effects and hemodynamically normal heart in a 7 year old. (*a*) *Electrocardiogram.* The following features are shown: abnormally deep Q wave in lead III; left axis deviation; and reversal of normal precordial Q wave pattern. (*b*) *Vectorcardiogram* (Frank lead system). The following features are shown: clockwise inscription of QRS loop in frontal plane (*F.*) with left axis deviation; direction of initial QRS vectors to left and slightly anterior in horizontal plane (*H.*). *L.S.*, left sagittal. (*c*) *Vectorcardiogram* (Grishman cube lead system) demonstrating posterior direction of initial QRS vectors with this lead system, as compared to the Frank system. *R.S.*, right sagittal.

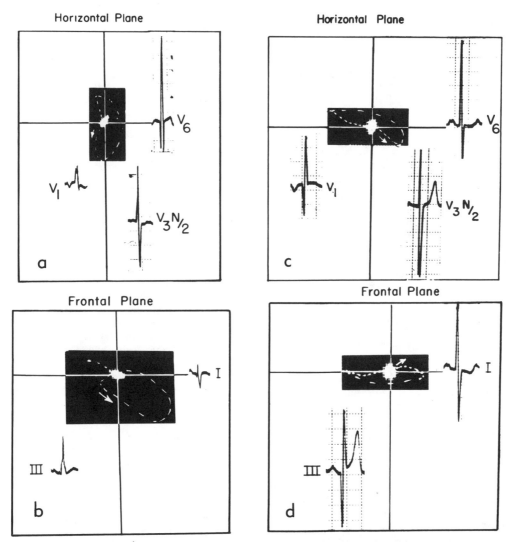

Fig. 22.4 Comparative electrocardiographic and vectorcardiographic findings in a case without transposition (*a*), and in a case with corrected transposition (*b*), each with ventricular septal defect, large left to right shunt, and pulmonary hypertension. (Schmitt vector lead system). (*a*) 1.5 year old with no transposition. *Upper left*, a large Q loop is represented by a large Q wave in V6. Combined ventricular hypertrophy demonstrated by QRS loop (reduced ½ standard size) and QRS complexes, (V3 reduced ½ standard size = N/2). *Lower left*, note the counterclockwise inscription of QRS loop and absence of Q wave in lead III. (*b*) 2.5 year old with corrected transposition. *Upper right*, the typical features are: straight line contour of the initial segment of the QRS loop (¼ standard size), initial QRS vectors directed to the left and anteriorly (absence of Q loop), absence of Q wave in V6, and presence of Q wave in V1. Combined ventricular hypertrophy demonstrated by QRS loop and QRS complexes. *Lower right*, typical features are superior direction of initial QRS vectors with abnormally large Q wave in III. (Reproduced with permission from The American Journal of Cardiology and Reuben H. Donnelley, publisher.)

judged by the RS complexes of the electrocardiogram and the contour and size of the QRS loop of the vectorcardiogram, correlate well with the ventricular overload. In a few cases, however, an indeterminate hypertrophy pattern is present,[16] and the QRS loop is oriented posteriorly in the midline. The ECG manifestations are rS patterns in the standard precordial leads. While the right precordial leads suggest left ventricular hypertrophy, the left precordial leads suggest right ventricular hypertrophy. Thus, the hypertrophy pattern is indeterminate. The terms *right* and *left* ventricular hypertrophy or pressure, as used in this section, refer to the venous and arterial ventricles, respectively.

Left axis deviation, clockwise loop in the frontal plane, and left ventricular hypertrophy patterns are present in the infrequent case of corrected transposition with either isolated left-sided lesion or VSD and normal right ventricular pressures. Most cases of corrected transposition have right axis deviation with clockwise loops in the frontal plane.

The electrocardiographic and vectorcardiographic features of corrected transposition with visceral-atrial situs inversus are the mirror image of those with visceral-atrial situs solitus. Thus, there are Q waves in leads V2 (V1R), V4 (V4R), and lead II (IIIR), with no Q waves in V6R.

When corrected transposition is associated with malposition of the cardiac apex (dextroversion or levoversion), the direction of the initial QRS vectors is variable. The direction depends, in part, on the degree of dextroversion or levoversion present. Dextroversion is usually accompanied by VSD, pulmonary arterial obstruction, and hemodynamic overload of the venous ventricle. In these cases, the initial QRS vectors are usually directed anteriorly and to the left, and either inferiorly or superiorly. The vector loop in the horizontal plane shows absence of the Q loop. Most cases show a leftward convexity of the initial segment of the QRS loop, which appears as the reverse of a Q loop. The electrocardiographic findings are absence of the Q wave in Leads V2 through V6. The QRS loop is usually a long narrow posterior clockwise loop directed toward the left, superior quadrant.

Disturbances in conduction and rhythm occur in about 60% of the cases. First degree block occurs in about 50%, and complete AV block occurs in 10 to 55%. Other degrees of AV dissociation occur as well as paroxysmal atrial tachycardia and the Wolff-Parkinson-White syndrome. AV dissociation tends to be progressive.

Phonocardiographic Features

There are no specific phonocardiographic features. However, Kraus et al.,[30] using the phonocardiogram, electrocardiogram, and percordial pulsations, found a reversal of precordial pulsations in 10 of 13 cases of corrected transposition. This finding was substantiated by data obtained at cardiac catheterization in three patients with corrected transposition and hemodynamically normal hearts.[48] Analysis of simultaneously recorded right and left ventricular high fidelity pressure tracings showed a reversal of pressure rise in these cases. This was in contrast to normal children, in whom left ventricular pressure rise precedes that of the right ventricle by an average of 13 milliseconds.

Echocardiographic Features

The diagnosis of corrected transposition is easily made with 2D echocardiography. In the short axial sweep from apex to base, the posterior medial great artery is seen to bifurcate into right and left pulmonary arteries while the other great artery (aorta) is visualized to the left and anteriorly. The ventricular septum is well seen in the apical or subxiphoid four-chamber view. The anatomy of the AV valves and ventricles may also be determined during the short axis sweep. The fishmouth appearance identifies the mitral valve on the right side. The left-sided ventricle may show the morphology of a right ventricle: it may appear coarsely trabeculated with an infundibular chamber located on the left and anteriorly. Single ventricle with L-transposition usually can be differentiated from corrected transposition when, in these views, the AV valve is seen to connect to their respective ventricular chambers. In some cases of single ventricle, the inverted (levo) infundibular chamber may be large and extended caudally. This appearance may mimic corrected transposition (in which two ventricles are present). Additionally, it may be difficult to be sure whether or not the left-sided AV valve is functionally related to the left-sided ventricle. In these instances, ventricular angiograms should define the anatomy and differentiate single ventricle from corrected transposition.

2D echocardiography is also helpful in determining the size and location of associated defects. It may also be possible to define Epstein's malformation of the systemic valve. The closure interval between the mitral and tricuspid valve have been shown to be abnormally long in Epstein's anomaly with or without ventricular inversion.[2]

Radiologic Features

Roentgenograms may suggest the presence of corrected transposition in some instances[8]; however, when it is not associated with other cardiac lesions or when there are minimal anomalies, the appearance of the heart may be within normal limits (Fig. 22.5a). In the right oblique view, however, the descending aorta does *not* cause an indentation of the barium-filled esophagus.

In cases with right to left shunts, the ascending aorta is enlarged and produces a prominent bulge at the upper left cardiac border (Fig. 22.5d). It should be appreciated, however, that the prominent ascending aorta is essentially only found when a predominant right to left shunt is present.

In cases with left to right shunts, the ascending aorta is normal in size and does not produce the characteristic prominence to the left upper cardiac border (Fig. 22.5c). The absence of a prominent bulge at the expected site of the main pulmonary artery in cases with increased pulmonary flow, therefore, should suggest corrected transposition. Actually, the pulmonary trunk is very large but its midline position hides it within the cardiac silhouette. Frequently, the enlarged main pulmonary artery produces an indentation in the left lateral wall of the barium-filled esophagus. Less frequently, the right pulmonary hilus is prominent and appears elevated with respect to the left hilus. This produces a "waterfall" appearance to the right hilus (Fig. 22.5c).

The presence of dextroversion or levoversion should suggest associated corrected transposition. When dextroversion is an additional anomaly in cases with right to left shunts, the enlarged aorta at the left upper cardiac border is helpful in establishing the diagnosis of corrected transposition (Fig. 22.5d). This sign is absent, however, in the rare case of corrected transposition with a right aortic arch.

In cases with visceral-atrial situs inversus and levoversion, the most commonly associated malformations are VSD and pulmonary stenosis or atresia with right to left shunt. In these, the enlarged ascending aorta produces a prominence at the upper right cardiac border.

CARDIAC CATHETERIZATION

The course of the catheter is a good method for establishing the diagnosis of corrected transposition. Although it is frequently difficult to pass the catheter from the venous ventricle into the pulmonary trunk, once entered, the posterior and midline position of this structure is an important diagnostic feature. It is necessary to view the position of the catheter in the lateral projection to note the posterior location of the pulmonary trunk since midline right ventricular outflow tracts are also seen in cases with mesoversion and no corrected transposition. In these, however, the pulmonary trunk originates anteriorly.

Retrograde passage of the catheter into the arterial ventricle establishes the typical position of the aorta and aortic valve in corrected transposition (Fig. 22.6c and d). This procedure demonstrates the superior location of the aortic valve and the course of the ascending aorta as it forms the upper left cardiac border. Once inside the left-sided ventricle, it is usually easy to pass the catheter into the left atrium.

Abnormalities in hemodynamic data are dependent on the associated lesions. The majority of cases have systemic pressures in the venous ventricle owing to a large VSD with pulmonary hypertension or pulmonary stenosis. His bundle recordings can be useful in the diagnosis and management of dysrhythmias so common in this condition.[22]

ANGIOCARDIOGRAPHY

Angiocardiography is the most accurate method in the diagnosis of corrected transposition and associated lesions. Not only do the position of the great arteries become obvious, but also the typical inverted architecture of the ventricle may be seen (Fig. 22.6). The ventricles tend to lie side by side with the ventricular septum oriented in an anterior-posterior direction, slanting obliquely from right-superior to left-inferior (Fig. 22.2). The venous ventricle in the frontal projection appears triangular with a tail-like projection to the left which forms the inferior margin of the ventricular

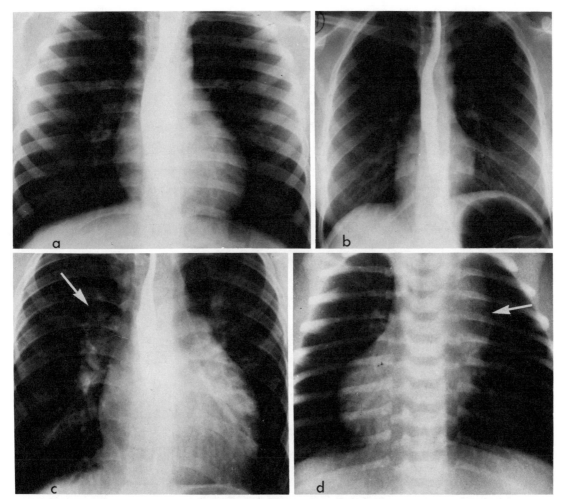

Fig. 22.5 Roentgenograms in corrected transposition with visceral-atrial situs solitus. (a) 7 year old with no associated defects and hemodynamically normal heart. (b) 14 year old with no associated defects and hemodynamically normal heart and mild dextroversion (mesoversion). (c) 8 year old with ventricular septal defect, left to right shunt, and pulmonary hypertension. Prominence of right pulmonary artery ("waterfall" appearance) denoted by *arrow*. (d) 2 day old with dextroversion, ventricular septal defect, pulmonary atresia, and right to left shunt. Dilated ascending aorta forms the prominence at upper left cardiac border (*arrow*).

mass (Fig. 22.6a). The arterial ventricle forms a round mass to the left of the venous ventricle and "sits" on the tail of the venous ventricle (Fig. 22.6c). The pulmonary trunk arises in the midline while the aorta originates from a more superior position and forms the left upper border of the cardiac silhouette.

In the lateral projection, the venous ventricle extends to the anterior limit of the ventricular mass and has the appearance of an inverted cone (Fig. 22.6b). Anteriorly, the cavity ends in a superior blind recess, while posteriorly the superior aspect of the inverted cone feeds into the posteriorly located pulmonary trunk. The arterial ventricle shows the characteristics of a right ventricle: an anterior-superior infundibular chamber bordered posteriorly by a crista superventricularis and a posteriorly located inflow portion of the ventricle. The aorta takes origin from the superiorly located aortic valve and ascends steeply superiorly before arching posteriorly (Fig. 22.6d).

In cases with dextroversion, the angiographic findings depend on the degree of dextroversion. Most cases are mild (mesoversion). In these, the arterial ventricle lies on the left while the venous ventricle lies either directly over or slightly to the right of the spine (Fig. 22.7). The venous ventricle

appears oval in contour with no "tail." The great arteries remain essentially in the characteristic position. The pulmonary trunk may originate to the right of the spine and ascend obliquely to the left while the aorta remains to the left of the pulmonary trunk. In extreme dextroversion, the arterial ventricle may be completely to the right and form the right-sided apex, whereas the venous ventricle lies posterior and to the right. The pulmonary trunk arises posteriorly and to the right of the aorta while the aorta arises to the right of the midline and ascends obliquely to the left, still anterior to the pulmonary trunk. When a right aortic arch is present with dextroversion, the diagnosis of corrected transposition is more difficult. In the lateral view, however, the aorta still remains anterior to the pulmonary trunk.

Selective ventriculography is the most effective procedure to demonstrate the anatomic characteristics. In cases with single ventricle and L-transposition, however, the angiographic appearance of the ventricular chamber may be misleading.[9] Occasionally, the large infundibular chamber in common ventricle is mistaken for the arterial ventricle, Left atrial injections may be required to demonstrate the common ventricle. Also, in most cases of common ventricle, the aortic and pulmonary valves are located near to or in the

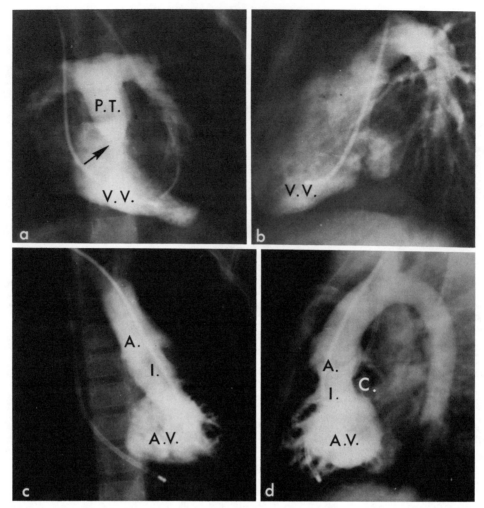

Fig. 22.6 Angiocardiographic features of corrected transposition with no associated malformation and hemodynamically normal heart. (*a* and *b*) Selective angiogram from venous ventricle (*V.V.*) in diastole: (*a*) anterior view and (*b*) lateral view demonstrating smooth-walled ventricular chamber with medial and posterior pulmonary trunk (*P.T.*). *Arrow* points to septal leaflet of mitral valve. "Inverted cone" appearance of venous ventricle seen in the lateral. (*c* and *d*) Selective angiogram from arterial ventricle (*A.V.*). (*c*) Anterior view and (*d*) lateral view demonstrate the inverted nature of the left-sided arterial ventricle. It is coarsely trabeculated and possesses an infundibular chamber (*I.*) and crista supraventricularis (*C.*). The typical course of the ascending aorta (*A.*) is shown as it arises anteriorly and forms the left upper cardiac border.

same transverse plane, a finding which is in contrast to the relationship of the semilunar valves in corrected transposition.

Selective aortography may demonstrate the inverted coronary arterial pattern, which is virtually always present in corrected transposition. Although this pattern may also be present in common ventricle with L-transposition, the absence of the inverted coronary pattern excludes the diagnosis of corrected transposition.

An arterial ventriculogram should *always* be obtained because of the high frequency of insufficiency of the arterial atrioventricular valve. Adequate ventriculograms not only allow for estimation of the degree of insufficiency but also may permit identification of the type of valvular malformation.[29] Angiographic differentiation between Ebstein's anomaly and the less common deformed but normally positioned arterial AV valve is dependent upon the position of the true tricuspid annulus and the leaflets, which is best seen in the frontal view. In Ebstein's, the leaflets are displaced distal to the true valve annulus. The level of the annulus may be identified by opacification of the circumflex branch of the

transposed left coronary artery which passes posteriorly in the AV groove.

DIFFERENTIAL DIAGNOSIS

It is easy to differentiate corrected transposition from other malformations when 2D echocardiography is combined with cardiac catheterization and selective angiography. Those conditions which may mimic corrected transposition are: L-transposition with single ventricle and double outlet left or right ventricle with L-malposition.

TREATMENT

Appropriate medical and surgical treatment depend on the clinical manifestations of associated lesions, dysrrhythmias, and conduction disturbances. The basic malformation of ventricular inversion (or atrial-ventricular discordance) and L-transposition presents specific problems to the surgeons. The problems are related, in part, to the AV conduction system, the coronary arterial pattern, and the frequent

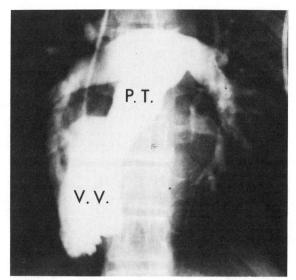

Fig. 22.7 Corrected transposition with mild dextroversion, no associated lesions, and hemodynamically normal heart (see Fig. 22.5b). Selective angiogram from the venous ventricle (*V.V.*) demonstrating position of ventricle to right of spine with medially located pulmonary trunk (P.T.).

occurrence of cardiac malposition. Problems created by passage of the right coronary artery across the pulmonary outflow tract, the location of the pulmonary outflow tract deeply wedged into the ventricular chamber between the AV valves, the location of the AV conduction pathway, the presence of malrotation of the ventricles, and the high frequency of systemic AV valve insufficiency have led to alternative approaches to surgical repair. The triad of ventricular septal defect, pulmonary outflow tract obstruction, and systemic AV valve insufficiency account for almost all open heart operations in patients with corrected transposition. Each of the problems will be discussed separately in regards to surgical treatment.

Ventricular Septal Defect. When ventricular septal defect is isolated or associated with pulmonary stenosis, the safest and most effective surgical approaches are: through the right atrium (in which case it may be necessary to detach the septal leaflet of the mitral valve) and through the root of the aorta in older children. When extreme dextroversion is present, the atrial approach may not allow for adequate exposure, and an approach through the pulmonary ventricle is recommended.[35] Repair of the VSD through the systemic ventricle is not recommended because of the reportedly high mortality rate.[35] Some surgeons have used a pulmonary ventriculotomy and placed the patch on the left (systemic) side of the septum. This technique is used to avoid the AV conduction system, which courses anterior to the pulmonary outflow tract around the anterior rim of the defect on the right (pulmonary) side of the septum.[13]

Ventricular Septal Defect and Pulmonary Stenosis. The forms of pulmonary outflow tract obstruction which are easily relieved by conventional techniques are pulmonary valvular stenosis, pulmonary band, and subpulmonic redundant tissue. Severe subpulmonic stenosis, however, is not successfully relieved by the conventional techniques of infundibulectomy and outflow tract patch because of problems discussed earlier. It is recommended that with severe subpulmonic stenosis, the VSD is closed through a pulmonary ventriculotomy, and the subpulmonic stenosis is bypassed with an external valved conduit.[35]

Systemic AV Valvular Insufficiency. The common association of clinically significant systemic AV valvular insufficiency may further complicate cardiac surgery for corrected transposition. In addition to patching the ventricular septal defect and/or relieving the pulmonary stenosis, the surgeon may find it necessary to repair the AV valve. This increases the risk of the procedure and may make the risk unacceptably high. This possibility may necessitate an alternative approach other than complete repair.

AV Conduction System. Intraoperative mapping of the conduction system has reduced the complication of complete heart block after open heart surgery in this condition.[31, 33, 35, 57] Marcelleti et al.[35] reported successful mapping in 27 of 32 patients in which electrograms of the common bundle were recorded along the anterior edge of the junction between the pulmonary (right-sided) AV valve annulus and the anterior rightward border of the pulmonary valve annulus in 24 patients with situs solitus.[35] In these, the bundle passed leftward and descended along the anterior rim of the septal defect. In the remaining three patients (two with situs inversus and one with dextroversion), the intraventricular course of the bundle was along the posterior rim of the septal defect. Seventeen of the 27 patients had normal sinus rhythm postoperatively, which suggests that mapping may have avoided AV block in 60% of the patients. Some have recommended that permanent pacing wires be left in all patients with corrected transposition at surgery since development of AV dissociation is a common occurrence.[14] The Wolff-Parkinson-White syndrome is common in corrected transposition but intraoperative mapping of the accessory pathways has been less successful in these patients.[35]

Prognosis. In general, the prognosis for children with corrected transposition is not as favorable as for those patients without it but with similar associated defects. Not only are the mortality and morbidity rates higher for cardiac surgery patients, but also, even without surgery, these patients tend to develop AV dissociation and tachyarrhythmias. Sudden unexpected death is not uncommon and is usually associated with preexisting complete AV block.[14]

SYNDROME OF CONGENITAL CARDIAC DISEASE WITH ASPLENIA

The striking association of agenesis of the spleen (asplenia) with cyanotic congenital cardiac disease and malposition of the abdominal viscera has been well documented. The cardiac anomalies are complex and multiple and usually include a combination of the following: transposition of the great arteries; pulmonary atresia or severe stenosis; large defects or absence of the atrial and ventricular septae; atrioventricular canal; anomalous pulmonary venous connections; bulboventricular inversion; and persistence of both superior venae cavae with absence of the coronary sinus. The number and complexity of the cardiac lesions present in each case frequently preclude surgical correction with present techniques. It is important, therefore, for the physician to recognize this syndrome and distinguish it from other forms of cyanotic congenital cardiac disease, many of which are more amenable to surgical therapy.

Martin[36] first described the syndrome of absence of the spleen and cyanotic congenital cardiac disease. Since then, this syndrome has been reported with increasing frequency. Putschar and Manion[43] reviewed 77 cases of asplenia, among which were 53 cases with congenital cardiac disease. Ivemark[28] reported 69 cases of this syndrome, 14 of which were his own. In these two large reviews, many cases were common to both series so that 80 cases were reviewed in all.

Ivemark commented that this syndrome was found in 11 of 7032 necropsies at the Boston Children's Hospital, which indicated a prevalence of about 0.1%. Gasser and Willi[21] found a prevalence of 1% of neonatal deaths which occurred over a 5-year period.

PATHOLOGY

The abdominal and cardiac malpositions and complex cardiac malformations characteristic of the asplenia syndrome suggest an early arrest in development of these organs. Gasser and Willi[21] and Ivemark[28] suggested that gestation occurs at the time during which the anlage of the spleen, the endocardial cushions, and the conotruncal area develop. Towers and Middleton,[52] however, reasoned that since systemic venous abnormalities occur, the process must start in the 24th to 27th days of postovulatory embryogenesis. The reader is referred to Freedom's extensive discussion of the embryology of this syndrome.[19]

In the typical case of asplenia, there is a persistence of early fetal bilaterality. The dorsal mesentery persists and is associated with malrotation of the intestines, including the duodenum and pancreas. Each lung has three lobes with eparterial bronchi,[54] the cardiac apex and/or stomach are often located on the right, and the liver is large and transverse as if there were two right lobes. Moreover, cor biloculare is commonly present with a functionally single great vessel supplying the circulation. The right and left atrial chambers have been shown to have the anatomic characteristics of a right atrium (atrial isomerism).[53] The three-lobed lungs and the appearance of the atria and liver have led some to describe this syndrome as demonstrating bilateral right-sidedness. In addition to the above complexities, the presence of bilateral superior vena cava and anomalous pulmonary venous connections produces a confused hemodynamic and anatomic situation in which it becomes very difficult to classify the type of cardiac malposition present. In asplenia, there is no constant relation between the arterial atrium. Each atrium resembles a right atrium and is supplied by a superior vena cava. Moreover, anomalous pulmonary venous connections further complicate identification of venous and arterial atrium. The absence of an atrial septum further ensures the complete mixing of systemic and pulmonary venous blood so that there is no hemodynamic basis for identifying arterial or venous chambers.

The uncertainty of the type of situs present in this syndrome creates difficulties in the classification of cases of asplenia. For example, many cases of asplenia have two ventricles and are classified as corrected transposition in the forthcoming section. In each of these, there is dextrocardia and a right-sided stomach. The additional fact that the ventricles are inverted (the right-sided ventricle is an anatomic left ventricle and the left-sided ventricle is an anatomic right ventricle) suggests that this arrangement may be a mirror image dextrocardia with complete transposition rather than a dextroversion with corrected transposition.

A pathologic classification for cases of asplenia is presented in this chapter while the uncertainties of classification based on situs and hemodynamics is recognized. This classification has been established because of the variations which exist within this syndrome and in order to relate these malformations to similar forms of cyanotic congenital cardiac disease that occur without asplenia. This classification, listed in Table 22.1, includes 17 cases previously reported[49] and six additional cases from the UCLA Hospital. The malformations in these cases conform with those reported in other series.

Case reports of the asplenia syndrome with no pulmonary

stenosis are rare. Truncus arteriosus has been reported,[28] but there is reason to believe that these cases actually had pulmonary atresia with no central pulmonary arteries (pseudotruncus).[19] Other rare cardiac malformations reported with the asplenia syndrome are hypoplastic left heart with aortic atresia, aortic stenosis, and coarctation of the aorta.[19]

Noncardiac anomalies include genitourinary in 15% and *bilateral trilobed* lungs in the majority of cases, while some have bilateral bilobed lungs or situs inversus of the lungs imperforate anus, and fused or horseshoe adrenals.[45] Abdominal heterotaxia is found in 90% of patients with the asplenia syndrome.

In a review of 32 necropsied cases, Rose *et al.*[45] found the following frequencies of cardiovascular anomalies: atrial septal defect in 100%, absent coronary sinus and defects in the ventricular septum in 90%, single AV valve in 87%, anomalous pulmonary venous connection in 84%, transposition of the great arteries in 81%, pulmonary stenosis or atresia in 78%, bilateral SVC in 53%, dextrocardia and single ventricle in 44%, and single coronary artery in 19%.

About one-half of the cases reviewed in this section have common atrial and ventricular chambers. When the ventricular septum is absent, an infundibulum is present at the base of the common ventricular chamber. When the infundibulum lies in the approximate position of the right ventricular infundibulum of a normal heart, the term *common ventricle with noninversion of the infundibulum* is used. *Common ventricle with inversion of the infundibulum* is the term applied when the infundibular chamber lies in the position of that found in the arterial ventricle under the conditions of inversion of the ventricles. This is commonly called single or common ventricle with L-transposition[55] since the position of the great vessels is similar to that in corrected transposition (in which a septum is present and the ventricles are inverted).

The malposition of the abdominal viscera is variable with respect to position of the stomach. Terms applied to abdominal malpositions such as *partial situs inversus* or *abdominal situs inversus* include all varieties. The term *abdominal heterotaxia* is preferred since the other terms imply a mirror image arrangement of the abdominal organs. Abdominal heterotaxia, as used here, applied to those cases with a right-sided stomach and a transverse or nearly symmetrical liver (Fig. 22.8). Additional malpositions, such as malrotation, may be present. In none of the cases reviewed was a complete abdominal situs inversus present.

TABLE 22.1   CLASSIFICATION OF MAJOR CARDIAC MALFOR-MATIONS IN 23 CASES WITH AGENESIS OF THE SPLEEN

Group I. Two ventricles: large ventricular septal defect	
A. Inversion of ventricles	
1. Origin of transposed aorta from arterial ventricle; pulmonary trunk from venous ventricle (corrected transposition of the great arteries); pulmonary atresia	5 cases
2. Origin of both great arteries from the arterial ventricle: pulmonary stenosis	
(a) Patent atrioventricular valves	3 cases
(b) Atresia of arterial atrioventricular valve	1 case
B. Noninversion of ventricles; complete transposition of great arteries; pulmonary stenosis or atresia	3 cases
Group II. Common ventricle.	
A. Great arteries transposed: pulmonary stenosis or atresia	10 cases
B. Great arteries normally related: pulmonary stenosis	1 case

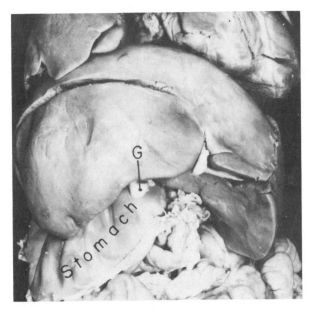

Fig. 22.8 Abdominal heterotaxia in case of asplenia. Upper abdominal viscera and lower thoracic organs (diaphragm removed). Abdominal heterotaxia indicated by right-sided stomach located under large transverse liver. Cardiac apex on left side (case of common ventricle). The gallbladder (G) lies just to right of midline. (Reproduced with permission from the American Journal of Cardiology and Reuben H. Donnelley, publisher.)

The pathologic features in each of 23 cases are summarized in Table 22.2. Certain features will be covered in detail.

The Atrial Septum and the Atrioventricular Valves

In 19 of 23 cases, there were two large distinct atrial septal defects (Fig. 22.9c). The first lay in the general region of the fossa ovalis, while the second occupied the position seen in atrioventricular canal. The only remnant of the atrial septum in these cases was a thin strand of tissue extending into the midline from the posterior to the anterior walls of the atrial portion of the heart between the coexistent large atrial defects. Two atrial appendages were present. This type of atrial arrangement has often been termed a *common atrium.* The lower part of the septum was absent in each ("ostium primum" defect). In 22 of the 23 cases, there was a common atrioventricular valve, regardless of the presence or absence of a ventricular septum.

The Ventricles and Great Arteries

Malformations of the ventricles and great arteries were present in each case. The 23 cases are divided into two main groups as shown in Table 22.1. In group I are placed those cases with two ventricles, while group II consists of those cases in which a common ventricle was present. The cases in these two groups are further divided into subgroups, depending on the presence or absence of ventricular inversion (L-transposition) in group I, and the presence or absence of transposition of the great arteries in group II.

Group I: Two Ventricles

This group, composed of 12 cases, was characterized by the presence of a large ventricular septal defect, transposition of the great arteries, and pulmonary stenosis or atresia. In nine of these, ventricular inversion (L-transposition) was

present. These cases were further subdivided according to the pattern of arterial origin.

Subgroup A1. Inversion of Ventricles: Large Ventricular Septal Defect, L-Transposition, Pulmonary Atresia, and Dextroversion. This pattern, which is identical with that of corrected transposition of the great arteries, represents one of the two most commonly observed anomalous arrangements in the cases studied. In each case, a large VSD lay beneath a common atrioventricular valve (Fig. 22.9c and d). The internal architecture of each ventricle was, in essence, a mirror image of the contralateral ventricle of normal hearts. The pulmonary valve arose from the right-sided ventricle and was atretic in each case. Atrioventricular valvular tissue appeared to be continuous with the atretic pulmonary valve. In each instance the ascending aorta curved above the left margin of the heart as in corrected transposition of the great arteries (L-malposition) (Fig. 22.9a).

Subgroup A2. Inversion of Ventricles: Origin of Both Great Arteries from Arterial Ventricles, Large Ventricular Septal Defect, Pulmonary Stenosis, and Dextrocardia. In each of the four hearts in this subgroup, the ventricular portion of the heart was similar to that in subgroup A1. In contrast to that subgroup, both great arteries arose from the arterial ventricle (Fig. 20.9). The aorta arose anteriorly from the infundibulum as in corrected transposition (L-transposition). The pulmonary trunk arose from behind the crista supraventricularis. The only outlet for the venous ventricle was the large VSD.

In each case the pulmonary valve was bicuspid and stenotic (Fig. 22.9d). In addition, a zone of stenosis beneath the pulmonary valve was present within the arterial ventricle in each.

Subgroup B. Two Ventricles without Inversion: D-Transposition, Pulmonary Atresia, or Stenosis. This subdivision, in which there were three cases, is essentially the condition called complete D-transposition of the great arteries. The pulmonary valve was atretic in two and stenotic in the other. Only one case was associated with abdominal heterotaxia.

Group II: Common Ventricle

The 11 cases forming the second major division were characterized by a common ventricle with pulmonary stenosis or atresia. In 10 of these, the great arteries were transposed (subgroup A), and in the remaining case (subgroup B) were normally related.

Subgroup A. Common Ventricle: Transposed Great Arteries, Pulmonary Stenosis, or Atresia. The second group was characterized by a common atrioventricular valve leading into a common ventricle, and transposition of the great arteries (Fig. 22.10). In each of the 10 cases the aorta arose anteriorly from the infundibular subdivision of the common ventricular chamber.

The infundibulum was considered to be inverted in six of this subgroup since it was located at the left anterior basal aspect of the common ventricle (Fig. 22.10). In the remaining four, the infundibulum was not inverted. The aorta lay anterior and to the left of the pulmonary trunk in each of the 10 cases (L-transposition). In two, the relatively large size of the infundibulum suggested that it was a second ventricular chamber (Fig. 22.10a). In no case, however, was there a direct communication between the infundibular chamber and atrioventricular valvular elements.

Severe pulmonary stenosis occurred in five cases and valvular atresia in five cases. The aortic arch was on the left side in six instances. The cardiac apex was on the left side in

TABLE 22.2   SUMMARY OF FINDINGS IN 23 PATIENTS WITH AGENESIS OF THE SPLEEN

Case No.	Age	Sex	Pulmonary Valve	AV Valves	Atrial Septum	Card. Apex	Abdom. Organs	Aortic Arch	Duct. Art.	Bilat. SVC	APVC to
							Position				
Group I. Two Ventricles (VSD)											

Group I. Two Ventricles (VSD)
Subgroup A1. Transposed Great Arteries Arising from Inverted Ventricles

Case No.	Age	Sex	Pulmonary Valve	AV Valves	Atrial Septum	Card. Apex	Abdom. Organs	Aortic Arch	Duct. Art.	Bilat. SVC	APVC to
1	36 hr	M	PA[f]	C	S, P	D	H	L	LP	+	0
2	2 mo	F	PA	C	S, P	D	H	L	LP	+	0[a]
3	6 mo	F	PA	C	S, P	D	H	L	LP	0	Port. vein
4	7 wk	F	PA	C	S, P	D	H	R	LL	+	RSVC
5	3 wk	M	PA	C	S, P	D	H	L	RL	+	0

Subgroup A2. Transposed Great Arteries Arising from Inverted Arterial Ventricle

6	2 mo	M	PS	C	S, P	D	S	L	RP	+	0[b]
7	16 hr	M	PS	C	S, P	D	H	L	LL	+	RSVC
8	10 days	M	PS	C	S, P	D	H	L	0?	+	0
9	4 yr	M	PS	AA	S, P	I	H	R	LL	+	0

Subgroup B. Complete Transposition without Ventricular Inversion

10	6 wk	F	PA	C	S, P	S	S	L	0	+	Port. vein
11	3 mo	M	PA	C	S, P	S	H	R	?	+	Port. vein
12	19 yr	M	PS	C	S, P	S	S	L	0	+	0

Group II. Common Ventricle
Subgroup A. Transposed Great Arteries (Infundibular Inversion: Cases 13–18)

13	3 wk	M	PS	C	P[c]	D	S	L	LP	+	LSVC
14	1 yr	M	PS	C	S, P	S	H	L	LL	0	0
15	2 yr	M	PS	C	P[d]	D	H	L	0	+	†
16	2 mo	F	PA	C	P[c]	S	H	R	LP	+	RSVC
17	9 days	F	PA	C	S, P	S	H	L	LP	+	RSVC
18	3 days	M	PA	C	S, P	S	H	R	RP	+	RA
19	6 hr	M	PA	C	S, P	S	H	R	RP	+	RSVC
20	5 wk	F	PA	C	S, P	S	H	L	LP	+	Port. vein
21	1 mo	M	PA	C	S, P	S	H	L	LP	0	Port. vein
22	19 days	F	PA	C	S, P	S	H	R	RP	+	RA, RSVC

Subgroup B. Great Arteries Normally Related

| 23 | 10 yr | M | PS | C | P[e] | S | H | L | LL | + | RA |

[a] Left upper pulmonary vein to arterial side, common trunk for all other pulmonary veins to venous side of common atrium.

[b] Common pulmonary vein to arterial atrium.

[c] Foramen ovale probe patent.

[d] Foramen ovale closed.

[e] Three small defects in foramen ovale.

[f] PA, pulmonary atresia; PS pulmonary stenosis; C, common AV canal; AA, atresia of arterial AV valve; S, P, coexisting superior (S, ostium secundum) and inferior (P, ostium primum) defects with rudimentary strand, the only remnant of atrial septum (common atrium); APVC, anomalous pulmonary venous connection; D, dextroversion; H, heterotaxia; I, normal situs inversus position; S, normal situs solitus position; L, left; R, right; 0, absent; RP, right patent ductus; LP, left patent ductus; RL, right ligamentous ductus; LL, left ligamentous ductus.

eight and on the right in two cases (dextroversion). Abdominal heterotaxia was present in 9 of 10 instances, while in the 10th case the stomach was on the left side.

Subgroup B. Common Ventricle: Great Arteries Normally Related and Pulmonary Stenosis. In the 23rd case in the series, a common atrioventricular valve led into a common ventricle, and a normal external relationship existed between the great arteries. From the noninverted infundibular chamber of the common ventricle, the narrow pulmonary trunk arose in a normal position. The pulmonary valve was bicuspid and stenotic. The aortic valve lay to the right, slightly posterior and inferior to the plane of the pulmonary valve. Neither semilunar valve was in continuity with atrioventricular valvular tissue.

The aortic arch was on the left side, while the ascending aorta curved to the right above the base of the heart. The cardiac apex was on the left side, while the stomach lay on the right.

Associated Anomalies (Table 22.3)

Anomalies of systemic veins were a common finding in 22 cases. In 21, there was absence of the coronary sinus and bilateral superior venae cavae. The right and left superior venae cavae connected directly to the atria or to corresponding aspects of a common atrium.

The inferior vena cava joined the arterial side of the common atrium in four cases, and bilateral inferior venae cavae were present in one case with a common atrium.

Anomalous pulmonary venous connection of classic variety was observed in 15 instances (14 total and 1 partial). The sites of termination of the anomalous pulmonary veins are shown in Table 22.2. In addition to the 15 cases described above, two cases had a common pulmonary vein connected with the arterial atrium, and at this junction there was minimal obstruction. This condition is considered to be a mild form of cor triatriatum.

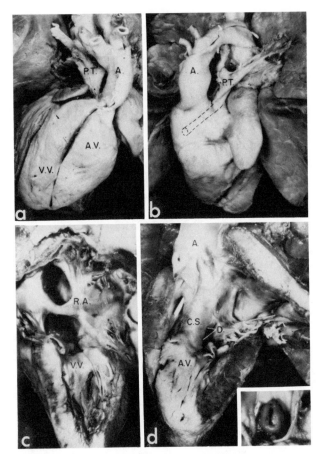

Fig. 22.9 Group 1, subgroup A2: origin of both great arteries from left-sided arterial ventricle. (*a*) Anterior view of arteries showing dextroversion and arrangement of great arteries as in corrected transposition. *P.T.*, pulmonary trunk; *A.*, aorta; *V.V.*, venous ventricle; *A.V.*, arterial ventricle. (*b*) Left lateral view showing aorta arising anterior to hypoplastic pulmonary trunk. *Dotted lines* are a diagrammatic representation of subpulmonary channel. (*c*) Right lateral interior view showing right side of common atrium (*R.A.*) and inverted venous ventricle. The only outlet of this chamber is the defect formed by the common atrioventricular canal. (*d*) Left lateral interior view of inverted arterial ventricle. The aorta arises anterior to the crista supraventricularis (*C.S.*). The probe is in the stenotic subpulmonary channel which courses obliquely posteriorly and superiorly to the stenotic pulmonary valve (*inset*). *D.*, ventrical septal defect. (Reproduced with permission from the British Heart Journal and B.M.A. House.)

Positional anomalies of the cardiac apex and other organs were present in each patient. It is apparent from Table 22.2 that abdominal heterotaxia was common, occurring in 19 cases, while transverse, nearly symmetrical livers were present in all cases in this study.

MANIFESTATIONS

Clinical Features

The usual infant with the asplenia syndrome has intense cyanosis from birth and dies within the first few months of life. Of the 23 cases reviewed in this chapter, 16 died within 2 months and six within the first 10 days of life. Historical and physical findings are nonspecific in defining the type of cyanotic cardiac disease. The syndrome is more common in males (2:1) than females.[54]

Detection of dextroversion and palpation of a transverse liver may suggest the syndrome. Systolic ejection murmurs of moderate intensity are usually heard along the left or right sternal border. The second sound is single and loud and maximal at the lower sternal border.

When absence of the spleen is suspected, a presumptive but not definitive diagnosis may be made by studies of the *peripheral blood* which should reveal Howell-Jolly and Heinz bodies in the red blood cells. Radioactive scan of the abdomen may demonstrate a transverse liver and is very useful in ruling out the presence of a spleen.[18]

Electrovectorcardiographic Features

The presence of a superior counterclockwise QRS loop in the frontal plane ("left axis deviation") in a cyanotic infant with decreased pulmonary flow may be helpful. The P-wave axis is usually inferior and anterior.

The QRS complexes of the precordial leads are strongly influenced by the malposition of the cardiac apex and by the presence of abnormal ventricular conduction associated with common ventricle[16] or ventricular inversion.[47] Dextroversion is associated with large RS complexes in the right precordial leads and progressively smaller complexes toward V6. The majority of cases have ventricular inversion or common ventricle, two conditions which are associated with distinctly abnormal initial QRS vectors. The initial vectors in these cases are usually directed to the left and are represented in the electrocardiogram by Q waves in the right precordial leads and absence of a Q wave in V6. The hypertrophy patterns are variable; the most common, however, is the indeterminate hypertrophy pattern.[16]

Echocardiographic Features

2D echocardiography is useful in defining the multiple and complex cardiovascular anomalies found in the asplenia syndrome. The long axial view should reveal a large single AV valve which is located in a large single ventricle or straddling a ventricular septum. There is no continuity between the AV valve and the semilunar valve or valves. When the transducer is moved superiorly to a transverse plane, a right and left superior vena cava may be imaged, as well as a large right or left aortic arch. The short axis view should demonstrate a large single ventricle or septal defect, a single AV valve, and an anterior infundibular chamber from which a large semilunar valve originates. The main pulmonary artery appears hypoplastic or cannot be imaged, and the pulmonary arterial branches are hypoplastic. The subxiphoid four-chamber view reveals an inferior vena cava and/or hepatic veins connecting to the right atrium. Hepatic veins may also be seen connecting to the left atrium. If infradiaphragmatic total anomalous pulmonary venous return is present, the common pulmonary vein may be imaged as it descends caudally through the diaphragm. Anomalous pulmonary veins may also be suspected when the pulmonary veins are not seen to connect to the left atrium. Abdominal ultrasonography may reveal the abdominal aorta and inferior vena cava on the same side.

Radiologic Features

The chest roentgenogram frequently presents a picture which is characteristic of the asplenia syndrome (Fig. 22.11): decreased pulmonary flow, normal to slightly enlarged heart, malposition of the cardiac apex and/or stomach, and a transverse liver. A striking feature is the presence of a homogeneous density, often with a sharply defined lower margin, that occupies the major portion of the left upper abdominal quadrant. This density, representing a large left hepatic lobe, blends with the density of the right hepatic lobe to form a transverse orientation of the lower hepatic margin. Dextrocardia is present in about one-half of the

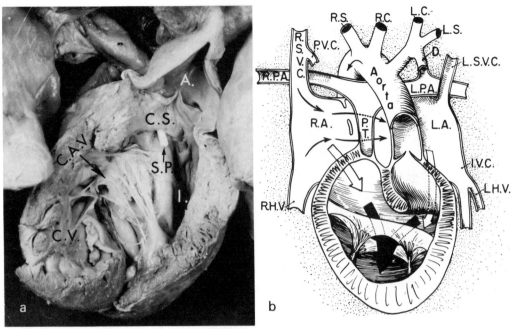

Fig. 22.10 Group II, subgroup A: common ventricle with transposition of the great arteries, L-transposition, and pulmonary atresia. (*A*) Anterior view of common ventricle (*C.V.*) with dextroversion. The aorta (*A.*) arises from a large inverted infundibular chamber (*I.*) and anterior to the crista supraventricularis (*C.S.*). The probe (*S.P.*) is in the subpulmonary stenotic chamber, which takes origin from the common ventricle posterior to the crista. A common atrioventricular (*C.A.V.*) valve leads into the common chamber. (*B*) Diagrammatic representation of case from group II, subgroup A: common ventricle with transposition of great arteries and pulmonary atresia. In addition to total anomalous pulmonary venous connection (*P.V.C.*) to the right superior vena cava (*R.S.V.C.*), there is a left superior vena cava (*L.S.V.C.*) and an inferior vena cava (*I.V.C.*) entering the left side of the common atrium (*L.A.*) after receiving the left hepatic veins (*L.H.V.*). The right hepatic vein (*R.H.V.*) enters the right side of the common atrium (*R.A.*). *Large arrows* show pathway of blood as it passes through atrioventricular canal into a common ventricle and out an inverted infundibular chamber to the aorta. A right aortic arch with mirror image branching is shown. A patent ductus (*D.*) connects the innominate and left pulmonary artery (*L.P.A.*). *R.S. and R.C.*, right subclavian and right common carotid arteries; *L.C. and L.S.*, left common carotid and left subclavian arteries which arise from a left innominate artery; *R.P.A.*, right pulmonary artery; *P.T.*, pulmonary trunk. (Reproduced with permission from The American Journal of Cardiology and Reuben H. Donnelley, publisher.)

cases. The main pulmonary artery segment is often difficult to visualize. The large aorta frequently produces a prominent convex density in the upper mediastinum, either to the right or left. If the tracheobronchial tree is well visualized on the frontal chest film, isometric bilateral eparterial bronchi may be identified, which suggests bilateral trilobed lungs.[54]

Cardiac Catheterization and Angiocardiography

Since these infants are critically ill, it is the obligation of the cardiologist to prepare a well thought out plan of catheterization and angiocardiography. Precise physiologic data are difficult to obtain. It is usually impossible to pass the catheter tip into the pulmonary trunk, so angiographic demonstration of the pulmonary veins cannot be accomplished in the usual manner and pulmonary venous obstruction and anomalous connection cannot be ruled out. The pulmonary arterial flow is greatly reduced and is usually supplied by a long, frequently abnormally located patent ductus arteriosus. If aortography doesn't adequately opacify the pulmonary artery, selective angiocardiography of the pulmonary arterial tree via the ductus arteriosus is the most effective method of delineating pulmonary venous drainage. Since the ductus may be the only source of pulmonary flow, this approach is dangerous. This procedure might be less dangerous if the ductus is dilated with prostaglandin E_1. If pulmonary stenosis is not severe, ventriculography may opacify the pulmonary arteries sufficiently to visualize the pulmonary veins during the levogram. The course of the catheter and/or opacification of the abdominal aorta and inferior vena cava may demonstrate both of these structures on the same side of the spine. This is an exclusive feature of asplenia[15] and polysplenia.

TREATMENT AND COURSE

In the majority of cases, palliative surgery offers some hope. Typically, complete intracardiac mixing is associated with inadequate pulmonary flow. Prostaglandin E_1 can improve oxygenation and allow for optimal stabilization before cardiac catheterization and surgery. Aortic-pulmonary shunts are effective in improving systemic oxygenation to the point where growth and development are satisfactory. When pulmonary venous obstruction is present, the situation is virtually hopeless.

If the infant has successful palliative surgery, then infection is the next hurdle the baby must overcome. The asplenia syndrome is associated with an increased risk of overwhelming infection. Waldman *et al.*[56] reported a frequency of 21% in 52 children with the asplenia syndrome. In their report, the etiologic agents in infants less than 6 months old were *Escherichia coli* and *Klebsiella. Streptococcus pneumoniae* and *H. influenza* were common in older children. Biggar *et al.*[7] reported immunologic deficiencies in the majority of eight children with asplenia syndrome. These authors recommended that, in all cases in which there is hope for survival, splenic function be assessed, prophylactic antibiotics be given when the diagnosis is established, and bacterial vaccines be given to children over 2 years of age.

SYNDROME OF CONGENITAL CARDIAC DISEASE WITH POLYSPLENIA

The presence of ectopic or accessory spleens is not necessarily associated with congenital cardiac disease. Polysplenia, however, is usually associated with complex cardiac

TABLE 22.3 SUMMARY OF FINDINGS IN 31 CASES WITH POLYSPLENIA SYNDROME[a]

Series	Total Cases	Interrupt. of IVC	APVC	Bilat. SVC	ASD[b]	AV Canal	VSD	DORV	PS	Abdominal Situs			Cardiac Apex		Other Cardiac Lesions
										Sol.	Inv.	Mixed	Left	Right	
Isabel-Jones et al.[27]	14	9	10	7	10	7	5	6	6	6	0	8	7	7	Hypoplastic left heart[6], single ventricle with TGA[1], DOLU[1]
Ongley et al.[41]	5	5	4	3	4	1	1	0	0	1	4	0	4	1	None
Moller et al.[37]	12	7	10	6	7	6	5	3	1	4	5	3	7‡	5	PDA[5] subaortic stenosis,[2] TGA[1]
Total	31	21	24	16	21	14	11	9	7	11	9	11	18	13	

[a] Abbreviations: IVC, inferior vena cava; APVC, anomalous pulmonary venous connection; SVC, superior vena cava; ASD, atrial septal defect; AV, atrioventricular; VSD, ventricular septal defect; DORV, double outlet right ventricle; PS, pulmonary stenosis; Sol, solitus; Inv, inversus; TGA, D-transposition of great arteries; PDA, patent ductus arteriosus.

[b] Not part of AV canal.

[c] One case has levoversion with situs inversus.

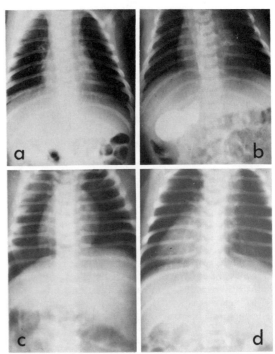

Fig. 22.11 Roentgenograms in three cases of asplenia. (a and b) Common ventricle with transposition of the great arteries (group II, subgroup A). The pulmonary vasculature is decreased, and there is a slight prominence of right superior mediastinum owing to the enlarged ascending aorta. The lower edge of the liver lacks the normal oblique orientation and tends toward the horizontal. (b) Barium in stomach demonstrates abdominal heterotaxia. (c) Corrected transposition with dextroversion and pulmonary atresia (group I, subgroup A1). The pulmonary vasculature is decreased, and the liver is represented by a large transverse density in upper abdomen. (d) Origin of both great arteries from the arterial ventricle with dextroversion and pulmonary stenosis (group 1, subgroup A2). The pulmonary vasculature is decreased. Enlarged aorta produces prominence of superior mediastinum on left. The shadow of the liver is transverse, and the barium-filled stomach is seen on left.

malformations and malpositions of the abdominal viscera. In a review of this subject, Moller and coworkers[37] defined the term polysplenia as that state in which splenic tissue is divided into two or more spleens of nearly equal size so that the total splenic mass approximates that of a single normal spleen. Certain malformations occur often enough in combination with multiple spleens to suggest a syndrome or clinical entity. Ongley and associates,[41] for example, reported five cases of a complex consisting of anomalous pulmonary venous connection to the right atrium, absence of the hepatic portion of the inferior vena cava with azygous continuation, atrial septal defect, situs inversus of abdominal organs, and multiple spleens. Moller and coworkers[37] studied 12 cases and found similar cardiac malformations in association with polysplenia. In addition, they brought attention to the tendency for isomerism or symmetry of organs. They contrasted the tendency in asplenia for bilateral right-sidedness (bilateral trilobed lungs with eparterial bronchi and bilateral right atria) with the tendency in polysplenia for bilateral left-sidedness (bilateral bilobed lungs with hyparterial bronchi and bilateral left atria).

PATHOLOGY

Pertinent pathologic findings in 31 cases of polysplenia are listed in Table 22.3. Malpositions of the liver, stomach, and cardiac apex are common in this syndrome, and abdominal heterotaxia is the rule. Van Mierop *et al.*[54] state that bilateral bilobed lungs with hyparterial bronchi are found in two-thirds of the cases. Peoples *et al.*,[42] in a review of 41 cases, reported similar findings and reported that 18% had bilateral trilobed lungs; also they noted that there were abdominal heterotaxia in 57% and abdominal situs inversus in 22%. The liver is frequently either transverse or has an abnormally large minor lobe. Isabel-Jones *et al.*,[27] in an unpublished review of 14 cases, found abnormalities of the gall bladder and extrahepatic bile ducts in seven cases: the gall bladder was absent in three cases, hypoplastic in two, and midline in three, and biliary atresia was present in two. The stomach is right-sided in about two-thirds of the cases, and malrotation of the intestines is very common.

The cardiovascular anomalies are complex and usually involve systemic and pulmonary veins, with atrial septal and endocardial cushion defects. Typically present are: absence of the hepatic portion of the inferior vena cava with azygous continuation on the right or left side (hereafter referred to as absent IVC); bilateral superior vena cava; anomalous pulmonary venous connection (usually veins from each lung drain into the ipsilateral atrium); bilateral left-sided atria (atrial isomerism); and atrial septal defect. Pulmonary stenosis occurs in one-third of the cases and is usually not severe. Nevertheless, pulmonary atresia has been reported in 9%.[42] Double outlet right ventricle occurs in 15 to 25% of the cases while D-transposition of the great arteries and single ventricle are very uncommon. Hypoplasia of the left-sided chambers is probably more common than previously believed. Isabel-Jones *et al.*[27] found varying degrees of hypoplasia of the left atrium and/or left ventricle in 6 of 14 cases. Peoples *et al.* reported left-sided obstruction in 50% and aortic atresia in 11%. In one-fourth of the cases of polysplenia, there is absence of significant cardiac anomalies.[54] These are usually patients with abdominal heterotaxia

who may have absent IVC as their only cardiovascular anomaly. Genitourinary anomalies occur in 15% of cases.[45]

MANIFESTATIONS

Clinical Features

The clinical features of the polysplenia syndrome are as variable as the combination of associated anomalies. The syndrome occurs equally often in males and females.[54] There does not appear to be a hereditary tendency in this syndrome.[45] Symptoms usually appear in infancy with signs of heart failure. Cyanosis is uncommon.[45] Dextrocardia and a transverse liver can be detected on physical examination, but the syndrome is usually suspected after reviewing the chest films and electrocardiogram.

Electrocardiographic Features

The most striking electrovectorcardiographic feature is the superior P axis (negative P waves in leads II, III and AVF), which is found in the majority of cases[38] and which may be associated with left atrial isomerism. A superior counterclockwise QRS loop in the frontal plane is often present and reflects the frequent occurrence of endocardial cushion defects. Atrioventricular dissociation is not common.

Radiologic Features

The roentgenographic features of the frontal and lateral chest films usually alert the clinician to the presence of the polysplenia syndrome, especially if the upper abdomen is included in the frontal film (Fig. 22.12). In general the pulmonary vascular markings are normal or increased. These features include a combination of right-sided stomach, a transverse liver, absent IVC, and less frequently dextrocardia. Absent IVC is suspected when, on the lateral film, the

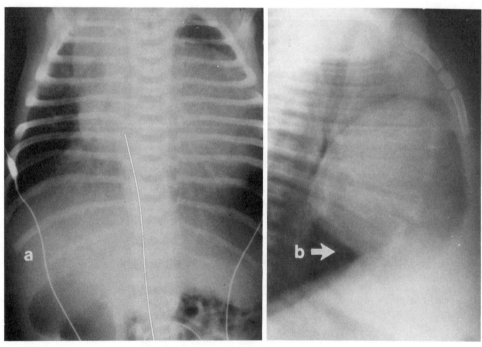

Fig. 22.12 Roentgenograms of thorax and upper abdomen in case of polysplenia with complete atrioventricular canal, severe pulmonary stenosis, absence of hepatic portion of inferior vena cava with azygous continuation to the left atrium, right aortic arch, and complete heart block. (*A*) Frontal view. Abdominal heterotaxia is suggested by the right-sided stomach and transverse liver. An umbilical arterial catheter demonstrates the right-sided aorta (the abdominal inferior vena cava was on the left). The heart is greatly enlarged, and the pulmonary vascular markings are decreased. (*B*) Lateral view: *arrow* points to junction of the diaphragm and cardiac silhouette where the expected curvilinear density of the hepatic portion of the inferior vena cava is absent.

normal inferior vena cava density is absent (Fig. 22.12b). With azygous continuation, the enlarged azygous arch, as it enters the superior vena cava, appears as a smooth, round prominence at the upper right or left base of the heart. This finding may be masked by the aortic arch if it is on the same side as the azygous arch. If the tracheobronchial tree is well visualized on the frontal chest film, isometric bilateral bronchi may be identified and may suggest bilateral bilobed lungs. An upper GI series may identify varying degrees of malrotation as well as a malpositioned stomach. *Radioactive scans* have been reported as helpful in demonstrating multiple spleens, a transverse liver, and abnormalities of the inferior vena cava.[18]

Echocardiographic Features

As in the asplenia syndrome, 2D echocardiography is very useful in defining the cardiovascular abnormalities. The usual views easily define the presence or absence of atrial and ventricular septal defects and AV canal. Hypoplasia of the left-sided structures can be detected. In the subxiphoid four-chamber view, the hepatic veins are seen to connect to the right atrium. Absence of the hepatic portion of the inferior vena cava is likely if the inferior vena cava cannot be found in its usual location caudal to the junction of hepatic veins and right atrium.

CARDIAC CATHETERIZATION AND ANGIOCARDIOGRAPHY

Because the cardiovascular malformations may be complex, the cardiologist should be as well informed as possible from the noninvasive studies and have a well thought out plan of attack, in order to perform a safe and thorough study. For example, if absent IVC is suspected, the cardiologist should be prepared to approach the heart from the arm veins. The use of a flow-directed catheter from below may overcome this problem. The primary goal of cardiac catheterization should be to rule in or rule out the cardiovascular anomalies commonly found in this syndrome, as well as the less common but serious malformations such as double outlet right ventricle and hypoplastic left-sided chambers.

DIFFERENTIAL DIAGNOSIS

This is primarily between the polysplenia and asplenia syndrome. The similarities between the syndromes are apparent. In general, the polysplenia syndrome is less severe, and the prognosis is better than for the asplenia syndrome. In contrast to asplenia, pulmonary arterial obstruction and maldevelopment of the ventricular septum and great arteries are less common in polysplenia and, when present, are less severe. Specific points of differentiation are the characteristic findings in the polysplenia syndrome of hyparterial bronchi, bilobed lungs, absent IVC, and superior P-wave axis. This is in contrast to a splenic syndrome in which is found eparterial bronchi and trilobed lungs, presence of the hepatic portion of the inferior vena cava, normal or rightward P-wave axis, and cyanosis associated with severe pulmonary arterial obstruction.

TREATMENT AND PROGNOSIS

The treatment and prognosis will depend on the combination and severity of the cardiovascular lesions present, as well as the degree to which the cardiovascular anomalies are delineated. In general, the prognosis is better for patients with polysplenia syndrome than for patients with asplenia syndrome. A greater proportion of patients with polysplenia syndrome are operable than those with asplenia. Yet, most of the infants with polysplenia and severely complicated cardiac malformations die within the first few years of life.[45]

In general, children with congenital heart disease and polysplenia have a higher mortality than children with similar cardiac anomalies but without polysplenia. In contrast to asplenia, severe infections do not appear to occur any more commonly in the polysplenia syndrome than in congenital heart disease without polysplenia.

REFERENCES

1. Allwork, S. P., Bentall, H. H., Becker, A. E., Cameron, H., Gerlis, L. M., Wilkinson, J. L., and Anderson, R. H.: Congenitally corrected transposition of the great arteries: Morphologic study of 22 cases. Am. J. Cardiol. 38:910, 1976.
2. Anderson, K. R., Danielson, G. K., McGoon, D. C., and Lie, J. T.: Ebstein's anomaly of the left-sided tricuspid valve. Circulation (Suppl. 1) 58:87–91, 1973.
3. Anderson, R. C., Lillehei, C. W., and Lester, R. G.: Corrected transposition of the great vessels of the heart: A review of 17 cases. Pediatrics 20:626, 1957.
4. Anderson, R. H., Becker, A. G., Arnold, R., and Wilkinsen, J. L.: The conduction tissues in congenitally corrected transposition. Circulation 50:911–923, 1974.
5. Anderson, R. H., Becker, A. G., and Gerlis, L. M.: The pulmonary outflow tract in classically corrected transpositions. J. Thorac. Cardiovasc. Surg. 747–757, 1975.
6. Anderson, R. H., Becker, A. E., Losekoof, T. G., and Gerlis, L. M.: Anatomically corrected transposition of the great arteries. Br. Heart J. 37:993, 1975.
7. Biggar, W. D., Ramirez, R. A., and Rose, V.: Congenital asplenia: Immunologic assessment and a clinical review of eight surviving patients. Pediatrics 67:548–551, 1981.
8. Carey, L. S., and Ruttenberg, H. D.: Roentgenographic features of congenital corrected transposition of the great vessels: A comparative study of 33 cases with roentgenographic classification based on the associated malformations and hemodynamic states. Am. J. Roentgenol. 92:623, 1964.
9. Carey, L. S., and Ruttenberg, H. D.: Roentgenographic features of common ventricle with inversion of the infundibulum. Corrected transposition with rudimentary left ventricle. Am. J. Roentgenol. 92:652, 1964.
10. Cummings, G. R.: Congenital corrected transposition of the great vessels without intracardiac anomalies: A clinical hemodynamic and angiographic study. Am. J. Cardiol. 10:605, 1962.
11. de la Cruz, M. V., Anselmi, G., Cisneros, F., Reinhold, M., Portillo, B., and Espino-Vela, J.: An embryologic explanation for the corrected transposition of the great vessels. Additional description of the main anatomic features of this malformation and its varieties. Am. Heart J. 57:104, 1959.
12. de la Cruz, M. V., and Miller, B. L.: Double inlet left ventricle. Circulation 37:249–262, 1968.
13. De Leval, M. R., Bastos, P., Stark, J., Taylor, F. N., Macartney, F. J., and Anderson, R. H.: Surgical techniques to reduce the risk of heart block following closure of ventricular septal defect in atrioventricular discordance. J. Thorac. Cardiovasc. Surg. 78:515–526, 1979.
14. Egloff, M., Rothlin, J., Schneider, G., Arbenz, V., Schönbeck, M., Senning, O., and Turina, M.: Congenitally corrected transposition of the great arteries: A clinical and surgical study. Thorac. Cardiovasc. Surg. 28(4):228–232, 1980.
15. Elliott, L. P., Cramer, C. G., and Amplatz, K.: The anomalous relationship of the inferior vena cava and abdominal aorta as a specific angiocardiographic sign in asplenia. Radiology 87:859, 1968.
16. Elliot, L. P., Ruttenberg, H. D., Eliot, R. S., and Anderson, R. C.: Vectorial analysis of the electrocardiogram in common ventricle. Br. Heart J. 26:302, 1964.
17. Fontana, R. S., and Edwards, J. E.: Congenital cardiac disease: A review of 357 cases studied pathologically. W. B. Saunders, Philadelphia, 1962, p. 40.
18. Freedom, R. M., and Treve, S.: Splenic scintigraphy and radionucleotide venography in the heterotaxy syndrome. Radiology 107:381–386, 1973.
19. Freedom, R. M.: Aortic valve and arch anomalies in the congenital asplenia syndrome. Case report, literative review and re-examination of the embryology of the congenital asplenia syndrome. Johns Hopkins Med. J. 135:124–135, 1974.
20. Friedberg, D. Z., and Nadas, A. S.: Clinical profile of patients with congenital corrected transposition of the great arteries: A study of

60 cases. N. Engl. J. Med. 282:1053–1059, 1970.

21. Gasser, C. V., and Willi, H.: Spontane Innenkörperbildung bei Milzagenesie. Helv. Paediatr. Acta, 7:369, 1952.

22. Gillette, P. C., Busch, V., Mullins, C. E., and McNamara, D. G.: Electrophysiologic studies in patients with ventricular inversion and "corrected transposition." Circulation 60:939–945, 1979.

23. Goodman, A. H., and Kuzman, W. J.: Functionally corrected transposition of the great vessels without significant associated defects. Am. Heart J. 61:811, 1961.

24. Grant, R. P.: The syndrome of dextroversion of the heart. Circulation 18:25, 1958.

25. Grant, R. P.: Morphogenesis of corrected transposition and other anomalies of cardiac polarity. Circulation 29:71, 1964.

26. Henry, J. G., Gordon, S., and Timmis, G. V.: Corrected transposition of great vessels and Ebstein's anomaly of tricuspid valve. Echocardiographic findings. Br. Heart J. 41:249–252, 1979.

27. Isabel-Jones, J. B., Ruttenberg, H. D., Jue, K. L., Linde, L. M., and Hurwitz, R. B.: The polysplenia syndrome: Observation in 14 cases. Unpublished data.

28. Ivemark, B. I.: Implications of agenesis of the spleen on the pathogenesis of conotruncus anomalies in childhood: An analysis of the heart malformations in the splenic agenesis syndrome, with fourteen new cases. Acta Paediatr. Scand. 104(Suppl.):1, 1955.

29. Jaffe, R. B.: Systemic atrioventricular regurgitation in corrected transposition of the great vessels. Angiographic differentiation of operable and nonoperable valve deformities. Am. J. Cardiol. 37:395, 1976.

30. Kraus, Y., Yahini, J. H., Shem-Tov, A., and Neufeld, H. N.: Precordial pulsations in corrected transposition of the great vessels. Am. J. Cardiol. 23:684–698, 1969.

31. Kuppersmith, J., Krongrad, E., Gersony, W. M., and Bowman, F. O., Jr.: Electrophysiologic identification of the specialized conduction system in corrected transposition of the great arteries. Circulation 50:795–800, 1974.

32. Lev, M., and Rowlatt, U. F.: The pathologic anatomy of mixed levocardia. A review of thirteen cases of atrial or ventricular inversion with or without corrected transposition. Am. J. Cardiol. 8:216, 1961.

33. Lev, M., Licata, R. H., and May, R. C.: The conduction system in mixed levocardia with ventricular inversion (corrected transposition). Circulation 28:232, 1963.

34. Levy, M. J., Lillehei, C. W., Elliott, L. P.,

Carey, L. S., Adams, P., Jr., and Edwards, J. E.: Accessory valvular tissue causing subpulmonary stenosis in corrected transposition of great vessels. Circulation 27:494, 1963.

35. Marcelleti, C., Maloney, J. D., Ritter, D. G., Danielson, G. K., McGoon, D. C., and Wallace, R. B.: Corrected transposition and ventricular septal defect. Surgical experience. Ann. Surg. 191:751–759, 1980.

36. Martin, M. G.: Observation d'une déviation organique de l'estomac, d'une anomalie dans la situation, dans la configuration du coeur et des vaisseaux qui en partent ou qui s'y redent. Bull Soc. Anat. Paris 1:39, 1826.

37. Moller, J. H., Nakib, A., Anderson, R. C., and Edwards, J. E.: Congenital cardiac disease associated with polysplenia: A developmental complex of bilateral "left-sidedness." Circulation 36:789, 1967.

38. Momma, K., and Linde, L. M.: Abnormal p-wave axis in congenital heart disease associated with asplenia and polysplenia. J. Electrocardiol. 2:395, 1969.

39. Morgan, A. D., Krovetz, L. J., Bartley, T. D., Green, J. R., Jr., Shanklin, D. R., Wheat, M. W., Jr., and Schiebler, G. L.: Clinical features of single ventricle with congenitally corrected transposition. Am. J. Cardiol. 17:379, 1966.

40. Okamura, K., and Konno, S.: Two types of ventricular septal defect in corrected transposition of the great arteries: Reference to surgical approaches. Am. Heart J. 55:483–489, 1973.

41. Ongley, P. A., Titus, J. L., Khoury, G. H., Rahimtoola, S. H., Marchall, H. J., and Edwards, J. E.: Anomalous connection of pulmonary veins to right atrium associated with anomalous inferior vena cava, situs inversus and multiple spleens: A developmental complex. Mayo Clin. Proc. 40:609, 1965.

42. Peoples, W. M., Moller, J. H., and Edwards, J. E.: The spectrum of polysplenia. Unpublished data.

43. Putschar, W. G. J., and Manion, W. C.: Congenital absence of the spleen and associated anomalies. Am. J. Clin. Pathol. 26:429, 1956.

44. Rokitansky, K. F. V.: Die Defekte der Scheidewande des Herzens: Pathologisch-anatomische Abhandlung. Vienna, W. Braumuller, 1875, pp. 83–86.

45. Rose, V., Izukawa, T., and Moes, C. A. F.: Syndrome of asplenia and polysplenia: A review of cardiac and non-cardiac malformations in 60 cases with special reference to diagnosis and prognosis. Br. Heart J. 37:840–852, 1975.

46. Rotem, C. E., and Hultgren, H. M.: Corrected transposition of the great vessels without as-

sociated defects. Am. Heart J. 70:305, 1965.

47. Ruttenberg, H. D., Elliot, L. P., Anderson, R. C., Adams, P., Jr., and Tuna, N.: Congenital corrected transposition of the great vessels: Correlation of electrocardiograms and vectorcardiograms with associated cardiac malformations and hemodynamic states. Am. J. Cardiol. 17:339, 1966.

48. Ruttenberg, H. D., Higashino, S. M., and Moss, A. J.: Ventricular function in congenital corrected transposition of the great arteries: Observations on ventricular asyndrony. Unpublished data.

49. Ruttenberg, H. D., Neufeld, H. M., Lucas, R. V., Jr., Carey, L. S., Adams, P., Jr., Anderson, R. C., and Edwards, J. E.: Syndrome of congenital cardiac disease with asplenia: Distinction from other forms of congenital cyanotic cardiac disease. Am. J. Cardiol. 13:387, 1964.

50. Schiebler, G. L., Edwards, J. E., Burchell, H. B., DuShane, J. W., Ongley, P. A., and Wood, E. H.: Congenital corrected transposition of the great vessels: A study of 33 cases. Pediatrics 27(Suppl.):851, 1961.

51. Spitzer, A.: The architecture of normal and malformed hearts: A phylogenetic theory of their development, edited by M. Lev and A. Vass. Charles C Thomas, Springfield, Ill., 1951, p. 72.

52. Towers, B., and Middleton, H.: Congenital absence of the spleen associated with malformations of the heart and transposition of the viscera. J. Pathol. 72:553, 1956.

53. Van Mierop, L. H. S., Patterson, P. R., and Reynolds, R. W.: Two cases of congenital asplenia with isomerism of the cardiac atria and the sinoatrial nodes. Am. J. Cardiol. 13:407, 1964.

54. Van Mierop, L. H. S., Gessner, I. H., and Schiebler, G. L.: Asplenia and polysplenia syndromes. The Fourth Conference on the Clinical Delineation of Birth Defects. XV. The cardiovascular system. 8:36–44, 1972.

55. Van Praagh, R.: The segmental approach to diagnosis in congenital heart disease. The fourth conference on the clinical delineation of birth defects. Part XV. The cardiovascular system. Birth Defects 8:4–23, 1972.

56. Waldman, J. D., Rosenthal, A., Smith, A. L., Shurin, S., and Nadas, A. S.: Sepsis and congenital asplenia. J. Pediatr. 90:555–559, 1977.

57. Waldo, A. L., Pacifico, A. D., Bargeron, L. M., James, T. N., and Kirklin, J. W.: Electrophysiological delineation of the specialized A-V conduction system in patients with corrected transposition of the great vessels and ventricular septal defect. Circulation 52:435–441, 1975.

23

Double-Outlet Right Ventricle

Donald J. Hagler, M.D., Donald G. Ritter, M.D., and Francisco J. Puga, M.D.

Basically recognized by the origin of both great arteries from the morphologic right ventricle, double-outlet right ventricle (DORV) encompasses clinical features of a variety of entities, ranging from simple ventricular septal defect (VSD) to tetralogy of Fallot (TF) and to transposition of the great arteries (TGA). This congenital malformation is a rare anomaly; its frequency has been reported as approximately 0.09 case per 1000 births.[1, 54] No racial or sexual predilection is evident.

In recent years, progress in corrective surgery of complex congenital heart disease has been possible, in part because of a better understanding of the variety of the pathologic features and an increased ability to make the exact diagnosis, with recognition of associated defects, by noninvasive techniques and by cardiac catheterization and selective angiography.[13, 22, 23, 31, 40, 49, 52, 62, 71]

In 1949, Taussig and Bing[75] first described a patient whose transposed aorta and the pulmonary artery originated from the right ventricle. There was also a supracristal VSD which allowed the pulmonary artery to override the ventricular septum. This condition has been considered the Taussig-Bing complex or the Taussig-Bing type of DORV. In 1957, Witham[82] first applied the term double-outlet right ventricle to a condition considered a partial transposition complex, in which both great arteries arose from the right ventricle. He divided his cases into two groups, the Fallot type and the Eisenmenger type, depending on the presence or absence of pulmonary stenosis (PS).

In 1961, Neufeld et al.[56, 57] developed the classification of double-outlet right ventricle with and without PS. Later, Neufeld et al.[58] subcategorized the group without PS on the basis of the position of the VSD in relation to the crista supraventricularis and the great arteries.

In 1972, Lev et al.[47] emphasized the variations in location of the VSD in relation to the great arteries. In 1975, Zamora et al.[84] classified DORV into five types on the basis of the position of the VSD.

Zamora et al.,[84] Cameron et al.,[7] and Sondheimer et al.[69] separately reviewed a number of associated defects observed in their autopsied series. They both noted the frequent occurrence of mitral valve anomalies. In 1976, Sridaromont et al.[71] reported a classification based on the location of the VSD and the great-artery relationships.

Patrick and McGoon[62] proposed a surgical classification of DORV according to the location of the VSD and the relation of the great arteries, including the presence or absence of PS.

In 1965, Carey, Edwards and associates[8, 16] first reported the angiocardiographic features of DORV. They emphasized the following diagnostic criteria: opacification of both great arteries from the right ventricle, visualization of the aortic and pulmonary valves in the same horizontal plane, frequent malposition of the aorta in the lateral view, and a "tongue-like" filling defect in the frontal view, at the base of the right ventricle representing the parietal limb of the crista supra-

ventricularis and forming a division for two outflow tracts. In 1970, Hallermann et al.[31, 32] studied the angiocardiographic and anatomic findings in DORV. They recognized the criteria proposed by Carey and Edwards and considered that in the lateral view the mitral valve was not in continuity with either semilunar valve.

In 1978, Sridaromont et al.[73] emphasized the importance of selective biplane angiocardiography of both right and left ventricles in order to recognize great artery relationships and the location of the VSD.

In the physiologic classification of Neufeld et al.,[56, 57] double-outlet right ventricle was categorized into two major groups, depending on the presence or absence of pulmonary stenosis. In the presence of PS, the features closely resembled those of tetralogy of Fallot. In patients without PS, the findings resembled those in patients who have a large VSD and a dominant left-to-right shunt or in those who have a right-to-left shunt and pulmonary vascular obstructive disease. Neufeld et al. suggested that the position of the VSD was a major factor in determining intracardiac streaming. In 1967, Hazell et al.[33] and later Sridaromont et al.[71] reported the physiologic and pathologic correlations observed in a large series of patients.

PATHOLOGY

Double-outlet right ventricle has been variably defined by different workers. Neufeld et al.[56, 57] defined it as follows: both great arteries and arterial trunks arise exclusively from the morphologic right ventricle; neither semilunar valve is in fibrous continuity with either atrioventricular valve; and usually a VSD is present and represents the only outlet from the left ventricle. Pulmonary valvular or subpulmonary stenosis may be present or absent. The definition proposed by Lev et al.[47] and by Anderson et al.,[3, 4, 80] however, requires less rigid criteria. They indicate that one complete arterial trunk and at least half of the other arterial trunk emerge from the right ventricle, and there may or may not be mitral-aortic or mitral-pulmonary continuity.

In this chapter, we have tried to require adherence to the original criteria of Witham's[82] and Neufeld's[56] definitions in an attempt to provide a group of cases that represent classic examples of DORV. Although we recognize that in many cases pronounced arterial override without mitral semilunar valve discontinuity and instances of bilateral conus without origin of both great arteries from the right ventricle may represent gray areas of uncertain diagnosis, we believe that their inclusion as DORV would dilute the significance of the basic combination of pathologic features as originally described. We have accepted that minor degrees of arterial override would not substantially detract from the basic definition of exclusive origin of the great arteries from the morphologic right ventricle with persistence of bilateral conus muscle (subaortic and subpulmonary) to separate both semilunar valves from both atrioventricular valves.

RELATION OF THE GREAT ARTERIES

There are four types of relation of the great arteries at the level of the semilunar valves: normal relation—the pulmonary artery arterial trunk is anterior and to the left of the aorta; side-by-side relation—the aorta is to the right of the pulmonary artery, and the semilunar valves lie approximately in the same transverse plane, which is the classic and true relation of the great arteries in DORV; dextroposition—the aorta is to the right and anterior to the pulmonary artery, which may include some cases with the aorta directly anterior; and levoposition—the aorta is to the left and anterior to the pulmonary artery, which may include some cases with the aorta nearly entirely to the left of the pulmonary artery.

POSITION OF THE VENTRICULAR SEPTAL DEFECT

There are four types of ventricular septal defects in DORV: the subaortic type, characterized by a VSD that is related more closely to the aortic valve than to the pulmonary valve; the subpulmonary type, in which the VSD is related more closely to the pulmonary valve—when this defect is located above the septal limb of the crista supraventricularis (supracristal VSD) this type of DORV is considered synonymous with the Taussig-Bing complex; the doubly committed or subaortic and subpulmonary type of VSD, in which the defect is very large and is closely related to both semilunar valves; and the remote type, in which the VSD is distant from both semilunar valves and may represent a posterior VSD, a defect of the atrioventricular canal type, or an isolated muscular VSD.

EMBRYOLOGY

Goor and Edwards[24] included double-outlet right ventricle within a "spectrum of transposition complexes." On the basis of their embryologic and pathologic studies, DORV would appear to repesent a relatively primitive embryologic condition. With subsequent development, failure to achieve conotruncal inversion (rotation) and leftward shift of the conus (aortic or pulmonary) results in persistence of this condition, with complete origin of both great arteries from the morphologic right ventricle.

Anderson et al.[3, 4] expanded Goor's and Edwards' conclusions and discussed a spectrum of entities ranging from tetralogy of Fallot to complete transposition of the great arteries. In such an analysis, one can explain DORV as an initial embryologic condition, whereas TF results if there is a leftward shift of the aortic conus, and TGA results if there is a leftward shift of the pulmonary conus. Since many variations in the pathologic findings of TF and TGA may be evident, it seems reasonable to accept these anomalies as a spectrum, but a spectrum that is centered about a more definitive and primitive embryologic state with origin of both great arteries from the morphologic right ventricle.

ANGIOGRAPHIC-PATHOLOGIC CORRELATIONS

The angiographic-pathologic review by Sridaromont et al.,[73] as well as others,[47, 84] allows a categorization of double-outlet right ventricle with 16 possible variations based on the great artery relationships and the location of the VSD. Figure 23.1 illustrates the possible combinations of these variations. In addition, an intact ventricular septum allows four other possible types of DORV, depending on the great artery relationships.

SIDE-BY-SIDE RELATIONSHIP OF THE GREAT ARTERIES

Subaortic Ventricular Septal Defect

Pathologic Observations. The most frequently encountered type of DORV in the Sridaromont series,[73] accounting for slightly less than half of the cases, was that of side-by-side relationship of the great arteries and subaortic VSD. In this type, the aorta and the pulmonary artery are side by side, and the aorta is to the right of the pulmonary artery (Fig. 23.2). Viewed from the right ventricle, the aortic outflow penetrates the parietal limb of the aortic conus. The VSD, which is in a posteroinferior position, is more closely related to the aorta than to the pulmonary artery (subaortic VSD). The aortic valve and the pulmonary valve are at approximately the same horizontal level (Fig. 23.2). The aortic conus to the right of the aorta, the conus septum (between two great arteries), and the pulmonary conus to the left of the pulmonary trunk are well demonstrated. The presence of bilateral conus separates both semilunar valves from both atrioventricular valves. The VSD is the only outlet from the left ventricle, and the aortic conus is the structure between the aortic valve and the anterior leaflet of the mitral valve (Fig. 23.2).

Angiographic Observations. The classic angiographic features of this type are the demonstration that the great arteries are side by side, with the aorta to the right of the pulmonary artery (Fig. 23.2). The aortic and pulmonary valves are in the same horizontal plane. The aortic conus, the conus septum, and the pulmonary conus (bilateral conus) are well demonstrated on the frontal view. The conus separates both semilunar valves from both atrioventricular valves, as is also noted on the lateral view. On the lateral view the VSD is below the aortic conus.

Subpulmonary Ventricular Septal Defect (Taussig-Bing Anomaly)

Pathologic Observations. The true Taussig-Bing anomaly is relatively rare. In the same series,[73] it accounted for approximately 8% of the cases. The great arteries are in a side-by-side relationship (Fig. 23.3). Since pulmonary stenosis does not occur in these cases, the pulmonary trunk is markedly dilated. The VSD is anterosuperior (supracristal) and immediately subjacent to the pulmonary valve (subpulmonary VSD). The VSD is more anterior than it is in the subaortic type, and it is the only exit by which blood from the left side of the heart enters the pulmonary trunk. The pulmonary conus is the structure between the pulmonary valve and the anterior leaflet of the mitral valve.

Angiographic Observations. The frontal view of the right ventricular angiocardiogram demonstrates that the great arteries are in a side-by-side relationship (Fig. 23.3). The aortic conus, conus septum, and pulmonary conus (bilateral conus) are well demonstrated on the frontal view. Usually, the conus septum is less prominent than it is in cases having side-by-side great artery relationships and subaortic VSD. The classic finding on the early phase of the right ventricular angiogram is a high VSD related directly to the pulmonary valve. There is no conus between the VSD and the pulmonary valve. The pulmonary conus is the structure between the pulmonary valve and the anterior mitral leaflet.

Doubly Committed (Subaortic and Subpulmonary) Ventricular Septal Defect

Pathologic Observations. In this type of DORV, the VSD is closely related to both semilunar valves and lies in

Relation of great arteries	Location of VSD (%)				Total
	Subaortic	Subpulmonary	Subaortic & Subpulmonary	Remote	
Normal	3%	0	0	0	3%
Side-by-side	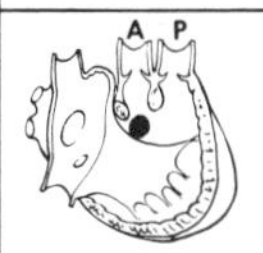 46%	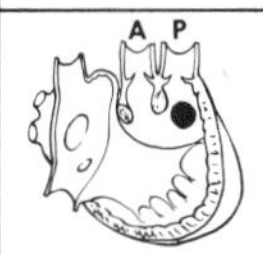 8%	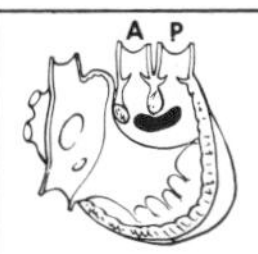 3%	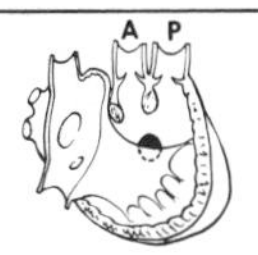 7%	64%
d – MGA	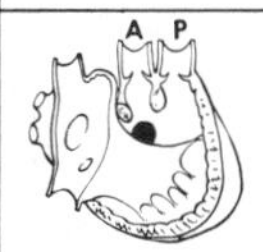 16%	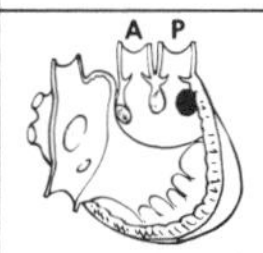 10%	0	0	26%
l – MGA	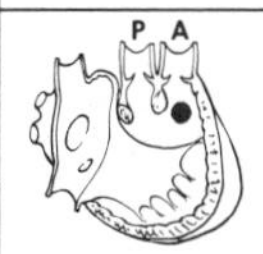 3%	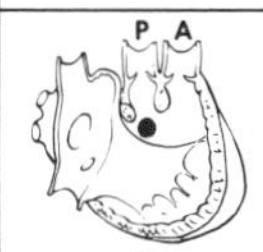 4%	0	0	7%
Total	68%	22%	3%	7%	

Fig. 23.1 Relationship of great arteries and location of ventricular septal defect (VSD) in 70 patients with double-outlet right ventricle. *d-MGA* and *l-MGA*, dextromalposition and levomalposition of great arteries, respectively; *A*, aorta; *P*, pulmonary artery.

a superior position, usually above the crista supraventricularis. The VSD is quite large and extends in an oblique course beneath both great arteries (Fig. 23.4). Thus, there is deficiency of the conus septum, but the aortic conus and pulmonary conus remain.

Angiographic Observations. The right ventricular angiocardiogram cannot differentiate this type from the Taussig-Bing anomaly because on the lateral view this VSD is high and anterior superiorly and directly related to both semilunar valves (Fig. 23.4). It is impossible to recognize whether the VSD is related to the pulmonary valve or to both semilunar valves.

Remote Ventricular Septal Defect

Pathologic Observations. The most common form recognized as a remote VSD is that of a complete atrioventricular canal defect with DORV[72] (Fig. 23.5). Splenic anomalies, common atrium, and visceral heterotaxia are common, along with anomalies of systemic and pulmonary venous connections. In these patients with complete atrioventricular canal defect, the anterior common leaflet of the common atrioventricular canal is undivided and is not attached to the crest of the ventricular septum (Rastelli type C complete atrioventricular canal defect[65]).

In addition, posteroinferiorly located VSDs involving the inflow portion of the ventricular septum and located between the atrioventricular valves or isolated VSDs of the atrioventricular canal type should be considered as remote types of VSDs, since usually in this situation the defect is not suitable for routing the left ventricular blood to either great artery. Such a remote VSD was reported by Ciaravella et al.[10] in association with side-by-side great arteries in one case and with dextromalpositioned great arteries in another. Because of the posterior location of the VSD, the tricuspid valve prevented accessibility of the defect to either great artery. Also, single or multiple muscular VSDs may be observed in DORV, and they should be considered a form of remote

VSD because of their inferior position in the trabeculated septum.

Angiographic Observations. The classic features observed with complete atrioventricular canal defect are the deformity of the left ventricular outflow tract caused by abnormal insertion of the left atrioventricular valve and deficiency of the ventricular septum. However, because of the right ventricular origin of both great arteries, a classic goose-neck deformity may not be observed (Fig. 23.5).

DEXTROMALPOSITION OF THE GREAT ARTERIES

Subaortic Ventricular Septal Defect

Pathologic Observations. This is a somewhat unusual form of DORV but was observed in 16% of the series reported.[73] The surgical findings have been described with typical dextromalpositioned great arteries. The VSD is located in an anterior and superior position adjacent to the malpositioned aortic valve above the septal limb of the crista supraventricularis.

Angiographic Observations. The right ventricular angiocardiogram demonstrates malpositioned great arteries arising from the right ventricle (Fig. 23.6 A and B). The aortic conus, conus septum, and pulmonary conus (bilateral conus) are well demonstrated in the lateral view.

Subpulmonary Ventricular Septal Defect

Pathologic Observations. This form of DORV occurred in 10% of the cases.[73] Because of the dextromalposition of the great arteries, the VSD is more closely related to the posterior pulmonary trunk.[36] However, the VSD is not as anterior and superior in location as that observed in the classic Taussig-Bing anomaly. This defect is in the more typical subcristal location involving the paramembranous portion of the ventricular septum.

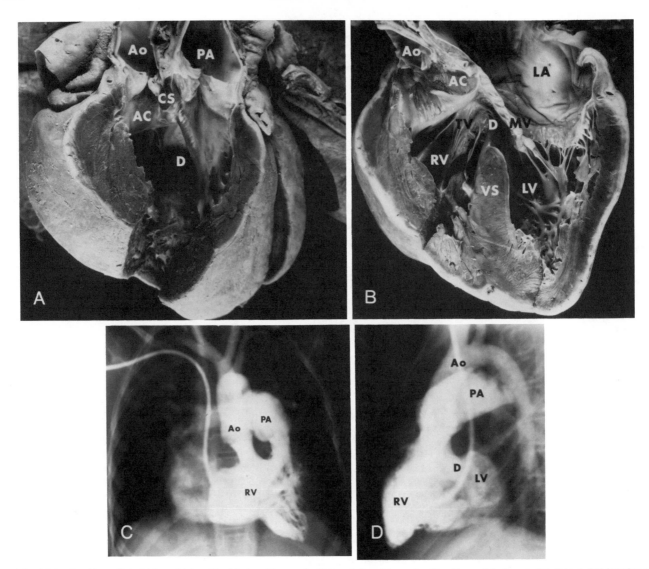

Fig. 23.2 Double-outlet right ventricle with side-by-side great-artery relationship and subaortic ventricular septal defect. (*A*) Interior of right ventricle, showing side-by-side relationship of great vessels. (*Ao* and *PA*) Coronal section has been made through valves and great arteries. Removal of part of conus septum (ventral limb) leaves aortic conus (*AC*) (dorsal limb). Conus septum (*CS*) is clearly demonstrated between great arteries. VSD (*D*) is immediately beneath conus. (*B*) Section through heart in sagittal plane carried across VSD (*D*) which is the only outlet of left ventricle (*LV*); it is more closely related to aortic orifice (*Ao*). Aortic conus (*AC*) is interposed between aortic valve and anterior leaflet of mitral valve (*MV*). *LA*, left atrium; *TV*, tricuspid valve; *VS*, ventricular septum; *RV*, right ventricle. (*C* and *D*) Right ventricular (*RV*) angiocardiogram. On frontal view, aortic conus (right of aorta, *Ao*), conus septum (between aorta and pulmonary artery, *PA*), and pulmonary conus (left of pulmonary artery) are well demonstrated. In lateral view, anterior wall of aorta is in about the same plane as anterior wall of pulmonary trunk. VSD (*D*) is below conus. *RV*, right ventricle; *LV*, left ventricle; *MV*, mitral valve. (*A* and *B*, reproduced with permission from H. N. Neufeld et al.[57] *C* and *D*, reproduced with permission from F. J. Hallerman et al.[31])

Angiographic Observations. Because the aorta is anterior to the pulmonary trunk, the lateral view is necessary to demonstrate the aortic conus (anterior to the aorta), conus septum (between the great arteries), and pulmonary consus (posterior to the pulmonary trunk). Pulmonary stenosis of the subvalvular and valvular types is commonly observed in cases with malposition of the great arteries. The subpulmonary location of the VSD is usually well demonstrated on the lateral view of the left ventricular angiocardiogram below the aortic conus (subpulmonary, subcristal VSD) (Fig. 23.7).

Remote Ventricular Septal Defect

A remote posterior VSD associated with dextromalposition of the great arteries was reported by Ciaravella et al.[10]

The anatomic and angiographic findings other than the great artery relationships were not different from those observed with side-by-side great arteries and remote VSD.

LEVOMALPOSITION OF THE GREAT ARTERIES

Subaortic Ventricular Septal Defect

Pathologic Observations. This form of DORV occurred in less than 5% of the series reported by Sridaromont et al.[73] However, it has been reported by a number of investigators.[77, 78] On the external surface of the heart, the aorta is anterior and to the left of the pulmonary trunk. The aortic conus is interposed between the aortic valve and both the

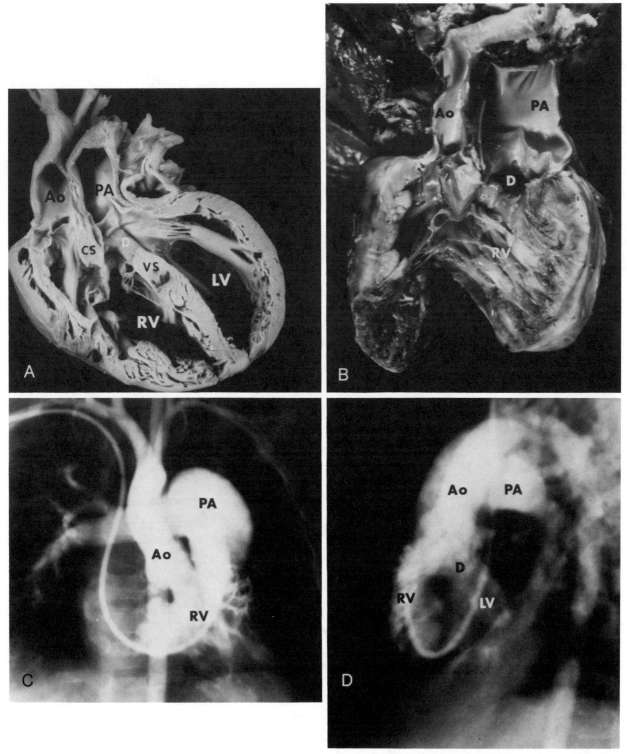

Fig. 23.3 Double-outlet right ventricle with side-by-side great artery relationship and subpulmonary ventricular septal defect, or Taussig-Bing anomaly. (*A*) Sagittal section VSD (*D*) is only outlet of left ventricle (*LV*) and is directly related to subpulmonary ventricular septal defect. *PA*, pulmonary artery; *CS*, conus septum; *Ao*, aorta; *VS*, ventricular septum; *RV*, right ventricle. (*B*) Interior of right ventricle (*RV*), aorta (*Ao*), and main pulmonary artery (*PA*) in another case. Ventricular septal defect (*D*) is beneath pulmonary valve and lies anterosuperior in ventricular septum. (*C* and *D*) Frontal and lateral angiocardiograms. On lateral view, VSD (*D*) is high and is adjacent to large pulmonary valve and main pulmonary artery (*PA*), without conus in between. Mitral valve is separated from pulmonary valve by pulmonary conus, and pulmonary trunk is markedly dilated. Aortic conus is well demonstrated. Conus septum is less prominent, compared with type having double-outlet right ventricle with side-by-side great artery relationship and subaortic VSD. *Ao*, aorta; *RV*, right ventricle; *LV*, left ventricle. (*A* provided courtesy of William D. Edwards. *B*, *C*, and *D* reproduced with permission from S. Sridaromont et al.[73])

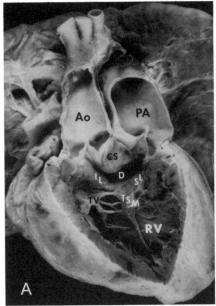
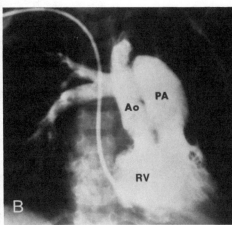
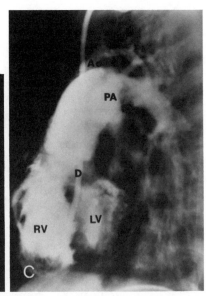

Fig. 23.4 Double-outlet right ventricle with side-by-side great artery relationship and doubly committed (subaortic and subpulmonary) ventricular septal defect. (*A*) Interior of right ventricle (*RV*) and great arteries, showing that great arteries are in side-by-side relationship. VSD (*D*) is doubly committed and is cradled between the inferior and superior limbs (*IL* and *SL*) of the trabecula septomarginalis (*TSM*). *CS*, conus septum; *Ao*, aorta; *PA*, pulmonary artery; *TV*, tricuspid valve. Frontal (*B*) and lateral (*C*) views of right ventricular (*RV*) angiocardiogram, demonstrating simultaneous opacification of great arteries (*Ao* and *PA*) in side-by-side relationship. Aortic and pulmonary conus are well demonstrated on frontal view. Conus septum is less prominent. On lateral view, VSD (*D*) is located high and is closely related to semilunar valves. *LV*, left ventricle. (*A* reproduced courtesy of William D. Edwards. *B* and *C* reproduced with permission from S. Sridaromont et al.[73])

VSD and the anterior leaflet of the mitral valve. The VSD, however, is located in an anterior and superior position, which allows exit of blood from the left ventricle into the aorta (Fig. 23.8). Pulmonary stenosis was commonly observed in these patients with malposition of the great arteries. We have also observed some cases with extreme leftward rotation of the aorta so that the great arteries are nearly in a side-by-side relationship with the aorta to the left.

Angiographic Observations. The frontal and lateral views of the left ventricular angiocardiogram best demonstrate the location of the VSD below the aorta. Levomalposition of the aorta can be seen in both frontal and lateral views. The left ventricular angiogram also demonstrates that the VSD is the only outlet from the left ventricle (Fig. 23.8).

Subpulmonary Ventricular Septal Defect

Pathologic Observations. This variety represents an uncommon form of DORV and was observed in only 4% of the cases in the same series.[73] Surgical descriptions have noted the VSD located posteroinferiorly in a typical paramembranous position. Again, because of the malposition of the great arteries, the VSD is more closely related to the posterior pulmonary trunk and is below the pulmonary conus.

Angiographic Observations. The right ventricular angiocardiogram demonstrates that the malpositioned great arteries arise entirely from the right ventricle, with the aorta anterior and to the left of the pulmonary trunk (Fig. 23.9). The aortic conus (left of the aorta), conus septum (between the great arteries), and pulmonary conus (right of the pulmonary trunk) are best demonstrated on the anteroposterior view. In some cases, the bilateral conus can be seen on the lateral view. The VSD is below the pulmonary conus (subpulmonary, subcristal VSD).

NORMAL RELATIONSHIP OF THE GREAT ARTERIES

Normally related great arteries were unusual in the series reported by Sridaromont et al.[73] Only two patients had normally related great arteries. In both cases, a subaortic VSD was present and was located in a posteroinferior location and was more closely related to the aorta. Bilateral conus was present.

The presence of the aortic conus septum can be seen in the frontal view of the right ventricular angiocardiogram. The lateral view shows the aorta arising from the right ventricle, with the normal relationship of the aorta to the pulmonary trunk. The VSD is located posteriorly and is more closely related to the posterior aorta (subaortic VSD) (Fig. 23.10).

UNUSUAL FORMS OF DOUBLE-OUTLET RIGHT VENTRICLE

Intact Ventricular Septum

A number of instances have been reported of DORV with intact ventricular septum.[2, 14, 50, 73, 84] However, a review of the literature through 1979[15] revealed only seven cases. Most often, it has been associated with varying degrees of hypoplasia of the left ventricle and with anomalies of the mitral valve. In these cases, the only outlet from the left ventricle is through the mitral valve and via the atrial septal defect. Great artery relationships have been described, ranging from normally related great arteries to dextromalpositioned and levomalpositioned great arteries. The right ventricular angiocardiogram demonstrates origin of both great arteries from the right ventricle and the presence of bilateral conus. Left atrial or left ventricular angiography may demonstrate the mitral valve deformity and hypoplasia of the left ventricle (Fig. 23.11).

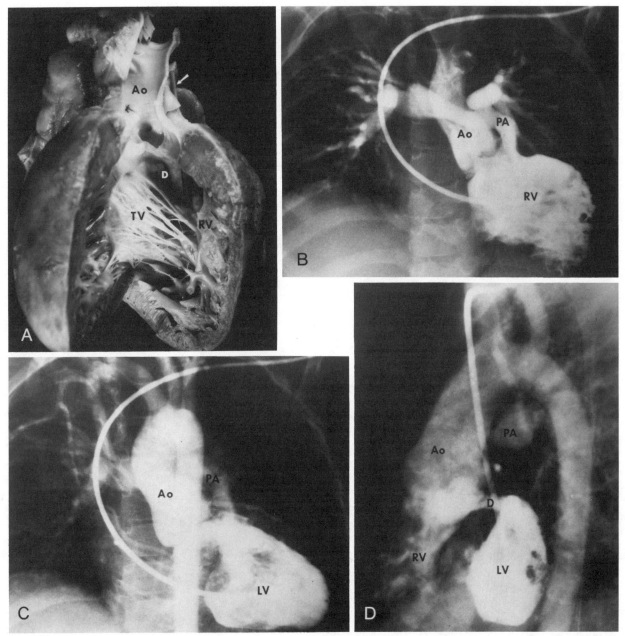

Fig. 23.5 Double-outlet right ventricle with side-by-side great artery relationship and remote VSD (complete atrioventricular canal defect). (*A*) View from right ventricle (*RV*) demonstrates that both aorta (*Ao*) and stenotic pulmonary trunk (with small probe, *arrow*) arise from right ventricle. Tricuspid valve (*TV*) is part of common atrioventricular valve. *D*, defect. (*B*) Frontal view of right ventricular angiocardiogram, showing that both great arteries (*Ao* and *PA*) arise from morphologic right ventricle (*RV*) in side-by-side relationship. (*C*) Frontal view of left ventriculogram demonstrating deformity of left ventricular (*LV*) outflow tract caused by abnormal insertion of left atrioventricular valve and deficiency of ventricular septum. *Ao*, aortic root; *PA*, main pulmonary artery. (*D*) Lateral view showing that VSD (*D*) is only outlet of left ventricle (*LV*). Mitral valve is not in fibrous continuity with either semilunar valve. Right ventricle (*RV*), aortic root (*Ao*), and main pulmonary artery (*PA*) are also opacified. (*A, C,* and *D* reproduced with permission from S. Sridaromont *et al.*[72] and the American Heart Association; *B* reproduced with permission from S. Sridaromont *et al.*[73])

Double-Chambered Right Ventricle

Ciaravella *et al.*[10] described an unusual associated anomaly in two cases of DORV with remote VSD. In these cases a double-chambered right ventricle was observed in which the accessory chamber received portions of the tricuspid valve attachments and prevented access of the great arteries to the VSD. Collan and Pesonen[11] reported one case of DORV associated with a two-chambered right ventricle. Markedly hypertrophied muscle bundles within the right

ventricle effectively divided the right ventricle into two portions. A narrow communication at the apex of the right ventricle provided the only access to the subpulmonary chamber, and a subaortic VSD was present. Judson *et al.*[39] have recently reported successful repair in two such cases.

Tricuspid Atresia

Rarely, tricuspid atresia has been reported with associated DORV. Both great arteries originate exclusively from the

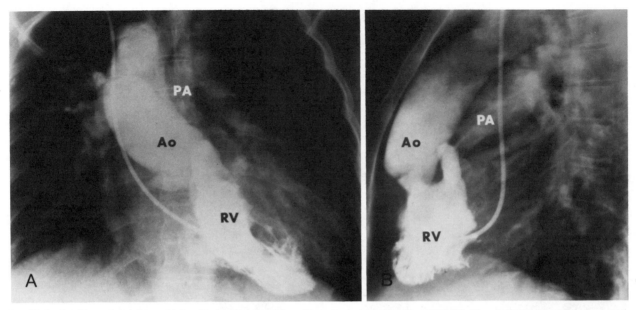

Fig. 23.6 Double-outlet right ventricle with dextromalposition of great arteries and subaortic VSD. (*A* and *B*) Frontal and lateral views of right ventricular (*RV*) angiocardiogram, demonstrating aorta (*Ao*) directly anterior to main pulmonary artery (*PA*) and arising completely from this ventricle. Pulmonary valve is markedly stenosed. Subaortic VSD, which was confirmed at operation, is not clearly demonstrated from right ventricular angiocardiogram but is suggested by small puff of dye crossing defect in frontal view. (*A* and *B* reproduced with permission from S. Sridaromont et al.[73])

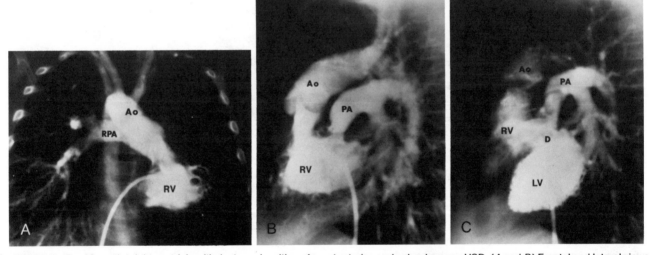

Fig. 23.7 Double-outlet right ventricle with dextromalposition of great arteries and subpulmonary VSD. (*A* and *B*) Frontal and lateral views of right ventricular angiocardiogram, demonstrating both aorta (*Ao*) and main pulmonary artery (*PA*) arising from right ventricle (*RV*) in dextromalposition. Aorta is directly anterior to right pulmonary artery (*RPA*). Aortic conus (anterior to aorta), conus septum (between two great arteries), and pulmonary conus (posterior to main pulmonary artery) are well demonstrated on lateral view. With right aortic arch and pulmonary stenosis and dextromalposition of great artery relationship, aortic valve often appears to be shifted leftward (more directly anterior), as in this situation. (*C*) Lateral view of left ventricular angiocardiogram. After opacification of left ventricle (*LV*) and part of right ventricular outflow tract (*RV*), aorta (*Ao*) and main pulmonary artery (*PA*) opacify through VSD (*D*), which is located beneath pulmonary conus (subpulmonary ventricular septal defect). *RPA*, right pulmonary artery. Note proximity of pulmonary artery to ventricular septal defect. (Reproduced with permission from S. Sridaromont, et al.[73])

hypoplastic right ventricular cavity, and bilateral conus is present.

DOUBLE-OUTLET RIGHT VENTRICLE ASSOCIATED WITH DEXTROCARDIA AND ATRIOVENTRICULAR DISCORDANCE

A constellation of defects, including situs solitus of the atria and viscera with dextrocardia, atrioventricular discord-

ance, PS, and VSD, have been commonly associated with DORV.[70] The great arteries in the levomalpositioned relationship originate exclusively from the morphologic right ventricle. There is usually severe subvalvular and valvular PS, and the VSD is subpulmonary in position (Fig. 23.12). There is bilateral conus, which separates both of the semilunar valves from the atrioventricular valves. Angiocardiography of the morphologic right and left ventricular cavities demonstrates the exclusive origin of both great arteries from

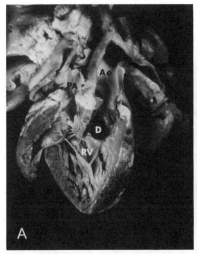
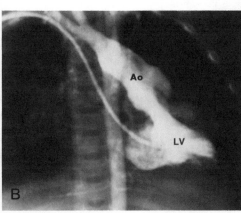
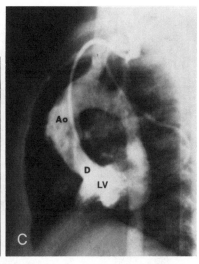

Fig. 23.8 Double-outlet right ventricle with levomalposition of great arteries and subaortic VSD. (*A*) Interior of right ventricle (*RV*) and great arteries. Because of malposition, aorta (*Ao*) is anterior to main pulmonary artery (*PA*) in this view. VSD (*D*) lies anterosuperior to septal limb of crista supraventricularis and immediately beneath transposed aortic valve (subaortic ventricular septal defect), as seen in case of side-by-side great artery relationship and subpulmonary VSD. Pulmonary outflow tract penetrates parietal limb of crista supraventricularis in same way as in side-by-side great artery relationship. Pulmonary conus is dorsal limb and is to right of pulmonary trunk, and conus septum is ventral limb and is between two great arteries. (*B* and *C*) Frontal and lateral views of left ventricular angiocardiogram, showing catheter through ASD and left atrioventricular valve. After opacification of left ventricle (*LV*), aorta (*Ao*) was opacified through VSD (*D*), which is only outlet of left ventricle. Aortic valve is far distant from left atrioventricular valve, with aortic conus interposed. (Reproduced with permission from S. Sridaromont *et al.*[73])

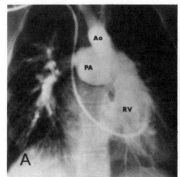
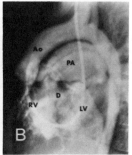

Fig. 23.9 Double-outlet right ventricle with levomalposition of great arteries and subpulmonary VSD. (*A* and *B*) Frontal and lateral views of right ventricular (*RV*) angiocardiogram. Bilateral conus is clearly demonstrated on lateral view, and VSD (*D*) is below pulmonary conus. Left ventricle (*LV*) was opacified via VSD. Both semilunar valves are at same level. The aorta (*Ao*) is anterior and to the left of the main pulmonary artery (*PA*). (Reproduced with permission from S. Sridaromont *et al.*[73])

the morphologic right ventricle. The lateral view demonstrates the side-by-side great artery relationship with the aorta anterior and to the left.

ASSOCIATED CARDIAC ANOMALIES

Pulmonary stenosis is the most commonly encountered associated anomaly.[7, 69, 71] It is seen in approximately 70% of patients with malposition of the great arteries. Pulmonary stenosis can often be clearly demonstrated angiocardiographically. Rarely, the pulmonary valve may be absent or rudimentary and may demonstrate features typically associated with absent pulmonary valve syndrome.

Atrial septal defect of the secundum type is a commonly associated anomaly. It represents the only outlet of the left

side of the heart in patients with intact ventricular septum.

Varying degrees of left ventricular outflow obstruction may be observed in patients with double-outlet right ventricle.[45, 51, 53, 55, 63] In only two patients reviewed by Sridaromont *et al.*[73] was an obstructive VSD observed with restriction of left ventricular outflow (Fig. 23.13). With the advent of 2D echocardiography, a small VSD was observed with significant frequency (approximately 17%).[30] In these cases, surgical enlargement of the VSD was required at the time of correction.

Subaortic stenosis occurs in 3% of the cases, and it appears to result from extensive hypertrophy of the aortic conus and conus septum (Fig. 23.14). Angiographic evidence of subaortic obstruction may be suggested, although not hemodynamically recognized. Less commonly, aortic valve stenosis or atresia has been reported.[7, 69, 84]

An association has been described with interruption of the aortic arch or coarctation of the aorta in patients with DORV and subpulmonary VSD.[48] Coarctation of the aorta, however, has also been described in instances of subaortic, doubly committed, and remote VSD.

Mitral valve abnormalities have been described. In addition to mitral atresia, Zamora *et al.*[84] described associated anomalies of parachute mitral valve and supravalvular stenosing mitral ring. Tandon *et al.*[74] and Quero Jiménez *et al.*[64] reported cases of DORV with straddling mitral valve. In most of the cases, the VSD was a subcristal, subpulmonary defect with dextromalposition of the great arteries and also with a remote posterior VSD.

Other associated anomalies with DORV include persistence of the left superior vena cava with drainage to the coronary sinus or left atrium and left juxtaposed position of the atrial appendages. As mentioned, splenic anomalies and abdominal heterotaxia represent complex lesions with anomalies of pulmonary and systemic venous connection and are often associated with DORV with complete atrioventricular canal defect. There appears to be an increased association with the trisomy-18 syndrome.[12, 17, 44, 61, 66]

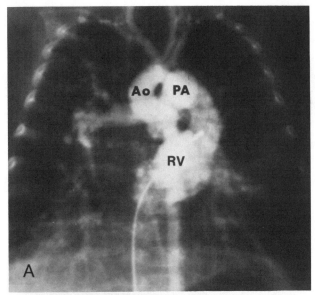

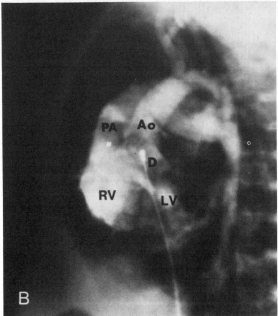

Fig. 23.10 Double-outlet right ventricle with great arteries in normal relationship and subaortic VSD. (*A* and *B*) Frontal and lateral views of right ventricular (*RV*) angiogram. Catheter was advanced across right atrioventricular (tricuspid) valve. Aorta (*Ao*) and main pulmonary artery (*PA*) arise entirely from right ventricle in normal relationship, in which aorta is posterior and to right of main pulmonary artery. Aortic conus and conus septum are well demonstrated in frontal view. VSD (*D*) is beneath aorta, and part of left ventricle (*LV*) is opacified. (Reproduced with permission from S. Sridaromont et al.[73])

Varying degrees of left ventricular hypoplasia may be observed, and, most often, the hypoplasia is mild if the left ventricular inflow is nonobstructed. Mild left ventricular hypoplasia may be observed in any type of DORV but may be more commonly seen with decreased pulmonary flow and restrictive VSD with associated large ASD. Special angulated cineangiograms, particularly those utilizing the long-axial oblique projection, may be helpful in assessing left ventricular size and VSD size, and position, and may be helpful in excluding associated muscular VSD. However,

caution must be advised in interpreting great artery position in reference to the ventricular septum when these angulated views are used. Since the superior portion of the ventricular septum may lie in a plane separate from the lower septum,

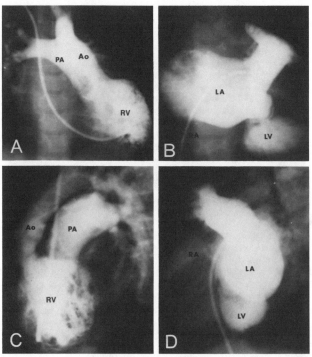

Fig. 23.11 Double-outlet right ventricle with levomalposition of great artery and intact ventricular septum. (*A* and *C*) Frontal and lateral views of right ventricular angiocardiogram, demonstrating simultaneous opacification of aorta (*Ao*) and main pulmonary artery (*PA*). Aorta is anterior and to left of pulmonary artery in levomalposition. *RV*, right ventricle. (*B* and *D*) Frontal and lateral views of left atrial angiocardiogram, demonstrating pronounced dilatation of left atrium. Left atrioventricular (mitral) valve is severely deformed. Left ventricle is also hypoplastic, and ventricular septum is intact. *RA*, right atrium; *LA*, left atrium; *LV*, left ventricle. (Reproduced with permission from S. Sridaromont.[73])

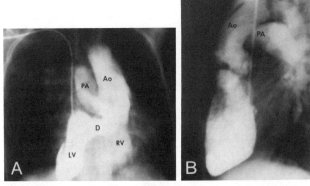

Fig. 23.12 Double-outlet right ventricle with dextrocardia and atrioventricular discordance. (*A*) Frontal view of morphologic left ventricular angiogram shows morphologic characteristics of respective ventricles; both great arteries arise from the morphologic right ventricle. (*B*) Lateral view shows both great arteries in side-by-side relationship. *Ao*, aorta; *PA*, pulmonary artery; *D*, VSD; *RA*, right atrium; *RV*, right ventricle; *LA*, left atrium; *LV*, left ventricle; *P*, probe.

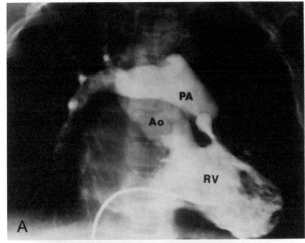

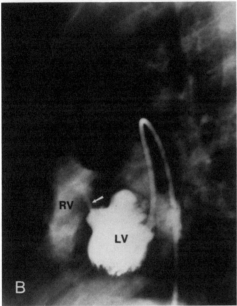

Fig. 23.13 Double-outlet right ventricle with side-by-side great artery relationship and obstructive subaortic VSD with severe subvalvular and valvular PS. (*A*) Frontal view of right ventricular (*RV*) angiocardiogram, demonstrating simultaneous opacification of aorta (*Ao*) and severe subvalvular and valvular PS. Great arteries are more or less in side-by-side relationship, and both arise completely from this ventricle. *PA*, main pulmonary artery. (*B*) Lateral view of left ventricular (*LV*) angiocardiogram. Part of left atrium (LA) was opacified from catheter-induced mitral insufficiency. Left ventricle is hypoplastic, and part of right ventricle (*RV*) was opacified via severely obstructive VSD (*arrow*). VSD is subaortic in position.

the position of the great arteries may be incorrectly related to the lower septum. It is important to relate the great artery position and conus septum to the superior ventricular septum since it is this malalignment that determines the origin of the great arteries.

CONDUCTION SYSTEM

The location of the atrioventricular node, bundle of His, and proximal portions of the right and left bundle branches was first reported by Titus *et al.*[76] in patients with subaortic VSD and side-by-side great arteries. In addition, the conduction system[49] in a case of DORV with subaortic VSD and

levomalposition of the aorta, and in patients with DORV with subpulmonary VSD and dextromalposition of the great arteries has been described.[5] In all cases, the atrioventricular node was in a normal posterior position, and the conduction system subsequently penetrated the right side of the central fibrous body. The atrioventricular bundle was noted to lie in the inferior (posterior) wall of the defect and passed beneath the crest of the ventricular septum in the fashion usually noted with an uncomplicated VSD.[80]

CORONARY ARTERY ANATOMY

Elliott *et al.*[18] and Vlodaver *et al.*[79] reported that the typical coronary artery pattern in DORV was normal, but in one case the origin of the left anterior descending artery was from the right coronary artery. This represents an anomaly similar to that observed in tetralogy of Fallot. Also, in another case, the origin of the right circumflex branch was from the left coronary artery.

Sridaromont *et al.*[73] described five patients with DORV with PS who had anomalous origin of the left anterior descending coronary artery from the right coronary artery. All of these patients had a subaortic VSD. Three had great arteries in a side-by-side relationship, and two had malposition.

Lev and Bharati[46] reported that in patients with dextromalposition of the great arteries and subpulmonary VSD, the branching of the coronary arterial pattern was similar to that observed in patients with TGA with origin of the right coronary artery from the posterior aortic cusp and origin of the left coronary artery from the left cusp.

PHYSIOLOGY

The physiology noted in DORV depends on the 16 pathologic variations noted above and is based primarily on the

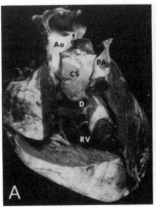
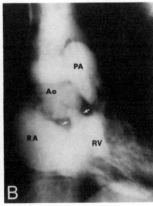

Fig. 23.14 Double-outlet right ventricle with side-by-side great artery relationship and subaortic VSD with subaortic stenosis. (*A*) Interior of right ventricle (*RV*) and side-by-side great arteries. Aortic outflow tract is markedly narrowed because of severely hypertrophied aortic conus and conus septum (*CS*). Subaortic VSD (*D*) is also an obstructive type. Main pulmonary artery (*PA*) and aortic root (*Ao*) are also seen. (*B*) Frontal right ventricular (*RV*) angiocardiogram with simultaneous opacification of side-by-side great arteries. Subaortic stenosis (between *arrows*) is well demonstrated. Right atrium (*RA*) was also opacified from catheter-induced tricuspid insufficiency. Aorta (*Ao*) and main pulmonary artery (*PA*) are also opacified. (*B*, reproduced with permission from F. J. Hallermann *et al.*[31])

four positions of the VSD and the four great artery relationships. The physiology is also affected by other associated conditions, most notably, pulmonary stenosis, the presence of pulmonary vascular obstructive disease, ASD, common atrium, atrioventricular canal, and subaortic stenosis, and the size of the VSD.

Tables 23.1 and 23.2 present data from 62 cases of DORV reported by Sridaromont et al.[71] The patients were divided into three groups: with pulmonary stenosis; without pulmonary stenosis but with pulmonary vascular obstructive disease; and without pulmonary stenosis or pulmonary vascular obstructive disease. Three additional categories of patients are reported in Table 23.1, namely, those with pulmonary artery saturation greater than systemic arterial saturation (25 patients); systemic arterial saturation greater than pulmonary artery saturation (27 patients); and pulmonary arterial saturation equal to systemic arterial saturation (10 patients). These hemodynamic patterns were not related to such factors as the relationship of the great arteries, the presence or absence of pulmonary stenosis, the presence or absence of pulmonary vascular obstructive disease, or functioning systemic pulmonary arterial shunts. However, there was a tendency toward a relationship between the systemic saturation and the position of the VSD.

POSITION OF THE VENTRICULAR SEPTAL DEFECT AND OXYGEN SATURATIONS

In all of the patients with subpulmonary VSD, the pulmonary arterial saturation was greater than the systemic arterial saturation, regardless of the presence or absence of PS or pulmonary vascular obstructive disease. When the VSD was subaortic, the saturation varied. In 60% of patients with subaortic VSD, the systemic arterial saturation was greater than the pulmonary arterial saturation (40% had pulmonary arterial saturation greater than systemic arterial saturation). The presence or absence of PS or pulmonary vascular obstruction had no consistent effect on systemic and pulmonary arterial saturation. Patients who had subaortic and subpulmonary VSD had pulmonary artery saturation greater than systemic arterial saturation.

Patients with a VSD that was remote from the semilunar valve had dissimilar arterial saturation levels. In patients with intact ventricular septum, the level of oxygen saturation was equal in the pulmonary and systemic arteries. From these data, one can conclude that patients who have systemic arterial saturation higher than pulmonary arterial saturation do not have subpulmonary ventricular septal defects, regardless of the presence or absence of pulmonary stenosis or pulmonary vascular obstructive disease. On the other hand, when the pulmonary arterial saturation is greater than systemic arterial saturation, the VSD location cannot be predicted.

PRESSURE RELATIONSHIPS

Because the aorta originates from the right ventricle, the right ventricular cavity must of necessity generate systemic pressures. In the presence of subvalvular or valvular PS, the pulmonary arterial pressure will be reduced. Of 65 patients reviewed by Sridaromont et al.,[71] 29 had PS. Three patients who had mild degrees of PS had significant elevation of pulmonary vascular resistance or histologic evidence of pulmonary vascular obstructive disease (Heath-Edwards grade 3 to 4).

In the same series, there were two patients who had intact ventricular septum and one patient with a severely restrictive VSD resulting in suprasystemic left ventricular pressures. In addition, patients who have severe degrees of subaortic stenosis in the presence of either PS or pulmonary vascular obstructive disease can be expected to have severe degrees of ventricular hypertrophy and suprasystemic ventricular pressures.

MANIFESTATIONS

The manifestations of DORV can be appreciated best as a spectrum outlining a diverse group of anomalies, all sharing

TABLE 23.1.   DIFFERENCES IN OXYGEN SATURATION IN 62 CASES OF DOUBLE-OUTLET RIGHT VENTRICLE[a]

Oxygen saturation	Cases (no.)	Range of oxygen saturation (%)[b]		Difference (%)	
		PA	SA	Range	Mean
PA > SA	25	71–93	54–88	3–23	8.2
SA > PA	27	52–94	69–97	2–20	8.8
PA = SA	10	57–92	57–92	<2	<2

[a] From S. Sridaromont et al.[71]

[b] PA, pulmonary arterial; SA, systemic arterial.

TABLE 23.2   RELATION OF VENTRICULAR SEPTAL DEFECT, OXYGEN SATURATION, PULMONARY STENOSIS, AND PULMONARY VASCULAR OBSTRUCTIVE DISEASE IN 62 CASES OF DOUBLE-OUTLET RIGHT VENTRICLE[a]

Location of VSD	Cases (no.)	Oxygen saturation	With PS	Without PS[b]		Total
				PVOD	No PVOD	
Subpulmonary	13	PA > SA	5	3	5	13
Subaortic	40	PA > SA	1	7	1	9
		SA > PA	16	5	3	24
		PA = SA	5	1	1	7
Subaortic and subpulmonary	2	PA > SA	0	2	0	2
Remote (atrioventricular canal)	5	PA > SA	0	0	1	1
		SA > PA	2	1	0	3
		PA = SA	0	1	0	1
No VSD (intact septum)	2	PA = SA	0	1	1	2
Total	62		29	21	12	62

[a] From S. Sridaromont, et al.[71]

[b] PA, pulmonary arterial; PS, pulmonary stenosis; PVOD, pulmonary vascular obstructive disease; SA, systemic arterial; VSD, ventricular septal defect.

a common pathologic feature of right ventricular origin of both great arteries. Clinically, DORV can be divided into four groups: subaortic VSD and PS, presenting features similar to those of tetralogy of Fallot; subpulmonary VSD with or without PS, resembling the picture in TGA; subaortic VSD without PS, presenting as simple VSD with pulmonary hypertension; and subaortic VSD without PS but with pulmonary vascular obstructive disease, demonstrating features of Eisenmenger's syndrome.

GROUP 1: SUBAORTIC VENTRICULAR SEPTAL DEFECT AND PULMONARY STENOSIS

With a clinical presentation similar to that in tetralogy of Fallot, these patients exhibit varying degrees of cyanosis. Depending on the severity of pulmonary stenosis, the cyanosis may become evident in the first year of life. When the PS is severe, early cyanosis, failure to thrive, exertional dyspnea, squatting, and polycythemia may be present. On examination, cyanosis and clubbing may be evident. The precordium may show evidence of a right ventricular impulse at the left sternal border, and a prominent systolic thrill is often palpable over the upper left sternal border. This is associated with a loud grade 4 to 5/6 systolic ejection murmur, which radiates into the lung fields. The first heart sound is normal, and usually the second heart sound is single. A third heart sound may be noted at the cardiac apex.

GROUP 2: SUBPULMONARY VENTRICULAR SEPTAL DEFECT WITH OR WITHOUT PULMONARY STENOSIS

These patients present clinically with features resembling those in TGA with VSD. Commonly, these patients present with cyanosis and heart failure in early infancy. When PS is also present, the cyanosis and polycythemia may be more severe and may be apparent earlier and with less evidence of heart failure. Patients in this group who have associated coarctation of the aorta may present in infancy with heart failure, cyanosis, and diminished or absent femoral pulses. As in patients with TGA, these patients also exhibit more severe failure to thrive and, with pulmonary plethora, may have frequent respiratory tract infections. On examination, there is typically severe cyanosis and clubbing. The height and weight may be markedly below normal. The precordial bulge and the right ventricular impulse are noted at the left sternal border. A grade 2 to 3/6 high-pitched systolic murmur may be present at the upper left sternal border. When PS is present, a systolic thrill may be associated, and the murmur is louder in quality (grade 3 to 4/6). The second heart sound is loud and single and is most notably related to the proximity of the aorta. With increased pulmonary flow, an apical diastolic rumble may be present.

GROUP 3: SUBAORTIC VENTRICULAR SEPTAL DEFECT WITHOUT PULMONARY STENOSIS

These patients present features typical of those with a large VSD and pulmonary hypertension. Usually, little cyanosis will be evident, but failure to thrive and heart failure are dominant features.[19] Similarly, with increased pulmonary flow, respiratory tract infections are frequent. On examination, the heart is overactive. A systolic thrill may be present at the upper left sternal border and a grade 3 to 4/6 holosystolic murmur may be evident at the left sternal border. An apical diastolic rumble and a third heart sound are audible at the cardiac apex.

GROUP 4: SUBAORTIC VENTRICULAR SEPTAL DEFECT WITH PULMONARY VASCULAR OBSTRUCTIVE DISEASE

These patients present as older Group 3 patients in whom pulmonary vascular obstructive disease has developed. Pulmonary flow is reduced, and heart failure and frequent respiratory infections are less evident. Now cyanosis and clubbing may be present. On examination, the systolic murmur may be markedly diminished or absent. The second sound is very loud and single. A decrescendo diastolic murmur of pulmonary valve insufficiency may be present.

Electrovectorcardiographic Features

A number of electrocardiographic abnormalities are typically present in most patients with DORV.[43, 56, 57] Right ventricular hypertrophy and right axis deviation are the most common features and are related primarily to the systemic work imposed on the right ventricle (Fig. 23.15). Left ventricular forces are usually normal in patients with PS, but combined ventricular hypertrophy may be present in patients with markedly increased pulmonary flow, as frequently observed in patients with subpulmonary VSD. In addition, a pronounced increase in left ventricular forces may be evident in instances of restrictive VSD. First-degree atrioventricular conduction delay is a common feature; however, it is not uniformly observed. A number of patients with DORV may have left axis deviation with a counterclockwise frontal plane loop.[43] It has been less commonly observed in DORV without PS.

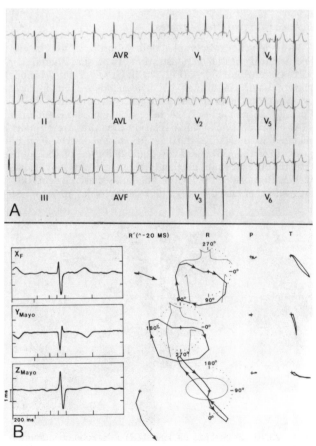

Fig. 23.15 Scalar (A) and vector (B) electrocardiograms (modified Frank lead system) demonstrate right axis deviation and right ventricular hypertrophy in patient with double-outlet right ventricle with pulmonary stenosis.

Right atrial enlargement is often observed, particularly in patients with PS, whereas left atrial enlargement may be observed in instances of increased pulmonary flow with intact atrial septum. Patients with complete atrioventricular canal defect associated with DORV would also be expected to have left axis deviation, combined ventricular hypertrophy, atrial enlargement, and first-degree atrioventricular conduction delay.[59, 72] Patients with complex associated anomalies such as abdominal heterotaxia may have anomalies of the P wave axis associated with the heterotaxia.

Radiologic Features

The roentgenographic features correspond to the physiological and clincal manifestations. In patients with PS, the features may resemble those seen in patients with tetraology of Fallot, but one may more commonly observe a mild degree of cardiomegaly. The pulmonary vascularlity is diminished. The main pulmonary artery segment is absent, which results in a concave upper-left border of the heart. When a subpulmonary VSD is present, the roentgenographic features may resemble those of TGA, especially when, in the absence of PS, a pronounced increase in pulmonary vascularity may be observed along with cardiomegaly (Fig. 23.16).

In cases of subaortic VSD without PS, with or without pulmonary vascular obstructive disease, there is generalized cardiomegaly and prominent main pulmonary artery segment and increased pulmonary vascularity. When pulmonary vascular obstructive disease is present, the central vessels may be prominent, with "prunning" of the peripheral arterial vasculature.

Echocardiographic Features

M-mode echocardiographic delineation of DORV has relied primarily on the demonstration of mitral and semilunar valve discontinuity[9, 21, 83] (Fig. 23.17). However, this M-mode feature has been limited by its dependence on operator interpretation and spatial anatomic relationships.[20, 25, 67, 81] Formidable obstacles have been the complex semilunar valve-atrioventricular valve relationships that are often associated with DORV, the inability to localize clearly the position of the VSD, and the poor definition of the conus that produces a semilunar and atrioventricular valve separation. Because of the lack of adequate spatial orientation, even in experienced hands, the rapidity of an apex-to-base

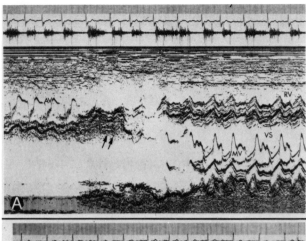

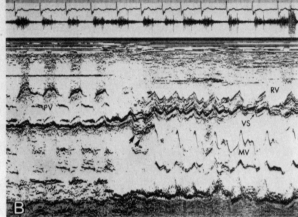

Fig. 23.17   M-mode echocardiogram in patient with double-outlet right ventricle (side-by-side great arteries), showing scans from aortic (A) and pulmonary (B) valves to left ventricle. Both appear to be separated from mitral valve by muscle (arrows). AV, aortic valve; PV, pulmonary valve; RV, right ventricle; VS, ventricular septum; MV, mitral valve. (Reproduced with permission from J. B. Seward and A. J. Tajik, Current status of echocardiography in cyanotic congenital heart diseases. Cardiovasc. Clin. 9 (2):269, 1978, and with permission from the F. A. Davis Co.)

scan and the angle of beam projection could produce false-positive and false-negative results in M-mode echocardiography.

Two-dimensional echocardiographic findings for the diagnosis of DORV have been reported.[27, 30, 35, 41] Three observations were noted for the diagnosis: origin of both great arteries from the anterior right ventricle; mitral-semilunar valve discontinuity; and absence of left ventricular outflow other than the VSD. In a series of 36 patients studied by 2D echocardiography, both great arteries were observed to originate predominantly from the anterior right ventricle. If one great artery overrode the VSD, nearly exclusive or predominant commitment to the right ventricle was required for diagnosis. An associated observation was a parallel course of the great arteries in their origin. This was recognized by simultaneous observation of both semilunar valves originating from the right ventricle, as noted in the same parasternal or subcostal long-axis scan (Fig. 23.18).

In about two-thirds of the cases, both great arteries can be observed originating anteriorly from the right ventricle but without clear visualization of both semilunar valves. However, the semilunar valves may be demonstrated with slight right or left transducer angulation. Less commonly, all cardiac chambers, atrioventricular valves, and semilunar

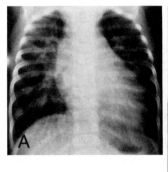

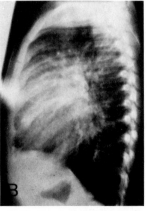

Fig. 23.16   Frontal (A) and lateral (B) chest roentgenograms in 7-month-old with double-outlet right ventricle, subpulmonary VSD, and pulmonary hypertension. Pulmonary vascularity is increased, and there is moderate cardiomegaly. Moderate cyanosis was present clinically.

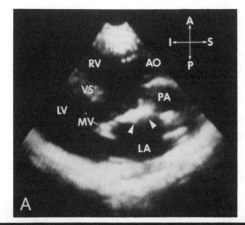

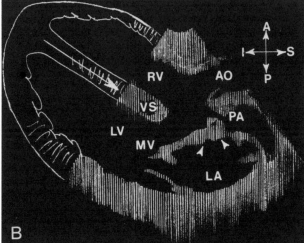

Fig. 23.18 (*A*) Parasternal long-axis scan in a patient who had double-outlet right ventricle with pulmonary artery (*PA*) posterior and to right of aorta (*AO*). Both great arteries originate entirely from anterior right ventricular cavity. (Both great arteries fall anterior to a line projected superiorly along plane of ventricular septum (*VS*) indicated by *arrow* on accompanying line drawing.) (*B*) Parallel orientation of great arteries is observed with simultaneous visualization of both semilunar valves in same long-axis plane. Pulmonary artery is recognized by its course posterior to lungs, and pulmonary stenosis is apparent. Large subpulmonary ventricular septal defect is observed. *Arrowheads* point to moderate subpulmonary conus tissue that separates mitral valve (*MV*) from pulmonary artery. Depth markers are present across top and down left side of figures. *RV*, right ventricle; *LV*, left ventricle; *LA*, left atrium. (Reproduced with permission from D. J. Hagler *et al.*[30] and the American Heart Association.)

valves can be demonstrated in the same parasternal long-axis scan (Fig. 23.19).

Short axis scans from apex to base are also helpful in demonstrating the commitment of both great arteries to the right ventricular cavity, as observed by their anterior position with reference to the plane of the ventricular septum[34, 35] (Fig. 23.20). With the use of a short axis scan at the cardiac base, a double-circle appearance of the great arteries was consistent with a parallel orientation of the great arteries.

Parasternal long-axis scans, often from a slightly more superior position at the left sternal edge, also demonstrate the initial parallel course of the great arteries[26, 29] (Fig. 23.21). The pulmonary artery may be recognized by its course posterior to the lungs, as observed on the long-axis scan, and by its bifurcation at the right and left pulmonary arteries, as noted with short-axis or subcostal scans.[6, 37, 38] A more ante-

rior and superior course of the great artery allows its identification as the aorta. Short-axis scans at the base allow recognition of the great artery spatial relationships (Fig. 23.22).

Parasternal long axis scans demonstrate mitral-semilunar valve discontinuity with the presence of muscular conus separation (Fig. 23.23). Mitral-semilunar valve discontinuity as observed by 2D echocardiography appears as a dense echo separating the two valves. The degree of separation is variable but can be recognized even when 0.5 to 1.0 cm in size.

Two-dimensional echocardioagraphy can accurately predict the position of the VSD in reference to the great arteries. In most patients, typical subaortic or subpulmonary defects can be demonstrated by parasternal or subcostal long and short axis scans. Utilizing both long and short axis scans allows confirmation of the VSD-great artery relationships. Very large defects or doubly committed defects are recognized as appearing nearly equally committed to both great arteries. Remote defects or noncommitted defects are usu-

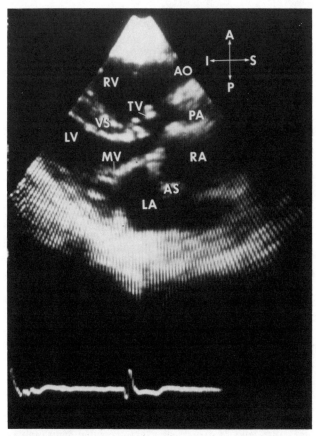

Fig. 23.19 Parasternal long-axis scan in a patient who had double-outlet right ventricle, with aorta (*AO*) anterior and to left of pulmonary artery (*PA*). Both great arteries are entirely committed to right ventricular cavity and are observed in parallel orientation originating from right ventricle (*RV*). In this standard long-axis scan, all four cardiac chambers and both great arteries are observed simultaneously. As identified, cardiac chambers and great artery locations were verified at cardiac catheterization with 2D echocardiographic contrast studies. Pulmonary valve appeared slightly thickened, and in real time valve domed during systole, consistent with PS. Mitral valve (*MV*) is markedly separated from semilunar valves. *LV*, left ventricle; *VS*, ventricular septum; *AS*, atrial septum; *LA*, left atrium; *RA*, right atrium; *TV*, tricuspid valve. (Reproduced with permission from D. J. Hagler *et al.*[30] and the American Heart Association.)

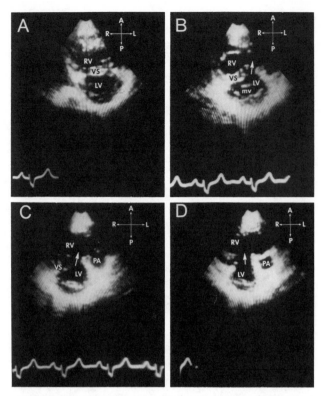

Fig. 23.20 Short-axis scan of heart from apex to base in a patient with double-outlet right ventricle. As scan progresses up through atrioventricular valves, VSD is observed. At cardiac base, it is apparent that the VSD is the only outlet from left ventricular cavity and that both great arteries originate entirely from the anterior right ventricular cavity. Pulmonary artery (PA) is to the left and is separated from LV by bridge of muscular tissue. Thus, VSD is noted to be subaortic at cardiac base. Aorta (AO) is anterior and to right of pulmonary artery, and large conus is observed posterior to both great arteries. Pulmonary valve appears bicuspid and small in this patient with associated PS. VSD is indicated by *arrow*. RV, right ventricle; VS, ventricular septum; LV, left ventricle; RA, right atrium; LA, left atrium; mv, mitral valve. (Reproduced with permission from D. J. Hagler et al.[30] and the American Heart Association.)

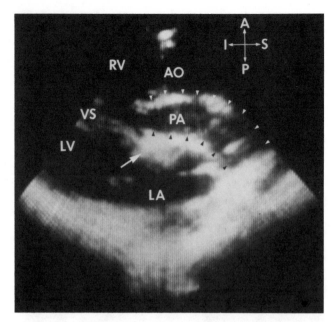

Fig. 23.21 Parasternal long-axis scan from slightly more superior position at left sternal edge in same patient as in Figure 23.18 demonstrates posterior angulation of pulmonary artery (PA) to lungs, which allows its identification as pulmonary artery. *Arrowheads* indicate posterior course of pulmonary artery. Both great arteries are entirely committed to right ventricular cavity (RV). Subpulmonary conus is demonstrated by *large arrow*. AO, aorta; VS, ventricular septum; LV, left ventricle; LA, left atrium. (Reproduced with permission from D. J. Hagler et al.[30] and the American Heart Association.)

ally complete atrioventricular canal defects. Complete atrioventricular canal defects are best recognized by apical or subcostal four-chamber views.[28] 2D echocardiography can also demonstrate small or restrictive VSDs. Contrast 2D echocardiography is helpful in demonstrating associated muscular VSDs.

Double-outlet right ventricle may be associated with a number of atrioventricular valve anomalies, including: complete atrioventricular canal defect[28, 30, 72]; isolated cleft of the anterior mitral leaflet; straddling left and right atrioventricular valves; and atrioventricular septal malalignment (anular override). These abnormalities may be diagnosed primarily by 2D echocardiography.[28, 68] Most are detected by utilizing short axis or apical four-chamber views. Short axis scans of the mitral valve can demonstrate the cleft in the anterior mitral leaflet associated with an atrioventricular canal type of VSD.

DIFFERENTIAL DIAGNOSIS

The clinical features of DORV span a wide spectrum from simple VSD to TGA and TF. There obviously are very few clinical, electrocardiographic, or radiographic features that allow distinction of these anomalies on a clinical basis.

2D echocardiography currently provides an ideal noninvasive method for the recognition of this complex form of congenital heart disease. In addition, 2D echocardiography has been particularly accurate in the demonstration of great artery relationships and the relationship of the VSD to the great arteries; it allows recognition of the presence or absence of PS, and it provides direct clues to the presence of associated complex atrioventricular valve abnormalities that may not be demonstrable by other means.

Cardiac catheterization and selective angiography require right and left ventricular injections to allow the best delineation of the ventricular and great artery anatomy and relationships. The presence or absence of PS may be clearly demonstrated, as may the status of the pulmonary vascular tree. Combined use of 2D echocardiography, cardiac catheterization, and selective angiography provides the most complete diagnosis of this complex anomaly.

SURGICAL TREATMENT

The surgical repair of the group of anomalies included under the heading of double-outlet right ventricle is complicated by the great variability in intracardiac and extracardiac morphology evidenced by these hearts.[80] Because of the complexity of intracardiac repair of these anomalies, we prefer to palliate infants and small children who become severely symptomatic in the first year of life. Pulmonary arterial banding in DORV without PS will reduce pulmonary flow and protect the pulmonary arterioles from obstructive pulmonary arteriopathy; systemic-to-pulmonary artery shunting will increase pulmonary flow and reduce cyanosis in patients with PS.

Complete correction of DORV depends on the complexity

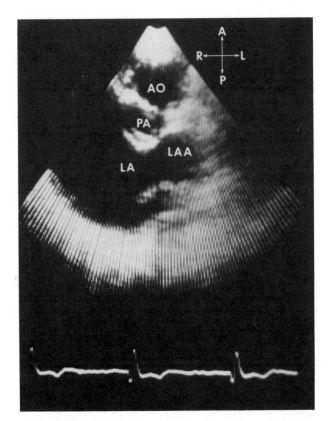

Fig. 23.22 Short-axis scan at cardiac base in patient with double-outlet right ventricle. Double-circle appearance of great arteries is noted. Scan shows aorta (*AO*) anterior and slightly to left of pulmonary artery (*PA*). The pulmonary valve appears bicuspid and stenotic. *LA*, left atrium; *LAA*, left atrial appendage. (Reproduced with permission from D. J. Hagler et al.[30] and the American Heart Association.)

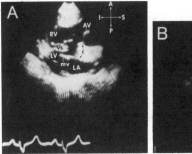
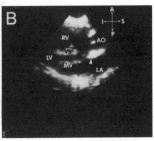

Fig. 23.23 (*A*) Parasternal long-axis scan in same patient as in Figure 23.20 demonstrates large conus (*c*) separating mitral valve (*mv*) from aortic valve (*AV*), which originates entirely from right ventricular cavity (*RV*) and is superiorly displaced by conus tissue. VSD is the only outlet from left ventricular cavity (*LV*) and is subaortic in position. *vs*, ventricular septum. (*B*) Parasternal long-axis scan in another patient with double-outlet right ventricle and subaortic VSD. Aorta (*AO*) is nearly entirely committed to anterior right ventricle. VSD is sole outlet from left ventricle. Smaller subaortic conus (*arrowhead*, approximately 1 cm) separates mitral valve (*MV*) from aortic valve. *LA*, left atrium; *VS*, ventricular septum. (Reproduced with permission from D. J. Hagler et al.[30] and the American Heart Association.)

of the intracardiac anatomy. Ideally, this may be attempted when the patient is about 2 years old but may be deferred in asymptomatic patients until 4 years if an extracardiac conduit is anticipated.

The objectives of the operation are as follows.

1. Establishment of Left Ventricle-to-Aorta Continuity. In general, this is accomplished by creating a tunnel between the VSD and the subaortic outflow tract by means of a patch of Dacron (Fig. 23.24). Care must be exercised to prevent obstruction of this connection, and because of this, some VSDs need to be enlarged in such a manner as to avoid injury to the conduction tissue. The location of the conduction bundle in reference to the type of VSD has recently been outlined.[80]

2. Establishment of Adequate Right Ventricle-to-Pulmonary Artery Continuity. In the simple forms of the anomaly—with situs solitus and atrioventricular concordance in which PS is absent—this requires care in preventing the subaortic tunnel from encroaching on the subpulmonary outflow tract. In patients with PS, this may require pulmonary valvotomy, infundibular resection, patch enlargement of the right ventricular outflow tract, or insertion of an extracardiac valved conduit and bringing the right ventricle into communication with the pulmonary artery.

3. Repair of Associated Lesions. In the surgical correction of DORV, the position of the VSD and its relationship to the great vessels is of paramount importance. The classic form of repair is possible only in those patients with subaortic VSD. When the defect is positioned at a distance

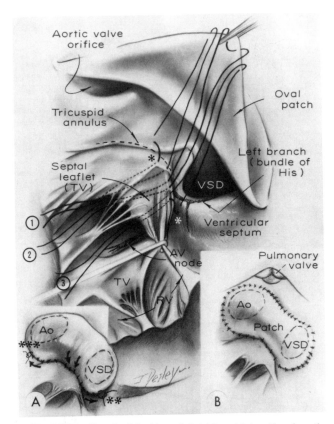

Fig. 23.24 Repair of double-outlet right ventricle with subaortic ventricular septal defect. The creation of the intracardiac tunnel establishing continuity between the left ventricle and aorta is shown. *VSD*, ventricular septal defect; *TV*, tricuspid valve; *RV*, right ventricle; *AV*, atrioventricular; *Ao*, aorta. The *circled numbers* indicate the three crucial sutures which attach the large oval patch to the base of the septal leaflet of the tricuspid valve (between single *). After these sutures are tied, the patch is attached to the ventricular septum caudally (**) and the muscle leading from the tricuspid annulus to the orifice of the aortic valve (***). (Reproduced with permission from M. M. R. Gomes[22] and the American Heart Association.)

from the aortic outflow tract, that is, in the muscular septum posteriorly or below the pulmonary outflow tract, tunneling from the VSD to the aortic outflow tract is not possible. Under these circumstances, other surgical solutions are required. In subpulmonary VSD, closure of the defect in such a manner as to divert left ventricular blood to the pulmonary artery creates TGA, which is then corrected by an inflow procedure (Mustard or Senning procedure) or by an outflow procedure (Jatene, Kaye-Damus-Stansel, or Aubert procedure[60, 80]). In DORV with levomalposition of the aorta, the repair proposed and achieved by Danielson et al.[13]—diverting left ventricular blood to the subaortic outflow tract and establishing right ventricle-to-pulmonary continuity—appears to be the method of choice.

In some patients in whom straddling of the right or left atrioventricular valve complicates the anatomy of the VSD, septation may not be possible without replacement of the straddling valve. Alternatively, if the pulmonary pressure and resistance are low, definitive palliation (as opposed to correction) can be achieved by obliteration of the right-sided atrioventricular valve and closure of any atrial septal defect, interruption of ventriculopulmonary arterial continuity, and establishment of an atriopulmonary connection (modified Fontan procedure).[10]

Other, more complex, forms of DORV have also been successfully repaired. Double-outlet right ventricle with atrioventricular discordance can be corrected by closure of the VSD, transsection of the pulmonary artery, and establishment of morphologic left ventricle-to-pulmonary artery continuity with an extracardiac conduit; in these patients, the right ventricle remains as the systemic ventricle. Kiser et al.[42] reported repair of dextrocardia, atrioventricular discordance, VSD, and double-origin right ventricle. Gomes et al.[23] reported on the results of complete repair of DORV without PS in 18 patients. The overall operative mortality rate was 22%; higher mortality rates were encountered in patients with elevated pulmonary arterial resistance and in those with associated lesions, especially atrioventricular canal defects. The authors concluded that patients with these conditions should have early operation before the onset of severe obstructive pulmonary arteriopathy. The same authors[22] reported on 22 patients with DORV and PS who underwent complete repair. The overall mortality was 32%, but in patients operated on after 1960, the mortality had decreased to 16%. A higher risk was associated in patients with anomalies of coronary distribution, multiple VSD, or residual PS. The use of extracardiac conduits becomes necessary in many cases in which there is complicated anatomy.

References

1. Abbott, M. E. Atlas of Congenital Cardiac Disease. American Heart Association, New York, 1936.
2. Ainger, L. E. Double-outlet right ventricle: Intact ventricular septum, mitral stenosis, and blind left ventricle. Am. Heart J. 70:521, 1965.
3. Anderson, R. H., Wilkinson, J. L., Arnold, R. Becker, A. E., and Lubkiewicz, K. Morphogenesis of bulboventricular malformations. II. Observations on malformed hearts. Br. Heart J. 36:948, 1974.
4. Anderson, R. H., Wilkinson, J. L., Arnold, R., and Lubkiewicz, K. Morphogenesis of bulboventricular malformations. I. Consideration of embryogenesis in the normal heart. Br. Heart J. 36:242, 1974.
5. Bharati, S., and Lev, M. The conduction system in double outlet right ventricle with subpulmonic ventricular septal defect and related hearts (the Taussig-Bing group). Circulation 54:459, 1976.
6. Bierman, F. Z., and Williams, R. G. Prospective diagnosis of transposition of the great arteries by subxyphoid two dimensional echocardiography in neonates (abstr.). Circulation 58 (Suppl. 2):201, 1978.
7. Cameron, A. H., Acerete, F., Quero, M., and Castro, M. C. Double outlet right ventricle: Study of 27 cases. Br. Heart J. 38:1124, 1976.
8. Carey, L. S., and Edwards, J. E. Roentgenographic features in cases with origin of both great vessels from the right ventricle without pulmonary stenosis. Am. J. Roentgenol., Radium Ther. Nucl. Med. 93:269, 1965.
9. Chesler, E., Joffe, H. S., Beck, W., and Schrire, V. Echocardiographic recognition of mitral-semilunar valve discontinuity: An aid to the diagnosis of origin of both great vessels from the right ventricle. Circulation 43:725, 1971.
10. Ciaravella, J. M., Jr., McGoon, D. C., Hagler, D. J., and Fulton, R. E. Caplike double-horned double-outlet right ventricle: Report of two cases. J. Thorac. Cardiovasc. Surg. 77:536, 1979.
11. Collan, Y., and Pesonen, E. Double outlet right ventricle with extreme hypertrophy of muscle bundles associated with crista supraventricularis: A heart with three ventricles. Helv. Paediatr. Acta 31:521, 1976.
12. Crawford, M. d'A. Multiple congenital anomaly associated with an extra autosome. Lancet 2:22, 1961.
13. Danielson, G. K., Ritter, D. G., Coleman, H. N., III, and DuShane, J. W. Successful repair of double-outlet right ventricle with transposition of the great arteries (aorta anterior and to the left), pulmonary stenosis, and subaortic ventricular septal defect. J. Thorac. Cardiovasc. Surg. 63:741, 1972.
14. Davachi, F., Moller, J. H., and Edwards, J. E. Origin of both great vessels from right ventricle with intact ventricular septum. Am. Heart J. 75:790, 1968.
15. Descalzo, A., Cañadas, M., Cintado, C., Castillo, J. A., Miralles, J., and Ariza, S. Ventricule droit à double issue avec septum interventriculaire intact: Présentation d'un cas et révision de la littérature. Arch. Maladies Coeur Vaisseaux 72:899, 1979.
16. Edwards, J. E., Carey, L. S., Neufeld, H. N., and Lester, R. G. Congenital Heart Disease: Correlation of Pathologic Anatomy and Angiocardiography. W. B. Saunders, Philadelphia, 1965.
17. Edwards, J. H., Harnden, D. G., Cameron, A. H., Crosse, V. M., and Wolff, O. H. A new trisomic syndrome. Lancet 1:787, 1960.
18. Elliott, L. P., Amplatz, K., and Edwards, J. E. Coronary arterial patterns in transposition complexes: Anatomic and angiocardiographic studies. Am. J. Cardiol. 17:362, 1966.
19. Engle, M. A., Steinberg, I., Lukas, D. S., and Goldberg, H. P. Acyanotic ventricular septal defect with both great vessels from the right ventricle. Am. Heart J. 66:755, 1963.
20. French, J. W., and Popp, R. Variability of echocardiographic discontinuity in double outlet right ventricle and truncus arteriosus. Circulation 51:848, 1975.
21. Goldberg, S. J., Allen, H. D., and Sahn, D. J. Pediatric and Adolescent Echocardiography. Year Book Medical Publishers, Chicago, 1975, p. 134.
22. Gomes, M. M. R., Weidman, W. H., McGoon, D. C., and Danielson, G. K. Double-outlet right ventricle with pulmonic stenosis: Surgical considerations and results of operation. Circulation 43:889, 1971.
23. Gomes, M. M. R., Weidman, W. H., McGoon, D. C., and Danielson, G. K. Double-outlet right ventricle without pulmonic stenosis: Surgical considerations and results of operation. Circulation 43 (Suppl. 1):31, 1971.
24. Goor, D. A., and Edwards, J. E. The spectrum of transposition of the great arteries: With specific reference to developmental anatomy of the conus. Circulation 48:406, 1973.
25. Gutgesell, H. P. [Echocardiographic vs anatomical "discontinuity"]. And continued (letter to the editor). Circulation 53:203, 1976.
26. Hagler, D. J., Tajik, A. J., Seward, J. B., Mair, D. D., and Ritter, D. G. 80-Degree sector echocardiographic profiles of patients with cono-truncal abnormalities. In Abstracts of the 8th World Congress of Cardiology. September 1978, p. 502.
27. Hagler, D. J., Tajik, A. J., Seward, J. B., Mair, D. D., and Ritter, D. G. Wide-angle sector echocardiographic assessment of double-outlet right ventricle (abstr.). Circulation 58 (Suppl. 2):202, 1978.
28. Hagler, D. J., Tajik, A. J., Seward, J. B., Mair, D. D., and Ritter, D. G. Real-time wide-angle sector echocardiography: Atrioventricular canal defects. Circulation 59:140, 1979.
29. Hagler, D. J., Tajik, A. J., Seward, J. B., Mair, D. D., and Ritter, D. G. Wide-angle two-dimensional echocardiographic profiles of conotruncal abnormalities. Mayo Clin. Proc. 55:73, 1980.
30. Hagler, D. J., Tajik, A. J., Seward, J. B., Mair, D. D., and Ritter, D. G. Double-outlet right ventricle: Wide-angle two-dimensional echocardiographic observations. Circulation 63: 419, 1981.
31. Hallermann, F. J., Kincaid, O. W., Ritter, D. G., Ongley, P. A., and Titus, J. L. Angiocardiographic and anatomic findings in origin of both great arteries from the right ventricle. Am. J. Roentgenol. Radium Ther. Nucl. Med. 109:51, 1970.
32. Hallermann, F. J., Kincaid, O. W., Ritter, D. G., and Titus, J. L. Mitral-semilunar valve relationships in the angiography of cardiac malformations. Radiology 94:63, 1970.
33. Hazell, S. G., Ritter, D. G., Ongley, P. A., and Hallermann, F. J. Hemodynamics in cases of origin of both great vessels from the right ventricle (P) (abstr.). Circulation 36 (Suppl. 2):138, 1967.

34. Henry, W. L., Maron, B. J., and Griffith, J. M. Cross-sectional echocardiography in the diagnosis of congenital heart disease: Identification of the relation of the ventricles and great arteries. Circulation 56:267, 1977.

35. Henry, W. L., Maron, B. J., Griffith, J. M., Redwood, D. R., and Epstein, S. E. Differential diagnosis of anomalies of the great arteries by real-time two-dimensional echocardiography. Circulation 51:283, 1975.

36. Hightower, B. M., Barcia, A., Bargeron, L. M., Jr., and Kirklin, J. W. Double-outlet right ventricle with transposed great arteries and subpulmonary ventricular septal defect: The Taussig-Bing malformation. Circulation 39 (Suppl. 1):207, 1969.

37. Houston, A. B., Gregory, N. L., and Coleman, E. N. Two-dimensional sector scanner echocardiography in cyanotic congenital heart disease. Br. Heart J. 39:1076, 1977.

38. Houston, A. B., Gregory, N. L., and Coleman, E. N. Echocardiographic identification of aorta and main pulmonary artery in complete transposition. Br. Heart J. 40:377, 1978.

39. Judson, J. P., Danielson, G. K., Ritter, D. G., and Hagler, D. J. Successful repair of co-existing double outlet right ventricle and two-chamber right ventricle. J. Thorac. Cardiovasc. Surg. 84:113, 1982.

40. Kawashima, Y., Fujita, T., Miyamoto, T., and Manabe, H. Intraventricular rerouting of blood for the correction of Taussig-Bing malformation. J. Thorac. Cardiovasc. Surg. 62:825, 1971.

41. King, D. L., Steeg, C. N., and Ellis, K. Demonstration of transposition of the great arteries by cardiac ultrasonography. Radiology 107:181, 1973.

42. Kiser, J. C., Ongley, P. A., Kirklin, J. W., Clarkson, P. M., and McGoon, D. C. Surgical treatment of dextrocardia with inversion of ventricles and double-outlet right ventricle. J. Thorac. Cardiovasc. Surg. 55:6, 1968.

43. Krongrad, E., Ritter, D. G., Weidman, W. H., and DuShane, J. W. Hemodynamic and anatomic correlation of electrocardiogram in double-outlet right ventricle. Circulation 46:995, 1972.

44. Kurien, V. A., and Duke, M. Trisomy 17-18 syndrome: Report of a case with diffuse myocardial fibrosis and review of cardiovascular abnormalities. Am. J. Cardiol. 21:431, 1968.

45. Lavoie, R., Sestier, F., Gilbert, G., Chameides, L., Van Praagh, R., and Grondin, P. Double outlet right ventricle with left ventricular outflow tract obstruction due to small ventricular septal defect. Am. Heart J. 82:290, 1971.

46. Lev, M., and Bharati, S. Transposition of the arterial truncus in levocardia. In Cardiovascular Pathology Decennial, 1966–1975, edited by S. C. Sommers. Appleton-Century-Crofts, New York, 1975, p. 30.

47. Lev, M., Bharati, S., Meng, L., Liberthson, R. R., Paul, M. H., and Idriss, F. A concept of double-outlet right ventricle. J. Thorac. Cardiovasc. Surg. 64:271, 1972.

48. Lev, M., Rimoldi, H. J. A., Eckner, F. A. O., Melhuish, B. P., Meng, L., and Paul, M. H. The Taussig-Bing heart: Qualitative and quantitative anatomy. Arch. Pathol. 81:24, 1966.

49. Lincoln, C. Total correction of D-loop double-outlet right ventricle with bilateral conus, L-transposition, and pulmonic stenosis. J. Thorac. Cardiovasc. Surg. 64:435, 1972.

50. MacMahon, H. E., and Lipa, M. Double-outlet right ventricle with intact interventricular septum. Circulation 30:745, 1964.

51. Mason, D. T., Morrow, A. G., Elkins, R. C., and Friedman, W. F. Origin of both great vessels from the right ventricle associated with severe obstruction to left ventricular outflow. Am. J. Cardiol. 24:118, 1969.

52. McGoon, D. C. Origin of both great vessels from the right ventricle. Surg. Clin. North Am. 41 (4):1113, 1961.

53. Megarity, A. L., Chambers, R. G., Calder, A. L., Van Praagh, S., and Van Praagh, R. Double-outlet right ventricle with left ventricular-right atrial communication: Fibrous obstruction of left ventricular outlet by membranous septum and tricuspid leaflet tissue. Am. Heart J. 84:242, 1972.

54. Mitchell, S. C., Korones, S. B., and Berendes, H. W. Congenital heart disease in 56,109 births: Incidence and natural history. Circulation 43:323, 1971.

55. Nadal-Ginard, B., Sanz, G., and Froufe, J. Total dextroposition of the great vessels with obstruction of the left ventricular outlet. Chest 64:270, 1973.

56. Neufeld, H. N., DuShane, J. W., and Edwards, J. E. Origin of both great vessels from the right ventricle. II. With pulmonary stenosis. Circulation 23:603, 1961.

57. Neufeld, H. N., DuShane, J. W., Wood, E. H., Kirklin, J. W., and Edwards, J. E. Origin of both great vessels from the right ventricle. I. Without pulmonary stenosis. Circulation 23:399, 1961.

58. Neufeld, H. N., Lucas, R. V., Jr., Lester, R. G., Adams, P., Jr., Anderson, R. C., and Edwards, J. E. Origin of both great vessels from the right ventricle without pulmonary stenosis. Br. Heart J. 24:393, 1962.

59. Neufeld, H. N., Titus, J. L., DuShane, J. W., Burchell, H. B., and Edwards, J. E. Isolated ventricular septal defect of the persistent common atrioventricular canal type. Circulation 23:685, 1961.

60. Pacifico, A. D., Kirklin, J. W., and Bargeron, L. M., Jr. Complex congenital malformations: Surgical treatment of double-outlet right ventricle and double-outlet left ventricle. In Adv. Cardiovascular Surgery, edited by J. W. Kirklin. Grune & Stratton, New York, 1973, p. 57.

61. Patau, K., Smith, D. W., Therman, E., Inhorn, S. L., and Wagner, H. P. Multiple congenital anomaly caused by an extra autosome. Lancet 1:790, 1960.

62. Patrick, D. L., and McGoon, D. C. An operation for double-outlet right ventricle with transposition of the great arteries. J. Cardiovasc. Surg. (Torino) 9:537, 1968.

63. Pellegrino, P. A., Eckner, F. A., Meier, M. A., Long, D. M., Hastreiter, A. R., and Serratto, M. Double outlet right ventricle with fibromuscular obstruction to left ventricular outlet. J. Cardiovasc. Surg. (Torino) 14:253, 1973.

64. Quero Jiménez, M., Pérez Martínez, V. M., Maitre Azcárate, M. J., Merino Batres, G., and Moreno Granados, F. Exaggerated displacement of the atrioventricular canal towards the bulbus cordis (rightward displacement of the mitral valve). Br. Heart J. 35:65, 1973.

65. Rastelli, G. C., Kirklin, J. W., and Titus, J. L. Anatomic observations on complete form of persistent common atrioventricular canal with special reference to atrioventricular valves. Mayo Clin. Proc. 41:296, 1966.

66. Rogers, T. R., Hagstrom, J. W. C., and Engle, M. A. Origin of both great vessels from the right ventricle associated with the trisomy-18 syndrome. Circulation 32:802, 1965.

67. Sahn, D. J., Allen, H. D., and Goldberg, S. J. Echocardiographic vs anatomical "discontinuity" (letter to the editor). Circulation 53:200, 1976.

68. Seward, J. B., Tajik, A. J., Hagler, D. J., and Mair, D. D. Straddling atrioventricular valve: Diagnostic two-dimensional echocardiographic features (abstr.). Am. J. Cardiol. 41:354, 1978.

69. Sondheimer, H. M., Freedom, R. M., and Olley, P. M. Double outlet right ventricle: Clinical spectrum and prognosis. Am. J. Cardiol. 39:709, 1977.

70. Squarcia, U., Ritter, D. G., and Kincaid, O. W. Dextrocardia: Angiocardiographic study and classification. Am. J. Cardiol. 32:965, 1973.

71. Sridaromont, S., Feldt, R. H., Ritter, D. G., Davis, G. D., and Edwards, J. E. Double outlet right ventricle: Hemodynamic and anatomic correlations. Am. J. Cardiol. 38:85, 1976.

72. Sridaromont, S., Feldt, R. H., Ritter, D. G., Davis, G. D., McGoon, D. C., and Edwards, J. E. Double-outlet right ventricle associated with persistent common atrioventricular canal. Circulation 52:933, 1975.

73. Sridaromont, S., Ritter, D. G., Feldt, R. H., Davis, G. D., and Edwards, J. E. Double-outlet right ventricle: Anatomic and angiocardiographic correlations. Mayo Clin. Proc. 53:555, 1978.

74. Tandon, R., Moller, J. H., and Edwards, J. E. Communication of mitral valve with both ventricles associated with double outlet right ventricle. Circulation 48:904, 1973.

75. Taussig, H. B., and Bing, R. J. Complete transposition of the aorta and a levoposition of the pulmonary artery: Clinical, physiological, and pathological findings. Am. Heart J. 37:551, 1949.

76. Titus, J. L., Neufeld, H. N., and Edwards, J. E. The atrioventricular conduction system in hearts with both great vessels originating from the right ventricle. Am. Heart J. 67:588, 1964.

77. Van Praagh, R., Pérez-Trevino, C., Reynolds, J. L., Moes, C. A. F., Keith, J. D., Roy, D. L., Belcourt, C., Weinberg, P. M., and Parisi, L. F. Double outlet right ventricle [S,D,L] with subaortic ventricular septal defect and pulmonary stenosis: Report of six cases. Am. J. Cardiol. 35:42, 1975.

78. Venables, A. W., and Campbell, P. E. Double outlet right ventricle: A review of 16 cases with 10 necropsy specimens. Br. Heart J. 28:461, 1966.

79. Vlodaver, Z., Neufeld, H. N., and Edwards, J. E. Coronary Arterial Variations in the Normal Heart and in Congenital Heart Disease. Academic Press, New York, 1975, p. 121.

80. Wilcox, B. R., Ho, S. Y., Macartney, F. J., Becker, A. E., Gerlis, L. M., and Anderson, R. H. Surgical anatomy of double-outlet right ventricle with situs solitus and atrioventricular concordance. J. Thorac. Cardiovasc. Surg. 82:405, 1981.

81. Williams, R. G., LaCorte, M., and Harada, K. Discontinuity continued (letter to the editor). Circulation 53:202, 1976.

82. Witham, A. C. Double outlet right ventricle: A partial transposition complex. Am. Heart J. 53:928, 1957.

83. Yeh, H.-C., Steinfeld, L., and Baron, M. Echocardiography of double outlet right ventricle (DORV)—A new diagnostic criteria. Circulation 52 (Suppl. 2):120, 1975.

84. Zamora, R., Moller, J. H., and Edwards, J. E. Double-outlet right ventricle: Anatomic types and associated anomalies. Chest 68:672, 1975.

24

Double-Outlet Left Ventricle

Richard Van Praagh, M.D., and Paul M. Weinberg, M.D.

Among the rarest and least well understood of the abnormal ventriculoarterial alignments, double-outlet left ventricle (DOLV) is nonetheless of practical importance because many of its types are now surgically correctable. To our knowledge, 111 well-documented cases of DOLV have been published as of January, 1982.[1-7, 10-15, 18, 21-24, 26-44, 46, 47, 49-52] This chapter is based in part on 36 well-studied cases of DOLV (Table 24.1),[49] which would not have been possible without the help of friends and colleagues* from many parts of the world.

DOLV was described first by Maréchal in 1819.[24] His patient was a cyanotic infant who died at 113 days of age. This infant had a single left ventricle with an infundibular outlet chamber, double-inlet left ventricle, double-outlet left ventricle, and absence of pulmonary valve leaflets. It is noteworthy that double-outlet right ventricle (DORV) with ventricular inversion (L-loop) has occasionally been misleadingly reported as DOLV.[9, 20, 25] The earliest report of DOLV with two ventricles was in 1967.[42]

DEFINITION

DOLV means that both great arteries arise entirely, or predominantly, above the morphologically left ventricle (LV). Or, as Kirklin et al.[16] have put it, double-outlet left or right ventricle (LV or RV) is present when more than 1½ great arteries arise above the same ventricle. Although the

---

* Alan B. Gazzaniga, M.D., Donald R. Sperling, M. D., and Marshall Rowen, M. D., Medical Center, University of California, Irvine, and Children's Hospital and St. Joseph's Hospital, Orange, Calif.; Teruo Izukawa, M. D., Hospital for Sick Children, Toronto, Canada; Billy Hightower, M. D., and Jerry D. Jordan, M.D., Mobile General Hospital, Mobile, Ala.; A. Louise Calder, M. D., Peter W. T. Brandt, M. D., Sir Brian G. Barratt-Boyes, M. D., and John M. Neutze, M. D., Green Lane Hospital, Auckland, New Zealand; K. Diane Vaughan, M. D., and Neil Finer, M. D., Royal Alexandra Hospital, Edmonton, Canada; William W. Miller, M. D., and Arthur G. Weinberg, M. D., Children's Medical Center of Dallas, Dallas, Texas; Ina Bhan, M. D., Marshall B. Kreidberg, M. D., and M. A. Ali Khan, M. D., New England Medical Center Hospital, Boston, Mass.; Carlos Lozano-Sainz, M. D., Joaquin Simon-Lamuela, M.D., José M. Revuelta, M. D., and José M. Arqué, M. D., Clinica Infantil "Francisco Franco," Barcelona, Spain; Dominique Métras, M. D., Hôpital de Treichville, Abidjan, Ivory Coast, Africa; Manuel Quero Jimenez, M. D., Ciudad Sanitaria de la Seguridad Social "La Paz," Madrid, Spain; Milton H. Paul, M. D., and Alex J. Muster, M. D., Children's Memorial Hospital, Chicago, Ill.; Kareem Minhas, M. D., Children's Hospital, Louisville, Ky.; Atsuyoshi Takao, M. D., Tokyo Women's Medical College, Tokyo, Japan; Ichiro Nihmura, M. D., Kanagawa Children's Medical Center, Yokohama, Japan; Frederick Levine, M. D., Alan Goldblatt, M. D., and Mortimer Buckley, M. D., Massachusetts General Hospital, Boston, Mass.; S. Bert Litwin, M. D., Milwaukee Children's Hospital, Milwaukee, Wisc.; Edmond J. Sacks, M. D., Wilford Hall USAF Medical Center, Lackland Air Force Base, Texas; and David T. Kelly, M. D., Johns Hopkins Hospital, Baltimore, Md.

foregoing seems appealingly simple, abnormal ventriculoarterial (VA) alignments may be far from simple to diagnose and classify satisfactorily. Overriding of a great artery may be difficult to judge at surgery and even at autopsy. We have found the following three points to be helpful.

1. When the aorta (Ao) is located normally, or approximately normally, above a ventricular septal defect (VSD), as in the tetralogy of Fallot, the aortic valve is mainly above the ventricular septum, not predominantly above the left ventricular cavity. Consequently, when the aorta is located normally, or nearly normally, and when aortic-mitral fibrous continuity is present, it is customary to regard the Ao as being related to the LV, even though the Ao is in fact mainly above the ventricular septum. Thus, when the Ao occupies it usual overriding position and the pulmonary artery arises above the LV, DOLV is considered to be present. This convention is generally accepted[1, 3-6, 14, 18, 34] It is noteworthy that in this situation, the criterion of 1½ great arteries[16] does not apply with accuracy because the normally located Ao with a subaortic VSD overrides the ventricular septum predominantly, not the LV cavity. This difficulty is solved by conventionally assigning the normally located Ao to the LV.

2. When the aorta is abnormally located above a VSD, the criterion of 1½ great arteries does apply accurately. For example, when the pulmonary artery (PA) arises above the LV and an anterior Ao overrides a VSD, DOLV is considered to be present if the Ao is predominantly above the LV. However, if the Ao overrides the LV and the RV equally, then the diagnosis is not DOLV, but transposition of the great arteries (TGA) with overriding Ao. This convention is also used by others[6] and is implicit in the aforementioned definition of DOLV.

3. When the pulmonary artery is abnormally located and overrides a VSD, and the Ao is normally located, the criterion of 1½ great arteries also applies accurately. DOLV is considered to be present only if the PA arises predominantly above the LV. If the PA is not displaced abnormally above the LV, then the diagnosis of DOLV is not made. The diagnosis may be conal septal defect, or tetralogy of Fallot with hypoplasia of the conal septum, etc.

To summarize, the criterion of more than 1½ great arteries[16] applies quite well to DOLV, except when the Ao is located normally or nearly normally above a VSD, in which case the Ao is conventionally assigned to the LV.

ALIGNMENTS AND CONNECTIONS

The great arteries and the ventricles are aligned, but not connected, because of the interposed infundibulum (conus). Similarly, the atria and the ventricles are aligned, but not connected, because of the interposed atrioventricular (AV) canal (junction). The infundibulum is connected with the great arteries above and with the ventricles below. When the infundibular free wall is absorbed, then a great artery is

TABLE 24.1   FINDINGS IN 36 CASES OF DOLV[a]

1. DOLV {S,D,D} with IVS and no outflow tract stenosis

(1) Paul, *et al.*,[36] 1970, autopsy, 2½ year-old boy, blind suprasystemic RV, fistula from RV apex to AD coronary artery (Figs. 24.1 and 24.2).

2. DOLV {S,D,D} with subaortic VSD and no outflow tract stenosis.

(2) Pacifico *et al.*,[34] case 3, 1973, angio and surgery, 9 years, Ao overrode RV by 20%, no outflow tract stenosis, successful surgical repair.

(3) Métras,[26] 1975, autopsy, 5-month-old boy, Ao overriding VSD as in T/F, tenuous Ao V-MV fibrous continuity, short nonstenotic sub PA conus, no outflow tract stenosis, PA entirely above LV (Figs. 24.1 and 24.6*a*).

3. DOLV {S,D,D} with subaortic VSD and PS

(4) Kerr *et al.*,[14] 1971, angio and surgery, 3½-year-old boy, overriding Ao, AoV-MV and PV-MV fibrous continuity, PS (valv), PA entirely above LV, successful surgical repair.

(5) Pacifico *et al.*,[34] 1973, case 2, angio and surgery, 26 years, PS (severe, at os inf), successful surgical repair.

(6) Van Praagh,[46] 1973, case of Gazzaniga *et al.*,[10] autopsy, 6⁴/₁₂ year-old girl, overriding Ao, AoV-MV fibrous continuity, short stenotic sub PA conus, PS (inf and valv), PA entirely above LV (Figs. 24.1 and 24.3).

(7) Anderson, *et al.*,[1] 1974, angio, 5-year-old boy.

(8) Miller and Weinberg,[27] 1972, autopsy, 15-day-old boy, overriding Ao, AoV-MV fibrous continuity, short stenotic sub PA conus, PS (inf and valv), PA entirely above LV, AD coronary from RCA, tricuspid atresia, ASD II.

(9) Arqué *et al.*,[2, 3] 1975, autopsy, 11-month-old boy, overriding Ao, AoV-MV fibrous continuity, short stenotic sub PA conus, PS (inf and annular), absence of PV leaflets, PA entirely above LV (Fig. 24.6*j*).

(10) Conti *et al.*,[6] 1974, angio and surgery, 12-year-old boy, successful surgical repair with patch closure of VSD, suture closure of pulmonary valve and annulus, 20-mm valveless Dacron conduit from RV to distal PA.

(11) Krongrad *et al.*,[18, 19] 1974, angio and surgery, 10 year old boy, successful surgical repair using aortic homograft from RV to PA on October 12, 1972. Successful reoperation on August 3, 1976, to replace calcified and stenotic homograft with a Dacron conduit containing a porcine aortic valve (Hancock).

(12) Brandt *et al.*,[6] 1976, autopsy, case 1, 3½-year-old boy, corrective surgery on Nov. 7, 1966, with VSD closure, closure of proximal PA, and aortic homograft conduit from RV to distal PA. Hospital death postoperatively.

(13) Brandt *et al.*,[6] 1976, surgery, case 4, 1½-year-old boy, successful surgical repair on March 26, 1973, with closure of VSD, proximal PA, and ASD, and aortic homograft conduit from RV to distal PA. Well 1 year postop.

4. DOLV, {S,D,D} with subaortic VSD and bilaterally absent conus

(14) Bhan *et al.*,[4] 1975, autopsy, 7-day-old girl, subaortic VSD, bilaterally absent conus with AoV-MV, AoV-TV and PV-MV fibrous continuity, Ao overriding VS, PA entirely above LV, no PS, subaortic stenosis (crowding, small subaortic outflow tract), tubular hypoplasia of transverse aortic arch, preductal coarc (Figs. 24.1 and 24.6*b*).

(15) Brandt *et al.*,[6] 1976, autopsy, case 2, 5¼-month-old girl, pulmonary stenosis (valvular), bicuspid AoV, AoV-MV, AoV-TV and PV-MV fibrous continuity, small RV with Ebstein's anomaly of TV.

5. DOLV {S,D,A} with subaortic VSD and TAt

(16) Leriche *et al.*,[21] 1974, angio, 21-year-old woman, tricuspid atresia, PA entirely above LV with PV-MV fibrous continuity, Ao arising from infundibular outlet chamber, AoV overriding inf and LV via VSD (Fig. 24.1).

6. DOLV {S,D,D} with subaortic VSD and TAt

(17) Quero Jiménez et al.,[38, 39] 1975, autopsy, 8-month-old girl, tricuspid atresia, bilateral conus, no outflow tract stenosis (figs. 24.1 and 24.6*c*).

7. DOLV {S,D,D} with subaortic VSD, MAt, and large LV

(18) A69-9, CHMC, autopsy, 2½-month-old girl, left AV valve atresia, large LV with inf outlet chamber, bilateral conus, bulboventricular foramen ("VSD") subaortic, subaortic stenosis produced by right AV valve tissue, preductal coarc, large closing PDA (Figs. 24.1 and 24.6*d* to *f*).

8. DOLV {S,D,L} with subaortic VSD and PS

(19) Pacifico Wet al.,[33, 34] 1972 and 1973, angio and surgery, 3½ years old, restrictively small VSD, successful surgical repair.

(20) Van Praagh *et al.*,[47] 1972, autopsy, case 1, 8½-year-old girl, overriding Ao, PA entirely above LV, small subaortic conus with tenuous AoV-MV fibrous continuity, PS (valv and subvalv) due to malalignment of the conotruncus (Figs. 24.1 and 24.4).

(21) Van Praagh *et al.*,[47] 1972, autopsy, case 2, A52-88, CHMC, 10-month-old boy, very similar to preceding case.

(22) Kelly,[13] 1970, angio, 2-year-old boy, with apparent atresia of LPA, collaterals from Ao to left lung, ASD II.

(23) Minhas,[28] 1970, 5-year-old boy.

(24) Sharratt *et al.*,[43] 1976, autopsy, 2-year-old boy, very hypoplastic RV, tricuspid stenosis, ASD II.

(25) Brandt *et al.*,[6] 1976, angio and surgery, case 3, 2¹⁰/₁₂-year-old girl, pulmonary stenosis (annular and leaflets), dextrocardia, successful surgical repair on February 13, 1973, with closure of VSD, proximal PA and ASD, with aortic homograft conduit from RV to distal PA.

---

[a] angio, angiography; AD, anterior descending coronary artery; Ao, aorta; AoV, aortic valve; ASD II, atrial defect, secundum type; AV, atrioventricular; CHMC, Children's Hospital Medical Center, Boston, Mass.; coarc, coarctation of the aorta; DOLV, double outlet left ventricle; {I,D,D}, situs inversus of the viscera and atria, D-loop, D-malposition of the great arteries; {I,L,D}, situs inversus of the viscera and atria, L-loop, D-malposition of the great arteries; inf, infundibulum; IVS, intact ventricular septum; LCA, left coronary artery; LPA, left pulmonary artery; LV, morphologically left ventricle; MAt, mitral atresia; MS, mitral stenosis; MV, mitral valve; os inf, os infundibuli; PA, pulmonary artery; PAt, pulmonary atresia; PDA, patent ductus arteriosus; postop, postoperatively; PS, pulmonary stenosis; PV, pulmonary valve; RCA, right coronary artery; RPA, right pulmonary artery; RV, morphologically right ventricle {S,D,A}, situs solitus of the viscera and atria, D-loop, A-malposition of the great arteries; {S,D,D}, situs solitus of the viscera and atria, D-loop, D-malposition of the great arteries; {S,D,L}, situs solitus of the viscera and atria, D-loop, L-malposition of the great arteries; {S,L,L}, situs solitus of the viscera and atria, L-loop, L-malposition of the great arteries; subvalv, subvalvular; VS, ventricular septum; T/F, tetralogy of Fallot; TV, tricuspid valve; TAt, tricuspid atresia; type B interrupted aortic arch, interruption distal to the left common carotid artery; valv, valvular; VS, ventricular septum; VSD, ventricular septal defect.

TABLE 24.1 *continued*

9. **DOLV {S,D,L} with subpulmonary VSD and preductal coarc**

   (26) Muster,[30] 1973, autopsy, 11-day-old girl, no PS, Ebstein's anomaly of TV, mild MS, bilateral conus, tubular hypoplasia of aortic arch and preductal coarc, PDA (Figs. 24.1 and 24.6g and h).

10. **DOLV {S,D,D} with subpulmonary VSD**

   (27) Sakakibara et al.,[42] 1967, angio and surgery, 12-year-old boy, conal septal defect with leftward displacement of PA, successful surgical repair.

   (28) Hightower and Jordan,[11] 1972, autopsy, 2½-month-old girl, subpulmonary conal septal defect, deficient subpulmonary conus, leftward displacement of PA, PV-MV and AoV-MV fibrous continuity, subaortic stenosis due to malalignment of truncal septum, hypoplasia of aortic arch, preductal coarc of Ao, PDA (figs. 24.1 and 24.5).

   (29) Litwin,[23] 1974, angio and surgery, 4½-year-old boy, PA overrides LV cavity 60% and overrides VS 39% and overrides RV cavity an average of 1%, PS, ASD II, single LCA, successful surgical repair with closure of VSD and 20 mm Hancock conduit from RV to PA.

   (30) Nihmura,[31] 1971, autopsy, 4-month-old girl, overriding PA, AoV-MV and PV-MV fibrous continuity, interrupted Ao arch (type B), aberrant right subclavian artery from descending thoracic Ao.

   (31) Vaughan and Finer,[51] 1976, autopsy, 4-day-old girl, overriding PA, severe subaortic stenosis due to deviation of conal septum toward mitral valve, bicuspid AoV (absence of septal commissure), interrupted aortic arch (type B), quadricuspid PV, no PV-MV fibrous continuity, AoV-MV fibrous continuity, PDA.

11. **DOLV {S,L,L} with subaortic VSD and PAt**

   (32) Paul,[35] autopsy, A59-71, Children's Memorial Hospital, Chicago, 5-day-old girl, long PDA to RPA (Figs. 24.1 and 24.6i)

12. **DOLV {I,L,L} with subaortic VSD and PS**

   (33) Davignon et al.,[49] 1977, 2-month-old boy with autopsy confirmation of dextrocardia with DOLV {I,L,L}, subaortic VSD, PS (infundibular and valvular), subpulmonary infundibulum, aortic-mitral and aortic-tricuspid fibrous continuity, unicuspid pulmonary valve (right septal leaflet present, others absent), right aortic arch, and aberrant left subclavian artery used at 2 weeks of age for left Blalock-Taussig anastomosis. Death apparently from hypoxemia, at home. This is tetralogy of Fallott type of DOLV in situs inversus totalis.

13. **DOLV {I,L,D} with subaortic VSD and PS or PAt**

   (34) Sacks,[41] 1974, angio, 12-year-old girl, ASD II, pulmonary outflow tract atresia.

   (35) Levine et al.,[22] 1976, angio and surgery, 10-year-old boy, PS (subvalv and valv), successfully corrected surgically (Fig. 24.1).

14. **DOLV {I,D,D} with subaortic VSD and PS**

   (36) Brandt et al.,[6] 1976, angio and surgery, case 5, 28-year-old man, bilaterally deficient conus, right aortic arch, complete heart block preoperatively. Surgical repair on August 16, 1972, with closure of VSD, connecting Ao to RV, and direct relief, PS. Late death 2 years postop, no autopsy.

---

connected to the AV canal via the intervalvular fibrosa, as in the normal aortic-mitral fibrous continuity. Similarly, the AV canal or junction is connected both to the atria and to the ventricles. Normally, the atria and the ventricles connect directly only at the bundle of His. As a rule, therefore, the major cardiac segments—the atria, the ventricles, and the great arteries—do not connect directly. Instead, the major cardiac segments are connected by means of the junctional cardiac segments—the AV junction, and the infundibulum. **This distinction between alignments and connections** is of fundamental importance. (Please see chapter 28 for a fuller explanation of why this distinction between alignments and connection is important anatomically, embryologically, etiologically, and physiologically.)

Great arteries do not in fact arise from the ventricles, but above them. The great arteries originate from the infundibulum (conus) and/or from the AV canal (Fig. 28.3 and 28.8). Although the great arteries arise above the ventricles, they often are not directly above them. This is why the great arteries are often said to be "related" to the ventricles in this or that manner. These distinctions, which may initially seem trivial, are in fact very helpful in understanding DOLV and other ventriculoarterial alignments.

The true ventricles—the RV and the LV—from the embryologic and anatomic standpoints are the ventricular sinuses, bodies, or inflow tracts—not the infundibulum, conus, or outflow tract. For example, in double-chambered RV (also known as anomalous muscle bundles of the RV), the proximal chamber or inflow tract is the true RV, whereas the distal chamber is the infundibulum, conus, or outflow tract. Similarly, in single LV with an outlet chamber, the true RV—the RV inflow tract—is the structure that is absent, whereas the outlet chamber is the infundibulum or conus. The distinction between the ventricles and the conus is basic. (Please see chapter 28 for a somewhat fuller consid-

eration of this distinction between the RV and the LV, on the one hand, and the infundibulum or conus, on the other.)

Since the great arteries arise from the conus and/or the AV canal (Figs. 28.3 and 28.8), rather than from the ventricular sinuses directly, the relationships between the great arteries and the ventricles are secondary, not primary, and are almost infinitely variable. If the PA normally arose directly *from* the RV sinus and if the Ao normally originated directly *from* the LV sinus, it seems highly probable that most of the abnormal ventriculoarterial alignments, including DOLV, would then not occur.

Normal and abnormal ventriculoarterial alignments form a spectrum in which one entity gradually merges with another. Nonetheless, it remains useful to distinguish one part of this spectrum, such as DOLV, from other closely related parts of the spectrum, particularly when such distinctions are of physiologic and surgical significance.

To summarize, the fact that the great arteries arise from the conus and from the AV canal if the subsemilunar conus is absorbed, rather than from the ventricles, explains why arterioventricular relationships are almost infinetly variable, why they form a spectrum, and why DOLV is possible.

CLASSIFICATION

DOLV is classified, as are DORV and TGA, in terms of the following criteria.

1. The Situs of the Major Cardiac Segments, i.e., the Atria, the Ventricles, and the Great Arteries. Examples include {S,D,D}, {S,D,L}, {I,L,L}, {I,L,D}, and {I,D,D} (Fig. 24.1).†

---

†For those unfamiliar with segmental diagnosis and symbols, please see Chapter 28, in particular Table 28.1 and Figures 28.1 to 28.7.

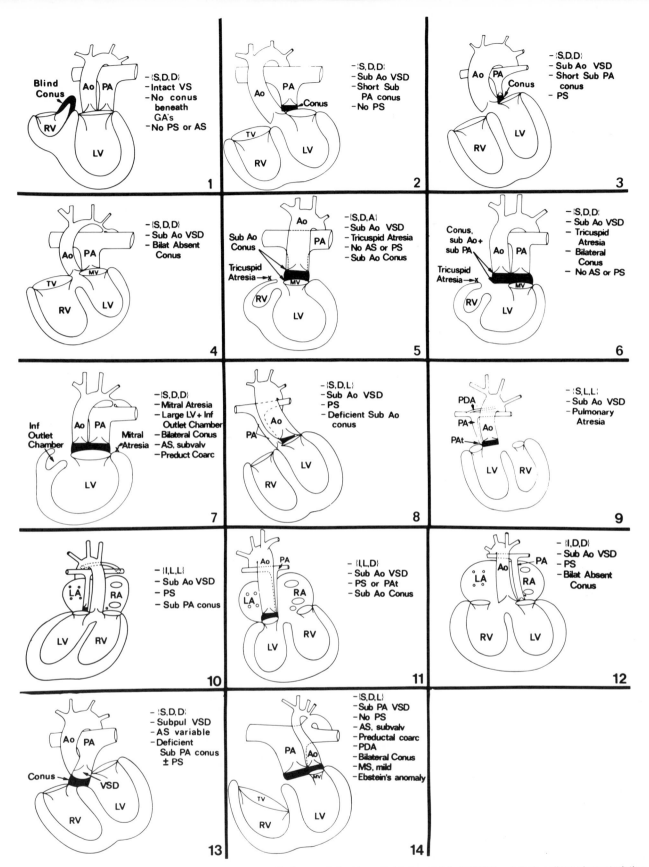

Fig. 24.1 Diagrams of the 14 presently known anatomic types of double-outlet left ventricle (DOLV) and their salient characteristics. Conal muscle is shown in *black*. Type 4 is a diagram of Case 14 (Table 24.1); hence, the subaortic narrowing, preductal coarctation, and small patent ductus arteriosus (*PDA*). Ao, aorta; *AS*, aortic stenosis; *Bilat*, bilateral; *coarc*, coarctation of the aorta; *GA's*, great arteries; {I,D,D}, situs inversus of the viscera and atria, D-loop, D-malposition of the great arteries; {I,L,D}, situs inversus of the viscera and atria, L-loop, D-malposition of the great arteries; *inf*, infundibulum; *LA*, left atrium; *LV*, morphologically left ventricle; *MS*, mitral stenosis; *MV*, mitral valve; *PA*, pulmonary artery; *PAt*, pulmonary atresia; *PDA*, patent ductus arteriosus; *Preduct*, preductal; *PS*, pulmonary stenosis; *RA*, right atrium; *RV*, morphologically right ventricle; {S,D,A}, situs solitus of the viscera and atria, D-loop, A-malposition of the great arteries; {S,D,D}, situs solitus of the viscera and atria, D-loop, D-malposition of the great arteries; {S,D,L}, situs solitus of the viscera and atria, D-loop, L-malposition of the great arteries; {S,L,L}, situs solitus of the viscera and atria, L-loop, L-malposition of the great arteries; *Subpul*, subpulmonary; *subvalv*, subvalvular; *TV*, tricuspid valve; *VS*, ventricular septum; *VSD*, ventricular septal defect.

373

2. The Alignments of the Atria, Ventricles, and Great Arteries. DOLV, double-outlet right ventricle (DORV), and transposition of the great arteries (TGA) are abnormal ventriculoarterial (VA) alignments (Figs. 24.1 and 28.6), while double-inlet LV, straddling tricuspid valve, and tricuspid atresia exemplify abnormal atrioventricular (AV) alignments. Alignments may be *concordant* (appropriate, or normal) or *discordant* (inappropriate, or the opposite of appropriate or normal). Normally related great arteries (NRGA) exemplify a concordant VA alignment, whereas TGA has a discordant VA alignment (Fig. 28.6). Solitus atria and solitus (D-loop) ventricles usually have a concordant AV alignment—RA to RV and LA to LV (Fig. 24.1 and 28.6), whereas solitus atria and inverted (L-loop) ventricles usually have a discordant AV alignment—RA to LV and LA to RV (Fig. 24.1 and 28.6). Since the concept of AV concordance or discordance often is inapplicable (situs ambiguus, straddling AV valves, double-inlet LV, double-inlet RV, tricuspid atresia, mitral atresia, etc.), it is therefore necessary to diagnose the ventricular situs (solitus or D-loop/inversus or L-loop) specifically. The AV alignments ("connections") often cannot be used to imply, or to ascertain, what the ventricular situs is. Thus, segmental situs and alignments *both* must be diagnosed specifically, particularly in complex congenital heart disease such as DOLV (Fig. 24.1).

3. Associated Cardiovascular and Noncardiovascular Anomalies. Examples include atrial septal defect, ventricular septal defect, pulmonary outflow tract stenosis, the asplenia syndrome, etc. In all abnormal VA alignments, the relationship of the ventricular septal defect (VSD) to the aorta (Ao), or to the pulmonary artery (PA), is very important clinically, physiologically, and surgically. Hence, in DOLV, whether the VSD is subAo, subPA, beneath both, beneath neither, or absent is noted with care (Fig. 24.1).

ANATOMIC TYPES OF DOLV

We reviewed the material at the Children's Hospital Medical Center in Boston, the literature, and all consultations that have been sent to R.VP. over the past 15 years. It was found that DOLV is not one disease. Instead, DOLV is a heterogeneous group of different diseases with only one thing in common: both great arteries arise above, or are related to, the LV. In 36 cases of DOLV, 14 different anatomic types were found (Fig. 24.1 and Table 24.1):

1. DOLV {S,D,D} with intact ventricular septum and no outflow tract obstruction was represented by the unique case of Paul et al.[36] (case 1 in Table 24.1 and Figs. 24.1 and 24.2). In the designation DOLV {S,D,D}, the braces indicate a subset of DOLV, in the mathematical sense of set theory. The members of the subset are the three major cardiac segments that are represented by symbols in the following order: {visceroatrial situs, ventricular loop, conotruncus} or, more briefly, {atria, ventricles, great arteries}. DOLV {S,D,D} indicates origin of both great arteries above the morphologically left ventricle with situs solitus (S) of the viscera and atria, a ventricular D-loop (D) in which the RV sinus or inflow tract is right-sided, and D-malposition of the great arteries (D), in which the malposed aortic valve lies to the right of the malposed pulmonary valve.

Surgically, this type of DOLV might be amenable to a Fontan procedure, i.e., an external valved conduit from right atrium to PA,[8, 17] ligation of the PA above the pulmonary valve, closure of the atrial septum, and surgical closure of the tricuspid ostium, probably with a prosthetic patch. An external valved conduit from RV to PA would probably be contraindicated by the smallness of the tricuspid orifice and

RV cavity, plus the absence of a VSD, all of which would produce tricuspid and subtricuspid stenosis.

Embryologically, this type of DOLV appears to result from excessive conal absorption beneath both semilunar valves and leftward displacement of the truncus relative to the ventricles, ventricular septum, and AV canal; hence, the observed aortic-mitral and pulmonary-mitral fibrous continuity (Figs. 24.1 and 24.2d). Not only were the subaortic and subpulmonary conal free walls absorbed, as the semilunar-mitral fibrous continuities indicate, even the conal septum was absorbed, or failed to form, between the subaortic and subpulmonary outflow tracts; hence, the fibroelastic truncal septum, devoid of conal musculature, extended approximately a millimeter below the semilunar valves (Fig. 24.2d).

How did the interventricular foramen close? Conal musculature appeared to be connected to the RV, forming a blind RV outflow tract (Figs. 24.1 and 24.2c) and contributing to closure of the interventricular foramen. Hence, the anatomic findings indicated a remarkable degree of conotruncal dissociation: a right ventricular conus and a left ventricular truncus (Figs. 24.1 and 24.2).

Hemodynamically, the fistula between the RV apex and the anterior descending coronary artery (Fig. 24.2a) permitted a major degree of bypassing of the myocardium by oxygenated blood: contrast from the suprasystemic RV (220/20 mm Hg) flowed retrogradely up the anterior descending coronary artery and into the aortic root via a single coronary ostium (Fig. 24.2a). Hence, the "myocardial factor" appears important in this type of DOLV and is similar to that seen in pulmonary atresia with intact ventricular septum and sinusoids between the cavity of the suprasystemic RV and the coronary arteries.

2. DOLV {S,D,D} with subaortic VSD and no outflow tract stenosis was represented by two patients (cases 2 and 3 in Table 24.1, Figs. 24.1, and 24.6a).[26, 34] The features of this type of DOLV are: (a) a subaortic VSD, (b) an overriding aorta, as in tetralogy of Fallot, and (c) a short but not stenotic subpulmonary conus. Since the subpulmonary conus is very short, the pulmonary valve is much too close to the mitral valve. This appears to explain why the PA arises entirely above the LV.

Diagnostically, the findings may suggest TGA with VSD. However, selective biventriculography should indicate the correct diagnosis because: the aortic valve is in "tetralogy location"; there is aortic-mitral contiguity; the Ao fills well from both ventricles; and the PA arises entirely above the LV, from a short, wide, nonstenotic subpulmonary conus.

Surgically, the VSD may be patched to the right of the aortic valve, placing the Ao into continuity with the LV. Continuity may be established between the RV and the PA by an external valve conduit and by interruption of the PA at or above the pulmonary valve.

3. DOLV {S,D,D} with subaortic VSD and pulmonary stenosis (PS) was found in 10 patients (cases 4 to 13 in Table 24.1, Figs. 24.1 and 24.3)[1–3, 6, 7, 14, 18, 19, 27, 34, 38] This was the commonest type of DOLV (Table 24.1). There is one important difference between this type of DOLV and the preceding one: pulmonary stenosis, infundibular and valvular. The very short subpulmonary conus is poorly expanded, resulting in PS.

Diagnostically, DOLV of this type is very likely to be mistaken preoperatively for tetralogy of Fallot. Indeed, this may be called the "tetralogy type" of DOLV. However, once one is aware of this entity, angiocardiography—preferably selective left ventriculography (Fig. 24.3b)—should facilitate the diagnosis by showing the aortic valve in tetralogy location and the origin of the PA entirely above the LV, from a short and stenotic subpulmonary conus.

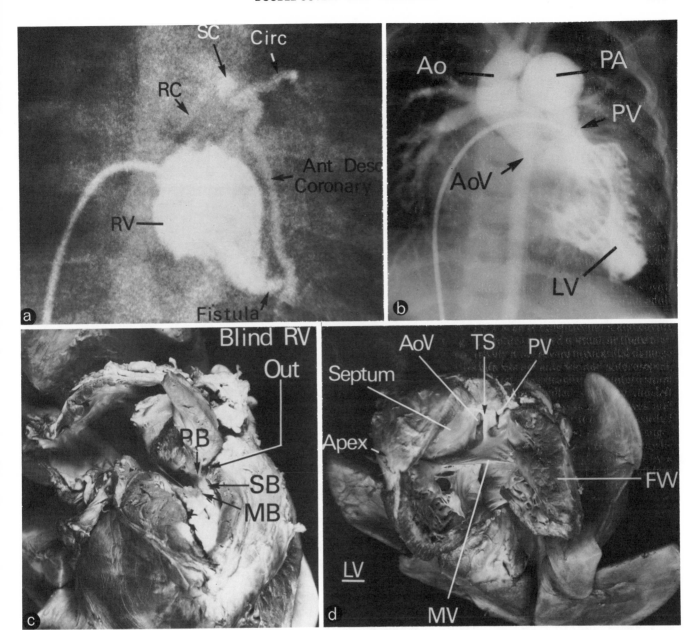

Fig. 24.2 DOLV {S,D,D} with intact ventricular septum (type 1, Fig. 24.1), a patient of Paul *et al.*[36] (case 1, Table 24.1). (*a*) Selective right ventricular injection in the posteroanterior projection demonstrates that the only outlet from the small-chambered morphologically right ventricle (*RV*) is via an apical fistula that connects with the anterior descending coronary artery (*Ant Desc Coronary*). Contrast passes retrogradely up the anterior descending coronary and demonstrates the single coronary (*SC*) artery arising from the aortic root and giving origin to the right coronary (*RC*) and left circumflex (*Circ*) branches. Hence, the heart is perfused by a considerable amount of unoxygenated blood. (*b*) Selective left ventricular injection in the posteroanterior projection shows that both the aorta (*Ao*) and the pulmonary artery (*PA*) arise above the morphologically left ventricle (*LV*). The great arteries are side by side, with the aortic valve (*AoV*) slightly lower than the pulmonary valve (*PV*). (*c*) The small-chambered right ventricle is opened in right lateral view and shows an intact ventricular septum, endocardial fibroelastosis toward the ventricular apex, and a blind right ventricular outflow tract (*Blind RV Out*). (*d*) Apical view of the opened left ventricle (*LV*) showing the intact ventricular septum (*Septum*), the left ventricular free wall (*FW*), and fibrous continuity between the aortic valve (*AoV*) and the anterior leaflet of the mitral valve (*MV*) and between the pulmonary valve (*PV*) and the anterior leaflet of the *MV*. *TS*, truncal septum. (Reproduced with permission from M. H. Paul *et al.*[36] and the American Heart Association.)

Regarding differential diagnosis, it is noteworthy that this type of DOLV and the preceding one are closely related, both anatomically and developmentally, to *TGA {S,D,D} with posterior aorta,* subaortic VSD, and short subpulmonary conus, with or without PS.[48] In these types of DOLV (types 2 and 3 in Fig. 24.1), the aortic valve is in tetraology location, and the VSD is relatively large; hence the Ao communicates readily with the LV. However, in TGA with a posterior Ao,[48] the aortic valve is further to the right, and

the VSD is relatively small[48]; consequently, the Ao communicates more readily with the RV than with the LV. This difference in VSD size can be important surgically, as, for example, in the Rastelli procedure. In TGA with posterior Ao, VSD, and PS, the VSD may well be too small to permit a Rastelli procedure; unless enlarged, the VSD would constitute subaortic stenosis.[48] This difficulty does not exist in this type of DOLV because the VSD is relatively large (Fig. 24.3*d*).

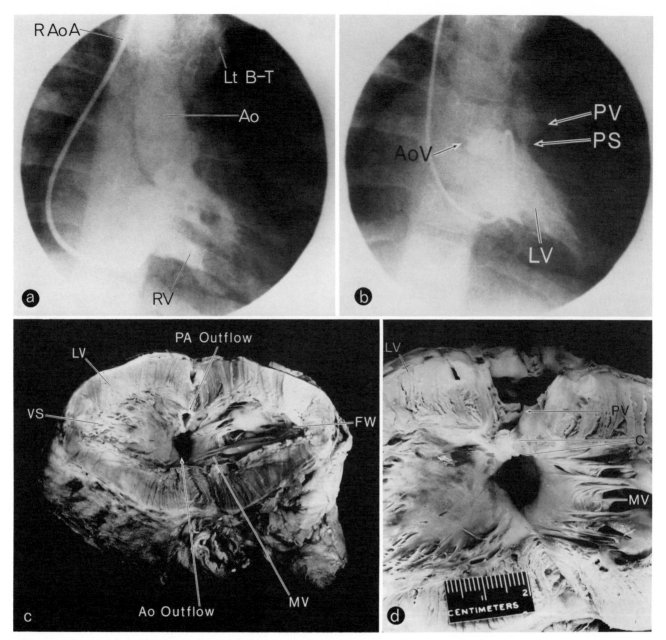

Fig. 24.3 DOLV {S,D,D} with subaortic ventricular septal defect and pulmonary stenosis (type 3, Fig. 24.1), i.e., the "tetralogy type" of DOLV, in a patient of Gazzaniga *et al.*[10] (case 6, Table 24.1). (*a*) Selective right ventricular injection in the posteroanterior projection reveals the ascending aorta (*Ao*) in "tetralogy" position, a left Blalock-Taussig anastomosis (*Lt B-T*) and a right aortic arch (*RAoA*). (*b*) Selective left ventricular injection in posteroanterior projection shows that the pulmonary artery arises above the left ventricle (*LV*). Pulmonary stenosis (*PS*) is produced by the short and poorly expanded infundibulum beneath the pulmonary valve (*PV*). Contrast also outlines the inferior surface of the aortic valve (*AoV*). (*c*) Apical view of the opened *LV* showing the ventricular septum (*VS*), the left ventricular free wall (*FW*), the widely patent aortic outflow tract (*Ao Outflow*), the stenotic pulmonary outflow tract (*PA Outflow*) that is surrounded by a cuff of thickened and white endocardium, and a normally formed mitral valve (*MV*). (*d*) A closeup of the outflow tracts showing the now opened stenotic pulmonary outflow tract, the stenotic pulmonary valve (*PV*), the very short and obstructive subpulmonary conus (*C*), and the resultant pulmonary-mitral fibrous discontinuity. Aortic-mitral fibrous continuity is present because the subaortic conal free wall has been absorbed normally. *RV*, right ventricle. (Reproduced with permission from R. Van Praagh.[46])

Embryologically, this type of DOLV appears to be produced by normal, or nearly normal, absorption of the subaortic conal free wall, resulting in essentially normal aortic-mitral approximation, and by marked shortening and failure of expansion of the subpulmonary conus. This could be due either to excessive absorption of the subpulmonary part of the conus, or failure of the normal growth of the subpulmonary conus, or both. Marked hypoplasia of the subpulmonary conus appears to result in a left ventricular PA because the

pulmonary valve is abnormally close to the mitral valve (Fig. 24.3*d*). The conal septum leaves the VSD wide open in this type of DOLV because the conal septum is hypoplastic and it is anterior and to the left of the ventricular septum (Fig. 24.3*d*); whereas in TGA with posterior Ao and subpulmonary conus,[48] the conal septum is less hypoplastic and is approximately parallel to the underlying ventricular septum.

Successful surgical correction of this type of DOLV was first reported in 1971.[14] The VSD is closed, as in tetralogy of

Fallot, placing the Ao into continuity with the LV. Continuity is established between the RV and the PA via an external valved conduit, and the PA is interrupted at or just above the pulmonary valve.

4. DOLV {S,D,D} with subaortic VSD and bilaterally absent conus was found in two patients (cases 14 and 15 in Table 24.1, Figs. 24.1 and 24.6b). This was a previously unreported type of congenital heart disease that had been observed by Brandt et al.[6] and by us.[4]

Embryologically, the key feature of this type of DOLV appears to be absorption or failure of formation of the entire subsemilunar conus, including the conal septum, thereby resulting in a subaortic VSD and permitting aortic-tricuspid, aortic-mitral, and pulmonary-mitral fibrous continuity (Figs. 24.1 and 24.6b).

Surgically, neither patient appears operable at the present time because of associated cardiovascular anomalies (cases 14 and 15, Table 24.1).

5. DOLV {S,D,A} with subaortic VSD and tricuspid atresia was found in one patient (case 16 in Table 24.1 and Fig. 24.1)[21] The segmental subset of DOLV {S,D,A} indicates the presence of situs solitus (S) of the viscera and atria, D-loop (D), and A-malposition (A) of the great arteries, the malposed aortic valve lying directly in front (*antero*, or A) relative to the malposed pulmonary valve. The salient features of this type of DOLV are the coexistence of triscuspid atresia and the smallness of the RV. In tricuspid atresia, the true RV—the sinus, body, or inflow tract—is absent. The small "RV" in typical tricuspid atresia is the infundibulum. The other finding is the presence of a subaortic conus with pulmonary-mitral fibrous continuity, as in typical TGA (Fig. 24.1). Since the Ao is very anterior, as opposed to the usual rightward position, the Ao overrides the LV above the subaortic VSD.

Surgically, in this type of DOLV (type 5, Fig. 24.1), the present management would probably be to band the PA to avoid heart failure and the development of hypertensive pulmonary vascular changes, and subsequently to perform a Fontan procedure.[8]

6. DOLV {S,D,D} with subaortic VSD and tricuspid atresia was found in one patient (case 17 in Table 24.1; Figs. 24.1 and 24.6c).[38] This type of DOLV is different in three respects from the preceding one: D-malposition of the great arteries is present, instead of A-malposition. There is a bilateral conus instead of a subaortic conus. There is more leftward displacement of the conotruncus relative to the ventricles, ventricular septum and AV canal; hence, DOLV (Figs. 24.1 and 24.6c). Otherwise, this type of DOLV and the preceding one are identical.

7. DOLV {S,D,D} with subaortic VSD, mitral atresia, large LV and infundibular outlet chamber was found in one patient (Case 18 in Table 24.1 and Fig. 24.1 and 24.6d to f). This type of DOLV had not been reported previously. The salient feature is the coexistence of mitral atresia with a large LV and an infundibular outlet chamber. The rare association of mitral atresia with a large LV and an infundibular outlet chamber was first reported in 1972.[37] (Usually, mitral atresia is associated with a small or absent LV and a large RV.)

Surgically, this type of patient (case 18, Table 24.1) would not now be regarded as correctable because of the coexistence of subaortic stenosis and preductal coarctation of the aorta.

8. DOLV {S,D,L} with subaortic VSD and PS occurred in seven patients (Cases 19 to 25 in Table 24.1 and Figs. 24.1 and 24.4)[6, 13, 28, 34, 43, 47] This was the second commonest type of DOLV (Table 24.1). L-Malposition of the great arteries in association with a D-loop indicates malalignment of the conotruncus relative to the ventricles, the ventricular septum, and the AV canal. The principal effects of this conotruncal malalignment are: the Ao overrides the LV, hence, DOLV (Fig. 24.4c), and the pulmonary outflow tract is squeezed between the truncal septum anteriorly and the mitral valve posteriorly (Fig. 24.4d), hence, PS. It is noteworthy that this is not malalignment of the conotruncal septum only. The *entire* conotruncus—septum and free wall—is malaligned relative to the ventricles and the AV canal. In other words, the malalignment of the truncal septum that produces PS in this type of DOLV is merely a reflection of malalignment of the entire conotruncus relative to the ventricles and the AV canal.

Embryologically, why the conotruncus and the ventricles twisted in opposite directions is unknown. However, the fact that this occurred appears basic to the development of this rare type of ventriculoarterial alignment. Had the conotruncus twisted to the right, as usually occurs with a D-loop, then the results would have been typical D-TGA without PS.

Surgically, the Ao is placed into continuity with the LV by patching the VSD to the right of the aortic valve, and continuity between the RV and the PA is established by an external valved conduit and by interruption of the PA above the pulmonary valve.[33, 34]

9. DOLV {S,L,L} with subaortic VSD and pulmonary atresia occurred in one patient (case 32, Table 24.1; Figs. 24.1 and 24.6i)[35] This type of DOLV‡ which had not been reported previously, is characterized by situs solitus (S) of the viscera and atria, a discordant L-loop (L) resulting in ventricular inversion, and L-malposition (L) of the great arteries, the malposed aorta lying to the left (levo or L) relative to the malposed and atretic pulmonary outflow tract. The anatomic findings suggested that conotruncal malalignment—rightward displacement—obliterated the pulmonary outflow tract. There was no space between the conal septum (anteriorly and to the left) and the mitral valve (posteriorly and to the right); hence, pulmonary outflow tract atresia.

Surgically, this type of DOLV might be correctable as follows: one could use a Waterston shunt early and a definitive repair later by patching the Ao into the left-sided RV and by an external valved conduit from the right-sided LV to the PA, if the latter is large enough to accept a conduit and if the pulmonary resistance is not prohibitively elevated.

10. DOLV {I,L,L} with Subaortic VSD, PS, and Subpulmonary Infundibulum with Aortic-Atrioventricular Fibrous Continuity was found in one patient, a 2-month-old boy (case 33 of Davignon et al.[49]; Table 24.1 and Fig. 24.1). This type had not been reported prior to our chapter in 1977.[49] Briefly, this is the "tetralogy of Fallot" type of DOLV in situs inversus totalis. This form of DOLV should be amenable to complete surgical repair using the same principles as in DOLV type 3 (Fig. 24.1) and applying them in mirror image. The aorta should be patched into the right-sided LV, thereby closing the VSD, and an external conduit from the left-sided RV to the pulmonary artery should make it possible to place the RV and the PA into continuity. The pulmonary artery would be interrupted at its origin (Fig. 24.1, type 10).

11. DOLV {I,L,D} with subaortic VSD and pulmonary outflow tract obstruction was found in two patients (cases 33 and 34, Table 24.1 and Fig. 24.1). This type of DOLV, which had not been reported previously, is characterized by situs inversus (I) of the viscera and atria, a

---

‡DOLV with pulmonary atresia is not regarded as a contradiction in terms because double-outlet left ventricle is merely a brief way of indicating that both great arteries arise above the LV. Both great arteries need not be patent.

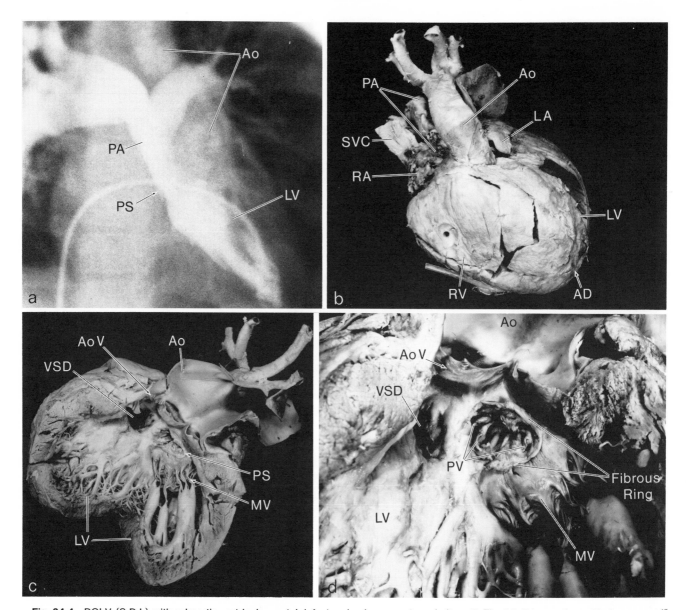

Fig. 24.4 DOLV {S,D,L} with subaortic ventricular septal defect and pulmonary stenosis (type 8, Fig. 24.1) in a patient of Izukawa *et al.*[47] (case 20, Table 24.1). (*a*) Selective left ventriculography, posteroanterior projection, showing normally located left ventricle (*LV*) giving rise to the pulmonary artery (*PA*) and to the overriding aorta (*Ao*). L-Malposition of the great arteries is present. Note the subvalvular pulmonary stenosis (*PS*). (*b*) Heart specimen, anteroposterior view, showing normally located superior vena cava (*SVC*), morphologically right atrium (*RA*), left atrium (*LA*), right ventricle (*RV*), and left ventricle (*LV*). L-Malposition of the great arteries is present, with the aorta (*Ao*) anterior and to the left, and the pulmonary artery (*PA*) posterior and to the right. (*c*) The opened *LV*, in left lateral view, gives rise to the aorta (*Ao*) and to the pulmonary artery. The aortic valve (*AoV*) overrides a ventricular septal defect (*VSD*). The stenotic pulmonary outflow tract (*PS*) is squeezed between the *Ao*, which is anterior and to the left, and the mitral valve (*MV*), which is posterior and somewhat to the right. (*d*) A closeup of the outflow tracts shows the pulmonary leaflets and the subvalvular fibrous ring. There is a small subaortic conus beneath the rightward portion of the aortic valve, as the diagram in Figure 24.1 (type 8) indicates. However, as this closeup shows, the muscular conus is absent beneath the leftward portion of the aortic valve, permitting fibrous continuity between the leftward portion of the aortic valve, the compressed pulmonary valve (*PV*), and the normal mitral valve. The pulmonary outflow tract is compressed by the truncoconal septum because of the malalignment of the conotruncus (L-malposition of the great arteries) relative to the normally located ventricles, ventricular septum, and atrioventricular canal (concordant D-loop). *AD*, anterior descending coronary artery.

concordant L-loop (L) with ventricular inversion and D-malposition (D) of the great arteries, the malposed aortic valve lying to the right (dextro or D) relative to the malposed pulmonary valve. Instead of the usual L-TGA with an L-loop, for reasons unknown, this transposition type of conotruncus has rotated to the right, resulting in: a subaortic VSD, due to malalignment of the conal septum relative to the ventricular septum; and DOLV, because not only does the PA arise above the LV close to the mitral valve, but also

the Ao originates predominantly above the LV because of the dextrorotation of the conotruncus; and pulmonary outflow tract stenosis or atresia, because malalignment of the conotruncus causes the conotruncal septum to encroach upon, or to obliterate, the pulmonary outflow tract. It is worthy of note that DOLV {I,L,D} is a mirror image of DOLV {S,D,L} (Fig. 24.1).

Surgically, the VSD is patched to the left of the aortic valve. This places the right-sided LA (morphologically left atrium), LV, and Ao into appropriate alignment. Continuity between the left-sided RA (morphologically right atrium), RV, and PA is established by an external valved conduit from RV to distal PA, with interruption of the proximal PA above the valve. This operation has recently been successfully performed for the first time in case 34 (Table 24.1).[22]

12. DOLV {I,D,D} with subaortic VSD and PS was found in one patient (case 35 in Table 24.1 and Fig. 24.1). This type of DOLV had not been reported previously. *Surgically,* the Ao was patched into the RV in order to convert this case into physiologically corrected transposition in situs inversus (Fig. 24.1), and the PS was relieved directly.

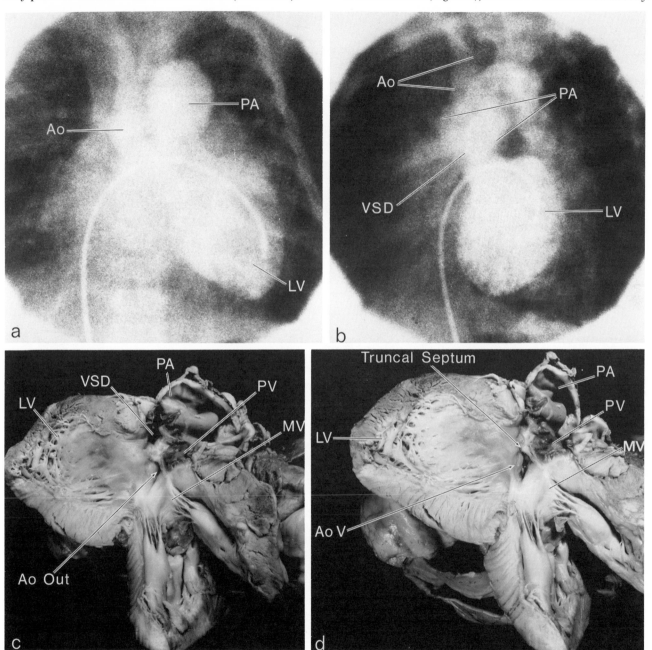

Fig. 24.5 DOLV {S,D,D} with subpulmonary ventricular septal defect (type 10, Fig. 24.1), patient of Hightower and Jordan[11] (case 28, Table 24.1). (a) Selective left ventricular injection in the posteroanterior projection showing simultaneous opacification of a large pulmonary artery (*PA*) and a relatively small ascending aorta (*Ao*). (b) Selective left ventricular injection in the left anterior oblique projection reveals that the *Ao* arises above the left ventricle (*LV*) and that the *PA* overrides a ventricular septal defect (*VSD*). (c) Opened left ventricle, left lateral view, shows that the large *PA* overrides a *VSD*. The *PA* is displaced abnormally leftward. The subpulmonary conus is absent beneath the leftward portion of the pulmonary valve (*PV*), permitting tenuous fibrous continuity between the darkly stained *PV* leaflets and the mitral valve (*MV*). The aorta arises entirely above the *LV* via a very stenotic outflow tract (*Ao Out*). (d) In this view, one can see that there is direct fibrous continuity between the hypoplastic and compressed aortic valve (*Ao V*) and the anterior leaflet of the mitral valve. The truncal septum, devoid of conal musculature, extends somewhat below the pulmonary leaflets (*PV*). The aortic outflow tract and *Ao V* is compressed between the truncal septum anteriorly and to the left because of the malalignment of the conotruncus relative to the ventricles, ventricular septum, and atrioventricular canal. The pulmonary valve and artery are abnormally levoposed. Consequently the truncoconal septum is malpositioned, resulting in a subpulmonary *VSD* and in compression of the aortic outflow tract, valve, and ascending aorta. Compression of the aortic outflow tract is reflected by hypoplasia of the aortic arch and preductal coarctation of the aorta, indicating reduced antegrade aortic blood flow, and by the enlarged pulmonary artery and patent ductus arteriosus, indicating increased antegrade pulmonary blood flow.

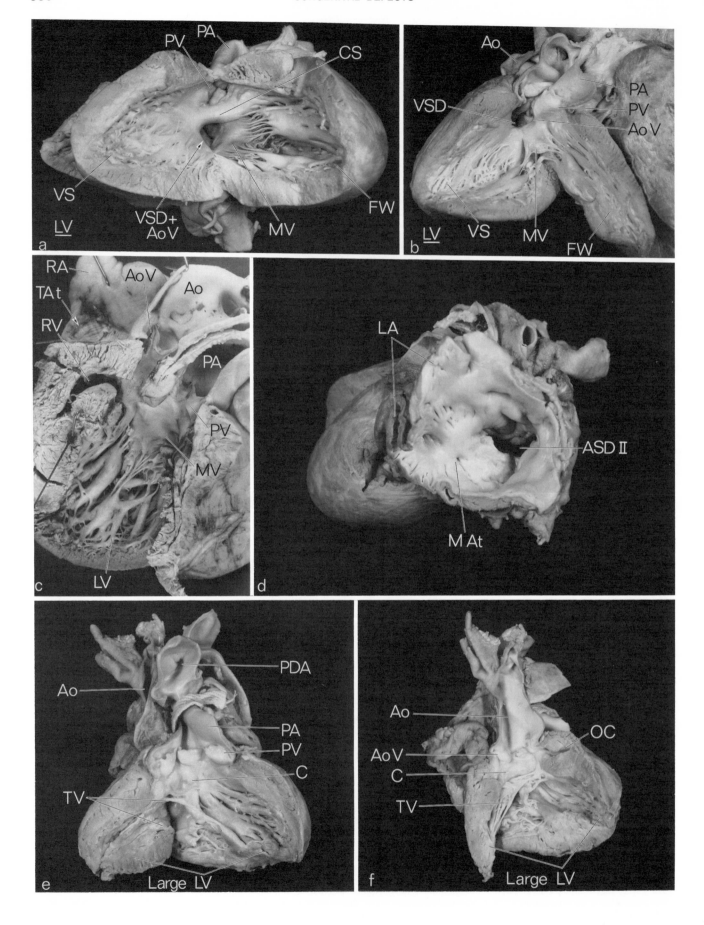

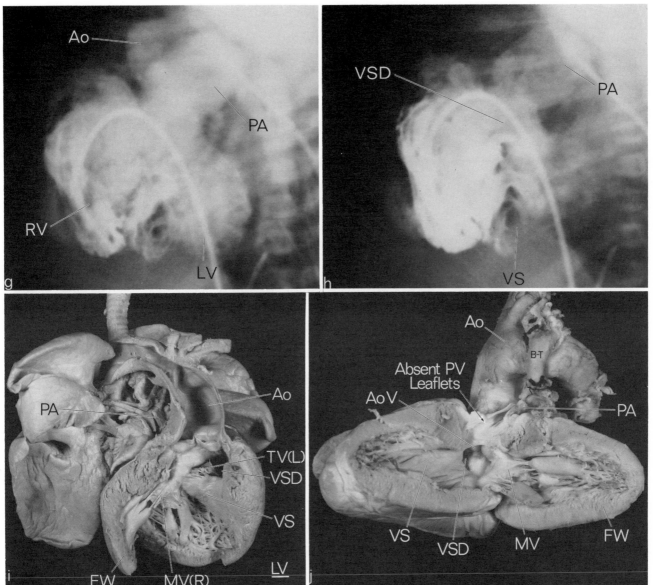

Fig. 24.6 Other anatomic types of double-outlet left ventricle (DOLV). (a) DOLV {S,D,D} with subaortic ventricular septal defect (*VSD*) and no pulmonary stenosis (*PS*) (type 2, Fig. 24.1) in patient of Métras[20] (case 3, Table 24.1), anterolateral view of opened left ventricle (*LV*). There is fibrous continuity between the aortic valve (*AoV*) and the mitral valve (*MV*), but no fibrous continuity between the pulmonary valve (*PV*) and the *MV* because of a short interposed conal septum (*CS*). (b) DOLV {S,D,D} with subaortic VSD and bilaterally absent conus (type 4, Fig. 24.1) in a patient of Bhan et al.[4] (case 14, Table 24.1), opened *LV*, left lateral view. There is fibrous continuity between the pulmonary valve and the anterior leaflet of the mitral valve and between the Ao V and the MV. (c) DOLV {S,D,D} with tricuspid atresia (*TAt*) and small right ventricle (*RV*) (really infundibulum) (type 6, Fig. 24.1), in a patient of Quero Jiménez et al.[33, 34] (case 17, Table 24.1), left anterolateral view of opened ventricles and great arteries. There is fibrous continuity between the pulmonary valve and the mitral valve. A muscular conus beneath the aortic valve precludes aortic-mitral fibrous continuity. The pulmonary artery (*PA*) arises entirely above the *LV*, whereas the overriding aorta (*Ao*) originates predominantly above the *LV*. (d–f) DOLV {S,D,D} with mitral atresia, large LV, and infundibular outlet chamber (type 7, Fig. 24.1; case 18, Table 24.1). (d) Left posterolateral view of the opened left atrium (*LA*), revealing mitral atresia (*MAt*) and a secundum atrial septal defect (*ASD II*). (e) Anterolateral view of the opened large *LV*, banded pulmonary artery, and patent ductus arteriosus (*PDA*). A well-developed subpulmonary conus (*C*) separates the pulmonary valve from the tricuspid valve (*TV*). (f) Anterior view of the opened large LV, the infundibular outlet chamber (*OC*), and the aorta. The subaortic conus (*C*) separates the aortic valve from the tricuspid valve. (g and h) DOLV {S,D,L} with subpulmonary VSD (type 14, Fig. 24.1), in a patient of Muster[30] (case 26, Table 24.1), selective right ventriculography in left lateral projection. The pulmonary artery overrides a ventricular septal defect, predominantly above the posterior LV, and the aorta originates entirely above the *LV*; these findings were confirmed at autopsy. Ebstein's anomaly, mild congenital mitral stenosis, preductal coarctation of the aorta, and a patent ductus arteriosus were also found. (i) DOLV {S,L,L} with subaortic VSD and pulmonary atresia (type 9, Fig. 24.1), in a patient of Paul[35] (case 32, Table 24.1), right anterior oblique view of opened *LV* (right-sided), aorta, and the relatively small pulmonary artery with an atretic pulmonary outflow tract. A long and tortuous patent ductus arteriosus can be seen leading to the right pulmonary artery. The aortic arch is right-sided. The subaortic conus separates the aortic valve from the right-sided mitral valve (*MV(R)*) and from the left-sided tricuspid valve (*TV(L)*). (j) DOLV {S,D,D} with subaortic *VSD*, PS, and absence of the leaflets of the pulmonary valve, without aneurysmal enlargement of the PA (type 3, Fig. 24.1), in a patient of Arqué et al.[2, 3] (case 9, Table 24.1). The rare feature of this case is complete absence of the pulmonary valve leaflets, this also having been reported by Maréchal[24] in 1819 in the earliest known case of apparently genuine DOLV. (c reproduced with the permission of M. Quero Jiménez and M. J. Maître Azcárate and the Revista Española de Cardiología[38] and Quero Jiménez et al., and the European Journal of Cardiology[39]; j reproduced with the permission of J. M. Arqué et al. and the Revista Española de Cardiologia[3] RA, right atrium; VS, ventricular septum; FW, free wall.

This patient had complete heart block preoperatively, which is not surprising in view of the presence of a discordant ventricular loop (a D-loop in situs inversus). The death of this 28-year-old man 2 years postoperatively may well have been due to a dysrhythmia.[6]

13. DOLV {S,D,D} with subpulmonary VSD occurred in five patients (cases 27 to 31 in Table 24.1; Figs. 24.1 and 24.5).[11, 23, 31, 42, 51] It occurs with and without aortic stenosis, and with or without pulmonary stenosis (Table 24.1). The conotruncus is malaligned relative to the ventricles and the AV canal, the PA being displaced abnormally far to the left (Fig. 24.5, c and d). A subpulmonary or conal septal defect is present, and deficiency of the subpulmonary conus may permit tenuous pulmonary-mitral fibrous continuity (case 28 in Table 24.1 and Fig. 24.5, c and d)[11] Conotruncal malalignment may result in significant aortic outflow tract obstruction by squeezing the aortic annulus between the abnormally located truncal septum anteriorly and the normally located mitral valve and ventricular septum posteriorly (Fig. 24.5c and d).

Surgically, this type of DOLV was first recognized and surgically repaired by Sakakibara, *et al.*[42] Repair was accomplished by patch closure of the subpulmonary VSD, their patient having neither aortic nor pulmonary stenosis (case 27, Table 24.1). Litwin[23] successfully corrected pulmonary outflow tract stenosis in this type of DOLV by an external valved conduit from RV to PA (case 29, Table 24.1).

14. DOLV{S,D,L} with subpulmonary VSD was found in one patient (case 26 in Table 24.1 and Figs. 24.1 and 24.6g and h).[30] This type has not been reported previously.

Surgically, we think that this type of DOLV is not correctable at the present time in view of the associated cardiovascular malformations: Ebstein's anomaly, mild mitral stenosis, and preductal coarctation of the aorta.

UPDATE

The foregoing is essentially what was known about DOLV as of 1977.[49] What have we learned over the past 5 years?

First of all, most serious students of congenital heart disease have felt a strong urge to reduce, somehow or other, these 14 different anatomic types (Fig. 24.1). There is a certain absurdity in the view that among 36 cases of DOLV, there are 14 different anatomic types. Yet, that is what we found (Fig. 24.1). In retrospect, one wonders whether we "split" too much, or did not "lump" enough?

Consequently, the diagram of the anatomic types of DOLV has been reorganized in a more physiologic and surgical way (Fig. 24.1). Note that types 1 to 12 inclusive all have a subaortic VSD, whereas only types 13 and 14 have a subpulmonary VSD. We have reorganized these anatomic types in terms of VSD site (subaortic or subpulmonary) because of the physiologic and surgical importance of this consideration.

Another thing that DOLV urgently needs for most cardiologists, radiologists, and surgeons is "familiarization." We are now going to attempt to accomplish this, even though we are fully aware that it is difficult to feel familiar with something that one may never have seen. Nonetheless, it is important to make DOLV seem less alien because, if understood, many forms are amenable to surgical management.

Type I. DOLV with Solitus Atria, Solitus Ventricles (Both Well-developed), and Subaortic VSD. This is much the commonest type of DOLV. There are several subtypes.

a. With Pulmonary Stenosis and D-positioned Aorta. This is the **"tetralogy of Fallot type" of DOLV** (Fig. 24.1,

diagram 3). This is probably the commonest form of DOLV and has often been mistaken for tetralogy of Fallot. Indeed, the only major difference between this type of DOLV and tetralogy of Fallot is that in the "tetralogy" type of DOLV, the pulmonary artery arises entirely from the LV (Fig. 24.3). It is noteworthy that in "the tetralogy type" of DOLV, the pulmonary leaflets occasionally can be absent (Fig. 24.6j)—as may occur in typical tetralogy of Fallot.

Parenthetically, it is noteworthy that *solitus* ventricles and D-*loop* ventricles are synonyms. *Inverted* ventricles and L-loop ventricles also are synonyms (see Chapter 25).

b. With Pulmonary Stenosis and an A-positioned or L-positioned Aorta (Fig. 24.1, Diagram 8). This is the **"transposition type" of DOLV** (Fig. 24.4).

c. Without Pulmonary Stenosis and D-positioned Aorta (Fig. 24.1, Diagram 2). This is the **"high-flow VSD type" of DOLV** (Fig. 24.6a and b).

d. With Subaortic Narrowing, Preductal Coarctation of the Aorta, and D-positioned Aorta (Fig. 24.1, diagram 4). This is the **"preductal coarctation type" of DOLV.**

Type II. DOLV with Solitus Atria, Solitus Ventricles (Both Well-Developed), and Subpulmonary VSD. There are several subtypes.

a. With D-positioned and Posterior Aorta (Fig. 24.1, Diagram 13). This is the relatively common **"conal septal defect type" of DOLV.** This is the type that Sakakibara *et al.*[42] corrected, thereby rediscovering DOLV in 1967.

b. With Ebstein's Anomaly, and Very Rare (Fig. 24.1, Diagram 14). This is **"Ebstein's type" of DOLV.** (Fig. 24.6g and h).

Type III. DOLV with Solitus Atria, Solitus Ventricles, and Ventricular Septal Defect, Both Subaortic and Subpulmonary. Although logically predictable, this type was not observed by us (Fig. 24.1) but was subsequently reported by Bharati *et al.*[5]

Type IV: DOLV with Solitus Atria, Solitus Ventricles, AV Valve Anomalies, and Only One Well-developed Ventricle.

a. The most frequent subset is **the "tricuspid atresia type" of DOLV** (Fig. 24.1, diagrams 5 and 6, and Fig. 24.6c).

b. Mitral atresia with a large LV and an infundibular outlet chamber (Fig. 24.1, diagram 7, and 24.6 d to f) is the **"mitral atresia with large LV type" of DOLV.**

c. The **"small, blind RV type" of DOLV** is the Paul type[36] DOLV with an intact ventricular septum (Fig. 24.1, diagram 1, and 24.2). This unique case was considered to have tricuspid stenosis by Bharati *et al.*[5] We prefer to view this as tricuspid hypoplasia because the tricuspid valve was small—consistent with the small size of the RV cavity—but was not otherwise malformed.

Type V. DOLV with solitus atria, inversus ventricles, and subaortic VSD.

a. With Pulmonary Outflow Tract Obstruction (Atresia, as in Fig. 24.1, Diagram 9). This is **"the corrected transposition type" of DOLV** (Fig. 24.6i).

Type VI. DOLV with Inversus Atria, Inversus Ventricles, and Subaortic VSD (Fig. 24.1, Diagrams 10 and 11).

a. The aorta may be in L-position, with pulmonary outflow tract obstruction (stenosis, diagram 10, Fig. 24.1), **"the tetralogy of Fallot in situs inversus type" of DOLV.**

Type VII. DOLV with Inversus Atria, Solitus Ventricles, and Subaortic VSD. *a. With pulmonary stenosis (diagram 12, Fig. 24.1).* This is **"the corrected transposition in situs inversus type" of DOLV.**

Type VIII. DOLV with Situs Ambiguus. This was not observed by us (Fig. 24.1) but has been reported by Otero Coto *et al.*[32]

TABLE 24.2   TYPES OF DOLV

Types	Subtypes	Features	Informal Name	Figures
I		DOLV {S,D,-} with subaortic VSD		
	a	DOLV {S,D,*D*} with subaortic VSD and PS	Tetralogy type	24.1 diagram 3, 24.3, and 24.6*j*
	b	DOLV {S,D,*A*} and {S,D,*L*} with subaortic VSD and PS	Transposition type	24.1 diagram 8, and 24.4
	c	DOLV {S,D,*D*} with subaortic VSD and *no PS*	High flow VSD type	24.1 diagram 2, and 24.6*a* and *b*
	d	DOLV {S,D,D} with subaortic VSD, subaortic narrowing, and preductal coarctation of Ao	Preductal coarctation type	24.1 diagram 4
II		DOLV {S,D,-}, with subpulmonary VSD		
	a	DOLV {S,D,D} with subpulmonary VSD	Conal septal defect type	24.1 diagram 13
	b	Ebstein's anomaly	Ebstein's type	24.1 diagram 14, and 24.6*g* and *h*
III		DOLV {S,D,-} with subaortic and subpulmonary VSD		
	a	DOLV {S,D,*D*}	Doubly committed VSD type	
IV		DOLV {S,D,-} with AV valve anomalies and only one well-developed ventricle.		
	a	DOLV {S,D,D} or {S,D,A}, or {S,D,L} with tricuspid atresia	Tricuspid atresia type	24.1 diagrams 5 and 6, and 24.6*c*
	b	DOLV {S,D,D} with mitral atresia	Mitral atresia type	24.1 diagram 7, and 24.6*g* and *f*
	c	DOLV {S,D,D} with intact ventricular septum and small blind RV	Small blind RV type with intact ventricular septum	24.1, diagram 1, and 24.2
V		DOLV {S,L,-} and subaortic VSD		
	a	DOLV {S,L,L} with subaortic VSD and pulmonary outflow tract obstruction	"Corrected" transposition type	24.1 diagram 9 and 24.6*i*
VI		DOLV {I,L,-} with subaortic VSD		
	a	DOLV {I,L,L} with subaortic VSD and PS	Tetralogy in situs inversus totalis type	24.1 diagram 10
	b	DOLV {I,L,D} with subaortic VSD and PS or PAt	Transposition in situs inversus type	24.1 diagram 11.
VII		DOLV {I,D,-} with subaortic VSD		
	a	DOLV {I,D,D} with subaortic VSD and PS	"Corrected" transposition in situs inversus type	24.1 diagram 12
VIII		DOLV {A,-,-} with asplenia		
	a	DOLV {A,L,L} with asplenia	Asplenia type	

The purpose of the aforementioned informal "types" of DOLV is to suggest similarities in order to aid comprehension. For example, "the tetralogy type" of DOLV is intended to suggest that DOLV is present and that the anatomy is similar to and, hence, reminiscent of the tetralogy of Fallot. In this way it is hoped that these informal "types" of DOLV will make the various anatomic sets and subsets more readily comprehensible—by pointing out the more familiar "cousins" of the various anatomic types of DOLV. (*It is most emphatically not being suggested that tetralogy of Fallot and DOLV in fact coexist.*) Thus, the "tetralogy type" of DOLV means *similar* to tetralogy but of course not identical to tetralogy.

Thus, eight main anatomic types of DOLV are known at the present time, each main type having one or more subtypes (as above).

In addition, a number of studies of DOLV have been published since the second edition of this book.[5, 12, 15, 29, 32, 40, 44, 45, 50, 52] The study of Bharati *et al.*[5] is noteworthy not only because of its large data base (45 cases), but also because it contains some previously unreported anatomic subtypes:

1. *DOLV {S,D,D} with subpulmonary VSD and anterior aorta.* To our knowledge, DOLV with a subpulmonary VSD has always previously had a posterior aortic valve, as in Figure 24.1, diagram 13. This increases our understanding of DOLV Type II.

2. *DOLV {S,D,D} with a VSD Both Subpulmonary and Subaortic.* DOLV with a doubly committed VSD is, to our knowledge, a new observation and is regarded as a newly recognized form of DOLV: Type III (above-mentioned).

3. *DOLV {S,D,A} or {S,D,L} with Double-Inlet LV, with Small RV Present.* DOLV with double-inlet LV is, to our knowledge, a newly reported finding. This is a contribution to our knowledge of DOLV with only one well-formed ventricle (Type IV, mentioned heretofore).

Although Bharati *et al.*[5] considered only DOLV with solitus atria and solitus ventricles, they found 10 different anatomic types. These workers excluded DOLV in situs solitus with AV discordance, DOLV in situs inversus, and DOLV in situs ambiguus. Although the findings of Bharati *et al.*[5] were complex enough, the full spectrum of DOLV—which this chapter seeks to present—is even more complex.

Otero Coto and his colleagues[32] reported five cases which are noteworthy for the following additions to our understanding of DOLV:

1. DOLV can occur with *situs ambiguus* and asplenia, hence, Type VIII above.

2. DOLV can occur with *straddling tricuspid valve* (left-sided), in a patient of the {S,L,A} type. This is a newly recognized subset of DOLV Type V (above).

We think that the case reported by Urban *et al.*[45] probably is not an example of DOLV but of TGA. We strongly suspect that what these authors identified as the VSD was in fact

the RV outflow tract. It can be very difficult to decide
whether a case is a genuine example of DOLV or not. Kinsley
et al.[15] reported a case in point. Although the aorta was
described as arising entirely above the RV, the VSD was
subaortic such that the aorta also overrode the LV via the
VSD. We prefer not to make the diagnosis of DOLV unless
this diagnosis is unequivocal. When it is a very "close call,"
we think that one should *not* make the diagnosis of DOLV.
In this way, when the enthusiasms of the moment subside,
one will be able to trust one's diagnoses of DOLV.

The case reported by Vaseenon *et al.*[50] is unique: DOLV
{*S,D,L*} with tricuspid atresia and a bilateral conus. Previously, only cases with D-positioned or *A*-positioned aorta
had been reported, to our knowledge. Hence, this case report[50] extends the understanding of DOLV Type IV (above).

Parenthetically, it should be added that we favor segmental diagnosis, as in Figure 24.1 and Table 24.1. We are *not*
proposing that the segmental diagnosis of DOLV be supplanted by Types I to VIII, inclusive. On the contrary, these
main types are viewed as a summary and simplification of
the segmental diagnostic data. We suspect that even Types
I to VIII are too much for most people to remember for long
and, hence, be able to use in their daily work. Thus, for easy
reference, these main types will be summarized in tabular
form (Table 24.2).

From the therapeutic standpoint, the papers of Rivera
et al.[40] and Murphy *et al.*[29] both emphasized the advantages,
when feasible, of intraventricular repair in order to avoid
extracardiac conduits.

Four different surgical procedures have been used in
the management of DOLV (Fig. 24.7):

1. An intraventricular conduit via the subpulmonary VSD
was employed by Sakakibara *et al.*[42] in their successful
treatment of DOLV with subpulmonary VSD (Fig. 24.1,
diagram 13).

2. Patch closure of the VSD, aligning the LV with the
aorta, ligation of the proximal pulmonary artery, and the use
of an external valved conduit from RV to PA have been
employed for DOLV of the "tetralogy" type (Fig. 24.1, diagram 3).[6, 14, 34]

3. A Fontan type of procedure has been used for cases of
DOLV with tricuspid atresia or "stenosis"[12, 43] (Fig. 24.1,
diagrams 6, 5, and 1).

4. When the VSD is subaortic and the pulmonary artery
arises entirely from the LV, the pulmonary artery may be
left arising from the LV, and the aorta can be aligned with
the RV by means of a subaortic patch-conduit. This can be
employed in the "corrected" transposition type of DOLV,
such as DOLV [I,D,D] (Fig. 24.1, diagram 12).[6] If the DOLV
is of the "transposition" (uncorrected) variety with a subaortic VSD, then in addition to patching the aorta into the
RV, an atrial baffle procedure (Senning or Mustard) also
would be necessary.[40] At least half of the known types of
DOLV are thought now to be surgically correctable (Fig.
24.1).

Regarding embryonic morphogenesis, the available anatomic data suggest that there are at least three factors of
importance in the morphogenesis of DOLV: excessive conal
absorption beneath both semilunar valves, permitting not
only aortic-mitral but also pulmonary-mitral approximation;

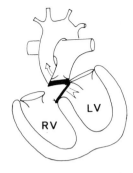
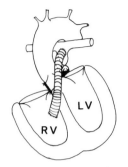

KERR, et al.   – '71   SAKAKIBARA, et al. – '67
PACIFICO, et al. – '72

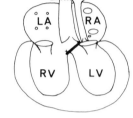
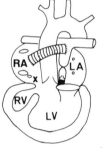

SHARRATT, et al. – '76   BRANDT, et al. – '76

Fig. 24.7 Surgical management of various anatomic types of
DOLV. (*Top left*) "Tetralogy" type with subaortic VSD. (*Top right*)
Conal septal defect type with subpulmonary VSD. (*Lower left*)
Tricuspid atresia type. (*Lower right*) "Corrected transposition"
type. See text for further details. See Brandt *et al.*,[6] Kerr *et al.*,[14]
Pacifico *et al.*,[33, 34] Sakakibara *et al.*,[42] and Sharratt *et al.*[43]

underdevelopment of the RV, so that both great arteries
tend to arise, *perforce*, above the LV; and conotruncal malalignment.

Idiopathic conotruncal malalignment is an important
developmental principle and anatomic fact that applies to
many types of abnormal ventriculoarterial alignments: TGA,
DORV, DOLV, and anatomically corrected malposition (Fig.
28.8). We are not referring to the classical concept of conotruncal *malseptation*. Rather, we seek to focus attention on
the widespread importance of malalignment of the *entire*
conotruncus-septum and free wall.

The principle of malalignment applies to all of the three
major cardiac segments, not just to the conotruncus. One of
the reasons that *the segmental approach* to the understanding of congenital heart disease is so helpful is that there are
many anomalies in which one cardiac segment is malaligned
relative to an adjacent segment (Fig. 28.6).

In conclusion, DOLV is characterized by anomalies of all
five of the diagnostically important cardiac segments—the
atria, the AV junction, the ventricles, the infundibulum, and
the great arteries. In view of the complexity and variability
of these malformations, a segment-by-segment and alignment-by-alignment diagnostic method is necessary. When
well understood, DOLV usually is amenable to surgical
correction or palliation.

REFERENCES

1. Anderson, R., Galbraith, R., Gibson, R., and
   Miller, G.: Double outlet left ventricle. Br.
   Heart J. 36:554, 1974.
2. Arqué, J. M.: Personal communication, Nov.
   5, 1975.
3. Arqué, J. M., Revuelta, J. M., Sanchez, C.,

Simon-Lamuela, J., and Lozano-Sainz, C.:
Tratamiento quirurgico del ventriculo derecho
de doble salida y del ventriculo izquierdo de
doble salida. Rev. Esp. Cardiol. 29:305, 1976.
4. Bhan, I., Kriedberg, M., and Khan, A.: Personal communication, Nov. 12, 1975.

5. Bharati, S., Lev, M., Stewart, R., McAllister,
   H. A., and Kirklin, J. W.: The morphologic
   spectrum of double outlet left ventricle and its
   surgical significance. Circulation 58:558, 1978.
6. Brandt, P. W. T., Calder, A. L., Barratt-Boyes,
   B. G., and Neutze, J. M.: Double outlet left

ventricle. Morphology, cineangiocardiographic diagnosis and surgical treatment. Am. J. Cardiol. 38:897, 1976.

7. Conti, V., Adams, F., and Mulder, D. G.: Double outlet left ventricle. Ann. Thorac. Surg. 18:402, 1974.

8. Fontan, F., Mounico, F. B., Baudet, E., Siminneau, S., Gordo, J., and Goufrant, P.: "Correction" de l'atrésie triscupidienne: Rapport de deux cas "corrigés" par l'utilisation d'une technique chirurgicale nouvelle. Ann. Chir. Thorac. Cardiovas. 10:39, 1971.

9. Fragoyannis, S., amd Kardalinos, A.: Transposition of the great vessels, both arising from the left ventricle (juxtaposition of pulmonary artery): Tricuspid atresia, atrial septal defect and ventricular septal defect. Am. J. Cardiol. 10:601, 1962.

10. Gazzaniga, A. B., Sperling, D. R., and Rowen, M.: Personal communication, Nov. 30, 1971.

11. Hightower, W., and Jordan, J. D.: Personal communication, March 23, 1972.

12. Katogi, T., Takenchi, S., Katsumoto, K., Fukuda, T., Morishita, M., and Inoue, T.; Surgical correction of double outlet left ventricle associated with hypoplastic right ventricle: Direct anastomosis of right atrial appendage and pulmonary artery. Jap. Circulation J. 43:768, 1979.

13. Kelly, D.: Personal communication, Sept. 30, 1970.

14. Kerr, A. R., Barcia, A., Bargeron, L. M., and Kirklin, J. W.: Double-outlet left ventricle with ventricular septal defect and pulmonary stenosis: Report of surgical repair. Am. Heart J. 81:688, 1971.

15. Kinsley, R. H., Levin, S. E., and O'Donovan, T. G.: Transposition of the great arteries associated with a double left ventricular outflow tract. Br. Heart J. 42:483, 1979.

16. Kirklin, J. W., Pacifico, A. D., Bargeron, L. M., and Soto, B.: Cardiac repair in anatomically corrected malposition of the great arteries. Circulation 48:153, 1973.

17. Kreutzer, G., Galíndez, E., Bono, H., de Palma, C., and Laura, J. P.: An operation for the correction of tricuspid atresia. J. Thorac. Cardiovasc. Surg. 66:613, 1973.

18. Krongrad, E., Malm, J. R., Bowman, F. O., Hoffman, B. F., and Waldo, A. L.: Electrophysiologic delineation of the specialized A-V conduction system in patients with congenital heart disease. II. Delineation of the distal His bundle and the right bundle branch. Circulation 49:1232, 1974.

19. Krongrad, E.: Personal communication, Aug. 24, 1976.

20. Kussmaul: Ueber angeborene Enge und Vershluss der Lungenarterien-Bahn. Z. rationelle Med. 26:99, 1866.

21. Leriche, H., Toussaint, M., and Piot, C.: Ventricule gauche á double issue: A propos d'un cas reconnu à l'angiographie (aspects clinique, angiocardiographique et embryologique). Coeur 5:167, 1974.

22. Levine, F., Goldblatt, A., and Buckley, M.: Personal communication, March 3, 1976.

23. Litwin, S. B.: Personal communication, October 31, 1974.

24. Maréchal.: Conformation vicieuse du coeur d'un enfant affecté de la maladie bleue. J. Gén. de Méd. 69:354, 1819 (Oct.).

25. Mery.: Diverses observations anatomiques. Hist. de l'Acad. Roy. des Sciences, p. 42, obs. 42, 1703, Paris.

26. Métras, D.: Personal communication, Aug. 8, 1975.

27. Miller, W. W., and Weinberg, A. G.: Personal communication, Oct. 4, 1972.

28. Minhas, K.: Personal communication, Oct. 7, 1970.

29. Murphy, D. A., Gillis, D. A., and Sridhara, K. S.: Intraventricular repair of double-outlet left ventricle. Ann. Thorac. Surg. 31:364, 1981.

30. Muster, A. J.: Personal communication, March 29, 1973.

31. Nihmura, I.: Personal communication, June 18, 1971.

32. Otero Coto, E., Quero Jimenez, M., Castaneda, A. R., Rufilanchas, J. J., and Deverall, P. B.: Double outlet from chambers of left ventricular morphology. Br. Heart J. 42:15, 1979.

33. Pacifico, A. D., Bargeron, L. M., Kirklin, J. W., and Barcia, A.: Surgical treatment of double outlet left ventricle. Circulation 46 (Suppl. II):35, 1972.

34. Pacifico, A. D., Kirklin, J. W., Bargeron, L. M., and Soto, B.: Surgical treatment of double-outlet left ventricle: Report of four cases. Circulation 48: (Suppl. III):19, 1973.

35. Paul, M. H.: Personal communication, Sept. 30, 1965.

36. Paul, M. H., Sinha, S. N., Muster, A. J., Cole, R. B., and Van Praagh, R.: Double outlet left ventricle. Report of an autopsy case with an intact ventricular septum and consideration of its developmental implications. Circulation 41:129, 1970.

37. Quero, M.: Coexistence of single ventricle with atresia of one atrioventricular orifice. Circulation 46:794, 1972.

38. Quero Jiménez, M., and Maître Azcárate, M. J.: Ventriculo izquierdo de doble salida: Estudio de un caso y revision de la literatura. Rev. Esp. Cardiol. 28:587, 1975.

39. Quero Jiménez, M., Maître Azcárate, M. J., Alvarez Bejarano, H., and Vázquez Martul, E.: Tricuspid atresia: An anatomical study of 17 cases. Eur. J. Cardiol. 3:337, 1975.

40. Rivera, R., Infantes, C., and Gil de la Peña, M.: Double outlet left ventricle. Report of a case with intraventricular surgical repair. J. Cardiovasc. Surg. 21:361, 1980.

41. Sacks, E.: Personal communication, May 6, 1974.

42. Sakakibara, S., Takao, A., Arai, T., Hashimoto, A., and Nogi, M.: Both great vessels arising from the left ventricle (double outlet left ventricle) (origin of both great vessels from the left ventricle). Bull. Heart Inst. Japan, p. 66, 1967.

43. Sharratt, G. P., Sbokos, C. G., Johnson, A. M., Anderson, R. H., and Monro, J. L.: Surgical "correction" of solitus-concordant, double-outlet left ventricle with L-malposition and tricuspid stenosis with hypoplastic right ventricle. J. Thorac. Cardiovasc. Surg. 71:853, 1976.

44. Stegmann, T., Oster, H., Bissenden, J., Kallfelz, H. C., and Oelert, H.: Surgical treatment of double-outlet left ventricle in 2 patients with D-position and L-position of the aorta. Ann. Thorac. Surg. 27:121, 1979.

45. Urban, A. E., Anderson, R. H., and Stark, J.: Double outlet left ventricle associated with situs inversus and atrioventricular concordance. Am. Heart J. 94:91, 1977.

46. Van Praagh, R.: Conotruncal malformations. In Heart Disease in Infancy, edited by B. G. Barratt-Boyes, J. M. Neutze, and E. A. Harris, p. 141. Churchill & Livingstone, Edinburgh and London, 1973.

47. Van Praagh, R., Calder, A. L., Delisle, G., and Izukawa, T.: Transposition of the great arteries with overriding aorta and pulmonary stenosis: New entity and its surgical management. Circulation 46: (Suppl. II):96, 1972.

48. Van Praagh, R., Pérez-Treviño, C., López-Cuellar, M., Baker, F. W., Zuberbuhler, J. F., Quero, M., Pérez, V. M., Moreno, F., and Van Praagh, S.: Transposition of the great arteries with posterior aorta, anterior pulmonary artery, subpulmonary conus and fibrous continuity between aortic and atrioventricular valves. Am. J. Cardiol. 28:621, 1971.

49. Van Praagh, R., and Weinberg, P. M.: Double outlet left ventricle. In Heart Disease in Infants, Children and Adolescents, 2nd ed., Chap. 22, edited by A. J. Moss, F. H. Adams, and G. C. Emmanouilides, Williams & Wilkins, Baltimore, p. 367.

50. Vaseenon, T., Diehl, A. M., and Mattioli, L.: Tricuspid atresia with double-outlet left ventricle and bilateral conus. Chest 74:676, 1978.

51. Vaughan, K. D., and Finer, N.: Personal communication, March 3, 1976.

52. Villani, M., Lipscombe, S., and Ross, D. N.: Double outlet left ventricle: How should we repair it? Anatomical details and report of two successful surgical cases. J. Cardiovasc. Surg. 20:413, 1979.

25

Single or Univentricular Heart

Larry P. Elliott, M.D., Robert H. Anderson, M.D., Lionel M. Bargeron, Jr., M.D.,
James K. Kirklin, M.D.

Hearts with both atria connected to the same ventricular chamber have long fascinated investigators of congenital heart disease and have been described by a bewildering variety of names.[15, 38, 40, 46, 54, 62] Of late there has been considerable debate[60, 61] as to whether hearts with double inlet to a right ventricular chamber in the presence of a rudimentary left ventricular chamber[37, 44, 48, 53] should properly be considered as "single" ventricle, along with the more common anomaly in which both atria are connected to a left ventricular chamber in the presence of a rudimentary right ventricular chamber. Semantic arguments along this line are nonproductive. All hearts with double inlet atrioventricular connection are unified by the connection, irrespective of their ventricular morphology. It is the different morphology of this *dominant* ventricle, along with the ventriculoarterial connections and associated lesions present, which serve to subcategorize the group. In this chapter, therefore, we will describe the features of those hearts unified by the atrioventricular connection of *double inlet ventricle*, regardless of the dominant ventricle morphology.

Although hearts with absent atrioventricular connection (atrioventricular valve atresia) have comparable ventricular morphologies to the hearts with double inlet,[2, 3, 15, 56] they will not be described in this chapter. It is our opinion, however, that the single or univentricular heart with atresia of an atrioventricular valve is as fundamental to the entity single ventricle or univentricular heart as those with two atrioventricular valves.[1, 13, 15]

GENERAL PRINCIPLES OF MORPHOLOGIC DESCRIPTION

The hearts to be described can exist with any of the four possible arrangements of the atrial chambers, that is, situs solitus (normally related atria), situs inversus (mirror image atria), right atrial isomerism, or left atrial isomerism (Fig. 25.1).[13, 39] Unless specified to the contrary, our description will be confined to cases with situs solitus.

The majority of hearts described herein will have double inlet atrioventricular (AV) connection, but when describing the connection, we account only for the way in which the *atrial myocardium is connected to the ventricular myocardium* at the AV junction. Thus, double inlet connection may occur through two separate AV valves or a common valve. When there are two valves, then usually both are perforated, but rarely one or the other valve may be imperforate. Because in the majority of the cases with double inlet, the AV valves (when two are present) cannot be distinguished as mitral or tricuspid in morphology,[13] we will describe them simply as right or left AV valves, irrespective of the atrial situs or ventricular morphology. One or both valves may be found to straddle the ventricular septum. Hearts with *straddling valves* will be described in this chapter, providing the

degree of *overriding** of the valve annulus is such as to preserve the double inlet atrioventricular connection.[59] A common valve may also straddle the septum. These cases will also be included when the overriding is such that the connection is still double inlet.

We will differentiate the ventricular chambers according to their *trabecular* characteristics. When two ventricular chambers are present, almost invariably they are of complementary trabecular pattern. Thus, when the atria are connected to a chamber with left ventricular pattern, almost always there is a second ventricular chamber present which lacks an AV connection, but which is of unequivocally *right ventricular* trabecular pattern. Contrawise, when the atria are connected to a right ventricular chamber, then the chamber without an AV connection is of *left ventricular* trabecular pattern. When there is a *sole* ventricular chamber, it is almost always of neither right nor left, but of *indeterminate* trabecular pattern. On occasion, hearts may be found with only one right or left ventricular chamber in which it is not possible on gross study to identify a second chamber. In our experience, a second chamber has been found in such cases following histological examination. Clinically and angiocardiographically, however, it is extremely difficult to distinguish these latter hearts from the indeterminate form of single ventricle.

When double inlet is found in hearts with two ventricular chambers, the chamber lacking the AV connection is the rudimentary or nondominant ventricular chamber. Of necessity, the septum separating the chambers cannot be an inlet septum. It is the trabecular septum.

The connections between the ventricular chambers and the great arteries will be defined according to the trabecular morphology. Thus, the ventriculoarterial connections will be described as *concordant* (normal connections) when the pulmonary trunk is connected to the right ventricular chamber and the aorta to the left ventricular chamber, regardless of the size of the chambers. *Discordant* connections (transposition) is the reverse. *Double outlet* can occur from main or rudimentary chambers of right or left type or from an indeterminate chamber. *Single outlet* can be found in any of its combination. Of necessity, when there is a sole ventricular chamber, only double outlet or single outlet connections are possible. Of all these variables, the most significant point in differentiating the heart with double inlet is ventricular morphology. This then will be the main basis for our subdivision, and we will recognize three groups: those with double inlet to a *left ventricular* (DILV) chamber, to a *right ven-*

---

*Overriding valve: when the valve *annulus* overrides the ventricular septum to varying degrees. Straddling valve: when the papillary muscles or tensor apparatus arise from both the dominant ventricle and rudimentary ventricle. In other words, an overriding and straddling valve don't necessarily coexist.

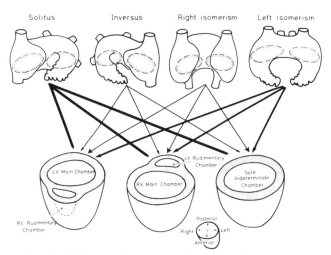

Fig. 25.1 Diagram showing how double inlet can exist with any arrangement of atrial chambers and with one of three ventricular morphologies. In the hearts with two ventricular chambers, the relationship of the rudimentary chamber to the main chamber is also variable. (Reproduced with permission from Churchill Livingstone, Edinburgh.)

tricular (DIRV) chamber, and to an *indeterminate* ventricular chamber (Fig. 25.1).

ANATOMY AND ANGIOCARDIOGRAPHY

Traditionally, anatomy and angiocardiography are presented as distinct topics. With the advent of axial cineangiography in children, the heart as viewed with this technique is not limited by obscuration and foreshortening of structures as seen with conventional views. Axial or angled angiography allows the heart to be viewed as if "held in hand."[4, 16, 17, 24] As a result, it became appropriate to portray the pathologic and angiographic findings simultaneously. Techniques and intrinsic advantages of axial cineangiography will be presented subsequently.

I. WITH DOUBLE INLET TO A LEFT VENTRICULAR CHAMBER

This is characterized by both AV valves (or a common valve) posterior to a trabecular septum (Fig. 25.2). The orientation of this trabecular septum varies according to the position of the rudimentary right ventricular chamber, its anatomic hallmark being that *the septum never extends to the crux.*

The two major positions of the rudimentary right ventricular chamber are anterosuperior on the right shoulder of the main chamber (normally related) (Fig. 25.3A and C) or anterosuperior on the left shoulder (inverted) (Fig. 25.3B and D). On occasion, however, the rudimentary chamber may be directly anterior. Irrespective of rudimentary chamber position, the main or dominant chamber is unequivocally of left ventricular pattern, and the posterior surface of the trabecular septum is characteristically smooth (Figs. 25.2C and 25.3C).

Anomalies of the valves entering this chamber are frequent, including stenosis, and overriding and/or straddling (Fig. 25.4). Rarely one valve may be imperforate, or a "parachute" deformity of the left valve may occur.[47] The rudimentary ventricular chamber possesses a trabecular component of unequivocally right ventricular pattern (Fig. 25.2B and D). It is usually hypoplastic but may attain considerable size, particularly when there is straddling and/

or overriding of an AV valve. When the papillary muscles of a valve straddle the septum it almost always does so on the same side as a rudimentary chamber (Fig. 25.4). Angiographically, this is shown best by the "four chamber" view (Fig. 25.4D). The posterior-anterior view is of no help (Fig. 25.4B).

Subpulmonary obstruction occurs within the left ventricular chamber most frequently due to posterior deviation of the infundibular septum (Fig. 25.5A). Alternatively, it may be due to anomalous attachment of the AV valves across the outflow tract or herniation of fibrous tissue tags into the subpulmonary artery. The pulmonary valve itself is often stenotic as well. The valve is usually thickened and often bicuspid.

Subaortic obstruction occurs most frequently from a restrictive type ventricular septal defect (Fig. 25.5B), and almost always is associated with coarctation of the aortic arch. There is a higher frequency of subaortic stenosis in patients with right AV valve atresia.

The *conduction tissue* disposition is grossly abnormal (Fig. 25.6).[1, 5, 21] The ventricular conduction tissues, carried on the trabecular septum, are connected to an anomalous node situated anterolaterally in the right atrioventricular orifice, irrespective of the position of the rudimentary chamber. When the chamber is *normally related*, the nonbranching bundle is inferior to the pulmonary valve annulus, or superior when viewed by the surgeon through a right atriotomy (Fig. 25.6A). The important point is that there is no relation between bundle and pulmonary valve attachment.[65]

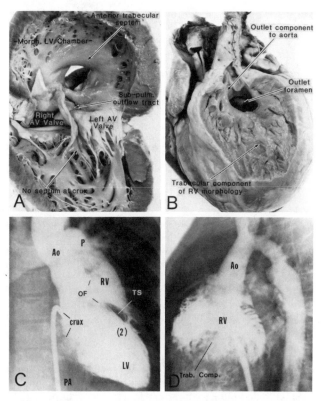

Fig. 25.2 (A) The morphology of double inlet to a left ventricular chamber. (B) With a rudimentary right ventricular chamber. (C) Posterior-anterior (*PA*) left ventriculogram. Double inlet left ventricle with an inverted rudimentary right ventricle (*RV*). There are two ventricular septal defects in the trabecular septum (*TS*). The superior outlet foramen (*OF*) defect and second muscular defect (*2*). *P*, pulmonary trunk. (D) Lateral right ventriculogram. Morphology of the rudimentary right ventricle. Note the trabeculated component (*Trab. Comp.*). *Ao*, ascending aorta.

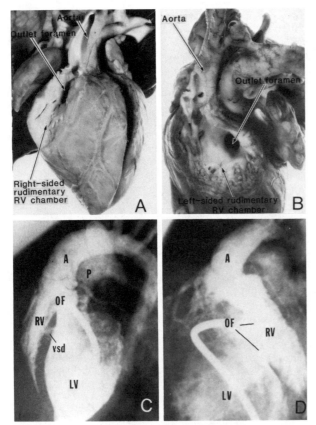

Fig. 25.3 The rudimentary right ventricular chamber is always anterior, but is usually either right-sided (normally related) (*A*) or left-sided (inverted) (*B*). Note that in each chamber there is an unequivocal trabecular component of right ventricular type. (*C*) Long axial oblique view showing the rudimentary right ventricle (*RV*) in normal position. Note the profiling of the entire trabecular septum. A second smaller ventricular septal defect (*vSD*) is shown. There is ventriculoarterial discordance (transposition). Note the characteristic smoothness of the left ventricle (*LV*). (*D*) Long axial oblique view. The rudimentary right ventricle (*RV*) is in the inverted position. Note how the trabecular septum is shown in better profile in the PA view in Figure 25.2*C*. *OF*, outlet foramen; *A*, ascending aorta; *P*, pulmonary trunk.

In contrast, when the rudimentary chamber is *inverted*, the bundle encircles the subpulmonary outflow tract, being intimately related to the pulmonary valve attachment, before reaching the trabecular septum on the crest of the outlet foramen (Fig. 25.6*B*).

In over 90% of cases of DILV, the *ventriculoarterial connections* are discordant (transposition) (Fig. 25.7*A*).[3, 15, 38, 62] Obstruction of one or other great artery is frequent.

Other ventriculoarterial connections can be found. Ventriculoarterial concordance (normal connections), although rare,[14] is found most frequently when the rudimentary chamber is normally related, the infundibulum then swinging up to a left-sided pulmonary artery in a fashion comparable to the normal heart. Subpulmonary obstruction is the rule, usually due to a restrictive ventricular septal defect, but further obstruction may be found between trabecular and infundibular components of the rudimentary chamber or at the pulmonary valve itself. Ventriculoarterial concordance can rarely occur when the rudimentary chamber is inverted (Fig. 25.2*C*); in most cases described,[26] the rudimentary chamber attained considerable size.

As in hearts with two equally dominant ventricles, a spectrum of arterial connections can exist between an artery arising entirely from one ventricle (Fig. 25.7*A*), overriding the ventricular septum approximately 50% (Fig. 25.7*B*), and double outlet connection (Fig. 25.7*C*). Angiographically, the ventriculoarterial connections are shown best by axial views.

Double outlet connection can occur either from the rudimentary right ventricular chamber or from the main left ventricular chamber (Fig. 25.7*C*). With the latter connection, the right ventricular rudimentary chamber persists simply as a trabecular pouch (Fig. 25.7*C*). *Single outlet* of the heart is found most frequently as pulmonary atresia; the solitary

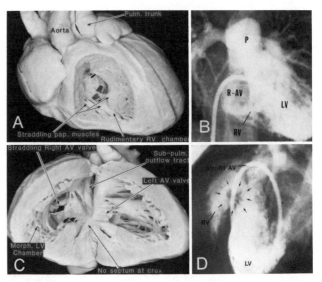

Fig. 25.4 DILV with overriding and straddling of the right atrioventricular (*RAV*) valve. (*A* and *B*) Anterior view of a specimen and left ventriculogram of another patient. In neither *A* or *B* can the true relationship of the AV valve to the septum be determined. *P*, pulmonary trunk. (*C*) Apical view showing overriding and straddling. (*D*) "Four chamber" left ventriculogram correlates well with the specimen and shows a clear view of the overriding of the right AV valve to the ventricular septum. The straddling papillary muscle was not seen. (Specimen photographed and reproduced with permission of L. H. S. Van Mierop, Gainesville, Fla.)

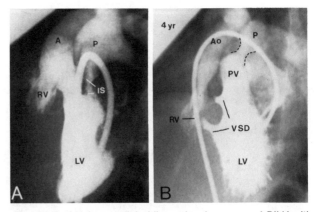

Fig. 25.5 (*A*) Long axial oblique view in a case of DILV with subpulmonary stenosis secondary to posterior deviation of the infundibular septum (*IS*) (comma shaped muscle bundle between the aortic and pulmonary valves). *A*, ascending aorta. (*B*) "Four chamber" view. There are two restrictive ventricular septal defects (*VSD*). The upper one has closed since banding of the pulmonary trunk (*P*). The lower one has become smaller. *PV*, pulmonary valve; *Ao*, ascending aorta.

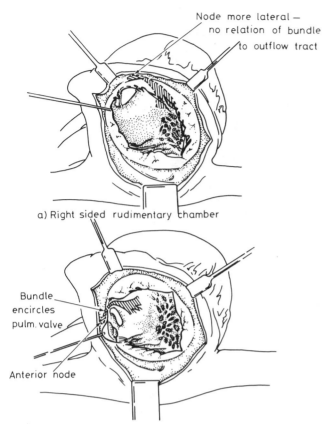

Node more lateral —
no relation of bundle
to outflow tract

a) Right sided rudimentary chamber

Bundle
encircles
pulm. valve

Anterior node

b) Left sided rudimentary chamber

Fig. 25.6 The conduction tissue disposition in hearts with double inlet to a left ventricular chamber as might be viewed by the surgeon through a right atriotomy when the rudimentary chamber is right-sided (*upper panel*) and when the rudimentary chamber is left-sided (*lower panel*).

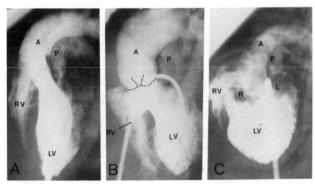

Fig. 25.7 Variations in ventriculoarterial connections in univentricular hearts. Each is a double inlet left ventricle with a normally related rudimentary right ventricle. (A) Ventriculoarterial discordance, long axial oblique view. A, ascending aorta: P, pulmonary trunk. (B) 50% overriding aortic valve; long axial oblique view. (C) Double outlet left ventricle; "four chamber" view. Note the reduced size of the pouch-like right ventricle (*RV*). Right (*R*) and left (*L*) AV valves are clearly shown.

aortic trunk arises from the rudimentary chambers, but any form can occur, including rare examples of truncus arteriosus.

The AV valves in this chapter are, by definition, of dual, common, or overriding type. To understand the total picture of the single or univentricular entity, one has to recognize the potential for atresia of the right or left AV valves as well.

Figure 25.8 shows three cases of univentricular heart. Double inlet ventricle of the left ventricular type is shown in Figure 25.8A. Note not only presence of two AV rings, but their respective size as related to the base of the ventricle. The other two cases show *single inlet* univentricular hearts: right AV valve atresia with the left AV valve entering a dominant left ventricle (Fig. 25.8B) and a case of left AV valve atresia with the right AV valve entering a dominant right ventricular chamber (Fig. 25.8C). The important point is the angiocardiographic manifestation of single inlet versus double inlet. A single inlet univentricular heart (or hypoplastic AV valve) should always be suspected when only one AV valve annulus is visualized or the AV valve occupies the majority of the base of the ventricle (Fig. 8D). This is obviously important, since the morphology of the ventricles and great arteries may be identical in those SV with and without AV valve atresia.

II. WITH DOUBLE INLET TO A RIGHT VENTRICULAR CHAMBER

In this variety, both AV valves (or a common valve) are anterior to the trabecular septum, which extends to the crux.

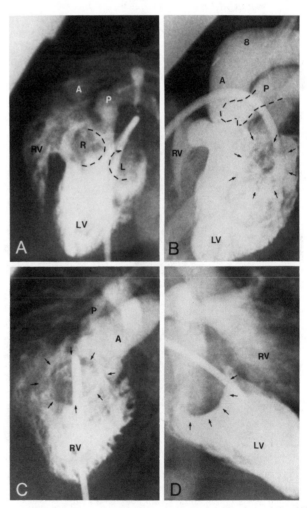

Fig. 25.8 "Four chamber" angiocardiographic view of the AV valves in univentricular hearts. (A) Two AV valves shown as circular radiolucencies. A, ascending aorta; P, pulmonary trunk. (B) Right and (C) left AV valve atresia. Note the larger circumference of the radiolucent annuli in B and C. (D) PA view. The left AV valve annulus (*arrows*) encompasses the entire base of the left ventricle. In SV, this should always suggest atresia or severe hypoplasia of the other AV valve.

(Again, as shown in Figure 25.8C, atresia of either AV valve can occur). The univentricular right ventricle shows coarser trabeculations than the univentricular left ventricle (Compare the specimens and angiograms in Figure 25.9A and B with Figure 25.2A and C).

The rudimentary left ventricular chamber is usually located in one of three positions: on the left posterior aspect of the heart, termed *normally related* (Fig. 25.9); on the anterior-inferior aspect of the heart, termed *inverted* (Fig. 25.10B); and a midline posterior position between the other two (Fig. 25.10A). The rudimentary chamber shows variations in size from a well defined hypoplastic chamber (Fig. 25.9D) to a tiny slit-like structure that may resemble a trabeculation (Fig. 25.9B) (additional views were obtained to confirm the fact that this questionable chamber in Figure 25.9B was a rudimentary left ventricle). This type of double inlet is found more frequently with right or left atrial isomerism[37, 53] than is DILV, but does occur with about equal frequency in situs solitus.

Straddling and overriding of the valves is common (Figs. 25.9C and D and 25.10B). As in DILV, it is usually found on the same side as the rudimentary chamber, which in this case is a morphologic left ventricle. The "four chamber" view depicts the straddling to best advantage in DIRV with the normally related rudimentary left ventricle, whereas a shallow right anterior oblique is the best view in the "inverted" type (Fig. 25.10B).

The ventriculoarterial connection most frequently encountered is double outlet from the main right ventricular

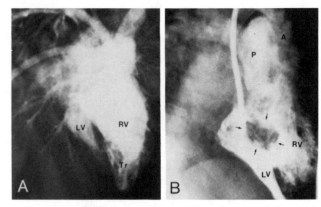

Fig. 25.10 DIRV. Two positions of the rudimentary left ventricle (*LV*). (*A*) 45° right anterior oblique (RAO) view. The left ventricle is in a posterior midline position. (*B*) 30° RAO view. The LV is in the inverted position, anterior and to the right of the dominant right ventricle (*RV*). There is overriding of the right AV valve. *Tr*, trabeculation.

chamber, usually with bilateral infundibulae (Fig. 25.9A, B, and D). The rudimentary left ventricular chamber forms a finely trabeculated pouch (Figs. 25.9 and 25.10). More rarely, there may be ventriculoarterial concordance, with the aorta arising from the rudimentary left ventricular chamber. Although we have yet to see it with DIRV, ventriculoarterial discordance (pulmonary trunk from rudimentary left ventricular chamber) must not be discounted as a possible ventriculoarterial connection. Pulmonary stenosis is the most frequent outflow tract problem, and in the severest cases the subpulmonary outflow tract may be atretic.

The *conduction tissue* disposition is dictated by the fact that the trabecular septum extends to the curx.[5] When the rudimentary chamber is normally related, the ventricular conduction tissues on the trabecular septum are connected to a regular AV node, the bundle passing posteroinferior to the interventricular communication. When the rudimentary chamber is inverted, the arrangement is comparable with corrected transposition of the great arteries, and in the only case studied histologically, there was a sling of conduction tissue between regular and anterolateral nodes.[21]

III. DOUBLE INLET TO AN INDETERMINATE VENTRICULAR CHAMBER

In our experience with hearts with double inlet to a sole ventricular chamber, the ventricle has been of neither right nor left trabecular pattern, but instead has had particularly loose apical trabeculations, often with large criss-crossing trabeculae, and much smoother walled inlet and outlet portions (Fig. 25.11). Often one trabecula is prominent, running up towards the atrial septum and giving rise to tension apparatus for both AV valves. The "four chamber" view is usually the projection of choice (Fig. 25.11B). The atrial situs is usually solitus, but isomerism is frequent. With isometric atria, there is usually a common AV valve. The only possible ventriculoarterial connections from a sole chamber are double outlet or single outlet, but there is great variability in arterial relationships. The aorta is usually anterior to the pulmonary trunk (Fig. 25.11B). When the arteries are normally related, the outflow part of the ventricle may become portioned from the sinus portion, resulting in pulmonary stenosis. If stenosis is found it is more usually owing to eccentric positioning of the infundibular septum. Because there is no septal structure present in this type of double inlet (apart from the infundibular septum), the con-

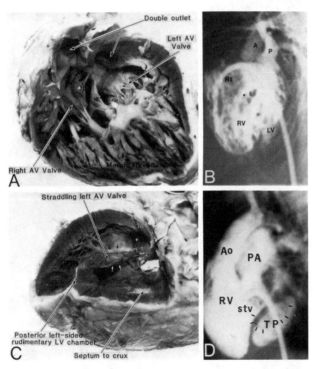

Fig. 25.9 DIRV. (*A*) Specimen and (*B*) "four chamber" right ventriculogram of another patient. Both depict the coarse trabeculations of the dominant right ventricle and double outlet from the same chamber. The rudimentary left ventricle (*LV*) is questionably seen in normal relationship of the left, posterior base of the heart. (*C*) Lateral view of specimen and (*D*) right ventriculogram. The rudimentary left ventricle is a pouch-like chamber in a normal position. Both specimen and the angio case show an overriding and straddling (*stv*) of the left AV valve. In *A*, the straddling papillary muscle is outlined by *arrows*. In *B*, it creates a filling defect into the left ventricle.

duction tissue disposition is of necessity anomalous. In some cases studied an anterolateral bundle descended directly into the parietal wall of the ventricle. In others, a bundle extended from an anterior node onto a prominent free-standing trabeculum or originated from a regular AV node.[5] In this context, we should emphasize that we have not included patients with huge ventricular septal defects. In the latter anomaly, an apical rim of septum separates right and left ventricular trabecular components. This rim ascends to the crux and carries a regular conduction system. Some have referred to this entity as common ventricle.

EMBRYOLOGY

The formation of the ventricular mass in hearts with double inlet ventricles depends on the way the ventricular trabecular components develop. In normal development the left ventricular trabecular component is formed from the inlet segment of the ventricular portion of the primary heart tube ("primitive ventricle"), while the right ventricular trabecular component is derived from the outlet segment ("bulbus," Fig. 25.12). Should the two trabecular components fail to develop, it is reasonable to presume that the ventricular mass will then form a sole unseptated chamber of indeterminate morphology, which of necessity can exist only with double inlet AV connection or with absence of one AV connection. This, then, is the mode of development of the indeterminate ventricle with double inlet (Fig. 12, *upper right*).

Usually the ventricular mass develops so that the inlet portions (AV junction) are shared between the trabecular components (Fig. 25.12, *upper left*). Failure of this normal sharing explains the other forms of double inlet, along with the different types of straddling AV valves.[9, 43, 48] If the AV junction retains its initial connection to the left ventricular trabecular zone, then there will be double inlet to the left ventricular chamber, the trabecular component of right ventricular type forming the basis of the rudimentary chamber (Fig. 25.12, *bottom left*). If the connection of the junction to the right ventricular component is exaggerated, then double inlet to a right ventricular chamber will ensue, the trabecular component of left ventricular type then forming a rudimentary ventricular chamber (Fig. 25.12, *bottom right*). The degree of connection of the AV junction then forms a series starting at double inlet to the left ventricular chamber, progressing through the normal and ending in double inlet to the right ventricular chamber. This series in the presence

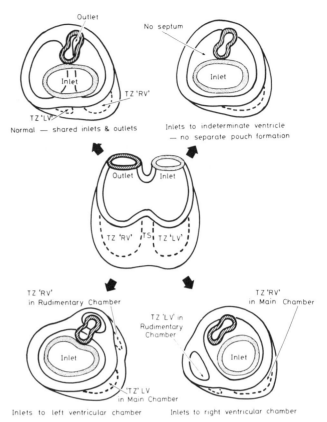

Fig. 25.12 The way in which the ventricular inlet components are usually shared between the ventricular trabecular components, with panels showing how abnormal sharing of the inlets can produce the different types of double inlet ventricle.

of right-hand ("d") ventricular looping explains the anomalies illustrated in Fig. 25.13, while the same series in presence of left-hand ("l") looping explains the anomalies in Fig. 25.14.

MANIFESTATIONS

Clinical Features

Patients presenting *without obstruction to pulmonary blood flow* demonstrate features typical of large left-to-right shunts. The most common clinical profile is a small infant, growing poorly with repeated upper respiratory infections, manifesting severe heart failure, including hyperpnea, sweating, tachycardia, and hepatomegaly. There is minimal cyanosis, a systolic thrill, and a harsh holosystolic murmur along the left sternal border. If mild to moderate pulmonic obstruction is present, the murmur will be low in frequency, more ejection in type, and located nearer the base. The systolic thrill may extend into the suprasternal notch. Without pulmonic obstruction, the second sound is single or narrowly split, and the pulmonic component is loud. A mitral type middiastolic flow murmur is heard between the lower left sternal border and the apex. Occasionally, an early diastolic murmur of pulmonic insufficiency is audible. In the presence of *mild to moderate pulmonic obstruction*, the second sound may be more clearly split with the pulmonic component of variable intensity. A mitral flow rumble will generally be present.

If severe pulmonary obstruction or *pulmonary atresia* exists, the clinical condition is dominated by that feature. While a lift may be palpated along the left sternal border,

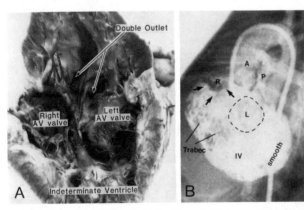

Fig. 25.11 Double inlet and double outlet from a sole ventricular chamber of indeterminate morphology. (*A*) Apical view of the specimen. (*B*) "Four chamber" view of another case depicting both AV valves, trabeculations (*Trabec.*) on the right side, and double outlet of the aorta (*A*) and pulmonary trunk (*P*). *IV*, indeterminate ventricle.

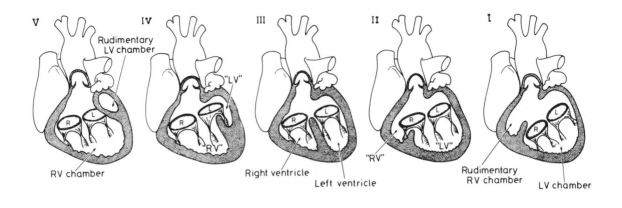

Fig. 25.13 The series of anomalies which link the different types of double inlet ventricles with the normal heart when there has been right-hand ("ᴅ") embryonic ventricular looping.

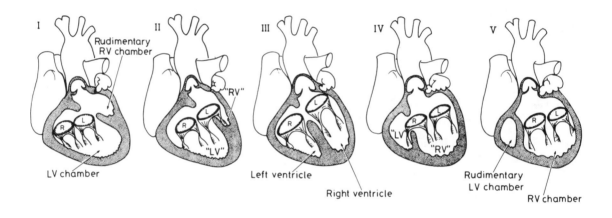

Fig. 25.14 The comparable series to that shown in Fig. 25.10 after left-hand ("ʟ") embryonic looping.

there is no precordial or suprasternal notch thrill, and no significant systolic murmur is heard. The second sound is single, and there is no mitral flow murmur. A continuous murmur of ductal flow may be appreciated. In those patients who develop severe *pulmonary arteriolar obstruction*, the second sound is single, but quite loud, and the early decrescendo diastolic murmur of pulmonic insufficiency is present.

Electrovectorcardiographic Features

The electrovectorcardiographic features of single ventricle in the past have been obscured by lumping together the various forms of this condition. In recent years, however, some orderliness has become apparent, and not surprisingly, characteristic electrovectorcardiographic features are now being recognized.[19, 29, 30] The most clearly understood form is DILV since it is the most common. Double inlet left ventricles with inverted or normally related rudimentary right ventricle have characteristic patterns which are of considerable assistance in making the clinical diagnosis.[29]

Electrical depolarization proceeds first through the central portion of the left side of the ventricular septum. The spread of excitation then follows in a left to right direction. As a

result, the initial qRs forces are directed anteriorly and leftward in the heart with a normally related rudimentary right ventricle (Fig. 25.15A). In ventricular inversion, the initial qRs forces are directed leftward and posteriorly (Fig. 25.15B).[63] The remainder of the qRs forces reflect the pattern of ventricular hypertrophy.

The electrocardiogram and vectorcardiogram in DILV with *normally related* rudimentary right ventricle show features characteristic of severe left ventricular hypertrophy (Fig. 25.15A).[29] The initial qRs forces are shifted slightly to the left and are directed straight anteriorly and usually inferiorly, resulting in the absence of a precordial Q wave. The major qRs forces are oriented leftward, posteriorly, and inferiorly, resulting in a pattern of left ventricular hypertrophy exemplified in Figure 25.15A. Superior qRs orientation will occur if a common AV valve is also present. Right ventricular hypertrophy is not seen. The horizontal qRs vectorcardiographic loop is directed counterclockwise and is located leftward and posteriorly. The frontal qRs vector loop is usually clockwise and directed leftward and inferiorly.

In DILV with an *inverted* rudimentary right ventricle, the initial qRs forces are directed leftward, posterior and superiorly, as they are in ventricular inversion without associated defects, that is, they are relatively normal for that heart. Since the single left ventricle is no located anteriorly and rightward the major qRs forces are so directed. The result is a qR pattern in right precordial leads and an Rs pattern in the left precordial leads (Fig. 25.15B). Note also that the T wave is generally upright in the right precordium. Q waves are usually seen in standard leads III and AVF. The QRS loop is directed clockwise in both the horizontal and frontal planes. The major portion of the qRs loop is located rightward, anteriorly and inferiorly. Thus the pattern seen in ventricular inversion with DILV is characteristic of right-sided ventricular hypertrophy for that type heart. Furthermore, varying forms of conduction disturbance, including *heart block* are not uncommon in the presence of ventricular inversion. One interesting finding characteristic for both forms of DILV is the direction of the initial qRs forces. They rarely course in an anterior-rightward direction as viewed in the horizontal plane. In other words, normal Q waves confined to the left precordial leads is a rare finding in both forms of DILV. From the opposite point of view, normal Q waves in the left precordial leads strongly imply *two ventricles which are normally related*.[20]

There are so few cases of indeterminate ventricle and double inlet right ventricle with clinical data that prevailing electrocardiographic patterns have not been established.

Echocardiographic Features

The experience at the University of Alabama and the Brompton Hospital of London[49] shows that the distinction between the various classifications is readily made using 2D echocardiography. Posterior chambers in univentricular

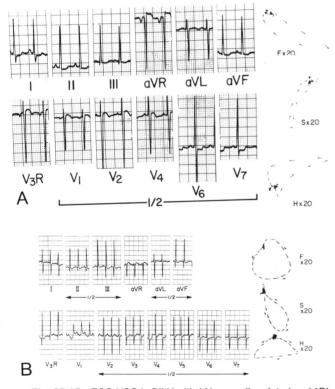

A

B

Fig. 25.15 ECG-VCG in DILV with (*A*) normally related and (*B*) inverted rudimentary right ventricle. Electrocardiograms in both cases recorded at 1 mv = 10 mm except where indicated "½" where 1 mv = 5 mm. Vectorcardiograms are Grisham cube method. The degree of magnification is indicated. (Reproduced with permission from I. H. Gessner *et al.*[29])

hearts of right ventricular type are the most easily seen. Anterior chambers in hearts of left ventricular trabecular pattern are also readily identified in the majority of cases, although a painstaking search using multiple echocardiographic planes is sometimes required.

The unequivocal demonstration of a rudimentary second chamber, and in particular, identifying its position can be difficult. In some, the second chamber can be seen only in one echocardiographic plane, and therefore a detailed systematic approach using each tomographic plane is essential. The apical and subcostal views are the most useful in identifying a rudimentary ventricle. However, it is important to obtain an image with the ultrasonic plane both at right angles to and parallel to the interatrial septum, or in similar positions when there is no septum.[49] In single ventricle (SV) of right ventricular morphology, posterior left ventricular rudimentary chambers are almost always to the left or directly posterior and can therefore be identified when the echocardiographic plane is at right angles to the interatrial septum in the classical apical and subcostal views. In SV of left ventricular morphology, a similar view will allow the identification of a right-sided anterior right ventricular rudimentary chamber. To demonstrate a left-sided rudimentary chamber in SV of the right ventricular type, the echocardiographic plane should be approximately parallel to the interatrial septum.

When a seond rudimentary ventricular chamber is seen on a short axis view at or just below the level of the AV valves, its position relative to the main chamber is easily defined.[49] Unfortunately, in infants an anterior chamber is frequently not identified when this view is used to examine SV of left ventricular morphology. Failure to demonstrate an anterior chamber in small infants in some echocardiographic planes reflects the resolution of the instrument used. When it is impossible by either angiography or echocardiography to define a second chamber within the ventricular mass, then it is most likely that the ventricular morphology is of indeterminate type. Both echocardiography and angiography may fail to demonstrate a small second chamber which may subsequently be found at autopsy. In such cases, from a clinical standpoint, hearts of left or right ventricular type effectively exist without a rudimentary chamber. Nonetheless, with a 5-megahertz transducer the modern ultrasonoscope will allow the delineation of exceedingly hypoplastic chambers, as lateral resolution 2 to 3 mm should be possible.[49]

Confusion can arise in diagnosis when, in some instances, thickened chordae are seen in the main chamber. They can be mistaken for an interventricular septum, unless their attachment to the AV valve leaflets is positively identified.

In hearts with a common AV valve we consider SV to exist when there is malalignment between the atrial septum and the trabecular septum. In the presence of a common atrium more than 75% of the AV valve should be committed to the main ventricular chamber. In the majority of hearts 2D echocardiography unequivocally demonstrates the type and mode of AV connection far more consistently than conventional selective angiography and is slightly superior to axial cineangiography. It is the most reliable method of distinguishing overriding from straddling valves. In the former, although the AV valve is related to both the main and rudimentary chambers, all the tensor apparatus arises from the main chamber, and the leaflets are seen within it during diastole. In contrast, straddling valves have their tensor apparatus attached in both main and rudimentary chambers, and one leaflet is sometimes, but not invariably, seen within the outlet chamber or trabecular pouch when the valve is open.

Radiologic Features

The first step in film analysis in a patient suspected of single or univentricular heart[18] is to determine whether or not the roentgenogram indicates an alteration in the position of the great arteries. This is because the vast majority of patients with SV show abnormal ventriculoarterial connections and relationships.

Signs of Transposition of the Great Arteries. Information regarding the position of the great arteries resides primarily in an analysis of the *mediastinum*. In the patient with normally related great arteries, the superior mediastinum often shows a *"triad of densities."*[13, 20, 57] In the posterior-anterior (PA) view, this includes: the *ascending aorta*; the *transverse arch* and *descending aorta* continuum; and the *pulmonary trunk*.

The Pulmonary Trunk in Single Ventricle. Among all forms of complex heart disease, especially SV, the most important great artery from an x-ray point of view is the *pulmonary trunk*. In SV with transposition of the great arteries, the posterior, midcardiac origin of the pulmonary trunk prohibits it from being a border-forming structure adjacent to the lung (Fig. 25.16*A*). Therefore, the premier x-ray sign is absence of a distinct pulmonary trunk on the PA chest film (Fig. 25.16).[13, 20, 57] This sign by itself is of relative value, but its significance depends on the *clinical* situation and the *age* of the patient. In an infant with thymic tissue covering the great arteries, it is worthless; however, in a cyanotic patient without thymic tissue, regardless of age, and especially with *shunt vascularity*, absence of a pulmonary trunk assumes added significance when correlated with the position of the thoracic aorta. DILV with a normally related rudimentary right ventricle and normally connected and related great arteries is the one instance in which SV can present with a normal pulmonary trunk and thoracic aorta.

The Thoracic Aorta in Transposition of the Great Arteries. There are three basic configurations of the ascending aorta in transposition of the great arteries: convex to the right; midline course or convexity to neither side; and convex to the left. There is a prevailing tendency for the truncus to divide so that the convexity of the ascending aorta is toward the side of the morphologic right ventricle, regardless of its size. In patients with SV of the left ventricular type and a normally related rudimentary RV, the aorta tends to be convex to the right. This of course also results in a visable left-sided transverse aortic arch as well.

In SV of the LV type with the rudimentary right ventricle in the inverted position, the ascending aorta usually shows varying degrees of convexity to the left. When this occurs in SV, the pulmonary trunk, normal right-sided ascending aorta, and left-sided transverse arch are absent. The ascending aorta produces a relatively straight (Fig. 25.16*B*) or overtly convex density in the left superior mediastinum (Fig. 25.16*C*), supplanting the familiar pulmonary trunk and thoracic aorta densities.

The Left Heart Border in Patients with SV and Inversion. In SV of the LV type with an inverted rudimentary right ventricle, the right ventricle forms the upper one-half to one-third of the left cardiac border. Therefore, the rudimentary right ventricle creates a localized bulge confined to the upper one-half of the left heart border (Fig. 25.16*B* and *C*). The notch in the left heart border represents the site of insertion of the trabecular septum into the lateral wall (Fig. 25.2*C*).

Pulmonary Vascularity. Once the great arteries have been evaluated, determination of the pulmonary flow is next. In the *absence* of pulmonary stenosis, there are usually signs of overcirculation (shunt) or a mixed pattern of shunt and

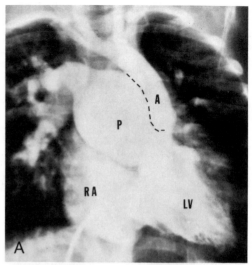

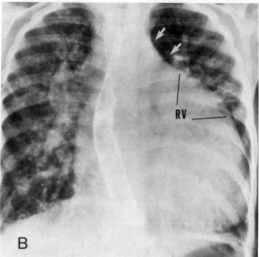

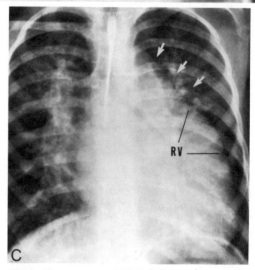

Fig. 25.16 Three cases of DILV. (*A*) Anterior-posterior seriographic film showing marked dilatation of the pulmonary trunk (*P*) to such a degree that it lifts the dilated right pulmonary artery and creates a "water-fall" hilum. *A*, ascending aorta; *RA*, right atrium. (*B*) PA chest film. The pulmonary trunk and transverse aortic arch shadows are absent. The ascending aorta (*arrows*) forms the upper left mediastinal shadow and the inverted rudimentary right ventricle (*RV*) a bulge below this. (*C*) PA chest film, companion to angiogram in (*A*). The ascending aorta is convex to the left (*arrows*) along with the classic bulge of the inverted right ventricle (RV).

venous congestion. Double inlet left ventricle shows a higher frequency of shunt vascularity than do DIRV and indeterminate ventricle. The latter two show a higher frequency of pulmonary and subpulmonary stenosis or atresia which is reflected as normal, diminished, or systemic collateral pulmonary vascularity. It becomes obvious that SV has many variations in presentation. In SV with shunt vascularity, there is almost invariably mild to moderate cardiomegaly, regardless of age. As a result of increased pulmonary flow, the *left atrium* is usually enlarged (Fig. 25.16C).

In cases with a *moderate degree of pulmonary stenosis*, the pulmonary vacularity may be within normal limits or slightly diminished. The heart size is normal or only mildly enlarged. Only in cases of severe stenosis is there *decreased* pulmonary vascularity. Single ventricle with decreased vascularity may mimic tetralogy of Fallot and other lesions with pulmonary stenosis. Only in cases of SV with inversion may the diagnosis be specific by showing a bulge created by the rudimentary right ventricle along the upper left heart border.

In cases with *pulmonary valve atresia*, the pulmonary vasculature usually shows systemic collateral flow. The heart size is varied. These patients are indistinguishable from tetralogy of Fallot with pulmonary atresia. The characteristic feature of systemic collateral vascularity is that the vessels appear prominent in a disorganized manner. The pathognomonic sign is absence of a normally formed right and left pulmonary artery in the lateral view.

Additional Signs Caused by the Dilated Pulmonary Trunk. In all forms of univentricular heart without obstruction to pulmonary flow, the pulmonary trunk may become exceedingly dilated (Fig. 25.16A). This dilatation causes deviation, unusual densities, or displacement of certain structures, namely the right and left pulmonary arteries and the superior vena cava. The dilated pulmonary artery is lifted superiorly. This together with the dilated branch arteries causes a "waterfall" appearance (Fig. 25.16).[18] This is not unique for SV but may occur uncommonly in other admixture lesions with a large ventricular septal defect and high pulmonary flow. The *left pulmonary artery* may cause an indentation on the left side of the esophagus at or just below the level of the carina. This finding is produced by the enlarged pulmonary trunk and/or main pulmonary arteries.

The right lateral wall of the dilated pulmonary trunk may displace the superior vena cava to the right. This results in a widened mediastinum to the right. Also, the right wall may project to the right side of the spine and create a pseudo-descending aorta, mimicking a right arch on plain film.

The *aortic arch* is left-sided in the majority of patients with SV. There is however, a tendency for *right aortic arch* in cases of *indeterminate ventricle. Malpositions of the heart* are unusual in SV unless there is an added complication, such as atresia or hypoplasia of the right AV valve or right or left atrial isomerism (asplenia or polysplenia).

CARDIAC CATHETERIZATION

Single ventricles belong in the category of cyanotic malformations, termed *admixture* lesions. By this we mean those conditions in which the nature of the malformation is responsible for mixing of venous and arterial blood within the heart and great arteries. The physiology is not affected by the position of the rudimentary chambers nor by whether one is dealing with a DILV, DIRV, or indeterminate ventricle. Similarly, a common AV valve, if competent, will not manifest itself hemodynamically. Neither are great vessel interrelationships a factor in the fundamental physiology in patients. Thus, all of these varied anatomic situations can be discussed as a group. A major determinant of the hemo-dynamic presentation is the presence and degree of obstruction to pulmonary blood flow. In the absence of pulmonary obstruction, cyanosis is mild or absent. The hematocrit is minimally elevated, and the aortic oxygen saturation is in the range of 80 to 93%. All of this is consistent with high pulmonary blood flow. Although measurement of aortic and pulmonary blood flow is difficult in admixture lesions, pulmonary to systemic flow ratios are in the range of 2.5:1 or more, unless the patient has developed pulmonary arteriolar disease. With obstruction to pulmonary blood flow, cyanosis deepens, and the pulmonary to systemic flow ratio becomes smaller.

Systolic pressure measurements in the ventricle and great arteries will be similar, unless one is dealing with either subpulmonic (Fig. 25.5B) or aortic obstruction, which will have the obvious effect of lowering pressure distal to the obstruction. Determination of the presence of two AV valves is important. At catheterization, this is accomplished by a combination of 2D ultrasound and cineangiography in axial views. Although the atrial septum may be patent, shunting in either direction at the atrial level should be detectable. In addition, left atrial pressure should be higher than right atrial pressures.

If **pulmonary obstruction** is present, systemic arterial saturation will be reduced proportionate to the degree of obstruction. Left atrial pressure may also be reduced. The presence of additional defects such as AV valve insufficiency, patent ductus arteriosus, coarctation of the aorta, etc., may affect the hemodynamics; however, discussion of these is beyond the scope of this chapter. Entrance into the pulmonary artery should be attempted at catheterization in all cases, but may be quite difficult. Use of guided catheters and the baloon-tipped flow-directed catheters has greatly increased the ability to obtain this information.

ANGIOCARDIOGRAPHY

The procedures of choice to delineate the anatomic abnormalities in all forms of SV and to make sound judgements regarding operability are 2D ultrasound followed by biplane cineangiography.

Because of the advancements in cardiovascular surgical techniques, it is simply no longer tenable to make a generalized diagnosis of SV of one type or another from routine angiography. It is now necessary to establish a "surgical diagnosis," which by definition is one that demands more accuracy and refinement than that offered by conventional angiography. This accuracy and refinement can only be achieved with biplane cineangiography systems.[4, 16, 17, 24]

The development of a filming system that is capable of such a consistent and accurate diagnosis requires an organized and knowledgeable approach to the intricacies of cineangiography. Our approach encompasses two major areas: precise and consistent techniques in film exposure and development and the development of projection techniques that place the pathologic lesion at right angle to the x-ray beam. The term that best describes these projection techniques is "axial" or angled cineangiography.[4, 16, 17, 24]

Space does not permit a detailed discussion of these techniques etc., but the principles and techniques of positioning will be reviewed briefly.

PRINCIPLES OF AXIAL CINEANGIOGRAPHY

The first principle of axial cineangiography is axial alignment of the heart, which is defined as placing the long axis of the heart perpendicular to an x-ray beam. The equipment configuration and size of the patient will determine which x-ray tube is utilized.[4]

The second principle involves rotation of the heart (in reality, the patient) on this long axis so as to place in profile those pathologic areas inside the heart that are of particular importance.

Axial alignment of the heart and rotation of the long axis can be accomplished angiographically by any one of three imaging techniques: rotation and movement of the patient in relationship to fixed anteroposterior and lateral tubes; movement of both equipment and patient; and movement of the equipment alone.[4, 16]

"Four Chamber" View

Since the posterior septum separates the two atrioventricular valves, and since the atrial septum is in roughly the same plane as the posterior ventricular septum, this view not only demonstrates well the posterior septum and the defects located in this region, but also clearly demonstrates the relationship of the AV valves to one another and to the septum. In SV, the inlet septum is absent by definition, but the "four chamber" view is superb in demonstrating the position of the AV valves and their relationship to the trabecular septum. The atria are also well separated from the ventricles and from one another in this view. Consequently, the four chambers resemble the leaves of a four-leaf clover, hence the term "four chamber" view. In infants and young children, this projection is obtained by elevating the patient's thorax at a 35 to 45° angle to the table, elevating the left shoulder 35 to 45°, and using the vertical x-ray tube.[16] In older children and adults, the patient is rotated into a left anterior oblique position of about 20 to 25°, and the image intensifier (C or Z arm) is moved 20 to 25° leftward and is tilted 30 to 40° cranially.[16] This view is uncommonly necessary in adults.

Long Axial Oblique View

In infants and most children, this is readily accomplished by positioning the patient obliquely 30° on the table (principle 1), raising the right shoulder 15 to 20°, and using the lateral x-ray tube as the primary diagnostic unit (principle 2). When the long axial oblique view is compared with the "four chamber" view, a left anterior oblique view of the ventricular septum that is 20 to 30° steeper is obtained with the long axial oblique projection. This results in the trabecular ventricular septum, rather than the inlet ventricular septum (as in the "four chamber" view), being viewed in profile (Figs. 25.3C and 25.4D).

In the patient with two normally related ventricles, the left ventricular outflow tract and the region of the subaortic valve are emphasized. The free edge of the anterior leaflet of the mitral valve is also seen in profile. The primary reason that this area is so well demonstrated is because the left outer shoulder of the left ventricle has been displaced inferiorly and no longer overlies the outflow area as in the conventional left anterior oblique view; the latter is a *worthless* view.

In patients with SV heart with the rudimentary right ventricle in the normal position, the long axial oblique is the superior one in profiling the outlet foramen in the subaortic region, as well as depicting additional muscular defects (Figs. 25.3C, 25.5A, and 25.7A). A conventional left anterior oblique view would result in a foreshortening of the septum, and the two defects would probably superimpose one on the other. In patients with the rudimentary right ventricle in the inverted position, the long axial oblique view does not profile the ventricular septum.

Ironically, axial cineangiography has not made as large a contribution to the diagnosis of single or univentricular heart

as it has to malformations superimposed on conditions with two equally dominant ventricles. It has, however, been critical in determining certain associated findings that are fundamental to the planning of a successful operation. These findings include: the number, size, and position of the AV valves (Figs. 25.4D, 25.8 and 25.9D); the size and number of defects between the dominant ventricle and often associated rudimentary one (Figs. 25.3C, 25.5B and 25.7A and B); the location of the common associated rudimentary ventricle (Figs. 25.3C, 25.4D, 25.7 and 25.8A and C); the type and degree of pulmonary stenosis (Figs. 25.5A and 25.11B); the precise origins of the great arteries (Fig. 25.7); and the relationship of the flow from the venous and arterial atria to the great arteries.

Ideally, a 2D echocardiogram should be performed prior to the catheterization. As mentioned previously, the absence of an inlet septum, the position of the rudimentary chamber, and presence or absence of two AV valves and their position in relation to the septum is usually well defined. This study can be performed in an office setting or immediately prior to the catheterization in the laboratory itself. In the latter site, the infant is much more cooperative owing to sedation.

The following cineangiographic views are recommended for the following types of SV heart, based upon an electrocardiographic chest film and 2D ultrasound profile. The advocated positions depend primarily on the position of the rudimentary chamber. The suggested views for angiography when the rudimentary chamber is in doubt will also be discussed.

DILV with Normally Related Rudimentary Right Ventricle. The initial angiogram should be a "four chamber" view in virtually all forms of SV, regardless of the position of the rudimentary chamber. This is for two reasons: all the information may be derived from this view along with its companion 45° right anterior oblique view (provided a biplane cine system is utilized); and more importantly, the x-ray beam passes through the greatest amount of liver tissue in this view. In other words, if another projection has been performed prior to the "four chamber" one, the contrast material from the initial injection remaining in the circulating blood pool and recirculating through the liver offers an added barrier to the x-ray beam. This barrier in effect increases the kilovoltage, which in turn degrades the cine image.

The "four chamber" view is the superior one in depicting the position of the AV valves (Figs. 25.4D and 25.8A to C). The ventriculoarterial connections are usually well defined, but this view may create a pseudooverriding of whichever artery arises from the rudimentary chamber. Moreover, the ventricular septum and infundibular septum are not as well profiled in this view as the long axial oblique (Figs. 25.3C and 25.5). Therefore, for precise analysis of the ventricular septum, infundibular septum (hence the region below the great artery arising from the dominant ventricle), and the ventriculoarterial connections, a long axial oblique projection is also recommended.

DILV with Inverted Rudimentary Right Ventricle. Ironically, this is one of the few entities for which the conventional frontal and lateral views remain as accurate as the axial ones in analyzing the ventricular septum (Fig. 25.2C). This is because of the leftward, semihorizontal position of the ventricular septum. The septum is profiled, and the size and number of ventricular septal defects are accurately visualized (Fig. 25.2C). The subarterial region in the dominant left ventricle is well defined. The "four chamber" view, however, remains the best for depicting the size, number, and position of the AV valves and should be the initial view.

DIRV with Posterior Leftward Rudimentary Left Ventricle (Normally Related). The "four chamber" view should be the initial cine projection. A long axial oblique view is also recommended. The rudimentary left ventricle together with an overriding AV valve will be less likely to be missed if both projections are performed (Fig. 25.9*B* and *D*). The rudimentary left ventricle is often shown on the companion 30° right anterior oblique view (Fig. 25.10*A*).

DIRV with Anterior Rightward Rudimentary Left Ventricle (Inverted Relationships). In this rare entity, the long axial oblique is the view of choice; however, it is the 30° right anterior oblique companion view from which most of the data are derived (Fig. 25.10*B*). The right anterior oblique view (Fig. 25.10*B*) shows the inverted rudimentary left ventricle together with an overriding right AV valve. Again, no one view is the only one and at least one other ventriculogram should be performed. Whether it is a posterior-anterior and lateral combination or a "four chamber" view and its companion 45° right anterior oblique is dependent upon what is determined from the video disc replay following the initial injection. This is one situation a four chamber view may be omitted or performed as the second or third injection.

Single Ventricle Heart without Demonstration of a Rudimentary Chamber by 2D Echocardiogram. The diagnostic possibilities here are several. This may be a SV of the indeterminate type or of left or right ventricular type in which the rudimentary chamber was not visualized by ultrasonography. The *initial* injection should be a "four chamber" ventriculogram for the reasons mentioned. Careful study of the videotape replay in both planes may define the rudimentary chamber. If not, a conventional posterior-anterior and lateral combination of views should be performed. If the rudimentary chamber and AV valve relationships are not clear-cut from these two injections, a long axial oblique should be contemplated if the renal and clinical status allow.

These multiple (up to three) ventriculograms result in a *radiographic sectioning* of the heart at 30° angles. Such sectioning may be the only way to distinguish between a SV of the indeterminate type and one of the right ventricular type in which the rudimentary left ventricle is faintly opacified or minuscule in size (Fig. 25.9*B*).

DIFFERENTIAL DIAGNOSIS

The SV or univentricular heart is the great mimicker of more common lesions, such as large left-to-right shunts in failure such as VSD, corrected transposition of the great arteries with a VSD, AV canal etc., and the admixture lesions, such as complete transposition of the great arteries, truncus arteriosus, double outlet right ventricle, etc. Lesions with *pulmonic obstruction* of varying degrees, including pulmonary atresia, tetralogy of Fallot, double outlet right ventricle, transposition of the great arteries, etc. may show many similar features. The 2D echocardiogram has made the other more conventional noninvasive tests nearly obsolete in terms of accurately assessing intracardiac anatomy. There is, however, a chest film-electrovectorcardiographic profile that is quite useful in the diagnosis of SV. In other words, regardless of the type of blood flow, position of the great arteries, number of AV valves etc., there is a nearly consistent profile presented by most SV hearts.

Chest Film and Electrocardiographic Profile

On the posterior-anterior chest film signs of alteration of the great arteries is almost invariably present. The most consistent sign is absence of a pulmonary trunk. The classic leftward ascending aorta and bulge of the upper left ventricular border is the most specific finding (Fig. 25.16).† Electrocardiographically, there is almost always an absence of normally formed Q waves in the left precordial leads or Q waves isolated to the right precordial leads (Fig. 25.15).

From another point of view, the presence of a pulmonary trunk on a chest film strongly implies that the great arteries are normally related, a rare finding in SV hearts of all types. Likewise, normal left precordial Q waves and/or a normal Q loop in the horizontal plane of the vectorcardiogram strongly imply the presence of two ventricles that are normally related.

TREATMENT

In 1956, Kirklin performed a septation operation in a 12-year-old boy with SV.[41] Despite this early success, subsequent attempts at surgical correction have been accompanied by a high operative mortality and uncertain long-term results. Moreover, palliative operations have not provided good long-term functional results.

PALLIATIVE OPERATIONS

Pulmonary Artery Banding. Banding of the main pulmonary artery in patients with SV without pulmonary stenosis has been recommended for patients with symptoms of heart failure and cardiomegaly when medical therapy has been ineffective. Mortality rates have generally ranged from 25 to 50%.[10, 32, 33, 45] The late results have not been well studied, but serious concern exists over possible late outlet chamber obstruction as well as progressive ventricular hypertrophy after pulmonary artery banding. Somerville[52] and Freedom[27] reported six cases of acquired subaortic stenosis in the rudimentary right ventricle after pulmonary artery banding. The morphologic result is severe hypertrophy of the ventricle with marked decrease in cavity size, decreased ventricular compliance, and marked narrowing of the outlet foramen with proliferation of fibrous tissue at its orifice (Fig. 25.5*B*).

Systemic-to-Pulmonary Artery Shunt. Systemic-to-pulmonary artery shunt procedures have been recommended when severe or progressive cyanosis occurs, usually associated with pulmonary stenosis, either congenital or acquired, secondary to previous pulmonary artery banding. Most commonly, a Blalock-Taussig operation is performed. Mortality is quite variable, but should be less than 20%. The long-term results are generally less good than for shunting procedures in tetralogy of Fallot.[55, 58] Taussig reported the long-term follow-up on 18 patients who survived systemic-to-pulmonary artery shunt procedures for SV performed between 1945 and 1951.[55] Only six of these 18 patients (33%) survived 25 years after operation, and four of the six required procedures to augment pulmonary blood flow. Thus, palliative operations have not provided optimal long-term results.

Fontan Operation. The concept of utilizing a direct right atrium-to-pulmonary artery connection as the source of pulmonary blood flow has been well studied experimentally,[34, 50, 64] and extensive experience with this operation has been accumulated in patients with tricuspid atresia.[6, 7, 25] The largest published experience in the treatment of SV

---

† One entity which may mimic the classic chest film of SV with the inverted rudimentary right ventricle is the anomaly of juxtaposition of the atrial appendages, an anomaly that is often associated with SV of the single inlet left ventricle, normally related rudimentary right ventricle, transposition of the great arteries, and right AV valve atresia.

with the Fontan operation is from the Mayo Clinic.[16] From 1974 to 1979, 14 patients aged 5 to 23 years underwent a Fontan operation for univentricular heart. Seven patients had DILV with an inverted rudimentary right ventricular chamber (no deaths), four patients had other subsets of DILV (two deaths), and three patients had indeterminate ventricle (two deaths). When compared to all other anatomic types, patients with SV of the inverted type had a lower operative mortality (0/7 versus 4/7).[28] Yacoub has reported on nine patients with SV and pulmonary stenosis with four hospital deaths (44%).[66] The usual mode of death in both series was low cardiac output. The intermediate-term results (2 to 17 months) from the Mayo Clinic indicate a good functional result (asymptomatic) in 50% of hospital survivors (5/10), a fair result (mild symptoms with medications) in 40% (4/10), and a poor result (persistent heart failure) in 10% (1/10).[28] All five hospital survivors in Yacoub's group had a good functional result up to 18 months after operation.[66] No late deaths occurred during the period of follow-up in either series.

Factors associated with a favorable outcome after the Fontan operation are difficult to isolate. Ideal candidates should have normal ventricular function, normal pulmonary vascular resistance,[2] and a mean pulmonary artery pressure less than 20 mm Hg. Considerable controversy exists over the need to insert a valve when doing the Fontan operation. Sufficient information is not yet available for a secure recommendation. Thus, the intermediate-term results in properly selected patients are usually satisfactory. Many patients, however, with SV have elevation of pulmonary vascular resistance by the time operation is undertaken[23]; the results of the Fontan operation in this subset would be compromised.

Septation Operation. The septation operation consists of separating the univentricular heart into two distinct pumping chambers utilizing a Dacron patch for the interventricular septum. Although first successfully performed in 1956,[41] the septation operation continues to have a mortality of nearly 50%.[11, 23, 41, 42] Analysis of results from the Mayo Clinic and the University of Alabama in Birmingham (UAB) suggests that good long-term results may be expected with certain subsets of single ventricle. Other subsets, however, have a poor outcome after septation.

McGoon and colleagues[41] have reported their experience with the septation operation between 1973 and 1977, and the mortality was 43% (13/30). McKay and colleagues have reported a mortality of 44% (8/18).[42] The usual mode of death was acute cardiac failure.

Of the various **anatomic subsets**, the largest experience is among patients with DILV and an inverted rudimentary right ventricle. At UAB, the mortality among this group is 44% (7/16), but no late deaths have occurred among hospital survivors.[42] The Mayo Clinic reported an unsatisfactory result in 42% (8/19) of patients with DILV and inversion of the rudimentary right ventricle versus 82% (9/11) with other anatomic types.[41] Only isolated case reports are available concerning surgical treatment in other anatomic subsets of SV.[12, 25, 26, 51]

The presence of **pulmonary outflow obstruction**, either congenital or acquired through pulmonary artery banding, may increase the risk of septation. Previous pulmonary artery banding has been associated with an increased early mortality after septation in the combined Mayo Clinic and UAB experience. As noted by Freedom et al.[27] and Somerville et al.,[52] pulmonary artery banding may promote ventricular hypertrophy and outlet foramen obstruction (subaortic stenosis in patients with transposition of the great arteries), both of which are deleterious to later septation

(Fig. 25.5B). The effect of congenital pulmonary outflow obstruction is less certain. The Mayo Clinic results suggest a favorable effect of congenital pulmonary outflow obstruction (9/16 with pulmonary stenosis versus 4/14 without pulmonary stenosis had a satisfactory late result).[1] At UAB, the presence of pulmonary stenosis and the use of valved external conduit were related to the development of low cardiac output postoperatively and subsequent hospital death.[42]

The presence of **subaortic stenosis** results in the most significant incremental risk.[42] **Ventricular size** was the second significant incremental risk factor in the same analysis: the smaller the ventricle the greater the risk.[42] Thus, the mortality was 18% (2/11) if the dominant ventricle was large and without obstruction of the outlet foramen, versus 100% (5/5) if the ventricle was small and the outlet foramen was narrowed.

Although optimal criteria for septation have generally included the presence of two normal AV valves, sufficient information is unavailable at present to clearly define the role of septation in this subset. No incremental risk has been demonstrated in the UAB or Mayo Clinic experience with AV valve repair or replacement.[23, 42]

No definite relationship between **age at operation** and mortality has been demonstrated; however, all patients in the UAB experience under 5 years of age or over 23 years of age at operation died, and all patients between these ages survived.[42]

Preoperative condition of the patient is a significant determinant of survival in both the UAB[42] and Mayo Clinic experience.[41] At UAB, the hospital mortality was 0% (0/2) among patients in NYHA Class I, 33% (2/6) in Class II, 50% (2/4) in Class III, and 75% (3/4) in Class IV.

Heart block and the need for permanent pacing has been common after operation, even with intraoperative mapping of the conduction system.[41] No relationship exists, however, between the need for a permanent pacemaker and early or late mortality.[23, 42]

Limited information is available on the *long-term results* of patients after septation operation, but recent information gathered on the intermediate term fate of patients at UAB is encouraging. Among nine survivors of the septation operation, no late deaths have occurred, and all patients are in New York Heart Association Functional Class I. Later postoperative exercise testing has demonstrated a near normal exercise tolerance.[42]

A comparison of available intermediate-term results of hospital survivors following the Fontan operation (Mayo Clinic experience)[28] and the septation operation (UAB experience)[42] for SV indicates that patients after septation are more likely to be in NYHA Class I and free of digitalis and diuretics. All patients (9/9) were in NYHA Class I after septation versus 50% (5/10) after the Fontan procedure. Only 11% (1/11) of patients continued to take digitalis and/or diuretics after septation versus 100% (10/10) after the Fontan procedure.[42]

RECOMMENDATIONS FOR THERAPY

Although the experience with the surgical treatment of SV remains limited, we believe there is sufficient experience to make the following recommendations. The septation operation should be recommended for patients with DILV with inversion of the rudimentary right ventricle with a large nonobstructive outlet foramen or ventricular septal defect. The ventricle should be enlarged and the AV valves normal. In the presence of pulmonary stenosis or previous pulmonary artery banding, a systemic-to-pulmonary artery shunt should be performed and operation delayed until ventricular dilatation has occurred. Optimal age for repair is approximately 5 to 15 years of age.

With other anatomic subsets, or in the presence of outlet foramen obstruction of a small hypertrophied ventricle, a modified Fontan operation is advisable as long as the mean pulmonary artery pressure is less than 20 mm Hg, the pulmonary vascular resistance is less than 5 units/m^2, and

the ventricular end diastolic pressure is normal. Patients younger than 3 to 5 years who have symptoms owing to cyanosis should have an initial systemic-to-pulmonary artery shunt in preparation for later septation if the anatomy is favorable. Infants in the first year of life with favorable anatomy and severe heart failure who are refractory to medical therapy should be considered for an initial septation operation due to the poor results of septation procedures following pulmonary artery banding.

REFERENCES

1. Anderson, R. H., Arnold, R., Thaper, M. K., Jones, R. S., and Hamilton, D. I.: Cardiac specialized tissues in hearts with an apparently single ventricular chamber. (Double inlet left ventricle.) Am. J. Cardiol. 33:95, 1974.
2. Anderson, R. H., Becker, A. E., Macartney, F. J., Shinebourne, E. A., Wilkinson, J. L., and Tynan, M. J.: Is "tricuspid atresia" a univentricular heart. Pediatr. Cardiol. 1:51, 1979.
3. Anderson, R. H., Tynan, M. J., Freedom, R. M., Quero-Jimenez, M., Macartney, F. J., Shinebourne, E. A., Wilkinson, J. L., and Becker, A. E.: Ventricular morphology in the univentricular heart. Herz. 4:184, 1979.
4. Bargeron, L. M., Jr., Elliott, L. P., Soto, B., Bream, P. R., and Curry, G. C.: Axial cineangiography in congenital heart disease. Section I. Concept, technical and anatomic considerations. Circulation 56:1075, 1977.
5. Becker, A. E., Wilkinson, J. L., and Anderson, R. H.: Atrioventricular conduction tissues: A guide in understanding the morphogenesis of the univentricular heart. In Etiology and Morphogenesis of Congenital Heart Disease, edited by R. Van Praagh and A. Takao. Futura Publishing Company, Mount Kisco, NY, 1980, p. 489.
6. Bjork, V. O., Olin, C. L., Bjork, B. B., and Thoren, C. A.: Right atrial-right ventricular anastomosis for correction of tricuspid atresia. J. Thorac. Cardiovasc. Surg. 77:452, 1979.
7. Breman, F. O., Jr., Malm, J. R., Hayes, C. J., and Gersony, W. M.: Physiological approach to surgery for tricuspid atresia. Circulation 58(Suppl I):I-83, 1978.
8. Davachi, F., and Moller, J. H.: The electrocardiogram and vectorcardiogram in single ventricle. Anatomic correlations. Am. J. Cardiol. 23:19, 1969.
9. De la Cruz, M. V., and Miller, B. L.: Double inlet left ventricle. Two pathological specimens with comments on the embryology and on the relation to single ventricle. Circulation 37:249, 1968.
10. Dooley, K. J., Paris-Buckler, L., Flyer, D. C., and Nadas, A. S.: Results of pulmonary arterial banding in infancy: Survey of 5 years' experience in the New England Regional Infant Cardiac Program. Am. J. Cardiol. 36:484, 1975.
11. Doty, D. B., Schieken, R. M., and Lauer, R. M.: Septation of the univentricular heart. J. Thorac. Cardiovasc. Surg. 78:423, 1979.
12. Edie, R. N., Ellis, K., Gersony, W. M., Krongrad, R., Bowman, F. O., Jr., and Malm, J. R.: Surgical repair of single ventricle. J. Thorac. Cardiovasc. Surg. 66:350, 1973.
13. Elliott, L. P.: An angiographic and plain film approach to complex congenital heart disease: Classification and simplified nomenclature. Curr. Probl. Cardiol. 3:47, 1978.
14. Elliott, L. P., Amplatz, K., Anderson, R. C., and Edwards, J. E.: Cor triloculare biatriatum with pulmonary stenosis and normally related great vessels. Am. J. Cardiol. 11:469, 1963.
15. Elliott, L. P., Anderson, R. C., and Edwards, J. E.: The common cardiac ventricle with transposition of the great vessels. Br. Heart J. 26:289, 1964.

16. Elliott, L. P., Bargeron, L. M., Jr., Soto, B., and Bream, P. R.: Axial cineangiography in congenital heart disease. Radiol. Clin. North Am. 18:515, 1980.
17. Elliott, L. P., Bargeron, L. M., Jr., Bream, P. R., Soto, B., and Curry, G. C.: Axial cineangiography in congenital heart disease. Section II. Specific lesions. Circulation 56:1084, 1977.
18. Elliott, L. P., and Gedgaudas, E.: The roentgenologic findings in common ventricle with transposition of the great vessels. Radiology 82:850, 1964.
19. Elliott, L. P., Ruttenberg, H. D., Ellot, R. S., and Anderson, R. C.: Vectorial analysis of the electrocardiogram in common ventricle. Br. Heart J. 26:302, 1964.
20. Elliott, L. P., and Schiebler, G. L.: In The X-Ray Diagnosis of Congenital Heart Disease In Infants, Children and Adults: Pathologic, Hemodynamic, and Clinical Correlations as Related to Chest Film, 2nd ed., chap. 5, 7. Charles C Thomas, Springfield, Ill., 1979.
21. Essed, C. E., Ho, S. Y., Hunter, S., and Anderson, R. H.: Atrioventricular conduction system in univentricular heart of right ventricular type with right-sided rudimentary chamber. Thorax 35:123, 1980.
22. Essed, C. E., Ho, S. Y., Shinebourne, E. A., Joseph, M. C., and Anderson, R. H.: Further observations on conduction tissues in univentricular hearts—surgical implications. Eur. Heart J. 2:87, 1981.
23. Feldt, R. H., Mair, D. D., Danielson, G. K., Wallace, R. B., and McGoon, D. C.: Current status of the septation procedure for univentricular heart. J. Thorac. Cardiovasc. Surg. 82:93, 1981.
24. Fellows, K. E., Keane, J. F., and Freed, M. O.: Angled views in cineangiography of congenital heart disease. Circulation 56:485, 1977.
25. Fontan, F., and Baudet, E.: Surgical repair of tricuspid atresia. Thorax 26:240, 1971.
26. Freedom, R. M., Nanton, M., and Dische, M. R.: Isolated ventricular inversion with double inlet left ventricle. Eur. J. Cardiol. 5:63, 1977.
27. Freedom, R. M., Sondheimer, H., Dische, R., and Rowe, R. D.: Development of "subaortic stenosis" after pulmonary arterial banding for common ventricle. Am. J. Cardiol. 39:78, 1977.
28. Gale, A. W., Danielson, G. K., McGoon, D. C., and Mair, D. D.: Modified Fontan operation for univentricular heart and complicated congenital lesions. J. Thorac. Cardiovasc. Surg. 78:831, 1979.
29. Gessner, I. H., Elliott, L. P., Schiebler, G. L., Van Mierop, L. H. S., and Miller, B. L.: The vectorcardiogram in double inlet left ventricle with and without inversion. Proceedings of the XIth International Vectorcardiogram Symposium.
30. Guller, B., Mair, D. D., Ritter, D. G., and Smith, R. E.: Frank vectorcardiogram in common ventricle: Correlation with anatomic findings. Am. Heart J. 90:290, 1975.
31. Holmes, W. F.: Case of malformation of the heart. Trans. Med. Chir. Soc. Edin. 1:252, 1824.
32. Horsley, B. L., Zuberbuhler, J. R., and Bahnson, H. T.: Factors influencing survival after

banding of the pulmonary artery: A review of 89 cases. Arch. Surg. 101:776, 1970.
33. Hunt, C. E., Formanek, G., Levine, M. A., Castaneda, A., and Moller, J. H.: Banding of the pulmonary artery: Results in 111 children. Circulation 43:395, 1971.
34. Hurwitt, E. S., Young, D., and Escher, D. J. W.: The rationale of anastomosis of the right auricular appendage to the pulmonary artery in the treatment of tricuspid atresia. J. Thorac. Cardiovasc. Surg. 30:503, 1955.
35. Ionescu, M. I., Macartney, F. J., and Wooler, G. H.: Intracardiac repair of single ventricle with pulmonary stenosis. J. Thorac. Cardiovasc. Surg. 65:602, 1973.
36. Kawashima, Y., Mori, T., Matsuda, H., Miyamoto, K., Kozuke, T., and Manabe, H.: Intraventricular repair of single ventricle associated with transposition of the greater arteries. J. Thorac. Cardiovasc. Surg. 72:21, 1976.
37. Keeton, B. R., Macartney, F. J., Hunter, S., Mortera, C., Rees, P., Shinebourne, E. A., Tynan, M. J., Wilkinson, J. L., and Anderson, R. H.: Univentricular heart of right ventricular type with double or common inlet. Circulation 29:403, 1979.
38. Lev, M., Liberthson, R. R., Kirkpatrick, J. R., Eckner, F. A. O., and Arcilla, R. A.: Single (primitive) ventricle. Circulation 39:577, 1969.
39. Macartney, F. J., Zuberbuhler, J. R., and Anderson, R. H.: Morphological considerations pertaining to recognition of atrial isomerism. Consequences for sequential chamber localisation. Br. Heart J. 44:657, 1980.
40. Mann, J. D.: Cor triloculare biatriatum. Br. Med. J. 1:614, 1907.
41. McGoon, D. C., Danielson, G. K., Ritter, D. G., Wallace, R. B., Maloney, J. D., and Marcelletti, C.: Correction of the univentricular heart having two atrioventricular valves. J. Thorac. Cardiovasc. Surg. 74:218, 1977.
42. McKay, R., Pacifico, A. D., Blackstone, E. H., Kirklin, J. W., and Bargeron, L. M., Jr.: Septation of the univentricular heart with left anterior subaortic outlet chamber, in press, 1982.
43. Mehrizi, A., McMurphy, D. M., Otteson, O. E., and Rowe, R. D.: Syndrome of double inlet left ventricle. Angiographic differentiation from single ventricle with rudimentary outlet chamber. Bull. Johns Hopkins Hosp. 119:225, 1966.
44. Munoz-Castellanos, L., De la Cruz, M. V., and Cieslinski, A.: Double inlet right ventricle: Two pathological specimens; with comments on embryology. Br. Heart J. 35:292, 1973.
45. Oldham, H. N., Jr., Kakos, G. S., Jarmakani, M. M., and Sabiston, D. C., Jr.: Pulmonary artery banding in infants with complex congenital heart defects. Ann. Thorac. Surg. 13:342, 1972.
46. Peacock, T. B.: Case of malformation of the heart. Both auricles opening into the left ventricle, and transposition of the aorta and pulmonary artery. Trans. Pathol. Soc. (Lond.) 6:177, 1855.
47. Quero-Jimenez, M., Cameron, A., Acerete, F., and Quero-Jimenez, C.: Univentricular hearts: Pathology of the atrioventricular valves. Herz.

4:161, 1979.
48. Quero-Jimenez, M., Perez Martinez, V. M., Maitre Azcarte, M. J., Merino-Batres, G., and Moreno Granados, F.: Exaggerated displacement of the atrioventricular canal towards the bulbus cordis (rightward displacement of the mitral valve). Br. Heart J. 35:65, 1973.
49. Rigby, M. L., Anderson, R. H., Gibson, D., Jones, O. D. H., Joseph, M. C., and Shinebourne, E. A.: Two dimensional echocardiographic categorisation of the univentricular heart: Ventricular morphology, type and mode of atrioventricular connexion. Br. Heart J., in press, 1982.
50. Rodhard, S., and Wagner, D.: Bypassing the right ventricle. Proc. Soc. Exp. Biol. Med. 71:69, 1949.
51. Sakakibara, S., Tominaga, S., Imai, Y., Uehara, K., and Matsumuro, M.: Successful total correction of common ventricle. Chest 61:192, 1972.
52. Somerville, J., Becu, L., and Ross, D.: Common ventricle with acquired subaortic obstruction. Am. J. Cardiol. 34:206, 1974.
53. Soto, B., Bertranou, E. G., Bream, P. R., Souza, A., Jr., and Bargeron, L. M., Jr.: Angiographic study of univentricular heart of right

ventricular type. Circulation 60:1325, 1979.
54. Taussig, H. B.: A single ventricle with a diminutive outlet chamber. J. Tech. Meth. 19:120, 1939.
55. Taussig, H. B.: Long-time observations on the Blalock-Taussig operation. IX. Single ventricle (with apex to the left). Johns Hopkins Med. J. 139:69, 1976.
56. Thiene, G., Daliento, L., Frescura, C., De Tommasi, M., Macartney, F. J., and Anderson, R. H.: Atresia of the left atrioventricular orifice. Anatomical investigation of 62 cases. Br. Heart J. 45:393, 1981.
57. Tonkin, I. L., Kelley, M. J., Bream, P. R., and Elliott, L. P.: The frontal chest film as a method of suspecting transposition complexes. Circulation 53:1016, 1976.
58. Truccone, N. J., Bowman, F. O., Jr., Malm, J. R., and Gersony, W. M.: Systemic-pulmonary arterial shunts in the first year of life. Circulation 49:508, 1974.
59. Tynan, M. J., Becker, A. E., Macartney, F. J., Quero-Jimenez, M., Shinebourne, E. A., and Anderson, R. H.: Nomenclature and classification of congenital heart disease. Br. Heart J. 41:544, 1979.
60. Van Praagh, R., David, I., Wright, G. B., and

Van Praagh, S.: Large RV plus small LV is not single LV. Circulation 61:1057, 1980.
61. Van Praagh, R., Leidenfrost, R. D., Lee, S. K., Marx, G., Wright, G. B., and Van Praagh, S.: The morphologic method applied to the problem of "single" right ventricle. Am. J. Cardiol., in press, 1982.
62. Van Praagh, R., Ongley, P. A., and Swan, H. J. C. Anatomic types of single or common ventricle in man: Morphologic and geometric aspects of sixty necropsied cases. Am. J. Cardiol. 13:367, 1964.
63. Victorica, B. E., Miller, B. L., and Gessner, I. H.: Electrocardiogram and vectorcardiogram in ventricular inversion (corrected transposition). Am. Heart J. 86:733, 1973.
64. Warden, H. E., DeWall, R. A., and Varco, R. L.: Use of the right auricle as a pump for the pulmonary circuit. Surg. Forum 5:16, 1954.
65. Wenink, A. C. G.: The conduction tissues in primitive ventricle with outlet chamber: Two different possibilities. J. Thorac. Cardiovasc. Surg. 75:747, 1978.
66. Yacoub, M. H., and Radley-Smith, R.: Use of a valved conduit from right atrium to pulmonary artery for "correction" of single ventricle. Circulation 54 (Suppl 3):III-63, 1976.

26

Truncus Arteriosus

Douglas D. Mair, M.D., William D. Edwards, M.D., Valentin Fuster, M.D., James B. Seward, M.D., and Gordon K. Danielson, M.D.

Persistent truncus arteriosus (TA) is an uncommon congenital cardiovascular malformation comprising 1 to 4% of the cardiac deformities found in a number of large autopsy series.[15, 22, 41] There is no striking sex difference in frequency, although most series have contained more males than females. With the advent of a corrective operation for this malformation in 1967,[21] the understanding of its physiology assumed greater importance if patients were to be successfully managed. With a number of patients who are alive more than 10 years after operation for correction and who presently are adolescents or young adults, truncus arteriosus has become a lesion of interest to the adult cardiologist as well, a change from the period when few of these patients survived childhood. During the past 5 years, surgical correction during infancy, at an acceptable risk, has become possible, and this development has further heightened interest in this deformity and brightened the outlook for afflicted children.

EMBRYOLOGY AND PATHOLOGY

The embryonic truncus arteriosus lies between the conus cordis proximally, and the aortic sac and aortic arch system distally. Partitioning of the TA, which is intimately associated with conal and aortopulmonary septation, has been reviewed by Van Mierop and illustrated by Netter.[23]

Truncus swellings, similar in appearance to endocardial cushions, divide the truncal lumen into two channels, the proximal ascending aorta and the pulmonary trunk. As the proximal portion of this truncal septum fuses with the developing conal septum (derived from conal swellings), right ventricular origin of the pulmonary trunk and left ventricular origin of the aorta are established. From truncal tissue at this line of fusion, valve swellings develop, the excavation of which leads to formation of the aortic and pulmonary valves and their respective sinuses of Valsalva. Along the aortic sac, the paired sixth aortic arches (primitive pulmonary arteries) migrate leftward, and the paired fourth aortic arches shift rightward. Invagination of the aortic sac roof thereby forms an aortopulmonary septum, which eventually fuses with the distal extent of the truncal septum. Accordingly, the right and left pulmonary arteries originate from the pulmonary trunk, and the aortic arch emanates from the ascending aorta. The spiral course of the truncoaortic partition results in the normal intertwinement of the great arteries.

When conotruncal or truncoaortic septation does not proceed normally, a variety of congenital ventriculoarterial anomalies may result,[40] one of which is truncus arteriosus, whereby a single arterial trunk exits from the heart. The conal (infundibular) septum is also either deficient or absent, resulting in a large ventricular septal defect (VSD). Since the conal septum also contributes, in part, to the development of the anterior tricuspid leaflet and medial tricuspid papillary muscle, these latter structures also may be malformed. The single truncal valve may be deformed and functionally insufficient or, less commonly, stenotic. If vestiges of distal truncoaortic septation develop, the pulmonary arteries may arise together from a short pulmonary trunk; otherwise, they arise separately from the truncal root.

The pathology of TA is characterized by a single arterial

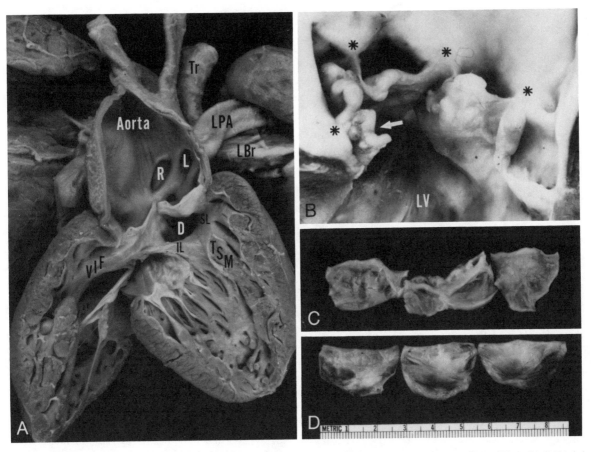

Fig. 26.1 Pathology of truncus arteriosus. (A) Right ventricular view, showing truncal origin of aorta, right (R) and left (L) pulmonary arteries (type II), and coronary arteries. Ventricular septal defect (D) is cradled between superior (SL) and inferior (IL) limbs of trabecula septomarginalis (TSM). Fusion of inferior limb with ventriculoinfundibular fold (VIF) separates tricuspid valve from bicuspid truncal valve and from mitral valve. Infundibular septum and medial tricuspid papillary muscle are absent. Aortic arch is right-sided. LBr, left bronchus; LPA, left pulmonary artery; Tr, trachea. (B) Insufficient quadricuspid truncal valve, with thickened, nodular, and deformed cusps. Ventricular septal defect (arrow) is obscured by cusps. LV, left ventricle; *, truncal valve commissures. C and D, Range of insufficient tricuspid truncal valves (surgically excised). Cusps may be deformed and thickened (C) or may simply have dilated annulus (D).

vessel arising from the base of the heart which gives origin to the coronary, pulmonary, and systemic arteries (Fig. 26.1A). A single semilunar valve is found in truncus arteriosus, and this valve differentiates TA from aortic and pulmonary valve atresia, conditions in which a single arterial vessel also receives the entire output of both ventricles but in which a second atretic semilunar valve is present.

Collett and Edwards[8] recognized four types of truncus arteriosus on the basis of the anatomic origin of the pulmonary arteries (Fig. 26.2). In type I, a short pulmonary trunk has its origin from the TA and gives rise to both pulmonary arteries. When both pulmonary arteries arise separately from the TA, with no vestige of pulmonary trunk, they may arise closely to one another (type II) or at some distance from one another (type III). Type IV truncus arteriosus is now considered to represent a form of pulmonary atresia with VSD, rather than TA.[9, 34]

The ventricular septal defect in truncus arteriosus is generally large and results from either absence or pronounced deficiency of the infundibular septum.[2] The defect is cradled between the two limbs of the trabecula septomarginalis and is roofed by the truncal valve cusps (Fig. 26.1A). In most instances, the fusion of the inferior limb and the ventriculoinfundibular fold results in muscular discontinuity between the tricuspid and the truncal valves.[9] Accordingly, the membranous septum is intact and the defect is of infundibular type. When such fusion fails to occur, tricuspid-truncal valvular continuity is present, and the defect (which now involves the membranous septum) is of combined paramembranous-infundibular types. Very rarely, the VSD in truncus arteriosus may be small and restrictive.[30]

The semilunar valve is tricuspid in 61 to 72% of patients, quadricuspid in 15 to 31%, bicuspid in 6 to 12%, and either

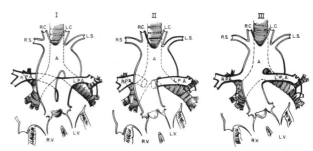

Fig. 26.2 Three types of truncus arteriosus. Type I, pulmonary trunk arises from truncus. Type II, right (R.P.A.) and left (L.P.A.) pulmonary arteries arise separately, but close to one another, from left posterolateral aspect of truncus. Type III, pulmonary arteries each arise from respective lateral aspects of truncus. Pulmonary trunk is absent in types II and III. (Reproduced with permission from J. E. Edwards and D. C. McGoon: Circulation 47:393, 1973, by permission of the American Heart Association.)

pentacuspid or hexacuspid in 0 to 2%.[7-9, 41] The semilunar valve is in fibrous continuity with the mitral valve in all patients but is continuous with a tricuspid valve in a minority. By overriding the ventricular septum, biventricular origin of the TA is observed in 68 to 83% of patients.[6, 8] In 11 to 29% of patients, the truncal valve is committed entirely to the right ventricle, whereas in 4 to 6% of patients, it is entirely left ventricular in origin. The anatomic cause for truncal valve insufficiency is variable and includes thickened and nodular dysplastic cusps (Fig. 26.1B and C), prolapse of unsupported cusps or conjoined cusps containing a shallow raphe, inequality of cusp size, minor commissural abnormalities, or anular dilatation[5, 11] (Fig. 26.1D). Truncal valve stenosis, when present, is usually associated with nodular and dysplastic cusps.[16, 26] The truncal root is frequently dilated, and the truncal sinuses of Valsalva are often poorly developed.

A right aortic arch with mirror-image brachiocephalic branching is more commonly associated with TA, occurring in 21 to 34% of patients,[7, 9, 19, 41] than with any other congenital cardiac malformation. Very rarely, a double aortic arch may persist. Hypoplasia of the arch, either with or without coarctation of the aorta, occurs in 3% of patients.[6, 9] Interrupted aortic arch, which forms a distinct category in Van Praagh's classification of truncus arteriosus,[41] occurs relatively frequently (11 to 19% of patients)[7, 9, 41] and is accompanied by ductal continuity of the descending thoracic aorta.

The ductus arteriosus is absent in approximately half the patients with TA but, in patients in whom it is present, will remain patent postnatally in nearly two-thirds.[7, 41] The relative sizes of the aorta and the ductus arteriosus tend to vary inversely.

The pulmonary arteries most commonly arise from the left posterolateral aspect of the TA, a small distance above the truncal valve. A short common pulmonary trunk (type I) is observed in 48 to 68% of patients, while type II accounts for 29 to 34%, and type III represents 6 to 10%.[6-9] In type II, the left pulmonary ostium is generally somewhat higher than the right.[41] Rarely in the setting of interrupted aortic arch, this ostium may arise to the right of the right pulmonary artery ostium, resulting in crossing of the pulmonary arteries posterior to the TA.[4]

Stenosis of the pulmonary artery ostia or arteries is uncommon, so that unless pulmonary arterial banding is performed, the pulmonary vascular bed will be exposed to systemic arterial pressure. In rare instances, deformed truncal valvular tissue may obstruct the pulmonary ostia during ventricular systole.[7]

In truncus arteriosus, there may be unilateral complete absence of one pulmonary artery. Sixteen percent (11 of 70 patients) of the Mayo Clinic's previously published series of patients with TA had only a single pulmonary artery.[18] In 9 of the 11 patients, the pulmonary artery was absent on the side of the aortic arch. Thus, in TA the pulmonary artery is most frequently absent on the side of the aortic arch, in contrast to the finding in tetralogy of Fallot, in which the pulmonary artery is more frequently absent on the side opposite the aortic arch.

This chapter will not deal with so-called pseudotruncus arteriosus, which in actuality is a form of pulmonary valve atresia with VSD, or with hemitruncus, in which one pulmonary artery arises from the ascending aorta while the other emanates from the right ventricle and has a well-developed pulmonary valve at its origin. Clearly, the embryologic basis for these deformities appears to be different from that for true persistent truncus arteriosus,[9] and it is unfortunate that the misnomers of pseudotruncus and hemitruncus enjoy such widespread use.

Knowledge of variations in coronary arterial origin and distribution, which are common in TA, is important to the surgeon. Since the left anterior descending coronary artery is frequently relatively small and displaced leftward, the conus branch of the right coronary artery, in a compensatory manner, is usually prominent and supplies several large branches to the right ventricular outflow tract.[1, 6] The posterior descending coronary artery arises from the left circumflex (so-called left coronary dominance) in 27%,[31] or approximately three times the frequency of this variation in the normal population. Anomalies of coronary ostial origin, involving 37 to 49% of patients with TA,[7, 41] are common, regardless of the number of truncal valve cusps. In general, however, the left coronary artery tends to arise from the left posterolateral truncal surface and the right from the right anterolateral surface.[1, 6, 31] In the setting of a single coronary ostium, frequently associated with left coronary dominance, all three major epicardial branches may originate from this common site, or the right coronary artery may be absent. When two ostia exist, both may arise from the same truncal sinus, one may take origin from the anticipated site of the noncoronary sinus, or both may arise normally. High ostial origin, above the truncal sinotubular junction, is common, but when origin is at or slightly above a truncal valve commissure, the involved ostium (most commonly the left) may be slitlike and functionally stenotic. Conceivably, dysplastic valvular tissue also could obstruct an otherwise normal coronary ostium. Rarely, the left coronary artery may originate from the pulmonary trunk.[6] Combinations of the above-mentioned coronary anomalies are common.

The location of the conduction tissue in truncus arteriosus is also of surgical importance. The sinus node and the atrioventricular node are normal in location and structure. The atrioventricular bundle courses to the left of the central fibrous body, and the left bundle branch emanates along the left ventricular septal subendocardium just beneath the membranous septum.[39] The right bundle branch travels within the myocardium of the ventricular septal summit, only attaining a subendocardial course at the level of the moderator band. In most instances in which the VSD is truly infundibular and the membranous septum is intact, the atrioventricular conduction tissue is somewhat distant from the rim of the defect. However, in patients with combined paramembranous-infundibular VSD, the conduction tissue passes along the left aspect of the posteroinferior rim of the defect.

The most commonly associated anomalies with truncus arteriosus which have been previously discussed include right aortic arch, interrupted aortic arch, absent ductus arteriosus, PDA, unilateral absence of a pulmonary artery, coronary ostial anomalies, and an incompetent truncal valve. A secundum atrial septal defect has been noted in 9 to 20% of patients, an aberrant subclavian artery in 4 to 10%, a persistent left superior vena cava draining into the coronary sinus in 4 to 9%, and mild tricuspid stenosis in 6%.[6, 19, 41] Partial anomalous pulmonary venous connection in association with TA also has been seen.[18]

Extracardiac anomalies are present in 21 to 30% of autopsy cases of TA and include skeletal deformities, hydroureter, bowel malrotation, and multiple complex anomalies. An association with splenic anomalies is very rare. Among the secondary complications of the basic pathology of TA, biventricular hypertrophy is frequent and dilatation of ventricular chambers is prominent when truncal valve insufficiency exists. In the setting of massive cardiac hypertrophy, chronic subendocardial myocardial ischemia may develop (even with normal epicardial coronary arteries). As a result of chronic exposure of the pulmonary vasculature to sys-

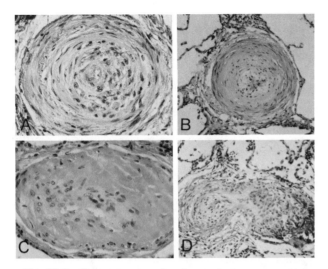

Fig. 26.3 Pulmonary vascular disease in truncus arteriosus. (*A*) Intimal cellular proliferation (grade 2) in 11-year-old. (*B*) Concentric intimal fibrosis (grade 3) in 11-year-old. (*C*) Necrotizing arteritis (grade 6) in 5-year-old. (*D*) Plexiform lesion (grade 4) in 18-month-old.

temic arterial pressure, hypertensive pulmonary vascular disease (plexogenic pulmonary arteriopathy) may develop (Fig. 26.3). The arteriolar lesions, as described by Heath and Edwards,[13] often develop more rapidly and to a more severe extent in TA than in isolated VSD. With chronic truncal valve insufficiency, pulmonary venous hypertension also may develop.

MANIFESTATIONS

Clinical Features

Most patients with truncus arteriosus are recognized to have congenital heart disease during early infancy, many during the neonatal period. The clinical features are largely dependent on the volume of pulmonary blood flow and the presence or absence of associated significant truncal valve insufficiency.

During the first few weeks of life, persistence of the increased pulmonary arteriolar resistance present during fetal life may result in mild cyanosis but little evidence of cardiac decompensation, unless severe truncal valve insufficiency is also present. As pulmonary resistance gradually decreases and flow through the lungs increases, the cyanosis may disappear. However, tachypnea, tachycardia, excessive sweating, poor feeding, and other signs of heart failure may then begin to appear secondary to the increased volume load on the heart produced by the excessive blood flow through the pulmonary circulation. If truncal valve insufficiency is severe, the signs and symptoms of heart failure may appear shortly after birth, and the additional volume load produced by this associated problem will always add to the increasing demands placed on the heart as pulmonary flow increases.

In the uncommon situation in which the infant has naturally occurring stenosis of the pulmonary arteries, obvious cyanosis may be present at birth and may intensify with increasing age. Such stenosis, however, protects the child from heart failure as a result of the large pulmonary blood flow as the pulmonary arterioles involute. Severe cyanosis in addition to the signs of heart failure may be present very early in the rare situation in which the child has both naturally occurring stenosis of the pulmonary artery and severe insufficiency of the truncal valve.

Physical Examination

Physical findings are also related primarily to the volume of pulmonary blood flow and the presence or absence of truncal valve insufficiency. The patient with a large pulmonary blood flow will have minimal or no cyanosis. The peripheral pulses are accentuated and may be bounding. The pulse pressure is usually increased. A left precordial bulge may be noted, and a systolic thrill is often palpable along the left sternal border. The heart is usually overactive. The first heart sound is normal and is frequently followed by a loud ejection click, which echophonocardiographic studies have demonstrated to coincide with maximal opening of the truncal valve.[29] The second heart sound is usually loud and single. The occasional auscultatory or phonocardiographic observation of a split second sound in these patients with a single semilunar valve may be due to delayed closure of some of the cusps of the abnormal truncal valve.[42] An apical third heart sound is often present. A loud pansystolic murmur maximal at the lower left sternal border which radiates to the entire precordium is most often heard. An apical diastolic low-pitched murmur secondary to increased flow across the normal mitral valve is frequently audible.

The patient with truncal valve insufficiency will usually have a blowing diastolic high-pitched murmur which is heard best along the left sternal border. A truly continuous murmur is uncommon in TA and, when present, usually is suggestive of pulmonary artery ostial stenosis. Continuous murmurs are very common, however, in the patient with pulmonary valve atresia and either a PDA or systemic collateral arteries providing pulmonary blood flow; and because the differential diagnosis of TA includes this lesion, the presence of such a murmur is strongly suggestive of pulmonary atresia rather than TA. Patients in heart failure may exhibit the additional signs of tachypnea, crepitant rales, hepatomegaly, and neck-vein distention.

Obvious cyanosis is present, and clubbing of the fingers and toes may be seen in the patient with decreased pulmonary blood flow secondary to naturally occurring pulmonary artery stenosis, pulmonary artery banding, or pulmonary vascular disease. If there is no associated truncal valve insufficiency, the peripheral pulses and pulse pressure are near normal. The apical diastolic murmur is often not present. This patient is less likely to have signs and symptoms of cardiac decompensation.

Electrovectorcardiographic Features

The electrocardiogram and vectorcardiogram commonly show a normal frontal plane QRS axis or minimal right axis deviation. Generally, normal sinus rhythm is present, and the conduction times are not prolonged. Combined ventricular hypertrophy is seen most often, and left ventricular forces are particularly prominent in patients with large pulmonary blood flow. Left atrial enlargement is also common in this group. Patients with normal or decreased pulmonary blood flow may exhibit right ventricular hypertrophy only. An example of a characteristic electrocardiogram and vectorcardiogram (Frank lead system) is seen in Figure 26.4.

Radiologic Features

Typically, the roentgenogram of the chest shows moderate cardiomegaly with an increase in pulmonary vascular markings (Fig. 26.5). The aortic arch is right-sided in approximately one-third of patients, and the combination of a right aortic arch and an increased pulmonary vascularity is strongly suggestive of truncus arteriosus. An abnormally high origin of the left pulmonary artery may be seen, and no main pulmonary artery segment is visualized. A dilated

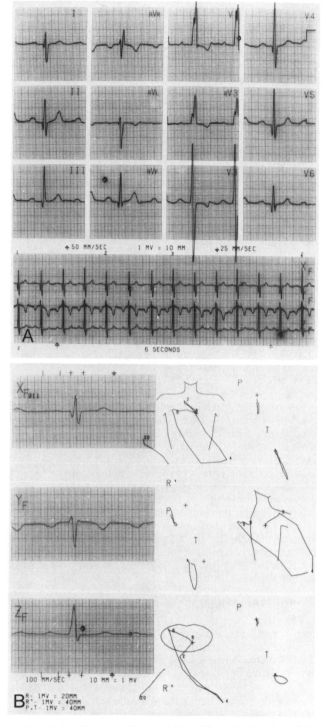

Fig. 26.4 Electrocardiogram (*A*) and Frank lead vectorcardiogram (*B*) from patient with truncus arteriosus. There is evidence of combined ventricular hypertrophy.

truncal root is common. Patients with decreased pulmonary blood flow may have minimal cardiomegaly, and the pulmonary vascular markings may be normal or decreased. A pronounced discrepancy in vascularity, increased on one side and decreased on the other, suggests the occasionally associated anomaly of unilateral absence of a pulmonary artery.

Echocardiographic Features

The use of 2D sector echocardiography[38] has greatly increased the ability to determine accurately the cardiac anat-

omy in malformations of the conotruncus.[12] Three defects that have a somewhat similar echocardiographic appearance when visualized from the parasternal view are truncus arteriosus, tetralogy of Fallot, and pulmonary atresia with VSD (Fig. 26.7). However, direct visualization of the origin of the pulmonary arteries using high parasternal short-axis views, scanning superiorly from the semilunar valve, usually can differentiate TA from tetralogy of Fallot and pulmonary atresia with ventricular septal defect (Fig. 26.6). In truncus arteriosus, the pulmonary arteries arise directly from the posterolateral aspect of the truncal root and bifurcate into the right and the left pulmonary artery. Examples of 2D echocardiograms obtained in patients with TA are illustrated in Figures 26.8 and 26.9.

Aortopulmonary window is in the differential diagnosis of truncus arteriosus and angiocardiographically may on occasion be confused with TA. However, echocardiographically these two entities can be easily differentiated. Aortopulmonary window usually is not associated with a VSD, and the right ventricular outflow tract and pulmonary valve are in

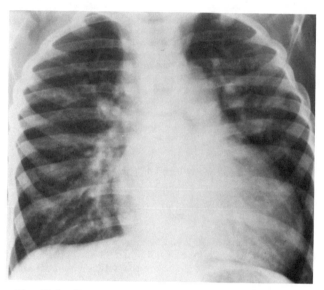

Fig. 26.5 Roentgenogram demonstrating typical features of truncus arteriosus. Note cardiomegaly, increased pulmonary vascularity, and right-sided aortic arch. A high left pulmonary artery origin is also evident.

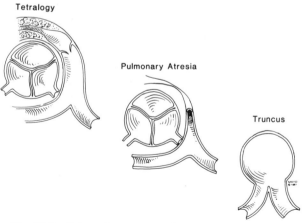

Fig. 26.6 Schematic representation of ultrasonic visualization of origin of pulmonary arteries using high parasternal short-axis views in tetralogy of Fallot, pulmonary atresia, and truncus. Note that in truncus arteriosus the pulmonary arteries arise directly from truncal root.

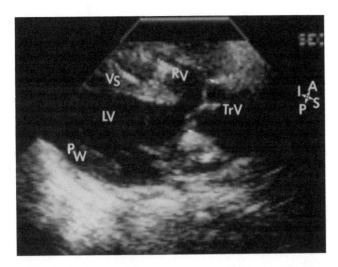

Fig. 26.7 Parasternal long-axis view in patient with truncus arteriosus showing large truncal root overriding ventricular septal defect. Margins of truncal valve are indicated by *arrows*. *TrV*, truncal valve; *RV*, right ventricle; *VS*, ventricular septum; *LV*, left ventricle; *PW*, posterior wall.

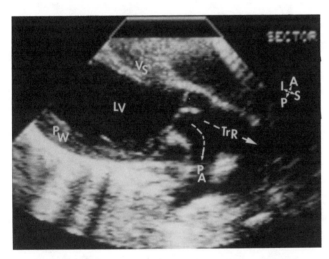

Fig. 26.8 A more superiorly oriented parasternal long-axis view in same patient as in Figure 26.7. In this view, pulmonary artery (*PA*) is originating from posterior aspect of truncal root (*TrR*).

the expected position. These features usually are easily recognized by sector echocardiography. Moreover, in aortopulmonary window using a high parasternal short-axis view, the aortopulmonary window usually can be visualized directly.

CARDIAC CATHETERIZATION AND ANGIOCARDIOGRAPHY

Cardiac catheterization and angiocardiography are necessary in truncus arteriosus if the pathologic and physiologic status are to be assessed precisely. These studies must be performed under stable conditions and with close attention to the patient's ventilatory status and acid-base balance if meaningful data are to be obtained. In most instances, all the necessary information can be obtained by use of the venous approach alone. This has been particularly true since the introduction of the flow-directed balloon catheters (Swan-Ganz), which have greatly facilitated entry into the pulmonary arteries from this approach. Occasionally, how-

ever, the retrograde arterial approach is used, particularly if an angiocardiogram of the truncal root is used to assess truncal valve insufficiency.

In our laboratory, a femoral arterial needle is placed to allow the continual monitoring of systemic blood pressure and as a sampling site for determination of arterial blood gases and dye-dilution curves. Anatomic diagnosis is established angiocardiographically. In larger patients, biplane roll film is used to demonstrate anatomic detail, but in infants and young children, cineangiography will give excellent results. The patient with TA often has a large heart and may have a large runoff of blood from the truncus into the pulmonary circulation. These conditions dictate that a large dose of contrast material be injected through a catheter whose size is adequate to allow a delivery rate that will give good delineation of anatomic detail. We use contrast material in doses as large as 2.0 ml/kg for each injection delivered in larger patients at rates as high as 50 ml/second to obtain this visualization. Often a right ventricular injection alone demonstrates the anatomic features accurately, but in some patients, a second dose is injected into the truncal root. In patients in whom previous surgery, usually pulmonary artery banding, has been performed and the pericardial space entered, epicardial adhesions may obscure the coronary arteries from direct visualization by the surgeon at the time of surgical correction. In such patients, if injection into the truncal root does not satisfactorily demonstrate the location of these arteries, selective coronary arteriography is performed to define their position for the surgeon, as it is critical that the ventriculotomy and proximal conduit anastomosis do not compromise a major coronary vessel. Characteristic biplane angiocardiograms are demonstrated in Figures 26.10 and 26.11.

The initial series of pressure and oximetric data is obtained with the patient breathing room air. Caval and right atrial pressures are usually normal, although they may be elevated if the patient is in heart failure. An increase in oxygen content at the atrial level is indicative of an atrial septal defect or partial anomalous pulmonary venous connection, both of which are occasionally found with truncus. When the catheter is advanced into the right ventricle, a pressure at systemic level is recorded, and an increase in oxygen content is noted high in the ventricle (opposite the VSD). Usually, the catheter can be manipulated easily into the truncal root, to the arch, and into the descending aorta.

For the accurate physiologic assessment of the patient with TA, the pulmonary arteries must be catheterized so that the pressure and oxygen content of the blood within

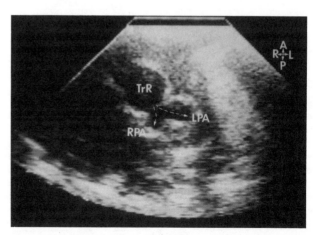

Fig. 26.9 High parasternal short-axis view in patient with truncus arteriosus. Note left pulmonary artery (*LPA*) and right pulmonary artery (*RPA*) originating from truncal root (*TrR*).

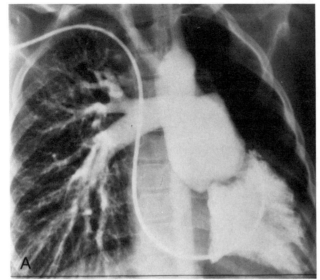

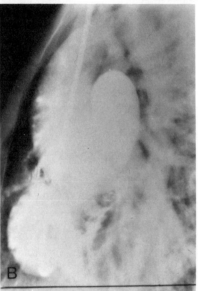

Fig. 26.10 Anteroposterior (A) and lateral (B) views of right ventricular angiocardiogram of patient with truncus arteriosus. Note complete absence of left pulmonary artery.

them can be determined. Naturally occurring pulmonary ostial stenosis is occasionally found, and if present, the pressure in the pulmonary arteries will be less than the systemic level pressure in the truncal root.

In the previously banded patient who is being evaluated, a pressure decrease in the pulmonary arteries is also expected if the banding has been effective. In patients without ostial stenosis or prior banding, the pressure in the pulmonary arteries is equal to systemic arterial pressure. Although, in TA, blood from both the right and left ventricles is ejected into the truncal root, which gives origin to the pulmonary arteries, the oxygen content in the pulmonary arteries cannot be assumed to be the same as that in the aorta. Considerable streaming may occur, and in our laboratory, two patients have exhibited an aortic oxygen saturation that was 12% greater than the saturation of blood in the pulmonary arteries. Such streaming is usually favorable (that is, aortic saturation greater than pulmonary artery saturation), but we have also recorded lesser degrees of unfavorable streaming. If two pulmonary arteries are present, they should both be

catheterized, because variations in pressure and oxygen content between the two arteries are possible.[20]

Patients with truncus arteriosus are at risk of developing pulmonary vascular obstructive disease at an early age, and pulmonary resistance must be assessed accurately in the evaluation of these patients if proper selection for the corrective operation now available is to be accomplished. Although the direct measurement of pulmonary resistance is not possible, the calculated indirect value, obtained by dividing the mean driving pressure across the pulmonary bed (mm Hg) by total pulmonary flow index (liter/minute/m^2) expressed as units/m^2, provides a reliable estimation of the status of the pulmonary arterioles.

Two publications from the Mayo Clinic[18, 19] have documented that patients with truncus who have two pulmonary arteries and a pulmonary arteriolar resistance of greater than 8.0 units/m^2 are at higher operative risk than are patients with resistances below that level. Of the initial 70 patients with TA who underwent correction,[19] 42 had pulmonary arteriolar resistances of less than 8.0 units/m^2. Among these 42, there were six operative deaths (14%). However, among the 28 patients with pulmonary arteriolar resistances higher than 8.0 units/m^2, there were 11 hospital

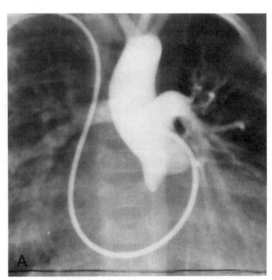

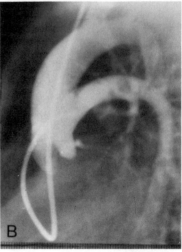

Fig. 26.11 Anteroposterior (A) and lateral (B) views of truncal root angiocardiogram in 10-month-old patient with truncus. Note common pulmonary trunk originating from posterolateral aspect of truncal root and bifurcating into right and left pulmonary arteries. Truncal valve is totally competent.

deaths (39%). Follow-up revealed that, among the group with resistances greater than 8.0 units/m^2, there were five late deaths, which were due to progression of pulmonary vascular obstructive disease with secondary severe pulmonary hypertension and right heart failure. Among the 36 operative survivors in the group with preoperative resistances less than 8.0 units/m^2, there have been no late deaths secondary to advancing pulmonary hypertension.

These data have led to our present policy of not offering surgery to patients with TA who have two pulmonary arteries and whose pulmonary arteriolar resistance is greater than 8.0 units/m^2, the exception being the child less than 2 years of age whose resistance decreases below 8.0 units/m^2 while breathing 100% oxygen or after the administration of a pharmacologic pulmonary vasodilator. In such young patients, surgery is still offered, if the parents are willing to accept a higher surgical risk, as there appears to be a good chance that the increased resistance is often a result primarily of arteriolar medial smooth muscle hypertrophy and vasoconstriction rather than advanced intimal occlusive disease. Because in such young patients there is a chance, based on our past experience, that the pulmonary resistance may stabilize or even decrease after corrective operation, it is considered reasonable to proceed with surgery—recognizing the risk of operation is probably 25 to 30%—as the natural history of this condition is very bad.[19]

Different physiologic criteria must be used to assess the operability of patients with unilateral absence of a pulmonary artery if pulmonary flow and resistance are calculated in the usual manner and if these parameters are correlated with the degree of pulmonary vascular disease present.[17] For a given degree of pulmonary vascular disease, the patient with only one pulmonary arteriolar bed exposed to systemic driving pressure would be expected to have approximately half the pulmonary flow and, hence, twice the calculated pulmonary resistance that the patient with comparable pulmonary vascular disease but two pulmonary arteries would have. Because of collateral supply to the lung with absent pulmonary artery, this is clearly an oversimplification, but certainly different physiologic criteria for operability are necessary. The convention of halving the calculated pulmonary resistance in such patients to determine operability based on criteria derived from patients who have TA and two pulmonary arteries, as proposed previously, has worked well. Thus, patients with a single pulmonary artery who had pulmonary arteriolar resistances as high as 16 units/m^2 may still have reactive pulmonary arterioles and may be surgical candidates. However, patients with a single pulmonary artery are likely to develop severe pulmonary vascular disease at an early age.[18] To achieve good results in this group, corrective operation should be performed before the patient is 1 year old. Even in this subset of patients who survive corrective operation, pulmonary vascular disease tends to progress after surgery more often than it does in patients with corrected TA who have two pulmonary arteries. This difference may be related to the fact that the entire cardiac output must still pass through one lung, and therefore the rate of flow through each arteriole remains approximately doubled, a potential stimulus for the progression of pulmonary vascular changes.

In the patient with truncus arteriosus, the systemic arterial saturation decreases as pulmonary blood flow decreases secondary to increasing pulmonary vascular disease. Systemic arterial saturation, therefore, reflects, in part, the status of the pulmonary vascular bed. Table 26.1 shows the systemic arterial saturation, while breathing room air, of 47 patients with TA who had two pulmonary arteries and who had neither a pulmonary artery band nor naturally occurring pulmonary stenosis—that is, they had systemic levels of

TABLE 26.1   SYSTEMIC ARTERIAL OXYGEN SATURATION (BREATHING ROOM AIR) RELATED TO PULMONARY RESISTANCE IN 47 PATIENTS[a] WITH TRUNCUS ARTERIOSUS AND TWO PULMONARY ARTERIES (1967–1972)

Rp (units/m^2)	No. of Patients	Systemic Arterial Saturation (%)	
		Range	Mean
<8.0	12	88–94	91
8.0–12.0	13	85–89	88
>12.0	22	61–85	79

[a] Excluding 12 patients with pulmonary artery banding or stenosis. (Reproduced with permission from D. D. Mair et al.[18] by permission of the American Heart Association).

pressure in the two pulmonary arteries. The data suggest that patients who are favorable for operation, those with pulmonary arteriolar resistances less than 8.0 units/m^2, have a systemic arterial saturation of 88% or greater. Conversely, a systemic saturation less than 85% in a patient with two pulmonary arteries and without a pulmonary artery band or pulmonary artery stenosis indicates that the patient probably is inoperable.

Occasionally, a patient with truncus arteriosus has systemic pressure in one pulmonary artery and a lower pressure in the other pulmonary artery, because of ostial stenosis or a previous unilateral pulmonary artery banding. In this patient, pulmonary arteriolar resistance cannot be estimated in each lung separately unless the blood flow to each lung is determined. Radioisotope injection and lung scanning may accomplish this determination. However, a review of patients who had different pressures in their two pulmonary arteries and who were operated on at our institution[20] indicates that, if the pressure in the pulmonary artery with the ostial stenosis or previous banding is less than one-half the systemic pressure, this pulmonary artery does not have pulmonary vascular obstructive disease and the patient is a good surgical candidate.

An accurate laboratory assessment of truncal valve insufficiency may be difficult. The commonly used method is injection of contrast material into the truncal root. However, because the pulmonary arteries also arise from the truncal root, preferential runoff into the pulmonary circulation may mask insufficiency of the truncal valve. In our experience, if the angiogram indicates that incompetence of the truncal valve is severe, severe incompetence is found at surgery. Occasionally, however, a patient whose angiocardiogram indicates only mild or moderate insufficiency is found to have severe insufficiency at surgery and may require valve replacement.

DIFFERENTIAL DIAGNOSIS

In the infant with truncus arteriosus and large pulmonary blood flow, the differential diagnosis includes the other congenital cardiac conditions that cause early heart failure and are associated with either mild or no cyanosis. Such malformations are: VSD, PDA, aorticopulmonary window, pulmonary atresia with VSD and PDA or large collateral arteries, double-outlet right ventricle, univentricular heart, and total anomalous pulmonary venous connection. Although certain physical findings, chest roentgenographic evidence, and electrocardiographic features may suggest the increased likelihood of a particular lesion, and the echocardiographic findings previously described may establish the diagnosis of TA, cardiac catheterization and angiocardiography are necessary to establish a complete assessment.

In truncus arteriosus with decreased pulmonary flow, the

other conditions to be considered include pulmonary atresia, tricuspid atresia, tetralogy of Fallot, univentricular heart with pulmonary stenosis, and double-outlet right ventricle with pulmonary stenosis.

The establishment of the diagnosis of TA by angiocardiography usually is not difficult. Aorticopulmonary window occasionally presents a similar appearance, but in this condition, the demonstration of two distinct semilunar valves establishes this, rather than TA, as the diagnosis. Aortography also will allow differentiation between TA and pulmonary valve atresia and a VSD. Careful analysis of the catheterization data and angiocardiograms should enable any associated malformation, such as atrial septal defect, partial anomalous pulmonary venous connection, and interrupted aortic arch, to be identified in the patient with TA.

NATURAL HISTORY

Although patients with truncus arteriosus occasionally survive to adulthood without surgery,[14, 32] the natural history of the condition usually runs a much shorter course. In an autopsy series of 57 cases reported by Van Praagh and Van Praagh,[41] the mean age of death was 5 weeks. Keith *et al.*[15] reported a survival of approximately 15% beyond 1 year of age, whereas Nadas and Fyler[22] reported 30%. Death in infancy is most commonly secondary to intractable heart failure. In patients who survive the first few years, death may occur from volume overload and cardiac decompensation, but it more frequently results from the complications of severe pulmonary vascular disease and occasionally after endocarditis develops.

Recently, Fuster has reviewed the subsequent clinical course of 76 truncus patients catheterized at the Mayo Clinic between 1960 and 1978 in whom a pulmonary arteriolar resistance of greater than 8 units/m^2 was found. The ages of these patients at catheterization ranged from 6 months to 19 years, with a median of 6 years. Follow-up after catheterization ranged from 1 to 20 years, with a median of 9 years. Forty-four of these patients either were not suitable surgical candidates because of the degree of pulmonary vascular disease or declined operation when the risk was considered. Of the 44 patients, 11 (25%) had subsequently died. Furthermore, the surviving 33 patients all had significant further deterioration in their condition, all being New York Heart Association Class III or IV at follow-up. Thus, once significant pulmonary vascular changes have occurred in patients with TA, generally there is continued rapid deterioration. This dismal natural history gives further impetus to the approach of early surgical intervention now advocated for these patients.

TREATMENT

Cardiac failure is managed by the use of digitalis and diuretic agents. If the infant responds to the medical regimen, our policy is to observe the patient with the prospect of performing surgical correction some time between 6 and 9 months of age. During this period, close observation must be maintained for signs of increasing pulmonary vascular resistance. Such signs may include less prominent peripheral pulses and a narrowing of the pulse pressure, disappearance of the apical middiastolic flow murmur, the development of cyanosis and polycythemia, decreasing heart size, and the improvement in the state of cardiac compensation with less need for digitalis. In follow-up of these patients, we find it useful to obtain systemic arterial oxygen saturation at intervals. A decrease in systemic arterial saturation, particularly if it has decreased below 88%, is an indication for prompt recatheterization to assess the pulmonary resistance.

Although medical therapy may be effective in alleviating the symptoms of heart failure, thereby allowing operative intervention to be delayed for a time in young infants, surgery is mandatory at an early age if any realistic hope for a long-term survival is to be offered. Because these patients tend to develop pulmonary arteriolar changes early in life, surgery aimed at reducing pulmonary artery pressure and flow must be done during the first year of life.

The choice of operation is between correction and pulmonary artery banding. Although pulmonary artery banding may provide palliation for the young patient with TA and may protect the pulmonary vascular bed so that correction will be feasible later, the risks and potential complications of banding for this condition have been well documented.[24, 27, 33, 36] In addition, successful banding has not guaranteed that these patients will be good candidates for later correction at reduced risk. A previous report from our laboratory concerning 27 patients with TA who were banded[20] disclosed that in two patients the band had been

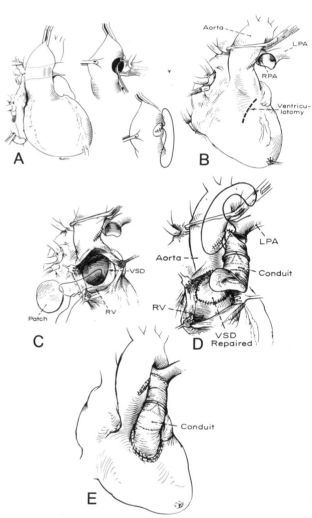

Fig. 26.12   Surgical repair. (*A*) Cardiopulmonary bypass; origin of pulmonary arteries excised from truncus; defect in truncus closed. (Reproduced with permission from D. C. McGoon *et al.*,[2] published by American Medical Association.) (*B*) Incision made high in right ventricle. (*C*) Ventricular septal defect closed with Teflon patch. (*D*) Dacron conduit with porcine valve sutured to pulmonary arteries. (*E*) Proximal end of conduit anastomosed to right ventricle. (Reproduced with permission from R. B. Wallace: *Gibbon's Surgery of the Chest*, edited by D. C. Sabiston, Jr. and F. G. Spencer, 3rd ed. W. B. Saunders, Philadelphia, 1976, pp. 1066–1075.

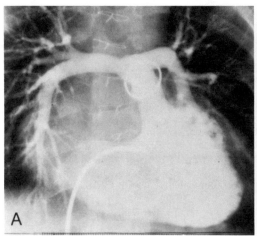
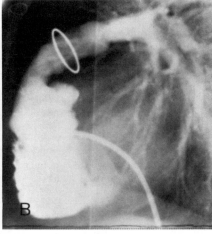
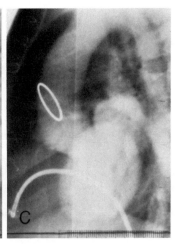

Fig. 26.13 Postoperative right ventricular angiocardiogram and later levophase from the same injection in the same patient as Figure 26.11. Anteroposterior (*A*) and lateral (*B*) views show Hancock conduit containing stinted porcine valve. Excellent filling of both pulmonary arteries is apparent. Late levophase (*C*) shows filling of left atria and left ventricle and unobstructed pathway constructed from left ventricle through ventricular septal defect to truncal root. No residual shunt is present.

ineffective in preventing the development of severe pulmonary vascular disease. An even more frequent complication of early banding has been the production of severe distortion of the pulmonary arteries at the band site and of hypoplasia beyond, seriously compromising the chances of achieving a good result with later correction. During the past 5 years, improved surgical techniques and postoperative care have made correction of truncus arteriosus during infancy possible at an operative risk no greater than that reported previously for banding.[3, 25, 35, 37] Because of this, the policy at the Mayo Clinic and most other large centers is to perform correction, rather than pulmonary artery banding, in most infants with TA. In so doing, however, a second operation will be required because the size of the conduit initially inserted will gradually become inadequate and will need to be replaced with a larger one.

SURGICAL CORRECTION

Successful definitive surgical correction of a patient with truncus arteriosus was first accomplished by McGoon *et al.*[21] in 1967. In the original operation, based on the experimental work of Rastelli *et al.*[28] continuity between the right ventricle and the pulmonary arteries was established by use of a conduit of a homograft aorta and aortic valve. In 1972, however, because of problems with calcification and secondary obstruction associated with the aortic homograft conduit, a switch was made to the use of a Dacron conduit containing a porcine semilunar valve (Hancock Laboratories), and since that time, this has been the conduit used in the operation. The steps of the operative repair are illustrated in Figure 26.12. A postoperative angiocardiogram is shown in Figure 26.13.

The early and late results experienced by the initial 92 patients who underwent correction at the Mayo Clinic were reported in 1977.[19] Although overall hospital mortality was 25%, the operative mortality decreased to 9% in the 33 patients operated on during the last 2½ years of the series, after the switch to the Hancock conduit. This operative mortality of approximately 10% has been maintained in the subsequent patients who have undergone correction after this initially reported series.

During the past 5 years, progress has also been achieved in the surgical management of the young infant. Because these patients tend to develop pulmonary vascular changes

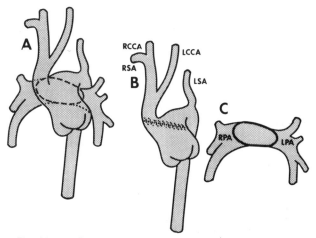

Fig. 26.14 Repair of truncus arteriosus in which there is interrupted aortic arch. (*A*) Excision of pulmonary arteries from posterior aspect of truncus. (*B*) Repair of resulting defect in truncus, leaving ductus arteriosus (now functioning as part of aortic arch) in continuity with truncus. (*C*) Orifice at pulmonary arteries to which conduit is sutured to establish continuity between right ventricle and pulmonary artery. *RCCA* and *LCCA*, right and left common carotid arteries; *RSA* and *LSA*, right and left subclavian arteries; *RPA* and *LPA*, right and left pulmonary arteries. (Reproduced with permission from M. M. R. Gomes and D. C. McGoon: *Mayo Clinic Proceedings* 46:40, 1971.)

at a young age, early surgical intervention is necessary to optimize the chance of a good long-term result. Excellent results have been obtained with corrective operation during infancy,[35, 37] and for patients without complicating features, the surgical risk now approaches the operative mortality achieved with the older patients.[19] In such patients successfully corrected during infancy, the small conduit inserted eventually needs to be replaced with a larger one, but this reoperation also seems to carry a low risk.

Severe incompetence of the truncal valve adds significantly to the risk of operation,[10, 11] particularly in the infant in whom valve replacement, even as an isolated operation, is associated with a high mortality and an uncertain late result. Because no really satisfactory prosthetic valve is now available for such small infants, our policy is to offer the corrective operation, at which time the surgeon inspects the truncal valve and performs a valvuloplasty to lessen the insufficiency. In such infants, the risk of corrective operation remains greater than 50%.

In the patient with TA who is beyond infancy, if severe insufficiency of the truncal valve is present, the valve can be replaced with only a moderate increase in risk. Our policy for these older patients is to replace the valve at the time of correction, if the insufficiency is moderate or severe. In patients with only mild insufficiency the valve is not replaced.

The operative repair of TA in association with arch interruption is illustrated in Figure 26.14. In older patients, this additional anomaly has not seemed to increase the risk of operation or compromise the late results. In infants, however, the operative risk has been greater than for the group as a whole.

Marcelletti et al.[19] reported follow-up information obtained for the 69 operative survivors of the initial Mayo Clinic surgical series of 92 patients with TA who underwent correction. At that time, the postoperative follow-up ranged from 6 months to 7½ years. There were eight late deaths (12%). Four patients died of pulmonary vascular disease, and two of these were from the small subset (eight operative survivors) of patients with single pulmonary artery, substantiating the tendency of this group to have progression of pulmonary vascular changes even after successful repair. One patient died of sudden ventricular fibrillation, one of dehiscence of a prosthetic truncal valve, and one secondary to mediastinal hemorrhage after rupture of a calcified aortic homograft conduit. The eighth patient died of injuries suffered in an automobile accident. Of the 61 patients still surviving at follow-up, 37 were in Class I, 23 in Class II, and 1 in Class IV.

REFERENCES

1. Anderson, K. R., McGoon, D. C., and Lie, J. T.: Surgical significance of the coronary arterial anatomy in truncus arteriosus communis. Am. J. Cardiol. 41:76, 1978.
2. Anderson, R. H., Becker, A. E., and Van Mierop, L. H. S.: What should we call the crista? Br. Heart J. 39:856, 1977.
3. Appelbaum, A., Bargeron, L. M., Jr., Pacifico, A. D., and Kirklin, J. W.: Surgical treatment of truncus arteriosus, with emphasis on infants and small children. J. Thorac. Cardiovasc. Surg. 71:436, 1976.
4. Becker, A. E., Becker, M. J., and Edwards, J. E.: Malposition of pulmonary arteries (crossed pulmonary arteries) in persistent truncus arteriosus. Am. J. Roentgenol. Radiol. Ther. Nucl. Med. 110:509, 1970.
5. Becker, A. E., Becker, M. J., and Edwards, J. E.: Pathology of the semilunar valve in persistent truncus arteriosus. J. Thorac. Cardiovasc. Surg. 62:16, 1971.
6. Bharati, S., McAllister, H. A., Jr., Rosenquist, G. C., Miller, R. A., Tatooles, C. J., and Lev, M.: The surgical anatomy of truncus arteriosus communis. J. Thorac. Cardiovasc. Surg. 67:501, 1974.
7. Calder, L., Van Praagh, R., Van Praagh, S., Sears, W. P., Corwin, R., Levy, A., Keith, J. D., and Paul, M. H.: Truncus arteriosus communis: Clinical, angiocardiographic, and pathologic findings in 100 patients. Am. Heart J. 92:23, 1976.
8. Collett, R. W., and Edwards, J. E.: Persistent truncus arteriosus: A classification according to anatomic types. Surg. Clin. North Am., August: 1245, 1949.
9. Crupi, G., Macartney, F. J., and Anderson, R. H.: Persistent truncus arteriosus: A study of 66 autopsy cases with special reference to definition and morphogenesis. Am. J. Cardiol. 40:569, 1977.
10. De Leval, M. R., McGoon, D. C., Wallace, R. B., Danielson, G. K., and Mair, D. D.: Management of truncal valvular regurgitation. Ann. Surg. 180:427, 1974.
11. Gelband, H., Van Meter, S., and Gersony, W. M.: Truncal valve abnormalities in infants with persistent truncus arteriosus: A clinicopathologic study. Circulation 45:397, 1972.
12. Hagler, D. J., Tajik, A. J., Seward, J. B., Mair, D. D., and Ritter, D. G.: Wide-angle two-dimensional echocardiographic profiles of conotruncal abnormalities. Mayo Clin. Proc. 55:73, 1980.
13. Heath, D., and Edwards, J. E.: The pathology of hypertensive pulmonary vascular disease: A description of six grades of structural changes in the pulmonary arteries with special reference to congenital cardiac septal defects. Circulation 18:533, 1958.
14. Hicken, P., Evans, D., and Heath, D.: Persistent truncus arteriosus with survival to the age of 38 years. Br. Heart J. 28:284, 1966.

15. Keith, J. D., Rowe, R. D., and Vlad, P.: Heart Disease in Infancy and Childhood, 3rd ed. Macmillan, New York, 1978.
16. Ledbetter, M. K., Tandon, R., Titus, J. L., and Edwards, J. E.: Stenotic semilunar valve in persistent truncus arteriosus. Chest 69:182, 1976.
17. Mair, D. D., Ritter, D. G., Danielson, G. K., Wallace, R. B., and McGoon, D. C.: Truncus arteriosus with unilateral absence of a pulmonary artery: Criteria for operability and surgical results. Circulation 55:641, 1977.
18. Mair, D. D., Ritter, D. G., Davis, G. D., Wallace, R. B., Danielson, G. K., and McGoon, D. C.: Selection of patients with truncus arteriosus for surgical correction: Anatomic and hemodynamic considerations. Circulation 49:144, 1974.
19. Marcelletti, C., McGoon, D. C., Danielson, G. K., Wallace, R. B., and Mair, D. D.: Early and late results of surgical repair of truncus arteriosus. Circulation 55:636, 1977.
20. McFaul, R. C., Mair, D. D., Feldt, R. H., Ritter, D. G., and McGoon, D. C.: Truncus arteriosus and previous pulmonary arterial banding: Clinical and hemodynamic assessment. Am. J. Cardiol. 38:626, 1976.
21. McGoon, D. C., Rastelli, G. C., and Ongley, P. A.: An operation for the correction of truncus arteriosus. J.A.M.A. 205:69, 1968.
22. Nadas, A. S., and Fyler, D. C.: Pediatric Cardiology, 3rd ed. W. B. Saunders, Philadelphia, 1972, p. 438.
23. Netter, F. H.: The Ciba Collection of Medical Illustrations, Vol. 5, Heart, edited by F. F. Yonkman, Ciba Pharmaceutical Company, Division of Ciba Corporation, Summit, N.J., 1969, pp. 122–123, 126–128.
24. Oldham, H. N., Jr., Kakos, G. S., Jarmakani, M. M., and Sabiston, D. C., Jr.: Pulmonary artery banding in infants with complex congenital heart defects. Ann. Thorac. Surg. 13:342, 1972.
25. Parenzan, L., Crupi, G., Alfieri, O., Bianchi, T., Vanini, V., Locatelli, G., Tiraboschi, R., Di Benedetto, G., Villani, M., Annecchino, F. P., and Ferrazzi, P.: Surgical repair of persistent truncus arteriosus in infancy. J. Thorac. Cardiovasc. Surg. 28:18, 1980.
26. Patel, R. G., Freedom, R. M., Bloom, K. R., and Rowe, R. D.: Truncal or aortic valve stenosis in functionally single arterial trunk: A clinical, hemodynamic and pathologic study of six cases. Am. J. Cardiol. 42:800, 1978.
27. Poirier, R. A., Berman, M. A., and Stansel, H. C., Jr.: Current status of the surgical treatment of truncus arteriosus. J. Thorac. Cardiovasc. Surg. 69:169, 1975.
28. Rastelli, G. C., Titus, J. L., and McGoon, D. C.: Homograft of ascending aorta and aortic valve as a right ventricular outflow: An experimental approach to the repair of truncus arteriosus. Arch. Surg. 95:698, 1967.

29. Ritter, D. G., Assad-Morell, J. L., Seward, J. B., Giuliani, E. R., and Tajik, A. J.: Echophonocardiographic correlates of ejection click in patients with systemic arterial trunk overriding the ventricular septum (abstr.). Circulation 52(Suppl 2):231, 1975.
30. Rosenquist, G. C., Bharati, S., McAllister, H. A., and Lev, M.: Truncus arteriosus communis: Truncal valve anomalies associated with small conal or truncal septal defects. Am. J. Cardiol. 37:410, 1976.
31. Shrivastava, S., and Edwards, J. E.: Coronary arterial origin in persistent truncus arteriosus. Circulation 55:551, 1977.
32. Silverman, J. J., and Scheinesson, G. P.: Persistent truncus arteriosus in a 43 year old man. Am. J. Cardiol. 17:94, 1966.
33. Singh, A. K., De Leval, M. R., Pincott, J. R., and Stark, J.: Pulmonary artery banding for truncus arteriosus in the first year of life. Circulation 54(Suppl 3):17, 1976.
34. Sotomora, R. F., and Edwards, J. E.: Anatomic identification of so-called absent pulmonary artery. Circulation 57:624, 1978.
35. Stanger, P., Robinson, S. J., Engle, M. A., and Ebert, P. A.: "Corrective surgery" for truncus arteriosus in the first year of life (abstr.). Am. J. Cardiol. 39:293, 1977.
36. Stark, J., Aberdeen, E., Waterston, D. J., Bonham-Carter, R. E., and Tynan, M.: Pulmonary artery constriction (banding): A report of 146 cases. Surgery 65:808, 1969.
37. Stark, J., Gandhi, D., De Leval, M., Macartney, F., and Taylor, J. F. N.: Surgical treatment of persistent truncus arteriosus in the first year of life. Br. Heart J. 40:1280, 1978.
38. Tajik, A. J., Seward, J. B., Hagler, D. J., Mair, D. D., and Lie, J. T.: Two-dimensional real-time ultrasonic imaging of the heart and great vessels: Technique, image orientation, structure identification, and validation. Mayo Clin. Proc. 53:271, 1978.
39. Thiene, G., Bortolotti, U., Gallucci, V., Terribile, V., and Pellegrino, P. A.: Anatomical study of truncus arteriosus communis with embryological and surgical considerations. Br. Heart J. 38:1109, 1976.
40. Van Mierop, L. H. S., Patterson, D. F., and Schnarr, W. R.: Pathogenesis of persistent truncus arteriosus in light of observations made in a dog embryo with the anomaly. Am. J. Cardiol. 41:755, 1978.
41. Van Praagh, R., and Van Praagh, S.: The anatomy of common aorticopulmonary trunk (truncus arteriosus communis) and its embryologic implications: A study of 57 necropsy cases. Am. J. Cardiol. 16:406, 1965.
42. Victorica, B. E., Gessner, I. H., and Schiebler, G. L.: Phonocardiographic findings in persistent truncus arteriosus. Br. Heart J. 30:812, 1968.

27

Hypoplastic Left Heart Syndrome

Robert M. Freedom, M.D.

The term *hypoplastic left heart syndrome* embraces a continuum of congenital cardiac anomalies characterized by underdevelopment of the aorta, aortic valve, left ventricle, mitral valve, and left atrium. Although the terms aortic atresia or hypoplastic left ventricle syndrome have been used synonymously, there are important exceptions to this.

PATHOLOGY

The majority of patients with the typical form of hypoplastic left heart syndrome (Fig. 27.1) have levocardia, visceroatrial situs solitus, and concordant atrioventricular and ventriculoarterial connections.[15, 17, 28, 55, 96] Much less commonly, significant underdevelopment of the left atrium, left ventricle, and aorta will be found in patients with dextrocardia or mesocardia or in patients exhibiting features of either right or left atrial isomerism.[16, 27] Such patients with atrial isomerism usually have splenic anomalies; thoracic symmetry and their abnormal viscera are heterotaxic.[40, 50, 97] That is, the disposition of the abdominal viscera indicates a lack of lateralization.

The morphologic right atrium is dilated, and external inspection reveals that the blunt right atrial appendage is considerably larger than the left atrial appendage, which is often inconspicuous.[15, 17, 28, 51, 55, 96, 101] The superior and inferior vena cavae usually terminate normally, as does the coronary sinus. The coronary sinus may appear dilated, reflecting either heart failure or anomalous connection of either systemic or pulmonary veins, or a left atrial-coronary sinus fenestration.

The tricuspid valve annulus is invariably dilated, and although the morphological tricuspid valve is usually normal, it may exhibit mild dysplasia. The morphological right ventricle is both dilated and hypertrophied. The internal organization of the right ventricle conforms to a "D"-ventricular loop with the inlet-trabecular-outlet axis oriented right-to-left.[109] The infundibular landmarks are usually accentuated in response to right ventricular hypertrophy. The pulmonary artery is invariably dilated and is supported by the right ventricular infundibulum with discontinuity between tricuspid valve and pulmonary valve.

The right and left pulmonary arteries are usually larger than normal, and it is extremely uncommon to demonstrate major anatomical abnormalities in the major branches of the pulmonary arteries. The pulmonary veins usually terminate in the left atrium and may appear dilated, reflecting some degree of left atrial hypertension. The left atrium is hypoplastic. This is certainly true in neonates dying with this disorder. Even among those patients who survive a month or longer, the left atrium rarely appears dilated. The left atrial endocardium may appear thickened, especially when compared to the right atrial endocardium, but in the neonate, endocardial sclerosis or elastosis is only rarely conspicuous.

A true defect of the fossa ovalis is evident in about 20% of patients with the hypoplastic left heart syndrome. Usually, the interatrial communication is restrictive, and it is common for the septum primum to herniate from left-to-right, forming a so-called aneurysm of the atrial septum. When a true defect of the atrial septum is present, it may rarely be of the sinus venous type, or of the ostium primum type.[114] The atrial septum will be intact in about 10% of patients with hypoplastic left heart syndrome indicative of so-called

premature closure of the foramen ovale.[56] The patient with aortic and mitral atresia, intact atrial septum, and absence of an alternate pathway for pulmonary venous return can exhibit conspicuous pulmonary lymphangiectasia. When mitral atresia is present and the atrial septum intact, an alternative pathway for pulmonary venous flow may be present. Such alternative routes include: anomalous pulmonary venous connections[48, 97]; the levoatriocardinal vein[58]; a venous channel connecting a pulmonary vein to a systemic vein[21]; or left atrial-coronary sinus fenestration (so-called unroofed coronary sinus).[5, 34, 73, 90] One or more pulmonary veins may terminate in the right atrium, coronary sinus, or systemic vein. In the presence of mitral atresia, or extreme stenosis, and a very restrictive interatrial communication, such anomalous pulmonary venous connections may provide an alternative route to the systemic circulation.[5, 59] If the alternate anomalous pulmonary venous connection is not obstructive, the lobe or segment of lung drained by the anomalously connected but not obstructed pulmonary vein may exhibit less pulmonary edema on the chest radiograph. The levoatriocardial vein connects the left atrium to the brachiocephalic vein. The anatomy of this unusual systemic venous connection suggests persistence of the left superior vena cava terminating in the left atrium. A similar left atrial bypass is provided by a systemic vein that connects a normally terminating left upper pulmonary vein to the brachiocephalic vein. The pathologic and clinical recognition of the partially unroofed coronary sinus has received considerable attention. Though this congenital fenestration can occur in isolation, its most frequent association has been in the patient with severe left atrial obstruction. This fenestration is circular or elliptical, is usually less than 2.0 cm in its greatest dimension, and is situated in the posterior aspect of the floor of the left atrium.

The mitral valve is either atretic or stenotic (Fig. 27.2) in more than 95% of patients with hypoplastic left heart syndrome. When mitral atresia is present, this takes either the form of an imperforate connection or an absent connection.[104] Mitral stenosis is extremely common among patients exhibiting hypoplasia of the left ventricle and aorta. All components of the valve, including the annulus, mitral valve tissue, interchordal spaces, chordae tendineae, and papillary muscles participate in rendering the mitral valve obstructive.[94]

The left ventricle usually exhibits some degree of hypoplasia (Fig. 27.3).[15, 17, 22, 28, 51, 55, 56, 77, 93, 96, 101] There are important exceptions to this which will be discussed later. The left ventricle may be absent, and this is the situation when both aortic and mitral valves are atretic. A perforate, though stenotic mitral valve, almost always implies hypoplasia of the left ventricular cavity. There is frequently a disparity between the left ventricular cavity and left ventricular free wall (Fig. 27.4). The left ventricular myocardium is often rather spectacularly hypertrophied, and buried within the myocardium is a small slit-like cavity.

The left ventricular endocardium may be thickened and opaque, and histologic examination provides evidence of endocardial sclerosis.[10, 22] The papillary muscles of the mitral valve are underdeveloped, which is in distinct contrast to the degree of free wall left ventricular hypertrophy. The left ventricle usually exhibits hypoplasia, with its inlet, trabecular, and outlet zones affected.

The ductus arteriosus is usually left-sided and may appear con-

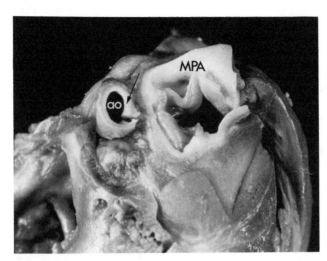

Fig. 27.1 Magnified transverse section of aortic (*ao*) and pulmonary roots (*MPA*) 0.5 cm distal to atretic aortic valve in a neonate with associated mitral atresia. Note the diminutive (2.0 mm), but thick-walled (*arrow*), ascending aorta (*ao*).

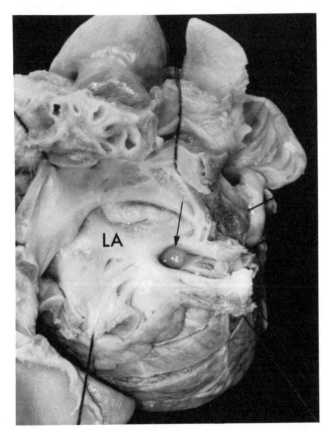

Fig. 27.2 Internal view of left atrium (*LA*) demonstrating a very stenotic but perforate mitral valve (*arrow*) in a neonate with aortic atresia.

a pattern that is theorized to result from sustained isometric contraction.[12] In other patients, the histologic features of the left ventricle are consistent with so-called persistence of spongy myocardium.[14] This disorder is characterized by the focal presence of the embryonic pattern of myoarchitecture with persistence of inter-

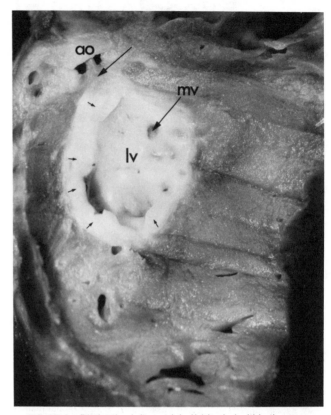

Fig. 27.3 Diminutive left ventricle (*lv*) buried within the myocardial mass in a neonate with aortic atresia. The subaortic infundibulum is atretic (*arrow*), separating the tiny left ventricle from the ascending aorta (*ao*). The endocardium of the left ventricle is sclerotic, and markedly thickened (*small black arrows*). The mitral valve (*mv*) is extremely stenotic.

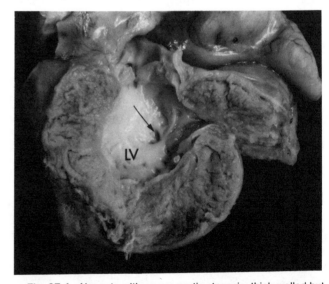

Fig. 27.4 Neonate with severe aortic stenosis, thick-walled but small left ventricle (*LV*); the endocardium is opaque and markedly thickened. This patient also had severe mitral stenosis (*arrow*).

stricted. In the rare situation of aortic atresia complicating atrial isomerism, a right-sided ductus might be encountered.

Some attention has been focused on the histologic appearance of the left ventricular endomyocardium.[22, 87] When the mitral valve is perforate, endocardial sclerosis is common, which may involve the left atrium as well. The left ventricular myocardial architecture is often disorganized, and the myocardial fiber disarray has suggested to some the features of hypertrophic obstructive cardiomyopathy, trabecular spaces and sinusoids which communicate both the ventricular lumen and coronary artery.[11, 19, 25, 37, 87]

Papillary muscle infarction and left ventricular subendocardial ischemia and infarction have also been observed,[69] which seems more common in patients with perforate aortic and mitral valves but with left ventricular hypoplasia. It is these patients who fall into the continuum of critical aortic stenosis and, in some patients, the left ventricular dimensions may approach the normal.[20]

The ascending aorta can vary in size, but is usually considerably smaller than the pulmonary artery.[15, 17, 22, 28, 51, 55, 56, 77, 93, 96, 101, 107, 108]

Anomalies of the Aortic Arch

Coarctation of the aorta (CA) can complicate hearts with aortic and mitral atresia or lesser forms of this disorder. Van Rueden et al.[111] studied the aortas of 41 specimens with aortic atresia to determine the frequency of CA.[111] Thirty-one instances were evident, but in 24 instances, the CA was considered mild, and in only seven was the obstruction considered major.

Interruption of the aortic arch can also complicate aortic valve atresia. Rosenquist et al.[92] first described this association in a neonate with a large ventricular septal defect (VSD) and a nearly normal left ventricle. This patient also had a congenital aorticopulmonary window that provided flow to the ascending aorta. Continuity with the descending aorta was provided by a left-sided patent ductus arteriosus (PDA). More recently, Neye-Bock and Fellows[76] have provided angiographic demonstration of aortic atresia, type C interruption of the aortic arch (between the innominate and left common carotid arteries), a large, probably infundibular VSD, and a normal left ventricle. This infant had bilateral ducti. The right PDA provided flow to the ascending aorta and in a retrograde direction to the coronary arteries and the innominate artery and its branches. A left PDA provided continuity with the descending thoracic aorta.

A right-sided aortic arch is extremely uncommon in the patient with the usual form of hypoplastic left heart syndrome. Indeed, we have not identified such a situation in over 200 necropsied patients. However, among some patients with visceroatrial heterotaxy and left atrial isomerism and dominant form of atrioventricular defect, a right aortic arch has been identified.

The Coronary Arteries

The aortic origins of the coronary arteries in this disorder are probably normal. Among some patients with aortic atresia, the ascending aorta and root are so diminutive that the aorta appears to terminate in the ramification of the coronary arteries. Left ventricular myocardial sinusoids connecting with the coronary arteries have been observed grossly and histologically; these have been demonstrated by selective left ventricular angiography. Yet, unlike the frequency of the comparable abnormality in patients with pulmonary atresia and intact ventricular septum,[83] this finding in patients with hypoplastic left heart syndrome is distinctly uncommon.

Disposition of the Conduction Tissue

There is little data on the disposition of the specialized conduction tissue among patients with the hypoplastic left heart syndrome. Bharati and Lev[7] have studied the course of the conduction system in two cases of "hypoplasia of the aortic tract complex," one with mitral stenosis and the other with mitral atresia.[7] Both demonstrated a posterior atrioventricular node which formed the AV bundle. In one, the bundle was short and bifurcated early. The branching bundle gave origin to a large left bundle branch, many Mahain fibers to the septum, and a small right bundle branch. In the other case, the AV node consisted of two parts which formed two posterior bundles which joined together to form a short branch-

ing bundle. The right bundle branch was large but inserted a discrete left bundle branch, and there were profuse Mahain fibers passing from the branching bundle to the depths of the ventricular septum.

Aortic Atresia and Normal Left Ventricle

A normal left ventricle is found in from 2 to 7% of patients with aortic atresia.[33, 35, 84, 85, 89, 105] With one well-documented exception,[23] a VSD has been present. Similarly, with one exception,[89] the mitral valve has been perforate.

Considerable attention has been focused on the morphology of the VSD among patients with aortic atresia and normal left ventricle. Although the VSD may involve the membranous or perimembranous septum, or the inlet septum (in the patient with atrioventricular defect),[39] our experience and that of others would suggest that in the majority of such patients, the VSD results from malalignment between the infundibular septum and the trabecula septomarginalis.[35] The caudally deviated infundibular septum is fused with the ventriculoinfundibular fold, virtually obliterating the subaortic vestibule (Fig. 27.5). Yet, in other patients, the VSD clearly results from a deficiency of the infundibular septum, without malalignment. Complete occlusion of the subaortic vestibule in these patients appears to result at least in part from persistence of the ventriculoinfundibular fold. The left ventricle in these patients is normally excavated, and left ventricular endocardial fibroelastosis

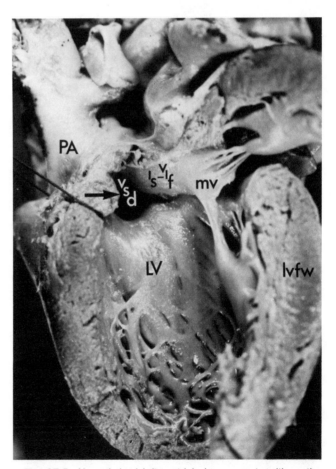

Fig. 27.5 Normal-sized left ventricle is a neonate with aortic atresia. Internal view of left ventricle (*LV*). The ventricular septal defect (*vsd*) results from fusion of the malaligned infundibular septum (*is*) with the ventriculoinfundibular fold (*vif*). The mitral valve (*mv*) inserts onto this muscular band. *PA*, pulmonary artery; *lvfw*, hypertrophied left ventricular free wall. (Modified from R. M. Freedom et al.[35])

has not been a feature. With the exception of the patient with mitral atresia reported by Roberts *et al.*[89] and the patient with complete form of atrioventricular defect reported by Freedom *et al.*,[39] the mitral valve has been consistently normal.

The left atrium is better developed in the patient with aortic atresia and normal left ventricle than in the patient with aortic atresia and hypoplasia of the left ventricle.[33, 35, 84, 85, 89, 105] We have not identified premature closure of the foramen ovale in the patient with aortic atresia and normal left ventricle. Among our 10 patients with this disorder, the aortic root and ascending aorta have been consistently diminutive.[33, 35]

Aortic Atresia and Atrioventricular Septal Defect

Aortic atresia (AA) can complicate the patient with atrioventricular septal defect.[6, 50, 52, 98, 100] Usually, the left ventricle is small, and the type of heart would conform to that characterized as having a dominant right form of atrioventricular orifice. In this constellation, the majority of the common atrioventricular orifice is committed to the morphologic right ventricle.[6, 29, 86] The mitral component of the common atrioventricular orifice is either stenotic or atretic (or, rarely, imperforate). The subaortic vestibule is occluded by maladherent and attached anterior leaflet of the mitral component of the common orifice, and accessory tissue tags may also participate in compromising flow through the subaortic ventibule.[29]

The ventricular component of the atrioventricular septal defect in this situation is usually small, and the interatrial communication is not usually restrictive. As in the patient with the usual form of hypoplastic left heart syndrome, systemic blood flow is dependent on the PDA. Isomeric left atria and splenic anomalies have been identified in some patients.

Aortic Atresia and Transposition of the Great Arteries

Only one such case has been reported. The patient was 4 years of age, mildly cyanosed and not in gross heart failure.[63] This patient had an enlarged heart with pulmonary plethora, and the electrocardiogram demonstrated right atrial enlargement, left ventricular hypertrophy, and an interventricular conduction delay. Hemodynamic investigation demonstrated an oxygen saturation of 90% in the ascending aorta, a right ventricular pressure of 230/20 mm Hg, and a left ventricular pressure of 75/8 mm Hg. The peak systolic pressure in the ascending aorta was 70 mm Hg, and that in the descending aorta was 80 mm Hg.

Angiocardiography revealed atrioventricular concordance. The morphological right ventricle supported the discordantly connected transposed aorta. The right ventricle was underdeveloped, and the right ventricular infundibulum was severely hypoplastic with atresia of the aortic valve. The ascending aorta opacified via right ventricular myocardial sinusoids which connected with the coronary arteries. The morphological left ventricle supported the transposed pulmonary artery, and the ductus arteriosus was widely patent. The ventricular septum was intact in this patient.

Aortic Atresia and Univentricular Heart

Aortic atresia can complicate the univentricular heart, but this association is very uncommon (Fig. 27.6). The most convincing examples of this constellation have been in the patient with single left ventricle, an infundibular outlet chamber, and discordantly connected, transposed great arteries.[36, 38, 110] The pertinent morphologic features in such hearts have previously been recorded. The outlet foramen (the foramen between the main left ventricle and the infundibular outlet chamber) is sealed or diminutive, and systemic blood flow is ductal dependent. The infundibular chamber is tiny, and the aortic valve is imperforate. McCartney and Anderson[61] have reported the angiographic features in such a patient. The diminutive ascending aorta occupies the leftward and superior heart border, and in the lateral projection is clearly anterior to the dilated

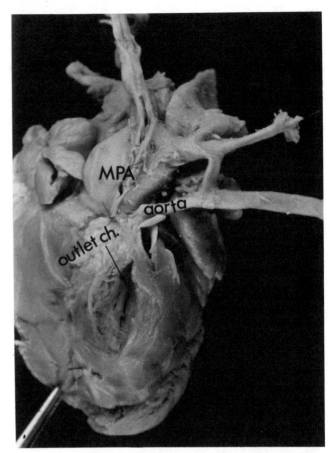

Fig. 27.6 External view of heart with single left ventricle, left-sided outlet chamber (*outlet ch.*) supporting a levo-positioned discordantly connected transposed aorta. The main pulmonary artery (*MPA*) is considerably larger than the ascending aorta (*ao*). There is aortic atresia and an intact outlet foramen. (Modified from R. M. Freedom *et al.*[36])

pulmonary artery. Only one such patient has been identified at the Hospital for Sick Children in Toronto. Both atrioventricular valves were normally formed, and they were connected to the left ventricle. The left atrium was enlarged, and a small defect of the fossa ovalis was present.

Aortic Atresia and Corrected Transposition of the Great Arteries

Brenner *et al.*[9] first described aortic atresia complicating corrected transposition of the great arteries (discordant atrioventricular and ventriculoarterial connections). This patient also had a congenitally unguarded left (tricuspid) atrioventricular orifice, and the right ventricular free-wall myocardium (left-sided) exhibited a Uhl-like deformity.

The Pulmonary Circulation in Aortic Atresia

Haworth and Reid[46] have established that the structure of the pulmonary circulation is modified by antenatal abnormalities in blood flow that occur through the heart and great vessels in the presence of congenital heart disease.[46] These authors have demonstrated that fetal multiplication in intra-acinar arteries in aortic atresia and stenosis is increased as in the muscularity of both pre- and intra-acinar arteries and veins. The muscularity represents both an increase in the wall thickness of normally muscular vessels as well as, by extension, an increase of muscle in vessels that do not normally contain it at this age.[44, 75]

FREQUENCY

Data from The New England Regional Infant Cardiac Program indicates a case discovery rate of 0.163/1000 live births.[41] The frequency of this malformation in infants in the New England study was 7.4%, and 9% in data from our institution.[49]

GENETICS

Several examples of hypoplastic left heart syndrome have been reported in siblings,[8, 88, 99] and autosomal recessive transmission has been suggested as the mode of inheritance on the basis of one study. However, Holmes et al.[47] suggest that a multifactorial mode of inheritance is most compatible with their data. Furthermore, their data revealed a recurrence risk in sibs of 0.5% for hypoplastic left heart syndrome, and 2.2% for all types of congenital heart defects.[47, 78] An experimental model has also been reported.[45]

MANIFESTATIONS

Clinical Features

There is a male predominance (67%) among patients with hypoplastic left ventricle, and slightly over 10% have associated extracardiac malformations. The birth weight is usually normal. Nearly 40% of babies with hypoplastic left syndrome come to medical attention within the first 2 days of life, another 35% by 6 days, and by 13 days, 86% of such patients will have come to medical attention. Nearly 95% of all such affected infants will have died within the first month of life.[42]

Cyanosis is rarely conspicuous at delivery but usually appears within hours or several days.[70, 77, 113] The nailbeds may appear even duskier than the mucous membranes, reflecting an inadequate systemic output. One-third of these babies present in a state of vascular collapse. They exhibit tachypnea and dyspnea, with some having agonal respirations. The blood pressures in all extremities may be 40 mm Hg or less. The babies are hypothermic and grunting, with flaring of the ala nasae, and they have an ashen color.

Heart failure is inevitable in this disorder, and tachycardia, tachypnea, enlargement of the liver, and a gallop rhythm are present in most babies. A left precordial bulge is present in nearly all of the patients but is conspicuous in one-third.

Auscultation usually reveals crisp, loud heart sounds. The second sound is single, and a pulmonary ejection click reflecting pulmonary artery hypertension and a dilated pulmonary artery may be present. Nearly all of the patients have a soft systolic ejection murmur, and some have an apical mid-diastolic murmur, indicative of high flow across the tricuspid valve.

The femoral pulses are certainly variable in volume and reflect the general circulatory status, unless there is a coexistent thoracic coarctation. In those babies not in vascular collapse, the brachial and femoral pulses have equal amplitude. Pulses may be absent in all extremities in these babies exhibiting vascular collapse. Varying degrees of metabolic acidosis, hypoglycemia, and hyperkalemia may be present, due to restricted systemic perfusion.

Electrocardiographic Features

Most show sinus tachycardia. The mean frontal QRS axis is usually +90 to +210°. Unless there is right or left atrial isomerism, the mean frontal P axis is about +60°, and the P waves are greater than 2.0 mm and peaked, indicative of right atrial enlargement.

Right ventricular hypertrophy is almost always present, and in about 40%, a qR pattern is present in the right precordial leads. The left precordial leads usually display a paucity of left ventricular forces, and rS pattern is typical (Fig. 27.7)[112] Left ventricular hypertrophy is distinctly uncommon.[103] Even among those patients with aortic atresia, large VSD, and normal left ventricle, a pattern of right ventricular hypertrophy is more consistently observed.[85]

Because many of these babies are seen in the first 24 hours of life, it is not surprising that a positive T wave is observed in the right precordial leads. Diffuse ST-T wave segment abnormalities may be observed, and these usually reflect coronary insufficiency resulting from ductal restriction and inadequate retrograde aortic blood flow.[93] Wolff-Parkinson-White syndrome is occasionally observed, and complete right bundle branch block has also been observed.

The Frank vectorcardiogram will demonstrate a clockwise frontal loop, with the loop in the horizontal plane clockwise, rightward, and anterior. It is distinctly unusual to record significant posterior and inferior vectors in this group of infants.

Radiological Features

No single radiographic pattern is diagnostic of aortic or mitral atresia or the somewhat less severe forms of this disorder. Most patients demonstrate levocardia and visceral situs solitus. The heart is enlarged, often to a moderate or severe degree. The heart exhibits a globular shape, and the right heart border is frequently conspicuous, indicative of right atrial enlargement (Fig. 27.8). Folger and Saied[26] called attention to a feature which they felt to be diagnostic of aortic atresia. This was the absence of the shadow of the ascending aorta, which produced in the right aspect of the cardiac silhouette an angulation at the junction of the superior vena cava and the right atrial shadow. This configuration resulted in the appearance of the numeral 5 in reverse. While the radiographs published by these authors were quite

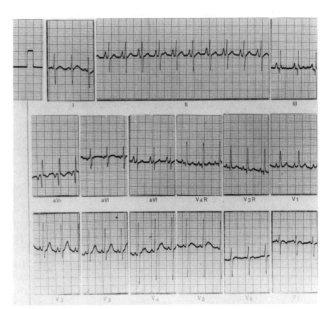

Fig. 27.7 Electrocardiogram of a 5 day old with aortic and mitral atresia. Right axis deviation of +150° is evident. Peaked P waves in *lead II* are consistent with right atrial enlargement. A qR pattern is evident in the right precordial leads, but the left chest leads do not exhibit septal q-waves. The T wave is positive in the right chest leads, and is diphasic in *V₇*.

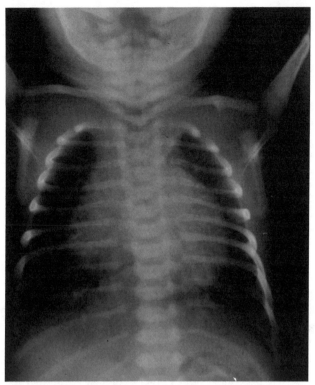

Fig. 27.8 Radiograph of same patient as in Figure 27.6. The heart is enlarged and pulmonary plethora is conspicuous.

convincing, this sign has not been frequently observed among our patients.

The pattern of pulmonary vascular markings in these patients is variable. They may appear nearly normal, especially among those babies presenting within a few hours of birth. However, it is more common to find evidence of both pulmonary plethora as well as pulmonary edema. Some patients may exhibit intense pulmonary edema. When only mild cardiomegaly is present in the patient with intense pulmonary edema, the chest radiograph may be indistinguishable from the patient with the obstructed form of total anomalous pulmonary venous connection.

Rarely, mesocardia or dextrocardia with evidence of thoracic isomerism and visceral heterotaxia will be observed. Such patients may have associated splenic anomalies, with polysplenia more common than asplenia.

Echocardiographic Features

The echocardiographic findings reflect the basic anatomic heterogeneity of this syndrome.[2, 4, 24, 43, 54, 60, 64, 72, 95] With the severest form of this disorder, M-mode echocardiographic examination reveals an enlarged right ventricle, increased tricuspid valve excursion, and a large pulmonary artery. The mitral vavle often cannot be visualized. When mitral valve tissue is present, and the valve is perforate but stenotic, these features are reflected in the recording. The left ventricle is usually absent in patients with aortic and mitral atresia. An absent or minute left ventricle and an anterior mitral leaflet excursion of 5.0 mm or less is diagnostic of hypoplastic left ventricle. Among most patients with aortic atresia, some aortic valve motion can be recorded (Fig. 27.9). The presence of an aortic root of 5.0 mm or less is consistent with aortic atresia, although in some patients with necropsy-proven aortic atresia, the dimensions of the aortic root are normal.

The left atrium is usually small in the neonate with aortic and mitral atresia.

With 2D echocardiography, one can readily image the greatly enlarged right heart chambers and pulmonary artery, and the grossly underdeveloped left heart chambers and aorta. The apical long axis views have readily allowed visualization of the aortic root size, dimensions of the left ventricle, and function of the mitral valve. The apical short axis projection provides a good view of the size of the left ventricle (Fig. 27.10).

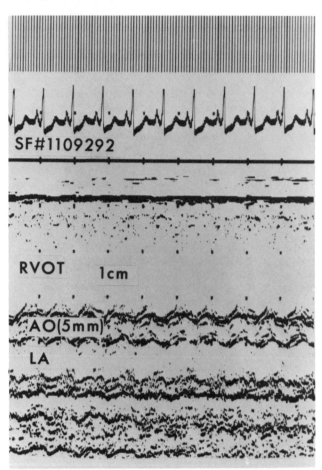

Fig. 27.9 M-mode echocardiogram consistent with hypoplastic left heart syndrome with a 5.0-mm aortic root (*AO*) and small left atrium (*LA*). RVOT, right ventricular outflow tract. (Courtesy of Walter J. Duncan, M.D., formerly Director of Section of Echocardiography, Division of Cardiology, The Hospital for Sick Children, Toronto.)

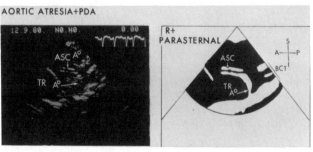

Fig. 27.10 2D echocardiogram performed in the right parasternal projection demonstrating a diminutive ascending aorta (*Asc. A°*) and small transverse aortic arch (*TRA°*).

CARDIAC CATHETERIZATION

The hemodynamic findings are quite variable, reflecting the heterogeneity of the cardiac malformations embraced by the term hypoplastic left heart syndrome, as well as by the clinical status of the patient.[53] Some patients may appear reasonably comfortable and stable, while others are moribund, intubated, and receiving continuous pressure applied to the airway, as well as supplemental oxygen.

When aortic and mitral atresia are present, obligatory left-to-right shunting at atrial level and right-to-left shunting through the PDA are present. The systemic venous saturations are frequently low, indicating a low cardiac output and heart failure. A rise in oxygen saturation is appreciated in the right atrium, right ventricule and pulmonary artery. The ascending and descending aortic saturations reflect the pulmonary artery saturation, but there is considerable variability. When marked pulmonary venous obstruction is present, right-to-left intrapulmonary shunting may be profound, and the systemic arterial oxygen saturation will be considerably lower than when pulmonary venous obstruction is less severe. When both aortic and mitral valves are perforate (though obstructive), the systemic arterial oxygen saturation is usually higher. Thus, systemic arterial oxygen saturation is higher in those patients with the highest pulmonary-systemic blood flow ratios.

Right heart pressures are usually markedly elevated, with right atrial pressures reflecting the degree of heart failure. Right ventricular and main pulmonary artery peak systolic pressures are equal to or exceed systemic arterial pressure. This observation reflects a degree of narrowing of the ductus arteriosus.

Miller[65] called attention to episodes of severe bradycardia which occurred when the catheter traversed a restrictive ductus arteriosus or when a retrograde arterial catheter was advanced into the ascending aorta towards the aortic root. Both maneuvers resulted in inadequate coronary blood flow, further myocardial ischemia, and bradycardia. Van der Horst and Hastreiter[106] have provided hemodynamic evidence that the diminutive ascending aorta may by itself obstruct retrograde coronary blood flow in some patients with aortic atresia.

Left atrial pressure usually reflects the adequacy of the interatrial communication. It may not be possible to probe the left atrium when the atrial communication is diminutive. The pulmonary capillary wedge pressure in this situation should provide the same information.

Finally, the hemodynamics in some patients with perforate though obstructive aortic and mitral valves can be consistent with severe aortic stenosis. A pressure gradient may be recorded between left ventricle and aorta, while right ventricular and pulmonary artery pressures are systemic, or higher. Left atrial or wedge pressures will reflect the degree of mitral valve disease, heart failure, or both.

ANGIOCARDIOGRAPHY

A number of papers and textbooks have addressed themselves to the angiocardiographic diagnosis of aortic atresia and the syndrome,[17, 30, 31, 32, 74, 91, 93] Selective injections of contrast material into the right ventricle and main pulmonary artery may allow diagnosis of aortic atresia by demonstrating late opacification of a small ascending aorta to the right of the pulmonary artery. Similarly, a venous catheter positioned in the descending thoracic aorta at ductal level should provide definition of the caliber of the descending aorta, as well as demonstrate a possible associated coarctation of aorta. However, retrograde aortography should provide the

clearest demonstration of the ascending aorta, its root, and the epicardial distribution of the coronary arteries.[74]

The aortic root exhibits considerable heterogeneity in appearance (Figs. 27.11 and 27.12).[31] The dimensions of the aortic root may appear nearly normal, or the aortic root may

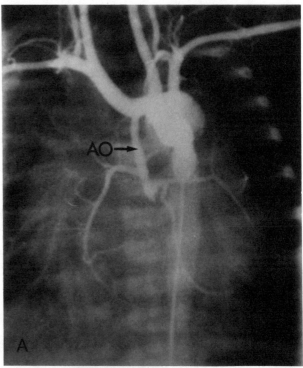

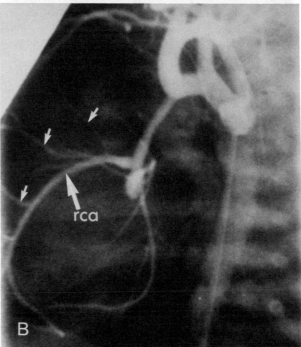

Fig. 27.11 Frontal (*A*) and lateral (*B*) retrograde aortogram in a neonate with necropsy-proven aortic atresia. (*A*) Note the diminutive ascending aorta (*AO*) that seems to terminate in the coronary arteries. (*B*) This lateral aortogram opacifies the atretic aortic root and the dominant right coronary artery (*rca*) with enlarged infundibular or conal branches (*small white arrows*).

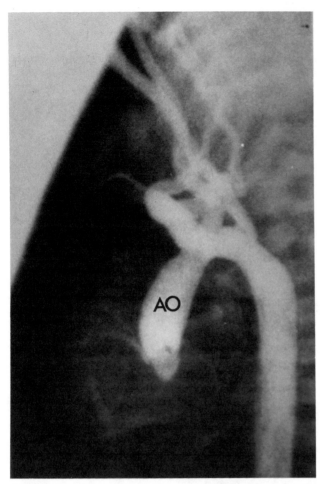

Fig. 27.12 Aortic atresia with nearly normal-sized aortic root (*AO*) with bicuspid imperforate aortic valve and mitral stenosis.

appear diminutive, virtually terminating in the coronary arteries. Usually, the aorta begins to taper at the level of the innominate artery, having its smallest dimension at the root itself. Less commonly, the aortic root appears bulbous, tapering towards the brachiocephalic vessels. Among some patients with aortic atresia, the imperforate but membranous valve demonstrates systolic and diastolic excursion. This observation is consistent with a perforate, though usually stenotic, mitral valve and functional left ventricle.

The epicardial distribution of the coronary arteries can give some idea of the dimensions of the left ventricle. However, the epicardial distribution of the left anterior descending coronary artery and the circumflex give only an estimate of the entire left ventricle—not the functional cavity. Thus, among some patients with a small left ventricular cavity but markedly hypertrophied free wall, the epicardial distribution may suggest normal dimension when, in reality, the cavity is small. Single plane umbilical aortography may be diagnostic of aortic atresia, but a biplane mode is necessary to define the epicardial distribution of the coronary arteries.[91] Rarely, myocardial sinusoids connecting with the left ventricle may terminate in the coronary artery, analogous to the same situation among patients with pulmonary atresia with intact ventricular septum. Because coarctation of the aorta can complicate aortic atresia, it may be necessary to perform an aortogram in the descending aorta at the ductal level. In the uncommon situation of aortic atresia and complete interruption of the aortic arch, one must define how the ascending aorta is perfused, i.e., via an aorticopulmonary window, or via a right-sided PDA.[26]

Biplane left atriography filmed in frontal and lateral or in the hepatoclavicular four-chamber projections[3] should demonstrate: the size of the left atrium and its true anlage, the left atrial apendage; the functional status of the mitral valve[62]; the site and size of the interatrial communication; and the presence of anomalous systemic venous connections. Unlike the right atrium in patients with pulmonary atresia with intact ventricular septum or tricuspid atresia, the left atrium is rarely enlarged. Rather, it is often small and thick walled. In the presence of an absent or imperforate mitral connection, left atrial angiography will show a flat or curvilinear appearance to the left atrial floor. Reflux of contrast material into distended pulmonary veins is indicative of a small interatrial communication. The presence of the so-called unroofed coronary sinus (left atrial-coronary sinus) can be demonstrated by left atriography.[34]

Selective left atriography is ideal to identify the functional status of the mitral valve. The levophase of a pulmonary arteriogram rarely provides enough detail about the mitral valve. Among most patients with hypoplastic left heart syndrome and a perforate but stenotic mitral valve, the mitral annulus is small, and leaflet, chordae, and papillary muscles are abnormal, all participating in the obstruction to left ventricular filling.

The left ventricle can vary in size from absent to normal in size (Fig. 27.13). With aortic and mitral atresia, the left ventricle is almost never opacified. The one exception here is the rare situation in which the presence of a VSD allows some development of the left ventricle. However, among patients with aortic atresia and a normal left ventricle, nearly all will have a perforate mitral valve and a large VSD. The VSD is often infundibular, and thus it can be profiled in the right and left long axial oblique projections (Fig. 27.14). For the rare patient with aortic atresia, normal left ventricle, and atrioventricular defect,[39] the inlet portion of the ventricular

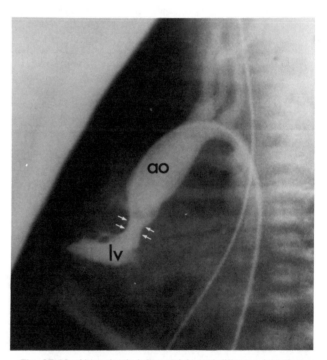

Fig. 27.13 Hypoplastic left ventricle and diffuse subaortic narrowing in a neonate with hypoplastic transverse aortic arch and large PDA who clinically was considered to have aortic atresia. This diastolic right posterior oblique left ventriculogram (*lv*) demonstrates the small left ventricle, diffuse subaortic narrowing (*white arrows*), and a slightly larger ascending aorta (*ao*).

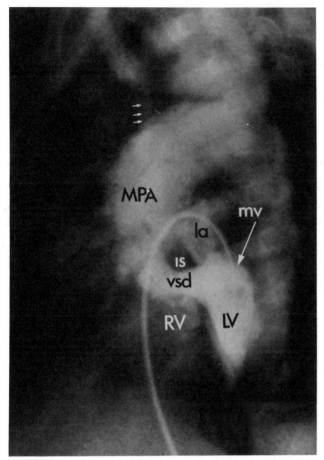

Fig. 27.14 Normal left ventricle in an infant with aortic atresia, malalignment-type VSD, and normal left ventricle. This long axial oblique left ventriculogram (*LV*) via the mitral valve (*mv*) demonstrates the posteriorly deviated infundibular septum (*is*) with the VSD immediately below. The right ventricle (*RV*) is opacified by left-to-right shunting at ventricular level. The main pulmonary trunk (*MPA*) is much enlarged. There is faint opacification of the small ascending aorta (*white arrows*). *la*, left atrium.

septum can best be profiled in the hepatoclavicular four-chamber projection.[102]

The rare variants of aortic atresia with complete[63] or corrected transposition[9] of the great arteries will have to be defined by selective right and left ventriculography, as well as by selective aortography.

DIFFERENTIAL DIAGNOSIS

Among neonates presenting in the first few days of life with intractable heart failure and varying degrees of cyanosis, any structural cardiac anomaly producing severe impedance to systemic blood flow must be considered in the differential diagnosis.[66] Thus, coarctation of the aorta or interruption of the aortic arch, critical aortic stenosis, and combinations must be considered. In all these conditions, a shock-like clinical picture can be seen, virtually indistinguishable from that observed in the patient with aortic and mitral atresia. Occasionally, a neonate with severely obstructed total anomalous pulmonary venous connection may have a similar presentation.

Nonstructural cardiac disorders must also be anticipated. These include: neonatal myocarditis, transient myocardial ischemia, intrauterine supraventricular tachycardia, and large systemic arteriovenous fistula. Each of these conditions

can mimic the hypoplastic left heart syndrome. Similarly, cardiac neoplasms, especially the rhabdomyoma which can obstruct the left ventricular outflow or the mitral orifice, must be considered. This clinical differential diagnosis is usually easily resolved by M-mode and 2D echocardiographic techniques, and cardiac catheterization can thus be avoided in neonates with nonstructural heart disease.

TREATMENT

For many years, the patient with hypoplastic left heart syndrome has been considered to have inoperable and thus fatal congenital heart disease—despite a few surviving past their first birthday and case reports of short-term palliative surgery. Recently, there has been a resurgence of interest in the palliation of these infants.[1, 13, 18, 57, 67, 68, 71, 79–81] There are at least several factors which may have influenced this posture. First, the hypoplastic left heart syndrome accounts for about 10% of neonates dying with structural congenital heart disease. Secondly, one can view the pathology of many patients with hypoplastic left heart syndrome as similar to that of the patient with a univentricular heart and, finally, the surgical concept of atriopulmonary diversion allows flexibility in the treatment of patients with complex congenital heart disease.

Certain patients will not be candidates for palliation. Those neonates with severe metabolic acidosis and shock, hypotension, hemorrhagic diathesis, or coexisting severe extracardiac anomalies should probably not be considered as surgical candidates. Because those cardiac malformations embraced by the term hypoplastic left heart syndrome are so heterogeneous, some patients solely on anatomic grounds might prove better candidates for palliation. Thus, the patient with aortic and mitral atresia (and absent left ventricle) could be viewed as a better candidate than the patient with aortic atresia, perforate but stenotic mitral valve, and diminutive and presumably hypertensive left ventricle. In this latter situation, the small and hypertensive left ventricle is unlikely to ever be satisfactorily decompressed, and the sustained pattern of isometric contraction[12] with its myocardial fiber disarray may jeopardize the integrity of both right and left ventricular myocardium (analogous to the patient with pulmonary atresia, intact ventricular septum, and diminutive and hypertensive right ventricle).

The immediate medical therapy must be directed at the treatment of heart failure and maintenance of patency of the ductus arteriosus. The judicious use of digoxin and diuretics themselves is but an important adjuvant to endotracheal intubation and the application of continued positive pressure to the airway. The administration of an E-type prostaglandin is essential to short-term maintenance of ductal patency. When possible, one would like to perform a balloon atrioseptostomy to decompress the small and restrictive left atrium.

Surgical therapy in the neonate must be directed at maintenance of adequate systemic perfusion, protection of the pulmonary vascular bed, and decompression of the left atrium by using balloon atrioseptostomy, blade atrioseptectomy,[82] or open or closed atrial septectomy.

Adequate systemic perfusion necessitates bypassing the constricting ductus arteriosus. This can be achieved by interposing a conduit between the right ventricle and the descending thoracic aorta, by interposing a conduit between the main pulmonary artery and descending thoracic aorta, or by anastomosis of the proximal end of the divided main pulmonary artery to a longitudinal incision in the ascending aorta and aortic arch. Pulmonary blood flow for this third procedure is established with a Gortex tube graft central shunt from the newly constructed ascending aorta to the confluence of the pulmonary arteries. Protection of the

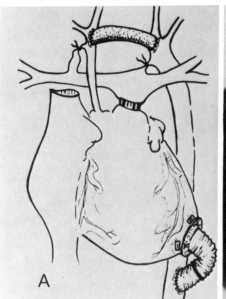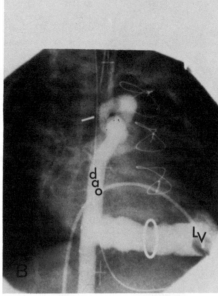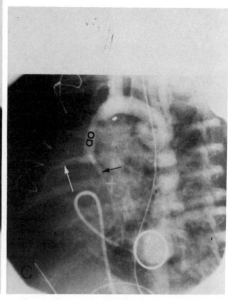

Fig. 27.15 Palliative surgery in an infant with aortic atresia, VSD, and type C interruption of the aortic arch. Palliation was accomplished by interposition of a 12-mm Hancock composite valved conduit between the apex of the left ventricle and the descending thoracic aorta; by interposition of an 8.0-mm graft between the ascending aorta and descending thoracic aorta at the level of the left ductus arteriosus; and by ligation of both ductus arteriosi and pulmonary artery banding. At a later date, the VSD was closed, and the pulmonary artery was debanded. The initial palliative operation is depicted in schematic form in A. (B) Injection of contrast material through a catheter positioned in the apex of the left ventricle (LV) fills the apical-aortic conduit and the descending thoracic aorta (dao). (C) A later frame shows retrograde flow to the ascending aorta (ao), with opacification of the coronary arteries (arrows). (Courtesy of Dr. William Norwood and modified from W. I. Norwood and G. I. Stellin.[81])

pulmonary arteries in the first two palliative approaches is accomplished by banding of the pulmonary artery (Fig. 27.15). Other palliative procedures designed to maintain systemic blood flow have included construction of a descending thoracic aorta-pulmonary artery anastomosis with banding of the individual pulmonary arteries, a similar procedure utilizing a more proximal (i.e., Waterston-like) approach. In all of these procedures, systemic venous blood flow will

eventually be diverted to the pulmonary arteries (modified Fontan procedure), and the pulmonary venous blood will be directed through the tricuspid valve with an interatrial baffle to the anatomic right ventricle and, thence, to the aorta. This approach effectively bypasses the left ventricle, but the morphologic right ventricle will support the systemic circulation.

REFERENCES

1. Albert, H. M., and Bryant, L. R.: A proposed technique for treatment of hypoplastic left heart syndrome. J. Cardiovasc. Surg. 19:257, 1978.
2. Allen, H. D., Sahn, D. J., and Goldberg, S. J.: Caveats in echocardiographic diagnosis, the hypoplastic left heart syndrome (abstr.). Circulation 56 (Suppl. 3):III–40, 1977.
3. Bargeron, L. M., Jr., Elliott, L. P., Soto, B., Bream, P. R., and Curry, G. C.: Axial cineangiography in congenital heart disease. Section I. Concept, technical, and anatomic considerations. Circulation, 56:1075, 1977.
4. Bass, J. L., Ben-Shachar, C., and Edwards, J. E.: Comparison of M-mode echocardiography and pathologic findings in the hypoplastic left heart syndrome. Am. J. Cardiol. 45:79, 1980.
5. Beckman, C. B., Moller, J. H., and Edwards, J. E.: Alternate pathways to pulmonary venous flow in left-sided obstructive anomalies. Circulation 52:509, 1975.
6. Bharati, S., and Lev, M.: The spectrum of common atrioventricular orifice (canal). Am. Heart J. 86:553, 1973.
7. Bharati, S., and Lev, M.: The conduction system in hypoplasia of the aortic tract complex. Circulation 59:1324, 1979.
8. Bjornstad, P. G., and Michalsen, H.: Coexistent mitral and aortic valve atresia with intact ventricular septum in sibs. Br. Heart J. 36:302, 1974.

9. Brenner, J. I., Bharati, S., Winn, W. C., Jr., and Lev, M.: Absent tricuspid valve with aortic atresia in mixed levocardia (atria situs solitus, L-loop). Circulation, 57:836, 1978.
10. Bryan, C. S., and Oppenheimer, E. H.: Ventricular endocardial fibroelastosis. Basis for its presence or absence in cases of pulmonic and aortic atresia. Arch. Pathol. 87:82, 1969.
11. Buhlmeyer, K., Simon, B., Mocellin, R., and Sauer, U.: Clinical angiocardiographic and functional studies in the assessment of critical valvular aortic stenosis. In Paediatric Cardiology, Vol. 2, Heart Disease in the Newborn, edited by M. J. Godman and R. M. Marquis, Churchill Livingstone, Edinburgh, 1979, p. 220.
12. Bulkley, B. H., Weisfeld, M. L., and Hutchins, G. M.: Isometric cardiac contraction. A possible cause of the disorganized myocardial pattern of idiopathic hypertrophic subaortic stenosis. N. Engl. J. Med. 296:135, 1977.
13. Cayler, G. C., Smeloff, E. A., and Miller, G. E., Jr.: Surgical palliation of hypoplastic left side of the heart. N. Engl. J. Med. 282:780, 1970.
14. Chenard, J., Samson, M., and Beaulieu, M.: Embryonal sinusoids in the myocardium. Report of a case successfully treated surgically. Can. Med. Assoc. J. 92:1356, 1965.
15. Deely, W. J., Ehlers, K. H., Levin, A., and Engle, M. A.: Hypoplastic left heart syn-

drome. Anatomic, physiologic, and therapeutic considerations. Am. J. Dis. Child. 121:168, 1971.
16. De Tommasi, S. M., Daliento, L., Ho, S. Y., Macartney, F. J., and Anderson, R. H.: Analysis of atrioventricular junction, ventricular mass, and ventriculoarterial junction in 43 specimens with atrial isomerism. Br. Heart J. 45:236, 1981.
17. Didier, F., Hoeffel, J-C., Worms, A-M., Henry, M., Lerbier, N., and Pernot, C.: Etude anatomo-radiologique du syndrome d'hypoplasie du coeur gauche. A propos de 72 observations. Ann. Radiol., 19:673, 1976.
18. Doty, D. B., Marvin, W. J., Jr., Schieken, R. M., and Lauer, R. M.: Hypoplastic left heart syndrome. Successful palliation with a new operation. J. Thorac. Cardiovasc. Surg. 80: 148, 1980.
19. Dusek, J., Ostadal, B., and Duskova, M.: Postnatal persistence of spongy myocardium with embryonic blood supply. Arch. Pathol. 99:312, 1975.
20. Edmunds, L. H., Jr., Wagner, H. R., and Heymann, M. A.: Aortic valvulotomy in neonates. Circulation 61:421, 1980.
21. Edwards, J. E., and Dushane, J. W.: Thoracic venous anomalies. Arch. Pathol. 49:517, 1950.
22. Essed, C. E., Klein, H. W., Krediet, P., and Vorst, E. J.: Coronary and endocardial fibroelastosis of the ventricles in the hypoplastic

left and right heart syndromes. Virchows Arch. Path. Anat. Histol. 368:87, 1975.
23. Esteban, I., and Cabrera, A.: Aortic atresia with normal left ventricle and intact ventricular septum. Chest 73:883, 1978.
24. Farooki, Z. Q., Henry, J. G., and Green, E. W.: Echocardiographic spectrum of the hypoplastic left heart syndrome. A clinicopathologic correlation in 19 newborns. Am. J. Cardiol. 38:337, 1976.
25. Feldt, R. H., Rahimtoola, S. H., Davis, G. D., Swan, H. J. C., and Titus, J. L.: Anomalous ventricular myocardial patterns in a child with complex congenital heart disease. Am. J. Cardiol. 23:732, 1969.
26. Folger, G. M., Jr., and Saied, A.: A new roentgenographic sign of hypoplastic left heart. Chest 64:298, 1973.
27. Freedom, R. M.: Aortic valve and arch anomalies in the congenital asplenia syndrome. Case report, literature review and re-examination of the embryology of the congenital asplenia syndrome. Johns Hopkins Med. J. 135:124, 1974.
28. Freedom, R. M.: Aortic atresia. In Heart Disease in Infancy and Childhood edited by J. D. Keith, R. D. Rowe, and P. Vlad. MacMillan, New York, 1978, p. 542.
29. Freedom, R. M., Bini, M., and Rowe, R. D.: Endocardial cushion defect and significant hypoplasia of the left ventricle: A distinct clinical and pathological entity. Eur. J. Cardiol., 7:263, 1978.
30. Freedom, R. M., Culham, J. A. G., and Moes, C. A. F.: The Angiocardiography of Congenital Heart Disease. MacMillan, New York, in press, 1982.
31. Freedom, R. M., Culham, J. A. G., Moes, C. A. F., and Harrington, D. P.: Selective aortic root angiography in the hypoplastic left heart syndrome. Eur. J. Cardiol. 4:25, 1976.
32. Freedom, R. M., Culham, J. A. G., and Rowe, R. D.: Angiocardiography of subaortic obstruction in infancy. Am. J. Roentgenol. 129:813, 1977.
33. Freedom, R. M., Culham, J. A. G., and Rowe, R. D.: Aortic atresia with normal left ventricle. Distinctive angiocardiographic findings. Cath. Cardiovasc. Diagn. 3:283, 1972.
34. Freedom, R. M., Culham, J. A. G., and Rowe, R. D.: Left atrial-coronary sinus fenestration (partially unroofed coronary sinus): Morphological and angiocardiographic observations. Br. Heart J. 46:63, 1981.
35. Freedom, R. M., Dische, M. R., and Rowe, R. D.: Conal anatomy in aortic atresia, ventricular septal defect, and normally developed left ventricle. Am. Heart J. 94:689, 1977.
36. Freedom, R. M., Dische, M. R., and Rowe, R. D.: Pathologic anatomy of subaortic stenosis and atresia in the first year of life. Am. J. Cardiol. 39:1035, 1977.
37. Freedom, R. M., Patel, R. G., Bloom, K. R., Duckworth, J. W. A., Silver, M. M., Dische, R., and Rowe, R. D.: Congenital absence of the pulmonary valve associated with imperforate membrane type of tricuspid atresia, right ventricular tensor apparatus and intact ventricular septum: A curious development complex. Eur. J. Cardiol. 10:171, 1979.
38. Freedom, R. M., and Rowe, R. D.: Morphological and topographical variations of the outlet chamber in complex congenital heart disease: An angiocardiographic study. Cath. Cardiovasc. Diagn. 4:345, 1978.
39. Freedom, R. M., Williams, W. G., Dische, M. R., and Rowe, R. D.: Anatomical variants in aortic atresia. Potential candidates for ventriculoaortic reconstitution. Br. Heart J. 38:821, 1976.
40. Friedberg, D. Z., Gallen, W. J., Oechler, H., and Glicklich, M.: Ivemark syndrome with aortic atresia. Am. J. Dis. Child. 126:106, 1973.
41. Fyler, D. C.: Report of the New England

Regional Infant Cardiac Program. Pediatrics 65 (No. 2, Part 2) (Suppl.):436, 1980.
42. Fyler, D. C., Rothman, K. J., Bulkley, L. P., Cohn, H. E., Hellenbrand, W. E., and Castaneda, A.: The determinants of five year survival of infants with critical congenital heart disease. In Pediatric Cardiovascular Disease, Cardiovascular Clinics, edited by M. A. Engle. F. A. Davis, Philadelphia, 1981, p. 393.
43. Goldberg, S. J., Allen, H. D., and Sahn, D. J.: Pediatric and adolescent echocardiography. Year Book Medical Publishers, Chicago, 1980, p. 243.
44. Grant, C. A., Robertson, B.: Microangiography of the pulmonary arterial system in "hypoplastic left heart syndrome." Circulation 45:382, 1972.
45. Harh, J. Y., Paul, M. H., Gallen, W. J., Friedberg, D. Z., and Kaplan, S.: Experimental production of hypoplastic left heart syndrome in the chick embryo. Am. J. Cardiol. 31:51, 1973.
46. Haworth, S. G., and Reid, L.: Quantitative structural study of pulmonary circulation in the newborn with aortic atresia, stenosis, or coarctation. Thorax 32:121, 1977.
47. Holmes, L. B., Rose, V., and Child, A. H.: Comment on hypoplastic left heart syndrome, in clinical delineation of birth defects. XVI. Urinary system and others. Baltimore, Williams & Wilkins, 1972, pp. 228–230.
48. Hunt, C. E., Rao, S., Moller, J. H., and Edwards, J. E.: Anomalous pulmonary vein serving as collateral channel in aortic stenosis with hypoplastic left ventricle and endocardial fibroelastosis. Chest, 57:185, 1970.
49. Izukawa, T., Mulholland, H. C., Rowe, R. D., Cook, D. H., Bloom, K. R., Trusler, G. A., Wiliams, W. G., and Chance, G. W.: Structural heart disease in the newborn. Changing profile: Comparison of 1975 with 1965. Arch. Dis. Child., 54:281, 1979.
50. Jue, K. L., and Edwards, J. E.: Anomalous attachment of mitral valve causing subaortic atresia. Observations in a case with other cardiac anomalies and multiple spleens. Circulation 35:928, 1976.
51. Kanjuh, V. I., Eliot, R. S., and Edwards, J. E.: Coexistent mitral and aortic valvular atresia. A pathologic study of 14 cases. Am. J. Cardiol., 15:611, 1965.
52. Keeton, B. R., Macartney, F. J., Hunter, S., Mortera, C., and Rees, P.: Shinebourne, E. A., Tynan, M., Wilkinson, J. L., and Anderson, R. H.: Univentricular heart of right ventricular type with double or common inlet. Circulation 59:403, 1979.
53. Krovetz, L. J., Rowe, R. D., and Schiebler, G. L.: Hemodynamics of aortic valve atresia. Circulation, 42:953, 1970.
54. Lance, L., Sahn, D. J., Allen, H. D., Ovitt, T. W., and Goldberg, S. J.: Cross-sectional echocardiography in hypoplastic left ventricle: Echocardiographic-angiographic-anatomic correlations. Pediatr. Cardiol., 1:287, 1980.
55. Lev, M.: Pathologic anatomy and interrelationship of hypoplasia of the aortic tract complexes. Lab Invest., 1:61, 1952.
56. Lev, M., Arcilla, R., Rimoldi, H. J. A., Licata, R. H., and Gasul, B. M.: Premature narrowing or closure of the foramen ovale. Am. Heart J., 65:638, 1963.
57. Levitsky, S., Van der Horst, R. L., Hastreiter, A. R., Eckner, R. A. O., and Bennett, E. J.: Surgical palliation in aortic atresia. J. Thorac. Cardiovasc. Surg. 79:456, 1980.
58. Lucas, R. V., Jr., Lester, R. G., Lillehei, C. W., and Edwards, J. E.: Mitral atresia with levoatriocardinal vein. A form of congenital pulmonary venous obstruction. Am. J. Cardiol., 9:607, 1962.
59. Lucas, R. V., Jr., Anderson, R. C., Amplatz, K., Adams, P., Jr., and Edwards, J. E.: Congenital causes of pulmonary venous obstruction. Pediatr. Clin. North Am. 10:781, 1963.

60. Lundstrom, N-R.: Ultrasound cardiographic studies of the mitral valve region in young infants with mitral atresia, mitral stenosis, hypoplasia of the left ventricle, and cor triatriatum. Circulation, 45:324, 1972.
61. Macartney, F. J., and Anderson, R. H.: Angiocardiography and haemodynamics of the univentricular heart with two atrioventricular valves or a common atrioventricular valve. In, Paediatric Cardiology, 1977, edited by R. H. Anderson and E. A. Shinebourne. Churchill Livingstone, Edinburgh, 1978, p. 353.
62. Macartney, F. J., Bain, H. H., Ionescu, M. I., Deverall, P. B., and Scott, O.: Angiocardiographic/pathologic correlations in congenital mitral valve anomalies. Eur. J. Cardiol., 4:191, 1976.
63. McGarry, K. M., Taylor, J. F. N., and Macartney, F. J.: Aortic atresia occurring with complete transposition of the great arteries. Br. Heart J., 44:711, 1980.
64. Meyer, R. A., and Kaplan, S.: Echocardiography in the diagnosis of hypoplasia of the left or right ventricles in the neonate. Circulation 46:55, 1972.
65. Miller, G. A. H.: Aortic atresia. Diagnostic cardiac catheterization in the first week of life. Br. Heart J. 33:367, 1971.
66. Miller, G. A. H.: Congenital heart disease in the first week of life. Br. Heart J. 36:1160, 1974.
67. Milo, S., Yen Ho, S., and Anderson, R. H.: Hypoplastic left heart syndrome: Can this malformation be treated surgically? Thorax 35:351, 1980.
68. Mohri, H., Horiuchi, T., Haneda, K., Sato, S., Kahata, O., Ohmi, M., Ishizawa, E., Kagawa, Y., Fukuda, M., Yoshida, Y., and Shima, T.: Surgical treatment for hypoplastic left heart syndrome. Case reports. J. Thorac. Cardiovasc. Surg., 78:223, 1979.
69. Moller, J. H., Nakib, A., and Edwards, J. E.: Infarction of papillary muscles and mitral insufficiency associated with congenital aortic stenosis. Circulation 34:87, 1966.
70. Moller, J. H., and Neal, W. A.: Heart Disease in Infancy. Appleton-Century-Crofts. New York, 1981, p. 5.
71. Moodie, D. S., Gallen, W. J., and Friedberg, D. Z.: Congenital aortic atresia. Report of long survival and some speculations about surgical approaches. J. Thorac. Cardiovasc. Surg. 63:726, 1972.
72. Mortera, C., and Leon, G.: Detection of persistent ductus in hypoplastic left heart syndrome by contrast echocardiography. Br. Heart J. 44:596, 1980.
73. Nath, P. H., Delaney, D. J., Zollikofer, C., Ben-Sachar, G., Castaneda-Zuniga, W., Formanek, A., and Amplatz, K.: Coronary sinusleft atrial window. Radiology 135:319, 1980.
74. Neufeld, H. N., Adams, P., Jr., Edwards, J. E., and Lester, R. G.: Diagnosis of aortic atresia by retrograde aortography. Circulation 25:278, 1962.
75. Neumann, M. P., Heidelberger, K. P., Dick, M., II, and Rosenthal, A.: Pulmonary vascular changes associated with hypoplastic left ventricle syndrome. Pediatr. Cardiol. 1:301, 1980.
76. Neye-Bock, S., and Fellows, K. E.: Aortic arch interruption in infancy: Radio-and angiographic features. Am. J. Roentgenol. 135:1005, 1980.
77. Noonan, J. A., and Nadas, A. S.: The hypoplastic left heart syndrome. An analysis of 101 cases. Pediatr. Clin. North Am. 5:1029, 1958.
78. Nora, J. J., and Nora, A. H.: Genetics and counseling in cardiovascular diseases. Charles C Thomas, Springfield, Ill., 1978, p. 181.
79. Norwood, W. I., Kirklin, J. K., and Sanders, S. P.: Hypoplastic left heart syndrome: Experience with palliative surgery. Am. J. Car-

diol. 45:87, 1980.

80. Norwood, W. I., Lang, P., Castaneda, A. R., and Campbell, D. N.: Experience with surgery for hypoplastic left heart syndrome. J. Thorac. Cardiovasc. Surg. 82:511, 1981.

81. Norwood, W. I., and Stellin, G. J.: Aortic atresia with interrupted aortic arch. Reparative operation. J. Thorac. Cardiovasc. Surg. 81:239, 1981.

82. Park, S. C., Neches, W. H., Zuberbuhler, J. R., Lenox, C. C., Mathews, R. A., Fricker, F. J., and Zoltun, R. A.: Clinical use of blade atrial septostomy. Circulation 58:600, 1978.

83. Patel, R. G., Freedom, R. M., Moes, C. A. F., Bloom, K. R., Olley, P. M., Williams, W. G., Trusler, G. A., and Rowe, R. D.: Right ventricular volume determinations in 18 patients with pulmonary atresia and intact ventricular septum. Analysis of factors influencing ventricular growth. Circulation 61:428, 1980.

84. Pellegrino, P. A., and Thiene, G.: Aortic valve atresia with a normally developed left ventricle. Chest 69:121, 1976.

85. Perry, L. W., Scott, L. P., III, Shapiro, S. R., Chandra, R. S., and Roberts, W. C.: Atresia of the aortic valve with ventricular septal defect. A clinicopathologic study of four newborns. Chest 72:757, 1977.

86. Quero Jiminez, M., Perez Martinez, V. M., Maitre Azcarate, M. J., Merino Batres, G., and Moreno Granados, F.: Exaggerated displacement of the atrioventricular canal towards the bulbus cordis (rightward displacement of the mitral valve). Br. Heart J. 35:65, 1973.

87. Raghib, G., Bloemendaal, R. D., Kanjuh, V. I., and Edwards, J. E.: Aortic atresia and premature closure of foramen ovale. Myocardial sinusoids and coronary arteriovenous fistula serving as outflow channel. Am. Heart J. 70:476, 1965.

88. Rao, S. S., Gootman, N., and Platt, N.: Familial aortic atresia. Report of a case of aortic atresia in siblings. Am. J. Dis. Child. 118:919, 1969.

89. Roberts, W. C., Perry, L. W., Chandra, R. S., Myers, G. E., Shapiro, S. R., and Scott, L. P.: Aortic valve atresia: A new classification based on necropsy study of 73 cases. Am. J. Cardiol. 37:753, 1976.

90. Rose, A. G., Beckman, C. B., and Edwards, J. E.: Communications between coronary sinus and left atrium. Br. Heart J. 36:182, 1974.

91. Rosenqart, R., Jarmakani, J. M., and Emmanouilides, G. C.: Single film retrograde

umbilical aortography in the diagnosis of hypoplastic left heart syndrome with aortic atresia. Circulation 54:345, 1976.

92. Rosenquist, G. C., Taylor, J. F. N., and Stark, J.: Aortopulmonary fenestration and aortic atresia. Report of an infant with ventricular septal defect, persistent ductus arteriosus, and interrupted aortic arch. Br. Heart J. 36:1146, 1974.

93. Rowe, R. D., Freedom, R. M., Mehrizi, A., and Bloom, K. R.: The Neonate with Congenital Heart Disease. W. B. Saunders, Philadelphia, 1981, p. 204.

94. Ruckman, R. N., and Van Praagh, R.: Anatomic types of congenital mitral stenosis: Report of 49 autopsy cases with consideration of diagnosis and surgical implications. Am. J. Cardiol. 42:592, 1978.

95. Ruschhaupt, D. G., Moshire, M., Lev, M., and Bharati, S.: Echocardiogram in mitral-aortic atresia: False identification of the ventricular septum and left ventricular septum and left ventricle. Pediatr. Cardiol. 1:281, 1980.

96. Saied, A., and Folger, G. M., Jr.: Hypoplastic left heart syndrome. Am. J. Cardiol. 29:190, 1972.

97. Salazar, J., Martinez, F., Valero, M. I., and Casado de Frias, E.: Polysplenia with left ventricular hypoplasia and partial anomalous pulmonary venous connection. Acta Cardiol. 6:483, 1976.

98. Shinebourne, E. A., Lau, K-C., Calcaterra, G., and Anderson, R. H.: Univentricular heart of right ventricular type: Clinical, angiographic and electrocardiographic features. Am. J. Cardiol. 46:439, 1980.

99. Shokeir, M. H. K.: Hypoplastic left heart syndrome: An autosomal recessive disorder. Clin. Genet. 2:7, 1971.

100. Silberberg, B.: Coexistent aortic and mitral atresia associated with persistent common atrioventricular canal. Am. J. Cardiol. 16:754, 1965.

101. Sinha, S. N., Rusnak, S. L., Sommers, H. M., Cole, R. B., Muster, A. J., and Paul, M. H.: Hypoplastic left ventricle syndrome. Analysis of thirty autopsy cases in infants with surgical considerations. Am. J. Cardiol. 21:166, 1968.

102. Soto, B., Bertranou, E. G., Bream, P. R., Souza, A., Jr., Bargeron, L. M., Jr.: Angiographic study of univentricular heart of right ventricular type. Circulation 60:1325, 1979.

103. Strong, W. B., Liebman, J., and Perrin, E.: Hypoplastic left ventricle syndrome. Electrocardiographic evidence of left ventricular hy-

pertrophy. Am. J. Dis. Child. 120:511, 1970.

104. Thiene, G., Daliento, L., Frescura, C., De Tommasi, M., Macartney, F. J., and Anderson, R. H.: Atresia of left atrioventricular orifice. Anatomical investigation in 62 cases. Br. Heart J. 45:393, 1981.

105. Thiene, G., Gallucci, V., Macartney, F. J., Del Torso, S., Pellegrino, P. A., and Anderson, R. H.: Anatomy of aortic atresia. Cases presenting with a ventricular septal defect. Circulation 59:173, 1979.

106. Van der Horst, R. L., and Hastreiter, A. R.: Ascending aortic obstruction of retrograde coronary blood flow in aortic atresia. Am. Heart J. 101:345, 1981.

107. Van Meurs-Van Woezik, H., and Werner Klein, H.: Calibres of aorta and pulmonary artery in hypoplastic left and right heart syndromes: Effects of abnormal blood flow. Virchows Arch. Pathol. Anat. Histol. 364:357, 1974.

108. Van Meurs-Van Woezik, H., Werner Klein, H., and Krediet, P.: Tunica media of aorta and pulmonary trunk in relation to internal calibres in transposition of great arteries, in aortic and pulmonary atresia and in normal hearts. Virchows Arch. Pathol. Histol. 386:306, 1980.

109. Van Praagh, S., LaCorte, M., Fellows, K. E., Bossina, K., Busch, H. J., Keck, E. W., Weinberg, P. M., and Van Praagh, R.: Superoinferior ventricles: Anatomic and angiocardiographic findings in ten postmortem cases. In Etiology and Morphogenesis of Congenital Heart Disease, edited by R. Van Praagh and A. Takao. Futura Publishing, Mount Kisco, N.Y., 1980, p. 317.

110. Van Praagh, R., Plett, J. A., and Van Praagh, S.: Single ventricle. Pathology, embryology, terminology and classification. Herz 4:113, 1979.

111. Von Rueden, T. J., Knight, L., Moller, J. H., and Edwards, J. E.: Coarctation of the aorta associated with aortic valvular atresia. Circulation 52:951, 1975.

112. Von Rueden, T. J., and Moller, J. H.: The electrocardiogram in aortic valvular atresia. Chest 73:66, 1978.

113. Watson, D. G., and Rowe, R. D.: Aortic-valve atresia. J.A.M.A. 179:14, 1962.

114. Williams, H. J., Tandon, R., and Edwards, J. E.: Persistent ostium primum coexisting with mitral or tricuspid atresia. Chest 66:39, 1974.

28

Malpositions of the Heart

Richard Van Praagh, M.D., Paul M. Weinberg, M.D., Rumiko Matsuoka, M.D., and Stella Van Praagh, M.D.

One of the fascinations of congenital heart disease is that the heart can be virtually "anywhere"—left-sided (levocardia), right-sided (dextrocardia), in the middle of the thorax (mesocardia), or extrathoracic (ectopia cordis).

Cardiac malposition denotes that the location of the heart as a whole is abnormal. The various parts of the heart (the cardiac segments) may be malpositioned individually or collectively, but unless the location of the heart as a whole is abnormal, cardiac malposition is not considered to be present.

The principal cardiac malpositions are dextrocardia, mesocardia, isolated levocardia pericardial defect,[5, 7, 11, 13, 18, 20, 32, 42, 46, 53, 72–74, 78–80, 83, 89, 90, 101, 121, 124] and ectopia cordis.

The segmental approach to the diagnosis of congenital heart disease[106, 66, 87, 31, 77, 103] is included in this chapter because it is the key to the diagnostic understanding of dextrocardia and the other cardiac malpositions, and also of the normally located heart.

SEGMENTAL DIAGNOSIS

The segmental approach to the diagnosis of congenital heart disease has aptly been called the *systematic approach*.[77] It has also been called the *sequential approach*[86] because the anatomic states of the viscera, the atria, the atrioventricular valves, the ventricles, the infundibulum, and the great arteries are determined in this venous-to-arterial sequence.

The cardiac segments are the anatomic and developmental components that together make up all human hearts. From the embryologic standpoint, there are at least 10 cardiac segments:[106] (1) the sinus venosus, (2) the primitive atrium, (3) the common pulmonary vein, (4) the atrioventricular canal, (5) the primitive ventricle (proampulla), (6) the proximal bulbus cordis (meta-ampulla), (7) the infundibulum (conus), (8) the truncus arteriosus, (9) the aortic sac, and (10) the arterial arches.

These ten cardiac segments may be greatly simplified for the purposes of clinical diagnosis. Diagnostically, it may be said that there are **three major cardiac segments**[106, 110, 118]: (1) the visceroatrial situs, which is important for the diagnostic localization of the atria (Fig. 28.1); (2) the ventricular loop, which is important for ventricular localization (Fig. 28.2 to 28.6); and (3) the truncus arteriosus, which is important for the diagnostic understanding of the various types of relationships between the great arteries and the ventricles (Fig. 28.6 to 28.8). The three major cardiac segments, expressed in anatomic terms, are: the atria; the ventricles; and the great arteries.

There are two diagnostically important junctional cardiac segments that lie between the atria and the ventricles, and between the ventricles and the great arteries.[75] The **two junctional cardiac segments** are: the atrioventricular canal (Fig. 28.6) and the infundibulum (conus) (Figs. 28.7 and 28.8). The two junctional cardiac segments, expressed in anatomic terms, are: the atrioventricular valves (tricuspid valve, mitral valve, and common atrioventricular valve) (Fig.

28.6) and the infundibulum (which may be subpulmonary, subaortic, bilateral—subaortic and subpulmonary, or absent) (Fig. 28.7 and 28.8).

Hence, there are five diagnostically important cardiac segments,[75] the three major cardiac segments (atria, ventricles, and great arteries), and the two junctional cardiac segments (atrioventricular valves, and infundibulum). The five diagnostically important cardiac segments, in veno-arterial sequence, are: the atria; the atrioventricular valves; the ventricles; the infundibulum; and the great arteries.

No matter where the heart may be located—within the thorax, within the abdomen, or outside the body—**the essence of the diagnostic problem posed by congenital heart disease** is: to establish the anatomic status of each of the five diagnostically **important** cardiac segments; to ascertain how the various cardiac segments are aligned, or are connected, with each other; to delineate the presence or absence of associated malformations; and to assess the function of the five cardiac segments, with their variable alignments, connections, and associated anomalies. This segment-by-segment or step-by-step diagnostic approach applies accurately and easily to all forms of congenital heart disease, no matter how complex.

The anatomic status of each of the five cardiac segments may be expressed in terms of their situs. *Situs* is a Latin word meaning place or location. The body as a whole may be in *situs solitus*, i.e., with normal visceral locations, or in *situs inversus*, i.e., with visceral locations that are a mirror image of normal, or in *situs ambiguus*, i.e., with visceral locations that are ambiguus—neither solitus nor inversus.

Just as the visceral organizational pattern (the situs) of the body as a whole may be solitus (normal), inversus (mirror image), or ambiguus (uncertain), so too the organizational pattern (situs) of each of the five cardiac segments may be solitus (normal), inversus (a mirror-image of solitus), or ambiguus (uncertain).

THE ATRIA

There are three types of visceroatrial situs (Fig. 28.1): situs solitus, situs inversus, and situs ambiguus.

Situs solitus is the normal, noninverted type of viscer-

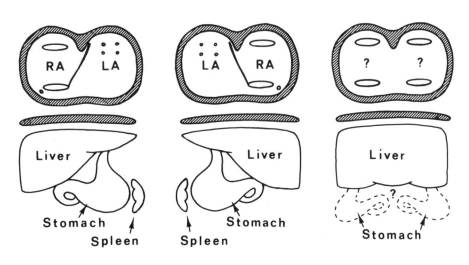

Situs Solitus   **Situs Inversus**   **"Situs Ambiguus"**

Fig. 28.1   **The three types of visceroatrial situs:** situs solitus, situs inversus, and situs ambiguus. For localizing the atria, note that the situs of the viscera and the situs of the atria almost always are the same: both solitus, both inversus, or both ambiguous. These are the visceroatrial concordances. (Reproduced with permission R. Van Praagh and P. Vlad.[118])

oatrial situs. The morphologically right atrium (RA) is right-sided, and its anatomic organizational pattern is noninverted. The morphologically left atrium (LA) is left-sided, and its anatomic organizational pattern is noninverted.

Situs inversus is the mirror-image or inverted type of visceroatrial situs. The RA is left-sided with an inverted anatomic organizational pattern, and the LA is right-sided with an inverted anatomic pattern.

Inversion in anatomy means right-left reversal without anteroposterior change, as in an image in a mirror.

Situs ambiguus[104] is the anatomically uncertain or indeterminate type of visceroatrial situs that typically is associated with the asplenia syndrome and with the polysplenia syndrome but which occasionally can occur with a normally formed spleen.

Situs ambiguus with the asplenia syndrome often has what may be called *bilateral "right-sidedness"* or *right "isomerism,"* while situs ambiguus with the polysplenia syndrome often has what may be referred to as *bilateral "left-sidedness"* or *left "isomerism."* Such bilateral "right-sidedness" and bilateral "left-sidedness" are regarded as helpful teaching mnemonics but not as accurate basic biology. As will be seen, there is considerable crossover of "typical" findings between these two syndromes. Moreover, there really is no such thing as bilateral LA, accurately speaking. The atrial findings in polysplenia often are somewhat suggestive of bilateral LA—particularly the ipsilateral pulmonary veins and the finger-like appendages. However, truly bilateral left atria—with four pulmonary veins on each side, and with two septa prima forming the septal surface on each side—has never been described. Nonetheless, bilateral "right-sidedness" with the asplenia syndrome and bilateral "left-sidedness" with the polysplenia syndrome are helpful summarizing mnemonics.[93]

The **visceroatrial concordances** and the **inferior vena cava to right atrial concordances** are also summarized in Figure 28.1. For the purposes of diagnostic localization of the RA, it is helpful to know that the situs of the viscera and the situs of the atria almost always are the same: both solitus, both inversus, or both ambiguus. Consequently, the visceroatrial concordances usually make it possible to diagnose the locations of the RA and the LA by means of the plain chest x-rays. The stomach bubble, liver shadow, and air bronchogram indicate the visceral situs and, hence, usually the atrial situs, with accuracy. The inferior vena cava (IVC) almost always returns to the RA, with apparent exceptions very rare.[36, 38] IVC-RA concordance is even more reliable diagnostically than is visceroatrial concordance. The IVC may ascend on the right side and then switch from right to left at the level of the liver in order to enter a left-sided RA.[45] Conversely, the IVC may ascend on the left and then switch from left to right at the level of the liver and so enter a right-sided RA.[45] Thus, IVC-to-RA concordance is diagnostically accurate, even when there is **visceroatrial discordance**, whereas visceroatrial concordance is not.

IVC-to-RA concordance is even accurate diagnostically concerning the localization of the atria when the IVC is "absent." Even when the IVC is interrupted between the renal veins and the RA, the hepatic segment of the IVC is always present and may be used to identify the RA. The hepatic segment of the IVC may be demonstrated by angiocardiography (e.g., by reflux of contrast into the hepatic IVC following selective RA injection), or by two-dimensional echocardiography.

THE ATRIOVENTRICULAR CANAL

The atrioventricular (AV) canal is the junctional segment between the atria and the ventricles. Anatomically, the AV canal consists of the tricuspid valve (TV), the mitral valve (MV), and the septum of the AV canal. The septum of the AV canal is missing in complete common AV canal. Hence, the septum of the AV canal consists of the ostium primum part of the atrial septum (that is absent in the ostium primum type of atrial septal defect), plus the canal part of the ventricular septum (that is absent in ventricular septal defect on the AV canal type in typical complete common AV canal).

The situs of the AV valves can be solitus, or inversus, or ambiguus. Typically, the situs of the AV valves corresponds to that of the ventricles of entry, not to that of the atria of exit. Usually, the TV and the MV are noninverted when the ventricles are noninverted and inverted when the ventricles are inverted, no matter what the atrial situs may be. The situs of the AV valves also can be uncertain. For example, with double-inlet LV, both AV valves often appear morphologically to be mitral in type.

The AV canal serves at least three different functions: the prevention of ventriculoatrial regurgitation by means of the MV and TV; the separation of the systemic and pulmonary circulations by means of the septum of the AV canal; and the electrical insulation of the atria from the ventricles, except at the bundle of His. In this regard, it is noteworthy that *the concept of AV connections* (concordant, or discordant, etc.) is anatomically erroneous. The atria and the ventricles normally do not connect because of the interposition of the AV canal. The AV canal or junctional tissue connects both with the ventricles and with the atria, but the atria and the ventricles normally do not connect directly, except at the bundle of His. In the interests of anatomic accuracy, therefore, we prefer the concept of AV *alignments* (concordant, or discordant, etc.) to that of AV connections. The atria and the ventricles can have virtually any alignment (Fig. 28.6) because there are no necessary AV connections. The junctional cardiac segments (AV canal and infundibulum) prevent direct connections between the primary cardiac segments (atria, ventricles, and great arteries).

This separation function of the junctional cardiac segments is of profound anatomic and developmental significance. For example, if the RA were connected of necessity to the morphologically right ventricle (RV) and if the LA were connected of necessity to the morphologically left ventricle (LV), then AV discordance (Fig. 28.6) would be developmentally impossible.

Since accuracy is so important to the clear understanding of congenital heart disease, we prefer the concept of AV alignments to that of AV "connections."

The anatomic types of AV alignment are the following.

1. Concordant.[56, 87, 112] The RA opens into the RV, and the LA opens into the LV. This usually happens when the situs of the atria and the situs of the ventricles both are the same—both solitus or both inversus—and when the atria and the ventricles both are well developed (Fig. 28.6).

2. Discordant.[56, 87, 112] The RA opens into the LV, and the LA opens into the RV. This usually occurs when the situs of the atria and the ventricles are different—one solitus and the other inversus, and both are well developed (Fig. 28.6).

3. Atresia. Either the TV or the MV can be atretic. The TV is right-sided with ventricular noninversion (D-loop) and left-sided with ventricular inversion (L-loop) (Fig. 28.2 and 28.6). Hence, tricuspid atresia is right-sided or left-sided, depending on the ventricular situs. Conversely, mitral atresia is left-sided or right-sided, depending on the ventricular situs.

4. Straddling. Either the TV or the MV may straddle the ventricular septum, i.e., either valve may have bicameral chordal insertions and papillary muscles. A *straddling TV* may have chordal insertions into the RV and into the LV or, when associated with a single LV and an infundibular outlet chamber, a straddling TV can insert into the single LV and also into the infundibular outlet chamber. A *straddling MV* may have chordal and papillary muscle insertions into the LV and into the RV, or into the LV and into the infundibulum. *Straddling MV and TV* is rare but does occur.[120]

Note that straddling AV valve is defined as *bicameral* insertion, not as biventricular insertion, because the infundibulum is not a ventricle (RV or LV).[117] Note also that *overriding AV valve* is distinguished from straddling AV valve. In overriding AV valve, the annulus overrides the ventricular septum, but without bicameral chordal and papillary muscular insertions. Thus, in overriding AV valves, the tensor apparatus is unicameral, not bicameral.

5. Double-Inlet. Both the TV and the MV can open predominantly or entirely into one ventricle, resulting in double-inlet LV or in double-inlet RV. Double-inlet LV or double-inlet RV may or may not be associated with single LV or with single RV, respectively. Double-inlet LV usually is associated with single LV.[109, 117] However, single LV can be associated with a tricuspid valve that opens predominantly or entirely into the infundibular outlet chamber.[119] Double-inlet RV often is not associated with single RV, a small LV being the rule in this situation.[117] Whether single LV or single RV is present is determined not by the atrioventricular alignments, nor by the attachments of the AV valves, but rather by myocardial morphologic analysis.[109, 112, 114, 117, 119]

6. Common-Inlet. A common AV valve may open predominantly or entirely into one ventricle, resulting in common-inlet LV or common-inlet RV. Common-inlet may or may not be associated with single ventricle.

One variable, such as the anatomic status of the AV valves, cannot be used to define another variable, such as the anatomic status of the ventricles. Instead, each variable should be defined primarily in terms of itself. Thus, the AV valves cannot be used to decide the presence or absence of single ventricle, nor can the AV valves be used to ascertain reliably what the ventricular situs is, i.e., D-loop or L-loop (Fig. 28.2 and 28.6). The anatomic status of the ventricles can only be ascertained with certainty by morphologic anatomic examination of the ventricular part of the heart.[117-120]

THE VENTRICLES

There are two types of ventricular situs (Figs. 28.2 to 28.5)[109, 112, 114]: solitus ventricles or D-loop ventricles and inversus ventricles or L-loop ventricles.

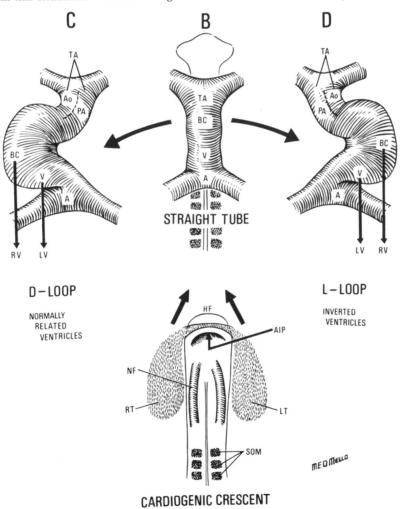

Fig. 28.2 Cardiac loop formation. D-loop formation results in normally interrelated (noninverted) ventricles, with noninverted right ventricular (*RV*) sinus to the right, noninverted left ventricular (*LV*) sinus to the left. L-loop formation results in inverted ventricles, with inverted RV sinus to the left and inverted LV sinus to the right. *A*, atrium; *AIP*, anterior intestinal portal; *Ao*, aorta; *BC*, bulbus cordis; *HF*, head fold; *LT*, left; *LV*, morphologically left ventricle; *NF*, neural fold; *PA*, pulmonary artery; *RT*, right; *RV*, morphologically right ventricle; *SOM*, somites; *TA*, truncus arteriosus; *V*, ventricles. (Reproduced with permission from R. Van Praagh.[110])

Situs ambiguus of the ventricles or X-loop ventricles indicates that the ventricular situs is undiagnosed, with X standing for the unknown.[112] Ventricular X-loop is not a characteristic type of ventricular anatomic organization and hence is not analogous to situs ambiguus of the atria..

Solitus Ventricles or D-Loop Ventricles. From the embryologic standpoint (Fig. 28.2),[96-99, 106, 29, 23, 26, 58, 59, 63, 115] the cardiogenic crescent of precardiac mesoderm forms a straight tube, which then normally loops convexly to the right, forming a D-loop (*dextro*, or D = right). D-loop formation places the developing morphologically right ventricle (RV) to the right (*dextro*, or D) relative to the developing morphologically left ventricle (LV). The RV is derived from the proximal bulbus cordis (meta-ampulla), whereas the LV develops from the ventricle (proampulla) or the bulboventricular loop (Fig. 28.2).

From the anatomic standpoint,[109, 111, 112, 114, 120] D-loop is defined as solitus or noninverted ventricles (Fig. 28.3, 28.5, and 28.8). This means that the ventricular anatomic pattern is as in situs solitus totalis. It is noteworthy that we are using *solitus* or *noninverted* ventricles in an absolute, or situs-independent way, rather than in the conventional situs-dependent way. Thus, solitus (noninverted) ventricles are D-loop ventricles. We are *not* using the designations *solitus* or

inversus ventricles in a situs-dependent way, i.e., in a way that depends for its specific meaning on what the type of visceroatrial situs happens to be. For example, in this conventional, situs-dependent approach, when there is situs solitus of the viscera and atria, ventricular *noninversion* means D-loop and ventricular *inversion* means L-loop. However, with situs inversus of the viscera and atria, ventricular noninversion means L-loop and ventricular inversion denotes D-loop. With situs ambiguus of the viscera and atria, ventricular *noninversion* and ventricular *inversion* both are meaningless because the frame of reference, the type of visceroatrial situs, itself is unknown.

Briefly, then, we suggest that the terms ventricular *noninversion* and *inversion* be used in a situs-independent way in order to avoid the problems inherent in the conventional situs-dependent usage of these designations.

Thus, in solitus, or noninverted, or D-loop ventricles, the RV is to the right of the LV. This is true even with superoinferior ventricles (Fig. 28.3).[120] However, it is important to understand what the **RV** really is: The RV is the RV inflow tract only. The "RV" outflow tract really is the infundibulum or conus.[1, 117] More precisely, the **RV** is the sinus, or body, or inflow tract that lies proximal or upstream to, and usually inferior and posterior to, the ring of infundibular muscle that is formed by the septal band, the moderator band, and the parietal band. The **infundibulum** extends from the septal, moderator, and parietal bands inferiorly to the semilunar valve (or valves) superiorly.[1, 117]

There are many reasons underlying the aforementioned conclusions concerning *what the RV and the infundibulum really are*. Several of the most important considerations are the following.

1. Anomalous muscle bundles of the RV, also known as **double-*chambered RV*,** is perhaps the most clear-cut natural experiment illustrating what RV is and what infundibulum is. We think that the inflow chamber is the true RV, the outflow chamber is the infundibulum, and the anomalous muscle bundles demarcate and partly separate the RV from the infundibulum.[1]

2. Single LV with an infundibular outlet chamber[109, 117] also supports the abovementioned interpretation. The RV (inflow tract) is absent, whereas the infundibulum (outflow tract) is present and forms the outlet chamber.

3. Typical tricuspid atresia also is consistent with this view. In typical tricuspid atresia, we think that both the tricuspid valve and the RV (the inflow tract) are atretic, and that the infundibulum (the outflow tract) is present. The infundibulum often is referred to inaccurately in this situation as "the small RV." Although single LV with double-inlet LV and an infundibular outlet chamber (referred to above) and typical tricuspid atresia are anatomically very similar, there are enough anatomic differences to merit continuation of the diagnostic distinction between these two conditions.

4. In Ebstein's anomaly of the tricuspid valve and RV, the septal leaflet of the tricuspid valve typically is "displaced down" to where? To the septal and moderator bands, where the RV stops and the infundibulum begins. Ebstein's anomaly is a malformation of the tricuspid valve and the RV (inflow tract), but the infundibulum (outflow tract) typically is spared. Thus, the findings of Ebstein's anomaly also support the aforementioned interpretation.

The difficulty at the present time concerning the definition of the RV and the infundibulum is related in part to the **tetralogy of Fallot.** Because of tetralogy, many people think that the infundibulum is synonymous with the characteristic infundibular outlet chamber of this anomaly, i.e.,

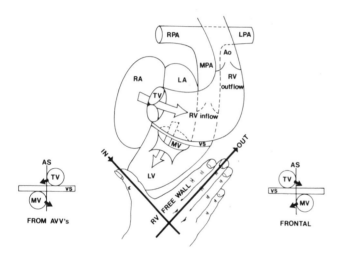

Fig. 28.3 Superoinferior ventricles with crisscross atrioventricular (AV) relations in a patient with physiologically uncorrected *TGA* {S,D,L}. The morphologically right ventricle (*RV*) is superior to the morphologically left ventricle (*LV*). The ventricular septum (*vs*) is horizontal, and the atrial septum (*AS*) is vertical. The viscera and atria are in situs solitus (*S*), the morphologically right atrium (*RA*) being right-sided relative to the morphologically left atrium (*LA*). The situs or intrinsic anatomic organization of *RA* and *LA* is solitus or noninverted. The situs or intrinsic anatomic organization of the RV and LV is solitus or noninverted, i.e., D-loop (D). The situs of the great arteries is inverted, i.e., in L-position (L), the ascending aorta (*Ao*) being to the left (*levo*, or L) relative to the main pulmonary artery (*MPA*). The atrioventricular alignments are concordant: *RA* to *RV* and *LA* to *LV*. The ventriculoarterial alignments are discordant: *RV* to *Ao* and *LV* to *MPA*; hence, transposition of the great arteries (*TGA*) is present. The vectors of the atrioventricular inflow tracts are markedly angulated relative to each other (*arrows*), i.e., crisscross AV relations are present. AV relations normally are approximately parallel. The tricuspid valve (*TV*) is superior and to the right of the mitral valve (*MV*). The intrinsic anatomic organization of the superior *RV* is right-handed (see text). Hence, this patient has physiologically uncorrected **TGA** {**S,D,L**} with superoinferior ventricles and crisscross AV relations. (Reproduced with permission from S. Van Praagh et al.[120])

from the parietal band below to the semilunar valve level above. Although the tetralogy concept of the infundibulum defines the infundibulum on its septal side—from the lower rim of the infundibular septum (the parietal band) to the semilunar valve—this concept leaves the infundibulum mysteriously undefined on its free wall side. It leaves unanswered the following question: Where does the infundibular free wall stop and where does the RV free wall begin?

We think that the concept of the infundibulum suggested by tetralogy of Fallot is the **distal infundibulum** only. This is the part of the infundibulum that lies above the level of the muscular ventricular septal crest and above the top of the septal band from the right ventricular aspect. In single LV, the distal infundibulum extends from the level of the bulboventricular foramen below to the level of the semilunar valve or valves above.[117]

The proximal part of the infundibulum[1, 117] lies below the crest of the muscular ventricular septum—for example in anomalous muscle bundles of the RV—and below the level of the bulboventricular foramen—in single LV. This proximal portion of the infundibulum, (which is prominent in double-chambered RV and in single LV) also is known as the **infundibular apical recess.**[117]

On the right side of the heart, there normally are two apices: the RV apex and the infundibular apex.[117] The RV apex is proximal to the moderator band, while the infundibular apex is distal to the moderator band. These two different apices are most obvious in double-chambered RV (anomalous muscle bundles of the RV).

The concept of the proximal and distal infundibulum answers many other questions. Where does the infundibular free wall end? It goes right down to the apex, as double-chambered RV makes clear. Why is the infundibular outlet chamber sometimes quite large with single LV? Because the infundibulum consists not only of its distal, subsemilunar part but also of its proximal, apical part. What are the developmental functions of the distal and proximal portions of the infundibulum? We think that the distal part of the infundibulum is where the circulations normally are crossed (Fig. 28.8).[115, 118] The proximal part of the infundibulum appears to be the "mother" of the RV: the septal and moderator bands are the parts beneath which the RV evaginates or outpouches. Thus, both the proximal infundibulum and the distal infundibulum are essential adaptations to air breathing.

The advantages of the double-chambered RV concept of what the RV and the infundibulum are: no imaginary junctions are invoked; the infundibulo-RV junction is defined both septally and parietally; and this concept of RV and infundibulum is both real and explains all known pathologic states, including so-called double-chambered RV, the infundibular outlet chamber with single LV, and the infundibular outlet chamber with tricuspid atresia.

"Double-chambered RV" is a misnomer. The RV is not really divided into two chambers. Instead, the RV is separated from the infundibulum.

"Anomalous muscle bundles of the RV" also is a misnomer. These anomalous muscle bundles are infundibular (conal or bulbar), not right ventricular, i.e., the parietal band, septal band, and moderator band are outflow tract (infundibular) musculature, not inflow tract (right ventricular) musculature. This infundibular ring of musculature is at the RV-infundibular junction, and demarcates this junction.

It is interesting that most of the papillary muscles of the tricuspid valve are infundibular (conal), not right ventricular: the papillary muscle of the conus; the attachments of the septal leaflet to the septal band; and the anterior papillary muscle, which usually is connected with the septal and moderator bands and which is an integral part of the aforementioned infundibular ring. Only the posterior papillary muscle group of the RV typically inserts into the RV (inflow tract). Consequently, the tensor apparatus (chordae tendineae and papillary muscles) of the tricuspid valve cannot be used to identify the RV. Instead, the RV should be identified by means of its characteristic and different gross myocardial morphologic characteristics.[117, 118] Hence, it is no surprise that the tricuspid valve may open partially, or entirely, into the infundibulum.[119]

The aforementioned discussion is relevant to the understanding of ventricular D-loops (Fig. 28.2 and 28.3) and ventricular L-loops (Fig. 28.2 and 28.4). It is noteworthy that the RV and the infundibulum are contralateral. In a D-loop, the RV is right-sided, and the infundibulum is left-sided (Figs. 28.3 and 28.5). In an L-loop, the RV is left-sided, and the infundibulum is right-sided (Fig. 28.4 and 28.5). This understanding of the *contralaterality of the RV and the infundibulum* is important to the understanding of **superoinferior ventricles** and **crisscross atrioventricular relations.**[120] Thus, the presence of a D-loop (or an L-loop) is judged by the position of the RV inflow tract, not by the position of the infundibular outflow tract.

In the past, it has been customary to regard the infundibulum as part of the RV. Normally, of course, the infundibulum and the RV are so well incorporated into each other that the infundibulum appears to be an integral part of the RV. Basically, however, this is not so, and complex congenital heart disease—as with the cardiac malpositions—makes this obvious. The infundibulum can straddle the ventricular septum to any degree, which is known as **straddling infundibulum** or **straddling conus.** Knowing that the RV and the infundibulum are different structures helps to explain how it is possible for the RV to be absent and the infundibulum to be present, as with single LV.

The above-described understanding of the distinction between the RV and the infundibulum is very helpful in the diagnostic understanding of complex congenital heart disease, as is diagrammed in Figures 28.3 and 28.4.[120]

Situs really is a question of intrinsic anatomic organization, not of extrinsic spatial relations (such as right-left, superior-inferior, and anterior-posterior). Such spatial relations relative to extrinsic spatial coordinates often are useful and convenient, but they are not basic (Fig. 28.3 and 28.4).

Chirality (handedness)[114, 120] is helpful in order to describe what is a D-loop and what is an L-loop, but in a fashion that is independent of external spatial referents such as right and left. It is noteworthy, for example, that the concepts of ventricular noninversion and ventricular inversion are meaningless as classically defined (in right-left terms, relative to the sagittal plane) when the ventricles are superoinferior and have crisscross AV relations.[120] When the RV is more or less directly superior to the LV, the ventricles cannot be described in right-left terms, i.e., using noninversion and inversion as these terms are conventionally employed. However, ventricular noninversion and inversion can be used, even in these situations, when it is understood that ventricular noninversion equals ventricular D-loop and that ventricular inversion equals ventricular L-loop. D-loop is the **noninverted isomer** of ventricular anatomic organization. L-loop is the **inverted isomer** of ventricular anatomic organization. Which anatomic isomer of ventricular anatomy is present can be recognized, no matter where the ventricles may be located in space, because which ventricular anatomic isomer is present is a question of the pattern of intrinsic anatomic organization, not extrinsic spatial relationships.

The following may be viewed as an expanded understanding of ventricular noninversion and inversion which is essential to the diagnostic understanding of the ventricular segment in complex congenital heart disease. An understanding of ventricular situs is as important as an undertanding of atrial situs.

The noninverted ventricular D-loop has a "right-handed" RV (Fig. 28.3).[114, 120] The thumb represents the RV inflow tract, and the fingers represent the infundibular outflow tract. The palm of the right hand faces the RV septal surface, while the dorsum of the right hand is adjacent to the RV free wall. **The D-loop LV is "left-handed."** The thumb of one's left hand represents the LV inflow tract. The fingers represent the LV outflow tract. The palm of one's left hand faces the noninverted LV septal surface, and the dorsum of the left hand is adjacent to the LV free wall.

The inverted ventricular L-loop has a left-handed RV (Fig. 28.4).[114, 120] The thumb of one's left hand represents the RV inflow tract, and the fingers of one's left hand symbolize the infundibular outflow tract. The palm of the left hand faces the inverted RV septal surface, while the dorsum of one's left hand is adjacent to the RV free wall. **The L-loop LV is "right handed".** The right thumb represents the inverted LV's inflow tract. The right fingers stand for the LV outflow tract. The palm of one's right hand faces the inverted LV's septal surface, and the dorsum of the right hand is adjacent to the inverted LV's free wall.

The D-loop (noninverted) RV and the L-loop (inverted)

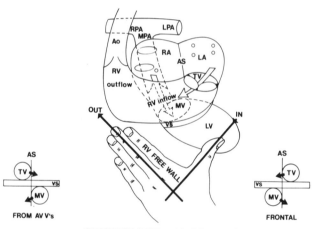

CRISSCROSS AV RELATIONS
TGA {S,L,D}

Fig. 28.4 Superoinferior ventricles with crisscross AV relations and physiologically "corrected" transposition of the great arteries {S,L,D}. There is situs solitus (S) of the viscera and atria. The morphologically right atrium (*RA*) is to the right of the morphologically left atrium (*LA*). The situs or intrinsic anatomic organization of the *RA* and *LA* is solitus (noninverted). The situs or intrinsic anatomic organization of the morphologically right ventricle (*RV*) and of the morphologically left ventricle (*LV*) is inverted or L-loop (L). The *RV* is left-handed (see text). The atrioventricular (*AV*) alignments are discordant: *RA* to *LV*, and *LA* to *RV*. The vectors of the AV inflow tracts are markedly angulated relative to each other (arrows), i.e., they are crisscross, instead of being approximately parallel. The tricuspid valve (*TV*) is superior and to the left of the mitral valve (*MV*). The situs of the great arteries is solitus or noninverted, i.e., in D-position, with the ascending aorta (*Ao*) to the right (*dextro*, or D) relative to the main pulmonary artery (*MPA*). The ventriculoarterial alignments are discordant: *RV* to *Ao* and *LV* to *MPA*, i.e., transposition of the great arteries (*TGA*) is present. Hence, this patient has physiologically "corrected" **TGA {S,L,D} with superoinferior ventricles and crisscross AV relations.** (Reproduced with permission from S. Van Praagh et al.[120])

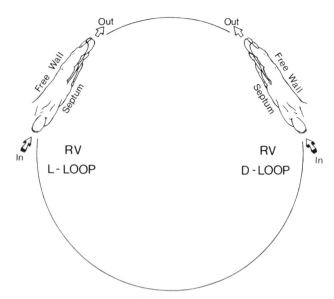

Fig. 28.5 The morphologically right ventricle (RV) of D-loop (noninverted) ventricles is right-handed. The RV of L-loop (inverted) ventricles is left-handed. The D-loop RV and the L-loop RV are stereoisomers or spatial mirror images, just as are the right and left hands. Hence, it is readily possible to diagnose the situs of the ventricles (D-loop or L-loop), no matter what the spatial relations of the ventricles may be, as in Figures 28.3 and 28.4.

RV are **stereoisomers** or spatial mirror images (Fig. 28.5). Similarly, the D-loop (noninverted) LV and the L-loop (inverted) LV are stereoisomers or spatial mirror images. One's right and left hands are also stereoisomers.

It should be understood that the inverted (L-loop) RV and LV are exact mirror images of their noninverted (D-loop) counterparts only under certain conditions: The L-loop ventricles must be "normally" positioned for an L-loop, i.e., dextrocardia with rightward pointing ventricular apex must be present. The L-loop ventricles must be "normally" formed, i.e., apart from their inversion, they must have no additional anomalies. For the L-loop atrioventricular conduction system to be a mirror image of the normal D-loop atrioventricular conduction system, the L-loop ventricles also must have atrioventricular concordance (situs inversus of the viscera and atria with an L-loop). Thus, the ventricles of classical corrected transposition with an L-loop will not be perfect mirror images of normal D-loop ventricles if the ventricles of the heart with corrected transposition are in levocardia (instead of being in dextrocardia, as they "should" be because an L-loop is present), or if the left-sided RV is underdeveloped or malformed (as it often is with L-loop ventricles and L-transposition of the great arteries). Nonetheless, if appropriately positioned and not otherwise malformed, D-loop (noninverted) ventricles and L-loop (inverted) ventricles are stereoisomers or spatial mirror images of each other.

The key to the understanding of the ventricular anatomy in superoinferior ventricles, crisscross AV relations, and single ventricle is the D-loop/L-loop concept. In complex ventricular anomalies, the conventional ventricular noninversion-inversion concept breaks down. However, when ventricular noninversion and inversion are redefined in terms of chirality,[120] these familiar conventional concepts regain their validity.

Intrinsic anatomic organization (situs) is different from, and more basic than, spatial relations (such as right-sided/left-sided). Indeed, situs is more basic than is looping. With superoinferior ventricles, with or without crisscross AV relations, ventricular looping is abnormal and very incomplete.[120] The RV has failed to descend to the right of the LV (Fig. 28.3), as it "should" in a normal D-loop, or has failed to descend to the left of the LV (Fig. 28.4), as it "should" in the typical L-loop. Thus, although D-loop is a way of expressing solitus ventricles and L-loop is a way of expressing inverted ventricles, ventricular situs really is more basic than is ventricular loop formation. This is why ventricular situs can readily be diagnosed, even when looping per se is very abnormal. Situs is one of the basic concepts in biology. Ventricular loop formation and ventricular spatial relations both are expressions of ventricular situs.

Others have thought that ventricular D-loop and ventricular L-loop are embryologic hypotheses and, hence, are unsuitable as clinical and anatomical diagnoses. Consequently, efforts have been made to *imply* the type of ventricular loop that is present by means of atrioventricular concordance or discordance, while avoiding the use of the terms D-loop and L-loop.

Over the past several years, however, new understanding has helped to clarify this problem. It has now been well documented that both ventricular D- and L-loops exist;[57-59, 106, 115] consequently, they can no longer be regarded as embryologic hypotheses. D-loop and L-loop have now been defined anatomically in terms of chirality.[114, 120] Hence, there is now a growing consensus that ventricular D-loop and L-loop are acceptable designations both embryologically and anatomically. For this there is ample precedent. **Many of our diagnostic designations are both embryologic and anatomic terms**: patent ductus arteriosus, ostium secundum type of atrial septal defect, ostium primum type of atrial septal defect, common atrioventricular canal, truncus arteriosus, etc. An anatomic term is satisfactory if it is well defined anatomically; embryologic provenance, or meaning, is not a disqualification.

It should also be understood that the term ventricular D-loop and L-loop were introduced[109] because of the inadequacies of the classical concepts of ventricular noninversion and inversion mentioned above. The clinical diagnoses of ventricular D-loop and L-loop have always been used in an anatomic sense.[69, 109, 112] It is only recently, however, that satisfactory anatomic definitions have been formulated in terms of chirality (Fig. 28.3 to 28.5)[114, 120] which apply to virtually all ventricular malpositions and malformations.

It is also only very recently that we have become aware of **the importance of situs to the understanding of all of the cardiac segments.** This is not merely for the purposes of clinical anatomic diagnosis. As will be seen, both embryology and etiology appear to be illuminated by this new understanding of segmental situs.

Ventricular situs may be expressed in many ways: looping (D-/L-), AV alignments (concordant-discordant), and handedness (right-left). Another way of expressing a solitus or D-loop organizational pattern is to say that, when viewed from the free wall aspect, *the D-loop RV is organized from right to left* (Fig. 28.3).[114, 120] Furthest to the right is the tricuspid valve. Somewhat to the left is the RV inflow tract. Further to the left are the septal and moderator bands. Furthest to the left is the infundibulum leading up to a great artery.[117] When viewed from the free wall perspective, *the L-loop RV is organized from left to right* (Fig. 28.4).[114, 120] Furthest to the left is the tricuspid valve. Somewhat to the right is the RV inflow tract. Further to the right are the septal and moderator bands. Furthest to the right is the infundibulum leading up to a great artery.[117]

Chirality is thought to be the best expression of ventricular situs because it is independent of external points of reference (such as right-left). It is noteworthy that chirality is important in the physics of elementary particles.[114]

It has been asked: **What difference does the type of ventricular loop (D- or L-) really make?** Surely, all one needs to know diagnostically is whether the atrioventricular alignments ("connections") are concordant or discordant. The answer to this critique is in several parts, as follows.

1. The concordance or discordance of AV alignments usually is very helpful diagnostically in indicating what type of ventricular loop is present. For example, in situs solitus of the viscera and atria with concordant AV alignments, D-loop ventricles almost always are present (Fig. 28.6). With situs inversus of the viscera and atria and concordant AV alignments, L-loop ventricles almost always coexist. Conversely, with situs solitus of the viscera and atria and discordant AV alignments, a ventricular L-loop almost always is present. With situs inversus of the viscera and atria and discordant AV alignments, a ventricular D-loop almost always is found. The foregoing are *the usual atrioventricular alignments*; hence, their understanding is diagnostically very important.

2. However, there are rare situations in which the atrioventricular alignments ("connections") are diagnostically misleading concerning the type of ventricular loop that is present. Concordant AV alignments can occur between solitus atria and inversus ventricles.[114] Discordant AV alignments can exist between solitus atria and solitus ventricles.[114]

3. A statistically much more important problem associated with the view that all one needs to know is the concordance or discordance of the AV alignments and therefore that the type of ventricular situs (D-loop/L-loop) need not be diagnosed specifically is the well documented fact that **there are many forms of congenital heart disease in which the concept of concordance or discordance of the atrioventricular alignments does not apply.**

a. In situs ambiguus, the type of ventricular situs (solitus or D-loop, inversus or L-loop) cannot be implied by means of the AV alignments. In situs ambiguus of the viscera and atria, concordant and discordant AV alignments both are meaningless. To say that the AV alignments are ambiguous, while accurate, is to make a nondiagnosis. In situs ambiguus (with asplenia, polysplenia, or occasionally with a normal spleen), the ventricular situs, must be diagnosed specifically.

Those who may wish to avoid the terms D-loop and L-loop because of their embryologic connotations may well prefer to use the designations *solitus (or noninverted) ventricles* and *inversus (or inverted) ventricles* instead, because the latter terms have anatomic connotations. We have no particular preference and use these designations interchangeably. Although we view anatomic designations as the primary requisite, we regard additional embryologic meaning as an asset.

b. With straddling AV valves, the AV alignments are neither concordant nor discordant. For example, with straddling tricuspid valve, the AV alignments are both concordant (RA-RV and LA-LV) and discordant (RA-LV).

c. With atresia of an AV valve, the AV alignments are only half concordant. In tricuspid atresia, for example, the LA opens into the LV (concordant), but the RA opens into nothing.

d. In double-inlet LV or RV, the AV alignments are both concordant and discordant. **In double-inlet** LV, for example, the LA opens into the LV (concordant), and the RA opens into the LV (discordant).

e. In double-outlet right atrium,[14] the RA opens into the RV (concordant) and into the LV (discordant).

Thus, there are many forms of congenital heart disease in which the concept of atrioventricular concordance or discordance does not apply. Hence, there are many situations in which the situs of the ventricles cannot be implied by means of the AV alignments ("connections"). Consequently, AV concordance or discordance is not a satisfactory basis for the classification of congenital heart disease as a whole. Instead, it is necessary to diagnose the ventricular situs specifically. No other method of classification of congenital heart disease applies accurately and simply in all cases. It should be added that we are not at all opposed to the concept of AV concordance or discordance; indeed, we proposed it.[112]

There are two different kinds of concordance and discordance: *alignment* concordance-discordance and *situs* concordance-discordance.

In a given patient, usually they are the same, but occasionally they are not. For example, we have studied an autopsied case of double-outlet right ventricle that had situs solitus of the viscera and atria, a ventricular L-loop (inversion), but with concordant AV alignments (RA-RV and LA-LV).[114] This patient had AV alignment concordance, but AV situs discordance.

We have also studied an autopsied case with situs solitus of the viscera and atria, solitus ventricles (D-loop), but with discordance of the AV alignments (RA-LV and LA-RV).[114] This patient had AV alignment discordance, with AV situs concordance.

Both of the aforementioned patients[114] had juxtaposition of the atrial appendages, i.e., both the atria and the ventricles were malposed. We think that this is why the AV alignments were unusual—the opposites of what one would expect based on the situs of the atrial and ventricular segments. In congenital heart disease, usually only the ventricles are malposed, with the atria relatively fixed in position by the systemic and pulmonary veins. However, when both the atrial segment and the ventricular segment are malposed, then the AV alignments can be surprising, as in these two patients. When we speak of AV concordance or discordance without other qualification, it is alignment (not situs) concordance or discordance that is meant. Segmental situs and segmental alignments both are important. These are two different considerations, as the above mentioned cases illustrate.

Segmental situs usually determines segmental alignments. As will be seen, this is an important principle. Alignments do not determine situs. Segmental situs is primary, and the resulting segmental alignments—which are physiologically of importance—are nonetheles anatomically and embryologically secondary. For example, when the atria and the ventricles both are solitus, then the AV alignments typically are concordant. When the atria are solitus and the ventricles are inversus, then the AV alignments typically are discordant (Fig. 28.6). The situs of the atria and the ventricles determines the AV alignments ("connections"), not vice versa. This is one of the reasons why, in the segmental approach to the diagnosis of congenital heart disease, the situs of the three major cardiac segments—the atria, the ventricles, and the great arteries—is noted specifically. The alignments, atrioventricular (AV) and ventriculoarterial (VA), are specified only when they are not otherwise understood. For example, when the atria and the ventricles both are in the situs solitus, it usually may be assumed that the AV alignment is concordant and, hence, this ordinarilly need not be specified. However, when the nature of the AV alignments is *not* what one would ordinarily assume, then it must be stated specifically. For example, with solitus atria and ventricles, if the tricuspid valve straddles, this must be specified.

In a well-formulated diagnosis, that which is normal and that which is understood are customarily omitted. Thus, with situs solitus of the atria and solitus (D-loop) ventricles,

it ordinarily is unnecessary to say that there is AV concordance because this is understood. Similarly, with transposition of the great arteries (TGA), it is unnecessary to say that there is ventriculoarterial (VA) discordance because this, too, is understood. Indeed, since TGA means VA discordance, saying that there is TGA with VA discordance is redundant.

THE INFUNDIBULUM

An understanding of situs also is of importance at the infundibular level. The infundibulum is the other diagnostically important junctional segment (the first being the atrioventricular junction or canal). The infundibulum connects the ventricles below with the great arteries above. The infundibulum (conus) has been defined heretofore. Suffice it to say that the part of the infundibulum that is involved in so-called conotruncal malformations (malformations of the infundibulum and great arteries) is the distal or subsemilunar part of the infundibulum (Fig. 28.7), whereas the part that is involved in anomalous muscle bundles (or double-chambered RV) is the proximal or apical part of the infundibulum. The distal or subsemilunar part of the infundibulum is the parietal band part, whereas the proximal or apical part is the septal band part. The parietal band is essentially synonymous with the infundibular septum, while the septal and moderator bands together have also been termed the trabecular septomarginalis.

In this section we are concerned with the distal or subsemilunar part of the infundibulum because of its importance in conotruncal anomalies. When we refer to the infundibulum without other qualification, it is always the distal infundibulum that is meant.

The infundibulum is the crucial connector between the ventricles and the great arteries. The concept of ventriculoarterial *alignments* (Fig. 28.6) is preferred to that of the ventriculoarterial connections, in the interests of anatomic and embryologic accuracy. The ventricles do not connect directly with the great arteries because of the interposition of the infundibulum. The infundibulum connects directly both with the great arteries above and with the ventricles below. However, it is anatomically accurate to say that the ventricles and the great arteries *are connected* concordantly or discordantly.

The four main anatomic types of infundibulum are summarized schematically in Figure 28.7.

1. Subpulmonary. The normal infundibulum is subpulmonary, left-sided, and anterior. It prevents fibrous continuity between the pulmonary valve and the atrioventricular valves. The subaortic part of the normal infundibulum is right-sided, posterior, and absorbed. The normally absorbed (essentially absent) subaortic infundibular free wall permits aortic-mitral fibrous continuity, and it also permits aortic-tricuspid fibrous continuity via the *pars membranacea septi*. The normal subpulmonary infundibulum is the solitus (or noninverted) infundibulum.

2. Subaortic. The subaortic infundibulum of typical D-transposition of the great arteries (Fig. 28.6, TGA, diagram 1) is right-sided and anterior. It prevents aortic-atrioventricular fibrous continuity (Fig. 28.7). The subpulmonary infundibular free wall is left-sided, posterior, and absorbed. The absorption of the subpulmonary infundibular free wall in typical transposition of the great arteries (both D- and L) permits pulmonary-mitral fibrous continuity, and pulmonary-tricuspid fibrous continuity via the membranous portion of the ventricular septum (*pars membranacea septi*). The subaortic infundibulum and the absence of the subpulmonary infundibular free wall of typical D-transposition of the great arteries (D-TGA) is infundibular inversion. The

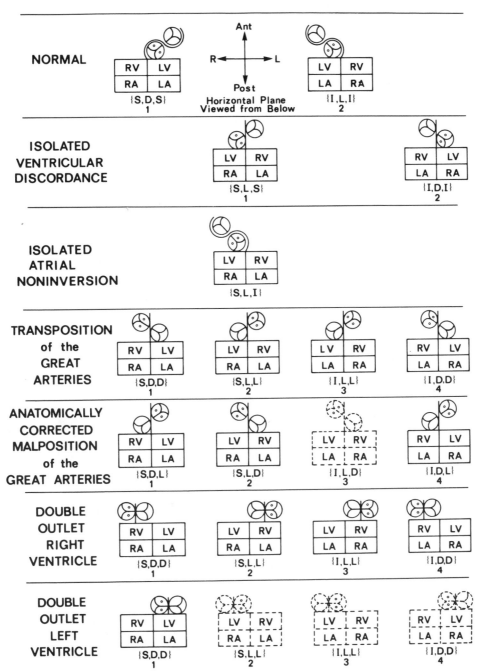

Fig. 28.6 How many types of human heart are there? By "type" of human heart we mean situs and alignments of the major cardiac segments. Examples of abnormal segmental situs are {S,D,D} and {S,L,L}. Examples of abnormal segmental alignments are transposition of the great arteries and double-outlet right ventricle. This diagram shows some common and some rare types of human heart but by no means all types. For example, situs ambiguus, double-inlet left ventricle (*LV*), double-inlet right ventricle (*RV*), and other forms of single or common ventricle have been omitted. *Broken lines* indicate types of heart (cardiotypes) that had not been documented when this diagram was made. It is noteworthy that this chart is organized in vertical columns and in horizontal rows. The *vertical columns* are organized in terms of the concordance or discordance of the AV alignments: column 1, {S,D,-}, and column 3, {I,L,-}, have concordant AV alignments; column 2, {S,L,-}, and column 4, {I,D,-}, have discordant AV alignments. The *horizontal rows* are organized in terms of the various types of ventriculoarterial alignments. Heart diagrams are viewed from below in order to facilitate correlation with angiocardiographic, echocardiographic, and surgical findings. All associated cardiovascular malformations are omitted for simplicity and brevity.

right-sided subaortic infundibulum of typical D-TGA is a mirror image of the left-sided subpulmonary infundibulum of solitus normally related great arteries, with the mirror in the sagittal plane.

3. Bilateral. The infundibulum can be both subpulmon-

ary and subaortic, i.e., in this sense bilateral, as in the Taussig-Bing malformation[107, 108] (Fig. 28.7). The bilateral infundibulum typically prevents all semilunar-atrioventricular fibrous continuity. The bilateral infundibulum may be viewed as one form of situs ambiguus infundibuli: the left-

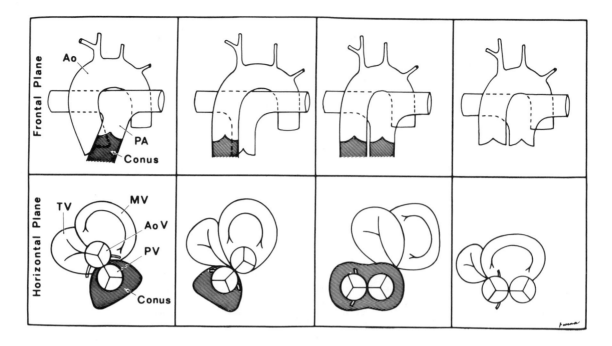

Subpulmonary Conus:

Normally related
great arteries

Tetralogy of Fallot

Truncus arteriosus
communis

Interrupted aortic arch

Isolated ventricular
discordance

Double outlet right
ventricle

Double outlet left
ventricle

Transposition with
posterior aorta

Subaortic Conus:

Typical transposition,
complete and
corrected

Anatomically
corrected
malposition of the
great arteries

Double outlet left
ventricle

Truncus arteriosus
communis

Bilateral Conus:

Double outlet right
ventricle

Transposition ±
pulmonary infun-
dibular stenosis
or atresia

Asplenia syndrome

Juxtaposition of
atrial appendages
syndrome

Anatomically corrected
malposition of the
great arteries

Transposition with
posterior aorta

Normally related great
arteries (rare)

Absent or Very Deficient Conus:

Double outlet left
ventricle

Transposition

Fig. 28.7 What kind of conus (subpulmonary, subaortic, bilateral, or absent) **is associated with what kind of relationship between the great arteries** (truncus arteriosus)? This diagram summarizes most of the known conotruncal-ventricular correlations. The great arteries are viewed from the front in the upper panel and from above in the lower panel. Conal (infundibular) musculature is indicated by cross-hatching. The aortic valve (*AoV*) is indicated by the coronary arteries. *MV*, mitral valve; *PV*, pulmonary valve; *TV*, tricuspid valve. (Reproduced with permission from R. Van Praagh.[108])

sided subpulmonary part of the infundibulum in the typical Taussig-Bing malformation is the solitus (noninverted) infundibulum, but the right-sided subaortic part of the infundibulum is the inverted (mirror image) infundibulum. When bilateral, the infundibular situs is both solitus (left-sided and subpulmonary) and inversus (right-sided and subaortic). Thus, the situs of the bilateral conus is ambiguous (both solitus and inversus).

4. Absent or Very Deficient. The infundibulum may

be absent or very deficient bilaterally, as in some forms of double-outlet left ventricle,[76] thereby permitting both aortic-atrioventricular and pulmonary-atrioventricular fibrous continuity (Fig. 28.7). Absence of the subaortic infundibular free wall is a characteristic of the noninverted (solitus) infundibulum. Absence (absorption) of the subpulmonary infundibular free wall is a feature of the inverted infundibulum, as in typical D-TGA. Thus, the bilaterally absent infundibulum may also be considered to have features both of the solitus conus and of the inverted conus and, hence, to have a form of situs ambiguus coni. Or, one may say that the bilaterally absent conus is neither solitus (left-sided and subpulmonary), nor inversus (right-sided and subaortic), i.e., that the bilaterally absent infundibulum is neither solitus nor inversus. Since the infundibulum always is bilateral (subpulmonary and subaortic), with one or other half unabsorbed or absorbed, we prefer the view that the bilaterally absent infundibulum is a form of situs ambiguus infundibuli. We think that both parts of the infundibulum always should be considered diagnostically, not just that part which is anatomically present (unabsorbed). The absorbed infundibular free wall that is anatomically absent and permits semilunar-atrioventricular approximation and fibrous continuity is as important as the unabsorbed part of the infundibular free wall that prevents semilunar-atrioventricular fibrous continuity (Fig. 28.8).

It is noteworthy that neither form of infundibular situs ambiguus (bilaterally present or bilaterally absent) can be expressed in terms of the concept of noninversion-inversion. This difficulty is solved by the concept of situs ambiguus, and by straightforward anatomic description.

THE GREAT ARTERIES

The great arteries may be related normally or abnormally to each other, to the ventricles, to the ventricular septum, and to the atrioventricular valves (Fig. 28.6). Normally and abnormally related great arteries customarily are designated in terms of their ventriculoarterial alignments ("connections"): normally related, transposed, double-outlet RV, double-outlet LV, etc. As will be seen, the situs of the great arteries is of fundamental importance. The various types of situs of the great arterial segment are as follows.

1. **Normally Related Great Arteries.** There are two kinds of normally related great arteries: solitus normally related and inversus normally related. In solitus normally related great arteries—the usual or noninverted normal—the pulmonary valve (PV) is anterior, superior, and to the left of the aortic valve (AoV). Since the AoV and the ascending aorta (Ao) are to the right (*dextro* or D) relative to the pulmonary valve (PV) and main pulmonary artery (MPA), respectively, solitus normally related great arteries have been referred to by some echocardiographers as D-normally related great arteries (Fig. 28.6 to 28.8).

In inverted normally related great arteries (Fig. 28.6 and 28.8), the PV is anterior, superior, and to the right relative to the AoV. Since the AoV and the ascending Ao are to the left (*levo*, or L) relative to the PV and MPA, inverted normally related great arteries also have been called L-normally related great arteries.

2. **Abnormally Related Great Arteries.** These may be in D-position, L-position, or A-position, depending on whether the abnormally related AoV is to the right (D-position), to the left (L-position), or directly anterior (A-position) relative to the PV.

The D-position is solitus or noninverted in situs, as in solitus normally related great arteries. The L-position of the semilunar valves is inverted in situs, as in inversus normally related great arteries. The A-position is ambiguus in situs, being neither solitus (noninverted) nor inversus (mirror image).

Transposition of the great arteries (TGA) may be D-TGA, L-TGA, or A-TGA (Fig. 28.6 to 28.8). Malposition of the great arteries (MGA) may be D-MGA, L-MGA, or A-MGA, as in double-outlet right ventricle (DORV), double-outlet left ventricle (DOLV), and anatomically corrected malposi-

tion (ACM) of the great arteries (Fig. 28.6). Indeed, TGA is a specific type of MGA.

What difference does an understanding of situs make at the infundibular and the great arterial levels? We have recently come to understand a principle that appears to be of anatomic and developmental significance. When the situs of the infundibulum and the situs of the great arteries are the same, both solitus or both inversus, then the great arteries always are normally related to the ventricles, no matter what the ventricular situs may be. When the situs of the infundibulum and the situs of the great arteries are different, then the great arteries always are abnormally related.

When the infundibulum and the great arteries both are in situs solitus (Fig. 28.7 and 28.8), then the great arteries always are **solitus normally related** (Fig. 28.6). This is true even when the ventricles are inverted, as in isolated ventricular inversion[111] (Fig. 28.6, Isolated Ventricular Discordance, diagram 1).

When the infundibulum and the great arteries both are in situs inversus (Fig. 28.8), then the great arteries are **inverted normally related** (Fig. 28.6). This is true even when the ventricles are noninverted, as in isolated ventricular noninversion (Fig. 28.6, Isolated Ventricular Discordance, diagram 2).

When the situs of the infundibulum and the situs of the great arteries are opposites, **transposition of the great arteries** results—if the situs of the ventricles and of the great arteries is the same. For example, in typical physiologically uncorrected D-TGA, the situs of the infundibulum is inverted, whereas the situs of the great arteries and the ventricles is noninverted (solitus) (Fig. 28.6 to 28.8). In classical physiologically corrected transposition, the situs of the infundibulum is noninverted, whereas the situs of the great arteries and the ventricles is inverted.

When the situs of the infundibulum is different from the situs of the great arteries, and when the situs of the great arteries and the ventricles also is different, then **anatomically corrected malposition of the great arteries** can occur (Fig. 28.6). The commonest form is shown in Figure 28.6, diagram 1: the great arteries are in L-position (inverted); the infundibular situs is not inverted, either being left-sided and subaortic (solitus), or bilateral (ambiguus); and the ventricles are solitus.

When the situs of the infundibulum is ambiguus and bilaterally present, and the situs of the great arteries and the ventricles is the same, then **double-outlet right ventricle** frequently occurs (Fig. 28.6).

When the situs of the infundibulum is ambiguus and bilaterally absent or very deficient, then **double-outlet left ventricle** may occur (Fig. 28.6).

Transposition of the great arteries is perhaps the clearest illustration of the importance of an understanding of ventricular, infundibular, and great arterial situs. When ventricular situs and great arterial situs are the same, as they almost always are, then TGA results from discordance of the infundibular situs, relative to the situs of the ventricles and the great arteries. The infundibulum is the crucial connector between the great arteries and the ventricles. When the infundibular situs is discordant ("backwards") relative to the situs of the great arteries, the great arteries therefore are connected "backwards" to the ventricles. The inverted subaortic infundibulum prevents aortic-mitral approximation, while the absent subpulmonary infundibular free wall permits pulmonary-mitral approximation, resulting in the ventriculoarterial alignments of TGA (Fig. 28.6 and 28.8). Ventriculoarterial alignment discordance (TGA) is due

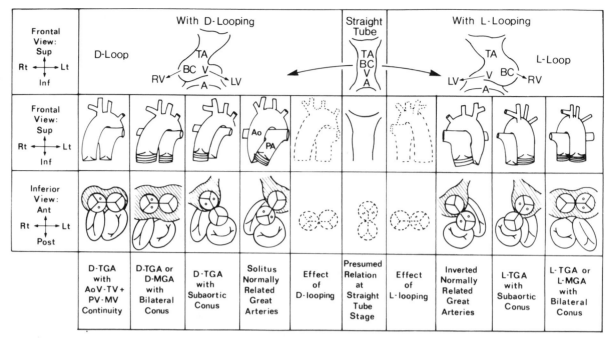

	With D-Looping				Straight Tube			With L-Looping		
	D-TGA with AoV-TV + PV-MV Continuity	D-TGA or D-MGA with Bilateral Conus	D-TGA with Subaortic Conus	Solitus Normally Related Great Arteries	Effect of D-looping	Presumed Relation at Straight Tube Stage	Effect of L-looping	Inverted Normally Related Great Arteries	L-TGA with Subaortic Conus	L-TGA or L-MGA with Bilateral Conus

Fig. 28.8 The differential conal development hypothesis concerning the morphogenesis of normally and abnormally related great arteries. Briefly, D-looping carries the developing aorta to the right, whereas L-looping carries the developing aorta to the left. Initially, there is a bilateral or combined conus beneath both developing semilunar valves. Normally with a D-loop, the subpulmonary part of the conus persists and grows, whereas the subaortic part of the conus is absorbed. This results in superior elevation and anterior protrusion of the developing pulmonary artery above the anterior and right-sided ventricle (RV), and permits the aortic valve to descend inferiorly, posteriorly and to the left, to come into fibrous continuity with the developing mitral valve, and to drain the posterior and left-sided left ventricle (LV), thereby resulting in normally related great arteries. Typical D-transposition of great arteries (TGA) results from the opposite development of the conus. When the right-sided subaortic part of the conus persists and develops, and the left-sided subpulmonary part of the conus is absorbed, the aortic valve is carried superiorly and anteriorly by the subaortic conus and so is located above the anterior and right-sided RV, whereas absorption of the subpulmonary part of the conus permits the pulmonary valve to descend posteriorly and to the left, to come into fibrous continuity with the developing mitral valve, and to drain the posterior and left-sided LV, thereby resulting in typical D-TGA. Hence, D-TGA results from conal inversion; development of the right-sided subaortic part and absorption of the left-sided subpulmonary part, instead of vice versa, which is normal. When both the subaortic and the subpulmonary parts of the conus persist and grow, i.e., when neither part of the conus undergoes absorption, often the result is double-outlet right ventricle, as in the Taussig-Bing malformation,[107, 108] in which both semilunar valves are elevated superiorly and protruded anteriorly above the anterior and right-sided RV, both semilunar valves being widely separated from the mitral valve and left ventricle by the persistence and growth of subsemilunar conal myocardium. When both the subaortic and the subpulmonary parts of the conus are absorbed, both semilunar valves may sink inferiorly and posteriorly, with both coming into fibrous continuity with the mitral valve and draining the posterior and left-sided LV, as in Paul's[76] unique case of double-outlet left ventricle. TA, truncus arteriosus; BC, bulbus cordis; A, atrium; V, ventricle; PA, pulmonary artery; Ao, aorta; AV, atrioventricular; AoV, aortic valve; MV, mitral valve; PV, pulmonary valve; D-TGAs and L-TGAs, dextro- and levotransposition of the great arteries. (Reproduced with permission from R. Van Praagh and S. Van Praagh.[111])

to infundibuloarterial situs discordance (when the situs of the great arteries and the situs of the ventricles are the same). Thus, it is noteworthy that alignment discordance (ventriculoarterial) is produced by situs discordance (infundibuloarterial).

Etiology of D-TGA. Since typical D-TGA (Fig. 28.6, diagram 1) appears to result from *isolated infundibular inversion* (the atria, ventricles, and great arteries being noninverted), an understanding of the etiology of inversion therefore seems to be relevant to the *etiology of D-TGA*. The recent findings of Layton[57–59] have clarified the etiology of situs inversus. Briefly, situs solitus totalis appears to result from the presence of a dominant gene that controls visceral situs. Layton[57, 58] found in mice with situs inversus that when the dominant gene for situs solitus was absent, the bodily situs developed at random, obeying the laws of chance. When many matings were done between male and female mice that were homozygous for the situs inversus (iv) gene, approximately 50% of the offspring had situs inversus, and approximately 50% had situs solitus; there was some heterotaxy in both groups.

These situs inversus mice appear to illustrate that the absence of genetic information can be teratogenic. Genetic anomalies are usually conceived to be *positive* abnormalities, either dominant or recessive, but situs inversus appears to result from a *negative* abnormality, a lack of genetic information.

If the concept that typical D-TGA results from isolated infundibular inversion[111, 115] is correct, then one would expect this colony of situs inversus mice to have cases of spontaneously occurring TGA. This is exactly what was found; the frequency of TGA was approximately 20%. Double-outlet right ventricle was found in another 20% of the offspring. Hence, the frequency of spontaneously occurring conotruncal anomalies is very high. There is also a high frequency of common atrioventricular canal (type C of Rastelli). Thus, these iv/iv mice are a mutant gene model not only of situs inversus, TGA, DORV, and common AV canal, but also these animals have features resembling situs ambiguus, but with normal motility of the tracheobronchial cilia and normal spermatic motility.

Also consistent with the hypothesis that situs inversus is

due to a lack of genetic information (absence of the dominant gene for situs solitus) is the finding that the bronchiectasis of Kartagener's syndrome (situs inversus, dextrocardia, and bronchiectasis)[51, 52] is due to hypomotility of the tracheobronchial cilia.[30] These cilia beat poorly and fail to clear the tracheobronchial tree of debris, resulting in bronchiectasis. These hypomotile cilia have been found to lack dynein side arms, accounting for their hypomotility.[30] The absence of a specific protein such as dynein strongly suggests that it is not being coded for. This in turn is consistent with the hypothesis that absence of DNA may well be the etiology of situs inversus and of hypomotile tracheobronchial cilia, explaining the bronchiectasis of Kartagener's triad.

Similarly, it has been found that patients with situs inversus may have infertility due to spermatic immotility.[2, 30] Such immotility in turn is due to absence of dynein side arms in the sperm tails, a lack of flagellar motion explaining the spermatic immotility, and the consequent infertility. Again, the absence of a specific protein (dynein) in the sperm tails suggests that it is not being coded for, such genetic absence being consistent with the Layton hypothesis[57, 58] concerning the genetic etiology of situs inversus.

It has long been thought that situs inversus totalis is due to a simple Mendelian autosomal recessive abnormality of variable penetrance. The degree of penetrance is different from strain to strain in a given laboratory animal such as the mouse. Although Layton now has several different strains of *iv/iv* mice, the results of the mating experiments are the same in all strains thus far examined: approximately 50% of the offspring have situs inversus, and approximately 50% have situs solitus. Thus, variability of penetrance appears not to play a role in the etiology of situs inversus in Layton's mice.

This new work concerning the etiology of situs inversus appears to be relevant to the understanding of the etiology of those forms of congenital heart disease that are characterized by total or segmental situs inversus. Typical D-TGA is just one form of congenital heart disease that has a segmental inversion (infundibular). Many other forms of congenital heart disease also have one or more segmental inversions that may be at the atrial, ventricular, infundibular, or great arterial levels. The Layton hypothesis[57, 58] suggests that segmental inversion may also reflect a lack of dominant genetic control over the development of the various cardiac segments.

CARDIOTYPES

By type of heart, cardiotype, in congenital heart disease one ordinarily means the following: the situs of the major cardiac segments—the atria, the ventricles, and the great arteries; the alignments of the major cardiac segments—the atrioventricular (AV) alignments and the ventriculoarterial (VA) alignments; the associated cardiac malformations within each of the three major cardiac segments, and between them; and the function of the combination of cardiac segments and alignments, with or without associated malformations. Thus, the cardiotype is primarily concerned with the *anatomic diagnosis*. However, the *physiologic diagnosis*, which usually is a sequela of the anatomic diagnosis, is nonetheless of clinical and surgical importance.

In order to facilitate the expression of, and the study of, the many combinations of cardiac segments and alignments, it is helpful to view the three major cardiac segments—the atria, ventricles, and great arteries—as the members of a set.[69, 118] In the mathematical sense of set theory, a set is indicated by braces { } (Fig. 28.6). The three major cardiac segments are expressed in venoarterial sequence: {atria,

ventricles, great arteries}. Note that the members of the segmental set are separated by commas, this being conventional set notation.

The *situs* of each of the major cardiac segments is expressed *inside* the braces. The *alignments* of the major cardiac segments are expressed *outside* the braces, as are the *associated malformations*.

The situs of each of the three major cardiac segments may be symbolized for ease of expression and manipulation of the variable segmental combinations. The segmental situs symbols that we have used in the past are summarized below:

Atrial Situs. S (solitus), I (inversus), A (ambiguus).

Ventricular Situs. D (D-loop, or solitus), L (L-loop, or inversus), X (X-loop, or ambiguus).

Arterial Situs. S (solitus normal), D (D-transposition or D-malposition, i.e., solitus transposition or solitus malposition), L (L-transposition or L-malposition, i.e., inverted transposition or inverted malposition), I (inversus normal), and A (A-transposition or A-malposition, i.e., ambiguus transposition or ambiguus malposition).

Thus, this **symbolic cardiac anatomy** uses set notation and is a form of **symbolic logic** applied to the diagnosis of congenital heart disease (Fig. 28.6 and Table 28.1). Examples of how this notation works, and how convenient it is, are as follows.

Typical complete physiologically uncorrected D-transposition of the great arteries is TGA {S,D,D}, which is read: transposition of the great arteries (TGA) with situs solitus of the viscera and atria (S), ventricular D-loop (D), and D-position of the semilunar valves (D). If the transposed aortic valve (AoV) happens to lie directly anteriorly to the transposed pulmonary valve (PV), then it may be expressed as TGA {S,D,A}. If the transposed AoV lies somewhat to the left of the transposed PV, it is TGA {S,D,L}. Associated malformations are expressed as follows: TGA {S,D,D} with ventricular septal defect (VSD) of the AV canal type, straddling tricuspid valve (TV), and small RV.

TABLE 28.1   NOTATION

{Visceroatrial Situs, Ventricular Loop, Conotruncus}, i.e., {Atria, Ventricles, Great Arteries}

Types of visceroatrial situs
  Situs solitus = S
  Situs inversus = I
  Situs ambiguus = A
Type of ventricular loop
  D-Loop = D
  L-Loop = L
  X-Loop = X (X = unknown)
Types of conotruncus
  Solitus normally related great arteries = S
  Inverted normally related great arteries = I
  D-Transposition or D-malposition = D
  L-Transposition or L-malposition = L
  A-Transposition or *A*-malposition = A[a]
Examples (see Fig. 28.6)
  Normal type of heart = NRGA {S, D, S}
  Inverted normal type of heart = NRGA {I, L, I}
  Typical D-TGA = TGA {S, D, D}
  Typical L-TGA = TGA {S, L, L}
  Typical DORV = DORV {S, D, D}[b]

[a] A = antero = the transposed or malposed aortic valve is directly anterior to the transposed or malposed pulmonary valve.

[b] DORV, double-outlet right ventricle; D-TGA, D-transposition of the great arteries; L-TGA, L-transposition of the great arteries; NRGA, normally related great arteries.

Thus, the situs of the three major cardiac segments—atria, ventricles, and great arteries—are expressed inside the braces by means of symbols, as in {**S,D,D**}. Major abnormal segmental alignments are expressed outside the braces, as in **TGA** {S,D,D} with **straddling TV.** Associated anomalies also are expressed outside the braces, and customarily after them, as in TGA {S,D,D} with straddling TV, **VSD of the AV canal type, and small RV.**

The foregoing is the method of diagnostic description that we have used for the past decade. We have found it to be satisfactory because it is accurate, brief, and convenient. Also, it applies to all forms of congenital heart disease, no matter how complex. Thus we have found no reason to modify this **method of notation.** However, there are, of course, many ways in which the diagnostic data could be expressed. In view of the importance of segmental situs, one could, for example, express **the situs of the {atria, ventricles, infundibulum, arteries}** as S (solitus), I (inversus), or A (ambiguus). Several examples follow.

TGA {S,D,D} = TGA {**S,S,I,S**}. The latter would be read as transposition of the great arteries (TGA) with situs solitus of the viscera and atria (S), solitus ventricles (S), inversus infundibulum (I), and solitus great arteries (S).

TGA {S,L,L} = TGA {**S,I,S,I**}. The latter would be read as transposition of the great arteries (TGA) with solitus viscera and atria (S), inversus ventricles (I), solitus infundibulum (S), and inversus great arteries (I).

Although we prefer the older, briefer, more descriptive symbols used in Figure 28.6 and in Table 28.1, we think that one should understand the foregoing **segmental situs analysis**; hence, its inclusion here. We are suggesting not a change in terminology but an enrichment of understanding. Much more important than the terms one may prefer is the systematic, segment-by-segment and alignment-by-alignment method of diagnosing complex congenital heart disease.

One should be aware that **there is no anatomically and embryologically valid connections-based alternative to the segmental approach**, for several reasons:

1. The atria do not connect directly with the ventricles, because the atria and the ventricles normally are separated by the atrioventricular junction, except at the bundle of His.

2. The ventricles do not connect directly with the great arteries, because of the interposition of the infundibulum (conus).

3. Hence, the concepts of atrioventricular connections and ventriculoarterial connections are anatomically and developmentally erroneous.

4. The structures that truly do connect the atria and the ventricles (the AV junction), and the ventricles and the great arteries (the infundibulum), are themselves junctional cardiac segments.[75]

5. Segments determine alignments, not vice versa. For example, whether the AV alignments ("connections") are discordant or not is usually determined by the adjacent cardiac segments, i.e., by the situs of the atria compared with the situs of the ventricles. Vice versa is not the case: the AV alignments ("connections") do not determine the situs of the atria and/or the situs of the ventricles. Thus, segmental situs is primary, whereas segmental alignments ("connections"), although very important, are nonetheless secondary.

However, in the segmental approach to the diagnosis of congenital heart disease, both segmental situs (inside the braces) and segmental alignments (outside the braces) are accorded *equal emphasis*, as is illustrated by the diagnosis TGA {S,D,D}. We therefore think that it is an unsatisfactory diagnostic approach to emphasize the AV and VA "connections" (alignments) but to omit the situs of the ventricles, infundibulum, and great arteries. As has been shown, understanding of the situs of the ventricles, infundibulum, and great arteries is diagnostically essential. For example, one cannot consider a case intelligently, particularly from the surgical standpoint, until one knows what the ventricular situs is. The segmental approach to the diagnosis of congenital heart disease thus is basic and has won general acceptance.[16, 103, 110, 118]

DEXTROCARDIA

First described in man by Fabricius[33] in 1606, dextrocardia means that the heart is predominantly right-sided. How many anatomic types of congenital dextrocardia are there? In an effort to answer this question, we reviewed 136 autopsied cases from three sources (Table 28.2).

The findings in this large series of anatomically confirmed cases are summarized in Table 28.3.

It will be seen that right-sided hearts can have any kind of congenital heart disease, just as left-sided hearts can. Indeed, one of the fundamental themes of this chapter is that the position of the heart within the thorax is not a basic biologic consideration. For example, in quadripeds, the heart is centrally located within the thorax, which is deep in the ventral-to-dorsal direction. One of the adaptations associated with man's bipedal locomotion and upright posture is considerable ventrodorsal flattening of the thorax, which makes cardiac lateralization advantageous. Thus, in most forms of life, mesocardia is normal. It is in this sense that cardiac laterality (levocardia or dextrocardia) is not a biologically basic consideration and, hence, it is not surprising that the same anatomic and developmental principles apply, no matter where the heart may be located. Consequently, the segmental approach to diagnosis applies to all of the cardiac malpositions because the principles of segmental diagnosis are independent of cardiac position.

The same diagnostic and surgical approach used for left-sided hearts may therefore be used for right-sided ones. In dextrocardia, chest x-rays should not be reversed. Similarly, the limb leads of the electrocardiogram should not be reversed in order to "correct for dextrocardia." Angiocardiograms should not be inverted as an aid to diagnostic understanding. The anatomic data should be viewed as they really are (Table 28.3) because the assumption underlying these various methods of "correcting" for dextrocardia is that all of the cardiac segments are inverted. This, however, usually is not the case. Indeed, mirror-image dextrocardia {I,L,I} was present in only 7 of these 136 autopsied cases. Hence, "correction" for dextrocardia usually introduces far more confusion that clarification into diagnostic thinking. The highly disadvantageous introduction of mental mirrors and spits for the diagnosis of dextrocardia is why right-sided hearts have been a diagnostic *bête noire*. The segmental approach has largely supplanted the old mirrors-and-spits approach to dextrocardia because segmental analysis is the

TABLE 28.2　DEXTROCARDIA MATERIAL

Source	No. of Cases
CHMC[a]	46
Van Praagh *et al.*[112]	51
Lev *et al.*[60]	39[b]
Total autopsied cases	136

[a] Children's Hospital Medical Center, Boston, Mass.

[b] Of the 41 cases of Lev et al.,[60] two were omitted because of insufficient data (cases 36 and 40).

TABLE 28.3   TYPES OF CONGENITAL DEXTROCARDIA IN 136 AUTOPSIED CASES

Type	No. of Cases
In situs solitus	
1. NRGA {S,D,S} [a]	24
2. TGA {S,D,D}	4
3. DORV {S,D,L}	1
4. ACM {S,D,L}	1
5. TGA {S,L,L}	28
6. DORV {S,L,L}	4
7. NRGA {S,L,I}	2
8. DOCV {S,X,D}	2
In situs inversus	
1. NRGA {I,L,I}	7
2. TGA {I,L,L}	7
3. TGA {I,L,D}	1
4. DORV {I,L,L}	3
5. DORV {I,L,L (I)}	1
6. TGA {I,D,D}	3
7. TGA {I,D,L}	1
8. NRGA {I,D,I}	1
In situs ambiguus	
With asplenia	
1. TGA {A,D,D}	4
2. DORV {A,D,D}	1
3. ACM {A,D,L}	2
4. TGA {A,L,L}	8
5. DORV {A,L,L}	6
6. DORV {A,L,D}	2
7. NRGA {A,L,I}	2
8. DOSV {A,X,L}	2
With polysplenia	
1. NRGA {A,D,S}	2
2. TGA {A,L,L}	6
3. NRGA {A,L,I}	10
With normally formed spleen	
1. NRGA {A,L,I}	1

[a] Letters within braces are explained in text.

[b] ACM, anatomically corrected malposition of the great arteries; DOCV, double-outlet common ventricle; DORV, double-outlet right ventricle; DOSV, double-outlet single ventricle; MGA, malposition of the great arteries; NRGA, normally related great arteries; TGA, transposition of the great arteries.

best way in which right-sided hearts can be understood. The difficulty with mental mirrors and spits in dextrocardia is that usually, some segments are inverted, whereas others are not. The solution to this diagnostic confusion is to use a more basic diagnostic approach, one that always works, namely, segment-by-segment and alignment-by-alignment analysis (Fig. 28.6). In the operating room, the surgeon must look at reality as it is. So, too, should the cardiologist and the radiologist. When one does this, what does one find? Table 28.3 will repay careful study.

Atria. The commonest type of visceroatrial situs was situs solitus, in 66 cases. Second in frequency was situs ambiguus, in 46 patients. Least frequent was situs inversus, in 24 cases. It will now be clear why we have thought it important to develop a diagnostic approach that works in situs ambiguus. Any diagnostic approach that does not apply in situs ambiguus (e.g., AV concordance-discordance) is unsatisfactory.

Ventricles. In the series as a whole, L-loop ventricles were twice as common as D-loop ventricles: D-loop, 44 patients; L-loop, 89 patients; and X-loop, 3 patients. The preponderance of L-loop becomes understandable when one

recalls that the L-loop "belongs" in the right chest, as in mirror-image dextrocardia, whereas the D-loop "belongs" in the left chest, as in normal levocardia.

It is, however, interesting that in situs solitus of the viscera and atria, the frequency of D-loops and L-loops was approximately equal: D-loop was found in 30/64 cases and L-loop was found in 34/64 cases. However, in situs inversus of the viscera and atria, L-loops were much commoner than D-loops: D-loop was found in 5/24 patients and L-loop was found in 19/24 patients. Similarly, in situs ambiguus of the viscera and atria, L-loops greatly predominated: D-loop was found in 9/45 cases, and L-loop was found in 36/45 cases.

These data suggest that in dextrocardia with situs solitus, D-loop ventricles and L-loop ventricles occur at random (approximately 50/50), whereas in dextrocardia with situs inversus and in dextrocardia with situs ambiguus, L-loops are approximately four times as common as D-loops.

Great Arteries. In this series of 136 cases of dextrocardia, the types of relationships between the great arteries and the ventricles were as follows (Table 28.3): L-TGA was by far the commonest, in 50 patients; solitus normally related great arteries were second in frequency, in 26 cases; inverted normally related great arteries were third, in 23 patients; DORV with L-MGA was fourth in frequency, in 15 cases; D-TGA was fifth, in 14 patients; ACM with L-MGA and DORV with D-MGA were tied for sixth place, each in 3 cases; and L-MGA was least frequent, in 2 patients. Both patients had morphologically undiagnosed single or common ventricle. The great arteries were L-malposed, but the type of VA alignment could not be specified further since the ventricular myocardial anatomy was regarded as morphologically uncertain or indeterminate.

Somewhat further simplified, the ventriculoarterial alignments in dextrocardia, in order of decreasing frequency, were: transposition of the great arteries (D- and L-), 64 cases; normally related great arteries (solitus and inversus), 49 cases; double-outlet right ventricle (D- and L-malposition) 18 cases; anatomically corrected malposition (L-malposition only), 3 cases; and malposition of the great arteries with morphologically undiagnosed single ventricle, 2 patients.

Since the type of visceroatrial situs is the body's statement of what is positionally "normal" for all asymmetric viscera, at least in situs solitus and in situs inversus, the question therefore arises: **Are the VA alignments related in any way to the type of visceroatrial situs that is present?** The data (Table 28.3) suggest that the type of situs and the types of VA alignment are interrelated.

In situs solitus, the VA alignments were: L-TGA, 28 cases; solitus normally related great arteries, 24 cases; D-TGA, 6 cases; DORV with L-MGA, 5 cases; inverted normally related great arteries, 2 patients; and ACM, 1 case.

In situs inversus, the VA alignments were: L-TGA, eight cases; inverted normally related great arteries, eight cases; D-TGA, four cases; and DORV with L-MGA, four cases.

In asplenia, the VA alignments were: L-TGA, eight patients; DORV with L-MGA, six patients; D-TGA, four cases; DORV with D-MGA, three cases; and inverted normally related great arteries, ACM with L-MGA, and L-MGA with undiagnosed single ventricle, 2 patients each.

In polysplenia, the AV alignments were: inverted normally related great arteries, 10 patients; L-TGA, six patients; and solitus normally related great arteries, two cases.

In situs ambiguus with a normally formed spleen, this patient had inverted normally related great arteries.

It is noteworthy that only in situs solitus was the frequency of solitus normally related great arteries appreciable (24 cases). In situs inversus, the frequency of solitus normally related great arteries was zero, as it also was with asplenia.

Only in situs inversus and with polysplenia was the frequency of inverted normally related great arteries considerable: in situs inversus, eight cases, and in polysplenia, 10 cases. These data (and others mentioned previously)[57-59] suggest that situs inversus and polysplenia may well be interrelated etiologically and embryologically.

Now we must consider in greater detail **the types of heart that occur in the right chest.** Specifically, how many anatomic types of heart occur in the right hemithorax? To the best of our knowledge, the answer is 29. Can these 29 anatomic types of right-sided heart be simplified in some valid way? Yes, they can. **The three major groups of dextrocardia** are (Table 28.3): in situs solitus, 66/136 cases; in situs inversus, 24/136 cases; and in situs ambiguus, 46/136 cases.

However, within each kind of situs, we still must consider the various anatomic types of heart (cardiotypes) that occur.

DEXTROCARDIA IN SITUS SOLITUS

Dextrocardia in situs solitus has classically been known as *isolated dextrocardia.* This designation indicates that the heart is right-sided (dextrocardia), but that this right-sided cardiac position is not associated with situs inversus viscerum and, hence, that the dextrocardia is "isolated" or unaccompanied by other evidence of visceral inversion. There are several very different types of dextrocardia in situs solitus (Table 28.3).

1. **Dextrocardia with Normally Related Atria, Ventricles, and Great Arteries.** This is a right-sided heart with situs solitus of the viscera and atria (S), D-loop ventricles (D), and normally related great arteries (NRGA) of the solitus (S) type, i.e., **dextrocardia with NRGA {S,D,S}.** This kind of dextrocardia has been called pivotal dextrocardia,[60] because it is as though the apex of a normal left-sided heart had pivoted horizontally to the right about a superoinferior axis. This is the kind of heart that also has been referred to as dextroversion[112] because it is as though a normal heart had turned to the right.

NRGA {S,D,S} was the second commonest type of dextrocardia in this series as a whole (24/136 cases) and the second commonest type of dextrocardia in situs solitus (24/66 cases).

An illustrative case is shown in Figures 28.9 and 28.10. This patient had *congenital secondary dextrocardia,* i.e., the right-sidedness of the heart was secondary to marked hypoplasia of the right lung. Because the heart was markedly right-sided and somewhat posterior, the normal left aortic arch (normal in situs solitus) passed transversely from the right to left, immediately anterior to the trachea. The normal transverse aortic arch severely indented the trachea anteriorly, producing symptoms and signs indistinguishable from those of a vascular ring. Dr. William Mustard performed an aortopexy, attaching the transverse aortic arch to the chest wall anteriorly. This immediately relieved the patient's stridor and dyspnea that had been produced by the marked anterior tracheal compression. Unfortunately, the aortopexy sutures did not hold. The aorta receded posteriorly to its

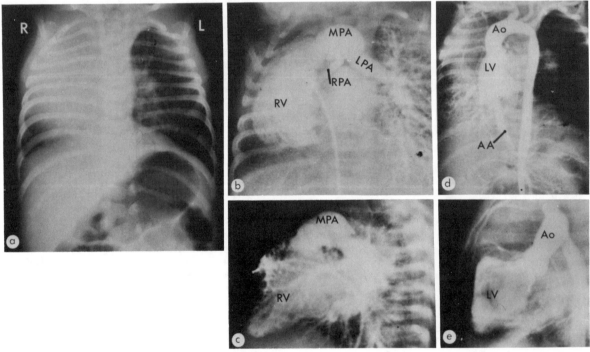

Fig. 28.9 Dextrocardia NRGA {S,D,S}. Situs solitus of the viscera and atria (S) is indicated by the right-sided liver shadow and the left-sided stomach bubble in *a* and by the catheter course in the right-sided inferior vena cava and right atrium in *b.* A D-loop is present (D), with right ventricle (*RV*) to the right (in *b*) and with left ventricle (*LV*) to the left (in *d*). An anomalous artery (*AA*) from the celiac axis supplies the lower right lung, and a hypoplastic right pulmonary artery (*RPA*) supplies the upper portion of the right lung. The right pulmonary veins connected anomalously into the inferior vena cava. The scimitar-shaped pulmonary veins were obscured by the right-sided heart shadow. Dextrocardia was secondary to hypoplasia of the right lung, that in turn is associated with hemivertebrae (seen through the stomach bubble in *a*). The right-sided location of the heart resulted in a normal left aortic arch producing severe anterior tracheal compression (seen in *e*) that claimed this patient's life. Hence, a normal aortic arch mimicked a fatal vascular ring, because of dextrocardia secondary to hypoplasia of the right lung. This was a normal heart in the right chest. *Ao,* aorta; *R,* right; *L,* left; *LPA,* left pulmonary artery; *MPA,* main pulmonary artery. (Reproduced with permission from R. Van Praagh *et al.*[113] and the Reuben H. Donnelley Corp.)

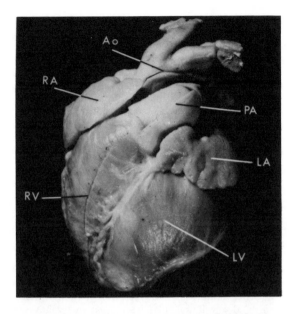
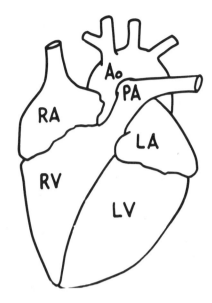
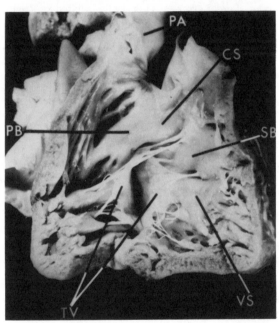
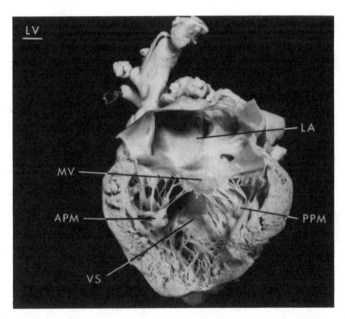

Fig. 28.10 Dextrocardia NRGA {S,D,S}. Heart specimen. Many of the normal gross morphologic characteristics of each ventricle are evident. *Ao,* aorta; *RA,* right atrium; *PA,* pulmonary artery; *TV,* tricuspid valve; *MV,* mitral valve; *SVC,* superior vena cava: *IVC,* inferior vena cava; *CS,* crista supraventricularis; *PB,* parietal band; *SB,* septal band; *VS,* ventricular septum; *APM,* anterolateral papillary muscle; *PPM,* posteromedial papillary muscle; *LA,* left atrium; *RV,* right ventricle; *LV,* left ventricle. (Reproduced with permission from R. Van Praagh *et al.*[112] and The Reuben H. Donnelley Corp.)

preoperative position, and the patient died of asphyxia on the way back to the operating room. Severe hypoplasia of the right lung was associated with the scimitar syndrome[112] and with hemivertebrae.

The heart was structurally normal (Fig. 28.10) but was positionally abnormal secondary to the right pulmonary hypoplasia. Consequently, this was a case of lung disease with other congenital anomalies. This really was not a case of congenital heart disease; rather, this was a structurally normal heart that had been secondarily attracted into the right hemithorax.

Multiple congenital anomalies were present in 17 of the 23 patients in whom this information was available:

hypoplasia of the right lung in seven cases, with scimitar syndrome in five; agenesis of the right lung in four; left diaphragmatic eventration in three; renal dysgenesis in two; tracheoesophageal fistula in two.

Apart from dextrocardia with the asplenia syndrome and dextrocardia with the polysplenia syndrome, dextrocardia with NRGA {S,D,S} was the only type of right-sided heart that was associated with multiple congenital anomalies.

Although this kind of right-sided heart can be structurally normal, congenital heart disease is the rule in dextrocardia with NRGA {S,D,S}, present in 17/24 such cases: ventricular septal defect in seven patients; left superior vena cava to coronary sinus in 6; coarctation of the aorta in four; secundum type of atrial septal defect in four; anomalous pulmonary venous connection in three; and complete common atrioventricular canal with common atrium in two.

2. Dextrocardia with Normally Related Atria, Ventricles, and Transposition of the Great Arteries. This is typical complete, physiologically uncorrected TGA in the right chest with situs solitus of the viscera and atria (S), D-loop ventricles (D), and D-transposition of the great arteries (D), i.e., **dextrocardia with TGA {S,D,D}** (Fig. 28.6). This was found in only four patients (Table 28.3). **Extracardiac anomalies** were present in only 1 of these four patients: microcephaly, hemivertebrae, and bilateral choanal atresia. **Associated cardiac malformations** were found in three of these four patients: ventricular septal defect in three cases and left juxtaposition of the atrial appendages[69] in three cases.

3. Dextrocardia with Normally Related Atria, Ventricles, and Double-Outlet Right Ventricle with Leftward Aorta. There was one such patient in this series with situs solitus of the viscera and atria (S), ventricular D-loop (D), and double-outlet right ventricle (DORV) with L-malposition of the great arteries (L), i.e., **dextrocardia with DORV {S,D,L}**. This 27-year-old woman (case 34 of Lev *et al.*[60]) also had left juxtaposition of the atrial appendages, a secundum atrial septal defect, pulmonary outflow tract stenosis, and a single coronary artery.

4. Dextrocardia with Normally Related Atria, Ventricles, and Anatomically Corrected Malposition of the Great Arteries with Leftward Aorta. This was a case with situs solitus of the viscera and atria (S), D-loop ventricles (D), and anatomically corrected malposition of the great arteries (ACM) with L-malposition (L), ie., this was **dextrocardia with ACM {S,D,L}** (Fig. 28.6). The patient, a 17-year-old boy, had **the juxaposition of the atrial appendages syndrome**[69]: left juxtaposition of the atrial appendages (JAA), tricuspid atresia which was membranous and transilluminated brightly, secundum atrial septal defect, ventricular septal defect, thick-walled and small-chamber "RV" (infundibulum), bilateral subsemilunar infundibulum with no semilunar-mitral fibrous continuity, and pulmonary outflow tract stenosis. An additional finding of interest, not part of the JAA syndrome,[69] was fibrous subaortic stenosis produced by a spinnaker of endocardial cushion tissue.

5. Dextrocardia with Normally Related Atria, Ventricular Inversion, and Physiologically "Corrected" Transposition of the Great Arteries. The commonest type of right-sided heart found in this study, occurring in 28 patients, was dextrocardia with situs solitus of the viscera and atria (S), L-loop ventricles (L), and L-transposition of the great arteries (L), i.e., **dextrocardia with TGA {S,L,L}** (Figs. 28.6, 28.11, and 28.12).

Associated cardiac anomalies in these 28 cases of classical L-TGA included: pulmonary outflow tract atresia in 13; pulmonary outflow tract stenosis in 10; single left ventricle with infundibular outlet chamber in 5; small right ventricle (left-sided) in 3; ventricular septal defect (with two ventricles present) in 16; common atrioventricular canal in 4; mitral atresia (right-sided) in 4; persistent left superior vena cava to coronary sinus to right atrium in 4.

This study of 28 autopsy-proved cases of so-called physiologically "corrected" TGA illustrates the very high frequency of associated cardiovascular anomalies that is found with this form of TGA. Of the eight associated cardiac malformations above-mentioned, seven are important clinically. Associated anomalies usually make a cruel joke out of the concept of physiologic correction of such a TGA. This is why we prefer to designate this anomaly segmentally, i.e., TGA {S,L,L}, rather than using the often physiologically

erroneous designation corrected TGA. Nowadays, "corrected TGA" also can be confused with surgically corrected TGA. Thus, we prefer anatomic designations that are not encumbered by erroneous physiologic connotations, nor by variably applicable surgical implications. The term physiologically corrected TGA is used above because it is in widespread usage and because not everyone may share our preferences.

Why is TGA {S,L,L} the commonest form of dextrocardia that the pediatric cardiologist and the cardiac surgeon are likely to see? We think that the answer is as follows.

Situs solitus of the viscera and atria is the most common type of visceroatrial situs, with situs solitus at least 5000 times more frequent than situs inversus.[65, 70, 125, 126]

L-loop ventricles "should" all have dextrocardia. Just as normal ventricles loop first to the right and then swing to the left, resulting in normal levocardia, so too inverted ventricles first loop to the left and then swing to the right, resulting in dextrocardia. Levocardia is an anomaly in classical "corrected" TGA; dextrocardia should be present, as in these 28 cases.

Discordant ventricles almost always are associated with TGA or other abnormal ventriculoarterial alignment. In other words, discordant ventricles almost never have normally related great arteries. This is why isolated ventricular inversion, NRGA {S,L,S}, and isolated ventricular noninversion, NRGA {I,D,I}, are so very rare.

Thus, TGA {S,L,L} appears to be the commonest form of dextrocardia because situs solitus is so common, because L-loops belong in the right chest, and because AV discordance almost always is associated with TGA. L-TGA is the rule (as opposed to D-TGA or A-TGA) because the transposed aorta arises above the *left-sided* RV, and the transposed pulmonary artery originates above the *right-sided* LV. Extracardiac anomalies did not occur in these 28 patients.

6. Dextrocardia with Normally Related Atria, Ventricular Inversion, and Double-Outlet Right Ventricle with Leftward Aorta. Four patients with right-sided hearts in this series had double-outlet right ventricle (DORV) with situs solitus of the viscera and atria (S), L-loop ventricles (L), and L-malposition of the great arteries (L), *i.e.*, *dextrocardia with DORV {S,L,L}* (Fig. 28.6). Associated cardiac anomalies were: pulmonary stenosis in 2; pulmonary atresia in 1; ventricular septal defect in 3; and common atrioventricular canal in 2.

7. Dextrocardia with Normally Related Atria, Inverted Ventricles, and Inverted Normally Related Great Arteries. This is dextrocardia with situs solitus of the viscera and atria (S), L-loop ventricles (L), and normally related great arteries (NRGA) of the inverted (I) type, i.e., *dextrocardia with NRGA {S,L,I}* (Fig. 28.6). This is an exceedingly rare cardiotype that was found in a 2-day-old boy and in a 6-week-old girl. This anomaly is so uncommon that even its name, expressed in words, is not well established. It may be called *ventricular inversion with inverted normally related great arteries in situs solitus.* Or it may be called *isolated atrial noninversion,* meaning that only the atria are not inverted. This type of heart also may simply be designated segmentally, with words or with symbols, as above.

Physiologically, there is **"transposition" of the circulations,** even though the great arteries themselves are not transposed. Physiologic uncorrection ("transposition") of the circulations occurs when only *one* of the major cardiac segments has an inversive or right-left switching error. Typical D-TGA, i.e., TGA {S,D,D}, is the most familiar example of a single segmental right-left switching error, at the great arteries only. Typical L-TGA, i.e., TGA {S,L,L}, is the most familar example of a *double* segmental right-left switching

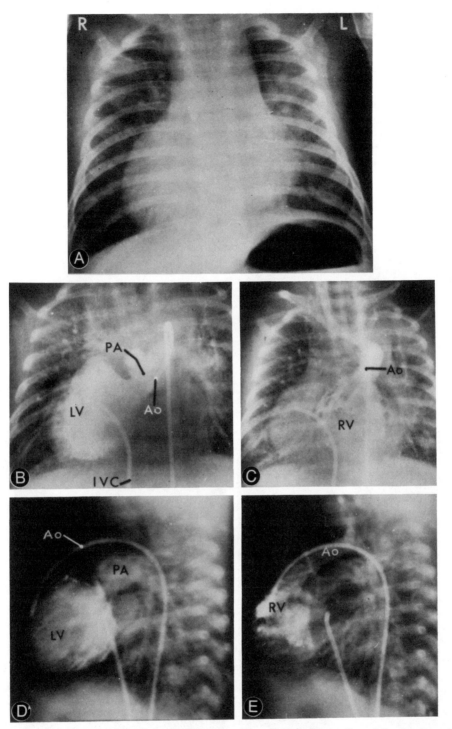

Fig. 28.11 **Dextrocardia with physiologically "corrected" transposition {S,L,L}.** Situs solitus of the viscera and atria (S) is indicated by the right-sided liver shadow and left-sided stomach bubble (a) and by the right-sided inferior vena cava (*IVC*) (b). An L-loop is indicated by the morphology of the right-sided left ventricle (LV) in b and c, by the discordant atrioventricular (AV) alignment, right atrium to LV (b and c), and by the presence of L-TGA (b to e). The left-sided right ventricle (*RV*) is visualized only well enough to exclude a single LV with an infundibular outlet chamber, with the RV appearing too large to be an outlet chamber. However, a selective RV injection (left-sided) is wise in this type of case, via a retrograde aortic catheter, to establish whether an RV is present, or is just an outlet chamber, and to assess the status of the left-sided tricuspid valve, which is frequently abnormal in form and function, i.e., regurgitation, stenosis, or atresia. *Ao,* aorta; *PA,* pulmonary artery; *IVC,* inferior vena cava. (Reproduced with permission from R. Van Praagh et al.[113] and The Reuben H. Donnelley Corp.)

error, at both the ventricular and at the great arterial levels. Double inversive errors cancel each other physiologically, associated anomalies permitting. Since NRGA {S,L,I} has only a single segmental right-left switching error relative to the other two cardiac segments, therefore physiologic uncorrection of the circulations is to be expected.

Surgically, NRGA {S,L,I} should be treated as though physiologically uncorrected TGA were present. The Sen-

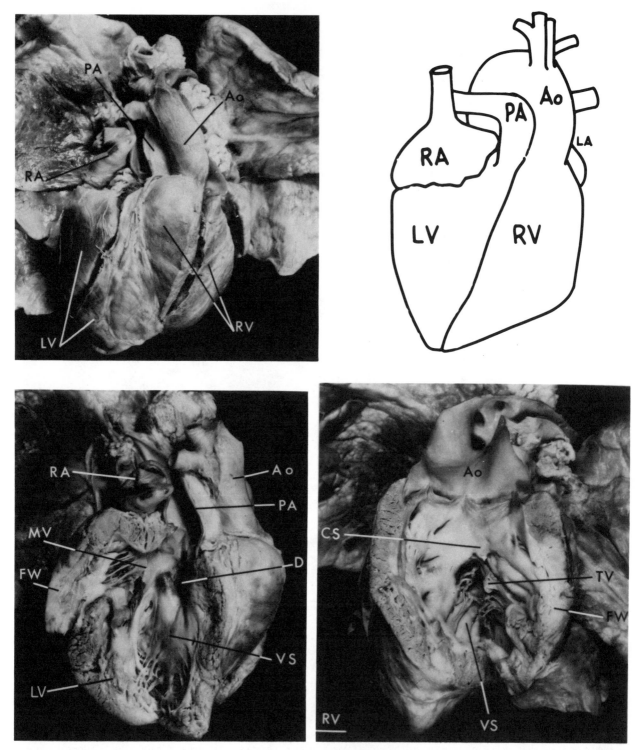

Fig. 28.12   Dextrocardia with physiologically "corrected" transposition {S,L,L}. Heart specimen. Note the typical morphologies of *RV* (left-sided) and *LV* (right-sided), the well-developed subaortic conus, the absent subpulmonary conus with pulmonary-mitral continuity, and a subpulmonary ventricular septal defect (VSD). *FW*, free wall. For other symbols, see Figure 28.10. (Reproduced with permission from R. Van Praagh *et al.*[112] and the Reuben H. Donnelley Corp.)

ning, Mustard, and Jatene operations are procedures for the physiologic correction of transposition of the *circulations*, not just for transposition of the great arteries. Transposition of the circulations means that the destinations of the venous blood streams are transposed: venae cavae return to the aorta, and pulmonary venous return to the pulmonary artery. The aforementioned operations for transposition of the

circulations are applicable no matter at what level the single inversive error has occurred: at the great arterial level only, as in TGA {S,D,D}; or at the ventricular level only, as in NRGA {S,L,S}; or at the atrial level only on comparison with the ventricles and the great arteries, as in this rare anomaly NRGA {S,L,I}.

Regarding associated cardiac malformations in dextrocardia with NRGA {S,L,I}, the girl had a single left ventricle with an infundibular outlet chamber. Both patients had a conotruncus like inverted tetralogy of Fallot.

8. Dextrocardia with Normally Related Atria, Uncertain Ventricular Situs with Common Ventricle, and Double-Outlet Common Ventricle with Rightward Aorta. There were two patients with right-sided hearts (cases 10 and 11 of Van Praagh *et al.*)[112] with situs solitus of the viscera and atria (S), uncertain ventricular situs (X-loop) because the ventricular apex pointed very posteriorly and somewhat to the right, and double-outlet common ventricle (DOCV) with D-malposition of the great arteries, i.e., *dextrocardia with DOCV {S,X,D}*. Since the ventricular situs was uncertain, the AV alignments could be described neither as concordant, nor as discordant.

Both patients had absence of the interventricular septum, resulting in a very rare form of common ventricle (type C)[109] in which the RV myocardium and the LV myocardium were in common (not separated). Both patients also had pulmonary outflow tract stenosis.

DEXTROCARDIA IN SITUS INVERSUS

Dextrocardia in situs inversus is often referred to as **mirror-image dextrocardia**. This term accurately suggests that the atria are inverted. The difficulty with this designation is that it also suggests that the ventricles are inverted, which may or may not be the case. The ventricles were inverted (L-loop) in 19/24 cases but were noninverted (D-loop) in 5/24 cases.* It is the erroneous notion that mirror-image dextrocardia always has ventricular inversion that has led in the past to "correcting" chest x-rays, electrocardiograms, and angiocardiograms for mirror-like dextrocardia. However, when the atrial and the ventricular segments both are inverted, such correction can be helpful in the interpretation of the date by "eliminating" the atrioventricular inversion.

What is mirror-image dextrocardia? In these 24 cases of dextrocardia in situs inversus, eight different types of heart were found (Table 28.3).

1. Dextrocardia with Inverted Atria, Inverted Ventricles, and Inverted Normally Related Great Arteries. This is classical mirror-image dextrocardia in which everything is inverted. There are situs inversus of the viscera and atria (I), L-loop ventricles (L), and normally related great arteries (NRGA) of the inverted (I) type, i.e., **dextrocardia with NRGA {I,L,I}**. This, the mirror-image normal type of heart, and complete transposition in situs inversus were tied for the commonest form of dextrocardia in situs inversus, each occurring in 7 of these 24 cases. Dextrocardia with NRGA {I,L,I} is shown schematically in Figure 28.6 and anatomically in Figure 28.13.

Although dextrocardia with NRGA {I,L,I} is the inverted normal type of heart, meaning that all of the cardiac segments are inverted and that the AV and VA alignments are concordant, only two of these seven patients had entirely "normal" inverted hearts. **Associated cardiac anomalies** occurred in five of these seven cases: inverted tetralogy of

---

* Whenever we use the term *ventricular noninversion*, we always mean D-loop ventricles, as in situs solitus totalis. Whenever we use the term *ventricular inversion*, we always mean L-loop ventricles, as in situs inversus totalis. Hence, we are not using the term ventricular noninversion and inversion in the conventional situs-dependent sense. By using these designations in a situs-independent way, ventricular noninversion and inversion have meanings that are specific and unchanging, no matter what the atrial situs may be.

Fallot in one; ventricular septal defect in one; secundum type of atrial septal defect in one; and polysplenia in two patients, with one having pulmonary atresia with intact ventricular septum and the other having common AV canal with common atrium.

2. Dextrocardia with Inverted Atria, Inverted Ventricles, and Inverted Complete Transposition of the Great Arteries. This is dextrocardia with situs inversus of the viscera and atria (I), L-loop ventricles (L), and L-transposition of the great arteries (L), i.e., *dextrocardia with TGA {I,L,L}*. TGA {I,L,L} is physiologically uncorrected ("complete") because the RA and the Ao are ipsilateral, and the LA and the PA are ipsilateral (Fig. 28.6, TGA 3). RA-Ao and LA-PA alignments result in physiologic uncorrection of the systemic and pulmonary circulations. As was mentioned previously, physiologically uncorrected TGA, as in TGA {I,L,L}, and physiologically corrected TGA, as in TGA {I,D,D}, *are both complete TGAs* in the anatomic sense: in both, the Ao and the PA are transposed completely across the plane of the ventricular septum, resulting in VA discordance. Nonetheless, usage has sanctioned that *complete* TGA should refer to physiologically uncorrected TGA, as opposed to physiologically corrected TGA. Hence, despite the aforementioned anatomic reservations, whenever we use the term *complete* TGA, physiologically uncorrected TGA is meant. Further anatomic precision may be conferred by the designations D-, L-, or A-TGA.

Dextrocardia with TGA {I,L,L} was one of the two commonest forms of right-sided heart in situs inversus.

Associated cardiac anomalies occurred in six of these seven patients: secundum type of atrial septal defect in two; pulmonary atresia with ventricular septal defect and hypoplastic left ventricle in one; pulmonary stenosis with intact ventricular septum and secundum type of atrial septal defect in one; bilateral superior venae cavae, each draining into the ipsilateral atrium, in one; and right coronary ostium originating from left coronary sinus of Valsalva in one.

3. Dextrocardia with Inverted Atria, Inverted Ventricles, Crisscross AV Relations, and Complete Transposition of the Great Arteries with Rightward Aorta. This was a rare case of dextrocardia with situs inversus of the viscera and atria (I), L-loop ventricles (L), and D-transposition of the great arteries (D), i.e., *dextrocardia with TGA {I,L,D}*. There were crisscross AV relations.[4, 120] This heart was very similar to the one diagrammed in Fig. 28.4, except that in this case there was situs inversus of the viscera and atria. In TGA {I,L,D}, the TGA is physiologically uncorrected: RA (left-sided) opens into RV (that begins on the left side but extends toward the right), and the RV ejects into the transposed aorta (which is right-sided because of the ventricular malposition that also results in crisscross AV relations); the LA (right-sided) opens into the LV (which begins on the right but extends toward the left), and the LV ejects into the transposed pulmonary artery (which is left-sided because of the ventricular malposition that also results in crisscross AV relations).

Thus, physiologically uncorrected TGA in situs inversus usually is L-TGA, as in TGA {I,L,L} (Fig. 28.6, TGA 3), but physiologically uncorrected TGA in situs inversus can be D-TGA, as in the present case of TGA {I,L,D}, if the ventricles are malpositioned such that the transposed aorta arises to the right of the transposed pulmonary artery.

Note that the designation *TGA {I,L,D}* is entirely clear and unequivocal in meaning. *I* indicates situs inversus atriorum. L denotes ventricular inversion. A concordant AV alignment is to be assumed, unless otherwise specified. *TGA* indicates that the VA alignments are RV to Ao and LV to PA. D-TGA specifies that the Ao arises to the right of the

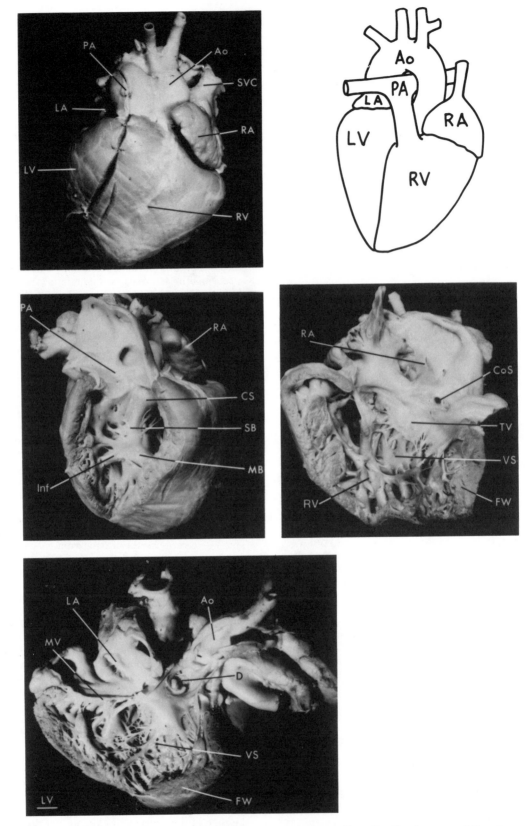

Fig. 28.13 Dextrocardia NRGA {I,L,I}, i.e., **classical mirror image dextrocardia,** with situs inversus of the viscera and atria (I), concordant L-loop (*L*), and inverted normally related great arteries (I). Note the normal subpulmonary conus, the absence of a subaortic conus, the aortic-mitral continuity, the subaortic ventricular septal defect, and the contrasting right and left ventricular morphologies. CoS, coronary sinus; *MB*, moderator band. For other symbols, see Figure 28.10. (Reproduced with permission from R. Van Praagh *et al.*[112] and The Reuben H. Donnelley Corp.)

PA. Hence, this is a physiologically uncorrected TGA in situs inversus in which the aorta is in an unusual D-position, instead of being in the usual L-position.

This patient, a 2-day-old girl, also had a ventricular septal defect, overriding mitral valve, absent anterolateral papillary muscle group of the LV, and pulmonary outflow tract atresia.

4. Dextrocardia with Inverted Atria, Inverted Ventricles, and Double-Outlet Right Ventricle with Leftward Aorta. This is dextrocardia with situs inversus of the atria (I), L-loop ventricles (L), and double-outlet right ventricle (DORV) with L-malposition of the great arteries (L), i.e., **dextrocardia with DORV {I,L,L}** (Fig. 28.6, DORV 3). DORV {I,L,L} occurred in 3 of these 24 patients with situs inversus viscerum.

Associated cardiac anomalies occurred in all three patients. One had common AV canal with hypoplasia of the LV (right-sided). A second had pulmonary outflow tract stenosis, ventricular septal defects (two), secundum atrial septal defect, and right-sided patent ductus arterious. The third patient had bilateral superior venae cavae, ipsilateral pulmonary veins, common atrium, common atrioventricular canal, pulmonary outflow tract stenosis, persistence of stratum spongiosum of both ventricles, with the latter an exceedingly rare anomaly (see Fig. 3 of Van Praagh et al.[112]).

5. Dextrocardia with Inverted Atria, Inverted Ventricles, and Double-Outlet Right Ventricle with Inverted "Normally" Related Great Arteries. This is dextrocardia with situs inversus of the viscera and atria (I), L-loop ventricles (L), and double-outlet right ventricle (DORV) with L-malposition of the great arteries (L), i.e., **dextrocardia with DORV {I,L,L}**. The difference between this rare case and the preceding type was that the conotruncus was of the inverted tetralogy of Fallot type, i.e., the great arteries were of the approximately normal, but inverted, type (I). This may briefly be represented as **DORV {I,L,L (I)}**. There was direct fibrous continuity between the right coronary leaflet of the aortic valve and the superior leaflet of a common AV valve. DORV was present apparently because of the marked hypoplasia of the right-sided LV, plus the aortic overriding that is characteristic of tetralogy of Fallot, both noninverted and inverted. Since both great arteries arise above the large left-sided RV, i.e., since DORV is present, we think these great arteries must be reported as an L-*malposition*, not as inverted normally related great arteries. However, the conotruncus *per se* is of the inverted normal type. The italicized *L* in DORV {I,L,*L*} indicates L-malposition of the great arteries. The following parenthetical (*I*) in DORV {I,L,L (*I*)} indicates that the L-malposed great arteries are very similar to inverted normally related great arteries.

DORV does not always have a bilateral infundibulum, as this case illustrates. Particularly when the LV is small, the infundibulum can be unilateral, subaortic only, or subpulmonary only, as in this case.

6. Dextrocardia with Atrial Inversion, Ventricular Noninversion, and Corrected Transposition of the Great Arteries. This is dextrocardia with situs inversus of the viscera and atria (I), D-loop ventricles (D), and D-transposition of the great arteries (D), i.e., **dextrocardia with TGA {I,D,D}**. TGA {I,D,D} is presented diagrammatically in Figure 28.6 (TGA 4), angiocardiographically in Figure 28.14, and anatomically in Figure 28.15. In TGA {I,D,D}, the circulations are physiologically "corrected"—associated anomalies permitting—because the **atrioarterial (AA) alignments** are concordant (LA to Ao, and RA to PA). In "corrected" TGA {I,D,D}, it is understood that the AV alignments are discordant (RA to LV, and LA to RV), unless

specifically stated to the contrary. In the patient shown in Figures 28.14 and 28.15, for example, the AV alignments are not purely discordant. There is a straddling tricuspid valve (TV) and a ventricular septal defect (VSD) of the AV canal type. Consequently, the diagnosis is: TGA {I,D,D} with straddling TV and VSD of the AV canal type.

Associated cardiac anomalies were present in all three patients with "corrected" TGA {I,D,D}: atresia of left AV valve; large LV with infundibular outlet chamber, small bulboventricular foramen producing severe subaortic stenosis, atresia of the aortic isthmus, and patent ductus arteriosus; right superior vena cava to coronary sinus, ventricular septal defect, single left coronary artery, and pulmonary outflow tract atresia; and straddling tricuspid valve, ventricular septal defect of the AV canal type, small right ventricle, and pulmonary outflow tract stenosis. Extracardiac anomalies were present in the first case abovementioned, a patient who also had the Klippel-Feil syndrome.

As usual, therefore, associated cardiac anomalies made **the concept of "physiologically corrected" TGA** to appear ludicrous.

Is **the concept of "complete" TGA** any better? Not really. **Complete** TGA, be it physiologically uncorrected or corrected, is simply redundant. All transpositions are complete; if not, the VA alignment is called something else. In all TGAs, as this term is now used, the Ao arises above the RV, and the PA originates above the LV. Both great arteries are transposed completely across the ventricular septum, resulting in VA discordance. When a TGA is **partial**, as opposed to complete, only one great artery is transposed across the plane of the ventricular septum. There are two kinds of **partial transposition** (Fig. 28.6): **DORV,** in which only the Ao is transposed above the RV; and **DOLV,** in which only the PA is transposed across the plane of the ventricular septum.

7. Dextrocardia with Atrial Inversion, Ventricular Noninversion, and Corrected Transposition with Leftward Aorta. This is dextrocardia with situs inversus of viscera and atria (I), D-loop ventricles (D), and L-transposition of the great arteries (L), i.e., **dextrocardia with "corrected" TGA {I,D,L}**. Thus, situs inversus of the viscera and atria is associated with AV and VA discordance. This double discordance indicates two right-left switching errors, hence, "corrected" TGA. In this "corrected" TGA in situs inversus, the ventricles are sufficiently malposed so that L-TGA is present, instead of the expected D-TGA, as in the previous cardiotype. Consequently, this patient has "corrected" TGA {I,D,L}.

This segmental set, TGA {I,D,L}, indicates that the ventricles are malpositioned; otherwise, the transposed aortic valve would be in the more usual D-position. This patient, a boy 2 years and 9 months old, had left juxtaposition of the atrial appendages,[69] which also correctly suggests ventricular malposition.

Associated cardiac anomalies in this case of "corrected" TGA also included complete common AV canal, severe pulmonary outflow tract stenosis, and a left aortic arch (abnormal in situs inversus).

8. Dextrocardia with Atrial Inversion, Ventricular Noninversion, and Inverted Normally Related Great Arteries. This is a very rare anomaly—dextrocardia with situs inversus of the viscera and atria (I), D-loop ventricles (D), and normally related great arteries (NRGA) of the inverted (I) type, i.e., **dextrocardia with NRGA {I,D,I}**. In words, this anomaly may be called *isolated ventricular noninversion*, which means that only the ventricles are noninverted (solitus), whereas the atria and the great arter-

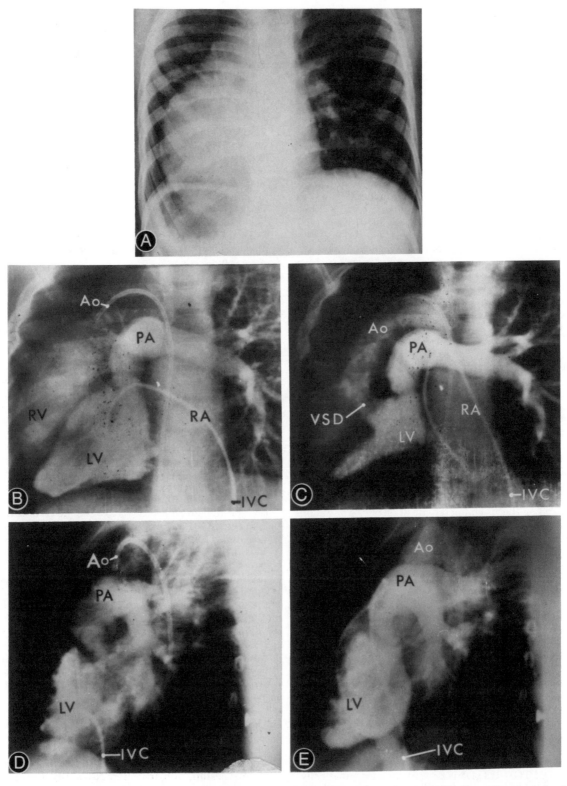

Fig. 28.14 Dextrocardia with physiologically "corrected" transposition of the great arteries {I,D,D}. The patient had situs inversus of the viscera and atria (I), with a discordant D-loop (D), and with D-TGA (D). Note the right-sided stomach bubble (a), the left-sided IVC (b and d), the typical morphology of the left-sided *LV*, indicating a D-loop (b and d), the discordant RA to LV alignment revealed by the catheter course (b), the presence of D-TGA (b to e), the fact that the transposed aorta (Ao) is somewhat posterior to the transposed pulmonary artery (*PA*), which can be seen in c and e, and the coexistence of a *VSD*, subpulmonary stenosis, and a right aortic arch. For explanation of symbols, see Figure 28.10. (Reproduced with permission from R. Van Praagh *et al.*[113] and The Reuben H. Donnelley Corp.)

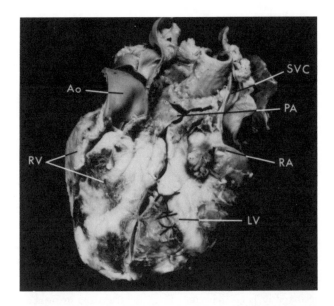
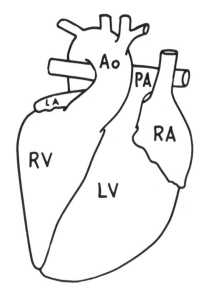
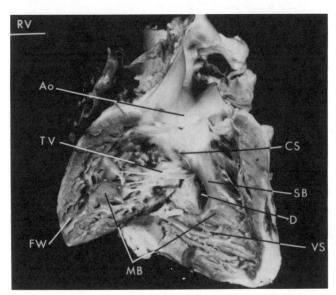
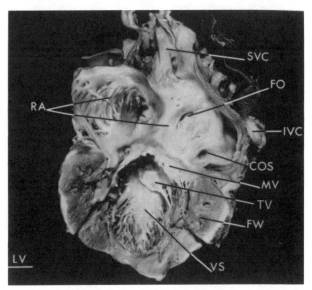

Fig. 28.15 Dextrocardia with physiologically "corrected" transposition of the great arteries {I,D,D}. Heart specimen. Note the hypertrophy and enlargement of the *RA* (left-sided), the discordant AV alignments, the small-chambered and thick-walled *RV*, the *VSD* of the AV canal type, and the overriding tricuspid valve (evident in both the *RV* and *LV* views). FO, foramen ovale. For explanation of symbols, see Figure 28.10. (Reproduced with permission from R. Van Praagh *et al.*[112] and The Reuben H. Donnelley Corp.)

ies are inverted. NRGA {I,D,I} is one of the two forms of **isolated ventricular discordance** (Fig. 28.6).

In terms of the segmental alignments, there is AV discordance and VA concordance. One discordance indicates that there is only a single right-left switching error or discordance, at the ventricular level. When only one of the segmental alignments is discordant, the circulations are transposed: RA to LV to Ao, and LA to RV to PA. Such cases should therefore be treated as though they have transposition of the great arteries. Instead, they have "transposition" of the ventricles. Again, this very rare case illustrates that discordance of any one major cardiac segment—atria only, or ventricles only, or great arteries only—physiologically uncorrects the systemic and pulmonary circulations by transposing their arterial destinations.

However, the rare aspect of NRGA {I,D,I} is that *solitus* ventricles are associated with an *inverted* conotruncus. Despite the fact that the situs of the ventricles and the situs of

the conotruncus are opposites, nonetheless, the VA alignments are concordant. Two normal but opposite segments at the ventricular and infundibular levels can connect approximately normally, resulting in approximately normal VA alignments.

In NRGA {I,D,I}, are the VA alignments truly normal? They are only approximately normal, but they are as close to normal as it is possible for them to be, bearing in mind that the situs of the ventricles and the situs of the conotruncus are opposites.

A 4-year-old boy with isolated ventricular noninversion had many associated cardiovascular anomalies: bilateral superior venae cavae with right superior vena cava returning directly to the LA (right-sided), common atrium, complete common AV canal, marked hypoplasia of the RV, pulmonary atresia, including atresia of the main pulmonary artery, and bilateral patent ductus arteriosi.

What, then, is dextrocardia in situs inversus? Based

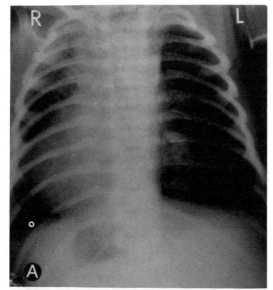

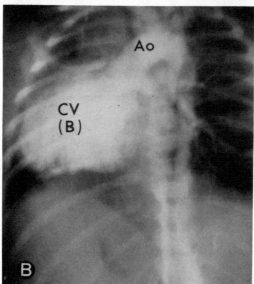

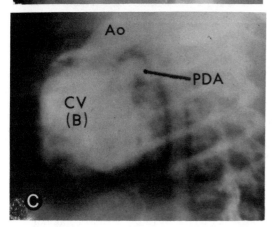

Fig. 28.16 Dextrocardia with double-outlet right ventricle (DORV) {A,D,D} and asplenia. Situs ambiguus (A) is indicated by the symmetrical liver shadow (B) and the midline stomach bubble (A). Note the presence of a single right ventricle without an outlet chamber (common ventricle type B, CV (B),[109] autopsy proved), and origin of both great arteries, perforce, above the single RV. However, the pulmonary arterial outflow tract was atretic, which is

common with asplenia, the pulmonary artery filling retrogradely via a patent ductus arteriosus (PDA). Ao, aorta. (Reproduced with permission from R. Van Praagh et al.[113] and The Reuben H. Donnelley Corp.)

on this series of 24 cases, the answer to this question, in order of decreasing frequency, was (Table 28.3): physiologically uncorrected TGA, either {I,L,L} or {I,L,D}, in 8; inverted normal type of heart, {I,L,I}, in 7; double-outlet right ventricle, either {I,L,L} or {I,L,L(I)}, in 4; physiologically "corrected" TGA, either {I,D,D} or {I,D,L}, in 4; and isolated noninversion of the ventricles, {I,D,I}, in 1.

DEXTROCARDIA IN SITUS AMBIGUUS

Based on this series of 136 autopsied cases of right-sided hearts, dextrocardia in situs ambiguus occurred in 46 patients (Table 28.3). Thus, dextrocardia in situs ambiguus was commoner than the classical form of dextrocardia in situs inversus (24/136 patients). Indeed, dextrocardia as part of the **asplenia syndrome**[92, 93] occurred in 27/136 patients and was commoner than dextrocardia in situs inversus. Dextrocardia as part of the **polysplenia syndrome**[92, 93] was found in 18/136 patients, and was almost as common as dextrocardia in situs inversus. Dextrocardia rarely can occur **in situs ambiguus with a normally formed spleen,** as occurred in 1/136 patients. Thus, dextrocardia in situs ambiguus is of considerable numerical importance.

Eight different types of heart were found in the right chest in association with the *asplenia syndrome* which, in order of decreasing frequency, were as follows.

1. Transposition of the Great Arteries with Uncertain Atrial Situs, Ventricular Inversion, and Leftward Aorta. This is dextrocardia in situs ambiguus of the viscera and atria (A), with L-loop ventricles (L) and L-transposition of the great arteries (L); i.e., briefly, this is **dextrocardia with the asplenia syndrome and TGA {A,L,L}.** This was the commonest kind of heart in these 27 patients with the asplenia syndrome, being present in eight cases.

2. Dextrocardia with Uncertain Atrial Situs, Ventricular Inversion, and Double-Outlet Right Ventricles with Leftward Aorta. The second commonest form of dextrocardia associated with the asplenia syndrome, which occurred in 6/27 patients, had situs ambiguus of viscera and atria (A), L-loop ventricles (L), and double-outlet right ventricle (DORV) with L-malposition of the great arteries (L); briefly, this is *dextrocardia with the asplenia syndrome and with DORV {A,L,L}.*

3. Dextrocardia with Uncertain Atrial Situs, Ventricular Noninversion and Transposition of the Great Arteries with Rightward Aorta. The third commonest type of heart found in these dextrocardias with the asplenia syndrome, which occurred in 4/27 patients, had situs ambiguus of the viscera and atria (A), D-loop ventricles (D), and D-transposition of the great arteries; briefly, this is **dextrocardia with the aplenia syndrome with TGA {A,D,D}.**

4. Dextrocardia with Uncertain Atrial Situs, Ventricular Inversion, and Double-Outlet Right Ventricle with Rightward Aorta. Fourth in frequency, found in 2/27 patients with asplenia, was a form of double-outlet right ventricle (DORV) with situs ambiguus of the viscera and atria (A), ventricular L-loop (L), and D-malposition of the great arteries (D); briefly, this is **dextrocardia with the asplenia syndrome and DORV {A,L,D}.**

5. Dextrocardia with Uncertain Atrial Situs, Noninverted Ventricles, and Anatomically Corrected Malposition of the Great Arteries with Leftward Aorta. Tied for fourth in frequency was a type of anatomically corrected malposition (ACM) of the great arteries (Fig. 28.6) with situs ambiguus of the viscera and atria (A), D-loop ventricles (D), and L-malposition of the great arteries (L). Briefly, this anomaly is **dextrocardia with the asplenia syndrome and ACM {A,D,L}.**

6. Dextrocardia with Uncertain Atrial Situs, Ventricular Inversion, and Inverted Normally Related Great Arteries. Also tied for fourth in frequency and affecting 2 of these 27 patients with dextrocardia and asplenia was a rare anomaly. The atrial situs was ambiguus (A). The ventricular situs was L-loop (L). Most surprisingly, the great arteries were of the inverted normally related type (I). Briefly, this anomaly is *dextrocardia with the asplenia syndrome and NRGA {A,L,I}*. In our experience, normally related great arteries in the asplenia syndrome are exceedingly infrequent.

7. Dextrocardia with Uncertain Atrial Situs, Uncertain Ventricular Situs with Single Ventricle, and Double-Outlet Single Ventricle with Leftward Aorta. Also affecting 2 of the 27 dextrocardias with the asplenia syndrome was the following cardiac anomaly: situs ambiguus of the viscera and atria (A), indeterminate ventricular situs (X-loop) with single ventricle of morphologically uncertain type (type D),[109] and double-outlet single ventricle (DOSV) with L-malposition of the great arteries (L). Briefly, this is **dextrocardia with the asplenia syndrome and DOSV {A,X,L}.**

8. Dextrocardia with Uncertain Atrial Situs, Ventricular Noninversion, and Double-Outlet Right Ventricle with Rightward Aorta. This was the least frequent type of heart encountered in these 27 dextrocardias with asplenia, affecting only 1 patient: situs ambiguus of the viscera and atria (A), D-loop ventricles (D), and double-outlet right ventricle (DORV) with D-malposition of the great arteries. Briefly, this is **dextrocardia with the asplenia syndrome and DORV {A,D,D}.**

Thus, in this series of 27 cases of asplenia with dextrocardia, TGA was the commonest VA alignment, followed by DORV. Together they accounted for more than three-quarters of the cases. The remaining quarter was equally divided among inverted NRGA, L-ACM, and L-DOSV.

Associated cardiovascular malformations are very important clinically, physiologically, and surgically in the asplenia syndrome (Table 28.4). Only 1 of these 27 patients had normally formed AV valves. All of the others had common AV canal (24 cases) or right-sided mitral atresia (two cases). Totally anomalous pulmonary venous connection was also very frequent (19 patients). Surgically important ventricular malformations (hypoplasia of LV, or of RV, or single LV, or morphologically undiagnosed single ventricle) were present in more than half of these patients (14 patients). Pulmonary outflow tract stenosis or atresia was the rule (24 patients). Aortic atresia—a rare finding in asplenia—occurred in one patient with inverted normally related great arteries {A,L,I}.

Three different anatomic types of heart occurred in the right chest in association with 18 cases of the **polysplenia syndrome** (Table 28.3).

1. Dextrocardia with Uncertain Atrial Situs, Inverted Ventricles, and Inverted Normally Related Great Arteries. Dextrocardia with NRGA {A,L,I} was the commonest form of congenital heart disease associated with the polysplenia syndrome[92, 93] (10/18 patients).

2. Dextrocardia with Uncertain Atrial Situs, Ventricular Inversion, and Transposition of the Great Arteries with Leftward Aorta. TGA {A,L,L} was the second commonest form of dextrocardia associated with the polysplenia syndrome (6/18 cases).

3. Dextrocardia with Uncertain Atrial Situs, Normally Related Ventricles, and Normally Related Great Arteries. NRGA {A,D,S} was the least frequent type of dextrocardia associated with the polysplenia syndrome (2/18 patients).

The abovementioned data suggest that polysplenia occurs both in noninverted and inverted people, but that it is much commoner in individuals whose type of visceroatrial situs probably is situs inversus. Hence, the classical designation *partial* (i.e., heterotaxic form of) *situs inversus* applies to many more cases than would its counterpart, *partial situs solitus*. Normally related great arteries are much commoner in the polysplenia sydnrome (12/18 patients) than in the asplenia syndrome (2/27 patients).

The associated cardiovascular malformations found in the polysplenia syndrome (Table 28.5) are similar to, but less severe than, those found in the asplenia syndrome (cf. Table 28.4). For example, only complete common AV canal was found in the asplenia syndrome (24/27 patients), but in the polysplenia syndrome, incomplete common AV canal (primum atrial septal defect) was approximately as frequent (4/18 cases) as complete common AV canal (5/18 cases). In polysplenia, only half the patients had common AV canal (complete or incomplete), whereas in asplenia, almost 90% had the complete form of common AV canal. Pulmonary outflow tract obstruction (stenosis or atresia) occurred in 5/18 patients with polysplenia, whereas pulmonary outflow tract obstruction was present with asplenia in 24/27 patients.

Features characteristic of the polysplenia syndrome such as interruption of the inferior vena cava with azygos extension to a superior vena cava (8/18 patients) and "partially" anomalous pulmonary venous connection (ipsilateral pul-

TABLE 28.4   ASSOCIATED CARDIOVASCULAR MALFORMATIONS IN DEXTROCARDIA WITH THE ASPLENIA SYNDROME

Anomaly	No. of Cases (N = 27)
Bilateral SVC	13
TAPVC	19
Supracardiac = 7	
Cardiac = 5	
Infracardiac = 5	
Uncertain = 2	
Common atrium	13
Complete common AV canal	24
Mitral atresia (right-sided)	2
Hypoplasia of LV	7
Hypoplasia of RV	2
Single LV	2
Single ventricle (morphology NOS)	3
Pulmonary atresia	11
Pulmonary stenosis	12
Tetralogy of Fallot with PS	1
Ao At	1
Double aortic arch (ring)	1
Coronary ostial anomalies	4
Single left = 1	
Single right = 1	
Both above LC sinus = 1	
High ostium = 1	

a Ao At, aortic atresia; AV, atrioventricular; LC, left coronary; LV, morphologically left ventricle; NOS, not otherwise specified; PS, pulmonary stenosis; RV, morphologically right ventricle; SVC, superior vena cava; TAPVC, totally anomalous pulmonary venous connection.

TABLE 28.5   ASSOCIATED CARDIOVASCULAR MALFORMATIONS IN DEXTROCARDIA WITH POLYSPLENIA SYNDROME

Anomaly	No. of Cases (N = 18)
Bilateral SVC[a]	7
Interrupted IVC	8
TAPVC	2
Supracardiac = 1	
Cardiac = 1	
"Partial" APVC (ipsilateral)	7
Common atrium	4
Complete common AV canal	5
Incomplete common AV canal (ASD I)	4
Secundum atrial septal defect	5
Sinus venosus atrial septal defect	1
VSD (infundiboloventricular)	2
Single LV	1
Pulmonary atresia	2
Pulmonary stenosis	3
Coarctation of the aorta	3

[a] APVC, anomalous pulmonary venous connection; ASD I, atrial septal defect of the persistent ostium primum type; AV, atrioventricular; IVC, inferior vena cava; LV, morphologically left ventricle; SVC, superior vena cava; TAPVC, totally anomalous pulmonary venous connection; VSD, ventricular septal defect.

monary veins) (7/18 patients) also are noteworthy (Table 28.5).

Polysplenia was associated with Noonan's syndrome in one patient, and with neurofibromatosis in another. Asplenia is never associated with another syndrome, to our knowledge, whereas polysplenia can be.

PROPHYLAXIS FOR ASPLENIA

Following the study of Waldman et al.[123] that showed a greatly increased frequency of fulminating and fatal septicemia produced by encapsulated bacteria in patients with the asplenia syndrome compared with appropriate controls, it is now generally agreed that some form of prophylaxis for congenitally asplenic patients is indicated. *Klebsiella* and *Escherichia coli* were the principle pathogens under 6 months of age, whereas *Diplococcus pneumoniae* (pneumococcus) and *Hemophilus influenzae* predominated from 6 months of age onward.

Consequently, we have recommended continuous antibiotic prophylaxis in infants, children, and adults with the asplenia syndrome: amoxicillin, 25 mg/kg/day in two divided doses, maximum 1 gm/day, or ampicillin, 50 mg/kg/day in four divided doses, maximum 2 gm/day. Use of pneumococcal vaccine is also under consideration as a possible method of protecting congenitally asplenic individuals from the pneumococcus—which can be fulminating and fatal in less than 24 hours.

If one decides not to give prophylaxis to patients with the asplenia syndrome, we think that at the first suggestion of an infection, such patients should receive antibiotic coverage as above.

MESOCARDIA

Mesocardia means that the heart is in the middle of the thorax, predominantly neither to the right nor to the left. Mesocardia is very infrequent, being found in only 0.2% of our autopsied cases of congenital heart disease (4/1716 cases).

What is congenital mesocardia? In an effort to answer this question, we did a study based on our four autopsied cases, plus 13 autopsied cases of Lev et al.[61] (Table 28.6). In order of decreasing frequency, congenital mesocardial was found to be: the normal type of heart, NRGA {S,D,S}, in five; physiologically "corrected" TGA {S,L,L} in three; physiologically uncorrected TGA {S,D,D} in two; and seven other kinds of heart, occurring in one patient each.

ISOLATED LEVOCARDIA

First reported in 1826 by Breschet[12] and Martin[68] isolated levocardia indicates that the heart is left-sided and that the viscera and atria are not in situs solitus. Either situs inversus or situs ambiguus is present.

What is isolated levocardia? To clarify this question, the findings in 37 autopsied cases from the Children's Hospital Medical Center in Boston were combined with those in 28 autopsied cases reported by Liberthson et al.,[64] and the data from these 65 cases are summarized in Table 28.7.

Situs inversus totalis occurred in only 9 of these 65 cases of isolated levocardia. Only two types of heart were found: "corrected" TGA in situs inversus, i.e., TGA {I,D,D}, in seven (Fig. 28.6); and DORV similar to "corrected" TGA in situs inversus, i.e., DORV {I,D,D}, in two patients with levocardia in situs inversus.

Situs ambiguus accounted for the great majority of cases of isolated levocardia, occurring in 56 of 65 cases. Situs ambiguus was associated with the asplenia syndrome in 33/56 cases, with the polysplenia syndrome in 13, with small accessory spleen or spleens plus a normal spleen in nine, and with a normally formed spleen without accessory spleen(s) in one.

Ventricles. In isolated levocardia, ventricular noninversion (D-loop) was much more frequent than was ventricular inversion (L-loop): D-loop in 55/65 patients; L-loop in 6/65 cases, and X-loop in 4/65 patients.

It is noteworthy that this is very different from isolated dextrocardia (Table 28.3) in which the frequencies of ventricular D-loops (47%) and L-loops (53%) were approximately equal.

Great Arteries. In order of diminishing frequency, the ventriculoarterial alignments in isolated levocardia were (Table 28.7): double-outlet right ventricle in 25; transposition of the great arteries in 23; normally related great arteries in 16; and anatomically corrected malposition of the great arteries in one.

TABLE 28.6   TYPES OF CONGENITAL MESOCARDIA IN 17 AUTOPSIED CASES

Type	No. of Cases
In situs solitus	
1. NRGA[a] {S,D,S}	5
2. TGA {S,D,D}	2
3. DORV {S,D,D}	1
4. TGA {S,L,L}	3
5. DORV {S,L,L}	1
In situs inversus	
1. TGA {I,D,D}	1
2. DORV {I,D,D}	1
In situs ambiguus	
With asplenia	
1. TGA {A,D,D}	1
2. DORV {A,L,L}	1
With polysplenia	
1. DORV {A,L,D}	1

[a] Abbreviations as in footnote of Table 28.3.

In greater detail, the findings were as follows.

1. Double-outlet right ventricle occurred in three basically different types of heart in isolated levocardia: {A,D,D}, {A,D,A}, and {A,D,L} in 22 and {I,D,D} in two.

2. Transposition of the great arteries occurred in four basically different kinds of heart in isolated levocardia: {A,D,D} and {A,D,L} in 10; {I,D,D} in seven; {A,X,D} in three; and {A,L,L} and {A,L,D} in three.

3. Normally related great arteries were present in three different types of heart in isolated levocardia: {A,D,S} in 14; {A,X,S} in one; and {A,L,I} in one.

4. Anatomically corrected malposition of the great arteries occurred in only one patient with the unusual segmental combination of {A,L,D}.

Associated malformations were very prominent in isolated levocardia. Those found in situs inversus (Table 28.8) were very similar to those found in situs ambiguus with asplenia (Table 28.9), polysplenia (Table 28.10), and accessory spleen (Table 28.11). Situs ambiguus rarely can occur with a normally formed spleen and without an accessory spleen, as in the patient with TGA {A,D,D} (Table 28.7). This patient also had visceroatrial discordance with situs inversus abdominis and situs solitus atriorum, malrotation of the bowel, bilaterally trilobed lungs, common atrium, complete common AV canal, common-inlet LV, RV hypoplasia, and pulmonary outflow tract atresia.

The fact that the associated malformations in situs inversus and in situs ambiguus were very similar in consistent with the **Layton hypothesis,**[57, 58] namely, that absence of the dominant gene for situs solitus permits bodily situs to develop at random. Layton's *iv/iv* mice are a model not only of situs inversus but also of situs ambiguus. The gene symbol

TABLE 28.7   TYPES OF ISOLATED LEVOCARDIA IN 65 AUTOPSIED CASES

Type	No. of Cases
In situs inversus	
1. TGA[a] {I,D,D}	7
2. DORV {I,D,D}	2
In situs ambiguus	
With asplenia	
1. NRGA {A,D,S}	3
2. TGA {A,D,D}	3
3. TGA {A,D,L}	2
4. DORV {A,D,D}	16
5. DORV {A,D,A}	1
6. TGA {A,L,L}	2
7. TGA {A,L,D}	1
8. DORV {A,L,L}	1
9. ACM {A,L,D}	1
10. NRGA {A,X,S}	1
11.TGA {A,X,D}	2
With polysplenia	
1. NRGA {A,D,S}	8
2. TGA {A,D,D}	1
3. DORV {A,D,D}	3
4. DORV {A,D,L}	1
With accessory spleen	
1. NRGA {A,D,S}	3
2. TGA {A,D,D}	3
3. DORV {A,D,D}	1
4. NRGA {A,L,I}	1
5. TGA {A,X,D}	1
With normally formed spleen	
1. TGA {A,D,D}	1

[a] Abbreviations as in footnote of Table 24.3.

TABLE 28.8   ASSOCIATED MALFORMATION WITH ISOLATED LEVOCARDIA IN SITUS INVERSUS (N = 9)

Type	No. of Cases
Complete common AV canal	6
Common atrium	3
Tricuspid stenosis	1
Totally anomalous pulmonary venous connection	4
Ipsilateral pulmonary veins	1
Ventricular septal defect	1
Hypoplastic LV	2
Single RV	2
Single LV	1
Pulmonary outflow tract stenosis	4
Pulmonary outflow tract atresia	4
Bilaterally trilobed lungs	2
Common gastrointestinal mesentery	4
Symmetrical liver	3

[a] Abbreviations as in footnote to Table 28.3.

iv stands for the inversus "gene." *iv/iv* indicates homozygosity for the situs inversus "gene." The situs inversus "gene" is hypothesized to be an absence of DNA. Hence, the situs inversus gene is thought not to be the presence of abnormal DNA, but rather the absence of normal DNA. Consequently, we hypothesize that human beings with situs inversus and situs ambiguus, like Layton's iv/iv mice, lack the dominant gene for situs soltus, permitting bodily organization (situs) to develop at random. This may well explain why the associated malformations in man with situs inversus and with situs ambiguus are so very similar.

In view of the foregoing, it is also noteworthy and comprehensible that the asplenia syndrome of bilateral "right-sidedness" (Table 28.9) and the polysplenia syndrome of bilateral "left-sidedness" (Table 28.10) are not as distinct and different, as has often been suggested. The asplenia syndrome has been said to have **right isomerism** (i.e., bilateral right-sidedness), while the polysplenia syndrome has been considered to have **left isomerism** (i.e., bilateral left-sidedness). In these 33 cases of the asplenia syndrome, although bilaterally trilobed lungs occurred in the majority (23 patients), five other patterns of lung lobation also were found (Table 28.9). In these 13 cases of polysplenia, bilaterally bilobed lungs did *not* predominate (four patients, Table 28.10). Similarly, interruption ("absence") of the inferior vena cava, with an azygos extension to a superior vena cava, did *not* occur in the majority (five cases, Table 28.10). Patients with a normally formed spleen, plus one or more accessory splenuli, also often had interruption of the inferior vena cava (6/9 cases, Table 28.11). In our experience, therefore, interruption of the inferior vena cava was commoner with accessory spleen (Table 28.11) than with polysplenia (Table 28.10).

There is considerable overlap of findings in situs inversus, asplenia, polysplenia, and accessory spleen. This overlap of findings is understandable if these syndromes are due to **genetic decontrol,** resulting in randomness of development.

CONGENITAL PERICARDIAL DEFECT

Since first reported by Columbus[20] in 1559, more than 140 cases of congenital pericardial defect have been reported. This is a rare form of congenital heart disease that was found in only 3 of 1716 autopsied cases in our Cardiac Registry. Congenital pericardial defect may be left-sided (much the commonest), right-sided, or diaphragmatic, and in any of

TABLE 28.9. ASSOCIATED MALFORMATIONS WITH ISOLATED LEVOCARDIA IN SITUS AMBIGUUS WITH ASPLENIA (N = 33)

Type		No. of Cases
Inferior vena cava		
Right-sided		19
Left-sided		13
Midline		1
Double below the liver		1
Switch from right to left at liver		1
Switch from left to right at liver		4
Interrupted ("absent")		0
Pulmonary veins		
Totally anomalous		23
To right SVC	11	
To left SVC	4	
Below diaphragm	6	
To right-sided atrium	1	
To unknown site	1	
Ipsilateral		2
Atrial septum		
Secundum ASD		9
Common atrium		17
Atrioventricular valves		
Complete common AV canal		27
Incomplete common AV canal (ASD I)		4
Tricuspid atresia		2
Ventricular septum		
VSD of infundibuloventricular type		1
VSD of AV canal type (without CAVC)		1
Ventricles		
Hypoplasia of LV (marked)		8
Hypoplasia of RV (marked)		2
Single LV		2
Single RV		7
Single ventricle (undiagnosed)		2
Pulmonary outflow tract		
Stenosis		14
Atresia		13
Tetralogy of Fallot		1
Lungs		
Bilaterally trilobed		23
Bilaterally quadrilobed		3
Bilaterally bilobed		1
Inverted lobation		2
Solitus lobation		1
Right = 7 lobes, left = 8 lobes		1
Unknown		2
Liver		
Symmetrical		21
Inverted		6
Solitus		4
Unknown		2
Stomach		
Right-sided		18
Left-sided		12
Unknown		3
Gut		
Common mesentery		20
Malrotation with cecum in RUQ[a]		6
Septicemia		3
Pneumococcus	2	
E. coli	1	
Familial congenital heart disease		3
Brother with asplenia	2	
Brother with PS	1	
Normal twin (probably identical)		1

[a] RUQ, right upper quadrant. Other abbreviations as previously.

TABLE 28.10 ASSOCIATED MALFORMATIONS WITH ISOLATED LEVOCARDIA IN SITUS AMBIGUUS WITH POLYSPLENIA (N = 13)

Type		No. of Cases
Inferior vena cava		
Right-sided		6
Left-sided		2
Interrupted ("absent")		5
Azygos to left SVC		5
Pulmonary veins		
Totally anomalous		3
To right SVC	1	
Below diaphragm	1	
To unknown site	1	
Ispilateral		3
Cor triatriatum		1
Atrial septum		
Secundum ASD		1
Common atrium		1
Atrioventricular valves		
Complete common AV canal		5
Incomplete common AV canal (ASD I)		1
Mitral atresia		1
Ventricular septum		
VSD of infundibuloventricular type		2
Ventricles		
Hypoplasia of LV (marked)		2
Pulmonary Outflow Tract		
Pulmonary stenosis		4
Pulmonary atresia		1
Aortic outflow tract		
Aortic stenosis		1
Coarctation of aorta		2
Preductal	1	
Unknown	1	
Lungs		
Solitus lobation		5
Bilaterally bilobed		4
Bilaterally trilobed		2
Bilaterally unilobed		1
Inverted lobation		1
Pulmonary veno-occlusive disease		1
Liver		
Symmetrical		6
Inverted		4
Solitus		2
Unknown		1
Biliary atresia		1
Stomach		
Right-sided		11
Left-sided		1
Unknown		1
Gut		
Common mesentery		8
Malrotation		4
Inverted		1
Absence of celiac and mesenteric arteries		1

these three sites it may be small or large; total absence of the pericardium also occurs (Table 28.12).[32] Pericardial defect represents defective formation of the pleuropericardial membrane[53] or, if diaphragmatic, defective formation of the septum transversum.[17]

MANIFESTATIONS

If pericardial defect is associated with other congenital anomalies such as diaphragmatic hernia or congenital heart

TABLE 28.11 ASSOCIATED MALFORMATION WITH ISOLATED LEVOCARDIA IN SITUS AMBIGUUS WITH ACCESSORY SPLEEN (N = 9)

Type	No. of Cases
Inferior vena cava	
Right-sided	1
Left-sided	2
Interrupted ("absent")	6
Azygos to left SVC	4
Azygos to right SVC	2
Pulmonary veins	
Ipsilateral	3
Atrial septum	
Common atrium	5
Atrioventricular valves	
Complete common AV canal	5
Mitral stenosis	1
Ventricular septum	
VSD (infundibuloventricular)	2
Pulmonary outflow tract	
Stenosis	1
Atresia	3
Tetralogy of Fallot	1
Aortic outflow tract	
Stenosis	1
Coarctation of aorta	2
Lungs	
Solitus lobation	4
Bilaterally bilobed	3
Bilaterally trilobed	2
Liver	
Inverted	7
Symmetrical	2
Stomach	
Right-sided	7
Symmetrical	2
Gut	
Malrotation	5
Solitus	2
Inversus	1
Common mesentery	1
Visceroatrial discordance	
Situs inversus abdominis and situs solitus atriorum	1

TABLE 28.12 CLASSIFICATION OF CONGENITAL PERICARDIAL DEFECTS (N = 85)[a]

Type	No. of Cases
A. Deficiency of pericardium and adjacent pleura	
1. Left side	
a. Partial defects (foramen type)	18
b. Complete defects	48
2. Right side	
a. Partial defects (foramen type)	2
b. Complete defects	1
3. Both sides	
a. Partial and complete defects	3
B. Deficiency of pericardium with adjacent pleura normally formed	3
C. Deficiency of diaphragmatic pericardium	10

[a] Modified from K. Ellis et al.[32] Cases with ectopia cordis excluded.

levoposed, and the left upper heart border shows three unusually prominent convexities (Fig. 28.17a), the aortic knob, the pulmonary artery, and the ventricles.[32] With a partial left pericardial defect, the heart is normally located, and there is a prominent bulge in the region of the pulmonary artery, produced by the herniating left atrial appendage (Fig. 28.18).[7]

Diagnostic pneumothorax results in pneumopericardium (Fig. 28.17b). Angiocardiography establishes that the left atrial appendage is herniating, producing the bulge in the region of the pulmonary artery, or that the heart is widely separated from the pericardium if the omentum or lung has herniated into the pericardial sac.[42, 73] Computed tomography now permits direct visualization of absence of the pericardium.[5]

TREATMENT

Only partial forms of pericardial defect (left-sided, right-sided, or diaphragmatic) require surgical treatment. Only with the partial forms is there the danger of herniation and strangulation of the ventricles, or the risk of herniation and strangulation of the left atrial appendage, or the possibility of the superior vena cava obstructive syndrome, or the problem of cardiac compression by abdominal contents. Complete left, complete right, and total pericardial defects ordinarily do not require surgical treatment.

It is noteworthy, however, that complete absence of the pericardium, or complete absence of half of the pericardium (typically of the left half), appears to predispose to posttraumatic cardiac lesions such as apical left ventricular myocardial infarction complicated by posttraumatic mitral insufficiency and apical ventricular septal defect.[78] The pericardial sac is the heart's restraining device or "seat belt." Following the impact of an automobile accident, it appears that if the heart is not restrained by its "seat belt"—the pericardial sac—then the heart is more prone to injury by the chest wall.[78] The heart also is not protected from the lung, which may be important in the event of pneumonia, and the lung is not protected from the beating of the heart. Thus, total absence of the pericardium is not entirely benign; nonetheless, these conditions usually are not treated by surgical repair.

Surgical treatment of partial pericardial defect has been of two types: enlargement, to avoid the risk of strangulation; or closure, usually with a flap of mediastinal pleura. The latter is considered preferable. A defect of the diaphragmatic pericardium requires reduction of the abdominal contents into the abdomen and repair of the diaphragmatic defect.

disease, these associated anomalies dominate the clinical picture. If pericardial defect is isolated, such patients may be asymptomatic, or they may have chest pain that may or may not be angina-like.[18, 79, 80, 124]

Partial left-sided pericardial defects may be associated with herniation of the ventricles through the patent pleuropericardial foramen, resulting in strangulation of the ventricles and leading to death.[11, 13, 24, 101] Herniation and strangulation of the left atrial appendage also can occur.[18, 79] Right-sided partial pericardial defect can be associated with obstruction of the superior vena cava, due to compression by the right lung that has herniated into the pericardial cavity.[73] Diaphragmatic pericardial defect usually is associated with a diaphragmatic defect, which may permit herniation of the greater omentum into the pericardial cavity, leading to chest pain and the radiologic appearance of cardiomegaly.[42]

DIAGNOSIS

The chest x-ray is often highly suggestive of this diagnosis.[32] With complete left pericardial defect, the heart is

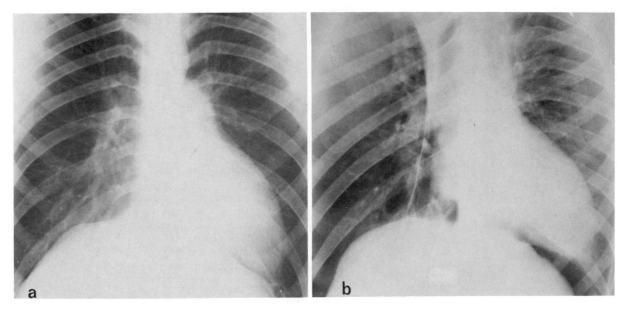

Fig. 28.17 Complete left-sided pericardial defect. (*a*) Posteroanterior chest x-ray showing left shift of the heart and three unusually prominent convexities of the elongated left heart border formed by the aortic knob, the pulmonary artery, and the ventricles. (*b*) Following the introduction of 500 of air into the left pleural space, a right posterior oblique chest film was taken with the horizontal beam, with the patient's left side down. Air separating the heart from the diaphragm and the right pneumopericardium indicates the presence of a left pericardial defect. That it is a complete left pericardial defect, rather than a partial defect, is indicated by the levoposition of the whole heart (*a*), that can be misread as cardiomegaly of obscure cause. (Reproduced with permission from K. Ellis *et al.*[32])

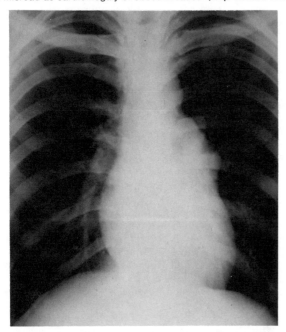

Fig. 28.18 Partial left pericardial defect. In this posteroanterior chest x-ray, note the characteristic prominence of the left heart border that could not be separated from the pulmonary artery shadow by fluoroscopy, with this prominence produced by herniation of the left atrial appendage through the left pleuropericardial foramen. Note that the location of the heart as a whole is normal, rather than being levoposed, as in Figure 28.17. (Reproduced with permission from W. P. Baker *et al.*[7] and The Reuben H. Donnelley Corp.)

ECTOPIA CORDIS

First reported in 1671 by Stensen[94] (this also being the earliest known case of the tetralogy of Fallot), ectopia cordis means that the heart is partially or totally outside the thorax.

CLASSIFICATION

There are essentially four types of ectopia cordis: cervical, in malformed fetuses only, found in 4 of 143 cases[85]; thoracic, found in 84 of 143 cases (Fig. 24.19)[85]; thoracoabdominal, occurring in 54 of 143 cases[85] (Fig. 28.20); and abdominal, represented to date only by Deschamps' case that was reported in 1806 by Cullerier,[21] in which the heart was described as being entirely within the abdomen (as opposed to being thoracoabdominal). This patient was a previously healthy French soldier, the father of three children. He died of pyelonephritis and autopsy showed that the left kidney was absent, and in its place was the heart, surrounded by the pericardial sac. The vessels arising from the heart passed upward through the diaphragm to reach the lungs.

With the exception of Deschamps' case, all cases of ectopia cordis that are reported as abdominal in fact had thoracoabdominal ectopia cordis. The thoracocervical[49] and partial thoracic[49] types are considered to be errors; both types have cleft sternum and intact skin, and the heart is basically intrathoracic. Cleft sternum should be distinguished from real ectopia cordis. Thus, for practical purposes, there are essentially only **two types of ectopia cordis: thoracic and thoracoabdominal.** The frequency of ectopia cordis in our Cardiac Registry of autopsied congenital cardiovascular disease is 2 of 1716 cases.

The thoracic type is the classical form of ectopia cordis (Fig. 28.19).[15] There is a sternal defect, absence of the parietal pericardium, cephalic orientation of the cardiac apex that often beats against the infant's chin, epigastric omphalocele or diastasis recti, and a small thoracic cavity.

Thoracoabdominal ectopia cordis (Fig. 28.20) is characterized by: partial absence or cleft of the lower sternum; almost always a half-moon-shaped anterior diaphragmatic defect (septum transversum defect); almost always a defect of the diaphragmatic parietal pericardium; omphalocele or diastasis recti; partial displacement of the ventricular portion of the heart through the diaphragmatic defect into the epigastrium; displacement of other viscera into the omphal-

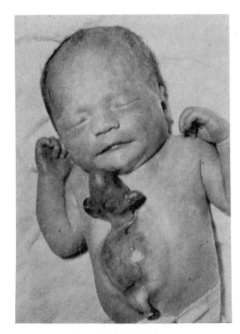

Fig. 28.19 Thoracic ectopia cordis in a newborn female infant. Note the cephalic orientation of the ventricular apex that beats against the infant's chin, the evident sternal defect, the absence of a pericardial sac, and the characteristic epigastric omphalocele. (Reproduced with permission from F. Byron[15])

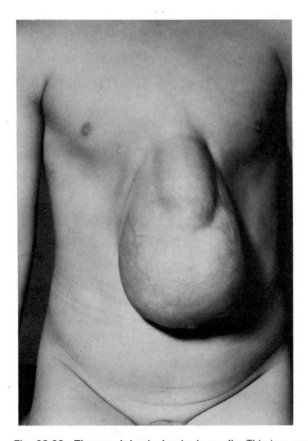

Fig. 28.20 Thoracoabdominal ectopia cordis. This is a preoperative photograph. The heart, in diastole, forms a conical epigastric bulge above a large epigastric hernia. This patient, a 3-year-old boy, was the first with thoracoabdominal ectopia cordis to be successfully repaired surgically, by Sir Russell Brock, in 1950. (Reproduced with permission from G. W. Scott.[85])

ocele, depending on its size; and other congenital anomalies, cardiac and extracardiac, almost all having congenital heart disease.[17, 67, 71, 85, 102] Many different types of congenital heart disease have been reported, including tetralogy of Fallot, VSD, ASD, tricuspid atresia, Ebstein's anomaly, common atrium, common AV canal, mitral atresia, persistent left superior vena cava, anomalous pulmonary veins, single ventricle, pulmonary stenosis, pulmonary atresia, aortic stenosis, coarctation of the aorta, TGA, diverticulum of LV, and diverticulum of both ventricles. There are at least five cases of thoracoabdominal ectopia cordis that have had no congenital heart disease.[102]

TREATMENT

For the first time, a case of thoracic ectopia cordis appears to have been successfully treated surgically by Saxena, Kettrick, Koop and their colleagues at the Children's Hospital of Philadelphia.[81, 82] The first operation that was performed on this 5-hour-old male infant on August 10, 1975 was essentially as follows:

Under general endotracheal anesthesia, an incision was made from the suprasternal notch to the umbilicus, curving around the chest wall defect. The heart was carefully dissected from the margins of the chest defect. In order to create space in the mediastinum for the heart, the diaphragm was detached from the lower border of the defect and from the anterior ribs. The falciform ligament was divided, and the liver was displaced downwards. Both pleural spaces were opened and mobilized. All great vessels connecting to the heart were mobilized to prevent kinking. The diaphragm was reattached at a lower level. The sternal bands were separated by 5 cm (2 inches). All attempts to approximate the two sternal bands directly or with a Dacron patch were abandoned because of resulting tamponade. Skin flaps were then mobilized to the midaxillary lines. After closure of the anterior abdominal wall, the skin flaps were closed over the heart with interrupted sutures. The patient was placed on a respirator.

He was kept paralyzed for 3 days in order to prevent suture line stress and to facilitate controlled ventilation with a volume ventilator. During the first 3 days he required a constant infusion of catecholamines in order to maintain a good blood pressure and urinary output. After 72 hours, the catecholamines were discontinued, and the patient was placed on digoxin and furosemide. Curare was discontinued, and the patient was changed to intermittent mandatory ventilation for a short while. Since he was unable to maintain good blood gases, controlled ventilation was reinstituted. A tracheostomy was performed on September 13, 1975. Cardiac catheterization of September 29 showed a very small VSD.

It was decided to postpone the second surgical operation until the infant was in better condition. He was bottle fed and hyperalimented.

On February 18, 1976, when the patient was 7 months of age, Koop and Saxena[82] performed a chest wall reconstruction operation.[82] This procedure took 4 hours. One of the more difficult aspects of this operation was the initial incision and exposure that took an hour to achieve because the skin was stretched immediately over the heart and was adherent to it. The manubrium was widened with an acrylic resin prosthesis that was shaped into a manubrium and was sutured to the sternal cartilage with wire sutures. The gap between the two halves of the body of the sternum was bridged with a two-layered prosthetic patch, the deeper layer of dacron, and the superficial layer of mylex mesh. The skin was closed primarily over the prosthetic material with interrupted sutures.

It was only following this chest reconstruction operation, that Koop had performed only twice before on infants with thoracic dystrophy, that it was possible to wean the patient from the respirator.

Unfortunately, the postoperative course[82] of this patient was complicated by the development of necrosis of the skin flap and infection of the prosthetic material. Consequently, the prosthetic material was surgically removed on April 2, 1976. After the skin infection and subcutaneous wound infection had been cleared up with the assistance of betadine irrigation, the patient underwent rotation of skin flaps to bridge the area over the heart. The heart had been covered with a thick layer of granulation tissue following the chest reconstruction operation. In July, 1976, the patient was 11 months of age, was gaining weight very slowly, and weighed only 9 kg. He still required some ventilatory support in order to keep his PCO_2 within normal limits.

Over the subsequent 5 years, the patient did well and now (September, 1981) is described as a "a cute kid." The patient still has a tracheostomy, and it is planned to close it soon.

It is noteworthy that smallness of the chest cavity may be the basic problem in thoracic ectopia cordis. This may explain why the chest cannot close anteriorly. Due to smallness of the thorax, the anterior chest wall attempts to come together beside the heart, instead of in front of it, thereby resulting in thoracic ectopia cordis. Koop and Saxena essentially built the chest around the heart, rather than attempting to put the heart into the abnormally small thorax. Efforts to put the heart into the small chest cavity have been made in the past but have never succeeded because of the development of tamponade or kinking of the vessels.

Jones et al.[48] suggested in 1979 that all cases of complete thoracic ectopia cordis should undergo *immediate* surgery (a) for their congenital heart disease and (b) for their anterior chest wall defect. Koop, and Jones et al.[48] favor the use of an acrylic prosthesis for anterior chest wall reconstruction. Detachment of the diaphragm from the thoracic wall, with reattachment of the diaphragm lower down, to the abdominal wall, also was suggested.[48]

Chromosomal abnormalities can be associated with complete thoracic ectopia cordis[54] and may be of significance etiologically.

Thoracoabdominal ectopia cordis was first successfully treated by Brock on October 5, 1950, as was reported by Scott[85] in 1955. The two essential steps in this surgical procedure are: repair of the anterior diaphragmatic defect and repair of the omphalocele or epigastric hernia.

REFERENCES

1. Abbott, M. E.: Pulmonary conus stenosis at lower bulbar orifice, all cardiac septa closed. In Atlas of Congenital Cardiac Disease. American Heart Association, New York, 1936, p. 42.
2. Afzelius, B. A., Eliasson, R., Johnsen, O., and Lindholmer, C.: Lack of dynein arms in immotile human spermatozoa. J. Cell Biol. 66:225, 1975.
3. Anderson, R. H., Shinebourne, E. R., and Gerlis, L. M.: Criss-cross atrioventricular relationships producing paradoxical atrioventricular concordance or discordance: Their significance to nomenclature of congenital heart disease. Circulation 50:176, 1974.
4. Ando, M., Satomi, G., and Takao, A.: Atresia of tricuspid or mitral orifice: Anatomic spectrum and morphogenetic hypothesis. In, Etiology and Morphogenesis of Congenital Heart Disease, edited by R. Van Praagh and A. Takao. Futura, Mt. Kisco, N.Y., 1980, p. 421.
5. Baim, R. S., MacDonald, I. L., Wise, D. J., and Lenkei, S. C.: Computed tomography of absent left pericardium. Radiology 135:127, 1980.
6. Bairov, G. A., Leibov, S. L., and Popov, A. A.: Ectocardia. Vestn. Khir. 122:63, 1979.
7. Baker, W. P., Schlang, H. A., and Ballenger, F. P.: Congenital partial absence of the pericardium. Am. J. Cardiol. 16:133, 1965.
8. Bharati, S., and Lev, M.: The course of the conduction system in dextrocardia. Circulation 57:163, 1978.
9. Bharati, S., and Lev, M.: Positional variations of the heart and its component chambers. Circulation 59:886, 1979.
10. Bhat, P. S., Ojha, J. P., Sinha, V. K., Srivastava, P. K., Avasthey, P., and Somani, P. N.: Myocardial infarction with dextrocardia and situs inversus. A rare case report. Indian Heart J. 32:190, 1980.
11. Boxall, R.: Incomplete pericardial sac: Escape of heart into left pleural cavity. Trans. Obstet. Soc. Lond. 28:209, 1887.
12. Breschet, G.: Mémoir sur l'ectopie de l'appareil de la circulation et particulièrement sur celle du coeur. Rep. Gén. d'Anat. et de la Physiol. Pathologiques et de Clinique Chirurg. (Paris) 2:1, 1826.
13. Bruning, E. G. H.: Congenital defect of the pericardium. J. Clin. Pathol. 15:133, 1962.
14. Büchler, J., Rabelo, R., Marino, R., David, I., and Van Praagh, R.: Double-outlet right atrium: Autopsied case of newly recognized entity. Abstracts, World Congress of Paediatric Cardiology, London, 1980, p. 223.
15. Byron, F.: Ectopia cordis. Report of a case with attempted operative correction. J. Thorac. Surg. 17:717, 1948.
16. Calcaterra, G., Anderson, R. H., Lau, K. C., and Shinebourne, E. A.: Dextrocardia—Value of segmental analysis in its categorisation. Br. Heart J. 42:497, 1979.
17. Cantrell, J. R., Haller, J. A., and Ravitch, M. M.: A syndrome of congenital defects involving the abdominal wall, sternum, diaphragm, pericardium, and heart. Surg. Gynecol. Obstet. 107:602, 1958.
18. Carty, J. E., Deverell, P. B., and Losowsky, M. S.: Pericardial defect presenting as acute pericarditis. Br. Heart J. 37:98, 1975.
19. Chandramouly, B. S., Kihn, R. H., and Flesh, L. H.: Dextrocardia with total situs inversus, radionuclide imaging and ultrasonography of liver and spleen. N.Y. State J. Med. 80:655, 1980.
20. Columbus, R.: De Re Anatomica, Book 15. Nicolai Beuilacquae, Venice, 1559, p. 265.
21. Cullerier: Observation sur un déplacement remarquable du coeur; par M. Deschamps, médecin à Laval. J. Gén. de Médecine, de Chirurgie et de Pharmacie 26:275, 1806.
22. Danielson, G. K., Tabry, I. F., Ritter, D. G., and Fulton, R. E.: Surgical repair of criss-cross heart with straddling atrioventricular valve. J. Thorac. Cardiovasc. Surg. 77:847, 1979.
23. Davis, C. L.: Development of the human heart from its first appearance to the stage found in embryos of twenty paired somites. Contrib. Embryol. 19:245, 1927.
24. De Garis, C. F.: Pericardial patency and partial ectocardia in a newborn organ-utan. Anat. Rec. 59:69, 1934.
25. De Haan, R. L.: Morphogenesis of the vertebrate heart. In Organogenesis, edited by R. L. De Haan and H. Ursprung. Holt, Rinehart, & Winston, New York, 1965, p. 377.
26. De la Cruz, M. V., Anselmi, C., Cisneros, F., Reinhold, M., Portillo, B., and Espino-Vela, J.: An embryologic explanation for the corrected transposition of the great vessels: Additional description of the main anatomic features of this malformation and its varieties. Am. Heart J. 57:104, 1959.
27. De la Cruz, M. V., and da Rocha, J. P.: An ontogenetic theory for the explanation of congenital malformations involving the truncus and conus. Am. Heart J. 51:782, 1956.
28. De Tommasi, S. M., Carminati, M., Invernizzi, P., Troiani, P., Velitti, F., and Tiraboschi, R.: Situs inversus con destrocardia, anàlisi delle cardiopatie congenite associate. G. Ital. Cardiol. 10:1192, 1980.
29. De Vries, P. A.: Evolution of precardiac and splanchnic mesoderm in relationship to the infundibulum and truncus. Perspect. Cardiovasc. Res. 5:31, 1981.
30. Eliasson, R., Mossberg, B., Cammer, P., and Afzelius, B.: The immotile-cilia syndrome, a congenital ciliary abnormality as an etiologic factor in chronic airway infections and male sterility. N. Engl. J. Med. 297:1, 1977.
31. Elliott, L. P.: An angiocardiographic and plain film approach to complex congenital heart disease: Simplified nomenclature. Curr. Probl. Cardiol. 3:1, 1978.
32. Ellis, K., Leeds, N. E., and Himmelstein, A.: Congenital deficiencies in the parietal pericardium. A review with 2 new cases including successful diagnosis by plain roentgenography. Am. J. Roentgenol. 82:125, 1959.
33. Fabricius, cited by Cleveland, M.: Situs inversus viscerum: Anatomic study. Arch. Surg. 13:343, 1926.
34. Fischer, T. J., McAdams, J. A., Entis, G. N., Cotton, R., Ghory, J. E., and Ausdenmoore, R. W.: Middle ear ciliary defect in Kartagener's syndrome. Pediatrics 62:443, 1978.
35. Freedom, R. M., Culham, G., and Rowe, R. D.: The criss-cross and superoinferior ventricular heart: An angiocardiographic study. Am. J. Cardiol. 42:620, 1978.
36. Gardner, D. L., and Cole, L.: Long survival with inferior vena cava draining into left atrium. Br. Heart J. 17:93, 1955.
37. Garson, A., Hawkins, E. P., Mullins, C. E., Edwards, S. B. Sabiston, D. C., and Cooley, D. A.: Thoracoabdominal ectopia cordis with mosaic Turner's syndrome: Report of a case. Pediatrics 62:218, 1978.
38. Gautam, H. P.: Left atrial inferior vena cava with atrial septal defect. J. Thorac. Cardiovasc. Surg. 55:827, 1968.
39. Goor, D. A., Dische, R., and Lillehei, C. W.: The conotruncus. I. Its normal inversion and conus absorption. Circulation 46:375, 1972.
40. Goor, D. A.: The conotruncus. I. Its normal inversion and conus absorption, the author's reply. Circulation 46:635, 1972.
41. Guthaner, D., Higgins, C. B., Silverman, J. F., Hayden, W. G., and Wexler, L.: An unusual form of the transposition complex, uncorrected levo-transposition with horizontal ventricular septum: Report of two cases. Circulation 53:190, 1976.
42. Haider, R., Thomas, D. G. T., Ziady, G., Cleland, W. P., and Goodwin, J. F.: Congenital pericardio-peritoneal communications with herniation of omentum into the pericardium: A rare cause of cardiomegaly. Br. Heart

J. 35:981, 1973.
43. Hamilton, W. J., and Mossman, H. W.: Growth and rotation of the gut. In Hamilton, Boyd, and Mossman's Human Embryology: Prenatal Development of Form and Function. Williams & Wilkins, Baltimore, 1972, p. 356.
44. Harris, T. R., and Rainey, R. L.: Ideal isolated levocardia. Am. Heart J. 70:440, 1965.
45. Hastreiter, A. R., and Rodriguez-Coronel, A.: Discordant situs of thoracic and abdominal viscera. Am. J. Cardiol. 22:111, 1968.
46. Inoue, H., Mashima, S., Takayanagi, K., Murayama, M., Matsuo, H. Sakamoto, T., and Murao, S.: Postural changes of vectorcardiogram in defect of the left pericardium. J. Electrocardiol. 14:21, 1981.
47. Jennings, R. B., Crisler, C., Johnson, D. H., and Brickman, R. D.: Tricuspid atresia with dextrotransposition, dextrocardia, and mitral insufficiency: successful circulatory correction. Ann. Thorac. Surg. 29:369, 1980.
48. Jones, A. F., McGrath, R. S., Edwards, S. M., and Lilly, J. R.: Immediate operation for ectopia cordis. Ann. Thorac. Surg. 28:484, 1979.
49. Kanagasuntheram, R., and Verzin, J. A.: Ectopia cordis in man. Thorax 17:159, 1962.
50. Karczenski, K., and Wozniewicz, B.: Congenital heart diseases and types of position of viscera. Pediatr. Pol. 53:1382, 1978 (in Polish).
51. Kartagener, M.: Zur Pathogenese der Bronchiektasian: Bronchiektasian bei situs viscerum inversus. Beitr. Klin. Tuberk., 83:489, 1933.
52. Kartagener, M., and Strucki, P.: Bronchiectasis with situs inversus. Arch. Pediatr. 79:193, 1962.
53. Keith, A.: Partial deficiency of the pericardium. J. Anat. Physiol. 41:6, 1907.
54. King, C. R.: Ectopia cordis and chromosomal errors. Pediatrics 66:328, 1980.
55. Kinsley, R. H., McGoon, D. C., and Danielson, G. K.: Corrected transposition of the great arteries: Associated ventricular rotation. Circulation 49:574, 1974.
56. Kirklin, J. W., Pacifico, A. D., Bargeron, L. M., and Soto, B.: Cardiac repair in anatomically corrected malposition of the great arteries. Circulation 48:253, 1973.
57. Layton, W. M.: Random determination of a developmental process: Reversal of normal visceral asymmetry in the mouse. J. Heredity 67:336, 1976.
58. Layton, W. M.: Heart malformations in mice homozygous for a gene causing situs inversus. In Morphogenesis and Malformation of the Cardiovascular System, edited by G. Rosenquist and D. Bergsma, Vol. 14. Alan R. Liss for the National Foundation March of Dimes, New York, 1980, p. 277.
59. Layton, W. M., and Manasek, F.: Cardiac looping of early *iv/iv* mouse embryos. In Etiology and Morphogenesis of Congenital Heart Disease, edited by R. Van Praagh and A. Takao. Futura, Mt. Kisco, 1980, p. 109.
60. Lev, M., Liberthson, R. R., Eckner, F. A. O., and Arcilla, R. A.: Pathologic anatomy of dextrocardia and its clinical implications. Circulation 37:979, 1968.
61. Lev, M., Liberthson, R. R., Golden, J. G., Eckner, F. A. O., and Arcilla, R. A.: The pathologic anatomy of mesocardia. Am. J. Cardiol. 28:428, 1971.
62. Lev, M., and Rowlatt, U. F.: The pathologic anatomy of mixed levocardia: a review of thirteen cases of atrial or ventricular inversion with or without corrected transposition. Am. J. Cardiol. 8:216, 1961.
63. Lewis, F. T., and Abbott, M. E.: Reversed torsion of the ventricular band of the embryonic heart in the explanation of certain forms of cardiac anomaly. Bull. Intern. Assoc. Med. Museums 61:111, 1916.
64. Liberthson, R. R., Hastreiter, A. R., Sinha, S.

N., Bharati, S., Novak, G. M., and Lev, M.: Levocardia with visceral heterotaxy—Isolated levocardia: Pathologic anatomy and its clinical implications. Am. Heart J. 85:40, 1973.
65. Logan, W. D., Abbott, O. A., and Hatcher, C. R.: Kartagener's triad. Dis. Chest 48:613, 1965.
66. Macartney, F. J., Shinebourne, E. A., and Anderson, R. H.: Connexions, relations, discordance, and distorsions. Br. Heart J. 38:323, 1976.
67. Major, J. W.: Thoracoabdominal ectopia cordis: Report of a case successfully treated by surgery. J. Thorac. Surg. 26:309, 1953.
68. Martin, G.: Observation d'une déviation organique de l'estomac, d'une anomalie dans la situation, dans la configuration du coeur et des vaisseaux qui en partant ou qui s'y rendent. Bull Soc. Anat. Paris 1:39, 1826.
69. Melhuish, B. P. P., and Van Praagh, R.: Juxtaposition of the atrial appendages: A sign of severe cyanotic congenital heart disease. Br. Heart J. 30:269, 1968.
70. Miller, R. D., and Divertie, M. B.: Kartagener's syndrome. Chest 62:130, 1972.
71. Milhouse, R. F., and Joos, H. A.: Extrathoracic ectopia cordis: Report of case and review of literature. Am. Heart J. 57:470, 1959.
72. Minocha, G. K., Falicov, R. E., and Nijensohn, E.: Partial right-sided congenital pericardial defect with herniation of right atrium and right ventricle. Chest 76:484, 1979.
73. Moene, R. J., Dekker, A., and van der Harten, H. J.: Congenital right-sided pericardial defect with herniation of part of the lung into the pericardial cavity. Am. J. Cardiol. 31:519, 1973.
74. Ochoteco, A., Figueroa, A., Pagola, M. A., Gallo, J. I., Martinez De Ubaga, J. L., and Gomez-Daran, C. M.: Agenesia parcial de pericardio con herniación de la oregjuela izquierda. Rev. Espan. Cardiol. 32:99, 1979.
75. Otero Coto, E., Quero Jimenez, M.: Aproximacion segmentaria al diagnostico y clasificacion de las cardiopatias congenitas. Fundamentos y utilidad. Rev. Espan. Cardiol. 30:557, 1977.
76. Paul, M. H., Sinha, S. N., Muster, A. J., Cole, R. B., and Van Praagh, R.: Double outlet left ventricle: Report of an autopsy case with an intact ventricular septum and consideration of its developmental implications. Circulation 41:129, 1970.
77. Rao, P. S.: Systematic approach to differential diagnosis. Am. Heart J. 102:389, 1981.
78. Reginato, E., Speroni, E., Riccardi, M., Verunelli, F., and Eufrate, S.: Post-traumatic mitral regurgitation and ventricular septal defect in absence of left pericardium. Thorac. Cardiovasc. Surg. 28:213, 1980.
79. Robin, E., Ganguly, S. N., and Fowler, M. S.: Strangulation of the left atrial appendage through a congenital partial pericardial defect. Chest 67:354, 1975.
80. Saito, R., and Hotta, F.: Congenital pericardial defect associated with cardiac incarceration: Case report. Am. Heart J. 100:866, 1980.
81. Saxena, N. C.: Personal communication, February 9, 1976, and Pediatric News, 9:1, 1975.
82. Saxena, N. C.: Personal communication, July 16, 1976, and Pediatric News, 10:3, 1976.
83. Shuster, P., and Eimermacher, H.: Difetto congenito parziale del pericardio con prolasso dell'orecchietta sinistra. G. Ital. Cardiol. 10:624, 1980.
84. Schwartz, H. A., and Wagner, P. I.: Corrected transposition of the great vessels in a 55-year-old woman: Diagnosis by coronary angiography. Chest 66:190, 1974.
85. Scott, G. W.: Ectopia cordis: Report of a case successfully treated by operation. Guys Hosp. Rep. 104:55, 1955.

86. Shah, C. V., Shah, K. D., Ashar, P. N., and Hansoti, R. C.: Mirror-image dextrocardia with thoraco-abdominal discordance and normal spleen. Chest 69:427, 1976.
87. Shinebourne, E. A., Macartney, F. J., and Anderson, R. H.: Sequential chamber localization—Logical approach to diagnosis in congenital heart disease. Br. Heart J. 38:327, 1976.
88. Silveira, S. R., Grinberg, M., Atik, E., Moffa, P. J., and Tranchesi, J.: Mesoposição associada à atresia tricúspide e transposição dos grandes vasos da base com aspectos eléctricos inusitados. Arq. Bras. Cardiol. 32:191, 1979.
89. Siman, J., Augustínová, A., and Čizmárová, E.: Congenital absence of the pericardium. Bratisl. Lek. Listy 71:554, 1979.
90. Siplovich, L., Bar-Ziv, J., Karplus, M., and Mares, A. J.: The pericardial "window": A rare etiologic factor in neonatal pneumopericardium. J. Pediatr. 94:975, 1979.
91. Squarcia, H., Ritter, D. G., and Kincaid, D. W.: Dextrocardia: Angiographic study and classification. Am. J. Cardiol. 32:965, 1973.
92. Stanger, P., Benassi, R. C., Korns, M. E., Jue, K. L., and Edwards, J. E.: Diagrammatic portrayal of variations in cardiac structure, reference to transposition, dextrocardia and the concept of four normal hearts. Circulation 37:iv-1, 1968.
93. Stanger, P., Rudolph, A. M., and Edwards, J. E.: Cardiac malpositions: An overview based on study of sixty-five necropsy specimens. Circulation 56:159, 1977.
94. Stensen, N.: In Acta Medica et Philosophica Hafniencia, Vol. 1, edited by T. Bartholin, 1671–1672, p. 202. Translated into English by F. A. Willius. An unusually early description of the so-called tetralogy of Fallot. Proc. Staff Meet. Mayo Clin. 23:316, 1948.
95. Stocker, F. P., Weber, J. W., Kinser, J., and Rösler, H.: The role of radio isotopes in the diagnosis of systemic vein abnormalities. Magyar Pediatr. (Suppl.) 12:4, 1978.
96. Streeter, G. L.: Developmental horizons in human embryos. Description of age group XI, 13 to 20 somites, and age group XII, 21 to 29 somites. Contrib. Embryol. 30:211, 1942.
97. Streeter, G. L.: Developmental horizons in human embryos. Description of age group XIII, embryos about 4 or 5 millimeters long, and age group XIV, period of indentation of the lens vesicle. Contrib. Embryol. 31:27, 1945.
98. Streeter, G. L.: Developmental horizons in human embryos. Description of age groups XV, XVI, XVII, and XVIII, being the third issue of a survey of the Carnegie Collection. Contrib. Embryol. 32:133, 1948.
99. Streeter, G. L.: Developmental horizons in human embryos. Description of age groups XIX, XX, XXI, XXII, and XXIII (the fifth issue of a survey of Carnegie Collection). Contrib. Embryol. 34:165, 1951.
100. Sturgess, J. M., Chao, J., Wong, J., Aspin, N., and Turner, J. A.: Cilia with defective radial spokes: A cause of human respiratory disease. N. Engl. J. Med. 300:53, 1979.
101. Sunderland, S., and Wright-Smith, R. J.: Congenital pericardial defects. Br. Heart J. 6:167, 1944.
102. Toyama, W. M.: Combined congenital defects of the anterior abdominal wall, sternum, diaphragm, pericardium and heart: A case report and review of the syndrome. Pediatrics 50:778, 1972.
103. Tynan, M. J., Becker, A. E., Macartney, F. J., Quero Jimenez, M., Shinebourne, E. A., and Anderson, R. H.: Nomenclature and classification of congenital heart disease. Br. Heart J. 41:544, 1979.
104. Van Mierop, L. H.: Asplenia and polysplenia syndromes. Birth Defects 8:36, 1972.
105. Van Mierop, L. H. S., and Wiglesworth, F.

W.: Pathogenesis of transposition complexes. III. True transposition of the great vessels. Am. J. Cardiol. 12:233, 1963.

106. Van Praagh, R.: The segmental approach to diagnosis in congenital heart disease. Birth Defects 8:4, 1972.

107. Van Praagh, R.: Conotruncal malformations. In Heart Disease in Infancy, edited by B. G. Barratt-Boyes, J. M. Neutze, and E. A. Harris. Churchill & Livingstone, Edinburgh and London, 1973, p. 141.

108. Van Praagh, R.: Les malformations conotroncales. Coeur Numéro Spécial:15, 1973.

109. Van Praagh, R., Ongley, P. A., and Swan, H. J. C.: Anatomic types of single or common ventricle in man: Morphologic and geometric aspects of 60 necropsied cases. Am. J. Cardiol. 13:367, 1964.

110. Van Praagh, R.: The segmental approach to understanding complex cardiac lesions. In Current Problems in Congenital Heart Disease, edited by Eldrege W. J., Lemole, G. M., Goldberg, H., Spectrum, New York, 1979, p. 1.

111. Van Praagh, R., and Van Praagh, S.: Isolated ventricular inversion: A consideration of the morphogenesis, definition and diagnosis of nontransposed and transposed great arteries. Am. J. Cardiol. 17:395, 1966.

112. Van Praagh, R., Van Praagh, S., Vlad, P., and Keith, J. D.: Anatomic types of congenital dextrocardia: Diagnostic and embryologic implications. Am. J. Cardiol. 13:510, 1964.

113. Van Praagh, R., Van Praagh, S., Vlad, P., and Keith, J. D.: Diagnosis of anatomic types congenital dextrocardia. Am. J. Cardiol.

15:234, 1965.

114. Van Praagh, R., David, I., Gordon, D., Wright, G. B., and Van Praagh, S.: Ventricular diagnosis and designation. In Pediatr. Cardiol., 1980. Churchill Livingstone, Edinburgh and London, 1982, p. 153.

115. Van Praagh, R., Layton, W. M., and Van Praagh, S.: The morphogenesis of normal and abnormal relationships between the great arteries and the ventricles: Pathologic and experimental data. In Etiology and Morphogenesis of Congenital Heart Disease, edited by R. Van Praagh and A. Takao. Futura, Mount Kisco, N.Y., 1980, p. 271.

116. Van Praagh, R., Pérez-Treviño, C., López-Cuellar, M., Baker, F., and Van Praagh, S.: Transposition of the great arteries with posterior aorta, anterior pulmonary artery, subpulmonary conus and fibrous continuity between aortic and atrioventricular valves. Am. J. Cardiol., 28:621, 1971.

117. Van Praagh, R., Plett, J. A., and Van Praagh, S.: Single ventricle: Pathology, embryology, terminology and classification. Herz 4:113, 1979.

118. Van Praagh, R., and Vlad, P.: Dextrocardia, mesocardia and levocardia. The segmental approach to diagnosis in congenital heart disease. In Heart Disease in Infancy and Childhood, 3rd ed., edited by J. D. Keith, R. D. Rowe, and P. Vlad. Macmillan, New York, 1978, p. 638.

119. Van Praagh, R., Wise, J. R., Dahl, B. A., and Van Praagh, S.: Single left ventricle with infundibular outlet chamber and tricuspid valve opening only into outlet chamber in a

44-year-old man with thoracoabdominal ectopia cordis without diaphragmatic or pericardial defect: Importance of myocardial morphologic method of chamber identification in congenital heart disease. In Etiology and Morphogenesis of Congenital Heart Disease, edited by R. Van Praagh, and A. Takao. Futura, Mount Kisco, N.Y., 1980, p. 379.

120. Van Praagh, S., LaCorte, M., Fellows, K. E., Bossina, K., Busch, H. J., Keck, E. W., Weinberg, P., and Van Praagh, R.: Supero-inferior ventricles, anatomic and angiocardiographic findings in 10 postmortem cases. In Etiology and Morphogenesis of Congenital Heart Disease, edited by R. Van Praagh, and A. Takao. Futura, Mount Kisco, N.Y., 1980, p. 317.

121. Victor, S., Rajesh, P. B., Daniel, I. D., Rajaram, S., and Lakshmikanthan, C.: Congenital pericardial defect with accessory lobules in the lung and patent ductus anteriosus: A case report. Indian Heart J. 31:61, 1979.

122. Von Rokitansky, C.: Die Defekte der Scheidwande des Herzens. Braumüller, Vienna, 1875.

123. Waldman, J. D., Rosenthal, A., Smith, A. L., Shurin, S., and Nadas, A. S.: Sepsis in congenital asplenia. J. Pediatr. 90:555, 1977.

124. Wallace, H. W., Shen, D., Baum, S., Blakemore, W. S., and Zinsser, H. F.: Angina pectoris associated with a pericardial defect. J. Thorac. Cardiovasc. Surg. 61:461, 1971.

125. Wellens, H. J. J., and Gorgels, A. P.: Mirror-image dextrocardia and the Wolff-Parkinson-White syndrome. Chest 76:91, 1979.

126. Wolfe, R. R.: Kartagener's syndrome: A pediatric responsibility. Chest 69:573, 1976.

29

Anomalous Venous Connections, Pulmonary and Systemic

Russell V. Lucas, Jr., M.D.

ANOMALIES OF THE PULMONARY VENOUS SYSTEM

Abnormalities of the pulmonary venous system are not common, although their real frequency is probably greater than that deduced from clinical and autopsy studies. These anomalies present in an almost endless variety and may be defined and classified on the basis of their anatomy, physiology, or embryology.

ANATOMY

In anatomic terms, the pulmonary venous anomalies may be: anomalous connections, stenotic connections, and abnormal numbers of pulmonary veins.

Anomalous Connections

One or more of the pulmonary veins may connect anomalously to the right atrium or one of its venous tributaries. The condition is termed total anomalous pulmonary venous connection (TAPVC) if all the veins connect anomalously,

and partial anomalous pulmonary venous connection (PAPVC) if one or more but not all the veins connect anomalously.

The physiologic consequence of anomalous pulmonary venous *connection* is anomalous pulmonary venous *drainage*. We agree with Edwards[23] that the term anomalous connection is preferable to anomalous drainage in the identification of these conditions. Use of the term anomalous connection clearly defines the anatomic feature. On the other hand, anomalous drainage, although a consequence of anomalous connection, also occurs in patients with atrial septal defect and common atrium.

Stenotic Connections

Stenosis may occur in one or more of the pulmonary veins or in the common pulmonary vein. Veins with normal connections may be stenosed (stenosis of one or more of the individual pulmonary veins, cor triatriatum). These produce obstruction to pulmonary venous return to the left atrium. Anomalously connected veins may also be stenosed, resulting in obstruction to pulmonary venous return to the *right* atrium. The physiologic feature common to these stenotic connections is obstruction to egress of pulmonary venous blood.

Abnormal Numbers of Pulmonary Veins

Normally, there are two right and two left pulmonary veins. The most common variation is the presence of a single pulmonary vein on either the right or left side, and these have a prevalence of about 24% in anatomic studies.[49] Rarely all pulmonary veins enter a common pulmonary vein which drains into the left atrium. The prevalence of a third pulmonary vein on either the right or left side is about 2%.[49] Rarely a fourth or even fifth vein may be present. An abnormal number of pulmonary veins imposes no physiologic handicap. They are primarily of interest to the thoracic surgeon.

EMBRYOLOGY

A classification based on embryologic principles introduces a unifying concept to the consideration of these anatomically and physiologically diverse conditions. Review of the embryologic development of the pulmonary venous system is a prerequisite.[68]

In the human embryo, the primordia of the lungs, larynx, and tracheobronchial tree are derived by a division of the foregut. In their early stages of development, the lungs are enmeshed by the vascular plexus of the foregut, the splanchnic plexus. As pulmonary differentiation progresses, part of the splanchnic plexus forms the pulmonary vascular bed. At this stage there is no direct connection to the heart. Instead, the pulmonary vascular bed shares the routes of drainage of the splanchnic plexus, i.e., the umbilicovitelline and cardinal systems of veins (Fig. 29.1A).

The definitive connection between the pulmonary vascular bed and the heart depends on the relatively late junction of an evagination from the sinoatrial region of the heart (common pulmonary vein) with the pulmonary portion of the splanchnic plexus (Fig. 29.1B). This outpouching originates to the left of the developing septum primum.[83] When the direct connection to the heart is established, the initial communications between the pulmonary portion of the splanchnic plexus and the cardinal and umbilicovitelline systems are, for the most part, lost. The pulmonary vascular bed then drains via four individual major pulmonary veins into the common pulmonary vein, which in turn empties into the left atrium (Fig. 29.1C). The common pulmonary vein is a transient anatomic structure; by a process of differential growth it becomes incorporated into the left atrium, resulting in the ultimate anatomic arrangement wherein the four individual pulmonary veins connect separately and directly to the left atrium (Fig. 29.1D).[23]

Imperfect development of the common pulmonary vein provides the embryologic basis for most anomalies of the pulmonary veins.[68] The following aberrations of development of the common pulmonary vein will serve to explain these anomalies and will be used as a means of classifying them (Table 29.1).

Early Atresia of the Common Pulmonary Vein while Pulmonary-Systemic Venous Connections Are Still Present

If atresia of the common pulmonary vein occurs early in its development, collateral channels for pulmonary venous drainage are available in the form of the primitive connections between the splanchnic plexus and the cardinal or umbilicovitelline systems of veins (Fig. 29.2). Any one of

these collateral channels may persist and enlarge; the result is TAPVC. Should only the right or left portion of the common pulmonary vein become atretic, persistence of the pulmonary venous-systemic venous connections on that side provides the etiologic basis for PAPVC[23] (Fig. 29.2).

Late Atresia of the Common Pulmonary Vein after Pulmonary-Systemic Connections Are Obliterated

When atresia of the common pulmonary vein occurs late, the collateral venous channels are already obliterated. The resulting anomaly has been termed atresia of the common pulmonary vein[69] (Fig. 29.3). The individual pulmonary veins empty into a blind cul-de-sac which has no direct connection to the left atrium or to the systemic venous systems.

Stenosis of the Common Pulmonary Vein

Cor triatriatum is the result of stenosis of the common pulmonary vein (Fig. 29.3). In the usual case the stenosis occurs late, after collateral venous connections have been lost; or else the severity of the obstruction produced by cor triatriatum is not sufficient to stimulate maintenance of the primitive routes of venous drainage. Occasionally, however, cor triatriatum may be associated with anomalous pulmonary venous connection, implying that in such cases the obstruction was early enough and sufficient to favor persistence of one of the primitive drainage channels.

Anamolous Incorporation of the Common Pulmonary Vein into the Left Atrium

Abnormal numbers of pulmonary veins are the result of imperfect incorporation of the common pulmonary vein into the left atrium. Incomplete absorption of the common pulmonary vein results in fewer than the normal number of pulmonary veins.[49] Rarely in the mature heart, a common pulmonary vein draining both lungs empties into the left atrium. More commonly a single pulmonary vein drains one lung. If more than the usual absorption takes place, there will be an increased number of pulmonary veins.

Stenosis in individual pulmonary veins at their junction with the left atrium is also a consequence of abnormal incorporation of the common pulmonary vein. One or more of the veins may be affected.

EARLY ATRESIA OF THE COMMON PULMONARY VEIN WHILE PULMONARY-SYSTEMIC VENOUS CONNECTIONS ARE STILL PRESENT

Partial Anomalous Pulmonary Venous Connection

Partial anomalous pulmonary venous connection defines the congenital anomaly in which one or more, but not all, of the pulmonary veins are connected to the right atrium or to one or more of its tributaries. Winslow is credited with the first description of this anomaly in 1739.[11] By 1942, Brody[11] was able to collect 65 cases from the literature. The advent of surgical correction of cardiac defects necessitated a more critical approach to diagnosis and has resulted in the identification and description of hundreds of cases.

Hughes and Rumore[51] found partial anomalous pulmonary venous connections in 0.7% of a series of 280 anatomic dissections, and Healy[49] found 0.6% in a series of 801 anatomic dissections. Both figures are higher than those deduced from clinical studies. This implies that a number of patients with PAPVC are not recognized.

Since an atrial septal defect (ASD) usually accompanies PAPVC, the frequency of the latter in patients with ASD is of interest. Gotsman and associates[39] reviewed 664 cases of

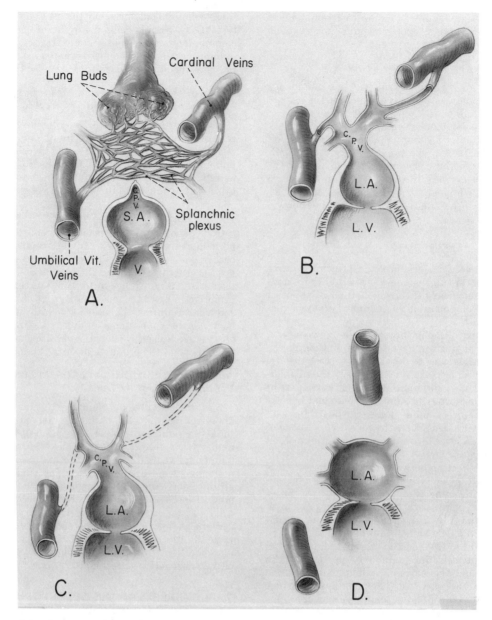

Fig. 29.1 Normal development of the pulmonary venous system. (*A*) Early, the splanchnic plexus drains the lung buds. This primitive pulmonary vascular bed has no direct connection with the heart; it shares the routes of drainage of the splanchnic plexus, the cardinal venous system, and the umbilicovitelline (*Umbilical Vit.*) systems. (*B*) The common pulmonary vein (*C.P.V.*) originates as an evagination from the left atrial (*L.A.*) side of the common atrium and establishes communication with the splanchnic plexus. Pulmonary venous blood may now drain directly to left atrium or indirectly to the heart via primitive venous connections. (*C*) No longer necessary, the primitive pulmonary venous connections disappear. (*D*) Finally, by means of the differential growth of the left atrium, the individual pulmonary veins are incorporated into the left atrium, and the common pulmonary vein no longer exists as an anatomic structure. L.V., left ventricle. (Reproduced with permission from R. V. Lucas, Jr., *et al.*[68])

ASD in the literature; 9% had associated PAPVC. Both sexes are affected equally.[74]

The etiology is unknown. The embryologic basis for PAPVC is partial: early obliteration of the common pulmonary vein, and persistence of one of the still present pulmonary-systemic venous channels as a route for pulmonary venous drainage.

Anatomy. PAPVC exhibits a wide anatomic spectrum. Almost every conceivable connection between the pulmonary veins, on the one hand, and the various systemic venous tributaries, on the other hand, has been reported (Fig. 29.4). Left-sided pulmonary veins usually connect anomalously to

derivatives of the left cardinal system, i.e., the coronary sinus and the left innominate vein. Anomalous connections of the right pulmonary veins are usually to derivatives of the right cardinal system, i.e., superior vena cava and inferior vena cava or the right atrium. However, the embryologic splanchnic plexus is a midline structure, and this explains the developmental possibility for crossed drainage of left-sided pulmonary veins to derivatives of the right cardinal system and vice versa.

Brody's review[11] of autopsy cases indicated the most common anomalous connections to be: right pulmonary veins to superior vena cava, right pulmonary veins to right atrium,

TABLE 29.1 EMBRYOLOGIC CLASSIFICATION OF PULMONARY VENOUS ANOMALIES

I. Atresia of common pulmonary vein (early) while pulmonary-systemic venous connections are still present
   A. Partial anomalous pulmonary venous connection
   B. Total anomalous pulmonary venous connection
      1. Without pulmonary venous obstruction
      2. With pulmonary venous obstruction
II. Atresia of the common pulmonary vein (late) after pulmonary-systemic venous connections are obliterated
   A. Atresia of the common pulmonary vein
III. Stenosis of the common pulmonary vein
   A. Cor triatriatum
IV. Abnormal absorption of the common pulmonary vein into the left atrium
   A. Stenosis of individual pulmonary veins
   B. Abnormal number of pulmonary veins

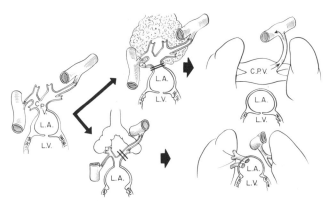

Fig. 29.2 Embryologic basis of anomalous pulmonary venous connection. (*Left*) The common pulmonary vein has joined the left atrium, but primitive venous connections still exist. (*Upper right*) If atresia of the common pulmonary vein occurs at this time, pulmonary venous blood can no longer drain directly into the left atrium. One, or occasionally more than one, of the primitive venous connections may persist and enlarge. This is total anomalous pulmonary venous connection. (*Lower right*) Atresia of a major branch of the common pulmonary vein results in partial anomalous pulmonary venous connection.

and left pulmonary veins to left innominate vein. Subsequent experience suggests that anomalous connection of the veins of the right lung to the inferior vena cava should rank third.[74]

Gross examination of the heart reveals features common to all cases, regardless of the specific site of anomalous connection. These include mild to moderate dilatation and hypertrophy of the right atrium and right ventricle and dilatation of the pulmonary artery. The left-sided chambers are normal. Specific anatomic features vary, according to the site of connection.

Right Pulmonary Veins to Superior Vena Cava (SVC) (Fig. 29.4A). Connection of veins of the right upper and middle lobes to the SVC is the usual form of this anomaly. The upper lobe drains by one large or two or three smaller veins into the SVC below the azygos vein. A middle lobe vein enters the SVC at its junction with the right atrium. The vein from the right lower lobe usually enters the left atrium, but occasionally connects to the right atrium. The lower part of the SVC, between the azygos vein and right atrium, is dilated about twice normal.

In most cases, an atrial septal defect of the sinus venosus type is present. The defect has no superior margin and very

little posterior margin. Occasionally, a secundum ASD is present and, rarely, an ostium primum atrial septal defect exists or the atrial septum is intact.[11] Persistence of a left superior vena cava is an occasional accompanying defect.[44]

Right Pulmonary Veins to Right Atrium. The anomalous drainage is usually from the whole of the right lung, by way of two or three right pulmonary veins. These enter the right atrium just to the right of the atrial septum. An atrial septal defect is usually present, most often of the sinus venosus variety, sometimes of the secundum type, and rarely of the ostium primum type. Occasionally, only a valve competent foramen ovale is present or the atrial septum is intact.[74]

Right Pulmonary Veins to Inferior Vena Cava (IVC) (Fig. 29.4B). All the right pulmonary veins, or occasionally, the veins draining the right middle and right lower lobes, enter the IVC either just above or below the diaphragm. The normal pulmonary venous pattern of the right lung is altered in this condition, resulting in a "fir tree" configuration. The atrial septum is usually intact. This malformation, termed the "scimitar syndrome" by Neill and associates,[84] is frequently associated with other anomalies, including hypoplasia of the right lung and anomalies of the bronchial system; dextroposition of the heart; hypoplasia of the right pulmonary artery; and anomalous arterial connection to the right lung from the aorta. Additional cardiac anomalies are also common, i.e., VSD, PDA, coarctation of the aorta, and tetralogy of Fallot. Neill and associates consider this to be a more primitive anomaly than other instances of PAPVC and

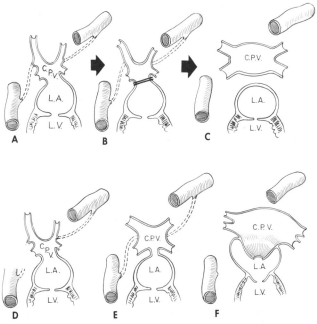

Fig. 29.3 Embryological basis of atresia of the common pulmonary vein (*A, B,* and *C*) and cor triatriatum (*D, E,* and *F*) (*A*) The common pulmonary vein (*C.P.V.*) has joined the left atrium (*L.A.*), and the primitive venous connections have disappeared. (*B*) Should atresia of the common pulmonary vein occur at this time, no significant alternative pathways for pulmonary venous drainage exist. (*C*) The result is atresia of the common pulmonary vein, wherein all pulmonary veins drain into a blind cul-de-sac. (*D*) The common pulmonary vein (*C.P.V.*) has joined the left atrium, and the primitive venous connections have disappeared (*E*) If stenosis occurs, pulmonary venous blood must drain through the narrow channel into left atrium. (*F*) The C.P.V. becomes markedly dilated and forms the accessory or third atrium. Anatomic variants of cor triatriatum may be explained by partial early stenosis of C.P.V.

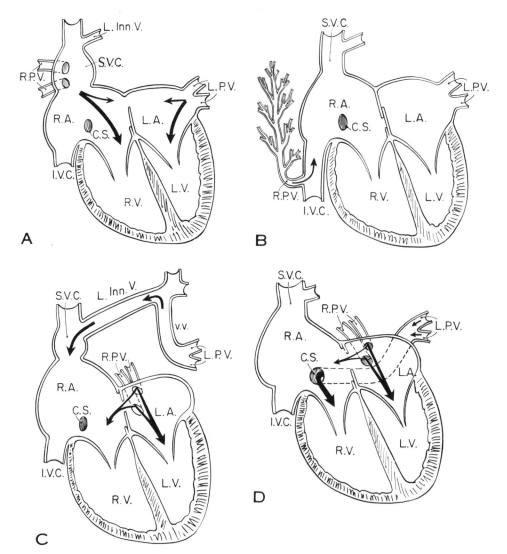

Fig. 29.4   Common forms of partial anomalous pulmonary venous connection (PAPVC). (*A*) Anomalous connection of the right pulmonary veins (*R.P.V.*) to superior vena cava (*S.V.C.*). A high or sinus venosus defect is usual in this anomaly. (*B*) Anomalous connections of the right pulmonary veins to the inferior vena cava (*I.V.C*). The right lung commonly drains by one pulmonary vein without its usual anatomic divisions. Parenchymal abnormalities of the right lung are common, and the atrial septum is usually intact. (*C*) Anomalous connection of the left pulmonary veins (*L.P.V.*) to the left innominate vein (*L. Inn. V.*) by way of a vertical vein (*v.v.*). An additional left to right shunt may occur through the atrial septal defect. (*D*) Anomalous connection of the left pulmonary veins to coronary sinus (*C.S.*). *R.A.*, right atrium; *L.A.*, left atrium; *R.V.*, right ventricle; *L.V.*, left ventricle.

suggest it represents an anomaly of development of the right lung.[84]

Left Pulmonary Veins to Left Innominate Vein (LIV) (Fig. 29.4C). The LIV is the usual site of anomalous connection of the left pulmonary veins.[11] The veins from the left upper lobe or from the whole left lung, connect to the LIV via a derivative of the left cardinal system. This connecting vein has been called a persistent left superior vena cava, but since it makes no direct connection to the heart, it cannot be so identified. A preferable term is anomalous vertical vein. An ASD of the secundum type is usual.[25] Rarely the septum is intact.[50]

Other Sites of PAPVC. Uncommon sites of PAPVC of the left pulmonary veins are coronary sinus (Fig. 29.4D), inferior vena cava, right superior vena cava, right atrium, and left subclavian vein. Unusual sites of drainage of the right pulmonary veins are azygos vein and coronary sinus.

In rare cases, veins of both lungs connect anomalously, while a small segment of the pulmonary venous system

connects normally to the left atrium. Edwards[25] has termed this situation subtotal anomalous pulmonary venous connection. Functionally, these patients closely resemble patients with total anomalous pulmonary venous connection.

Physiology. The fundamental physiologic disturbance of PAPVC is similar to that in atrial septal defect, i.e., increased pulmonary blood flow as a consequence of recirculation of oxygenated blood through the lungs. The factors determining the hemodynamic state include: the number of anomalously connected veins; the site of the anomalous connections; the presence or absence of atrial septal defect; and the size and location of the atrial septal defect.

PAPVC with Intact Atrial Septum. When the atrial septum is intact the factors determining the proportion of blood which drains through the anomalously connected veins are the number of veins anomalously connected, the relative resistances of the vascular beds normally and anomalously connected, and the compliance of the respective atria into which the normally and anomalously connected veins empty.

When a single pulmonary vein is anomalously connected, the anomalously draining blood flow is about 20% of total pulmonary blood flow.[108] It is of such slight hemodynamic significance that the lesion is rarely recognized clinically. When all save one of the pulmonary veins drain anomalously, the anomalously draining blood approximates 80% of the pulmonary blood flow. The physiology and clinical presentation of these patients are more comparable to the patient with total anomalous pulmonary venous connection.

When the veins of one lung drain anomalously, the factors of relative pulmonary resistance and relative atrial compliance modify the relative blood flows. In patients with partial anomalous pulmonary venous connection of the right pulmonary veins to the IVC with intact atrial septum (scimitar syndrome), calculated pulmonary blood flow to the anomalous connected vein is 24 to 32% of the pulmonary blood flow.[31] This low flow is related to abnormalities of parenchyma of the right lung and the frequently associated anomalies of arterial supply that are seen in the scimitar syndrome.[31] These result in an increase in pulmonary vascular resistance of the anomalously connected lung. On the other hand, when anomalous connection of one lung is the sole abnormality, the anomalously draining blood flow approximates 66% of the pulmonary blood flow.[74] This is due to the greater compliance of the right atrium to which the anomalous veins drain and the lesser compliance of the left atrium, the chamber receiving the normally draining blood. Thus right atrial pressure is lower than left atrial pressure. Since pulmonary artery pressures are equal the pressure gradient across the anomalously connected lung is greater than across the normally connected lung. The pulmonary vascular resistance in each lung is equal (except in scimitar syndrome); thus, blood flow is greater than the anomalously connected lung.[2]

Right to left shunting is prevented by the intact atrial septum. Pulmonary hypertension has not been reported in PAPVC with intact atrial septum, in the absence of complicating defects.

Since the intact atrial septum excludes blood from the anomalously connected lung from the systemic circulation, disease or surgical resection of the normally connected pulmonary parenchyma may be fatal.

PAPVC with Atrial Septal Defect. When the atrial septal defect is small, the hemodynamic state closely resembles that of PAPVC with intact septum. On the other hand, a large ASD significantly influences the hemodynamic picture. It is pertinent to review briefly the physiology of uncomplicated ASD, in particular the preferential shunting that occurs in this anomaly.

Utilizing indicator-dye dilution techniques, Swan and associates[105, 106] evaluated the relative contribution of each lung to the left to right shunt in patients with atrial septal defect. The average ratio of pulmonary blood flow to systemic blood flow was 3.5:1. The proportion of blood from the right lung shunted left to right averaged 84%, while the proportion of blood from the left lung that was shunted averaged 54%. Thus, blood from both lungs drained anomalously, but the right lung contributed more than the left lung to the left to right shunt (Fig. 29.5A). This preferential shunting from the right lung in ASD has been shown experimentally to result from the proximity of the right pulmonary venous orifices to the atrial septal defect.[101]

When PAPVC and ASD coexist, the hemodynamic picture may be identical to that of uncomplicated ASD. The left to right shunt may be large (PBF:SBF = 3:1, where PBF is the pulmonary blood flow, SBF the systemic blood flow). This shunt is the result of anomalous drainage of most of the blood from the anomalously connected lung, and of anomalous drainage of half or more of the blood from the normally connected lung via the ASD (Fig. 29.5B).[105, 106]

A small right to left shunt from the superior vena cava (both systemic venous blood and anomalously draining pulmonary venous blood) is usual in the presence of a high sinus venosus atrial septal defect. Likewise, a small right to left shunt from the IVC is commonly seen in a secundum ASD. Pulmonary hypertension has been reported in older patients with uncomplicated PAPVC.[50] While elevated pulmonary artery pressure is thought to be rare, its prevalence is not known.

Manifestations. *Clinical Features.* The anomalous con-

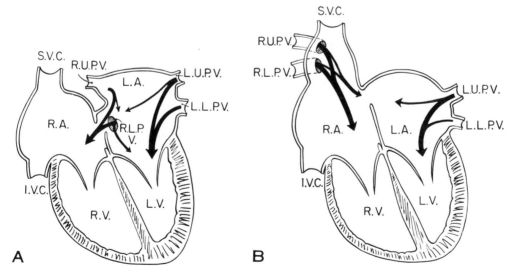

Fig. 29.5 Anomalous pulmonary venous drainage. (*A*) In atrial septal defect. The right pulmonary vein orifices are closer than the left to the atrial septal defect, and thus more of right pulmonary vein blood drains anomalously to right atrium. (*B*) In PAPVC. The major portion of blood from the right pulmonary veins drains anomalously while a small amount shunts right to left, and thus drains normally to the left atrium. A small portion of systemic venous blood from S.V.C. also reaches left atrium. The majority of blood from the normally connected left pulmonary veins reaches left ventricle, but some shunts left to right. *R.U.P.V.* and *L.U.P.V.*, right and left upper pulmonary vein; *R.L.P.V.* and *L.L.P.V.*, right and left lower pulmonary vein; other abbreviations as in Figure 29.4.

nection of one pulmonary vein is not apparent clinically. If all save one of the veins connect anomalously (subtotal TAPVC) the clinical features mimic those of TAPVC. The following features occur when the veins of one lung connect anomalously. Symptoms are uncommon in childhood, but there may be some dyspnea on exertion.[74]

Cyanosis is unusual during childhood, even though a small right to left shunt may exist. The frequency of patients presenting with cyanosis increases during the third and fourth decades, owing to changes in the pulmonary vascular bed, pulmonary hypertension, and increasing right to left shunt.[50]

Respiratory infections are commonly seen in patients with anomalous drainage of the right pulmonary veins to the inferior vena cava, as a consequence of the associated pulmonary parenchymal abnormalities. These same patients often show a small right hemithorax and evidence of dextroposition of the heart.

In the presence of an associated ASD, the physical findings are identical to those noted in uncomplicated ASD.

When the atrial septum is intact, splitting of the second sound is not marked, and there is normal variation of splitting on respiration. A pulmonary outflow murmur is usually present, and a diastolic tricuspid flow murmur may also be present.[74]

Electrocardiographic Features. The electrocardiographic findings are comparable to those seen in uncomplicated ASD.[61] The rR′ pattern and the rSR′ pattern are most commonly seen; the electrocardiogram is occasionally normal. Peaked P waves and right ventricular hypertrophy of the systolic overload pattern occur in the older patients exhibiting pulmonary hypertension. A frontal P-wave axis of 15° or less (inverted P wave in lead III) was noted in 8 of 10 patients with sinus venosus type atrial septal defect by Hancock.[44] The electrocardiogram is often normal in the patient with intact atrial septum.

Echocardiographic Features. The findings in PAPVC are dependent on the magnitude of the pulmonary blood flow (left to right shunt). When one pulmonary vein connects anomalously, the left to right shunt is small and the echocardiogram is normal.[108] When the veins of one lung connect anomalously the left to right shunt is equivalent to that of an uncomplicated large ASD and the echocardiogram is similar to that of an ASD. The right ventricular dimension index is increased, and the ventricular septum moves paradoxically.[108]

Cross-sectional (2D) echocardiography can identify the entry site of one or more pulmonary veins in the majority of infants and children with increased pulmonary blood flow. In some patients this procedure may allow a definitive diagnosis.[97]

Radiologic Features. The routine roentgenogram reflects the increased pulmonary blood flow and right ventricular dilatation. In addition, there may be distinctive roentgenographic features dependent on the site of anomalous connection.

The patient with anomalous connection of the right pulmonary veins to the inferior vena cava has a crescent-like shadow in the right lower lung field. This characteristic shadow prompted Neill and associates[84] to coin the term "scimitar syndrome" for this group of patients. Hypoplasia of the right chest, dextrocardia, and pulmonary parenchymal abnormalities may also be seen on the roentgenogram when drainage is into the IVC.

When the SVC is the site of the anomalous connection, dilatation of the lower portion of the SVC is often recognized just above the right atrial contour, or as a double density just inside the upper right atrial border. When the anomalous connection is to the azygos vein, this structure is enlarged and can be recognized on the plain roentgenogram as a rounded bulge in the right superior mediastinum at the right cardiac border.

When the left innominate vein is the site of connection of the left pulmonary veins, the chest roentgenograms reveal a prominent supracardiac shadow composed of the vertical vein on the left, the innominate vein above, and the superior vena cava at the right. These structures are the same ones that account for the characteristic "snowman" appearance when there is total anomalous pulmoanry venous connection to the innominate vein, but the enlargement is not as prominent.

Cardiac Catheterization. The routine use of extracorporeal circulation in the correction of secundum ASD and partial anomalous pulmonary venous connection has greatly diminished the need for invasive study. The authors' practice is to send to operation, without cardiac catheterization, those patients who have the typical clinical features of atrial septal defect. Thus, the majority of patients with PAPVC and ASD are unrecognized preoperatively and are identified and managed by the surgeon at the time of operation.

When cardiac catheterization is performed, frequent oximetry sampling usually allows identification of anomalous pulmonary venous connection to the coronary sinus, to the azygos vein, and to the superior vena cava. Oximetry is usually of little value when the anomalous connection is to the IVC, since blood flow through the right lung is diminished and because of the contribution of highly oxygenated blood by the renal veins.

Inability to pass the catheter from the right atrium to left atrium or a difference between the right atrial pressure and the pulmonary wedge pressure is suggestive of PAPVC with intact atrial septum.

Indicator Dilution Studies. These techniques have been considered at length by Swan and co-workers.[105, 106] Our experience and Hawker et al.[48] suggest that the reliability of indicator dilution studies is not sufficient to allow separation of PAPVC and atrial septal defect from an isolated ASD. On the other hand, PAPVC of veins from one lung and intact atrial septum can be separated from ASD by indicator dilution studies.

Contrast Echocardiography. Danilowicz and Kronzon[19] used this technique to differentiate between ASD with normal venous connection and ASD with anomalous connection of the RPV to the RA. The method was not useful if a right to left atrial shunt was present.

Angiocardiography. Selective angiography is of a limited value if the anomalously connected veins enter the right atrium or close to it. However, when the anomalous connections are to more peripheral vessels, angiography often clearly defines the site of anomalous connection; for example, PAPVC to the inferior vena cava, left innominate vein, and azygos vein.

Differential Diagnosis. The difficult diagnostic problem is separating PAPVC from uncomplicated secundum ASD. This differential is academic, since current surgical approach utilizes cardiopulmonary bypass, thus allowing the surgeon to identify precisely the anomalously connected veins if they coexist.

Ostium primum atrial septal defect and single atrium also result in left to right shunt at the atrial level; these may be differentiated on the basis of their characteristic electrocardiographic pattern, i.e., counterclockwise frontal vector loop and left axis deviation.

Total anomalous pulmonary venous connection presents

a strikingly different clinical picture with severe pulmonary congestion and cardiac failure, usually leading to death prior to 6 months of age. Cyanosis is an additional distinguishing feature.

Treatment. *Medical Management.* When failure occurs, either as a result of increased pulmonary blood flow or as a consequence of pulmonary vascular disease, the usual measures are indicated. When pulmonary parenchymal anomalies are associated, as in anomalous connection to the IVC, medical measures may be of temporary benefit. However, the only definitive therapy in partial anomalous venous connection is surgical correction.

Surgical Treatment. At the present time, extracorporeal circulation is used exclusively in the repair of partial anomalous pulmonary venous connection. The current surgical techniques are briefly summarized below.

PAPVC to right atrium. An atrial septal defect is almost always associated. The free margin of the ASD may be directly sutured to the wall of the right atrium to the right of the entrance of the anomalous veins or a patch may be utilized.

PAPVC to SVC. At the present time, the preferred procedure is utilization of a Teflon, Ivalon, or pericardial patch which is sewn along the wall of the superior vena cava so as to include the anomalously connected veins; suturing of the patch is then carried down into the right atrium, and it is sewn about the ASD. In this way, the anomalously connected pulmonary veins may drain through a tunnel, whose posterior wall is composed of the superior vena cava and whose anterior wall is composed of the patch, through the ASD into the left atrium. To prevent the occurrence of obstruction to the superior vena cava, a plastic or pericardial gusset is placed in the superior vena cava and upper right atrium. The right atrial appendage may be used in a plastic procedure to enlarge the SVC-right atrium RA junction.

The identical surgical approach has been utilized in the repair of PAPVC to the right lung to the azygos vein.

PAPVC to IVC. Repair has been accomplished in the presence of an atrial septal defect by transecting the anomalously connecting vein at its inferior vena caval junction and reanastomosing it to the right atrial wall opposite the ASD. Repair can then be continued as in partial anomalous pulmonary venous connection to the right atrium. When, as is usually the case, the atrial septum is intact, the anomalously connected vein is transplanted to the right atrial wall. Then an atrial septal defect is created and made contiguous to the anomalously connected vein by patching. When an anomalous vein is occluded during its correction, fatal pulmonary edema may occur unless the pulmonary artery to the affected part is also temporarily occluded.

PAPVC to coronary sinus. When this anomaly is present, it may be repaired utilizing the technique described for repair of total anomalous pulmonary venous connection to the coronary sinus.

PAPVC left pulmonary veins to innominate vein. Kirklin[57] corrected this anomaly by anastomosing the common left pulmonary vein to the base of the amputated left atrial appendage. Others have also successfully utilized this technique.[54] It is essential to occlude the appropriate pulmonary artery at the time the pulmonary vein is occluded. The ASD, if present, must also be closed.

Prognosis. *Untreated.* There is a paucity of information upon which to base an accurate prognosis in this defect. Studies based on anatomic material[11, 51] indicate that patients with one pulmonary vein connected anomalously and with an intact septum have an excellent prognosis and do not present with problems.

It would be erroneous, however, to apply this excellent prognosis to patients who present with symptoms. The natural history in these patients appears comparable to that in uncomplicated ASD.

Postoperative. The impact of operative intervention of PAPVC depends in part on the state of the pulmonary vascular bed at the time of surgery. In patients with high pulmonary blood flow, symptoms are dramatically reduced, postoperative studies reflect a normal physiology, and a near normal longevity may be assumed. These favorable results cannot be anticipated in the patient who has developed pulmonary hypertension.

Total Anomalous Pulmonary Venous Connection

Total anomalous pulmonary venous connection defines the anomaly in which the pulmonary veins have no connection with the left atrium. Rather, the pulmonary veins connect directly to the right atrium or to one of the systemic veins.

The frequency of TAPVC is difficult to define. In Abbott's[1] series of one thousand cases of congenital heart disease, there were four instances of TAPVC. Other recorded figures are 2% of 800 autopsied cases of congenital cardiac disease[18] and 2% of the deaths from congenital cardiac disease in the 1st year of life.[79] There is a marked male preponderance in TAPVC to the portal vein (3:6:1),[67] whereas the sex prevalence in the other sites of connection seems to be equal.

Anatomy. All pulmonary veins from both lungs connect anomalously to the right atrium or to a systemic venous tributary. In about one-third of patients, TAPVC is associated with an additional major cardiac malformation, while in two-thirds it exists as an isolated anomaly. Numerous classifications of TAPVC have been advanced. Darling and associates[18] divided them as follows: type I, anomalous connection at the supracardiac level; type II, anomalous connection at the cardiac level; type III, anomalous connection at the infracardiac level; and type IV, anomalous connection at two or more of the above levels. Smith and coworkers[102] suggested a simplified classification: supradiaphragmatic (without pulmonary venous obstruction) and infradiaphragmatic (with pulmonary venous obstruction).

Burroughs and Edwards[13] suggested a classification with prognostic implication based on the length of the anomalous channel, i.e., long, intermediate, or short. However, the prognostic and physiologic implications suggested by these classifications are not universally true, and it seems best to utilize the embryologic and anatomic classification proposed by Neill.[83] This, modified by the substitution of "connection" for "drainage," follows: connection to the right atrium, connection to the right common cardinal system (superior vena cava, azygos vein), connection to the left common cardinal system (left innominate vein, coronary sinus), and connection to the umbilicovitelline system (portal vein, ductus venosus).

The frequency of the various sites of total anomalous pulmonary venous connection is seen in Table 29.2. More than one-third of the cases had the anomalous connection to the left innominate vein.

The presence of interatrial communication is necessary to sustain life, and therefore an ASD or patent foramen ovale is considered part of the complex. Also, the young age of the patients makes the presence of a probe patent ductus arteriosus usual, and this is not considered a complicating defect.

Gross examination of the heart reveals several features common to all cases, regardless of the site of the anomalous connection. These include dilatation and hypertrophy of the

TABLE 29.2   SITE OF CONNECTION IN 113 CASES OF UNCOMPLICATED TOTAL ANOMALOUS PULMONARY VENOUS CONNECTION [a]

I. Connection to right atrium	15%
II. Connection to right common cardinal system	
A. (Right) superior vena cava	11%
B. Azygos vein	0%
III. Connection to left common cardinal system	
A. Left innominate vein	36%
B. Coronary sinus	16%
IV. Connection to umbilicovitelline system	
A. Portal vein	6%
B. Ductus venosus	4%
C. Inferior vena cava	2%
D. Hepatic vein	1%
Multiple sites	7%
Unknown	2%

[a] Modified from Burroughs and Edwards.[13]

right ventricle and right atrium, and dilatation of the pulmonary artery.

The left ventricle is of normal size, and left ventricular volume measured in life is in the normal range. Left atrial size has been considered diminished by most observers. Recent in vivo measurements indicate the left atrial volume to be 53% of predicted normal.[73]

In addition to these common findings, specific anatomic features vary as to the site of the anomalous connection as follows:

Connection to the Right Atrium (Fig. 29.6C). The site of connection is usually located in the posteroinferior portion of the right atrium. A common pulmonary vein draining both lungs may connect to the right atrium; or two, three, or four pulmonary veins may drain separately into the right atrium. Stenosis in the anomalous connection is rarely seen. Associated cardiac anomalies are common.

Connection to the Right Common Cardinal System. Right Superior Vena Cava. The pulmonary veins from each lung join to form a confluence posterior to the left atrium. An anomalous trunk originating from the right side of this confluence ascends, passes anterior to the hilus of the right lung, and enters the posterior aspect of the right superior vena cava. In a rare case, the right-sided ascending pulmonary venous trunk connects to the azygos vein.

Connection to the Left Common Cardinal System. Left Innominate Vein (Fig. 29.6A). In this, the most common site of anomalous pulmonary venous connection, the pulmonary veins from both lungs form a confluence immediately posterior to the left atrium. A venous trunk originates from the left portion of the confluence, usually passes anterior to the left pulmonary artery and main stem bronchus, ascends into the superior mediastinum, passes anterior to the aortic arch, and joins the left innominate vein proximal to its origin from the left jugular and subclavian veins (Fig. 29.7A). The left innominate vein then joins the superior vena cava in normal fashion. Less commonly, the ascending trunk passes between the left pulmonary artery and left main stem bronchus; the latter structures produce an extrinsic obstruction to pulmonary venous flow (Fig. 29.7B). The venous channel connecting the pulmonary vein to the left innominate vein has been called a persistent left superior vena cava, as well as an anomalous vertical vein.

Coronary Sinus (Fig. 29.6B). The entire anomalous pathway is situated within the pericardium. The pulmonary veins join a common trunk which connects to the coronary sinus in the region of the atrioventricular groove. The coronary

sinus then follows its normal course to the right atrium, the orifice of the coronary sinus being normally placed between the orifices of the inferior vena cava and tricuspid valve. The cardiac veins drain normally into the coronary sinus, and the coronary sinus is covered with left atrial fibers. The coronary sinus shares a common wall with the left atrium throughout the greater portion of its length. Stenosis at the junction of common pulmonary vein with the coronary sinus or within the coronary sinus occurs rarely.[68]

Connection to the Umbilicovitelline System (Fig. 29.6D). The distal site of connection is situated below the diaphragm. The pulmonary veins from both lungs join to form a confluence immediately behind the left atrium. A common trunk originates from the midportion of this confluence, descends immediately anterior to the esophagus, and penetrates the diaphragm through the esophageal hiatus. Most commonly, the anomalous trunk then joins the portal vein at the confluence of the splenic and superior mesenteric veins (Fig. 29.6D). Less often, the anomalous trunk connects to the ductus venosus or to one of the hepatic veins, or to the inferior vena cava. When the anomalous connection is to the umbilicovitelline system, pulmonary venous obstruction is usually present.

Anatomic Sites of Obstruction to Pulmonary Venous Drainage. Presence of an obstructive lesion in the anomalous pulmonary venous channel profoundly influences the hemodynamic state and clinical features in a case of TAPVC. We list below some of the anatomic causes of obstruction.

Obstruction at the Interatrial Septum. Burchell[12] suggested that a small interatrial communication might result in inadequate blood flow to the left atrium, and thus obstruction to pulmonary venous drainage. Burroughs and Edwards[13] clearly related longevity in TAPVC to the size of the ASD. Those patients with large defects survived longer than the patients with restricted interatrial openings.

Obstruction in the Anomalous Venous Channel. Obstruction in the anomalous venous channel is related primarily to factors which produce narrowing of the channel. Intrinsic narrowing in the walls of the anomalous vessels frequently occurs.[99] Extrinsic pressure also results in narrowing of the venous structure. The latter is commonly seen when the anomalous vein traverses the diaphragm through the esophageal hiatus[67] and may also be produced by thoracic structures. For example, when the vertical vein in TAPVC to the innominate vein passes between the left main pulmonary artery and left main stem bronchus the latter structures may obstruct the former (Fig. 29.7B). Similarly, the anomalous pulmonary vein in TAPVC to the SVC may be obstructed by the right pulmonary artery and trachea (Fig. 29.7C). Since the ductus venosus normally undergoes constriction, anomalous connection to this structure results in pulmonary venous obstruction. Finally, when the anomalous connection is to the portal vein or one of its tributaries, the hepatic sinusoids are interposed in the pulmonary venous channel and result in increased resistance to pulmonary venous return.

Associated Cardiac Anomalies. In about one third of patients with total anomalous pulmonary venous connection, there is an associated major cardiac malformation. Among these are cor biloculare, single ventricle, truncus arteriosus, transposition of the great arteries, pulmonary atresia, coarctation of the aorta, and anomalies of the systemic veins. A particularly high frequency of TAPVC occurs in patients with congenital cardiac disease and asplenia.[52, 96] The hemodynamic state and clinical picture are usually dominated by the associated cardiac anomaly. These complex lesions will not be considered further.

Microscopic Anatomy. *Anomalous Trunks.* Sherman

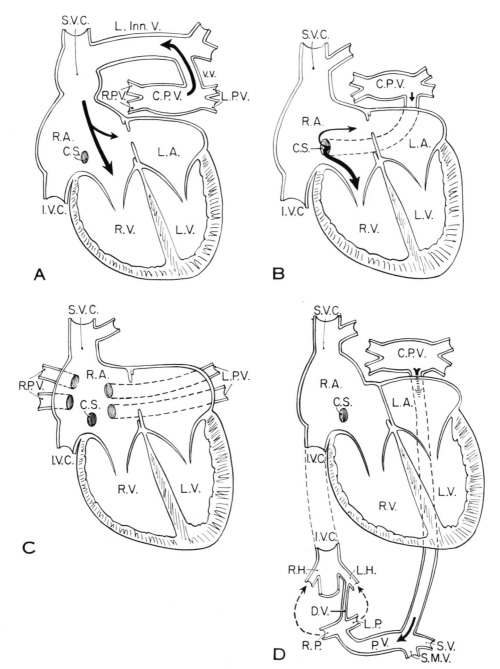

Fig. 29.6 Common forms of total anomalous pulmonary venous connection (TAPVC). (*A*) TAPVC to the left innominate vein (*L. Inn. V.*) by way of a vertical vein (*v.v.*). (*B*) TAPVC to coronary sinus (*C.S.*). The pulmonary veins join to form a confluence designated common pulmonary vein (*C.P.V.*), which connects to the coronary sinus. (*C*) TAPVC to right atrium. The right and left pulmonary veins (*L.P.V.* and *R.P.V.*) usually enter the right atrium separately. (*D*) TAPVC to the portal vein (*P.V.*). The pulmonary veins form a confluence, from which an anomalous channel arises. This connects to the portal vein, which communicates with the inferior vena cava (*I.V.C.*) by way of ductus venosus (*D.V.*) or the hepatic sinusoids. *S.V.*, splenic vein; *S.M.V.*, superior mesenteric vein; *R.P.* and *L.P.*, right and left portal veins; *R.H.* and *L.H.*, right and left hepatic veins; *S.V.C.*, superior vena cava; *R.A.* and *L.A.*, right and left atrium; *R.V.* and *L.V.*, right and left ventricle.

and Bauersfeld[99] examined the anomalous trunk in eight patients and reported each to be altered by scarring. Fibrosis was abundant in the adventitia, and in some cases there were focal areas of severe medial fibrosis. An intimal fibrous scar was noted in one.

Left Atrium. Sherman and Bauersfeld reported that the histologic picture of the left atrium in 13 patients was atrophy rather than aplasia. Although the muscle fibers were narrow with scanty cytoplasm, they had abundant nuclei. The authors found that the number of muscle fibers in the left atrium in TAPVC approximated controls.

Lungs. The microscopic findings in the lungs vary depending on whether pulmonary venous obstruction is present.

TAPVC without Obstruction. In the absence of pulmonary venous obstruction, the muscular arteries and arterioles generally have prominent medial hypertrophy. Intimal lesions in the arterioles are uncommon in the infant but usual in the older child and adult.

TAPVC with Obstruction. There is medial hypertrophy within the anomalous venous channels, the extrapulmonary veins, and the small veins of the lungs[68] (Fig. 29.8*A* and *B*).

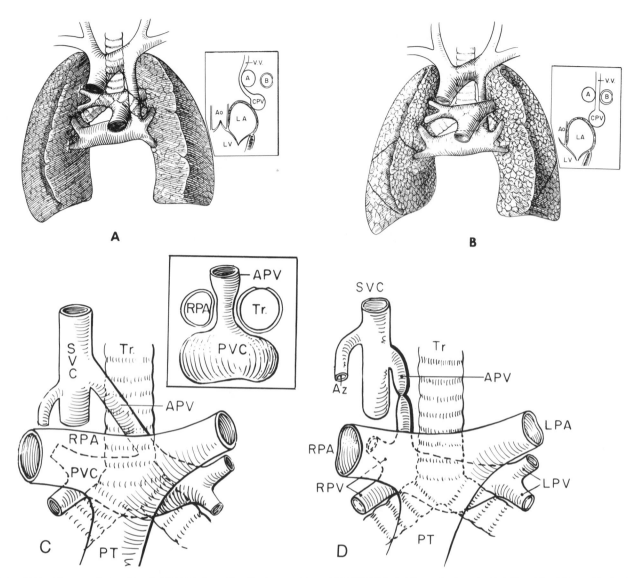

Fig. 29.7 Venous obstructions in TAPVC above the diaphragm. (*A* and *B*) TAPVC to left innominate vein. Relationship of the vertical vein to thoracic structures (*A*). More commonly the vertical vein (*V.V.*) ascends from the confluence of the four pulmonary veins (*CPV*) and passes *anterior* to the left pulmonary artery (*A*) to join the left innominate vein. (*B*) Less often, the vertical vein ascends and passes *behind* the left pulmonary artery to join the left innominate vein. The vertical vein is thus confined between the left pulmonary artery and the left main stem bronchus (*B*); the extrinsic pressure of these two structures results in pulmonary venous obstruction. Intrinsic narrowing of the vertical vein also occurs. (*C* and *D*) TAPVC to the right superior vena cava. (*C*) The anomalous venous trunk (*APV*) passes between the right pulmonary artery (*RPA*) and the trachea (*Tr*) and is compressed. (*D*) Intrinsic narrowing of the anomalous venous trunk. This produced high grade pulmonary venous obstruction in a 2-day-old child. See Figure 29.10*B* for the selective pulmonary venous angiogram in this patient. (*A* and *B*, reproduced with permission from L. P. Elliot and J. E. Edwards: Circulation 25:913, 1962, by permission of the American Heart Association, Inc.)

Pulmonary edema and extravasation of red cells into the alveolar spaces is pronounced (Fig. 29.8). There is prominent dilatation of the subpleural and interlobular lymphatics (Fig. 29.8*C*). Medial hypertrophy of the pulmonary arterioles and pulmonary arteries is pronounced (Fig. 29.8*D*). Intimal proliferation within the arterioles is common, and necrotizing arteritis is rarely seen.

Physiology. All venous blood, pulmonary as well as systemic, returns to the right atrium. [107] The physiologic features depend on the distribution of this mixed venous blood between the pulmonary and systemic circuits. The state of the interatrial septum is of primary importance in this distribution. When the interatrial communication is small, the amount of blood reaching the left atrium is limited, and systemic output is reduced. Elevation of right atrial pressure

is an attempt at compensation for this low output state. Since pulmonary and systemic veins all connect to the right atrium, increased right atrial pressure results in pressure elevation in both venous circuits.

On the other hand, the presence of a widely patent foramen ovale or ASD allows free communication between the two atria. In this circumstance, the distribution of mixed venous blood depends on the relative compliance of the atria and ventricles and on the relative resistances imposed by the pulmonary and systemic arterial circuits. The major variable is the state of the pulmonary vascular bed, which initially depends on the presence or absence of pulmonary venous obstruction.

TAPVC without Pulmonary Venous Obstruction. At birth, the distribution of blood between the pulmonary and

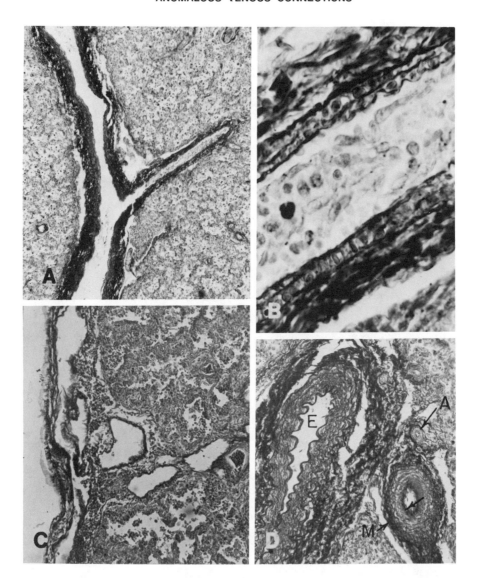

Fig. 29.8 Photographs of the lung in pulmonary venous obstruction. (*A*) A venous channel receives a tributary in a 5-week-old infant with total anomalous pulmonary venous connection to portal vein. Elastic tissue stain, ×150. (*B*) Magnification of the tributary shown in *A*. The prominence of the muscle in the media resembles that seen in arteries. Characteristic interdigitating of the elastic fibers identifies the structure as venous. Elastic tissue stain, ×380. (*C*) Dilatation of subpleural and interlobular lymphatic channels in an infant with atresia of the common pulmonary vein. Hematoxylin and eosin stain, ×25. (*D*) Medial hypertrophy of an elastic artery (*E*), a muscular artery (*M*) and an arteriole (*A*) in a 4½-month-old child with TAPVC to portal vein. Elastic tissue stain, ×125. (*A*, *B*, and *D*, reproduced with permission from R. V. Lucas, Jr., *et al.*[67] *C*, reproduced with permission from R. V. Lucas *et al.*[68]

systemic circuits is approximately equal, since resistance in these two vascular beds is equal. In the first few days of life, maturation of the pulmonary vascular bed produces a decrease in pulmonary vascular resistance, and a larger and larger proportion of the mixed venous blood traverses the pulmonary circuit. Pulmonary blood flow is commonly three to five times systemic blood flow. Systemic blood flow is usually normal. Since the mixed venous pool receives three to five parts of fully saturated blood for each part of desaturated systemic venous blood, oxygen saturation in the right atrium may be 90% or higher.[40] Adequate mixing in the right atrium is the rule; thus, oxygen saturations in right ventricle, pulmonary artery, left atrium, left ventricle, and aorta are equal to those in the right atrium.

Dilatation and hypertrophy of the right ventricle and dilatation of the pulmonary artery occur. Right heart failure is commonly seen.

Pulmonary artery pressure in infants ranges from slightly elevated to systemic. In the few who survive to older childhood or early adulthood, the pulmonary artery pressure is only slightly elevated. As time goes on, medial hypertrophy and intimal proliferation occur in the pulmonary arterioles; these result in more severe pulmonary hypertension in the third and fourth decades.

TAPVC with Pulmonary Venous Obstruction. Elevated pressure in the pulmonary venous channels is freely transmitted to the pulmonary capillary bed. Pulmonary edema results when the osmotic pressure of the blood is exceeded by the hydrostatic pressure in the capillaries. Mechanisms which tend to prevent pulmonary edema include increased pulmonary lymphatic flow, alternative pulmonary venous bypass channels, such as pulmonary venous-bronchial venous anastomoses, altered permeability of the pulmonary capillary wall, and reflex pulmonary arteriolar constriction.[68]

The latter results in a decrease in pulmonary blood flow, pulmonary artery hypertension, right ventricular hypertension and hypertrophy, and, ultimately, right heart failure.

While saturations in right atrium, left atrium, pulmonary artery, and aorta are still approximately equal, the decrease in pulmonary blood flow results in a smaller proportion of fully saturated blood entering the mixed venous sample and significant desaturation in these sites.

Manifestations. The signs and symptoms in TAPVC are variable, depending on the underlying hemodynamics. When the interatrial communication is inadequate, symptoms occur at birth or shortly thereafter. The hemodynamic consequences of inadequate interatrial communication include pulmonary venous obstruction. The presence of intrinsic or extrinsic narrowing in the connecting vein also produces pulmonary venous obstruction. Thus, the clinical manifestations may be conveniently divided according to whether pulmonary venous obstruction is absent or present.

TAPVC without Pulmonary Venous Obstruction. Clinical Features. The patients are usually asymptomatic at birth. However, in the latter part of the 1st month, tachypnea and feeding difficulties occur. From that point on, the infants do not thrive, are subject to repeated respiratory infections, and usually have cardiac failure by 6 months of age. Cyanosis may be so mild as to be clinically inapparent, except in the presence of cardiac failure and in the patient who survives long enough to acquire secondary pulmonary vascular changes.[56] Seventy-five to eighty-five percent of these infants are dead by 1 year of age, the majority in the first 3 months of life.[13, 56]

The infants are scrawny and irritable, and may exhibit slight duskiness on crying and exertion. Dyspnea, tachypnea, and tachycardia are almost always present. A right ventricular heave is usual.

A characteristic feature is the presence of multiple cardiac sounds. The first sound is loud and distinct and followed by a systolic ejection click. The second sound is widely split and does not vary with respiration. The pulmonary component of the second sound is accentuated. A third heart sound, maximal at the apex, is almost always present. A fourth heart sound is frequently heard in older patients.

A cardiac murmur is occasionally absent.[56] A thrill is rarely felt. Characteristically, a grade 2/6 soft, blowing, systolic murmur is heard in the pulmonic area. This murmur is often well heard over the xiphoid and at the lower left sternal border. Turbulence in the pulmonary outflow tract and tricuspid valve insufficiency, or both, account for the systolic murmurs. A diastolic tricuspid flow murmur at the lower left sternal border is present i about 50% of cases.[56]

When the anomalous connection is to the left innominate vein, a venous hum at the left or right base may be heard.[56] Unlike the innocent venous hum, this murmur is not louder during diastole and is not altered by change in position or pressure on the neck veins. Cardiac failure occurs in the majority of patients prior to 6 months of age. In cardiac failure, hepatomegaly is constantly present and peripheral edema is present in about one-half the cases. Clubbing is occasionally seen in the patient who survives infancy.

Electrocardiographic Features. A tall, peaked P wave in lead II or the right precordial leads characteristic of right atrial enlargement is a constant finding. Right axis deviation is usual. Right ventricular hypertrophy is invariably present, usually manifested by high voltage in the right precordial leads, occasionally as an incomplete right bundle branch block pattern.

Gessner and associates[35] reported vectorcardiograms in 10 patients with TAPVC. All were diagnostic of right ventricular hypertrophy.

Echocardiographic Features. TAPVC is one of the entities that produces the echocardiographic signs of right ventricular diastolic volume overload.[108] These are increased right ventricular dimension index and paradoxical ventricular septal movement. Decreased left atrial size has been reported but is not consistent enough to be of diagnostic usefulness.

The finding of an echo-free space posterior to the left atrium appears to be a highly reliable sign of the venous confluence (common pulmonary vein) almost always present in TAPVC (Fig. 29.9). Paquet and Gutgesell[87] reported this finding in all seven patients with TAPVC. Our experience confirms the reliability of the constant and easily reproducible echo-free space posterior to the left atrium in TAPVC. Rarely, there may be no venous confluence posterior to the left atrium in TAPVC, and the sign would be absent. In addition, since atresia of the common pulmonary vein has a venous confluence, an echo-free space posterior to the left atrium would be expected in this condition. From anatomic considerations, some forms of cor triatriatum might also have this feature.

Sahn and associates[97] have demonstrated that cross-sectional echocardiography is a reliable tool to diagnose TAPVC. In a prospective study they showed that 2D echocardiography correctly identified seven patients with TAPVC without a false negative. TAPVC was ruled out in 15 patients with persistence of the fetal circulation without a false postive.

Orsmond and associates[86] reported that five of six patients with TAPVC to coronary sinus had a mobile linear echo behind the aortic wall in the left atrial cavity that extended behind the mitral valve. This echo has two peaks per cardiac cycle. When combined with the echo-free space behind the left atrium the linear echo is a highly reliable diagnostic sign (Fig. 29.9B). Left superior vena cava connecting to the coronary sinus may simulate TAPVC to coronary sinus on echo (Fig. 29.15B).

Radiologic Features. Certain roentgenographic features are common to all cases. The lung fields reflect increased pulmonary blood flow. Right atrium and right ventricle are dilated and hypertrophied, and the pulmonary artery segment is prominent. The left-sided chambers are not enlarged.

In addition, the specific site of anomalous connection may result in characteristic roentgenographic signs. A figure-of-eight or snowman appearance of the cardiac shadow is seen in patients with TAPVC to the left innominate vein. The upper portion of the figure-of-eight is composed of the anomalous vertical vein on the left, the left innominate vein superiorly, and the superior vena cava at the right. This diagnostic sign is not usually present in the first few months of life, but is usually present in the older child and adult. When the anomalous connection is to the right superior vena cava, dilatation of this structure results in a prominence at the upper right cardiac border.

Cardiac Catheterization. The venous site of anomalous connection may be identified if highly saturated blood is obtained from the left innominate vein, right superior vena cava, or coronary sinus. Anomalous connection directly to the right atrium results in a step-up of oxygen saturation at right atrial level, as do other left to right shunts into the right atrium. In TAPVC, however, the oxygen saturation in right atrium usually ranges between 80 and 95%, and saturations in right atrium, right ventricle, pulmonary artery, left atrium, left ventricle, and systemic arteries are nearly identical. When TAPVC is to the left innominate vein or right superior vena cava, superior vena cava blood preferentially flows into the tricuspid orifice, and inferior vena cava blood preferentially shunts into the left atrium, resulting in a pulmonary artery oxygen saturation that may be

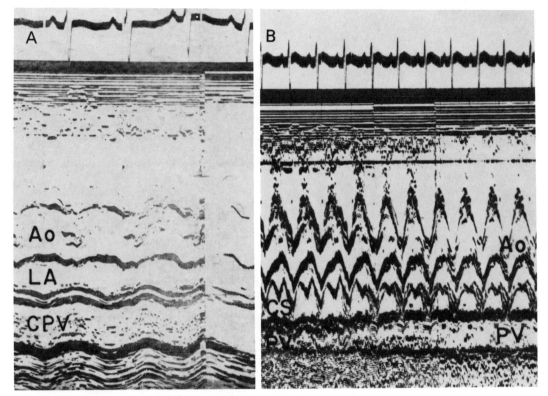

Fig. 29.9 (*A*) Echocardiogram in a 3-week-old girl with total anomalous pulmonary venous connection to innominate vein. The echo beam passes through aorta (*Ao*) and left atrium (*LA*). The echo-free space posterior to the left atrium is clearly seen and represents the pulmonary confluence or common pulmonary vein (*CPV*). (*B*) Echocardiogram in a 2-month-old boy with subtotal anomalous pulmonary venous connection to coronary sinus (the right upper pulmonary vein connected normally to LA). The echo-free space representing the pulmonary venous confluence (*PV*) is present posterior to the left atrium. Additionally, there is a distinct and persistent line that appears to lie within the left atrium. We believe this line represents the posterior wall of left atrium and anterior wall of the enlarged coronary sinus. Thus the echo beam passes from anterior to posterior through aorta, left atrium, coronary sinus (*CS*), and pulmonary venous confluence. At operation there was no membrane within left atrium and the coronary sinus bulged into LA. The contiguous walls of LA and CS were excised to allow a large opening between CS and LA. A postop echocardiogram revealed persistence of the most posterior venous confluence, but the line separating CS and LA was absent.

somewhat higher than that in the systemic artery.

Pressures in the right ventricle and pulmonary artery range from slightly elevated to equality with systemic pressure. Interpretation of atrial pressures, particularly in an attempt to determine the adequacy of the interatrial communication, is difficult. In our experience, the presence of equal pressures in the two atria is an unreliable sign of a nonobstructive interatrial communication. This phenomenon is most likely due to the fact that the compliances of the two ventricles are usually comparable, and thus their filling pressures are equal even in the face of a restrictive interatrial communication. A right atrial pressure 2 mm Hg or more in excess of left atrial pressure is more reliable in predicting a restrictive interatrial communication but too often occurs in the face of free communication between the atria. The only reliable way to assess the size of the interatrial communication is to measure it with a balloon catheter.

Selective pulmonary arteriography is usually diagnostic. Following injection and passage of opaque dye through the pulmonary fields, it collects in the pulmonary venous channels and clearly outlines the anomalous connection. In TAPVC to the left innominate vein (Fig. 29.10*A*), the vertical vein can be seen originating from the area of the common pulmonary vein and ascending to join the left innominate vein. The latter is outlined in its course to the superior vena cava. The opaque material then outlines the superior vena cava.

When the anomalous connection is to the coronary sinus,

the opaque material collects in the common pulmonary vein and enters the coronary sinus at the posterior portion of the heart.[78] In posteroanterior projection, the sinus appears as an egg-shaped mass at the medial, inferior portion of the right atrium. The anatomic features of the coronary sinus are more clearly defined in a lateral view (Fig. 29.10*B*).

When anomalous connection is directly to the right atrium, no extracardiac structures are visualized, and opaque dye promptly enters the right atrial cavity.

If the cardiac catheter enters the anomalous venous connection the oxygen saturation of the blood approximates 100%. Selective angiography is then usually diagnostic. However, since intrinsic or extrinsic obstructions may occur in any connecting vein, the potential of the cardiac catheter to produce high grade obstruction must be always in mind (Fig. 29.10*B*).

TAPVC with Pulmonary Venous Obstruction. Clinical Features. Pulmonary venous obstruction is usual when the venous connection is to the umbilicovitelline venous system but occasionally occurs when the connection is to other sites, such as the left innominate vein, the coronary sinus, the right superior vena cava, or the right atrium directly. Regardless of the site of pulmonary venous obstruction, the clinical profile is the same.

Cyanosis and tachypnea are present at birth or occur within the first few days of life. There is rather rapid progression to dyspnea, feeding difficulties, and cardiac failure. Age at death ranges from 2 days to 4.5 months.[67] When the

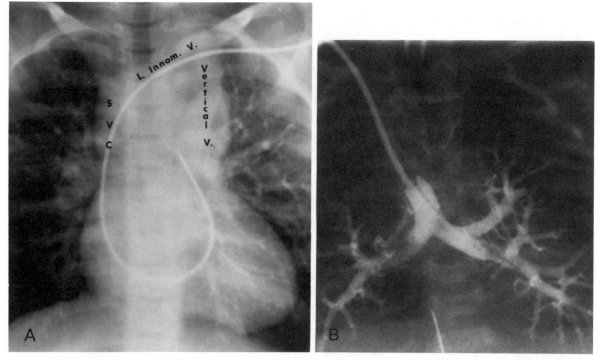

Fig. 29.10 (A) Late film in anteroposterior projection of a pulmonary arteriogram in a 10-year-old girl with TAPVC to innominate vein (*L. Innom. V.*). Contrast material has collected from the pulmonary veins and has emptied into the vertical vein (*Vertical V.*) along the left cardiac border. The left innominate vein and superior vena cava (*S.V.C.*) are also well outlined. (B) Selective pulmonary arteriogram in a 2-day-old male with TAPVC to the superior vena cava. In this late cine frame the small pulmonary veins, the major pulmonary venous branches, and the proximal portion of the anomalous venous trunk are well opacified. The cardiac catheter has traversed an intrinsic narrowing in the anomalous venous trunk, completely occluding the trunk.

anomalous connection is below the diaphragm, cyanosis and dyspnea may be accentuated by straining and swallowing, as a consequence of interference of pulmonary venous outflow by increased intraabdominal pressure or impingement of the esophagus on the common pulmonary vein as it exits through the esophageal hiatus.

In spite of the alarming symptoms, the cardiovascular findings may be minimal. The heart is not enlarged and has no significant right ventricular heave. The second sounds are usually split and the pulmonary component is accentuated. A cardiac murmur is often absent; when present it is usually a soft, blowing, systolic murmur in the pulmonic area. Moist rales are usual at the lung bases. Hepatomegaly is almost always present, and peripheral edema is often associated.

Electrocardiographic Features. Right ventricular hypertrophy is invariably present. Unlike TAPVC without venous obstruction, however, right atrial enlargement is not a usual feature.

Echocardiographic Features. The echo-free space posterior to left atrium is an expected finding. On the other hand, right ventricular diastolic overload is not present. Cross-sectional echocardiography often allows identification of the anomalous connection.

Radiologic Features. Harris and associates[46] have stressed the features of the chest roentgenogram in patients with TAPVC to the portal vein; these findings have been confirmed in pulmonary venous obstruction at other sites.[68] The cardiac size is normal or nearly so. The lung fields reveal abnormal pulmonary vascular markings, characterized by diffuse, stippled densities that form a reticular pattern which fans out from the hilar regions. The cardiac borders are often obscured. Kerley B lines have been described, and prominence of the superior pulmonary veins is usual.[68] The roent-

gen appearance is not diagnostic of TAPVC with obstruction, since it also is associated with other causes of pulmonary venous obstruction.

Cardiac Catheterization. Oximetry may be helpful if fully saturated blood is obtained from the inferior vena cava or the superior vena cava. Interpretation of oximetry must be cautious, however, since on the one hand, pulmonary blood flow is decreased and its volume may not be sufficient to allow high saturation when mixed with systemic venous blood; and on the other hand, streaming of renal venous blood may result in the appearance of highly oxygenated blood in the inferior vena cava.

Right ventricular presures are usually systemic or higher.[68] Pressures in right atrium are usually normal. Left atrial pressure is also normal, but contrasts strikingly to the elevated pulmonary artery wedge pressure.

Angiocardiography. When the pulmonary arteriogram demonstrates TAPVC to the portal venous system, pulmonary venous obstruction may be assumed (Fig. 29.11A). Sites of obstruction may be also outlined when the anomalous connection is to other venous channels. In view of the marked delay in passage of opaque material through the pulmonary vasculature, the angiogram must be programmed so as to allow films to be obtained up to 12 seconds after initial injection.

If the cardiac catheter enters the anomalous venous channel it may traverse the area of obstruction, thereby creating high grade or complete obstruction to venous return (Fig. 29.10B). If selective injection of contrast material into the anomalous venous channel is contemplaed in the patient with TAPVC with obstruction the injection should be done by hand and without delay.

Differential Diagnosis. *TAPVC without Pulmonary Venous Obstruction.* In the infant with this condition, the

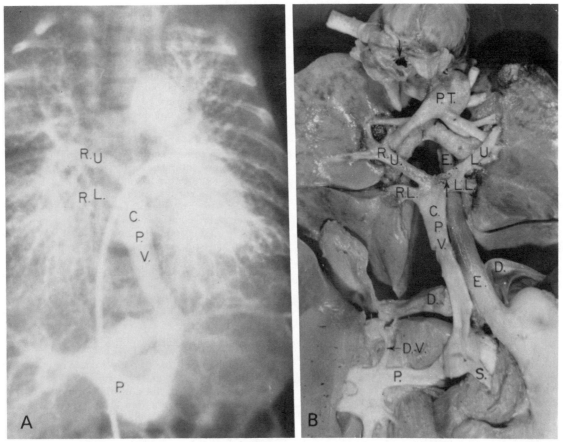

Fig. 29.11 Total anomalous pulmonary venous connection to portal vein in a 6-week-old boy. (*A*) Selective right ventriculogram 3 seconds after injection. Opaque material still outlines right ventricle and pulmonary trunk. The left pulmonary veins are obscured behind the heart, but the right pulmonary veins (*R.U.* and *R.L.*) are visualized. The pulmonary veins empty into an anomalous channel (*C.P.V.*) which descends below the diaphragm to join the portal vein (*P.*). Filling of hepatic veins has occurred. (*B*) Corresponding view of the thoracic and abdominal organs from in front. The heart has been raised and the liver rotated posteriorly. The four pulmonary veins (*R.U., R.L., LU.,* and *L.L.*) join the common pulmonary vein behind the heart. The latter descends in association with the esophagus (*E.*), penetrates the diaphragm (*D.*) through the esophageal hiatus and joins the portal vein (*P.*). The ductus venosus (*D.V.*) is atretic. *P.T.*, pulmonary trunk; *S.*, splenic vein. *Arrows* indicate the site of surgical anastomosis between common pulmonary vein and left atrium. (Reproduced with permission from R. V. Lucas, Jr., et al.[68])

differential diagnosis must include large VSD, PDA, truncus arteriosus, atrioventricular canal, and single ventricle without pulmonary stenosis. Unlike TAPVC, all these anomalies have roentgen and electrocardiograph evidences of left atrial and left ventricular hypertrophy. Multiple heart sounds are not usual, and the cardiac murmur is harsher and usually associated with a thrill. The counterclockwise frontal vector loop identifies atrioventricular canal, as does the murmur of mitral insufficiency. The severity of the illness in the infants suspected of having TAPVC warrants echocardiography and/or cardiac catheterization which will provide a definitive diagnosis.

In the older child or adult with TAPVC, the differential diagnosis must include ASD, common atrium, and partial anomalous pulmonary venous connection. Common atrium and ostium primum ASD may be differentiated on the basis of a counterclockwise frontal vector loop. In the older patient, at least mild cyanosis is usually present in TAPVC, and this feature is absent in the usual case of secundum atrial septal defect or PAPVC. Nonetheless, a clinical distinction may be difficult in the older patient and require special studies.

TAPVC with Pulmonary Venous Obstruction. Differential diagnosis in these infants includes first the other causes of pulmonary venous obstruction, and, in addition, hypo-

plastic left heart syndrome, tricuspid atresia, pulmonary atresia, coarctation of the aorta, transposition of the great arteries, respiratory distress syndrome, and persistence of the fetal circulation. Gross cardiomegaly is usual in atresia of any of the valves and in coarctation of the aorta, and thus allows these anomalies to be separated from TAPVC with pulmonary venous obstruction. Increased arterial vascular markings are characteristic of transposition of the great arteries and hypoplastic left heart syndrome, and diminished pulmonary vascularity is present in pulmonic or tricuspid atresia.

Differential Diagnosis of the Causes of Pulmonary Venous Obstruction.[68] Pulmonary venous obstruction may be the result of mitral insufficiency or left ventricular failure. These causes are readily identified, since they cause left ventricular hypertrophy as well as right ventricular hypertrophy. Absence of left ventricular hypertrophy indicates that the obstructing anomaly is mitral stenosis or one more proximally located. Further separation is then possible on the basis of left atrial size. The presence of left atrial hypertrophy indicates that the obstruction is close to the mitral valve, specifically, mitral valve stenosis and supravalvular stenosing ring of the left atrium. Left atrial pressures are elevated in these two anomalies.

When only right ventricular hypertrophy is present, differential diagnosis lies among stenosis of the individual pulmonary veins, cor triatriatum, atresia of the common pulmonary vein, and total anomalous pulmonary venous connection with obstruction. In all these, pulmonary arterial wedge pressure is elevated, while left atrial pressure is normal.

Selective angiography usually allows identification of the specific obstructing lesions. In addition to outlining the anomalous venous channels, angiography defines the presence or absence of an atrial right to left shunt and the duration of opacification of left atrium.

Echocardiography is particularly useful in identifying TAPVC in the acutely ill infant when the differential is among persistence of the fetal circulation, respiratory distress syndrome, and TAPVC with obstruction.

Treatment. Intensive treatment of cardiac failure is usually of only temporary benefit and does not prevent the majority of infants from dying prior to 6 months of age. Providing optimal treatment for patients with TAPVC continues to challenge surgical teams. The patient who survives past 12 months of age usually has a widely patent interatrial communication, no obstruction in the venous pathways, and pulmonary arteriolar resistance that restricts the pulmonary blood flow to an óptimal amount. These children may be operated on electively after 1 year of age with a mortality of about 10%.[115]

Unfortunately these patients represent less than 20% of patients with TAPVC. The majority die prior to 12 months and thus require surgery for survival.

Operation for correction of TAPVC in infants under 1 year of age was associated with a mortality of about 50% through the early 1970s.[7, 9, 88, 115] Reports in the last 5 years show a reduction in surgical mortality to 30% and lower.[17, 112] While this is encouraging, continued improvement in management is still sought.

Why do infants with TAPVC fare less well at operation than infants with other cardiac conditions? The small size of the left atrium has been offered as a cause. Surgeons have recognized this possibility and have created a large left atrial reservoir by making a large anastomosis between the common pulmonary vein and left atrium, and by appropriate reconstruction of the atrial septum. The specific technique for gaining intracardiac access does not appear critical to the operative mortality rate,[17] though most surgeons utilize deep hypothermia.

In our opinion, a major factor in survival has been the timing of operative intervention. In prior years a high operative mortality resulted in a fair amount of procrastination before operation was recommended. Now, infants with TAPVC are rapidly stabilized, a definitive diagnosis is established on an emergency basis, and the patient is operated on without delay.

Operative mortality is much higher when the anomalous venous channel is obstructed, for example, TAPVC to portal venous system.[7, 115] Since the intraoperative approach is no different, the higher mortality in these infants may be related to the younger age at operation, the severe pulmonary edema, the increased pulmonary vascular resistance, and the critically ill preoperative status.

In the unoperated patient, survival is longer when the interatrial communication is large. This observation has led to the use of balloon atrial septostomy at the time of diagnostic catheterization. Mullins et al.[81] prospectively evaluated the use of balloon septostomy in 20 patients with TAPVC. Septostomy was felt not advisable in eight (five were over one year, two had a large ASD, and one had TAPVC to the portal system). Of the 12 having balloon septostomy, nine improved and were followed medically.

One of these died suddenly. The others were adequately palliated for several months. The remaining three did not improve and had early surgery. In our opinion, balloon septostomy should be done at the time of cardiac catheterization in infants under 6 months of age, not with the goal of long-term palliation but to improve cardiovascular function so as to provide a better operative candidate. We then recommend operative correction within 48 hours.

The surgical techniques for the specific anomalies are as follows:

TAPVC to Right Atrium. The right atrium is opened and the atrial septum excised. A patch is then sewn so as to create a new interatrial septum which diverts pulmonary venous blood into the left atrium.

Modification of this technique is applicable to the correction of TAPVC to the coronary sinus. The common wall of the coronary sinus and left atrium is generously excised through a right atriotomy approach. The enlarged interatrial defect, consisting of coronary sinus orifice, original atrial septal defect, and the intervening excised tissue, is then closed with a patch. Some surgeons prefer to widely excise the common wall between left atrium and coronary sinus without enlarging the ASD. Then the ASD and coronary sinus orifice are closed by direct suturing. These repairs result in drainage of coronary sinus blood from the heart into the left atrium, but this minor hemodynamic abnormality is well tolerated.

TAPVC to Left Innominate Vein. The basis of this correction is the creation of a large side to side anastomosis between the left atrium and the common pulmonary vein. Subsequent to the creation of the anastomosis, the atrial septal defect is closed, and the site of anomalous connection is ligated. A patch is usually utilized in ASD closure so as to ensure that the postoperative left atrial volume is normal. With minor modifications, this technique is utilized in the correction of TAPVC to the right superior vena cava and TAPVC to the umbilicovitelline system.

An end to side anastomosis of common pulmonary vein to left atrium often kinks. Use of the stump of the amputated left atrial appendage as a site for anastomosis often results in an inadequate opening, since the diameter of the waist of the left atrial appendage is significantly smaller than the diameter of the common pulmonary vein.[56]

Prognosis. *Untreated.* The prognosis in TAPVC is influenced by the size of the interatrial communication and by the presence of obstructing lesions in the anomalous venous pathways. The state of the pulmonary vascular bed by determining the magnitude of the pulmonary blood flow during infancy, and through the development of obstructive pulmonary vascular changes in the fortunate patients who survive to older life, also plays a significant role.

In the survey by Keith et al.[56] of 58 patients with TAPVC of all types, 50% were dead at 3 months and 80% had succumbed by 1 year of age. The figures reported by Burroughs and Edwards[13] are comparable. Those patients with inadequate interatrial communication had an even poorer prognosis.[13, 56] When obstruction exists in the anomalous venous channel, the prognosis is grim. Death usually occurs within the first few weeks of life, and in a series of 33 cases of TAPVC with obstruction, the oldest survivor was 4.5 months.[67] Those patients who survive infancy often do so as a consequence of the protection provided by increased pulmonary vascular resistance. This is a mixed blessing and may jeopardize subsequent attempts at surgery. Far advanced intimal lesions have been described as early as 8 months of age.[62]

Postoperative. The long-term prognosis appears to depend mainly on the state of the pulmonary vascular bed at the time of operation and the adequacy of the venous-left atrial anastomosis. Both of these are influenced by growth and maturation, and sufficient time has not yet elapsed to allow accurate assessment of these factors.

ATRESIA OF THE COMMON PULMONARY VEIN AFTER THE PULMONARY SYSTEMIC CONNECTIONS ARE OBLITERATED

Atresia of the Common Pulmonary Vein

In this anomaly, no communication exists between the normally formed pulmonary veins and the left atrium. In addition, there is no anomalous connection between the confluence of the pulmonary veins, on the one hand, and the heart or any systemic vein, on the other. The physiologic consequence is severe obstruction to pulmonary blood flow.[69] The condition appears to be quite rare. In addition to the three original cases,[69] additional cases are known.[47]

Anatomy. The characteristic anatomic feature is the absence of a functional connection between the pulmonary veins and the left atrium or any other cardiac chamber or systemic vein (Fig. 29.12). The normally formed pulmonary veins converge immediately behind the left atrium to form a blind cul-de-sac which has no outlet for pulmonary venous blood. Minor anatomic variations in the pulmonary venous system exist in some cases as follows: an atretic strand of tissue may extend from one of the pulmonary veins to the right atrium or left atrium[68]; an atretic fibrous strand may connect the common pulmonary vein to a systemic vein.[47]

The lungs are firm and congested, and their pleural surfaces are remarkable in that the lobules are prominently outlined by edematous interlobular tissue and dilated lymphatic channels and appear as though chicken wire had been pressed against the surface (Fig. 29.12).

On microscopic examination the pulmonary veins are thick-walled, as a result of medial hypertrophy. The pul-

monary arteries also reflect medial hypertrophy (Fig. 29.8). The subpleural and interlobular lymphatics are markedly dilated and the interlobular connective tissue is edematous. Large dilated irregular venous channels are also present in the parenchyma and interlobular areas. The alveoli contain many erythrocytes and iron-containing macrophages.

Physiology. Severe obstruction to pulmonary venous flow is present in this anomaly. Since these patients live a few days to a few weeks, some means of flow of blood from the lungs must exist. One must assume that an exit, however restricted, is provided by the bronchopulmonary veins carrying blood from the lungs to the systemic venous system.[89] The features of severe pulmonary venous obstruction are comparable to those in TAPVC with venous obstruction.[47, 69]

Manifestations. *Clinical Features.* Dyspnea and cyanosis appear on the 1st day of life. Death occurs in the 1st month. A thrill is not present. A grade 1 to 2, soft, systolic murmur along the left sternal border is usual, although a murmur may be absent.

Electrocardiographic Features. The electrocardiogram may be normal or show evidence of right ventricular hypertrophy.

Radiologic Features. The usual picture of severe pulmonary venous obstruction is present. The pulmonary vascular markings have a diffuse reticular character. Cardiomegaly is minimal or absent.

Cardiac Catheterization. Cardiac catheterization reveals severe pulmonary hypertension and marked systemic desaturation.[47, 69] Selective injection of contrast material into the right ventricle results in persistence of the contrast material in the pulmonary vascular bed and failure of opacification of the left atrium.[47, 69]

Differential Diagnosis. This anomaly represents a severe form of pulmonary venous obstruction. The differential features are discussed in the section on total anomalous pulmonary venous connection.

Treatment. Some factors seem favorable for successful surgical intervention. The anatomic problems are similar to those in cases of TAPVC, and anastomosis of the confluence of the pulmonary veins and the left atrium would afford a direct route of pulmonary venous drainage. The confluence of pulmonary veins is ample in size and is located directly behind the left atrium. The left atrium and left ventricle seem to be of adequate size, and complex cardiac anomalies are not present. Hawker, *et al.*[47] made a premortem diagnosis in two infants 24 hours old and operated on one of them. The common pulmonary vein-LA anastomosis was accomplished and appeared adequate, but the infant did not survive.

Prognosis. Symptoms occur on the 1st day of life, and these patients follow a progressive downhill course to death within the 1st month of life.

STENOSIS OF THE COMMON PULMONARY VEIN

Cor Triatriatum

In cor triatriatum, the pulmonary veins enter an accessory chamber, which joins the left atrium through a narrow opening. Alternatively, the accessory chamber may communicate with the right atrium directly, or indirectly, by way of an anomalous channel. The classic form was clearly described by Church[16] in 1868.

Cor triatriatum is an unusual congenital anomaly, but it is probably not as rare as reports indicate. Jegier *et al.*[53] reported a frequency of 0.4% in 474 autopsied patients with congenital cardiac disease. In Niwayama's study,[85] the ratio of males to females was 1.5:1. The etiology is unknown.

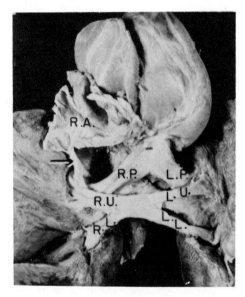

Fig. 29.12 Atresia of the common pulmonary vein in a 28-day-old boy. Viewed from in front; the heart has been reflected upward. Four pulmonary veins (*R.U., R.L., L.U., L.L.*) converge to form a pulmonary venous confluence which has no outlet. An atretic strand of tissue (*arrow*) extends from right upper pulmonary vein to the wall of right atrium (*R.A.*) and represents an atretic anomalous venous connection between these two structures. *R.P.*, right pulmonary artery; *L. P.*, left pulmonary artery. (Reproduced with permission from R. V. Lucas, Jr., *et al.*[69])

The variety of anatomic expressions of cor triatriatum defeats an attempt to define a unified embryogenesis for all of them. The theory that abnormal growth of the septum primum accounts for cor triatriatum is difficult to reconcile with the observations of most workers in this field.

Failure of incorporation of the common pulmonary vein into the left atrium is the most widely accepted theory of the embryogenesis of cor triatriatum.[27] However, some of the variants of cor triatriatum did not appear consistent with this theory.

Other reports amplify the embryogentic complexities of this group of cardiac defects.[36, 110]

Anatomy. The number of variants of cor triatriatum recently described demands a more inclusive classification than that proposed by Loeffler.[65] The following classification (Table 29.3) is based on the contributions of Loeffler,[65] Edwards,[27] Niwayama,[85] and Grondin and associates.[41]

Accessory Left Atrial Chamber Receives All Pulmonary Veins and Communicates with Left Atrium. No Other Connections—Classic Cor Triatriatum (Fig. 29.13A). In classic cor triatriatum, a membranous partition having the shape of a windsock separates the more proximal chamber which receives the pulmonary veins from the more distal left atrium which communicates with the mitral valve (Fig. 29.14). The windsock is directed toward the mitral valve. The orifice at its tip (or eccentrically placed) ranges from less than 3 mm in diameter to about 1 cm in diameter. There may be several small defects in the septum.[85] The anomalous septum contains cardiac muscle fibers and is occasionally calcified.

The more distal, true left atrium communicates with the left atrial appendage and in almost all cases has the fossa ovalis lying between it and the right atrium. In the majority of patients, there is no communication between either of the left atrial chambers and the right atrium.[85] Occasionally, a patent foramen ovale or an atrial septal defect allows the lower left atrial chamber to communicate with the right atrium. Right ventricular hypertrophy and dilatation is almost invariably found and right atrial hypertrophy, and dilatation is present in about one-quarter of cases.[85]

Other Anomalous Connections. In a few cases, the proximal accessory atrial chamber communicates with the more distal true left atrium via a stenotic opening in the interatrial membrane and, additionally, with the right atrium through a defect between the right atrium and the accessory atrial chamber (Fig. 29.13B).[41]

TABLE 29.3   ANATOMIC CLASSIFICATION OF COR TRIATRIATUM

I. Accessory atrial chamber receives all pulmonary veins and communicates with left atrium.
   A. No other connections—*classic cor triatriatum*
   B. Other anomalous connections
      1. To right atrium directly
      2. With total anomalous pulmonary venous connection
II. Accessory atrial chamber receives all pulmonary veins and does not communicate with left atrium
   A. Anomalous connection to right atrium directly
   B. With total anomalous pulmonary venous connection
III. Subtotal cor triatriatum
   A. Accessory atrial chamber receives part of pulmonary veins and connects to left atrium
      1. Remaining pulmonary veins connect normally
      2. Remaining pulmonary veins connect anomalously
   B. Accessory atrial chamber receives part of the pulmonary veins and connects to right atrium
      1. Remaining pulmonary veins connect normally

The accessory left atrial chamber may communicate indirectly with the right atrium via anomalous venous connections (Fig. 29.13C). Marin-Garcia and associates[72] reported findings on 20 patients with complete cor triatriatum communicating with left atrium. In 12 patients a classic diaphragm divided left atrium. In three patients an extrinsic constriction separated the accessory chamber from the left atrium (hourglass type), and in three there was obstructive tubular narrowing of the channel connecting the common venous confluence with the left atrium (tubular type). The hourglass and tubular types were all associated with complex cardiac lesions.

Accessory Atrial Chamber Receives All Pulmonary Veins and Does not Communicate with Left Atrium. In this anomaly, the septum separating the accessory atrial chamber from the left atrium is intact and prevents the direct flow of pulmonary venous blood to the left atrium. A defect exists between the accessory atrial chamber and the right atrium, and another defect or patent foramen ovale allows communication between the right atrium and the lower, true left atrium (Fig. 29.13D). Pulmonary venous blood thus enters the accessory left atrium, crosses the defect into the right atrium, and then traverses the second defect to reach the true left atrium. In three of the six cases reported by Lam,[60] the defect was successfully corrected by excising the anomalous septum and closing the atrial defects.

The other alternative, when the accessory atrial chamber receiving the pulmonary veins is completely divided from the true left atrium, is total anomalous pulmonary venous connection[67] (Fig. 29.13E). Pulmonary venous blood entering the accessory atrial chamber reaches the right atrium via the anomalous connecting vein and then enters the left atrium via a patent foramen ovale or atrial septal defect. This condition is usually classified as TAPVC.

Subtotal Cor Triatriatum. The accessory atrial chamber receives part of the pulmonary veins and connects to the left atrium. In this anomaly, the veins from one lung empty into a small accessory atrial chamber which communicates with the true left atrium via a stenotic opening. The remaining pulmonary veins may connect normally to the left atrium[41] (Fig. 29.13F), or they may connect anomalously to a systemic vein (Fig. 29.13G).

The accessory chamber receives part of the pulmonary veins and connects to the right atrium (Fig. 29.13H). In this circumstance the pulmonary veins from one lung empty into a small accessory atrial chamber which communicates via a small accessory atrial chamber which communicates via a stenotic opening with the right atrium. The remaining pulmonary veins connect normally to the left atrium.[41]

Microscopic Anatomy. When cor triatriatum obstructs pulmonary venus flow, the lungs reflect varying degrees of pulmonary edema and intraalveolar hemorrhage. There is medial hypertrophy of the pulmonary veins, and lymphatic channels are dilated. Pulmonary arterial lesions range from medial hypertrophy alone, to medial hypertrophy with intimal proliferation, to necrotizing arteriolitis.

Physiology. In those defects where the blood from the accessory atrial chamber either directly or indirectly drains to the right atrium, the hemodynamic features are comparable to those seen in TAPVC and will not be further considered. On the other hand, when there is no alternative pathway for pulmonary venous blood, the stenotic opening in the intraatrial membrane dividing the accessory atrium from the left atrium results in elevated pressure in the accessory atrial chamber, which is transmitted to the pulmonary veins. The features of pulmonary venous obstruction pertain.

In the patient with subtotal cor triatriatum, the obstruc-

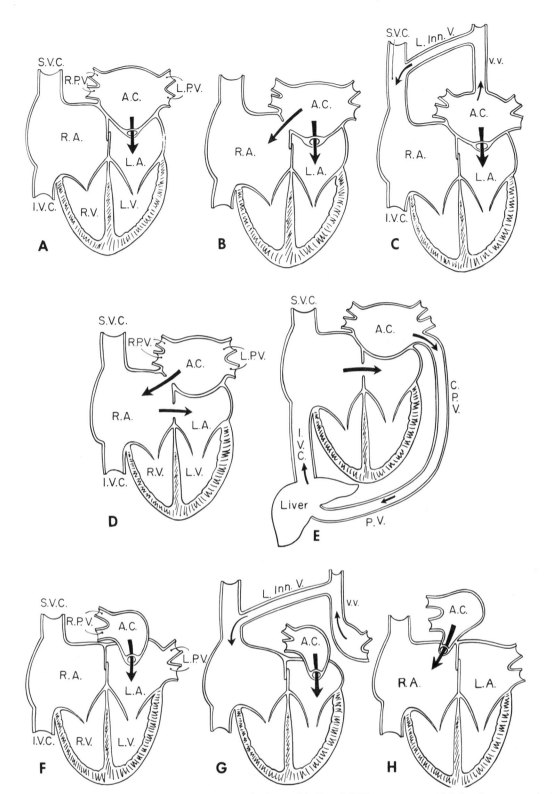

Fig. 29.13 Diagrammatic representation of variants of cor triatriatum. (*A, B,* and *C*) The accessory atrial chamber communicates with left atrium (*L.A.*). (*A*) Classic cor triatriatum. The accessory chamber (*A.C.*) receives all pulmonary veins (*R.P.V.* and *L.P.V.*). The only outlet for pulmonary venous blood is the orifice in the intraatrial membrane. (*B*) Cor triatriatum with anomalous connection between the accessory atrial chamber and the right atrium (*R.A.*). This communication decompresses the accessory atrial chamber and results in a left to right shunt at atrial level. (*C*) Cor triatriatum with anomalous pulmonary venous connection. In this example, the accessory atrial chamber is decompressed by way of a vertical vein (*v.v.*) to the left innominate vein (*L. Inn. V.*). (*D.* and *E*) The accessory atrial chamber does not communicate with left atrium. (*D*) The accessory atrial chamber (*A.C.*) communicates directly with right atrium (*R.A.*). Blood reaches the true left atrium (*L.A.*) by way of a patent foramen ovale or atrial septal defect. (*E*) The accessory atrial chamber connects with a common pulmonary vein (*C.P.V.*) which joins the portal vein (*P.V.*). Pulmonary venous blood traverses the hepatic vascular bed, *I.V.C.*, and ultimately reaches left atrium through an atrial septal defect or patent foramen ovale. (*F, G,* and *H*) Subtotal cor triatriatum. (*F*) The accessory atrial chamber (*A.C.*) receives the right pulmonary veins (*R.P.V.*) and communicates via a stenotic opening to left atrium (*L.A.*). The left pulmonary veins (*L.P.V.*) connect normally to left atrium. (*G*) Subtotal connection of right pulmonary veins to left atrium by means of a stenotic opening, and PAPVC of left pulmonary veins to left innominate vein (*L. Inn. V.*). (*H*) Subtotal connection of right pulmonary veins to right atrium via a stenotic opening and normal connection of left pulmonary veins.

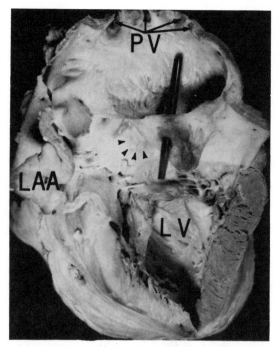

Fig. 29.14 Anatomy in classic cor triatriatum. The pulmonary veins (*PV*) empty into a large, thick-walled, accessory chamber. The only outlet for this chamber is a small eccentrically located orifice (probe) in the membrane separating the accessory atrial chamber from the true left atrium. The left atrial appendage (*LAA*) and the foramen ovale (*arrowheads*) communicate with the true left atrium. The mitral valve and left ventricle (*LV*) are normal in size and structure.

tive phenomenon affects only one lung. Reflex pulmonary arterial constriction in the affected lung will result in diminished flow through that lung. However, the remaining unobstructed lung is usually capable of accepting increased blood flow, and thus pulmonary arterial pressure is not elevated.

Manifestations. The following sections consider only the features of classic cor triatriatum.

Clinical Features. Most patients with classic cor triatriatum have the onset of symptoms within the first few years of life.[86] Nonetheless, a number of patients are asymptomatic until the second and third decades of life. Usually the patients present with a history of breathlessness, frequent respiratory infections, and pneumonia. More often than not they are considered to have primary pulmonary disease.

The signs of pulmonary hypertension, i.e., loud pulmonary component of the second sound, right ventricular heave, and pulmonary ejection systolic click are most characteristic. Right heart failure is usual. Pulmonary rales are not infrequent. The usual cardiac murmur is a soft, blowing, systolic murmur along the left sternal border. Less often, a diastolic murmur is detected at the mitral area or a continuous murmur is heard.

Echocardiographic Features. The multiple anatomic expressions of cor triatriatum account for the difficulty in defining pathognomic echo features. In classic cor triatriatum, the membrane may form a windsock which hangs down into the mitral valve orifice (Fig. 29.14). In this case the abnormal echo is usually seen near the anterior left atrial wall, closely approximating the mitral valve (Fig. 29.15*A*).[38, 64] This echo moves briskly with atrial events. We cannot differentiate this echo from the echoes recorded in TAPVC to coronary sinus (Fig. 29.9*B*) or persistent left superior vena cava (LSVC) connecting to coronary sinus (Fig. 29.15*B*). The atrial membrane may be taut in classic

cor triatriatum. This results in a middle left atrial echo with less motion. Since the membrane lies more parallel to the echo beam it may be less persistent and could be missed entirely. A similar echo has been reported in supravalvar stenosing ring of the left atrium.[64] It may also be mimicked by the thin intermittent middle left atrial echo sometimes seen in normal patients when the echo beam is aimed laterally and cephalad.

Cross-section (2D) echocardiography improves our ability to define the anomalous membrane and to differentiate cor triatriatum from the other anatomic conditions which may mimic it. Despite improved technology and expanded experience, the variety of form and position of the membranes, accessory chambers, and anomalous venous pathways in cor triatriatum should be sufficient to create a sense of humility when the echocardiographer aims the beam at the left atrium.

Electrocardiographic Features. The typical electrocardiographic findings are systolic overload of the right ventricle. Right atrial hypertrophy results in tall, peaked P waves in some of the cases. Broad, notched P waves are present in some cases, presumably as a consequence of the dilated accessory atrial chamber, but are absent in others.

Radiologic Features. The routine chest roentgenogram reflects pulmonary venous obstruction. Fine, diffuse, reticular pulmonary markings fan out from the pulmonary hilus to involve the lower lung fields. Kerley B lines may be present. Prominent venous engorgement of the upper pulmonary veins results in the staghorn sign. The roentgenogram also reveals enlargement of the main pulmonary artery, right ventricular hypertrophy, and signs of "left atrial" enlargement, including posterior deviation of the barium-filled esophagus and a double density at the right cardiac border. These latter features are due to the dilated accessory atrial chamber (Fig. 29.16*A* and *B*).

Cardiac Catheterization. Pulmonary hypertension is routinely found. Oximetry will rule out a left to right shunt. Thus, the cause of pulmonary hypertension is either primary pulmonary vascular disease or secondary to pulmonary venous obstruction. The pulmonary aterial wedge pressure is elevated, and left atrial pressure is normal.

Selective pulmonary arteriography usually demonstrates cor triatriatum. Pulmonary transit time is prolonged. As the pulmonary veins opacify, they drain into an accessory left atrial chamber (Fig. 29.16*C* and *D*). There is usually a significant delay between the opacification of this chamber and the opacification of the true left atrium and left ventricle. Moreover, in some cases, the intraatrial diaphragm can be identified as a linear or cone-shaped filling defect between the accessory atrial chamber and the true left atrium. The accessory atrial chamber remains opacified for a period of time and does not change size or contour with cardiac contractions as does a normal left atrium.[75]

Differential Diagnosis. The differential diagnosis differs somewhat in relation to the age of the patient. In the infant or young child, the differential lies within the group of congenital cardiac anomalies which produce pulmonary venous obstruction.

In the adult a somewhat different differential diagnosis pertains. It includes rheumatic mitral stenosis, left atrial tumor, and left atrial thrombus. In the adults with cor triatriatum reviewed by McGuire *et al.*[75] four of eight had a mitral diastolic murmur, but none had the typical presystolic crescendo rumble of mitral stenosis. Likewise, no case had an opening snap. The absence of broad and notched P waves was another feature distinguishing cor triatriatum from mitral stenosis. Atrial fibrillation, commonly seen in mitral stenoses of comparable severity, was observed in only one of eight patients with cor triatriatum.

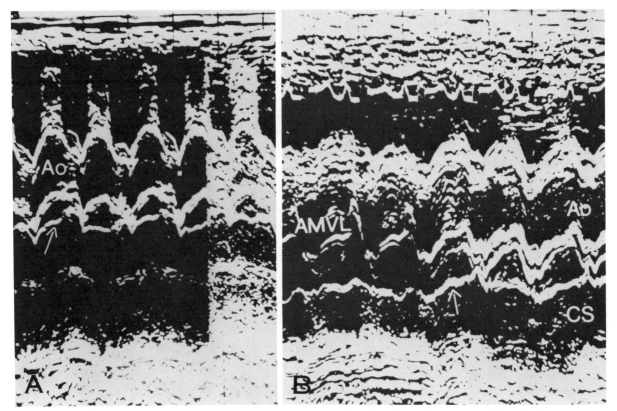

Fig. 29.15 (A) Echocardiogram in a 12-month-old boy with classic cor triatriatum. The echo beam is directed through aorta (Ao) and left atrium. There is a dense persistent echo (arrow) within the left atrial cavity just posterior to aorta. The fainter echo in midleft atrium is often seen in normal left atria. (B) Echocardiogram is a 3½-year-old boy with persistent left superior vena cava connecting to coronary sinus. The echo beam has been swept from high left ventricle through aortic root (Ao). A dense persistent echo (arrow) is present posterior to aorta. This echo extends a short distance into left ventricle. Our initial echo diagnosis of our triatriatum was incorrect. There was no membrane within the left atrium. We believe the line represents the contiguous wall of coronary sinus (CS) and left atrium. See Figure 29.20 for location and size of coronary sinus when it receives the left superior vena cava. See Figure 29.9 for echocardiogram of anomalous pulmonary venous connection to coronary sinus. AMVL, anterior mitral valve leaflet.

Treatment. In the patient with pulmonary edema or right heart failure, the usual medical management should be instituted. Once the patient has reached this stage, the disease usually pursues a relentless downhill course despite medical management. Surgical intervention should be planned as soon as possible.

Numerous patients have undergone successful surgical correction by open or closed methods.[4, 15, 60] The great variety of cor triatriatum configurations that may be encountered makes the utilization of cardiopulmonary bypass and correction under direct vision the operation of choice.

Prognosis. The prognosis of cor triatriatum is related to the size of the orifice in the obstructing membrane. In Niwayama's survey,[85] average survival was 3.3 months when the opening was less than 3 mm, and 16 years when the opening was greater than 3 mm. When pulmonary edema and right heart failure occur, survival is usually only a matter of months.

In those patients surviving operative correction, the prognosis seems excellent. The severe pulmonary arterial changes which result in pulmonary hypertension have been reversible in those patients studied postoperatively.[4, 37]

ABNORMAL ABSORPTION OF THE COMMON PULMONARY VEIN INTO LEFT ATRIUM

Stenosis of the Individual Pulmonary Veins

Two varieties of this unusual cardiac anomaly are recognized. In localized stenosis of the pulmonary veins, one or more of the pulmonary veins has a localized stenosis at its junction with the left atrium. The other variety is characterized by narrowing of the lumen of the pulmonary veins for a considerable distance in their intra- and extrapulmonary portions; this may be termed hypoplasia of the pulmonary veins.

Localized stenosis of the individual pulmonary veins may be an isolated phenomenon or it may be associated with a minor or major cardiac anomaly. Reye[93] first clearly described this anomaly in 1951. Shone and associates[100] have defined a characteristic angiographic feature which should allow a premortem diagnosis of this condition.

Hypoplasia of the individual pulmonary veins has been described as an isolated phenomenon in one case and is occasionally present in patients having pulmonary artery atresia or hypoplastic left heart syndrome. The clinical manifestations are those of the major cardiac anomaly when one is present. In the one case in which hypoplasia of the pulmonary veins was an isolated anomaly, the manifestations and hemodynamic features were identical to those patients with localized stenosis of the individual pulmonary veins. The following discussion will consider only localized stenosis of the individual pulmonary veins.

We have been able to find adequate descriptions of 11 cases of this anomaly, five with localized stenosis or localized atresia of all the pulmonary veins and six with localized stenosis or localized atresia of the pulmonary veins of only one lung.

The factors favoring a congenital etiology are summarized by Shone and associates.[100] The embryologic basis for ste-

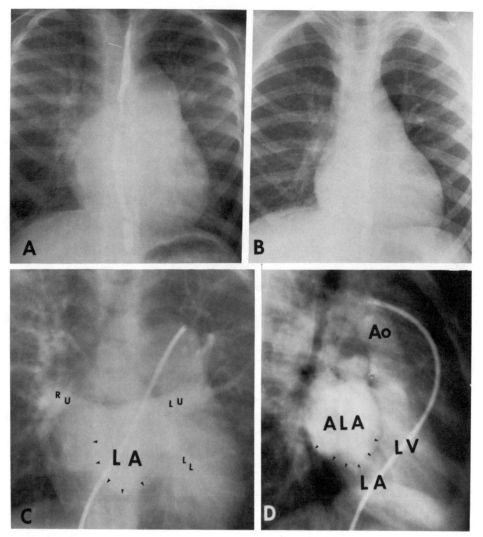

Fig. 29.16 Roentgenograms and pulmonary arteriogram in a 6-year-old girl with cor triatriatum. (*A*) Before operation. Prominent dilatation of the pulmonary artery, right ventricle, and right atrium is present. The following features of the lung fields indicate pulmonary venous obstruction: diffuse reticular markings fanning out from the hilar regions, prominent upper pulmonary veins in a staghorn appearance, and Kerley B lines. (*B*) Roentgenogram 1 year after corrective surgery. Normal cardiac size and lung fields. (*C*) Four seconds after injection, opacification of pulmonary veins has occurred (*RU, LU,* and *LL*). These drain into a large box-shaped chamber. The left atrium is seen as an overlying double density (*arrowheads*). (*D*) Lateral projection 6 seconds after injection. The accessory left atrium (*ALA*) is still densely opacified and extends as a cone-shaped protuberance (*arrowheads*) into the left atrium (*LA*). The mitral valve plane between left atrium and left ventricle (*LV*) is clearly seen. *Ao,* aorta.

nosis of the individual pulmonary veins appears to be abnormal incorporation of the common pulmonary vein into the left atrium.

Anatomy. In five patients all the pulmonary veins had localized obstructive lesions.[24, 93] Each of the individual pulmonary veins had a normal site of connection with the left atrium. At each pulmonary vein-left atrial junction, a circumferential protrusion of intimal fibrous tissue extended into the venous lumen, producing severe localized narrowing (Fig. 29.17*B*). Two patients had an ASD and a third had tetralogy of Fallot.

In six additional patients, the obstructive lesion involved the veins of only one lung. In three, the veins from one lung were atretic at the pulmonary vein-left fibrous tissue at the venous-left atrial junction. In two, a localized protrusion of intimal fibrous tissue at the venous-left atrial junction resulted in stenosis of the common pulmonary vein of one lung. In the remaining case, the left upper pulmonary vein was stenotic, while the left lower pulmonary vein was atretic.

Complex congenital cardiac lesions were associated in four patients.

In those cases without other cardiovascular anomalies, the lungs were congested, the pulmonary artery dilated and thick-walled, and there was right ventricular and right atrial hypertrophy. Atheromatous plaques were noted in the pulmonary artery in some instances.[93, 100] The typical hemodynamic features of severe pulmonary venous obstruction were present.

Manifestations. *Clinical Features.* The children present with a long history of respiratory symptoms, which ultimately progresses to right heart failure. The majority are cyanotic. A short systolic murmur is the usual finding. The pulmonary second sound is accentuated and, in the case of Shone *et al.*[100] a pulmonary systolic click was heard.

Electrocardiographic Features. Right ventricular hypertrophy is usual, and right atrial hypertrophy may be present.

Radiologic Features. The heart is not greatly enlarged, but reflects right ventricular hypertrophy. The pulmonary

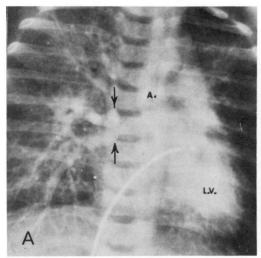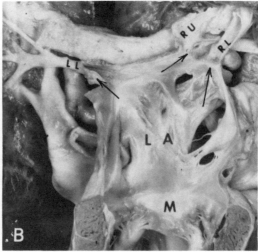

Fig. 29.17 Localized stenosis of the individual pulmonary veins in a 7-month-old boy. (*A*) Late film in a right ventriculogram. The right upper and right lower pulmonary veins are well outlined (*arrows*). Individual stenosis of the pulmonary veins is suggested by the constriction just distal to the arrows and persistence of opaque dye in the pulmonary veins proximal to the site of constriction. *L.V.*, left ventricle; *A.*, aorta. (*B*) The left ventricle and left atrium (*LA*) have been opened. Three moderate-sized defects are seen in the area of the fossa ovalis. At the junction of pulmonary veins (*RU, RL,* and *LL*) with left atrium, localized thickening and protrusion of the epithelium has produced a stenotic orifice. The left upper pulmonary vein (*LL*) has been transected. *M*, mitral valve. (Modified from J. D. Shone *et al.*,[100])

artery segment is enlarged, and the characteristic reticular markings of pulmonary venous obstruction are usual.[100]

Cardiac Catheterization. Right heart catheterization reflects pulmonary hypertension. Angiography reveals prolonged transit time of opaque dye through the lung. The angiogram in the case reported by Shone *et al.*[100] clearly demonstrated the constriction at the pulmonary vein-left atrial junction and delayed emptying of the pulmonary veins (Fig. 29.17*A*).

Treatment. The usual treatment for cardiac failure has been of little value in these patients. To our knowledge, successful surgical correction of this defect has not been reported. Patients with stenosis of the individual pulmonary veins exhibit a slow but progressive downhill course. The average age at death is 4 years, with a range of 5 months to 10 years.

ANOMALIES OF THE SYSTEMIC VENOUS SYSTEM

The wide range of the abnormalities of the systemic venous system has long fascinated the anatomist. Moreover, the embryologist has shown how clearly these anomalies reflect fundamental embryologic processes. Recent developments in the diagnosis and treatment of cardiovascular disorders have brought anomalies of the systemic veins to the attention of the cardiologist and thoracic surgeon.

In considering these diverse conditions, an anatomic classification tends to be cumbersome, whereas one based solely on physiology excludes conditions which result in no hemodynamic derangement. A classification based on embryologic principles provides a more inclusive framework for their discussion. This classification includes: anomalies of the cardinal venous system, anomalies of the inferior vena cava, and anomalies of the valves of the sinus venosus.

ANOMALIES OF THE CARDINAL VENOUS SYSTEM

These include developmental aberrations of the right and left superior vena cava and of the coronary sinus.

Embryology

The first veins to appear in the human embryo are the umbilicals (Fig. 29.18*A*). At 3 weeks these can be identified emptying into the caudal portion of the heart, while the vitelline veins are present only in the form of a plexus at the junction of embryo and yolk sac. The cardinal veins develop next (Fig. 29.18*B*).[104] These serve the fast-growing central nervous system. The anterior cardinal veins, which drain the head and neck, and the arms are recognizable early in the 4th week. Soon the posterior cardinal veins appear; lateral to the spinal cord. The anterior and posterior cardinals unite on each side to form a common cardinal vein. The common cardinals join the umbilical and vitelline veins to enter the heart as the right and left horns of the sinus venosus. By this time, the heart has begun to beat.[104]

Each sinus horn might be expected to empty into its own side of the developing common atrium. This does not occur, even as a normal stage in development.[83] During the 4th week an invagination appears (Fig. 29.18*B*) between the left sinus horn and left atrium. Ultimately this invagination completely separates the left sinus horn from the left atrium.[90] A rightward shift of the transverse portion of the sinus venosus, into which both sinus horns empty, completes the anatomic isolation of the left atrium from the systemic veins (Fig. 29.18*C*). This right-sided asymmetry of the systemic veins results in drainage of all systemic venous blood into the right atrium.

With the exception that both common cardinal veins empty into the right atrium, the cardinal venous system is bilaterally symmetrical at this stage. This is the final stage of development for venous return in birds. All the mammalia modify this primitive plan. The final form in humans calls for all the blood from the head and arms to enter the anterior cardinal on the right. On the left, the anterior cardinal obliterates, and the common cardinal remains to drain only the coronary circulation (Fig. 29.18*D*).

This is accomplished by development of the left innominate vein, early in the 8th week, to connect the two anterior cardinal veins. As blood flow through the left innominate increases, flow through the left anterior cardinal diminishes.

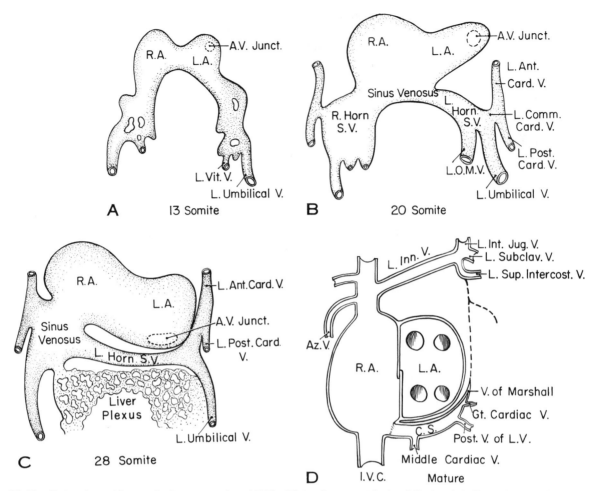

Fig. 29.18 Embryology of the cardinal venous system. (*A*) The bilaterally symmetrical umbilical and vitelline veins drain into the right and left sides of the common atrium. Asymmetry is already apparent in that the atrioventricular junction is located on the left side of the developing atrium. (*B*) The anterior and posterior cardinals have appeared. Asymmetrical development in continued by the occurrence of an invagination between the left horn of the sinus venosus and the left atrium. (*C*) Ultimately, the invagination completely separates the left horn of the sinus venosus from the left atrium and results in drainage of all systemic venosus blood into the right atrium. (*D*) Asymmetry is continued by the development of the left innominate vein (*L. Inn. V.*). As the left innominate vein enlarges, the left anterior cardinal vein diminishes until it becomes atretic. The common cardinal vein persists and, receiving the coronary veins, becomes the coronary sinus (*C.S.*). *L. Ant. Card. V.*, left anterior carotid vein; *L. Post. Card. V.*, left posterior carotid vein; *L. Comm. Card. V.*, left common carotid vein; *L. Umbilical V.*, left umbilical vein; *R.A.*, right atrium; *L.A.* left atrium; *L. Int. Jug. V.*, left internal jugular vein; *L. Subclav. V.*, left subclavian vein; *L. Sup. Intercost. V.*, left superior intercostal vein; *V. of Marshall*, Marshall's vein; *Gt. Cardiac V.*, great cardiac vein; *Post. V. of L.V.*, posterior vein of the left ventricle; *Middle Cardiac V.*, middle cardiac vein; *I.V.C.*, inferior vena cava; *Az. V.*, azygos vein; *L. Vit. V.*, left vitelline vein; *R. Horn S.V.* and *L. Horn S.V.*, right and left horn of the sinus venosus; *A.V. Junct.*, atrioventricular junction; *L.O.M.V.*, left omphalomesenteric vein. (Modified from G. L. Streeter.[104])

By the 6th fetal month, the latter vein has become obliterated. Its uppermost portion persists as the superior left intercostal vein. Occasionally, an additional portion remains as a fibrous cord attached to the posterior left aspect of the pericardium and coronary sinus. This is the oblique ligament of Marshall of the left atrium. Sometimes a small vein extends a variable distance from the coronary sinus into the fibrous cord (the oblique vein of Marshall of the left atrium). The left common cardinal persists and empties into the right atrium. When it receives the cardiac veins, relatively late in embryologic development, it assumes the function of coronary sinus.

Anomalies of the cardinal venous system result from the following embryologic aberrations:

Failure of Obliteration of the Left Anterior Cardinal Vein. Simple failure of obliteration of the left anterior cardinal vein results in persistence of the LSVC. If the normal invagination which separates the left sinus horn from

the left atrium has occurred, a coronary sinus is formed, which serves as a conduit between LSVC and right atrium.

Failure of Invagination Between Left Sinus Horn and Left Atrium. Should this invagination fail to occur, a coronary sinus cannot develop, since the cardiac veins alone are incapable of forming a coronary sinus. LSVC then connects directly to the superior pole of the left atrium.

Persistent Left Superior Vena Cava Connecting to Right Atrium (Normal Formation of Coronary Sinus)

In this anomaly, the LSVC connects to coronary sinus, which in turn joins right atrium. The physiology is normal. Its importance lies in the frequent coexistence of other congenital cardiac defects, and in the technical complications it may engender during cardiac catheterization or cardiac surgery.

Persistent LSVC is the only common anomaly of the superior caval system. In over 4,000 unselected autopsies, the prevalence was 0.3%.[34] The persistent LSVC connected to the right atrium in 92% of cases and to the left atrium in the remainder.[77] In patients with additional cardiac defects, the prevalence of LSVC was higher, ranging from 2.8 to 4.3%.[66]

Anatomy. From the junction of the left subclavian and the left internal jugular, the LSVC descends vertically in front of the aortic arch. A short distance from its origin, it receives the superior left intercostal vein. It then passes in front of the left pulmonary veins or between these vessels.[113] It usually receives a hemiazygos vein, then penetrates the pericardium and crosses the posterior wall of left atrium obliquely to approach the posterior atrioventricular sulcus. There it receives the great cardiac vein and becomes the coronary sinus. The coronary sinus and its right atrial ostium are larger than normal. The Thebesian valve is often small or absent.

As a rule, persistent LSVC is part of a *bilateral superior caval system* (Fig. 29.19*A*). Bilateral superior cavae are a normal stage in evolutionary development, as well as in the growth of the human embryo. When no communication has been formed between the right and left superior vena cava, the two veins tend to be equal in caliber. When a bridging

innominate is present (in 60%), the innominate and the LSVC vary inversely in caliber.[113]

Rarely, the right superior vena cava (RSVC) may be *absent* (Fig. 29.19*B*). Karnegis *et al.*[55] reviewed 30 known cases in 1964. When RSVC is absent, LSVC receives a right innominate, and thus the entire venous return from the head and arms. The LSVC, coronary sinus, and ostium of coronary sinus are greatly enlarged. In four cases the obliterated RSVC was identified as a fibrous cord running to the upper pole of the right atrium. When RSVC is absent, the azygos system is ordinarily found on the left, but may be right-sided or bilateral.

Associated Anomalies. Wood[114] found persistent LSVC in 20% of tetralogy of Fallot and in 8% of patients with Eisenmenger's syndrome. A high frequency occurs with the sinus venosus atrial septal defect.[32] LSVC is not uncommonly associated with cyanotic cardiac defects, and with malposition of the heart or abdominal viscera.[14]

Manifestations. *Clinical Features.* None.

Echocardiographic Features. The enlarged coronary sinus may produce an abnormal echo in left atrium (Fig. 29.15*B*).

Electrocardiographic Features. Hancock[44] reported a

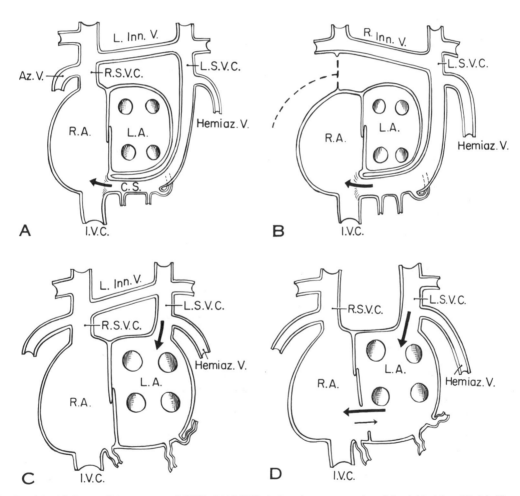

Fig. 29.19 Persistent left superior vena cava (LSVC). (*A*) LSVC drains via coronary sinus into right atrium (*R.A.*). The sizes of the left innominate vein (*L. Inn. V.*) and LSVC vary inversely; the former is often absent. (*B*) Uncommonly, RSVC may be atretic. (*C*) The coronary sinus is absent and LSVC drains directly into left atrium (*L.A.*). The atrial septum is intact. Coronary veins drain directly into the atria. The bridging innominate vein may be present (*C*) or absent (*D*). (*D*) LSVC connects to LA, and there is a posterior atrial septal defect, which allows a left to right shunt at atrial level. Some systemic venous blood from LSVC crosses the atrial septal defect, and thus drains normally. *R.S.V.C.*, right superior vena cava; *Hemiaz. V.*, hemiazygous vein; *R. Inn. V.*, right innominate vein; *C.S.*, coronary sinus. Other abbreviations as in Figure 29.18.

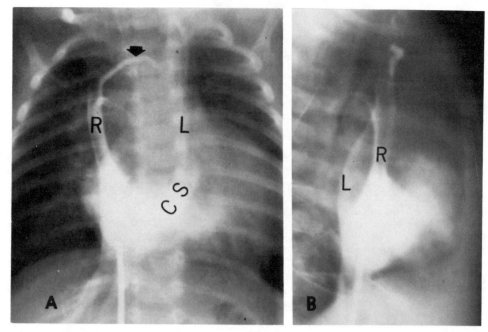

Fig. 29.20   Right atrial injection is persistent left superior vena cava draining via coronary sinus into right atrium. (*A*) Anteroposterior view. (*L*) and coronary sinus (*CS*) are large, while the left innominate vein (*arrow*) is small. The azygous vein can be seen just below the junction of left innominate vein and right superior vena cava (*R*). (*B*) Lateral projection. The characteristic posterior location of the left superior vena cava (*L*) is evident.

high prevalence of leftward P axis (15° or less) with a normal PR interval. Others have mentioned this finding, but its significance has not been clarified.

Radiologic Features. The shadow of the LSVC may be seen along the left upper border of the mediastinum.

Cardiac Catheterization. Persistent LSVC may make catheterization more difficult from the left arm approach. A higher than expected coronary sinus oxygen saturation is usual. Angiocardiography is diagnostic. It may reveal the size of the LSVC and the presence or absence of a bridging innominate, important factors in surgical management of associated cardiac defects (Fig. 29.20).

Treatment. None required.

Persistent Left Superior Vena Cava Connecting to Left Atrium (Failure of Coronary Sinus Development)

When the invagination which isolates the left sinus horn from the left atrium fails to occur, the coronary sinus does not develop, and the LSVC connects directly to the left atrium (Fig. 29.19*C* and *D*). This occurs rarely as an isolated defect, occasionally in association with defects of the atrial septum, and commonly with primitive cardiovascular defects, such as cor biloculare and the cardiac defects associated with asplenia syndrome.[91] Connection is to left atrium in 8% of cases of persistent LSVC.

Anatomy. The LSVC takes its usual course anterior to the aortic arch and the left pulmonary vessels. Then, instead of crossing the back of the left atrium to enter the coronary sinus, it connects to the upper pole of the left atrium between the left superior pulmonary vein posteriorly and the left atrial appendage anteriorly. Since the LSVC is not in proximity to the cardiac veins, the latter must drain individually into their corresponding atria. The coronary sinus is absent.

Associated Cardiac Anomalies. Associated cardiac anomalies are almost invariably present. Persistent LSVC connecting to the left atrium is rarely associated with simple cardiovascular anomalies[1] but is commonly associated with complex defects.

Defects of the Atrial Septum. Defects of the atrial septum are occasionally associated.[42] These include absence of the atrial septum (single atrium), primum ASD, secundum ASD, and a specific type of atrial septal defect considered by Raghib and associates[90] to be embryologically related to failure of development of the coronary sinus.

Primitive Cyanotic Congenital Cardiac Defects. The invagination which separates left sinus horn from left atrium is an early embryologic event, and it is not surprising that failure of this invagination is often associated with other primitive cardiovascular anomalies, such as cor biloculare, anomalies of conotruncal development, and the syndrome of splenic agenesis.[14]

In splenic agenesis, bilateral symmetry is the rule.[91, 109] In 15 of 17 cases of this syndrome,[96] a persistent LSVC entered the left atrium, and the coronary sinus was absent, thus confirming the tendency toward bilateral symmetry as far as the cardinal venous system is concerned.

Physiology. In the normal individual, superior vena cava flow represents approximately 40% of total systemic venous return. A persistent LSVC would generally carry one-half or less of the superior vena cava flow (except when RSVC is absent). Connection of LSVC to the left atrium would thus result in a relatively small right to left shunt of perhaps 20% of systemic blood flow.

When the LSVC to the left atrium is an isolated anomaly, the small right to left shunt is the only significant hemodynamic abnormality (Fig. 29.19*C*). Cardiac chamber hypertrophy is unusual, cardiac failure does not occur, and these patients have peripheral cyanosis out of proportion to other cardiovascular findings.

When an ASD is associated, it results in a left to right shunt at the atrial level (Fig. 29.19*D*). As a consequence, some of the systemic venous blood from the anomalously connected LSVC crosses the atrial septal defect and thus drains normally. Systemic venous blood reaching the peripheral arterial circulation may be minimal, and arterial saturations in five of six patients ranged between 88 and 96%.

Thus, the major hemodynamic findings are those secondary to the left to right shunt.

When the LSVC to the left atrium is associated with a complex cyanotic cardiac defect, the physiologic derangements due to anomalous LSVC are dwarfed by those of the more serious defect.

Manifestations. Features of a complex defect obscure the clinical effects of LSVC to left atrium. When a defect in the atrial septum is associated, the primary manifestations are those found in ASD. The following features suggest the coexistence of the LSVC to the left atrium: presence of mild arterial desaturation, left P-wave axis, and a prominent upper left cardiac border on the roentgenogram.

When the LSVC to the left atrium is an isolated phenomenon, cyanosis begins early in infancy. Clubbing and polycythemia are usual. There are no other significant symptoms, and the heart is usually normal on auscultation. The electrocardiogram and chest roentgenogram may show mild left ventricular hypertrophy. As with other forms of LSVC, left P-wave axis and a prominent shadow at the left cardiac border may be present.

Cardiac Catheterization. The course of the cardiac catheter through the LSVC allows the diagnosis. Right heart catheterization is normal or reflects an atrial left to right shunt. This in the face of peripheral cyanosis suggests a systemic vein draining anomalously into the left atrium.

Precise definition is possible utilizing peripheral angiography. In the case of LSVC to left atrium, injection should be made into a left arm vein.

Treatment. Treatment is surgical.[92] There are two options. The LSVC may simply be ligated. In this case it is necessary that the RSVC be present and that adequate bridging veins connect the RSVC and the LSVC. If the RSVC is absent or if collateral circulation is inadequate, the LSVC must be transposed to the right atrium.

When the LSVC to the left atrium is associated with an atrial septal defect, closure of the ASD eliminates the left to right shunt but results in greater arterial desaturation, because the LSVC blood is no longer permitted to drain normally through the ASD. The LSVC must then be handled as outlined above.

Prognosis. Prognosis is difficult to define on the basis of the few cases reported. The hemodynamic load is easily carried. On the other hand, drainage of systemic venous blood into the left side of the heart predisposes to peripheral embolization. Cerebral complications due to emboli have been reported in two patients. In one, death was related to unilateral acute encephalomalacia and thrombic occlusion of the right internal carotid artery.[90]

Right Superior Vena Cava Connecting to Left Atrium

This anomaly has been described in several patients[58, 111, 113] as an isolated condition. The clinical features were comparable to LSVC to left atrium. Diagnosis was accomplished with selective angiography. In one patient, the RSVC was successfully surgically transposed to the right atrium.[58] Persistence of the valves of the sinus venosus may also produce drainage of the RSVC to left atrium.

Anomalies of the Coronary Sinus

These are rare. A variety of abnormalities have been described, largely at postmortem examination. Although some cause alterations in coronary sinus drainage there is no evidence that they affect cardiac function adversely.

Anatomy. The abnormalities of the coronary sinus are: absence of coronary sinus, hypoplasia of the coronary sinus, atresia or stenosis of coronary sinus, communication of coronary sinus with both atria, and connection of coronary sinus to inferior vena cava. In addition, an otherwise normal coronary sinus may continue to receive a left hepatic vein, as evidence that it once functioned as the left horn of the embryonic sinus venosus.

Absence of the Coronary Sinus. Absent coronary sinus is never an isolated anomaly. It always is associated with a persistent LSVC draining into left atrium.

Hypoplasia of the Coronary Sinus. Hypoplasia of the coronary sinus occurs when one or more of the cardiac veins fails to join the coronary sinus and empties instead into one of the atria through an enlarged Thebesian vein.[71]

Atresia or Stenosis of Ostium of Coronary Sinus. In coronary sinus obstruction, alternative routes of drainage exist. Coronary venous blood may drain into the left atrium through a defect in the wall separating the left atrium from the coronary sinus (Fig. 29.21A).[70] The coronary sinus may drain via a persistent LSVC, left innominate vein, and RSVC to the right atrium[26, 45] (Fig. 29.21B).

Several patients have been described with atresia of the coronary sinus ostium, in whom no gross channel of egress existed. Instead, many enlarged Thebesian veins connected the coronary sinus to the left atrium.[26, 71]

Communication of Coronary Sinus with Both Atria. In this anomaly, the coronary sinus connects normally to the right atrium and additionally, communicates with the left atrium through a defect in their common wall (Fig. 29.21C). The coronary sinus may be otherwise normal,[28] or the LSVC may be continuous with the coronary sinus.[71] A left to right shunt at the atrial level is the major hemodynamic consequence.

Connection of Coronary Sinus to Inferior Vena Cava. Occasionally, the coronary sinus is normally located in the coronary atrioventricular sulcus and receives the cardiac veins in the usual way, but rather than connecting directly to the right atrium, it joins the inferior vena cava just below its junction with the right atrium.[6] This imposes no physiological handicap.

Physiology. In those conditions in which the coronary sinus blood ultimately reaches the right atrium, the physiology is normal. In other cases, the anatomic features suggest coronary sinus obstruction. However, there is no evidence that a physiologic derangement exists. Presumably Thebesian veins enlarge in the face of chronic obstruction and provide adequate coronary sinus drainage.

When coronary sinus drainage is into the left atrium, a small (10%) right to left shunt exists. This has no significant impact on cardiac function. If coronary sinus communicates with both right and left atrium, it serves as a conduit between the atria and is thus comparable to an atrial septal defect.

Treatment. Surgical correction is usually not indicated and has not been described. Theoretically, the coronary sinus communicating with both atria is amenable to correction by closing the coronary sinus ostium and ligating the LSVC if present.

ANOMALIES OF THE INFERIOR VENA CAVA

Many variations in formation of the inferior vena cava (IVC) have been described. These include double IVC,[94] left IVC,[80] and a host of lesser aberrations.[22] These occasionally present problems to the abdominal surgeon but have no other importance. Significant anomalies of the inferior vena cava are: infrahepatic interruption of the IVC with azygous continuation and anomalous drainage of the IVC into the left atrium.

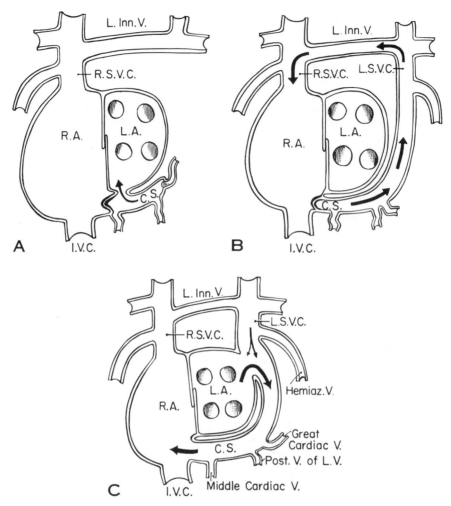

Fig. 29.21 Anomalies of the coronary sinus. *A* and *B*. Atresia of the ostium of the coronary sinus. (*A*) Drainage of coronary sinus blood may be into the left atrium through a defect between the coronary sinus and left atrium. (*B*) Alternatively, coronary sinus blood may drain in a retrograde fashion by way of LSVC to left innominate vein and into right atrium. (*C*) Coronary sinus communicating with both atria. The coronary sinus (*C.S.*) serves as a conduit between left atrium (*L.A.*) and right atrium (*R.A.*), resulting in a left to right shunt at atrial level. The volume of LSVC blood reaching the left atrium is small. See Figure 29.19 for explanation of other abbreviations.

Infrahepatic Interruption of IVC with Azygous Continuation

In this condition, the IVC is interrupted below the hepatic veins, and the systemic venous drainage from below the interruption is via an enlarged azygous vein to the SVC. Anderson *et al.*[3] reported 15 patients with interruption of IVC with azygous continuation among 2,500 cases of congenital heart disease studied by cardiac catheterization. In 170 patients catheterized by the saphenous route, so that the defect could not be missed, Dupuis *et al.*[21] found a prevalence of 2.9%. In normal hearts, the condition is very rare.

Embryology of the IVC and Azygous Vein. The caudal portion of the body continues to drain through the primitive posterior cardinal venous system until late in cardiac embryogenesis. The definitive IVC is formed during the 6th to 8th weeks (Fig. 29.22). Important steps in this development are listed below.

Transfer of Venous Return from Posterior Cardinal Veins to More Centrally Located Venous Systems. The first of these centrally located systems, the subcardinal, forms *ventral* and medial to the posterior cardinal veins. Anastomoses develop between the posterior cardinals and the subcardinals, and venous return is diverted to the subcardinal

system. Subsequently, the supracardinal system develops *dorsal* and medial to the posterior cardinal veins, and the remaining posterior cardinal venous flow is transferred to the supracardinals. No significant remnant of the posterior cardinal system persists between the diaphragm and the junction of the iliac veins.

Development of Right-Sided Dominance. Anastomoses develop between the right and left subcardinal veins and between the right and left supracardinal veins. Venous return is preferentially channeled to the right side; the left subcardinal system atrophies and the left supracardinal (hemiazygos) vein joins the right supracardinal (azygos) vein.

Junction of Right Subcardinal Vein with Hepatic Vein. This junction establishes the central venous route to right atrium and completes the development of IVC above the level of the kidneys. The definitive IVC is thus derived from above downward from hepatic vein, right subcardinal vein, subcardinal anastomoses, and right supracardinal vein (Fig. 29.22, *center*).

Failure of junction of the right subcardinal vein to the hepatic vein results in interruption of the IVC with azygous continuation. When this occurs, multiple anastomoses between the right subcardinal system (IVC) and the right

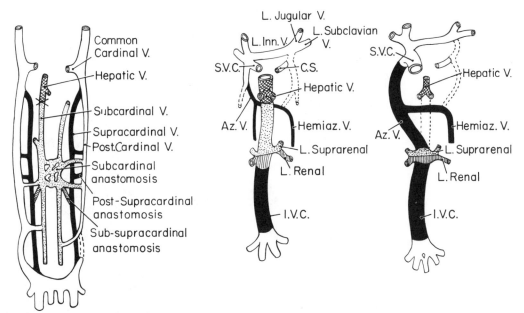

Fig. 29.22 Embryologic development of the inferior vena cava (*IVC*). (*Left*) Early stage. Venous blood from the lower body may reach the heart by way of the posterior cardinal veins (*Post. Cardinal V.*), supracardinal veins, and the upper portion of the IVC, derived from hepatic and subcardinal veins. Multiple anastomotic sites between these venous systems exist in the renal area as shown. (*Center*) Normal development of IVC. The major venous drainage channel from the lower body is by way of the IVC, derived, from below upward, from the posterior cardinal system (*white*), the supracardinal system (*black*), the renal collar (*lines*), the subcardinal system (*stippled*), and the hepatic veins (*cross-hatched*). A small accessory venous channel is provided by persistence of the supracardinal veins, as hemiazygous and azygous veins. (*Right*) Interruption of the IVC with azygos continuation. Failure of junction of the right subcardinal vein and hepatic vein occurs and results in absence of the IVC from the region of the renal veins upward. The hepatic veins drain directly into the right atrium. All other blood from the lower body drains normally to the junction of the renal veins with the IVC and then continues by way of a greatly dilated azygous vein into SVC. *L.*, left; *V.*, vein; *Inn.*, innominate; *Az*, azygous; *S.V.C.*, superior vena cava; *C.S.*, coronary sinus; *Hemiaz.*, hemiazygous.

supracardinal veins (azygus system) allow diversion of all venous blood from the lower portion of the body into the supracardinal or azygous system (Fig. 29.22, *right*).

Anatomy. The IVC below the level of the renal veins is unaltered. The hepatic veins connect directly to the right atrium (Fig. 29.23*C*). The IVC is absent between the renal veins and hepatic veins. In the usual case, the renal veins join the normal lower portion of the IVC. Systemic venous drainage then continues via an enlarged azygous vein. The latter is in its usual position to the right of the spine. The azygos enters the thorax through the aortic hiatus of the diaphragm and stays posterior until it arches forward over the root of the right lung to join the SVC just above the SVC-RA junction. The azygos receives the hemiazygos in normal fashion. Less often, the hemiazygous vein is the alternative venous pathway, and empties into a persistent LSVC (hemiazygous continuation).

Associated Cardiac Anomalies. Azygous continuation is often associated with complex cyanotic cardiovascular defects. Frequently encountered are cor biloculare, atrioventricular canal, anomalies of pulmonary venous return, origin of both great arteries from the right ventricle, pulmonary stenosis or atresia, and combinations of the above.[3] Less often a simple cardiac defect is associated. No case has been reported with associated asplenia, but multiple spleens are occasionally present.[3, 91] (Fig. 29.23*C*).

In 40 cases reviewed by Anderson *et al.*,[3] abnormal cardiac situs was noted in 11 and isolated abdominal situs inversus in six. Bilateral SVC was also common; in some of these, the azygous vein joined RSVC, and the hemiazygos persisted to connect to LSVC.

Physiology. Since the size of the azygous vein is inadequate to obviate venous obstruction and the azygos empties into right atrium, the physiology is normal, whether the condition exists as an isolated anomaly or is associated with other cardiac defects.

Manifestations. Interruption of the IVC with azygos continuation is of clinical importance only insofar as it suggests the possibility of an associated cardiac defect, many complicate cardiac catheterization, and can render surgical correction of an underlying defect more difficult.

Cardiac Catheterization. When the saphenous approach is used, the catheter enters the azygous vein. From this approach the catheter may be manipulated into right atrium, but manipulation into more distal chambers may be difficult.

Venous angiography from the lower extremities is diagnostic (Fig. 29.23).[103] In children with normal IVC, venous angiography from the lower extremities often results in opacification of the azygous vein. Occasionally, sufficient spasm of the IVC exists to divert most of the dye to the azygous vein. This may lead to an erroneous diagnosis of interruption of the IVC with azygous continuation.

Treatment. There is no need for surgical correction of interrupted IVC with azygous continuation. Inadvertent ligation of the azygous vein may lead to death.[29] During cardiopulmonary bypass, the surgeon must recognize and deal with the altered systemic venous drainage.[10]

In the absence of associated cardiac abnormalities, longevity is normal. Interruption of the IVC with azygous continuation does not influence the prognosis of other conditions which may be associated.

IVC Connecting to Left Atrium

A distinction must be made between *connection* of the IVC to the left atrium with intact atrial septum and cases in which a low atrial septal defect allows *drainage* of IVC blood into the left atrium. In the latter cases, the Eustachian

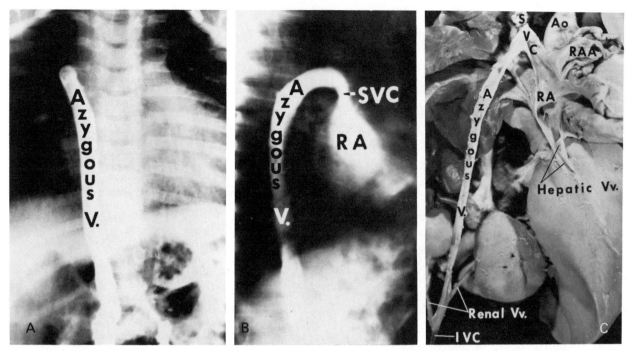

Fig. 29.23 Interruption of inferior vena cava (*IVC*) with azygous continuation. (*A*) Venous angiography. Anteroposterior projection. The dilated azygous vein can be seen just to the right of the spine in its characteristic location. (*B*) Right lateral view. The azygous vein ascends in the posterior mediastinum, curves anteriorly, and joins the superior vena cava (*SVC*). It has a characteristic "candy cane" configuration. (*C*) Thoracic and abdominal organs viewed from the right. The renal veins connect to IVC which drains the caudal portion of the body normally. Then IVC continues as the azygous vein to join SVC. The hepatic veins drain directly into the right atrium (*RA*). *RAA*, right atrial appendage; *Ao*, aorta. Three of numerous spleens may be identified posterior to the azygous vein, just above the left kidney. *Vv.*, vertical vein.

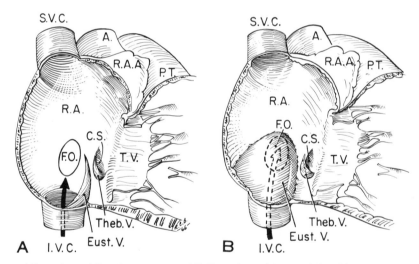

Fig. 29.24 Persistence of the valves of the sinus venosus. (*A*) Normal persistence of the valves of the sinus venosus results in the Eustachian valve (*Eust. V.*) and the (*Theb. V.*) Thebesian valve. (*B*) Pathologic persistence of the valves of the sinus venosus has resulted in a membrane which completely excludes inferior vena cava (*I.V.C.*) from right atrium (*R.A.*). Blood from the IVC is channeled through the foramen ovale (*F.O.*) into the left atrium. In similar fashion, the ostium of the coronary sinus, the superior vena cava (*SVC*) orifice, or all three orifices may be isolated from the true right atrium by abnormal persistence of the valves of the sinus venosus. *R.A.A.*, right atrial appendage; *T.V.*, tricuspid valve. *A.*, atrium; *P.T.*, pulmonary trunk; *C.S.*, coronary sinus.

valve may be mistaken for the lower margin of the atrial septal defect.[63] Closure may then divert IVC blood into left atrium.[30, 82]

In cases of connection of the IVC to the left atrium, some are due to persistent valves of the sinus venosus and are described in the subsequent section.[8, 98] Others have not been well defined embryologically.[76]

The clinical features in these cases are comparable to those of SVC connecting to the left atrium.[33] Cerebral acci-

dents have occurred. Surgical cure has been accomplished.[8, 98]

PERSISTENT VALVES OF THE SINUS VENOSUS

In the normal heart, remnants of the valves of the sinus venosus are the Eustachian and Thebesian valves and crista terminalis (Fig. 29.24*A*). Minor abnormal persistence of the valves of the sinus venosus results in larger than usual

Eustachian and Thebesian valves and in Chiari's networks. The latter are fine, filamentous structures which may represent persistence of either the right or left valves. Usually Chiari's networks are persistent right valves and extend from the crista terminalis or tuberculum Loweri to Eustachian and/or Thebesian valves. Networks derived from the left valves are inconspicuously located at the posterior rim of the limbus fossae ovalis and on the medial wall of the IVC as it enters the right atrium. None of these are of hemodynamic consequence.

Pathologic overgrowth of the valves of the sinus venosus may produce complete subdivision of the right atrium or lesser degrees of subdivision. As a consequence, the SVC, IVC, coronary sinus, or combinations of these may be excluded from the true right atrium. The result may be obstruction to systemic venous return or channeling of systemic venous blood into left atrium. Pathologic persistence of the right valve of the sinus venosus is an uncommon lesion.

Anatomy. Four anatomic patterns of pathologic persistence of the valves were recognized by Doucette and Knoblich[20] and the patients of Schölmerich et al.,[98] and Rossall and Caldwell[95] represent a fifth and sixth. These are summarized below.

In the complete form, the right valve persists as a membrane which extends across the right atrium, from the crista terminalis laterally to the medial wall of right atrium, and from the SVC above to a point below the coronary sinus. The right atrium is thereby divided into two chambers: the sinus venarum and right atrium proper.[20] The sinus venarum receives the IVC, SVC, and coronary sinus. The true right atrium has the right atrial appendage and communicates with the right ventricle by way of the tricuspid valve.

If the persistent valve were intact, the systemic venous blood would be excluded from right atrium. However, variable-sized defects in the valve allow communication between the sinus venarum and the true right atrium. The foramen ovale also allows communication from the sinus venarum to the left atrium. Because the membrane is formed from the right valve of the sinus venosus, these hearts do not have Eustachian or Thebesian valves.

In a second type, the membrane covers the orifices of the SVC and IVC, but the coronary sinus empties into the right atrium in the usual manner. Thus, the SVC and IVC empty into the sinus venarum and communicate with the true right atrium only through defects in the membrane. The foramen ovale allows communication of the sinus venarum with the left atrium. Since the lowermost portion of the right venous valve does not contribute to the membrane, the Thebesian valve is present.

In a third form, the persistent right valve of the sinus venosus excludes only the IVC; the SVC and coronary sinus drain normally into the true right atrium (Fig. 29.24B).[8] The persistent valve fuses with the septum secundum at the foramen ovale, and the blood from the IVC drains through this opening into the left atrium.

In a fourth type, only the ostium of coronary sinus was excluded from the right atrium; the SVC and IVC drained normally.[59]

In another, the IVC and coronary sinus were both excluded from right atrium while SVC drained normally.[98]

Rossall and Caldwell[95] reported a patient in whom a persistent right venous valve caused nearly complete obstruction of the IVC. The valve was not within the right atrium, but at the junction of IVC and right atrium.

The patients reported as having RSVC connecting to left atrium[58, 113] may represent persistence of the cephalic option of the right valve of the sinus venosus which has fused to the atrial septum, thus excluding the RSVC from the right atrium. The RSVC blood reaches the left atrium via an atrial septal defect in the cephalic portion of the septum.

Associated Cardiac Anomalies. One half the patients with persistence of the valves of the sinus venosus have severe associated cardiac defects. The anomaly in five of seven reported cases took the form of severe obstruction to right ventricular outflow.[20] Right to left shunt at the atrial level is obligatory in these patients. Since the persistent valve favors such a shunt, its presence incurs no additional hemodynamic handicap.

Physiology. Evidence exists for the following hemodynamic abnormalities: systemic venous obstruction, right to left shunt, and left to right shunt.

Manifestations. Symptoms due to persistence of sinus venosus valves are the result of systemic venous obstruction and right to left shunting. A nonobstructive valve associated with ASD produces no symptoms but may complicate surgical repair.

Treatment. The therapy of these anomalies is surgical. The precise anatomic relationships of abnormal sinus venosus valves are rarely defined preoperatively; thus the burden of precise diagnosis as well as surgical repair falls on the surgeon. At operation, the first clue to the presence of abnormal valves may be difficulty in cannulating the vena cava from the right atrium. The affected cava must then be cannulated more peripherally and occluded by tourniquet at its junction at the heart.[8] Then the interior of the right atrium is inspected for its usual landmarks, including the ostia of the IVC, SVC, coronary sinus, fossa ovalis, right atrial appendage, and tricuspid valve. Presence of a persistent valve will obscure one or more of these landmarks. Once recognized, the valve is incised, and its precise anatomic relationships are then apparent. Repair may be completed by excision of redundant valve tissue and closure of the usually associated atrial septal defect.

It is appropriate to emphasize the need to close an ASD from the bottom up. We are aware of several patients in whom total diversion of the IVC blood into the left atrium was accomplished at the time of ASD repair. In these patients the patch was sutured from above downward, and the lower portion of the patch was sutured to a valve of the IVC.

REFERENCES

1. Abbott, M. E.: Atlas of Congenital Cardiac Disease. American Heart Association, New York, 1936.
2. Alpert, J. S., Dexter, L., Vieweg, W. V. R., Haynes, F. U., and Dalen, J. E.: Anomalous pulmonary venous return with intact atrial septum. Circulation 56:870, 1977.
3. Anderson, R. C., Adams, P., Jr., and Burke, B.: Anomalous inferior vena cava with azygos continuation (infrahepatic interruption of the inferior vena cava). J. Pediatr. 59:370, 1961.
4. Anderson, R. C., and Varco, R. L.: Cor triatriatum: Successful diagnosis and surgical correction in a 3-year-old girl. Am. J. Cardiol. 7:436, 1961.
5. Bardeleben. Über vena azygos, hemiazygos und coronaria cordis bei Säugethieren. Müller's Arch., 1848, p. 497.
6. Basu, B. N.: Persistent "left superior vena cava," "left duct of Cuvier," and "left horn of the sinus venosus." J. Anat. 66:268, 1932.
7. Behrendt, D. M., Aberdeen, E., Waterson, D. J., and Bonham-Carter, R. E.: Total anomalous pulmonary venous drainage in infants. I. Clinical and hemodynamic findings, methods, and results of operation in 37 cases. Circula-

tion 47:347, 1972.
8. Black, H., Smith, G. T., and Goodale, W. T.: Anomalous inferior vena cava draining into the left atrium associated with intact interatrial septum and multiple pulmonary arteriovenous fistulae. Circulation 29:258, 1964.
9. Bonchek, L. P., Anderson, R. P., Wood, J. A., Chapman, R. D., and Starr, A.: Intracardiac surgery with extracorporeal circulation in infants. Ann. Thorac. Surg. 17:280, 1974.
10. Bosher, L. H.: Problems in extracorporeal circulation relating to venous cannulation and drainage. Ann. Surg. 149:652, 1959.

11. Brody, H.: Drainage of the pulmonary veins into the right side of the heart. Arch. Pathol. 33:221, 1942.

12. Burchell, H. B.: Total anomalous pulmonary venous drainage: Clinical and physiologic patterns. Mayo Clin. Proc. 31:161, 1956.

13. Burroughs, J. T., and Edwards, J. E.: Total anomalous pulmonary venous connection. Am. Heart J. 59:913, 1960.

14. Campbell, M., and Deuchar, D. C.: The left-sided superior vena cava. Br. Heart J. 16:423, 1954.

15. Carpena, C., Colokathis, B., and Subramanian, S.: Cor triatriatum successful correction in 4 patients including 2 under 1 year of age. Ann. Thorac. Surg. 17:325, 19974.

16. Church, W. S.: Congenital malformation of the heart: Abnormal septum in left auricle. Trans. Pathol. Soc. (Lond.) 19:188, 1868.

17. Clarke, D. R., Stark, J., Deheval, M., Pincott, J. R., and Taylor, J. F. N.: TAPVD in infancy. Br. Heart J. 39:436, 1977.

18. Darling, R. C., Rothney, W. B., and Craig, J. M.: Total pulmonary venous drainage into the right side of the heart: Report of 17 autopsied cases not associated with other major cardiovascular anomalies. Lab. Invest. 6:44, 1957.

19. Danilowicz, D., and Kronzon, I.: Use of contrast echocardiography in the diagnosis of PAPVC. Am. J. Cardiol. 43:248, 1979.

20. Doucette, J., and Knoblich, R.: Persistent right valve of the sinus venosus. Arch. Pathol. 75:105, 1963.

21. Dupuis, C., Nuyts, J. P., and Christiaens, L.: "Continuation azygos" de la veine cave inférieure. Arch. Mal. Coeur 57:28, 1964.

22. Edwards, E. A.: Clinical anatomy of lesser variations of the inferior vena cava, and a proposal for classifying the anomalies of this vessel. Angiology 2:85, 1951.

23. Edwards, J. E.: Pathologic and developmental considerations in anomalous pulmonary venous connection. Mayo Clin. Proc. 28:441, 1953.

24. Edwards, J. E.: Congenital stenosis of pulmonary veins: Pathological and developmental considerations. Lab. Invest. 9:46, 1960.

25. Edwards, J. E.: Malformations of the thoracic veins. In Pathology of the Heart, 2nd ed., edited by S. E. Gould. Charles C Thomas, Springfield, Ill., 1960, p. 492.

26. Edwards, J. E.: Malformations of the thoracic veins. In Pathology of the Heart, 2nd ed., edited by S. E. Gould. Charles C Thomas, Springfield, Ill., 1960, p. 484.

27. Edwards, J. E.: Malformations of the coronary vessels: Anomalies of the coronary sinus. In Pathology of the Heart, 2nd ed., edited by S. E. Gould. Charles C Thomas, Springfield, Ill., 1960, p. 431.

28. Edwards, J. E.: Malformations of the atrial septal complex. In Pathology of the Heart, 2nd ed., edited by S. E. Gould. Charles C Thomas, Springfield, Ill., 1960, p. 275.

29. Effler, D. B., Greer, A. E., and Sifers, E. C.: Anomaly of the vena cava inferior. Report of fatality after ligation. J.A.M.A. 146:1321, 1951.

30. Effler, D. B., and Groves, L. K.: Pitfalls in the surgical closure of atrial septal defect. Cleve. Clin. Q. 28:166, 1961.

31. Fiandra, O., Barcia, A., Cortes, R., and Stanham, J.: Partial anomalous pulmonary venous drainage into the inferior vena cava. Acta Radiol. [Diagn.] [Suppl.] (Stockh.), 57:301, 1961.

32. Fleming, J. S., and Gibson, R. V.: Absent right superior vena cava as an isolated anomaly. Br. J. Radiol. 37:696, 1964.

33. Gardner, D. L., and Cole, L.: Long survival with inferior vena cava draining into left atrium. Br. Heart J. 17:93, 1955.

34. Geissler, W., and Albert, M.: Persistierende linke obere Hohlvene und Mitralstenose. Z. Gesamte Inn. Med. 11:865, 1956.

35. Gessner, I. H., Krovetz, L. J., Wheat, M. W., Jr., Shanklin, D. R., and Schiebler, G. L.: Total anomalous pulmonary venous connection. Am. Heart J. 68:459, 1964.

36. Gharagozloo, F., Bulkley, B. H., and Hutchins, G. M.: A proposed pathogenesis of cor triatriatum. Am. Heart J. 94:618, 1977.

37. Gialloreto, O. P., and Vineberg, A.: A case of cor triatriatum studied five years after surgery. Am. J. Cardiol. 9:598, 1962.

38. Gibson, D. G., Honey, M., and Lennox, S. C.: Cor triatriatum: Diagnosis by echocardiography. Br. Heart J. 36:835, 1974.

39. Gotsman, M. S., Astley, R., and Parsons, C. G.: Partial anomalous pulmonary venous drainage in association with atrial septal defect. Br. Heart J. 27:566, 1965.

40. Gott, V. L., Lester, R. G., Lillehei, C. W., and Varco, R. L.: Total anomalous pulmonary return: An analysis of thirty cases. Circulation 13:543, 1956.

41. Grondin, C., Leonard, A. S., Anderson, R. C., Amplatz, K. A., Edwards, J. E., and Varco, R. L.: Cor triatriatum: A diagnostic surgical enigma. J. Thorac. Cardiovasc. Surg. 48:527, 1964.

42. Gruber, W.: Anatomische Mittheilungen. Vjschr. Prakt. Heilk. 9:78, 1846.

43. Haeger, K., Juhlin, I., and Krook, H.: Eisenmenger's complex accompanied by double superior venae cavae, the left draining into left atrium. Am. Heart J. 50:471, 1955.

44. Hancock, E. W.: Coronary sinus rhythm in sinus venosus defect and persistent left superior vena cava. Am. J. Cardiol. 14:608, 1964.

45. Harris, G. B. C., Neuhauser, E. B. C., and Giedion, A.: Total anomalous pulmonary venous return below the diaphragm. Am. J. Roentgenol. Radium Ther. Nucl. Med. 84:436, 1960.

46. Harris, W. G.: A case of bilateral superior venae cavae with a closed coronary sinus. Thorax 15:172, 1960.

47. Hawker, R. E., Celermajer, J. M., Gengos, D. C., Cartmill, T. M., and Bowdler, J. D.: Common pulmonary vein atresia, premortem diagnosis in two children. Circulation 46:368, 1972.

48. Hawker, R. E., Freedom, R. J., and Krovetz, L. J.: Preferential shunting of venous return from normally connected left pulmonary veins in secundum atrial septal defect. Am. J. Cardiol. 34:339, 1974.

49. Healy, J. E., Jr.: An anatomic survey of anomalous pulmonary veins: Their clinical significance. J. Thorac. Cardiovasc. Surg. 23:433, 1952.

50. Hickie, J. B., Gimlette, T. D. M., and Bacon, A. P. C.: Anomalous pulmonary venous drainage. Br. Heart J. 18:365, 1956.

51. Hughes, C., and Rumore, P.: Anomalous pulmonary veins. Arch. Pathol. 37:365, 1944.

52. Ivemark, B. I.: Implications of agenesis of the spleen on the pathogenesis of conotruncus anomalies in childhood: An analysis of the heart malformations in the splenic agenesis syndrome, with fourteen new cases. Acta Paediatr. Scand. Suppl. 104:1, 1955.

53. Jegier, W., Gibbons, J. E., and Wiglesworth, F. W.: Cor triatriatum: Clinical, hemodynamic, and pathologic studies: Surgical correction in early life. Pediatrics 31:255, 1963.

54. Kalmansohn, R. B., Maloney, J. V., Jr., and Kalmansohn, R. W.: Partial anomalous pulmonary venous connection with unusual variations. N. Engl. J. Med. 264:1233, 1961.

55. Karnegis, J. N., Wang, Y., Winchell, P., and Edwards, J. E.: Persistent left superior vena cava, fibrous remnant of the right superior vena cava and ventricular septal defect. Am. J. Cardiol. 14:573, 1964.

56. Keith, J. D., Rowe, R. D., Vlad, P., and O'Hanley, J. H.: Complete anomalous pulmonary venous drainage. Am. J. Med. 16:23, 1954.

57. Kirklin, J. W.: Surgical treatment of anomalous pulmonary venous connection (partial anomalous pulmonary venous drainage). Mayo Clin. Proc. 28:476, 1953.

58. Kirsch, W. M., Carlsson, E., and Hartmann, A. F., Jr.: A case of anomalous drainage of the superior vena cava into the left atrium. J. Thorac. Cardiovasc. Surg. 41:550, 1961.

59. Kjellberg, S. R., Mannheimer, E., Rudhe, U., and Jonsson, B.: Diagnosis of Congenital Heart Disease, 2nd ed. Year Book Medical Publishers, Chicago, 1959, pp. 26, 167.

60. Lam, C. R., Green, E., and Drake, E.: Diagnosis and surgical correction of two types of triatrial heart. Surgery 51:127, 1962.

61. Lee, Y., and Scherlis, L.: Atrial septal defect: Electrocardiographic, vectorcardiographic and catheterization date. Circulation 25:1024, 1962.

62. Levy, A. M., Naeye, R. L., Tabakin, B. S., and Hanson, J. S.: Far-advanced intimal proliferation and severe pulmonary hypertension secondary to total anomalous pulmonary venous drainage. Am. J. Cardiol. 16:280, 1965.

63. Lewis, F. J., Varco, R. L., and Taufic, M.: Repair of atrial septal defects in man under direct vision with the aid of hypothermia. Surgery 36:538, 1954.

64. Lindstrom, N. R.: Ultrasound cardiographic studies of the mitral valve region in young infants with mitral atresia, mitral stenosis, hypoplasia of the left ventricle and cor triatriatum. Circulation 45:325, 1972.

65. Loeffler, E.: Unusual malformation of the left atrium: Pulmonary sinus. Arch. Pathol. 48:371, 1949.

66. Loogen, F., and Rippert, R.: Anomalien der grossen Körper und Lungenvenen. Z. Kreislaufforsch. 47:677, 1958.

67. Lucas, R. V., Jr., Adams, P., Jr., Anderson, R. C., Varco, R. L., Edwards, J. E., and Lester, R. G.: Total anomalous pulmonary venous connection to the portal venous system: A cause of pulmonary venous obstruction. Am. J. Roentgenol. Radium Ther. Nucl. Med. 86:561, 1961.

68. Lucas, R. V., Jr., Anderson, R. C., Amplatz, K., Adams, P., Jr., and Edwards, J. E.: Congenital causes of pulmonary venous obstruction. Pediatr. Clin. North Am. 10:781, 1963.

69. Lucas, R. V., Jr., Woolfrey, B. F., Anderson, R. C., Lester, R. G., and Edwards, J. E.: Atresia of the common pulmonary vein. Pediatrics 29:729, 1962.

70. MacMahon, H. E.: Communication of the coronary sinus with the left atrium. Circulation 28:947, 1963.

71. Mantini, E., Grondin, C. M., Lillehei, C. W., and Edwards, J. E.: Congenital anomalies involving the coronary sinus. Circulation 33:317, 1966.

72. Marin-Garcia, J., Tandon, R., Lucas, R. V., Jr., and Edwards, J. E.: Cor triatriatum: Study of 20 cases. Am. J. Cardiol. 35:59, 1975.

73. Matthew, R., Thilenius, O. B., Replogle, R. L., and Arcilla, R. A.: Cardiac function in total anomalous pulmonary venous return before and after surgery. Circulation 55:361, 1977.

74. McCormack, R. J. M., Marquis, R. M., Julian, D. G., and Griffiths, H. W. C.: Partial anomalous pulmonary venous drainage and its surgical correction. Scott. Med. J. 5:367, 1960.

75. McGuire, L. B., Nolan, T. B., Reeve, R., and Dammann, J. F., Jr.: Cor triatriatum as a problem of adult heart disease. Circulation 31:263, 1965.

76. Meadows, W. R., Bergstrand, I., and Sharp, J. T.: Isolated anomalous connection of a great vein to the left atrium. Circulation 24:669, 1961.

77. Meadows, W. R., and Sharp, J. T.: Persistent left superior vena cava draining into the left atrium without arterial oxygen unsaturation. Am. J. Cardiol. 16:273, 1965.

78. Mehrizi, A., Dekker, A., and Ottesen, O. E.: Angiocardiographic feature of total anomalous venous return into coronary sinus simulating tricuspid atresia or stenosis. J. Pediatr. 65:615, 1964.

79. Mehrizi, A., Hirsch, M. S., and Taussig, H. B.: Congenital heart disease in the neonatal period: Autopsy study of 170 cases. J. Pediatr. 65:721, 1964.

80. Milloy, F. J., Anson, B. J., and Cauldwell, E. W.: Variations in the inferior vena caval veins and in their renal and lumbar communications. Surg. Gynecol. Obstet. 115:131, 1962.

81. Mullins, C. E., El-Said, G. M., Neches, W. H., Williams, R. L., Vargs, T. A., Nihill, M. R., and McNamara, D. G.: Balloon atrial septostomy for TAPVR. Br. Heart J. 35:752, 1973.

82. Mustard, W. T., Firor, W. B., and Kidd, L.: Diversion of the venae cavae into the left atrium during closure of atrial septal defects. J. Thorac. Cardiovasc. Surg. 47:317, 1964.

83. Neill, C. A.: Development of the pulmonary veins, with reference to the embryology of anomalies of pulmonary venous return. Pediatrics 18:880, 1956.

84. Neill, C. A., Ferencz, C., Sabiston, D. C., and Sheldon, H.: The familial occurrence of hypoplastic right lung with systemic arterial supply and venous drainage: "Scimitar syndrome." Johns Hopkins Med. J. 107:1, 1960.

85. Niwayama, G.: Cor triatriatum. Am. Heart J. 59:291, 1960.

86. Orsmond, G. S., Ruttenberg, H. D., Bessinger, F. B., and Moller, J. H.: Echocardiographic features of TAPVC to the coronary sinus. Am. J. Cardiol. 41:597, 1978.

87. Paquet, M., and Gutgesell, H.: Echocardiographic features of total anomalous pulmonary venous connection. Circulation 51:599, 1975.

88. Parr, G. V. S., Kirklin, J. W., Pacifico, A. D., Blackstone, E. H., and Lauridsen, P.: Cardiac performance in infants after repair of TAPVC. Ann. Thorac. Surg. 17:561, 1974.

89. Rabin, E. R., and Meyer, E. C.: Cardiopulmonary effects of pulmonary venous hypertension, with special reference to pulmonary lymphatic flow. Circ. Res. 8:324, 1960.

90. Raghib, G., Ruttenberg, H. D., Anderson, R. C., Amplatz, K., Adams, P., Jr., and Edwards, J. E.: Termination of left superior vena cava in left atrium, atrial septal defect, and absence of coronary sinus. Circulation 31:906, 1965.

91. Randall, P. A., Moller, J. H., and Amplatz, K.: The spleen and congenital heart disease. Am. J. Roentgenol. Radium Ther. Nucl. Med. 119:551, 1973.

92. Rastelli, G. C., Ongley, P. A., and Kirklin, J. W.: Surgical correction of common atrium with anomalously connected persistent left superior vena cava: Report of case. Mayo Clin. Proc. 40:528, 1965.

93. Reye, R. D. K.: Congenital stenosis of the pulmonary veins in their extrapulmonary course. Med. J. Aust. 1:801, 1951.

94. Rischbieth, H.: Anomaly of the inferior vena cava: Duplication of the post-renal segment. J. Anat. 48:287, 1914.

95. Rossall, R. E., and Caldwell, R. A.: Obstruction of inferior vena cava by a persistent eustachian valve in a young adult. J. Clin. Pathol. 10:40, 1957.

96. Ruttenberg, H. D., Neufeld, H. N., Lucas, R. V., Jr., Carey, L. S., Adams, P., Jr., Anderson, R. C., and Edwards, J. E.: Syndrome of congenital cardiac disease with asplenia: Distinction from other forms of congenital cardiac disease. Am. J. Cardiol. 13:387, 1964.

97. Sahn, D. J., Allen, H. D., Lange, L. W., and Goldberg, S. J.: Cross sectional echocardiographic diagnosis of the sites of TAPV drainage. Circulation 60:1317, 1979.

98. Schölmerich, P., Stein, E., Klinner, W., and Zenker, R.: Transposition der unteren Hohlvene mit Zyanose und Linkshypertrophie. Verh. Deutsch. Ges. Kreislaufforsch. 28:321, 1962.

99. Sherman, F. E., and Bauersfeld, S. R.: Total, uncomplicated, anomalous pulmonary venous connection: Morphologic observations on 13 necropsy specimens from infants. Pediatrics 25:656, 1960.

100. Shone, J. D., Amplatz, M. D., Anderson, R. C., Adams, P., Jr., and Edwards, J. E.: Congenital stenosis of individual pulmonary veins. Circulation 26:574, 1962.

101. Silver, A. W., Kirklin, J. W., and Wood, E. H.: Demonstration of preferential flow of blood from inferior vena cava and from right pulmonary veins through experimental atrial septal defects in dogs. Circ. Res. 4:413, 1956.

102. Smith, B., Frye, T. R., and Newton, W. A., Jr.: Total anomalous pulmonary venous return: Diagnostic criteria and a new classification. Am. J. Dis. Child. 101:41, 1961.

103. Stackelberg, B., Lind, J., and Wegelius, C.: Absence of inferior vena cava diagnosed by angiocardiography. Cardiologia (Basel) 21:583, 1952.

104. Streeter, G. L.: Developmental horizons in human embryos. Description of age group XI, 13 to 20 somites, and age group XII, 21 to 29 somites. Carnegie Inst. Contrib. Embryol. 30(197):211, 1942.

105. Swan, H. J. C., Hetzel, P. S., Burchell, H. B., and Wood, E. H.: Relative contribution of blood from each lung to the left-to-right shunt in atrial septal defect. Circulation 14:200, 1956.

106. Swan, H. J. C., Hetzel, P. S., and Wood, E. H.: Quantitative estimation by indicator dilution techniques of the contribution of blood from each lung to the left-to-right shunt in atrial septal defect. Circulation 14:212, 1956.

107. Swan, H. J. C., Toscano-Barboza, E., and Wood, E. H.: Hemodynamic findings in total anomalous pulmonary venous drainage. Mayo Clin. Proc. 31:177, 1956.

108. Tajik, A. J., Gau, G. T., Ritter, D. G., and Schattenberg, T. T.: Echocardiographic pattern of right ventricular diastolic volume overload in children. Circulation 46:36, 1972.

109. Van Mierop, L. H. S., and Wiglesworth, F. W.: Isomerism of the cardiac atria in the asplenia syndrome. Lab. Invest. 11:1303, 1962.

110. Van Praagh, R., and Corsini, I.: Cor triatriatum: Pathologic anatomy and a consideration of morphogenesis based on 13 postmortem cases and a study of normal development of the pulmonary and atrial septum in 83 human embryos. Am. Heart J. 78:379, 1969.

111. Vazquez-Perez, J., Frontera-Izquierdo, P.: Anomalous drainage of the right superior vena cava into the left atrium as an isolated anomaly. Am. Heart J. 97:89, 1979.

112. Whight, C. M., Barratt-Boyes, B. G., Calder, A. L., Neutze, J. M., and Brandt, P. W. T.: TAPVC. Long term results following repair in infancy. J. Thorac. Cardiovasc. Surg. 75:52, 1978.

113. Winter, F. S.: Persistent left superior vena cava: Survey of world literature and report of thirty additional cases. Angiology 5:90, 1954.

114. Wood, P.: Diseases of the Heart and Circulation, 2nd ed. J. B. Lippincott, Philadelphia, 1956, p. 457.

115. Wukasch, D. C., Deutsch, M., Reul, G. J., Hallman, G. L., and Cooley, D. A.: Total anomalous pulmonary venous return. Ann. Thorac. Surg. 19:622, 1975.

30

Arteriovenous Fistulas

M. Quero Jiménez, M.D., and F. Acerete Guillén, M.D.

An arteriovenous fistula is an abnormal vascular structure that establishes a communication between an artery and a vein without the interposition of the capillary bed. There are two main groups, according to their location in the *systemic* or *pulmonary* circulation. Fistulas involving the coronary vessels constitute a special group, and are dealt with in Chapter 31.

SYSTEMIC FISTULAS

Systemic arteriovenous fistulas may be *congenital* or *acquired*. The persistence of modified vascular channels pertaining to the primitive capillary network, from which arteries and veins derive, forms the embryologic basis of the systemic arteriovenous fistulas. Important etiologic factors giving rise to acquired arteriovenous fistulas are: trauma, diagnostic puncture of vessels, atherosclerosis, and syphilis. Most arteriovenous fistulas in the pediatric age group are congenital.

PATHOLOGY

There are two groups of vascular anomalies[54] giving rise to an arteriovenous fistula: vascular channels communicating arterial and venous trunks; and angiomas, which owing to their relationships with arterial and venous branches, behave as an arteriovenous communication. They can be single or multiple. The afferent artery and the efferent vein become dilated and elongated, tortuous and coiled. The wall of the artery becomes thinner, and there is reduction in its elastic and muscular elements. This may result in the formation of aneurysms and the rupture of its wall.[22] A collateral circulation develops as a response to the diminution of the capillary blood flow. The vessels forming the fistula are dilated channels from capillary size upwards. The veins show arterialization and degenerative changes in their walls.

Most congenital systemic fistulas are located in the brain, neck, thoracic wall, heart, liver, and extremities. Occasionally several regions are involved. In some patients, the fistula is a manifestation of hemorrhagic hereditary telangiectasia[22, 52, 58, 79] This is a hereditary disorder characterized by a simple dominant type of transmission, affecting males and females equally. The elementary lesion is a small arteriovenous fistula, widespread throughout the skin, below the fingernails, lips, mucous membranes, liver, kidneys, and brain.[32, 47, 67]

Half of the cerebral fistulas involve the middle and posterior cerebral arteries, the vertebral artery, and the vein of Galen.[23, 26, 35, 41] However, other vessels may be involved. As the vein of Galen is usually very dilated, the flow of cerebrospinal fluid through the aqueduct of Sylvius may be hindered, giving rise to hydrocephalus.[22] Cerebellar arteriovenous fistulas are uncommon.[2]

Cervical fistulas are rare. In a reported case[57] the fistula affected the vertebral artery and the internal jugular vein. In one of our cases the vessels of the mandible were involved. Fistulas located proximal to the region of the aortic isthmus may be associated with preductal coarctation of the aorta, a fact probably related to the diminished blood flow through the aortic isthmus during embryonic life.[60]

Thoracic fistulas frequently involve the internal mammary artery.[45] The connection may be established with the mammary veins[3, 65] and the ductus venosus.[25, 66] Anomalous connections between the intercostal arteries and the azygous vein,[5] between the epicardial and pulmonary arteries,[29] and between the right subclavian artery and right iliac vein have been described.[1]

Hepatic fistulas are often multiple. They may be the local expression of the Rendu-Osler-Weber syndrome or part of a hemangioendothelioma of the liver.[35] The vascular structures of this tumor may be undifferentiated, which has created a controversy concerning its potential malignancy.[12] Anomalous communications between the hepatic artery and the ductus venosus are possible.[44]

Congenital arteriovenosus fistulas of the *extremities* are often associated with: hypertrophy and disfigurement of the involved extremity; cutaneous and subcutaneous hemangiomas; and hypertrophy or dystrophy of bones.[54]

PHYSIOLOGY

The main physiological derangement is the passage of blood from the artery to the vein. The amount of the blood shunted will depend on the size of the vessels involved, the size and length of the channels between them, and the situation of the fistula. The resulting diminished capillary blood flow is compensated by an increased cardiac output and the development of collateral circulation supplying the territory distal to the fistula.[23] The cardiac output increases due to tachycardia and an augmented stroke volume.[22, 33, 59] The latter results from diminished peripheral vascular resistance and, therefore, increased venous return.[35, 42, 80] The association of increased stroke volume and diminished peripheral resistance results in a wide pulse pressure. The increased venous return results in a volume overload of the heart and, sometimes, augmented central venous pressure, even in the presence of normal or increased myocardial contractility. The combination of rapid heart rate, wide pulse pressure, and increased cardiac output characterizes the hyperkinetic circulatory state. The association of an increased venous pressure with an increased cardiac output has been named high output heart failure.[42, 80] The hyperkinetic circulation and high output are maintained as long as the heart is able to cope with the volume overload. Otherwise, true cardiac failure, with a low cardiac output, appears.

The coronary blood flow is increased due to diminished resistances of the coronary circulation and increased myocardial oxygen consumption resulting from increased cardiac work.[59]

MANIFESTATIONS

In the pediatric age group, congenital arteriovenous fistulas may manifest themselves in the following ways: neonatal heart failure, hyperkinetic circulatory state, and local manifestations.

Neonatal Heart Failure

Fistulas located in the brain or in the liver are often large enough to cause heart failure in newborns.[13, 15, 26, 28, 33, 35, 60, 63, 76] The same may be provoked by fistulas located between the subclavian artery and the innominate vein,[78] the internal mammary artery and the ductus venosus,[25] the vertebral vessels,[49] and by multiple cutaneous and visceral hemangiomas.[12] Symptoms begin within the first month of life, mainly during the first days. Respiratory distress and vomiting are frequent. A central cyanosis appears in at least 70% of the cases.[55]

Cerebral arteriovenous fistulas affect males more frequently than females.[50] Peripheral pulses are bounding[22, 23, 41], unless they are in gross heart failure.[22, 41, 60] The bounding pulse is very prominent in the neck. This quality may be present only in the carotid vessels[41, 60] and not in the femoral arteries.[17]

The scalp and the skin of the neck and abdomen should be carefully examined for increased venous circulation, telangiectasias, and cutaneous angiomas, which may be associated with arteriovenous fistulas. A nodular hepatomegaly without signs of liver involvement suggests the possibility of hemangioendothelioma of the liver.[23] Systolic or continuous murmurs (Fig. 30.1C) caused by turbulent blood flow through the fistula may be heard over the region overlying the anomaly.[22, 23, 35, 72] This sign is neither constant nor pathognomonic. It may be absent during the first weeks of life,[22, 28] in the presence of heart failure,[41, 60] or in fistulas deeply situated in the brain. On the other hand, murmurs of congenital heart lesions may have good transmission to the skull.[23, 28, 35, 72] Fistulas which are superficially situated in the neck and thoracic wall give rise, however, to conspicuous continuous murmurs.[25, 78]

The heart is enlarged by palpation.[23, 60] Auscultation shows systolic murmurs, due to either tricuspid insufficiency or

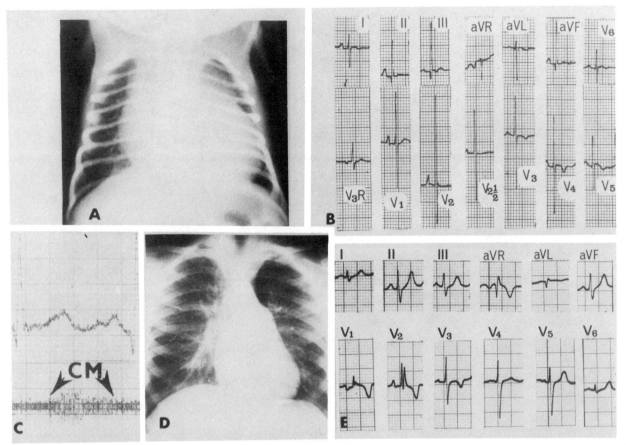

Fig. 30.1 (*A*) Chest x-ray of a newborn with a large cerebral fistula, showing cardiomegaly and pulmonary venous congestion. (*B*) Electrocardiogram of a newborn with a huge hepatic fistula 15 days old. Right atrial enlargement. T wave is positive in V_1 and negative in *I*, *aVL*, and V_3 to V_6. (*C*) Case of a newborn with a large fistula involving the medial cerebral arteries and the vein of Galen. Continuous murmur (*CM*) over left parietal region. (*D*) Chest x-ray of a case with a medium sized cerebral fistula revealing a prominent pulmonary artery. (*E*) Electrocardiogram of the same case. Shows right bundle branch block.

increased blood flow through the pulmonary and aortic valves.[22, 23] A third heart sound[23] or a gallop rhythm[22] may be present. There are two components in the second heart sound,[60] with the pulmonary one accentuated.

Convulsions, opisthotonus, and increased head size have been described as initial symptoms in newborns with cerebral fistulas.[22, 50]

Roentgenograms reveal generalized cardiomegaly and increased pulmonary circulation[22, 23, 35, 60] owing to pulmonary congestion and plethora (Fig. 30.1*A*). The electrocardiogram may show enlargement of the right heart cavities[23, 35, 41, 60] or biventricular hypertrophy.[23] In newborns with heart failure, the T wave in the left precordial leads may be negative during the first month of life (Fig. 30.1*B*).

Cardiac catheterization shows an important difference in the oxygen saturation between both venae cavae.[22, 41] The oxygen saturation is higher in the superior vena cava in fistulas located in the brain or in the neck. It is higher in the suprahepatic segment of the inferior vena cava when the fistula is situated in the liver or lower extremities.[23, 35] The oxygen saturation in the mixed venous blood and the cardiac output are, therefore, increased.[23] The pressure in the pulmonary artery is increased,[41] sometimes above systemic levels.[60] In cases with heart failure, the pulmonary wedge pressure is elevated.[35] In newborns it is not exceptional to find low arterial oxygen saturation, owing to a venoarterial shunt across the foramen ovale caused by pulmonary hypertension.[41, 60] A pressure gradient between the ascending and descending aorta has been encountered in one case of arte-

riovenous fistula of the brain.[17] Maneuvers aiming the catheter into the fistula are discouraged, because of the danger of rupture of the fistula's wall.[23]

Angiography shows dilatation, elongation, and tortuosity of the afferent arteries. When the fistula is located in the brain, the vein of Galen is clearly seen (Fig. 30.2) and there is an early opacification of the jugular veins and superior vena cava. When the draining vein is the longitudinal sinus, it is also clearly opacified (Fig. 30.2,*C* and *D*). Figure 30.3*A* and *B* shows the angiographic features in one case of multiple fistulas of the liver.

Hyperkinetic Circulatory State

Children with fistulas, where the volume of blood shunted through the anomaly is not sufficient to cause heart failure, may have a hyperkinetic circulatory state: tachycardia, bounding peripheral pulses, systolic murmur, and third heart sound.[80] These fistulas frequently involve the vessels located in the thoracic wall or in the neighboring structures. A few fistulas situated in the extremities[35, 70] and cerebral or hepatic fistulas may behave similarly. Local manifestations are usually present: a pulsatile mass, a thrill, and a continuous or systolic murmur over the fistulous region. Digital compression of the afferent vessel makes the murmur disappear and the heart rate slows down.[6, 48] This sign is more conspicuous in acquired fistulas. Chest roentgenogram may be normal[22] or show slight cardiomegaly. The aortic or pulmonary artery segments may be prominent (Fig. 30.1*D*). Electrocardiograms may be normal, or show right bundle branch block

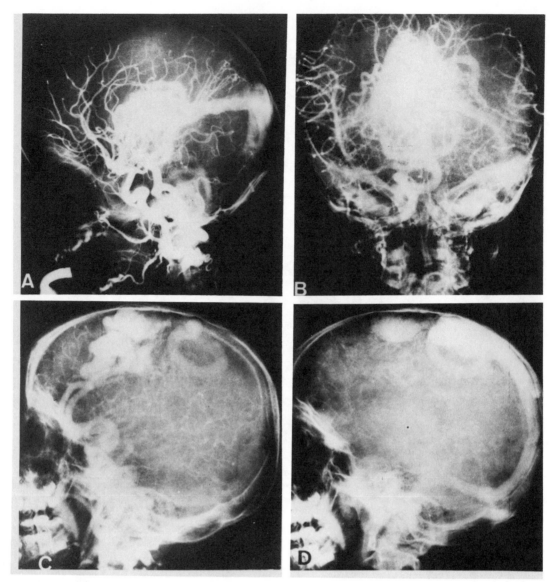

Fig. 30.2 (*A* and *B*) Large arteriovenous fistula located in the midline and fed by branches from anterior, middle, and posterior cerebral arteries. Venous drainage into the straight sinus. (*C* and *D*) Abnormal anterior cerebral arteries feeding an aneurysmal communication with the sagittal sinus. The latter forms a loop. (*A*, reproduced with permission from M. Quero Jiménez *et al.* and *Editorial Científico Médica*.

(Fig. 30.1*E*) or a moderate degree of left or biventricular hypertrophy.[23] Cardiac catheterization reveals normal pressures, a slight increase in the oxygen saturation in the corresponding venous collector, and a proportional increase in the cardiac output. Selective angiography is the procedure of choice to establish the diagnosis.[54]

Local Manifestations

Cutaneous angiomas, derangement in the growth of extremities, neurologic symptomatology, tendency to bleed, or discovery of a murmur may be the main manifestations in patients with small fistulas at various locations. Signs of increased local circulation (with or without swelling), bleeding and pain must arouse the suspicion of a fistula. Vomiting, headache, diplopia, seizures, paresthesias, and hemiparesis are common symptoms in patients with intracranial fistulas. Hematuria and hypertension may characterize fistulas involving the renal vessels.[14] Portal hypertension has been reported in cases with fistulas involving the vena porta.[69] During the first 3 months of life, a congenital hemangioma

may show profuse intratumural bleeding. Plasma fibrinogen and platelets are low, suggesting both being consumed within the hemangioma.[51]

DIFFERENTIAL DIAGNOSIS

Neonates with Heart Failure

In aortic atresia the second sound is single. The diagnosis may be very difficult in fistulas with severe heart failure, cyanosis, and very weak or absent peripheral pulses.

In preductal coarctation of the aorta, as well as in systemic fistulas, peripheral pulses may be strong in the neck and upper extremities and weak in the lower extremities. In both situations, chest x-ray may show cardiomegaly and increased pulmonary circulation. The discovery of a continuous murmur over the area of the fistula favors its diagnosis.

Total anomalous pulmonary venous connection with pulmonary venous obstruction characteristically shows a chest x-ray with a normal-sized cardiac shadow and a very typical pattern of pulmonary venous congestion, in contrast to the

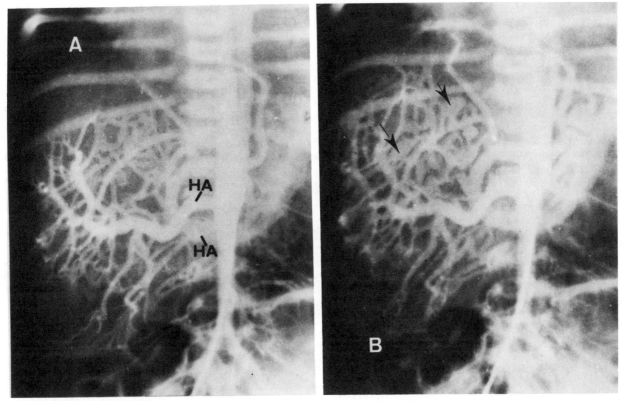

Fig. 30.3 (*A* and *B*) Aortogram of a case with an hemangioendothelioma of the liver. Note two separate hepatic arteries (*HA*) and an abnormal vascular pattern with multiple blood pools (*arrows*).

pattern of cardiomegaly and pulmonary plethora present in large fistulas. Heart failure is not so early in the same anomaly without pulmonary venous obstruction.

Congenital beriberi may mimic the clinical picture of large systemic fistulas. Babies with this disease dramatically improve with the intravenous injection of 10 mg of thiamine every 6 hours.[62]

Myocarditis and fibroelastosis have to be considered in the differential diagnosis, since there are cases of systemic fistulas showing inverted T waves in V_5–V_6 beyond the first week of life. Weak peripheral pulses and muffled heart sounds favor the diagnosis of myocardial disease.

Left to right shunts in premature babies may provoke early heart failure. Consequently they have to be considered in the differential diagnosis.

Other conditions giving rise to heart failure in newborns are: fetal hypoxemia; respiratory distress syndrome; fetal to fetal transfusion; mother to fetal transfusion; hypoglycemia; and the metabolic derangements of babies of diabetic mothers.

Children with Hyperkinetic Circulatory State

There is no problem in differentiating arteriovenous fistulas from fever and anemia, which are the two main causes giving rise to a hyperkinetic circulatory state in infancy and childhood. Left to right shunts in children usually have specific murmurs allowing their recognition.[23] Otherwise, chest x-ray and electrocardiograms of some patients with systemic fistulas may closely resemble those of patients with a moderate left to right shunt. In this regard, the chest x-ray and electrocardiogram of patient D. P. (Fig. 30.1*D* and *E*) are similar to the ones usually encountered in atrial septal defect.

Other Manifestations

Patent ductus arteriosus and fistulas of the coronary vessels have to be differentiated from cases of systemic fistulas involving the vessels of the chest wall. In these situations, the presence of a continuous murmur over the chest wall may be the sole abnormality. The superficial nature and high pitch quality of the murmur are common to fistulas involving the vessels of the thoracic wall and to those affecting the coronary vessels. The continuous murmur produced by a patent ductus arteriosus is well localized in both pulmonary and the left subclavicular areas. When the murmur is heard away from these areas the diagnosis of arteriovenous fistula must be suspected.

Children with systemic fistulas, in whom the main manifestations are neurological, present very specific differential diagnostic problems which lie beyond the scope of this book. The same happens with cases whose manifestations are hematuria, systemic hypertension, or portal hypertension.

TREATMENT AND COURSE

Most of the patients with large cerebral arteriovenous fistulas die in the neonatal period, due to cardiac failure or neurologic complications (convulsions and intracranial hemorrhage).[41, 60] In the few patients overcoming this phase, hydrocephalus, mental retardation, and intracranial hemorrhage may occur. Hepatic fistulas also succumb frequently to heart failure during the neonatal period.[41] A spontaneous regression with improvement and even cure is possible.[10] The treatment of cerebral fistulas by the ligation or clipping of afferent arteries is difficult and of questionable result.[22, 41, 60] The outcome has been surprisingly good in one of our patients in whom, 5 years after the operation, the hyperkinetic circulation and the murmurs had completely disappeared. Surgical treatment is impossible in most cases of hepatic fistulas because they are small and widespread throughout the organ. Radiotherapy has been used with some hope.[41] Excellent results have been reported with corticosteroids.[27, 73] Surgery is feasible in fistulas involving the vessels of the neck and thoracic wall, due to their accessibility and limited nature. Embolization of the feeding arteries has been applied with success, as well.[20]

Three kinds of surgical procedures have been proposed for fistulas of the extremities.[43] (a) Radical operations eliminate the arteriovenous shunt and the angiomatous formations, preserving the systemic vessels and other important structures. They are indicated in localized fistulas, in forms with visible anastomotic foci, and in angiomas located in muscular regions. Limited amputations may be indicated in cirsoid aneurysms of the hand and foot. (b) Hemodynamic operations diminish the flow of blood to the fistula by interrupting the afferent arteries. They are indicated in extensive fistulas and angiomas in which a radical excision is impossible. (c) Complementary measures such as varicectomy, sclerotherapy, radiotherapy, and elastic bandage are of great utility, both alone and associated with surgery. A complete cure is not always obtained with these operations. Recurrences are common. Nevertheless, a satisfactory result was obtained in 72% of 43 operated patients in a recent review.[43]

PULMONARY FISTULAS

The origin of pulmonary arteriovenous fistulas is almost always congenital, although there exists the possibility of this disease being acquired,[34] due to schistosomiasis,[39] juvenile hepatic cirrhosis,[61] metastatic carcinoma of the thyroid,[53] or trauma. When congenital, its origin seems to be the abnormal development of pulmonary arteries and veins in a common vascular complex.[47] A special type of pulmonary arteriovenous fistula is the direct communication between the right pulmonary artery and the left atrium. Its embryologic origin seems to be an abnormal connection between a pulmonary arteriovenous fistula and the left atrium.[21, 40, 46] It is an uncommon malformation.

PATHOLOGY

This anomaly is a complex malformation, in which a variable number of pulmonary arteries of different sizes connect, without the interposition of the pulmonary capillary bed, with a variable number of pulmonary veins.

The pulmonary fistula is a sacciform vascular structure in direct communication with branches of pulmonary arteries and pulmonary veins.[74] Both vessels are tortuous and dilated. The wall of the artery is thinner and that of the vein thicker than normal.[18, 22, 37, 74, 77] The aneurysmal sac has a rounded morphology. Its interior may be partially occupied by thrombus.[74, 77] In cavernous angiomas, the aneurysmal sac is divided by septa in multiple compartments. The name of cirsoid aneurysm refers to a simple continuation of the arteries into the veins.[74] Simple fistulas are those in which arteries and veins are communicated side by side by a simple connection.[74]

The thickness and structure of the wall of the aneurysm varies from place to place. In some areas the wall is reduced to an endothelial layer[32, 47]; in others it shows degenerative changes[23, 24, 77] and even calcification.[74] These changes are responsible for the occasional rupture of the aneurysm,[32, 47, 77] which, in turn, may give rise to hemosiderosis of the lung[77] and hemothorax. Although in some cases areas of atelectasis have been described,[74] alterations of the lung tissue around

the fistula are very scarce, suggesting a slow growth of the anomaly.

The dimensions of these anomalies vary between 1 mm in diameter and those of one entire lung.[22, 23, 31, 74] They are single or multiple, unilateral or bilateral.[18, 47, 72] Small lesions tend to be widespread throughout the entire lung. Larger fistulas are less numerous and most commonly located in the subpleural regions of both lower lobes and the middle right lobe.[4, 18, 37, 47, 74, 77] Lesions of different sizes may coexist in the same individual.[77]

In some cases, the fistula receives, in addition to the pulmonary artery blood supply, systemic arterial branches coming either from the aorta, or from the intercostal, pericardiophrenic, or internal mammary arteries.[4, 72, 74] When the arterial supply to the fistula exclusively derives from the systemic circulation, the name of systemic-pulmonary arterioarterial fistula is more appropriate.[16]

About 60% of patients with pulmonary arteriovenous fistulas have an associated Rendu-Osler-Weber syndrome.[4, 18, 23, 32, 47, 52, 58, 68, 74, 79] This association is more common when the fistulas are multiple.[4] Other lesions which have been described in association with pulmonary fistulas are: bronchiectasis and other malformations of the bronchial tree,[8, 74] absence of the right lower lobe,[40] and congenital heart disease.[71]

PHYSIOLOGY

The essential physiologic disturbance is the shunt of venous blood from the pulmonary arteries to the pulmonary veins, which results in arterial oxygen unsaturation. The volume of the shunt varies between 18 and 89%.[21, 22, 47] The systemic arterial blood saturation ranges between 50 and 85%.[22, 47] As ventilation is not impaired, arterial PCO_2 is kept within normal levels. The rapid pulmonary circulation may be demonstrated by contrast echocardiography and radioisotopes.[38]

The pulmonary blood flow[47] and pressure[21, 22] remain unchanged. Exceptional cases with volume overload of the left heart have been reported.[30] Most cases develop polycythemia in response to the arterial hypoxemia. As a consequence, the total blood volume is increased at the expense of its cellular element.[47] The cardiac output is normal.[21] The lack of the filter function of the lung makes easier the passage of bacteria to the systemic circulation. The development of brain abscess is, therefore, a possible complication.

MANIFESTATIONS

Clinical Features

Pulmonary arteriovenous fistulas affect equally both sexes. Cyanosis is almost always present since childhood[18, 21, 22, 32, 36, 47, 74] and occasionally since birth.[30] Some cases may be acyanotic. A progressive increase in cyanosis has been reported.[19, 37] This is attributed to an increase in the fistula's size, opening of latent fistulas,[47] and development of secondary polycythemia. Dyspnea on effort, of a moderate degree, due to hypoxemia may be present.[22, 23, 36, 74] An abnormal roentgenologic shadow can be the only finding in acyanotic patients.

In 25% of the patients,[36] neurologic symptoms (convulsions, speech disorders, diplopia, transitory numbness, etc.) may dominate the clinical picture. Responsible factors for this are: brain abscess,[32, 36, 37] hypoxemia, polycythemia, thrombosis of small vessels,[36, 72] and repeated hemorrhages originating in the telangiectatic lesions in the brain.[72]

Personal or family symptomatology related to hereditary hemorrhagic telangiectasis (nosebleeds, hemoptysis, hematuria, and vaginal or gastrointestinal hemorrhage) has been obtained in 35 to 50% of the patients.[4, 18, 22, 24, 31, 36, 47, 72] Hemoptysis is due either to telangiectatic lesions of the bronchial mucosa, or to the rupture of the fistula. It may be slight, intermittent, relapsing, or frank and even fatal.[36, 72] Pulmonary fistulas may be present in more than one member of the family.[47] Thoracic pain is a prominent symptom in patients in whom the rupture of a fistula located in subpleural region of the lung has given rise to a hemothorax.[32, 37, 71] Endocarditis may complicate the fistula.[22, 37] A few patients remain completely asymptomatic.[36]

Cyanosis and clubbing are common.[22, 32, 36, 72] They are less obvious in patients with hereditary hemorrhagic telangiectasis who have anemia, due to repeated blood loss.[32, 72] Arterial pulse and precordial palpation are normal. Increased amplitude of the peripheral pulses and hyperactivity of the precordium were reported in a newborn with a huge pulmonary arteriovenous fistula.[30]

Careful auscultation of the entire thoracic wall[23, 74] shows a faint[37] systolic or continuous murmur[64] over a limited area overlying the fistula[22, 74] in about 50% of the patients. Only in one patient,[30] the continuous murmur was louder than grade 3/6. Very small lesions,[32, 68] or those deeply situated inside the thoracic cavity[46] do not give rise to audible murmurs. Pure diastolic murmurs are exceptional.[47] The intensity of the murmur increases during inspiration and diminishes during expiration.[22, 23, 36, 68]

Lesions of hereditary hemorrhagic telangiectasis associated with a pulmonary arteriovenous fistula may be absent in infants and young children.[30]

Radiologic Features

The size of the heart shadow is usually normal.[18, 22, 23, 37, 47, 72, 74] Cardiomegaly is only present when the fistula is very large.[18, 30, 37] There are no significant alterations in the configuration of the cardiac silhouette.[22, 23, 37, 47, 72, 74]

In 50% of the cases,[23, 47] the frontal and lateral chest x-ray films[23, 68, 72, 74] show one or more rounded opacities, of variable size, in one or both lung fields (Fig. 30.4A and B).[18, 32, 47, 68] The afferent and efferent vessels may be seen as a strand-like opacity going from the fistula to the hilum.[18, 32, 37, 47, 68, 74] Calcification of the fistula is uncommon.[68] A pleural effusion may be present.[32, 47] Costal erosion, due to enlargement of the intercostal arteries, is uncommon.[37, 74] A rounded opacity adjacent to the right posterior border of the heart silhouette may be seen in cases of direct communication between the right pulmonary artery and the left atrium (Fig. 30.4A and B). Tomography may help to localize the radiologic features described above.[72, 74] Fluoroscopy shows the pulsatility of the mass[72, 74] and its enlargement with the Valsalva's maneuver.[36, 37, 47, 68, 74]

Electrocardiographic Features

The electrocardiogram is usually normal. Left axis deviation and left ventricular enlargement have been reported in one case with a huge pulmonary arteriovenous fistula[30] and in another one with a direct communication between the right pulmonary artery and the left atrium.[40] Left atrial and ventricular hypertrophy have been encountered as well (Fig. 30.5C and D).[55]

CARDIAC CATHETERIZATION

There is a decrease in systemic arterial oxygen saturation, which is detected in samples obtained in the left atrium[72] or in the involved pulmonary vein. Maneuvers aiming to catheterize the fistula should be avoided because of the danger of rupture of its wall.[23] The pressures and the cardiac output are normal.[21, 23, 74] Nevertheless, the pressure in the pulmonary artery on some occasions has been reported to be lower than normal,[23] a fact that could be due to a diminution of the vascular resistance in the region of the fistula. The hematocrit and hemoglobin values are usually higher than normal. Dye dilution studies have been used to localize and quantify the shunt.[7]

ANGIOCARDIOGRAPHY

Since the first clinical diagnosis of this anomaly was made by Smith and Horton[64] in 1939, angiocardiography has been considered to be the optimal means to recognize the anomaly.[9, 22] The injection of contrast material into the appropriate pulmonary artery will show the fistula, the dilated, elongated, and tortuous afferent and efferent vessels, the early opacification of the left atrium, and the scarce opacification of the uninvolved lung.[18, 36, 56] It may also reveal other smaller lesions which had not been visualized in plain roentgenograms (Figs. 30.4C and D, and 30.5B).[72, 74]

An aortogram is necessary to discover a possible systemic arterial supply.[23] Angiocardiography may fail to show the lesions when they are very small. In these cases, the diagnosis could be made by radioisotopes and, if necessary, by a biopsy of the lung.[11]

DIFFERENTIAL DIAGNOSIS

The diagnosis of pulmonary arteriovenous fistula should be considered in: relatively asymptomatic, cyanotic patients, with normal heart sounds, a chest roentgenogram showing a normal heart, and a normal electrocardiogram; acyanotic patients coming to consultation because of the discovery of abnormal opacities in the lung fields; and symptomatic newborns with cardiac enlargement, left axis deviation, left ventricular hypertrophy, and abnormal shadows in the lung fields.[30] In any of these situations, the diagnosis of a pulmonary arteriovenous fistula is favored by the presence of: hereditary hemorrhagic telangiectatic lesions; a faint continuous murmur over the thoracic wall; the roentgenologic alterations of the lung fields described above; and persistent low arterial oxygen content.

Other conditions giving rise to cyanosis without modifications in the heart sounds, cardiac silhouette, and electrocardiogram have been thoroughly summarized.[22] These are all sorts of anomalous connections of the venae cavae with the left atrium, acquired and congenital metahemoglobinemia, and polycythemia. Anomalous connection of the venae cavae with the left atrium is rarely an isolated anomaly and its diagnosis is obtained by angiocardiography. The ingestion of food or water which are rich in nitrates or other toxic agents (anilines, phenacetins, acetanilides, sulfonamides, etc.) is in favor of the diagnosis of acquired metahemoglobinemia. The tests with methylene blue and ascorbic acid, and the study of the spectrography of the hemoglobin are definite in proving the diagnosis of metahemoglobinemia. The arterial oxygen saturation is normal in the different forms of polycythemia which are not secondary to hypoxemia.

Hepatic cirrhosis,[61] metastatic carcinoma of the thyroid,[53] and pulmonary schistosomiasis[39] are conditions which may be accompanied by the development of acquired arteriovenous fistulas. Patients suffering from these conditions will show, in addition to cyanosis, all the other symptoms derived from the main disease.

Tuberculosis, coccidioidomycosis, histoplasmosis, tumors of the lung,[22, 23, 74] and isolated varicose dilatations of the

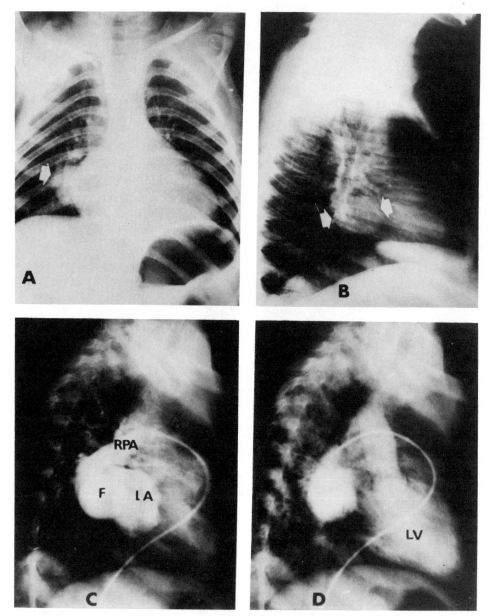

Fig. 30.4 (*A* and *B*) A case with a direct communication between the right pulmonary artery and the left atrium. Chest x-ray. Rounded opacity (*arrows*) adjacent to the right posterior heart border. (*C* and *D*) Angiography into the right pulmonary artery (*RPA*) with immediate filling of the fistula (*F*), left atrium (*LA*), and left ventricle (*LV*). (Reproduced with permission from M. Quero Jiménez *et al.* and *Editorial Cientifico Médica.*)

pulmonary veins[30] have to be considered in the differential diagnosis of patients in whom the main complaint is an abnormal pulmonary opacity in a chest roentgenogram. Selective angiography will determine whether pulmonary arteriovenous fistulas are present.

TREATMENT AND COURSE

Most of the patients with pulmonary arteriovenous fistulas remain asymptomatic during infancy and childhood.[22] Beyond this age, the frequency of fatal complications is high enough to make one seriously consider surgical treatment. Rupture of the aneurysm,[23, 36] massive hemorrhage,[23, 32] endocarditis,[23] and cerebral abscess[18, 22, 23, 36, 40, 56, 74, 77] are important complications frequently leading to the patient's death. It seems, therefore, reasonable to state that all symp-

tomatic patients with pulmonary fistulas should be operated upon.[22, 56, 72] An exception are those patients, in whom the lesions are small and widespread throughout both lungs.[11] A zero mortality rate has been reported in a recent review of the problem.[56]

The surgical technique should aim at the removal of the lesions, trying to preserve as much healthy lung tissue as possible.[4, 56, 74] Dissection and division of the afferent pulmonary artery and resection of the aneurysm is the procedure of choice for those instances where there is communication of the right pulmonary artery with the left atrium.[21, 46] The segmental resection consists in the isolation and division of the segmental artery, vein, and bronchus and the removal of the involved pulmonary segment. It is a safe procedure, easier than the previous one, but it has the disadvantage of removing uninvolved lung tissue.[56] The endoaneurysmorrha-

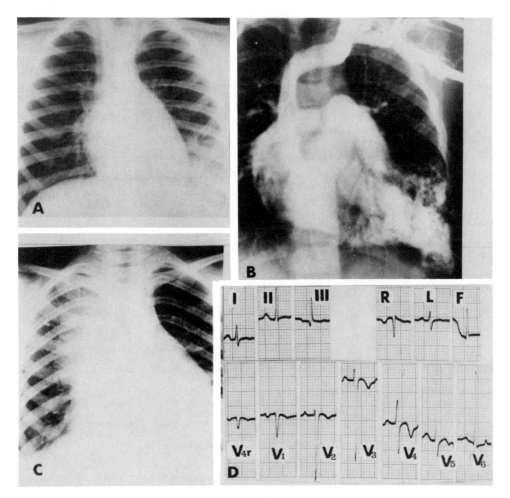

Fig. 30.5 (A) Ill-defined opacity with nondescriptive pattern in the lower lobe. (B) Venous angiocardiography of same case. Dilated left pulmonary artery filling a complicated network of vessels. (C) Chest x-ray of a case with a systemicopulmonary cirsoid fistula located in the right upper lobe. Opacity in right upper lobe, moderate cardiomegaly, prominent aortic arch, and right pleural effusion. (D) Electrocardiogram of same cases. Shows enlargement of left heart cavities.

phy with temporary ischemia is also a good method which has been used with good results.[4, 56] Lobectomy or pneumectomy should be reserved for cases in which the previous operations are not feasible.[31, 56] The simple ligature of the afferent artery should be avoided, since the posterior development of new collateral arteries feeding the aneurysm reproduces a situation which is very similar to the preoperative one.[56] The obliteration of the aneurysm with iron perchloride was used by the first surgeon who operated upon a patient with a pulmonary arteriovenous aneurysm.[75]

REFERENCES

1. Atwood, G. F., King, T. D., Graham, T. P., Jr., Canent, R. V., Jr., Ebert, F. A., and Spach, M. S.: Thoracic arteriovenous fistula. Am. J. Dis. Child. 129:233, 1975.
2. Baird, W. F., and Stitt, D. G.: Arteriovenous aneurysm of the cerebellum in a premature infant: Report of a case. Pediatrics 24:455, 1959.
3. Boontje, A. H., and Kruyswijk, H. H.: Arteriovenous fistula of the internal mammary vessels. J. Thorac. Cardiovasc. Surg. 62:618, 1971.
4. Bosher, L. H., Blake, A., and Byrd, B. R.: An analysis of the pathologic anatomy of pulmonary arteriovenous aneurysms with particular reference to the applicability of local excision. Surgery 45:91, 1959.
5. Bouhour, J. B., Dupon, H., Nicolas, G., Godin, J. F., and Horeau, J.: Fistule artérioveineuse systémique congénitale: Cause inhabituelle de souffle continu thoracique. Arch. Mal. Coeur 67:345, 1974.
6. Branham, H. H.: Aneurysmal varix of the femoral artery and vein, following a gunshot wound. Int. J. Surg. 3:250, 1890.
7. Callahan, J. A., Helmholtz, H. F., and Kirklin, J. W.: Pulmonary arteriovenous fistula located by indicator dilution studies. Am. Heart J. 52:916, 1956.
8. Caralps, A., and Martinez Bordíu, C.: Adenomas de los bronquios y fistulas arteriovenosas del pulmón. Editorial Paz Montalvo, Madrid, 1953.
9. Castellanos, A., García, C., Rodríguez Díaz, A., *et al.*: Intern. de Chir. 10:223, 1950.
10. Clatworthy, H. W., Boles, E. T., and Newton, W. A.: Primary tumors of the liver in infants and children. Arch. Dis. Child. 35:22, 1960.
11. Cooley, D. A., and McNamara, D. G.: Pulmonary telangiectasis: Report of a case proved by pulmonary biopsy. J. Thorac. Surg. 27:614, 1954.
12. Cooper, A. G., and Bolande, R. P.: Multiple hemangiomas in an infant with cardiac hypertrophy: Post mortem angiography demonstrations of the arteriovenous fistulae. Pediatrics 35:27, 1965.
13. Corrin, B.: Three cases of intracranial vascular malformation in infants. J. Clin. Pathol. 12:412, 1959.
14. Crummey, A. B., Atkinson, R. J., and Caruthers, S. B.: Congenital renal arteriovenous fistulas. J. Urol. 93:24, 1965.
15. Cunliffe, P. N.: Cerebral arteriovenous aneurysm presenting with heart failure: Report of three cases. Br. Heart J. 36:919, 1974.
16. Davilea, J. C., Hamilton, G. B., and Charbonneau, A.: Systemic-pulmonary arterioarterial fistula. Arch. Surg. 76:496, 1958.
17. Deverall, P. B., Taylor, J. F. N., Sturrock, G. S., and Aberdeen, E.: Coarctation-like physiology with cerebral arterio-venous fistula. Pediatrics 44:1024, 1969.
18. Edwards, J. E., Carey, L. A., Neufeld, H. N., and Lester, R. G.: Congenital Heart Disease: Correlation of Pathologic Anatomy and Angiocardiography. W. B. Saunders, Philadelphia, 1965, p. 648.
19. Espino Vela, J., Anselmi, G., *et al.* Fistula arteriovenosa pulmonar congenita. Arch. Inst.

Cardiol. Mex. 30:245, 1960.
20. Fabiani, J. N., Mercier, J. N., Ribierre, M.: Traitement pour embolisation d'une fistule arterioveineuse vertebrale congenitale. Arch. Fr. Pediatr. 36:34, 1979.
21. Friedlich, A., Bing, R. J., and Blount, S. G., Jr.: Physiologic studies in congenital heart disease. IX. Bull. Johns Hopkins Hosp. 86:20, 1950.
22. Fyler, D. C.: Arteriovenous fistulas. In Heart Disease in Infants, Children and Adolescents, edited by A. J. Moss and F. H. Adams. Williams & Wilkins, Baltimore, 1968, p. 728.
23. Gasul, B., Arcilla, R., and Lev, M.: Heart Disease in Children: Diagnosis and Treatment. Pittman Publishing Company and J. B. Lippincott, London and Philadelphia, 1966, pp. 442 and 459.
24. Giampalmo, A.: The arteriovenous angiomatosis of the lung with hypoxaemia. Acta Med. Scand. 139(Suppl. I), 1950.
25. Glass, H., Rowe, R. D., and Duckworth, J. W. A.: Congenital arteriovenous fistula between the left internal mammary artery and the ductus venosus: An unusual cause of congestive heart failure in the newborn infant. Pediatrics. 26:604, 1960.
26. Glatt, B. S., and Rowe, R. D.: Cerebral arteriovenous fistula associated with congestive heart failure in the newborn: Report of two cases. Pediatrics 26:596, 1960.
27. Goldberg, S. J., and Fonkalsrud, E.: Successful treatment of hepatic hemangioma with corticosteroids. J.A.M.A. 208:2473, 1969.
28. Gómez, M. R., Whitten, C. F., Nolke, A., Bernstein, J., and Meyer, J. S.: Aneurysmal malformation of the great vein of Galen causing heart failure in early infancy: Report of five cases. Pediatrics 21:400, 1963.
29. Greenberg, B. H., Stasikowski, J. J., Harrison, C. E., Jr., and McGoon, D. C.: Epicardial artery-pulmonary artery fistula. Presentation as a continuous precordial murmur. Am. J. Cardiol. 22:893, 1968.
30. Hall, R. J., Nelson, W. P. Blake, H. A., and Geiger, J. P.: Massive pulmonary arteriovenous fistula in the newborn. A correctable form of "cyanotic heart disease": An additional cause of polycythemia. Circulation 31:762, 1965.
31. Hepburn, J., and Dauphinée, J. A.: Successful removal of hemangioma of the lung followed by the disappearance of polycythemia. Am. J. Med. Sci. 204:681, 1942.
32. Hodgson, C. H., Burchell, H. B., Good, C. A., and Clagett, O. T.: Hereditary hemorrhagic telangiectasia and pulmonary arteriovenous fistula: Survey of a large family. N. Engl. J. Med. 261:625, 1959.
33. Holman, E.: The physiology of an arteriovenous fistula. Arch. Surg. 7:64, 1922.
34. Jiménez Díaz, C.: Rev. Clin. Esp. 44:41, 1952. Quoted in reference 56.
35. Kaplan, S.: Pulmonary arteriovenous fistula and systemic arteriovenous fistula. In Paediatric Cardiology, edited by H. Watson. C. V. Mosby, St. Louis, 1968, p. 316 and 320.
36. Keith, J. D., Rowe, R., and Mehrizi, A.: Heart Disease in Infancy and Childhood, 2nd ed. MacMillan, New York, 1967, p. 888.
37. LeRoux, B. T.: Pulmonary arteriovenous fistulae. Q. J. Med. 28:1, 1959.
38. Lewis, A., Gates, G., and Stanley, P. H.: Echocardiography and perfusion scintigraphy in the diagnosis of pulmonary arteriovenous fistula. Chest 73:675, 1978.
39. Lopes de Faria, J.: Pulmonary arteriovenous fistulas and arterial distribution of eggs of Schistosoma mansoni. Am. J. Trop. Med. Hyg.

5:860, 1956.
40. Lucas, R. V., Jr., Lund, G. W., and Edwards, J. E.: Direct communication of a pulmonary artery with the left atrium: An unusual variant of the pulmonary arteriovenous fistula. Circulation 24:1409, 1961.
41. Lucet, Ph.: Fistules artério-veineuses systémiques. In Précis de Cardiologie de l'Enfant, edited by R. Gérard and E. Louchet. Masson et Cíe., Paris, 1973, p. 428.
42. MacMichael, J.: Circulatory failure studies by means of venous catheterization. Adv. Int. Med. 2:64, 1947.
43. Malan, E.: The treatment of congenital arteriovenous fistulas of the limbs. J. Cardiovasc. Surg. 2:433, 1961.
44. Martin, L. W., Benzing, G., and Kaplan, S.: Congenital intrahepatic arteriovenous fistula. Ann. Surg. 161:209, 1965.
45. Massumi, R. A.: Internal mammary arteriovenous fistulas. Med. Ann. D.C. 36:163, 1967.
46. Moreno, F., Quero, M., Pérez, V., and Alvarez, F.: Direct communication of a pulmonary artery with the left atrium. Bull. Am. Coll. Chest Physicians 14:39, 1975.
47. Moyer, J. H., Glantz, G., and Brest, A. N.: Pulmonary arteriovenous fistulas. Am. J. Med. 32:417, 1962.
48. Nicoladoni, C.: Phlebarteriectasie der rechten oberen Extremität. Arch. Klin. Chir. 18:252, 1875.
49. Norman, J. A., Schmidt, K. W., and Grow, J. B.: Congenital arteriovenous fistula of the cervical vertebral vessels with heart failure in an infant. J. Pediatr. 36:598, 1950.
50. Olivecrona, H., and Riives, J.: Arteriovenous aneurysms of brain: Their diagnosis and treatment. Arch. Neurol. Psychiatry 59:567, 1948.
51. Oski, F. A., and Noriman, J. L.: Hematologic problems in the newborn. Major Problems in Clinical Pediatrics, Vol. 4. W. B. Saunders, Philadelphia, 1966, p. 221.
52. Osler, W.: On family form of recurring epistaxis, associated with multiple telangiectasis of skin and mucous membranes. Bull. Johns Hopkins Hosp. 12:333, 1901.
53. Pierce, J. A., Reagan, W. P., and Kimball, R. W.: Unusual cases of pulmonary arteriovenous fistulas, with a note of thyroid carcinoma as a cause. N. Engl. J. Med. 260:901, 1959.
54. Puglionisi, A.: Congenital arterio-venous fistulae of the limbs: Classification and anatomoclinical forms. J. Cardiovasc. Surg. (Suppl.) 7th Congress International Vascular Society Philadelphia, 1965, p. 231.
55. Quero Jiménez, M., Acerete Guillén, F., and Castro Gussoni, M. C.: Arteriovenous fistulas. In Heart Disease in Infants, Children and Adolescents, 2nd ed., edited by A. J. Moss, F. H. Adams, and G. C. Emmanouilides. Williams & Wilkins, Baltimore, 1977, pp. 470–482.
56. Quijano Pitman, F.: Fístulas arteriovenosas del pulmón. Arch. Inst. Cardiol. Mex. 44:4, 1974.
57. Rashkind, R., Weiss, S. R., and Doria, A.: Non traumatic fistula, cervical portion vertebral artery-internal jugular vein. Vasc. Surg. 1:221, 1967.
58. Rendu, H.: Epistaxis répétée chez un sujet porteur de petit angiomes cutanés et muqueaux. Bull. Mem. Soc. Med. d'Hôp. Paris 13:731, 1896.
59. Rowe, G. G., Castillo, C. A., Alfonso, S., and Crumpton, C. W.: The systemic and coronary hemodynamic effect of arteriovenous fistulas. Am. Heart J. 64:44, 1962.
60. Row, R., and Mehrizi, A.: The neonate with congenital heart disease. W. B. Saunders, Philadelphia, 1968, p. 374.
61. Rydell, R., and Hoffbauer, F. W.: Multiple

pulmonary arteriovenous fistulas in juvenile cirrhosis. Am. J. Med. 21:450, 1956.
62. Schaffer, A. J.: Diseases of the Newborn. W. B. Saunders, Philadelphia, 1960, p. 713.
63. Silverman, B. K., Breckx, T., Craig, J., and Nadas, A. S.: Congestive failure in the newborn caused by cerebral A-V fistula. Am. J. Cardiol. 24:414, 1969.
64. Smith, H. L., and Horton, B. T.: Arteriovenous fistula of lung associated with polycythemia vera: Report of a case in which diagnosis was made clinically. Am. Heart J. 18:589, 1939.
65. Stafford, R. V., Kronenberg, M. W., Dunbar, J. D., and Wooley, C. F.: Continuous precordial murmurs due to internal mammary artery fistulas. Including internal mammary to pulmonary artery fistulas. Am. J. Cardiol. 24:414, 1969.
66. Stanford, W., Fixler, D. E., Armstrong, R. G., Lindberg, E. F., and Johnson, R. H.: Congenital arteriovenous fistula between the left internal mammary artery and the ductus venosus: A case report. J. Thorac. Cardiovasc. Surg. 60:248, 1970.
67. Steinberg, I., Miscall, B., and Vogel, F. S.: Pulmonary arteriovenous fistula associated with capillary telangiectasia (Rendu-Osler-Weber disease): Report of a case illustrating use of metal casting for demonstrating the lesion. J. Thorac. Cardiovasc. Surg. 35:517, 1958.
68. Steinberg, I.: Diagnosis and surgical treatment of pulmonary arterio-venous fistulas: A report of three cases and a review of nineteen consecutive cases. Surg. Clin. North Am. 41:523, 1961.
69. Stone, H. H., Jordan, W. D., Acker, J. J., and Martin, J. D.: Portal arterio-venous fistulas. Review and case report. Am. J. Surg. 109:191, 1955.
70. Szilagyi, D. E., Elliott, J. P., DeRusso, F. J., and Smith, R. F.: Peripheral congenital arteriovenous fistulas. Surgery 57:61, 1965.
71. Taiana, J. A., Schiappati, E., and Pini, A.: Arteriovenous fistula of lung: Surgical treatment of 2 cases. Ann. Surg. 141:417, 1955.
72. Taussig, H. B.: Congenital Malformations of the Heart, 2nd ed. Commonwealth Fund, New York, 1960, p. 364.
73. Toulokian, R. J.: Hepatic hemangioendothelioma during infancy: Pathology, diagnosis and treatment with prednisone. Pediatrics 45:71, 1970.
74. Tricot, R., and Vernant, P.: Les angiomes pulmonaires. In Cardiopathies Congénitales, edited by P. Soulié. L'Expansion Scientifique Française, Paris, 1956, pp. 374–383.
75. Tufier, T.: Bull. Mem. Soc. Chir. Paris 34:897, 1908. Quoted in reference 56.
76. Vinh, L.T., Rivron, Obaldía, A. G., Canlorbe, P., and Lelong, M.: Hémangiome multi-nodulaire cardiaque progressive et mortelle. Démonstration de la fistule artério-veineuse intra-hépatique. Arch. Fr. Pédiatr. 16:808, 1959.
77. Wagenvoort, C. A., Heath, D., and Edwards, J. E.: The pathology of the pulmonary vasculature. Charles C Thomas, Springfield, Ill., 1964, pp. 441.
78. Walker, W. J. Mullins, C. E., and Knovich, G. C.: Cyanosis, cardiomegaly, and weak pulse manifestation of massive congenital systemic arteriovenous fistula. Circulation 29:777, 1964.
79. Weber, F. P.: Multiple hereditary developmental angiomata (telangiectasis) of the skin and mucous membranes associated with recurring hemorrhages. Lancet 2:160, 1907.
80. Wood, P.: Diseases of the heart and the circulation, 2nd ed. Eyre and Spottiswoode, London, 1962, p. 897.

31

Abnormalities and Diseases of the Coronary Vessels

Paul R. Lurie, M.D., and Masato Takahashi, M.D.

EMBRYOLOGY

The hearts of very young mammalian embryos have no coronary circulation. Like the adult hearts of primitive vertebrates, their loosely interwoven muscle fibers are bathed in the blood which they pump. During development, the myocardium condenses, and the spaces between muscle strands disappear or remain as flattened sinusoids. Veins, arteries, and capillaries grow in, connecting with the sinusoids. In the 7th week human embryo, shortly after the aorta has been partitioned from the truncus, minute buds appear at the base of the aorta and rapidly mature as coronary arteries. In an appreciable number of embryos studied at this stage, similar buds were seen in the pulmonary artery.[26] They usually involute, but various patterns of abnormal persistence and involution can explain most of the anomalies of origin of the coronary arteries, other than those determined by more extensive cardiac malformations. Tortuous fistulas between coronary arteries and veins or cardiac chambers which may form anomalously may be interpreted as localized failures of development from the primitive sinusoidal condition of the myocardium.

ANATOMY

The unique microcirculation of the heart is presented schematically in Figure 31.1. It shows the interconnection of the coronary arteries with pericardial arteries, vasa vasorum of the great vessels, extracardiac arteries, and also the many normal routes of blood flow through the wall of the heart and the anastomoses among arterioles, sinusoids, venules, and capillaries. At birth when the two ventricles are both thick-walled, the finer structure of the coronary artery branches is in the form of perforating, broom-like projections arising at the epicardial surface from the coronary arteries and plunging perpendicularly to the endocardium. During the first 6 months of life as the right ventricle gradually becomes relatively thinner, a more oblique course is assumed by the branches on that side while the left retains the broomlike perpendicular arrangement. Furthermore in the course of the second decade of life, the richness of the branches per unit of myocardium becomes noticeably less on the right.[24]

Collateral circulation in the coronary arterial bed has been studied extensively. The review by Bloor[9] is comprehensive. The most significant collateral is between the small branches of the right and left coronary in those parts of the heart where their distributions overlap. Although connections between these vessels are normally quite small (about 70 μm), permitting infarction if a large vessel is suddenly occluded, they open widely over varying periods of time in the face of local pressure gradients such as may occur with stenoses or smaller occlusions. These potential connections occur even in the neonate.[54] The microscopic anatomy of an individual coronary artery is similar to that of any medium-sized artery.

Coronary Arteries

The coronary arteries[28] arise from orifices approximately in the middle of the right and left aortic sinuses of Valsalva and are named according to the sinus of origin. They never arise from the posterior sinus. The ostia are round, ovoid, or elliptical. Sometimes they are as high as the supravalvar ridge or even above the sinus. The left coronary artery (Fig. 31.2) passes behind the pulmonary trunk and beneath the left atrial appendage for a few millimeters to a point of bifurcation, where it gives off the anterior descending branch which descends to the apex of the heart in the anterior longitudinal sulcus. Its other branch curves around to the back of the heart in the atrioventricular sulcus as the circumflex branch.

The right coronary artery passes backward in the atrioventricular groove. Its first branch is the branch to the right ventricular outflow tract or conus, but in about 50% of hearts a separate conus artery arises from a diminutive secondary ostium next to the main ostium and replaces this branch (Fig. 31.4A). When the right coronary artery reaches the posterior longitudinal sulcus, it frequently gives off one posterior descending artery, then makes a U-shaped curve toward the junction of the mitral and tricuspid annuli. From the apex of the U, the artery to the atrioventricular node arises, then the U returns to the atrioventricular groove and thence the artery courses down the posterior longitudinal sulcus as a second posterior descending artery. In 10% of individuals, the posterior descending artery is the termination of the circumflex branch of the left coronary artery. It is the variance in supply of the posterior longitudinal sulcus which determines whether a given coronary circulation is considered to be "right dominant" or "left dominant," a clinical classification which is useful in the interpretation of coronary arteriograms (Fig. 31.3).

The essentially circular course of the principal coronaries in the atrioventricular groove gives them their superficial resemblance to a crown, hence, the name "coronary." The circle is completed anteriorly by connections between the conus artery and branches of the anterior descending artery, known collectively as the circle of Vieussens. This general distribution is retained even when there are major variations in the origin and proximal courses of the arteries. Thus, there will be a vessel in the distribution of the right, the anterior descending, and the circumflex arteries in almost all hearts. Some of the variations in origin and proximal course are shown in diagrammatic form in Figure 31.4. Perhaps the commonest variation is the origin of the left circumflex artery as a first branch from the right coronary artery which winds around the back of the aorta to the left atrioventricular groove and then travels its normal course.[49]

Single coronary arteries in hearts not otherwise significantly malformed usually have a large artery forming a complete circle of Vieussens with normal branch distribution

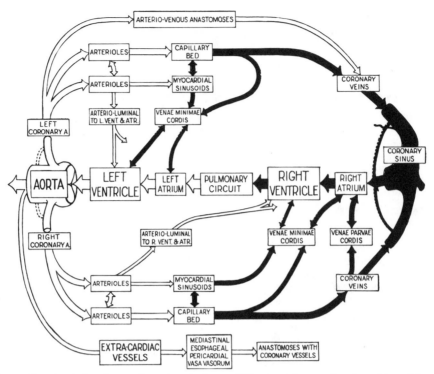

Fig. 31.1 Schema of the cardiac circulation. Among the unique features of this circulation are the sinusoids and the direct communications of arterioles and venules with the lumina of the cardiac chambers. Also, note the anastomoses of the extracardiac vessels with coronary vessels. (Reproduced with permission from B. M. Patten: *Pathology of the Heart*, edited by S. E. Gould. Charles C Thomas, Springfield, Ill., 1953.)

(Fig. 31.4*C*). There may or may not be an atrophic relic present where one coronary artery bud regressed. This normal variation must be contrasted to the more significant congenital stenosis or atresia of a coronary ostium discussed later, in which the circle is incomplete and supply to the deficient side is by distal collaterals from the other coronary artery.

The circumflex and left anterior descending arteries may originate from separate ostia (Fig. 31.4*D*).

The anterior half of the left ventricle is almost exclusively supplied by the left coronary artery. The posterior half of the right ventricle is usually predominantly supplied by the right coronary. The apex of the heart is usually supplied by the anterior descending branch of the left coronary. The anterior half of the right ventricle gets contributions from both right and left coronaries. The posterior half of the left ventricle has an extremely variable supply with more or less from the left circumflex, the terminal end of the left anterior descending coming from the apex, and the right coronary artery. The interventricular septum is predominantly supplied by long penetrating branches of the anterior descending artery.

Cardiac Veins

The great cardiac vein drains upward in the anterior longitudinal sulcus and follows the atrioventricular groove around to a point beneath the left lower pulmonary vein where it becomes continuous with the coronary sinus. The middle cardiac vein drains upward in the posterior longitudinal sulcus to empty into the coronary sinus just before the sinus drains into the right atrium. The small cardiac vein drains backward in the atrioventricular groove in the right side to enter the coronary sinus just before it enters the right atrium.

The anterior cardiac veins on the anterior aspect of the

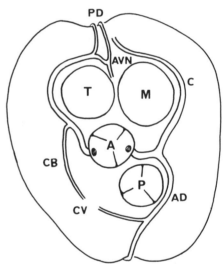

Fig. 31.2 Normal anatomy of the coronary arteries, in diagrammatic form, viewed from above, with atria removed. *A*, aortic valve; *P*, pulmonic valve; *T*, tricuspid valve; *M*, mitral valve; *C*, circumflex branch of left coronary artery; *AD*, anterior descending branch of left coronary artery; *CBN*, conus branch of the right coronary artery *CV*, circle of Vieussens, formed by anastomosis of branches of right and left coronary arteries over the right ventricular outflow tract; *PD*, posterior descending arteries in the posterior interventricular groove; *AVN*, atrioventricular nodal artery arising from the apex of the U-shaped bend in the right coronary artery.

right ventricle empty into the small cardiac vein or directly into the right atrium. The oblique vein of the left atrium drains down from the posterior wall of the left atrium, just to the left of the left pulmonary vein to enter the distal end of the coronary sinus. This vein is the remnant of the left

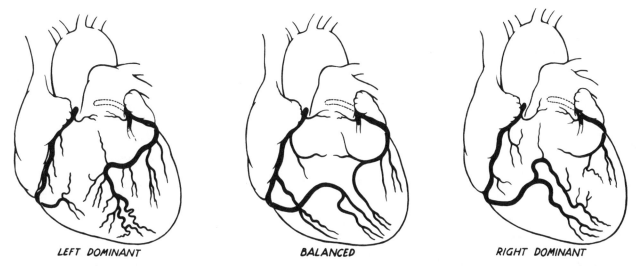

LEFT DOMINANT   BALANCED   RIGHT DOMINANT

Fig. 31.3 Dominance of coronary arteries is determined by the contribution of ventricular branches made by the left and right coronary arteries in the region of the intersection of the atrioventricular sulcus and the posterior longitudinal sulcus. The diagram looks through the heart from the front, emphasizing the arterial distribution over the posterior surface. (Reproduced with permission from Q. R. Stiles, B. L. Tucker, G. D. Lindesmith, and B. W. Meyer: *Revascularization of the Myocardium*. Little, Brown, Boston, 1976.)

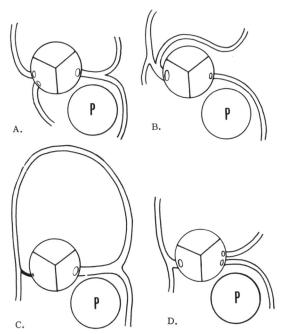

Fig. 31.4 Some variations in origin and course of the coronary arteries. (*A.*) Conus artery with separate orifice. (*B.*) Circumflex artery arising from right coronary artery, passing behind aorta; only the anterior descending arises from the left coronary artery. (*C.*) Involution of right coronary bud with circumflex artery taking over its distribution, a small nonpatent cord remaining. (*D.*) Separate origin of circumflex and anterior descending arteries.

common cardinal vein of the embryo and forms the terminal portion of the left superior vena cava when it persists. The Thebesian, or minimal cardiac veins, as shown in the schema of the microcirculation above, are terminal communications between veins of the myocardium and the lumen of a chamber.

PHYSIOLOGY

The pattern of flow through the coronary bed is unlike that of any other organ, and significant differences even occur between the right and left ventricular coronary flows.[23] Pressure within the wall of the left ventricle quickly rises slightly above that within the coronary arteries, during isovolumic contraction. In the inner third of the myocardium, pressure remains higher throughout the early part of the systolic ejection phase, forcing blood out of the perforating branches and halting inflow at the coronary ostia. There is then a brief peak of forward flow as ejection progresses and aortic pressure rises. Most of the flow in this phase is merely into the portion of the coronaries on the epicardial surface, and into the outer layers of the myocardium where peak intramural pressures are about one-third as high as in the subendocardial layers.[5] Flow ceases later in the ejection phase when the capacity of these arteries has been reached. At the end of ejection, when diastolic relaxation begins, blood again rushes forward from the aorta into the coronaries. At this moment, the deep layers of the left ventricle start to be perfused while aortic diastolic pressure exceeds left ventricular pressure and the wall is subjected only to passive stretch. Flow continues until it is throttled by the rising intramural tension of the next isovolumic contraction. Flow through the right ventricular wall in the heart with normal pressures differs from that of the left in that there is a continuous excess of coronary arterial over right ventricular pressure so that flow is continuous throughout the cardiac cycle.

Two teleologic advantages in the anatomy of the coronary arteries are evident: the epicardial position frees them of intramural tension over most of their course and the broom-like perpendicular penetration of branches through high pressure ventricles enables the most direct possible route of flow through the portion of the vascular bed where phasic obstruction occurs.

CONGENITAL ANOMALIES

ANOMALOUS ORIGIN OF THE CORONARY ARTERIES

Variations of normal anatomy discussed earlier may attain pathologic significance under certain circumstances. A single coronary supply, of course, increases vulnerability to infarction after onset of atherosclerosis. Coronary arteriographic studies in adults with angina have in rare instances shown such situations as a single coronary of aortic origin or another artery with anomalous origin, where the artery is compressed just at its origin[13, 33, 63] as it traverses the wall of the aorta obliquely rather than radially. We have observed at postmortem a left coronary arising from the internal mammary artery compressed between the aorta and the pulmonary artery in a 12-year-old girl who died suddenly.

When the left coronary artery arises from the right sinus of Valsalva, whether from a separate ostium or as a branch of a single right coronary artery, it may course leftward between the anterior aspect of the aorta and the posterior side of the right ventricular outlet or pulmonary trunk. In such a case, flattening of the coronary may occur in systole.[13, 33, 37] This has been identified as a cause of death in three of 29 competitive athletes between the ages of 13 and 30.[40]

A single coronary artery of pulmonary origin has not been reported, but both coronaries coming from the pulmonary artery is a rare occurrence,[57] compatible with life beyond early infancy only if associated with pulmonary hypertension. Accessory coronary arteries from the pulmonary artery usually are small and supply a limited part of the right ventricle without ill effect. Larger ones tend to form fistulous anastomoses with branches of the normal coronaries so the blood shunts from aorta to pulmonary artery. Such fistulas are discussed later.

Origin of the right coronary artery from the pulmonary trunk is a lesion found incidentally on postmortem examination. It permits flow from the aorta to the pulmonary artery via anastomoses between the left and right coronaries. The lesion is benign since the ventricular areas supplied under low pressure from pulmonary artery are parts of the right ventricle with a low intramural tension to match. Since there is no ischemia, there is little stimulus to development of anastomoses with the left coronary arterial distribution.

LEFT CORONARY ARTERY FROM PULMONARY TRUNK

In this anomaly the left coronary artery arises from the left sinus of Valsalva of the pulmonary trunk and then assumes the course and distribution of a coronary artery of normal origin. It is a rare lesion but one of great physiological and clinical importance since it produces symptoms, is diagnosable during life, and is surgically treatable.

This abnormality was first described by Abbott[1] in a 60-year-old woman, and later Abrikosoff[2] reported it in a 5-month-old infant. Bland and co-workers[8] showed that the condition could be diagnosed early in life and described the clinical syndrome; it is often referred to as the Bland-White-Garland syndrome. The terms adult type and infantile type were first used by Gouley[20] to distinguish between the patients who survived for many years with few or no symptoms and those who died in infancy with profound symptoms. More accurate physiological characterization of the individual case is now demanded.[4] Surgical therapy was first proposed in 1955 with the report of pericardial poudrage by Paul and Robbins.[50]

Anatomy and Physiology

The myocardium is a muscle which is specialized metabolically to pay its oxygen debt continually from beat to beat. Its unusual avidity for oxygen permits it to extract virtually all of the available oxygen from the blood in the coronary arteries. Low tensions of oxygen in the blood perfusing the coronaries are well tolerated within rather broad limits. Rarely, patients with rather severe cyanotic congenital cardiac malformations develop myocardial dysfunction or damage because of perfusion of the coronaries with blood of low oxygen content.

The problem in this disease is the low perfusing pressure in the left coronary artery. In fetal and neonatal life when the right ventricle is a systemic ventricle, the left coronary perfusion pressures are normal. The left ventricular myocardium is well nourished, so that intercoronary anastomoses, although present, are not highly developed. In the postnatal period, when pulmonary arterial pressure falls, an intermediate phase is entered which varies in length. The tendency for pulmonary arterial pressure to fall leads to decreased perfusion of the left ventricular myocardium, which must develop the high intramural tensions associated with production of systemic pressures despite the fact that it is perfused by coronary arteries under a lower pressure. However, the decreased perfusion of the left ventricle results in poorer output with a tendency to elevation of left atrial pressure and secondary pulmonary hypertension. This reactive pulmonary hypertension, to which the young infant is especially subject, prevents the pressure in the pulmonary and left coronary arteries from dropping precipitously and provides time for the development of increasing collateral circulation from the right coronary to the ischemic left coronary bed. This collateral circulation, if adequate, may be life-saving; if inadequate, it may not prevent infarction and, if large, it may have the disadvantage of causing a left to right shunt with volume overload of the heart.

Since some patients have been shown to have large left to right shunts, ligature of the left coronary at its pulmonary arterial origin has been proposed[12] to reduce volume work and to raise perfusion pressure in the coronary arterial distribution over the left ventricle. While some patients are helped greatly, others suffer from aggravated myocardial ischemia.[34, 41, 51] The mechanism of these varied effects will be discussed under Treatment.

As the left ventricular myocardium and endocardium suffer ischemia and infarctions, permanent changes in and around the mitral valve occur with secondary endocardial fibroelastosis, contraction of chordae tendineae, and infarction of papillary muscles.[17] This can result in mitral insufficiency, so that, if sufficient myocardial function remains for survival, the left atrial pressure rises, and the consequent pulmonary hypertension maintains left coronary artery pressure.

The minority of patients whose collateral circulation is developed and effectively distributed may never show symptoms; such patients have been discovered at autopsy in adult life. The majority of patients do not have such a course and, after 1 or 2 months of age, enter a stormy period in which there are manifestations of myocardial ischemia and heart failure, usually ending fatally before the end of 2 years.

The adult heart with this anomaly will usually have a very large, thick-walled, at times mildly aneurysmal, right coronary artery with very large branches which taper gradually over the course normally occupied by distal branches of the left coronary artery. The distribution is likely to be typical of a dominant right coronary artery. The proximal branches of the left coronary artery are smaller than normal and thin-walled, with the gross appearance of veins. After traversing only short distances, they enlarge and lose their identity, merging with the distal branches of the right coronary. The heart is small or only slightly enlarged, and there is only slight fibrosis of the myocardium.

The hearts of infants who die of the disease are large, with dilated left ventricles. The evidences of myocardial ischemia, past and present, are there in the form of infarcts, scars and thinning of the apex, papillary muscles, and septum, as well as endocardial fibrosis in and around the mitral valve. The fibrotic areas may include foci of calcification and may radiate deeply into the myocardium. The size of collaterals varies greatly. Some infants show no evidence of intercoronary anastomoses, while others may have some large but localized communications remote from the infarcted areas. Infants who survive longer tend to have more scarring and more mitral valve involvement with retractions of chordae and endocardial sclerosis.

Manifestations

Clinical Features. The classic description of the syndrome by Bland et al.[8] is still unchallenged:

Nothing remarkable was noted about the patient until the tenth week; while nursing from the bottle, the onset of an unusual group of symptoms occurred which consisted of paroxysmal attacks of acute discomfort precipitated by the exertion of nursing. The infant appeared at first to be in obvious distress, as indicated by short inspiratory grunts, followed immediately by marked pallor and cold sweat with a general appearance of severe shock. Occasionally, with unusually severe attacks there appeared to be a transient loss of consciousness. The eructation of gas at times seemed to relieve the discomfort and to shorten the duration of an attack which usually lasted from 5 to 10 minutes, and following which the infant might proceed to nurse without difficulty and remain free of symptoms for several days.... It seems probable that in this infant the curious attacks of paroxysmal discomfort.... were those of angina pectoris. If this be true, it represents the earliest age at which this condition has been recorded.

Such episodes occur usually with increasing frequency and then are gradually replaced by chronic dyspnea as heart failure becomes evident. Most infants who reach this stage succumb within a few weeks but a few improve. The children who develop adequate collateral circulation may show no symptoms and pass unrecognized. Others with suboptimal collateral development may have increasing episodes for a time which gradually decrease in frequency until the episodes finally disappear. Some of the older children who survive have an occasional anginal attack under the influence of emotion or exertion. Others may present a picture of mitral insufficiency and borderline heart failure.

The appearance of the infant during the attack of angina has been described. Other physical findings depend on the pathophysiology. There may be extreme cardiomegaly with a large but very inactive thin-walled left ventricle in cases in which there is very little or no effective collateral circulation. Paradoxical pulsations due to ventricular aneurysm should be looked for. On the other hand, the heart of an older child with good collaterals might be normal in size. The pansystolic murmur of mitral insufficiency might be associated with an enlarged heart or might be present in a heart with good compensation but with damage around the mitral valve or chordae tendineae. In the presence of excessive collaterals with aortic-pulmonary shunting through the coronary arteries, there may be a continuous murmur similar to that heard in coronary arterial aneurysms of other types.

Electrovectorcardiographic Features. In cases with infarction, the electrocardiogram resembles that of an adult with arteriosclerotic heart disease. There may be phases of infarction with severe S-T segment displacement and coving followed by healing with return toward normal, or there may be evidence of progressively more severe myocardial damage (Fig. 31.5). Often, the infarcts are anterior and anteroseptal, which is related to the fact that usually the anteroseptal aspect of the left ventricle is supplied solely by the left coronary artery. Commonly, there are deep Q waves and inverted T waves in Leads I, AVL, and the left precordial leads. In the vectorcardiogram, the most striking changes are seen in the horizontal QRSe loop in which there may be initial forces oriented anteriorly to the right followed by a clockwise deeply posterior terminal loop. In older children with good myocardial nutrition, signs of infarction or ischemia are usually absent, but there may be minor clues sug-

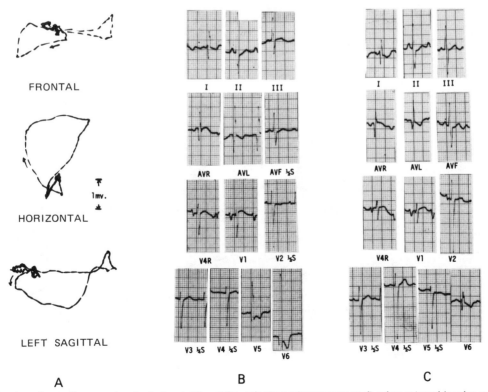

FRONTAL

HORIZONTAL

LEFT SAGITTAL

I   II   III

AVR   AVL   AVF ½S

V4R   V1   V2 ½S

V3 ½S   V4 ½S   V5   V6

I   II   III

AVR   AVL   AVF

V4R   V1   V2

V3 ½S   V4 ½S   V5 ½S   V6

A   B   C

Fig. 31.5 (A) Frank vectorcardiogram of patient at age 20 months, prior to aortocoronary graft using external jugular vein. Also ECG (B) prior to surgery and (C) after clotting of graft and progressive infarction.

gesting left ventricular hypertrophy, such as Q waves in Leads I, AVL, V5, and V6; deep S in the right precordial leads; and tall R in the left precordium, sometimes with T inversion.

Radiologic Features. The plain films will vary with the pathophysiology. They may show a large left ventricle and left atrium with passive pulmonary congestion in the patient in failure without adequate collateral circulation (Fig. 31.6). In patients with large aortic-pulmonary shunting, there may be pulmonary engorgement. Older children and adults may have only slight cardiomegaly involving the left heart. Fluoroscopically, the dilated heart with a thinned-out left ventricle will show little movement.

Thallium-201 myocardial perfusion imaging is quite sensitive, showing abnormalities of perfusion when they occur.[14] Since some patients with cardiomyopathy have diminished perfusion, the study is not specific.[25]

Echocardiographic Features. M-mode studies yield information on myocardial contractility but are not specifically diagnostic. 2D has, in some cases, permitted direct observation of the anomalous origin of the left coronary artery.[15]

Cardiac Catheterization

Selective angiocardiography is the most definitive study. Injection into the pulmonary artery in cases with little or no collateral circulation will delineate the left coronary artery directly (Fig. 31.7), while in cases with aortic-pulmonary shunting a negative jet from the left coronary orifice may be found in the pulmonary artery injection sequence. In some cases, forward flow into the coronary bed may be seen in diastole, while shunt flow into the pulmonary trunk occurs in systole. Aortic injection will always show only the right coronary artery arising from the aorta. In the cases with good collateral development, as well as in those with aortic-pulmonary shunts, the right coronary artery is large, while in cases without collateral circulation, it is normal in size. The progress of contrast through the dilated right coronary, through anastomoses and retrograde through the left coronary into the pulmonary artery, can be followed when it occurs. Its absence is strong evidence against good collateral circulation, though its presence does not guarantee adequate collateral blood flow to permit coronary artery ligation without danger of infarction. The size and origin of each major branch should be analyzed for associated anomalies which might influence the outcome. Although selective injection into the right coronary would produce a beautiful picture, it is not recommended in infants with life-threatening myocardial ischemia. The ejection fraction should be estimated from the left ventricular measurements.

Patients with no collateral circulation tend to show pulmonary hypertension, elevated left atrial pressure, and elevated left ventricular end-diastolic pressure, but no shunt either left to right or right to left. Patients with large left to right shunts with good myocardial function may only show admixture of oxygenated blood at the pulmonary artery level. These shunts tend to be of small to moderate size. The largest pulmonary-systemic flow ratio reported is 2:1. In

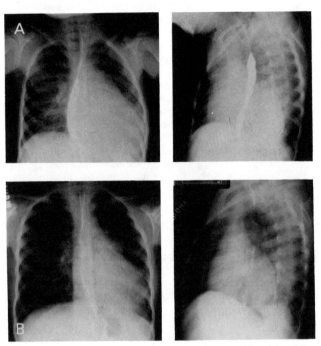

Fig. 31.6 Roentgenograms of a patient, age 5, with origin of the left coronary artery from the pulmonary artery before (*A*) and 1 year after (*B*) successful left subclavian to coronary graft. Posterior-anterior and left anterior oblique views with barium esophagram. Ejection fraction changed from <10% to 45%.

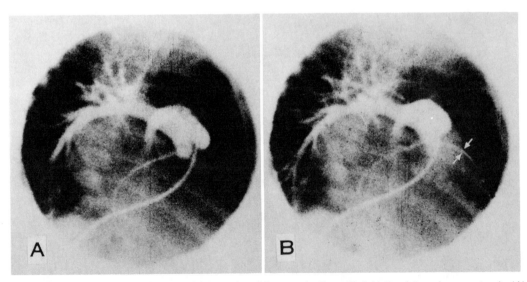

Fig. 31.7 Frames of selective cineangiocardiogram, right anterior oblique projection with injection into pulmonary trunk. (*A*) Filling of the circumflex branch of the left coronary artery. (*B*) A few frames later, the anterior descending branch fills (*arrows*). (Reproduced with permission from Armer *et al.*: Pediatrics 32:588, 1963 and from the American Academy of Pediatrics.)

patients with excellent myocardial function and very well-distributed collateral circulation, little left to right flow may reach the pulmonary artery.

Differential Diagnosis

The episodes of acute distress may superficially suggest a cyanotic malformation or paroxysmal tachycardia. Occasionally, acute myocarditis or endocardial fibroelastosis may cause episodic distress. Of these entities, the last two are the ones which require consideration after the initial steps in diagnosis. It may be very difficult to distinguish these various diseases clinically. The development of changes suggesting myocardial infarction is strongly suggestive of anomalous coronary artery but can occur in myocarditis. The frequency of dysrhythmias with fulminating myocarditis is contrasted with their rarity in anomalous origin of the left coronary artery.

If the most striking feature of the illness is left heart failure with low voltages throughout the electrocardiogram, myocarditis is more likely, while the same circumstances with evidences of left ventricular hypertrophy without ischemic changes favor endocardial fibroelastosis. In the experience of Noren and colleagues,[48] the vectorcardiogram (VCG) was very helpful in the differentiation between anomalous coronary and endocardial fibroelastosis, as all seven cases of anomalous coronary showed clockwise posterior loops in the horizontal plane, a finding not seen in their experience with endocardial fibroelastosis. Another patient with a cardiomyopathy[59] displayed this type of VCG, however, and a similar infarction-like VCG might be expected in calcification of the coronaries or premature atherosclerosis. Cardiac catheterization and angiocardiography are essential in cases of cardiomyopathy in order to rule out anomalous left coronary.

Other causes of myocardial disease leading to heart failure in infancy are calcification of the coronary arteries and glycogen storage disease; both are generalized disorders. In the former, calcification of the arteries of the neck and extremities may be seen in roentgenograms, or the retinal arteries may show the abnormality upon ophthalmoscopy; in the latter, the involvement of skeletal muscle and tongue are usually evident when the heart disease is noted. Evidences of infarction in the electrocardiogram are seen in calcification. Glycogen storage disease produces bizarre QRS wave forms, usually quite large, often with Wolff-Parkinson-White conduction.

If a continuous murmur is audible over the precordium at any age, a coronary vascular fistula must be considered, and this in turn must be distinguished from anomalous left coronary artery with a murmur arising from a left to right aortic-pulmonary shunt. Evidence of myocardial ischemia in the true fistulas adds to the difficulty. 2D echocardiography in some instances may enable differentiation of these entities. Before surgical correction, aortography will still be necessary.

In the older child with or without cardiac failure, anomalous coronary is a diagnosis which deserves more consideration if a continuous murmur is present over the midprecordium, or if symptoms suggesting angina are present. This lesion should also be considered in cases of mitral insufficiency without satisfactory clues to etiology, both in decompensated infants and in older children with relatively mild evidence of disease.

Treatment

The variable nature of the presentation requires individualized treatment. Infants suffering from classic Bland-White-Garland syndrome are at risk of sudden death from coronary insufficiency and require catheterization and surgery without delay. Interim treatment with morphine for pain and restlessness and oxygen to raise myocardial tissue PO_2 as much as possible are helpful. Intensive care with electrocardiographic monitoring may be lifesaving if cardiac dysrhythmia can be detected and treated in time.

Infants suffering only from heart failure require digitalis and diuretics. An impressive response to treatment suggests that surgery may be deferred in the expectation that collateral circulation may enlarge and myocardial function may improve. Deterioration despite treatment calls urgently for a surgical solution.

A specific point should be made regarding infants who show symptoms of both myocardial ischemia and heart failure. When an inotropic agent is mandatory, dopamine or dobutamine, with their transient action and lack of interaction with electrolyte levels, are preferable to digoxin in the period of diagnosis and preparation for surgery. Digitalis aggravates dysrhythmias at the time of coming off bypass when there is usually hypokalemia plus the irritability of previously ischemic myocardium which is reperfused.

Rarely, a child or adolescent with this anomaly who has never been ill and presumably has had adequate collateral circulation dies suddenly. For this reason, it would seem logical that a patient with anginal symptoms who is discovered to have the disease be treated not merely with nitroglycerin or propranolol but by surgery as soon as possible.

Once the need for surgical intervention has been determined, what operation should it be? The answer is still not clear, but an effort will be made to deal with the advantages and disadvantages of the various procedures. It must be reemphasized that the natural course of individual cases varies so much as to make it unwise to draw hasty conclusions as to the efficacy of an intervention.

The current procedures are several.

Ligation of the Artery at Its Origin from the Pulmonary Trunk. The advantages of this operation are speed and lack of need for complex equipment; cardiopulmonary bypass is not used. Disadvantages are that the heart and circulation cannot be controlled well if ventricular fibrillation occurs and that a proportion of patients needs the blood flow which they are getting from the pulmonary trunk to their left coronary to the extent that they will worsen or die if it is ligated. The outcome of ligation is not always predictable. On angiography when the pulmonary artery is injected, the finding of flow into a left coronary artery of normal caliber, whether this occurs in diastole only or in both phases, warns of a bad outcome. Even a large shunt does not ensure a good outcome, since the fistulous flow may occur only in systole through some large but localized connections while other areas located remotely from these connections remain dependent upon the pulmonary artery for their perfusion. Ligation is most likely to succeed: when there is a large shunt from left to right in both systole and diastole; when there is widely distributed adequate collateral circulation; and when there is volume overload without evidence of myocardial ischemia.

Ligation plus Graft. *End of Left Subclavian Artery to Left Coronary Artery.* The coronary artery is dissected from its bed proximal to the bifurcation and ligated where it emerges from the pulmonary artery. Either it is divided and the distal end is lifted outward for the anastomosis, as described by Meyer et al.,[44] or it may be left in situ, and an end to side anastomosis may be performed. In Meyer's case, it was performed on the beating heart through a left thoracotomy. The advantage of working without cardiopulmonary bypass is offset by the disadvantage of poor control of the circulation should the heart fibrillate. The operation has the advantage that if the anastomosis remains patent, the patient has a systemic level of pressure in the left coronary artery and a two coronary system. Should it clot, the patient may still be one of the 75% who would have been helped by a ligation only. Not all of these grafts have remained open in the experience at our clinic, and those in smaller infants have clotted.

Ligations plus Various Types of Grafts Using Cardiopulmonary Bypass. These procedures are more complex operations but have the advantages of control of circulation should the heart fibrillate and a quiet heart which permits more precise surgery. The approach is midline, making either subclavian less accessible, and the distance is so great in some instances as to require using the artery as a free graft. The external jugular vein has been used in our clinic as an aorta to coronary bypass graft in a toddler at the age of 20 months. It clotted about 2 weeks postoperative. In the same child on a second attempt at the age of 24 months, the saphenous vein was used. In our experience saphenous vein grafts have remained open in older patients with this malformation.

Newer Operations Using Cardiopulmonary Bypass. Excision of a cuff of the pulmonary trunk containing the ostium of the anomalous artery has been described by Neches et al.[47] In this way the size of the coronary artery anastomosis can be fashioned to be as large as the end of the subclavian artery which can be either turned down or detached and used as a free graft. Their experience included an infant who had marked ischemia when operated upon at 6 months of age with angiographic proof of patency of the graft one month later and excellent clinical follow-up for 1 year after surgery.

Recently, several operations have been designed for restoration of a 2-coronary system in even the youngest patients. One of these begins with transsection of the pulmonary trunk just above the coronary ostium. The ostium is excised with a cone of pulmonary artery which can be attached directly to a hole in the aorta. The aorta can be reached with ease with the pulmonary trunk out of the way. Should the distance to the aorta be too great, an extension can be fashioned from a strip of pulmonary artery taken off with the ostium. Finally, continuity of the pulmonary trunk is reestablished without graft material. This operation has been reported successfully in small infants.[21, 64]

Another series of operations[3, 27, 66] begins with the creation, through a pulmonary arteriotomy, of an aortic-pulmonary window. This is followed by a transpulmonary arterial baffle or free graft of pericardium or subclavian artery from that window to the coronary ostium which remains *in situ*. The pulmonary artery is closed with a gusset to avoid stenosis.

Though it is too early to be certain, it is clear that several alternatives to ligation now exist. It is the authors' opinion that: ligation will soon become obsolete due to its unpredictable early result and its failure to establish a 2-coronary system and the risky period of waiting for the patient to become sicker or to respond to medical management should be eliminated and one of the aggressive procedures should be performed.

STENOSIS OR ATRESIA OF A CORONARY OSTIUM

Though rare, this is a potentially lethal and sometimes treatable condition. The ostium and sometimes a few millimeters of the artery either fail to canalize or involute. There may be a normally formed set of peripheral branches. These develop multiple collateral connections with the distal branches of the opposite coronary artery. Physiologically, these patients are in a precarious state as they are dependent on collateral flow. Our one patient, a 3-month-old with near

atresia of the left ostium, presented with failure and angina. The 6-month-old of Byrum et al.[11] with atretic left ositum went into sudden failure with an acute myocardial infarction. The patient of Mullins et al.[46] also with atretic left ostium developed angina with effort at 10 years, and the patient of Fortuin and Roberts[16] died suddenly at age 60.

Angiographically, in left-sided involvement, it is easy to be misled into the diagnosis of left coronary from pulmonary trunk as the left coronary distribution fills late by numerous connections from the right. No contrast enters the pulmonary artery, however, which is a warning of the possibility of this diagnosis. If the patient's clinical status is severe enough to demand surgery, it should be undertaken despite the fact that there are no reports of a successful bypass graft in infancy for this rare condition. The most likely operation to succeed would be a subclavian artery free graft placed during cardiopulmonary bypass. Mullins' 14-year-old had an excellent result from a saphenous vein graft.

CORONARY ARTERIES IN SPECIFIC MALFORMATIONS

The origin and course of the coronaries in some of the common malformations will be briefly mentioned here.

TETRALOGY OF FALLOT

A common associated peculiarity involves the conus artery which, instead of being short and high, tends to be long and swings low over the right ventricular outflow tract with a richer branching distribution than usual (Fig. 31.8A). A very important anomaly associated with tetralogy is a single right coronary artery, the anterior branch of which swings around

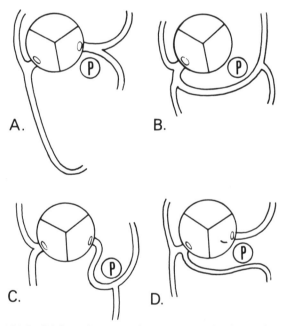

Fig. 31.8 Origin and course of coronary arteries in tetralogy of Fallot. (*A.*) Long low-branching conus artery. (*B.*) Single coronary artery arises from right sinus of Valsalva, anterior branch of which loops in front of pulmonary trunk to take the position of anterior descending and circumflex arteries. (*C.*) Left coronary artery loops between aorta and pulmonary trunk, then loops in front of pulmonary trunk, where it bifurcates into anterior descending and circumflex arteries. (*D.*) Anterior descending artery arises from bifurcation of right coronary artery and passes in front of pulmonary trunk.

in front of the pulmonary artery to supply the anterior descending artery and then the circumflex (Fig. 31.8*B*). In a case reported by Longenecker *et al.*,[36] the left coronary artery coursed in front of the pulmonary trunk (Fig. 31.8*C*). Another pattern of distribution occurs when the anterior descending artery arises from the right coronary artery and crosses the right ventricular outflow tract before descending in the anterior interventricular sulcus (Fig. 31.8*D*). In these instances surgical repair of the obstructive right ventricular outflow tract is limited by the need to avoid section of this vital vessel. Although in most cases the anomalous artery is clearly visible to the surgeon,[18, 36, 53] in a case reported by Senning,[61] the anomalous left coronary originating from the single right coronary artery coursed within the myocardium of the right ventricular outflow tract and was severed in the initial ventriculotomy.

TRANSPOSITION OF THE GREAT ARTERIES

In Shaber and Puddu's[62] study of 149 specimens, 89 showed origin of the left coronary artery from the left sinus of Valsalva and the right coronary from the posterior sinus. The left gave off the anterior descending and circumflex branches (Fig. 31.9*A*). In 31 cases, the right coronary artery and the left circumflex originated from the posterior sinus, either from one or separate ostia (Fig. 31.9*B* and *C*). The left circumflex artery then passed behind the pulmonary artery. In both of these situations, the right sinus was the noncoronary sinus. Many other variations occur, but much less often.

CORRECTED TRANSPOSITION OF THE GREAT ARTERIES

The right coronary artery usually arises above the right aortic sinus, gives rise to the anterior descending branch, and then continues in the right atrioventricular groove. The left coronary artery has only the circumflex distribution. It arises from the left coronary sinus. The anterior is the noncoronary sinus (Fig. 31.10).

ANEURYSMS OF THE SINUSES OF VALSALVA

This is a congenital weakness resulting in a gradual downward bulge of a sinus of Valsalva. The bulge herniates into an atrium or ventricle and may rupture. Thurnam[67] reported the first case, and Meyer[45] reported 45 patients treated

surgically. It is still a rare problem in infancy and childhood, becoming more frequent in adolescence, with most of the cases occurring in adults. About three-fourths of the patients are males. It occurs in coincidence with ventricular septal defect and less often with coarctation of the aorta.

ANATOMY AND PHYSIOLOGY

Sakakibara and Konno[60] classified the manifestations of these lesions and proposed a theory to explain their pathogenesis. They observed a linear translucency in normal hearts along the line of fusion between the dextrodorsal and sinistroventral conus ridges and assumed that fragile tissue in this area was stretched by aortic pressure resulting in herniation and ultimately in rupture. Their classification included aneurysms of the right sinus protruding into the right ventricle and right atrium and from the noncoronary cusp sinus into the right atrium but excluded cases where there was protrusion from the left cusp or from any cusp into the left ventricle, all of which they denied were of congenital origin. Subsequent authors have not made this distinction, as protrusions which look otherwise identical are also observed in these locations. The lesions are often associated with ventricular septal defects (VSD), and the commonest aneurysm of all is that from the right sinus to the right ventricle in association with a VSD. This group ruptures into the right ventricular outflow or penetrates the crista supraventricularis.

The aneurysms of the sinuses of Valsalva occurring in Marfan's syndrome are not related to this entity. They are diffusely dilated sinuses which stretch in all directions but do not rupture. The dissecting aneurysms of the aortic wall which also occur with Marfan's syndrome are still another entity.

Endocarditis may involve a congenital sinus of Valsalva aneurysm. However, whenever endocarditis involves the aortic root, regardless of the nature of the primary abnormality, mycotic aneurysm, dissection, and acquired VSD may occur. After some progression of such damage, it may become impossible to determine the primary disease.

The unruptured aneurysm may produce no manifestations and may be discovered by chance during angiography for another lesion, most often a VSD. However, right ventricular outflow obstruction with symptoms from the pressure of the unruptured aneurysm has been reported, and obstruction of the tricuspid valve as well as dysrhythmias due to compression of atrioventricular junctional tissues may be postulated.

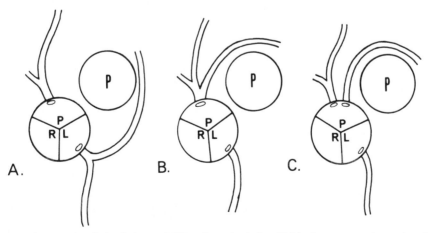

Fig. 31.9 Origin and course of coronary arteries in transposition of great arteries. (*A.*) Left coronary artery arises from left sinus and right coronary artery from posterior sinus, with both anterior descending and circumflex branches from the left coronary. (*B.* and *C.*) Right coronary artery and left circumflex arise from posterior sinus, from one or separate ostia. Left circumflex passes behind pulmonary trunk.

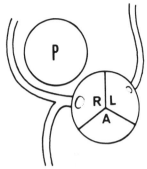

Fig. 31.10 Origin and course of coronary arteries in corrected transposition of great arteries. Right coronary artery arises from right sinus (R) and also gives rise to the anterior descending branch. Left coronary artery arises from left sinus (L) and has only the circumflex distribution.

Few data are available on the time required for a congenital weakness to progress to the point of symptomatic compression, or to rupture. In part this is due to rarity of the lesion, in part to the fact that only in cases in which another recognizable congenital cardiac lesion coexists would there be reason for angiography. Finally, an angiographer faced with the wide range of normal is unwilling to pronounce a small protrusion as abnormal. The authors' experience includes many such small protrusions without a single one becoming known later as a ruptured sinus aneurysm. In cases of a sinus rupture occurring after previous angiography, aortography had not been performed, and review of other earlier studies was unrevealing. Mayer et al.[42] described a patient who had a normal aortic root prior to correction of a coarctation of the aorta at the age of 10 years, and who, 8 years later, had repeat aortography showing a large protrusion from the noncoronary sinus.

Once rupture has occurred, the effects are those of sudden onset of aortic runoff and left to right shunting at right atrial or right ventricular level, or aortic insufficiency in case of rupture into the left ventricle. Infundibular stenosis produced by the bulge may balance the left to right shunting at the expense of acutely increased systolic loading of the right ventricle. Rupture into the pericardial sac with tamponade and rupture into the pulmonary trunk have both been reported but are extremely rare.

MANIFESTATIONS

Clinical Features

Rupture of the aneurysm may occur at rest or during activity. The moment of rupture is often associated with violent symptoms. An interesting patient of ours was a 15-year-old boy who had had a coarctation of the aorta resected 18 months earlier. He had made an uneventful recovery from surgery. While watching television one evening he noted a sudden tearing pain in the midchest, followed immediately by a sensation he described as a "waterfall" inside his chest. Within a few minutes, he became short of breath, and within 24 hours he had advanced heart failure. This is a typical history of rupture into the right ventricle.

In cases with rupture into the right atrium the pain may be upper abdominal. Occasionally, there is no dramatic onset of symptoms, as in cases with right ventricular outflow tract obstruction. Commonly after rupture, there follows a recovery of cardiac compensation for a few weeks to months, but ultimately sudden deterioration and death occur.

In all types, wide pulse pressures and left ventricular overactivity result from marked diastolic runoff from the aorta and from diastolic overload of the left ventricle. In the rare case with rupture into the left ventricle, only left ventricular overload occurs. In the usual case, the right ventricle is also overactive. The location and type of murmurs and thrills vary with location of rupture. There may be separate systolic and diastolic peaks in the intensity of the murmur, or a holosystolic murmur of the VSD, plus an ejection murmur of infundibular stenosis, plus a regurgitant murmur, all maximal at the pulmonic area or more toward the right. There may be a continuous murmur with systolic accentuation close to the sternum at the right or left third to fifth rib, or at the xiphoid or in the epigastrium.

Electrovectorcardiographic Features

Findings secondary to the hemodynamics such as biventricular diastolic overload are to be expected. There may be incomplete atrioventricular (AV) block and Wenckebach's phenomenon, or AV nodal rhythm due to compression of the AV junction by the aneurysm.

Radiologic Features

The findings of pulmonary vascular engorgement, dilated widely pulsating aorta, and enlargement of the heart are confirmatory, though not specific. The findings on selective aortography are diagnostic. The coronary arteries are visible and uninvolved. The right or the noncoronary aortic sinus is malformed and, if ruptured, contrast is seen pouring from the lower end of the elongated sinus, directly into the right atrium or ventricle. Associated aortic insufficiency may be found. The frequently associated VSD should, of course, be sought.

Echocardiographic Features

It is possible to suspect a sinus of Valsalva aneurysm by M-mode, and to delineate some quite well by 2D. We have also experienced failure to demonstrate a large, thin-walled ruptured aneurysm presenting in the outflow tract of the right ventricle.

CARDIAC CATHETERIZATION

A pressure gradient suggestive of infundibular pulmonic stenosis and evidence of left to right shunt at right atrial or right ventricular level may be encountered and there may be a mild to severe increase in right heart pressure.

DIFFERENTIAL DIAGNOSIS

The history at the time of rupture may suggest a myocardial infarction, or the rupture of a valve cusp or of chordae tendineae. The associated signs of left to right shunt should make the correct diagnosis evident in all except the rare case with rupture into the left ventricle. This may be impossible to distinguish from rupture of an aortic cusp without resorting to selective aortography.

TREATMENT

Heart failure must be treated, and the patient must be subjected to cardiac catheterization and selective aortography, followed by corrective surgery without delay. The surgery must be performed with the aid of cardiopulmonary bypass. Direct closure is usually through an aortotomy, plus a right ventriculotomy or right atriotomy.

With few exceptions these lesions ultimately cause death if surgical correction is not made. After surgical correction the prognosis must be guarded, as residual aortic insufficiency is common and the lesions may recur due to the necessity of placing sutures in abnormally fragile tissues. Surgical correction of the asymptomatic, accidentally discovered aneurysm is debatable.

ANEURYSMS AND FISTULAS OF THE CORONARY CIRCULATION

A number of different aneurysmal dilatations of the coronary vasculature occur, some of which are the result of acquired disease and of no importance in pediatrics. This discussion will be devoted to those dilatations characterized by congenitally abnormal circulatory connections.

These lesions often have an impressive gross anatomic appearance and therefore were considered as curiosities by early pathologists. The first report is probably that of Brooks[10] in 1886. Grant[22] pointed out the relationship of this malformation to the early stage of embryogenesis of the myocardium when musculature is loose and sinusoids communicating with the ventricular cavity are the prime element in its circulation. Most subsequent writers have ascribed the genesis of these defects to a partial localized retention of the fetal noncondensed vascular relationship, although some cases resemble the fetal state more than others. When it became feasible to operate upon patent ductus arteriosus, similarities in physical findings led to unintentional exploration of a few patients with coronary fistulas. The first of these to be successfully ligated was reported by Biörck and Crafoord.[6] With the advent of selective aortography, precise clinical diagnosis became possible. These are rare lesions. Nothing is known of their etiology.

Typically, the dilated, often tortuous fistulas form communications between a dilated main or branch coronary artery and one or several routes of drainage. McNamara and Gross[38] classified 163 cases from the literature and added eight new cases. Over one-half originate from the right coronary. Of all fistulas, from either coronary 92% enter the right side of the heart. Entry may occur into the right atrium or its tributaries, right ventricle, pulmonary artery, left atrium, or left ventricle. In communications between the aorta and the right side of the heart the physiologic effect is that of a left to right shunt producing runoff from the aorta, increased volume loading of the left atrium and ventricle, the pulmonary vascular bed, and those right heart chambers through which the shunted blood flows. Fistulas which enter the left atrium and ventricle do not increase pulmonary blood flow but cause excessive runoff from the aorta and volume overloading of the chambers receiving the shunt.

All degrees of shunting have been found with these lesions with a tendency to follow a pattern that the shortest, smallest, and most direct fistulas have large orifices of communication and large flows while the longest fistulas tend to be tortuous and large and have little flow. Some of the largest have been found to have multiple channels and very small orifices of communication to their final outlets, and sometimes rather large sections are involved in antemortem clot (Fig. 31.11). Some have been as large as the heart itself. It is possible that the tortuosity of the longer fistulas is in part due to undifferentiation between sinusoidal and arterial structure, since such tortuosity has been found in fistulas in the newborn. It is also reasonable to postulate a tendency for the dilatation and tortuosity to increase with time, as the epicardial position of the major coronary arteries permits them to store blood under aortic pressure during systole, when the outlets from the aneurysm may be virtually closed. This closure would be expected to be most effective in the

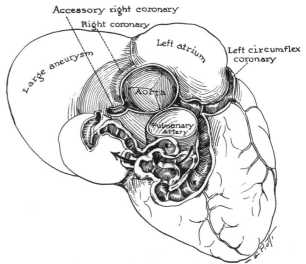

Fig. 31.11 Heart with multiple connecting aneurysms to illustrate large size, little blood flow, and small orifices of communication. In this instance, the conus artery (*Accessory right coronary*) directly entered the largest aneurysm, measuring 10 by 8 by 8 cm, from which another vessel connected by a tortuous course to an aneurysm 3 cm in diameter. The vessel then passed through four small saccular enlargements, received a communication branch from the anterior descending branch of the left coronary artery, and terminated in a saccular dilatation 1.6 cm in diameter. This connected with the pulmonary artery through an opening less than 2 mm in diameter. The large aneurysm overlies and hides the right atrium.

left ventricle, less in the right ventricle, least of all in the atria, and not at all in the pulmonary artery. There may be sufficient deviation of coronary artery blood through a fistula so that ischemia is produced in neighboring parts of the coronary bed.

In a few fistulas, the direction of blood flow is reversed. In association with pulmonary[31] or aortic[52] atresia with intact ventricular septum or small VSD and competent atrioventricular valve, the sinusoidal structure may be preserved, and a moderate flow of blood occurs from the lumen of the ventricle to the coronary artery and thence to the aorta or the coronary sinus.

MANIFESTATIONS

Appreciation of these lesions will be dependent upon their pathologic details. Many of the reported cases were discovered incidentally at postmortem. Others were noted on routine physical examination in asymptomatic individuals with a murmur suggestive of patent ductus arteriosus. Some with very little flow have had no murmur but have shown a large mass on x-ray which has been thought to be the heart itself, or a paracardiac mass. Some of the fistulas with a large shunt have symptoms and signs of heart failure and excessive pulmonary perfusion. Some have symptoms and electrocardiographic signs of myocardial ischemia. The murmur is most often "close to the ear" and heard in an area centered over the midprecordium or slightly to the right of the sternum. It is often diphasic, although continuous, with the middiastolic phase louder than the midsystolic.

The electrocardiogram and vectorcardiogram show the effects of volume overload of the left ventricle and left atrium as well as of affected right-sided chambers. Ischemic changes have also been reported. 2D echocardiography may permit tracing a dilated coronary artery into a fistulous mass.

Aortography or coronary arteriography gives the essential

diagnostic information, in cases where the flow is forward through the dilated coronary artery. Injection into the appropriate ventricle may outline the fistula in aortic or pulmonary atresia after retrograde flow through sinusoids. Cardiac catheterization gives the information on the size of the shunt as well as intracardiac and vascular pressures. In most instances the shunt is not great and the pressures tend to be normal, but a few cases with large shunts have been associated with elevation of pulmonary arterial pressure. This results in part from left heart failure due to volume overload and in part from equalization of the ejectile force of the two ventricles via a large communicating orifice.

DIFFERENTIAL DIAGNOSIS

The lesion should be suspected whenever a patient is referred with the diagnosis of patent ductus arteriosus and the murmur is not typical. The timing of the ductus murmur with late systolic accentuation is in contrast to that of some fistulas which have their greatest peak in early diastole but may have both systolic and diastolic peaks. The location of the murmur of the ductus is usually maximal at the second left interspace somewhat lateral to the midline. Coronary aneurysms may resemble ruptured sinus of Valsalva aneurysm, VSD with aortic insufficiency, intrathoracic venous hums, systemic arteriovenous fistulas of the chest wall, and pulmonary arteriovenous fistulas. The aortogram in ruptured sinus of Valsalva aneurysm shows both coronary arteries to be uninvolved. Furthermore, the channel tends to avoid the exterior surface of the heart, whereas in coronary artery fistula, the superficial location of the anomalous channel is apparent.

TREATMENT AND COURSE

This is a disturbing abnormality even when its hemodynamic effects are mild, as it presents some risk from endocarditis. The possibilities of progressive enlargement, secondary atherosclerotic involvement with rupture, and thromboembolic complications add to the arguments favoring surgical closure. The operative results are good, and the surgical mortality in some series is zero. Though most of the fistulas have been corrected by clamping and suture-ligation without extracorporeal circulation total cardiopulmonary bypass should be available should it be necessary to enter a chamber to close a fistula from within, or should a bypass graft be necessary to maintain viability of myocardium distal to ligation of the artery.

At birth, a fistula with potentially large left to right flow may be kept in check by the neonatal elevated pulmonary vascular resistance. As this resistance falls and as the fistula orifice enlarges, a dramatic increase in shunting may occur, leading to failure and pulmonary engorgement. At the other extreme some lesions are associated with small orifices which never enlarge to permit significant shunt. However, progressive enlargement of the shunt, secondary atherosclerotic changes, clotting and endocarditis, and ischemic changes in the surrounding myocardium may complicate the otherwise mild lesion. It is difficult to evaluate the relative importance of these complications in view of the low frequency of the anomalies.

AORTIC-LEFT VENTRICULAR TUNNEL

In this extremely rare condition, an endothelialized vascular connection between the aorta and the left ventricle simulates aortic insufficiency. The tunnel is thought to be present at birth. Its aortic origin is above the right sinus of

Valsalva and right coronary ostium, both of which remain normal except for displacement (Fig. 31.12). There is usually a sharp ridge separating the sinus below and the orifice above. The tunnel passes behind the infundibulum of the right ventricle and through the anterior upper part of the ventricular septum to enter the left ventricle just below the right and left aortic cusps. It is usually short and direct, though it may be dilated aneurysmally. Severe insufficiency is produced, with wide pulse pressure, loud systolic and diastolic murmurs, usually with a momentary interval separating them, marked left ventricular enlargement and overactivity, and a dilated ascending aorta. The aortographic demonstration of normal coronary arteries arising separately differentiates this malformation from coronary artery fistula to the left ventricle, whereas the anterior location of the abnormal channel and the normal sinus of Valsalva distinguish it from ruptured aneurysm of a sinus of Valsalva into the left ventricle.

Levy et al.[32] first reported the entity as a congenital disease requiring surgery in early life. Most of the patients are males. Björk et al.[7] reviewed the 31 cases which had been recorded and added one. There is a consistent pattern of "aortic regurgitation" being noted at birth with early heart failure. Medical therapy is usually inadequate, and surgical treatment often results in residual aortic insufficiency. To combat this, Björk recommended patching the aortic orifice of the tunnel so as to preserve the support of the right coronary cusp without distortion.

ANOMALIES OF THE CORONARY SINUS

Most of the following anomalies are dealt with in other contexts in this and other chapters, but they are brought together here in summary form for convenient reference. The classification of Mantini et al.[39] has been adopted.

The anomalies of the coronary sinus are chiefly divided into enlargements, absence, atresia of the right atrial ostium, and hypoplasia.

ENLARGEMENTS

This group of anomalies may be subdivided into those with and those without left to right shunt. Enlargements without left to right shunts imply the presence of some additional systemic venous tributary. The most common of these, and indeed the most frequent thoracic venous anom-

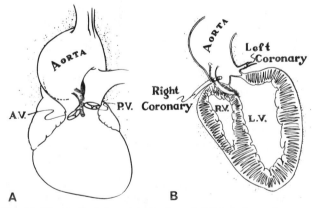

Fig. 31.12 Aortic-left ventricular tunnel. (A) Anterior surface relation. (B) Sagittal section showing the tunnel burrowing through the septal wall of the right ventricle to enter the left ventricle. (Reproduced with permission from M. J. Levy et al.[32] and the American Heart Association.)

aly, is the persistent left superior vena cava which empties into the coronary sinus. Its chief importance is in the planning of cardiac surgery. Its presence must be recognized in venous inflow occlusion and cardiopulmonary bypass techniques. Such an additional communication must be ruled out before right superior vena cava-right pulmonary artery anastomosis. Another venous tributary, either alone or together with a left superior vena cava, is an anomalous hepatic vein, usually from a left lobe of the liver, which perforates the diaphragm and pericardium. Still another condition is an anomalous inferior vena cava which connects with the hemiazygos vein and passes forward above the heart to enter the left superior vena cava and coronary sinus.

Enlargements with left to right shunt include both low-pressure and high-pressure shunts. The low pressure shunts include communication with the left atrium, which mimics an atrial defect, as well as total and partial anomalous pulmonary venous connection to the coronary sinus. The high pressure shunts are the coronary artery fistulas. Two types have been described: a more common one, in which a tortuous coronary artery enters the coronary sinus directly or via a dilated cardiac vein, and a less common situation in which a blind ventricle discharges blood from its lumen via intramural sinusoids into a coronary artery which then connects to the coronary sinus. Such a patient with aortic atresia and premature closure of the foramen ovale has been reported. The pulmonary venous return found its way via this route to a systemic right ventricle.

ABSENCE OF THE CORONARY SINUS

This lesion is associated with atrial septal defects of two types. One is a defect which lies in the normal location of the coronary sinus. The other is a large defect involving the entire lowermost portion of the atrial septum: either an atrioventricular canal or one of the even more primitive cor biloculare defects.

ATRESIA OF THE RIGHT ATRIAL OSTIUM OF THE CORONARY SINUS

This may be associated with three alternatives: either the coronary sinus empties retrogradely into a left superior vena cava, or there is a large communication between the sinus and the left atrium, or there are several small orifices between the sinus and the right and left atria.

HYPOPLASIA OF THE CORONARY SINUS

In this situation, most of the normal venous outflow from the heart is via very small cardiac (Thebesian) veins, so that the sinus is diminutive, but with normal position and orifice location.

DISEASES OF THE CORONARY ARTERIES

Generalized arterial calcification of infancy is a very rare lesion which may be one of a group of abnormalities with different pathogeneses. In the few descriptions, the histology varies from medial arterial calcification to a predominance of intimal connective tissue proliferation with small amounts of calcium in the internal elastic lamina. The etiology is unknown. Severe arterial calcification has been reported in one infant overfed with vitamin D.[35] This resembled pathologically the state produced in animals by overfeeding mother or infant vitamin D and calcium, which differs from this disease in many respects. Furthermore, in most patients, excessive ingestion of vitamin D has been denied. Williams[70]

found PAS-positive material encrusting and replacing fibers of the internal elastic lamina in the earliest lesions. Calcium seemed to be present in this material in more advanced lesions. He suggested that the disease might be an anomaly of mucopolysaccharide metabolism, not one of calcium metabolism.

The process begins before birth and progresses rapidly, involving peripheral, retinal, renal, and coronary arteries. Usually, death occurs by the age of 6 months from cardiac or cerebellar involvement. The diagnosis may be made from soft tissue radiographs[69] and from examination of the retinal arteries. The cardiac symptoms may be anginal, followed quickly by evidence of infarction and heart failure. No treatment has been successful.[68]

Localized intimal fibrous proliferations in the coronary and other arteries have been seen often in neonates. The internal elastic lamella is interrupted and reduplicated at the site of the thickenings. They are usually small and produce no disturbance. Robertson[58] found them in about half the newborn coronaries he examined. However, others have found such thickenings associated with myocardial infarction in utero and in early infancy. Witzleben[71] found at autopsy in a 7-month-old numerous foci of intimal fibrous proliferation, many of which were associated with disruption of the internal elastic lamella, and some of which also showed elastic tissue degeneration and beginning calcification. On that basis, he suggested that generalized arterial calcification may be an advanced form of the same disease, and he proposed a new provisional term—"occlusive infantile arteriopathy"—to embrace this wider concept.

Richart and Benirschke[55] point out that myocardial infarction may occur in the perinatal period or in utero, unrelated to coronary artery disease. Papillary muscle infarction has become a recognized but infrequent complication of severe congenital heart disease with chronic overloading of the heart, presumably due to the fact that the circulation to the papillary muscle is "at the end of the line." No structural abnormality has been found in this terminal artery.

Occlusive fibroelastosis of the coronary arteries was described by MacMahon and Dickinson[37] in a newborn infant. It seemed to be an anomaly of development resulting in extreme stenosis of the proximal portion of both right and left coronary artery with a gradual transition to normalcy of the rest of the tree. The histology was more compatible with malorganization than an inflammatory disease, and it occurred in a malformed heart with tricuspid atresia. There was no involvement of arteries in other parts of the body. It probably fits better under the category of congenital ostial stenosis.

Premature coronary atherosclerosis is discussed in Chapter 40. The various types of *coronary arteritis* which are part of more *generalized* processes may be infectious or immunologic, and may include infantile polyarteritis nodosa[56] and mucocutaneous lymph node syndrome.

MUCOCUTANEOUS LYMPH NODE SYNDROME (KAWASAKI'S DISEASE)

This syndrome, first described in Japan in 1967,[29, 30] has become widely recognized in the Western world, where it has occurred in many small clusters in the past decade. The etiology is unknown, but the epidemiology suggests an idiosyncratic immunologic response triggered by an infection.[43] The hallmarks of the acute early phase of the disease are fever lasting over 5 days, generalized erythematous rash, and erythema and edema of palms and soles progressing to desquamation, conjunctivitis, stomatitis, glossitis, and non-suppurative lymphadenitis. It may affect newborn infants and adults, but the peak frequency is in the 6-month to 5-year age group.

PATHOLOGY[19]

There is a generalized microvasculitis which underlies all of the early clinical findings and provides the basis for the late sequelae. In the early inflammatory phase there may be myocarditis and pericarditis. The vasculitis often involves the walls of muscular arteries and, most importantly, the coronaries. There it produces focal destructive lesions, similar to those of infantile polyarteritis nodosum, resulting in the formation of saccular and cylindrical aneurysms, often with narrow areas interspersed so as to suggest beads on a string. The aneurysms may leak, clot, or disturb flow by compression. As the arteries heal, flow may be reduced by scar formation. These complications due to involvement of the coronary arteries have been recorded as early as the first week of the disease and as late as 16 years later. Though the few very late complications of coronary aneurysms have resulted in great concern, most aneurysms begin to resolve within 6 months to a year after the acute onset and only a small minority enlarge late in the course of the disease.

MANIFESTATIONS

The early myocarditis is difficult to diagnose in these patients, who are febrile, very irritable, and difficult to approach. While excessive tachycardia and gallop rhythm may be suggestive of cardiac involvement, definite evidence may occur in the form of dysrhythmias, conduction disturbances, and T wave abnormalities on the electrocardiogram, as well as cardiomegaly by x-ray and evidence of enlargement and reduced contractility on the M-mode echocardiogram.

The coronary arteritis is silent until a critical narrowing or occlusion occurs, resulting in infarction or angina diagnosable by electrocardiography. A vast amount of coronary pathology may be present in the asymptomatic patient with a normal electrocardiogram, however. Since the worst and most frequent aneurysm formation tends to occur close to the origin of the coronary arteries, two-dimensional echocardiography is quite useful in revealing and following the course of aneurysms. Aortography is necessary to confirm the findings of aneurysm on echo and to demonstrate the aneurysm more than 2 to 3 cm beyond the ostia. When numerous aneurysms occur, selective coronary arteriography (Fig 31.13) with careful multiple positioning provides the most definitive information, by avoidance of superimposition of involved branches. Selective arteriography in this age group[65] requires specially sized and shaped catheters. It is unsafe to enter these diseased arteries with a guide wire.

TREATMENT

Early in the disease, bedrest is required. Sedation may be necessary as these patients are so irritable. Aspirin is given for its antipyretic, anti-inflammatory, and anticoagulant effects.

If no coronary artery aneurysm or stenosis is demonstrable in a patient who seems clinically recovered three to 6 months after the onset of the disease, the aspirin can be discontinued. On the other hand, if the presence of aneurysm or stenosis is established, the family must be warned of the possible need for cardiopulmonary resuscitation and instructed in it. Aspirin should not be discontinued unless the aneurysms resolve. In high risk cases, aspirin is combined with dipyridamole. The frequency and extent of follow-up studies of the

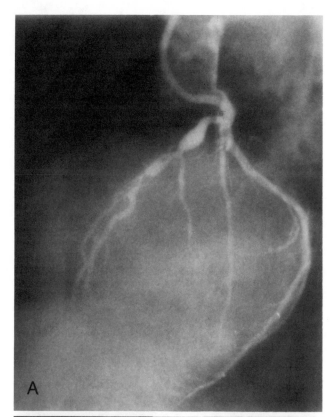

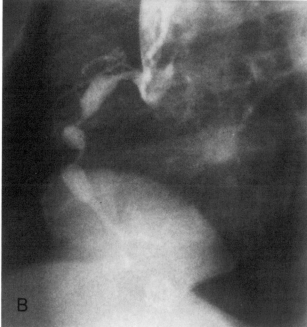

Fig. 31.13 Selective coronary arteriograms of a 17-month-old studied 2 months after onset of Kawasaki disease. (A.) Two aneurysms of left anterior descending with narrowing between them; normal left main and circumflex arteries. (B.) Three aneurysms of right coronary artery.

aneurysms may be individualized. Two-dimensional echocardiography and electrocardiogram should be part of the follow-up evaluation. When aneurysms are present which cannot be seen echocardiographically, aortography should be done annually until a stable state has occurred.

In cases where infarction or angina occur early in the

disease, these are best treated medically. Bypass graft surgery has been successful in a small number of subjects who developed myocardial infarction late in the course of the disease.

REFERENCES

1. Abbott, M. E. Congenital cardiac disease. In *Osler's Modern Medicine* vol. 4. Lea & Febiger, Philadelphia, 1908 p. 420.
2. Abrikossoff, A.: Aneurysma des linken Herzventrikels mit abnormer Abgangsstelle der linken Koreonararterie von der Pulmonalis bei einem fünfmonatlichen Kinde. Virchows Arch. Pathol. Anat. Phys. 203:413, 1911.
3. Arciniegas, E., Farooki, Z. Q., Hakimi, M., and Green, E. W.: Management of anomalous left coronary artery from the pulmonary artery. Circulation 62 (Suppl I)180, 1980.
4. Askenazi, J., and Nadas, A. S.: Anomalous left coronary artery originating from the pulmonary artery: Report on 15 cases. Circulation 51:976, 1975.
5. Baird, R. J. Manktelow, R. T., Shah, P. A., and Ameli, F. M.: Intramyocardial pressure. A study of its regional variations and its relationship to intraventricular pressure. J. Thorac. Cardiovasc. Surg 59:810, 1970.
6. Biörck, G., and Crafoord, C.: Arteriovenous aneurysm on the pulmonary artery simulating patent ductus arteriosus botalli. Thorax 2:65, 1947.
7. Björk, V. O., Ekjlöf, G. and Zetterqvist, P.: Successful surgical treatment of an aortic-left ventricular tunnel in a four-month-old infant. J. Thorac. Cardiovasc. Surg. 78:35, 1979.
8. Bland, E. F., White, P.D., and Garland, J.: Congenital anomalies of the coronary arteries. Am. Heart J. 8:787, 1933.
9. Bloor, C. M.: Functional significance of the coronary collateral circulation. A review. Am. J. Pathol. 76:562, 1974.
10. Brooks, H. St. J.: Two cases of abnormal coronary artery of the heart arising from the pulmonary artery. J. Anat. Physiol. 20:26, 1866.
11. Byrum, C. J., Blackman, M. S., Schneider, B., Sondheimer, H. M., and Kavey, R. W.: Congenital atresia of the left coronary ostium and hypoplasia of the left main coronary artery. Am. Heart J. 99:354, 1980.
12. Case, R, B., Morrow, A. G., Stainsby, W., and Nestor, J. O.: Anomalous origin of the left coronary artery: The physiologic defect and suggested surgical treatment. Circulation 17:1062, 1958.
13. Cheitlin, M. D., De Castro, C. M., and McAllister, H. A.: Sudden death as a complication of anomalous left coronary origin from the anterior sinus of Valsalva: A not-so-minor congenital anomaly. Circulation 50:780, 1974.
14. Finley, J. P., Holman-Giles, R., Gilday, D. L., Olley, P. M., and Rowe, R. D.: Thallium-201 myocardial imaging in anomalous left coronary artery arising from the pulmonary artery. Applications before and after medical and surgical treatment. Am. J. Cardiol. 41:675, 1978.
15. Fisher, E. A., Sepehri, B., Lendrum, B., Luken, J., and Levitzky, S.: Two-dimensional echocardiographic visualization of the left coronary artery in anomalous origin of the left coronary artery from the pulmonary artery: Pre-and postoperative studies. Circulation 63:698, 1981.
16. Fortuin, N. J., and Roberts, W. C.: Congenital atresia of the left main coronary artery. Am. J. Med. 50:385, 1971.
17. Foster, H. R., Jr., Hagstrom, J. W. C., Ehlers, K. H., and Engle, M. A.: Mitral insufficiency due to anomalous origin of the left coronary artery from the pulmonary artery. Pediatrics 34:649, 1964.
18. Friedman, S., Ash, R., Klein, D., and Johnson, J.: Anomalous single coronary artery complicating ventriculotomy in a child with cyanotic congenital heart disease. Am. Heart J. 59:140, 1960.
   Gault, M. H., and Usher, R.: Coronary throm-

bosis with myocardial infarction in a newborn infant. N. Engl. J. Med. 263:382, 1960.
19. Fujiwara, H., and Hamashima, Y.: Pathology of the heart in Kawasaki disease. Pediatrics 61:100, 1978.
20. Gouley, B. A.: Anomalous left coronary artery arising from the pulmonary artery (adult type). Am. Heart J. 40:630, 1950.
21. Grace, R. R., Angelini, P., and Cooley, D. A.: Aortic implantation of anomalous left coronary artery arising from pulmonary artery. Am. J. Cardiol. 39:608, 1977.
22. Grant, R. T.: An unusual anomaly of the coronary vessels in the malformed heart of a child. Heart 13:285, 1926.
23. Gregg, D. E., and Fisher, L. C.: Blood supply to the heart. In Handbook of Physiology, Section 2. Circulation. American Physiological Society, Washington, D. C., 1963.
24. Gross, L., and Kugel, M. A.: Arterial blood vascular distribution to the left and right ventricles of the human heart. Am. J. 9:165, 1933.
25. Gutgesell, H. P., Pinsky, W. W., and DePuey, E. G.: Thallium-201 myocardial perfusion imaging in infants children: Value in distinguishing anomalous left coronary artery from congestive cardiomyopathy. Circulation 61:596, 1980.
26. Hackensellner, H. A.: Aksessorische Kranzgefässanlagen der Arteria pulmonalis unter 63 menschlichen Embryonenserien mit einer grössten Länge von 12 bis 36 mm. Mikroscopischanat. Forsch. 62:153, 1956.
27. Hamilton, D. J., Ghosh, P. K., and Donnelly, R. J.: An operation for anomalous origin of left coronary artery. Brit. Heart J. 41:12, 1979.
28. James, T. N.: *Anatomy of the Coronary Arteries.* P. B. Hoeber, Inc. New York, 1961.
29. Kawasaki, T.: M. C. L. S.—Clinical observation of 50 cases (in Japanese). Jap. J. Allerg. 16:178, 1967.
30. Kawasaki, T., Kosaki, F., Okawa, S., Shigematsu, I., and Yanagawa, HJ.: A new infantile acute febrile mucocutaneous lymph node syndrome (MLNS) prevailing in Japan. Pediatrics 54:271, 1974.
31. Lauer, R. M., Fink, H. P., Petry, W. L., Dunn, M. I., and Diehl, A. M.: Angiographic demonstration of intramyocardial sinusoids in pulmonary-valve atresia with intact ventricular septum and hypoplastic right ventricle. N. Engl. J. Med. 271:68, 1964.
32. Levy, M. J., Lillehei, C. W., Anderson, R. C. Amplatz, K., and Edwards, J. E.: Aortico-left ventricular tunnel. Circulation 27:841, 1963.
33. Liberthson, R. R., Dinsmore, R. E., Bharati, S., Rubenstein, J. J., Caulfield, J. Wheeler, E. O. Harthorne, J.W., and Lev, M.: Aberrant coronary artery origin from the aorta: Diagnosis and clinical significance. Circulation 50:774, 1974.
34. Liebman, J., Hellerstein, H. D., Ankeney, J. L., and Tucker, A.: The problem of the anomalous left coronary artery arising from the pulmonary artery in older children. Report of three cases. N. Engl. J. Med., 269:486, 1963.
35. Lippincott, S. W.: Histopathological study of a fatal case of hypervitaminosis D. Am. J. Pathol. 16:665, 1940.
36. Longenecker, C. G., Reemstma, K., and Creech, O., Jr.: Anomalous coronary artery distribution associated with tetralogy of Fallot: A hazard in open cardiac repair. J. Thorac. and Cardiovasc. Surg. 42:258, 1961.
37. MacMahon, H. E., and Dickinson, P. C. T.: Occlusive fibroelastosis of coronary arteries in the newborn. Circulation 35:3, 1967.
38. McNamara, J. J. and Gross, R. E.: Congenital coronary artery fistula. Surgery 65:59, 1969.
39. Mantini, E., Grondin, C. M., Lillehei, C. W.,

and Edwards, J. W.: Congenital anomalies involving the coronary sinus. Circulation 33:317, 1966.
40. Maron, B. J., Roberts, W. C., McAllister, H. A., Rosing, D. R., and Epstein, S. E.: Sudden death in young athletes. Circulation 62:218, 1980.
41. Massih, N. A., Lawler, J., and Vermillion, M.: Myocardial ischemia after ligation of an anomalous left coronary artery arising from the pulmonary artery. N. Engl. J. Med., 269:483, 1963.
42. Mayer, J. H., Holder, T. M., and Canent, R. V.: Isolated, unruptured sinus of Valsalva aneurysm: Serendipitous detection and correction. J. Thorac. Cardiovasc. Surg. 69:429, 1975.
43. Melish, M. E.: Kawasaki syndrome: A new infectious disease? J. Infect. Dis. 143:317, 1981.
44. Meyer, B. W., Stefanik, G., Stiles,, Q. R., Lindesmith, G. G., and Jones, J. C.: A method of definitive surgical treatment of anomalous origin of left coronary artery. J. Thorac. Cardiovasc. Surg. 56:104, 1968.
45. Meyer, J., Wukasch, D. C., Malloy, K. P., Sanford, F. M., Reul, G. J. Jr., Hallman, G. L., and Cooley, D. A.: Aneurysms of the sinus of Valsalva: Surgical treatment in 45 patients. Circulation 50 (Suppl. IIII):192, 1974.(abstr.).
46. Mullins, C. E. El-Said, G., McNamara, D. G., Cooley, D. A., Treistman, B., and Garcia, E.: Atresia of the left coronary artery ostium: Repair by saphenous vein graft. Circulation 46:989, 1972.
47. Neches, W. H., Mathews, R. A., Park, S. C., Lenox, C. C. Zuberbuhler, J. R. Siewers, R., D., and Bahnson, H. T.: Anomalous origin of the left coronary artery from the pulmonary artery: A new method of surgical repair. Circulation 50:582, 1974.
48. Noren, G. R., Raghib, G., Moller, J. H. Amplatz, K., Adams, P., Jr., and Edwards, J. E.: Anomalous origin of the left coronary artery from the pulmonary trunk with special reference to the occurrence of mitral insufficiency. Circulation 30:171, 1964.
49. Ogden, J. A.: Congenital anomalies of the coronary arteries. Am. J. Cardiol. 25:474, 1970.
50. Paul, R. N., and Robbins, S. G.: A surgical treatment proposed for either endocardial fibroelastosis or anomalous left coronary artery. Pediatrics 16:147, 1955.
51. Perry, L. W., and Scott, L. P.: Anomalous left coronary artery from pulmonary artery: Report of 11 cases; review of indications for and results of surgery. Circulation 41:1043, 1970.
52. Raghib, G., Bloemendaal, R. D., Kanjuh, V. I., and Edwards, J. E.: Aortic atresia and premature closure of foramen ovale: Myocardial sinusoids and coronary arterio-venous fistula serving as outflow channel. Am. Heart J. 70:476, 1965.
53. Reemstma, K., Longenecker, C. G., and Creech, O., Jr.: Surgical anatomy of the coronary artery distribution in congenital heart disease. Circulation 24:782, 1961.
54. Freudenthal, R. R.: Inter-arterial coronary anastomoses in neonates. Arch. Pathol. 71:103, 1961.
55. Richart, R., and Benirschke, K.: Myocardial infarction in the perinatal period. J. Pediatr. 55:706, 1959.
56. Roberts, F. B., and Fetterman, G. H.: Polyarteritis nodosa in infancy. J. Pediatr. 63:519, 1963.
57. Roberts, W. C.: Anomalous origin of both coronary arteries from the pulmonary artery. Am. J. Cardiol. 10:595, 1962.
58. Robertson, J. H.: Significance of intimal thickening in the arteries of the newborn. Arch Dis.

Child. 35:598, 1960.
59. Ruttenberg, H. D., Jue, K. L., Elliott, L. P. Anderson, R. C., and Edwards, J. E. Cardiac myopathy, probably of congenital origin: A case simulating anomalous origin of the left coronary artery from the pulmonary trunk. Circulation 29:768, 1964.
60. Sakakibara, S., and Konno, S.: Congenital aneurysm of the sinuses of Valsalva: Anatomy and classification. Am. Heart J. 63:405, 1962.
61. Senning, A.: Surgical treatment of right ventricular outflow stenosis combined with ventricular septal defect and right-left shunt (Fallot's tetralogy). Acta Chir. Scand. 117:73, 1959.
62. Shaher, R. M., and Puddu, G. C.: Coronary arterial anatomy in complete transposition of the great vessels. Am. J. Cardiol. 17:355, 1966.
63. Sharbaugh, A. H., and White, R. S.: Single

coronary artery: Analysis of the anatomic variation, clinical importance, and report of five cases. J.A.M.A. 230:243, 1974.
64. Stiles, Q. R.: Surgery for anomalous origin of the left coronary artery from the pulmonary artery. In Congenital Heart Disease, edited by B. L. Tucker and G. G. Lindesmith, New York, Grune & Stratton, 1979
65. Takahashi, M., Schieber, R. A., Wishner, S. H., Ritchie, G. W., and Francis, P. S.: Selective coronary arteriography in infants and children. Amer. J. Cardiol., in press, 1982.
66. Takeuchi, S., Imamura, H., Katsumoko, K., Hayashi, I., Katohgi, T., Yozu, R., Okura, M., and Inouye, T.: New surgical method for repair of anomalous left coronary artery from pulmonary artery. J. Thorac. Cardiovasc. Surg. 78:7, 1979.

67. Thurnam, J.: On aneurysms, and especially spontaneous aneurysms of the ascending aorta, and sinus of Valsalva. Med. Chir. Tr., 23:323, 1840.
68. Traisman, H. S., Limperis, N. M., and Traisman, A. S.: Myocardial infarction due to calcification of the arteries in an infant. Am. J. Dis. Child. 91:34, 1956.
69. Weens, H. S.,, and Marin, C. A.: Infantile arteriosclerosis. Radiology 67:168, 1956.
70. Williams, A. L.: Quoted in McKusick, V. A., Hereditable Disorders of Connective Tissue, 2nd ed. C. V. Mosby Company, St. Louis, 1960, pp. 310–312.
71. Witzleben, C. L.: Idiopathic infantile arterial calcification—A misnomer? Am. J. Cardiol. 26:305, 1970.

32

Diseases of the Mitral Valve

Barry G. Baylen, M.D., and J. Michael Criley, M.D.

A comprehensive description of mitral valve anatomy and the integrated function of its components is required in order to appreciate the clinical and pathophysiological manifestations of diseases of the mitral valve in children.

EMBRYOLOGY AND PATHOLOGY

The embryonic mitral valve is formed primarily from the endocardial cushions that lie on the left side of the atrioventricular orifice and from ventricular muscle which is separated from the ventricular wall by a process of undermining and diverticulation.[94] The four primary components of the mitral valve apparatus are: the anulus; anterior and posterior valve leaflets; chordae tendineae; and papillary muscles.[23, 46, 62, 67, 102] The integrated function of these components in concert is required in order that the valve may perform its primary functions, namely to allow unobstructed diastolic flow of pulmonary venous blood from the left atrium into the left ventricle, and to maintain a competent seal of the inlet of the left ventricle during systole.

The mitral anulus is formed from the fibrous skeleton of the heart. A fibromuscular component of the anulus attaches at the base of the anterior leaflet and constricts the anulus at the onset of atrial systole and throughout ventricular contraction, allowing greater systolic overlap of the leaflets.[91]

The mitral leaflets consist of a collagenous peripheral fibrosa and a mucoid myxomatous central tissue, the spongiosa.[70] A sail-shaped anterior leaflet attaches in a hinge-like manner to approximately one-third of the anteromedial portion of the ring. The C-shaped posterior leaflet hinges upon the posterolateral two-thirds of the ring. The leaflets are separated at the anterolateral and posteromedial commissures where they are attached to the fibrous trigones. The anterior leaflet forms the semicircular posterior border of the left ventricular outflow tract. It is in direct continuity with one-half the noncoronary cusp and most of the left coronary cusp. However, a spectrum of discontinuity between the anterior leaflet and coronary cusps may be present in some forms of congenital heart disease associated with

left ventricular outflow tract obstruction.[73] The posterior leaflet is attached to the remaining two-thirds of the anulus extending along the posterolateral free wall of the left ventricle. The posterior mitral leaflet is longer at its base and shorter in its basal to apical length than the anterior leaflet, although both have approximately the same area.[67] The leaflets possess approximately 20% more cross-sectional area than the mitral orifice, which allows the leaflets to overlap during systolic closure.[23] During closure the sail-like anterior leaflet is enveloped by the gusset-like C-shaped posterior leaflet.[18] The posterior leaflet is generally subdivided by medial and lateral clefts into scallop-shaped areas designated the posteromedial, middle, and anterolateral scallops.

The chordae tendineae consist of a complex network of flexible cord-like structures consisting primarily of collagen.[46, 70] These originate from the papillary muscles and/or posterior ventricular wall and diverge in a pattern of increasing orders of branches to their insertion at the free edges or ventricular surfaces of the leaflets.[46]

The anterolateral and posteromedial papillary muscles serve to secure and tense the chordae and mitral leaflets at the onset of ventricular systole. The former is supplied by the left, and the latter by the left and/or right coronary artery. The interpapillary distance is relatively constant.[74] However, the posteromedial papillary muscle is frequently bifid.

Several anatomical, cellular, and physiological factors are required for the mitral valve to function normally. Cellular factors include the normal development of the myxomatous elements of the leaflets and the collagen matrix of the chordae. Abnormal or excessive deposition of fibrous tissue or myxomatous material can lead to relative inflexibility or weakness of these components and cause stenosis and/or insufficiency of the valve.[20, 70, 71, 76] Malalignment of the mitral valve anulus and straddling or anomalous insertion of the chordae can cause obstruction or incompetence of the leaflets along with abnormal diversion of the systemic or pulmonary venous blood flow. Hypoplasia of one or more components of the mitral valve apparatus may cause narrowing of the effective orifice area and obstruction to ventricular inflow. Isolated or combined fusion of the leaflets, fibrosis and shortening of the chordae, anomalous chordal attachment or insertion, and variable papillary muscle fusion may also lead to left ventricular inflow obstruction. In addition, these anomalies may lead to insufficient overlap and coaptation of the leaflets causing mitral insufficiency as well.

It is difficult to extrapolate functional integrity of the mitral valve from postmortem specimens.[76] It has been postulated that abnormal fetal blood flow patterns which lead to a reduction of work or flow through the left heart cause downstream developmental hypoplasia of the cardiac chambers, valves, and aorta.[77] In view of its central location, it is hardly surprising that major mitral anomalies are rarely isolated. It is reasonable to propose that congenital mitral valve malformations should generally be considered but one component of a variably expressed developmental abnormality involving most of the left ventricle. Thus, the functional integrity of the mitral valve and clinical physiological correlations must generally be inferred in the context of coexistent cardiac malformations. Furthermore, little pathologic material is available from children with less functionally significant but important mitral valve abnormalities, such as mitral valve prolapse.[70] The ensuing discussion will describe diseases of the mitral valve in terms of their dominant functional or clinical manifestations. Diseases of the mitral valve included under other major congenital or acquired cardiac conditions, such as endocardial cushion defect and rheumatic heart disease, are discussed elsewhere in this text.

CONGENITAL MITRAL VALVE MALFORMATIONS ASSOCIATED WITH OBSTRUCTION TO LEFT VENTRICULAR INFLOW

PHYSIOLOGY

Functional obstruction of the mitral valve apparatus at any level interferes with pulmonary venous flow from the left atrium into the left ventricle. Associated reduction of left ventricular volume, ischemia, fibrosis, and left ventricular dysfunction may further compromise cardiac output. Consequently, left atrial, pulmonary venous, and capillary pressures rise. In accordance with Starling's concept of transvascular fluid exchange, net exchange of capillary water into the interstitial and alveolar spaces occurs when the hydrostatic pressure gradient exceeds that of plasma oncotic pressure. Congested bronchial veins encroach upon the small bronchiolar airways causing an increase of airway resistance. These factors and others adversely affect mechanical and gas-exchanging properties of the lung and manifest clinically by increased effort of breathing and marked abnormalities of arterial blood gas tensions, such as hypoxemia and hypercapnia. Hypoxic and/or reflexly mediated pulmonary vasoconstriction and hypertension may be present. Critical reduction of cardiac output and mismatch of organ and tissue demand versus supply of oxygen and other nutrients lead to metabolic insufficiency, anaerobic metabolism, and systemic acidemia. Finally, renal insufficiency, imbalance of fluid, and electrolyte metabolism and fluid retention is caused by abnormal intake, renal hypoperfusion, and hormonal factors.

CLINICAL FEATURES

The timing and manifestations of symptoms of mitral valve stenosis vary with the degree of obstruction to left ventricular inflow, the presence and type of associated le-

sions, and with the nutritional status and growth rate of the infant.[19, 76] Mitral valve obstruction is of no apparent hemodynamic consequence in the fetus, since newborns with complete mitral atresia are normally developed, and there is no evidence of intrauterine cardiac failure at birth.[60] A detailed presentation of the manifestations of the most severe forms of mitral atresia or hypoplasia associated with the hypoplastic left heart complex is discussed elsewhere in this text. Briefly, symptoms and signs appear shortly after birth and are primarily related to constriction of the ductus arteriosus, reduction of systemic blood flow, and respiratory distress associated with pulmonary edema.[60] Infants with less severe mitral valve obstruction and/or less significant associated lesions present beyond the neonatal period often with a history of antecedent pulmonary infection and failure to gain weight appropriately. Other features include irritability, exhaustion at feeding, diaphoresis, tachypnea, and chronic cough.[19] Clinical features associated with a particularly poor outcome are presentation early in infancy and signs of low systemic cardiac output and right cardiac failure.[19]

Severe mitral valve obstruction is associated with diminished peripheral perfusion and pulses. An active right ventricular impulse is palpated when pulmonary hypertension is present. In most cases, the first heart sound is relatively soft, and mitral valve opening sound is usually absent, as the mitral valve leaflets are relatively inflexible and immobile.[19] This finding contrasts with those of acquired rheumatic mitral stenosis in childhood. The second heart sound varies from widely split to narrowly split with an accentuated pulmonic component when pulmonary hypertension is present. Although left ventricular inflow tract obstruction should preclude auscultation of ventricular filling sounds, right ventricular third or fourth heart sounds may be present. A low-frequency, low intensity diastolic murmur often with presystolic accentuation is auscultated at the apex. However, in some cases, a loud, high-frequency diastolic murmur may be present and its timing suspected only by palpation of the peripheral pulses. The murmur may diminish in intensity or be completely absent when cardiac output is markedly reduced. The murmur of mitral insufficiency, pulmonary valve insufficiency, and findings characteristic of associated cardiac malformations may be present.

CONGENITAL MITRAL STENOSIS

Congenital mitral valve stenosis has been traditionally classified according to which component of the mitral valve apparatus was abnormal.[20, 58] However, most cases involve diffuse abnormalities of several components of the valve, and some have proposed that congenital mitral stenosis be considered a continuous spectrum of malformations involving several components of the valve apparatus.[74, 76] For example, a wide spectrum of representative mitral valve anomalies has been observed in postmortem specimens of patients presenting with coarctation of the aorta[74] (Fig. 32.1).

Congenital mitral stenosis is characterized by variable combinations of anomalies including: thickened rolled leaflet margins; shortened and thickened chordae tendineae; fibrous obliteration of the interchordal spaces; abnormal chordal insertions; papillary muscle hypoplasia; and decreased interpapillary muscle distance or fusion.[19, 20, 25, 58, 76] The most commonly accompanying malformations are coarctation of the aorta and aortic valve stenosis.[76] Left ventricular endocardial sclerosis is usually present, but left ventricular size is usually normal to mildly reduced (greater than 70% of normal) in most patients. The median survival in one series was $2^{11}/_{12}$ years and was unrelated to mitral orifice or left ventric-

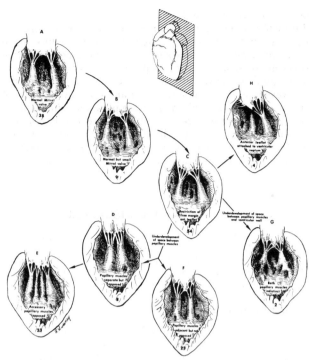

Fig. 32.1 Illustration of the spectrum of mitral valve anomalies associated with coarctation of the aorta.[74] Three basic anomalies of various components of the mitral valve are shown by arrows radiating from C. (Reproduced with permission from G. C. Rosenquist.[74])

ular size but primarily to the presence of complicating associated lesions.[76]

HYPOPLASIA OF THE MITRAL VALVE AND MITRAL VALVE ATRESIA

In hypoplasia of the mitral valve all components of the valve apparatus are relatively small. The individual components are relatively normally formed in relation to the smaller valve and ventricle.[76] Minimal mitral valve sclerosis and shortening of the chordae tendineae are often present. Narrowing of the mitral anulus, severe hypoplasia of the left ventricle, and significant left ventricular outflow tract obstruction are universally present. A small left ventricle is observed in 80%. Such infants represent a portion of the spectrum of hypoplastic left heart syndrome.[60] Generally, those infants with left ventricular size less than 70% do not survive beyond the neonatal period, while the majority of those with values greater than 70% of normal survive beyond the neonatal period.[76]

Mitral valve atresia with normal aortic valve is a rare malformation often included in the spectrum of "hypoplastic left heart syndrome."[59] It has been suggested that those forms of this condition with normal aortic valve and left ventricle be considered a distinct entity since the course differs from that of classical hypoplastic left heart syndrome, and recent surgical developments may potentially lead to effective palliation and ultimately to successful repair.[45] Approximately 12% of patients have a "normal left ventricle" often associated with a large ventricular septal defect (VSD) or straddling tricuspid valve. Some have proposed that this malformation be classified as univentricular heart.[2] Timing of presentation and severity of symptoms vary with associated lesions, patency of the foramen ovale, the presence of left atrial hypertension, the size of the VSD, and pulmonary blood flow.

PARACHUTE MITRAL VALVE

This condition is characterized by insertion of all the chordae tendineae into a single papillary muscle group.[6, 20, 31, 58, 74, 76] The chordae are generally shortened and thickened, and the anatomy of the papillary muscles is highly variable. The anterolateral papillary muscle may be completely absent, or two identifiable but partially fused papillary muscles may be present. Commonly associated conditions include isolated or combined supramitral ring, aortic subvalvular and/or valvular stenosis, coarctation of the aorta (CA), or the complete "Shone complex" of anomalies.[85] Right ventricular outflow tract obstruction has also been described. Median longevity approaches 10 years of age, correlating best with left ventricular size and poorly with mitral valve orifice size.[76]

SUPRAMITRAL RING

This condition is caused by accumulations of connective tissue which arise from the atrial surface of the mitral leaflets and consequently encroach upon the mitral valve orifice. Isolated supramitral ring is a rare condition, and the anomalies mentioned above are present in most instances.[20, 52, 58, 72, 76, 85]

MITRAL VALVE STENOSIS ASSOCIATED WITH OTHER CONGENITAL ANOMALIES

Mitral valve stenosis has been reported in association with a wide variety of congenital cardiac malformations. Rosenquist *et al.* demonstrated a wide variety of mitral valve disease generally of minor functional importance in patients with transposition of the great arteries.[73] A relatively high frequency of mitral valve stenosis is present in patients with double outlet right ventricle, occurring in as many as 28% of those individuals with VSD in the subaortic position.[87] Duplication of the mitral valve orifice caused by an accessory bridge crossing the mitral inlet is usually associated with stenosis.[69] Malalignment of the atrioventricular valve orifice (override) or straddling of the ventricular septum by chordal or papillary muscle components occasionally causes significant mitral valve obstruction.[21, 48] Finally, congenital mitral valve stenosis has been associated with secundum and primum atrial septal defect.[88]

Electrocardiographic Features

The ECG usually demonstrates left atrial enlargement; right ventricular and atrial enlargement suggest severe stenosis associated with pulmonary hypertension. The QRS axis is generally rightward (90 to 150°), and left ventricular forces are usually reduced. However, the QRS axis and ventricular forces vary with the associated lesions and the development of the left ventricle.[19, 35, 92]

Radiologic Features

Radiologic findings include left atrial enlargement, prominence of the pulmonary vasculature, and right cardiac enlargement.[19, 92]

Echocardiographic Features

Echocardiography has been an extremely useful method for the evaluation of the mitral valve in adults and older children. However, little echocardiographic experience has been available from children with congenital mitral stenosis.[32, 44, 49, 50] Typically, in acquired mitral valve stenosis, mitral valve opening, D-E excursion, and E-F slope are decreased. Posterior leaflet diastolic motion is generally abnormal, that is, anterior. Other M-mode echo findings include left atrial enlargement and reduced aortic wall motion, indicative of impaired left atrial emptying and low cardiac output. Left ventricular dimensions are decreased. It must be emphasized that M-mode echocardiography has been less reliable in infants and children with congenital mitral valve stenosis, since valve leaflet motion may not reveal obstruction at distal levels within the mitral apparatus.[32] However, it has been suggested that parachute mitral valve deformity can be differentiated from supramitral stenosing ring.[44] Two-dimensional echocardiography provides superior imaging of the mitral valve in the long and short axis orientations.

The long axis view provides assessment of the mobility of the body of the mitral valve leaflets, as well as chordal length and insertion. Anomalies of the papillary muscles may be observed in the short axis orientation.[98] Estimation of the valve orifice area is limited, since obstruction may be distal to the leaflets themselves, and the valve area varies with transducer angulation.[32]

CARDIAC CATHETERIZATION

Analyses of blood gases may demonstrate mild systemic desaturation and hypercapnea in the presence of pulmonary edema. Oximetry may demonstrate a left-right shunt at the atrial level through a patent foramen ovale when valvular stenosis is severe. Pulmonary arterial and capillary wedge pressures may be elevated. Direct left atrial pressure recording should be obtained in the presence of pulmonary hypertension in order to rule out pulmonary venous obstruction, cor triatriatum, severe left ventricular dysfunction, or left ventricular outflow tract obstruction. It should be noted that pulmonary vein obstruction may coexist with mitral valve malformations.[51, 84] Catheter withdrawal from the left ventricle to atrium or simultaneous pressure recordings demonstrate increased left atrial A and V pressure waves and a diastolic pressure gradient between the left atrium and ventricle. Cineangiocardiography with injections in the left atrium or ventricle in the right anterior oblique projection may demonstrate thickening and reduced mobility of the mitral valve leaflets in patients with isolated mitral valve stenosis or an hourglass shaped diastolic left ventricular filling defect characteristic of parachute mitral valve malformation.[51] Mitral insufficiency may be present. Associated congenital cardiac malformations, particularly those of the left ventricular outflow tract, should be actively sought.[10, 20, 76] In rare instances of mitral atresia with normally developed left ventricle and aortic valve, selective left atrial injection is required to establish the diagnosis, and balloon or blade atrial septostomy should be performed to decompress the obstructed left atrium.[59]

TREATMENT

Medical management of infants and children with mild to moderate congenital mitral valve stenosis includes conventional therapy for cardiac failure, and attention to common complications, such as pulmonary infection, endocarditis, and atrial fibrillation with embolization. Theoretically, digoxin should not relieve cardiac "failure" in patients with mitral stenosis, since the elevated left atrial pressure is caused by mechanical obstruction. When cardiac failure is not responsive to medical management, surgical relief of obstruction by valvotomy or replacement is necessary. Although isolated cases of successful mitral valve replacement have been achieved in infancy, mitral valvotomy or fenestration remains the initial procedure of choice.[5, 16, 28, 35, 45, 51, 81, 93, 99] Median survival is generally related to left ventricular development and associated congenital malformations rather than mitral valve orifice size.[35, 76] Palliative mitral valvotomy or fenestration procedures have been employed with some success. A 10-year postoperative survival rate of 50% has been reported for children primarily undergoing mitral valvotomy.[35] A recent report described a 32% operative mortality and actuarial 5-year survival rate of 50% in infants and children following prosthetic mitral valve replacement.[99] Operative mortality was greatest in children under 10 years of age and those with associated congenital cardiac defects. Currently all efforts should be directed at optimum medical therapy and preservation of the mitral valve at surgery.

CONGENITAL MITRAL INSUFFICIENCY

Congenital mitral insufficiency (MI) is an extremely rare isolated defect. It is most frequently found in association with other congenital cardiac defects or cardiomyopathy, metabolic disorders, and mucocutaneous lymph node (Kawasaki) syndrome.[20, 27, 33, 35, 38, 41, 65]

Clinical Features

Increased precordial activity and a diffuse apical impulse may be palpated. The first heart sound is diminished, and the pulmonic component is loud and narrowly split when pulmonary hypertension is present. A high frequency, plateau-type blowing or harsh holosystolic murmur is auscultated at the apex with radiation to the axilla and back. The harsh murmur may sound like the murmur of a VSD. A low-frequency, apical diastolic murmur and third heart sound may be present with more severe degrees of valvular insufficiency.

ABNORMAL CLEFT POSTERIOR LEAFLET

This condition has been associated with significant MI.[20, 26, 54] However, such clefts are apparently present in normal individuals.[67] Patients with significant MI may represent a more extreme form or have associated abnormalities of the mitral valve apparatus, such as anomalies of the papillary muscles or chordae tendineae.[7, 54]

ANOMALOUS MITRAL ARCADE

The complex of anomalous mitral arcade has been variably described.[12, 20, 47, 58, 76] Generally, the free margins of the mitral valve are thickened and rolled, and the chordae tendineae are shortened and fused. Together these form an arcade-like structure which appears to connect directly with the papillary muscles. Anomalies of the papillary muscles are usually present. In most cases, limited coaptation of the valve leaflets causes predominant MI; however, stenosis may be present as well.[12, 47]

Finally, MI may be associated with a wide variety of congenital and acquired cardiac conditions. These include endocardial cushion defect, CA, VSD and ASD, PDA, left ventricular diverticulum, anomalous origin of left coronary artery from the pulmonary artery, coronary arteritis, congestive and hypertrophic cardiomyopathies, cardiac tumor, rheumatic and viral myocarditis, collagen diseases, metabolic disorders (Hurler's disease), homocystinuria, and connective tissue disorders (Marfan's disease and Ehlers-Danlos' syndrome.[27, 33, 38, 65] MI in these conditions is secondarily related to left ventricular dysfunction and/or mitral anular dilatation, which ultimately leads to insufficient systolic overlap of the leaflets.

Electrocardiographic Features

The electrocardiogram demonstrates left atrial and left ventricular enlargement when significant MI is present.

Radiographic Features

The chest radiograph demonstrates left atrial and ventricular enlargement and engorgement of the pulmonary vasculature.

Echocardiographic Features

M-mode echocardiography may suggest abnormal mitral valve anatomy, such as thickened leaflets and valve preclosure.[32] Secondary findings include increased left atrial and ventricular dimensions and normal to increased systolic function indices when cardiac failure is absent. These findings vary with the presence of associated cardiac malformations. Two dimensional echocardiograms in the long and short axis orientations may demonstrate abnormalities of the valve apparatus similar to those mentioned for congenital mitral valve stenosis. The long axis orientation may additionally demonstrate insufficient overlapping of the anterior and posterior leaflets. The short axis orientation may show insufficient coaptation of the leaflets at various portions of the valve; however, this finding may be produced artifactually. A break in the anterior or posterior leaflet echogram suggests the possibility of cleft mitral valve leaflet.

TREATMENT

Prognosis of congenital MI varies with the timing of presentation and with the severity of associated congenital cardiac malformations. Management in young infants and children with mild to moderate MI remains primarily that of medical management of cardiac failure. In those instances when cardiac failure is unresponsive to medical management, initial surgical attempts should be made to preserve the valve either by mitral valvuloplasty or annuloplasty.[28, 93, 99]

MITRAL VALVE PROLAPSE

The clinical constellation of nonejection click and late systolic murmur has been termed Barlow's syndrome in recognition of his pioneering work.[3] Angiographic correlations with mitral valve prolapse were demonstrated relatively recently in the mid-sixties.[17] Early observations in children, an increasing awareness of the clinical features of this condition, and widespread availability of echocardiography have suggested a frequency in the pediatric population similar to that reported for adults (6.3%).[8, 13, 30, 56, 66] A frequency of 1.4% was detected during a routine screening of predominantly black South African school children.[56] However, it was noted that rheumatic fever was commonly present in this population. At one major center, 10% of the population referred for cardiac evaluation had evidence of mitral valve prolapse either as an isolated condition or in association with other congenital heart diseases.[30] For example, in patients with secundum ASD, estimates of associated prolapse vary from 15 to 41%.[22, 40, 96] Other associated conditions include Ebstein's anomaly of the tricuspid valve, L transposition of the great arteries, connective tissue disorders (Marfan's syndrome, Ehlers-Danlos' syndrome), Turner's syndrome, metabolic disorders (homocystinuria), rheumatic fever, Kawasaki's syndrome, anomalous origin of left coronary artery from the pulmonary artery, and cardiomyopathy.[11, 18, 57, 70, 80, 89, 95] In view of the frequency of this condition in the general population, it has been difficult to conclude whether such observations represent more than a chance association of mitral valve prolapse with the underlying cardiac disorder.

PATHOLOGY

The etiology of "idiopathic" or isolated mitral valve prolapse in children and adults remains unknown. It has been proposed that a condition so ubiquitous as mitral valve prolapse may represent a "silent form of congenital heart disease" which is ultimately manifested by a characteristic constellation of clinical findings and valvular dysfunction.[70] Some have proposed that a basic abnormality of the myxomatous matrix of the mitral valve leaflet or of the collagenous structure of the chordae may be the primary cause of this disorder.[70] Others have suggested that the developmental abnormality proposed for Ebstein's anomaly of the tricuspid valve could similarly explain the redundant mitral valve tissue and elongated chordae characteristic of mitral prolapse.[90] A congenital or developmental malformation is presumably involved in those individuals with familial forms of mitral valve prolapse or in those with hereditary connective tissue disorders such as Marfan's syndrome.[68, 78] Others have proposed cardiomyopathy, myocardial dysfunction, and coronary insufficiency as causes.[42, 57, 95] Finally, it is most likely that "secondary" mitral valve prolapse associated with underlying cardiac conditions may be related to myocardial and hemodynamic abnormalities or to changes of ventricular geometry.

Because mitral valve prolapse is a relatively benign condition in childhood, little clinical and pathological correlation is available.[8, 30, 56, 70] However, abundant anatomical information is available regarding later stages of the disease in adults.[70] The major anatomical findings consist of focal or diffusely redundant valve tissue involving one or both valve leaflets with or without associated lengthening of the chordae tendineae. Commissure to commissure width and base to free edge length are generally greater than normal. The leaflet diameter at the base becomes greater than that of the anulus. Less commonly, the length is increased. Three clinical pathological stages have been proposed: Stage 1. Nonejection mitral click may be associated with grossly normal mitral leaflets; Stage 2. Nonejection click and late systolic murmur may be related to scalloping of the leaflets but normal anulus; Stage 3. Holosystolic murmur alone may be related to anular dilatation and stretching (rather than scalloping) of the leaflets.[70] It is noteworthy that pathological changes characteristic of mitral valve prolapse, such as anular dilatation and myxomatous degeneration of the leaflets, occur commonly in other forms of cardiac disease, such as rheumatic carditis. However, the diameter of the mitral anulus is usually less than 25% larger than normal values, whereas in mitral valve prolapse it is frequently greater than 50% larger than normal. Furthermore, in rheumatic carditis the mitral leaflet and chordal length are generally decreased.

Microscopy demonstrates an increase of acid mucopolysaccharide or myxomatous material in the central portion of the leaflets. The atrial aspects of the leaflet are focally thickened, and this is probably caused by increased sliding and friction between the leaflets during systole. Connective tissue pads form on the ventricular surface of the leaflets, often extending to the ventricular endocardium behind the posterior leaflet. Ultrastructural studies have demonstrated abnormalities of collagen in the leaflets and chordae.

PHYSIOLOGY

Mitral systolic closure normally occurs in the subanular position. The prolapsing mitral leaflets, however, undergo a sudden systolic tension following closure, much like an "unfurled sail" snapping in the wind.[14, 18] Initially closure may be in the subanular position, but slippage places the leaflets in a supranular position. The slippage imposes stress upon the leaflets and tensor apparatus. In addition, the mitral anulus contracts less in patients with mitral valve prolapse than in normals.[61] In diastole, the prolapsing redundant areas of the leaflets virtually "dump" into the left ventricle. The stressed areas of the mitral valve appear to ultimately provide a focus for thrombi or vegetations.[70] Hemodynamic and clinical abnormalities associated with mitral valve prolapse are conveniently described in terms of ventriculovalvular disproportion.[18] Consequently, the reduction of left ventricular diastolic volume causes the mitral leaflets to prolapse to a greater degreee and earlier in systole, producing an earlier click and longer murmur.

Clinical Features

Mitral valve prolapse is a relatively common condition in childhood and adolescence.[8, 13, 30, 56, 66] However, few infants have been described without underlying connective tissue disorder or congenital cardiac disease.[13] The youngest child with isolated mitral valve prolapse reported in one large series of pediatric patients was 2.5 years of age, with the mean age at presentation 9.9 years.[8] As in adults, the female to male ratio was 2:1. The majority of patients (34%) were referred for atypical auscultatory findings first noted after a febrile illness. Another third of the patients were referred primarily for auscultatory findings noted on routine physical examination. The commonest presenting complaint was poorly defined nonexertional chest pain (18%). Others described common complaints of atypical chest pain and exertional intolerance.[10] Dizziness and syncope occurred less frequently. Dysrhythmia (3%) and fatigue (3%) were rarely the primary reason for referral.[8] The occurrence of clinically "silent" mitral valve prolapse in children remains controversial.[32]

Physical Examination

A slendor gracile habitus and various thoracic cage abnormalities, such as pectus excavatum, have been described in adults.[9, 55, 79, 90] However, these findings are less common in children.[8, 10, 30] High arched palate, increased joint laxity, or abnormal dermatoglyphic patterns may be present. The auscultatory findings of isolated mitral valve prolapse often vary from examination to examination and even during the examination.[18, 30] The clinical diagnosis requires a high degree of suspicion in order to elicit the characteristic auscultatory findings. The click associated with mitral valve prolapse is best heard at the left sternal border and is described as midsystolic or "nonejection." However, it may vary from early to late systolic and may even fuse with the first or second heart sound. Multiple systolic clicks may be present, producing a staccato or grating sound. The click may originate from the sudden prolapsing of the valve leaflets or from the tensing of the chordae tendineae. The characteristic auscultatory feature relates to change in the timing of the click and response to pharmacologic or postural maneuvers which alter left ventricular volume[3, 18] (Table 32.1, Fig. 32.2). Interventions which reduce ventricular volume increase the degree of mitral valve prolapse and, therefore, the click moves toward the first heart sound. Conversely, those which increase the ventricular volume move the click toward the second heart sound (Fig. 32.2). The second heart sound may be widely split due to early aortic valve closure. An early diastolic sound which may resemble fixed split second sound or second sound opening snap is frequently heard. The finding may be due to recoaptation when the prolapsed

TABLE 32.1 EFFECTS OF POSTURAL AND PHYSIOLOGICAL INTERVENTIONS UPON CLICK-MURMUR OF PROLAPSED MITRAL VALVE SYNDROME

Click (earlier)	Click (later)
Mumur (louder, longer)	Murmur (softer, shorter)
↓ Left ventricular size	↑ Left ventricular size
↓ Preload, afterload	↑ Preload, afterload
Supine to sitting	Sitting to supine
Sitting to standing	Standing to squatting
Squatting to standing	Passive leg raising
Tachycardia	Phenylephrine
Amyl nitrite	
Valsalva	

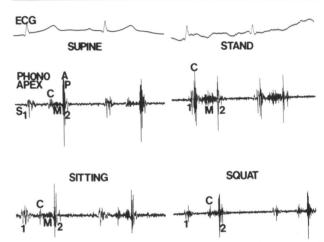

Fig. 32.2 Phonocardiogram of postural interventions recorded in an 8-year-old boy with familial prolapsed mitral valve syndrome. Excerpts of medium frequency apex recordings were obtained at constant amplification and paperspeed. *Supine,* A "nonejection" click (c) is followed by low intensity murmur at approximately two-thirds systole. *Sitting,* The click and murmur occur earlier (midsystole), and the intensity of the murmur is increased. *Standing,* The click and murmur occur at early systole. The murmur is of maximum intensity and had a "honking" quality. *Squatting,* The cardiac rate slows, the click and murmur occur earlier, and the intensity of the murmur is decreased.

posterior leaflet hits the anterior leaflet as it is "unprolapsed" prior to opening.[97]

The cardiac murmur of mitral valve prolapse is generally but not always preceded by the click and is classically described as late systolic in timing.[3, 18] The murmur, like the click, varies in timing, intensity, and duration in response to postural and pharmacologic maneuvers (Table 32.1 and Fig. 32.2). The murmur occurs earlier and the intensity and duration increase with those interventions which decrease left ventricular volume.[14, 18, 53] It is best heard at the apex with radiation to the midprecordium but is occasionally auscultated at the base and in the neck. The character is crescendo-decrescendo, and the intensity may vary dramatically with changes of posture from nondetectable to audible without a stethoscope.[26] Occasionally the murmur may have a "honking" or "whooping" quality.[63]

Generally the harsh musical qualities and the paradoxical responses to pharmacologic and postural maneuvers distinguish the murmur from that of acquired rheumatic mitral valve insufficiency.[89] In one series, the majority of children with isolated mitral valve prolapse had a nonejection click and late systolic murmur (62%), whereas 24% had an isolated systolic murmur, and 13% had isolated click or series of clicks.[8] A pansystolic murmur without click was generally but not necessarily associated with significant degrees of MI.[8, 30] A noteworthy atypical finding was the auscultation of a vibratory murmur with the character of Still's murmur.[30] However, the nonejection click and the apical location suggested the diagnosis of mitral valve prolapse. It is worth reemphasizing that the diagnosis of mitral valve prolapse requires a high degree of suspicion and cannot be ruled out in any child without carefully performing the described postural maneuvers (Table 32.1, Fig. 32.2).

Radiologic Features

The chest radiograph of isolated mitral valve prolapse is generally normal, and thoracoskeletal abnormalities, including narrow anteroposterior diameter, are infrequent in the pediatric population.[8, 9, 10, 30, 79]

Electrocardiographic Features

Electrocardiographic features may vary from time to time within a given patient. Abnormalities of repolarization, conduction, and cardiac rhythm may be variably present at rest, at exercise, during amyl nitrate inhalation, or on ambulatory ECG (Holter) monitoring. Repolarization abnormalities described include prolongation of the QT interval and T wave inversion in the inferolateral leads (II, III, AVF and V_4 to V_6).[8, 10, 30, 36, 39, 64] Generally, ST segment changes are absent at rest but often are induced during exercise.[8] Various reports have cited abnormal ECG findings in 49 to 63% of children; the majority (21 to 48%) had the classic pattern of isolated T wave inversion.[8, 30] Smaller numbers exhibited cardiac dysrhythmia (unifocal PVCs) and/or conduction disturbances. Others found echocardiographic evidence of mitral valve prolapse in six of 51 patients referred for evaluation of ventricular dysrhythmia of undetermined etiology. However, it is noteworthy that all of these patients initially had clinically "silent" mitral valve prolapse; two ultimately manifested the classical auscultatory findings.[64]

Echocardiographic Features

M-mode echocardiography characteristically demonstrates a dorsal systolic movement of the posterior and/or anterior leaflet of the mitral valve (Fig. 32.3). False positive and negative results are readily produced.[32, 78] Proper positioning of the transducer on the lower precordium, and horizontal to superior angulation is essential in order to eliminate these artifacts. Optimal recordings are obtained from the free edges of the leaflets. False posterior mitral systolic motion is produced when the transducer has been positioned too high or is angulated inferiorly. The normal basal to apical movement of the mitral apparatus away from the superiorly placed transducer causes the artifactual posterior systolic mitral motion.

Several echocardiographic criteria have been proposed as diagnostic of mitral valve prolapse. Pansystolic posterior displacement (hammocking) of the valve greater than 2 mm dorsal to the closure point or a distinct late systolic displacement are the generally accepted echocardiographic features in adults. Others have suggested a pediatric criterion of any systolic mitral valve motion posterior to a reference line drawn parallel to the chest wall from the closure (C) point of the mitral valve.[8] It is our belief that the isolated pattern of late systolic posterior motion (dip) or combined systolic hammocking and late systolic dip of either leaflet are more reliable echocardiographic criteria than holosystolic hammocking alone. The latter may represent exaggerated systolic concavity of the anterior leaflet occurring when it is

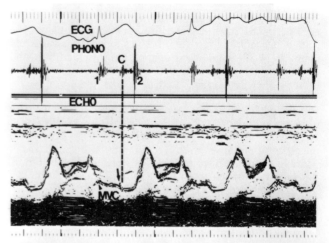

Fig. 32.3 M-mode echocardiogram and apical phonocardiogram. The mitral valve appears thickened, and opening excursion appears increased. Following mitral valve closure (*MVC*), early gradual posterior systolic mitral motion is interrupted by abrupt posterior systolic motion at midsystole. A "nonejection" click (*C*) and murmur are recorded concomitant with the midsystolic prolapse.

engulfed by the gusset-like posterior leaflet and constricting anulus.[17, 18, 91] Additional helpful findings include thickening of the leaflets or multiple leaflet echoes and increased mitral D-E excursion.

In those children with equivocal M-mode echocardiographic findings, a 2D study provides the advantage of assuring transducer angulation and/or obtaining M-mode recordings from selected portions of the mitral valve leaflets.[29] Positioning of the bodies of the anterior and/or posterior valve leaflets superior to the atrioventricular junction is a relatively specific diagnostic criteria of mitral valve prolapse.[32] This finding may be observed either in the long axis or four chamber orientation (Figs. 32.4 and 32.5). Currently we, as others, remain reluctant to diagnose clinically "silent" mitral valve prolapse on the basis of M-mode echocardiography alone, particularly if the findings cannot be confirmed by 2D echocardiography.[32]

Phonocardiographic Features

Phonocardiography remains the most objective method of demonstrating the auscultatory findings of mitral valve prolapse, namely the characteristic mobile nonejection click and murmur previously described (Fig. 32.2, Table 32.1). Since the diagnosis of mitral valve prolapse should not be established on the basis of echocardiographic findings alone, and because physical signs may be variably present, validation and documentation of the auscultatory findings by phonocardiography remain important. We would accept the diagnosis of mitral prolapse based on auscultatory features even if the echocardiogram fails to demonstrate a characteristic pattern.

CARDIAC CATHETERIZATION

Diagnostic catheterization and angiocardiography are infrequently required in children with uncomplicated mitral valve prolapse as combined physical, phonocardiographic, and echocardiographic findings are sufficient to establish the diagnosis. Hemodynamic measurements are generally normal unless significant mitral insufficiency is present.[18] Left ventriculography demonstrates the body of the mitral valve leaflets prolapsing superior to the valvular anulus. In the right anterior oblique projection, the anterior commissural

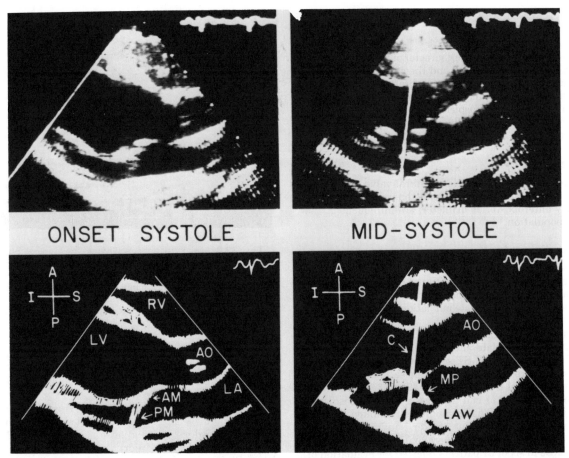

Fig. 32.4 Single frame two-dimensional echocardiograms (*above*) and corresponding diagrams (*below*) from same patient (Figs. 32.2 and 32.3). Long axis orientation. *Onset systole*, Anterior (*AM*) and posterior (*PM*) mitral leaflets coapt remaining below the plane of the atrioventricular junction. *Midsystole*, The posterior mitral leaflet arches or prolapses (*MP*) superior to the plane of the atrioventricular junction indicated by the cursor (*C*). The posterior mitral leaflet strikes the left atrial wall (*LAW*) in later frames. The mitral leaflets appear thickened. *A*, anterior; *P*, posterior; *S*, superior; *I*, inferior; *AO*, aorta; *LA*, left atrium; *LV*, left ventricle; *RV*, right ventricle.

scallop of the posterior mitral leaflet appears to protrude as "hump" below the anterior sinuses of the aortic valve.[17] The prolapse may be present throughout all phases of the cardiac cycle but is generally greatest during systole. Tricuspid valve prolapse and Ebstein's anomaly of the tricuspid valve have been associated with mitral valve prolapse in adults. Abnormalities of left ventricular contraction observed in adults include hyper- or hypocontractility and an indentation at the base of the posteromedial papillary muscle (ballerina foot deformity).[18] The latter findings have been infrequently observed in children.

Various methods have been proposed for quantification of mitral valve prolapse in children.[22] Optimum visualization of the mitral leaflets and anulus by cineventriculography requires proper angulation in order to view the mitral valve leaflets and anulus en face (approximately 60° right anterior oblique; 45° left anterior oblique).[17] Proper patient angulation is mandatory to establish the diagnosis of mitral valve prolapse when associated with congenital heart disease, such as ASD. Recent observations suggest a falsely high frequency of angiographic mitral valve prolapse in such patients which may be related primarily to alteration of left ventricular position and distortion of ventricular geometry.[22, 86]

NATURAL HISTORY

The natural history of mitral valve prolapse has been extensively documented in adults.[1, 18] Major, albeit infre-

quent, complications reported include endocarditis, chordal rupture, progressive MI, transient cerebral ischemic attacks, ventricular dysrhythmias, and sudden death.[4, 34, 43, 83, 100] Although the history of mitral valve prolapse is incompletely understood, it appears that mitral valve prolapse is a relatively benign condition in children.[8, 10, 30, 56] Cardiac dysrhythmia at rest or during exercise is common. Sudden death has not yet been reported but has been narrowly averted in two older children.[30] Chordal rupture has not been reported in children. Progression from mild to severe MI occurred most commonly in those with familial history or with connective tissue disorders.[18] Endocarditis and cerebrovascular accidents have been rare events in children.[8, 30] Currently, no consistent risk factors have been identified in children. However, morbidity and mortality appears greater in familial cases, connective tissue disorders, or cardiomyopathy.[1, 18, 83]

TREATMENT

The asymptomatic child with uncomplicated mitral valve prolapse requires occasional cardiac evaluation to ensure that symptoms and physical findings remain unchanged and to reinforce the necessity for prophylaxis against endocarditis. Initial evaluation includes chest radiograph and resting ECG. Phonocardiogram and echocardiogram are recommended in those cases with equivocal or atypical auscultatory findings. Children with a history of palpitations, dizziness, syncope, chest pain, or dysrhythmia on resting ECG

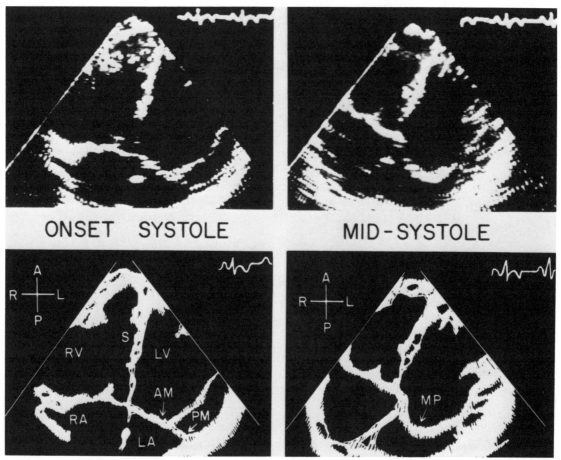

Fig. 32.5 Two-dimensional echocardiograms (*above*) and illustrations (*below*) from same patient. Four chamber apex orientation. *Onset systole*, Both mitral and tricuspid valves close below the planes of their respective atrioventricular junctions. The chordae tendineae of the mitral valve appear elongated and serpentine. *Midsystole*, The T-shaped tricuspid valve arches slightly superiorly but maintains a normal subanular position. In contrast, the mitral valve arches superior to the plane of its atrioventricular junction or anulus prolapsing (*MP*) nearly to the wall of the left atrium (*LA*). *A*, anteroinferior; *P*, posterosuperior; *S*, septum.

require ambulatory ECG (Holter) monitoring and exercise ECG. The latter is particularly recommended in those who routinely perform exhaustive or competitive athletics, as it is speculated that life-threatening dysrhythmias might be provoked under such circumstances.[8, 18, 39, 64, 100] In view of the potential likelihood of such dysrhythmias, we discourage participation in strenuous or competitive athletics.

We currently recommend antibiotic prophylaxis for endocarditis in all patients with mitral valve prolapse, even in those with isolated nonejection click. Symptomatic dysrhythmias should be treated with appropriate antiarrhythmic agents.[64] Recurrent or debilitating atypical precordial chest pain may respond to propranolol, and in these instances reassurance is essential.[101] Cerebral vascular episodes may be treated with anticoagulants or inhibitors of platelet aggregation.[4] It is noteworthy that these medications are contraindicated during pregnancy.[28, 93]

Surgical management is rarely required in children. However, mitral valvuloplasty or annuloplasty are effective and preferred in children with severe MI. We, as well as others, have experienced the complication of dislodgement of su-

tures and valve prosthesis in patients with connective tissue disorders.[30] Mitral valve replacement has been reported to be beneficial in some adult patients with life-threatening dysrhythmias but has not been required in children.

Finally, family counseling and reassurance are essential. Unless directly questioned, we do not discuss the morbid complications of mitral valve prolapse since they occur infrequently in adults and are particularly unusual in children. Nevertheless, we do mention the slight possibility of dysrhythmia and the necessity of reporting symptoms to the physician. Because the prognosis is less favorable in those families with an autosomal dominant mode of inheritance, cardiac evaluation of first degree relatives is indicated.

In view of the common prevalance of this condition in adults, it is apparent that pediatricians have merely exposed the tip of a prolapsing iceberg. Because of the economic, human, and social implications of this condition, it is important that pediatricians, in particular, exercise a wide degree of diagnostic suspicion and interest in the investigation of this important "congenital" cardiac condition.

REFERENCES

1. Allen, H., Harris, A., and Leatham, A.: Significance and prognosis of an isolated late systolic murmur: A 9 to 22 year follow-up. Br. Heart J. 36:525, 1974.

2. Anderson, R. H., Becker, A. E., Macartney, F. J., Shinebourne, E. A., Wilkinson, J. L., and Tynan, M. J.: A question of definition. Is "Tricuspid Atresia" a univentricular heart?

Pediatr. Cardiol. 1:51, 1979.

3. Barlow, J. B., and Bosman, C. K.: Aneurysmal protrusion of the posterior leaflet of the mitral valve. An auscultatory-electrocardio-

graphic syndrome. Am. Heart J. 1:166, 1966.
4. Barnett, H. J. M., Jones, M. W., Boughner, D. R., and Kostuk, W. J.: Cerebral ischemic events associated with prolapsing mitral valve. Arch. Neurol. 33:777, 1976.
5. Bernhard, W. F., and Litwin, S. B.: The surgical treatment of unusual congenital mitral valve anomalies. Circulation 45(Suppl. II):46, 1972.
6. Bett, J. H. N., and Storin, P. G. I.: Parachute deformity of the mitral valve. Thorax 24:632, 1969.
7. Bevilacqua, G.: Congenital mitral regurgitation due to "posterior reinsertion" of chordae tendineae. Br. Heart J. 36:520, 1974.
8. Bisset, G. S., III, Schwartz, D. C., Meyer, R. A., James, F. W., and Kaplan, S.: Clinical spectrum and long term follow-up of isolated mitral valve prolapse in 119 children. Circulation 62:423, 1980.
9. Bon Tempo, C. P., Ronan, J. A., Jr., De Leon, A. C., et al.: Radiographic appearance of the thorax in systolic click-late systolic murmur syndrome. Am. J. Cardiol. 36:27, 1975.
10. Brown, L. M.: Mitral valve prolapse in children. Adv. Pediatr. 24:327, 1978.
11. Brown, O. R., De Mots, H., Kloster, F. E., Roberts, A., Menashe, V. D., and Beals, R. K.: Aortic root dilatation and mitral valve prolapse in Marfan's syndrome. Circulation 52:651, 1975.
12. Castenada, A. R., Anderson, R. C., and Edwards, J. E.: Congenital mitral stenosis resulting from anomalous arcade and obstructing papillary muscles. Am. J. Cardiol. 24:237, 1969.
13. Chandraratna, P. A., Vlahovich, G., Kong, Y., and Wilson, D.: Incidence of mitral valve prolapse in one hundred clinically stable newborn baby girls. Br. Heart J. 98:312, 1979.
14. Cobbs, B. W., and King, S. B.: Ventricular buckling: A factor in the abnormal ventriculogram and peculiar hemodynamics associated with mitral valve prolapse. Am. Heart J. 93:741, 1977.
15. Collins-Nakai, R. L., Rosenthal, A., Castenada, A. R., Bernhard, W. F., and Nadas, A. S.: Congenital mitral stenosis: A review of twenty years experience. Circulation 56:1039, 1977.
16. Crawford, F. A., Jr., Selby, J. H., Jr., and Joransen, J. A. Mitral valve replacement with a porcine heterograft in an infant. J. Thorac. Cardiovasc. Surg. 75:705, 1978.
17. Criley, J. M., Lewis, K. B., Humphries, J. E., and Ross, R. S.: Prolapse of the mitral valve: Clinical and cine-angiocardiographic findings Br. Heart J. 28:482, 1966.
18. Criley, J. M., and Heger, J.: Prolapsed mitral leaflet syndrome. Cardiovasc. Clin. 10:213, 1979.
19. Daoud, G., Kaplan, S., Perrin, E. V., Dorst, J. P., and Edwards, K. F.: Congenital mitral stenosis. Circulation 27:185, 1963.
20. Davachi, R., Moller, J. H., and Edwards, J. E.: Diseases of the mitral valve in infancy: Anatomic analysis of 55 cases. Circulation 43:565, 1971.
21. De La Cruz, M. V., and Miller, B. L.: Double inlet left ventricle. Circulation 37:249, 1968.
22. Duncan, W. J., Moes, F. C., Rose, V., Bloom, K. R., and Olley, P. M.: Angiographic quantification of mitral valve prolapse in children with secundum atrial septal defect. A new method. Pediatr. Cardiol. 1:29, 1979.
23. Du Plessis, L. A., and Marchand, P.: The anatomy of the mitral valve and its associated structures. Thorax 19:221, 1964.
24. Edwards, J. E., and Burchell, H. B.: Pathologic anatomy of mitral insufficiency. Proc. Mayo Clin. 33:497, 1958.
25. Ferencz, C., Johnson, A. L., and Wigglesworth, F. W.: Congenital mitral stenosis. Circulation 9:161, 1954.

26. Fiddler, G. I., and Scott, O.: Heart murmurs audible across the room in children with mitral valve prolapse. Br. Heart J. 44:201, 1980.
27. Freed, M. D., Kenae, J. F., Van Praagh, R., Castenada, A. R., Bernhard, W. F., and Nadas, A. S.: Coarctation of the aorta with congenital mitral regurgitation. Circulation 49:1175, 1974.
28. Friedman, S., Edmunds, L. H., Jr., and Causo, C. C.: Long term mitral replacement in young children. Influence of somatic growth and prosthetic valve adequacy. Circulation 57:981, 1978.
29. Gilbert, B. W., Schatz, R. A., Von Ramm, O. T., Behar, V. S., and Kisslo, J. S.: Mitral valve prolapse: Two-dimensional echocardiographic and angiographic correlation. Circulation 54:716, 1976.
30. Gingell, R. L., and Vlad, P.: Mitral valve prolapse. In Heart Disease in Infancy and Childhood, edited by J. D. Keith, R. D. Rowe, and P. Vlad. Macmillan, New York, 1978, p. 810.
31. Glancy, D. L., Chang, M. Y., Dorney, E. R., and Roberts, W. D.: Parachute mitral valve. Further observations and associated lesions. Am. J. Cardiol. 27:309, 1971.
32. Goldberg, S. J., Allen, H. D., and Sahn, D. J.: Pediatric and Adolescent Echocardiography. Year Book Medical Publishers, New York, 1980, p. 214.
33. Goodman, D. J., and Hancock, E. W.: Secundum atrial septal defect associated with a cleft mitral valve. Br. Heart J. 35:1315, 1973.
34. Goodman, D., Kimbiris, D., and Linhart, J. W.: Chordae tendineae rupture complicating the systolic click-late systolic murmur syndrome. Am. J. Cardiol. 33:681, 1974.
35. Gueron, M., Hirsch, M., Opschitzer, I., and Mogel, P.: Left ventricular diverticulum and mitral incompetence in asymptomatic children. Circulation 53:181, 1976.
36. Hancock, W. E., and Cohn, K.: The syndrome associated with midsystolic click and late systolic murmur. Am. J. Med. 41:183, 1966.
37. Hunt, D., and Sloman, G.: Prolapse of the posterior leaflet of the mitral valve occurring in eleven members of a family. Am. Heart J. 78:149, 1969.
38. Iwa, T., Watanabe, Y., Misaki, T., and Yoshida, H.: Simultaneous repair of anomalous origin of the left coronary artery from the pulmonary artery and mitral regurgitation. Ann. Thorac. Surg. 29:562, 1980.
39. Kavey, R. E., Sondheimer, H. M., and Blackman, M. S.: Detection of dysrhythmia in pediatric patients with mitral valve prolapse. Circulation 62:582, 1980.
40. Keck, E. W., Henschel, W. G., and Gruh, L.: Mitral valve prolapse in children with secundum-type atrial septal defect. Eur. J. Pediatr. 121:89, 1976.
41. Kitamura, S., Kawashima, Y., Kawachi, K., Harima, R., Ihara, K., Nakano, S., Shimazaki, Y., and Mori, T.: Severe mitral regurgitation due to coronary arteritis of mucocutaneous lymph node syndrome. A new surgical entity. J. Thorac. Cardiovasc. Surg. 80:629, 1980.
42. Koch, F. H., Billingham, M. E., Mason, J. W., et al.: Pathogenesis of the click-murmur-prolapse syndrome: Biopsy evidence supporting an underlying cardiomyopathic process. Am. J. Cardiol. 39:272, 1977.
43. Lachman, A. S., Braunwell-Jones, D. M., Lakier, J. B., Pocock, W. A., and Barlow, J. B.: Infective endocarditis in the billowing mitral leaflet syndrome. Br. Heart J. 37:326, 1975.
44. La Corte, M., Harada, K., and Williams, R.: Echocardiographic features of left ventricular inflow obstruction. Circulation 54:562, 1976.
45. Laks, H., Hellenbrand, W. E., Kleinman, C., and Talner, N. S.: Left atrial-left ventricular conduit for relief of congenital mitral stenosis

in infancy. J. Thorac. Cardiovasc. Surg. 80:782, 1980.
46. Lam, J. H. C., Ranganathan, M., Wigle, E. D., and Silvers, M. D.: Morphology of the human mitral valve: Chordae tendineae. Circulation 35:389, 1967.
47. Layan, T. E., and Edwards, J. E.: Anomalous mitral arcade: A type of congenital mitral insufficiency. Circulation 35:389, 1967.
48. Lieberthson, R. R., Paul, M. H., Muster, A. J., Arcilla, R. A., Eckner, F. A. O., and Lev, M.: Straddling and displaced atrioventricular orifices and valves with primitive ventricles. Circulation 43:213, 1971.
49. Lundstrom, N. R.: Echocardiography in the diagnosis of congenital mitral stenosis and in evaluation of the results of mitral valvotomy. Circulation 46:44, 1972.
50. Lundstrom, N. R.: Value of echocardiography in diagnosis of congenital mitral stenosis. Br. Heart J. 38:534, 1976.
51. Macartney, F. J., Scott, O., Ionescu, M. I., and Deverall, P.: Diagnosis and management of parachute mitral valve and supravalvar ring. Br. Heart J. 36:641, 1974.
52. Manubens, R., Krovetz, L. J., and Adams, P., Jr.: Supravalvar stenosing ring of the left atrium. Am. Heart J. 60:286, 1960.
53. Mathey, D. G., DeCoodt, P. R., Allen, H. N., and Swan, H. J. C.: The determinants of onset of mitral valve prolapse in the systolic click-late systolic murmur syndrome. Circulation 53:872, 1976.
54. McEnany, M. T., English, T. A., and Ross, D. M.: The congenitally cleft posterior mitral valve leaflet. Ann. Thorac. Surg. 16:281, 1973.
55. McKusick, V. A.: Heritable Disorders of Connective Tissue, 4th ed. C. V. Mosby, St. Louis, 1972.
56. McLaren, M. J., Hawkins, D. M., Lachman, A. S., Lakier, J. B., Pocock, W. A., and Barlow, J. B.: Non-ejection systolic clicks and mitral systolic murmurs in black children in Soweto, Johannesburg. Br. Heart J. 38:718, 1976.
57. Mercer, E. N., Frye, R. L., and Giulani, E. R.: Late systolic click in nonobstructive cardiomyopathy. Br. Heart J. 32:681, 1970.
58. Moller, H.: Congenital causes of left ventricular inflow obstruction. In The Heart, edited by J. E. Edwards. Williams & Wilkins, Baltimore, 1974.
59. Moreno, F., Quero, M., and Diaz, L. P.: Mitral atresia with normal aortic valve. A study of eighteen cases and a review of the literature. Circulation 53:1004, 1976.
60. Noonan, J. A., and Nadas, A. S.: The hypoplastic left heart syndrome. Pediatr. Clin. North Am. 5:1029, 1958.
61. Ormiston, J. A., Shah, P. M., Tei, C., and Wong, M.: Mitral valve annulus abnormalities in mitral valve prolapse (MVP). Circulation 62(Suppl. III):301, 1980.
62. Perloff, J. K., and Roberts, W. D.: The mitral apparatus: Functional anatomy of mitral regurgitation. Circulation 46:227, 1972.
63. Pickering, P.: Clicks, whoops and honks. Arch. Dis. Child. 47:731, 1972.
64. Pickoff, A. S., Gelband, H., Ferrer, P., Garcia, O., and Tamer, D.: Premature ventricular contractions as the presenting feature of mitral valve prolapse in childhood. J. Pediatr. 94:615, 1979.
65. Pliego, J., Martin-Infante, A., and Arcas-Meca, R.: Myxoma of the left atrium associated with congenital mitral insufficiency. Report of a case successfully operated on. Arch. Inst. Cardiol. Mex. 42:982, 1972.
66. Procacci, P. M., Savran, S. V., and Streiter, S. L.: Prevalence of clinical mitral valve prolapse in 1169 young women. N. Engl. J. Med. 294:1086, 1976.
67. Ranganathan, M., Lam, J. H. C., Wigle, E. D., and Silvers, M. D.: Morphology of the

human mitral valve. II. The valve leaflets. Circulation 41:459, 1970.

68. Read, R. C., Thal, A. P., and Vernon, E. W.: Symptomatic valvular myxomatous transformation (the floppy valve syndrome): A possible forme fruste of the Marfan syndrome. Circulation 32:897, 1965.

69. Reid, G. E., Cortes, L. E., Clauss, R. H., and Reppert, E. H.: The surgical repair of duplication of the mitral orifice. Ann. Thorac. Surg. 9:81, 1970.

70. Roberts, W. C.: Congenital cardiovascular abnormalities usually "silent" until adulthood: Morphologic features of the floppy mitral valve, valvular aortic stenosis, discrete subvalvular aortic stenosis, hypertrophic cardiomyopathy, sinus of Valsalva aneurysm, and the Marfan syndrome. Cardiovasc. Clin. 10:407, 1979.

71. Roberts, W. C., Dangel, J. C., and Bulkley, B. H.: Nonrheumatic valvular cardiac disease: A clinico-pathological survey of twenty-seven different conditions causing valvular dysfunction. Cardiovasc. Clin. 5:346, 1973.

72. Rogers, H. M., Waldron, B. R., and Murphy, D. F. H.: Supravalvular stenosing ring of the left atrium in association with endocardial sclerosis (E.F.E.) and mitral insufficiency. Am. Heart J. 50:777, 1955.

73. Rosenquist, G. C., Clark, E. B., McAllister, H. A., Bharati, S., and Edwards, J. E.: Increased mitral-aortic separation in discrete subaortic stenosis. Circulation 60:70, 1979.

74. Rosenquist, G. C.: Congenital mitral valve disease associated with coarctation of the aorta. Circulation 49:985, 1974.

75. Rosenquist, G. C., Stark, J., and Taylor, J. F. N.: Congenital mitral valve disease in transposition of the great arteries. Circulation 41:731, 1975.

76. Ruckman, R. N., and Van Praagh, R.: Anatomic types of congenital mitral stenosis: Report of 49 autopsy cases with consideration of diagnosis and surgical implications. Am. J. Cardiol. 42:592, 1978.

77. Rudolph, A. M., Heymann, M. A., and Spitznas, U.: Hemodynamic considerations in the development of narrowing of the aorta. Am. J. Cardiol. 30:514, 1972.

78. Sahn, D. J., Wood, J., Allen, H. D., Peoples, W., and Goldberg, S. J.: Echocardiographic spectrum of mitral valve motion in children with and without mitral valve prolapse: The nature of false positive diagnosis. Am. J. Cardiol. 39:442, 1977.

79. Salomon, J., Shah, P. M., and Heinle, R. A.: Thoracic skeletal abnormalities in idiopathic mitral valve prolapse. Am. J. Cardiol. 36:32, 1975.

80. Sanyal, S. K., Johnson, W. W., Dische, M. R., Pitner, S. E., and Beard, C.: Dystrophic degeneration of papillary muscle and ventricular myocardium. A basis for mitral valve prolapse in Duchenne's muscular dystrophy. Circulation 62:430, 1980.

81. Schachner, A., Varsano, I., and Levy, M. J.: The parachute mitral valve complex. Case report and review of the literature. J. Thorac. Cardiovasc. Surg. 70:451, 1975.

82. Schieken, R. M., Friedman, S., Waldhausen, J., and Johnson, J.: Isolated congenital mitral insufficiency: Pathological and surgical variations in five children. J. Pediatr. Surg. 6:49, 1971.

83. Shappell, S. D., Marshall, C. E., Brown, R. E., et al.: Sudden death and the familial occurrence of mid-systolic click, late systolic murmur syndrome. Circulation 48:1128, 1973.

84. Shone, J. D., Anderson, R. C., Amplatz, K., Varco, R. L., Leonard, A. S., and Edwards, J. E.: Pulmonary venous obstruction from two separate co-existent anomalies. Am. J. Cardiol. 11:525, 1963.

85. Shone, J. D., Sellers, R. D., Anderson, R. C., Adams, P., Jr., Lillehei, C., and Edwards, J. E.: The developmental complex of "parachute mitral valve," supravalvular ring of left atrium, subaortic stenosis and coarctation of the aorta. Am. J. Cardiol. 11:714, 1963.

86. Sommerville, J., Kaku, S., and Saravelli, O.: Prolapsed mitral cusps in atrial septal defect: An erroneous radiological interpretation. Br. Heart J. 40:58, 1978.

87. Sondheimer, H. M., Freedom, R. M., and Olley, P. M.: Double outlet right ventricle: Clinical spectrum and prognosis. Am. J. Cardiol. 39:709, 1977.

88. Steinbrunn, W., Chon, K. E., and Selzer, A.: Atrial septal defect associated with mitral stenosis. The Lutembacher syndrome revisited. Am. J. Med. 48:295, 1970.

89. Steinfeld, L., Dimich, I., Rappaport, H., and Baron, M.: Late systolic murmur of rheumatic mitral insufficiency. Am. J. Cardiol. 34:397, 1975.

90. Swartz, M. H., Herman, M. V., and Teicholz, L. E.: Dermatoglyphic patterns in patients with mitral valve prolapse. A clue in pathogenesis. Am. J. Cardiol. 38:588, 1976.

91. Tsakiris, A. G., Von Bernuth, R. G. C., Bourgeois, M. J., Titas, J. L., and Wood, E. H.: Size and motion of the mitral valve annulus in anesthetized intact dogs. J. Appl. Physiol. 39:611, 1971.

92. van der Horst, R. L., and Hastreiter, A. R.: Congenital mitral stenosis. Am. J. Cardiol. 20:773, 1967.

93. van der Horst, R. L., Le Roux, B. T., Rogers, N. M. A., and Gotsman, M. S.: Mitral valve replacement in childhood. A report of 51 patients. Am. Heart J. 24:624, 1973.

94. Van Mierop, L. H. S., Alley, R. D., Kausel, H. W., and Stranahan, A.: The anatomy and embryology of endocardial cushion defect. J. Thorac. Cardiovasc. Surg. 74:71, 1962.

95. Verani, M. S., Carroll, R. J., and Falsetti, H. L.: Mitral valve prolapse in coronary artery disease. Am. J. Cardiol. 37:1, 1976.

96. Victorica, B., Elliot, L., and Gessner, I.: Ostium secundum atrial septal defect associated with balloon mitral valve in children. Am. J. Cardiol. 33:668, 1974.

97. Wei, J. Y., and Fortuin, N. J.: Diastolic sounds and murmurs associated with mitral valve prolapse. Circulation 63:559, 1981.

98. Williams, D. E., Sahn, D. J., and Friedman, W. F.: Cross-sectional echocardiographic localization of sites of left ventricular outflow tract obstruction. Am. J. Cardiol. 37(2):250, 1976.

99. Williams, W. G., Pollock, J. C., Geiss, D. M., Trusler, G. A., and Fowler, R. S.: Experience with aortic and mitral valve replacement in children. J. Thorac. Cardiovasc. Surg. 81:326, 1981.

100. Winkle, R. A., Lopes, M. G., Popp, R. L., and Hancock, E. W.: Life-threatening arrythmias with mitral valve prolapse syndrome. Am. J. Med. 60:961, 1976.

101. Winkle, R. A., and Harrison, D.: Propranolol for patients with mitral valve prolapse. Am. Heart J. 93:422, 1977.

102. Zimmerman, J., and Bailey, C. P.: The surgical significance of the fibrous skeleton of the heart. Thorac. Cardiovasc. Surg. 44:701, 1962.

33

The Adolescent and Young Adult with Congenital Heart Disease

Catherine A. Neill, M.D., and Lulu M. Haroutunian, M.D.

In the adolescent and young adult, congenital heart disease manifests different diagnostic groupings, problems, and psychosocial consequences from those seen in infancy. In the 1980s, with three decades of open heart surgery behind us, cardiac diagnosis has already been long established and surgical repair undertaken in the majority of patients seen. The cardiologist trained in the swift decisive dramas of infancy, the emergency cardiac catheterizations and balloon atrial septostomies, is confronted by questions on athletics, vocation, contraception, and pregnancy. Aware of the difficulties modern teenagers with normal hearts encounter in reaching maturity,[9] one must be mindful of the injunction "non nocere." The physician to be helpful and supportive to the patient, his family, and his future, needs to consider both the effect of the cardiac defect itself on the developmental years and also ancillary problems, whether congenital or acquired, which may influence the difficult and exciting road from childhood to maturity.

In the present analysis, we have reviewed patients followed in our weekly cardiac clinic for adolescents and young adults whose records are in our current file. We established the clinic in 1963, and patients are seen jointly by cardiologists trained in pediatrics and in internal medicine.[5] Because the problems of career choice, establishing a new family base, and others continue beyond adolescence, we have included patients seen in the second and third decades of life, namely from 10 to 29 years of age. Of 2,639 persons in this age group, 1,924 have congenital malformations of the heart and form the major basis of this review (Table 33.1).

Many congenital cardiac defects causing major problems in infancy are associated with a high mortality and are not seen in our group: for example, hypoplastic left heart syndrome, present in 13% of critically ill infants 0 to 30 days of age,[21] is represented by only two individuals with mitral atresia who survived to their late teens. By contrast in the 1970s children with uncomplicated patent ductus (PDA) or atrial septal defect (ASD) have usually undergone successful heart surgery before 10 years of age, and many have been discharged from follow-up. It is of interest to compare the 10 defects most frequently encountered in our series with those reported by Rowe and Mehrizi[21] in 93 consecutive infants seen in and surviving the newborn period (Table 33.2).

Although superficially the frequency of pulmonic stenosis is the same at all ages, when this defect presents in the neonatal period it is usually extreme, often associated with hypoplasia of the right ventricle and has a high mortality, while milder degrees of pulmonic stenosis may not be recognized until long after the neonatal period.

TABLE 33.1   CARDIAC DIAGNOSES OF PATIENTS 10 TO 29 YEARS OF AGE

Congenital malformations	1924
Rheumatic heart disease	174
Dysrhythmias (heart otherwise normal)	49
Systemic hypertension; cardiomyopathy secondary to renal or neurologic disease and other	47
Normal heart, including straight back syndrome, murmur associated with pectus, "innocent" murmurs, LVH[a] by voltage without other abnormal findings, etc.	445
	2639

[a] LVH, left ventricular hypertrophy.

TABLE 33.2   MOST FREQUENT CARDIAC DIAGNOSES (%)

Defect	Abbreviation	A[a]	B[a]
Ventricular septal defect[14]	VSD	21	28
Tetralogy of Fallot	TF	20	13
Pulmonic stenosis	PS	10	10
Atrial septal defect	ASD	9	—
Aortic stenosis	AS	7	1
Coarctation of aorta	CA	6	9
Single ventricle	SV	4	5
Tricuspid atresia	TA		
Patent ductus arteriosus	PDA	4	2
Mitral insufficiency, stenosis	MI	4	1
Endocardial cushion defect	ECD	3	3
Transposition of the great arteries	TGA	2	13
All other		10	15
		100	100

[a] Present series of 1924 patients 10 to 29 years of age seen in clinic.

[b] Series of 93 consecutive infants seen in and surviving newborn period.

TABLE 33.3   PROBLEM LISTING

Cardiac problems
  Functional grouping
    Normal cardiac function
    Mild cardiac defect
    Moderate cardiac defect ± dysrhythmias
    Severe cardiac defect with cyanosis, failure or severe dysrhythmias
  Progressive changes
    Increasing stenosis or insufficiency-valve, outflow
    Calcification of valve, pulmonary outflow patch, pericardium
    Cardiac failure, cardiomegaly
    PVOD (pulmonary vascular obstructive disease)
  Complications and new developments
    Dysrhythmias
    Endocarditis
    Other
Problems of other systems
  Congenital, e.g., Down's, other syndromes
  Acquired
    Secondary to cardiac defect, e.g., hemoptysis
    Other, e.g., scoliosis
Psychosocial adaptation
  Schooling, exercise
  Marriage, pregnancy, contraception
  Self-acceptance
  Other

Another major difference between our series and those in infancy is in the frequency of prior surgery. At least 965 (50%) patients had undergone one or more cardiac operations. In attempting an organized approach to this apparently complex blend of unoperated and operated young people, we have found a problem list helpful (Table 33.3).

The problem listing for an individual patient includes: the cardiac diagnosis, both anatomic and physiologic; consideration of major extracardiac defects; and an analysis of the problems of psychosocial adaption which may be encountered.

CARDIAC PROBLEMS

Before one can begin to use the problem-oriented approach outlined in this chapter, each patient requires a definitive diagnosis. The methods of achieving this are described elsewhere in this textbook. If the cardiac defect is one requiring surgery, this should be undertaken. Whether or not surgery is indicated, the patient himself as well as his parents should clearly understand the lesion, the frequency of anticipated follow-ups or future studies, and the general nature of any progressive changes anticipated.

Once an accurate diagnosis is reached the cardiac problems can be considered under three main headings: the current *functional grouping*, any likely *progressive changes*, and the risk of *complications or new developments*, such as dysrhythmias.

FUNCTIONAL GROUPING

Symptoms alone are not adequate for this assessment, since an asymptomatic teenager may have severe aortic stenosis (AS) with major physiologic impairment. Four groups can be delineated ranging from group A with functionally normal hearts to group D with major functional impairment and major possibility of progressive changes (Table 33.4).

TABLE 33.4   FUNCTIONAL GROUPING

Group A. Normal functional cardiac status
PDA	Postoperative (PO) with no residual defect
ASD	(PO) no residual defect, normal sinus rhythm (NSR)
VSD	(PO) no residual defect, NSR
VSD	Spontaneous closure
TF	Corrected, no residual defect, NSR
Other	Anomalous subclavian artery, right aortic arch, dextrocardia and situs inversus, other defects of embryologic and possibly genetic significance, but not affecting cardiac function

Group B. Mild cardiac defect
VSD	Qp:Qs < 2:1 with normal PA pressure, NSR unoperated, or PO with residual shunt
PS	RV-PA pressure difference 50 mm or less (unoperated or PO)
CA	(PO) normal blood pressure, arm to leg BP difference < 20 mm Hg
ECD	(PO) with mild residual MI
MI	Congenital MI due to prolapse or other causes; mild, no severe dysrhythmia
TF	(PO) mild residual PS ± PI ± small VSD, ± RBBB
Other	Bicuspid aortic valve (BAV) with AI ± LV-aorta pressure difference of 20 mm or less: small atrial or other shunts (PO or unoperated) with Qp:Qs 1.5:1 or less; peripheral PS mild

Group C. Moderate cardiac defect
VSD	Qp:Qs > 2:1 and/or with AI, PS, or anomalous RV muscle bundle
PS	RV-PA pressure difference > 50 mm Hg (unoperated or PO)
CA	(Unoperated or PO) with BP differences arms and legs > 30 mm Hg and/or arm BP greater than 150/95
TF	(PO) with RV-PA pressure difference > 50 mm Hg, grossly dilated or calcified outflow patch, AI or TI or dysrhythmias
AS	(Unoperated or PO) with LV-aortic pressure difference 20 mm Hg ± AI
TGA	(Post-Mustard) ± residual shunts or dysrhythmias
Other	Unoperated (or PO) PDA, ASD, AV canal etc. requiring surgery or reoperation: AI, moderate. Dysrhythmias: sick sinus syndrome, other. Cardiomegaly with C/T ratio 60% ± with any congenital lesion

Group D. Severe cardiac defect

Cyanotic
TF	Unoperated or with palliative shunt, PO open repair with homograft, prosthetic valve, or with severe dysrhythmia
TGA	All not in Group C
SV	All types with or without prior shunts
TA	All types with or without prior shunts
PVOD	Eisenmenger reaction or primary pulmonary hypertension
Other	Truncus variants, pulmonary atresia with VSD, rare cyanotic lesions

Acyanotic

Cardiomyopathy including hypertrophic subaortic stenosis (IHSS) or following fibroelastosis or ligation anomalous left coronary artery, other

LV outflow obstruction, e.g., subaortic tunnel or other unrelieved AS with LV-aortic pressure differences of 80 mm Hg or greater

Dysrhythmias—associated syncope, or requiring pacemaker: prolonged or incapacitating + any cardiac defect

Prosthetic valves: severe AI or MI, other

The patients in group A have a cardiac murmur of grade II intensity or less, and except for the presence of a thoracic scar in some, their bodily appearance is normal and clinical course through adolescence is benign.

The patients in group B may have cardiac murmurs of grade III or more intensity, but their cardiothoracic ratio is less than 60%. The electrocardiogram may show right bundle branch block, but no major dysrhythmias or hemiblocks. Their course has been most gratifying, particularly patients with tetralogy of Fallot, who despite residual murmurs of pulmonic stenosis and insufficiency following open repairs, have shown a stable and excellent clinical course.

Group C appears heterogeneous, but all need very careful follow-up because of the risk of progression in severity.

Group D, though small in numbers (205 or 11% of our series), manifests a large number of progressive changes and other problems during the second and third decades of life and has a significant morbidity and mortality.

Multiple cardiac defects are rarer than in infancy, but occurred in 15% of the series. In the classification in Table 33.4, a patient is assigned to the functional grouping of his major residual defect: for example, a boy who underwent repair of coarctation of the aorta (CA) and PDA in infancy and now has moderate AS with a left ventricular to aortic pressure difference of 60 mm Hg, is included in group C.

PROGRESSIVE CHANGES (TABLE 33.5)

Favorable progression may occur; for example, spontaneous closure of a small VSD occurred in six of the 254 unoperated patients.

Unfavorable progression included increasing outflow obstruction, progressive cardiomegaly, development of cardiac failure, or increasing polycythemia. Except for four patients with VSDs and Qp:Qs ratios of 1.8:1, who developed an increase in heart size and required surgery, none of these changes occurred in groups A or B.

Some progressive changes seem related to the adolescent growth spurt: examples include systemic hypertension in CA, increasing outflow obstruction in AS or unoperated TF, or progressive cardiomegaly in moderate or severe AI. Other changes seem more specifically time related; for example, calcification of a grossly dilated pulmonary artery is rare under 20 years of age, and calcification of previously used prosthetic materials or homografts usually appears around 5 years after their insertion. Similarly, calcific pericarditis following hemopericardium is usually seen at least 3 years

TABLE 33.5   PROGRESSIVE CHANGES: RISKS AND METHODS OF ASSESSMENT[a]

	Group				Methods of Assessment
	A	B	C	D	
Stenosis or outflow obstruction	0	0	M	H	ECG, vector
Valvar insufficiency	0	0	M	M	Clinical, echo, x-ray
Cardiomegaly	0	L	L	M	X-ray, echo
Heart failure	0	0	L	L	Clinical, x-ray, echo
Calcification	0	0	L	L	X-ray
Polycythemia	0	0	0	M	Hematology, oximetry
PVOD[b]	0	0	L	M	Clinical + radionuclide scanning

[a] H, high risk (10% or greater); M, moderate (5–10%); L, low (less than 5%); 0, not observed in series.

[b] Other progressive changes may include systemic hypertension in coarctation.

after the surgery associated with the hemopericardium. Although calcification of bicuspid aortic valves probably occurs in the second decade, present methods have not allowed us to observe its occurrence in our patients who do not already have major AS. Progressive polycythemia in the cyanotic group seems both time related and also to have some relationship to the adolescent growth spurt.

COMPLICATIONS AND NEW DEVELOPMENTS

Complications of particular note in the series include endocarditis and dysrhythmias. Endocarditis occurred in 35 patients: one in a previously operated ASD, six in VSD, one in a previously operated AS, and the remainder in the cyanotic group. Cyanotic patients in group D, especially those with systemic pulmonary anastomoses, are at particular risk for endocarditis during these years.

The development of *dysrhythmias* during the second and third decade of life is arousing increasing interest and concern. A total of 48 patients had major dysrhythmias. The frequency ranged from 90% in the transposition group, virtually all of whom had junctional rhythm following Mustard repair, to less than 10% in patients with VSD or ASD in whom the dysrhythmias were mild, presenting with either brief episodes of supraventricular tachycardia or occasional premature contractions not requiring treatment. Dysrhythmias in TF patients following open heart surgery are still in the process of being defined and elucidated. At present it appears that somewhere between 1 and 2% of all such patients may show either trifascicular block or a right bundle branch block together with multiple premature ventricular contractions, and that these two groups are at risk for sudden death during early adult life. A high frequency of junctional rhythm following repair of sinus venosus defects has also been noted, but no untoward sequelae have been reported to date.

The complications of endocarditis and life-threatening dysrhythmias seem at present to be a particular threat to the cyanotic group included in group D.

PROBLEMS OF OTHER SYSTEMS

Cardiac patients may have congenital syndromes involving many systems such as trisomy 21 or Down's syndrome. In others, the cardiac lesion itself may have secondary effects which become apparent in the second or third decade of life.

Problems of the *respiratory system* show many interesting differences from those encountered earlier. Recurrent pneumonias and atelectasis, common in infancy, are now rare. Hemoptysis may occur either in pulmonary vascular obstructive disease or as a manifestation of extreme dilation of the bronchial arteries in severe and unrelieved pulmonic stenosis or atresia.[10, 11] Hemoptysis or pulmonary pseudofibrosis occurred in 19 patients, 1% of the total series or approximately 5% of group D. By the early teens, patients with absence of one pulmonary artery show marked compensatory emphysema of the contralateral lung. Radionuclide studies[12] may show reduced perfusion of the right lung in patients who have undergone banding of the pulmonary artery and later successful open repair of VSD. Other perfusion abnormalities without clinical manifestation are common in the cyanotic group, particularly those who have undergone multiple procedures, and their long-term significance is currently unknown. Pulmonary thromboembolism is a particular hazard in the Eisenmenger group.

Involvement of the *central nervous system* may be on a congenital basis or the result of a past brain abscess, cerebrovascular accident, or perioperative cerebral hypoxia (Ta-

TABLE 33.6 MENTAL RETARDATION[a]

Congenital	
Down's syndrome	31
Rubella embryopathy	19
Other	38
Congenital—acquired	
William's syndrome ("hypercalcemia")	9
Acquired	
Brain abscess, cerebrovascular accident, other	10
Total	107 (5.5%)

[a] Etiologic basis

ble 33.6). All these causes should become rarer in future years as rubella embryopathy and Williams' syndrome disappear and as successful uncomplicated intracardiac repair in early childhood becomes the norm. At present the transposition group surviving to the teens shows an 80% frequency of hyperactivity and difficulty in school, indicative of minimal brain damage, a much higher frequency than in other lesions.

Because mental retardation tends to be included in diagnostic coding only when it is severe and resulting in major schooling difficulties, it is likely that this tentative estimation of around 5% is an understatement of the problem and requires further study.

The *genitourinary system* may show congenital defects as in Turner's XO syndrome (nine patients) or in the phenotypically similar syndrome without ovarian agenesis known as Noonan's (13 patients). The cardiac lesions characteristic of the two syndromes, CA and PS, respectively, allow for survival to adult life usually following successful surgery, but each patient and family encounters a group of problems, including stunting of growth, abnormalities of body image, keloid scar formation, and others not generally shared by cardiac adolescents as a whole.

Recurrent urinary infections and congenital anomalies of the urinary tract have been reported as frequent in patients with VSD, but were rare in our series.

The *musculoskeletal system* may be involved from birth in those with Marfan's, Holt-Oram, or Ellis-van Creveld syndromes. The present series included 15 such patients. In others, scoliosis may become manifest in the teenage years, particularly in the cyanotic group. Scoliosis or other skeletal defects, usually of a minor degree, were present in approximately 10% of the present series; however, only four patients required surgery for scoliosis. Marked thinning of cortical bone and stunting of bone growth has been noted in the severely cyanotic.[24]

Abnormalities of the *gastrointestinal system* were noted in 31 patients (1.7%), including situs inversus, intestinal malrotation, repaired omphalocele, and imperforate anus. Gallstones necessitating cholecystectomy were encountered in six patients, five of them with cyanotic lesions, and may need to be considered as a cause of abdominal pain in this population.

Neoplastic disease has not been shown to have a higher than expected frequency,[17] but this question needs continuing study.* A major effort to avoid excessive radiation from fluoroscopy, frequent cardiac catheterizations, or repeated chest x-rays is warranted. *Metabolic disorders*, including gout and pheochromocytoma, seem to be a slightly increased risk, but only in severely cyanotic patients.

---

* Adams, F. H., Norman, A, Bass, D., and Oku. Chromosome damage in infants and children after cardiac catheterization and angiocardiography. Pediatrics 62:312, 1978.

PSYCHOSOCIAL ADAPTATION

SCHOOLING AND EXERCISE

On entering high school, the majority of patients have had corrective surgery and are strongly encouraged to attend school regularly and to reach their maximum academic potential. About 80% of our group were in the appropriate grade for age or had graduated from high school. Taussig et al.[23] have emphasized the good scholastic achievement that can occur despite cyanosis in the early years of life.

Exercise studies in postoperative patients have been rare but suggest that those who have had a ventriculotomy or who have had prior ventricular hypertension may show some limitation in cardiopulmonary reserve following satisfactory repair.[22] The reasons are not yet clear. It is postulated that early repair of a cardiac defect prior to 2 years of age will result in completely normal cardiorespiratory function, but this has yet to be proven.

Advice regarding physical activity has varied, but the tendency is toward less restriction than in the past.[2] *Normal activity* with no restriction is advised for those in our groups A and B. Restriction from *competitive sports*, particularly those involving strenuous contact, is advised for those with AS or AI of more than mild degree and for others in group Co.

Severe limiation is usually only advised for those with major dysrhythmias. The exercise electrocardiogram is proving helpful in distinguishing, for example, the majority of patients with partial or complete dissociation whose ventricular rate rises with exercise and who can safely be allowed to participate in sports, from those who develop ectopic foci or bradydysrhythmias and should probably be restricted.

Severe restriction (that is no physical education or sports) is necessary only in group D. The patient is usually grossly cyanotic or in heart failure, and it is clear to him and his family that he cannot participate.

Some teachers go to great lengths to assist a handicapped child, allowing him or her to participate and stop when tired, or allowing those with major limitations to assist with time keeping or organizing sports. Although there is debate as to whether the mother or father's role is greater in urging achievement in competitive sports, we have found it helpful to discuss the matter with both parents, dwelling on the temporary nature of the family's gratification in Little League baseball, for example, as compared with the longtime pleasures of golf, fishing, or other activities in which the father and his handicapped son can participate together.

VOCATION

The same should apply to future occupation as to exercise, namely, the minimal amount of restriction and the optimal freedom for the patient. However, a number of obstacles lie in the path of achieving this goal. These include the necessity of physical examination for some jobs, the question of insurability, and the lack of early realistic vocational guidance.[2]

At pre-employment examination, the patient with a small VSD may be equally in trouble whether or not he has had surgery. Without surgery he has a loud murmur, and with surgery he has a prominent scar on his chest and possibly also a "significant" murmur, an abnormal electrocardiogram with right bundle branch block, and a chest x-ray showing sternal wires and perhaps some pleuropericardial adhesions. If the company physician obtains a recent catheterization report, he may read some sinister-sounding phrase such as "aneurysm of the ventricular septum," which to a cardiologist carries a benign connotation, but this benignity is not universally recognized. Since large companies frequently join group insurance plans, the patient may be rejected as an insurance risk. Insurance companies have had several meetings with the American Heart Association on this topic and are reassessing information on long-term follow-up. Patients with operated PDA and small VSD are now not customarily rejected, and postoperative ASD are also recognized as good risks.

Vocational rehabilitation counselors can often be helpful in working with the school and family, and their help should be enrolled early in the teens.[2] A number of our patients have been assisted financially through college by vocational rehabilitation and have entered successful careers.

In summary, except for occupations involving prolonged heavy lifting or continued exposure to extremes of temperature, virtually all young cardiac patients should be encouraged and helped towards the career of their own choosing (Table 33.7). The cardiologist and family physician need to be closely involved by phone and letter with specific clear recommendations regarding employability.

MARRIAGE, PREGNANCY, AND CONTRACEPTION

Many parents with an infant girl who has a malformed heart will ask as an early question, "Will she be able to have children?" With the rare exception of those with Turner's syndrome, most patients with congenital heart disease are normally fertile. In girls who remain cyanotic into the teenage years, menstruation is often delayed 1 or 2 years beyond the family pattern and is often irregular for several years after menarche. There is a suggestion of a corresponding delay of a year or more in the onset of puberty in boys with slow growth during childhood. Precocious puberty, on the other hand, may occur in the retarded and seems a particular problem in those unfortunate children with the William's syndrome and in a few of those with Down's syndrome.

Marriage tends to occur later in those with congenital heart disease than in their peers,[20] though this discrepancy may change as marriage is now occuring later in the population as a whole than previously. There may be many years, whether pre- or postmartial, when contraception is needed. Although oral contraceptives, which carry an increased risk of thromboembolism in the normal population, should be avoided in the cyanotic woman,[10] there is no evidence that girls with murmurs, but without cyanosis or heart failure, face any unusual hazards. Most now reaching their reproductive years are acyanotic and free of heart failure or major venous thromboses, and there seems no reason to insist on their being at special risk. In the small but important group of young women in whom oral contraception is contraindicated, there is a special problem. If they are married or have a stable sexual relationship, their gynecologist can often help the two partners use a combined method of avoiding pregnancy. For the girl with varying partners, an intrauterine device may be the solution. Tubal ligation has a very restricted role for those with malformations not amenable to repair in the foreseeable future, who have themselves reached this decision after many conferences and consultations with family, qualified gynecological advisors, and reli-

TABLE 33.7   RESTRICTIONS

	Exercise	Vocation
Group A	None	None
Group B	None	None-mild
Group C	Mild	Moderate
Group D	Moderate-severe	Moderate-severe

TABLE 33.8 PREGNANCY RISKS

Maternal
  Thromboembolism
  Ruptured aneurysm
  Sudden death
  Other
Other
  Fetal wastage
  Prematurity
  Congenital malformations, cardiac or other

gious or other counsellors. The technique has proved valuable in some of those happily married with Eisenmenger's syndrome who have been unable to tolerate pregnancy and who have later successfully adopted children, and in a few cyanotic young women in whom other contraceptive methods have failed.

Sterilization by hysterectomy is never indicated on cardiac grounds alone. Parents may request it for the retarded cardiac patient with Down's or William's syndrome. The ethical problems of such a recommendation are great[3] and require consultation with a physician with special empathy for the retarded child and a long interval for consideration.

When contraception fails, the recent liberalization in abortion laws in the United States and other countries has made the previous familial stress much less than in the past. It seems clear that the unborn child of an unwilling or unmarried mother with congenital heart disease would face exceptional difficulty in life. However, the cardiologist must help the young mother reach the decision appropriate for herself and her child.

Pregnancy risks may affect either the mother or the fetus and are summarized in Table 33.8.

Pregnancy risks for the mother are now confined to those with pulmonary vascular obstructive disease and those with aneurysmal dilation of the aorta or pulmonary artery. The risk of major pulmonary thromboembolism in the Eisenmenger group is probably between 20 and 30%, and such an incident may occur during the pregnancy or during the first 2 weeks after delivery. If the couple is very desirous of going through a pregnancy in spite of this risk, close teamwork with the obstetrician, hospitalization for the last 4 to 6 weeks of pregnancy, and possible heparinization immediately postpartum, all need to be considered and discussed.

Fetal wastage is high only if the mother is cyanotic (Group D). If the mother's arterial oxygen saturation is 85% or less, or if the hematocrit is 65% or greater, there is only a 10% chance of the fetus being carried to term. With the hematocrit in the range of 55 to 65%, the fetal wastage approaches 50%. With lower hematocrits between 45 and 55%, there is a 60% chance of a live born infant, though almost invariably of low birth weight for gestational age.[18]

The risk of congenital heart disease in the infant depends on the family history and is discussed in detail elsewhere[19] and in Chapter 1. If either parent has Noonan's or Holt-Oram syndrome or idiopathic hypertrophic subaortic stenosis, all of which are inherited as Mendelian dominants, the risk to the fetus is 50%, even though the infant can be expected to be born alive and the cardiac lesion will rarely show manifestations until later in the perinatal period. In most cardiac lesions, the risk of recurrence in the infant is only between 2 and 5%. This risk increases if there are other affected family members, so a detailed family tree of both parents is essential. The type of congenital heart disease tends to be similar to that of the affected parent in about two-thirds of cases. Thus, a young adult with a VSD or TF who has no other affected family member has at most a 5% chance of having an affected child. Counsel on the risk of congenital heart disease in the offspring can only be given after obtaining a precise diagnosis and a detailed family tree. We have also strongly advised the future mother against the taking of any medications in pregnancy and recommended the discontinuance of oral contraceptives or other hormonal therapy for some weeks before attempting conception.

Self-acceptance seems to be much less of a problem in cardiac patients than in individuals with gross external malformations. Only 3% of patients in this series have required major psychiatric counseling during their teenage and early adult years, probably not much greater than for a similar age population without heart disease. Cosmetic problems of one or more scars are apparently well tolerated by most, although keloid formation may cause anxiety. Efforts to minimize the scar by using a right-sided inframammary thoracotomy in girls with ASD or other suitable lesions seem worth pursuing. A cosmetic problem frequently seen in cyanotic boys is severe acne, poorly responsive to any treatment except elimination of the cyanosis.

COMMENT

Adolescents and young adults with congenital heart disease in the 1980s are unlike those of past and probably also of future generations. Unlike past generations, they have benefited from the development of closed and open heart surgery, but in many cases have undergone several procedures, each during its own developmental years. They have usually been relieved of cyanosis, outflow obstruction, or intracardiac shunts. Nevertheless, they may have residua of their defects, and the long-term effect of these needs continuing follow-up. In the future, patients entering their teenage years will have had the benefit of early repair without multiple prior investigative procedures and palliative operations. In those who do not require surgery, appropriate decisions will have been reached and multiple childhood visits avoided. Their exposure to the hazards of radiation and repeated hospitalizations will be less than in our current group. The patient and family should be helped in the process of turning over responsibility for the taking of medications and for other health measures from the parents to the individual himself. Counseling on preventive medicine, such as avoidance of obesity, continuance of good exercise programs into adult life, the dangers of smoking, drug use, and other pitfalls all need to be discussed in an open an constructive way. Follow-up visits and all procedures should be kept to a minimum so that these fine adolescents and young adults and their families, who have undergone so much more than the normal polulation, may continue into maturity with as much confidence as possible.

REFERENCES

1. Braley, R. K., Gardner, T. J., Donahoo, J. S., Neill, C. A., Rowe, R. D., and Gott, V. L.: Late results after right ventricular outflow tract reconstruction with aortic root homografts. J. Thorac. Cardiovasc. Surg. 64:314, 1972.
2. Committee Report of the American Heart Association ad hoc Committee on Rehabilitation of the Young Cardiac: Recreational activity and career choice recommendations for use by physicians counseling physical education directors, vocational counselors, parents and young patients with heart disease. Circulation 43:459, 1971.
3. Editorial: Sterilization of handicapped minors. Lancet 2:352, 1975.
4. Engle, M. A.: Ventricular septal defect: Status report for the seventies. Cardiovasc. Clin. 4(3):281, 1972.
5. Engle, M. A., Adams, F. H., Betson, R., DuShane, J., Elliott, L., McNamara, D. G., Rashkind, W. J., and Talner, N. S.: Resources for

optimal long-term care of congenital heart disease: Report of Inter-Society Commission for Heart Disease Resources. Circulation 44:205, 1971.

6. Ferencz, C.: The quality of life of the adolescent cardiac patient. Postgrad. Med. 56(6):67, 1974.

7. Fyler, D. C., Parisi, L., and Bermann, M. A.: The regionalization of infant cardiac care in New England Cardiovasc. Clin. 4:340, 1972.

8. Gersony, W. M., and Krongrad, E.: Evaluation and management of patients after surgical repair of congenital heart diseases. Prog. Cardiovasc. Dis. 18:39, 1975.

9. Hammar, S. L.: The approach to the adolescent patient. Pediatr. Clin. North Am. 20:779, 1973.

10. Haroutunian, L. M., and Neill, C. A.: Pulmonary complications in congenital heart disease: Hemoptysis. Am. Heart J. 84:540, 1972.

11. Haroutunian, L. M., and Neill, C. A.: Pulmonary pseudofibrosis in cyanotic heart disease: A clinical syndrome mimicking tuberculosis in patients with extreme pulmonic stenosis. Chest 62:587, 1972.

12. Haroutunian, L. M., Neill, C. A., Wagner, H. N., Jr., and White, R. I., Jr.: Preoperative and postoperative assessment of congenital heart disease. In Pediatric Nuclear Medicine, edited by A. E. James, H. N. Wagner, Jr., and R. E. Cooke. W. B. Saunders, Philadelphia, 1974, p. 265.

13. Jones, E. L., Conti, C. R., Neill, C. A., Gott, V. L., Braley, R. K., and Haller, J. A., Jr.: Long-term evaluation of tetralogy patients with pulmonary valvular insufficiency resulting from outflow patch correction across the pulmonic annulus. Circulation 47(Suppl. III):11, 1973.

14. Krovetz, L. J.: A simple mnemonic code for cardiovascular data. Johns Hopkins Med. J., 127:344, 1970.

15. Maron, B. J., Humphries, J. O'N., Rowe, R. D., and Mellits, E. D.: Prognosis of surgically corrected coarctation of the aorta: A 20 year postoperative appraisal. Circulation 47:119, 1973.

16. Morriss, J. H., and McNamara, D. G.: Residuae, sequelae and complications of surgery for congenital heart disease. Prog. Cardiovasc. Dis. 18:1, 1975.

17. Mulvihill, J. J., Miller, R. W., and Taussig, H. B.: Longtime observations on the Blalock-Taussig operation. V. Neoplasms in tetralogy of Fallot. Johns Hopkins Med. J. 133:16, 1973.

18. Neill, C. A., and Swanson, S.: Outcome of pregnancy in congenital heart disease. Circulation 24:1003, 1961.

19. Neill, C. A.: Genetics of congenital heart disease. Annu. Rev. Med. 24:61, 1973.

20. Nora, J. J., Dodd, P. F., McNamara, D. G., Hattwick, M. A. W., Leachman, R. D., and Cooley, D. A.: Risk to offspring of parents with congenital heart defects. J.A.M.A. 209:2052, 1969.

21. Rowe, R. D., and Mehrizi, A.: The Neonate with Congenital Heart Disease. W. B. Saunders, Philadelphia, 1969, p. 79.

22. Stone, M. F., Bessinger, B., Lucas, R. V., and Moller, J. H.: Pre and postoperative rest and exercise hemodynamics in children with pulmonary stenosis. Circulation 49:1102, 1974.

23. Taussig, H. B., Kallman, C. H., Nagel, D., Baumgardner, R., Momberger, N., and Kirk, H.: Longtime observations in the Blalock-Taussig operation. VII. 20 to 28 year follow-up on patients with tetralogy of Fallot. Johns Hopkins Med. J. 137:13, 1975.

24. White, R. I., Jordan, C. E., Fischer, K. C., Lampton, L., Neill, C. A., and Dorst, J. P.: Skeletal changes associated with adolescent congenital heart disease. Am. J. Roentgenol. 141:531, 1972.

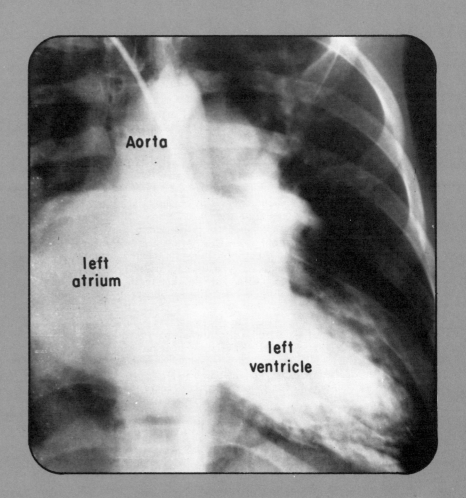

Aorta

left
atrium

left
ventricle

Part 3
INFECTIOUS
DISEASES

34

Acute Rheumatic Fever

Lewis W. Wannamaker, M.D., and Edward L. Kaplan, M.D.

Though less common now than previously, at least in its recurrent and most crippling forms, acute rheumatic fever maintains its position as the leading cause of postnatally acquired heart disease in children in the United States and Western Europe. In many other parts of the world, acute rheumatic fever is the predominant cause of all heart disease in the pediatric age group. Both here and abroad rheumatic fever is a significant contributor to heart disease among adults.

The term acute rheumatic fever, although useful and well entrenched, falls short of identifying the important features or the fundamental nature of the disease. The name is inadequate to describe a polymorphous clinical entity which may affect (sometimes exclusively) organ systems other than the joints, most prominently the central nervous system and the heart.

Acute rheumatic fever is best viewed as a complication of a specific infectious disease. Recognition of its relationship to infection with group A streptococci has resulted in a clearer understanding of the epidemiology and natural history of rheumatic fever, a more precise delineation of the clinical entity, and practical approaches to its control. Much has been written about acute rheumatic fever and streptococcal infections, including several symposia[71, 168, 187] and monographs.[117, 160] Historical considerations have been summarized in the first edition of this book.

EPIDEMIOLOGY

Many of the epidemiologic features of acute rheumatic fever are explicable in terms of the epidemiology of streptococcal infections of the upper respiratory tract.[136] Like streptococcal sore throat, acute rheumatic fever occurs most commonly in the young school age child and rarely in early infancy when streptococcal infections are relatively uncommon. When adults are exposed to increased risk of streptococcal sore throat, in military service or as parents of young children, more frequent occurrence of acute rheumatic fever can be anticipated. Crowding through inadequate housing is probably the chief reason for the magnified risk of streptococcal infection and acute rheumatic fever in certain ethnic and disadvantaged populations. The high incidence of streptococcal upper respiratory infections in the winter and spring months accounts for the frequency of onset of acute rheumatic fever in these seasons. Epidemics of scarlet fever or streptococcal pharyngitis, unless brought under control, result in an increased number of cases of acute rheumatic fever. One notable exception is streptococcal impetigo or pyoderma which does not lead to this complication. The differences between streptococcal infections of the skin and those of the throat and the possible reasons for the failure of rheumatic fever to appear after these skin infections have been reviewed elsewhere.[184, 185]

The natural habitat of the group A streptococcus is the upper respiratory tract of man.[182] Although these organisms may be found in large numbers and may persist for long periods of time in dust, clothing, and bedclothing, human rather than environmental reservoirs are the most important sources of upper respiratory tract infection.[131] Individuals harboring streptococci in the nose are especially likely to spread infection.[69] There is also some evidence to suggest that children with suppurative complications such as otitis media are more likely to spread infection.[21] Most spread occurs during the first 2 weeks after infection or parasitization[182]; chronic carriers are ordinarily not dangerous either to themselves or to others. Transmission occurs by direct physical contact of individuals or by projection of large droplets.[182] Food-borne epidemics are rare but when they occur may be dramatic.[72]

Type-specific antibodies (antibodies to M protein) protect against reinfection of the throat with the same serologic type.[182] Other factors which may influence resistance are ill-defined. Some evidence has been presented which suggests that certain strains of alpha streptococci and other throat flora may interfere with the establishment of throat infection by group A streptococci.[36]

A characteristic feature of the epidemiology of streptococcal pharyngitis and its nonsuppurative sequelae is the latent period, which in epidemics results in a lag between the peak incidence of streptococcal sore throat and the peak incidence of acute rheumatic fever. The latent period is commonly between 7 and 35 days, with an average of about 18 days,[137] but it may be as long as 2 to 6 months in patients with pure Sydenham's chorea.[162]

Approximately 3% of individuals with well-documented streptococcal sore throat will develop acute rheumatic fever.[136] This attack rate was obtained on young adults during military epidemics. Although some studies have suggested that attack rates among children in endemic situations may be lower,[153] it is not clear whether this is a true difference in attack rate caused by possible variations in the virulence of the infecting organism or in the reaction of the young host, or is a spuriously low attack rate caused by difficulties in distinguishing true streptococcal infection under these conditions. When streptococcal infections are strictly defined, attack rates are the same in civilian and military populations and in epidemic and endemic situations.

The frequency of occurrence of rheumatic fever after well-documented streptococcal sore throat does not appear to vary from year to year, from season to season, or between epidemic and nonepidemic periods. Most serotypes of group A streptococci which infect the pharynx appear to be able to produce this complication. The possibility has been entertained that certain serotypes or strains, notably those which primarily produce impetigo but may also appear in the upper respiratory tract, may lack the capacity to induce rheumatic fever, and some evidence has been obtained to support this view.[160]

More detailed reviews of the epidemiology of streptococcal infections are given elsewhere.[71, 135, 182] The epidemiology of recurrent rheumatic fever, including the increased attack rate following streptococcal infection, will be discussed under the section on Natural History and Prognosis.

THE ETIOLOGIC AGENT

The close association of group A beta-hemolytic streptococci with acute rheumatic fever has spurred on an intense examination of the biology of these organisms. These biologic features are important in the recognition and classification of streptococci pathogenic for man, in providing immunologic evidence of streptococcal infection, and in suggesting clues to the pathogenesis of such streptococcal sequelae as acute rheumatic fever and acute glomerulonephritis.

Group A beta-hemolytic streptococci are a complex group of organisms both with respect to their cellular composition and with respect to the wide variety of their extracellular products. A detailed discussion of the biologic characteristics and properties of group A beta-hemolytic streptococci is beyond the scope of this chapter. The interested reader is referred to recent reviews.[187, 194] However, several of the seemingly more important biological products are discussed below.

Most streptococci producing upper respiratory infection in man can be recognized by their clear (beta) hemolysis on blood agar but must be carefully differentiated from other hemolytic species such as staphylococci and gram-negative organisms by colony characteristics and gram stain. Differentiation from alpha-hemolytic (green) streptococci and *Haemophilus haemolyticus* can be most reliably made on sheep blood agar. Some strains of group A streptococci produce feeble or green hemolysis under the aerobic conditions on the surface of the plate but can be detected by the clear hemolysis produced anaerobically around a stab in the solid media. Hemolysis in blood agar is due primarily to streptolysin S, rather than to the oxygen-sensitive streptolysin O. Nonhemolytic group A streptococci are apparently rare but are difficult to recognize and can be associated with rheumatic fever.[79] Details on methods of identifying pathogenic streptococci in throat cultures are given elsewhere.[183]

Both streptolysin O and S are potentially capable of producing tissue damage by lysis of membranes and by disruption of lysosomes in mammalian cells.[192] Streptolysin O, which is lethal on intravenous injection in experimental animals, causes loss of myocardial contractility in the isolated mammalian heart[99] and has been shown to damage isolated myocardial cells in tissue culture.[171] The marked electrocardiographic changes[68] accompanying cardiotoxicity may be due in part to severe potassium toxicity secondary to hemolysis. In addition to being hemolytic and cardiotoxic, streptolysin O is also antigenic, providing the basis for one of the most commonly used streptococcal antibody tests. In contrast, streptolysin S is not antigenic.

In addition to streptolysin O, group A streptococci often produce a variety of other extracellular products, most of which are specific enzymes with known biochemical actions.[194] Many of these are antigenic in man, and specific neutralizing antibodies developed against them are useful in epidemiologic and clinical studies, providing additional methods for immunologic confirmation of streptococcal infection. Streptococcal deoxyribonuclease B, streptococcal nicotinamide adenine dinucleotidase (NADase), hyaluronidase, and streptokinase have been used clinically in this regard.

Although generally not available in a pure enough state for individual testing, most of the extracellular products are probably also capable of inducing a delayed type of skin hypersensitivity. Despite extensive studies and well-documented biochemical or physiologic effects, such as potent activation of the fibrinolytic system by streptokinase, it has not been possible to associate any of the extracellular enzymes with definite clinical manifestations of streptococcal disease or its complications. Only the erythrogenic toxins (streptococcal pyrogenic exotoxins) have been related to a definite clinical manifestation, the rash of scarlet fever, which apparently results from an enhancement by these toxins of hypersensitivity to streptococcal products.

Like many other organisms, streptococci may be infected with temperate bacteriophage. Production of erythrogenic toxin has been shown to be associated with the so-called lysogenic state.[199] This is analogous to the role of lysogeny in the production of diphtheria toxin and suggests the possibility that bacteriophage may play a role in the epidemiology of streptococcal infections or the pathogenesis of their complications.

Exploration of the cellular composition of hemolytic streptococci has provided a rational basis for serologic classification of these organisms. The streptococcal cell wall[101] is composed of (a) a rigid peptidoglycan skeleton, (b) a specific carbohydrate which is the basis for the serologic grouping in most streptococci (including group A), and (c) various surface proteins, including M protein (the serologic diversity of which is responsible for the type classification of group A streptococci).

The classical Lancefield method of identifying group A streptococci[105] is to boil them in acid and to place the acid extract in a capillary tube with specific group A antiserum, whereupon a cloudy precipitin reaction will appear. Maxted[121] has reported that group A strains are more sensitive than others to bacitracin, an observation which is the basis for a simple and reasonably accurate screening method. Group A strains can also be identified by fluorescent antibody techniques[30] and by countercurrent immunoelectrophoresis,[38] or by newer coagglutination techniques.

Outermost on the streptococcal cell is the hyaluronic acid capsule which is nonantigenic and chemically indistinguishable from the hyaluronic acid of man and other mammals. It is antiphagocytic but is of doubtful significance in human infections because most normal human sera contain a factor which neutralizes this effect.[73]

The group A carbohydrate moiety of the cell wall deserves some emphasis because of the fact that it has been shown to be antigenically similar to the glycoprotein of bovine and human cardiac valves.[61] This relationship has led to speculation regarding a role for this cell wall component in the pathogenesis of valvular damage in rheumatic fever.

The M protein coat[106] renders the streptococcal cell antiphagocytic. It is a primary virulence factor and induces the formation of type-specific antibodies which are the basis of type-specific immunity. M protein will also precipitate fibrinogen and may localize in the tissues and produce nephropathy in experimental animals.[83] M protein is a double alpha-helically coiled molecule, with striking physiochemical similarity to mammalian muscle tropomyosin.[113] Evidence has been presented that a protein closely associated with the M protein cross-reacts antigenically with an antigen(s) in heart muscle cells,[97] an observation of possibly great importance in understanding the pathogenesis of rheumatic carditis.

Electron microscopic studies[161] have indicated that group A streptococci have fimbriae on their surface and that the M protein is located on these hairlike projections. The fimbriae appear to be necessary for the attachment of streptococci to epithelial cells, an essential step in the initiation of infection. Attachment may occur via a lipoteichoic acid component of the fimbriae.[128] Because of its affinity for cell membranes, lipoteichoic acid may play a role in tissue injury.

Although differing chemically from endotoxin of gram-negative bacteria, the peptidoglycan or mucopeptide comprising the backbone of the streptococcus has many of the biologic and toxic properties of endotoxin and produces myocardial degeneration in rabbits.[144] Cell wall fragments of streptococci containing peptidoglycan produce recurrent subcutaneous nodular lesions in rabbits, resembling in some respects the nodules of rheumatic fever.[149]

The inner protoplast membrane of the streptococcal cell is the outer membrane of wall-less osmotically fragile forms. Multiplying wall-less forms, known as L forms, have been considered by some to be important in the pathogenesis of rheumatic fever. The protoplast membrane is a complex lipoprotein structure. An antigenic component of the cell membrane which cross-reacts immunologically with sarcolemmal antigen(s)[200] has been described; it may play a role in the pathogenesis of rheumatic carditis. The relationship of this cross-reacting antigen to the one associated with M protein has been a matter of some dispute.

PATHOGENESIS

The fragmentary state of our knowledge of the pathogenesis of acute rheumatic fever is due to: our inability to relate definitely any of the known components or products of the group A streptococcus to this disease; the lack of a suitable experimental model for the disease; and our failure to provide a provable hypothesis which encompasses possible factors contributed by the host as well as the organism. Some of the current views on the nature of rheumatic fever and the missing links in its pathogenesis have been critically reviewed.[112, 185]

Early concepts of rheumatic fever were drawn from an analogy to serum sickness, which may mimic many of the clinical features of rheumatic fever, including the latent period. The rarity of acute rheumatic fever among infants has suggested to some investigators[138] that it is necessary to experience repeated streptococcal infections to develop sufficient hypersensitivity for this complication to occur. However, type-specific antibody data[115] would suggest that the rheumatic host has not had more frequent streptococcal infections before the first attack than the nonrheumatic individual. An alternative explanation for the infrequency of rheumatic fever among infants, which is consistent with the sparse epidemiologic data available, is that streptococcal infections are relatively uncommon in this very young age group.

The demonstration that streptococcal antibodies are usually produced in larger amounts in individuals who develop acute rheumatic fever than in those who do not is consistent with an immunologic basis for the pathogenesis of this complication.[156] However, there are many exceptions in individual patients and with different antibodies. Moreover, rheumatic subjects do not respond with an exaggerated antibody response when injected with nonstreptococcal antigens.[135] The possibility that a delayed type of hypersensitivity may be involved in the pathogenesis of rheumatic fever has not been extensively explored, because the complex antigens have been difficult to separate and because normal individuals as well as rheumatic subjects may show striking skin reactions. Studies of inhibition of migration of human blood leukocytes by particulate antigens of streptococci, notably membrane antigens, have shown an exaggerated response in rheumatic subjects, supporting the possible role of hypersensitivity.[139]

Observations of antigenic cross-reactions between streptococcal components and human myocardium have revived interest in the possibility that rheumatic fever may be an autoimmune disease.[97, 200] A plethora of streptococcal cellular components cross-reacting with various mammalian tissues has been described which may account for the many different tissue sites manifesting injury in this disease.[8] As with other possible autoimmune diseases, the difficulties of distinguishing cause of injury from effect of injury has rendered these hypotheses unprovable. The additional fact that circulating cross-reacting antibodies may be found among individuals who fail to develop rheumatic fever following streptococcal infection as well as in those who do[98] makes it even more difficult to develop a satisfactory theory along these lines.

The notion has been entertained that some components of the streptococcus, cross-reacting or otherwise, may persist in the tissues, and it has been hypothesized that it may be relatively difficult for rheumatic individuals to remove certain components, of the cell wall for example, perhaps due to a host enzyme deficiency.[10] This hypothesis might put rheumatic fever in the group of enzyme deficiency diseases.

Streptolysin O has been shown to be cardiotoxic in animals.[99] Inhibition of streptolysin O by cholesterol or related lipids in skin appears to account for the feeble antistreptolysin O response in patients with streptococcal impetigo[93] and may relate to the failure of rheumatic fever to develop after group A streptococcal infections of the skin.[185]

Both streptolysin O and streptolysin S are toxic for isolated mammalian hearts.[75, 171] It has been shown that cholesterol can prevent myocardial cytotoxicity induced by streptolysin O.[56] It has been postulated that patients with acute rheumatic fever may be unable to neutralize streptolysin S during a streptococcal infection. Since this product is nonantigenic, protection from repeated damage by the development of neutralizing antibody would not occur.

Streptococci produce substances which stimulate blastogenesis in lymphocytes, including a glycopeptide,[6] blastogen A[65] and other streptococcal products. Some differences in response to streptococcal products have been observed in rheumatic subjects,[65] but the role which these responses may play in the pathogenesis of acute rheumatic fever has not been well defined.

The possibility that blood groups may play a role in the pathogenesis of acute rheumatic fever has also been suggested.[59] Reports of a small increase among rheumatic subjects of individuals who do not secrete blood group substances have been held to be consistent with the hypothesis that rheumatic fever occurs only in individuals who harbor the nonsecretor gene, in either a homozygous or a heterozygous state. Although this theory has been challenged,[45] it is attractive in that it may relate to the ability of streptococci to absorb haptenic polysaccharides and convert them to complete antigens. It is also consistent with the clinical observation that streptococcal infections in sites other than the throat do not result in rheumatic fever.[185]

It has been suggested that certain strains or serotypes of streptococci may be rheumatogenic,[159, 160] in the same sense that certain strains or serotypes have been shown to be nephritogenic. However, the epidemiologic evidence supports the view that most serotypes which commonly cause clinical pharyngitis can result in this complication. Nevertheless, it is possible that the so-called impetigo strains which can also be found in the throat but rarely cause clinical pharyngitis may lack some rheumatogenic factor.[160, 185]

The necessity for the preceding streptococcal infection to occur in the throat or upper respiratory tract rather than the skin is now well documented but poorly understood.[160, 184, 185] Perhaps this observation is due to a difference in strains which commonly infect these two sites. The feeble antistreptolysin O response following streptococcal infection of the skin,[17, 40, 87] and the demonstration of skin lipids which inhibit the biologic effects and the antigenicity of this cardiotoxic streptococcal product[93] may also explain why rheumatic fever does not occur after streptococcal impetigo. This and other possible explanations for this curious infection site specificity have been discussed elsewhere,[185] including the possibility that streptococci or some product of streptococci may travel by direct lymphatic channels from the throat to the heart. Recent studies have suggested that rheumatic fever-associated strains of group A streptococci adhere more avidly to pharyngeal cells of patients with acute rheumatic fever than strains not associated with rheumatic fever.[140]

The possibility of direct infection of the heart valves by streptococci was suggested by postmortem cultures reported by several groups in England and Scotland.[172] Although this view is supported by evidence of persistence of viable organisms in experimental animals,[39] the original postmortem observations were not confirmed when an effort was made to repeat them using strictly aseptic techniques.[190]

That living streptococci, whether located in the valve or confined to the upper respiratory tract, may play a role in the pathogenesis of rheumatic fever is cogently suggested by the observation that successful primary prevention depends on eradication rather than suppression of the infecting organism[26] and by the observation that penicillin treatment initiated after complete subsidence of the active streptococcal infection may abort the development of acute rheumatic fever.[27] Attempts to prove that massive penicillin treatment, started after the onset of acute rheumatic fever, will prevent the development of carditis or permanent heart disease[179] have been unsuccessful and have therefore failed to support this concept.

The possibility that streptococci may survive in the tissues as aberrant forms has received special attention, particularly since the demonstration that streptococci can be rather readily converted to L forms in vitro. Since L forms lack a cell wall, they would be resistant to the effects of antibiotics such as penicillin whose action depends on inhibition of cell wall formation. Although it has been shown that streptococci may be converted to L forms in experimental animals,[126] no convincing evidence has been produced that group A streptococcal L forms are present as such in either clinical or postmortem material.

The tendency for rheumatic fever to occur in families has led to consideration of a primary role of genetic factors in this disease, with the suggestion by some that rheumatic fever is transmitted by a recessive autosomal gene.[196] However, the use of somewhat unusual criteria for the diagnosis of acute rheumatic fever has made these studies difficult to interpret. Although other workers[175] have failed to find a consistent genetic pattern, this does not exclude genetic factors in view of the necessity of streptococcal stimulation for expression of the disease. Perhaps the best approach to this problem is the study of rheumatic fever in monozygotic and dizygotic twins. In one such study of twins,[166] less than one-fifth of the pairs of monozygotic twins was concordant for rheumatic fever. These findings were interpreted as consistent with, but not proof of, the hypothesis that genetic factors of limited penetrance may play a role in the etiology of rheumatic fever. Studies of histocompatibility antigens in rheumatic subjects have so far revealed no clear-cut distinctive patterns.[49]

The possible role of viruses in the pathogenesis of rheumatic fever has been entertained from time to time and has recently been re-emphasized by Burch and his colleagues[23] who have demonstrated valvular lesions in animals inoculated with Coxsackie viruses and have found evidence of viral antigens in the heart valves of patients at autopsy.

However, one study failed to show a higher prevalence of enterovirus antibodies present in the sera of individuals with rheumatic heart disease than in controls, suggesting that viruses are not associated with this syndrome.[109] Experimental data from a mouse model have raised additional questions.[48]

Definite proof has not been obtained for any of these concepts of the pathogenesis of rheumatic fever, but whatever concept is finally developed must fit with and explain all the aspects of the disease, including the multiformity of clinical manifestations as well as the various features of the epidemiology and natural history of the disease, the tendency to occur in families, the necessity for the precipitating streptococcal infection to be located in the upper respiratory tract, the development of this complication in only a small percentage of those infected, and the increased susceptibility of the rheumatic subject to recurrent attack following streptococcal infection.

NATURAL AND EXPERIMENTAL PATHOLOGY

The diverse clinical manifestations of acute rheumatic fever are reflected in pathologic lesions which most commonly involve the heart, blood vessels, joints, and subcutaneous tissues but may also involve the brain, the lungs, the pleura, and the kidney. The inflammatory reaction is of two types, exudative and proliferative. These two types of reactions may account for the transitory or permanent nature of the process in different affected anatomic parts and for differences in response of various manifestations to antiinflammatory agents.

The hallmark of rheumatic fever has long been the Aschoff body or nodule.[147, 180] From a pathologic point of view, this unique lesion sets rheumatic fever apart from a number of other so-called collagen diseases, just as the relationship to preceding streptococcal infection sets it apart clinically, epidemiologically, and bacteriologically. The unification of the pathologic process is not complete in the Aschoff body, however, since this lesion has not been consistently reported in relationship to lesions of the joints and has never been found in the brain. Histologic criteria for the identification of the Aschoff body have been reemphasized.[181] The lesion has generally been considered a form of granuloma, with the presence of focal swelling and fragmentation of collagen fibers and the appearance of typical Aschoff cells with serrated intranuclear bar-shaped chromatin and basophilic, indistinct cytoplasm. Fibrinoid and other inflammatory cells may or may not be present.

Classic interpretations of the origin and significance of Aschoff bodies have been questioned from several quarters. Murphy[127] has suggested that the primary lesion develops from injury to the myofibers rather than collagen fibers. This interpretation has not gained wide acceptance among pathologists. Recently Hutchins and Payne[77] have offered yet another interpretation for the origin of Aschoff bodies. These investigations suggest that these characteristic lesions arise from terminal branches of myocardial nerve cells. The concept of development of the Aschoff body as a result of blockage of lymphatic channels of the heart[191] also requires confirmation.

Uncertainty about the significance of Aschoff bodies as indicators of active rheumatic inflammation has arisen from the observation of many recent workers that auricular appendage biopsies taken from patients with quiescent rheumatic disease at the time of cardiac surgery often show Aschoff bodies.[94] An alternative interpretation is that the inflammatory process may be so subtle that it fails to provoke recognizable clinical or laboratory changes. This interpretation is consistent with the observation that rheumatic heart disease often develops silently, i.e., without overt evidence of an inflammatory process.

The demonstration of deposits of gamma globulin in rheumatic heart tissue,[95] together with the detection of streptococcal cross-reacting antigen(s) in normal human hearts and circulating cross-reacting antibodies in rheumatic patients' sera, supports the view that rheumatic fever is an autoimmune disease.[46, 94, 98, 201] Recently, this concept of autoimmunity has been extended to Sydenham's chorea by studies demonstrating antibody to human caudate and subthalamic nuclei in sera from patients with this rheumatic manifestation.[76] This antibody could be absorbed with group A streptococcal membranes. However the presence of these various cross-reacting antibodies in the sera of some individuals with uncomplicated streptococcal infection raises questions about the pathogenic significance of these antibodies.

Many attempts have been made to develop a pathologic model for acute rheumatic fever, but the lesions produced have in general resembled more closely those of focal or diffuse myocarditis and according to most pathologists do not meet the criteria for strict comparability with the human disease. The most successful model developed to date is that of Murphy,[127] who injected rabbits repeatedly with group A streptococci of different types and produced lesions which closely resemble those found in man. More detailed discussions of some of the other pathologic features of rheumatic fever and rheumatic heart disease and of experimental models are available.[94, 96, 127, 147, 160, 169]

INCIDENCE, PREVALENCE, AND MORTALITY

The general impression in the United States, Western Europe, and Japan that rheumatic fever and its sequelae are less of a problem than several decades ago seems well founded, although it is difficult to document all aspects with reliable statistics.[117, 164] Several factors contribute to this difficulty: acute rheumatic fever is not a reportable disease in many localities; definition and interpretation of the criteria used for diagnosis vary significantly; and reporting on death certificates is often incomplete or inaccurate.

The reasons for the decline are uncertain.[188] Since the incidence and the death rate were decreasing before widespread use of prophylaxis had been adopted, it seems unlikely that antibiotics have been the major determining factor. Changes in social conditions which made streptococcal infections less common may have contributed predominantly to the decline. Some data are available to suggest that improvement in the delivery of health care in defined populations may also be significant.[63] Other factors, such as change in the organism or host, are also possible, but little information is available to support these possibilities.

The decline in mortality is well documented. With chronic diseases in which incidence and survival rates are changing, the age pattern of mortality can be best determined by following through life the experience of a cohort of persons born in the same period of time (cohort analysis). Such studies[145] for rheumatic fever and rheumatic heart disease combined indicate that in the United States the death rate between 15 and 19 years of age was 11.5 per 100,000 population for males born in 1920 to 1924 and only 1.6 for males born in 1940 to 1944. The general pattern is similar for females. Other data[111] reveal approximately a twofold decline in deaths in the United States in the 15 to 24 year age group between 1920 (27.6 per 100,000 per year) and 1959 (15.6 per 100,000 per year) and a more than 70% reduction during the 1950s in children aged 5 to 14 years. The decline in death

rates for acute rheumatic fever is especially striking; the overall death rate for all ages has declined from 10.3 in 1920 to 0.4 per 100,000 population in 1960.[117] These figures are confirmed by reports from individual clinics or hospitals,[118] but must be interpreted with some caution in view of the known errors and omissions in reporting.[84, 117] Despite evidence of decreasing mortality, rheumatic fever and rheumatic heart disease are among the top causes of all deaths in the 15 to 24 year age group in the United States.[198]

A relative decrease in prevalence of rheumatic heart disease compared to other forms of heart disease is suggested by the data of White,[193] who compared 3000 cardiac cases seen in 1925 with an equal number drawn from similar sources seen in 1950 and found that rheumatic heart disease accounted for 39.5% of cases in 1925 and 23.5% of cases in 1950. Again, this comparison depends upon the accuracy of diagnoses and methods of reporting. While at one time, almost all valvular heart disease was considered to be rheumatic in origin, current data from the United States and Great Britain suggest that a significant proportion of damaged valves may be attributed to congenital defects or to acquired disease of other etiologies.[23, 25, 142] Prevalence surveys in more recent years[124, 154] indicate that congenital heart disease is more common by perhaps several fold than rheumatic heart disease in elementary school children and about twice as common among high school children. In these studies the prevalence rate for rheumatic heart disease in both age groups was 0.7 per 1,000. Other surveys[22, 123] have shown prevalence rates of 1.3 to 1.6 per 1000 school children. Less encouragingly, extensive studies in young men of military age[146] and among college students[114] suggest a prevalence of rheumatic heart disease of 8.8 and 5.7 per 1000, respectively. A still more recent study suggests that the prevalence may be somewhat less among college students in one geographic area.[129] In the earlier study of military selectees, the 8.8 per 1000 rate of rejections for rheumatic heart disease was more than sixfold greater than the 1.3 rate of rejections for congenital heart disease. Other studies in the United States have emphasized the decline in severity of first attacks.[122]

Data evaluating current trends in the incidence of acute rheumatic fever in the United States are also difficult to interpret. There has been a gradual decline in recurrence rates even in populations where antimicrobial therapy was not used routinely. During the period from 1937 to 1952 one such population showed a drop in age-adjusted recurrence rates from 12.9 to 8.8%.[195] A definite decline in the incidence of first attacks of rheumatic fever is less certain. In a 1962 symposium,[111] Stamler estimated the incidence in Chicago to be about 50 per 100,000 children. Unfortunately, no comparable studies were done in this same area at an earlier period, but Collins[31] reported an incidence of 100 to 120 per 100,000 children in a series of six surveys done in 1928 to 1943. Current incidence figures for the United States may not be meaningful since it is very apparent that acute rheumatic fever may be more of a problem in certain populations, and reporting from these populations may not be accurate. Careful studies in Baltimore have revealed incidence figures of at least 20 per 100,000 per year.[64] Thus, when one calculates overall incidence figures, the incidence in certain population subgroups may be disguised.

Surveys such as those conducted in Minnesota suggest that rheumatic fever has not disappeared.[57, 120] In 1 year approximately 1400 active cases were reported in children under 15 years with a rate for this age group of 1.53 per 1000 and for all ages of 0.73 per 1000. One report from North Dakota[203] indicates that acute rheumatic fever can still occur in epidemic proportions in civilian populations.

The common impression that rheumatic fever is completely dying out may be due not so much to a drop in the incidence of initial attacks but rather to a decline in severity and in number of recurrences of the disease. For example, in South America,[145] India,[130] and Egypt,[1] rheumatic heart disease is still the predominant form of heart disease in children. The declining prevalence and severity of rheumatic heart disease in a number of the more industrialized countries does not apply to many other parts of the world. Recent information indicates that rheumatic fever is the most common cause of heart disease in the 5 to 30 age group in developing countries.[3, 165] This impression is also likely influenced by the fact that relatively few rheumatic fever prevention/surveillance programs remain in operation.[86] Even in those that are still in operation, questions remain about the validity of collected data.

DIAGNOSIS

The diagnosis of acute rheumatic fever is complicated by the wide variations in qualitative and quantitative expression of the disease, resulting in clinical pictures which overlap and which may be mimicked by many other disease states, particularly in their initial stages.[43] Attempts to bring a degree of uniformity to the diagnosis have been partially resolved by general adoption of standardized clinical criteria and by the recognition that evidence of a preceding streptococcal infection sets this disease entity apart and is useful in differentiating it from other clinical states with similar manifestations.

Among the various criteria which have been proposed, those of Jones[81] have survived with modification[34] because of their generally recognized usefulness (see Table 34.1).

The arrangement of Table 34.1 emphasizes the source of the information required to meet the various criteria. It should be noted that all the major criteria are based on objective clinical findings, obtained primarily by a careful physical examination. The presence of two major or one major and two minor manifestations has been considered as necessary for establishing the diagnosis of acute rheumatic fever. The most recent revision of the criteria[34] stresses the additional importance of strengthening the diagnosis by requiring evidence of a preceding streptococcal infection.

Aside from the major and minor criteria listed in Table 34.1, other clinical features may suggest the possibility of acute rheumatic fever but are not sufficiently common or specific to be included in the Jones criteria. Tachycardia, which occurs in many other febrile diseases, is commonly present at the onset of acute rheumatic fever and may be disproportionate to the degree of fever. Anemia may also be present but is not helpful in suggesting the diagnosis, because it is not specific and does not usually become evident until after other manifestations of rheumatic fever are well developed. Epistaxis occurs in 5 to 10% of patients with acute rheumatic fever.[54] The declining frequency of bleeding from the nose and the virtual disappearance of exsanguinating episodes requiring transfusion have been an interesting change in the clinical picture of rheumatic fever.[82] This may be explained in part but not completely by better differentiation of disorders such as Henoch-Schönlein purpura. Since nosebleeds in children are common, an extensive work-up for the possibility of rheumatic fever is not indicated in such patients in the absence of other symptoms or signs suggestive of this disease. Abdominal pain may herald the onset of acute rheumatic fever and may be of sufficient degree to result in unnecessary appendectomy. In appendicitis, the fever and the sedimentation rate are usually not as

TABLE 34.1 JONES CRITERIA BY SOURCE OF INFORMATION[a]

History	Physical examination
Previous rheumatic fever or rheumatic heart disease	FEVER
Arthralgia	POLYARTHRITIS
Fever	CARDITIS
Recent scarlet fever	CHOREA
	ERYTHEMA MARGINATUM
	SUBCUTANEOUS NODULES

Laboratory findings
  Acute-phase reactants
    Erythrocyte sedimentation rate, C-reactive protein, leukocytosis
  Prolonged PR interval
  Elevated streptococcal antibodies:
    ASO (antistreptolysin O)
    Other specific antibodies (e.g., anti-DNAse B, anti-NADase, antihyaluronidase)
  Positive throat culture for group A streptococcus

[a] Adapted from the modified criteria of the American Heart Association.[34] Major criteria in capital letters; minor criteria in capital and lower case letters; support evidence of streptococcal infection in italic. One major criterion and 2 minor, *or* 2 major criteria *plus* evidence of a preceding streptococcal infection are required to establish a diagnosis.

high as in acute rheumatic fever. A careful physical examination and a short period of observation may be helpful in differentiating the two diseases. Rheumatic pneumonia, the specificity and incidence of which is debatable,[54, 60] may occur in patients with well-developed and often long-standing rheumatic disease, usually those with severe carditis and grave prognosis.[150]

Among the major criteria, *polyarthritis* is the one most often encountered, particularly in older children and adults. Arthralgia with indefinite physical findings is not sufficient to meet this criterion; the joints should manifest definite tenderness or painful limitation of motion. Joint symptoms which are alleviated by massage, as is frequently the case with so-called "growing pains," are particularly suspect; if they can be definitely localized to the joints, they should be labeled arthralgia at most and never polyarthritis. Swelling, heat, and redness are additional objective signs which are helpful when present. For this criterion to be met, objective findings must also involve more than one joint. Although patients with acute rheumatic fever may present with findings limited to a single joint, they usually progress to involve more than one joint, unless antiinflammatory agents are initiated prematurely. The migratory feature is often present in rheumatic arthritis and infrequently present in other forms of arthritis. Although the large joints of the extremities are most commonly involved, the small joints, including unusual ones such as the temporomandibular joint, and those of the vertebrae may be affected. The necessity for withholding antiinflammatory therapy until the physician has had sufficient time to observe that the signs and symptoms are compatible with migratory polyarthritis should be emphasized.

Carditis is perhaps the major manifestation which is most often overdiagnosed on the basis of misinterpretation or insufficient evidence. This is commonly due to confusion of innocent with pathologic murmurs, overinterpretation of the electrocardiographic findings, and failure to differentiate carefully the manifestations of preexisting congenital or acquired heart disease from active inflammatory disease, which the label carditis implies.

Significant murmurs in patients with carditis of acute rheumatic fever include the apical systolic murmur of mitral insufficiency and the basal diastolic decrescendo murmur of aortic insufficiency. In patients known to have or suspected of having previous rheumatic fever or rheumatic heart disease the physician needs to carefully document a change in established murmurs or the appearance of a new murmur. Valvular stenosis is usually due to preexisting acquired (predominately rheumatic) or congenital lesions and is seldom seen with an initial attack of acute rheumatic fever.

The additional presence of cardiac failure[56] with cardiomegaly, pericarditis, or pericardial effusion documented by physical findings or laboratory studies (roentgenogram, electrocardiogram, or echocardiogram) may be helpful in substantiating the diagnosis of rheumatic carditis (Fig. 34.1). However, other conditions including congenital heart disease, other so-called collagen diseases, and viral myopericarditis can produce similar clinical and laboratory findings and should not be dismissed as a possible cause of these findings.

Carditis is a common manifestation of acute rheumatic fever, occurring in more than one-third of the cases[176] and is frequently the sole major manifestation in infants or very young children. Since this major manifestation is the only one which results in permanent sequelae, it is heartening to note recent evidence that carditis is a less frequent finding in acute rheumatic fever.[118]

Chorea (Sydenham's chorea), which occurs in from one-fifth to one-half of patients with rheumatic fever,[20, 122] is a peculiar neurologic disorder resulting in involuntary purposeless movements which must be differentiated from fidgeting, tics, and athetosis. Emotional instability is often a prominent feature of this form of rheumatic fever, and many of these children are labeled as behavior problems until the true nature of the rheumatic process is recognized. Muscle weakness can usually be demonstrated if sought for.

Chorea often occurs without other clinical or laboratory evidence of rheumatic fever and may develop much later than other clinical manifestations. This is due, at least in part, to the long latent period of several months between streptococcal infection and onset of this complication.[162] Although symptoms and signs of chorea have been reported in other diseases, observations on the natural history of chorea[7] and streptococcal antibody data[12] would suggest that it is often associated with streptococcal infection. Evidence of other disease processes should be carefully sought, but in the absence of such evidence, Sydenham's chorea should be strongly considered.

Erythema marginatum, although uncommon in rheumatic fever, occurs so infrequently in association with other diseases that it has been granted major status in the modified Jones criteria. In its early stages it may appear as undifferentiated pink macules, most commonly over the trunk and inner proximal portions of the extremities, but in its fully developed form shows central blanching and fusion of individual lesions to form a serpiginous pattern, the appearance of which has reminded some observers of chicken wire (Fig. 34.2). It is characteristically evanescent and may be elicited or accentuated by the application of heat. The lesions do not

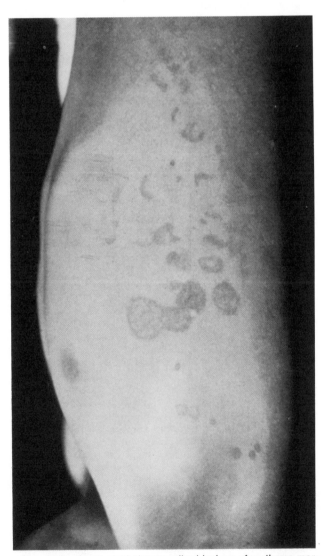

Fig. 34.2 The typical circumscribed lesions of erythema marginatum. (Reproduced with permission of C. B. Perry: *Archives of Disease in Childhood* 12:233, 1937).

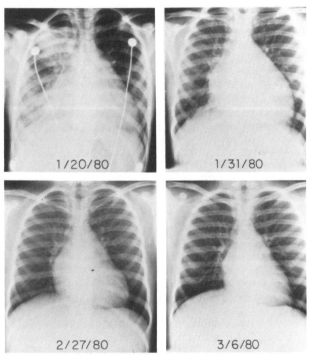

Fig. 34.1 Chest roentgenograms showing almost complete resolution of marked cardiomegaly and heart failure in a 12-year-old girl presenting with an initial attack of acute rheumatic fever and carditis. The echocardiogram revealed no evidence of pericardial effusion.

itch and show no induration, which distinguishes them from those associated with drug reactions and serum sickness. Erythema marginatum may appear late and without other evidence of rheumatic activity,[54] but often occurs with carditis.

Because of their relative infrequency and their rare presence in the early stages of the disease process *subcutaneous nodules* are not often helpful in the initial diagnosis of acute rheumatic fever. They are seen most commonly in longstanding rheumatic subjects, often with repeated attacks and severe carditis. Nodules almost never occur as an isolated manifestation of rheumatic fever.[163] They may be associated with the chronic joint involvement of rheumatoid arthritis, especially in adult patients. The British, perhaps because of their emphasis on clinical medicine, find more subcutaneous nodules in rheumatic fever than we do in the United States.[176] Nodules should be looked for over the extensor surfaces of joints, such as the elbows, knees, knuckles, and ankles, and also over the scalp and spinous processes of the vertebrae. Rheumatic nodules are firm and nontender and without attachment to or inflammation of the overlying skin. They are often quite small but may be large in patients with persistent disease.

The minor manifestations are so categorized because they are nonspecific. Arthralgia, although common in rheumatic fever, may be found in many other diseases and even with careful history may be difficult to differentiate from so-called "growing pains" or minor injury to the extremities.

Prolongation of the PR interval in the electrocardiogram is nonspecific and occurs in many infectious diseases as well as acute rheumatic fever. For this reason it is now generally agreed that carditis should not be diagnosed on the basis of this finding alone.

Fever and the acute phase reactants are nonspecific indicators of inflammation. Their absence in untreated patients with rheumatic polyarthritis and acute carditis is unusual and should prompt careful reconsideration of the diagnosis. High fever, of greater than 104° F, is also unusual; the fever of rheumatic fever is rarely accompanied by chills or seizures.

Two kinds of laboratory tests which give different kinds of information are commonly used in acute rheumatic fever. Neither is specific for this disease. The acute phase reactants confirm the presence of an inflammatory process, and streptococcal antibody tests provide specific evidence of a preceding illness which could have resulted in this complication. Because of their nonspecific nature, the acute phase reactants are considered as a minor manifestation in the revised Jones criteria. Evidence of streptococcal infection is too specific to be considered a minor criterion but not specific enough to be considered a major criterion. It is therefore listed as supporting evidence which greatly strengthens the possibility of rheumatic fever and should be sought in all patients suspected to have this disease.

Among the available acute phase reactants the erythrocyte sedimentation rate and C-reactive protein test are most commonly used.[197] Both of these tests are often normal in patients with pure chorea and may also be normal in patients with isolated erythema marginatum but are usually positive in other forms of acute rheumatic fever unless suppressed by salicylate or steroid therapy. The erythrocyte sedimentation rate has the disadvantage of being influenced by accompanying features of rheumatic fever, such as anemia, which results in a more rapid rate, and by heart failure, which may result in a slower rate, probably as a result of decreased fibrinogen production by a passively congested liver. Borderline sedimentation rates may also be difficult to interpret.

The C-reactive protein is an unusually sensitive indicator of inflammation. It was first recognized by its ability to react with the C polysaccharide of the pneumococcus but is now commonly measured in a semiquantitative fashion by precipitation with a specific immune rabbit antiserum[197] which is commercially available. It is completely absent from the sera of normal individuals and is not influenced by anemia. The problem of borderline values does not exist with the C-reactive protein test since even small amounts are abnormal. The chief difficulty with this test is its extreme sensitivity. A positive test may occur with heart failure regardless of cause and with mild inflammatory processes of nonrheumatic origin. Even the local inflammation which may follow an injection of benzathine penicillin may be a sufficient stimulus on occasion to result in the appearance of an abnormal test. Nevertheless, it is the generally preferred test because it is a more accurate and more readily interpreted index of rheumatic activity.

Other acute phase tests, such as the Weltmann reaction and serum mucoprotein tests, offer no certain advantage and have not been as widely used as the erythrocyte sedimentation rate and the C reactive protein test. Leukocytosis may occur but is too often absent to be of definite value.

Supporting evidence of streptococcal infection has received special emphasis in the latest revision of the Jones criteria[34] because of the conviction that acute rheumatic fever does not occur in the absence of streptococcal infection and that with sufficient examination all or almost all patients with active rheumatic polyarthritis or carditis should present evidence of this highly specific precipitating insult. Patients with chorea, and perhaps those with erythema marginatum, may be exceptions because the long interval before appearance of these complications may afford sufficient time for the clinical evidence of streptococcal infection to be forgotten or the laboratory evidence to disappear.

A history of scarlet fever is rarely obtained but when present is usually a reliable indication of preceding streptococcal infection. Sore throat, which may be of varying etiology, is less reliable unless substantiated by isolation of group A beta-hemolytic streptococci. By the time the patient presents with acute rheumatic fever, the number of streptococci in the throat may have declined to the point where it is difficult or impossible to isolate them. Patients in whom the diagnosis of acute rheumatic fever is being considered should have at least one and preferably two or three adequately obtained and properly interpreted throat cultures.

Specific antibody tests are generally a more reliable method of obtaining evidence of recent streptococcal infection. Titers obtained with these specific antibody tests may be elevated even in the absence of clinical or current bacteriologic evidence of streptococcal disease. Development of antibody responses may be suppressed by antibiotic therapy and may be suppressed or delayed by steroid therapy.

Whether streptococcal antibody titers are rising or falling will depend on the interval of time since the streptococcal infection. Occasionally patients are seen before peak titers are achieved. Serial titers are particularly valuable in such patients, as the initial titer may be borderline or low, and a significant increase in titer (usually two dilution increments or greater) on simultaneously run sera is indicative of a streptococcal infection regardless of the absolute titer levels. Patients seen late, such as those with chorea[12] or longstanding carditis, may have titers which have returned to normal or near normal levels by the time of recognizable onset.

The antistreptolysin O test (ASO) is most commonly used, not only because of tradition but also because it is well standardized and good commercial reagents are available. About 80% of patients with acute rheumatic fever and 20%

of normal individuals may have definitely elevated antistreptolysin O titers. Titers of 333 Todd units or greater in children over 5 years of age and of 250 units or greater in adults are commonly found in the early active phase of acute rheumatic fever.

Patients who present with low or borderline ASO titers, including those with chorea,[12] may show elevated antibody titers to other streptococcal antigens. An antibody test for a different streptococcal antigen is especially valuable in such patients. A wide choice of secondary antibody tests is available. Antistreptokinase tests present problems in standardization because of differences in reagents, and the assay is complicated by the existence of several different streptokinases.[41] Commercial reagents for the antihyaluronidase test have not been uniformly satisfactory and titers are difficult to reproduce at close dilution increments.

The antideoxyribonuclease B (anti-DNase B) test has proven to be a useful and highly reproducible streptococcal antibody determination.[11] In fact, in certain circumstances, such as patients with pyoderma,[17, 40, 87] the anti-DNase B test is preferable to the ASO test. Reagents for this test are commercially available.

The anti-nicotinamide-adenine-dinucleotidase (anti-NADase) test is yet another antibody test which may provide serologic evidence of streptococcal infection.[11, 12, 14] Although a preparation of the enzyme is not yet commercially available, the test has proven useful in those laboratories where the enzyme is made and carefully standardized. A comparison of the distribution of three streptococcal antibody tests in patients with acute rheumatic fever and pure chorea compared with normal control groups is shown in Figure 34.3.

Recently a simple agglutination test has become commercially available for testing for streptococcal antibodies. This test (Streptozyme®) has been referred to as a "universal" antibody test, i.e., one test which simultaneously determines antibodies to a number of streptococcal extracellular antigens. Some studies have demonstrated a generally good correlation between elevated titers using this agglutination test and the more established neutralization tests (most consistently the ASO test).[18, 100] In clinical studies the sensitivity of this test was equal to, but not better than conventional neutralization tests for streptococcal antibodies. However, questions were raised about the specificity of the test since some individuals with non-group A streptococci in their upper respiratory tract also showed rises in titer when using the Streptozyme test.[90] Further data are needed regarding preparation and standardization of the Streptozyme reagents before the value of this test for general usage can be accepted with certainty.[91]

Since patients with recent streptococcal infection who have escaped nonsuppurative sequelae also show elevated streptococcal antibody titers, these tests are specific only for streptococcal infection and not for acute rheumatic fever or acute nephritis. The major contribution which these antibody tests make is to provide assurance that the disease entity under consideration has been preceded by an illness which *could* have resulted in rheumatic fever.

The absence of elevated antibody titers should be a red flag that stimulates the physician to reconsider his diagnosis. In this way they are useful in eliminating disease states which may simulate acute rheumatic fever. They may be particularly helpful in the differential diagnosis of patients with isolated inflammatory disease of the heart or joints. It should again be emphasized that in acute rheumatic fever[11] as well as in uncomplicated streptococcal pharyngitis,[88] the performance of several streptococcal antibody tests will in-

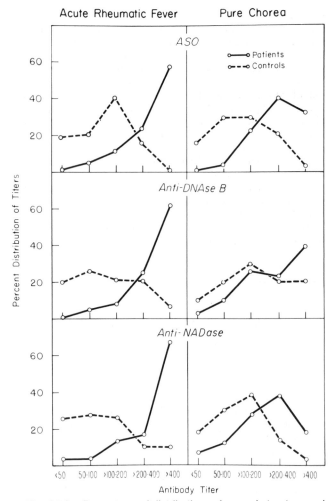

Fig. 34.3   Percentage of distributions of several streptococcal antibodies in patients with acute rheumatic fever or pure chorea as compared with matched controls (modified from previously published data[11, 12]). *AntiDNAse B*, antideoxyribonuclease B; *ASO*, antistreptolysin O; *anti-NADase*, antinicotinamide adenine dinucleotidase.

crease the percentage of those with documented serologic evidence of streptococcal infection when compared with patients whose sera are tested for only one antibody. A more extensive review of the dynamics of the immune response to streptococcal antigens and its relationship to rheumatic fever is given elsewhere.[186]

Recent studies indicate that so-called heart-reactive antibodies are present in the sera of a majority of patients with acute rheumatic fever.[98, 201] Tests for these antibodies make use of the cross-reactive antigens in the streptococcal cell membrane or wall and those in myocardial sarcolemma. The tests require special fluorescent techniques and are currently done in only a few laboratories. While helpful when demonstrated to be positive, it should be remembered that not all patients with acute rheumatic fever have such antibodies in their sera; some patients with only acute streptococcal pharyngitis—and not rheumatic fever—will also have these antibodies.

The determination of antibodies to the group A carbohydrate (A-CHO) moiety of the streptococcal cell wall has not been selectively helpful in making a diagnosis of acute rheumatic fever. These antibodies are elevated following uncomplicated streptococcal pharyngitis and may be used in a way similar to the ASO or anti-DNase B tests.[88] Encouraging reports have, however, suggested that anti-A-CHO levels remain elevated in patients with chronic rheumatic valvular heart disease (in the absence of evidence of recent streptococcal infection),[46] and this test may ultimately prove most useful for the differentiation of rheumatic heart disease from valvular heart disease of other etiologies.[152] However, it has been our experience that these antibodies are frequently elevated in the pediatric age group, thereby limiting its usefulness in differentiating rheumatic heart disease from other forms of valvular heart disease.[85]

Judicious use of the Jones criteria and streptococcal antibody tests will minimize incorrect diagnoses of rheumatic fever, but many other diseases may fit the Jones criteria, especially in their initial stages. Rheumatoid arthritis, reactions to penicillin and foreign serum, septic arthritis, endocarditis, Henoch-Schönlein purpura, acute leukemia, viral myocarditis and pericarditis, intracardiac tumors, lupus erythematosus, and other collagen-type diseases must be considered, as well as neurological and dermatological disorders which may resemble Sydenham's chorea and erythema marginatum.

CLINICAL COURSE AND TREATMENT

The clinical course of patients with acute or recurrent rheumatic fever may be quite variable. In patients whose initial manifestations are fever and arthritis, the illness may present abruptly with rapid appearance of inflammation in one or more joints. The disease begins much more insidiously in patients presenting with Sydenham's chorea. Symptoms often develop so gradually in these patients that they may be considered merely as nervous children or children with behavior problems for several weeks or months. Carditis may also be silent in its appearance and may not be suspected until a murmur is heard on physical examination. Patients with pericarditis may complain of chest pain, and occasionally patients may present in heart failure with only complaints of shortness of breath. The sinus tachycardia which may be present on admission may subside with the disappearance of fever or may convert to a sinus brachycardia lasting several days.[74] The complaint of sore throat, which sometimes develops or recurs at the onset of acute rheumatic fever,[174] may be accompanied by little physical and minimal bacteriologic evidence of acute infection, suggesting that this may be a delayed type of reaction of a nonsuppurative type.

The duration of the natural course of acute rheumatic fever varies considerably. Symptoms and signs characteristically develop in successive joints over a period of several days or weeks in the patient who has not yet received antiinflammatory agents. Arthritis ordinarily subsides in the untreated patient after a period of 1 to 4 weeks, with involvement of individual joints lasting 1 to several days, rarely longer than 1 week. Patients with carditis, particularly those with moderate or severe carditis, tend to run a more protracted course, often lasting 2 to 6 months and sometimes longer.[54] In most patients with chorea the manifestations gradually subside over a period of 2 to 3 months but may occasionally last for longer periods of time.

About 3% of patients show chronic activity lasting more than 6 months.[167] Such a protracted course occurs most often in patients with a history of previous bouts of rheumatic fever. So-called "chronic" rheumatic fever only rarely occurs, and prior to accepting this diagnosis, other diagnoses must be carefully excluded.

Treatment of individual cases is dependent upon the man-

ifestations. In general, patients should be put to bed for the duration of the acute and febrile portion of the illness until there is no remaining laboratory or clinical evidence of inflammation. Careful records of the pulse rate, particularly the sleeping pulse rate, should be maintained, since tachycardia during sleep in the afebrile patient may be an indication of carditis. Initial laboratory studies should include a hemoglobin, acute-phase reactants (white blood cell count, erythrocyte sedimentation rate, and C-reactive protein), throat cultures (preferably two or more taken before initiation of penicillin therapy since the number of group A streptococci may be few), streptococcal antibody titers (e.g., ASO or anti-DNAse B), a roentgenogram of the chest to evaluate heart size, and an electrocardiogram. An echocardiogram may be helpful, particularly if pericardial involvement is suspected.

The importance of delaying the initiation of antiinflammatory or suppressive therapy until the disease process is sufficiently manifest for definite diagnosis cannot be overstressed. A premature therapeutic trial of aspirin or steroids in a patient with early monoarticular arthritis or arthralgia and fever may suppress the disease process enough to eliminate any possibility of making a firm diagnosis.

Once the diagnosis is established, therapy can then be initiated. Antiinflammatory drugs are widely used in acute rheumatic fever and are usually effective in promptly suppressing many of the acute manifestations of the disease. Joint inflammation and fever subside rapidly, ordinarily within a few days and often sooner. The acute phase reactants, especially the sedimentation rate, may remain abnormal for several weeks after disappearance of fever and joint manifestations. The antiinflammatory agents have either no effect or questionable effect on erythema marginatum, Sydenham's chorea, subcutaneous nodules, and the development of valvular heart disease.

Both aspirin and corticosteroids are dramatically effective in suppressing the acute signs of inflammation. Steroids may bring these acute manifestations under control somewhat more rapidly than aspirin, but there is a greater tendency for them to reappear after discontinuation of treatment.[176] The debate in the choice of aspirin or steroids in the therapy of acute rheumatic fever centers around their possible effects on the cardiac manifestations of rheumatic fever, especially whether they can prevent residual rheumatic heart disease. Most carditis appears early in the course of rheumatic fever (76% in the 1st week)[54] and, regardless of treatment, the risk of developing subsequent heart disease is probably minimal in patients who do not have it at the time of admission to the hospital or at the time treatment is begun.[44, 176] Therefore, the principal question is not whether aspirin or steroids may prevent the development of carditis but whether they will influence the development of rheumatic valvulitis. Several studies[44, 78] indicate that aspirin treatment does not alter the frequency of residual heart disease, and a few[5, 24] have suggested that the increased oxygen consumption which occurs with salicylate therapy may result in a possible deleterious effect by increasing the work load of the heart, possibly fostering the development of heart failure.

A large scale cooperative study using relatively low dosages of steroids for 6 weeks failed to show any advantage of steroids over aspirin with respect to residual heart damage 1, 5, and 10 years after the acute attack.[176–178] A subsequent controlled study indicated that short-term therapy, even if quite intensive (1.5 mg/kg/day for 1 or 2 weeks), does not modify the frequency of residual heart disease 1 year later.[33] Moreover, especially if prolonged, such large doses may result in serious complications.[62] Differences of opinion are most marked about the use of moderately high doses of steroids for prolonged periods of time. In one study[32] in which prednisone (in a dosage of 60 mg daily for 3 weeks with gradual reduction over an additional 9-week period) was used, no superiority in cardiac status over control patients treated with aspirin was found 1 year later. A directly opposing result was suggested by another controlled study[44] in which hydrocortisone was used (200 to 250 mg/day for 4 days followed by 80 to 100 mg/day for 8 weeks with a gradual tapering over an additional 4-week period). In the latter study no additional advantage was found in combining aspirin with steroids. Whether the differences in results in these two studies are due to the kinds or schedules of steroids used or the selection of patients for study is not clear. The two studies agree that evidence of heart disease will disappear spontaneously in a substantial proportion (about one-half) of carditis patients treated with no suppressive drugs or with aspirin alone. The studies also agree that a variable but significant portion of carditis patients treated with steroids or with steroids plus aspirin must be classified as treatment failures on the basis of cardiac findings 1 year later. More detailed accounts and discussions of the many studies which have been carried out in an attempt to answer this question are given in the literature.[47, 50, 117, 158]

No final conclusions about the place of steroids in preventing the development of rheumatic heart disease can be reached from the data presently available from controlled studies. However, in view of the infrequency of late appearance of heart disease, it would seem reasonable to limit consideration of the use of steroids to patients who exhibit carditis of at least moderate degree, especially those with evidence of heart failure. Patients who have arthritic disease alone or only mild or questionable carditis can usually be handled well with aspirin.

There is a tendency to use steroids in patients with moderate to severe carditis. This is based on the observation that these drugs may bring the acute manifestations under control more rapidly. Many observers believe that steroids may sometimes be life-saving in the patient with overwhelming acute rheumatic myocarditis or pancarditis. In view of the disappearance of carditis in many patients regardless of the type of management used, the documented hazards of prolonged administration of steroids, and the indefinite and conflicting evidence that prolonged administration to patients with moderate or severe carditis results in decreased residual heart disease, discontinuation of steroids as soon as the acute disease is brought under control seems justified. To avoid rebounds, tapering of steroids with overlapping of salicylates is recommended in patients who have been on steroids for periods longer than 1 week. Salicylate therapy should be continued until both laboratory and clinical manifestations of activity have subsided.

Aspirin should be given in a dose sufficient to achieve blood levels of approximately 20 to 25 mg/100 ml. This can usually be reached with a daily dose of 90 to 120 mg/kg of body weight, but more or less may be needed in individual patients. The maximal daily dose should ordinarily not exceed 10 gm. Serum salicylate levels are desirable in following patients on aspirin therapy. Aspirin therapy, especially prolonged high dose therapy resulting in salicylate blood levels of greater than 25 mg/100 ml, may produce hepatic injury as reflected by increased blood levels of transaminases.[202] The injury is usually mild and reversible. The appearance of toxic symptoms, especially nausea and vomiting, may cause difficulties in maintaining adequate therapy. Sodium bicarbonate or antacids should not be prescribed or permitted for gastric distress because it reduces the effectiveness of aspirin

therapy. The use of enteric-coated drug or administration after meals may be helpful. Tinnitus is commonly present when fully suppressive salicylate levels are achieved and may be accompanied by some temporary deficiency in hearing. Hyperpnea may also occur. It is sometimes necessary to discontinue therapy for several days or reduce the dosage if toxic symptoms appear.

Adrenocorticotropic hormone (ACTH) is no longer employed, and prednisone is generally favored over other steroids because it is less likely to cause electrolyte problems. By using prednisone, low sodium diet and the need for added potassium are avoided.

Dosage of steroids should be no greater than that sufficient to cause suppression of acute manifestations. Some individualization of dosage may be required. A total dose of 2.5 mg/kg/day divided into two doses is usually adequate. With steroid therapy some Cushingoid changes should be expected, including moonface, abdominal fullness, and not infrequently, hirsutism. Hypertension and toxic psychoses may also occur. Susceptibility to infection is increased. Life-threatening bacteremia may develop with few or no clinical manifestations. Varicella may also be unusually severe. Gastric ulcers and compression fractures of the spine may develop during prolonged therapy. Although not studied in a controlled fashion, alternate day steroids have been used in patients with acute rheumatic fever.[67] This theoretically could reduce the untoward effects caused by these drugs.

Rebounds occur more often with steroids than with aspirin. They may be avoided or minimized by introducing salicylates just prior to discontinuing or tapering the steroids. Rebounds vary in intensity. Some are only detectable by laboratory indications of activity. Clinical rebounds usually show arthralgia, fever, and sometimes arthritis, but severe cardiac manifestations may occasionally be seen. Rebounds probably occur because the rheumatic episode has not finished running its natural course when suppressive drugs are withdrawn.[24] No treatment is required for mild rebounds since they usually subside spontaneously within a few days. Salicylates are preferable to steroids as suppressive therapy for more severe rebounds, since a second rebound is less likely if salicylates are used. Treatment of rebounds may increase the total period of time required for subsidence of active disease.[53]

Although opinions vary, there are no controlled studies and little general enthusiasm for the use of steroids in the treatment of Sydenham's chorea. Patients with concomitant rheumatic activity should be given salicylates. Patients should be removed to a quiet environment, should have understanding attendants, and should be protected against self-inflicted injury caused by uncontrollable movements. Phenobarbital or other sedatives may be helpful, but occasionally their use results in increased agitation. Some favorable reports have appeared on the use of chlorpromazine.[173] Recently two additional drugs have been utilized in the management of Sydenham's chorea.[110] Diazepam, a benzodiazepine derivative, is now the initial choice of many physicians. Although not yet officially approved or recommended for use in the pediatric age group, haloperidol, a butyrophenone has been used with encouraging results in some patients with chorea who prove difficult to manage. A note of caution should be given about the use of haloperidol in Sydenham's chorea since severe adverse reactions have been reported in children treated with this drug.[151] Antimicrobials should be used as in other forms of rheumatic fever.

Digitalis was formerly considered to be contraindicated in the treatment of heart failure associated with rheumatic carditis. Some patients may be inordinately sensitive to digitalis, requiring unusual caution in digitalization, but it is now generally agreed that digitalis should be used in rheumatic patients who have heart failure, regardless of the presence or absence of active disease. A more complete description of the treatment of heart failure including the use of diuretics is given in Chapter 44.

Antimicrobial agents are an important part of the management of acute rheumatic fever, including Sydenham's chorea.[7, 12] Secondary prophylaxis should be started as soon as the diagnosis is established and appropriate cultures have been taken. The risk of contracting a new streptococcal infection may be especially high in hospital environments. Therefore, initiation of prophylaxis should not be delayed until discharge from the hospital. Before starting prophylaxis, a therapeutic course of penicillin should be given to eradicate residual group A streptococci, which may be difficult to isolate. In the hope of altering the frequency of residual heart disease, massive penicillin treatment has been tried by some investigators, with negative results.[179]

Patients with arthritis who do not develop carditis in the 1st week or 2 of illness may begin to be ambulated; they may return to full activity, usually after 4 to 6 weeks.

Patients with carditis should be kept in bed for longer periods of time, depending on its severity. This is usually 3 to 6 months but may be longer in patients with protracted active carditis. It is customary to ambulate patients several weeks after all evidence of heart failure and inflammatory activity has subsided.[107] Resumption of full activity depends upon the clinical course. In patients with prolonged borderline elevated sedimentation rates, ambulation may be tried under careful observation.

NATURAL HISTORY AND PROGNOSIS

The case fatality rate for acute rheumatic fever and rheumatic heart disease in children has been estimated to be 2 to 3%.[4, 177] A few patients progress to death during or after a single attack.[4, 176] Arthritis is never permanently crippling. In many patients with carditis, the cardiac manifestations also regress either during the acute attack or over a period of 5 to 10 years.[119, 176-178] Disappearance of murmurs is more likely to occur after first attacks. The frequency of residual heart disease is related to the severity of the cardiac involvement at the time of acute attack.[177, 178] Cardiomegaly is a particularly unfavorable prognostic sign. The silent development of heart disease many years after the first attack of rheumatic fever, once thought to be common,[20] is now rarely seen.[4] Some observers have, in fact, raised the question as to whether these patients, many of whom do not have a good history of rheumatic fever, actually may have some other form of acquired valvular heart disease not related to the sequelae of streptococcal infection. In the opinion of many, penicillin prophylaxis is responsible for this improved outlook for delayed appearance of heart disease. Whether it acts by preventing additional subclinical attacks or by terminating or suppressing smoldering disease is uncertain.

Rheumatic fever is by nature a recurrent disease, and most chronic disability and deaths are related to recurrent attacks. In unprotected patients, the frequency of recurrences is high.[157] Roth and colleagues[143] reported that more than two-thirds of patients experienced at least one recurrence during an average of 8 years. A number of factors, both streptococcal and host factors, contribute to the frequency and epidemiology of rheumatic recurrences.

It has been well documented that recurrent attacks, like first attacks, are invariably preceded by streptococcal infection. Infection may be either clinical or subclinical. Each recurrence is due to infection with a new serologic type. Throat cultures and especially antibody tests are important in documenting the occurrence of streptococcal infection in these patients.

The risk of developing acute rheumatic fever following streptococcal infection is greatly increased among individuals who have experienced one or more previous attacks. Attack rates among rheumatic subjects vary from 16 to 50%.[4, 103] This is 5- to 15-fold greater than the 3% attack rate following epidemic streptococcal infection in nonrheumatic military populations.[136] It is not known whether these attack rates are higher because of some acquired host susceptibility in connection with the events leading to the first attack or whether the first attack selects out an inherently susceptible population group. The nature and interrelationships of these streptococcal and host factors are poorly understood.

The risk is highest in the first few years after an attack.[143] The studies of Bland and Jones[20] indicate that during the first 5 years the average attack rate is 19 attacks per 100 patients per year, during the second 5 years 11 per 100 per year, during the third 5 years 6 per 100 per year, and during the fourth 5 years 1.4 per 100 per year. Younger children are more likely to develop recurrences. Marienfeld and colleagues[114] showed that recurrence rates are highest in the 1st year after attack regardless of the age of the child. Since carditis is more common in younger age groups, this may contribute to the increased frequency of recurrences in this age group. The number of preceding attacks and the presence of heart disease are also interrelated,[4] and it is difficult to determine the extent to which each contributes to the risk of recurrence.

The incidence of streptococcal infection is known to vary with age, with generally diminishing frequency in older groups. This undoubtedly contributes to the declining frequency of recurrences in older individuals, but some data suggest that once streptococcal infection occurs, the attack rate for recurrence is greater among children than it is among adolescents and adults.[160]

A number of authors have emphasized the mimetic features of rheumatic recurrences,[52, 143] and in certain patients this may be quite striking, not only with regard to reappearance of similar major manifestations but also with recurrent involvement of identical joints. However, as Kuttner and Mayer[104] have pointed out, the pattern varies, with some patients showing a mimetic pattern and others developing new major manifestations, including carditis. A significant proportion of patients with chorea (approximately one-third) will ultimately develop heart disease.[7]

In addition to the severity of heart involvement and the number of recurrent attacks, the susceptibility to endocarditis is an important factor in the prognosis of those patients with acute rheumatic fever who develop rheumatic heart disease. Rheumatic heart disease and endocarditis are discussed in Chapters 35 and 36.

PREVENTION

The natural history of rheumatic fever can be dramatically altered by introduction of appropriate antimicrobials at several different points. Epidemics of streptococcal upper respiratory tract infection and rheumatic fever are promptly halted by mass penicillin prophylaxis. Adequate prolonged penicillin treatment initiated during the course of, or sometimes even after subsidence of, acute streptococcal upper respiratory tract infection will abort initial attacks of acute rheumatic fever and, less regularly, rheumatic recurrences. Prophylactic administration of sulfadiazine or penicillin in low doses on a continuous basis to patients with a well-documented history of rheumatic fever or established rheumatic heart disease is highly effective in protecting them from subsequent attacks. Apart from the practical implications of these observations, they provide important confirmation of the role of streptococcal infections in the pathogenesis of acute rheumatic fever and rheumatic heart disease.

The term *secondary prevention*, which is commonly used to describe protection against second or recurrent attacks by continuous antimicrobial prophylaxis, is somewhat misleading, because the prophylaxis is primary in the sense that it is the most important preventive approach available and is indispensable in the long-term treatment of patients with acute rheumatic fever and rheumatic heart disease. Since patients with pure chorea are prone to recurrences which may produce further periods of disability or may result in permanent cardiac sequelae,[7] they, too, should receive continuous antimicrobial prophylaxis.

It has been suggested that patients with a history of rheumatic fever or with established rheumatic heart disease may be managed by treating streptococcal infections as they occur.[108] This approach is hazardous in such a high-risk group, since many streptococcal infections which result in recurrences are subclinical or mild and since it is more difficult to abort recurrent attacks than first attacks. Acute streptococcal infections occurring in rheumatic individuals should be treated promptly and vigorously with full therapeutic doses of penicillin or other suitable antibiotics if the patient is allergic to penicillin, but reliance on prevention of recurrences should not rest solely on this approach.

After establishing a diagnosis of rheumatic fever, but before initiation of prophylaxis, residual streptococci which may or may not be detectable on admission throat cultures should be eradicated by a therapeutic course of penicillin as recommended in the section describing treatment of acute streptococcal infections. Although no effect of this procedure on the course of subsequent events has been proved, it seems reasonable to remove the causative agent, and from a practical standpoint it is less confusing in deciding whether future throat cultures are more likely to represent a persistent carrier state or new streptococcal infection.

Intramuscular benzathine penicillin G, injected once a month in a dosage of 1,200,000 units,[141] is the most effective form of prophylaxis. In the extensive studies reported by the Irvington House group,[4] an attack rate of less than 1 recurrence per 25,000 patient years was observed among patients using this form of prophylaxis. This method does not rely upon the patient's memory to take medication daily or depend upon possible variations in absorption of the drug from the gastrointestinal tract. Closer surveillance of the patient and of his prophylactic program is automatically achieved by the necessity to return at monthly intervals for injections. Studies on the use of intramuscular benzathine penicillin for mass prophylaxis in military populations have suggested that streptococcal infections rarely occur before 3 weeks after an injection of 1,200,000 units of benzathine penicillin G.[29] When they occur after this period in rheumatic subjects, the subsequent injection at 4 weeks probably serves as adequate therapy of this infection.

Practical experience in the United States has indicated that it is not necessary to administer injections more frequently than once a month. However, clinical observations of breakthroughs with every 4 week injections have led some rheumatic fever clinics, especially in developing countries, to adopt an every 3 week schedule for injection of benzathine penicillin G. Extension of the routine injection period to 6 weeks is probably risky, particularly since patients sometimes report a week late for injections. Although the reaction rate is higher for injectable forms of penicillin, regardless of kind,[66] than with oral penicillin, it is minimal and very rare after the first months of prophylaxis. In patients who have proved unreliable with respect to oral prophylaxis and in patients with well-established heart disease, monthly injections of benzathine penicillin are undoubtedly the preferred form of prophylaxis.

The recommended dosages for oral sulfadiazine prophylaxis are 0.5 gm once daily for patients under 60 pounds and 1 gm once a day for patients weighing more than 60 pounds and 1 gm once a day for patients weighing more than 60 pounds.[141] For oral penicillin prophylaxis, the recommended dose is 200,000 to 250,000 units twice daily.[141]

Oral prophylaxis is less reliable than repository penicillin prophylaxis. In the Irvington House studies,[4] considerable effort was expended to encourage taking of oral drug. Nevertheless, a recurrence rate of almost 1 per 2500 patient years was observed in patients on oral medication. Failure to take the antimicrobial is probably the major cause of prophylactic failure in patients on oral drug. In view of the widespread current use of oral penicillin in preference to oral sulfadiazine, it is of interest that in this study recurrence rates were higher in the group receiving oral penicillin. Even when oral penicillin was administered twice daily, no superiority over sulfadiazine could be demonstrated.[55] The fact that multiple recurrences were more common in the group receiving oral penicillin suggests individual differences in the effectiveness of this drug.[4] Oral penicillin G is more likely to be effective when the drug is taken at least ½ hour before or 1 hour after meals. Although other forms of penicillin may be taken with less attention to meals, they are generally more expensive and their superiority in the prevention of rheumatic fever is speculative. Strains of streptococci resistant to sulfonamide have appeared with mass sulfonamide prophylaxis in military populations but have never been a problem in secondary prophylaxis of rheumatic patients. Reaction rates are generally low with both oral sulfadiazine and oral penicillin and are very rare after the first months of prophylaxis.

Prophylaxis by the oral route is preferable only in patients with no or minimal heart disease, who have had a single attack of rheumatic fever, and who are responsible with respect to regular ingestion of the drug. Because of lack of necessity to orient ingestion around meals and possibly more dependable effectiveness, sulfadiazine may be the oral drug of choice. Caution should be used in prescribing sulfonamide for women during the last trimester of pregnancy because of possible hyperbilirubinemia in the fetus and newborn infant.[9] Oral penicillin should not be relied upon in patients who have experienced a recurrence while on this drug. In those in whom there is a question of compliance, some physicians make spot checks of the urine for the presence of penicillin.[116] Another method for evaluating the efficacy of secondary prophylaxis involves determination of serial streptrococcal antibody titers. The presence of increasing antibody titers can be used to convince the patient that repository penicillin prophylaxis is superior to the oral form.

Some investigators have reported an increased prevalence of penicillinase-producing staphylococci in patients receiving oral penicillin as prophylaxis for rheumatic fever,[70] but only on rare occasions does this appear to result in clinical problems. The possibility that penicillinase-producing staphylococci harbored in the upper respiratory tract may be responsible for prophylactic breakthroughs has not received adequate study. Because of the low dosage of drug, a mechanism of this kind seems more likely in this situation than when large doses of penicillin are administered for treatment of streptococcal infection (see below). Patients receiving oral penicillin prophylaxis are more likely to harbor resistant green or nonhemolytic streptococci in their oropharynx[102] and this should be taken into account when considering antibiotic prophylaxis for endocarditis in these patients.[35] Rare patients who are sensitive to both sulfadiazine and penicillin may be maintained on oral erythromycin,[155] 250 mg twice daily.[141]

Prophylaxis should be maintained year-round and should be continued during hospitalization, summer camps, and military service. Continuous prophylaxis should be withheld or discontinued in patients in whom the diagnosis of acute rheumatic fever or rheumatic heart disease is not well established.

Recommendations of the American Heart Association are that prophylaxis should be continued for a long period of time in patients who have had well-documented rheumatic fever or rheumatic heart disease.[141] Although risks of recurrence decline with age and with increased interval from onset or recurrence, a high risk continues for long periods of time. The studies of Bland and Jones[20] suggest that among patients who are more than 10 years since onset of rheumatic fever, each year 6 of 100 will experience a recurrence, and among those who are more than 15 years beyond onset 1 or 2 of 100 will develop a recurrence each year. These studies were performed before prophylaxis was routinely used and when rheumatic fever was a more severe disease. It is possible that protection against streptococcal infection for a long period of time, 5 to 10 years, may result in declining susceptibility to recurrence following streptococcal infection. Some objections to prolonged prophylaxis in adults have been raised, and attempts have been made to obtain reliable information on the risks involved in discontinuing prophylaxis after 5 or 10 years in adult patients without heart disease.[80]

Exceptions to prophylaxis should be made in adults only, and only after considering the evidence in regard to the factors involved, including the risk of being exposed to and developing streptococcal infection and the risk of developing rheumatic fever once infection occurs. Adults who are in close contact with school-age children, who are in the military service, or those who are employed in medical or allied health fields, are apt to be at high risk of developing streptococcal infection and should not be exempted from prophylaxis. Age is a factor not only in the frequency of streptococcal infections but also in the frequency of recurrence following streptococcal infection. Patients with significant degrees of rheumatic heart disease, with a history of several repeated attacks of rheumatic fever, or with a recent attack are more susceptible to recurrence after streptococcal infection and should be maintained on prophylaxis.

Prevention of first attacks of rheumatic fever by treatment of the streptococcal upper respiratory tract infection is known as *primary prophylaxis*. This approach has proved highly effective in military populations with a high frequency of streptococcal infections.[189] Studies in these population groups have indicated that with penicillin treatment it is possible to reduce the attack rate of acute rheumatic fever from 3 to 0.3%. The success of this approach depends upon the recognition and treatment of streptococcal infections. Recognition is a particular problem in both military and civilian populations since about one-half of the streptococcal infections are subclinical or so mild that they are not brought to the attention of a physician. These unrecognized infections may nevertheless lead to rheumatic fever.

Attempts to apply primary prevention measures to civilian populations, particularly children experiencing endemic streptococcal infections, have met with some difficulty, particularly with regard to diagnosis. Viral infections are common in children and may mimic streptococcal infections. Fever is common in nonbacterial as well as streptococcal upper respiratory infection in children. Leukocyte counts may be elevated in viral infections as well as in streptococcal infection. Pharyngeal exudate and tender cervical nodes are the most reliable physical signs suggestive of streptococcal infection. Throat cultures, carefully taken and processed, are especially helpful in eliminating patients with nonstreptococcal infection. However, even when positive for group A beta-hemolytic streptococci, throat cultures may be difficult to interpret because of the problem of differentiating streptococcal carriers with intercurrent nonstreptococcal infections from patients with true streptococcal infections. Quantitation of the number of colonies of group A streptococci on throat cultures may be helpful. Although a more strongly positive culture may suggest active infection, studies correlating the number of colonies with the antibody response have shown that quantitation is not a consistent indicator of the presence or absence of active streptococcal infection. Quantitation is more accurate when the sterile swab is directly planted on the agar plate than when desiccated swabs or transport media are used. Recent studies have indicated that a significant proportion of children harboring group A streptococci present with high streptococcal antibody titers at the onset of their acute pharyngitis, suggesting that the streptococci isolated on culture may only reflect that the patient is a carrier of residual streptococci.[89, 92] The existence of such patients may account, in part, for the low attack rates reported in civilian studies.[153]

Studies among children suggest that the risk of rheumatic fever may be small among patients harboring group A streptococci who exhibit nonexudative pharyngitis.[153] Therefore, patients should be carefully examined for pharyngeal exudate, which may not appear until the second day of illness.

Effective therapy depends upon eradication of the infecting organism, which is only achieved with regularity by prolonged penicillin therapy. Ten days of oral treatment are required. Many patients fail to take oral antibiotics after the acute symptoms of streptococcal infection subside. In such patients the organisms which have been suppressed by antibiotic therapy may reappear, usually without recurrent symptoms, and the patient is just as much at risk to rheumatic fever as if no antibiotic treatment had been given. A single injection of benzathine penicillin G (600,000 units in children under 60 pounds, 1,200,000 units in children over 60 pounds and in adults) is the treatment of choice.[141] Among the oral drugs, penicillin G (200,000 or 250,000 units three or four times daily for 10 days) is the antibiotic of choice, but erythromycin (250 mg four times a day for older children and adults, 40 mg/kg/day in younger children) may be used in patients sensitive to penicillin.[141] Rare strains of group A streptococci resistant to erythromycin have been recovered.[148] Since over 25% of strains of group A streptococci are resistant to tetracyclines, treatment with these antibiotics is unacceptable. Treatment of acute streptococcal infections with sulfadiazine does not reduce the attack rate of acute rheumatic fever.[125] Therefore, the sulfonamides, although effective as continuous prophylaxis, should not be used for treatment of acute infection.

Treatment failures (failure to eradicate the group A streptococcus from the upper respiratory tract) occur not infrequently among individuals adequately treated with antibiotics. Under most circumstances, it probably happens more often in patients treated orally than in those treated by intramuscular injection of benzathine penicillin G. There is some evidence that penicillinase-producing staphylococci may interfere with effective penicillin therapy by the oral route,[15] but their presence does not appear to explain failures which occur with parenteral therapy.[133] Some apparent treatment failures are due to persistance of non-group A carrier streptococci which may have been temporarily overgrown by the infecting group A organism. Others are due to reinfection with a new type or even with the same type (since type-specific antibody formation is suppressed by penicillin therapy). Recent studies suggest that most treatment failure episodes occur in streptococcal carriers and not in patients with bona fide infection.[89] Individuals who have harbored the same strains of streptococci for longer than 1 month are not likely to develop complications or to spread infection.[182] For this reason, a follow-up throat culture (taken 4 or 5 days after discontinuing oral therapy or 3 weeks after an injection of benzathine penicillin G) is not usually required in asymptomatic individuals, unless special epidemiologic circumstances (e.g., outbreak of scarlet fever, rheumatic fever, acute nephritis) are present or unless there is a known rheumatic fever-susceptible person in close contact with the patient. If group A streptococci are still present, a second course of penicillin should be given using intramuscular benzathine penicillin G. Alternative antimicrobial agents (e.g., erythromycin, β-lactamase-resistant penicillins, cephalosporins) may be tried, but at present there is no clear evidence of their superiority. Under the usual circumstances, multiple courses of antibiotics in an attempt to eradicate the carrier state are not warranted.

Studies of household contacts of index cases of streptococcal infection have shown that 25% or more may harbor streptococci.[21, 42] In families where there is a known rheumatic or in outbreaks of streptococcal infection, clinical studies and throat cultures may be indicated in other members of the family, followed by treatment of those with clinical evidence of infection or large numbers of beta-hemolytic streptococci on throat culture. Carriage of group A streptococci is common in school age children and may range from 5 to 50%.[134]

Mass antibiotic prophylaxis is effective in populations when streptococcal pharyngeal infections are epidemic.[29] This is rarely necessary in civilian populations[117, 203] but may occasionally be indicated if proved streptococcal respiratory infections are occurring at epidemic levels and especially if several cases of acute rheumatic fever have appeared within a few weeks.

Other approaches to prevention have been advocated but have either been abandoned or have not been developed sufficiently to be useful. Tonsillectomy was at one time almost a routine procedure in rheumatic subjects. Although there is some evidence that tonsillectomy may reduce the frequency of clinically apparent streptococcal infection[42] and large tonsils are associated with increased frequency of recurrences in rheumatics with poor prophylaxis compliance,[512] there is no evidence that tonsillectomy reduces the attack rate of rheumatic fever.[28] Indeed, this procedure may make clinical recognition of streptococcal infection more difficult since suppurative complications which may bring the patient to the attention of a physician are rare, and exudate is less frequent and more difficult to visualize in tonsillectomized patients.

The clinical and epidemiological efficacy of streptococcal vaccines has not been conclusively demonstrated. Recent studies have suggested that it may be possible to induce antibodies with small doses of purified M protein.[58] However, immunity to streptococcal infection is type-specific, and an effective vaccine would have to immunize against at least the majority of prevalent serotypes.[160, 187] Since it is apparent that antibiotics have not been successful in eradicating the rheumatic fever problem, interest continues in clinical and laboratory investigation of streptococcal vaccines. Recent advances in purifying M proteins and in defining their molecular structure have provided encouraging data which may ultimately make the approach to a group A streptococcal vaccine more feasible.[13, 113] Until a vaccine is available or more becomes known about the pathogenetic mechanisms responsible for rheumatic fever, control of rheumatic fever depends largely upon control of streptococcal infections by antimicrobial agents.

REFERENCES

1. Abdin, Z. H.: Rheumatic fever and rheumatic heart disease in Egyptian children. Gaz. Egypt. Paediatr. Assoc. 8:282, 1960.
2. Acheson, R. M.: The epidemiology of acute rheumatic fever. J. Chronic Dis. 18:723, 1965.
3. Agarwal, B. L.: Rheumatic heart disease unabated in developing countries. Lancet ii:910, 1981.
4. Albam, B., Epstein, J. A., Feinstein, A. R., Gavrin, J. B., Jonas, S., Kleinberg, E., Simpson, R., Spagnuolo, M., Stollerman, G. H., Taranta, A., Tursky, E., and Wood, H. F.: Rheumatic fever in children and adolescents: A long-term epidemiologic study of subsequent prophylaxis, streptococcal infections, and clinical sequelae. Ann. Intern. Med. 60 (Suppl. 5): no. 2, part II, 1964.
5. Alexander, W. D., and Smith, G.: Disadvantageous circulatory effects of salicylate in rheumatic fever. Lancet 1:768, 1962.
6. Amos, B., and Plate, J. M.: Lymphocyte stimulation by a glycopeptide isolated from S. pyogenes C203S. I. Isolation and partial purification. Cell. Immunol. 1:476, 1971.
7. Aron, A. M., Freeman, J. M., and Carter, S.: The natural history of Sydenham's chorea. Am. J. Med. 38:83, 1965.
8. Ayoub, E. M.: Cross-reacting antibodies in the pathogenesis of rheumatic myocardial

and valvular disease. In Streptococci and Streptococcal Diseases, edited by L. W. Wannamaker and J. M. Matsen. Academic Press, New York, 1972, p. 451.
9. Ayoub, E. M.: Use of sulfonamides for rheumatic fever prophylaxis during pregnancy. Circulation 46:1, 1972.
10. Ayoub, E. M., and McCarty, M.: Intraphagocytic beta-N-acetylglucosaminidase: Properties of the enzyme and its activity on group A streptococci carbohydrate in comparison with a soil bacillus enzyme. J. Exp. Med. 127:833, 1968.
11. Ayoub, E. M., and Wannamaker, L. W.: Evaluation of the streptococcal desoxyribonuclease B and diphosphopyridine nucleotidase antibody tests in acute rheumatic fever and acute glomerulonephritis. Pediatrics 29:527, 1962.
12. Ayoub, E. M., and Wannamaker, L. W.: Streptococcal antibody titers in Sydenham's chorea. Pediatrics 38:946, 1966.
13. Beachey, E. H., Seyer, J. M., Dale, J. B., Simpson, W. A., and Kang, A. H.: Type-specific protective immunity evoked by synthetic peptide of Streptococcus pyogenes M protein. Nature 292:457, 1981.
14. Bernhard, G. C., and Stollerman, G. H.: Serum inhibition of streptococcal diphospho-

pyridine nucleotidase in uncomplicated streptococcal pharyngitis and in rheumatic fever. J. Clin. Invest. 38:1942, 1959.
15. Bernstein, S. H., Stillerman, M., and Allerhand, J.: Demonstration of penicillin inhibition by pharyngeal microflora in patients treated for streptococcal pharyngitis. J. Lab. Clin. Med. 63:14, 1964.
16. Bisno, A. L.: The concept of rheumatogenic and nonrheumatogenic group A streptococci. In Streptococcal Diseases and the Immune Response, edited by S. E. Read and J. B. Zabriskie. Academic Press, New York, 1980, p. 789.
17. Bisno, A. L., Nelson, K. E., Waytz, P., and Brunt, J.: Factors influencing serum antibody responses in streptococcal pyoderma. J. Lab. Clin. Med. 81:410, 1973.
18. Bisno, A. L., and Ofek, I.: Serologic diagnosis of streptococcal infection. Am. J. Dis. Child. 127:676, 1974.
19. Bland, E. F.: The declining severity of rheumatic fever: A comparative study of the past four decades. Trans. Am. Clin. Climatol. Assoc. 71:136, 1959.
20. Bland, E. F., and Jones, T. D.: Rheumatic fever and rheumatic heart disease: A twenty year report on 1000 patients followed since childhood. Circulation 4:836, 1951.

21. Breese, B. B., and Disney, F. A.: Factors influencing the spread of beta-hemolytic streptococcal infections within the family group. Pediatrics 17:834, 1956.

22. Brownell, K. D., and Stix, R. K.: A public health program for children with heart disease or rheumatic fever. Am. J. Public Health 53:1587, 1963.

23. Burch, G. E., Giles, T. D., and Colcolough, H. L.: Pathogenesis of "rheumatic" heart disease: Critique and theory. Am. Heart J. 80:556, 1970.

24. Bywaters, E. G. L., and Thomas, G. T.: Bed rest, salicylates and steroid in rheumatic fever. Br. Med. J. 1:1628, 1961.

25. Campbell, M.: Calcific aortic stenosis and congenital biscuspid aortic valves. Br. Heart J. 30:606, 1968.

26. Catanzaro, F. J., Rammelkamp, C. H., Jr., and Chamovitz, R.: Prevention of rheumatic fever by treatment of streptococcal infections. II. Factors responsible for failures. N. Engl. J. Med. 259:51, 1958.

27. Catanzaro, F. J., Stetson, C. A., Morris, A. J., Chamovitz, R., Rammelkamp, C. H., Jr., Stolzer, B. L., and Perry, W. D.: The role of the streptococcus in the pathogenesis of rheumatic fever. Am. J. Med.. 17:749, 1954.

28. Chamovitz, R., Rammelkamp, C. H., Jr., Wannamaker, L. W., and Denny, F. W., Jr.: The effect of tonsillectomy on the incidence of streptococcal respiratory disease and its complications. Pediatrics 26:355, 1960.

29. Chancey, R. L., Morris, A. J., Conner, R. H., Catanzaro, F. J., Chamovitz, R., and Rammelkamp, C. H., Jr.: Studies of streptococcal prophylaxis. Comparison of oral penicillin and benzathine penicillin. Am. J. Med. Sci. 229:165, 1955.

30. Cherry, W. B., and Moody, M. D.: Fluorescent antibody techniques in diagnostic bacteriology. Bacteriol. Rev. 29:222, 1965.

31. Collins, S. D.: The incidence of rheumatic fever as recorded in general morbidity surveys of families. Public Health Rep. Suppl. 198, 1947.

32. Combined Rheumatic Fever Study Group: A comparison of the effect of prednisone and acetylsalicylic acid on the incidence of residual rheumatic heart disease. N. Engl. J. Med. 262:895, 1960.

33. Combined Rheumatic Fever Study Group: A comparison of short-term, intensive prednisone and acetylsalicylic acid therapy in the treatment of acute rheumatic fever. N. Engl. J. Med. 272:63, 1965.

34. Committee to Revise the Jones Criteria: American Heart Association. Jones criteria (revised) for guidance in the diagnosis of rheumatic fever. Circulation 32:664, 1965.

35. The Committee on Rheumatic Fever and the Committee on Congenital Cardiac Defects. American Heart Association. Report: Prevention of bacterial endocarditis. Circulation 46:3, 1972.

36. Crowe, C. C., Sanders, W. E., Jr., and Longley, S.: Bacterial interference. II. Role of normal throat flora in prevention of colonization by group A streptococcus. J. Infect. Dis. 128:527, 1973.

37. Cunningham, M. W., and Beachey, E. H.: Peptic digestion of streptococcal M protein. I. Effect of digestion at suboptimal pH upon the biological and immunochemical properties of purified M protein extracts. Infect. Immun. 9:244, 1974.

38. Dajani, A. S.: Rapid identification of beta hemolytic streptococci by counterimmunoelectrophoresis. J. Immunol. 110:1702, 1973.

39. Denny, F. W., Jr., and Thomas, L.: Persistence of group A streptococci in tissues of rabbits after infection. Proc. Soc. Exp. Biol. Med. 88:260, 1955.

40. Dillon, H. C., and Reeves, M. S. A.: Streptococcal immune responses in nephritis after skin infection. Am. J. Med. 56:333, 1974.

41. Dillon, H. C., Jr., and Wannamaker, L. W.: Physical and immunological differences among streptokinases. J. Exp. Med. 121:351, 1965.

42. Dingle, J. H., Badger, G. F., and Jordan, W. S., Jr.: Illness in the Home. A Study of 25,000 Illnesses in a Group of Cleveland Families. The Press of Western Reserve University, Cleveland, 1964.

43. DiSciasco, G., and Taranta, A.: Rheumatic fever in children: A review. Am. Heart J. 99:635, 1980.

44. Dorfman, A., Gross, J. I., and Lorincz, A. E.: The treatment of acute rheumatic fever. Pediatrics 27:692, 1961.

45. Dublin, T. D., Bernanke, A. D., Pitt, E. L., Massell, B. F., Allen, F. H., and Amezcula, F.: Red blood cell groups and ABH secretor system as genetic indicators of susceptibility to rheumatic fever and rheumatic heart disease. Br. Med. J. 2:775, 1964.

46. Dudding, B. A., and Ayoub, E. M.: Persistence of streptococcal group A antibody in patients with rheumatic valvular disease. J. Exp. Med. 128:1081, 1968.

47. Editorial: Treatment of rheumatic fever. N. Engl. J. Med. 272:101, 1965.

48. El Khatib, M. R., Chasen, J. L., Ho, K. L., Silberberg, B., and Lerner, A. M.: Coxsackie B4 myocarditis in mice: Valvular changes in virus-injected and control animals. J. Infect. Dis. 137:410, 1978.

49. Falk, J., A., Fleischman, J. L., Zabriskie, J. B., and Falk, R. E.: A study of HL-A antigen phenotype in rheumatic fever and rheumatic heart disease patients. Tissue Antigens 3:173, 1973.

50. Feinstein, A. R.: Standards, stethoscopes, steroids and statistics. The problem of evaluating treatment in acute rheumatic fever. Pediatrics 27:819, 1961.

51. Feinstein, A. R., and Arevalo, A. C.: Manifestations and treatment of congestive heart failure in young patients with rheumatic heart disease. Pediatrics 33:661, 1964.

51a. Feinstein, A. R., and Levitt, B. A.: The role of tonsils in predisposing to streptococcal infections and recurrences of rheumatic fever. N. Engl. J. Med. 282:285, 1970.

52. Feinstein, A. R., and Spagnuolo, M.: Mimetic features of rheumatic fever recurrences. N. Engl. J. Med. 262:533, 1960.

53. Feinstein, A. R., and Spagnuolo, M.: Experimental reactivation of subsiding rheumatic fever. J. Clin. Invest. 40:1891, 1961.

54. Feinstein, A. R., and Spagnuolo, M.: The clinical pattern of acute rheumatic fever: A reappraisal. Medicine (Baltimore) 41:279, 1962.

55. Feinstein, A. R., Wood, H. F., Spagnuolo, M., Taranta, A., Tursky, E., and Kleinberg, E.: Oral prophylaxis of recurrent rheumatic fever: Sulfadiazine vs. a double daily dose of penicillin. J. Am. Med. Assoc. 188:489, 1964.

56. Fisher, M., Kaplan, E. L., and Wannamaker, L. W.: Cholesterol inhibition of streptolysin O toxicity for myocardial cells in tissue culture. Proc. Soc. Exp. Biol. Med. 168:233, 1981.

57. Fleming, D. S., Hirschboeck, F. J., and Cosgriff, J. A.: Minnesota rheumatic fever survey. 1955. Minn. Med. 39:208, 1956.

58. Fox, E. N., Waldman, R. H., Wittner, M. K., Mauceri, A. A., and Dorfman, A.: Protective study with a group A streptococcal M protein vaccine. J. Clin Invest. 52:1885, 1973.

59. Glynn, L. E., and Holborow, E. J.: Relation between blood groups, secretor status and susceptibility to rheumatic fever. Arthritis Rheum. 4:203, 1961.

60. Goldring, D., Behrer, M. R., Brown, G., and Elliot, G.: Rheumatic pneumonitis. II. Report on the clinical and laboratory findings in twenty-three patients. J. Pediatr. 53:547, 1958.

61. Goldstein, I., Halpern, B., and Robert, L.: Immunological relationship between streptococcus A polysaccharide and the structural glycoproteins of heart valve. Nature 213:44, 1967.

62. Good, R. A., Vernier, R. L., and Smith, R. T.: Serious untoward reactions to therapy with cortisone adrenocorticotropin in pediatric practice (part I). Pediatrics 19:95, 1957.

63. Gordis, L.: Effectiveness of comprehensive-care programs in preventing rheumatic fever. N. Engl. J. Med. 289:331, 1973.

64. Gordis, L., Lilienfeld, A., and Rodriquez, R.: Studies in the epidemiology and preventability of rheumatic fever. I. Demographic factors and the incidence of acute attacks. J. Chronic Dis. 21:645, 1969.

65. Gray, E. D., Wannamaker, L. W., Ayoub, E. M., El Kholy, A., and Abdin, Z. H.: Cellular immune response to extracellular products in rheumatic heart disease. J. Clin. Invest. 68:665, 1981.

66. Guthe, T., Isdöe, O., and Willcox, R. R.: Untoward penicillin reactions. Bull. WHO 19:427, 1958.

67. Haim, S., Benderly, A., Shafrir, A., and Levy, J.: Alternate-day corticosteroid regimen. Dermatologica 142:171, 1971.

68. Halbert, S. P., Bircher, R., and Dahle, E.: The analysis of streptococcal infections. V. Cardiotoxicity of streptolysin O for rabbits in vivo. J. Exp. Med. 113:759, 1961.

69. Hamburger, M., Jr., Green, M. J., and Hamburger, V. G.: The problem of the "dangerous carrier" of hemolytic streptococci. II. Spread of infection by individuals with strongly positive nose cultures who expelled large numbers of hemolytic streptococci. J. Infect. Dis. 77:96, 1945.

70. Harris, T. N., Friedman, S., Hallidie-Smith, K. A., Coriell, L. L., and Fabrizio, D.: Occurrence of penicillin-resistant staphylococci in patients receiving penicillin orally for prophylaxis of recurrences of rheumatic fever. Am. J. Med. 32:545, 1962.

71. Haverkorn, M. J. (ed.): Streptococcal Disease and the Community. American Elsevier Publishing Company. New York, 1974.

72. Hill, H. R., Zimmerman, R. A., Reid, G. K., Wilson, E., and Kilton, R. M.: A food-borne epidemic of streptococcal pharyngitis at the United Air Force Academy. N. Engl. J. Med. 280:917, 1969.

73. Hirsch, J. G., and Church, A. B.: Studies of phagocytosis of group A streptococci by polymorphonuclear leukocytes in vitro. J. Exp. Med. 111:309, 1960.

74. Hirsch, J. G., and Flett, D. M.: Acute rheumatic fever in the young adult white male. Am. J. Med. Sci. 221:599, 1951.

75. Hryniewicz, W., Gray, E. D., Tagg, J. R., Wannamaker, L. W., Kanclerski, K., and Laible, N.: Streptolysin S: Purification and properties. Zbl. Bakt. Hyg., I. Abt. Orig. A., 242:327, 1978.

76. Husby, G., van de Rijn, I., Zabriskie, J. B., Abdin, Z. H., and Williams, R. C.: Antibodies reacting with cytoplasm of subthalamic and caudate nuclei neurons in chorea and acute rheumatic fever. J. Exp. Med. 144:1094, 1976.

77. Hutchins, G. N., and Payne, K. T.: Possible origin of myocardial Aschoff bodies of rheumatic heart fever from nerves. Johns Hopkins Med. J. 132:315, 1973.

78. Illingworth, R. S., Lorber, J., Holt, K. S., Rendle-Short, J., Jowett, G. H., and Gibson, W. M.: Acute rheumatic fever in children. A comparison of six forms of treatment in 200 cases. Lancet 2:653, 1957.

79. James, L., and McFarland, R. B.: An epidemic of pharyngitis due to a nonhemolytic group A streptococcus at Lowry Air Force

Base. N. Engl. J. Med. 284:750, 1971.

80. Johnson, E. E., Stollerman, G. H., and Grossman, B. J.: Rheumatic recurrences in patients not receiving continuous prophylaxis. J. Am. Med. Assoc. 190:407, 1964.

81. Jones, T. D.: The diagnosis of rheumatic fever. J. Am. Med. Assoc. 126:481, 1944.

82. Jones, T. D., and Bland, E. F.: The natural history of rheumatic fever. In Rheumatic Fever, edited by L. Thomas. University of Minnesota Press, Minneapolis, 1952.

83. Kantor, F. S.: Fibrinogen precipitation by streptococcal M protein. I. Renal lesions induced by intravenous injection of M protein into mice and rats. J. Exp. Med. 121:861, 1965.

84. Kaplan, E. L.: Epidemiology and pathogenesis of acute rheumatic fever. Minn. Med. 58:592, 1975.

85. Kaplan, E. L.: Observations on the clinical usefulness and theoretical implications of the immune response to streptococcal group A carbohydrate in man. In Streptococcal Diseases and the Immune Response, edited by S. E. Read and J. B. Zabriskie. Academic Press, New York, 1980

86. Kaplan, E. L.: Current status of rheumatic fever control programs in the United States. Public Health Rep. 96:267, 1981.

87. Kaplan, E. L., Anthony, B. F., Chapman, S. S., Ayoub, E. M., and Wannamaker, L. W.: The influence of the site of infection on the immune response to group A streptococci. J. Clin. Invest 49:1405, 1970.

88. Kaplan, E. L., Ferrieri, P., and Wannamaker, L. W.: Comparison of the antibody response to streptococcal cellular and extracellular antigens in acute pharyngitis. J. Pediatr. 84:21, 1974.

89. Kaplan, E. L., Gastanaduy, A. S., and Huwe, B. B.: The role of the carrier in treatment failures following antibiotic therapy for group A streptococci in the upper respiratory tract. J. Clin. Med. 98:326, 1981.

90. Kaplan, E. L., and Huwe, B. B.: The sensitivity and specificity of an agglutination test for antibodies to streptococcal extracellular antigens. J. Pediatr. 96:367, 1980.

91. Kaplan, E. L., and Kunde, C.: A quantitative evaluation of variation in composition of the streptozyme agglutination reagent for detection of antibodies to group A streptococcal extracellular antigens. J. Clin. Microbiol. 14:678, 1981.

92. Kaplan, E. L., Top, F. H., Dudding, B., and Wannamaker, L. W.: Diagnosis of streptococcal pharyngitis: Differentiation of active infection from the carrier state in the symptomatic child. J. Infect. Dis. 123:490, 1971.

93. Kaplan, E. L., and Wannamaker, L. W.: Suppression of the antistreptolysin O response by cholesterol and by lipid extracts of rabbit skin. J. Exp. Med. 144:754, 1976.

94. Kaplan, M. H.: The concept of autoantibodies in rheumatic fever and in the post commissurotomy state. Ann. N.Y. Acad. Sci. 86:974, 1960.

95. Kaplan, M. H., and Dallenbach, F. D.: Immunologic studies of heart tissue. III. Occurrence of bound gamma globulin in auricular appendages from rheumatic hearts. Relationship to certain histopathologic features of rheumatic heart disease. J. Exp. Med. 113:1, 1961.

96. Kaplan, M. H., and Frengley, J. D.: Autoimmunity to the heart in cardiac disease. Am. J. Cardiol. 24:459, 1969.

97. Kaplan, M. H., and Suchy, M. L.: Immunologic relation of streptococcal and tissue antigens. II. Cross-reaction of antisera to mammalian heart tissue with a cell wall constituent of certain strains of group A streptococci. J. Exp. Med. 119:643, 1964.

98. Kaplan, M. H., and Svec, K. H.: Immunologic relation of streptococcal and tissue antigens.

III. Presence in human sera of streptococcal antibody cross-reactive with heart tissue. Association with streptococcal infection, rheumatic fever, and glomerulonephritis. J. Exp. Med. 119:651, 1964.

99. Kellner, A., Bernheimer, A. W., Carlson, A. S., and Freeman, E. B.: Loss of myocardial contractility induced in isolated mammalian hearts by streptolysin O. J. Exp. Med. 104:361, 1956.

100. Klein, G. C., and Jones, W. L.: Comparison of the Streptozyme test with the antistreptolysin O, anti-deoxyribonuclease B, and anti-hyaluronidase tests. Appl. Microbiol. 21:257, 1971.

101. Krause, R. M.: Symposium on relationship of structure of microorganisms to their immunological properties. IV. Antigenic and biochemical composition of hemolytic streptococcal cell walls. Bacteriol. Rev. 27:369, 1963.

102. Krumwiede, E.: Penicillin resistance of nonhemolytic streptococci from rheumatic children receiving prophylactic penicillin. Pediatrics 4:634, 1949.

103. Kuttner, A. G., and Krumwiede, E.: Observations on the effect of streptococcal upper respiratory infection on rheumatic children: A three-year study. J. Clin. Invest. 20:273, 1941.

104. Kuttner, A. G., and Mayer, F. E.: Carditis during second attacks of rheumatic fever: Its incidence in patients without clinical evidence of cardiac involvement in their initial rheumatic episode. N. Engl. J. Med. 268:1259, 1963.

105. Lancefield, R. C.: Specific relationship of cell composition to biological activity of hemolytic streptococci. Harvey Lect. 36:251, 1940–1941.

106. Lancefield, R. C.: Current knowledge of type-specific M antigens of group A streptococci. J. Immunol. 89:307, 1962.

107. Lendrum, B. L., Simon, A. J., and Mack, I.: Relation of duration of bed rest in acute rheumatic fever to heart disease present 2 to 14 years later. Pediatrics 24:389, 1959.

108. Lim, W. N., and Wilson, M. G.: Comparison of the recurrence rate of rheumatic carditis among children receiving penicillin by mouth prophylactically or on indication. A six-year study. N Engl. J. Med. 262:321, 1960.

109. Limson, B. M., Chan, V. R., Guzman, S. U., Maaba, M. R., and Mendoza, M. T.: Occurrence of infection with group B coxsackie virus in rheumatic and non-rheumatic Filipino children. J. Infect. Dis. 140:415, 1979.

110. Lockman, L. A.: Movement disorders. In Practice of Pediatric Neurology, edited by K. Swaiman and F. Wright. C. V. Mosby, St. Louis, 1975.

111. Luisada, A. A. (ed.): Symposium on the epidemiology of heart disease. Am. J. Cardiol. 10:315, 1962.

112. McCarty, M.: Theories of pathogenesis of streptococcal complications. In Streptococci and Streptococcal Diseases, edited by L. W. Wannamaker and J. M. Matsen. Academic Press, New York, 1972, p. 517.

113. Manjula, B. N., and Fischetti, V. A.: Tropomyosin-like seven residue periodicity in three immunologically distinct streptococcal M proteins and its implications for antiphagocytic property of the molecule. J. Exp. Med. 151:695, 1980.

114. Marienfeld, C. J., Robins, M., Sandidge, R. P., and Findlan, C.: Rheumatic fever and rheumatic heart disease among U.S. college freshmen, 1956–1960. Public Health Rep. 79:789, 1964.

115. Markowitz, M.: Studies on type-specific streptococcal antibodies as indicators of previous streptococcal infections in rheumatic and nonrheumatic children. J. Clin. Invest. 42:409, 1963.

116. Markowitz, M., and Gordis, L.: A mail-in technique for detecting penicillin in urine: Application to the study of maintenance of prophylaxis in rheumatic fever patients. Pediatrics 41:151, 1968.

117. Markowitz, M., and Gordis, L.: Rheumatic Fever, 2nd ed. W. B. Saunders, Philadelphia, 1972.

118. Massell, B. F., Amezcua, F., and Pelargonio, S.: Evolving picture of rheumatic fever: Data from 40 years at the House of the Good Samaritan. J. Am. Med. Assoc. 188:287, 1964.

119. Massell, B. F., Jhaveri, S., and Czoniezer, G.: Therapy and other factors influencing the course of rheumatic heart disease. Circulation 20:737, 1959.

120. Mathy, W. E.: Rheumatic fever survey, 1958. Minn. Med. 42:930, 1959.

121. Maxted, W. R.: The use of bacitracin for identifying group A hemolytic streptococci. J. Clin. Pathol. 6:224, 1953.

122. Mayer, F. E., Doyle, E. F., Herrera, L., and Brownell, K. D.: Declining severity of first attack of rheumatic fever. Am. J. Dis. Child. 105:146, 1963.

123. Miller, R. A., Smith, J., Stamler, J., Hahneman, B., Paul, M. H., Abrams, I., Hait, G., Edelman, J., Willard, J., and Stevens, W.: The detection of heart disease in children. Results of a mass field trial with use of tape-recorded heart sounds. Circulation 25:85, 1962.

124. Miller, R. A., Stamler, J., Smith, J. M., Milne, W. S., Paul, M. H., Abrams, I., Hastreiter, A. R., Restivo, R. M., and deBoer, J.: The detection of heart disease in children. Results of mass trials with use of tape-recorded heart sounds. II. The Michigan City study. Circulation 32:956, 1965.

125. Morris, A. J., Chamovitz, R., Catanzaro, F. J., and Rammelkamp, C. H., Jr.: Prevention of rheumatic fever by treatment of previous streptococci infections: Effect of sulfadiazine. J. Am. Med. Assoc. 160:114, 1956.

126. Mortimer, E. A., Jr.: Production of L forms of group A streptococci in mice. Proc. Soc. Exp. Biol. Med. 119:159, 1965.

127. Murphy, G. E.: Nature of Rheumatic Heart Disease, with Special Reference to Myocardial Disease and Heart Failure. Williams & Wilkins, Baltimore, 1960.

128. Ofek, I., Beachey, E. H., Jefferson, W., and Campbell, G. L.: Cell membrane-binding properties of group A streptococcal lipoteichoic acid. J. Exp. Med. 141:990, 1975.

129. Osterud, H. T., McFadden, R. B., and Morton, W. E.: The frequency of rheumatic heart disease among freshmen at eight Oregon colleges in 1966. J. Am. Coll. Health Assoc. 19:293, 1971.

130. Padmavati, S.: Epidemiology of cardiovascular disease in India. I. Rheumatic heart disease. Circulation 25:703, 1962.

131. Perry, W. D., Siegel, A. C., Rammelkamp, C. H., Jr., Wannamaker, L. W., and Marple, E. C.: Transmission of group A streptococci. I. The role of contaminated bedding. Am. J. Hyg. 66:85, 1957.

132. Poskanzer, D. C., Feldman, H. A. Beadenkopf, W. G., Kuroda, K., Duslane, A., and Diamond, E. L.: Epidemiology of civilian streptococcal breakouts before and after penicillin prophylaxis. Am. J. Public. Health 46:1513, 1956.

133. Quie, P. G., Pierce, H. C., and Wannamaker, L. W.: Influence of penicillinase-producing staphylococci on the eradication of group A streptococci from the upper respiratory tract by penicillin treatment. Pediatrics 37:467, 1966.

134. Quinn, R. W., and Martin, M. P.: The natural occurrence of hemolytic streptococci in school children: A five-year study. Am. J. Hyg. 73:193, 1961.

135. Rammelkamp, C. H., Jr.: Epidemiology of streptococcal infections. Harvey Lect. 51:113, 1957.
136. Rammelkamp, C. H.,, Jr., Denny, F. W., Jr., and Wannamaker, L. W.: Studies on the epidemiology of rheumatic fever in the Armed Services. In Rheumatic Fever, edited by L. Thomas. University of Minnesota Press, Minneapolis, 1952.
137. Rammelkamp, C. H., Jr., and Stolzer, B. L.: The latent period before the onset of acute rheumatic fever. Yale J. Biol. Med. 34:386, 1961–1962.
138. Rantz, L. A., Maroney, M., and DeCaprio, J. M.: Infection and reinfection by hemolytic streptococci in early childhood. In Rheumatic Fever, edited by L. Thomas. University of Minnesota Press, Minneapolis, 1952.
139. Read, S. E., Fischetti, V. A., Utermohlen, V., Falk, R. E., and Zabriskie, J. B.: Cellular reactivity studies to streptococcal antigens. Migration inhibition studies in patients with streptococcal infections and rheumatic fever. J. Clin. Invest. 54:439, 1974.
140. Reed, W. P., Selinger, D. S., Albright, E. L., Abdin, Z. H., and Williams, R. C.: Streptococcal adherence to pharyngeal cells of children with rheumatic fever. J. Infect. Dis. 142:803, 1980.
141. Rheumatic Fever Committee of the Council on Cardiovascular Disease in the Young of the American Heart Association. Report: Prevention of rheumatic fever. Circulation 55:1, 1977.
142. Roberts, W. C.: Anatomically isolated aortic valvular disease. Am. J. Med. 49:151, 1970.
143. Roth, I. R., Lingg, C., and Whittemore, A.: Heart disease in children. A. Rheumatic group. I. Certain aspects of the age at onset and of recurrences in 488 cases of juvenile rheumatism ushered in by major clinical manifestations. Am. Heart J. 13:36, 1937.
144. Rotta, J., and Bednar, B.: Biological properties of cell wall mucopeptide of hemolytic streptococci. J. Exp. Med. 130:31, 1969.
145. Rudd, E.: Report of the meeting of the study group on Rheumatic Fever in the Americas. Santiago, Chile, October 1963.
146. RuDusky, B. M.: Heart murmurs in youths of military age. Evidence of inadequate rheumatic fever prophylaxis. J. Am. Med. Assoc. 185:96, 1963.
147. Sacks, B.: The pathology of rheumatic fever. A critical review. Am. Heart J. 1:750, 1926.
148. Sanders, E., Foster, M. T., and Scott, D.: Group A beta-hemolytic streptococci resistant to erythromycin and lincomycin. N. Engl. J. Med. 278:538, 1968.
149. Schwab, J. H., and Cromartie, W. J.: Immunological studies on a C polysaccharide complex of group A streptococci having a direct toxic effect on connective tissue. J. Exp. Med. 111:295, 1960.
150. Seldin, D. W., Kaplan, H. S., and Bunting, H.: Rheumatic pneumonia. Ann. Intern. Med. 26:496, 1947.
151. Shields, W. D., and Bray, P. F.: A danger of haloperidol therapy in children. J. Pediatr. 88:301, 1976.
152. Shulman, S. T., Ayoub, E. M., Victorica, B. C., Gessner, I. H., Tamer, D. F., and Hernandez, F. A.: Differences in antibody response to streptococcal antigens in children with rheumatic and non-rheumatic mitral valve disease. Circulation 50:1244, 1974.
153. Siegel, A. C., Johnson, E. E., and Stollerman, G. H.: Controlled studies of streptococcal pharyngitis in a pediatric population. I. Factors related to the attack rate of rheumatic fever. N. Engl. J. Med. 265:559, 1961.
154. Smith, J. M., Stamler, J., Miller, R. A., Paul, M. H., Abrams, I., Restivo, R. M., and deBoer, L.: The detection of heart disease in children: Results of mass field trials with use of tape recorded heart sounds. III. The Chicago area high school study. Circulation, 32:966, 1965.
155. Stahlman, M. T., and Denny, F. W., Jr.: The prophylaxis of streptococcal infection in patients with streptococcal infection. A comparison between sulfadiazine and erythromycin. Am. J. Dis. Child. 98:66, 1959.
156. Stetson, C. A., Jr.: The relation of antibody response to rheumatic fever. In Streptococcal Infections, edited by M. McCarty, Chap. 15. Columbia University Press, New York, 1954, p. 208.
157. Stollerman, G. H.: The use of antibiotics for the prevention of rheumatic fever. Am. J. Med. 17:757, 1954.
158. Stollerman, G. H.: Prognosis and treatment of acute rheumatic fever: The possible effect of treatment on subsequent heart disease. Prog. Cardiovasc. Dis. 3:193, 1960.
159. Stollerman, G. H.: The relative rheumatogenicity of strains of group A streptococci. Mod. Concepts Cardiovasc. Dis. 44:35, 1975.
160. Stollerman, G. H.: Rheumatic Fever and Streptococcal Infection. Grune & Stratton, New York, 1975.
161. Swanson, J., Konrad, H., and Gotschlich, E.: Electron microscopic studies on streptococci. I. M antigen. J. Exp. Med. 130:1063, 1969.
162. Taranta, A.: Relation of isolated recurrences of Sydenham's chorea to preceding streptococcal infections. N. Engl. J. Med.. 260:1204, 1959.
163. Taranta, A.: Occurrence of rheumatic-like subcutaneous nodules without evidence of joint or heart disease: Report of a case. N. Engl. J. Med. 266:19, 1962.
164. Taranta, A., Fiedler, J., Frank, C. W., Gilson, B. S., Gordis, L., Hufnagel, C., Markowitz, M., and Wannamaker, L. W.: Prevention of rheumatic fever and rheumatic heart disease. Report of Inter-Society Commission for Heart Disease Resources. Circulation 41:A-1, 1970.
165. Taranta, A., and Markowitz, M.: Rheumatic fever. A guide to its recognition, prevention and care. With special reference to developing countries. MTP Press, Lancaster, England, 1981.
166. Taranta, A., Metrakos, J., and Uchida, I.: Rheumatic fever in monozygotic and dizygotic twins. Circulation 20:778, 1959.
167. Taranta, A., Spagnuolo, M., and Feinstein, A. R.: "Chronic" rheumatic fever. Ann. Intern. Med. 56:367, 1962.
168. Thomas, L. (ed.): Rheumatic Fever. University of Minnesota Press, Minneapolis, 1952.
169. Thomas, L.: Experimental models for the pathogenesis of rheumatic heart disease. In Streptococci and Streptococcal Diseases, edited by L. W. Wannamaker and J. M. Matsen. Academic Press, New York, 1972, p. 465.
170. Thompkins, D. G., Boxerbaum, B., and Liebman, J.: Long-term prognosis of rheumatic fever patients receiving regular intramuscular benzathine penicillin. Circulation 45:543, 1972.
171. Thompson, A., Halbert, S. P., and Smith, U.: The toxicity of streptolysin O for beating mammalian heart cells in tissue culture. J. Exp. Med. 131:745, 1970.
172. Thomson, S., and Innes, J.: Haemolytic streptococci in the cardiac lesions of rheumatism. Br. Med. J. 2:733, 1940.
173. Tierney, R. C., and Kaplan, S.: Treatment of Sydenham's chorea. Am. J. Dis. Child. 109:408, 1965.
174. Trousseau, A.: Lectures on Clinical Medicine, Vol. 2. In The New Sydenham Society, edited by J. R. Cormack, Vol. 42, 3rd ed. Lecture XIX: Inflammatory sore throat. London, 1869, p. 460.
175. Uchida, I. A.: Possible genetic factors in the etiology of rheumatic fever. Am. J. Hum. Genet. 5:61, 1953.
176. United Kingdom and United States Joint Report. The treatment of acute rheumatic fever in children. A cooperative clinical trial of ACTH, cortisone and aspirin. Circulation 11:343, 1955.
177. United Kingdom and United States Joint Report: The evolution of rheumatic heart disease in children. Five-year report of a cooperative clinical trial of ACTH, cortisone and aspirin. Circulation 22:503, 1960.
178. United Kingdom and United States Joint Report: The natural history of rheumatic fever and rheumatic heart disease: Ten-year report of a cooperative clinical trial of ACTH, cortisone, and aspirin. Circulation 32:457, 1965.
179. Vaisman, S., Guasch, L., Vignau, A., Correa, E., Schuster, A., Mortimer, E. A., and Rammelkamp, C. H., Jr.: Failure of penicillin to alter acute rheumatic valvulitis. J. Am. Med Assoc. 194:116, 1965.
180. Von Glahn, W. C.: The pathology of rheumatism. Am. J. Med. 2:76, 1947.
181. Wagner, B. M.: Studies in rheumatic fever. III. Histochemical reactivity of the Aschoff body. Ann. N. Y. Acad. Sci. 86:992, 1960.
182. Wannamaker, L. W.: The epidemiology of streptococcal infections. In Streptococcal Infections, edited by M. McCarty. Columbia University Press, New York, 1954.
183. Wannamaker, L. W.: A method for culturing beta hemolytic streptococci from the throat. Circulation 32:1054, 1965.
184. Wannamaker, L. W.: Medical progress: Differences between streptococcal infections of the throat and of the skin. N. Engl. J. Med. 282:23, 78, 1970.
185. Wannamaker, L. W.: The chain that links the heart to the throat. (T. Duckett Jones Memorial Address) Circulation 48:9, 1973.
186. Wannamaker, L. W., and Ayoub, E. M.: Antibody titers in acute rheumatic fever. Circulation 21:598, 1960.
187. Wannamaker, L. W., and Matsen, J. M. (eds.): Streptococci and Streptococcal Diseases: Recognition, Understanding and Management. Academic Press, New York, 1972.
188. Wannamaker, L. W.: On the survival of streptococci and of rheumatic fever. Robert Koch Foundation Bulletin and Communications 3:23, 1981.
189. Wannamaker, L. W., Rammelkamp, C. H., Jr., Denny, F. W., Jr., Brink, W. R., Houser, H. B., Hahn, E. O., and Dingle, J. H.: Prophylaxis of acute rheumatic fever: By treatment of the preceding streptococcal infection with various amounts of depot penicillin. Am. J. Med. 10:673, 1951.
190. Watson, R. F., Hirst, G. K., and Lancefield, R. C.: Bacteriological studies of cardiac tissues obtained at autopsy from eleven patients dying with rheumatic fever. Arthritis Rheum. 4:74, 1961.
191. Wedum, B. G., and McGuire, J. W.: Origin of the Aschoff body. Ann. Rheum. Dis. 22:127, 1963.
192. Weissman, G., Keiser, H., and Bernheimer, A. W.: Studies on lysosomes. III. The effects of streptolysins O and S on the release of acid hydrolases from a granular fraction of rabbit liver. J. Exp. Med. 118:205, 1963.
193. White, P. D.: Changes in relative prevalence of various types of heart disease in New England: Contrast between 1925 and 1950. J. Am. Med. Assoc. 152:303, 1953.
194. Wilson, G. S., and Miles, A.: The streptococci. In Topley & Wilson's Principles of Bacteriology and Immunity. Williams & Wilkins, Baltimore, 1975, p. 712.
195. Wilson, M. G., Lim, W. N., and Birch, A. M.: The decline of rheumatic fever. Recurrence rates of rheumatic fever among 782 children for twenty-one consecutive calendar years

(1936–1956). J. Chronic Dis. 7:183, 1958.
196. Wilson, M. G., and Schweitzer, M.: Pattern of heredity susceptibility in rheumatic fever. Circulation 10:699, 1954.
197. Wood, H. F., and McCarty, M.: Laboratory aids in the diagnosis of rheumatic fever and in evaluation of disease activity. Am. J. Med. 17:768, 1954.
198. World Health Statistics Annual. World Health Organization, Geneva, 1971.
199. Zabriskie, J. B.: The role of temperate bac-teriophage in the production of erythrogenic toxin by group A streptococci. J. Exp. Med. 119:761, 1964.
200. Zabriskie, J. B., and Freimer, E. H.: An immunological relationship between the group A streptococcus and mammalian muscle. J. Exp. Med. 124:661, 1966.
201. Zabriskie, J., Hsu, K. C., and Seegal, B. C.: Heart-reactive antibody associated with rheumatic fever: Characterization and diag-nostic significance. Clin. Exp. Immunol. 7:147, 1970.
202. Zimmerman, H. J.: Effects of aspirin and acetaminophen on the liver. Arch. Intern. Med. 141:333, 1981.
203. Zimmerman, R. A., Siegel, A. C., and Steele, C. P.: An epidemiological investigation of a streptococcal and rheumatic fever epidemic in Dickinson, North Dakota. Pediatrics 30:712, 1962.

35

Chronic Rheumatic Heart Disease

Samuel Kaplan, M.D.

The clinical features of rheumatic fever and subsequent chronic rheumatic heart disease have great geographic variation, with a high frequency in certain parts of the world, including Africa, Asia, and in economically underprivileged areas in the western world. In these areas the course of the disease can be malignant and accelerated so that well-established mitral valve disease occurs in childhood,[18] and many of these patients succumb before the age of 20 years. However, in North America, the frequency and virulence of rheumatic fever has been decreasing, especially during the last 30 years.[27] Rheumatic heart disease has a greater frequency in patients who had severe cardiac involvement during their attack or recurrence of acute rheumatic fever,[27] and rheumatic valvular disease occurs in the following order of frequency: (a) mitral insufficiency (MI); (b) dominant mitral insufficiency with associated mitral stenosis (MS); (c) aortic insufficiency (AI) with mitral valve disease; (d) isolated aortic valve disease with dominant insufficiency and varying degrees of stenosis; (e) dominant MS with or without trivial MI; (f) tricuspid valve disease with insufficiency secondary to pulmonary hypertension due to left-sided valvular lesions; (g) tricuspid stenosis usually associated with mitral and aortic valve disease; and (h) pulmonary valve insufficiency secondary to pulmonary hypertension due to left-sided lesions. For practical purposes the pulmonary valve is not primarily affected. In all cases of chronic rheumatic heart disease in children and adolescents, the mitral valve is involved in 85%, the aortic valve in 54%, and the tricuspid and pulmonary valve in less than 5%.

Healing of rheumatic myocardial lesions results in varying degrees of interstitial fibrosis. However, subacute or chronic carditis may modify the course of the disease by intensifying myocardial dilatation which has resulted from the hemodynamic effects of valvular lesions. Acute rheumatic pericarditis may heal with a resultant normal pericardium. In some cases, fusion and thickening of the pericardium occur with the formation of adhesions, but these abnormalities seldom affect cardiac performance.

Rheumatic carditis may heal with few residua. These consist of minor degrees of fibrosis of the valvular endocardium, vascularization of the valve leaflets, some thickening of the chordae tendineae, and small myocardial perivascular scars. There is no evidence that these lesions are progressive or produce abnormal hemodynamic effects. However, these valves are susceptible to endocarditis. It is probable that episodes of subclinical carditis occur with resultant chronic rheumatic heart disease. Evidence to support this view is the fact that many adults with rheumatic heart disease deny an earlier acute episode. The frequency of subclinical attacks is difficult to evaluate.

MITRAL INSUFFICIENCY

PATHOLOGY

Mitral insufficiency (MI) is the commonest lesion found in children and adolescents with chronic rheumatic heart disease. Associated organic mitral stenosis (MS) is difficult to exclude in the majority of instances. Healing of acute rheumatic valvulitis results in fibrosis of valve leaflets with contracture.[20, 21] This process is usually more obvious at one commissure. Also some valvular shortening may occur so that the leaflets cannot coapt. Further separation of the leaflets occurs with left atrial enlargement, initiating a vicious circle with an increase in the degree of MI.[25] In these patients, the chordae tendineae restrain the posterior leaflet, which is displaced posteriorly over the base of the left ventricular wall. In some adolescents, calcification of the commissures may be found.

The severity of the lesion is variable. In the majority, it is mild or moderate with minor variations of the abnormalities described above. However, in patients with extreme MI and some associated stenosis, there is disorganization of the valve mechanism, shortening of the valve cusps, chordae tendineae, and papillary muscles, and dilatation of the valve ring. Secondary MI may result from left ventricular enlargement due to aortic valve disease. This occurs because of the displacement of the papillary muscles and elongation of the chordae tendineae which accompanies left ventricular dilatation.

PHYSIOLOGY

During left ventricular systole, blood regurgitates into the left atrium (Fig. 35.1). Relatively mild MI can result in a significant regurgitant flow because of the large systolic pressure gradient between the left ventricle and left atrium. However, mild MI is usually well tolerated without hemo-

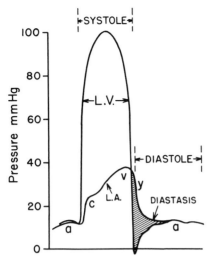

Fig. 35.1 Diagram of pressure changes in florid mitral insuffi- ciency. The left atrial (*L. A.*) pressure is increased due to a promi- nent regurgitant C-V wave. In some patients the C wave is not discernible and absence of X descent is usual. Opening of the mitral valve is followed by a rapid Y descent. The diastolic gradient (*shaded area*) is due to a high flow across the mitral valve, and the gradient can be high in the absence of major mitral stenosis. *L.V.*, left ventricle.

dynamic changes. In moderate or severe MI, the regurgitant flow increases the pressure and volume of the left atrium. The increased pressure is transmitted upstream to the pul- monary circulation, increasing the pulmonary venous and later pulmonary arterial pressures. Although the pulmonary vascular resistance is increased, it seldom reaches the high levels associated with tight mitral stenosis. Persistent pul- monary hypertension results in right ventricular hypertro- phy and dilatation with secondary tricuspid insufficiency and sometimes pulmonary valve insufficiency. In a small number of patients with florid MI, aneurysmal dilatation of the left atrium accommodates the regurgitant flow without increase in pressure.[6]

During diastole, the left ventricle is subjected to a high filling pressure, fills rapidly, and dilates to accommodate the blood which leaked during the previous systole in addition to the normal pulmonary venous return. This produces a flow murmur that can imitate MS even when the latter is absent. In chronic MI, there is an apparent increase in left ventricular diastolic compliance as the left ventricle en- larges.[35] The increase in end-diastolic volume brings the Frank-Starling mechanism into play which permits a large stroke output. The increase in end-diastolic fiber length is not reflected in an increase in end-diastolic pressure because of the increase in left ventricular compliance. Thus, a marked increase in pulmonary venous pressure is avoided. Patients with chronic MI may remain well for many years, and this has been attributed to systolic unloading of the left ventri- cle.[35] Since regurgitation occurs with the onset of systole, the isovolumic contraction period is absent, undue tension does not develop in the wall of the left ventricle, and the energy of contraction is expended in useful shortening.

MANIFESTATIONS

Clinical Features

The severity of the lesion determines the symptomatology. In many children and adolescents the lesion is mild, there are no symptoms, and the only abnormal sign is the murmur

of MI. In severe lesions, symptoms are dominated by fatigue, weakness, poor weight gain, pallor, palpitation, effort dysp- nea due to pulmonary congestion, and later by heart failure with or without pulmonary edema.

The jugular venous pulse is normal in the absence of heart failure. The peripheral pulse also is usually normal but may appear to be collapsing in type because of systolic leak into the left atrium. The precordium is normal to palpation in mild lesions; however, a heaving, hyperdynamic apical im- pulse is palpable in severe MI, owing to left ventricular hypertrophy and dilatation.

In patients with mild MI, the only abnormal physical sign may be the presence of an apical pansystolic murmur. How- ever, attention to auscultatory details gives important diag- nostic information in patients with moderate or severe MI.[34] The first heart sound is usually normal and seldom decreased in intensity because extensive disorganization of the valve with heavy calcification is rare in children. Similarly, the second heart sound is usually normal. However, wide expi- ratory splitting of the second sound may occur in florid MI (Fig. 35.2), possibly as a result of shortening of left ventric- ular systole.[33] Pulmonary valve closure is loud in the pres- ence of pulmonary hypertension. A low-pitched third heart sound is prominent and is produced by the large early diastolic filling of the ventricle.[32] The presence of this sound excludes the diagnosis of tight MS. The classical murmur is pansystolic, starts with the first sound, occupies all of systole, encroaches on aortic valve closure, has a maximal intensity at the apex, radiates to the left axilla and left sternal edge, and is unaffected by respiration. However, in some instances the murmur is short, occurring in early, mid-, or late systole. Late systolic murmurs, sometimes initiated by a click, may

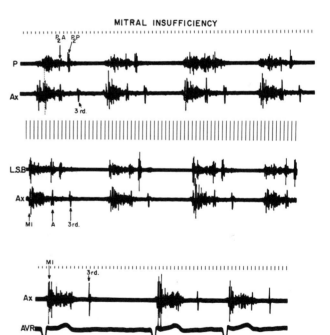

Fig. 35.2 Phonocardiograms in a child with chronic mitral in- sufficiency. The pansystolic murmur at the apex of the heart (*Ax*) is transmitted to the left sternal border (*L.S.B.*). In the second left intercostal space (*P*) the second heart sound is widely split (P_2A = aortic component and P_2P = pulmonic component of second heart sound). The prominent third heart sound (*3rd.*) is also shown. The rumbling middiastolic murmur which was present in this patient is not illustrated. *MI*, first heart sound; *AVR*, electrocardiogram; time lines = 0.04 second.

follow acute rheumatic fever (Fig. 35.3). These auscultatory findings are indistinguishable from the billowing mitral leaflet syndrome of unknown etiology.[2] In rare instances, florid MI is silent.[42] There is no correlation between the length and intensity of the systolic murmur and the severity of incompetence.

Acute changes in systemic resistance produced by drugs may be helpful in analysis of the typical and atypical systolic murmur of MI. Phenylephrine increases systemic resistance and augments the degree of MI, which results in an increase in the length and intensity of the systolic murmur. In contradistinction, inhalation of amyl nitrite decreases peripheral resistance and the degree of MI, so that the systolic murmur is shortened and softened.

Diastolic flow through the mitral valve is increased be-cause of the increment in volume added to left atrial blood during the previous systole. This increased flow results in a diastolic murmur which in severe MI is loud, rumbling, explosive, middiastole, and is shorter than the long rumbling murmur of MS.

Electrocardiographic Features

The electrocardiogram is normal if the lesion is mild. Even in the presence of moderate or marked MI, the electrocardiogram may be nondescript. The P waves may be notched and broad (Fig. 35.4). Atrial fibrillation occurs in patients with long-standing disease, especially with large left atria. Intermittent premature atrial or ventricular contractions may occur for many months and precede the establishment of atrial fibrillation. Voltage criteria compatible with left

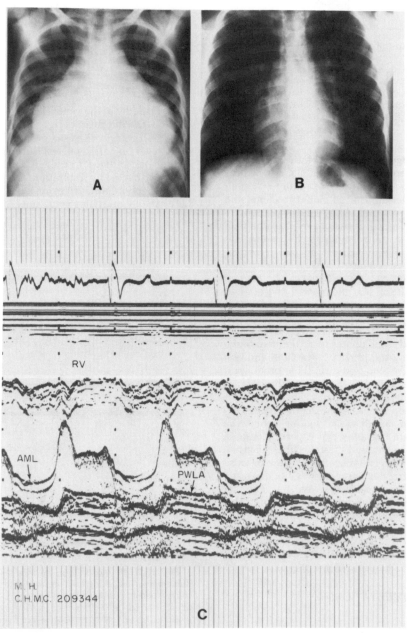

Fig. 35.3 Data from a 10-year-old with rheumatic heart disease. (A) During acute episode of classic rheumatic fever without pericardial effusion. At that time florid mitral insufficiency and heart failure were present. (B) Two years later the heart size was normal, and the only abnormal auscultatory finding was a late systolic murmur initiated by a click. At that time the echocardiogram in panel C was obtained and shows pansystolic mitral valve prolapse. RV, right ventricle; AML, anterior mitral leaflet; PWLA, posterior wall left atrium.

PRE·OPERATIVE

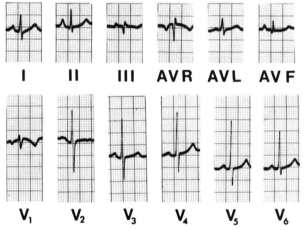

POST·OPERATIVE

Fig. 35.4 Pre- and postoperative electrocardiograms in a 12-year-old who required mitral valve replacement because of severe rheumatic MI. The preoperative tracing shows prominent notched P waves (left atrial enlargement) and tall R waves in V_5 and V_6 followed by inverted T waves. Note that V_3, V_5, and V_6 were taken at one-half sensitivity. The postoperative tracing is within normal limits.

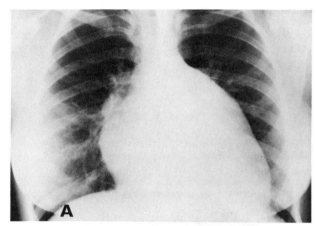

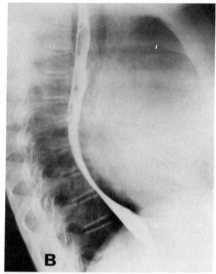

Fig. 35.5 Posteroanterior (A) and lateral (B) teleroentgenograms of a 13-year-old with chronic rheumatic mitral insufficiency and stenosis. She had maintained a normal sinus rhythm since her original episode of acute rheumatic fever at age 7 years. Note the generalized cardiomegaly and marked left atrial enlargement, as shown by the deviation of the barium-filled esophagus in the lateral projection.

ventricular hypertrophy are present in many patients with florid MI. ST segment and T wave changes may be due to left ventricular hypertrophy or digitalis therapy. Right ventricular hypertrophy is usually associated with pulmonary hypertension.

Radiologic Features

Roentgenographic examination is normal in patients with mild lesions. In well-developed MI, the left atrium is enlarged to varying degrees and is sometimes aneurysmal (Fig. 35.5). The silhouette of the left ventricle is usually prominent in moderate or severe lesions because of dilatation of this chamber. Prominence of the pulmonary artery, right ventricle, and right atrium occurs in association with heart failure or major pulmonary hypertension. Although signs of pulmonary venous hypertension may be present, these are not as obvious as in patients with MS. In the presence of left ventricular failure, septal lines may be prominent. Mitral valve calcification is not common in pure MI, but it occurs

with sufficient frequency in combined MI and MS to warrant a careful search for this sign using image intensification.

Echocardiographic Features

The echocardiogram[15] in pure moderate or severe MI shows a large left atrium and large left ventricle (Fig. 35.6). Mild MI usually does not result in chamber enlargement but may be detected by Doppler echocardiography (Fig. 35.6). This technique shows the regurgitant flow into the left atrium. Furthermore, the differentiation of mild MI from a small ventricular septal defect is facilitated by Doppler echocardiography which shows turbulence in the right ventricle across the ventricular defect. The EF slope of diastolic closure of the mitral valve is not specific for MI nor does its measurement indicate severity of the incompetence. This slope probably reflects the compliance of the left ventricle. Echocardiographic features of mitral valve prolapse may be found in chronic rheumatic heart disease (Fig. 35.3). In this situation the posterior and/or anterior mitral leaflets move posteriorly during systole after isovolumic contraction. This posterior movement may be pansystolic or discrete in late systole.

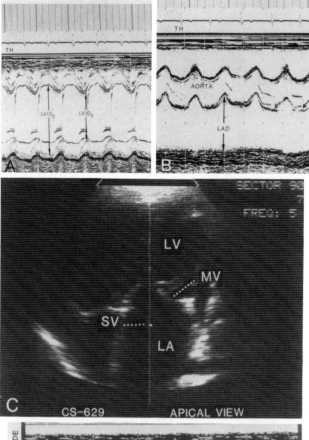

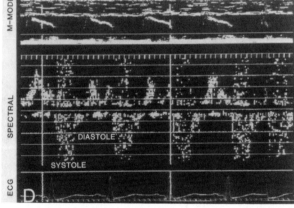

Fig. 35.6 (*A*) The left ventricular dimension in end diastole (*LVID*^d) is greatly enlarged (6.2 cm). The shortening fraction (LVID_d − LVID_s)/LVID_d × 100 = 31%, which suggests normal left ventricular function. *LVID*^s, left ventricular dimension in end systole. (*B*) The left atrial dimension (*LAD*) of 4.4 cm is much larger than normal. (*C*) Two dimensional apical view of patient with mitral insufficiency demonstrating location of the Doppler sample volume (*SV*). *LV*, left ventricle; *MV*, mitral valve; *LA*, left atrium. (*D*) Doppler signals from sample volume shown in *C*. Turbulent flow is seen during systole.

CARDIAC CATHETERIZATION

These studies are seldom indicated in children and adolescents. However, in a minority of patients rapid progression of the disease in the absence of clear-cut exacerbation of the rheumatic process warrants documentation of the hemodynamic effects of the lesion. The cardiac output remains relatively normal at rest in patients with moderate regurgitant flow but is frequently decreased in florid lesions.

The mean left atrial pressure is determined by the pressure and volume relationships in this chamber. Usually the pressure is increased, but in a minority an aneurysmally dilated left atrium can accommodate a large regurgitant flow without increase in pressure.[6] In patients with severe lesions, the left atrial pressure pulse curve shows a steep rise in early systole to the peak of the V wave (Fig. 35.1). This regurgitant wave is sometimes giant, with resultant ventricularization of the left atrial pressure curve.[45] As the mitral valve opens, a rapid Y descent is inscribed. A diastolic gradient across the mitral valve may be measurable even in the absence of significant MS and presumably is due to the large diastolic flow across the mitral valve.[31] At rest the left ventricular end-diastolic pressure may be normal. However, this rises during exercise or in the presence of left ventricular failure.

It is difficult to quantitate the degree of chronic MI from analysis of the left atrial pressure curve.[23, 30] Also Gorlin's formula for measurement of valve area is less accurate in presence of valvular incompetence. Presently used methods to quantitate MI include: comparison of angiographically derived left ventricular output with the forward output determined by the Fick method or by dye dilution[40, 41]; calculation of stroke volume of the right and left ventricles from cineangiocardiograms [the regurgitant volume is determined by subtracting right from left ventricular stroke volume[44]; the regurgitant fraction is the ratio of the regurgitant volume to total left ventricular stroke volume; these calculations can only be used in the absence of aortic or tricuspid valve insufficiency]; and the continuous infusion of xenon 133 in saline into the left ventricle.[29] After a constant concentration has been established and before recirculation has reached high values, left atrial and arterial blood are sampled.

Many clinicians rely on an estimation of the severity of MI by selective left ventricular angiocardiography.[19, 38] The degree of opacification of the left atrium from regurgitant contrast material gives a qualitative assessment of the severity (Fig. 35.7). However, this infrequently tells one more

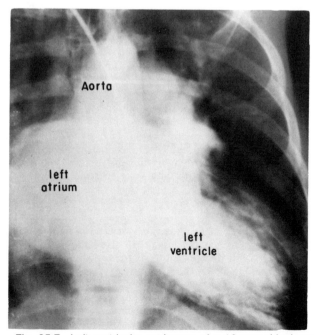

Fig. 35.7 Left ventricular angiogram of a 16-year-old whose mitral insufficiency was worsened markedly by an episode of endocarditis. Note that the left atrium is more densely opacified than the aorta, owing to massive regurgitation of contrast during left ventricular systole.

than the bedside estimation. It is usual to perform an aortogram in the course of left heart catheterization to exclude associated aortic valve disease.

COMPLICATIONS

Cardiac failure may occur from progressive MI arising from either recurrence of acute rheumatic fever or the relentless progression of subacute or subclinical rheumatic pancarditis. Intercurrent infection or the onset of atrial fibrillation with rapid ventricular response may herald the onset of heart failure. Although pulmonary congestion is common, episodes of frank pulmonary edema are not frequent. Right-sided heart failure may be accompanied by tricuspid or pulmonary insufficiency.

Lesions of the mitral valve which favor the onset of endocarditis usually consist of combined MI and MS with dominant MI. In these patients the bacterial infection may be cured, but further valve damage results. The progression of the degree of MI may be insidious after bacteriologic cure. However, in others there is a sudden and dramatic increase in severity of MI, owing to ruptured chordae tendineae or other parts of the valve complex. Endocarditis is rare in florid "pure" MI.

Infrequent atrial or ventricular premature contractions are well tolerated. First-degree heart block may develop during the recurrence of acute rheumatic fever, and may persist for many years after the initial episode, or it may be due to digitalis therapy. Atrial fibrillation is more common when MI is associated with MS and when the left atrium is large and hypertensive.[16]

MITRAL STENOSIS

Usually many years must elapse before narrowing of the mitral valve orifice reaches levels sufficient to produce symptoms. Therefore, isolated tight rheumatic mitral stenosis is not common in children and adolescents and is usually accompanied by MI. However, in some parts of the world, particularly Asia, Africa, and some western countries, severe rheumatic MS occurs in children under the age of 15 years, and frequently these patients deny a previous history of acute rheumatic fever.[18] In the normal adult the mitral valve orifice varies from 4 to 6 cm^2 (4 cm in the long axis). If this size is reduced to 2 to 2.5 cm^2, symptoms will occur on extreme effort, and with an orifice size of 1.5 to 2 cm^2, symptoms will occur with moderate exercise. With a valve orifice of about 1 cm^2 or less, mild exercise will cause symptoms. Therefore, major MS implies a mitral valve orifice of about 25% of the expected normal.

PATHOLOGY

Mitral stenosis results from fibrosis, commissural adhesions, and contracture of the valve leaflets and chordae tendineae. When viewed from the left atrium, the valve orifice has been described as "buttonhole" or "fishmouth." The whole valve mechanism becomes funnel-shaped, with the apex in the left ventricular cavity. Obstruction to left atrial flow results in hypertrophy and dilatation of the left atrium and right heart chambers. Continued and progressive pulmonary venous hypertension results in congestion, edema, and fibrosis of the alveolar walls, intimal fibrosis with medial hypertrophy of the pulmonary arterioles, and progressive loss of lung compliance.

PHYSIOLOGY

Minimal MS is well tolerated without measurable hemodynamic effects. However, critical obstruction at the mitral valve orifice (less than 25% of the expected normal) results in severe left atrial and pulmonary venous hypertension. The pulmonary artery pressure rises to maintain pulmonary flow. In patients with complicating pulmonary vascular disease, pulmonary hypertension may be extreme and in fact exceed systemic arterial pressure. Pulmonary arteriolar constriction produced by a combination of vasospasm and pulmonary arteriolar disease results in a raised pulmonary vascular resistance. Continued and progressive pulmonary arterial hypertension results in right ventricular failure.

In critical MS, pulmonary venous pressure during exercise may exceed the oncotic pressure of plasma (30 mm Hg). In this situation, protective mechanisms come into play to prevent an overwhelming increase in pulmonary venous pressure and the development of pulmonary edema. These protective mechanisms include: a high pulmonary vascular resistance; the development of a physical barrier at the capillary-alveolar interface from thickening of the capillary walls, interstitial tissue, and alveolar membrane; and some decompression of the pulmonary veins into the bronchial veins.

The pulmonary pressure-flow relationships vary in patients with MS. In some, pulmonary vascular disease is not extreme, so that the pulmonary circulation is maintained with only moderate elevation of pulmonary artery pressure. However, in patients who develop pulmonary vascular disease, the lesser circulation meets two areas of obstruction, the pulmonary arteriolar bed and the stenosed mitral valve. In these patients pulmonary hypertension is extreme.

During exercise, patients with mild or moderate MS raise the pressures in the left atrium and pulmonary circulation to maintain a normal cardiac output. However, in critical stenosis, the cardiac output is decreased at rest, and in this situation the heart is unable to increase forward flow by increasing left atrial pressure because of the rapid development of pulmonary edema. During exercise, the cardiac output may fall when severe pulmonary vascular disease is present.

MANIFESTATIONS

Clinical Features

Generally, symptoms correlate well with the severity of the obstruction.[22] Patients with minimal MS are asymptomatic. With more severe degrees of obstruction, effort intolerance is associated with dyspnea. Orthopnea and paroxysmal nocturnal dyspnea with or without attacks of pulmonary edema occur with critical MS. These symptoms occur with progressive degrees of stenosis and rheumatic myocarditis or are triggered by respiratory infections, or uncontrolled tachycardia, or atrial fibrillation.

Cardiac failure is usually associated with severe degrees of mitral obstruction and moderate to severe pulmonary hypertension. This complication may also be precipitated by intercurrent infections, reactivation of active carditis or uncontrolled tachycardia, or atrial fibrillation. The discomfort of hepatic engorgement may be an early clue to the diagnosis. Functional tricuspid insufficiency secondary to right ventricular dilatation will enhance hepatomegaly, hepatic angina, and the development of peripheral edema and ascites. Pulmonary valve insufficiency may complicate marked pulmonary artery dilatation secondary to pulmonary hypertension.

Hemoptysis may occur and is due to various causes. Blood-streaked sputum occurs during paroxysmal dyspnea or pulmonary edema. Sudden brisk and sometimes profuse hemoptysis has been attributed to rupture of a bronchial or pleurohilar vein. This frightening symptom is seldom fatal and usually lasts for less than 1 hour, although blood streaking of the sputum may occur for a few days. Hemoptysis usually does not occur in patients with marked elevation of pulmonary vascular resistance. Pulmonary infarctions due to emboli are not as common as in adults.

Endocarditis is uncommon in isolated tight MS and has a predilection for valves that have dominant insufficiency with associated stenosis. Systemic embolization secondary to left atrial thrombosis is uncommon in children even with atrial fibrillation. Hoarseness due to paralysis of the left vocal cord (Ortner's syndrome) and angina pectoris are also seldom seen in children.

Peripheral cyanosis and a malar flush are associated with severe MS with a low cardiac output and frequently a high pulmonary vascular resistance. The pulse volume is small. The jugular venous pressure is increased in the presence of heart failure, severe pulmonary hypertension, or associated tricuspid valve disease. The heart size varies according to the degree of mitral valve obstruction and is normal in patients with minimal disease. In others, significant degrees of obstruction can occur with only moderate cardiomegaly, especially in the presence of sinus rhythm. However, marked cardiac enlargement is usual in the presence of cardiac failure and atrial fibrillation. The apical impulse is either impalpable or brief and tapping in nature. An easily palpable thrusting apical impulse is usually associated with significant MI. A right parasternal lift is palpable if the pulmonary vascular resistance is high.

The cardinal auscultatory findings of mitral stenosis (Fig. 35.8) are a loud first heart sound, an opening snap of the mitral valve, and a long mitral diastolic murmur with presystolic accentuation.[13] An accentuated and sharp first heart sound may be the first clue to the diagnosis and alert the listener to evaluate more subtle auscultatory signs. The sharp first heart sound is due to a more rapid rate of left ventricular pressure rise (dp/dt) at the time of mitral valve closure.[11] The opening snap of the mitral valve is a sharp high-pitched sound which occurs during the maximal diastolic gradient across the mitral valve. The severity of mitral valve obstruction may be assessed by measuring: the Ql interval, which is the time interval between the onset of electrical systole (as seen by the Q wave of the electrocardiogram) and the first heart sound; and the 20S interval, which is the time interval between aortic valve closure and

the opening snap. In milder lesions, the Ql interval is short and the 20S interval long (up to 0.10 second). In severe degrees of mitral valve obstruction the Ql interval is long and the 20S interval short (down to 0.06 second). Absence of the opening snap should make one wary of the diagnosis of MS except in the presence of a fixed calcified valve, which is rare in children.

The apical diastolic murmur is low-pitched, rumbling, of low intensity, is initiated by the opening snap, and is best heard with a bell stethoscope lightly placed on the chest with the patient in a left lateral position. The presystolic murmur results from progressive narrowing of the mitral orifice with resulting increased velocity of flow as the valve closes.[11] Changes in the velocity of flow across the mitral valve as occurs with exercise and with the inhalation of amyl nitrite will augment the intensity of the murmur. In the absence of MI, the longer the diastolic murmur the more severe is the obstruction. However, in the presece of MI, this is no longer valid. In the presence of heart failure the mitral diastolic murmur may be absent only to return with the relief of this complication. A characteristic feature of the diastolic murmur is its presystolic accentuation. An apical systolic murmur may be present in patients with severe obstruction and does not necessarily indicate the presence of MI. In some instances the systolic murmur is due to complicating tricuspid insufficiency.

The second heart sound is normal except in the presence of pulmonary hypertension, when pulmonary valve closure is loud and may be followed by a high-pitched early diastolic murmur of pulmonary valve insufficiency. The latter may be difficult to differentiate from the more common early diastolic murmur of aortic insufficiency.[39] In tight MS without complicating tricuspid valve disease or cardiac failure, the third heart sound is absent.

Electrocardiographic Features

The electrocardiogram is normal if the stenosis is mild. In patients with more severe degrees of obstruction, the P waves are broad and notched, the so-called P mitrale, indicative of left atrial hypertrophy (Fig. 35.9). A tall spiked P wave, P pulmonale, usually associated with right atrial hypertrophy, may be found if the pulmonary vascular resistance is high or in the presence of associated tricuspid ste-

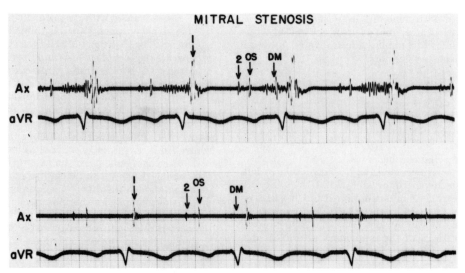

Fig. 35.8 Phonocardiograms in a patient with isolated tight mitral stenosis. *Ax*, apex; *aVR*, electrocardiogram; *1*, first sound; *2*, second sound; *OS*, opening snap of mitral valve, *DM*, diastolic murmur. Time lines, 0.04 sec. In the *upper tracing*, the rumbling diastolic murmur with presystolic accentuation is initiated by the opening snap. In the *lower tracing* the murmur has been filtered to exaggerate the sounds. The 20S interval is 0.07 second and the Q1 interval is 0.08 second. In this patient a systolic murmur is inaudible.

nosis. There is a marked overlap in these signs, in that many patients with left atrial hypertrophy will show tall spiked P waves in the absence of right atrial hypertrophy. Similarly, patients with broad notched P waves may have an increase of pulmonary vascular resistance. The degree of right ventricular hypertrophy is frequently proportional to the degree of pulmonary hypertension and may be marked if pulmonary vascular resistance is greatly elevated. However, patients with major MS but without severe pulmonary vascular disease may not demonstrate the electrocardiographic signs of right ventricular hypertrophy. Unequivocal evidence of gross left ventricular hypertrophy is most unusual and is seldom compatible with the diagnosis of isolated tight MS.

Radiologic Features

Roentgenographic examination is normal in mild cases but may be characteristic in patients with moderate or severe mitral valve obstruction (Fig. 35.10). In these in-

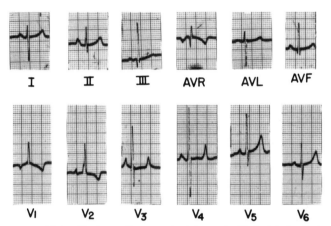

Fig. 35.9 Electrocardiogram of adolescent with isolated mitral stenosis. Note the notched P waves and marked right ventricular hypertrophy.

stances, the left atrium is enlarged to varying degrees, tending to be larger if there is associated MI or atrial fibrillation. The left ventricle is normal in size or displaced posteriorly by an enlarged right ventricle. The main pulmonary artery segment and the right heart chambers are enlarged, especially in the presence of pulmonary hypertension. The aorta is normal or small. Although valvular calcification is not common in children, careful examination for this sign with image intensification is warranted, especially in adolescents.

Changes in pulmonary blood flow occur in patients with major MS, and this can be appreciated on the x-ray film. In normal individuals in the upright position, the upper portions of the lung have less perfusion with blood than the lower segments.[46, 47] There is a more equal distribution to all parts of the lung if a normal individual lies flat. In the presence of severe MS and pulmonary hypertension, there is greater perfusion of the upper lobes.[14] If pulmonary hypertension is extreme, there may be more perfusion of the upper than the lower areas of the lung. The shift of area of blood flow may be related to the greater degree of pulmonary vascular disease in the lower segment of the lung. The redistribution of pulmonary flow can be appreciated on the x-ray by comparing the pulmonary vascular markings in the upper and lower pulmonary segments. This sign is more noteworthy in serial films with progression of the stenosis and pulmonary hypertension. In many patients with pulmonary venous hypetension, prominence of the pulmonary veins, especially at the lung apices, is seen on the x-ray. Septal lines, especially at the costophrenic angles, are also seen in this group of patients. Acute pulmonary edema is recognized by typical opacities radiating outward from the lung hilus to the periphery. Bilateral miliary shadows may be due to pulmonary hemosiderosis.

Echocardiographic Features

The echocardiogram shows a thick wave form of the anterior mitral leaflet. The posterior leaflet is also thick and its movement is generally anterior during diastole rather than posterior. The left atrium is large, and the size of the

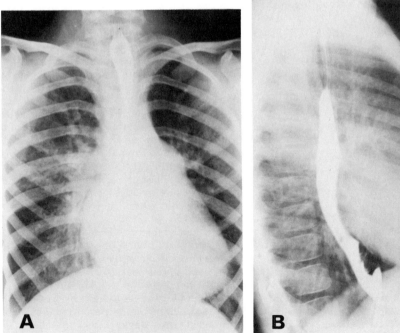
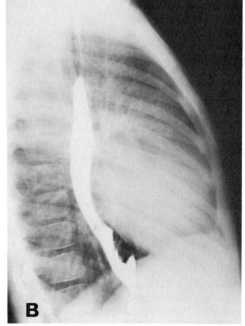

Fig. 35.10 Posteroanterior (A) and lateral (B) teleroentgenograms of an 8-year-old with isolated tight mitral stenosis. Cardiomegaly is evident, as is prominence of the main pulmonary artery. The enlarged left atrium impinges on the barium-filled esophagus, as seen in the lateral projection. Pulmonary flow is increased in the lung apices, especially the right.

left ventricle and aortic valve is normal. Echographic features of left ventricular function are within normal limits. Although the velocity of diastolic closure of the anterior mitral leaflet (EF slope) has previously been related to severity of obstruction, recent assessment shows poor correlation between the EF slope and calculated mitral valve area.[9] Two dimensional echocardiography demonstrates noncomplaint, thickened leaflets which open and close abruptly. In the short axis view, measurement of valve area is possible. Doppler turbulence during left ventricular filling across the stenotic mitral valve can be detected.

CARDIAC CATHETERIZATION

The basic abnormality at cardiac catheterization is the diastolic gradient across the mitral valve (Fig. 35.11). This is usually measured by simultaneous recording of pressures in the left ventricle and the pulmonary arterial wedge. If the obstruction is severe, the gradient is present throughout diastole, whereas in milder lesions the gradient is noted in early diastole or during atrial contraction.[30] In the presence of sinus rhythm, left atrial pressure curves show an elevated mean pressure and a narrow pulse pressure. In some patients the amplitude of the A, C, and V waves are similar, whereas in others the A is prominent or even giant, with a prominent V wave. In well-established lesions, a clear X descent is present, Y descent is slow, and diastasis is absent. In the presence of atrial fibrillation, the A wave disappears, the C wave may be prominent, and the X descent is not clearly discernible. These changes are probably related to the duration of the previous diastole rather than to the stenotic lesion per se. In some patients with severe MS, the pressure pulse curve appears normal, except that the mean left atrial pressure is increased.

Right heart catheterization determines the degree of elevation of pulmonary arterial pressure and resistance. Selective pulmonary arterial or left atrial angiocardiography confirms the degree of enlargement of the left atrium and indicates slow emptying of this chamber. Whenever there is doubt about the competence of the aortic valve, aortography should be performed.

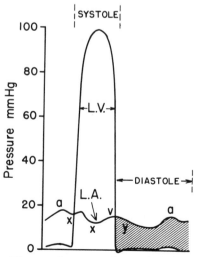

Fig. 35.11 Diagram of pressure changes in isolated tight mitral stenosis. The left atrial (*L.A.*) pressure curve shows a, c, and v waves with a slow Y descent. The diastolic pressure gradient is indicated by the *shaded area. LV*, left ventricle.

AORTIC VALVE DISEASE

In children and adolescents dominant aortic stenosis (AS) with or without aortic insufficiency (AI) is usually congenital. In this age group, rheumatic aortic valve disease presents as isolated or dominant AI with mild or moderate stenosis. The nature of healing of acute aortic valvulitis determines the resultant lesion. Insufficiency results from fibrous thickening and contracture of the leaflets so that they are unable to coapt during diastole. Fusion of the commissures results in stenosis. If only one commissure is involved, the aortic orifice is smaller than normal, but aortic flow is not greatly compromised. Fusion of two commissures usually results in dominant AS with little or no insufficiency. If all three commissures are fused, movement of the aortic leaflets is restricted, so that stenosis is associated with some degree of AI.

PHYSIOLOGY

Aortic insufficiency produces a large volume load on the left ventricle with resultant dilatation of this chamber. In chronic AI the left ventricle accommodates the large ejection fraction without an increase in end-diastolic pressure, which is presumably due to an increase in diastolic compliance as the left ventricle enlarges over a period of years. The left ventricle may perform efficiently for many years because of reduced aortic impedance due to associated peripheral vasodilation and because associated hypertrophy keeps the ventricular stress within the normal range.[35] This results in dilatation of the left ventricle with an increased stroke volume but with a normal or only slightly elevated end-diastolic pressure. When the left ventricle fails, the end-diastolic pressure rises with a concomitant rise in left atrial pressure. Progressive AI and left ventricular dilatation may result in secondary MI and a rapid downhill course. Cardiac failure may be preceded by episodes of frank pulmonary edema or occur insidiously. In these patients, elevation of pulmonary arterial pressure is slight or moderate and seldom extreme. The classic peripheral arterial pulse of free AI is due to a wide pulse pressure which is produced by the combination of peripheral vasodilatation and the aortic reflux. The pulse curve shows a rapid rise to a high peak with a collapsing descending limb, an insignificant dicrotic notch, and a low diastolic pressure. The central aortic pressure curve differs from that obtained in peripheral arteries. In the ascending aorta there is an uninterrupted rise of pressure to a sharp first peak, which is followed by a second peak of varying amplitude. The first peak of the central aortic pressure curve is not as prolonged as in AS and averages about 44% of total ejection time.[37] The position of the incisura can be related to the severity of the lesion and in gross AI is lower relative to the pulse amplitude (average is 41% of the pulse pressure). The wave following the incisura may be prominent. The ratio of the femoral to the central aortic pulse pressure averages 1.75 (normal average 1.58).[37] The hemodynamic effects of aortic stenosis are considered in Chapter 12.

The hemodynamic effects of combined lesions depend on whether insufficiency or stenosis dominates. The central aortic pressure curve may show an anacrotic shoulder with a delayed initial peak (suggesting a stenotic lesion) and a dicrotic notch low on the descending limb (suggesting AI). Although indirect carotid arterial pulse curves may show a pulsus bisferiens, intraarterial recording fails to show the prominent tidal wave. A peak systolic gradient of varying degree is measured across the aortic valve if stenosis is present.

MANIFESTATIONS

Clinical Features

In children and adolescents, chronic rheumatic aortic valve disease usually results in dominant AI with or without varying degrees of stenosis. Symptoms are unusual except in patients with gross AI. Palpitations may occur because of the large stroke volume and forceful left ventricular contraction. Excessive sweating and heat intolerance due to vasodilatation may be an early complaint and worsen with progression of AI. Effort dyspnea occurs early and progresses to orthopnea and pulmonary edema with the onset of left ventricular failure. Angina pectoris may be present during heavy exertion. The prognosis is poor if angina is nocturnal or associated with the onset of left ventricular failure. Distressing nocturnal symptoms may occur in adolescents in the late stage of the disease and consists of nightmares, tachycardia, sweating, paroxysmal hypertension, and chest pain. Sudden death may occur in these patients or in those whose course has been complicated by severe heart failure or uncontrollable angina pectoris.

AI is associated with vasodilatation and results in a wide pulse pressure. The peripheral pulse is usually normal in trivial AI but rises rapidly and collapses suddenly in free regurgitation. However, with moderate lesions the width of the pulse pressure is not necessarily proportional to the severity of the lesion. Many descriptions and eponyms have been applied to characterize the wide pulse pressure and its effects. The sharp rise of the pulse has been compared to that produced by a water hammer, a Victorian child's toy. Pistol shots may be audible over large arteries and a systolic and diastolic bruit when critical pressure is applied to the artery (Duroziez). The wide pulse pressure also results in visible carotid pulsations (Corrigan) and capillary pulsations. The blood pressure usually shows some systolic hypertension and a low diastolic pressure in established AI, but the diastolic pressure is not necessarily an index of the severity of the leak. Although the diastolic pressure in severe lesions is seldom less than 35 mm Hg, the pistol shot sounds over the artery give the impression that the diastolic pressure is zero. In these patients it is not possible to obtain an accurate reading of the diastolic pressure with the cuff method. The pulse pressure may narrow during severe heart failure because of a rise in diastolic pressure.

A lifting apical impulse due to left ventricular enlargement is easily palpable in the presence of moderate or severe lesions. The diagnostic sign of AI is an early high-pitched blowing diastolic murmur heard best at the upper and middle left sternal border (Fig. 35.12). This murmur may be transmitted to the apex, the second right interspace, and sometimes the right sternal border if there is associated aortic dilatation. Generally the diastolic murmur is more easily audible in full expiration with the patient leaning far forward. However, in some instances, this murmur is louder in the recumbent position. A systolic ejection type murmur, sometimes preceded by an ejection click, is usually present. It is a flow murmur caused by increased left ventricular stroke volume and does not indicate accompanying stenosis. An apical diastolic murmur (Austin-Flint) may be audible in severe AI in the absence of mitral valve disease. This murmur occurs in middiastole and in presystole and may be indistinguishable from that of MS. The murmur is presumably due to antegrade blood flow across a closing mitral orifice.[10] The distinction between combined AI and AS from free AI and an Austin-Flint murmur may be difficult. The effects of inhalation of amyl nitrite on the auscultatory events help in this differentiation. Amyl nitrite produces

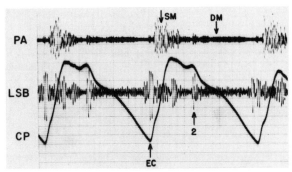

Fig. 35.12 Phonocardiograms in aortic insufficiency with associated aortic stenosis. *PA*, pulmonary area; *LSB*, lower left sternal border; *CP*, carotid pulse; *EC*, aortic ejection sound; *SM*, systolic ejection type murmur; *2*, second heart sound; *DM*, early diastolic murmur.

vasodilatation, tachycardia, and an increase in cardiac output. This diminishes the intensity of the early diastolic and Austin-Flint murmur but augments the murmur of organic MS. The echocardiogram usually resolves the issue as to the presence or absence of MS.

Electrocardiographic Features

The electrocardiogram is normal in mild lesions. In established free AI, left ventricular hypertrophy is usual. Notched or spiked P waves may be seen and are due to left atrial hypertrophy. Atrial fibrillation is rare in isolated AI without mitral valve disease.

Radiologic Features

Roentgenographic studies are abnormal in moderate or severe lesions. In these patients there is enlargement of the left ventricle. The ascending aorta and aortic knob are prominent and have an increased pulsation. Pulmonary congestion and generalized cardiac enlargement are seen in the presence of cardiac failure.

Echocardiographic Features

The echocardiogram[15] shows a large left ventricle with a normal left atrium. Flutter of the anterior mitral leaflet occurs in the presence of left ventricular volume overload and is due to the regurgitant jet striking the anterior leaflet. However, absence of mitral flutter does not exclude AI. Premature closure and delayed opening of the mitral valve are seen in severe acute AI and may complicate endocarditis. Doppler echocardiography detects the regurgitant jet in the left ventricular outflow tract.

CARDIAC CATHETERIZATION

It is seldom necessary to undertake cardiac catheterization and angiocardiography in children and adolescents with chronic rheumatic aortic valve disease. However, in patients with progressive lesions, these investigations usually precede surgical treatment. Details of abnormal pressures and flows have been described above. Selective angiography with injection of contrast in the aortic root will give a qualitative estimate of the degree of AI but in the presence of florid AI, this procedure adds little to the clinical evaluation.

COURSE AND PROGNOSIS

In children, mild and moderate lesions are well tolerated. However, a progressive downhill course may be initiated by recurrent acute episodes of rheumatic fever, smouldering subacute disease, or endocarditis. Unfavorable signs include the onset of heart failure, episodes of pulmonary edema, or angina pectoris. Many adolescents with severe AI are symptom-free and appear to tolerate advanced lesions well into the third and fourth decade. However, more than 50% succumb within 20 years after the onset of the disease.

TRICUSPID VALVE DISEASE

Tricuspid insufficiency is usually secondary to right ventricular dilatation, which complicates pulmonary hypertension. This implies that there are coexistent severe left-sided lesions, usually combined MS and MI. Symptoms are dominated by those produced by the left-sided lesions, although in some patients the onset of tricuspid insufficiency relieves severe dyspnea and orthopnea. Right upper quadrant discomfort is frequent and is due to hepatic engorgement. Physical signs are dominated by the raised venous pressure produced by the regurgitant flow. Prominent systolic C-V waves in the jugular venous pulse are accompanied by hepatic tenderness or enlargement. The murmur of tricuspid insufficiency is audible at the lower left sternal border, pansystolic in time, and louder in inspiration. Concomitant signs of mitral and/or aortic valve disease with or without atrial fibrillation are frequent. Signs attributable to tricuspid insufficiency improve or disappear in some patients when compensation from cardiac failure is restored. The electrocardiogram shows the effects of the left-sided lesion, and atrial fibrillation is frequent. Roentgenographic examination shows considerable generalized cardiomegaly with or without signs of pulmonary hypertension. Echocardiography confirms the presence of right volume overload. Mild tricuspid insufficiency may not result in right-sided chamber enlargement but may be detected by Doppler echocardiography. This technique shows the regurgitant flow into the right atrium. Cardiac catheterization shows an elevated right atrial pressure with a prominent C-V wave, the height of which increases with inspiration. The Y descent is rapid.

Isolated rheumatic tricuspid stenosis is extremely rare, and concomitant mitral and/or aortic valve disease is usual. Even with these lesions pure tricuspid stenosis is very rare, and usually combined stenosis and insufficiency are present. The major pathologic change in the tricuspid valve is commissural fusion, but chordal shortening and fibrosis are not marked. Symptoms are related to those produced by the associated left-sided lesions; however, dyspnea and orthopnea may not be prominent because tricuspid obstruction prevents sudden increases in pulmonary flow. In advanced lesions edema, ascites, and hepatomegaly are usual. The classical physical sign in tricuspid stenosis is the presence of a brief, sharp A wave in the jugular venous pulse if the patient is in sinus rhythm. The diastolic murmur of tricuspid stenosis mimics that of MS. However, it is usually best heard at the lower left sternal border, clearly augmented by inspiration and frequently higher pitched than the murmur of MS. Presystolic accentuation occurs in the presence of sinus rhythm, but the murmur occurs earlier in diastole in the presence of atrial fibrillation. An opening snap of the tricuspid valve may be audible but with associated MS is difficult to differentiate from a mitral opening snap. The echocardiogram usually resolves the issue as to the presence of associated mitral stenosis. Two dimensional echocardiography is preferable to M-mode for the diagnosis and shows noncompliant, thickened leaflets which open and close abruptly. In the short axis view, measurement of valve area is possible. Doppler turbulence during right ventricular filling across the stenotic tricuspid valve can be detected. The electrocardiogram may show tall spiked P waves in the presence of sinus

rhythm. Other electrocardiographic signs are produced by the associated left-sided lesions. Similarly, radiographic abnormalities of the cardiac silhouette and pulmonary circulation are usually those produced by the associated left-sided lesions. Cardiac catheterization demonstrates a diastolic gradient across the tricuspid valve. The right atrial pressure is increased with a giant A wave (in the presence of sinus rhythm) and a slow Y descent. The cardiac output is usually decreased.

TREATMENT

In North America, the majority of children and adolescents with chronic rheumatic heart disease are completely asymptomatic and have trivial or only moderate valvular disease with normal heart size or insignificant cardiomegaly. In these patients restriction of physical activity is unnecessary and, in fact, is harmful because of the possible development of cardiac neurosis. Furthermore, restriction of physical activities in the presence of moderate disease is also unnecessary, because the patient soon learns his own tolerance for effort. However, competitive and team sport and individual activities, such as weight lifting and other isometric exercises, should be discouraged if there has been a recent history of heart failure or if there is persistent moderate or severe cardiomegaly. Normal schooling should be encouraged when at all possible.

Prophylaxis

The time to stress the importance of long-term continuing prophylaxis is during the early association with the patient and his relatives, preferably during the early part of the initial acute episode of rheumatic fever. During these interviews, the recurrent nature of the disease should be stressed, and the importance of eradicating streptococcal infection emphasized. The patient and his family must be informed of the hazard of endocarditis. Emphasis on the details of prophylaxis during initial interviews and during subsequent outpatient visits appears to decrease the number of dropouts from a program of long-term chemoprophylaxis, especially in children and adolescents who are symptom-free. The advantages and problems associated with various forms of prophylaxis are discussed above in Chapter 34.

Cardiac Failure

Therapy for cardiac failure is described in Chapter 44. However, special problems arise in children and adolescents who are on therapy for many years. In patients who have an unaccountable downhill course, the following mechanisms should be considered:

1. Reactivation of rheumatic carditis. In many patients this problem is difficult to exclude, especially in the absence of overt signs of acute rheumatic fever.

2. Infection. Unrecognized and untreated endocarditis complicating chronic rheumatic heart disease is associated ultimately with uncontrollable heart failure. In patients who have recovered from endocarditis, destruction of valve mechanisms may initiate a downhill course. Inadequately treated endocarditis is also associated with a course which may result in heart failure. Breakdown while continuing previously successful therapy may be due to intercurrent infection, frequently pulmonary or urinary.

3. Electrolyte inbalance. Long-term diuretic therapy may be complicated by hypokalemia, hypochloremic alkalosis or hyponatremia.

4. Pulmonary embolism is not frequent in children and

adolescents but should be considered in the patient who is unresponsive to therapy.

5. Dysrhythmia, especially atrial fibrillation with rapid ventricular response. In these patients digitalis is the drug of choice, although direct-current countershock is effective in persistently unresponsive patients. Countershock is, however, unwise when atrial fibrillation is part of the natural course of the disease, as relapse is likely.

Other complications which are peculiar to patients with chronic rheumatic heart disease and which require specific therapy include: (1) Pulmonary edema. These episodes constitute a medical emergency and require the judicious use of oxygen, morphine, diuretics, rotating tourniquets, and digitalis. (2) Hemoptysis. This frightening complication is seldom exsanguinating or fatal and is treated with bed rest and morphine.

Surgery

Although surgical treatment for chronic rheumatic heart disease is available, it is seldom indicated in children or adolescents. In the majority of patients in this age group, the disease is stable, with only mild or moderate valvular deformity. It is difficult to evaluate the role of progressive but smouldering subacute or chronic rheumatic carditis in patients who are deteriorating. Nevertheless, in specific instances, great benefit can be derived from surgery, especially in patients in whom the rheumatic process is dormant.

The major indications for surgery in *dominant* MI include recurrent episodes of heart failure with inadequate response to medical measures, extreme dyspnea with moderate activity, progressive cardiomegaly, pulmonary venous or arterial hypertension, a regurgitant fraction of over 50%, and a left ventricular end-diastolic volume of 250% or more of the predicted normal.[44] In the preoperative period the patient may respond dramatically to digitalis and diuretics. However, this response is deceptive since symptoms may recur rapidly with resumption of normal activity.[12]

Although the above indications are generally accepted, there is no unanimity concerning the surgical method. A number of authors have reported good results from *annuloplasty*.[43, 44] Even though this technique is not popular, it is attractive for application in children because the valve is frequently still pliable and because of the concern of long-term complications from prostheses, such as thromboembolism, infection, hemolysis, and complications of anticoagulants. However, long-term results from annuloplasty are not clear since MI may recur or MS may develop consequent to the original rheumatic infection.[44] Successful mitral *valvuloplasty* with the use of specially designed prosthetic frames inserted into the mitral annulus was reported by Carpentier and his colleagues[8] who cited the following advantages for this technique: preservation of the normal configuration of the mitral annulus; absence of narrowing of the orifice area; retention of mobility of the leaflets; and prevention of recurrent dilatation of the annulus.

It is generally agreed that valve replacement is necessary if the valve is thick, scarred, and grossly deformed. The mitral valve may be replaced by a *prosthesis*. Although none of these prostheses is ideal and reluctance to use them in children is easily appreciated, brilliant results have been obtained with dramatic improvement in symptoms, regression of severity of MI, increased longevity, and an improved quality of life. The largest experience is with the caged ball prosthesis described by Starr and Edwards.[1] Evaluation of the late results of this prosthesis shows a substantial reduction in operative mortality and prosthesis-related complications.[5] In the United States, frequently used low profile prostheses include the Bjork-Shiley tilting disc[4] and the

Lillehei-Kaster pivoting disc.[2, 6] The low profile devices may be advantageous in patients with a small left ventricular cavity.

Although advances continue in surgical care and prosthetic design, substantial morbidity and mortality still occurs after prosthetic valve replacement.[3, 17, 24] Most evidence suggests that long-term postoperative anticoagulant therapy is indicated,[7] but frequently this therapy is erratic or ineffective. This results in thromboembolism, hemorrhage from anticoagulants, or prosthesis dysfunction due to thrombus. The latter is recognized by recurrence of symptoms of heart failure, syncope, altered prosthetic valve sounds or new murmurs, and requires reoperation. It is also recognized that coumadin, the most commonly used anticoagulant, is teratogenetic. This is an important consideration in the decision of which valve to use in young or adolescent girls. The onset of endocarditis within 3 months of surgery carries a poor prognosis and is treated vigorously with appropriate antimicrobial agents. Early surgical intervention is frequently necessary in these desperately ill patients. Late onset endocarditis has a better prognosis and frequently responds to antibiotic therapy alone, although reoperation is necessary in some instances. Intravascular hemolysis occurs with most prostheses, but usually this becomes significant when paravalvular leaks develops. This complication is treated with oral iron therapy, intermittent blood transfusion, or reoperation, if the leak is major.

The use of *tissue valves* has appeal in children because with these valves thromboembolic complications are infrequent. An inverted aortic tissue valve has been used to replace the mitral valve. Glutaraldehyde-preserved porcine xenografts enjoyed a period of popularity, but it is now recognized that their durability is limited especially in children.[12] Valve failure has resulted from stiffening, calcification, and stenosis of the valve cusps. Fresh antibiotic-sterilized homografts are used in centers abroad, who report excellent results and durability. To date, there is limited use of these valves in the United States.

The immediate surgical results for dominant MI are impressive, with regression of symptoms and signs associated with cardiomegaly (Figs. 35.4 and 35.13). If this does not occur, one should suspect associated rheumatic myocardial disease, progressive disease of other valves especially the aortic, and recurrence of rheumatic fever.

The timing of operation in isolated tight rheumatic MS is determined by the effects of the obstruction rather than the age of the patient.[18, 36] The major surgical indications are episodes of acute pulmonary edema and signs of a high pulmonary vascular resistance. Systemic embolization occurs rarely but is another indication for surgery. In children and adolescents, extreme valvular distortion and calcification is rare, so that a closed transventricular mitral valvotomy yields good immediate results. Many surgeons prefer to do the valvotomy under direct vision during cardiopulmonary bypass, and some prefer to have a pump oxygenator available as a standby during surgery in case of inadequate or too generous relief of obstruction. Surgery under direct vision is preferable when there is associated major MI, heavy valve calcification, or when surgery for restenosis is undertaken. In this age group restenosis is common, so it is wise to wait as long as practicable before the first valvotomy is undertaken. After operation, signs of pulmonary hypertension regress rapidly, with marked improvement in exercise tolerance and stamina.

Patients with dominant AI require surgery when there is a history of recurrent pulmonary edema and heart failure or uncontrollable angina pectoris. Although AI can be well tolerated for a number of years, every effort should be made

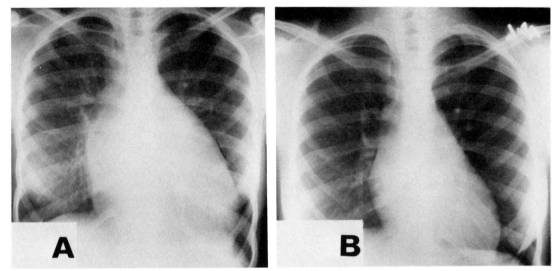

Fig. 35.13 Pre- (*A*) and post- (*B*) operative teleroentgenograms of a 13-year-old with severe rheumatic mitral insufficiency who required replacement of the mitral valve with a Bjork-Shiley prosthesis. Postoperatively there was a striking reduction of heart size.

to institute surgical therapy before serious left ventricular dysfunction occurs. Biplane left ventriculography is precise to determine left ventricular function but is impractical because the method cannot be used serially. Useful information can be obtained from serial echocardiograms and/or radionuclide ventriculograms. Assessment of left ventricular function is difficult in asymptomatic patients with chronic AI, especially when left ventricular end-diastolic pressures and ejection fractions are normal at rest. However, early signs of left ventricular dysfunction can be obtained during graded exercise testing, which can unmask a diminished left ventricular reserve and also detect decreased ejection fraction with radionuclide angiography and/or echocardiography. Surgical therapy of rheumatic aortic valve disease usually requires total valve replacement with a prosthesis or a tissue valve.

The preparation for cardiac surgery of all patients with chronic rheumatic heart disease includes adequate digitalization and diuresis. However, overzealous diuresis in the immediate preoperative period should be avoided, because electrolyte imbalance, especially hypokalemia, is associated with postoperative complications, such as severe dysrhythmias, digitalis intoxication, and psychoses. Emboli from prosthetic valves occur with sufficient frequency to require the long-term use of anticoagulants. The problems of controlling the dosage of these agents in children are self-evident. Careful follow-up after surgery is essential with emphasis on penicillin prophylaxis to prevent recurrences of rheumatic fever and prophylaxis against endocarditis. Evaluation of valve function also requires close follow-up to determine recurrences of valvular insufficiency or stenosis and to recognize prosthetic or tissue valve dysfunction.

REFERENCES

1. Barhorst, D. A., Oxman, H. A., Connolly, D. C., Pluth, J. R., Danielson, G. K., Wallace, R. B., and McGoon, D. C.: Long term follow up of isolated replacement of the aortic or mitral valve with the Starr-Edwards prosthesis. Am. J. Cardiol. 35:228, 1975.
2. Barlow, J. B., and Pocock, W. A.: The problems of nonejection systolic clicks and associated mitral systolic murmurs: Emphasis on the billowing mitral leaflet syndrome. Am. Heart J. 90:636, 1975.
3. Benzing, G., and Kaplan, S.: Late complications of cardiac surgery. Pediatr. Clin. North Am. 18:1225, 1971.
4. Bjork, V. O., and Olin, C.: A hydrodynamic comparison between the Bjork-Shiley tilting disc valve and the Lillihei-Kaster pivoting disc valve. Scand. J. Thorac. Cardiovasc. Surg. 7:107, 1973.
5. Bonchek, L. I., and Starr, A.: Ball valve prosthesis: Current appraisal and late results. Am. J. Cardiol. 35:843, 1975.
6. Braunwald, E., and Awe, W. C.: The syndrome of severe mitral regurgitation with normal left atrial pressure. Circulation 27:29, 1963.
7. Brawley, R. K., Donahoo, J. S., and Gott, V. L.: Current status of the Beall, Bjork-Shiley, Braunwald-Cutter, Lillehei-Kaster and Smellof-Cutter cardiac valve prosthesis. Am. J. Cardiol. 35:855, 1975.

8. Carpentier, A., Deloche, A., Dauptain, J., Soyer, R., Blondeau, P., Piwnica, A., and DuBost, Ch.: A new reconstructive operation for correction of mitral and tricuspid insufficiency. J. Thorac. Cardiovasc. Surg. 61:1, 1971.
9. Cope, G. D., Kisslo, J. A., Johnson, M. L., and Behar, V. S.: A reassessment of the echocardiogram in mitral stenosis. Circulation 52:664, 1975.
10. Craige, E.: The Austin Flint murmur. In Physiologic Principles of Heart Sounds and Murmurs. Am. Heart Assoc., Monograph 46, p. 160, New York, 1975.
11. Criley, M. J., Chambers, R. D., Blaufuss, A. H., and Friedman, N. J.: Mitral stenosis: Mechanico-acoustical events in Physiologic principles of heart sounds and murmurs. Am. Heart Assoc. Monograph 46, p. 149, 1975.
12. Curcio, C. A., Commerford, P. J., Rose, A. G., Stevens, J. E., Barnard, M. S.: Calcification of glutaraldehyde-preserved porcine xenografts in young patients. J. Thorac. Cardiovasc. Surg. 81:621, 1981.
13. Dack, S., Bleifer, S., Grishman, A., and Donoso, E.: Mitral stenosis: Auscultatory and phonocardiographic findings. Am. J. Cardiol. 5:815, 1960.
14. Dollery, C. T., and West, J. B.: Regional uptake of radioactive oxygen, carbon dioxide in the lungs and patients with mitral stenosis.

Circ. Res. 8:765, 1960.
15. Feigenbaum, H.: Echocardiography, 3rd ed. Lea & Febiger, Philadelphia, 1981.
16. Feinstein, A. R., Wood, H. F., Spagnuolo, M., Taranta, A., Jones, A., Kleinberg, E., and Tursky, E.: Rheumatic fever in children and adolescents. VII. Cardiac changes and sequelae. Ann. Intern. Med. 60 (Suppl. 5):87, 1964.
17. Freed, M. D., and Bernhard, W. F.: Prosthetic valve replacement in children. Prog. Cardiovasc. Dis. 17:475, 1975.
18. Gotsman, M. S., and Van der Horst, R. L.: Surgical management of severe mitral valve disease in childhood. Am. Heart J. 90:685, 1975.
19. Gray, I. R., Joshipura, C. S., and Mackinnon, J.: Retrograde left ventricular cardioangiography in the diagnosis of mitral regurgitation. Br. Heart J. 25:145, 1963.
20. Hudson, R. E. B.: Cardiovascular Pathology, Vol. 1. Edward Arnold, Ltd., London, 1965, pp. 919–1036.
21. Hudson, R. E. B.: Cardiovascular Pathology, Vol. 3. Williams & Wilkins, Baltimore, 1970, pp. 549–581.
22. Hugenholtz, P. G., Ryan, T. J., Stein, S. W., and Abelmann, W. H.: The spectrum of pure mitral stenosis. Am. J. Cardiol. 10:773, 1962.
23. Kaplan, S.: Pressure curve analysis. In Intravascular Catheterization, edited by H. A. Zim-

merman. Charles C Thomas, Springfield, Ill., 1966.

24. Kloster, F. E.: Diagnosis and management of complications of prosthetic heart valves. Am. J. Cardiol. 35:872, 1975.

25. Levy, M. J., and Edwards, J. E.: Anatomy of mitral insufficiency. Prog. Cardiovasc. Dis. 5:119, 1962.

26. Lillehei, C. W., Kaster, R. L., Coleman, M., and Bloch, J. H.: Heart valve replacement with the Lillehei-Kaster pivoting disc prosthesis. N.Y. State J. Med. 74:1426, 1974.

27. Markowitz, M., and Gordis, L.: Rheumatic fever. W. B. Saunders, Philadelphia, 1972.

28. McManus, Q., Grunkemeier, G. L., Lambert, L. E., Starr, A.: Non-cloth-covered caged-ball prostheses. The second decade. J. Thorac. Cardiovasc. Surg. 76:788, 1978.

29. Morch, J. E., Smith, H. J., and McGregor, M.: Quantitation of mitral regurgitation by constant infusion of xenon 133. Circulation 35:501, 1967.

30. Morrow, A. G., Braunwald, E., Haller, J. A., and Sharp, E. H.: Left atrial pressure pulse in mitral valve disease. Circulation 16:399, 1957.

31. Neustadt, J. E., and Shaffer, A. B.: Diagnostic value of the left atrial pressure pulse in mitral valvular disease. Am. Heart J. 58:675, 1959.

32. Nixon, P. G. F.: The third heart sound in mitral regurgitation. Br. Heart J. 23:677, 1961.

33. Nixon, P. G. F., and Wagner, G. R.: The duration of left ventricular systole in mitral incompetence. Br. Heart J. 24:464, 1962.

34. Perloff, J. K., and Harvey, W. P.: Auscultatory and phonocardiographic manifestations of pure mitral regurgitation. Progr. Cardiovasc. Dis. 5:172, 1962.

35. Rapaport, E.: Natural history of aortic and mitral valve disease. Am. J. Cardiol. 35:221, 1975.

36. Reale, A., Colella, C., and Bruno, A. M.: Mitral stenosis in childhood: Clinical and therapeutic aspects. Am. Heart J. 66:15, 1963.

37. Rosche, J., and Morrow, A. G.: Central and femoral pressure pulses in aortic valve disease: A quantitative and qualitative analysis. Am. Heart J. 55:599, 1958.

38. Ross, R. S., and Criley, J. M.: Cineangiocardiographic studies of the origin of cardiovascular physical signs. Circulation 30:255, 1964.

39. Runco, V., Molnar, W., Meckstroth, C. V., and Ryan, J. M.: The Graham Steell murmur versus aortic regurgitation in rheumatic heart disease. Am. J. Med. 31:71, 1961.

40. Sandler, H., Dodge, H. T., Hay, R. E., and Rackley, C. E.: Quantitation of valvular insufficiency in men by angiocardiography. Am. Heart J. 65:501, 1963.

41. Sauter, H. J., Dodge, H. T., Johnston, R. R., and Graham, T. P.: The relationship of left atrial pressure and volume in patients with heart disease. Am. Heart J. 67:635, 1964.

42. Schrire, V., Vogelpoel, L., Nellen, M., Swanepoel, A., and Beck, W.: Silent mitral incompetence. Am. Heart J. 61:723, 1961.

43. Spencer, F. C.: Acquired heart disease. In Principles of Surgery, 2nd ed. edited by S. I. Schwartz, G. T. Shires, F. C. Spencer, and E. H. Storer. New York, McGraw-Hill, 1979, p. 813.

44. Sulayman, R., Mathew, R., Thilenius, O. G., Replogle, R., and Arcilla, R. A.: Hemodynamics and annuloplasty in isolated mitral regurgitation in children. Circulation 52:1144, 1975.

45. Werko, L.: The dynamics and consequences of stenosis or insufficiency of the cardiac valves. In Handbook of Physiology, Sect. 2, Vol. 1. American Physiological Society, Washington, D.C., 1962.

46. West, J. B.: Regional differences in gas exchange in the lung of erect man. J. Appl. Physiol. 17:893, 1962.

47. West, J. B., and Dollery, C. T.: Distribution of blood flow and the pressure-flow relations of the whole lung. J. Appl. Physiol. 20:175, 1965.

36

Endocarditis

Edward L. Kaplan, M.D., and Stanford T. Shulman, M.D.

Infective endocarditis is one of the most feared complications of structural heart disease. Although a relatively rare problem if one considers the number of patients at risk, this infection continues to have a disproportionate influence on clinical practice. Reported mortality rates are much lower now than in the preantibiotic era, when the rate was virtually 100%, but the ultimate consequences, including morbidity and mortality and the expenses associated with prolonged and often intense medical and surgical therapy, remain formidable.

Significant advances in the understanding of this disease process have been made during the last decade or two. One of the most important contributions in furthering our concepts of this infectious disease was the important utilization, initially by Garrison and Freedman[28] and later by a number of other investigators, of a reliable experimental animal model for the study of the pathogenesis, treatment, and prevention of infective endocarditis. While extrapolation of some data from the animal model directly to clinical practice has been criticized, it still has provided important insight into the disease and its complications. This model has allowed modification of many of the older concepts of the disease. Since well-controlled prospective epidemiologic studies cannot be completed because of the large number of patients needed to conduct a definitive examination of this problem and because of ethical constraints, the experimental model has also proven invaluable. We will attempt to emphasize these newer concepts and recently reported data. A complete discussion is beyond the space limitations of this discussion; the reader is referred to the several recent monographs and reviews which are available.[6, 44, 47, 50, 64]

DEFINITION

For the purpose of this discussion, infective endocarditis is an inflammatory process resulting from infection of a valve, the mural endocardium, or vascular endothelium, with the infection caused by a bacterial or by a fungal agent. Using an inclusive definition, one might include pathologic processes in which viruses are the etiologic agent. However, the subjects of viral endocarditis and valvulitis are adequately discussed in Chapter 37. This definition is important because it limits consideration to infective processes which, at least in theory, are amenable to modern medical and surgical treatment.

At one time, convention dictated that endocarditis be classified as acute or subacute. While this distinction still frequents the vocabulary of many clinicians, the recent tendency has been to avoid this terminology. In its place, it seems preferable to describe the disease based upon the microorganism involved. For example, streptococci, especially the alpha-hemolytic streptococci, almost without exception caused a prolonged "subacute" form of the illness. On the other hand, *Staphylococcus aureus* and other pyogenic bacteria such as *Streptococcus pneumonia* (pneumococci) or beta-hemolytic streptococci usually are associated with a virulent, or "acute" clinical illness.

EPIDEMIOLOGY

Although much has been written about the epidemiology of endocarditis, documentation of epidemiologic trends has been somewhat imprecise. This has been related to two deficiencies: first, the lack of adequate epidemiologic data about the size and specific characteristics of the population at risk and, secondly, the lack of conclusive documentation of the diagnosis. Furthermore, because there are relatively few cases seen in any one institution, many authors have combined their clinical experience over several decades. This has frequently resulted in obscuring epidemiological trends.

There are three aspects of the epidemiology of endocarditis which are most relevant to this discussion: the incidence, the age of patients developing endocarditis, and the prevalence of the predisposing cardiovascular lesions. The responsible microorganisms are discussed elsewhere in this chapter.

There has been an impression among students of this disease that the incidence of endocarditis fell after the introduction of antibiotics, but conclusive epidemiologic data are difficult to locate, and some investigators have been unable to confirm this observation. There are data which would suggest that the incidence of the disease has increased somewhat in the pediatric age group. Data have usually been expressed with the denominator as the number of total admissions to a given hospital or medical center. Blumenthal et al.[8] reported an incidence of 1:2000 admissions to a children's hospital in the 1960s and noted no change during the two previous decades. A lower incidence for the same time period was noted by Zakrzewski and Keith[97] from Toronto. However, several reports published in the 1970s suggest that the incidence has, in fact, increased among pediatric patients with cardiovascular disease. In an extensive series from the Boston Children's Hospital, the apparent incidence rose from 1:4500 pediatric admissions during the period of the 1930s through the decade of the 1950s to an incidence of 1:1800 during the years 1963 to 1972.[39] This trend was confirmed by Edis and Venables[23] from the Royal Children's Hospital in Melbourne. The incidence reported in that institution rose from 1:4500 pediatric admissions to 1:2700 in more recent years. It should be recognized that these figures may well represent underestimates of the incidence of endocarditis since with more well-trained physicians in practice in smaller cities and towns—both specialists and primary physicians—a number of cases of endocarditis probably do not come to the attention of larger medical centers, especially if they are "uncomplicated." Whether this increase in endocarditis is due to the fact that, with advances in cardiovascular surgical approaches to congenital heart disease during the last 3 decades, more patients live longer (thus, increasing the population at risk to develop endocarditis) is difficult to determine.

It has been the impression of several investigators that the average age of patients with endocarditis has increased during the middle decades of the 20th century. Weinstein and Rubin[90] reported that the average age of onset was approximately 34 years, several decades ago, while within the last decade the average age of onset of endocarditis was approximately 50 years of age, with an increasing number of patients older than 60 years of age. All of the reasons for these are not evident, but it is quite likely that the observation is a reflection of improved medical and surgical management, causing more patients to live longer and allowing them to develop cardiovascular disease.

Clinicians have recognized that endocarditis affects all ages of children with underlying cardiovascular disease. For example, in a recent collaborative study of 30 large cardiovascular centers in North America, slightly over 20% of the patients were in their first two decades at onset of disease.[43] While relatively uncommon, endocarditis occurs in infants and young children,[54] but most of the cases appear to occur

among older children. This was true in an extensive review of the literature in the pediatric age group, for almost half of children with endocarditis were 10 years of age or older.[42] In a recent study of 50 children with endocarditis reported from the Mayo Clinic, this also was certainly the case.[37] Pediatricians also must be aware of cases recently reported in neonatal intensive care units which are related to the routine use of indwelling intravascular lines for monitoring and support of critically ill neonates.[7, 38]

One of the most complete and succinct summaries of these epidemiologic changes was recently published by Durack and Petersdorf.[21] They divided the last 4 decades into three eras: preantibiotic (before 1944), early antibiotic (1944–1965), and recent (after 1965)), and they categorized and compared the cardiac disease. The proportion of patients with congenital heart disease has remained stable throughout the 4 decades, while the proportion of patients with rheumatic heart disease has fallen. This is probably due to the falling incidence of rheumatic fever and the falling prevalence of rheumatic heart disease in industrialized countries. (It should be noted that this does not appear to be the case in developing countries where endocarditis remains an important complicating factor in the patients with rheumatic valvular heart disease.) Modern therapeutic advances, not only in cardiovascular medicine and surgery but also in patients with malignancies, have resulted in a large group of susceptible candidates (e.g., compromised hosts, cardiac surgery, intravascular lines, etc.). The propensity for individuals with prosthetic valves to contract endocarditis is a serious and common problem.[40] In addition, the "epidemic" of endocarditis associated with drug abuse has added a number of cases.[82] In fact, in some metropolitan medical centers the last category results in the largest group of endocarditis patients, and one of the most difficult to manage. If one examines a cross-section of all patients developing endocarditis in recent years, it should be recognized that most of them are individuals with valvular heart disease. In a recent survey of cases of endocarditis in 30 large medical centers in North America, 67% (41% rheumatic and 26% congenital) of the cases were related to valvular deformities.[43] Review of the pediatric literature, through the mid 1970s, reveals that between one-quarter and one-half of the cases of endocarditis were valve related.[42] The data from this latter series again suggest less rheumatic heart disease in the pediatric population in recent years.

Finally, there are a group of patients with endocarditis who are now seen who were seen very infrequently or not at all in the past. Individuals with prosthetic valves and intravascular lines make up a high percentage of this group. Patients with ventriculoatrial shunts, right atrial access lines for monitoring or medication, or transvenous pacemakers are among the best examples. The propensity for such individuals to develop endocarditis is easily understood when considering the rabbit model of endocarditis.

Microorganisms

The group of microorganisms isolated either from blood, from surgical specimens, or at necropsy of individuals with endocarditis includes most of the common bacterial and fungal pathogens. However, case reports continue to appear, describing unusual bacteria and fungi isolated from patients with this infection. In a recent cooperative study, the variety of bacterial species isolated was similar in patients with underlying heart disease and in those who did not have underlying cardiovascular pathology.[43]

Review of the literature indicates that the majority of

cases are associated with relatively few bacterial species. Although all of the reasons for this are not clear, data are available which suggest reasons for some bacteria to be more commonly associated with endocarditis. One of the most logical and intriguing concepts is that of bacterial adherence. Following careful in vitro studies, Gould et al.[32] presented data indicating that bacteria which most frequently were responsible for endocarditis (e.g., viridans streptococci) displayed a propensity for adherence to canine or human valves. Gram negative organisms which are seldom responsible for endocarditis adhered rather poorly in this in vitro system.

The impressions from these experimental data are confirmed when one evaluates the literature. In most large series, streptococci (viridans more frequently than enterococci) are responsible for most cases of endocarditis. Staphylococci (*Staphylococcus aureus* and *Staphylococcus epidermidis*) are usually the second largest group.[25, 52, 86] These ratios have changed only slightly in recent years. In a recent review, it was found that viridans streptococci were responsible for 63% in the preantibiotic era and 52% in the antibiotic era after 1965.[21] Staphylococci increased slightly from 12% in the former to just more than 20% in the latter period. In another report, Wilson et al.[94] noted that streptococci and staphylococci accounted for about 80% of organisms isolated from patients with this disease; the percentage of streptococci decreased slightly from the 1950s to the 1970s, and the number of staphylococcal cases increased slightly.

In the pediatric age group, similar trends have been noted. In a review of pediatric endocarditis during the last 3 decades, Kaplan[42] found that almost 80% of the cases were due to these two groups of organisms. Two recent tabulations of organisms isolated from pediatric cases of endocarditis at the Mayo Clinic and at the Boston Children's Hospital were similar.[37, 69]

In a recent review of 260 cases of endocarditis in the pediatric age group, less than 5% of organisms isolated were other than streptococci or staphylococci. About half of this 5% were gram negative organisms.[42] Although not exclusively from children, recent data from the Mayo Clinic suggest that gram negative endocarditis is frequent.[29] Geraci and Wilson[29] reviewed the experience at that institution during a 20-year period and found 56 cases; approximately one-third followed cardiac surgery. Of the 56 patients with gram negative endocarditis, almost a third were members of the *Haemophilus* group. Twenty other gram-negative bacterial species were identified. In contrast to some reports, the overall cure rate was over 80% in the Mayo series and was much better in those who did not contract the disease following cardiovascular surgery.

In narcotic addicts, in addition to *S. aureus*, other organisms commonly isolated include gram-negative organisms (especially pseudomonas species) and occasionally candida or other fungal species.[82] To some degree, the same can be said for prosthetic valve endocarditis. Although not as universally fatal as the early experience suggested, mortality rates of up to 60% are still evident. Both the mortality and the infective organisms are different, depending upon whether prosthetic valve endocarditis is classified as early (less than 2 to 3 months following surgical procedure) or late. The early onset disease is probably related to contamination during the surgical procedure, either directly or through resultant bacteremia.[27] Since virtually all of the patients are receiving prophylactic antibiotics at the time of the procedure, unusual and resistant organisms are frequently found. In contrast, the late form of the infection usually is related to staphylococcal (often *S. epidermidis*) or streptococcal species.

Another unusual group of microorganisms sometimes associated with endocarditis are the anaerobic organisms. At one time the view was commonly held that a large percentage of individuals with the clinical syndrome of endocarditis, but with sterile blood cultures, were likely infected with anaerobic organisms which could not be recovered by usual methods in the clinical laboratory. While there is little doubt that anaerobic organisms can cause endocarditis, it is unusual. Anaerobic organisms recovered from the blood of 33 patients, reviewed by Felner and Dowell[26] included bacteroides, fusobacterium, clostridium, propionibacterium, and peptostreptococcus. Only half of the patients in this series had preexisting underlying heart disease. Seven of the 33 patients (21%) died.

Fungal endocarditis is one of the most feared forms of endocarditis.[1, 75] Complications are frequent (especially embolization[33]), and both medical and surgical therapy present problems for the physician. *Candida albicans*, aspergillus species, and *Torulopsis glabrata* are among the most frequent organisms recovered,[70] but other species of candida and even more unusual fungi have been reported. While often associated with narcotic addicts or cardiac surgery, fungal endocarditis occurs in other compromised individuals. We have recently seen this infection as a complication in the newborn intensive care unit.[38] The mortality due to fungal endocarditis is high even with intensive therapy.[70]

It should be noted that in most series, about 5% of cases of endocarditis are recorded as culture negative. The possible reasons for this are many and are oftentimes related to previous treatment with antibiotics. Occasionally, the percentage of culture-negative cases is larger; in two recent series of postoperative pediatric cases, it was over 20%.[31, 43] The clinician should carefully evaluate such cases for the possibility of other diseases. The infection can be confused with other causes of postoperative fever (e.g., postpericardiotomy syndrome).

It is important to define the bacteria recovered for yet another reason. Antibiotic prophylactic regimens such as those recommended by the American Heart Association[10] have been based upon the frequency with which various organisms are recovered from individuals with endocarditis. The high incidence of viridans streptococci and the paucity of isolation of the gram negative organisms are examples. In addition, staphylococci are frequently recovered from patients developing endocarditis during the perioperative period.

PATHOGENESIS

The many organ systems involved and the multiple forms of involvement of each make endocarditis a fascinating study of pathology. Understanding the pathogenetic mechanisms which vary from aberrations in fluid dynamics, on the one hand, to immune complex formation and organ damage, on the other, is necessary for a comprehensive concept of this infective process. It is beyond the scope of this chapter to completely discuss all aspects, but recent comprehensive discussions are available for those seeking additional information.[64]

In virtually all instances two preexisting conditions must be present for endocarditis to develop. The first is the presence of the infective agent in the blood stream. The second is the presence of an acquired or congenital lesion in the heart or great vessels. In rare instances, endocarditis develops in the absence of cardiovascular abnormalities, but the mechanism(s) in these instances are poorly understood.

When considering the pathogenesis of endocarditis, not

only does one have to consider bacteremia induced by various dental and surgical procedures but also spontaneous bacteremia in individuals with competent host defense mechanisms deserves consideration.[36] Whether this is a common occurrence is not fully known. Even if spontaneous bacteremia occurs, we know little about its significance. It has been shown in animals that large doses of bacteria are frequently needed to colonize vegetations. In humans, it is likely that the dose in spontaneous bacteremia may be too small to lead to implantation of bacteria on cardiac lesions.

The bacteremia associated with various tissue manipulations, including dental and surgical procedures, has been carefully studied. Bacteremia has also been noted to occur with massaging carbuncles or chewing of candy. Almost every dental procedure has been associated with bacteremia. Among the most potentially dangerous inducers of bacteremia is extraction of abscessed teeth. In this instance the percent with subsequent bacteremia may reach 80%. In one study, 155 strains of bacteria were isolated from 100 patients undergoing dental extraction; seven different microorganisms were isolated from the blood of a single patient following tooth extraction.[51]

Careful clinical and pathologic studies of endocarditis have defined the underlying structural cardiac or greater vessel abnormalities which are most frequently the sites of infection. Virtually all vegetation occur in areas where there is a pressure gradient with resulting turbulence of blood flow. The hemodynamic mechanism responsible has been described by Rodbard.[68] Because of the hydrodynamic effect caused by the pressure gradient, turbulence against either the mural endocardium or vascular endothelium results in tissue damage.

Much has been learned about the pathogenesis of the developing nidus of infection by study in experimental animals of nonbacterial thrombotic endocarditis (often referred to as NBTE). By utilization of a polyethylene catheter in the rabbit model of endocarditis, important new data have been collected. Electron microscopic studies have shown that very shortly after the vascular endothelium is injured by the catheter, platelets and fibrin adhere to the site of injury.[9] This meshwork becomes larger and continues to grow with primarily platelets and fibrin; very few leukocytes are involved. Following the initial deposition of platelets and fibrin, thrombus formation occurs. The process is further influenced by the fact that certain bacteria, such as staphylococci and streptococci, which are commonly implicated in endocarditis, are potent stimuli of platelet aggregation.[9] In addition, the lysosomal granules of platelets may release hydrolytic enzymes or other active proteins which may potentiate the process.

Experimental studies show further that it is within this meshwork that circulating microorganisms become entrapped, becoming the nidus of the infection. This usually occurs distal to the pressure gradient. The exception to this is valvular aortic stenosis where the site of the vegetation is usually on the left ventricular side of the aortic valve. One explanation for this finding is the observation that in almost all instances of aortic stenosis there is some aortic insufficiency.

During the subsequent time interval, the original nidus of infection changes in character, depending upon several factors, including the microorganism involved. In what used to be referred to as the subacute form of the disease—the best example of which is caused by viridans streptococci—the large colonies of bacteria become encased in an organizing mass of fibrin. This is of considerable significance because of the effect of the fibrin barrier on two important factors in

defense against infection: the prevention of the invasion by phagocytic leukocytes and the difficulty in perfusion of the vegetation by antimicrobial agents. For reasons that are not fully appreciated, this type of vegetation formation does not frequently occur with some of the more virulent bacteria (best exemplified by *S. aureus*). This infection may be rapidly destructive of the valve or invasive of the myocardium with subsequent abscess formation.

Following successful medical therapy, the cardiac lesions of endocarditis usually heal. Experimental studies in the rabbit suggest that the process is one of endothelialization of the surface, phagocytosis of bacterial debris, sometimes with calcification, and subsequent organization by fibroblasts. Any resulting hemodynamic abnormality depends upon the location and damage caused by the active vegetation and/or abscess.

Physicians sometimes refer to spontaneous healing of endocarditis or to healing of lesions due to coincidental antibiotic therapy received for concomitant minor infections, such as otitis media. Supporting evidence for this concept is not impressive. In fact, a convincing case can be made against the occurrence of spontaneous healing. First, it was documented in the preantibiotic era that endocarditis was virtually 100% fatal. Secondly, from what is known about diffusion of antibiotics across the vegetation, high serum levels are usually required for a prolonged period of time to kill the bacteria and cure the lesions of endocarditis. Adequate therapy for endocarditis is seldom, if ever, given for minor respiratory infections. Finally, there is reason to believe that the healed lesions often described as residual of endocarditis probably represent nonbacterial thrombotic endocarditis (NBTE), which was never colonized by bacteria and which healed by the mechanisms described above.

The immediate consequences of endocarditis, including vegetation formation, hemodynamic alterations, and the clinical syndrome, make up only one part of what is evolving into a complex disease entity. Distal manifestations of the disease were considered to be the results of embolic phenomenon in the past. It is now recognized that other mechanisms are involved in the pathogenesis of endocarditis. One of the most fascinating manifestations of this disease process is the immunologic component.

It has become clear that important extracardiac manifestations in endocarditis are related to immunologic mechanisms.[12] The development of rheumatoid factor in the serum of about half of individuals with endocarditis present for 6 weeks or longer has generally been considered to be related to a gradual hyperimmunization of the host.[57, 77] Supporting evidence comes from reports of correlation of the duration of infection with the presence of rheumatoid factor and also reports that this antiglobulin is more frequently found in individuals with endocarditis due to viridans streptococci than in those due to *S. aureus* infection. This again seems to indicate the duration of the infection. Rheumatoid factor tends to disappear from the sera with successful therapy; this event has been used clinically as a method for following the progress of these patients.[55]

Another advance in our understanding of the immunologic sequelae has been the discovery of circulating immune complexes in the sera of patients with endocarditis.[2] This may not be surprising since there is an extended exposure to a foreign protein, which provides the antigen for production of immune complexes. That these immune complexes are related to the infection is difficult to argue, since they also disappear with successful antimicrobial therapy. However, their precise role in the pathogenetic mechanisms has not been fully defined. There are data, however, demonstrating deposition of immune complexes in renal parenchyma.

The kidney appears to be one of the most frequent extra-cardiac sites affected in patients with endocarditis. In the past, the most frequently described renal lesion has been both microscopic and macroscopic embolic disease. One series[64] reported evidence of this in almost 40% of autopsied cases of left-sided endocarditis. While many are reported to be sterile, abscess formation has been reported following septic embolization to the kidney.

The nephritis of endocarditis may manifest itself microscopically in two forms: a focal glomerulonephritis and a more diffuse form of nephritis.[34, 62] In the focal lesion there is often segmental fibrinoid necrosis of isolated lobules of the glomerular tuft. In the more diffuse form there is marked cellular proliferation with interstitial round cell infiltrates.[62] Immunofluorescent studies have shown granular deposits in the glomerular basement membrane and mesangium, usually associated with complement or IgG deposits, although IgA, IgM and fibrinogen have also been demonstrated. In such instances the urinalysis may be normal, but oftentimes, hematuria cylindruria, and pyuria have been reported. Compromise of renal function is known to occur and it would appear to be more common in adults than in children.

CLINICAL FEATURES

Infective endocarditis simulates a wide variety of diseases, including infectious diseases, malignancies, and connective tissue diseases. It appears in the differential diagnosis of almost any unusual or febrile illness in individuals with heart disease. Many times even a positive blood culture does not clarify the diagnosis; bacteremia or septicemia frequently accompany these other illnesses. Unless the clinician includes endocarditis in the differential diagnosis, the disease may escape detection until the process is far advanced with irreparable damage.

The clinical features differ greatly, depending on the site of the infection. In this regard, the findings may differ in children and in adults since the majority of cases of endocarditis in adults is valvular and since endocarditis in children with congenital heart lesions more often involves the right side of the heart.

In endocarditis involving the left heart, one of the more common findings is peripheral embolization, resulting in ischemia, infarction, or mycotic aneurysms. Specific clinical findings depend upon the localization of the emboli. While the frequency of embolization from endocarditis of the right side may be no less frequent, they likely are unrecognized clinically because of filtering by the lungs. This is not always the case; for example, consider the large infected emboli that may complicate endocarditis of the tricuspid valve in addicts.

Table 36.1 lists the common clinical findings and symptoms seen in individuals with endocarditis; usual laboratory findings are listed at the bottom of the table.

When diligently searched for, new or changing murmurs are almost always present. It may be difficult to recognize these in a patient who has a preexisting cardiac murmur. It is for this reason that frequent auscultation is essential. This is not only to assist with the diagnosis but also to assist with management. For example, increased intensity of aortic insufficiency murmur should warn of the possibility of impending cardiac failure and allow sufficient time to thoroughly discuss this with the cardiovascular surgeon in preparation for aortic valve replacement.

Except in acute endocarditis, where a toxic febrile course is the rule, children presenting with endocarditis due to

TABLE 36.1 MOST FREQUENT CLINICAL AND LABORATORY FINDINGS ASSOCIATED WITH ENDOCARDITIS

Clinical finding	
Fever	++++[a]
Heart murmur (new or changing)	++++
Nonspecific symptoms (myalgia, arthralgia, headache, malaise)	+++/++++
Heart failure	++/+++
Petechiae	+++
Embolic phenomena	++/+++
Splenomegaly	++/+++
Embolic pneumonia	++/+++
Osler nodes, Janeway lesions	+/++
Laboratory finding	
Positive blood culture (off antibiotics)	++++
Positive acute phase reactants	++++
Anemia	+++
Hematuria	+++
Presence of rheumatoid factor	++
Leukocytosis	++

[a] ++++, very common; +++, in a majority of instances; ++, infrequent; +, rare.

viridans streptococci or, in many instances, even the enterococcus, display nonspecific symptoms, including myalgias, arthralgias, headache, and general malaise. In children, there is often a marked diminution in appetite. In infections where viridans streptococci are responsible, the fever may often be low grade with the maximum 39°C. In contrast, for acute endocarditis, such as caused by S. aureus, high spiking fever elevations up to 40°C are common.

Embolic events have been commented upon previously. These are relatively common, especially with involvement of the left side of the heart. Their presence is an important observation, for many clinicians feel that embolic events are indications for cardiovascular surgery. Patients with suspected embolic events also are candidates for serial echocardiography to attempt to localize and define the lesion and the changes which may occur with time. Splenomegaly may be seen in a majority of instances when the disease has been present for weeks or months. Janeway lesions and Osler's nodes are relatively rare in children.

LABORATORY DIAGNOSIS

From the laboratory there is no more valuable aid in making the diagnosis of endocarditis than the blood culture. While it is true that every positive blood culture in a child with underlying or predisposing cardiac disease does not indicate endocarditis, it is imperative that the diagnosis be considered in such patients.

There are two major problems associated with using the blood culture as a diagnostic aid. The first is the frequent problem of previous administration of antibiotics to a patient who later in the clinical course is suspected of having endocarditis. Efforts to either inactivate antibiotics or to absorb them from the sera placed into the culture medium have proven helpful in some instances.[22] For patients suspected of having endocarditis who have been given antibiotics before microorganisms can be isolated and/or identified, it is often useful for the clinician to discuss the problem with the clinical microbiologist, as well as to review the pharmacokinetics of the antibiotic in question. Most clinical microbiology laboratories have their own procedures for handling such specimens. In addition, most will keep the cultures for a longer period of time before discarding them as negative.

The second major problem is associated with the patient with negative blood cultures (who has not received antibiotics), who clinically is suspected of having endocarditis. This presents a dilemma for the clinician. Approximately 5 to 8% of patients in any series with endocarditis are blood culture negative. Many of these individuals will demonstrate subsequent proof of endocarditis, either in the operating room or at necropsy.

The more blood cultures that are obtained, the more likely that one will grow a contaminant. Again, consultation with the clinical microbiology laboratory is indicated. It is not possible to specify the number of cultures that should be taken in each instance, but in this relatively rare situation one must begin either to question the diagnosis or arbitrarily begin therapy after six or eight cultures have been obtained over an appropriate time period. It should always be remembered that one important cause of "culture-negative" endocarditis is nutritionally deficient streptococcal strains (satellite streptococci) that survive only around other bacteria on blood agar.[67] It should also be recalled that blood cultures are only positive in about half of individuals with fungal endocarditis.[76]

While it is not always possible to wait for a positive blood culture in a very ill patient, careful observations and reculture before initiating antibiotic therapy are usually prudent. If only one or two blood cultures are taken, and antimicrobial agents are immediately started, and one culture subsequently grows an organism (which likely represents a contaminant), the clinician is faced with a difficult decision.

Faced with these problems, how should the blood culture be utilized? The bacteremia of endocarditis is continuous.[88, 91] Therefore, it is not necessary to obtain blood cultures only associated with a temperature elevation. Another consideration, especially in pediatrics, is the volume of blood to be collected. There are data to indicate the importance of the volume of blood, especially in instances where there is a low order of magnitude of bacteremia.[88] It is not unusual to recommend collection of 20 to 30 ml of blood from an adult, but this is not possible in a small child. While it is not possible to recommend specific amounts in infants and small children, the clinician should obtain as large a volume as reasonable, using about 10% blood per total volume of the blood culture media.

Data are available which suggest that the collection of two or three sets of blood cultures in a 24-hour period (shorter if the clinical situation dictates it) is adequate. Washington and colleagues[88] were able to show that three blood cultures detected over 97% of cases of bacterial endocarditis. Data are also available that suggest advantages of arterial blood cultures or even bone marrow cultures.[3, 53] While each of these techniques appears to have merit, it is generally agreed that, for most instances, culture of venous blood is sufficient.

With few exceptions, other laboratory tests are not specific for confirming a diagnosis of endocarditis, but they may be helpful in diagnosis and management of patients with this infection. As mentioned previously, about half of individuals with endocarditis will have rheumatoid factor or immune complexes present in their serum.[2, 55] These are not specific for endocarditis but may be helpful in both diagnosis and follow-up.

Acute phase reactants (erythrocyte sedimentation rate or C-reactive protein) are also helpful but in a nonspecific way. The physician must be aware of the fact that it is possible in a patient with very recent onset of the disease to find the sedimentation rate only minimally elevated. As the disease progresses, the value will increase. Another potential pitfall

in the use of the acute phase reactants is related to the fact that the sedimentation rate may remain elevated for a short time, even after documented bacteriologic cure. In order to avoid being misled in such a situation, the clinician should continue to search for evidence that the sedimentation rate is decreasing.

Other blood studies have been used in the diagnosis and management of patients with endocarditis. The value of finding phagocytic reticuloendothelial cells in blood obtained from the lobe of the ear has been commented upon.[15] Abnormal blood gas values, and the presence of inappropriate antidiuretic hormone secretion, have been noted in narcotics addicts with endocarditis who were compared with addicts who do not have the infection.[57, 58] It should be emphasized that all of these represent nonspecific but sometimes helpful findings.

Sophisticated tests for the presence of bacterial antigens have been reported but are not in general use. Example of this are tests for teichoic acid antibody and antibodies to cell wall peptidoglycan in severe staphylococcal infection.[13, 83] Myocardial imaging with gallium-67 or technetium have also been reported to be helpful in diagnosing endocarditis.[66, 95]

One of the frequently used newer advances has been echocardiography. The literature is filled with reports of the use of both M-mode and 2D echo in patients suspected of having this disease.[56, 78, 87] The present consensus regarding the use of echocardiography can best be summarized by stating that if a vegetation is clearly seen, it may be helpful to the clinician. However, if no vegetation is recognized, even after extensive examination, the diagnosis of endocarditis is not necessarily ruled out.

The electrocardiogram is usually not of help either in the diagnosis or localization of endocarditis. There is one important exception to this. In individuals with endocarditis of the aortic valve who show premature ventricular contractions, the association with infection of the noncoronary cusp with tunneling and abscess formation into the adjacent ventricular septum has been noted.

TREATMENT

General Principles

Complete eradication of infecting organisms in patients with endocarditis usually requires weeks of antibiotic therapy. This is not because the bacteria responsible are resistant to the antibiotics, but because within vegetations they are relatively protected from phagocytic and other host defense mechanisms. In addition, very high densities of bacteria are present at these sites.[18] Another factor which potentiates bacterial survival within vegetations involves relatively low rates of bacterial metabolism and cell division with resultant diminished susceptibility to the action of antimicrobial agents.[19]

Parenterally administered antibiotics are recommended because of the desirability of achieving high levels of drug consistently. Intravenous antibiotics are preferred to intramuscular agents because of the lack of muscle mass in small children. Use of heparin lock devices for intravenous therapy in older children and adults facilitates ambulation and activity. Bactericidal antibiotics are greatly preferred over bacteriostatic drugs which have been associated with frequent treatment failures or relapses.[41] When combinations of antibiotics are employed, they should be tested in the laboratory for definite synergistic bactericidal activity (e.g., as demonstrated by penicillin G with streptomycin or gentamicin against enterococci or alpha (viridans) streptococci).[71, 96]

Documentation of termination of bacteremia should be sought early in therapy as a means of measuring the adequacy of the antibiotic regimen. The adequacy of antibiotic therapy of endocarditis should also be monitored by periodic determination of serum bactericidal activity.[92] Peak serum bactericidal levels ≥1:8 are desirable, although the relatively poor standardization of these tests makes interpretation difficult at times unless standardized by the hospital microbiology laboratory.[72] A 1:8 titer has been associated with therapeutic success. Serum peak and trough aminoglycoside levels should be monitored when the agents are used to ensure that levels are adequate and have not reached the toxic range. All patients with endocarditis should have close follow-up, including periodic blood cultures during the first 8 weeks after cessation of treatment, since most relapses will become evident during this period of time.

Except in the rare patient with acute fulminant endocarditis (e.g., S. aureus), it is highly desirable to establish a bacteriologic diagnosis prior to initiation of antibiotic therapy. Failure to make a firm diagnosis of endocarditis or to isolate the infecting microorganisms prior to institution of antibiotics may result in prolonged or unnecessary hospitalization, exposure to iatrogenic and nosocomial hazards and risks of drug toxicity, and possible relapse of infection. Thus, in typical cases of endocarditis with a subacute course (e.g., viridans streptococci), initiation of therapy should be delayed until the diagnosis is secure and the organism has been isolated and identified. In contrast, patients with an acute toxic course should have therapy instituted promptly after blood cultures are obtained.

The role of cardiovascular surgery in the therapy of endocarditis is determined by the site of infection, and the clinical course, especially the hemodynamic status of the patient.[65] Decisions for surgical intervention must be individualized. Two indications for surgery which are almost always agreed upon include the presence of significant embolic events and progressive cardiac failure, especially when the aortic or mitral valve are involved. Clinical experience has proven that medical management of progressive valvular damage and resulting heart failure are suboptimal. It is not necessary or even desirable to complete a full course of antibiotic therapy prior to surgery.

Penicillin-sensitive Streptococcal Endocarditis

Streptococci with minimal inhibitory concentration (MICs) to penicillin ≤ 0.20 μg/ml are considered highly penicillin-sensitive and are the most common organisms causing endocarditis. In children the vast majority of these organisms are α-hemolytic (viridans) streptococci, with the rest being either Streptococcus bovis (nonenterococcal Group D streptococci) more rarely and Group A streptococci (Streptococcus pyogenes). For individuals who are not allergic to penicillin, at least three therapeutic regimens are associated with high cure rates in penicillin-sensitive streptococcal endocarditis: 4 weeks of intravenous penicillin G; 4 weeks of intravenous penicillin G or intramuscular procaine penicillin G together with 2 weeks of a parenteral aminoglycoside; and 2 weeks of intravenous penicillin G in combination with parenteral aminoglycoside. Each of these regimens has certain advantages and disadvantages.

Intravenous aqueous crystalline penicillin G (150,000 units/kg/day administered continuously or divided into six doses) for 4 weeks has been associated with very low relapse rates and avoids exposure to an aminoglycoside.[46] This regimen is preferred for patients with impaired renal function or at risk of aminoglycoside toxicity. Unacceptably high relapse rates have been reported for intravenous penicillin administered alone for 2 or 3 weeks.[35]

Because synergy between penicillin G and aminoglycosides (e.g., gentamicin, streptomycin, amikacin) is readily demonstrated for viridans streptococci and for nonenterococcal Group D organisms[96] and because combinations of penicillin G and an aminoglycoside are superior to penicillin alone in the treatment of experimental endocarditis in the animal model,[72] regimens of 4 weeks of penicillin combined with an aminoglycoside for the first 2 weeks are widely employed. Reported relapse rates are also very low with these regimens.[96] Most published experience with this regimen employ twice daily intramuscular streptomycin (7.5 mg/kg/dose up to 500 mg), rendering it unattractive for treating small children. Regimens of 4 weeks of intravenous penicillin with intravenous gentamicin (2.5 mg/kg/dose up to 80 mg every 8 hours) or amikacin (7.5 mg/kg/dose up to 240 mg, every 8 hours) are more acceptable for children.

Short-term (2-week) combined penicillin and aminoglycoside regimens have become increasingly popular in the treatment of highly penicillin-sensitive streptococcal endocarditis because reported relapse rates have been low and because of the very considerable savings associated with a shortened hospital stay.[93] Experience with 2-week regimens in children is limited, but these regimens appear promising. The Mayo Clinic series of adult patients receiving 2-week treatment with 1.2 million units of intramuscular procaine penicillin G every 6 hours and 500 mg of intramuscular streptomycin every 12 hours includes 124 subjects with penicillin-susceptible streptococcal endocarditis treated from 1970 to 1982 with only one relapse (0.8%).[93] For chidren, intravenous therapy appears preferable to intramuscular; either gentamicin or amikacin is preferred as the aminoglycoside of choice.

Consideration of a 2-week treatment regimen for streptococcal endocarditis should be limited to patients in whom clinical features, as well as characteristics of the bacterial isolate, strongly suggest a favorable outcome. Short-course therapy should not be used for patients infected with a "relatively penicillin-resistant" organism (see below) or a nutritionally deficient viridan streptococcus. Furthermore, it should not be used for patients who have any of the following clinical features: endocarditis of more than 3-months' duration; prosthetic valve infection; shock or decreased perfusion; extracardiac foci of infection; mycotic aneurysm or cerebritis; renal failure; vesticular dysfunction; or presence of vegetation visible by echocardiography. In general, relapses occurring following therapy have been readily detected and responsive to treatment.[93] The majority of such relapses occur within 2 months.

Penicillin-allergic individuals frequently can be desensitized successfully to enable treatment with the drug of choice, penicillin. Effective alternative regimens when penicillin cannot be employed safely include intravenous vancomycin (10 mg/kg up to 500 mg every 6 hours) for 4 weeks or cephalothin (100 to 150 mg/kg/day in four doses) for 4 weeks. Cephalosporins should be used cautiously in highly penicillin-allergic patients. In vitro sensitivity testing of the patient's organism should be performed with these agents before they are used.

"Relatively Penicillin-resistant" Streptococcal Endocarditis

Viridans streptococci with minimum inhibitory concentrations for penicillin ≥ 0.2 μg/ml are occasionally recovered from pediatric patients with endocarditis and are best treated with 4 weeks of combined penicillin and aminoglycoside therapy. Four weeks of vancomycin is a reasonable alternative for penicillin-allergic individuals; there are insufficient clinical data available to determine the advantages of the addition of an aminoglycoside to the latter agent.

Enterococci are fortunately uncommon causes of endocarditis in pediatric patients. Treatment of this infection is difficult, requiring combination therapy of penicillin G or ampicillin with either streptomycin or gentamicin for 4 to 6 weeks.[49] In penicillin-allergic patients who cannot be desensitized, 4 to 6 weeks of vancomycin combined with streptomycin or gentamicin is recommended. Patients receiving these regimens should be closely monitored for renal toxicity and ototoxicity.

Staphylococcal Endocarditis

Because only a small percentage of strains of *S. aureus* associated with endocarditis are penicillin sensitive, antibiotic therapy must include a penicillinase-resistant penicillin (nafcillin, oxacillin, or methicillin) or a cephalosporin (cephalothin or cefazolin) administered intravenously for 4 to 6 weeks. The 6-week regimen is more commonly used and is preferable. Some clinicians have used oral therapy (with careful monitoring of serum levels) during the last several weeks of therapy, but this should be undertaken with extreme caution.[59] In the unusual instance of endocarditis caused by a penicillin-sensitive *S. aureus*, large doses of intravenous penicillin G are indicated, for 4 to 6 weeks.

Data are available to suggest a theoretical advantage of using both an aminoglycoside and one of the penicillin-resistant penicillins. For this reason, a combination of gentamicin and methicillin given for the initial 5 days of therapy, and then completing the course with methacillin alone has been suggested.[72]

Reports have appeared of what has been called antibiotic tolerance. A tolerant organism has been defined as one in which there is a large discrepancy between the MIC (minimal inhibitory concentration) and the MBC (minimal bactericidal concentration). These organisms may be particularly difficult to treat with antibiotics. Successful therapy of tolerant *S. aureus* has been reported with a combination of vancomycin and rifampin, although this remains somewhat controversial.[24] Vancomycin has also been used for methicillin-resistant *S. aureus*.[4]

In the penicillin-allergic individual who cannot be desensitized or in the patient infected with methicillin-resistant *S. aureus* or *S. epidermidis*, intravenous vancomycin administered for 6 weeks is the drug of choice. An alternative for *S. epidermidis* is one of the appropriate cephalosporin antibiotics. Clindamycin has been associated with an unacceptedly high relapse rate and cannot be recommended.

Gram-Negative Endocarditis

Endocarditis caused by an aerobic enteric organism such as *Escherichia coli*, *Pseudomonas aeruginosa*, or *Serratia marcescens* is seen occasionally. Most such patients are intravenous drug abusers, although occasionally a postoperative cardiac patient, an immunocompromised individual or a neonate may develop endocarditis with one of these organisms. Therapy must be individualized and guided by in vitro antimicrobial sensitivity testing. The bulk of the scattered experience has been with carbenicillin or a cephalosporin together with an aminoglycoside such as gentamicin or amikacin.[29] Four to 6 weeks of therapy is recommended.

More common gram-negative bacteria causing endocarditis in children are the group of fastidious gram-negative coccalbacilli including *Haemophilus aphrophilus* and other haemophilus species, *Actinobacillus actinomycetemcomitans*, *Cardiobacterium hominis*, *Eikenella corrodens*, and *Kingella kingii*. These infections have most often been treated with penicillin G or ampicillin, frequently in combination with an aminoglycoside.[89] In this instance, the physician must be guided by the antibiotic sensitivities and by the use of bactericidal antibiotics when possible. Gonococcal endocarditis can be treated successfully with high dose penicillin.

Fungal Endocarditis

Endocarditis due to *Candida* or other fungi is seen in the setting of narcotic abuse, postcardiac surgery, prolonged antibiotic administration, central hyperalimentation, or immunocompromised patients and is associated with very high mortality.[1] Diagnosis is difficult because blood cultures positive for *Candida* do not necessarily indicate the presence of endocarditis, while endocarditis due to other fungi is rarely associated with positive blood cultures and is frequently diagnosed at surgery or autopsy.

Treatment of fungal endocarditis with antifungal agents alone is almost always unsuccessful. Surgical replacement of the infected valve, together with at least 6 weeks of amphotericin B therapy, is usually required. The role of adjunctive therapy with other antifungal agents such as 5-fluorocytosine or ketoconazole has not been clearly defined.[63] Surgery is probably best performed after 1 to 2 weeks of medical therapy if the patient's hemodynamic status permits and if there is no evidence of embolic phenomenon.

Culture-Negative Endocarditis

Therapy for the rare patient believed to have culture-negative endocarditis after careful work-up should include penicillin G or a penicillinase-resistant penicillin (nafcillin or oxacillin) together with streptomycin or gentamicin. For patients who are allergic to penicillin or for those with prosthetic valves, vancomycin with streptomycin or gentamicin should be used. Discontinuation of the aminoglycoside after 2 weeks may be considered if there has been a substantial response to therapy. Treatment should be continued for 6 full weeks.[60]

Prosthetic Valve Endocarditis

Antibiotic therapy for patients with infected prosthetic heart valves must be appropriate for the specific infecting agent and must be administered for at least 4 weeks, with treatment for 6 weeks being usual. For infections with penicillin-sensitive (MIC < 0.1 μg/ml) staphylococci, penicillin G is the preferred agent. Penicillin-resistant staphylococcal infections are treated with nafcillin, oxacillin, or methicillin, or one of these antibiotics in combination with an aminoglycoside. Methicillin-resistant *S. aureus* or *S. epidermidis* infections, or any staphylococcal infection in a penicillin-allergic individual should be treated with intravenous vancomycin 10 mg/kg every 6 hours (not to exceed 500 mg/dose).

Prosthetic valve infections due to highly penicillin-sensitive streptococci (MIC ≤ 0.2 μg/ml) should be treated with 6 weeks of intravenous penicillin and gentamicin, while those caused by "relatively penicillin-resistant" streptococci or enterococci should be treated for up to 8 weeks with the same drugs. For penicillin-allergic individuals who cannot be desensitized, vancomycin in combination with gentamicin or streptomycin is recommended. Prosthetic valve endocarditis caused by diphtheroids is best treated with penicillin and gentamicin, or with vancomycin for penicillin-allergic patients.[84] Therapy for gram-negative bacillary prosthetic valve endocarditis must be based upon the results of in vitro MIC and MBC tests and evaluation of synergy between several antibiotics. Common regimens include cephalothin and gentamicin, and carbenicillin and gentamicin, for at least 6 weeks. The role of newer cephalosporins in these infections remains to be clarified.

Recent experience in adults with prosthetic valve endocarditis has emphasized that early surgical replacement of the infected valve may reduce the excessively high mortality rate associated with such infections.[16] The timing of surgical removal and replacement of an infected prosthetic valve must be individualized; the clinician should establish that operative intervention is necessary but should not delay consideration of surgery in a deteriorating clinical situation until the risk becomes prohibitive. Some authorities recommend that most or all patients with staphylococcal or with early onset prosthetic valve infection should undergo valve replacement. Definite indications for operative intervention include: significant valvular obstruction; progressive heart failure secondary to valvular insufficiency or dehiscence; proved or suspected fungal endocarditis; persistently positive blood cultures after appropriate antibiotics for 10 to 14 days; bacteriologic relapse after an appropriate course of therapy; and recurrent major emboli. Less definite indications for surgery include: a single major embolus; echocardiographic demonstration of a large vegetation; and extension of infection to an annular abscess or myocardial abscess.[16]

PROPHYLAXIS

There are few topics in medicine today which are more controversial than antibiotic prophylaxis for prevention of endocarditis.[5, 48, 61] It is not simply a dispute of the merits of various antimicrobial agents or routes of administration. Because of the lack of adequate controlled studies of the efficacy of this form of antibiotic prophylaxis in the human and the relatively large percentage of cases of endocarditis which are not related to recognized dental or surgical procedures, the question of prophylaxis itself is perpetually on the minds of thoughtful clinicians. Add to these issues the problems which attempt to assign the relative risks to various cardiac lesions or dental or surgical procedures, and the current controversy becomes even more obvious.

If one accepts the necessity for bacteremia to occur to initiate the infection, it is logical then to formulate the concept that prevention of bacteremia is warranted whenever possible. As mentioned previously, prevention of all episodes of bacteremia is practically impossible. However, since certain procedures are known to initiate bacteremia, efforts can be taken to intervene to reduce the risk. Endocarditis prophylaxis with antibiotics is an attempt to reduce the patient's exposure to circulating bacteria in instances when bacteremia is likely to be unavoidable. However, it must be recognized that, practically speaking, there are instances when prevention is impossible.

Data, although indirect in some instances, are available to provide guidelines. These data are derived from several sources: epidemiologic data from reports of series of endocarditis; in vitro laboratory susceptibility testing; and studies in experimental animal models.[17] Detailed reviews of these data are available.[79]

The epidemiologic data provide several reasons for justification. The most obvious of these is the frequency with which specific bacteria are recovered from documented cases of endocarditis. Numerous reports of organisms recovered from patients with endocarditis consistently result in similar lists of bacteria involved.[76] Two species account for the majority of cases: streptococci and staphylococci. This allows the clinician to direct antibiotic prophylaxis against these organisms. Secondly, careful studies have provided at least strong implication of specific procedures for predisposing to endocarditis (for example, dental procedures). These data have then allowed clinical studies to determine the incidence of bacteremia following specific procedures in patients who do not have underlying cardiovascular disease (and thus not being at risk to develop endocarditis). From such controlled studies, the efficacy of antibiotics in preventing bacteremia (not necessarily in preventing endocarditis) can be carried out. For example, the risk of bacteremia following extraction of an abscessed tooth has been shown to be well over 50% in most studies. This risk of bacteremia can be reduced significantly with prophylaxis.[51] On the other hand, other studies have shown that in some instances the risk of bacteremia has been shown to be very small. For example, the risk of bacteremia following simple endotracheal intubation under direct vision (with suctioning) is small, less than 5%.[30] Such instances raise questions about the need for conventional endocarditis prophylaxis for all surgical procedures.

Isolation and identification of organisms from cases of endocarditis has provided the opportunity to study the antibiotic sensitivity patterns in the laboratory. Not only have such strains been tested with single antibiotics, but antibiotic synergy studies have also been performed.

Finally, these two types of data have allowed testing of certain hypotheses in the experimental animal model. While results of efficacy studies in the animal model require extrapolation for practical clinical application, these in vivo studies have provided important information in understanding the prevention of endocarditis.

The discussion of specific lesions and specific dental and surgical procedures should be prefaced with the warning that in all instances, careful thought is required by the physician or dentist. Secondly, it has been shown that prophylaxis failures do occur; these measures are not infallible.[20] For that reason the physician and the dentist must be ever watchful for signs and symptoms compatible with endocarditis, even following prophylaxis.

Table 36.2, modified from the most recent American Heart Association guidelines,[10] lists cardiac lesions for which antibiotic prophylaxis is currently recommended. Almost all congenital or acquired cardiac lesions are included, except secundum atrial septal defect. At the present time almost all repaired or corrected cardiovascular lesions are given prophylaxis after surgery, even though data to support this are

TABLE 36.2 INDICATIONS FOR ANTIBIOTIC PROPHYLAXIS TO PREVENT ENDOCARDITIS[a]

Prosthetic heart valves (high risk)
Rheumatic, calcific, or other acquired valvular heart disease
Structural congenital heart disease except ASD[b]
Idiopathic hypertrophic subaortic stenosis
Mitral valve prolapse syndrome
Postoperative patients (repair or palliation), except ASD and PDA
Unclear but probable
   Ventriculoatrial shunts for hydrocephalus
   Dialysis fistulae and shunts
   Transvenous pacemakers

[a] (Modified and adapted from: The Committee on Prevention of Rheumatic Fever and Bacterial Endocarditis of the American Heart Association.[10])

[b] ASD, atrial septal defect; PDA, patent ductus arteriosus.

less than ideal. Two postoperative states do not require prophylaxis—secundum atrial septal defect repaired without a patch (after 6 months) and patent ductus arteriosus. Three other lesions appear to be at especially high risk. Prosthetic valves are at extremely high risk, and current American Heart Association recommendations suggest parenteral antibiotics to ensure compliance and high levels of antibiotic in the serum at the time of bacteremia. Data from the natural history study of congenital cardiac defects indicate that patients with congenital aortic stenosis are at higher risk after surgery—perhaps due to the influence of resulting aortic insufficiency, which is a common finding.[31] Finally, in a recent evaluation of postoperative risk for endocarditis, the most common lesion among congenital heart disease was in children with systemic artery to pulmonary artery anastomoses.[43]

Antibiotic regimens for various procedures are listed in Table 36.3. The question of oral versus parenteral administration is frequently raised. A majority of authorities feel more comfortable with parenteral antibiotics, especially in high risk lesions or surgical procedures likely to cause a large bacterial dose to enter the bloodstream. However, this is often impractical and represents an added expense and inconvenience for the patient. Clinical judgment must be exercised.

Recent studies have suggested the usefulness of gingival degerming as an adjunct to antibiotic prophylaxis. Cutcher and colleagues,[14] using a phenolated mouthwash, and Scopp and Orvieto,[74] using povidone iodine mouthwash, have presented convincing evidence showing a decrease in bacteremia with tooth extraction following gingival degerming. However, it should be made quite clear that this is only to be used as an adjunct to antibiotics, not instead of antibiotics. It does, however, appear to be logical to consider the use of such agents in the maintenance of healthy oral hygiene in patients who have particular problems (such as adolescents with orthodontic appliances).

One of the most difficult aspects of endocarditis prophylaxis has been the confusion with secondary prophylaxis for prevention of rheumatic fever.[11] Many physicians and dental practitioners believe that simply increasing the dose for rheumatic fever prevention is sufficient for endocarditis prophylaxis. This is not true for several reasons. One reason is the emergence of penicillin-resistant oral streptococci in individuals receiving oral penicillin daily for prevention of rheumatic fever[80]; the other is the fact that adequate antibiotic blood levels are not attained with the small doses given for rheumatic fever prophylaxis.

Maintenance of optimal dental care and hygiene is important for the prevention of endocarditis in children with congenital or rheumatic heart disease. It is particularly important that those patients in whom prosthetic valves or other devices are to be placed undergo needed dental procedures prior to cardiac surgery to establish optimal oral hygiene. In this way, prevention of factors which predispose to prosthetic valve endocarditis can be effected.

Common errors in the use of antibiotics for prevention of endocarditis include: initiation of antibiotics too long before the procedure, prompting the selection of resistant organisms; continuing antibiotics longer than 48 hours after the procedure; using low dose oral antibiotics which result in inadequate serum levels; and failure to use prophylaxis for dental procedures, other than extractions, which are likely to cause gingival bleeding. Parenteral antibiotics should be used in all high risk patients, particularly those with prosthetic valves, and in other patients whenever practical.

Endocarditis prophylaxis is widely used for patients undergoing cardiac surgery with cardiopulmonary bypass to

TABLE 36.3   ANTIBIOTIC PROPHYLAXIS TO PREVENT ENDOCARDITIS[a, b]

I. For Dental, Otolaryngologic, and Bronchoscopic Procedures
  A. Single drug
    1. *Parenteral and oral penicillin*
      Aqueous penicillin G (30,000 units/kg) mixed with *procaine penicillin G* (600,000 units) intramuscularly 30–60 min before procedure followed by *penicillin V* orally 500 mg (250 mg for <60 lbs) every 6 hr for 8 doses.
    2. *Oral penicillin*
      Penicillin V (2.0 gm) orally 30–60 min before procedure and then 500 mg orally every 6 hr for 8 doses (half-doses for children <60 lbs)
    3. *For penicillin-allergic patients*
      a. *Vancomycin* (20 mg/kg) intravenously over 30–60 min beginning 30–60 min before procedure, followed by erythromycin (10 mg/kg) orally every 6 hr for 8 doses. Or
      b. *Erythromycin* (20 mg/kg) orally 1½ to 2 hr prior to procedure, followed by 10 mg/kg every 6 hr for 8 doses.
  B. Two drugs
    1. *Aqueous penicillin G* (30,000/kg) mixed with *Procaine penicillin* (600,000 units) intramuscularly *plus streptomycin* (20 mg/kg) intramuscularly, both given 30–60 min before procedure, followed by *penicillin V* 500 mg orally (250 mg for 60 lbs) every 6 hr for 8 doses.
    2. *For penicillin-allergic patients*
      Vancomycin (20 mg/kg) intravenously over 30–60 min, beginning 30–60 min before procedure followed by *erythromycin* (10 mg/kg) orally every 6 hr for 8 doses.
II. For Genitourinary or Gastrointestinal Tract Procedures
  A. *For nonpenicillin-allergic patient*
    1. *Aqueous penicillin* G (30,000 units/kg) IM or IV
    2. *Ampicillin* (50 mg/kg) IM or IV
                plus
    3. *Gentamicin* (2.0 mg/kg) IM or IV *or*
    4. *Streptomycin* (20 mg/kg) IM. Doses should be given 30–60 min prior to procedure and should be repeated every 8 hr times 2 if gentamicin is used, or every 12 hr times 2 if streptomycin is used.
  B. *For Penicillin-Allergic Patients*
    Vancomycin (20 mg/kg) given IV over 30–60 min beginning 30–60 min before procedure *plus* streptomycin (20 mg/kg) IM 30–60 min before the procedure and repeated once in 12 hr.

[a] (Modified from: The Committee on Prevention of Rheumatic Fever and Bacterial Endocarditis of the American Heart Association (10).)

[b] In no instance should the dose of drugs exceed the adult dosage (aqueous penicillin G, 1,000,000; streptomycin, 1 gm; vancomycin, 1 gm; erythromycin, 1 gm; ampicillin, 1 gm; gentamicin, 80 mg). Doses may need modification for patients with compromised renal function.

prevent perioperative and postoperative endocarditis. This is of particular importance for those undergoing placement of prosthetic valves or other intracardiac prosthetic material. Prominent among the agents which cause early postoperative endocarditis are *S. aureus* and *S. epidermidis*. Therefore, antibiotic prophylaxis at the time of open heart surgery should be directed primarily against these organisms and should be of relatively short duration to minimize the risk of superinfection with resistant organisms.[73] While the choice of antibiotic should be influenced by each individual hospital's sensitivity data, penicillinase-resistant penicillins or cephalosporins are most often utilized. Prophylaxis should be started shortly before the operative procedure and continued for no more than 3 to 5 days postoperatively.

REFERENCES

1. Andriole, V. T., Kravetz, H. M., Roberts, W. C., and Utz, J. P. *Candida* endocarditis. Am. J. Med. 32:251, 1962.
2. Bayer, A. S., Theofilopolos, A. N., Eisenberg, R., Dixon, F. J., and Guze, L. B. Circulating immune complexes in infective endocarditis. N. Engl. J. Med. 295:1500, 1976.
3. Beeson, P. B., Brannon, E. S., and Warren, J. V. Observations on the sites of removal of bacteria from the blood in patients with bacterial endocarditis. J. Exp. Med. 81:9, 1945.
4. Benner, E. J., and Morthland, V.: Methicillin-resistant *Staphylococcus aureus:* Antimicrobial susceptibility. N. Engl. J. Med. 277:678-680, 1967.
5. Bisno, A. L.: Antimicrobial prophylaxis of infective endocarditis. In Treatment of Infective Endocarditis, edited by A. L. Bisno. Grune & Stratton, New York, 1981, p. 281.
6. Bisno, A. L.: Antimicrobial prophylaxis of infective endocarditis. In Treatment of Infective Endocarditis, edited by A. L. Bisno. Grune & Stratton, New York, 1981.
7. Bleiden, L. C., Morhead, R. R., Burke, B., and Kaplan, E. L.: Bacterial endocarditis in the neonate. Am. J. Dis. Child. 124:747, 1972.
8. Blumenthal, S., Griffith, S. P., and Morgan, B. C.: Bacterial endocarditis in children with heart disease. A review based on the literature and experience with 58 cases. Pediatrics 26:993, 1960.
9. Clawson, C. C.: Role of platelets in the pathogenesis of endocarditis. In Infective Endocarditis: An American Heart Association Symposium, edited by E. L. Kaplan and A. V. Taranta. American Heart Association, Dallas, Texas, 1977, p. 24.
10. Committee on Prevention of Rheumatic Fever and Bacterial Endocarditis of the American Heart Association: Prevention of bacterial endocarditis. Circulation 56:139A, 1977.
11. Committee on Prevention of Rheumatic Fever and Bacterial Endocarditis of the American Heart Association: Prevention of rheumatic fever. Circulation 55:1, 1977.
12. Cordeiro A., Costa H., and Laginha F.: Immunologic phase of subacute bacterial endocarditis. A new concept and consideration. Am. J. Cardiol. 16:477, 1965.
13. Crowder J. C., and White A.: Teichoic acid antibodies in staphylococcal and nonstaphylococcal endocarditis. Ann. Intern. Med. 77:87, 1972.
14. Cutcher J. L., Goldberg, J. R., Lilly, G. E., and Jones, J. C.: Control of bacteremia associated with extraction of teeth. II. Oral Surg. 31:602, 1971.
15. Daland, G. A., Gottlieb, L., Wallerstein, R. O., and Castle, W. B.: Hematologic observations in bacterial endocarditis, especially the prevalence of histiocytes and the elevation and variation of the white cell count in blood from the earlobe. J. Lab. Clin. Med. 48:827, 1956.
16. Dismukes, W. E.: Prosthetic valve endocarditis: Factors influencing outcome and recommendations for therapy. In Treatment of Infective Endocarditis, edited by A. L. Bisno. Grune & Stratton, New York, 1981, p. 167.
17. Durack, D. T.: Experience with prevention of experimental endocarditis. In Infective Endocarditis: An American Heart Association Symposium, edited by E. L. Kaplan and A. V. Taranta, American Heart Association, Dallas, Texas, 1977, p. 28.
18. Durack, D. T., and Beeson, P. B.: Experimental bacterial endocarditis. I. Colonization of a sterile vegetation. Br. J. Exp. Pathol. 53:44-49, 1972.
19. Durack, D. T., and Beeson, P. B.: Experimental bacterial endocarditis. II. Survival of bacteria in endocardial vegetations. Br. J. Exp. Pathol. 53:50-53, 1972.
20. Durack, D. T., Kaplan, E. L., and Bisno, A. L.:

Twenty-five cases of apparent endocarditis prophylaxis failure: Results of a national survey. Clin. Res. 15:615, 1981.
21. Durack, D. T., and Petersdorf, R. G.: Changes in the epidemiology of endocarditis. In Infective Endocarditis: An American Heart Association Symposium, edited by E. L. Kaplan and A. V. Taranta. American Heart Association, Dallas, Texas, 1977, p. 3.
22. Dowling, H. F., and Hirsh, H. L.: The use of penicillinase in cultures of body fluids obtained from patients under treatment with penicillin. Am. J. Med. Science 210:756, 1945.
23. Edis, B., and Venables, A.: Unpublished observations.
24. Faville, R. J., Zaske, D. E., Kaplan, E. L., Crossley, K., Sabath, L. D., and Quie, P. G. *Staphylococcus aureus* endocarditis. Combined therapy with vancomycin and rifampin. J.A.M.A. 240:1963, 1978.
25. Fekety, F. R.: Staphylococcal bacteremia and endocarditis. In Textbook of Medicine, 14th ed., edited by P. B. Beeson and W. McDermott. W. B. Saunders, Philadelphia, 1975, p. 323.
26. Felner, J. M., and Dowell, V. R. Jr.: Anaerobic bacterial endocarditis. N. Engl. J. Med. 283:1188, 1970.
27. Foster, F. E.: Infective prosthetic valve endocarditis. In Infective Endocarditis, edited by S. H. Rahimtoola. Grune & Stratton, New York, 1978, p. 291.
28. Garrison, P. K., and Freedman, L. R.: Experimental endocarditis. I. Staphylococcal endocarditis in rabbits resulting from placement of polyethylene catheter on the right side of the heart. Yale J. Biol. Med. 42:394, 1970.
29. Geraci, J. E., and Wilson, W. R.: Endocarditis due to gram-negative bacteria: Report of 56 cases. Mayo Clinic Proc. 57:145, 1982.
30. Gerber, M. A., Gastanaduy, A., Buckley, J., and Kaplan, E. L.: The risk of bacteremia following endotracheal intubation for general anesthesia. South Med. J. 73:1428, 1980.
31. Gersony, W. M., and Hayes, C. J.: Bacterial endocarditis in patients with pulmonary stenosis, aortic stenosis, or ventricular septal defect. Circulation 56(Suppl. I):84, 1977.
32. Gould, K., Ramirez-Ronda, C. H., Holmes, R. K., and Sanford, J. P. Adherence of bacteria to heart valves in vitro. J. Clin. Invest. 56:1364, 1975.
33. Gulmen, S., and Anderson, W. R.: *Candida* endocarditis with distal aortic embolization. Minn. Med. 60:469, 1977.
34. Gutman, R. A., Striker, G. E., Gilliland, B. C., and Cutler, R. E.: The immune complex glomerulonephritis of bacterial endocarditis. Medicine 51:1, 1972.
35. Hamburger, M., and Stein, L.: *Streptococcus viridans* subacute bacterial endocarditis: Two week treatment schedule with penicillin. J.A.M.A. 149:542-545, 1952.
36. Hockett, R. N., Loesche, W. J., and Sodeman, T. M.: Bacteremia in asymptomatic individuals. Arch. Oral Biol. 22:451, 1977.
37. Johnson, C. M., and Rhodes, K. H.: Pediatric endocarditis. Mayo Clinic Proc. 57:86, 1982.
38. Johnson, D. E., Bass, J. L., Thompson, T. R., Foker, J. E., Speert, D. P., and Kaplan, E. L.: *Candida* septicemia and a right atrial mass in infancy secondary to umbilical vein catheterization. Am. J. Dis. Child 135:275, 1981.
39. Johnson, D. H., Rosenthal, A., and Nadas, A. S.: A forty-year review of bacterial endocarditis in infancy and childhood. Circulation 51:581, 1979.
40. Johnson, W. D., Jr.: Prosthetic valve endocarditis. In Infective Endocarditis, edited by D. Kaye. University Park Press, Baltimore, Md., 1976, p. 29.
41. Kane, L. W., and Finn, J. J.: The treatment of subacute bacterial endocarditis with aureo-

mycin and chloromycetin. N. Engl. J. Med. 244:623, 1951.
42. Kaplan, E. L.: Infective endocarditis in the pediatric age group. An overview. In Infective Endocarditis: An American Heart Association Symposium, edited by E. L. Kaplan and A. V. Taranta. American Heart Association, Dallax, Texas, 1976, p. 51.
43. Kaplan, E. L., Rich, H., Gersony, W., and Manning, J.: A collaborative study of infective endocarditis in the 1970's. Emphasis on infections in patients who have undergone cardiovascular surgery. Circulation 59:327, 1979.
44. Kaplan, E. L., and Taranta, A. V. (eds.): Infective Endocarditis Symposium. American Heart Association, Dallas, Texas, 1976.
45. Karchmer, A. W.: Issues in the treatment of endocarditis caused by viridans streptococci. In Treatment of Infective Endocarditis, edited by A. L. Bisno. Grune & Stratton, New York, 1981, p.31.
46. Karchmer, A. W., Moellering, R. C. Jr, Maki, D. G., and Swartz, M. N.: Single-antibiotic therapy for streptococcal endocarditis. J.A.M.A. 241:1801-1806, 1979.
47. Kaye, D., (ed.): Infective Endocarditis. University Park Press, Baltimore, Md., 1976.
48. Kaye, D.: Prophylaxis against bacterial endocarditis: A dilemma. In Infective Endocarditis: An American Heart Association Symposium, edited by E. L. Kaplan and A. V., Taranta. American Heart Association, Dallas, Texas, 1977, p. 67.
49. Kaye, D.: Treatment of enterococcal endocarditis in experimental animals and man. In Treatment of Infective Endocarditis, edited by A. L. Bisno. Grune & Stratton, New York, 1981, p. 97.
50. Kerr, A. Jr.: Subacute bacterial endocarditis. Charles C Thomas, Springfield, Ill., 1955.
51. Khairat, O.: An effective antibiotic cover for the prevention of endocarditis following dental and other postoperative bacteremias. J. Clin. Pathol. 19:561, 1961.
52. Lerner, P. I., and Weinstein, L.: Infective endocarditis in the antibiotic era. New Engl. J. Med. 274:199, 259, 323, 388, 1966.
53. Mallen, M. S., Hube, E. L., and Brenes, M.: Comparative studies of blood cultures made from artery, vein and bone marrow of patients with subacute bacterial endocarditis. Am. Heart J. 33:692, 1947.
54. McCauley, D.: Acute endocarditis in infancy and early childhood. Am. J. Dis. Child 88:715, 1954.
55. Messner, R. P., Laxdal, T., Quie, P. G., and Williams, R.: Rheumatoid factors in subacute bacterial endocarditis—Bacterium, duration of disease or genetic predisposition? Ann. Intern. Med. 68:746, 1968.
56. Mintz, G. S., Kotler, M. N., Segal, B. L., and Parry, W. R.: Comparison of two-dimensional and M-mode echocardiography in the evaluation of patients with infective endocarditis. Am. J. Cardiol 43:738, 1979.
57. Ogbuawa, O., Singleton, G., Williams, J. T., Henry, W. L., and Towsend, J. L.: Blood chemistry abnormalities in bacterial endocarditis of narcotics addicts. South. Med. J. 71:1526, 1978.
58. Ogbuawa, O., and Towsend, J. L.: Bacterial endocarditis in narcotic addicts: Analysis of arterial blood gases. South Med. J. 71:813, 1978.
59. Parker, R. H., and Fossieck, B. E., Jr.: Intravenous followed by oral antimicrobial therapy for staphylococcal endocarditis. Ann. Intern. Med. 93:832-834, 1980.
60. Pesanti, E. L., and Smith, I. M.: Infective endocarditis with negative blood cultures: An anslysis of 52 cases. Am. J. Med. 66:43, 1979.

61. Petersdorf, R. G.: Antimicrobial prophylaxis of bacterial endocarditis: Prudent caution or bacterial overkill? Am. J. Med. 65:220, 1978.

62. Porter, G. A., Bennett, W. M., and Wilson, J. W.: Renal consequences of valvular heart disease. Am. J. Cardiol. 35:886, 1975.

63. Rahal, J. J., Jr., and Simberkoff, M. S.: Treatment of fungal endocarditis. In Treatment of Infective Endocarditis, edited by A. L. Bisno. Grune & Stratton, New York, 1981, p.135.

64. Rahimtoola, S. H. (ed.): Infective Endocarditis. Clinical Cardiology Monographs. Grune & Stratton, New York, 1978.

65. Reitz, B. A., Baumgartner, W. A., Oyer, P. E., and Stinson, E. B.: Surgical treatment of infective endocarditis. In Treatment of Infective Endocarditis, edited by A. L. Bisno. Grune & Stratton, New York, 1981.

66. Riba, A. L., Downs, J., Thakur, M. L., Gottschalk, A., Andriole, V. T., and Zaret, B. L.: Technetium-99m stannous pyrophosphate imaging of experimental infective endocarditis. Circulation 58:111, 1978.

67. Roberts, K. B., and Sidlak, M. J.: Satellite streptococci. A major cause of negative blood cultures in bacterial endocarditis? J.A.M.A. 241:2293, 1979.

68. Rodbard, S.: Blood velocity and endocarditis. Circulation 27:18, 1963.

69. Rosenthal, A., and Nadas, A. S.: Infective endocarditis in infancy and childhood. In Infective Endocarditis, edited by S. H. Rahimtoola. Grune & Stratton, New York, 1978, p. 149.

70. Rubinstein, E., Noriega, E.R., Simberkoff, M. S., Holzman, R., Rahal, J. J., Jr.: Fungal endocarditis: Analysis of twenty-four cases and review of the literature. Medicine 54:331, 1975.

71. Sande, M. A., and Irvin, R. G.: Penicillin-aminoglycoside synergy in experimental *Streptococcus viridans* endocarditis. J. Infect. Dis. 129:572–576, 1974.

72. Sande, M. A., and Scheld, W. M.: Combination antibiotic therapy of bacterial endocarditis. Am. Intern. Med. 92:390, 1980.

73. Sanford, J. P.: Prophylactic use of antibiotics: Basic considerations. South Med. J. 70(Suppl. 1):2, 1977.

74. Scopp, I. W., and Orvieto, L. D.: Gingival degerming by povidone-iodine irrigation: Bacteremia reduction in extraction procedures. J. Am. Dent. Assoc. 83:1294, 1971.

75. Seelig, M. S., Goldberg, P., Kozinn, P. J., and Berger, A. R.: Fungal endocarditis: Patients at risk and their treatment. Postgrad. Med. J. 55:632, 1979.

76. Seelig, M. S., Speth, C. T., Kozinn, P. J., Toni, E. F., and Taschdjian, C. L.: *Candida* endocarditis after cardiac surgery: Clues to earlier detection. J. Thorac. Cardiovasc. Surg. 65:573, 1973.

77. Sheagren, J. N., Tuazon, C. U., Griffin, C., and Padmore, N.: Rheumatoid factor in acute bacterial endocarditis. Arthritis Rheum 19:887, 1976.

78. Sheikh, M. U., Covearrubias, E. A., Ali, N., Lee, W. R., Sheikh, N. M., and Roberts, W. C.: M-mode echocardiographic observations during and after healing of active bacterial endocarditis limited to the mitral valve. Am. Heart J. 101:37, 1981.

79. Sipes, J. N., Thompson, R. L., and Hook, E. W.: Prophylaxis of infective endocarditis: A reevaluation. Annu. Rev. Med. 28:371, 1977.

80. Sprunt, K., Redman, W., Leidy, G.: Penicillin resistant alpha streptococci in the pharynx of patients given oral penicillin. Pediatrics 42:957, 1968.

81. Starkebaum, M., Durack, D., and Beeson, P.: The "incubation period" of subacute bacterial endocarditis. Yale J. Biol. Med. 50:49, 1977.

82. Stimmel, B., and Dack, S.: Infective endocarditis in narcotic addicts. In Infective Endocarditis, edited by S. P. Rahimtoola. Grune & Stratton, New York, 1978, p. 195.

83. Tuazon, C. U., and Sheagren, J. N.: Teichoic acid antibodies in the diagnosis of serious infections with *Staphylococcus aureus*. Ann. Intern. Med. 84:543, 1976.

84. Van Scoy, R. E., Cohen, S. N., Geraci, J. E., *et al.*: Coryneform bacterial endocarditis. Mayo Clin. Proc. 52:216–219, 1977.

85. Verbrugh, H. A., Peters, R., Rozenberg-Arska, M., Peterson, P. K., and Verhoef, J.: Antibodies to cell wall peptidoglycan of *Staphylococcus aureus* in patients with serious staphylococcal infections. J. Infect. Dis. 144:1, 1981.

86. Von Reyn, C. F., Levi, B. S., Arbeit, R. D., Friedland, G., and Crumpacker, C. S.: Infective endocarditis: An analysis based on strict case definitions. Ann. Intern. Med. 94:505, 1981.

87. Wann, L. S., Hallam, C. C., Dillon, J. C., Weiman, A. E., and Feigenbaum, H.: Comparison of M-mode and cross-sectional echocardiography in infective endocarditis. Circulation 60:728, 1979.

88. Washington, J. A., II: Blood cultures: Principles and techniques. Mayo Clinic Proc. 50:91, 1975.

89. Watanakunakorn, C.: Antimicrobial therapy of endocarditis due to less common bacteria. In Treatment of Infective Endocarditis, edited by A. L. Bisno. Grune & Stratton, New York, 1981, p. 123.

90. Weinstein, L., and Rubin, R. H.: Infective endocarditis—1973. Prog. Cardiovasc. Dis. 16:239, 1973.

91. Werner, A. S., Cobbs, C. G., Kaye, D., and Hook, E. W.: Studies on the bacteremia of bacterial endocarditis. J.A.M.A. 202:127, 1967.

92. Williams, T. W., Jr, Viroslav, J., and Knight, V.: Management of bacterial endocarditis—1970. Am. J. Cardiol. 26:186, 1970.

93. Wilson, W. R., and Thompson, R. L.: Short-term therapy for streptococcal infective endocarditis: Combined intramuscular administration of penicillin and streptomycin. J.A.M.A. 245:360–363, 1981.

94. Wilson, W. R., Giuliani, E. R., Danielson, G. K., and Geraci, J. E.: General considerations in the diagnosis and treatment of infective endocarditis. Mayo Clinic Proc. 57:81, 1982.

95. Wiseman, J., Rouleau, J., Rigo, P., Strauss, H. W., and Pitt, B.: Gallium-67 myocardial imaging for the detection of bacterial endocarditis. Radiology 120:135, 1976.

96. Wolfe, J. C., and Johnson, W. D., Jr.: Penicillin-sensitive streptococcal endocarditis. *In vitro* and clinical observations on penicillin-streptomycin therapy. Ann. Intern. Med. 81:178–181, 1974.

97. Zakrzewski, T., and Keith, J. D.: Bacterial endocarditis in infants and children. J. Pediatr. 67:1179, 1975.

37

Nonrheumatic Inflammatory Diseases

George R. Noren, M.D., Edward L. Kaplan, M.D., and Nancy A. Staley, M.D.

In recent years, accumulated evidence has shown that nonrheumatic inflammatory disease of the heart is much more prevalent in children than was previously appreciated. However, because of the wide spectrum of clinical presentations and difficulty in establishing a rapid, definitive diagnosis without the use of invasive techniques, inflammatory cardiac disease remains as a rarely reported clinical event. Necropsy and animal data provide most of our current information.

Inflammatory diseases of the heart are rarely limited to the pericardium, myocardium, or endocardium alone. Pancarditis is the more frequent occurrence.[15, 209] However, for ease of presentation, this chapter will be arbitrarily divided into the inflammatory diseases of the pericardium and the myocardium. Endocarditis is discussed in Chapter 36.

INFECTIOUS MYOCARDITIS

Extensive reviews of myocarditis by Wegner[205] and by Abelman *et al.*[2, 3, 4] outline most known etiologic agents responsible for the production of myocarditis: bacteria, spirochetes, Rickettsia, virus, fungus, protozoa, and helminths. However, because of the very nature of the above etiologic agents, the symptoms and signs of myocarditis are often difficult to recognize. Not only may the infection be mild or subclinical and so temporally removed from the initial phase of the infection, it is often masked by the more overt signs and symptoms of the other organ involvement.

The prevalence of myocarditis in any given population is unknown, and occurrence rates must be generalized by retrospective reviews of necropsy material. In a review of 40,000 autopsies, Gore and Saphir[73] identified 1402 cases of myocarditis for an overall prevalence of 3.5%. Seventy cases were associated with viral illness, and an additional 80 cases of isolated myocarditis were presumed to have been of viral etiology, providing a maximal autopsy diagnosis of viral myocarditis of 0.38%.

Gormsen[75] reported only 17 cases of myocarditis among 1378 cases of sudden unexpected death, but histologic examination had been carried out in only 117 cases. Recent data from Stevens[191] suggest that asymptomatic focal myocarditis in British males, age 18 to 50 years, may be as high as 5%.

Our own 3-year review of pediatric cases submitted to a large medical examiner's office revealed a slightly different frequency of histologic myocarditis.[140] Of a total of 6582 cases, 353, or 5.2%, involved children through the age of 16 years. Sudden death accounted for 329 cases, 214 of which were violent and 115 of which were unexpected by history. Myocardial tissue was available for histologic examination in 90 of the 115 sudden unexpected deaths, and 48 of the 214 violent deaths. Myocarditis was present in 15 of the 90 sudden unexpected deaths, or 17%, while only 2 of 48 dying from accidents, suicide, or homicide demonstrated histologic myocarditis, or 4%. Eight of the cases with myocarditis in the sudden unexpected death group appeared in the birth to 1 year old age group, while seven were over 1 year of age. Both of the cases with myocarditis in the violent death group were over 1 year of age.

In recent years many cases of acute myocarditis appear to have a viral etiology and occur in conjunction with other organ involvement which may be the primary clinical feature.[65] Viral agents which have been implicated in myocarditis are numerous. The most predominant ones are Coxsackie A and B, influenza, ECHO, mumps, and rubella. Grist and Bell[77] in their review of 385 patients with suspected heart disease, determined that the Coxsackie group B virus infections were associated with at least one-half of the cases of acute myocarditis. In addition, Burch and co-workers[30] found evidence of Coxsackie B antigen in the myocardium, by immunofluorescent techniques, in 30.9% of routine autopsy specimens and in 29 of 50 hearts of children examined at necropsy, with types B_3 and B_5 being the most frequently identified.[29] Helin et al.[88] reports a 33% frequency of myocardial involvement in clinical Coxsackie B_1 infections, while Kitaura and Morita[112] found evidence of cardiac involvement in 49 of 263 children infected with Coxsackie B_3.

Hackel[80] first described focal myocarditis in seven cases of varicella. His report was followed by a review by Tobin[199] of 34 cases of fatal varicella infection in which 20 cases had microscopic material available for evaluation. He found that 10 of 20 cases had microscopic evidence of myopericarditis. In none of these 10 cases was myocarditis recognized prior to death. Sixteen of the 20 had pneumonitis, and of those 16, 6 had cardiac involvement. Three had additional central nervous system involvement and two had myocarditis alone without other histologic evidence of pathology.

In 102 cases of congestive cardiomyopathy, infection by influenza A was proven in 14. Coxsackie B, infectious mononucleosis, and infectious hepatitis viruses were also implicated in this series by Hall.[84] In addition, the ECHO viruses are also prominently associated with cardiac disease.[16, 47, 120] Focal interstitial myocarditis is reported to occur in 43.5% of necropsied cases of human rabies,[7] 40% in fatal poliomyelitis,[123] while 7 of 16 cases of Naegleria showed either diffuse or focal myocarditis, with myocardial necrosis present in two.[125]

As previously stated, myocarditis has been produced by almost all agents known to afflict mankind, and the bulk of myocardial inflammatory disease remains submerged through the more overt expression of the infectious process. Reports of the prevalence of myocarditis associated with additional pathogens are few but do give some insight into the "iceberg" phenomenon of this disease.[73, 87, 162]

From the foregoing discussion it becomes apparent that the conflicting data concerning the incidence of myocarditis in the general population is in part due to the inability of the clinician or pathologist to define the subclinical case and also to the difficulty in carrying out a well-controlled prospective study with the limited diagnostic tools which are presently available.

PATHOLOGY

Gross

At necropsy, the heart may display as great a spectrum of findings as the clinical presentations of inflammatory myocarditis. At one end is an entirely normal-appearing heart, particularly if death has occurred in the acute stage of the disease. A more frequent finding in viral myocarditis is a dilated heart with little or no hypertrophy (dilatation is general with evidence of atrial ventricular valve insufficiency, particularly of the mitral valve). The myocardium appears flabby to the touch and may have a slightly pale appearance on the cut surface. At the other end of the spectrum is a dilated heart in association with varying degrees of left ventricular hypertrophy and endocardial thickening. The mitral valve leaflets may be rolled and their chordae may be thickened, and they may have a foreshortened appearance. Gross scarring may be seen on cut section of the ventricular myocardium.[9, 74, 95, 144, 166]

In the hypereosinophilic syndrome of Löffler's endocarditis, the heart is generally enlarged with 41% of cases showing mural thrombi in the ventricles.[24, 40] Eighteen percent have valvular damage, usually mitral, and myocardial fibrosis is present in 15%.

Myocardial abscesses are seen with bacterial myocarditis, particularly with gram-positive cocci. Caseous nodules may be present in association with tuberculous myocarditis.[74, 95, 205] Petechiae and occasionally gross hemorrhage are seen in meningococcemia.[166, 205] Mycotic myocarditis frequently will demonstrate fibrocaseous abscesses, focal granulomas, or vegetations, while most protozoal lesions are evident only on microscopic examination.[65, 95, 205] Echinococcus demonstrates varying sized cysts within the myocardium, and in ascariasis abscess formation is present.[74, 205]

Microscopic

Myocarditis may be defined as an inflammatory lesion characterized by cellular infiltrate that is usually predominantly mononuclear. The infiltrates are often present in the perivascular area. Lesions are focal or diffuse or may show predilection for the subendocardial or subepicardial regions. Myocytolysis and necrosis are varied and are dependent on the agent involved (Figs. 37.1 and 37.2). The subepicardial lesions often are associated with pericarditis. Of considerable import is the fact that lesions are not usually limited to the interstitium and muscle but may also involve specialized tissue such as the conduction system.[73, 74, 95, 115, 166, 205] Therefore, the location, as well as the extent of the lesion, will be the determinant of functional impairment or clinical manifestations.[74, 174]

Stevens and Underwood Ground[191] have defined myocarditis as a single, focal inflammatory infiltrate of approximately 100 cells or more in the absence of ischemia. Lesions about one-half of that number are acceptable if additional

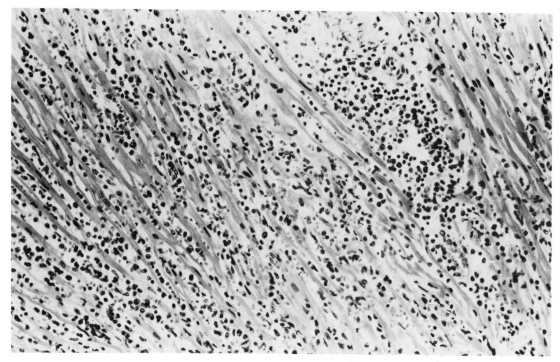

Fig. 37.1 Myocardium from a 7-year-old who, during an influenza A$_2$ virus epidemic, developed symptoms compatible with that disease. The child died suddenly at home 3 weeks following the onset of the "flu." Section demonstrates an intense infiltrate of eosinophiles and mononuclear cells. (Hematoxylin and eosin stain; original magnification, ×423).

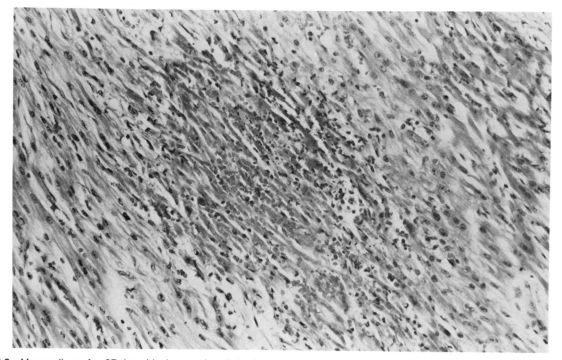

Fig. 37.2 Myocardium of a 27-day-old who was found dead in her crib. Section demonstrates a focal area of mononuclear infiltrate associated with myocytolysis, as is often observed in Coxsackie myocarditis. (Hematoxylin and eosin stain; original magnification, ×424).

foci can be found in other portions of the myocardium. These rigid criteria of Stevens' may produce false negative histologic diagnoses of viral myocarditis in some instances, particularly when only a few myocardial sections are available for study. In fact, Miranda *et al.*,[133] in their study of Coxsackie B$_5$ infection in mice, showed that despite a mortality rate of more than 50% at 4 weeks and approximately 70% at 12 weeks, histologic examination of the heart in these

animals revealed very small foci of necrosis involving only two or three muscle fibers at 3 days following inoculation, with very sparse or no cellular infiltration. Areas of necrosis increased in size and number but never involved more than 12 or 15 fibers. Cellular infiltration gradually increased with time and consisted almost entirely of mononuclear cells. By 15 days after inoculation, the necrotic muscle was being resorbed, lesions were reduced in size, and fibrous tissue appeared. Fibrous scars of varying size were still present at 270 days. Similar findings in mice infected with Coxsackie A and B virus have also been observed by Feinstone et al.[54] and Wilson et al.[207] (Fig. 37.3).

Diphtheria toxin frequently produces fatty changes with myocytolysis observed in the most severely affected heart.[74, 95] The interstitial exudate is predominantly of histiocytes, plasma cells, and lymphocytes. Marked distortion of mitochondria is also seen.[31] Fibrosis occurs by the end of the third week.[74] Fatty changes are also seen in *Salmonella* and *Clostridium* infections associated with varying degrees of cellular infiltrate.[74, 205] Leptospirosis is characterized by focal hemorrhage and edema with mononuclear infiltrate most prominently observed in the subendocardial area, conduction tissue, and papillary muscles.[74, 205]

Rickettsial lesions are somewhat nonspecific as in viral myocarditis but tend to produce more vasculitis with perivascular infiltrate.[74] Gore and Saphir[73] found evidence of myocarditis in 100% of 277 cases of scrub typhus and approximately 50% of 59 cases of epidemic typhus and 19 cases of Rocky Mountain spotted fever.

Mycotic myocarditis can usually be characterized by the observations of the etiologic agent in abscesses, granulomas, macrophages, or free in the myocardium. These findings are in association with the nonspecific changes of myocardial damage.[95, 205] Protozoal and helminthic myocarditis will also occasionally reveal the agent responsible on microscopic examination of the myocardium.[74, 95, 205]

PATHOGENESIS

Difficulties confronting the pathologist in elucidating the spectrum of myocarditis in man stem from the difficulty in identifying the virus involved and the frequent absence of significant histologic findings. As is known from experimental myocarditis in animals, viral cultures obtained at the time of death may be unrewarding unless appropriate cultures are collected during the early stages of the disease.[117, 133, 194] Adding to this logistics problem is the fact that in experimental animals, virus has been shown to replicate in cardiac tissue without clinical or light microscopic abnormalities.[131]

Sohal and Burch[181] have demonstrated in hearts of mice infected with Coxsackie B_4 virus that ultrastructural changes in the myocardial cell occur secondary to the viremia. These changes include cellular shedding, membrane vesicle complex formation, disappearance of Golgi bodies, nuclear shrinkage, disintegration of mitochondria, and increase in ribosomal population. Haas and Yunis,[79] however, have postulated that viral replication with Coxsackie virus occurs within endothelial cells and that endothelial infection occurs before myocardial damage. In their studies, the least altered myocardial fibers exhibited swelling of mitochondria with distortion of cristae and distention of sarcoplasmic reticulum. In the more obvious damaged areas, myofibril architecture was focally or diffusely affected, and myofibril collapse gave the impression of an excessive number of mitochondria. In addition, they felt that the phenomenon of damage ascribed by Rabin et al.[154] to the viral multiplication within myocytes has not been established and perhaps should not be equated with intracellular localization of viral antigen. Rabin also points out that the mitochondria swelling and distention of sarcoplasmic reticulum are similar to changes produced by ischemia, and that these alterations may be secondary to a single pattern of myocardial response to a variety of injurious agents. Nemetsehek–Gansler et al.[137] also suggest that Coxsackie B_1 virus affects newborn mice not by direct damage of heart muscle cells but by disturbance of myocardial circulation by aggregation of platelets.

The extensive studies of mumps myocarditis by St. Geme and co-workers[185, 186] have shown that the mumps virus can be isolated from the heart for a brief period of time in the

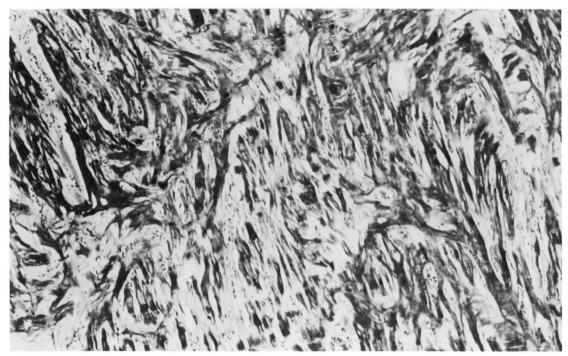

Fig. 37.3 Myocardium of a 15-year-old boy who developed a "sore throat" 4 weeks prior to dying suddenly at school. Section is representative of the generalized fibrosis and loss of cellular architecture that was present in both ventricular myocardia. Neutralizing antibody titres to Coxsackie B_4 were 1:32 in the 19 S fraction and 1:128 in the 7 S fraction. (Hematoxylin and eosin stain; original magnification, ×425).

hatchling chick following early embryonic inoculation of the virus. Although the organism can be recovered from all organs, the highest titres of virus are found within the heart. Gradual development of a lymphocytic inflammatory reaction in the heart occurs a few days prior to hatch and begins to subside within a week after hatch. Development of endocardial thickening is evident 1 year later. These workers have also demonstrated that chicken embryonic heart tissue is highly susceptible to mumps virus in vitro, as cultivated embryonic heart cells produce 10- to 20-fold more virus than cells cultivated from other organs. These data suggest that heart cells are more efficient in viral replication and release of new virions into the extracellular environment. Since interferon is not produced by mumps virus-infected chicken cells, and there is no significant change in the low titers of interferon detected in chicken embryonic organs, this regulator protein does not explain the differential organ and cellular susceptibility of the mumps virus. The lipid composition of the plasma membrane, in particular the ratio of cholesterol to phospholipid, may be the important factor in the terminal event of the host cell virus infection.

Diphtheritic myocarditis occurs as a result of the diphtheria exotoxin's effect on the myocardium. Microscopically, lipid accumulates and is seen in addition to inflammatory changes and loss of myofibers.[74, 205] Wittels and Bressler[208] suggest that the diphtheria toxin may cause depletion of carnitine, which in turn may interfere with normal transport of fatty acids into the cardiac mitochondria. In support of this, Challoner et al.[39] have shown that carnitine injection exerts a marked protective effect against LD_{50} doses of diphtheria toxin in guinea pigs. This group has also shown that when dogs are given diphtheria toxin until cardiovascular impairment develops, carnitine injections restored cardiac function to or towards normal in all animals treated.

In our studies of a naturally occurring congestive cardiomyopathy of turkeys (associated with C-type viral particles within the cardiac sarcoplasmic reticulum), we find a 50% prevalence of predominant left ventricular dilatation with varying degrees of left ventricular endocardial fibroelastosis.[50, 141, 189] This transition of myocarditis to endocardial fibroelastosis is also quite prominent in dengue fever and chikungunya fever,[144] and its association with other viral disease has been reported in humans by several authors.[9, 60, 96, 139, 170, 204]

Utilizing hatchling poults from our inbred flock of turkeys, treatment with three agents or procedures that apparently suppress humoral immunity (cortisone acetate, cyclophosphamide, or surgical removal of the bursa of Fabricius) significantly reduced early mortality in the treated birds when compared with the controls. Long-term morbidity, as reflected by the frequency of cardiac dilatation and hypertrophy in all birds dying or killed through 1 year of age, was lower after treatment with all three agents. Ca^{2+} transport studies of isolated sarcoplasmic reticulum in these birds reveal that Ca^{2+} uptake and Ca^{2+} binding are significantly reduced prior to the development of cardiac dilatation when compared to controls at 10 days of age. Immunosuppression of affected birds reversed the altered Ca^{2+} transport to normal values. These data suggest that the humoral immune system may function in the pathogenesis of this naturally occurring cardiomyopathy in the turkey.[188]

Immune mechanisms have been implicated in the pathogenesis of several human cardiac diseases. Heart-reactive antibodies have been identified in sera of patients with rheumatic fever, postpericardiotomy, and postinfarction syndromes, and in some "idiopathic" cardiomyopathies.[103, 107, 109, 117, 201] Lerner and Wilson[117] have reported several cases of acute myocarditis that have progressed to a

chronic myocarditis or cardiomyopathy characterized by cardiomegaly with recurrent episodes of heart failure. It has been speculated that these cases represent an autoimmune phenomenon in which altered myocardial proteins, virus, or viral-induced proteins may serve as a foreign protein to which specific heart-reactive antibodies are formed. This antigen-antibody reaction occurring in heart tissue could produce further damage to the myocardium.[57, 107, 117] However, the question remains as to whether these antibodies actually produce the myocardial injury or result from the injury.

In summary, mechanisms implicated or postulated to be involved in the production of myocardial injury by viruses and perhaps other agents include invasion of the myocardial cell by the virus, indirect involvement of the myocardial cell by the virus, indirect involvement of the myocardium from metabolic derangement, vascular disturbances with secondary myocardial injury, elaboration of toxins that damage the myocardium, and antigen-antibody reactions.[28, 57]

As must be surmised from the epidemiologic data presented earlier in this chapter, the vast majority of patients must recover from their acute episode of myocarditis with little or no sequelae. Of those individuals surviving this initial illness, there are some who retain evidence of myocardial damage such as persistent conduction defects or cardiac hypertrophy.[18] At the other end of the spectrum are those patients who progress from their acute episode to a chronic cardiomyopathy with left ventricular endocardial proliferation and mitral valve insufficiency (Fig. 37.4). This sequence of events from acute myocarditis to chronic cardiomyopathy remains as one of the most intriguing problems confronting the investigator.[54, 72, 170]

MANIFESTATIONS

Clinical Features

Because of the variety of manifestations of infectious myocarditis, the clinical diagnosis is often not made.[17] Only with awareness of its possible existence and dogged pursuit with the available diagnostic tools will its presence and etiologic agent be determined. As is usually the case, infections will often have systemic manifestations of organ involvement other than the heart, and cardiac pathology may be submerged. In addition, there may well be an asymptomatic period following the initial phase of the disease before cardiac manifestations develop.[3, 9, 110] The presence of a persistent tachycardia out of proportion to the fever, irregularities of the heart beat, presence of a gallop rhythm, tachypnea, dyspnea, and evidence of failure should alert the clinician to the possibility of involvement of the heart. Weakness and fatigue are also common complaints in the older child.[9]

Cardiomegaly may not be present in the mild cases but when it occurs, the classic auscultatory findings of cardiomyopathies are usually present. These include atrial or ventricular gallops or both, accentuation and wide splitting of the pulmonic component of the second sound secondary to increasing pulmonary hypertension, and the presence of a systolic murmur of mitral and, rarely, tricuspid insufficiency. It must be remembered that atrial and ventricular gallops may at times sound like the rumble of mitral stenosis and may confuse the listener. Paradoxical splitting of the second sound may be heard when left bundle branch block occurs. Premature beats of ventricular origin are common and atrial dysrhythmias may also occur.[10, 43, 55, 163, 174]

Elevated erythrocyte sedimentation rates and elevation of aspartate transaminase (AST), lactic dehydrogenase (LD)

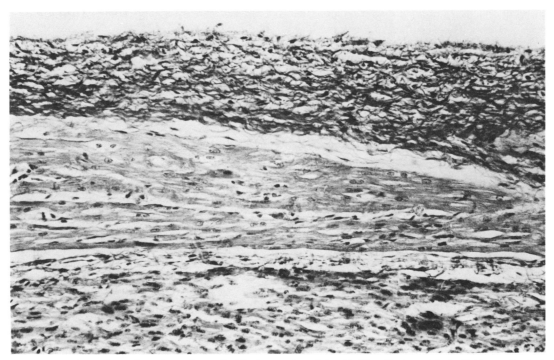

Fig. 37.4 Left ventricular endocardium of an 18-month-old who was found dead in his crib. Associated with the moderated endocardial fibroelastosis demonstrated here were focal areas within the myocardium of interstitial infiltrates, each containing 20 to 40 mononuclear cells. (Elastic van Gieson stain; original magnification, × 425).

(with LD, isoenzyme), and creatinine phosphokinase (CPK with MB fraction) levels are variably present and are usually dependent on the nature of the infection and extent of tissue damage.

As might be anticipated, the clinical manifestations of myocarditis vary from one etiologic agent to another and are dependent on the host's age, sex, and defense mechanisms.

Myocarditis in the newborn infant may be of sudden onset during the first 8 or 9 days of life and is sometimes preceded by a few hours or days of episodes of diarrhea and anorexia. Clinical features include lethargy, grayish pallor, mild icterus. Tachycardia, dyspnea, and cyanosis, if present early in the course, are evidence of cardiopulmonary failure. Cardiomegaly and hepatomegaly usually are present, and electrocardiograms often demonstrate conduction defects and, occasionally, ST segment abnormalities.[100] In an outbreak involving nine proven cases of ECHO 11 infections in newborns, myocarditis was thought to be present in five of the nine cases. Fever was the most frequent presenting feature, with rhinorrhea and acute collapse also noted. Symptoms began from the 6th to the 38th days of of life. Five of the babies presented with tachycardia out of proportion to their fever, and two infants developed vague systolic murmurs. An electrocardiogram was done in three cases and showed superventricular tachycardia in all and ST depression in two.[47]

Smith[179] presented 42 adults with Coxsackie heart disease. Twenty patients had clinical pericarditis, and 22 had myocarditis without evidence of pericarditis. There was a predominance of male patients. Chest pain was present in 67% of patients, with radiation to the throat. The pain could be relieved by sitting forward. Fever was present in 59% and 36% of patients had a flu-like illness with fever, malaise, myalgia, and sore throat. Twenty-three percent had troublesome palpitations, and 12% had shoddy lymph nodes, usually in the neck and axillae.

Coxsackie B infection was suggested by virus isolation,

and by a rising virus titer in 26 children reported by Dery et al.[46] The spectrum of illness associated with the five implicated Coxsackie B virus serotypes included gastroenteritis, pleurodynia, pharyngitis, meningitis, and pericarditis. One child had a friction rub and increased heart size on x-ray. He developed heart failure with a normal electrocardiogram and erythrocyte sedimentation rates of 30 to 52 mm/hour. Four of five patients with pericarditis were boys. Ayuthya et al.,[9] in a study of 18 cases of myocarditis in children, noted a male to female ratio of 2:1.

In *Mycoplasma pneumoniae* infection, Lewis et al.[121] found myalgia to be present in all patients with myocarditis due to that organism, and found that of 12 patients with normal electrocardiograms and proven viral or *M. pneumoniae* infections, only one complained of transitory muscle pains. They regard myalgia not only as a cardinal symptom presaging *M. pneumoniae* myocarditis, but also as an indication for an immediate electrocardiogram despite the absence of cardiac symptoms or signs.

Diphtheria toxin may cause peripheral circulatory failure during the first 7 to 10 days, and myocarditis from the 10th day to the 3rd week with damage to the nervous system from the 3rd to the 7th week. Clinically, the softening of the first heart sound, dysrhythmias, or heart block in association with nasopharyngeal or cutaneous ulcer with membrane formation in an unimmunized child should alert the clinician to the possibility of diphtheritic myocarditis. Clinically, the specialized myocardial conduction tissue is most affected by diphtheria toxin. Involvement of the bundle branches may be followed by partial or total heart block. Dysrhythmias may also be present. When cardiac failure occurs, it may be a consequence of heart block or dysrhythmia. With complete heart block, the mortality is 84 to 100%.[31, 74, 85, 95] The mortality in neonates ranges from 40 to 75%.[211]

The eosinophilic syndrome of Chusid et al.,[40] which has also been called Löffler's fibroplastic endocarditis, disseminated eosinophilic collagen disease, and eosinophilic leukemia, in all probability represents a clinicopathologic spectrum of multiple causes. This syndrome presents with a clinical diagnosis with varying features. There may be systemic illness with abdominal symptoms, or complaints of lower respiratory bronchospasm. The onset also may be vague with myalgia and loss of weight. The heart is frequently not enlarged, or if so, only slightly, thus resembling constrictive pericarditis. Murmurs of mitral insufficiency are frequent. Electrocardiogram shows changes in the ST segment and T wave with low voltage suggestive of myocardial damage such as found in myocarditis or constrictive pericarditis. Conduction defects are also occasionally seen. There are frequently leukoyctosis and eosinophilia present at one stage or another of the illness, and the erythrocyte sedimentation rate is frequently increased. Abnormal echocardiograms were noted by Chusid et al.[40] in 9 of 10 patients examined and demonstrated increased left ventricular muscle mass associated in many cases with left ventricular free wall or intraventricular septal thickening. Although this syndrome is predominantly a disease of adults, children have been reported with this syndrome, the youngest 5 years of age. Of interest is that in the series of Chusid et al.,[40] 90% of the patients were male.

Bacterial, spirochetal, rickettsial, protozoal, and helminthic myocarditis are also frequently masked by the systemic manifestations of the disease and may be only suspected by the presence of dysrhythmias. Laboratory findings are nonspecific, with the majority of cases demonstrating elevated erythrocyte sedimentation rates, leukocytosis, and elevation of AST or LD levels. Specific findings with individual agents such as eosinophilia with helminthic infections are valuable in determining the etiologic agent.

Electrocardiographic Features

Electrocardiographic evidence of myocarditis, although relatively nonspecific, include: ST segment abnormalities, dysrhythmias, and ectopic beats, secondary to atrial-ventricular or intraventricular conduction defects.[134, 171, 174, 202] Electrocardiographic abnormalities are often fleeting and display evolution or may be the most prominent residual of postinfection.[31, 55]

Hemodynamic Findings

As might be expected, hemodynamic data of acute myocarditis is not readily available.[2] However, reports of findings from chronic cases give valuable information about this disease spectrum.[70–72] Goodwin[70] studied eight patients with congestive cardiomyopathy and in addition reviewed the literature. He found that the right atrial pressure is usually elevated with moderate elevation of both ventricular systolic pressures and little or no elevation of right ventricular enddiastolic pressure. The pulmonary arterial pressure can be normal or slightly elevated, consistent with an elevation of the pulmonary arterial wedge pressure. In patients with diffuse myocardial disease, characteristic invasive and noninvasive findings of a congestive cardiomyopathy are evident. These include left atrial and left ventricular dilatation, reduced left ventricular shortening fraction, low cardiac output, and systemic hypotension.[62, 109, 145] Adesanya et al.[5] has described persistent depression of myocardial function after experimental Coxsackie B₃ viral myocarditis. Three months after inoculation, the hamsters appeared clinically healthy with few histologic lesions and no cardiac hypertrophy; however, left ventricular trabeculae carnae were found to have decreased compliance and depressed myocardial function, as compared to controls. In addition, Einzig et al.[50] have found relative subendocardial underperfusion to be a prominent feature in the cardiomyopathic turkey.

DIFFERENTIAL DIAGNOSIS

As it is frequently difficult to make a diagnosis of viral myocarditis with certainty during the acute phase, one must be diligent in exploring all possible avenues of diagnosis. In addition to the previously mentioned studies, attempts at pathogen isolation from throat washings, feces, blood, or pericardial fluid should be done early in the course of the illness. Isolation of a virus does not, however, establish its etiologic role.

Lerner and Wilson[117] have suggested criteria to establish the etiologic association of Coxsackie virus infections in patients with acute or chronic myocardiopathy which appear appropriate for most viral infections. High order association includes isolation of the virus from the myocardium, endocardium, or pericardial fluid. Moderate order association is present if virus is isolated from the pharynx or feces or a fourfold increase in type-specific neutralizing, hemagglutination-inhibiting, or complement-fixing antibody is demonstrated. Moderate order association is also present if virus is isolated from the pharynx or feces with a concomitant serum titer of 1:32 or greater of type-specific (IgM)-neutralizing or hemagglutination-inhibiting antibodies. Lower order association is present if the virus is isolated from pharynx or feces or a fourfold rise in type-specific neutralizing, hemaglutination-inhibiting, or complement-fixing antibodies is demonstrated. Single serum samples showing a titer of 1:32 or greater, or type-specific IgM-neutralizing or hemagglutination-inhibiting antibody is also considered to have a low order association.

Schmidt et al.[168, 169] have found that even in initial infections with a Coxsackie virus, complement-fixing antibodies are invariably demonstrable only in the 7 S immunoglobulin fraction. Neutralizing and hemagglutination-inhibiting antibodies which appear consist largely of 19 S immunoglobulins. They are replaced by 7 S antibody globulins in the convalescent phase sera. In addition, these workers performed IgM antibody tests to Group B Coxsackie viruses on sera from 259 patients with a clinical diagnosis of pericarditis, myocarditis, or pleurodynia. There were no definitive serologic virus isolation findings to establish a viral etiology. Another 259 patients with clinical diagnosis of viral or M. pneumoniae or pneumonitis served as controls. IgM antibodies to Coxsackie B₁, B₃, B₄, B₅, and B₆ were detected in 27% of the cardiac pulmonary disease group, as compared to 8% in the control group. In a retrospective review of the clinical diagnoses, some of the patients in the control group with IgM antibody were found to have additional findings which could be attributed to a Coxsackie virus infection. A greater number of pericarditis, myocarditis, or pleurodynia patients occurred in the 21 through 60 age group than in the younger group.

Within 3 days after the onset of virus infection, IgM-neutralizing antibodies may be detected in sera, but fourfold rises in titer are often not demonstrable. IgM antibodies normally disappear from sera about 39 days later. Considerable cross-reacting IgM neutralizing antibody occurs among the Coxsackie B sera types, and the possibility of demonstrating significant increases in neutralizing antibodies due to enteroviruses is greatly reduced if the titer in the acute phase serum is 1:32 or greater.[168, 169]

Identification of the offending agent in the myocardium is also potentially possible for the use of cardiac biopsy techniques in obtaining material for immunofluorescence, electronmicroscopy, and viral culture.[29, 30, 127]

The clinical diagnosis of nonrheumatic inflammatory myocarditis is often one of exclusion due to the latent period or invasive techniques that are required for definitive etiologic identification. Endocardial fibroelastosis, which may present a chronic form of myocarditis, glycogen storage disease type II, and anomalous origin of the left coronary artery, may present early in life in acute heart failure. Tissue biopsy for alpha-glucosidase deficiency will define Pompe's disease, whereas an anterior lateral infarct pattern on the electrocardiogram in association with angiographic demonstration of an aberrant left coronary artery will provide the diagnosis of anomalous origin of left coronary artery.

Dilatation of the heart secondary to systemic AV fistulas should be resolved by auscultation of the affected organ and subsequent angiography, while chronic anemias due to thalassemia major and sickle cell disease can be suggested on peripheral blood smears. Identification of acute rheumatic fever is discussed in Chapter 34.

TREATMENT AND COURSE

Norris and Loo[142] have shown in mice infected with Coxsackie B_3 virus that induction of interferon by interferon inducer had a significant protective effect when interferon was stimulated 12 to 48 hours before challenge with Coxsackie B_3 virus. There was also significant protection even when the stimulator poly IC was given 24 hours after challenge with Coxsackie virus. However, recent experiments by Rager-Zisman and Allison[155] have shown that type-specific neutralizing antibodies, probably in conjunction with macrophages, are most important in limiting enterovirus infections. Cellular immunity including interferon seems less important. In addition, Woodruff and Woodruff[210] postulated that in Coxsackie B_3 virus in mice, B-cell responsiveness determines the capability of the individual to terminate viral replication, whereas T-cell responsiveness influences the severity of inflammation and tissue injury in the heart.

Kilbourne et al.[111] have shown that when corticosteroids are given during the acute phase of Coxsackie virus disease, both viral replication and myocardial necrosis are increased. Rytel[160] has suggested that cortisone may act by impairing the production of interferon and, thus, Lerner and Wilson[117] have recommended that steroids be avoided, at least during the first 10 days of infection. If active disease continues, both they and Bell and Grist[16] recommended that patients severely ill and unresponsive to usual supportive therapies should receive steroids. Thus, on the basis of animal studies, the use of steroids in acute myocarditis has been questioned. However, recent reports in both humans and animals with acute inflammatory myocarditis, immunosuppressive therapy has been shown to improve cardiac function, resolve infiltrates in the myocardium, and reduce mortality and morbidity.[6, 100, 119, 128, 188 189] Asplen and Levin[8] describe two patients who, having responded to steroids, were unable to discontinue this therapy without exacerbation of symptoms. When the immunosuppressant azathioprine was added, first the steroid and finally the azathioprine could be discontinued.

Once the diagnosis of myocarditis is made, very careful observation of the patient, preferably in an intensive care setting with adequate monitoring, is mandatory, particularly if there is evidence of dysrhythmias, anginal pain, and cardiomegaly, with or without heart failure. This is because of the frequency with which sudden death is encountered.[43, 67, 120, 134, 140, 174, 191] Complete heart block may necessitate pacing, and strict attention to fluid administration should be maintained. Atrial flutter, atrial fibrillation, or heart failure may require digitalization, which should be done cautiously. A lowered threshhold for digitalis toxicity in patients with myocarditis has been postulated but not proved. Ventricular irritability may be treated with antiarrythmic agents which, however, may further depress myocardial contractility and should be used with caution. Bedrest is recommended for the acute phase of the disease, which is usually limited to 10 to 14 days in viral infections.

Many factors have been shown both clinically and experimentally to alter the outcome of viral myocarditis.[1, 117, 118] The deleterious effect of exercise on experimental Coxsackie A and B myocarditis has been well-established.[198] When mice are forced to swim in a preheated pool in the early infectious phase of this myocardiopathy, virulence is strikingly augmented, and replication of Coxsackie virus in the heart is increased 530 times.[63] Paulson and Abelmann[148] also found that *Trypanosoma cruzi* myocarditis is more severe, cellular infiltration is more diffuse, and parasites are more numerous in the myocardium with exercise.

Studies by Pearce[149] with experimental vaccinia and pseudorabies infection suggests that hypoxia increases both the incidence and severity of myocarditis. Clinically, hypoxia plays a major role in myocarditis seen in patients with influenza or poliomyelitis. Adequate oxygenation is desirable, especially in the presence of pulmonary infiltration, congestion, or an irritable myocardium. Hyperbaric conditions, on the other hand, have been shown to enhance replications of Coxsackie B_1 virus in mouse hearts and to double the mortality rate.[147]

In summary, one can no longer consider viral myocarditis to be a benign condition. For those who survive the acute episode, progression from the acute phase of infectious myocarditis to a chronic cardiomyopathy occurs, and its presence must be considered in the follow-up care of such patients.[65, 112, 161, 164]

NONINFECTIOUS INFLAMMATORY MYOCARDITIS

SYSTEMIC LUPUS ERYTHEMATOSUS

Cardiovascular manifestations in systemic lupus erythematosus are not a rare event, and approximately 40% of patients demonstrate signs and symptoms of cardiac disease. Pericarditis and pericardial effusion are most commonly encountered while myocarditis, conduction disturbances, and heart failure occur less frequently.[26, 45, 52, 150, 151]

Pathology

The classical atypical verrucous endocarditis, which occurs in the majority of patients with systemic lupus erythematosus, may be found on both surfaces of all four valves with involvement of the chordae tendineae. Focal or diffuse pericarditis also occurs in the majority of necropsied cases and is mainly fibrinous. Focal interstitial mononuclear cell infiltrates in the myocardium are also frequently seen and may be associated with necrotic foci. Bulkey and Roberts[26] describe myocardial scarring and hemorrhage of the proximal portion of the bundle branches in three of six patients who had electrocardiographic conduction disturbances.

Bulkey and Roberts[26] have also reported corticosteroid-induced changes in this disease. In steroid-treated lupus, endocarditis was confined mainly to the left-sided valves and mural endocardium and almost always affected only the underside of the mitral valve. Most verrucae showed evidence of healing, and three patients demonstrated calcification of the annular ring. The frequency of the pericarditis or endocarditis was not affected by steroid therapy. The pericarditis, however, was usually fibrous instead of fibrinous. In addition, the plasma cell and lymphocyte interstitial myocarditis was found to be much less frequent in the steroid-treated patients when compared to that of the nonsteroid group. Subepicardial myocardial fat was increased significantly in the steroid-treated patients.

Manifestations

Cardiac manifestations are more prominent in systemic lupus erythematosus than the other connective tissue diseases.[52, 150, 151] Pericarditis in association with a friction rub is most commonly seen. Pericardial tamponade or constrictive pericarditis is less frequent. The pericarditis is usually transient and may have no relation to the other activity of this disease.[150] Apical systolic murmurs of mitral insufficiency are frequently heard and may or may not be related to Libman-Sacks endocarditis.[26] Cardiac failure secondary to systemic lupus erythematosus myocarditis is infrequent and may relate more to the degree of valvular involvement. Electrocardiographic abnormalities, such as nonspecific ST changes, dysrhythmias, or conduction defects, are common, and with pericarditis T wave inversion and ST elevations are frequently seen. Demonstration of lupus erythematosus cells in the patient's pericardial fluid in association with low complement, if there is active disease elsewhere[89, 102] is helpful in the differential diagnosis. Heart-reactive antibodies are reported to be of variable significance in the diagnosis of this disease.[89]

Treatment and Course

As previously stated, corticosteroids have had a major impact on the cardiac pathology of systemic lupus erythematosus, but reversal has not been complete or without production of other abnormalities.[26]

One also must keep in mind that several cardiac drugs have been shown to produce the lupus syndrome and that these drugs may potentiate the cardiac disability. These drugs are hydralazine hydrochloride, procainamide hydrochloride, practolol, and diphenylhydantoin.[150]

POLYARTERITIS NODOSA

Although a relatively rare condition in children, polyarteritis nodosa has manifestations of which the clinician should be aware.

Pathology

The majority of cases demonstrate coronary arteritis, myocardial infarction, acute pericarditis, or cardiac hypertrophy alone or in combination. Myocarditis is rarely seen, and its extent is minimal.

The pathologic manifestations of periarteritis nodosa may also be seen in association with rheumatic fever, rheumatoid arthritis, systemic lupus erythematosus, or scleroderma.[87]

Manifestations

Hypertension, tachycardia, and heart failure are outstanding findings in periarteritis nodosa. Noncardiac signs are persistent fever, rash, and conjunctivitis.[61]

Systolic murmurs are not common and are usually mitral in origin when they are present. Dysrhythmias may occur, as can pericardial friction rubs, but neither is frequent. Electrocardiographic abnormalities occurred in 85% of Holsinger's[93] group and consisted commonly of nonspecific T wave abnormalities. Evidence of pericarditis or myocardial infarction by electrocardiography was rarely observed.

Periarteritis nodosa is seen more commonly in males, and its peak frequency is in the third to fifth decade. This disease can occur rarely in infants and children with a seemingly more fulminant course than is generally observed in the adult.[66, 93]

The pathogenesis is thought to be the deposition of immune complexes in the bifurcations of medium and small arteries with resultant degenerative and exudative changes in the arterial wall. Decreasing complement levels and circulating immune complexes have been identified in the adult.[66] Identification of the pathologic lesion in a peripheral artery may be of diagnostic value.

MUCOCUTANEOUS LYMPH NODE SYNDROME (KAWASAKI'S DISEASE)

PATHOLOGY

The frequency of cardiac involvement in a pathologic study of 13 cases of Kawasaki's disease by Fujiwara and Hamashima[62] revealed 100% with pericarditis and 69% with myocarditis of children dying in the first month of their illness. Angiitis of major, minor, and microscopic coronary arteries was present in the first 8 days. Angiitis of only major coronary arteries with aneurysm and thrombi was observed from the 10th to 30th days of illness. During this stage there may also be phlebitis of the larger veins as well as internal thickening and round cell infiltration of other small and medium-sized arteries.[61] Coronary stenosis, fibrosis of the pericardium and myocardium, and acute myocardial infarction was observed in children dying and after 40 days of illness. On gross inspection, the heart often demonstrates dilatation and hypertrophy with numerous small aneurysms of the major coronary arteries which may be tortuous and dilated.[196]

MANIFESTATIONS

Clinical Features

Kawasaki's disease presents as an acute inflammatory process consisting of an angiitis involving multiple organ systems. Diagnostic criteria are as follows: fever for 5 or more days; bilateral congestion of the conjunctivae; changes of the mucous membranes of the oral cavity, including erythema, dryness, and fissuring of lips, erythema of the tongue, prominence of the papillae, and diffuse reddening of the oropharyngeal mucosa; changes of the peripheral extremities, including reddening and indurative edema of the hands and feet, and membranous periungal desquamation; polymorphous exanthem; and acute nonsuppurative swelling of the cervical lymph nodes. The presence of prolonged fever and four of the remaining five criteria are required to establish the diagnosis of Kawasaki's disease.[212]

In a prospective study of 79 children with Kawasaki's disease, 40 had evidence of myocarditis during the first 3 weeks of the disease. Pericarditis was also present in 6 of the 40 patients with myocarditis. Signs of myocarditis resolved by the 4th week in all but three children. One or more coronary aneurysms developed in 11 patients. The occurrence of coronary aneurysm, however, does not appear to correlate with the presence or absence of carditis.[90] In another prospective study of 132 cases reported by Melish et al.,[130] 20% had carditis, 17% had coronary aneurysms, and 33% had arthritis.

Laboratory studies frequently reveal an elevated ESR and IgE levels with leukocytosis and a positive C-reactive protein.[212] Cultures for bacterial and nonbacterial agents are usually negative.

Abnormalities of the electrocardiogram include transient prolongation of the PR interval, flattening of the T waves, and depression of the ST segment. Abnormal Q waves in leads II, III, and aVF were correlated with myocardial infarction and fibrosis of more than 30% of myocardial wall thickness in four of five children studied retrospectively by Fujiwara.[61]

Abnormal M-mode echocardiographic findings are consistent with those observed in a congestive cardiomyopathy while 2D echocardiography may reveal coronary artery aneurysms by the 4th week of illness.[90, 130]

DIFFERENTIAL DIAGNOSIS

The differential diagnosis of Kawasaki's disease during the acute phase of the disease can usually be made by the process of elimination if one pays close attention to the features of this mucocutaneous disease. Other diseases which may have early similar features are: scarlet fever, Reiters syndrome, Stevens-Johnson syndrome, rubella, rubeola, ivy eruption, infectious mononucleosis, and rheumatoid arthritis. The similarities between infantile periarteritis nodosa and Kawasaki's disease have been detailed by Yanagihara and Todd[212] demonstrating few qualitative clinical pathologic differences between these two syndromes.

TREATMENT

The treatment of Kawasaki's disease remains controversial. It is currently recommended that aspirin, in anti-inflamatory doses during the early phase of the disease and then reduced to approximately 10 mg/kg/day until the disease process has subsided, be utilized in the therapy of this condition. In the event of the presence of aneurysms, salicylate therapy (in low doses) has been suggested for at least the first 12 months following the onset of Kawasaki's disease.[105, 130]

TAKAYASU'S DISEASE

PATHOLOGY

Four types of Takayasu's disease have been described.[124] Type I is characterized by acute and chronic inflammation of the ascending aorta, including the arch and great vessels. Type II has a segmental stenosis of the descending thoracic aorta while the most common form, type III, displays a mixture of involvement of the aortic arch and its branches and the abdominal aorta. Type IV is characterized as a combination of the first three types, with additional involvement of the pulmonary artery.

In an autopsy study of 16 cases of Takayasu's disease, Rose and Sinclair–Smith[157] described frequent internal fibrous plaques in all portions of the aorta. The plaques consisted of smooth muscle cells which often overlayed areas of medial destruction. Thrombi were rare, and aneurysms were commonly found, particularly in the lower thoracic and abdominal aorta. Coronary artery aneurysms were infrequent. Fatal complications due to hypertension were seen in eight patients while rupture of aneurysms accounted for three deaths. Microscopic evidence of active arteritis (presence of predominantly mononuclear cells) was observed more frequently in the adventitia than in the media or intima.[157]

MANIFESTATIONS

Takayasu's disease (pulseless disease) is a relatively rare form of arteritis that occurs predominantly in females in the second and third decades of life but may affect children as well.[124] Strachau[192a] has characterized the disease as having an acute and chronic phase. During the acute systemic stage there is an elevated sedimentation rate, weight loss, arthralgia, and localized chest tenderness. The chronic stage is characterized by signs and symptoms of progressive arterial destruction such as claudication, weakness, and paresthesia.

The cause of Takayasu's disease remains obscure, although there is evidence which suggests an autoimmune etiology[200] with a genetically related factor.[143] Diagnosis of Takayasu's disease is predominantly by arteriography which shows narrowing and/or dilatation of the affected arteries. Confirmatory histological diagnosis may be made at the time of surgical intervention for isolated arterial disease.

Treatment with corticosteroids and/or cytotoxic drugs has been suggested in the therapy of this disease.[108]

MISCELLANEOUS

Radiation, trauma, phosphorus ingestion, and drugs are all known to produce inflammatory changes in the myocardium.[25, 82, 156] Additional agents causing myocarditis are snake and scorpion venoms, heavy metals, antibiotics, and emetine.[102, 156, 165]

INFECTIOUS INFLAMMATORY DISEASE OF THE PERICARDIUM AND PERICARDIAL SPACE

The broad spectrum of inflammatory diseases—both infectious and noninfectious—which can involve the pericardium, the pericardial space, and the contiguous tissues and the proximity of these structures to the heart and the great veins and arteries contribute to the diagnostic and therapeutic dilemmas facing the physician. The potential for disaster requires expedient but accurate diagnosis and therapy. Numerous infectious agents may be responsible. This discussion will emphasize inflammatory pericardial disease due to pyogenic bacteria, *Mycobacterium tuberculosis* and idiopathic or "acute benign" pericarditis.

PHYSIOLOGY

Knowledge of the anatomic relationships of the pericardium is essential to understanding the pathology and physiology of pericarditis. This thin and semitransparent sac normally envelopes the heart and the proximal portion of the great arteries. There are two layers, the visceral and the parietal pericardium. Between them is a potential space—the pericardial space. The pericardium is in direct contact with the contiguous structures about it, the pleura, the mediastinum and its structures, and the sternum. These relationships are important to remember when considering the physiology of pericarditis. For details of the gross and microscopic anatomy of the pericardium and pericardial space, the reader is referred to the classical descriptions.[13, 182]

The deep infection of pericarditis, especially when pyogenic bacteria are involved, is in itself of concern, but with pericarditis it is the hemodynamic consequences, either of an abnormal accumulation of fluid in the pericardial sac or of a scarred and restrictive pericardium, that make this infection uniquely life-threatening. Normally, in the adult the pericardial space contains less than 50 ml of clear serous fluid.[104] With pericardial inflammation and/or infection, the volume of fluid in the pericardial sac may increase rapidly due to the influx of fluid containing leukocytes.

Pressure-volume curves have been constructed to show that large amounts of fluid may be infused acutely into the pericardial sac of animals with little change in pericardial pressure. However, at some point the pressure-volume curve bends sharply upward, and relatively small amounts of additional fluid cause a major rise in intrapericardial pressure.[135, 177]

The acute increase in volume in the pericardial space and the resultant rise in intrapericardial pressure may lead to tamponade and decreased cardiac output. When the rate of secretion of fluid into the pericardial space exceeds the rate of reabsorption, fluid accumulates. Although fluid which slowly accumulates seems to be reasonably well tolerated (probably because of the ability of the parietal pericardium to "stretch") an acute buildup of fluid interferes with diastolic filling of the heart and causes a decrease in cardiac output. The mechanisms involved remain somewhat controversial. Some emphasize the importance of abolishing the normal gradient between the pulmonary veins and the left atrium,[69] others mention a reduction in gradients across the AV valves caused by raising end-diastolic pressure in the ventricles which hinders atrial emptying and reduces cardiac output.[182] Both of the mechanisms may play important roles. The raised intrapericardial pressure interferes with ventricular filling, and AV valves close prematurely, leading to decreased stroke volume, cardiac output, and systolic pressure. It has also been suggested that the fall in cardiac output may be related to a shorter myocardial fiber length resulting from the premature termination of diastole.[97] This vicious circle may be enhanced by a decrease in coronary perfusion secondary to the decrease in cardiac output.

Several compensatory mechanisms are called upon in patients with pericardial tamponade. There is a reflex vasoconstriction which is an attempt to support the lowered blood pressure. An increase in venous pressure is helpful in attempting to increase diastolic filling of the ventricles. Perhaps the most effective compensatory mechanism is an increase in cardiac output secondary to tachycardia. However, the effectiveness of this is limited by the decreased filling resulting from the rapid heart rate.

Pulsus paradoxus is often present in patients with acute tamponade. Normally, in inspiration there is an increase in systemic venous blood return to the right atrium and augmented right ventricular output. However, inspiration also leads to increased capacitance in the pulmonary capillary bed. A thought to occur—despite the increased right ventricular output—causing a net decrease in systemic output. When one measures this in the normal human subject, the fall in pulse pressure during inspiration is usually less than 8 to 10 mm Hg. When there is tamponade because of the reasons previously stated, there is even more embarrassment of return to the left heart and a greater fall in pulse pressure during inspiration. Most cardiologists accept a fall of greater than 10 mm Hg as significant pulsus paradoxus. Pulsus paradoxus is present in acute tamponade but also may be seen in constrictive pericarditis, cardiac dilatation, advanced respiratory failure, and sometimes in patients on mechanical ventilators. Although the mechanisms vary somewhat, the effect on cardiac output in chronic constrictive pericarditis is similar. In the latter case, however, it is felt that restriction of the myocardium may play a more important role in decreased cardiac performance.

Several reviews of the physiology of pericardial disease have recently been published.[58, 59, 175]

PYOGENIC PERICARDITIS

Pyogenic pericarditis is less common since the advent of the antibiotic era.[53] Yet, it still occurs and is often associated with systemic infections. Purulent pericarditis occurs relatively frequently in the pediatric age group. Over half of the cases in a recent review were patients less than 20 years of age; approximately one-third were in children less than 6 years of age.[22]

Bacteriology

Pyogenic bacteria most commonly causing pericarditis include: staphylococci (primarily *Staphylococcus aureus*),

Streptococcus pneumoniae, Hemophilus influenzae, Neisseria meningitidis, and streptococci. A literature review of 425 patients with pericarditis revealed that 26% were due to staphylococci, 20% to pneumococci, 10% to streptococci, and smaller percentages to meningococci, *H. influenzae*, and other miscellaneous organisms.[22] As with several other bacterial infections, recent experience with pericarditis has revealed a higher proportion of unusual organisms recovered.[159]

In two reviews of patients with pericarditis in the pediatric age group, staphylococci accounted for 43 and 67% of the cases[56, 203] In Tunisia, staphylococci were responsible for 100% of the cases seen during a 6-year period.[98] A more recent report of 25 cases seen since 1962 revealed that less than 20% were caused by staphylococci.[146]

S. aureus pericarditis may be associated with lower respiratory tract infection, but this organism is especially recognized for its ability to gain entrance to the pericardial space by hematogenous spread from deep-seated infection at other sites, especially osteomyelitis. In the review by Boyle *et al.*,[22] over 60% of cases of staphylococcal pericarditis were thought to be secondary to spread from remote infections such as osteomyelitis; less than 20% came from lung or pleura.

An experimental animal model has provided insight into the pathogenesis of staphylococcus pericarditis. When rabbits were injected intravenously with staphylococci, the initial lesion was microscopic bacterial emboli to the smaller coronary arteries. Microabscess formation followed with development of a pericardial effusion. These abscesses eventually either ruptured into the pericardial space or spread into the epicardium without rupture.[138]

Pericarditis due to *S. pneumoniae* occurs less frequently since the introduction and the widespread use of antibiotics. Pneumococcal pericarditis was the most common agent from patients with purulent pericarditis prior to antibiotics.[106] Less than 10% of the 25 cases reported in children were caused by this organism.[146] In a review of over 100 cases, over 90% were associated with pneumonitis and almost half had empyema.[106] Studies have suggested that the earliest lesion following direct spread from the lungs may be inflammation of the parietal pericardium adjacent to the area of infected lung. A pericardial effusion results, and later becomes purulent.[192] Pneumococcal pericarditis may also result from hematogenous spread from distant sites.

H. influenzae pericarditis has been reported to be a disease of infants and children. A recent review found only three cases in adults; all others occurred in children less than 12 years of age.[44] Over 90% were associated with respiratory tract infection. Distant sites of simultaneous infection have been recognized (e.g., meningitis).[146]

N. meningitidis was responsible for less than 5% of 400 cases of pericarditis reviewed.[22] This was attributed to the fact that it is a relatively late complication of severe untreated meningococcemia. Cases of meningococcal pericarditis without meningitis have been reported.[136] In children, over 90% have been associated with meningitis.[203]

Streptococcal inflammatory disease of the pericardium and pericardial space was the third most common reported cause in an extensive review,[22] yet it seems to be uncommon in recent years. Most of the cases were associated with lower respiratory tract infections. The majority of the streptococci recovered were beta hemolytic streptococci; *Streptococcis viridans* was rare as a cause.

Many other bacteria have been associated with purulent pericarditis, including salmonella, *Escherichia coli, Pseudomonas*, gonococci, *Klebsiella, Proteus*, and bacteroides. Pericarditis with simultaneous recovery of more than one organism has been reported, but it is not common.[22]

Clinical Features

The signs and symptoms in patients with bacterial pericarditis may vary, depending upon the organism, the age of the patient, and the site of associated infection. Fever, tachycardia, chest pain, and dyspnea are almost always present. The fever usually is higher than 38°C and may range to 40°C or 41°C. Substernal chest pain is common, and it may be more severe with inspiration. The heart tones may be muffled, and there often is a friction rub. Tachypnea and dyspnea with flaring of the alae nasi are usual, especially in young children. Whether there is neck vein distention and hepatomegaly, pulsus paradoxus, and/or hypotension with a narrow pulse pressure is dependent upon the amount of pericardial exudate and the resulting degree of embarrassment of cardiac function. Cardiac tamponade is the reason for classifying acute suppurative pericarditis as a medical and/or surgical emergency. Spodick[183] has discussed the features of this finding in detail elsewhere. Clincial evidence for associated sites of infection should be searched for extensively so that effective therapeutic methods can be instituted.

Laboratory Evaluation

The laboratory evaluation of the patient suspected of having acute suppurative pericarditis is similar to the evaluation of patients with other life-threatening acute bacterial infections, but special studies are also indicated.

The peripheral white blood count is usually elevated; leukopenia in the face of severe infection is a poor prognostic sign. White counts of 18,000 to 25,000 are common. Immature polymorphonuclear leukocytes may be visible on the peripheral blood smear. In staphylococcal septicemia, microhematuria may be present, and there may be evidence of gram-positive cocci on gram stain of the urine.

Close collaboration with the hospital bacteriology laboratory is vital. Because of the importance of accurate identification of the organism, cultures should be obtained *prior* to beginning antibiotics if possible. Blood cultures have been reported to be positive in 40 to 80% of cases, depending upon the organism.[136, 203] Three to five blood cultures are usually sufficient to recover an organism if bacteremia is present. The addition of penicillinase to the blood culture media might be considered if the patient has already received penicillin; other specialized blood culture media are available which can absorb antibiotics. A urine culture may be useful, especially in staphylococcal septicemia, since small numbers of these organisms may be recovered from the urine following microabscess formation in the kidney. Clinical judgment must be exercised, but in those patients with appropriate signs or symptoms or in whom there is suspicion of a menigococcal or *H. influenzae* etiology, lumbar puncture may be necessary to eliminate the diagnosis of concomitant meningitis.

The sine qua non for establishing the diagnosis of suppurative pericarditis is culture and examination of pericardial fluid. This is obtained by pericardiocentesis. While this procedure is associated with morbidity and even mortality, it is essential in management; it may be both diagnostic and therapeutic.

Although pericardiocentesis can be done on the ward or in the emergency room, many prefer the catheterization laboratory or some other facility where fluoroscopy is available. This procedure should be carried out by an experienced physician. The patient is placed supine with the head elevated to about 20 to 40° above the horizontal. After infiltrating the skin and subcutaneous tissues with a local anesthetic and after making a small stab wound through the skin just below and to the left of the xiphoid process, an 18- to 20-gauge pericardial (or spinal) needle is advanced toward the left shoulder at an angle of approximately 30° to the ventral surface of the body. Constant electrocardiograph monitoring is necessary. The physician should attach the exploring electrode of the electrocardiogram to the needle by means of a sterile "alligator" clamp. Using this method an injury current is usually detected if the needle contacts the epicardial surface of the heart.[20, 180] By advancing the needle cautiously and constantly withdrawing on a 5- or 10-ml syringe attached to the needle, one usually feels a "pop" as the pericardial sac is entered. Loculation of the pericardial exudate may require several attempts before success is achieved. Withdrawal of grossly bloody fluid should prompt partial withdrawal of the needle since an intracardiac cavity may have been entered. All fluid which contains more than a trace of blood should be sent for hemoglobin and hematocrit, and this should be compared with the hemoglobin and hematocrit of venous blood obtained at the same time.

If the child is having distress, removal of as little as 50 to 100 ml of fluid will often result in marked clinical improvement. If the material is grossly purulent, it may not be possible to remove much fluid due to loculations. Total evacuation of the pericardial cavity is unnecessary since most agree that surgical pericardiotomy and drainage are indicated in patients with purulent pericarditis.

Pericardial fluid should be directly inoculated into culture media; most use bottles of media available from the bacteriology laboratory for blood cultures. Material for culture for *M. tuberculosis* and fungi should also be obtained. Fluid should also be sent to the laboratory for viral cultures (see below). A sterile tube should be sent for cell count and differential. The fluid should be smeared and gram stained; special stains for acid fast bacteria should be done. Inoculation of specific media for recovery of other microorganisms may be indicated, depending upon the clinical findings and the suspicion of the physician. Many physicians, since they do not have a definite diagnosis at the time, also send an aliquot for a cell block and cytology to eliminate malignancy as a cause of the effusion. Counterimmune electrophoresis is available in many hospital laboratories for identification of some bacterial antigens (e.g., *H. influenzae*, pneumococci, and group A and C meningococci). In the case of some bacteria, (e.g., *H. influenzae*), the antigens also may be present in urine. The test has proven to be very useful in rapid diagnosis of many bacterial infections.

Analysis of the pericardial fluid in patients with purulent pericarditis usually reveals a marked leukocytosis, often over 50,000 per mm.[3] Protein levels may vary, but glucose levels in the fluid are usually low.

In patients with acute suppurative pericarditis, the cardiac configuration is almost always abnormal on the chest roentgenogram if there is a major amount of fluid present. Figure 37.5A is the chest film of a 19 month old with *H. influenzae* pericarditis. Marked "cardiomegaly" is obvious. Figure 37.5B is the film from the same patient taken 1 month following combined medical and surgical therapy showing the cardiac configuration returning toward normal. The heart assumes a so-called "water bottle" configuration; the "cardiac" shadow is large. Evidence of pneumonitis, pleural effusions, or empyemas should be searched for. If the chest roentgenogram is suggestive of effusion, fluoroscopy may be helpful in that it is usually difficult to define variations in heart size during the cardiac cycle.

Confirmatory evidence of pericardial effusion may also be obtained by the use of several radioscintographic methods for evaluating the cardiac blood pool. These involve scanning the chest after intravenous infusion of radioactive-labeled compounds and are reliable methods for establishing pericardial effusions.[21, 41] Very helpful but more invasive meth-

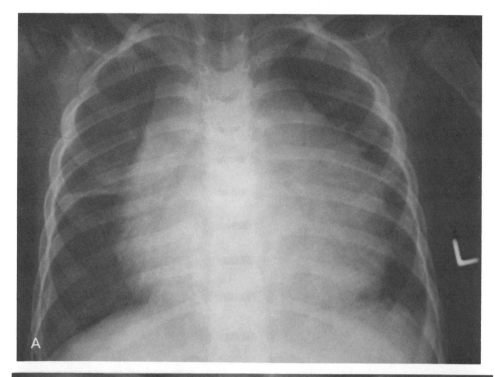

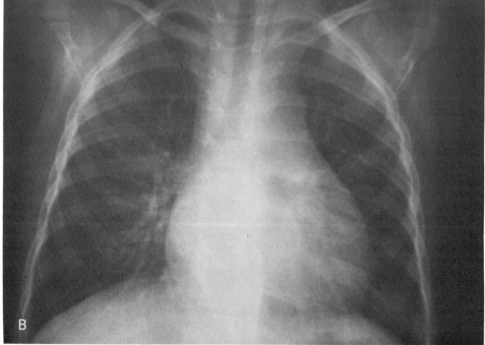

Fig. 37.5 X-ray of a 19-month-old infant with pericarditis due to *H. influenzae*. During the acute stage, before pericardiocentesis and prior to surgical drainage (Fig. 37.5*A*), the "cardiac" shadow is markedly enlarged. During the convalescent period, the "cardiac" configuration returned toward normal (Fig. 37.5*B*).

ods may involve either intravenous or intrapericardial injection of contrast material or carbon dioxide, allowing the radiologist and the clinician to differentiate the actual heart size from the entire "cardiac" shadow.[152, 167, 190] For additional information, the reader is referred to a recent review.[51]

Echocardiographic Features

Echocardiography has proven to be one of the most useful tools in establishing the diagnosis of fluid in the pericardial space.[132] In this situation the beam is passed through the heart and posteriorly into the lung. The presence of a space, usually devoid of echoes, between the pericardium and the epicardium alerts the echocardiographer to the presence of an effusion. More detailed discussions of the use of echocardiography in pericardial effusions are available.[19, 68, 173] Figure 37.6 shows an echocardiogram from a patient with pericarditis. Figure 37.6*A* reveals the presence of effusion (*PER. EFF.*) both anteriorly and posteriorly. Figure 37.6*B* is an

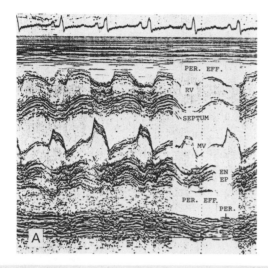

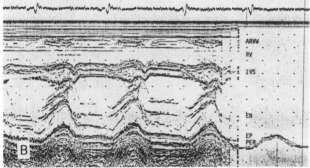

Fig. 37.6 An echocardiogram from a patient with pericarditis and pericardial effusion. *A* shows the presence of the pericardial effusion, both anteriorly and posteriorly during the acute stage. *B* shows the disappearance of the fluid following convalescence.

echocardiogram from the same patient taken following recovery. There is no evidence of fluid in the pericardial space.

Electrocardiographic Features

The electrocardiogram is often useful. However, some patients never demonstrate changes in the electrocardiogram. Although many comment on the diminution in amplitude of the QRS complex—thought to be related to the presence of pericardial fluid—this is not a constant finding. The presence of abnormalities in the ST segment and T waves is more consistent with pericarditis. Superficial myocarditis is usually present when ST segment elevation or depression occurs, both in man[182] and in the experimental animal.[32] Changes in the ST segments and T waves have been described in detail.[78, 122, 184] These changes, however, are not specific for pericarditis and have been described in other conditions. Although relatively rare, dysrhythmias may occur during acute pericarditis.[185]

Treatment

Data regarding therapy for acute purulent pericarditis support a combination of medical and surgical approaches. In two reports, greater than 75% of those treated by pericardial drainage alone (prior to antibiotic era) died. A very high mortality rate was seen in those treated with antibiotics alone, but less than 20% mortality occurred in those treated with both antibiotics and pericardial drainage.[64, 146] One group has suggested that in addition to antibiotics, one or two pericardiocenteses prior to surgical drainage may be adequate.[159]

Many feel that surgical drainage in addition to large doses of antibiotics is the method of choice. The frequent occurrence of loculations in the pericardial sac in patients with pyogenic pericarditis has made the practice of percutaneous insertion of a small polyethylene tube into the pericardial space unrewarding. The inability of the pericardium to absorb transudate and exudate has been recognized for some time.[48] Effective surgical drainage is warranted.[99] This either includes creation of a subxiphoid pericardial window[113] with placement of a tube or, in some cases, anterior pericardiectomy with tube drainage. Purulent pericarditis is a serious infection, yet the prognosis with early diagnostic and therapeutic measures can be good.

Careful identification of the organism responsible for the infection cannot be overemphasized. Broad spectrum antibiotics should be avoided if possible; the antibiotic should be in accordance with antibiotic sensitivities of the organism. Evidence suggests that adequate levels of several antibiotics (including penicillin, semisynthetic penicillins, at least one of the cephalosporin antibiotics, and aminoglycoside drugs) may be attained in infected pericardial fluid.[195] Even in the patient who has had a pericardial window with insertion of a tube, it is preferable to continue antibiotics after the patient has become afebrile. Total antibiotic therapy of 4 to 6 weeks has been suggested, but the duration depends upon the factors mentioned above and the patient's clinical response. The fever curve, peripheral leukocyte count, and sedimentation rate may be helpful in following the individual patient.

TUBERCULOUS PERICARDITIS

With the fall in the prevalence of tuberculosis, one might expect that pericarditis due to *M. tuberculosis* would be uncommon. In the early 1950s tuberculous pericarditis was responsible for 5 to 10% of all cases of acute pericarditis.[182] This infection was seen approximately once a year between 1948 and 1972 in a large midwestern medical center. Although largely a disease of adults, these same authors reported that 25% of the cases were less then 20 years of age.[56] The mortality has been reported to be as high as 90%,[78] but there is a striking decrease in the fatality rate with chemotherapy.[56, 182]

Tuberculous pericarditis usually occurs as the result of direct spread from the lymph nodes in the proximity. Tuberculous pericarditis occurs commonly without parenchymal lung disease. It may also seed into the pericardial space via the hematogenous route from a distant site.[182]

Although this disease is seen in patients with advanced miliary tuberculosis, pericarditis also may be the first manifestation of tuberculosis. The onset may be insidious. Cough, dyspnea, and chest pain are commonly seen, as are night sweats, orthopnea, and weight loss. Fever, tachycardia, pericardial friction rub, and pulsus paradoxus are uncommon findings.[56] Constrictive pericarditis is also observed. The chest x-rays often reveal "cardiomegaly," which often turns out to be pericardial effusion. Characteristic changes in S-T segments and T waves in the electrocardiogram are usually present.

The diagnosis of tuberculous pericarditis in a patient with pericarditis may be unexpected. Most patients have a positive reaction to purified protein derivative (PPD) skin tests. The diagnosis is established by examination of the pericardial fluid. The fluid is usually sanguinous, and there is a predominance of lymphocytes. Pericardial fluid obtained by pericardiocentesis is sent for the usual examination (see above) and, in addition, where there is a suspicion that the diagnosis is tuberculous pericarditis, fluid should be inoculated directly into guinea pigs. When Ziehl-Neelsen stains of pericardial fluid are negative, pericardial biopsy has been suggested as having a higher return.[182]

The frequency of cardiac tamponade makes rapid and adequate therapeutic measures necessary. Several different chemotherapeutic regimens have been used, varying from streptomycin alone to combinations of drugs (such as isoniazid, para-aminosalicylic acid, and streptomycin) to reduce the possibility of the development of drug resistance. Antituberculous drugs such as rifampin and ethambutol should also be considered. Streptomycin, in combination with other chemotherapeutic agents, would seem to be a good choice since it has been shown to diffuse into the pericardial space in patients with pericarditis.[195]

After pericardiocentesis there should be relief of symptoms of tamponade. If tamponade recurs, or if the patient does not improve, many advocate a direct surgical approach to remove the pericardium. It has been shown that the wounds will tend to heal despite active infection with *M. tuberculosis*.[92] Pericardiectomy is also necessary if the patient develops constrictive pericarditis.

VIRAL PERICARDITIS

The etiology of acute "benign" pericarditis has remained controversial. These patients often present with the classical signs and symptoms of pericarditis. Yet, even after extensive diagnostic studies, no etiology can be established. Whereas the mortality for bacterial infections of the pericardium and pericardial space approached 100% prior to the availability of antibiotics and therefore, rarely, if ever, went undetected, there is undoubtedly a proportion of viral infections of the pericardium which are "subclinical" and are not brought to the physician's attention. Prevalence figures, therefore, are difficult to interpret. A viral etiology for this syndrome was postulated over 30 years ago by Barnes and Burchell.[12] Most physicians classify this entity as part of the spectrum of viral myopericarditis, even though it is common that one cannot either isolate the responsible virus or show serologic evidence of viral infection. In two reports, evidence of a viral infection was found less than 20% of the time in patients with so-called "idiopathic acute pericarditis."[56, 101] Nonetheless, it seems likely this entity is related to a viral etiology.

The term myopericarditis seems appropriate since it has been shown that the myocardium, epicardium, and pericardium are often involved simultaneously.[91] This being the case, it seems logical to consider Lerner's hypothesis that there are alternating infectious and immunologic stages in viral myocarditis.[116] Perhaps the postinfectious stage is present when many of the negative studies are obtained.

Viral infection of the pericardium has been documented to occur with Coxsackie, ECHO, adenovirus, influenzae, mumps, varicella zoster, vaccinia, and infectious mononucleosis.[7, 27, 56, 129, 178, 203]

Clinical Features

The symptoms of viral pericarditis include: chest pain, fever, and a pericardial friction rub. Usually, the fever is low grade, and the patients do not appear to be toxic. Cardiac tamponade is rare in the acute stage but can occur. The disease is often preceded by evidence of an upper respiratory infection. Some patients have evidence of pulmonary infiltrates or pleural effusion. In contrast to most cases of bacterial pericarditis, the peripheral white cell count is usually normal, and the differential may show an increase in lymphocytes.

Cardiomegaly may or may not be evident upon roentgenographic evaluation. An echocardiogram is helpful to determine whether a pericardial effusion is present.

The electrocardiogram may be normal but ST segment and T wave changes are often seen. These changes are similar to those seen with bacterial pericarditis. ST segment depression may be more representative of the acute phase of the disease; the T wave changes may persist for years.[23]

Some do not feel a pericardiocentesis is always necessary in these patients. Certainly it is indicated in toxic patients to eliminate other causes of pericarditis and in those with evidence of pericardial tamponade. However, even those relatively asymptomatic patients with clinical or laboratory evidence of pericardial effusion in whom a diagnosis has not been established should be considered for diagnostic pericardiocentesis. The pericardial fluid may be serous or serosanguinous and may show polymorphonuclear leukocytes or mononuclear cells. A gram stain should be done. The fluid should be cultured for bacteria and for viruses. The virology laboratory should be informed in advance of the pericardiocentesis of the clinical picture so that appropriate cell lines can be used to recover the virus. Fluid also should be sent for cytology to eliminate a malignant process.

In making a diagnosis of viral infection of the pericardium, one should ideally require isolation of the virus and serologic confirmation of infection (two- to fourfold rise in serum antibody titer). It is important to obtain acute phase serum as soon as possible and a convalescent sample 3 or 4 weeks later. Schmidt and her colleagues have pointed out the usefulness of fractionation of the serum into specific IgM and IgG antibodies. The presence of IgM antibodies strongly suggests that the immune response to the virus in question is recent and therefore is related to the illness.[168]

Treatment

The treatment is symptomatic. Bedrest is imperative, usually for a period of several weeks until laboratory and clinical evidence of inflammation disappear. The importance of prolonged bedrest in patients with myocardial involvement has been stressed. The patient should be carefully observed for evidence of tamponade or cardiac decompensation. Salicylates may be used for fever and relief of pain. Salicylates are also used for their anti-inflammatory properties. Codeine or meperidine can be added if the chest pain is severe. Some have used left stellate ganglion block for intractable pericardial pain.[206] Cardiac glycosides may be used for appropriate dysrhythmias, but care should be taken in using these drugs if myocarditis or tamponade is suspected.

The use of steroids is controversial. Some have reported that acute and dramatic relief may be obtained by using moderate doses of steroids. However, rebounds have been seen after discontinuation of steroid therapy.[209] Although some advocate their use,[56] there is no convincing evidence that they reduce the frequency of sequelae (myocardial scarring or constrictive pericarditis). Complications of steroid therapy should also be considered when deciding whether to use them. Intrapericardial steroids have been successful in uremic pericarditis[34] and have been used in a few nonuremic patients, but there are no controlled studies to support their use.[33] In any person to be treated with steroids, the other infectious causes must be excluded.

The surgical construction of a pericardial window, or pericardiectomy, is usually reserved for those with recurrent disease or with constrictive pericarditis. Carmichael *et al.*[37] have reported that recurrent attacks were seen in 15% of cases.[37]

OTHER INFECTIOUS AGENTS

Mycotic infections, including those with *Aspergillus*, actinomycetes, *Blastomyces*, *Coccidioides*, and *Histoplasma* may produce pericarditis. Toxoplasma gondi[197] and *Entamoeba histolytica*[153] among the protozoan agents have been reported to infrequently cause pericarditis. Echinococcosis rarely causes the disease.[182]

CONSTRICTIVE PERICARDITIS

That constrictive pericarditis is a late sequela of purulent pericarditis is controversial. Boyle and colleagues[22] determined that between 3 and 6% of cases had a septic illness with signs of pericarditis which preceded constrictive disease.[22] Strauss *et al.* revealed that 2 of 12 cases of purulent pericarditis in children developed constriction (one presumably due to *H. influenzae* and one due to *S. aureus*).[193] Other reports have also implicated *H. influenzae*[35, 158] and *N. meningitidis*[172] as having the potential to lead to constrictive pericarditis. Constrictive pericarditis may take several weeks to several months to develop following the acute illness.

Constrictive pericarditis more commonly follows tuberculous pericarditis than other bacterial infections of the pericardial space. Constrictive pericarditis has been reported to occur in from 12 to 35% of patients with tuberculous pericarditis.[182] In over 50% of cases of constrictive pericarditis, the etiology cannot be determined.[182] Viral or acute benign pericarditis may be responsible for many of these cases, but other causes of constrictive pericarditis, including trauma, tumors, uremia, radiation, and rheumatic fever, have been mentioned.[81] The hemodynamics in constrictive pericarditis have been commented on in detail.[114, 176]

Symptomatic or hemodynamically significant constrictive pericarditis requires surgical relief.[42] Sometimes, the scar tissue so surrounds the heart that pericardiectomy becomes technically perilous.

OTHER CAUSES OF PERICARDITIS

Several other causes of pericarditis should be mentioned, as these may enter the differential diagnosis in a patient suspected of having infectious pericarditis. Patients with collagen diseases, especially lupus erythematosus and rheumatoid arthritis, often have pericarditis. In fact, pericarditis has been reported to occur in as many as 50% of patients with lupus, although it only rarely is present initially.[86] Its occurrence in rheumatic fever as a part of the pancarditis has been commented upon. Because of improved methods of management, patients with severe renal disease frequently develop uremic fibrous pericarditis. Therapeutic radiation to the mediastinum in patients with malignant tumors has made radiation-induced pericarditis common.[126] Pericardiectomy has been necessary for some patients both in uremic and in radiation-induced pericarditis. The reason for mentioning these three groups of patients: collagen diseases, uremic patients, and those with malignancies is that since these patients are often debilitated, the question of infection commonly enters the differential diagnosis.

REFERENCES

1. Abelmann, W. H.: Current concepts: Myocarditis. N. Engl. J. Med. 275:944, 1966.
2. Abelmann, W. H.: Virus and the heart. Circulation 44:950, 1971.
3. Abelmann, W. H.: Clinical aspects of viral cardiomyopathy. In Myocardial Diseases, edited by N. O. Fowler. Grune & Stratton, New York, 1973, p. 253.
4. Abelmann, W. H., Kumar, R., and Wagner, R. L.: Biventricular heart failure in experimental chagasic myocarditis. Circulation 40:33, 1969.
5. Adesanya, C. O., Phear, W. P., Goldberg, A. H., Young, N. A., and Abelmann, W. H.: Heart muscle performance after experimental myocarditis. J. Clin. Invest. 57:569, 1976.
6. Ainger, L. E.: Acute aseptic myocarditis: Corticosteroid therapy. J. Pediatr. 64:716, 1964.
7. Araujo, M. F., Brito, T., and Machedo, C. G.: Myocarditis in human rabies. Rev. Inst. Med. Trop. Sao Paulo 13:99, 1971.
8. Asplen, C. H., and Levin, H. D.: Azathioprine therapy of steroid-responsive pericarditis. Am. Heart J. 80:109, 1970.
9. Ayuthya, P. S. N., Jayavasu, J., and Pongpanich, B.: Coxsackie group B virus and primary myocardial disease in infants and children. Am. Heart J. 88:311, 1974.
10. Bairan, A. C., Cherry, J. D., Fagan, L. F., and Codd, J. E., Jr.: Complete heart block and respiratory syncytial virus. Am. J. Dis. Child. 127:264, 1974.
11. Bajusz, E.: A disease model of hereditary cardiomyopathy: Its usefulness and limitations. In Recent Advances in Studies on Cardiac Structure and Metabolism, edited by E. Bajusz and G. Rona, vol. 4. The University Park Press, Baltimore, 1973, p. 291.
12. Barnes, A. R., and Burchell, H. B.: Acute pericarditis simulating acute coronary occlusion: Report of 14 cases. Am. Heart J. 23:247, 1942.
13. Basmajian, J. V.: Grant's Method of Anatomy. Williams & Wilkins, Baltimore, 1972.
14. Bates, H. R., Jr.: Coxsackie virus B3 calcified pancarditis and hydrops fetalis. Am. J. Obstet. Gynecol. 106:629, 1970.
15. Bell, E. J., and Grist, N. R.: Coxsackie virus infections in patients with acute cardiac disease and chest pain. Scott. Med. J. 13:37, 1968.
16. Bell, E. J., and Grist, N. R.: ECHO viruses, carditis and acute pleurodynia. Am. Heart J. 82:133, 1971.
17. Bell, R. W., and Murphy, W. M.: Myocarditis in young military personnel. Am. Heart J. 74:309, 1967.
18. Bengtsson, B., and Lamberger, B.: Five year follow-up study of cases suggestive of acute myocarditis. Am. Heart J. 72:751, 1966.
19. Berger, M., Bolak, L., Jelvek, M., and Goldberg, E.: Pericardial effusion diagnosed by echocardiography. Chest 74:174, 1978.
20. Bishop, L. H., Estes, H., Jr., and McIntosh, H.: The electrocardiogram as a safeguard in pericardiocentesis. J.A.M.A. 162:264, 1956.
21. Bonte, F. J., Christensen, E., and Curry, T.: Tc99m pertechnetate angiocardiography in the diagnosis of superior mediastinal masses and pericardial effusions. Am. J. Roentgenol. Radium Ther. Nucl. Med. 107:404, 1969.
22. Boyle, J. D., Pearce, M. L., and Guze, L. B.: Purulent pericarditis: Review of literature and report of eleven cases. Medicine 40:119, 1967.
23. Bradley, E. C.: Acute benign pericarditis. Am. Heart J. 67:121, 1964.
24. Brink, A. J., and Weber, H. W.: Fibroplastic parietal endocarditis with eosinophilia. Am. J. Med. 34:52, 1963.
25. Buhler, F., Bersch, W., and Kreinsen, U.: Zur Pathomorphologie der Sogenannten Epinephrin-Myokarditis nach Gabe uon Hypertension, Lict und Elektronenmikroskopische Untersuchuagen. Virchows Arch. [Pathol. Anat.] 363:249, 1974.
26. Bulkey, B. H., and Roberts, W. C.: The heart in systemic lupus erythematosus and the changes induced in it by corticosteroid therapy. Am. J. Med. 58:243, 1975.
27. Burch, G., Walsh, J. J., and DeMasi, C.: Pericarditis due to infectious mononucleosis. Am. Heart J. 67:421, 1964.
28. Burch, G. E., and Giles, T. D.: Viral cardiomyopathy. In Recent Advances in Studies on Cardiac Structure and Metabolism, edited by E. Bajusz and G. Rona, vol. 2. University Park Press, Baltimore, 1973, p. 121.
29. Burch, G. E., Sun, S. C., Chu, K. C., Sohal, R. S., and Colcolough, H. L.: Interstitial and Coxsackievirus B myocarditis in infants and children. J.A.M.A. 203:1, 1968.
30. Burch, G. E., Sun, S. C., Colcolough, H. L., Sohal, R. S., and DePasquale, N. P.: Coxsackie B viral myocarditis and valvulitis identified on routine autopsy specimens by immunofluorescent techniques. Am. Heart J. 74:13, 1967.
31. Burch, G. E., Sun, S. C., Sohal, R. S., Chu, K., and Colcolough, H. L.: Diphtheritic myocarditis: A histologic and electronmicroscopic study. Am. J. Cardiol. 21:261, 1968.
32. Burchell, H. B., Barnes, A. R., and Mann, F.: The electrocardiographic picture of experimental localized pericarditis. Am. Heart J. 18:133, 1939.
33. Buselmeier, T. J., Simmons, R. L., Najarian, J. S., Burchell, H. B., and Kjellstrand, C. M.: Local steroid therapy of chronic pericarditis (abstr.). Circulation 52 (Suppl. II):79, 1975.
34. Buselmeier, T. J., Simmons, R. L., Najarian, J. S., Dietzman, R. H., von Hartitzsch, B., Mauer, S. M., Casali, R. E., and Kjellstrand, C. M.: Symptomatic pericardial effusion: Pericardial drainage and localized steroid instillations as definitive therapy. Proc. Clin. Dial. Transplant Forum 3:55, 1973.
35. Caird, R., Conway, N., and McMillan, I. K. R.: Purulent pericarditis followed by early constriction in young children. Br. Heart J. 35:201, 1973.
36. Cambridge, G., MacArthur, C. G. C., Water-

son, A. P., Goodwin, J. F., and Oakley, C. M.: Antibodies to Coxsackie B viruses in congestive cardiomyopathy. Br. Ht. J. 41:692, 1979.

37. Carmichael, D. B., Sprague, H., Wyman, D., and Bland, E. F.: Acute nonspecific pericarditis: Clinical, laboratory, and follow-up considerations. Circulation 3:321, 1951.

38. Carter, J. B., Blieden, L. C., and Edwards, J. E.: Congenital heart block: Anatomic correlations and review of the literature. Arch. Pathol. 97:51, 1974.

39. Challoner, D. R., Mandelbaum, I., and Elliot, W.: Protective effect of L-carnitine in experimental intoxication with diphtheria toxin. J. Lab. Clin. Med. 77:616, 1971.

40. Chusid, M. J., Dale, D. C., West, B. C., and Wolff, S. M.: The hypereosinophilic syndrome: Analysis of fourteen cases with review of the literature. Medicine 54:1, 1975.

41. Cook, C. B., Dunson, G. McFarland, P., and Godwin, I.: Single image pericardial effusion. Evaluation with technetium compounds. South. Med. J. 68:392, 1975.

42. Copeland, J. G., Stinson, E. B., Griepp, R. B., and Shumway, N.: Surgical treatment of chronic constrictive pericarditis using cardiopulmonary bypass. J. Thorac. Cardiovasc. Surg. 69:236, 1975.

43. Corby, C.: Isolated myocarditis as a cause of sudden obscure death. Med. Sci. Law 1:23, 1960.

44. Crossley, K., Bigos, T., and Joffe, C. D.: *Hemophilus influenzae* pericarditis. Am. Heart J. 85:246, 1973.

45. Decker, J. L., Steinberg, A. D., Gershwin, M. E., Seaman, W. DO, Klippel, J. H., Plotz, P. H., and Paget, S. A.: Systemic lupus erythematosus: Contrasts and comparisons. Ann. Intern. Med. 82:391, 1975.

46. Dery, P., Marks, M. I., and Shapera, R.: Clinical manifestations of Coxsackievirus infections in children. Am. J. Dis. Child. 128:464, 1974.

47. Drew, J. H.: ECHO 11 virus outbreak in a nursery associated with myocarditis. Aust. Paediatr. J. 9:90, 1973.

48. Drinker, C. K., and Field, M. E.: Absorption from the pericardial cavity. J. Exp. Med. 53:143, 1931.

49. Einzig, S., Jankus, E. F., and Moller, J. H.: Round heart disease in turkeys: A hemodynamic study. Am. J. Vet. Res. 33:557, 1972.

50. Einzig, S., Staley, N. A., Mettler, E., Nicoloff, D. M., and Noren, G. R.: Regional myocardial blood flow and cardiac function in a naturally occurring congestive cardiomyopathy of turkeys. Cardiovasc. Res. 14:396, 1980.

51.. Ellis, K., and King, D. L.: Pericarditis and pericardial effusion: Radiologic and echocardiographic diagnosis. Radiol. Clin. North Am. 11:393, 1973.

52. Estes, D., and Christian, C. L.: The natural history of systemic lupus erythematosus by prospective analysis. Medicine 50:85, 1971.

53. Evans, E.: Introduction to symposium on pericarditis. Am. J. Cardiol. 7:1, 1961.

54. Feinstone, S. M., Hensley, G. T., and Rytell, M. W.: Postcoxsackievirus B3 myocardiopathy in mice. Proc. Soc. Exp. Biol. Med. 144:345, 1973.

55. Forfang, K., and Lippestad, C. T.: Transient left posterior hemiblock in acute myocarditis. J. Electrocardiol. 7:83, 1974.

56. Fowler, N., and Manitsas, G.: Infectious pericarditis. Prog. Cardiovasc. Dis. 16:323, 1973.

57. Fowler, N. O.: Autoimmune heart disease. Circulation 44:159, 1971.

58. Fowler, N. O.: Physiology of cardiac tamponade and pulsus paradoxus. I. Mechanisms of pulsus paradoxus in cardiac tamponade. Mod. Concepts Cardiovasc. Dis. 47:109, 1978.

59. Fowler, N. O.: Physiology and cardiac tamponade and pulsus paradoxus. II. Physiology, circulatory, and pharmacological responses in cardiac tamponade. Mod. Concepts Cardiovasc. Dis. 47:115, 1978.

60. Fruhling, L., and Adam, C. H.: Etude anatomopathologique de la myo-endocardite chronique fibroelastique du Nourrisson. Ann. Anat. Pathol. 1:59, 1956.

61. Fujiwara, H., Chen, C., Fujiwara, T., Nishioka, K., Kawai, C. and Yoshihiro, H.: Clinicopathologic study of abnormal Q waves in Kawasaki disease. Am. J. Card. 45:797, 1980.

62. Fujiwara, H., and Hamashima, Y.: Pathology of the heart in Kawasaki disease. Ped. 61:100, 1978.

63. Gatmanitan, B. G., Chason, J. L., and Lerner, A. M.: Augmentation of the virulence of murine Coxsackie virus B3 myocardiopathy by exercise. J. Exp. Med. 131:1121, 1970.

64. Gersony, W. M., and McCracken, G. H.: Purulent pericarditis in infancy. Pediatrics 40:224, 1967.

65. Gerzen, P., Granath, A., Holmgren, B., and Zetterquist, S.: Acute myocarditis: A follow-up study. Br. Heart J. 34:575, 1972.

65a. Ghafour, A. S. and Gutgesell, H. P.: Echocardiographic evaluation of left ventricular function in children with congestive cardiomyopathy. Am. J. Card. 44:1332, 1979.

66. Gillespie, D. N., Burke, E. C., and Holley, K. E.: Polyarteritis nodosa in infancy: A diagnostic enigma. Mayo Clin. Proc. 48:773, 1973.

67. Gold, E., Carver, D. H., Heineberg, H., Adelson, L., and Robbins, F. C.: Viral infection: A possible cause of sudden unexpected death in infants. N. Engl. J. Med. 264:53, 1961.

68. Goldberg, S. J., Allen, H. D., and Sahn, D. J.: Pediatric and adolescent echocardiography. Year Book Medical Publishers, Chicago, 1975.

69. Golinko, R. J., Kaplan, N., and Rudolph, A.: The mechanism of pulsus paradoxus during acute pericardial tamponade. J. Clin. Invest. 42:249, 1963.

70. Goodwin, J. F.: Cardiac function in primary myocardial disorders. Br. Med. J., 1 (Part I):1527, 1964.

71. Goodwin, J. F.: Cardiac function in primary myocardial disorders. Br. Med. J., 1 (Part II):1595, 1964.

72. Goodwin, J. F.: Prospects and predictions for the cardiomyopathies. Circulation 50:210–219, 1974.

73. Gore, I., and Saphir, O.: Myocarditis: A classification of 1,402 cases. Am. Heart J. 38:827, 1947.

74. Gore, I., and Kline, I. K.: Myocarditis. In Pathology of the Heart, Ed. 3, edited by S. E. Gould. Charles C Thomas, Springfield, Ill., 1968, p. 731.

75. Gormsen, H.: Sudden unexpected death due to myocarditis. Acta Pathol. Microbiol. Scand. Suppl. 105:30, 1955.

76. Grist, N. R., and Bell, E. J.: Coxsackie viruses and the heart: Editorial. Am. Heart J. 77: 295, 1969.

77. Grist, N. R., and Bell, E. J.: A six-year study of Coxsackievirus B infections in heart disease. J. Hyg. (Camb.) 2:73, 1974.

78. Guntheroth, W. G.: Pediatric Electrocardiography: Normal and Abnormal Patterns, Incorporating the Vector Approach. W. B. Saunders, Philadelphia, 1965.

79. Haas, J. E., and Yunis, E. J.: Viral crystalline arrays in human Coxsackie myocarditis. Lab. Invest. 23:442, 1970.

80. Hackel, D. B.: Myocarditis in association with varicella. Am. J. Pathol. 29:369, 1953.

81. Hackel, D. B.: Diseases of the pericardium. Cardiovasc. Clin. 4:143, 1972.

82. Haft, J. I.: Cardiovascular injury induced by sympathetic catecholamines. Prog. Cardiovasc. Dis. 17:73, 1974.

83. Hageman, J. H., D'Esopo, N. D., and Glenn, W. L.: Tuberculosis of the pericardium: A long-term analysis of forty-four proved cases. N. Engl. J. Med. 270:327, 1964.

84. Hall, G. V.: The Cardiomyopathies in Sydney: A study of 129 cases, 1966–1971. Med. J. Aust. 2:597, 1973.

85. Harris, L. C., and Nghiem, Q. X.: Cardiomyopathies in infants and children. Prog. Cardiovasc. Dis. 15:285, 1972.

86. Harvey, A. M., Schulman, L. E., Tumulty, P. A., Conley, C. L., and Schoenrich, E. H.: Systemic lupus erythematosus: Review of the literature and clinical analysis of 138 cases. Medicine 33:291, 1954.

87. Harvey, W. P., and Segal, J. P.: The spectrum of primary myocardial disease. Prog. Cardiovasc. Dis. 7:17, 1964.

88. Helin, M. J., Savola, J., and Lapinleimu, K.: Cardiac manifestations during a Coxsackie B5 epidemic. Br. Med. J. 3:97, 1968.

89. Hess, E. V., and Kirsner, A.: Immunologic studies in myocardial diseases. In Myocardial Diseases, edited by N. O. Fowler. Grune & Stratton, New York, 1973, p. 281.

90. Hiraishi, S., Yashiro, K., Oguchi, K., Kusano, S., Katsumi, I., and Keiji, N.: Clinical course of cardiovascular involvement in the mucocutaneous lymph node syndrome. Am. J. Card. 47:323, 1981.

91. Hirschman, S., and Hammer, G.: Coxsackie virus myopericarditis: A microbiological and clinical review. Am. J. Cardiol. 34:224, 1974.

92. Holman, E., and Willett, F.: Treatment of active tuberculous pericarditis by pericardiectomy. J.A.M.A. 146:1, 1951.

93. Holsinger, D. R., Osmundson, P. J., and Edwards, J. E.: The heart in periarteritis nodosa. Circulation 25:610, 1972.

94. Holt, L. E.: Myocarditis. In The Diseases of Infancy and Childhood. D. Appleton and Company, 1897, p. 588.

95. Hudson, R. E. B.: Myocardial involvement (myocarditis) in infections and infestations. In Cardiovascular Pathology, vol. 3. Williams & Wilkins, Baltimore, 1970, p. 483.

96. Hutchins, G. M., and Vie, S. A.: The progression of interstitial myocarditis to idiopathic endocardial fibroelastosis. Am. J. Pathol. 66:483, 1972.

97. Isaacs, J. P., Berglund, E., and Sarnoff, S.: Ventricular function. III. The pathologic physiology of acute cardiac tamponade studied by means of ventricular function curves. Am. Heart J. 48:66, 1954.

98. Ismail, M. B., Saied, H., and Ghariani, M.: Pericarditis purulentes: A propos de 12 cas. Coeur Med. Interne 12:499, 1973.

99. Iturrino, J. L., and Holland, R. H.: The emergency surgical management of acute pericarditis. J. Thorac. Cardiovasc. Surg. 45:324, 1963.

99a. Jaskiewicz K.: Trials of treating myocarditis in mice infected with Coxsackie B3 virus. Arch. Immunol. Ther. Exp. (Warsz) 27:99, 1979.

100. Javett, S. N., Heymann, S., Mundel, B., Pepler, W. J., Lurie, H. I., Gear, J., Measroch, V., and Kirsch, Z.: Myocarditis in the newborn infant: A study of an outbreak associated with Coxsackie group B virus infection in a maternity home in Johannesburg. J. Pediatr. 48:1, 1956.

101. Johnson, R. T., Portnoy, B., Rogers, N., and Buescher, E.: Acute benign pericarditis. Arch. Intern. Med. 108:823, 1961.

102. Kalikshtein, D. B., Odinokova, V. A., Paleev, N. R., and Gurevich, M. A.: Hypersensitivity of delayed type manifested during the development of allergic lesions of the myocardium. Bull. Exp. Biol. Med. 77:789, 1975.

103. Kaplan, M. H., and Frengley, J. D.: Autoimmunity to the heart in cardiac disease. Am. J. Cardiol. 24:459, 1969.

104. Karsner, H. T.: Human Pathology. Lippincott, Philadelphia, 1955.

105. Kato, H., Koike, S., and Yokoyama, T.: Kawasaki disease: Effect of treatment on coronary artery involvement. Ped. 63:175, 1979.

106. Kauffman, C. A., Watanakunakorn, C., and Phair, J.: Purulent pneumococcal pericarditis: A continuing problem in the antibiotic era. Am. J. Med. 54:743, 1973.

107. Kawai, C.: Idiopathic cardiomyopathy: A study on the infectious immune theory as a cause of disease. Jap. Circ. J. 35:765, 1971.

108. Kawai, C., Ishikawa, K., Kato, M., Ishii, Y. and Nakao, K.: Clinical conference in cardiology. Pulmonary pulseless disease; pulmonary involvement in so-called Takayasu's disease. Chest 73:651, 1978.

109. Kawai, C., and Takatsu, T.: Clinical and experimental studies on cardiomyopathy. N. Eng. J. Med. 293:592, 1975.

110. Kibrick, S., and Bernirschke, K.: Acute aseptic myocarditis and meningoencephalitis in the newborn child infected with Coxsackie virus, group B, type 3. N. Engl. J. Med. 235:883, 1956.

111. Kilborne, E. D., Wilson, C. B., and Perrier, D.; The induction of gross myocardial lesions via Coxsackie (pleurodynic) virus and cortisone. J. Clin. Invest. 35:362, 1956.

112. Kitaura, Y., and Morita, H.: Secondary myocardial disease - virus myocarditis and cardiomyopathy. Jap. Circ. J. 43:1017, 1979.

113. Lajos T. Z., Black, H. E., Cooper, R. G., and Wanka, J.: Pericardial decompression. Ann. Thorac. Surg. 19:47, 1975.

114. Lange, R. L., Botticelli, J. T., Tsagaris, T. J., Walker, J. A., Gani, M., and Bustamante, R.: Diagnostic signs in compressive cardiac disorders. Constrictive pericarditis, pericardial effusion, and tamponade. Circulation 33:763, 1966.

115. Lebowitz, W. B.: The heart in rheumatoid arthritis: Rheumatoid disease. Ann. Intern. Med. 58:102, 1963.

116. Lerner, A. M.: Coxsackievirus myocardiopathy. J. Infect. Dis. 120:496, 1969.

117. Lerner, A. M., and Wilson, F. M.: Virus myocardiopathy. Prog. Med. Virol. 15:63, 1973.

118. Levenson, S. O., Milzer, A., and Lewin, P.: Effect of fatigue, chilling and mechanical trauma on resistance to experimental poliomyelitis. Am. J. Hyg. 42:204, 1945.

119. Levine, H. D.: Virus myocarditis, a critique of the literature from clinical, electrocardiographic, and pathologic standpoints. Am. J. Med. Sc. 277:132, 1979.

120. Lewis, D., and Rainford, D. J.: Echo viruses and carditis. Lancet 1:520, 1970.

121. Lewis, D., Rainford, D. J., and Lane, W. F.: Symptomless myocarditis and myalgin in viral and mycoplasma pneumoniae infections. Br. Heart J. 36:924, 1974.

122. Lipman, B. S., and Massie, E.: Clinical scalar electrocardiography. Year Book Publishers, Chicago, 1959.

123. Ludden, T., and Edwards, J. E.: Carditis in poliomyelitis: An anatomic study of thirty-five cases and a review of the literature. Am. J. Pathol. 25:357, 1949.

124. Lupi Herrera, E., Sanchez Torres, G., Marcushamer, J., Mispireta, J., Horwitz, S., and Espinovela, J.: Takayasu's arteritis. Clinical study of 107 cases. Am. Ht. J. 93:94, 1977.

125. Markowitz, S. M., Martinez, A. J., Duma, R. J., and Shiel, F. O. M.: Myocarditis associated with primary amebic (Naegleria) meningoencephalitis. Am. J. Clin. Pathol. 62:619, 1974.

126. Martin, R. G., Ruckdeschel, J. C., Chang, P., Byhardt, R., Bouchard, R. J., and Wiernik, P. H.: Radiation-related pericarditis. Am. J. Cardiol. 35:216, 1975.

127. Mason, J. W. and Billingham, M. E.: Myocardial biopsy. In Progress in Cardiology, Vol. 9, edited by P. N. Yu and G. F. Goodwin. Lea and Febiger, Philadelphia, 1980, p. 113.

128. Mason, J. W., Billingham, M. E. and Ricci, D. R.: Treatment of acute inflamatory myocarditis assisted by endomyocardial biopsy. Am. J. Card. 45:1037, 1980.

129. Matthews, A. W., and Griffiths, I. D.: Postvaccinal pericarditis and myocarditis. Br. Heart J. 36:1043, 1974.

130. Melish, M. E., Hicks, R. M., Dean, A. C. and Marchette, N. J.: Endemic and epidemic Kawasaki syndrome. Ped. Res. 15:617, 1981.

131. Melnick, J. L., and Godman, G. C.: Pathogenesis of Coxsackie virus infection: Multiplication of virus and evolution of the muscle lesion in mice. J. Exp. Med. 93:247, 1951.

132. Meyer, R. A., and Kaplan, S.: Radionuclide pericardial scan. Is it outmoded by echocardiography? Pediatrics 49:637, 1972.

133. Miranda, W. R., Kitck, R. S., Beswick, T. S., and Campbell, A. C. P.: Experimental Coxsackie B5 myocarditis in mice. J. Pathol. 109:175, 1973.

134. Morales, A. R., Adelman, S., and Fine, G.: Varicella myocarditis: A case of sudden death. Arch. Pathol. 91:29, 1971.

135. Morgan, B. C., Guntheroth, W. G., and Dillard, D. H.: Relationship of pericardial to pleural pressure during quiet respiration and cardiac tamponade. Circ. Res. 16:493, 1965.

136. Naraqui, S., and Kabins, S.: Acute meningococcal pericarditis without meningitis. Arch. Intern. Med. 135:314, 1975.

137. Nemetsehek–Gansler, H., Hofman, W., Hopker, W. W., and Heilmann, K.: Experimentelle Coxsackie-Virus-Myokarditis bei babymäusen. Virchows Arch. [Pathol. Anat.] 361:349, 1973.

138. Nikolaw, G. F.: La Pathogénie des péricardites suppurées. Presse Méd. 45:926, 1937.

139. Noren, G. R., Adams, P., Jr., and Anderson, R. C.: Positive skin reactivity to mumps virus antigen in endocardial fibroelastosis. J. Pediatr. 62:604, 1963.

140. Noren, G. R., Staley, N. A., Bandt, C. H., and Kaplan, E. L.: Occurrence of myocarditis in sudden death in children. J. Forensic Sci. 22:188, 1977.

141. Noren, G. R., Staley, N. A., Jankus, E. F., and Stevenson, J. E.: Myocarditis in round heart diseases of turkeys. Virchows. Arch. (Pathol. Anat.) 352:285, 1971.

142. Norris, D., and Loh, P. C.: Coxsackievirus myocarditis: Prophylaxis and therapy with an interferon stimulator. Proc. Soc. Exp. Biol. Med. 142:133, 1973.

143. Numano, F., Isohisa, I., Hidenori, M. and Takeo, J.: HL-A antigens in Takayasu's arteritis. Am. Ht. J. 98:153, 1979.

144. Obeyesekere, I., and Hermon, Y.: Myocarditis and cardiomyopathy after arbovirus infections (dengue and chikungunya fever). Br. Heart J. 34:821, 1972.

145. Oda, T., Hamamoto, K. and Morinaga, H.: Clinical aspects of non-rheumatic myocarditis in children. Jap. Circ. J. 43:433, 1979.

146. Okoroma, E. O., Perry, L. W., and Scott, L. P.: Acute bacterial pericarditis in children: Report of 25 cases. Am. Heart J. 90:709, 1975.

147. Orsi, E. B., Mancini, R., and Barriso, J.: Hyperbaric enhancement of Coxsackievirus infection in mice. Aerosp. Med. 41:1169, 1970.

148. Paulson, S. H., and Abelmann, W. H.: Effects of muscular activity upon the acute myocarditis of C3H mice infected with trypanosoma cruzi. Am. Heart J. 69:629, 1965.

149. Pearce, J. H.: Heart disease and filterable viruses. Circulation 21:448, 1960.

150. Perlroth, M. C.: Connective tissue diseases and the heart. J.A.M.A. 231:410, 1975.

151. Peterson, R. D. A., Vernier, R. L., and Good, R. A.: Lupus erythematosus. Pediatr. Clin. North Am. 10:941, 1963.

152. Pyle, R.: Diagnosis of pericardial effusion by intravenous atriography. N. Engl. J. Med. 275:816, 1966.

153. Rab, S. M., Alam, N., Hoda, A. N., and Yee, A.: Amoebic liver abscess. Am. J. Med. 44:811, 1967.

154. Rabin, E. R., Hassan, S. A., Jenson, A. B., and Melnick, J. L.: Coxsackievirus B3 myocarditis in mice: An electron microscopic, immunofluorescent and virus-assay study. Am. J. Pathol. 44:775, 1964.

155. Rager–Zisman, B., and Allison, A. C.: Role of antibody and host cells in resistance of mice against infection by Coxsackie B3 virus. J. Gen. Virol. 19:329, 1973.

156. Roberts, W. C., and Ferrans, W. J.: Morphologic observations in the cardiomyopathies. In Myocardial Diseases, edited by N. O. Fowler. Grune & Stratton, New York, 1973, p. 92.

157. Rose, A. G., and Sinclair–Smith, C. C.: Takayasu's arteritis—A study of 16 autopsy cases. Arch. Pathol. Lab. Med. 104:231, 1980.

158. Rubenstein, J., Goldblatt, A., and Daggett, W.: Acute constriction complicating purulent pericarditis in infancy. Am. J. Dis. Child. 124:591, 1972.

159. Rubin, R. H., and Moellering, R. C.: Clinical, microbiologic, and therapeutic aspects of purulent pericarditis. Am. J. Med. 59:68, 1975.

160. Rytel, M. W.: Interferon response during Coxsackie B3 infection in mice. I. The effect of cortisone. J. Infect. Dis. 120:379, 1969.

161. Sainani, G., Krompotic, E., and Slodki, S. J.: Adult heart disease due to the coxsackie virus B infection. Med. 47:133, 1967.

162. Sanders, V.: Viral myocarditis. Am. Heart J. 66:707, 1963.

163. Sanghvi, L. M., and Misra, S. N.: Electrocardiographic abnormalities in epidemic hepatitis. Circulation 16:88, 1957.

164. Sanner, E., Sigurdsson, G., Gislasson, D., Gudbrandsson, B., and Stefausson, M. Acute myopericarditis. Upsala J. Med Sci. 81:167, 1976.

165. Santhanakrishnan, B. R., and Raju, V. B.: Management of scorpion sting in children. J. Trop. Med. Hyg. 77:133, 1974.

166. Saphir, O.: Nonrheumatic inflammatory diseases of the heart. In Pathology of the Heart, ed. 2, edited by S. E. Gould. Charles C Thomas, Springfield, Ill., 1960, p. 779.

167. Scatliff, J. H., Kummer, A. J. and Janzen, A.: The diagnosis of pericardial effusion with intracardiac carbon dioxide. Radiology 73:871, 1959.

168. Schmidt, N. J., Lennette, E. H., and Dennis, J.: Characterization of antibodies produced in natural and experimental Coxsackievirus infections. J. Immunol. 100:99, 1968.

169. Schmidt, N. J., Magoffin, R. L., and Lennette, E. H.: Association of group B Coxsackieviruses with cases of pericarditis, myocarditis, or pleurodynia by demonstration of immunoglobulin M antibody. Infect. Immun. 8:341, 1973.

170. Schryer, M. J. P., and Karnauchow, P. N.: Endocardial fibroelastosis. Am. Heart J. 88:557, 1974.

171. Scott, L. P., Gutelius, M. F., and Parrott, R. H.: Children with acute respiratory tract infections: An electrocardiographic survey. Am. J. Dis. Child. 119:11, 1970.

172. Scott, L. P., Knox, D., Perry, L. W., Pineros–Torres, and Francisco, J.: Meningococcal pericarditis: Report of 2 cases, 1 complicated by acute constrictive pericarditis. Am. J. Cardiol. 29:104, 1972.

173. Settle, H. P., Adolph, R. J., Fowler, N. O., Engle, P., Agruss, N. S., and Levenson, N. I.: Echocardiographic study of cardiac tamponade. Circulation 56:951, 1977.

174. Sevy, S., Kelly, J., and Ernst, H.: Fatal paroxysmal tachycardia associated with focal myocarditis of the Purkinje system in a fourteen month old girl. J. Pediatr. 72:796, 1968.

175. Shabetai, R.: The pericardium: An essay on some recent developments. Am. J. Cardiol. 42:1036, 1978.

176. Shabetai, R., Fowler, N., and Fenton, J.: Restrictive cardiac disease: Pericarditis and the myocardiopathies. Am. Heart J. 69:271, 1965.

177. Shabetai, R., Fowler, N., and Guntheroth, W. G.: The hemodynamics of cardiac tamponade and constrictive pericarditis. Am. J. Cardiol. 26:480, 1970.

178. Shapiro, S. C., Dimich, I., and Steier, M.: Pericarditis as the only manifestation of infectious mononucleosis. Am. J. Dis. Child. 126:662, 1973.

179. Smith, W. G.: Coxsackie B myopericarditis in adults. Am. Heart J. 80:34, 1970.

180. Sobol, S. M., Thomas, H. M., and Evan, R. W.: Myocardial laceration not demonstrated by continuous electrocardiographic monitoring occurring during pericardiocentesis. N. Engl. J. Med. 292:1222, 1975.

181. Sohal, R. S., and Burch, G. E.: Ultrastructural lesions of the myocardial cell in Coxsackie B4 infected mice. Virchows Arch. (Pathol. Anat.) 346:361, 1969.

182. Spodick, D. H.: Acute Pericarditis. Grune & Stratton, New York, 1959.

183. Spodick, D. H.: Acute cardiac tamponade pathologic physiology, diagnosis, and management. Prog. Cardiovasc. Dis. 10:64, 1967.

183a. Spodick, D. H.: Arrhythmias during acute pericarditis. A prospective study of 100 cases. J. Am. Med. Assoc. 235:39, 1976.

184. Spodick, D. H.: Electrocardiogram in acute pericarditis: Distributions of morphologic and axial changes by stages. Am. J. Cardiol. 33:470, 1974.

185. St. Geme, J. W., Jr., Davis, C. W. C., and Noren, G. R.: An overview of primary endocardial fibroelastosis and chronic viral cardiomyopathy. Perspect. Biol. Med. 17:495, 1974.

186. St. Geme, J. W., Peralta, H., Farias, E., Davis, C. W. C., and Noren, G. R.: Experimental gestational mumps virus infection and endocardial fibroelastosis. Pediatrics 48:821, 1971.

187. Staley, N. A., Noren, G. R., and Einzig, S.: Early alterations in the function of sarcoplasmic reticulum in a naturally occurring model of congestive cardiomyopathy. Cardiovasc. Res. 15:276, 1981.

189. Staley, N. A., Noren, G. R., and Kaplan, E. L.: Alteration of early mortality in a naturally occurring cardiomyopathy. J. Lab. Clin. Med. 86:844, 1975.

190. Stauffer, H. M., Soloff, L., Zatuchni, J., and Carter, B.: Gas and opaque contrast in roentgenographic diagnosis of pericardial disease. J.A.M.A. 172:1122, 1960.

191. Stevens, P. J., and Underwood Ground, K. E.: Occurrence and significance of myocarditis in trauma. Aerosp. Med. 41:776, 1970.

192. Still, G. F.: Observations on suppurative pericarditis in children. Br. Med. J. 2:606, 1901.

192a. Strachau, R. W.: The natural history of Takayasu's arteriopathy. Quart. J. Med. 33:57, 1964.

193. Strauss, A. W., Santa–Maria, M., and Goldring, D.: Constrictive pericarditis in children. Am. J. Dis. Child. 129:822, 1975.

194. Sutton, G. C., Harding, H. B., Trueheart, R. P., and Clark, H. P.: Coxsackie B4 myocarditis in an adult: Successful isolation of virus from ventricular myocardium. Aerosp. Med. 38:66, 1967.

195. Tan, J. S., Holmes, J. C., Fowler, N. O., Manitsas, C., and Phair, J. P.: Antibiotic levels in pericardial fluid. J. Clin. Invest. 53:7, 1974.

196. Tanaka, N., Sekimoto, K. and Naoes, S.: Infantile periarteritis nodosa. Arch. Pathol. Lab. Med. 100:81, 1976.

197. Theologides, A., and Kennedy, B. J.: Toxoplasmic myocarditis and pericarditis. Am. J. Med. 47:169, 1969.

198. Tilles, J. G., Elson, S. H., Shaka, J. A., Abelmann, W. H., Lerner, A. M., and Finland, M.: Effects of exercise on Coxsackie A-9 myocarditis in adult mice. Proc. Soc. Exp. Biol. Med. 117:777, 1964.

199. Tobin, J.: Personal communication.

200. Ueda, H., Saito, Y., Morooka, S., Itoh, I., Yamaguchi, H. and Sugiuro, M.: Experimental arteritis produced immunologically in rabbits. Jap. Ht. J. 9:573, 1968.

201. Van der Geld, H.: Anti-heart antibodies in the post-pericardiotomies and the post-myocardial infarction syndromes. Lancet 2:617, 1964.

202. Van Kirk, J. E., Simon, A. B., and Armstrong, W. R.: Candida myocarditis causing complete atrio-ventricular block. J.A.M.A. 227:931, 1974.

203. Van Reken, D., Strauss, A., Hernandez, A., and Feigin, R. D.: Infectious pericarditis in children. J. Pediatr. 85:165, 1974.

204. Van Reken, D. E., Geffen, W. A., and Cramer, S. F.: Sudden congestive heart failure in a five-month old infant. J. Pediatr. 85:724, 1974.

205. Wegner, N. K.: Infectious myocarditis. Cardiovasc. Clin. 4:168, 1972.

206. Weissbein, A. S., and Heller, F. N.: A method of treatment for pericardial pain. Circulation 24:607, 1961.

207. Wilson, F. M., Miranda, W. R., Chason, J. L., and Lerner, A. M.: Residual pathologic changes following murine Coxsackie A and B myocarditis. Am. J. Pathol. 55:253, 1969.

208. Wittles, B., and Bressler, R. J.: Biochemical lesion of diphtherotoxin in the heart. J. Clin. Invest. 43:630, 1964.

209. Wolff, L., and Grunfeld, O.: Pericarditis. N. Engl. J. Med. 268:419, 1963.

210. Woodruff, J. F., and Woodruff, J. J.: Involvement of T lymphocytes in the pathogenesis of Coxsackie virus B3 heart disease. J. Immunol. 113:1726, 1974.

211. Wyatt, C. B.: Diphtheria. Trop. Doct. 4:110, 1974.

212. Yanagihara, R., and Todd, J. K.: Acute febrile mucocutaneous lymph node syndrome. Am. J. Dis. Child. 134:603, 1980.

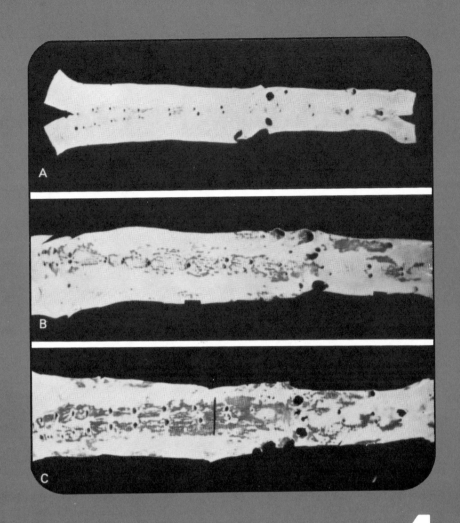

Part 4
CONNECTIVE TISSUE: METABOLIC AND DEGENERATIVE DISEASES

38

Metabolic and Nutritional Diseases

Joan L. Caddell, M.D.

This chapter reviews the cardiovascular aspects of the major metabolic and nutritional diseases of infants, children, and adolescents. It is divided into four sections: (I) inherited errors of metabolism; (II) syndromes resulting from deficiency or excess of nutrients; (III) cardiotoxic substances; and (IV) cardiovascular disease of the tropics and subtropics.

I. INHERITED ERRORS OF METABOLISM

ACROMEGALY

Acromegaly is a disorder marked by progressive enlargement of the head, distal extremities, and thorax because of hypersecretion of growth hormone by the anterior lobe of the pituitary gland. The disorder may be apparent during adolescence or early adulthood; cardiac symptoms usually develop during adulthood.[171, 124] Primary myocardial disease has been described in isolated case reports and as a rare finding in large series. There may be progressive enlargement of the heart, dilatation, and elongation of the thoracic aorta, and arteriosclerotic changes with premature coronary artery disease. The heart disease initially may be of no clinical importance, but the patient then may develop cardiac dysrhythmias, especially premature ventricular beats and intraventricular conduction defects. Systemic hypertension is sometimes found to be mild and responsive to drugs, but it may be intractable. Heart failure may develop.

Echocardiography offers a simple, noninvasive method of evaluating myocardial structure and functioning.[171] In one adult series of 27 patients, six met the criteria for asymmetrical septal hypertrophy, and eight had concentric left ventricular hypertrophy. Patients with asymmetric septal hypertrophy appeared to have increased ventricular ejection. However, many with left ventricular hypertrophy were asymptomatic, and their hypertrophy may have been related to higher initial growth hormone.[171]

The key to management of acromegaly would be effective treatment of the hypersecretion of growth hormone.[124] Reduction of the plasma hormone to normal values appeared to benefit a patient with poorly controlled heart failure.

ALCAPTONURIA

Alcaptonuria is a rare metabolic disease in which there is absence of the enzyme homogentisic acid oxidase. Homogentisic acid, produced during the metabolism of phenylalanine and tyrosine, cannot be further metabolized; it accumulates and is excreted in the urine. Ochronosis refers to the ochre-colored pigment that appears microscopically in alcaptonuric patients. Alcaptonuric patients have a high frequency of heart disease, including chronic mitral and aortic valvulitis; aneurysm of the aorta and left ventricle; generalized arteriosclerosis; calcification of the heart valves; and myocardial infarction, which is a common cause of death.[113]

CUSHING'S SYNDROME

Cushing's syndrome is a disorder resulting from persistent, chronically increased cortisol secretion by the adrenal cortex, either associated with acquired adrenal hyperplasia or caused by cortical neoplasm. The resultant clinical picture is one of combined obesity and virilization, and, if untreated, there is impaired growth, progressive muscle weakness, and debility. Hypertension usually progresses and may cause symptoms of cardiac insufficiency.[24] The therapy is surgical.[24, 61]

DIABETES MELLITUS

Infants Of Diabetic Mothers

Diabetic mothers produce an excess of high birth weight infants of all gestational ages, as well as an excess of low birth weight infants of 37 to 40 weeks gestational age. Cardiorespiratory distress and congenital heart lesions are prominent findings in such infants.

Pathophysiology

It is thought that maternal hyperglycemia provokes fetal hyperglycemia, which in turn leads to fetal hyperinsulinemia.[20] The increased fetal insulin and glucose leads to increased hepatic uptake of glucose and synthesis of glycogen. There is evidence of increased lipid and protein synthesis. Related pathologic findings are: hypertrophy and hyperplasia of the pancreatic islets and a disproportionate increase in the number of beta cells; increased amounts of cytoplasm in liver cells; and extramedullary hematopoiesis. At birth the maternal glucose infusion is interrupted while the hyperinsulinism persists, resulting in temporary hypoglycemia in the neonate. Infants may die in heart failure. Examination of the heart has shown septal hypertrophy and distortion of right and left ventricular cavities. Microscopic examination has revealed hypertrophic fibers and areas of cellular disarray in the septum.[82]

Clinical Features

Infants of diabetic mothers usually have puffy, plethoric faces, and they are often large, due to increased body fat and enlarged viscera. Some are prematurely born and have normal or low birth weight. For the first few days of life, the infants are usually tremulous and easily startled, but they may have lethargy, hypotonia, and a poor suck.[20]

Cardiorespiratory distress may be evident at birth and usually appears within the first week of life. Findings may include tachycarida, tachypnea, and systolic ejection murmurs.[196] Harsh murmurs are heard in infants with obstructive hypertrophic cardiomegaly. About 30% of infants develop cardiomegaly, while 5 to 10% develop heart failure.[117] The overall prevalence of congenital anomalies in diabetic pregnancy is 5 to 10%. Disorders of the heart, usually ventricular septal defects, are prominent among these.[71]

Electrocardiographic Features

The electrocardiogram does not correlate with the degree of distress or the degree of left ventricular septal hypertrophy seen on echocardiography. There may be no changes, right ventricular hypertrophy, or left ventricular hypertrophy.[20]

Radiologic Features

About 30% of infants show cardiomegaly. Venous congestion without pulmonary disease is usually found, although the frequency of hyaline membrane disease is higher in these infants than in infants of comparable gestational age who were born to nondiabetic mothers.

Echocardiographic and Cardiac Catheterization Features

Echocardiograms (Fig. 38.1) may reveal disproportionate thickening of the interventricular septum, sometimes with left ventricular outflow obstruction.[82, 117, 196] A few infants may show systolic anterior motion of the mitral valve leaflet. In one study, normal indices of left ventricular performance were found, despite heart failure. Cardiac catheterization may also reveal subaortic obstruction, which may improve after treatment with propranolol.[196]

Laboratory Data

About 75% of infants develop hypoglycemia. Other findings may include hypocalcemia and hypomagnesemia.[20]

Prevention, Treatment, and Prognosis

Diabetic mothers should be carefully monitored during pregnancy. There is some evidence that rigid control of maternal diabetes may reduce the frequency of myocardial abnormalities in the infant.[117]

The neonate should be closely observed, with hourly blood sugar determinations for the first 6 hours of life, and 2-hourly feedings of glucose water, followed by milk formula. Most of the infants found to have hypertrophic cardiomyopathy need only supportive care. However, if any of these infants develop heart failure, an echocardiogram should be performed to evaluate the left ventricular outflow tract for obstruction. Digitalis is contraindicated if obstruction if found.[117] If phar-

macologic intervention is necessary in such infants with subaortic stenosis, propranolol appears to be the drug of choice.[196]

The hypertrophic cardiomyopathy is transient, with a resolution of symptoms within 2 to 4 weeks[196] and a resolution of septal hyertrophy within 2 to 12 months, if the infant survives heart failure. Between 1 and 7% of infants of diabetic mothers subsequently develop diabetes mellitus.

JUVENILE DIABETES MELLITUS

Diabetes mellitus is a common disorder of energy metabolism which results from an absolute or functional deficiency of insulin.[65] It is inappropriate hyperglycemia,[148] resulting from one or more inborn errors of metabolism, the nature of which has not been established. It may be that diabetes mellitus is a syndrome of variable primary causes, genetic and nongenetic.[148]

The incidence has been estimated to 1.3 cases/1000 children under 17 years of age.[65] The peak incidence of new cases is in winter among two age groups: 5 to 6 years and 11 to 13 years. No striking sex difference is reported.

Pathophysiology

The susceptibility to diabetes mellitus is partly conditioned by inherited factors; however, the pathologic lesion suggests an autoimmune inflammatory process.[148] Early in the course of the disease, there is intense infiltration of lymphocytes around the islets of Langerhans in the pancreas.[65] There is gradual scarring of the inflamed tissue. As the insulin-producing beta cells are replaced by scar tissue, the production of insulin is reduced.

The long-term cardiovascular complications of diabetes account for the major morbidity and mortality of the disease. Two types are recognized: atherosclerosis and microangiopathy. Atherosclerosis affects large vessels and leads to disability and death from myocardial infarction, peripheral vascular disease, and cerebrovascular accidents. The atherosclerotic changes have been linked to abnormal lipid metabolism and are indistinguishable from those occurring in nondiabetics but usually occur earlier and more extensively in diabetics. Microangiopathy refers to the striking and specific alterations in small blood vessels: capillaries and the smallest arterioles and venules. In the capillaries, the basement membrane is thickened in direct relation to the duration of the disease. The thickening is more severe in the glomerulus of the kidney.[71] A peculiarity of juvenile onset diabetes of recent origin is increased permeability of vascular beds to protein. Microvascular permeability to both small and large molecules is increased during poor metabolic regulation in short-term juvenile diabetics. The mechanism appears to be increased filtration pressure in the microcirculation and increased porosity of the microvasculature.[141] Leakage of fluorescein during fluorescein angiography is an early sign of juvenile diabetic retinopathy.[64] Physiologic changes occur before morphologic changes. After 1½ to 5 years, findings may include increased thickness in the peripheral glomerular basement membrane and an increase in content of basement membrane-like material in mesangial regions of glomeruli.[83, 139]

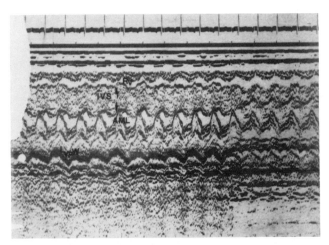

Fig. 38.1 An echocardiogram from a 2-day-old infant of a diabetic mother demonstrating a thickened interventricular septum (IVS) (10 mm) and a normal left ventricular posterior wall ($L_{VP}W$, 4mm). AML, anterior mitral valve leaflet; *RV*, right ventricle. (Reproduced with permission from G. L. Way *et al.*[196])

Clinical Features

The child with diabetes mellitus experiences polyuria, polydipsia, polyphagia, and weight loss. Additional symptoms may include fatigue, irritability, and moodiness. There may be acute metabolic derangement.[70]

Treatment and Prognosis

Depending upon the type of severity of diabetes, the disease may be controlled by diet, antidiabetic drugs, or injection of insulin, as discussed in detail elsewhere. Education is an important part of therapy.[71] Ordinary stress, well tolerated by nondiabetics, may greatly increase the metabolic abnormality of diabetes. Stress-induced hyperglycemia has been attributed to the synergistic action of anti-insulin hormones: epinephrine, glucagon, cortisol, and growth hormone. Increased insulin is often indicated during periods of stress.[71]

Vascular disease is the major problem of the diabetic patient.[101] Joslin Clinic studies have shown that retinopathy develops in 63% of juvenile diabetics by 30 years of age and in 87% by 50 years.[65] The life expectancy for the patient with diabetes is approximately two-thirds that of the general population matched for age at the time of diagnosis.[65]

FAMILIAL TYPE IIa HYPERLIPOPROTEINEMIA

Familial hypercholesterolemia is a well-defined familial disorder characterized chemically by an elevated plasma concentration of cholesterol carried by low density lipoproteins (LDL); clinically by xanthomas, arcus corneae, and premature coronary heart disease; and biochemically by deficiency in the cell surface receptor that regulates LDL degradation and cholesterol synthesis. It has autosomal dominant inheritance.[73] (See Chapter 40)

THE GLYCOGEN STORAGE DISEASES

The glycogen storage diseases (GSD) are uncommon inherited errors of metabolism that may lead to accumulation of glycogen in one or more tissues or may be associated with abnormal structure of glycogen.[94] These diseases are classified according to identified enzyme defects or distinctive clinical features. Some patients have multiple enzyme defects. Twelve main types have now been delineated (Table 38.1).[95] The following discussion concerns only those types that may affect the heart, Types II to V.[95]

GLYCOGEN STORAGE DISEASE IIa

Pathophysiology

Glycogen storage disease (GSD) type IIa, or Pompe's disease, is the classic form of infantile GSD, which is uniformly fatal within the first 2 years of life. It is characterized by progressive deposition of glycogen of normal structure in

TABLE 38.1   CLASSIFICATION OF GLYCOGEN STORAGE DISEASES[a, b]

Type	Eponyms or Familiar Terms	Tissue or Organ Involved	Enzyme Defect
0	Aglycogenosis GSD 0	Liver, not muscle	Deficiency of glycogen synthetase
I Pseudo	Von Gierke disease	Liver, kidney, intestine	Deficiency of glucose-6-phosphatase
Type I	Pseudo GSD I	Liver	Transport defect for glucose-6-phosphatase at microsomal membrane
IIA	Pompe disease Generalized glycogenosis Glycogen storage disease of the heart (infantile fatal form) GSD IIa	Generalized, especially heart, muscle, liver	Deficient activity of lysosomal enzyme alpha-1,4-glucosidase (lysosomal acid maltase) in involved tissues and in cultured amniotic fluid cells (normal activity in amniotic fluid)
IIb	Juvenile-adult form GSD IIb	Muscle and liver without cardiomegaly	
III	Forbes or Cori disease Limit dextrinosis, debrancher glycogenosis GSD III	Liver, heart, muscle, leukocytes	Amylo-1,6-glucosidase, "debrancher enzyme" deficiency in affected tissues and in cultured amniotic fluid cells (perhaps unnecessary; course usually benign)
IV	Andersen disease, amylopectinosis GSD IV	Generalized (?) Glycogen abnormal in structure	Amylo-1,4 → 1,6-transglucosidase, "brancher enzyme"
V	McArdle syndrome GSD V	Skeletal muscle	Congenital absence of skeletal muscle phosphorylase
VI	GSD VI	Liver	Deficiency of liver phosphorylase
VII	GSD VII	Skeletal muscle (severe) Erythrocytes (mild)	Reduction of phosphofructokinase activity
VIII	GSD VIII	Liver, brain	No enzymatic deficiency yet demonstrated; total liver phosphorylase normal but most is in inactive form
IX IXa and IXb	GSD IX	Liver	Deficiency of liver phosphorylase kinase; GSD IXa, autosomal recessive; GSD IXb, X-linked recessive
X	GSD X	Liver and muscle	Loss of activity of cyclic 3',5'-AMP-dependent kinase in muscle, presumably also in liver
	GSD XI (may include patients with glycogenosis with different enzyme defects.)	Liver, or liver and kidney	All enzymatic activities measured to date are normal.

[a] Modified with permission from G. Hug[95] and W. B. Saunders.

[b] This classification differs somewhat from that of Howell,[94] who recognizes eight types.

all tissues examined, especially the myocardium, skeletal muscle, and liver. There is deficient activity of the lysosomal enzyme, acid maltase, or alpha-1,4-glucosidase transmitted through a single recessive autosomal gene. The usual enzymes of glycogen synthesis and degradation are normal.[92, 94, 95, 123]

The lysosomal enzyme activity is diminished in all tissues examined except the kidney.[95] This accounts for the increased glycogen within lysosomes,[92, 123] but the cause of the accumulation of glycogen in the cytoplasm of the heart and skeletal muscle cells has not been explained. The liver glycogen can be mobilized by epinephrine, glucagon, or starvation, but this normalization of hepatic ultrastructure is of no apparent benefit to the patient.[95, 170]

In the final stages of the disease, the heart is globular and may be 3 to 10 times its normal weight.[92] The atria are relatively normal, but the ventricular walls, particularly those of the left heart, are massive. Sometimes, the left lung is collapsed. The liver, tongue, and diaphragm are usually enlarged. The brain is grossly normal.

Widespread glycogen deposits can be seen on examination by light microscopy, using periodic acid-Schiff reagent or Best's carmine staining. After digestion of glycogen with salivary amylase, the myocardium assumes a classical lacework pattern (Fig. 38.2). Individual muscle cells may be hypertrophied or fragmented and may reveal a severe vacuolar myopathy with large amounts of glycogen and some chemically unidentified basophilic material. Other sites of glycogen deposition include smooth muscle cells of blood vessels and intestines, hepatocytes, renal glomeruli, and tubules and neurones in both the peripheral and central nervous system.[30]

Analysis of tissues shows a marked increase in glycogen content. The normal concentration in skeletal muscle is usually under 1.5% of wet weight and that of the liver is 0 to 5%.[30] In patients with GSD IIa, glycogen is often found to be 5 to 10% of wet weight of these tissues.[30, 92]

The progressive deposition of glycogen in muscles and in the nervous system appears to be the direct cause of generalized muscular weakness. The massive glycogen infiltration in the cardiac muscle encroaches on the ventricular chamber size, as well as the left lung; the heart fails and there is respiratory embarassment. The enlarged tongue in the hypotonic child contributes to faulty deglutition and aspiration. Aspiration pneumonia results.[40]

Clinical Features

Most affected children appear clinically well at birth,[95] but the child may initially showed irritability and poor feeding.[30] The heart size and electrocardiogram at birth have been called marginally abnormal.[95] Physical signs and symptoms of the disease are usually noted in the early postnatal period: lethargy, poor weight gain, progressive hypotonia, difficulty in sucking, a feeble cry, and an enlarged protruding tongue. There may be cardiac murmurs, intermittent cyanosis, dyspnea, and cardiomegaly. As the disease progresses, heart sounds become distant and muffled, and an occasional episode of tachycardia or some other dysrhythmia may develop. A Wolff-Parkinson-White syndrome was noted in one.[30] Gallop rhythm is often present at the time of cardiac decompensation. Dysrhythmias may be readily induced by small doses of digitalis, suggesting an irritable myocardium.

Glycogenosis progressively leads to cardiomegaly, impaired myocardial function, and, finally, to cardiac failure. GSD IIa is reported to be uniformly fatal, usually by the 4th to 8th months of life. Aspiration or pneumonia is a terminal complication.[40] Death has been attributed to failure of respiratory muscles or to cardiac involvement.[30, 170]

Electrocardiographic Features

Characteristic electrocardiographic changes[40, 77] include a short PR interval, high QRS voltages, and evidence of left ventricular or biventricular hypertrophy. Less constant

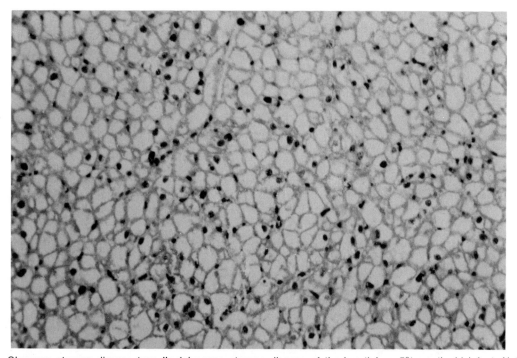

Fig. 38.2 Glycogen storage disease type IIa (glycogen storage disease of the heart) in a 5¾-month-old infant. Note the marked vacuolization of the left ventricle representing displaced glycogen. Formalin fixation, hematoxylin and eosin stain. (Reproduced with permission from J. L. Caddell and R. Whittemore[40] and The American Academy of Pediatrics.)

changes include slight prolongation of the QRS complexes; deep Q waves over the mid- or left precordium; transient T wave inversion; and ST segment elevation, depression, or bowing; and supraventricular tachycardia, nodal escapes, or other atrial dysrhythmias (Fig. 38.3). Vectorcardiograms are often compatible with bilateral ventricular enlargement and may have large QRSs E loops but with almost normal contour and orientation in the three conventional planes.

Gilette et al.[77] conducted intracardiac electrograms in an attempt to define the mechanism of the short PR interval. They found that the low right atrium to His bundle interval (LRA-H), a reflection of the artrioventricular conduction time, measured only 40% of the average for this age, and that there was slight lengthening following treatment with a glycolytic enzyme (Fig. 38.4). Caddell and Whittemore[40] had postulated that excess glycogen in the myocardium and

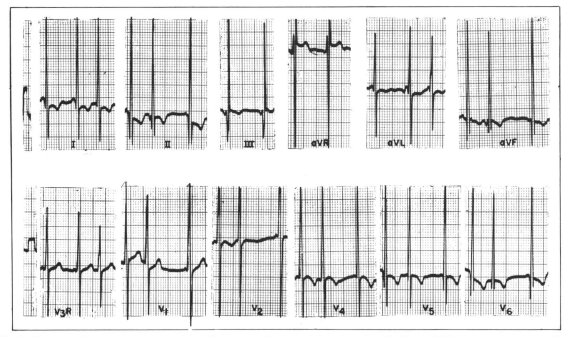

Fig. 38.3 Electrocardiogram in glycogen stage disease type IIa in the infant described in Figure 38.2 at 5 months of age. High voltage of QRS segments in all leads with evidence of combined ventricular hypertrophy is seen. The PR interval is shortened, with some evidence of a wandering of the pacemaker. T waves are inverted over the left precordium with reciprocal upright T waves in V_1 and in aVR. Calibration markers at the left of the figures indicate standardization.

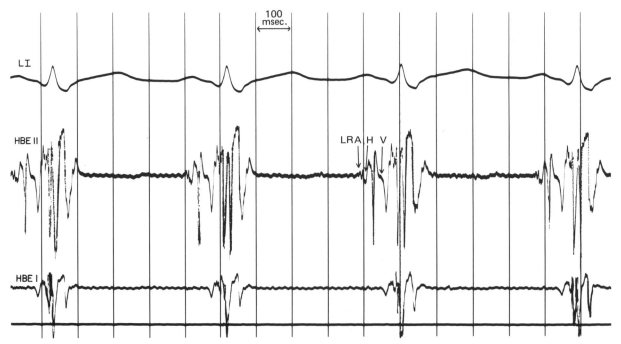

Fig. 38.4 His bundle electrogram with the intracardiac catheter withdrawn into the tricuspid valve area showing large His potential and abnormally short LRA-H interval. *LI*, surface standard lead I ECG; *HBE II*, His bundle electrogram with 11-mm interelectrode distance; *HBE I*, His bundle electrogram with 1-mm interelectrode distance; *LRA*, low right atrial depolarization; *H*, His bundle depolarization; *V*, ventricular depolarization. (Reproduced with permission from P. Gillette *et al.*[77] and the American Medical Association.)

conduction system might facilitate conduction in these patients. In a recent study,[30] glycogen accumulation was present in the specialized conduction tissue, as in the working myocardium.

Radiologic, Echocardiographic, and Angiocardiographic Features

The heart is enlarged and globular, the lungs are often congested, and pneumonia is a late complication.

The echocardiogram shows severe thickening of the intraventricular septum and the posterior left ventricular wall and a small left ventricular cavity.[30] Normal motion of the interventricular septum and anterior mitral valve leaflet has been noted. Other findings include a decreased E to F slope of the mitral valve associated with severe left ventricular hypertrophy, which is compatible with diminished left ventricular compliance.[30]

Hemodynamic and angiocardiographic studies have related normal ventricular ejection in some patients, and impaired ejection secondary to right or bilateral endocardial fibroelastosis in others. Isoproterenol injection may reveal a gradient between the left ventricle and the aorta not evident under basal conditions. Angiocardiographic findings in two infants indicated an abnormal trabecular pattern in the left ventricle.[60]

Differential Diagnosis

The diagnosis is suspected in the young infant who manifests progressively poor muscle tone with failure to thrive, has cardiomegaly with left ventricular hypertrophy, and has a short PR interval on the electrocardiogram. A skeletal muscle biopsy reveals histologic and histochemical evidence of glycogen deposition. The diagnosis is established by demonstrating glycogen in excess of 15% by wet weight of muscle and absence of α-1,4-glucosidase in the muscle.

The prenatal diagnosis of GSD IIa can be accomplished a few days after amniocentesis by the electron microscopic demonstration of abnormal lysosomes in *uncultured* amniotic fluid cells. *Cultured* amniotic fluid cells show deficient alpha-glucosidase activity.[95]

The differential diagnosis of glycogen storage disease of the heart includes congenital heart defects and metabolic or neurologic disease. Cardiac failure in this disease occurs in the early months of life and must be differentiated from other cardiac problems. Endocardial fibroelastosis is differentiated by the normal PR interval, as distinct from the short PR interval of glycogen storage disease of the heart. Coarctation of the aorta may be differentiated by blood pressure determinations. The murmur of aortic stenosis is usually far more distinct than that heard in glycogenosis. The aberrant coronary artery arising from the left pulmonary artery usually has a distinctive electrocardiographic pattern of an anterolateral myocardial infarction. The development of flaccid musculature may simulate amyotonia congenita. A floppy child with macroglossia must be differentiated from cretinism or mongolism.[40] The echocardiograms are similar to those of familial idiopathic hypertrophic subaortic stenosis associated with asymmetric septal hypertrophy, further illustrating the heterogeneous spectrum of diseases that comprise the group "hypertrophic cardiomyopathies."[30]

Treatment

Treatment is supportive. Digitalis may provoke dysrhythmias or aggravate obstruction of the ventricular outflow tract. Propranolol may be of benefit.[30] Although the lysosomal glycogen can be mobilized from hepatocytes by the administration of purified glycogen-degrading enzymes of fungal origin, the normalization of the hepatic ultrastructure does not benefit the patient.[95]

GLYCOGEN STORAGE DISEASE IIb

Juvenile and adult patients with GSD IIb[95] present weakness of skeletal muscle later in life. The condition develops progressively as a myopathy, beginning in the lower limbs and evolving slowly without cardiac signs or symptoms. The patients show difficulty walking which may demand a sedentary life-style that may be compatible with a normal life span. Some patients may die of respiratory failure during the third or fourth decade.

GLYCOGEN STORAGE DISEASES III, IV, AND V

Cardiac involvement has been reported in GSD III and IV, and a suggestive case of cardiomuscular glycogenosis was described in GSD V.

GSD III patients with deficiency of amylo-1,6-glucosidase may have abnormal glycogen deposition in cardiac muscle, as well as in skeletal muscle. It is recommended that they refrain from strenuous exercise and that anesthetics and cardiodepressant drugs be used cautiously. Death in one 4½-year-old child with this disorder was attributed to the cardiomyopathy.[155]

GSD IV infants appear normal at birth, but they soon fail to thrive. Only one is known to have survived until 4 years of age. No clinically significant heart disease has appeared, but nonspecific electrocardiographic abnormalities are found.[94, 170]

GSD V patients with muscle phosphorylase deficiency have not had clinical cardiac problems, but electrocardiographic abnormalities have been recorded.[94]

HYPERALDOSTERONISM

Chronic excessive aldosterone secretion by the adrenal (Conn's syndrome) rarely occurs in children and usually results from congenital bilateral adrenal hyperplasia. There is malignant hypertension, hypokalemia, hypernatremia, and metabolic alkalosis. Untreated, the childhood form progresses to chronic renal failure or to coronary artery disease in young adulthood. The treatment is surgical.[24, 61] Bongiovanni[24] estimates that the hypertension disappears in half of the surgically treated patients but persists in those with irreversible renal damage. The prognosis for life is guarded.

HYPOADRENALISM

Chronic adrenal insufficiency (Addison's disease) occurs rarely in childhood. The onset is usually insidious, with few symptoms such as increased pigmentation of the skin. There may be some degree of systemic and postural hypotension. The heart size in children is usually normal, in contrast to the thin cardiac silhouette of adult patients.[24] Under stress of infection or injury, the patient may develop symptoms of impending crisis: weakness, fatigability, anorexia, nausea, and vomitting. A crisis of acute adrenocortical insufficiency is characterized by shock, stupor, or coma and profound hypotension. Laboratory findings characteristically include electrolyte changes which may be reflected in the electrocardiogram: hyponatremia, hyperkalemia, and, sometimes, hypercalcemia. During therapy of the crisis, overtreatment with salt and mineralocorticoid therapy may cause edema, hypertension, cardiac failure, and death. Most children are restored to health and can be maintained on oral glucocorticoid and table salt.

PROGERIA

Progeria is an inborn error of metabolism apparent very early in childhood; no genetic basis has been proved. Characteristic features include a beak-like nose, small jaw, alopecia, retarded growth, scleroderma-like changes in connective tissue, and muscle contractures.[126] Systemic diastolic hypertension, cardiomegaly, and hypercholesterolemia develop around the age of 5 or 6 years. Atherosclerotic changes are premature and severe; death owing to myocardial infarction or cerebral vascular accident occurs on average at 14 years.

THE SALT-LOSING FORM OF CONGENITAL ADRENAL HYPERPLASIA

Approximately 50% of infants with deficiency of 21-hydroxylase exhibit salt losing; they have deficiency in the synthesis of both cortisol and aldosterone. Other causes are rare. Symptoms begin shortly after birth: virilization, failure to regain birth weight and progressive weight loss, anorexia, vomiting, and dehydration. Disturbances in cardiac rate and rhythm occur, with cyanosis and dyspnea. Treatment includes intravenous saline solutions and intramuscular desoxycorticosterone acetate, with biochemical monitoring.[24] Unless treated, the symptoms progress, and the patient collapses. Death may occur within a few weeks.[24] Normal growth and maturation can be achieved on adequate replacement therapy.[24, 61]

SICKLE CELL ANEMIA

Sickle cell anemia is a severe, chronic hemolytic anemia occurring in persons homozygous for the sickle gene.[142] In the United States, 1 in 500 blacks has sickle cell anemia,[85] which is about 50,000 patients.[199]

The basic defect is a mutant autosomal gene (the sickle gene) which causes an amino acid substitution in hemoglobin. As a result of this mutation, deoxygenated hemoglobin molecules aggregate and form fibers which cause the erythrocytes to become rigid and to "sickle."[142] This leads to capillary occlusion and to "crisis." The increased stroke volume of the heart compensates for the reduced oxygen-carrying capacity of the red cells. Very gradually, cardiac dilation and hypertrophy develop. Heart failure may sometimes be a late complication.

Clinical Features

Clinical symptoms of the anemia may be apparent in infants after 5 or 6 months,[142] but cardiovascular symptoms usually appear in older patients. Patients may show exertional dyspnea and palpitations. The diastolic blood pressure is lowered, and the pulse pressure is widened. The arterial pulse is brisk, there are commonly "pistol shot" sounds over the arteries, and the precordium is active. There is usually an ejection systolic murmur along the left sternal border, sometimes with an apical systolic thrill. Variable findings may include a middiastolic apical murmur and a gallop rhythm. The second sound is often widely split, with accentuation of the pulmonic component.[85]

The nonspecific electrocardiographic changes may include first degree AV block, left ventricular hypertrophy, and nonspecific T wave changes. Rarely, there may be right ventricular hypertrophy resulting from cor pulmonale or changes indicative of myocardial ischemia.[85]

The chest x-ray shows generalized cardiomegaly in nearly all patients.

Echocardiographic findings include vigorous left ventricular contraction, generalized chamber enlargement, and increased stroke volume. The velocity of circumferential fiber shortening, ejection fractions, and systolic time intervals is generally considered to be within normal limits.[85] The chronic volume overload of sickle cell anemia is well tolerated without development of left ventricular dysfunction.[76, 187]

Diagnosis

The most reliable evidence for the presence of a sickling disorder is the direct visualization of sickled cells after the addition of sodium metabisulfite. The presence of hemoglobin S cannot be established unless the typical hemoglobin electrophoretic pattern is obtained.[199] Blood cultures are necessary to rule out endocarditis.

Cardiovascular findings in sickle cell anemia may mimic rheumatic fever, mitral stenosis, congenital heart disease, or heart failure.[85] The subcutaneous nodules and erythema marginata, sometimes present in rheumatic fever, are not found in sickle cell crisis. In sickle cell crisis, there is pain over long bones as well as joints, and salicylate therapy is not effective. Cardiac catheterization is required for proof of coexisting congenital heart disease.

Treatment

There is no treatment for the anemia. Iron therapy is contraindicated unless iron deficiency can be diagnosed. During the acute episode, dehydration and acidosis should be vigorously corrected, and complicating bacterial infections should be treated with antibiotics. During the crisis, transfusions of packed red cells, sometimes as partial exchange transfusion, are valuable.

THALASSEMIA MAJOR

Thalassemia major (Cooley anemia) is the homozygous state for an inherited disorder which results from defective B-chain synthesis in hemoglobin.[197] In this anemia, regularly spaced blood transfusions are necessary to prevent severe anemia and hypertrophy of the erythropoietic tissues. For several reasons, hemochromatosis develops as the patients grow older (see Iron Excess and Secondary Hemochromatosis in this chapter). Pericarditis and chronic heart failure due to myocardial siderosis usually occur during the 2nd decade, and the patients usually die during the 2nd or 3rd decade. It is impossible to distinguish the effects of anemia from those of hemochromatosis. Despite intensive medical management that did not include chelation therapy, the mortality of thalassemia major in recent years[68] was essentially unchanged from that of a pre-1964 series.[69] It is concluded that the major findings in this syndrome are those of iron overload; hopefully, the use of iron chelators to retard or prevent iron deposition may modify the cause of heart disease in these subjects.[68, 90, 135]

THYROID DISEASES

Deficiency or excess of thyroid hormones produce syndromes that directly affect the cardiovascular system.

Pathophysiology

The main function of the thyroid gland is to synthesize thyroxine (T_4) and triiodothyronine (T_3).[62] Iodine is essential for the synthesis of these hormones, which takes place mainly within the thyroglobulin molecule.[150] Under normal conditions, most circulating T_3 is derived from T_4 rather than directly from the thyroid gland.[62] The synthesis, storage, accretion, delivery, and utilization of thyroid hormones involve a complex sequence of metabolic events, each of which probably depends on specific enzymatic activity. Thyroid disease may result from blockage at many steps in the metabolic process.[175] The metabolic potency of T_3 is three to four times that of T_4,[62] but in the blood, the level of T_3 is 1/50th that of T_4. Those circulating hormones are bound to thyroxine-binding globulins and other proteins.[62]

The anterior pituitary hormone, thyroid stimulating hormone (TSH), regulates the thyroid gland.[150] In states of decreased production of thyroid hormone, TSH is increased, producing hypertrophy and hyperplasia of thyroid cells. Synthesis of the thyroid hormones is increased; these, in turn, inhibit the production of TSH.[62, 175]

The thyroid hormones increase oxygen consumption, stimulate protein synthesis, influence growth and differentiation, and affect the metabolism of carbohydrates, lipids, minerals, and vitamins.[175] There are several possible mechanisms by which the thyroid hormones may influence the cardiovascular system. For example, they may increase the demand for cardiac output by increasing oxygen utilization and metabolic consumption, and they may increase myocardial sensitivity to catecholamines.

Thyroid disease may occur in the neonate. During pregnancy, only limited amounts of maternal thyroid hormones slowly cross the placenta to enter the fetal circulation.[175] However, transplacental passage of other substances may profoundly influence the fetal thyroid.[62, 96, 175] Thyroid stimulating immunoglobulin (TSI) or other maternal factors as yet unidentified may cause congenital hyperthyroidism; iodine and radioiodine (^{131}I) may damage the thyroid, causing hypothyroidism.[33, 62, 96]

Laboratory Tests

The most common screening test for hypo- and hyperthyroidism are serum levels of thyroxine (T_4) and triiodothyronine (T_3). A radioimmunoassay for T_4, referred to as T_4 (RIA), is an efficient micromethod for analysis. Normal levels of thyroxine are higher during the first weeks of life than subsequently. For example, values by RIA are 8 to 13 μg/dl in cord blood, 10 to 20.8 in the newborn, 7 to 15 in the infant, and 5 to 14 in the child.[62, 116] Levels of T_3 (RIA) are under 50 ng/dl of cord blood, increase to mean levels of 400 ng/dl by 24 hours, and by 3 days of age stabilize between 100 and 170 ng/dl, the level of older children and adults.[62, 116] Thyrotropin is also measured by radioimmunoassay TSH (RIA). Normal levels are less than 10 μU/ml; levels over 20 μU/ml indicate hypothyroidism. The use of ^{131}I is no longer recommended for children; it has been largely replaced by technetium (^{99m}Tc), which has a half-time of only 6 hours and is useful for thyroid scanning.[62]

Hypothyroidism results from deficiency of production of thyroid hormone or unresponsiveness of the thyroid gland to thyrotropin or to thyroid hormone. It may be congenital and clinically apparent in the perinatal period, or it may appear after a period of apparently normal thyroid function. At that time, symptoms may result from delayed manifestations of congenital hypothyroidism or from a newly acquired defect.

CONGENITAL HYPOTHYROIDISM

All expressions of congenital hypothyroidism, whether sporadic or familial, goitrous or nongoitrous, will be included in this section. The problem is most commonly caused by a developmental defect of the thyroid gland, thyroid dysgenesis, which occurs in about 1 of every 6000 births. Maternal

ingestion of iodides,[127] propylthiouracil,[62] methimazole, or radioactive sodium iodide (^{131}I) during pregnancy may result in congenital hypothyroidism. Deficiency of thyrotropin or thyroid hormone are among the other causes of congenital hypothyroidism. Published data on the influence of maternal hypothyroidism[62] on the offspring are controversial.[130] Several investigators studied the infants of hypothyroid women and found that they may be normal.[130]

Clinical Features

Regardless of the etiology, the clinical manifestations of cretinism are the same, and the severity of the syndrome appears to be directly related to the degree of thyroid hormone deficiency.[150] Congenital hypothyroidism is about three times as common in girls as in boys. The earliest signs are increased body weight and unusual prolongation of the physiologic jaundice.

The typical picture of hypothyroidism may not be apparent until the age of 3 months and may not be fully developed until 6 months. The infant has a normal or subnormal temperature and a normal or slow heart rate. There is persistence of infantile features, with a protuberant tongue and often a harsh cry. The skin is cool and mottled, and the hair is coarse and dry. Myxedema may develop in the skin of the eyelids, the back of the hands, and the external genitalia. Carotenemia causes a yellowish discoloration. Respirations may be noisy, and there may be apneic spells. Cardiac examination may initially show a normal rate and quality of heart sounds, except for variable murmurs. The murmur has been described as crescendo in nature, loudest over the base of the heart. As the child grows older, the heart rate slows, and the heart sounds become softer. The precordial pulsation may be difficult to localize. Untreated infants are mentally retarded and are late in sitting and standing.

Electrocardiographic Features

The electrocardiogram shows nonspecific changes; low voltage may occur in all of the complexes, most frequently in P waves, with flattening or inversion of T waves, especially in leads I and II. Low voltage of the QRS complex is a less constant finding.[74] These signs all revert toward normal with adequate thyroid replacement therapy.[74, 150]

Radiologic Features

An enlargement of the cardiac silhouette, due to cardiac enlargement or pericardial effusion, is common in hypothyroidism. There is rarely evidence of heart failure. Examination of bones of the cretin at term shows delayed epiphyseal development for the infant's chronological age with absence of distal femoral and proximal tibial epiphyses.

Echocardiographic Features

Recent echocardiographic studies in children with hypothyroidism showed frequent small pericardial effusions which were not related to the severity of the thyroid failure. Compared with euthyroid children, the hypothyroid children showed no abnormality in cardiac chamber or myocardial dimensions, systolic time intervals, or indices of myocardial contractility. Myocardial contractility was expressed by the percent of change in left ventricle diameter. Data for the velocity of circumferential fiber shortening also showed no change from normal. After normal thyroxine concentration was established with exogenous hormone, the children showed no changes in myocardial dimensions or contractility indices. Only heart rate showed a significant change, and the small pericardial effusions usually resolved.[88] This work is at variance with echocardiographic data from patients with long-standing hypothyroidism within an age range that includes adolescents and young adults. Echocardiographic studies showed an asymmetric septal hypertertrophy in 17 of 19 patients in one series.[159, 160] Additional abnormalities included reduced amplitude of systolic septal excursion and reduced percent of systolic anterior motion of the mitral valve. These abnormalities resolved in patients who returned to the euthyroid state after L-thyroxine therapy.

Laboratory Data

In primary hypothyroidism, serun levels of T_4 and T_3 are low or borderline, and serum levels of TSH exceed 20 μU/ml. Patients with thyroid enlargement (goitrous hypothyroidism) may require definitive testing, including perchlorate discharge tests, kinetic studies, chromatography, and studies of thyroid tissues. Technetium scanning may be indicated in other infants to determine whether there is any thyroid tissue.[62] Mass screening programs for congenital hypothyroidism have been employed.[66, 72] Thyroxine[66] and TSH[109] determinations are conducted from filter paper blood spots collected by heel stick on days 2 to 4 of life.

Differential Diagnosis

The presence of a murmur together with a prominent tongue may raise the question of 21-trisomy syndrome (Down syndrome), cardiac glycogenosis (glycogen storage disease IIa), or amyotonia congenita. The child with 21-trisomy, however, usually shows more interest in his surroundings and is usually more active than the hypothyroid infant. In general, the child with 21-trisomy has characteristic facies, including epicanthic folds, and has normal texture of skin and hair. Congenital heart defects are prominent findings in 21-trisomy children. On the other hand, the infant with cardiac glycogenosis has poor growth, nondescript cardiac murmurs, and distinctive electrocardiographic changes. These may include QRS complexes of high amplitude and shortening of the PR interval. Chemical and chromosomal studies are most helpful in establishing these diagnoses.

Prevention and Treatment

Prevention of congenital hypothyroidism should be the first consideration. This includes treatment of hypothyroid patients with iodine, enriching salt with iodine, and careful management of pregnant mothers, particularly in respect to any form of therapy that may affect the fetal thyroid gland. The aim of therapy in the hypothyroid child is to establish and maintain a euthyroid state at the earliest possible age to permit suitable mental and physical development; thyroid hormone is critical for normal cerebral development in the early months of life.[110, 127] Replacement therapy with thyroid hormone is indicated and is effective for hypothyroidism of all causes. Sodium L-thyroxine, given orally, is preferred to dessiccated thyroid because of its stability, long shelf-life, and constant biologic activity.[62] Larger doses relative to body weight are required during the first year of life. DiGeorge[62] treats infants with 50 μg/day, gradually doubling this dose after 6 months of age. Older children are begun on a dose of 100 to 150 μg/day. This dose is estimated to be 4 μg/kg of body weight.[62] Serum levels of T_4 and TSH should be monitored and maintained within the normal range. Rapid full replacement has been associated with sudden death in severely hypothyroid children with poor heart sounds and evidence of myxedema.[150] Excessive thyroid hormone in infants can lead to cranial synostosis. The metabolism of many drugs, including digitalis, barbiturates, narcotics, or tranquilizers, is delayed in hypothyrodism.[150] Digitalis is poorly tolerated and is rarely indicated in hypothyroidism of childhood.

Prognosis

The best results in severe cretinism, insofar as mental achievement and neurological sequelae are concerned, are obtained by early adequate thyroid replacement therapy.[172] Without treatment, affected infants may die of infections or respiratory obstruction, or they may survive and become mentally deficient dwarfs. The more profound the deprivation of thyroid hormone in the early months of life, the poorer the prognosis for mental development.

JUVENILE HYPOTHYROIDISM

Juvenile hypothyroidism refers to acquired thyroid deficiency during childhood and adolescence[129] in previously euthyroid subjects. Acquired hypothyroidism most commonly results from lymphocytic thyroiditis (Hashimoto's disease or autoimmune thyroiditis), which may have a prevalence as high as 1% of school children. It may or may not be associated with goiter. Other causes include subtotal or complete thyroidectomy for thyrotoxicosis or carcinoma, cystinosis, and protracted ingestion of goitrogens or of medications such as iodides or cobalt.

Clinical Features

The most striking manifestations of juvenile hypothyroidism are delayed skeletal growth and maturation. After 2 years of age, mental deficiency is not usually a feature of the syndrome,[172] although the untreated child may appear dull and lethargic, with myxedematous changes of the skin and constipation.[150] The degree of skeletal retardation and the presence of epiphyseal dysgenesis may be important clinical signs that date the onset of the disease.[150] Hypothyroidism occurring before puberty has been associated with a delay in pubescence.

Cardiac manifestations are few. Bradycardia is usually noted with a low pulse pressure, poor peripheral circulation, and an occasional variable systolic murmur which may be innocent. Heart failure rarely occurs.[150] However, pericardial effusion occurs in some cases of myxedematous cardiac enlargement. The effusion may be very large, but because of slow accumulation, it rarely produces tamponade.[150] There is no evidence of associated pericarditis.[74] The effusion has a high protein concentration and is associated with a pleural effusion in about 50% of cases.

The diagnostic studies for juvenile hypothyroidism during childhood, including electrocardiographic, radiologic, and echocardiographic features, are the same as described for congenital hypothyroidism.[62]

Differential Diagnosis

Since most of the signs and symptoms of hypothyroidism are nonspecific, one must have a high index of suspicion to make the diagnosis. In the presence of clinical signs and low serum thyroxine concentration, the diagnosis is not difficult.[150] Cessation or retardation of growth in a child whose growth has previously been normal should alert one to the possibility of hypothyroidism. The diagnosis of obesity in children has sometimes been mistaken for hypothyroidism. Most obese children are tall and have warm, moist skin and normal thyroid function.[62]

Treatment

The treatment is as described for congenital hypothyroidism.

GOITER

A goiter is an enlargement of the thyroid gland and may result in normal function of the thyroid gland, hypothyroidism, or hyperthyroidism. It may be congenital or acquired, endemic or sporadic.[62]

Congenital Goiter

Congenital goiter is usually sporadic and may result from the administration of antithyroid drugs and/or iodides to the mother during pregnancy. These drugs and iodides cross the placenta and interfere with synthesis of thyroid hormone in the fetus. The infants are often euthyroid but may be hypothyroid, as illustrated by Melvin and associates.[127] An infant of an asthmatic mother who received 160 mg of potassium iodide daily throughout pregnancy showed bilateral swelling of the anterior neck, labored respirations, and pallor at birth. Technetium scan of the neck revealed a massively enlarged thyroid. At 21 hours of age, serum T_4 and TSH were diagnostic of hypothyroidism with compensatory elevation of TSH. Chest roentgenograms at 24 hours showed cardiomegaly (Fig. 38.5), and the electrocardiogram showed combined ventricular hypertrophy. Because of tachypnea, cyanosis, and apneic episodes, the thyroid isthmus was re-

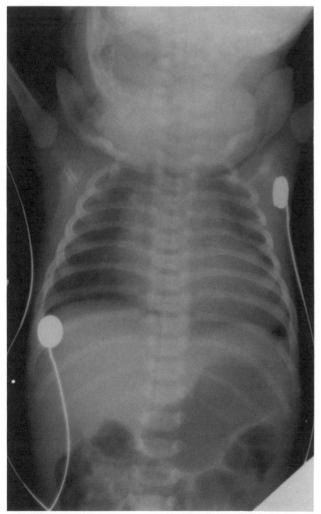

Fig. 38.5 Portable chest x-ray taken at 24 hours of age in a term infant with iatrogenic congenital goiter and hypothyroidism. Note the bilateral swelling of the anterior neck and the cardiac enlargement. (Reproduced with permission from G. R. Melvin et al.[127])

sected at 36 hours of age, and oral thyroid replacement therapy was begun. The microscopic examination revealed a diffuse thyroid hyperplasia. At 3 weeks, the child was clinically well, except for a small goiter, and showed a normal electrocardiogram and chest roentgenogram. Development was normal at 20 months.

Endemic Goiter and Cretinism

Endemic goiter has been associated with deficiency of environmental iodine since 1852 when Chatin, a French botanist, linked the condition to decreased iodine content of soils, waters, and foods in Europe.[184] In regions where deficiency of iodine is severe, decompensation of the thyroid gland and hypothyroidism may result. In mild iodine deficiency, thyroid enlargement may not be noted unless there is increased demand for the hormone, as during adolescent growth or pregnancy. Serum thyroxine levels may be low in endemic goiter, but clinical hypothyroidism is relatively rare. Endemic goiter has disappeared in areas where adequate dietary iodine is provided.

Endemic cretinism affects up to 10% of the people in an area where endemic goiter is prevalent, and most suffer from deaf mutism.[150] It occurs mainly in relatively isolated and socioeconomically retarded areas whose inhabitants are poorly nourished, which suggests that the pathogenesis may include interactions of genetic and environmental factors, including goitrogenic agents.[96] The treatment of endemic cretinism is generally unsatisfactory. Emphasis must be on prevention, since endemic cretinism related to iodine deficiency can be eliminated by appropriate iodine therapy to the affected population, or to women in the form of iodized oil.[150]

HYPERTHYROIDISM

Hyperthyroidism is the result of excessive secretion of the thyroid hormone. It may be congenital or acquired after a period of apparently normal thyroid function (juvenile).

CONGENITAL HYPERTHYROIDISM

When hyperthyroidism has its onset in the neonatal period, the most common cause is increased thyroid-stimulating immunoglobulin (TSI) in infants of mothers who had active or recently active Graves' disease during pregnancy. The condition is thought to be due to transplacental passage of TSI or of other thyroid-stimulating factors from the mother. Male and female infants are equally affected. The maternal supply of TSI terminates at birth.[150]

Clinical Manifestations

The infant is often premature and usually has a goiter. He appears anxious and is restless, alert, and irritable. The eyes are widely open and appear exophthalmic. The thyroid is enlarged, and the head may be hyperextended. Periorbital edema and acrocyanosis are frequently seen. Tachypnea, full and bounding pulses, and cardiomegaly may be presenting findings. A short, harsh, variable systolic murmur without a thrill and hepato- and splenomegaly are usually found.

Extremely affected infants may show a progression of symptoms. Despite a ravenous appetitie, the infants may lose weight. Hepatomegaly increases, and jaundice may develop. Cardiac decompensation is common. The infants may die if therapy is not instituted promptly. The condition usually resolves as the level of blood immunoglobulins decreases.

There is usually elevation and peaking of the P waves in standard lead II and in the leads from the right precordium, presumably due to increased atrial filling in an overactive heart and relatively high pulmonary vascular resistance of the newborn period. A series of dysrhythmias have been described: supraventricular tachycardia, nodal rhythm, complete heart block, and, occasionally, atrial arrest patterns. Right ventricular or combined ventricular hypertrophy is often found (Fig. 38.6).

Cardiac enlargement, which diminishes with improvement in compensation, is the main finding related to the heart. Advanced bone age, frontal bossing, and cranial synostosis are commonly found.

The serum level of thyroxine, T_4, is markedly elevated, as is thyroid stimulating-immunoglobulin (TSI). Other laboratory changes (Fig. 38.7) may be seen.

Treatment

The choice of drug depends upon the severity of the condition. In severe thyroid storm, a prompt-acting drug is required. Propranolol has a rapid effect and short duration but must be given cautiously. A dose of 2 mg/day in three divided doses is effective. The patient may also require digitalis therapy. In less urgent situations, Lugol's solution, in a dose of 1 drop every 8 hours, and propylthiouracil (10 mg every 8 hours) may be given, but this therapy is not completely effective until 4 to 6 weeks have passed. Other supportive measures include sedation and parenteral fluid therapy.

Congenital hyperthyroidism usually remits within 3 months, but it occasionally persists for up to 6 months and in some instances for many years. The latter group of infants usually occur in families with high frequency of hyperthyroidism in childhood or later life.

JUVENILE HYPERTHYROIDISM

Pathophysiology

Diffuse toxic goiter or Graves' disease, the commonest cause of hyperthyroidism in children, is believed to be caused

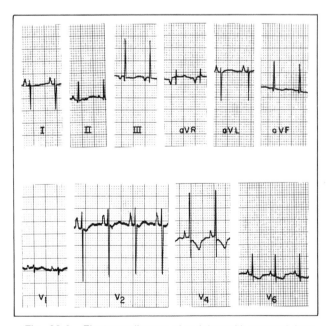

Fig. 38.6 Electrocardiogram of an infant with neonatal thyrotoxicosis at 48 hours of age, showing right axis deviation, tall peaked P waves suggesting right atrial enlargement, and nonspecific ST-T wave changes. (Reproduced with permission from R. Whittemore, Yale University School of Medicine.)

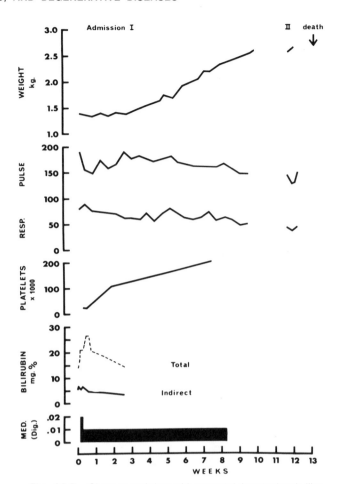

Fig. 38.7 Chart on an infant with neonatal thyrotoxicosis illustrating initial hyperbilirubinemia and thrombocytopenia with poor initial weight gain and variable tachycardia until the 5th week. (death was due to fire.) (Reproduced with permission from R. Whittemore, Yale University School of Medicine.)

by antibodies such as the long-acting thyroid stimulator (LATS) or LATS protector and human thyroid stimulator.[62] The condition is often associated with lymphocytic thyroiditis and other autoimmune disorders. "Pre-Graves' disease" refers to a dynamic state of disordered antithyroid immunity, sometimes leading to overt thyrotoxicosis and found in children of parents who have Graves' disease.[44] Hyperthyroidism in children may also be caused by thyroid carcinoma, acute suppurative thyroiditis, or toxic uninodular goiter.[62]

Clinical Manifestations

The peak frequency of Graves' disease occurs during adolescence[62] and is more common in females than in males.[183] The onset is gradual. The children become hyperactive, irritable, and excitable. The thyroid is enlarged, and there may be audible bruits over it. The child may have dyspnea. Cardiac findings may be life-threatening. There is an increase in heart rate, systolic blood pressure, and pulse pressure. Palpitation, cardiac enlargement, and cardiac insufficiency may occur. Atria fibrillation rarely occurs. Mitral insufficiency, resulting from papillary muscle dysfunction, may cause an apical systolic murmur. Growth is accelerated; osseous development is advanced.

There are two forms of hyperthyroidism that may rarely occur in childhood. The first, thyroid crisis or storm, is defined as the life-threatening or exacerbation of thyrotoxicosis characterized by fever and severe tachycardia and the exaggeration of all its metabolic manifestations.[193] There may be rapid progression to prostration and death. The second, "apathetic" hyperthyroidism,[62] is characterized by marked lethargy and progressive muscular weakness, symptoms that mask the hyperthyroidism.

Electrocardiographic Features and Noninvasive Techniques

The electrocardiogram may be normal, but findings suggestive of atrial and left ventricular hypertrophy are more common in children than in adults. Prominence of P waves in lead II and over the right precordium has been reported in over 25% of older patients. The QRS complex sometimes is abnormally tall. High T waves may be associated with increased myocardial contractility, low T waves with myocardial hypoxemia. A number of children may also show nonspecific ST and T changes. Sinus tachycardia is commonly seen,[45] while dysrhythmias are rare and are occasionally associated with reserpine therapy. Atrial fibrillation almost never occurs in children. Electrocardiographic abnormalities usually disappear soon after the patient becomes euthyroid.[58, 143]

Noninvasive techniques such as simultaneous carotid pulse, electrocardiography, and phonocardiography may reflect cardiac output and the rate of rise of left ventricular pressure. A decreased pre-ejection phase (PEP), due to shortened isovolumic contraction (ICT), is found in hyperthyroidism. Serial PEP may be useful to measure treatment response: the shortened pre-ejection period returns toward normal as serial T_4 measurements improve.[140]

M-mode echocardiography is the most direct means of demonstrating the hyperkinesia of the intraventricular septum and left ventricular posterior wall (Fig. 38.8A). This results in increased shortening fraction. Sinus tachycardia or dysrhythmia may be evident. In patients with incipient or clinical thyrotoxic heart failure, the left ventricular diameters ($LVID_d$ and $LVID_s$) and left atrial diameter are increased. The shortening fraction is often decreased (Fig. 38.8B).[136]

Radiologic Features

There is generalized cardiac enlargement, often with prominence of the pulmonary conus. Pulmonary vascular markings may be slightly engorged, especially in the presence of heart failure.

Ultrasound examination of the thyroid gland is now an established diagnostic technique.[163, 200] Abnormalities of the parenchymal texture are readily shown in diffuse lesions such as inflammatory and dysplastic conditions. Focal lesions such as cysts and adenomas as small as ½ to 1 cm in diameter may also be demonstrated with the newer high resolution small part scanners.[200]

Laboratory Data

Levels of both thyroxine (T_4) and triiodothyronine (T_3) are usually increased. Thyrotropic (TSH) levels are usually low, and there are usually elevated levels of thyroid-stimulating immunoglobulin.

Differential Diagnosis

Chorea and rheumatic carditis occasionally must be differentiated from the cardiac manifestations of hyperthyroidism. The emotional lability, restlessness, and irritability associated with tachycardia may suggest Sydenhams's chorea, but the excessive movements in hyperthyroidism are better coordinated than they are in chorea, where they are purposeless and uncontrollable. The systolic murmur referred to the apex in a child with tachycardia, and a hyperkinetic

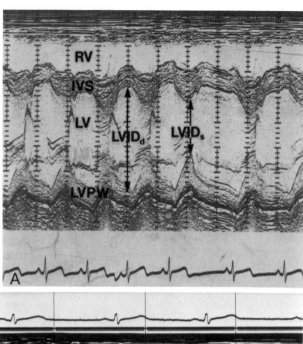

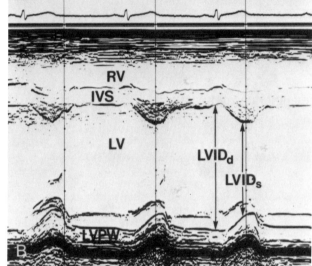

Fig. 38.8 (A) M-mode echocardiogram of a 12-year-old with thyrotoxicosis showing "hyperkinetic" heart with increased shortening fraction (49%). RV, right ventricle; IVS, interventricular septum; LV, left ventricle; $LVID_d$, left ventricular internal diameter during diastole; $LVID_s$, left ventricular internal diameter during systole. LVPW, left ventricular posterior wall. (B) M-mode echocardiogram of a 13-year-old with thyrotoxicosis and incipient heart failure showing increased $LVID_d$ with a shortening fraction of 30% that is at the lower limit of normal. (Reproduced with permission from S. Nouri.[136])

heart may suggest rheumatic carditis. Pheochromocytoma may resemble hyperthyroidism clinically, but the serum catecholamine level is elevated while the thyroid hormones are within normal range.

Treatment

There are two approaches to treatment, medical and surgical. Many physicians prefer a course of medical treatment before considering subtotal thyroidectomy. The recommended antithyroid drugs are propylthiouracil and methimazole (Tapazole), both of which produce a progressive decrease in the synthesis of thyroid hormone by inhibiting the incorporation of iodide into organic compounds. The dose of propylthiouracil is 100 to 150 mg three times daily;

the dose of methimazole is 10 to 15 mg three times daily. Smaller initial doses should be used in young children; overdosage may lead to hypothyroidism. The dose is individually adjusted to the needs of the patients. Toxic reactions may occur with either drug with about equal frequency. The most common toxic reactions are: transient urticarial skin rashes, leukopenia, and fever. Rarely, more serious reactions may occur.

A beta-adrenergic blocking agent such as propranolol is a useful supplement to the severely toxic patient to reduce the effect of catecholamines. Thyroid hormones potentiate the action of catecholamines, manifestations of which include tachycardia.

Surgical management, subtotal thyroidectomy, is sometimes indicated. This is relatively safe after a course of therapy with antithyroid drugs to bring the patient to a euthyroid state and after potassium iodide to reduce the vascularity of the gland. Careful and repeated evaluation of the cardiac status is essential in the postoperative period. There may be residual or recurrent hyperthyroidism, or hypothyroidism may develop after extensive surgery.[62] Recurrent laryngeal nerve injury and hypoparathyroidism may complicate postthyroidectomy.[42] Radioactivity therapy should be avoided because of the possible development of thyroid nodules.[150]

II. SYNDROMES RESULTING FROM DEFICIENCY OR EXCESS OF NUTRIENTS

DEFICIENCY OR EXCESS OF OVERALL NUTRITION

Obesity

In the United States, 15% of children are estimated to be greater than 40% above their ideal weight.[28] The cardiovascular implications of this are great.[188]

Cardiac output is increased in simple obesity. There is a close relationship between cardiac output and body weight, and between cardiac output and total blood volume. The high blood flow in obese subjects is largely distributed to fat droplets. The pulmonary blood volume increases in obese subjects in proportion to the increase in total blood volume.[152] The principal ventilatory consequences of obesity are: reduction of lung and chest wall compliance; normal airway resistance; an increase in work of breathing together with reduced respiratory muscle efficiency; and closure of peripheral lung units with consequent shunts and systemic arterial hypoxemia.[152]

The *Pickwickian Syndrome* named after Joe, the fat boy in Dicken's *Pickwick Papers*, is a rare complication of extreme exogenous obesity in which there is severe cardiorespiratory distress. Heart failure and pulmonary insufficiency are cardinal features.[17, 152] The patient is obese, somnolent, and cyanotic. He has tachycardia, cardiac dilatation with signs of tricuspid insufficiency, an enlarged liver, and peripheral edema. Laboratory tests reveal polycythemia and hypoxemia. There is sometimes an elevated left ventricular end-diastolic pressure. The pulmonary function tests reveal a decrease in pulmonary, tidal, and expiratory reserve.[17, 152] The aims of therapy are weight reduction, control of circulatory failure, and improvement of ventilation. The regimen includes strict dietary control, diuretics, venesection, and digitalis. The patient can restore blood gases to normal with voluntary overbreathing. Oxygen must be given with caution because the respiratory drive may depend upon the stimulatory effect of hypoxemia; uncontrolled administration of oxygen can lead to hypoventilation and CO_2 narcosis.[17, 152]

Children of obese parents and those with obese siblings should adhere to a program of energetic exercise and a nutritionally balanced diet low in calories with as much bulk as possible.[17] The prevention of morbid obesity (100 lbs. overweight) is of greatest importance.[188] There is a danger of sudden death from ventricular dysrhythmias in obese patients experiencing too rapid weight reduction by prolonged use of low calorie weight reduction regimens consisting largely of protein. In these patients, the electrocardiograms and pathological specimens revealed a pattern of cardiac changes previously described in starvation.[174] Jejunoileal bypass for morbid obesity is still an experimental procedure; the long-term effect on survival is not yet known.[138, 153] Severe complications have been reported,[153] many of which are related to malabsorption of essential nutrients, including vitamins and minerals. This procedure is not recommended.[153] The balance of essential nutrients in man is of growing concern.[7, 52, 151]

PROTEIN OR PROTEIN-CALORIE DEFICIENCY STATES

Protein allowances for infants, 2.2 gm/kg of body weight, decrease gradually to 0.8 gm/kg at the age of 18.[52] Protein or protein-calorie malnutrition states are primarily syndromes of technically underdeveloped countries in the tropics (see Section IV of this chapter), but there is an increased awareness of its occurrence among children of the new vegetarians[7] and in patients with heart failure and other chronic diseases.

DEFICIENCY OR EXCESS OF MINERALS

Calcium Deficiency

Hypocalcemic cardiomyopathy is a reversible syndrome that promptly responds to adequate calcium and vitamin D therapy.

Calcium is concerned in the "coupling mechanism"—in linking of electrical stimulation to the contractile process—and in the absence of calcium ions contraction does not take place despite electrical excitation.[182] The sarcoplasmic reticulum of cardiac muscle is reported to be unable to sequester sufficient quantities of calcium to trigger contraction and is therefore dependent on extracellular sources of ionic calcium. Acute heart failure has been reported in calcium-deficient dogs, in human neonates with low serum calcium the only finding, and in hypocalcemic children and adolescents with previously undiagnosed hypoparathyroidism.[12, 18, 132] Patients may sometimes show peripheral edema, cardiomegaly, pulmonary congestion, hepatomegaly, and positive Chvostek and Trousseau signs. The electrocardiogram may show prolongation of the QT interval, and the chest x-ray film shows generalized cardiomegaly and congested pulmonary vessels with acute pulmonary edema.[18] The heart failure is refractory to digitalis and diuretics, but responds when specific therapies such as those using calcium gluconate and vitamin D restore the serum calcium to normal.

Calcium Excess

Increased calcium deposition may occur in association with excessive vitamin D,[23,156] in magnesium deficiency,[89] and in a variety of metabolic disorders. Generalized aortic calcification of infancy is fundamentally a disorder of degeneration of elastic fiber, with calcification predominantly in the internal elastic lamina, followed by occlusion and rupture of the tunica intima and death from myocardial infarction during the first 6 months of life. Idiopathic hypercalcemia with failure to thrive is associated with hypertension and supravalvular aortic stenosis.[23,156] An infant with calcifications in medium-sized arteries and in arterioles has recently been described.[189]

Copper Deficiency

Copper deficiency in animals may result in lesions in the heart and arteries; there are species differences. Cattle develop a progressive degeneration of the myocardium with replacement by dense collagenous tissue and may die suddenly, presumably of heart failure. Copper treatment prevents the disease. Pigs may develop cardiac hypertrophy and failure.[185] Rat pups born to copper-deficient dams showed cardiac enlargement, sometimes with apical aneurysms, myocardial necrosis, and hemopericardium.[105] The integrity of the cardiovascular system, particularly of the great arteries, largely depends on the quantity and quality of elastin and collagen. Copper is required for the maturation of these connective tissue proteins. Copper-deficient chicks and pigs may develop structural defects in major arteries with rupture, hemorrhage, and death.[185]

Menkes' kinky hair syndrome, an X-linked genetic disorder in infants,[128] is a manifestation of copper deficiency resulting from defective intestinal absorption of the mineral.[55] The infants have pudgy cheeks, straight eyebrows, and hair that resembles steel wool (Fig. 38.9A). They show progressive degeneration of the brain, scurvy-like changes in long bones, and tortuosity of cerebral and other arteries (Fig. 38.9B). Menkes' syndrome proves[96] that copper is required for normal fetal and neonatal development; similar changes have been described[96] in an infant born to a woman who was treated during pregnancy with a copper-binding drug, penicillamine.

There are several copper deficiency syndromes of infancy and childhood related to low dietary copper. Premature infants less than 1500 g always have low copper reserves and may develop a copper deficiency syndrome of growth if they are fed a copper-poor food such as modified cow's milk for several months.[52] Copper deficiency was diagnosed in malnourished infants during prolonged parenteral alimenta-

tion.[102] Severely malnourished children with chronic diarrhea became deficient after being rehabilitated on cow's milk-based diets[52]; copper reabsorption is impaired during enteritis. Manifestations of copper deficiency may include anemia, neutropenia, and scurvy-like bone lesions, sometimes with pathological fractures. Serum copper and ceruloplasmin levels are decreased. It is recommended that infant formulas furnish 100 μg/kg body weight/day.[52]

Copper Excess

Work in experimental animals has shown that excessive copper may affect the mammalian heart. Sheep poisoned by dosing with copper sulfate showed hemolysis and ultrastructural changes in mitochondria of cardiac and skeletal muscle.[80] Pregnant golden hamsters injected intraperitoneally on the 8th day of gestation with copper citrate delivered 37 edematous embryos, 21 of which showed a total of 58 cardiac defects. Sixteen of the embryos were affected with double outlet right ventricle in association with a membranous ventricular septal defect.[59]

Wilson's disease is a rare autosomal recessively inherited disorder characterized by a lifelong tendency to accumulate copper, resulting in degenerative changes in the brain, particularly in the basal ganglions, cirrhosis of the liver, and greenish-brown Kayser-Fleischer rings of the cornea.[164] There is often an associated hemolytic anemia, and other organs may be affected.

Onset may be as early as 4 years, but most patients develop symptoms in adolescence or early adulthood. In two instances, a 10-year-old and a 17-year-old patient showed increased copper deposition in the myocardium with concomitant myocardial damage.[16] The lifelong administration of penicillamine (β-β-dimethylcysteine) to asymptomatic patients with the disease prevents all overt manifestations.[164]

Iron Deficiency

The clinical manifestation of iron deficiency is an anemia. It constitutes the most frequent hematologic disease of infancy and childhood in the United States.[142] The concentration of iron in milk is low (0.08 mg/100 gm), and relatively small quantities of iron-rich foods are fed during infancy. Should the diet be inadequate to meet the needs of young growing infants and children, or should abnormal external iron loss occur through bleeding, iron deficiency anemia may develop rapidly.

As iron deficiency anemia develops, stores of iron (as hemosiderin) in liver and bone marrow are reduced, levels of serum ferritin decrease from the normal 35 ng/ml to less than 10 ng/ml,[142] and total serum iron decreases from the normal range of 40 to 120 μg/dl[116] to less than 30 μg/dl. The red cells show microcytosis, hypochromia, and poikilocytosis. In severe anemia, there is hypervolemia, with cardiac dilatation.

The child is pale. When the hemoglobin level falls below 5.0 gm/dl, irritability and anorexia become prominent. Cardiovascular findings include tachycardia and cardiac dilatation. Systolic murmurs are often present. Heart failure may develop.

Iron deficiency anemia responds rapidly to adequate amounts of iron. The oral dose is 6 mg/kg of elemental iron, given as the sulfate (20% elemental iron, or the gluconate (10 to 12% elemental iron)).[142] Milk should be restricted to 1 pint/day, and iron-rich foods should be fed.[48]

There is a potential danger that transfusion of whole blood in severely anemic children may precipitate heart failure. Therefore, children with hemoglobins less than 4 gm/dl should be given packed cells in small transfusions of 2 to 3

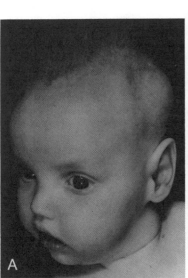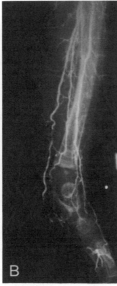

Fig. 38.9 (A) Typical appearance of the face and hair in Menkes' kinky hair syndrome. Note the pudgy cheeks and steel wool appearance of the hair in this 5-month-old. (B) Abnormal tortuosity of the arteries in the lower leg of an infant who died of Menkes' kinky hair syndrome at 10 months of age. (Reproduced with permission from D. M. Danks et al.[55] and The American Academy of Pediatrics.)

ml/kg. If heart failure has developed, a modified exchange transfusion employing fresh packed red cells may be indicated.

Iron Excess

Primary Hemochromatosis. Familial or primary hemochromatosis, a genetically determined error of metabolism, is a rare iron storage disease resulting from an increase in intestinal absorption of iron from a normal diet. It is characterized by excessive deposition of hemosiderin, an iron hydroxide-protein complex, in many organs, including the heart. The hemosiderin deposit in the heart is usually 10 to 15 times more than normal,[145] occurring in atria, ventricles, and the conduction system, with heaviest concentrations in the myocardium of the ventricles. There are varying degrees of fatty degeneration and fibrosis of the muscle fibers.

Unequivocal cases below 13 years of age have not been reported. The disorder is 10 to 20 times more common in males than in females, and the onset is delayed in females.[145] Symptoms in untreated adults are usually related to a triad of cirrhosis, diabetes mellitus, and bronze pigmentation of the skin.[46, 145] Cardiac dysrhythmias and heart failure may result from progressive myocardial hemosiderosis.

Electrocardiographic findings include supraventricular dysrhythmias, atrioventricular block, low voltage of the QRS complex, and flattened T waves.[145]

In heart failure, there is biventricular enlargement, and the roentgenographic shadow of the heart is globular, resembling that found in pericardial effusion.[145] There may be increased radiographic density of the liver due to increased nonfat tissue and iron deposition.

The diagnosis of primary hemochromatosis depends upon careful family history and laboratory studies. Serum iron levels become progressively increased. Plasma transferrin is decreased and is almost completely saturated with iron.

Removal of excess body iron, either by phlebotomy or by a chelating agent such as deferoxamine,[135, 142, 157] is the only effective treatment. Approximately one-third of the patients die in heart failure.

Secondary Hemochromatosis. Secondary, exogenous, or acquired hemochromatosis may result from excessive dietary iron or from increased absorption of iron from a normal dietary intake in various anemias with erythroid hyperplasia such as thalassemia major, vitamin B$_{12}$, or folic acid deficiency megaloblastic anemia.[46, 145] In these patients there is the combined effect of persistent increased iron absorption and increased intramedullary hemolysis.[69, 161] Multiple blood transfusions may cause exogenous hemochromatosis, as can parenteral iron therapy in hemodialysis patients.[78]

The characteristic findings include widespread iron deposition and fibrosis in tissues, especially in liver, spleen, pancreas, gonads, and heart. The iron deposits in the heart have been identified as particles of two closely related iron storage proteins, ferritin and hemosiderin.[103] There may be fluid in the pericardial sac.[69] The heart is dilated as well as hypertrophied, and is often more than twice the expected weight.[69, 161] In an electron microscopic study of secondary hemochromatosis, iron was detected in the myofiber nucleus (Fig. 38.10) and mitochondria. The concentration of iron was greatest within the outer thirds of the ventricular myocardium and in the interventricular septum.[161]

There is speckled pigmentation over the entire body, especially on the neck and back of the hands. The facial appearance is immature. Growth and weight gain are slowed; the expected adolescent growth spurt and development of sexual characteristics may be delayed or arrested. The liver and spleen are enlarged.[69]

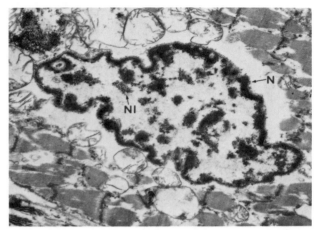

Fig. 38.10 Cardiac myofiber containing intranuclear and paranuclear deposits of iron (dark granules) from the heart of a 14-year-old girl who died from exogenous hemochromatosis. Because of chronic anemia, she had received a total of 140 units of blood transfusions (71 gm of elemental iron). She died in heart failure. Reduced from 30,000. N, nucleus; NI, nuclear iron. (Reproduced with permission from S. K. Sanyal et al.[161] and The American Academy of Pediatrics.)

The patients may develop cardiac complications such as acute benign pericarditis, which may be recurrent, and heart failure, often with dysrhythmias.[69] The appearance of heart failure may be insidious.

The heart size may begin to increase at about 10 years of age in patients with chronic refractory anemia and hemochromatosis.[69] First degree heart block may appear, and a left ventricular hypertrophy pattern may develop. Just before the onset of heart failure, there may be occasional atrial premature contractions and abnormalities of T wave.[69] Twenty-four-hour Holter recordings of the cardiac rhythm in patients under 14 years of age have shown rare atrial premature beats; over this age, ectopy is common. Patients over 19 years old often exhibited both frequent atrial and ventricular premature beats, which suggests that ectopy may antedate overt cardiac dysrhythmias and heart failure.[135] The more serious disturbances of rhythm and conduction develop with heart failure, including supraventricular tachycardia, atrial flutter and fibrillation, ventricular premature beats, and repetitive ventricular tachycardias. Some children develop atrioventricular block, including complete heart block.

Fluoroscopy reveals an enlarged heart, often with diminished pulsations.[69] Angiocardiography may distinguish cardiac dilatation from pericardial effusion; there may be a combination of these.[69] Echocardiography may reveal an increase in left ventricular wall thickness,[90, 135] which may be due to anemia or to iron deposition.[90, 135]

Beside the usual treatment for heart failure and anemia, children who require regular transfusions should receive an iron chelating agent such as deferoxamine[142] to prevent or reverse cardiac abnormalities.[135] Vitamin C levels may be reduced in leukocytes of patients receiving deferoxamine; therefore, vitamin C should be given to prevent deficiency and to maximize iron excretion. The Vitamin C dose should be minimal, since a high dose may be harmful in iron overload patients. Echocardiographic studies have shown a high frequency of cardiac deterioration in patients receiving 500 mg/day.[90, 135]

In a large series reported by Engle and associates,[69] cardiac failure with dysrhythmias often occurred during the 2nd decade of life, usually followed by death within months or years. These events were attributed to hemochromatosis rather than to anemia per se. This emphasizes the importance of iron chelating agents and the prevention of life-threatening hemochromatosis.[90, 135]

Magnesium Deficiency

Magnesium deficiency might develop in any child who has had prolonged losses of body fluids without magnesium replacement, or in any child who has grown rapidly while fed a diet adequate in protein, calcium, and phosphorus and relatively poor in magnesium (the magnesium deficiency syndrome of growth).[37, 38, 86] The morbidity and mortality from magnesium deficiency is most severe in the smallest and youngest members of any species.

The pathology of magnesium depletion in the child is not known. In acute severe deficiency, very young weanling rats first experience brief fleeting episodes of cyanosis or pallor, staring and rigidity. One or two days later, they may suddenly experience acute shock-like episodes characterized by apnea, tetany, and bradycardia, sometimes with ventricular beats originating from ectopic foci.[35] The animals may spontaneously recover, or they may die. The lungs of these animals show varying amounts of edema, hemorrhage, and congestion.[35] In chronic magnesium depletion in older animals, the earliest lesions are characterized by swelling and vacuolization of mitochondria, and distortion of christae.[89] Focal myocardial hemorrhage and necrosis may later be seen on light microscopy, followed by fibrosis and calcification.[89]

As in animals, there are several magnesium deficient syndromes in infants and children, with the clinical expressions depending on maturity and age of the infant and the time factors in the development of deficiency. For example, Harris and Wilkinson[86] described the magnesium-deficient infant as pale and limp, lying quietly, not interested in feeds, sometimes with twitching or convulsions. Three-year-old children with chronic deficiency resulting from high protein feedings that excluded magnesium but were otherwise nutritionally balanced became irritable, developed eye signs such as staring, nystagmus, and oculogyric crises, and tremors, twitching, and seizures. They became progressively weaker, with hypotension, hypothermia, weak pulses, and shallow respiration, sometimes with brief episodes of apnea.[37, 38] The electrocardiograms showed unstable cardiac rate and rhythm, low amplitude complexes, and progressive inversion of the T waves over the left precordial leads V_4 to V_6. All of the above signs usually began to normalize[37, 38, 86] after adding magnesium to the otherwise adequate nutritional therapy.[166]

The diagnosis of magnesium deficiency may be difficult to establish during life. Plasma values are helpful when low,[37] but they are labile,[35] and magnesium-depleted patients may have normal plasma levels.[38, 86] The parenteral magnesium load tests appear to be the most feasible and informative of the other diagnostic tests.[86]

Repletion of the severely depleted child should be accomplished slowly and gradually, with well-balanced therapy to avoid an electrolyte imbalance. Initial safe doses are 0.5 mEq magnesium/kg body weight/day parenterally, or 1 to 3 mEq/kg/day orally.[37] As soon as possible the child should receive natural sources of magnesium (nuts, legumes, and other green vegetables, and coarsely milled cereal grains).[166]

Magnesium Excess

Magnesium intoxication has been found in acute renal failure, in Addison's disease, and in the iatrogenic administration of magnesium for toxemia of pregnancy or hypertension. Magnesium produces peripheral vasodilatation and a fall in blood pressure. When serum values increase from the normal (1.4 to 2.4 mEq/liter to 5 to 10 mEq/liter), both normal and ectopic conduction mechanisms of the heart are depressed. Respiratory failure occurs at 15 mEq/liter, and at still higher levels, the heart stops in diastole.

It is recommended that 10% calcium gluconate in the dose of 2 ml/kg of body weight be given slowly with monitoring of the cardiac rate. One infant with magnesium intoxication was successfully treated by exchange transfusion.

Phosphorus Deficiency

Hypophosphatemia may result from binding of phosphates by aluminum hydroxide antacids, by prolonged administration of phosphate-free solutions,[137] or from vitamin D-resistant or dependent rickets.[114] Severe hypophosphatemia in man is associated with low intracellular stores of adenosine triphosphate (ATP), the energy-rich nucleotide; muscular weakness results. O'Connor and associates[137] recently showed that critically ill patients with hypophosphatemia had depressed myocardial contractility. Return of serum phosphate to normal improved myocardial stroke work independently of the Starling effect. The mechanism of this improvement in contractile force is unknown but may be related to intracellular availability of ATP.[137] Prevention should be practiced in intensive-care settings. However, when depressed cardiac work and hypophosphatemia are found to coexist, the serum phosphorus should be carefully increased to normal.

Phosphorus Excess

Excessive phosphorus causes an imbalance in the calcium-phosphorus ratio that may result in hypocalcemia and increased neuromuscular irritability, sometimes with tetany. It is recommended[52] that the dietary Ca to P ratio in infancy be 1.5:1, decreasing to 1:1 at 1 year of age.

Potassium Deficiency

Hypokalemia usually reflects potassium deficiency, but the serum potassium concentration may sometimes be elevated in relation to total body stores, as in acidosis.[165] Hypokalemia may result from diuretic therapy, or insufficient K^+ in parenteral fluids to replace losses such as those in gastroenteritis, in renal tubular acidosis, or in patients with edema and secondary hyperaldosteronism. Myocardial lesions have been observed in potassium depletion in man. There is an infiltration of neutrophils, lymphocytes, and macrophages associated with necrosis of muscle fibers.[167]

Potassium deficiency results in poor quality heart sounds, dysrhythmias, and potentiation of digitalis effects. There is weakness or paralysis of skeletal muscle, and hyporeflexia; the effect on smooth muscle is seen as abdominal distension or ileus. Electrocardiographic changes include prolongation of the QT interval, widening and lowering of the T waves, and U waves.

The treatment of potassium depletion must be individualized. The usual dose of potassium may range from 1 to 5 mEq/kg/day.[114] Potassium may be given orally as tablets of potassium chloride containing 4 mEq of K^+. Enteric-coated tablets should not be used because of their intestinal insolubility.[114] Fruit-flavored powders are available for pediatric use. Triamterene can aid in prevention of urinary K^+ losses. In Bartter syndrome, inhibition of prostaglandin synthetase such as aspirin have produced striking improvements in potassium balance.[114] Serum potassium levels must be monitored.

Potassium Excess

Hyperkalemia usually indicates potassium intoxication. Potassium given by mouth rarely causes severe hyperkalemia unless renal function is markedly impaired.[165] Hyperkalemia usually results from renal failure, hemolysis, tissue necrosis, and deficiency of adrenal mineralocorticoid, as in Addison's disease. The spironolactones impair the ability of the kidney to respond to a potassium load, and triamterene impairs the exchange of sodium for potassium by the tubule; these diuretics should not be given with potassium supplements.[165] Acidosis, hypocalcemia, and hyponatremia all exacerbate the toxic effects of hyperkalemia, which are chiefly cardiac and neuromuscular. Rising serum K^+ interferes with normal nodal and bundle conduction. The morphologic changes in the heart have not been defined.[167]

Rising serum K^+ interferes with normal nodal and bundle conduction. Electrocardiographic abnormalities are the earliest and most frequent signs of disturbed membrane excitability and are characterized by tall, "tent-shaped" T waves, decreased amplitude of the P waves, and later by atrial asystole.[165] These usually occur when the serum potassium concentration reaches 7 to 8 mEq/L; cardiac standstill may occur when the concentration reaches 9 to 10 mEq/L.[165]

A recommended sequence of therapy for children includes: sodium bicarbonate, 2.5 mEq/kg IV; calcium infusion (except in digitalized patients), to counteract the cardiac effects of severe hyperkalemia; and orally administered cation exchange resins such as Kayexalate (sodium polystyrene sulfonate) which accumulate in K^+ in exchange for Na^+. However, excessive use may produce hypocalcemia.[114] For older children and adolescents, the infusion of 10% glucose with insulin induces the cellular deposition of glycogen and a shift of K^+ to the intracellular space; profound hypoglycemia may result in infants.[114] Peritoneal dialysis should be initiated in the face of continued rising K^+, particularly if there is heart failure.[114]

Selenium Deficiency

Selenium is an essential component of the enzyme glutathione peroxidase, which protects vital components of the cell against oxidative damage.[52] Selenium deficiency in animals is well documented. The squirrel monkey, with dietary selenium deficiency, develops degeneration and necrosis of the cardiac and skeletal muscle and hepatic necrosis.[32]

Keshan Disease in Children. Recent reports from the Chinese Academy of Medical Sciences[106, 107] have described Keshan disease, a potentially fatal cardiomyopathy in children 1 to 9 years of age who live in a selenium-poor belt stretching across China from northeast to southwest. Children with the disease developed heart failure, and half of them died. In 1975 there were 52 cases in 5445 control children but only 7 in 6767 children treated with sodium selenite. There has been no evidence of side effects from the therapy. Selenium is thought to play an important role in the etiology of Keshan disease for three reasons: (1) Its occurrence is invariably associated with a lower hair selenium content of the population affected. (2) Results of selenium loading tests and whole blood glutathione peroxidase measurements reveal that the populations in the affected areas are in a selenium-poor status. (3) Sodium selenium supplements are effective in preventing Keshan disease.[106]

Selenium Excess

A warning that widespread use of sodium selenite may produce disease cites the chronic granulomatous hypersensitivity lung disease of selenium refiners as an example.[63] Selenium toxicity is a well-established phenomenon in animals grazing in selenium-rich areas, but no definite disease process has been found in humans living in those areas.[32]

DEFICIENCY OR EXCESS OF VITAMINS

Thiamine Deficiency

Beriberi is the most important and most common syndrome of thiamine (vitamin B_1) deficiency. The cardinal signs are edema and cardiovascular disturbances in the wet form and neurologic and trophic changes in the dry form.[191] Shoshin beriberi, the fulminating cardiovascular beriberi, has been called the ultimate consequence of the metabolic lesion of thiamine deficiency.[99] Beriberi is also classified according to age: infantile, juvenile, and adult.[97, 180]

Thiamine is a water-soluble vitamin that functions as thiamine pyrophosphate, a coenzyme in key reactions in energy metabolism, particularly carbohydrate metabolism.[194] The daily requirements for pregnant and lactating mothers are about 1.7 mg; for infants, 0.5 mg; and for older children, 0.7 to 1.5 mg.[17, 52] Requirements are increased with a high carbohydrate diet and during periods of hard physical labor. Much of the natural thiamine, which is found in the outer coating of the grain, is lost during milling and boiling of rice.[17] Because of rice enrichment programs, the disease in the Orient has largely disappeared, but beriberi is still an important cause of infant death in regions where enrichment of rice with thiamine has not been instituted.[158]

Beriberi heart disease now appears, usually in summer, among laboring Japanese adolescents whose diet is largely composed of sweet carbonated soft drinks, instant noodles, and powermill-polished rice.[104, 192]

The usual cardiovascular manifestations of thiamine deficiency in infants and adolescents are those of high output cardiac failure, the mechanisms of which are uncertain. The cardiovascular changes might be related to excessive epinephrine production; abnormally high concentrations of catecholamines and acetylcholine have been found in hearts of thiamine-deficient animals. States of low cardiac output that may occur are probably explained by the severely compromised cardiac metabolism of pyruvate due to lack of thiamine.[158]

The beriberi patient has reduced blood thiamine level and urinary excretion of thiamine, and a parenteral thiamine load test reveals abnormally high retention. High blood levels of pyruvic and lactic acid are found, particularly after administration of dextrose or after strenuous exercise; these normalize after thiamine therapy. The erythrocyte transketolase activity[194] correlates with thiamine status.

Infantile Beriberi. The pathologic findings of infantile beriberi include dilatation of the right side of the heart, edematous interstitial tissue, venous engorgement of viscera, and generalized edema. There are reversible changes; the heart is not permanently damaged.[97]

Infantile beriberi usually develops in an infant between 1 and 4 months of age who has been fed breast milk by a thiamine-deficient mother, but occasionally he has had feedings of cow's milk.[158] The Japanese classify this condition into five types: "shoshin," "edema," "paralytic," "cerebral," and "mixed," depending upon the predominant manifestations.[97] Beriberi infants are pale, edematous, irritable, and anorectic, and they frequently have some diarrhea and vomiting. Early in the disease, the infant becomes hoarse or aphonic, owing to involvement of the recurrent laryngeal nerve. About one-third of the cases have blepharoptosis. The infants appear apathetic and are weak, with poor head control, and reduced knee and ankle jerks. As edema increases, urinary output decreases.

Some trivial problem such as a slight infection may precipitate the sudden development of the "shoshin" state,[97] sometimes in apparently healthy infants with no previously recognized illness. The infant rapidly becomes acutely distressed with progressive symptomatology: tachycardia, dyspnea, rales, and rhonchi. The heart becomes enlarged due to dilatation of the right ventricle, there is marked accentuation of the second pulmonary sound, and there may be an apical systolic murmur. The systemic diastolic pressure decreases; a vascular murmur is often audible. The liver and spleen become enlarged and palpable. The child may die of heart failure within 36 to 48 hours if untreated, but if given thiamine intravenously, he usually improves within a few hours. Lesser degrees of thiamine deficiency may result in edema, or predominantly neurologic disturbances. Some develop the "cerebral" type, with convulsions and coma.[97, 158]

Only infants with the cardiovascular form of beriberi have electrocardiographic changes, which are nonspecific and usually include dwarfing of the complexes with prolongation of the Q T interval and low amplitude or inverted T waves over the left precordium.

There is cardiomegaly with right ventricular dilatation and evidence of pulmonary edema in the shoshin type.

The differential diagnosis of infantile beriberi includes congenital heart disease, myocarditis, encephalitis, meningitis, myasthenia gravis, and acute gastroenteritis, depending upon the predominant clinical manifestations.[97, 158] A sample of venous blood should be obtained for biochemical studies, followed by a therapeutic dose of thiamine chloride, the response to which remains the best diagnostic test.

For the treatment of severe fulminating cardiovascular beriberi, 50 mg of thiamine chloride should be given, half of it intramuscularly and half of it intravenously. The dose is then reduced to 10 mg/day, given parenterally for several days and then orally for several weeks. Treatment should include a multivitamin preparation since there may be deficiencies of several B vitamins. Oxygen is beneficial during the acute cardiovascular episode. Digitalis is of some benefit as a vasoconstrictor during the shoshin phase. Smaller doses of thiamine, usually 5 to 10 mg/day, are adequate for the less severe forms of beriberi; oral therapy is adequate if there is not severe gastroenteritis.

The mother of the breast-fed infant should receive diagnostic tests and prompt therapy with thiamine, multivitamins, and generally improved diet before resuming breast feeding. Adequate thiamine intake in the lactating mother prevents beriberi in the breast-fed infant.

Infantile beriberi may be rapidly fatal if untreated, but it responds to specific therapy. Biochemical changes normalize over the next few days; complete cure requires several weeks of therapy. There are no known sequelae.

Juvenile Beriberi. Beriberi in children beyond infancy, or juvenile beriberi, is essentially a "dry" beriberi in children fed chiefly polished overmilled rice. Gastroenteritis and physical exertion are contributory factors. It accounts for about 10% of beriberi in the Philippines.[97] The pathology of juvenile beriberi is muscle atrophy and degenerative lesions of the peripheral and cranial nerves. Cardiovascular involvement is rare.

The juvenile beriberi patient is a poorly nourished child who experiences anorexia, pallor, and weight loss. Features are peripheral neuritis, most often with pain or tenderness of the gastrocnemius muscle or muscles of the thigh with difficulty rising from the squatting position[180] and impaired gait. Cranial nerve involvement results in a nasal voice, hoarseness, deafness, or ocular signs such as strabismus, nystagmus, or ptosis. The facial appearance may suggest myasthenia gravis. Cardiovascular findings include an accentuated second pulmonic sound and a decreased diastolic blood pressure with a vascular murmur over the femoral

artery. However, edema and cardiac edema occur rarely, and there are no important electrocardiographic or radiologic features.

The differential diagnosis of juvenile beriberi is essentially the diagnosis of polyneuritis which may be caused by substances such as arsenic, lead, or cyanide, or other deficiency disorders such as vitamin B_{12} neuropathy or folic acid deficiency. The diagnosis must be established biochemically.[17, 194]

The specific therapy is thiamine in moderate doses, given orally, together with other vitamins of the B complex and an improved diet. Recovery from juvenile beriberi depends upon the chronicity and nature of the neurologic lesions which may be only slowly and incompletely reversible. Parts affected first are the last to recover.[97]

Beriberi in Adolescents. Beriberi in adolescents is grouped with adult cases. Half of a series from Thailand and three-quarters of recent Japanese cases were adolescents.[104, 192] Characteristic features among the adolescents were those of heart disease, infrequently combined with peripheral neuritis.[104, 180]

When the onset is subacute, peripheral edema, easy fatigability, general malaise, palpitation, and dyspnea are common features.[34] The pulse rate is usually high but rarely exceeds 120/minute.[104] The neck veins are engorged, and the venous pressure may exceed 200 mm H_2O. Increased pulse pressure, a gallop rhythm at the apex, nonspecific midsystolic murmurs between the left sternal border and the apex, and an accentuated second pulmonic sound are often found.[104]

Shoshin beriberi refers to the form characterized by fulminant cardiac failure, which may be precipitated by physiologic stress.[168] Patients may rapidly die of predominantly right-sided heart failure. Systolic hypertension, venous distension, and peripheral cyanosis, rapidly followed by pulmonary congestion, are the expected findings. The untreated patient dies in extreme agony and fully conscious.[158]

The electrocardiographic changes are nonspecific and variable. There is usually sinus tachycardia, but some patients have sinus dysrhythmia. The electrical voltage may be low[99, 180] or high.[97] There may be prolongation of the PR or QT interval.[180] Nonspecific ST changes[99] and low or inverted T waves over the left precordium are usually found.

The radiologic cardiothoracic ratio may be normal[104] but is often over 50%. The heart is hyperactive. Pulmonary congestion, sometimes with pleural effusion,[180] was common in the Thai series but not mentioned in the Japanese reports. In shoshin beriberi, there is marked cardiac enlargement, predominantly right-sided, and terminal pulmonary congestion, often with pleural effusion.

In contrast to patients over 20 years of age, adolescents may show markedly increased cardiac index,[111] stroke index and circulating blood volume, and markedly decreased peripheral vascular resistance.[4, 104] There is a low arteriovenous oxygen difference.

Adolescents with beriberi heart disease promptly respond to thiamine administration[97]; a favorable therapeutic effect may be obtained with rest alone.[104] The therapy should include rest, all B vitamins, and improved diet.[17, 97] Digitalis and diuretics are useful in heart failure. Diuresis may occur within 24 to 48 hours, gallop rhythm may disappear within 48 hours, and the electrocardiogram and chest radiologic changes may be normal within 30 to 40 days.[180]

Shoshin beriberi is a medical emergency; if untreated it is rapidly fatal. As soon as blood is obtained for diagnostic tests, thiamine chloride in the dose of 50 to 100 mg is given intravenously. Hypoxemia, acidosis, hyperventilation, and heart failure must be vigorously treated. Therapy must include oxygen, morphine sulfate, digoxin, and rotating tourniquets. Intravenous $NaHCO_3$ is recommended for severe acidosis.[99] A diuretic is sometimes used. Multiple vitamins, including other B complex vitamins, should be given. Such therapy may be followed by prompt reversal of the abnormal hemodynamic parameters. Emphasis is then directed at improving the patient's general nutrition with a well-balanced diet.[97, 99, 180] In adolescents and in adults, this may imply management of alcoholism.[14, 111, 119]

Vitamin B₂ (Riboflavin) Deficiency

Deficiency of riboflavin in pregnancy has been shown to produce congenital malformations in experimental animals, but such lesions have not been reported in man. When pregnant rats were fed a riboflavin-deficient diet and a riboflavin antagonist, galactoflavin, during pregnancy, the pups showed defects that included edema and cardiovascular anomalies.[96] Deficiency of the vitamin may cause corneal vascularization and poor growth in man. The recommended dietary allowance for riboflavin ranges from 0.4 mg/day for neonates to 1.5 mg/day for pregnant women.[52]

Vitamin B₁₂ and Folic Acid Deficiency States

A wide variety of congenital malformations were demonstrated in the offspring of rats treated during pregnancy with a folate-deficient diet in combination with an antagonist, X-methyl pteroylglutamic acid. The findings included marked edema and anemia and defects of the lungs and cardiovascular system.[96] In man, deficiency of either vitamin B₁₂ or folic acid may result in megaloblastic anemia. Vitamin B₁₂ deficiency has developed in strict vegetarians, and their breast-fed infants may be affected. Vitamin B₁₂ nutrition can be impaired by a deficiency of intrinsic factor, which results in pernicious anemia. Severely anemic patients may experience palpitations, dyspnea, and angina. The syndromes of deficiency of vitamin B₁₂ and folic acid have been fully discussed elsewhere.[91]

Vitamin C Deficiency

The biochemical functions of the water-soluble vitamin C, ascorbic acid, are not well defined, but the vitamin has been implicated in functions that include the formation of collagen, the synthesis of epinephrine and anti-inflammatory steroids, folic acid metabolism, leukocyte functions, and iron absorption.[52] The manifestation of the deficiency of vitamin C is scurvy. Scurvy can occur at any age, but infants rarely develop it before 6 months of age. Findings may include hemorrhage, skeletal changes, bone marrow depression, and degenerative changes in cardiac and skeletal muscle.[17] Sudden death in infants with evidence of severe vitamin C deficiency has been attributed to cardiac hypertrophy, particularly of the right ventricle.[167] Microscopic findings of the heart were not significant in those infants, but myocardial degeneration has been described in other patients with scurvy and in guinea pigs with vitamin C deficiency. The recommended dietary allowance for vitamin C ranges from 35 mg/day in infants to 60 mg/day in adolescents and adults, with an additional 20 mg for pregnancy and 40 mg for lactation.[52]

Vitamin C Excess

Intakes of ascorbic acid in excess of physiological requirements (1 gm/day or more) may have some pharmacological or drug-like effects that are not related to the normal functioning of the vitamin; examples include: lowering of serum cholesterol in *some* hypercholesterolemic subjects[52]; and in-

creasing human serum levels of IgA, IgM, and complement component C-3.[52] High doses of vitamin C may have a deleterious effect on myocardial function in children with secondary hemachromatosis and may promote undesirable intestinal absorption of iron.[90, 135] The excessive intake of vitamin C during pregnancy has been associated with termination of early pregnancy and "conditioned" scurvy in the offspring,[96] that is, a relative lack of responsiveness to normal doses. It may interfere with anticoagulant therapy, both with heparin and with coumadin drugs. Other effects may include impaired bactericidal activity of leukocytes.[52]

Vitamin D Deficiency

The importance of vitamin D in human nutrition lies in its role of regulating the metabolism of calcium and phosphate and, to a lesser extent, magnesium. Deficiency of vitamin D in children leads to rickets, a metabolic disorder of growing bone characterized by retarded formation of epiphyseal cartilage and impaired mineralization of the bone matrix resulting in bone deformities.[17, 52] The abnormal configuration of the chest in advanced rickets may lead to cor pulmonale. The recommended daily dose of this fat-soluble vitamin is 10 μg (400 International Units (IU)).[52] Care must be taken, as the concentration of the vitamin varies in different preparations.[17]

Vitamin D Excess

Vitamin D is a potentially toxic substance, particularly in young children.[52] Ingestion of excessive amounts for 1 to 3 months may lead to a symptom complex similar to idiopathic hypercalcemia. Possibly, a hypersensitivity phenomenon is involved. The child develops irritability, hypotonia, anorexia and, despite polydipsia and polyuria, usually appears dehydrated. The urine may contain albumin. Metastatic calcification and aortic valvular stenosis, renal damage, and generalized osteoporosis are among the findings. Prevention requires careful evaluation of vitamin D dosage. The treatment includes discontinuance of vitamin D intake and decreased dietary calcium. Severely affected infants may require aluminum hydroxide by mouth, cortisone, or sodium versenate therapy.[17]

Vitamin E Deficiency

Vitamin E, alpha-tocopherol, is a fat-soluble antioxidant. Premature infants absorb the vitamin poorly and may have low serum levels of tocopherol. Hemolytic anemia may develop at 6 to 10 weeks of age; this is corrected by administration of vitamin E. Deficiency may occur in malabsorption states and may contribute to the anemia of kwashiorkor. Some patients deficient in vitamin E complain of weakness and show creatinuria, ceroid deposition in smooth muscle, and focal necrosis of striated muscle. There may be some improvement after administration of vitamin E. The minimal daily requirements for vitamin E are not known. It is recommended that low birth weight infants receive 1 IU (1 mg) of vitamin E/gm linoleic acid in their formulas, as well as 5 IU of water-soluble alpha-tocopherol/day. About 10 IU/day is adequate for older children and adults, with an additional 2 IU for pregnancy.[52]

Vitamin E Excess

Compared with the fat-soluble vitamins A and D, vitamin E is relatively nontoxic. Most adults have appeared to tolerate large doses of 0.4 to 1.0 g (400 to 1000 IU) of alpha-tocopherol.[52] Adverse effects are known. Large doses of the vitamin in anemic children suppress the normal hematologic response to parenteral iron.[52] It has been shown that alphatocopherolquinone, an oxidation product of the vitamin, is an inhibitor of vitamin K. This may explain the observation that large doses of vitamin E potentiates the effect of the anticoagulant warfarin. This is of potential importance to cardiac patients who may be receiving anticoagulant therapy: care should be taken that patients receiving anticoagulants are not taking large amounts of vitamin E.

Vitamin K Deficiency

Vitamin K is the antihemorrhagic vitamin necessary for the synthesis of prothrombin and other blood-clotting factors in the liver.[52] A deficiency of this vitamin may result in defective blood coagulation; this should be considered in all patients with a hemorrhagic disturbance.[17] As noted above, large doses of vitamin E constitute a risk factor for vitamin K deficiency. Vitamin K deficiency may occur in newborn infants, because the placenta is a relatively poor organ for the transmission of lipids and because the gut is sterile, initially lacking the intestinal bacteria for synthesis of quinones with vitamin K activity. The incidence of hemorrhagic disease of the newborn has been markedly decreased by the prophylactic administration of vitamin K.[17] Vitamin K deficiency in childhood is usually due to factors affecting absorption or utilization of fat.[17] The total requirement for vitamin K (from all sources) appears to be about 2 μg/kg of body weight.[52]

Vitamin K Excess

Many therapeutic preparations of vitamin K are available. Menadione can be toxic and may cause hemolytic anemia and liver damage. Phylloquinone preparations are preferred for medical situations requiring pharmacological amounts of vitamin K; these include coumarin overdosage, liver disease, and severe malabsorption syndromes.[52]

III. CARDIOTOXIC SUBSTANCES

ALCOHOL

Cardiovascular depression that is observed in acute severe alcoholic intoxication has been attributed to central vasomotor factors and to respiratory depression. A direct depression of the heart by alcohol has been observed in experimental animals following acute administration that results in blood concentrations as low as 100 mg/dl. Both myocardial contractility and working efficiency are impaired.[134] The precise role of alcohol in the etiology of alcoholic cardiomyopathy is unclear because of frequent associated malnutrition and vitamin deficiency.[67] However, electron microscopic studies show that chronic excessive use of alcohol has a deleterious effect on the heart, leading to characteristic intracellular lesions in the myocardium, associated with heart failure. Prognosis for return of muscle function is guarded.[147, 149]

Fetal Alcohol Syndrome

> Behold, thou shalt conceive, and bear a son. Drink no more wine or strong drink . . . Judges 13:7.

Despite early writings,[49] the association of ethanol ingestion during pregnancy and teratogenic effects has only recently been fully appreciated.[84, 179] The fetal alcohol syndrome has been estimated to occur in 1 to 2/1000 live births, with partial expression in about 3 to 5/1000 live births.[49] Moderate or heavy ingestion of alcohol during early pregnancy may result in a characteristic cluster of abnormalities in the infant. These may include: low IQ and microcephaly;

intrauterine and postnatal growth failure; a distinctive facial appearance with short palpebral fissures, epicanthal folds, a low nasal bridge, maxillary hypoplasia, long upper lips with narrow vermillion borders, and hirsutism of the forehead and other parts of the body (Fig. 38.11); cardiac defects; and minor joint and limb abnormalities. In one series, cardiac defects, mostly septal defects, were noted in 20 of 41 patients (49%).[83] In one series the only infant examined at autopsy had a ventricular septal defect, but this diagnosis was made clinically in other infants.[100]

ANTIMONY

The antimony compounds that are used in chemotherapy of helminthiasis may result in untoward reactions, including some related to the cardiovascular and respiratory systems.[154] Dyspnea, apnea, and vascular collapse sometimes occur. Marked bradycardia, which occasionally develops late in the course of therapy, necessitates cessation of the medication.[87] A high percentage of patients treated with trivalent antimonials develop electrocardiographic changes. These are unassociated with cardiovascular symptoms and disappear within 30 to 60 days of discontinuing therapy.[87]

CHLOROQUINE

Overdosage of chloroquine, a drug used in the treatment of malaria, was first recognized as a fatal poisoning in children in 1961.[43] The drug has a myocardial depressant effect which may be the cause of the hypotension that is associated with toxicity.[26] Initial symptoms are gastrointestinal and

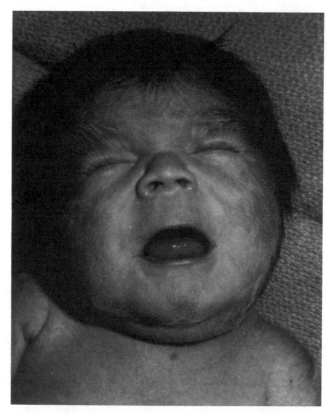

Fig. 38.11 Evidence of the fetal alcohol syndrome in a 1-day-old American Indian male born to a 30-year-old mother who was an alcoholic for 6 years before his birth. Note the infant's hirsutism and short palpebral fissures. (Reproduced with permission from Kenneth L. Jones and Lancet. Other photographs of this infant were published by K. L. Jones and D. W. Smith.[100]

neurological, followed by life-threatening cardiac dysrhythmias.[26] A review of 26 episodes in adolescents and young adults in Australia showed a 50% frequency of cardiac arrest and a 19% mortality resulting from ingestion of 2.25 gm or more of the drug. The toxicity of the drug and the inadequacy of current therapy for toxicity together constitute a special danger to children.[26]

COBALT

There is considerable evidence that cobalt is toxic to the myocardium.[112] Cobalt cardiomyopathy was diagnosed in a 17-year-old white girl on maintenance hemodialysis who had been given cobaltous chloride for 8 months to treat anemia. Biopsy specimens of the myocardium showed elevated cobalt.[121] In other reports, heavy intake of beer that contained cobalt resulted in cardiomyopathies characterized by a sudden onset of right-sided heart failure, frequently with pericardial effusion, polycythemia, lactic acidosis, and shock. The myocardial fiber degeneration was nonspecific.[122, 131]

DAUNORUBICIN AND DOXORUBICIN

Severe cardiomyopathy that may cause heart failure and death is the major complication of two of the newer and most effective antitumor agents used in oncology, daunorubicin and doxorubicin (Adriamycin). The risk of cardiotoxicity may occur in lower dose levels in younger children.[146] The cumulative dose may be more important than the dose schedules,[198] but severe early reactions may occur.[25] Cardiopulmonary-mediastinal irradiation and the combined effect of certain other chemotherapeutic agents may contribute to the cardiomyopathy. The drugs may produce a pericarditis and myocarditis. Electron microscopy reveals a decrease in the number of myocardial fibrils, mitochondrial changes, and cellular degeneration.

Early and late effects of the drugs are recognized.[25] *Early effects* include: pericarditis-myocarditis which can affect patients with no previous history of cardiac disease and which carries a mortality rate of about 20%[25]; left ventricular dysfunction, which may lead to heart failure; and dysrhythmias. *Late effects* may include subclinical left ventricular dysfunction and heart failure. The heart failure associated with these drugs is often refractory to medical treatment.[198]

Echocardiographic changes precede clinical and electrocardiographic evidence of cardiotoxicity. Using M-mode echocardiography, Nouri[136] found that reduction in left ventricular contractility and, hence, reduced shortening fraction[22, 136] was often first shown by septal and then posterior left ventricular wall hypokinesia. Administration of digoxin does not improve the shortening fraction.[22] An increase in the left ventricular internal diameter during diastole is also an early indicator of incipient left ventricular failure in these children.[136] Echocardiography is, therefore, an important guide to the therapy of patients receiving these drugs.

Electrocardiographic changes include a reduction in voltage in the limb leads, dysrhythmia, and nonspecific ST-T wave changes.[41, 136]

EMETINE AND IPECAC

Emetine, a widely used agent for treatment of intestinal ambiasis and amebic liver abscess,[201] is obtained from ipecac (Brazil root), and is used as an emetic; both have direct toxic effects on the myocardium. Both may result in cardiac dilatation, failure, and, rarely, death.[2, 201] Microscopic examination of the heart reveals separation of muscle fibers and myocardial fiber destruction. The lack of inflammatory cells suggest a toxic rather than an inflammatory response.[154] Clinical changes include hypotension, precordial pain, tachycardia, and electrocardiographic abnormalities. Therapeutic doses of emetine may produce flattening and inversion of the T waves in all leads and prolongation of the QT interval. The combination of emetine and chloroquine in conventional doses has resulted in ventricular tachycardia.[169] Even sequential use of these two drugs may be cardiotoxic. Therefore, electrocardiographic monitoring of therapy is important.

MARIJUANA

Smoking marijuana, cannabis, obtained from the flowering tops of *hemp* plants, produces several cardiovascular effects. These include an increase in heart rate, an increase in systolic blood pressure, and reddening of the conjunctivae. The tachycardia is dose related and may be prevented by propranolol.[98] One youth without a history of heart disease had severe sinus bradycardia and second degree AV block which was related to drug use and disappeared 72 hours after discontinuing the drug.[5] Electrocardiographic changes are neither consistent nor specific. With chronic use there is an unexplained increase in plasma volume.

QUININE

Quinine, the chief alkaloid from the bark of the cinchona tree, is still a necessary antimalarial drug. Oral therapeutic doses have little, if any, effect on the normal heart, but when given intravenously, hypotension may develop precipitiously.[154]

TOBACCO

The concept that tobacco smoking is harmful to health and to the vascular endothelium in particular is possibly of greatest importance to the human fetus. Fetal carboxyhemoglobin saturations due to smoking are about 1.8 times higher than corresponding maternal values. Due to low fetal oxygen saturation, the effect is relatively more serious on fetal blood oxygen transport than on maternal transport. Pronounced intimal changes have been found in human umbilical arteries from newborn children born to smoking mothers. These include degenerative changes of the endothelium such as swelling, bleeding, and subendothelial edema.[13]

IV. CARDIOVASCULAR DISEASES OF THE TROPICS AND SUBTROPICS

Cardiac problems of importance in children native to the tropics and subtropics are reviewed and compared to North America and Europe to give the cardiologist an overview of what he would encounter if he were practicing in the tropics.

CONGENITAL HEART DISEASE

The frequency and distribution of congenital heart disease in the tropics and subtropics appears to be no different from that of the temperate zones.[9, 36] However, the child with a congenital heart lesion has a poor prognosis; most of the 104 autopsied cases of congenital heart disease studied in Ibadan, Nigeria, were infants.[27]

ENDOCARDIAL FIBROSIS

Endomyocardial fibrosis (EMF) is an acquired progressive disease of indigenous children and young adults living in many regions of the tropics and subtropics. It has been described in East, West, and South Africa, India, South America,[11] and in other parts of the world, particularly where the climate is hot and humid.[115] The frequency is highest among peoples from specific regions within these areas, such as the Rwandan immigrants in Uganda[53] and persons from the Ijebu Province in Nigeria.[27] The etiology is unknown.

Pathophysiology

The pathological expression varies somewhat from region to region. In his study of five Ugandan children who died between 4 and 12 years old, Connor noted scarring of the endocardium at the usual sites in the right and left ventricles. There were pericardial fluid collections between 25 and 1500 ml in four, and ascitic fluid collections of 500 to 4500 ml in all. Histological examinations showed interstitial stellate scarring, evidence of burned out vasculitis, and degenerative changes such as deposits of calcium in the endocardial scars.[54] These lesions have been described in detail[27, 53] (Fig. 37.12A and B). The concomitant finding of Aschoff bodies and other evidence of rheumatic carditis in some Nigerian patients has been considered too frequent to be coincidental.[27] The hearts of South African patients showed multiple discrete mural thrombi; in hearts with long-standing disease, these had organized to patchy and sometimes diffuse mural scars.[53]

Clinical Features

Children with right-sided EMF show wasting, growth retardation, and evidence of right heart failure. There is high venous pressure, a large sometimes pulsatile liver due to tricuspid insufficiency, evidence of cardiac enlargement due to a dilated right atrium, massive ascites, and minimal dependent edema.

Late in the disease, they occasionally develop cyanosis, clubbing of the fingers, and jaundice. The presence of murmurs is variable. Quadruple rhythm has been found in some patients.

Children with left-sided EMF present with mitral insufficiency, pulmonary hypertension, and left heart failure. Signs and symptoms include cough, breathlessness, chest pain, a left ventricular heave, and an apical systolic murmur. Hemoptysis is occasionally a late manifestation. The manifestations of bilateral EMF largely depend on which side is more severely incapacitated.

Electrocardiographic Features

The electrocardiogram shows no consistent pattern. There may be P mitrale or P pulmonale. The QRS complexes may be low in voltage, and there may be T wave inversion. Varying degrees of right or left bundle branch block are often present.

Radiologic Features

Radiologic findings of right-sided EMF reveal a greatly enlarged globular heart with marked diminution of pulsations. There may be calcification of the infundibulum of the right ventricle. In advanced left ventricular EMF with pulmonary hypertension, the heart is enlarged with a straight left border, a small aorta, and a prominent pulmonary artery segment. The periphery of the lungs is strikingly clear.

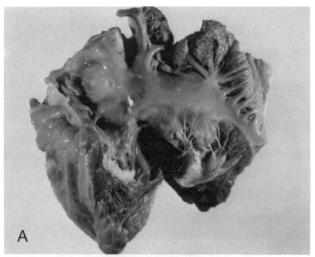

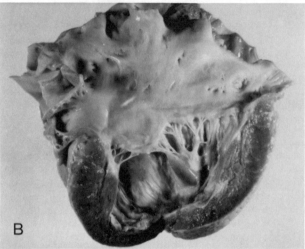

Fig. 38.12 (*A*) Dilated tricuspid ring with severe scarring of the endocardium of the right ventricular apex, papillary muscles, and chordae tendineae. There is an organizing thrombus in the atrial appendage. (*B*) Severe scarring of the endocardium of the left ventricle. The chordae tendineae of the posterior mitral leaflet are bound to the posterior wall. The endocardium of the apex is also severely scarred, and between the apex and the scar on the posterior wall there is a characteristic "skip area" of uninvolved endocardium around the base of the posterior papillary muscle.

Cardiac Catheterization

Cardiac catheterization is technically difficult in right-sided EMF because of distortion of the tricuspid valve and right heart chambers. Findings in severe tricuspid insufficiency include an attenuated right ventricular pressure, high right atrial and central venous pressures, and low cardiac output. In left-sided EMF, the left atrial and pulmonary wedge pressures are usually elevated, and the left ventricular end-diastolic pressure is raised.

Angiocardiography

Angiocardiography in right-sided EMF reveals severe distortion of the right heart; the thrombus formation prevents opacification of the ventricular apex, and the right ventricular outflow tract is often distended. In left ventricular EMF, there is little change in the ventricular volume throughout the cardiac cycle, and apical filling defects may be present.

Reflux of dye to an enlarged left atrium indicates mitral insufficiency (Fig. 38.13).[50]

Differential Diagnosis

Right ventricular EMF must be differentiated from Ebstein's anomaly, and left ventricular EMF shares many features of rheumatic heart disease, which may be coexistent.

Treatment

Treatment is supportive and is generally unsatisfactory. Digitalis and diuretics provide little benefit, and aspirating pericardial effusions or ascitic fluid provides only temporary relief. The course is usually one of progressive decompensation, with survival ranging from several weeks to several years.

ENDOCARDITIS

Endocarditis with and without pre-existing heart disease is common in the tropics.[178] Endocarditis is found in patients with pre-existing lesions, such as from congenital heart defects, EMF, or rheumatic heart disease, and an unusually high frequency of endocarditis is also found in patients without such defects. Reports from Nigeria[27] and Uganda[56] attest to the severity of this problem. The organisms most frequently responsible are: *Staphylococcus aureus*, beta-hemolytic streptococci, pneumococci, and *Escherichia coli*.[27, 56]

LEFT VENTRICULAR ANEURYSMS

Left ventricular aneurysms are classified according to the position of their opening in the internal ventricular surface. Aneurysms with an ostium beneath the aortic valve are termed subaortic; those opening beneath the mitral valve are submitral. The etiology is unknown, but finding the lesions in young children suggests a congenital weakness or defect in some cases.[51] Evidence of tuberculous infection was found in 23% of aneurysms studied in Nigeria.[27] The lesion most commonly becomes evident in the second and third decades.[51]

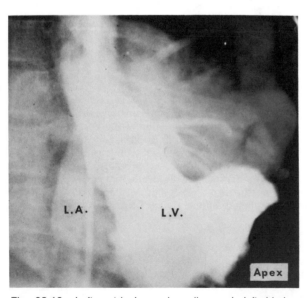

Fig. 38.13 Left ventricular angiocardiogram in left-sided endomyocardial fibrosis (EMF). Anteroposterior view shows an apical filling defect and reflux of contrast material into the left atrium. (Courtesy of Professor W. P. Cockshott.)

Clinical Features

Clinical findings depend on the size and location of the aneurysm. The patient usually presents in heart failure, with an enlarged, sometimes abnormally shaped heart on x-ray. Subaortic aneurysms lead to aortic insufficiency and left heart failure. Submitral aneurysms, the more common form in the Nigerian patients,[51] give rise to mitral insufficiency. Triple rhythm is common in these patients.[1] Electrocardiography may reveal first degree heart block, ST-T changes, and deep Q waves in the left ventricular leads.

X-rays are not helpful in diagnosing subaortic aneurysms, but the submitral aneurysm can be seen as a convex bulge high on the left border of the heart. Left ventricular aneurysms are best defined by left ventricular angiocardiography.

Treatment

Surgical excision may be necessary in patients with severe symptomatology resulting from valvular insufficiency.[181]

In some patients, thrombotic organization spontaneously obliterates the lesion, and the clinical course is good. However, untreated patients usually show progressive deterioration.

RHEUMATIC CARDITIS

Once thought rare, rheumatic fever has now been reported from numerous countries of the tropics and subtropics. Stanfield and Bracken[176] surveyed Ugandan children and found normal antistreptolysin titers at birth, followed by a rapid increase in the early months of life with titers exceeding 600 units during the second 6 months of life. Caddell et al.[39] described severe acute carditis in Ugandan children with a mean age of 6.7 years.[39] D'Arbela et al.[57] found that 10% of a series of 150 hospitalized Ugandan children with rheumatic fever were less than 5 years of age. Bhattacharya et al.[21] reported a 70% mortality during initial carditis in a group of Indian children. The most remarkable feature is the severity of pancarditis in very young children living in these areas. However, Sanyal and associates[162] reported findings and a mortality rate during the initial attack of acute rheumatic fever in children from North India to be similar to corresponding features of the disease in Western nations. They suggested that the severe pancarditis reported in developing nations resulted from recurrence of attacks in untreated previously undiagnosed patients.

There is a high frequency of chronic rheumatic carditis; this condition may be difficult to diagnose because it shares many features with EMF. Features of both diseases may be found in the same patient.

AFRICAN TRYPANOSOMIASIS (SLEEPING SICKNESS)

This disease is caused by *Trypanosoma gambiense* and *Trypanosoma rhodesiense* that are transmitted by the bite of the tsetse fly, genus *Glossina*, and may cause myo- and pericardiopathy as well as meningoencephalopathy. This disease is found in Tropical Africa between 15°N and 20°S. The well-documented findings of one 13-year-old Ugandan boy showed severe myocarditis, an endocarditis with occasional granulocytes, a moderate epicarditis, a generalized valvulitis, and lesions of the conducting system, thus establishing a diagnosis of pancarditis.[144]

AMERICAN TRYPANOSOMIASIS (CHAGAS' DISEASE)

This disease, caused by *Trypanosoma cruzi* and spread by blood-sucking species of reduviidae by blood transfusion or transplacentally, is an important cause of acute myocarditis in children in Central and South America,[11] with the highest frequency in Brazil, Venezuela, and Argentina. In the acute stage, the cardiac lesion is a myocardial reaction leading to dilatation, particularly of the pulmonary conus. The right heart becomes greatly enlarged. This is associated with high fever, malaise, tachycardia, cardiac dilatation and myocarditis, hepatosplenomegaly, and meningoencephalitis. Death is from cardiac failure. The chronic form, which may begin in late childhood, is marked by myocardial hyalinization and fibrosis, sometimes with infiltration of inflammatory cells. A myocardiopathy develops with steadily progressive cardiac failure and dysrhythmias. Disturbances in cardiac rhythm occur; right bundle branch block is a common conduction defect.[8, 81]

ANEMIC HEART DISEASE

Anemia is a complication of many cardiovascular disorders, compounding the patient's illness. Anemia headed the list of precipitating causes of heart failure in 132 Tanzanian patients.[120] The relative importance of anemia in the etiology of heart disease in tropical pediatrics varies greatly from region to region; the commonest causes are associated with: blood loss (hookworms, ritualistic practices); decreased or impaired production of erythrocytes (due to nutritional deficiency of iron, protein, pyridoxine, folic acid, vitamin B_{12}, vitamin E and, possibly, copper); and extensive blood destruction from congenital or acquired anemias. The most important of the congenital hemolytic anemias in the tropics is sickle cell anemia, and the commonest cause of acquired hemolytic anemia is malaria; all species of malarial parasites destroy the red blood cells and may cause malarial anemia.[29] Multiple causes are usually present in the very ill child. For example, anemia due to defective erythrocytes in a child with sickle cell disease may be associated with excessive blood loss due to hookworm infestation.[108]

A sudden loss of circulating hemoglobin causes cardiac dilatation; sudden loss of more than 20% of the circulating blood volume results in shock. A gradual loss of blood or a chronic anemic condition leads to myocardial hypertrophy, particularly of the left ventricle. According to Varat et al.,[190] cardiac enlargement occurs more commonly in sickle cell anemia than in other types of anemia and presents special problems because of chronicity, the increased viscosity of the blood, and the microthrombi that may result in tissue infarctions. Chronic anemia ordinarily decreases blood viscosity,[177, 190] accounting for booming heart sounds.[177]

COXSACKIE GROUP B VIRAL MYOCARDITIS

Most cases of heart disease due to Coxsackie viruses are caused by viruses of the B group.[31, 47, 93]

Neonatal Myocarditis

Myocarditis due to the Coxsackie B group may occur during the first 8 or 9 days of life.[93] Epidemics have been reported from South Africa and Southern Rhodesia.[93] The virus has worldwide distribution, but since the virus is excreted in the feces, serious outbreaks of illness are associated with hot weather, flies, and improper sewage disposal.[93] The essential lesion is an intense inflammatory infiltration with muscle necrosis. There may be mural endocarditis overlying subendocardial necrosis. It is frequently accompanied by encephalitis.[8]

The infant is lethargic, with grayish pallor, and may have mild icterus. Tachycardia, dyspnea, and cyanosis and evidence of cardiomegaly are often present. The electrocardiogram shows characteristics of myocarditis. Treatment is

symptomatic, including the cautious use of digitalis and diuretics.[47] When all the signs of heart failure are present, the prognosis is poor.[15, 47]

Myocarditis and Pericarditis in Older Age Groups

Older children and adults may develop myocarditis or myopericarditis due to Coxsackie B viruses 1 to 5.[47] Patients may be severely ill. Exercise aggravates the syndrome.[93] Most patients recover completely,[47] but fatalities have been reported.[93]

The treatment is bed rest and supportive therapy for relief of pain, heart failure, and cardiac dysrhythmias.[93, 133] Because pericardial effusion can be hemorrhagic, aspirin and anticoagulant therapy should be avoided.[93] Steroids may potentiate injury by viral agents to the myocardium through the suppression of interferon.[133] Conversely, interferon stimulators may protect against Coxsackie B_3 viral infection.[133] If fever is absent after 3 or 4 weeks and the cardiac silhouette returns to normal, the patient may gradually resume activity.[93]

DIPHTHERITIC HEART DISEASE

In areas of the world where the level of immunization is low, as in parts of Africa, Taiwan, Greece, Iran, and Jamaica, diphtheritic heart disease remains a health problem. Changes in the heart are common. In toxic cases the heart may be dilated and flabby, with fatty degeneration of myocardium, sometimes with infiltration of the interstitium with leukocytes which may involve the conducting fibers. This may be replaced by fibrosis and scarring which, if extensive, may lead to cardiac failure late in convalescence.[47]

Clinical cardiovascular changes may be peripheral or cardiac. Peripheral circulatory failure is shown by increasing pallor, rapid thready pulse, and a collapsed blood pressure. Patients who survive shock develop signs of cardiac damage: weak heart sounds, a triple or gallop rhythm, soft murmurs and, sometimes, the slow pulse of atrioventricular block.[47]

The electrocardiogram may show flattening or inversion of the T wave and lengthening of the PR or QT intervals. Bundle branch block, complete block with AV dissociation, and intraventricular block are evidence of severe cardiac damage.

Antitoxin should be administered on the basis of clinical diagnosis. Antimicrobial therapy is a valuable adjunct; penicillin and erythromycin are the drugs of choice.[8]

If the patient recovers, he apparently makes a complete clinical recovery. Examination of patients 15 to 20 years after severe diphtheria shows no evidence of permanent cardiac damage.[47]

IDIOPATHIC CARDIOMEGALY

The term "idiopathic cardiomegaly" is used here to describe an obscure form of heart disease which may occur in various parts of the world but is mainly found in the tropics and subtropics.[125] The cause is unknown. It presents clinically as cardiac dilatation and/or failure and has been given many other names, including primary myocardial disease, heart muscle disease, idiopathic hypertrophy of the heart, etc.[10, 79] The discussion here is confined to the disease as found among 13 children indigenous to Nigeria.[10]

The patients gave a history of fever at the onset of illness. All but one complained of cough. Dyspnea at rest and on exertion and edema were complaints in nearly all of the children. The duration of symptoms was usually under 1 month.

All 13 patients looked ill. Physical findings included tachycardia, normal blood pressures, evidence of cardiomegaly, and an enlarged tender liver. All children had gallop rhythms. On admission, about one-quarter had murmurs indicating moderate mitral insufficiency, dependent edema, and a moderate degree of malnutrition.

Some patients showed T inversion in the left chest leads of the electrocardiogram and nonspecific ST segment abnormalities. Chest x-rays showed cardiomegaly, with cardiothoracic ratios ranging from 60 to 75%. The cardiac silhouette was globular in all cases, without any suggestion of a particular chamber enlargement and without definite evidence of pericardial effusion.

Treatment is symptomatic. Of seven patients attending regularly for follow-up, all gradually recovered good health, and the heart size in the majority returned to normal.[10]

PROTEIN-CALORIE MALNUTRITION (PCM)

Protein-calorie malnutrition (PCM) or protein-energy malnutrition (PEM) is a collective term denoting a spectrum of nutritional deficiency syndromes ranging from marasmus to kwashiorkor. These are essentially disorders of artificially fed or weaned children that constitute a health problem of immense proportions in economically underdeveloped areas of the tropics and subtropics.[19] Marasmus, of dietary origin resulting from a symmetrical decrease of all nutrients, is the dry form of PCM. Kwashiorkor, which has classically been attributed to protein malnutrition, is the wet form, with pitting edema.[19] Modifying factors that are important in the development of the syndromes include: deficiency of essential minerals such as sodium, potassium, calcium, magnesium, zinc, chromium and, possibly, selenium; and deficiency of water- and fat-soluble vitamins and other essential nutrients.[6, 37] Environmental noxious factors such as: toxins and infectious agents, psychological stress, and large losses of nutrients through gastroenteritis are important contributory factors.[186] Some investigators view PCM as a continuum of syndromes ranging from marasmus at one end and kwashiorkor at the other, with the main differences between the two syndromes being the host's endocrine adaptation to the nutritional disorders: no edema occurs as long as the cardiac index is sufficient to provide adequate renal perfusion and as long as serum albumin levels remain in the normal range. When these fail, sodium is retained, and edema appears.[186]

PCM may be associated with other nutritional deficiency states, including juvenile beriberi, pellagra, and mineral imbalance, and there are often concomitant medical problems, including hookworm infestation, sickle cell anemia, or malaria. It is impossible to ascribe any given symptom to any single nutritional deficiency on initial examination.

Marasmus

There is general wasting of muscle, including heart muscle, loss of subcutaneous fat, and atrophy of most organs. The clinical appearance is that of an infant or young child with extreme emaciation and growth retardation. The skin is wrinkled and loose but there are no pellagroid lesions. Initially, the child is alert, but as the disease progresses, he becomes listless. The vital signs reflect clinical deterioration: hypothermia, low systolic blood pressure, narrow pulse pressure, and shallow respiratory excursions. Diarrhea may become an important problem.

The electrocardiogram usually has dwarfing of all electrical complexes (Fig. 38.14). The PR interval may be short. The T waves are often of low amplitude or are inverted over the left precordium. There may be premature ventricular contractions.

On x-ray, the heart is small or normal, and bronchopneu-

monia may be an associated finding. Cardiac function tests reveal some degree of circulatory failure with reduced cardiac output and prolonged circulation time. The reduced cardiac output is directly related to the weight deficit.[195]

The immediate goal on hospitalization of the PCM patient is to correct fluid and electrolyte imbalance and to treat infection and associated problems such as anemia and parasites, including malaria. A liquid diet is gradually introduced to provide the nutrients for optimal tissue repair and growth. Milk protein (3 to 4 gm/kg/day) and up to 200 calories/kg/day are fed. Extra mineral and vitamin supplements are required during this period. Because of slow and incomplete absorption of magnesium, it is recommended that the parenteral route be used during the 1st week.[38] A well-balanced natural diet should be gradually introduced as early as possible.

The treatment of the dehydrated or severely anemic PCM patient is precarious, because the heart is easily overloaded. Heart failure is infrequent if one avoids overloading with sodium, water, or blood transfusions.[195] The myocardium in PCM is sensitive to moderate doses of digitalis, possibly because of potassium and magnesium deficiency; digitalis must be given cautiously in heart failure.

Kwashiorkor

There is wasting of muscle but not of subcutaneous fat, and edema is usually generalized. The heart is thin-walled, pale, and flabby; it may appear small in the untreated child but may dilate after therapy has begun. The liver is enlarged because of fatty infiltration of the large droplet type. Histologic examination of the heart reveals thinning and atrophy of the muscle fibers, sometimes with interstitial edema or vacuolization of the myocardial fibers.

The child with kwashiorkor shows retarded growth, and edema ranging from pitting edema of the ankles to severe generalized edema with the eyes swollen shut. The child is apathetic, anorexic, and weak, and he may lie motionless, moaning or whimpering only when disturbed. He may appear pale or dusky and may be hypothermic and hypotensive, with poor peripheral pulses, poorly defined cardiac impulses, and barely perceptible respirations. The heart sounds may be muffled, and there may be transient dysrhythmias. Other changes include pellagroid skin lesions, hair changes, and liver enlargement (Fig. 38.15A).

Four or more days after beginning fluid and nutrition therapy, abrupt changes in heart rate and rhythm, brief periods of apnea, electrocardiographic changes,[37, 173] and a wide range of neurologic manifestations may develop.[38] In two separate series, these have been linked to hypomagnesemia,[37, 38] which developed when adequate magnesium supplements were not included in the initial therapy. Good recovery was achieved with nutritionally balanced therapy (Fig. 38.15B).

SCHISTOSOMIASIS (BILHARZIASIS)

Cor pulmonale, or chronic right ventricular failure secondary to pulmonary disease, occurs in children and adolescents throughout the world. In the Philippines, the main causes are tuberculosis, schistosomiasis, and asthmatic bronchitis with emphysema. In a Nigerian series, 23% were attributed to tuberculosis.[27] This discussion is limited to schistosomiasis due to *Schistosomiasis haematobium* and *Schistosomiasis mansoni*. Both of these forms may infect the same child.[75] *Schistosomiasis japonicum,* the third main form of these parasites, rarely causes cor pulmonale.

The agents of the schistosomiasis infestations are trematode worms that are distributed in many areas of the tropics.

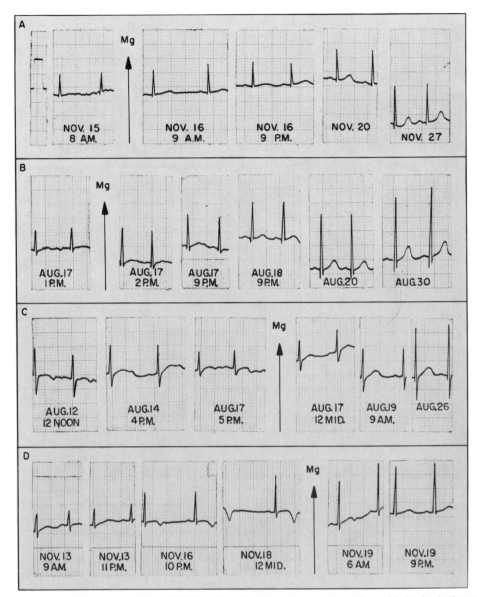

Fig. 38.14 Electrocardiographic changes in Lead V_5 illustrating the effect of magnesium when added to basic therapy in protein-calorie malnutrition. The children in *A* and *B* received daily magnesium therapy beginning soon after admission (*arrow*), whereas those in *C* and *D* did not receive magnesium therapy until after clinical signs of magnesium deficiency appeared. Note the deterioration of the T waves, with subsequent improvement after magnesium is administered.

The host passes eggs in stool and/or urine. This may infect certain fresh water snails where multiplication occurs and larvae (cercariae) emerge. These may penetrate the skin of humans in contact with fresh water, and they rapidly enter the cutaneous blood vessels. The migration of large numbers of schistosomulae through the lungs may result in pneumonic or diffuse infiltration of a miliary size. The form of lesion of most concern to the cardiologist is that associated with cardiac embarrassment due to obliterative endarteritis of the pulmonary arterioles, caused by the ova or by the adult worms. The ova of either *S. hemotobium* or *S. mansoni* may rarely settle in the heart muscle.

The patient is usually between 10 to 35 years of age. He complains of bronchitis-like symptoms and shortness of breath on exertion. He may have raised venous pressure and a swollen face. The cardiac impulse is weak and quiet. The second pulmonic sound is accentuated. The electrocardiographic changes are those of right ventricular hypertrophy.

On x-ray, the patient may show pneumonic or diffuse

infiltrations of a miliary size. In the more chronic forms, two main types of lesions result: nodules in the bronchopulmonary form or diffuse changes due to obliterative endarteritis of the pulmonary arterioles.[75]

The diagnosis of schistosomiasis is established by finding ova in either the urine or stool. Specimens should be taken between 10:00 a.m. and noon, when the output of ova is maximal. Other diagnostic procedures include serologic tests.[8] The nodules seen on x-ray must be differentiated from those of pulmonary tuberculosis. The filarial worm, *Onchocerca volvulus*,[8, 118] which affects 20 million people in the tropics, may also invade the lungs, lymphatics, and blood vessels.

Treatment with antimony-containing drugs and several other effective drugs are toxic. Current expert opinion should be sought at the Center for Disease Control, Atlanta, Ga. Newer drugs are being tested for the treatment of schistosomiasis.[8]

Prevention is unsatisfactory, because of illiteracy and lack

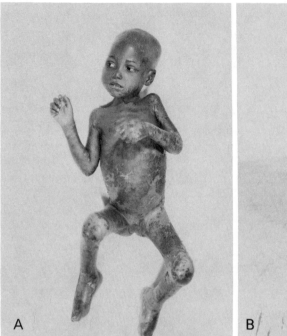
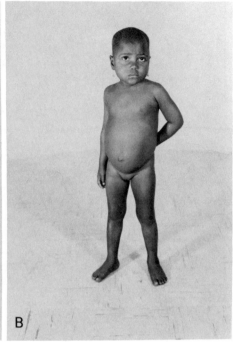

Fig. 38.15 (*A*) Protein-calorie malnutrition in a 3½-year-old Nigerian girl 48 hours after onset of therapy. Note peripheral edema, evidence of wasting in upper arm and thorax, exfoliative dermatitis, and gray hair stubble. (Head has been shaved.) (*B*) Two months later, the same child has black hair and dark healthy skin, and is sturdy, ambulatory, and vigorous.

of education among the majority of the indigenous population of the tropical areas where these parasites are most prevalent.

PURULENT PERICARDITIS

A high frequency of purulent pericarditis and of early constrictive pericarditis has been reported in young children from several regions of the tropics: Uganda, Ethiopia, and India. In a series of 154 cases of pericarditis in Uganda, 43% of cases were pyogenic, the commonest pathogens being *Staphylococcus aureus* and pneumococcus.[56] Constriction occurred in 32%, usually within a few weeks of illness.

Tuberculous pericarditis accounted for 27% of the pericarditis in the Ugandan series[56] and is a prominent cause of pericarditis in children in the tropics.

IDIOPATHIC ARTERITIS

Idiopathic arteritis is an inflammatory panarteritis of the aorta that occurs most commonly in warm climates. Histologic examination reveals round cell infiltration around the

vasa vasorum and a loss of elastic and muscle fibers. Aneurysms develop in the affected areas. A thoracic aortic aneurysm may lead to aortic insufficiency; an abdominal aortic aneurysm may lead to stenosis of the renal artery with secondary hypertension.

SYSTEMIC ARTERIAL HYPERTENSION

A 9-year retrospective study[3] of 138 cases of systemic arterial hypertension in Nigerian children revealed specific data about this important problem in West Africa. Hypertension was defined as a sustained diastolic blood pressure of 90 mm Hg or above. Most of the hypertensive children were between 5 and 10 years of age; there was no sex difference. Most of them presented as the nephrotic syndrome and had glomerulonephritis, which was considered a *Plasmodium malariae* nephropathy. Lesions were rapidly progressive and not influenced by steroids or immunosuppressive drugs. The mortality rate was 28%, with death occurring an average of 16 weeks after detection of hypertension.

REFERENCES

1. Abrahams, D. G., Barton, C. J., Cockshott, W. P., Edington, G. M., and Weaver, E. J. M.: Annular subvalvular left ventricular aneurysms. Q. J. Med. 31:345–360, 1962.
2. Adler, A. G., Walinsky, P., Krall, R. A., and Cho, S. Y.: Death resulting from ipecac syrup poisoning. J.A.M.A. 243:1927–1928, 1980.
3. Aderele, W. I., and Seriki, O.: Hypertension in Nigerian children. Arch. Dis. Child. 49:313–317, 1974.
4. Akbarian, M., Yankopoulos, N. A., and Abelmann, W. H.: Hemodynamic studies in beriberi heart disease. Am. J. Med. 41:197–212, 1966.
5. Akins, E., and Awdeh, M. R.: Marijuana and second-degree AV block. South. Med. J. 74:371–373, 1981.

6. Alleyne, G. A. O.: Mineral metabolism in protein-calorie malnutrition. In Protein-Calorie Malnutrition, edited by R. E. Olson. Academic Press, New York, 1975, pp. 201–227.
7. American Academy of Pediatrics, Committee on Nutrition: Pediatric Nutrition Handbook. Evanston, Illinois, 1979.
8. American Academy of Pediatrics Report of the Committee on Infectious Diseases. 18th ed. American Academy of Pediatics, Evanston, Ill., 1977.
9. Antia, A. U.: Congenital heart disease in Nigeria. Clinical and necropsy study of 260 cases. Arch. Dis. Child. 49:36–39, 1974.
10. Antia, A. U., Cockshott, W. P., and Thorpe, G. J.: Idiopathic cardiomegaly in Nigerian children. Br. Heart J. 31: 178–183, 1969.

11. Araújo, J., Sánchez, G., Gutiérrez, J., and Pérez, F.: Cardiomyopathies of obscure origin in Cali, Colombia. Am. Heart J. 80:162–170, 1970.
12. Aryanpur, I., Farhoudi, A., and Zangeneh, F.: Congestive heart failure secondary to idiopathic hypoparathyroidism. Am. J. Dis. Child. 127:738–739, 1974.
13. Asmussen, I., and Kjeldsen, K.: Intimal ultrastructure of human umbilical arteries. Observation on arteries from newborn children of smoking and nonsmoking mothers. Circ. Res. 36:579–589, 1975.
14. Attas, M., Hanley, H. G., Stultz, D., Jones, M. R., and McAllister, R. G.: Fulminant beriberi heart disease with lactic acidosis: Presentation of a case with evaluation of left

ventricular function and review of pathophysiologic mechanisms. Circulation 58:566–572, 1978.

15. Ayuthya, P., Jayavasu, J., and Pongpanich, B.: Coxsackie Group B virus and primary myocardial disease in infants and children. Am. Heart J. 88:311–314, 1974.

16. Azevedo, E. M., Scaff, M., Barbosa, E. R., Neto, A. E. G., and Canelas, H. M.: Heart involvement in hepatolenticular degeneration. Acta Neurol. Scand. 58:296–303, 1978.

17. Barness, L. A.: Nutrition and nutritional disorders. In Nelson Textbook of Pediatrics, 11th ed., edited by V. C. Vaughan, III, R. J. McKay, Jr., and R. E. Behrman. W. B. Saunders, Philadelphia, Pa., 1979, pp. 173–236.

18. Bashour, T., Basha, H. S., and Cheng, T. O.: Hypocalcemic cardiomyopathy. Chest 78:663–665, 1980.

19. Béhar, M., and Viteri, F. E.: Protein-energy malnutrition. In Diseases of Children in the Subtropics and Tropics, 3rd ed., edited by D. B. Jelliffe and J. P. Stanfield. Edward Arnold, London, 1978, pp. 197–221.

20. Behrman, R. E.: Infants of diabetic mothers. In Nelson Textbook of Pediatrics, 11th ed., edited by Victor C. Vaughan, III, R. J. McKay, Jr., and R. E. Behrman. W. B. Saunders Co., Philadelphia, Pa., 1979, pp. 464–466.

21. Bhattacharya, S. K., Jha, B. N., and Somani, P. N.: Carditis in acute rheumatic fever in Varanasi, India. Trop. Geogr. Med. 26:271–277, 1974.

22. Biancaniello, T., Meyer, R. A., Wong, K. Y., Sager, C., and Kaplan, S.: Doxorubicin cardiotoxicity in children. J. Pediatr. 97:45–50, 1980.

23. Bird, T.: Idiopathic arterial calcification in infancy. Arch. Dis. Child. 49:82–89, 1974.

24. Bongiovanni, A. M.: Action and metabolism of adrenocortical hormones. In Pediatrics, 15th ed., edited by H. L. Barnett. Appleton-Century-Crofts, New York, 1972, pp. 1093–1102.

25. Bristow, M. R., Billingham, M. E., Mason, J. W., and Daniels, J. R.: Clinical spectrum of anthracycline antibiotic cardiotoxicity. Cancer Treat. Rep. 62:873–879, 1978.

26. Britton, W. J., and Kevau, I. H.: Intentional chloroquine overdosage. Med. J. Aust. 21:407–410, 1978.

27. Brockington, I. F., and Edington, G. M.: Adult heart disease in western Nigeria: A clinicopathological synopsis. Am. Heart J. 83:27–40, 1972.

28. Brook, C. G. D.: Consequences of childhood obesity. World Med. J. 19:45–46, 1972.

29. Bruce-Chwatt, L. J.: Malaria. In Diseases of Children in the Subtropics and Tropics, 3rd ed., edited by D. B. Jelliffe and J. P. Stanfield, Edward Arnold, Ltd., London, 1978, pp. 827–856.

30. Buckley, B. H., and Hutchins, G. M.: Pompe's disease presenting as hypertrophic myocardiopathy with Wolff-Parkinson-White syndrome. Am. Heart J. 96:246–252, 1978.

31. Burch, G. E., and Giles, T. D.: The role of viruses in the production of heart disease. Am. J. Cardiol. 29:231–240, 1972.

32. Burk, R. F.: Selenium in man. In Trace Elements in Human Health and Disease, Vol. II, edited by A. S. Prasad. Academic Press, New York, 1976, pp. 105–133.

33. Burrow, G. N.: The thyroid in pregnancy. Med. Clin. North Am. 59:1089–1098, 1975.

34. Byrne-Quinne, E., and Fessas, C.: Beriberi heart disease in London. Br. Med. J. 4:25–28, 1969.

35. Caddell, J. L.: Exploring the magnesium-deficient weanling rat as an animal model for the sudden infant death syndrome: Physical, biochemical, electrocardiographic, and gross pathologic changes. Pediatr. Res. 12:1157–1166, 1978.

36. Caddell, J. L., and Connor, D. H.: Congenital

heart disease in Ugandan children. Br. Heart J. 28:766–767, 1966.

37. Caddell, J. L., and Goddard, D. R.: Studies in protein-calorie malnutrition. I and II. N. Engl. J. Med. 276:533–535 and 535–540, 1967.

38. Caddell, J. L., and Olson, R. E.: An evaluation of the electrolyte status of malnourished Thai children. J. Pediatr. 83:124–128, 1973.

39. Caddell, J. L., Warley, A., Connor, D. H., D'Arbela, P. G., and Billinghurst, J. R.: Acquired heart disease in Ugandan children. Br. Heart J. 28:759–765, 1966.

40. Caddell, J. L., and Whittemore, R.: Observations on generalized glycogenosis with emphasis on electrocardiographic changes. Pediatrics 29:743–763, 1962.

41. Calabresi, P., and Parks, R. E., Jr.: Antiproliferative agents and drugs used for immunosuppression. In Goodman and Gilman's The Pharmacological Basis of Therapeutics, 6th ed., edited by A. G. Gilman, L. S. Goodman, and A. Gilman. Macmillan, New York, 1980, pp. 1256–1313.

42. Caldarelli, D. D., and Holinger, L. D.: Complications and sequelae of thyroid surgery. Otolaryngol. Clin. North Am. 13:85–97, 1980.

43. Cann, H. M., and Verhulst, H. L.: Fatal acute chloroquine poisoning in children. Pediatrics 27:95–102, 1961.

44. Carey, C., Skosey, C., Pinnamaneni, K. M., Barsano, C. P., and DeGroot, L. J.: Thyroid abnormalities in children of parents who have Graves' disease: Possible pre-Graves' disease. Metabolism 29:369–376, 1980.

45. Chen, Su-chiung, Associate Professor of Pediatrics, St. Louis University, Personal Communication, 1981.

46. Chisolm, J. J., Jr.: Hemochromatosis. In Nelson Textbook of Pediatrics, 11th ed., edited by V. C. Vaughan, III, R. J. McKay, Jr., and R. E. Behrman. W. B. Saunders, Philadelphia, Pa., 1979, pp. 580–581.

47. Christie, A. B.: Infectious disease. In Epidemiology and Clinical Practice, 3rd ed., Churchill Livingstone, Edinburgh, 1980, pp. 532 and 868.

48. Chu, J-Y., O'Connor, D. M., and McElfresh, A. E.: Nutritional anemia. In The Clinical Practice of Adolescent Medicine, edited by J. T. Y. Shen, Appleton-Century-Crofts, New York, 1980, pp. 205–210.

49. Clarren, S. K., and Smith, D. W.: The fetal alcohol syndrome. N. Engl. J. Med. 298:1063–1067, 1978.

50. Cockshott, W. P.: Angiocardiography of endomyocardial fibrosis. Br. J. Radiol. 38:192–200, 1965.

51. Cockshott, W. P., Anita, A., Ikeme, A., and Uzodike, V. O.: Annular subvalvar left ventricular aneurysms. Br. J. Radiol. 40:424–435, 1967.

52. Committee on Dietary Allowances, the National Research Council: Recommended Dietary Allowances, 9th ed. National Academy of Sciences, Washington, D.C., 1980.

53. Connor, D. H., Somers, K., Hutt, M. S. R., Manion, W. C., and D'Arbela, P. G.: Endomyocardial fibrosis in Uganda (Davies' disease). Part I. Am. Heart J. 74:687–709, 1967; Part II, Am. Heart J. 75:107–124, 1968.

54. Connor, D. H.: Personal Communication (in Caddell, J. L.: Diseases of the Cardiovascular System). In Diseases of Children in the Subtropics and Tropics, 3rd ed., edited by D. B. Jelliffe and J. P. Stanfield. Edward Arnold, Ltd., London, 1978, p. 404.

55. Danks, D. M., Campbell, P. E., Stevens, B. J., Mayne, V., and Cartwright, E.: Menkes' kinky hair syndrome. An inherited defect in copper absorption with widespread effects. Pediatrics 50:188–201, 1972.

56. D'Arbela, P. G., Patel, A. K., Grigg, G. L., and Somers, K.: Pericarditis, with particular emphasis on pyogenic pericarditis: A Uganda experience. East Afr. Med. J. 49:803–816,

1972.

57. D'Arbela, P. G., Patel, A. K., and Somers, K.: Juvenile rheumatic fever and rheumatic heart disease at Mulago Hospital, Kampala, Uganda: Some aspects on the pattern of the disease. East Afr. Med. J. 51:710–714, 1974.

58. deGroot, W. J.: Cardiomyopathy associated with endocrine disorders. Cardiovasc. Clin. 4 (1):306–344, 1972.

59. DiCarlo, F. J., Jr.: Syndromes of cardiovascular malformations induced by copper citrate in hamsters. Teratology 21:89–101, 1980.

60. Dickinson, D. F., Houlsby, W. T., and Wilkinson, J. L.: Unusual angiographic appearances of the left ventricle in 2 cases of Pompe's disease (glycogenosis type II). Br. Heart J. 41:238–240, 1979.

61. Di George, A. M.: Adrenocortical hyperfunction. In Nelson Textbook of Pediatrics, 11th ed., edited by V. C. Vaughan, III, R. J. McKay, Jr., and R. E. Behrman. W. B. Saunders, Philadelphia, Pa., 1979, pp. 1668–1677.

62. Di George, A. M.: Disorders of the thyroid gland. In Nelson Textbook of Pediatrics, 11th ed., edited by V. C. Vaughan, III, R. J. McKay, Jr., and R. E. Behrman. W. B. Saunders, Philadelphia, Pa., 1979, pp. 1632–1650.

63. Diskin, C. J.: Caution with selenium replacement. Lancet 2:1249, 1979.

64. Dorchy, H., Toussaint, D., Vanderschueren-Lodeweyckx, M., Vandenbussche, E., De-Vroede, M., and Loeb, H.: Leakage of fluorescein: First sign of juvenile diabetic retinopathy. Role of diabetic control and of duration of diabetes. Acta Paediatr. Scand. (Suppl.) 277:47–53, 1979.

65. Drash, A. L.: Diabetes mellitus. In Nelson Textbook of Pediatrics, 11th ed., edited by V. C. Vaughan, III, R. J. McKay, Jr., and R. E. Behrman, W. B. Saunders, Philadelphia, Pa., 1979, pp. 1581–1597.

66. Dussault, J. H., Coulombe, P., Laberge, C., Letarte, J., Guyda, H., and Khoury, K.: Preliminary report on a mass screening program for neonatal hypothyroidism. J. Pediatr. 86:670–674, 1975.

67. Dyer, A. R., Stamler, J., Paul, O., Berkson, D. M., Lepper, M. H., McKean, H., Shekelle, R. B., Lindberg, H. A., and Garside, D.: Alcohol consumption, cardiovascular risk factors, and mortality in two Chicago epidemiologic studies. Circulation 56:1067–1074, 1977.

68. Ehlers, K. H., Levin, A. R., Markenson, A. L., Marcus, J. R., Klein, A. A., Hilgartner, M. W., and Engle, M. A.: Longitudinal study of cardiac function in thalassemia major. Ann. N.Y. Acad. Sci. 344:397–404, 1980.

69. Engle, M. A., Erlandson, M., and Smith, C. H.: Late cardiac complications of chronic, severe, refractory anemia with hemochromatosis. Circulation 30:698–705, 1964.

70. Erlich, R. M.: Diabetes mellitus in childhood. Pediatr. Clin. North Am. 21:871–884, 1974.

71. Felig, P.: Disorders of carbohydrate metabolism. In Metabolic Control and Disease, 8th ed., edited by P. K. Bondy and L. E. Rosenberg. W. B. Saunders, Philadelphia, Pa., 1980, pp. 276–392.

72. Fisher, D. A.: Advances in the laboratory diagnosis of thyroid disease. I and II. J. Pediatr. 82:1–9 and 187–191, 1973.

73. Fredrickson, D. S., Goldstein, J. L., and Brown, M. S.: The familial hyperlipoproteinemias. In The Metabolic Basis of Inherited Disease, 4th ed., edited by J. B. Stanbury, J. B. Wyngaarden, and D. S. Frederickson. McGraw-Hill Book Co., New York, 1978, pp. 604–669.

74. Friedberg, C. K.: The heart and circulation in myxedema. In Diseases of the Heart, 3rd ed., edited by C. K. Friedberg. W. B. Saunders, Philadelphia, Pa., 1966, pp. 1629–1641.

75. Gelfand, M.: Schistosomiasis. In Diseases of Children in the Subtropics and Tropics, 3rd ed., edited by D. B. Jelliffe and J. P. Stanfield.

Edward Arnold, Ltd., London, 1978, pp. 883–914.

76. Gerry, J. L., Baird, M. G., and Fortuin, N. J.: Evaluation of left ventricular function in patients with sickle cell anemia. Am. J. Med. 60:968–972, 1976.

77. Gillette, P. C., Nihill, M. R., and Singer, D. B.: Electrophysiological mechanism of the short PR interval in Pompe Disease. Am. J. Dis. Child. 128:622–626, 1974.

78. Gokal, R., Millard, P. R., Weatherall, D. J., Callender, S. T. E., Ledingham, J. G. G., and Oliver, D. O.: Iron metabolism in haemodialysis patients. Q. J. Med. 48:369–391, 1979.

79. Goodwin, J. F., and Oakley, C. M.: The cardiomyopathies. Br. Heart J. 34:545–552, 1972.

80. Gooneratne, S. R., and Howell, J. M.: Creatine kinase release and muscle changes in chronic copper poisoning in sheep. Res. Vet. Sci. 28:351–361, 1980.

81. Gurdiel, P., Páris, A., Alemán, C., Penso, M., Gordo, J., and Harris, A.: Low right ventricular endocardial potentials in chronic Chagas' disease. Br. Heart J. 36:1239–1243, 1974.

82. Gutgesell, H. P., Mullins, C. E., Gillette, P. C., Speer, M., Rudolph, A. J., and McNamara, D. G.: Transient hypertrophic subaortic stenosis in infants of diabetic mothers. J. Pediatr. 89:120–125, 1976.

83. Hanson, J. W., Jones, K. L., and Smith, D. W.: Fetal alcohol syndrome. Experience with 41 patients. J.A.M.A. 235:1458–1460, 1976.

84. Hanson, J. W., Streissguth, A. P., and Smith, D. W.: The effects of moderate alcohol consumption during pregnancy on fetal growth and morphogenesis. J. Pediatr. 92:457–460, 1978.

85. Hardison, J. E., and Rogers, C. M.: Cardiovascular manifestations of sickle cell anemia. In Update I: The Heart, edited by J. W. Hurst. McGraw-Hill, New York, 1979, pp. 185–190.

86. Harris, I., and Wilkinson, A. W.: Magnesium depletion in children. Lancet 2:735–736, 1971.

87. Harvey, S. C.: Heavy metals. In The Pharmacological Basis of Therapeutics, 4th ed., edited by L. Goodman and A. Gilman, Macmillan, New York, 1970, pp. 958–986.

88. Hayford, J. T., Schieken, R. M., and Thompson, R. G.: Cardiac function in primary hypothyroidism. Am. J. Dis. Child. 134:556–559, 1980.

89. Heggtveit, H. A., and Nadkarni, B. B.: Ultrastructural pathology of the myocardium. Methods Achiev. Exp. Pathol. 5:474–517, 1971.

90. Henry, W.: Echocardiographic evaluation of the heart in thalassemia major. In Thalassemia major: Molecular and clinical aspects (N.I.H. Conference). Ann. Intern. Med. 91:883–897, 1979.

91. Herbert, V., Colman, N., and Jacob, E.: Folic acid and vitamin B12. In Modern Nutrition in Health and Disease, 6th ed., edited by R. S. Goodhart and M. E. Shils, Lea & Febiger, Philadelphia, Pa., 1980, pp. 229–259.

92. Hers, H. G., and de Barsy, T.: Type II glycogenosis (acid maltase deficiency). In Lysosomes and Storage Diseases, edited by H. G. Hers and F. VanHoof. Academic Press, New York, 1973, pp. 197–216.

93. Hirschman, S. Z., and Hammer, G. S.: Coxsackie virus myopericarditis. A microbiological and clinical review. Am. J. Cardiol. 34:224–232, 1974.

94. Howell, R. R.: The glycogen storage diseases. In The Metabolic Basis of Inherited Disease, 4th ed., edited by J. B. Stanbury, J. B. Wyngaarden, and D. S. Fredrickson, McGraw-Hill, New York, 1978, pp. 137–159.

95. Hug, G.: Defects in metabolism of carbohydrates. In Nelson Textbook of Pediatrics, 11th ed., edited by V. C. Vaughan, III, R. J. McKay, and R. E. Behrman, W. B. Saunders, Philadelphia, Pa., 1979, pp. 520–548.

96. Hurley, L. S.: Developmental nutrition. Prentice-Hall, Englewood Cliffs, N.J., 1980.

97. Inouye, K., and Katsura, E.: Chapters I–III in Review of Japanese Literature on Beriberi and Thiamine, edited by N. Shimazono and E. Katsura. Vitamin B Research Committee of Japan, Igaku Shoin, Tokyo, 1965, pp. 1–80.

98. Jaffe, J. H.: Drug addiction and drug abuse. In Goodman and Gilman's The Pharmacological Basis of Therapeutics, 6th ed., edited by A. G. Gilman, L. S. Goodman, and A. Gilman, Macmillan, New York, 1980, pp. 535–584.

99. Jeffrey, F. E., and Abelmann, W. H.: Recovery from proved shoshin beriberi. Am. J. Med. 50:123–128, 1971.

100. Jones, K. L., and Smith, D. W.: Recognition of the fetal alcohol syndrome in early infancy. Lancet 2:999–1001, 1973.

101. Kannel, W. B., Hjortland, M., and Castelli, W. P.: Role of diabetes in congestive heart failure: The Framingham study. Am. J. Cardiol. 34:29–34, 1974.

102. Karpel, J. T., and Peden, V. H.: Copper deficiency in long-term parenteral nutrition. J. Pediatr. 80:32–36, 1972.

103. Kaufman, K. S. Papaefthymiou, G. C., Frankel, R. B., and Rosenthal, A.: Nature of iron deposits on the cardiac walls in β-thalassemia by Mössbauer spectroscopy. Biochim. Biophys. Acta 629:522–529, 1980.

104. Kawai, C., Wakabayashi, A., Matsumura, T., and Yui, Y.: Reappearance of beriberi heart disease in Japan. A study of 23 cases. Am. J. Med. 69:383–386, 1980.

105. Kelly, W. A., Kesterson, J. W., and Carlton, W. W.: Myocardial lesions in the offspring of female rats fed a copper deficient diet. Exp. Mol. Pathol. 20:40–56, 1974.

106. Keshan Disease Research Group of the Chinese Academy of Medical Sciences, Beijin, China: Epidemiologic studies on the etiologic relationship of selenium and Keshan disease. Chinese Med. J. 92:477–482, 1979.

107. Keshan Disease Research Group of the Chinese Academy of Medical Sciences, Beijin: Observations on effect of sodium selenite in prevention of Keshan disease. Chinese Med. J. 92:471–476, 1979.

108. Khan, A. A.: Disorders of the haemopoietic system. In Diseases of Children in the Subtropics and Tropics, 3rd ed., edited by D. B. Jelliffe and J. P. Stanfield. Edward Arnold, London, 1978, pp. 573–604.

109. Klein, A. H., Agustin, A. V., and Foley, T. P., Jr.: Successful laboratory screening for congenital hypothyroidism. Lancet 2:77–79, 1974.

110. Klein, A. H., Meltzer, S., and Kenny, F. M.: Improved prognosis in congenital hypothyroidism treated before age three months. J. Pediatr. 81:912–915, 1972.

111. Kozam, R. L., Esguerra, O. E., and Smith, J. J.: Cardiovascular beriberi. Am. J. Cardiol. 30:418–422, 1972.

112. Krumlovsky, F. A.: Cardiac function in the chronic dialysis patient. Intern. J. Artif. Organs 2:175–178, 1979.

113. La Du, B. N.: Alcaptonuria. In The Metabolic Basis of Inherited Disease, 4th ed., edited by J. B. Stanbury, J. B. Wyngaarden, and D. S. Fredrickson. McGraw-Hill, New York, 1978, pp. 268–282.

114. Link, D. A.: Fluid and electrolytes. In Manual of Pediatric Therapeutics, 2nd ed., edited by J. W. Graef and T. E. Cone, Jr., Little, Brown, Boston, 1980, pp. 177–204.

115. Lowenthal, M. N.: Endomyocardial fibrosis: Familial and other cases from Northern Zambia. Med. J. Zambia 12:2–7, 1978.

116. Mabry, C. C., and Tietz, N. W.: Tables of Normal Laboratory Values. In Nelson Textbook of Pediatrics, 11th ed., edited by V. C. Vaughan, III, R. J. McKay, and R. E. Behrman. W. B. Saunders, Philadelphia, Pa., 1979, pp. 2075–2093.

117. Mace, S., Hirschfield, S. S., Riggs, T., Fanaroff, A. A., and Merkatz, I. R.: Echocardiographic abnormalities in infants of diabetic mothers. J. Pediatr. 95:1013–1019, 1979.

118. Mahoney, J. L.: Onchocerciasis in expatriates on the Ivory Coast. Southern Med. J. 74:295–297, 1981.

119. Majoor, C. L. H.: Alcoholism as a cause of beriberi heart disease. J. Roy. Coll. Phys. 12:143–152, 1978.

120. Makene, W. J., and Muindi, J. R.: Some observations on congestive cardiac failure in African patients in Dar es Salaam. East Afr. Med. J. 53:326–331, 1976.

121. Manifold, I. H., Platts, M. M., and Kennedy, A.: Cobalt cardiomyopathy in a patient on maintenance haemodialysis. Br. Med. J. 2:1609, 1978.

122. Maron, B. J., and Ferrans, V. J.: Ultrastructural features of hypertrophied human ventricular myocardium. Prog. Cardiovasc. Dis. 21:207–238, 1978.

123. Martin, J. J., deBarsy, T., Van Hoff, F., and Palladini, G.: Pompe's disease: An inborn lysosomal disorder with storage of glycogen: A study of brain and striated muscle. Acta Neuropathol. (Berl.) 23:229–244, 1973.

124. McGuffin, W. L., Jr., Sherman, B. M., Roth, J., Gorden, P., Kahn, C. R., Roberts, W. C., and Frommer, P. L.: Acromegaly and cardiovascular disorders: A prospective study. Ann. Intern. Med. 81:11–18, 1974.

125. McKinney, B.: Cardiac muscle fiber size in African cardiomyopathies. Am. Heart J. 87:298–301, 1974.

126. McKusick, V. A.: Heritable Disorders of Connective Tissue, 4th ed. C. V. Mosby, St. Louis, 1972, pp. 725–727.

127. Melvin, G. R., Aceto, T., Jr., Barlow, J., Munson, D., and Wierda, D.: Iatrogenic congenital goiter and hypothyroidism with respiratory distress in a newborn. S. Dakota J. Med. 31:15–19, 1978.

128. Menkes, J. H., Alter, M., Steigleder, G. K., Weakley, D. R., and Sung, J. H.: A sex-linked recessive disorder with retardation of growth, peculiar hair, and focal cerebral and cerebellar degeneration. Pediatrics 29:764–779, 1962.

129. Montelone, J. A.: Thyroid disease in adolescence. In The Clinical Practice of Adolescent Medicine, edited by J. T. Y. Shen, Appleton-Century-Crofts, New York, 1980, pp. 284–292.

130. Montoro, M., Collea, J. V., Frasier, S. D., and Mestman, J. H.: Successful outcome of pregnancy in women with hypothyroidism. Ann. Intern. Med. 94:31–34, 1981.

131. Morin, Y., Têtu, A., and Mercier, G.: Cobalt cardiomyopathy: Clinical aspects. Br. Heart J. (Suppl.) 33:175–178, 1971.

132. Murros, J., and Luomanmäki, K.: A case of hypocalcemia, heart failure, and exceptional repolarization disturbances. Acta Med. Scand. 208:133–136, 1980.

133. Nankin, R. G., and Arensberg, D.: Viral myocarditis. In Update V, The Heart, edited by J. W. Hurst. McGraw-Hill, New York, 1981, pp. 245–251.

134. Newman, W. H., and Valicenti, J. F., Jr.: Ventricular function following acute alcohol administration. A strain gauge analysis of depressed ventricular dynamics. Am. Heart J. 81(1):61–68, 1971.

135. Nienhuis, A. W., Griffith, P., Strawczynski, H., Henry, W., Borer, J., Leon, M., and Anderson, W.: Evaluation of cardiac function in patients with thalassemia major. Ann. N.Y. Acad. Sci. 344:384–396, 1980.

136. Nouri, S.: Director of Pediatric Cardiology, Assistant Professor of Pediatrics, St. Louis University Medical Center, Personal Communication, 1981.

137. O'Connor, L. R., Wheeler, W. S., and Bethune, J. E.: Effect of hypophosphatemia on myocardial performance in man. N. Engl. J. Med. 297:901–903, 1977.

138. O'Leary, J. P.: Jejunoileal bypass in the treat-

ment of morbid obesity. Intern. J. Obesity 2:191–196, 1978.

139. Østerby, R.: Morphometric studies of the peripheral glomerular basement membrane in early juvenile diabetes. I. Development of initial basement thickening. Diabetologia 8:84–92, 1972.

140. Parisi, A. F., Hamilton, B. P., Thomas, C. N., and Mazzaferri, E. L.: The short cardiac preejection period. An index to thyrotoxicosis. Circulation 49:900–904, 1974.

141. Parving, H-H., Noer, I., Deckert, T., Ervin, P-E., Nielsen, S. L., Lyngsøe, J., Mongensen, C. E., Rorth, M., Svendsen, P., Trap-Jensen, J., and Lassen, N. A.: The effect of metabolic regulation on microvascular permeability to small and large molecules in short-term juvenile diabetics. Diabetologia 12:161–166, 1976.

142. Pearson, H. A.: Diseases of the blood. In Nelson Textbook of Pediatrics, 11th ed., edited by V. C. Vaughan, III, R. J. McKay, Jr., and R. E. Behrman. W. B. Saunders, Philadelphia, Pa., 1979, pp. 1363–1395.

143. Pilapil, V. P., and Watson, D. G.: Electrocardiogram in hyperthyroid children. Am. J. Dis. Child. 119:245–248, 1970.

144. Poltera, A. A., Cox, J. N., and Owor, R.: Pancarditis affecting the conducting system and all valves in human African trypanosomiasis. Br. Heart J. 38:827–837, 1976.

145. Polycove, M.: Hemochromatosis. In The Metabolic Basis of Inherited Disease, 4th ed., edited by J. B. Stanbury, J. B. Wyngaarden, and D. S. Frederickson. McGraw-Hill, New York, 1978, pp. 1127–1164.

146. Pratt, C. B., Ransom, J. L., and Evans, W. E.: Age-related adriamycin cardiotoxicity in children. Cancer Treatment Rep. 62:1381–1385, 1978.

147. Regan, T. J., and Ettinger, P. O.: Alcohol and the heart. In Update I: The Heart, edited by J. W. Hurst. McGraw-Hill, New York, 1979, pp. 259–274.

148. Renold, A. E., Mintz, D. H., Muller, W. A., and Cahill, G. F., Jr.: Diabetes mellitus. In The Metabolic Basis of Inherited Disease, 4th ed., edited by J. B. Stanbury, J. B. Wyngaarden, and D. S. Fredrickson. McGraw-Hill, New York, 1978, pp. 80–109.

149. Ritchie, J. M.: The aliphatic alcohols. In Goodman and Gilman's The Pharmacological Basis of Therapeutics, 6th ed., edited by A. G. Gilman, L. S. Goodman, and A. Gilman. Macmillan, New York, 1980, pp. 376–390.

150. Robbins, J., Rall, J. E., and Gorden, P.: The thyroid and iodine metabolism. In Metabolic Control and Disease, 8th ed., edited by P. K. Bondy and L. E. Rosenberg. W. B. Saunders, Philadelphia, Pa., 1980, pp. 1325–1425.

151. Robinson, M. F., McKenzie, J. M., Thomson, C. D., and Van Rij, A. L.: Metabolic balance of zinc, copper, cadmium, iron, molybdenum and selenium in young New Zealand women. Br. J. Nutr. 30:195–205, 1973.

152. Rochester, D. F., and Enson, Y.: Current concepts in the pathogenesis of the obesity-hypoventilation syndrome: Mechanical and circulatory factors. Am. J. Med. 57:402–420, 1974.

153. Rogers, E. L.: Surgery for morbid obesity: Indications, complications, alternatives. Southern Med. J. 74:47–52, 1981.

154. Rollo, I. M.: Chemotherapy of parasitic diseases. In Goodman and Gilman's The Pharmacological Basis of Therapeutics, 6th ed., edited by A. G. Gilman, L. S. Goodman, and A. Gilman. Macmillan, New York, 1980, pp. 1013–1079.

155. Rossignol, A. M., Meyer, M., Rossignol, B., Palcoux, M. P., Raynaud, E. J., and Bost, M.: La Myocardiopathie de la Glycogenose Type III. Arch. Franç. Pédiat. 36:303–309, 1979.

156. Rowe, R. D., and Cooke, R. E.: Vitamin D and craniofacial and dental anomalies of su-

pravalvular stenosis. Pediatrics 43:1–2, 1969.

157. Saddi, R., Feingold, J., Degrese, C. H., and Fagard, R.: Desferrioxamine utilisation for the quantitation of iron excess. Study of 24 patients having idiopathic haemochromatosis. Biomedicine 28:41–47, 1978.

158. Sandstead, H. H.: Clinical manifestations of certain classical deficiency diseases. In Modern Nutrition in Health and Disease, 6th ed., edited by R. S. Goodhart and M. E. Shils, Lea & Febiger, Philadelphia, Pa., 1980, pp. 685–696.

159. Santos, A. D., Mathew, P. K., and Miller, R. P.: The cardiomyopathy of hypothyroidism revisited. Am. J. Dis. Child. 134:547–549, 1980.

160. Santos, A. D., Miller, R. P., Mathew, P. K., Wallace, W. A., Cave, W. T., Jr., and Hinojosa, L.: Echocardiographic characterization of the reversible cardiomyopathy of hypothyroidism. Am. J. Med. 68:675–682, 1980.

161. Sanyal, S. K., Johnson, W., Jayalakshmamma, B., and Green, A. A.: Fatal "iron heart" in an adolescent: Biochemical and ultrastructural aspects of the heart. Pediatrics 55:336–341, 1975.

162. Sanyal, S. K., Thapar, M. K., Ahmed, S. H., Hooja, V., and Tewari, P.: The initial attack of acute rheumatic fever during childhood in North India. A prospective study of the clinical profile. Circulation 49:7–12, 1974.

163. Scheible, W., Leopold, G. R., Woo, V. L., and Gosink, B. B.: High-resolution real-time ultrasonography of thyroid nodules. Radiology 133:413–417, 1979.

164. Scheinberg, I. H., and Sternlieb, I.: Copper toxicity and Wilson's disease. In Trace Elements in Human Health and Disease, Vol. I, edited by A. S. Prasad. Academic Press, New York, 1976, pp. 415–438.

165. Schwartz, W. B.: Disorders of fluid, electrolyte, and acid-base balance. In Cecil Textbook of Medicine, Vol. 2, 15th ed., edited by P. B. Beeson, W. McDermott, and J. B. Wyngaarden. W. B. Saunders, Philadelphia, Pa., 1979, pp. 1950–1969.

166. Science and Education Administration's Agricultural Research Staff, U.S. Department of Agriculture: Composition of Foods. Baby Foods. Agriculture Handbook No. 8.3, U.S. Department of Agriculture. Washington, D.C., 1978.

167. Scotti, T., M.: Heart. In Pathology, Vol. I, 7th ed., edited by W. A. D. Anderson and J. M. Kissane. C. V. Mosby, St. Louis, 1977, pp. 737–855.

168. Seftel, H. C., Metz, J., and Lakier, J. B.: Cardiomyopathies in Johannesburg Bantu. I. Aetiology and characteristics of beriberi heart disease. S. Afr. Med. J. 46:1707–1713, 1972.

169. Seshadri, M. S., John, L., Varkey, K., and Koshy, T. S.: Ventricular tachycardia in a patient on dehydroemetine and chloroquine for amoebic liver abscess. Med. J. Aust. 1:406–407, 1979.

170. Sidbury, J. B., Jr., and Heick, H. M. C.: Glycogen storage diseases: A review with emphasis on gastrointestinal manifestations. South. Med. J. 61:915–922, 1968.

171. Smallridge, R. C., Rajfer, S., Davia, J., and Schaaf, M.: Acromegaly and the heart. An echocardiographic study. Am. J. Med. 66:22–27, 1979.

172. Smith, D. W., Blizzard, R. M., and Wilkins, L.: The mental prognosis in hypothyroidism of infancy and childhood. Pediatrics 19:1011–1022, 1957.

173. Smythe, P. M., Swanepoel, A., and Campbell, J. A. H.: The heart in kwashiorkor. Br. Med. J. 1:67–73, 1962.

174. Sours, H. E., Frattali, V. P., Brand, C. D., Feldman, R. A., Forbes, A. L., Swanson, R. C., and Paris, A. L.: Sudden death associated with very low calorie weight reduction regi-

mens. Am. J. Clin. Nutr. 34:453–461, 1981.

175. Stanbury, J. B.: Familial goiter. In The Metabolic Basis of Inherited Disease, 4th ed., edited by J. B. Stanbury, J. B. Wyngaarden, and D. S. Fredrickson. McGraw-Hill, New York, 1978, pp. 206–239.

176. Stanfield, J. P., and Bracken, P. M.: Antistreptolysin titres in the childhood population in rural and semi-rural Buganda. East Afr. Med. J. 50:153–158, 1973.

177. Stein, P. D., and Sabbah, H. N.: Accentuation of heart sounds in anemia: An effect of blood viscosity. Am. J. Physiol. 235:664–669, 1978.

178. Steiner, I., Patel, A. K., Hutt, M. S. R., and Somers, K.: Pathology of infective endocarditis: A postmortem evaluation. Br. Heart J. 35:159–164, 1973.

179. Streissguth, A. P., Herman, C. S., and Smith, D. W.: Intelligence, behavior, and dysmorphogenesis in the fetal alcohol syndrome: A report on 20 patients. J. Pediatr. 92:363–367, 1978.

180. Tanphaichitr, V., Vimokesant, S. L., Dhanamitta, S., and Valyasevi, A.: Clinical and biochemical studies of adult beriberi. Am. J. Clin. Nutr. 23:1017–1026, 1970.

181. Treistman, B., Cooley, D. A., Lufschanowski, R., and Leachman, R. D.: Diverticulum or aneurysm of left ventricle. Am. J. Cardiol. 32:119–123, 1973.

182. Troughton, O., and Singh, S. P.: Heart failure and neonatal hypocalcaemia. Br. Med. J. 4:76–79, 1972.

183. Tunbridge, W. M. G., Evered, D. C., Hall, R., Appleton, D., Brewis, M., Clark, F., Evans, J. G., Young, E., Bird, T., and Smith, P. A.: The spectrum of thyroid disease in a community: The Whickham survey. Clin. Endocrinol. 7:481–493, 1977.

184. Underwood, E. J.: Methodology of trace element research. In Trace Elements in Human Health and Disease, Vol. II, edited by A. S. Prasad. Academic Press, New York, 1976, pp. 269–279.

185. Underwood, E. J.: Trace Elements in Human and Animal Nutrition, 4th ed. Academic Press, New York, 1977, pp. 56–108, 196–242, and 302–346.

186. Unsigned: Adaptation in protein calorie malnutrition (PCM). Nutrition Rev. 37:250–252, 1979.

187. Val-Mejias, J., Lee, W. K., Weisse, A. B., and Regan, T. J.: Left ventricular performance during and after sickle cell crisis. Am. Heart J. 97:585–591, 1979.

188. Van Itallie, T. B.: Obesity: Adverse effects on health and longevity. Am. J. Clin. Nutr. 32:2723–2733, 1979.

189. Van Oort, A. M., Sengers, R. C. A., Stadhouders, A. M., and ter Haar, B. G. A.: Idiopathic arterial calcification of infancy. Helv. Paediatr. Acta 34:369–374, 1979.

190. Varat, M. A., Adolph, R. J., and Fowler, N. O.: Cardiovascular effects of anemia. Am. Heart J. 83:415–426, 1972.

191. Wagner, P. I.: Beriberi heart disease. Am. Heart J. 69:200–205, 1965.

192. Wakabayashi, A., Yui, Y., and Kawai, C.: A clinical study on thiamine deficiency. Jap. Circ. J. 43:995–999, 1979.

193. Waldstein, S. S.: Medical complications of thyroid surgery. Otolaryngol. Clin. North Am. 13:99–107, 1980.

194. Warnock, L. G.: A new approach to erythrocyte transketolase measurement. J. Nutr. 100:1057–1062, 1970.

195. Waterlow, J. C., and Alleyne, G. A. O.: Protein malnutrition in children: Advances in knowledge in the last ten years. Adv. Protein Chem. 25: 117–241, 1971.

196. Way, G. L., Wolfe, R. R., Eshaghpour, E., Bender, R. L., Jaffe, R. B., and Ruttenberg, H. D.: The natural history of hypertrophic cardiomyopathy in infants of diabetic mothers. J. Pediatr. 95:1020–1025, 1979.

197. Weatherall, D. J.: The thalassemias. In The Metabolic Basis of Inherited Disease, 4th ed., edited by J. B. Stanbury, J. B. Wyngaarden, and D. S. Fredrickson. McGraw-Hill, New York, 1978, pp. 1508–1523.
198. Weisburst, M. R., Pearlman, E. S., and Capone, R. J.: Doxorubicin (Adriamycin) cardiotoxicity. Conn. Med. 44:133–136, 1980.
199. Winslow, R. M., and Anderson, W. F.: The hemoglobinopathies. In The Metabolic Basis of Inherited Disease, 4th ed., edited by J. B. Stanbury, J. B. Wyngaarden, and D. S. Fredrickson. McGraw-Hill, New York, 1979, pp. 1465–1508.
200. Wolverson, M., Director of Ultrasound, Associate Professor of Radiology, St. Louis University Medical Center: Personal Communication, 1981.
201. Yang, W. C. T., and Dubick, M.: Mechanism of emetine cardiotoxicity. Pharmacol. Ther. 10:15–26, 1980.

39

Cardiac Manifestations of Systemic Disease

James H. Moller, M.D., and Mary Ella Mascia Pierpont, Ph.D., M.D.

MUCOPOLYSACCHARIDOSES

The mucopolysaccharidoses are a diverse group of inherited metabolic disorders which derive their name and classification from the fact that excessive amounts of mucopolysaccharides are stored in various tissues and excreted in the urine. Variation in the type of mucopolysaccharides (glycosaminoglycans) excreted in the urine is present among the different types of mucopolysaccharidoses.

In 1917, Hunter[90] described two brothers with the familiar features of the disorder which now bears his name. Two years later, Hurler[91] described two patients with similar features. Hunter's description was overlooked for many years, but subsequently the differences between these two groups of patients have become apparent. In 1952, Brante[30] found mucopolysaccharides in the liver of patients with Hurler syndrome and thus began usage of the term "mucopolysaccharidosis." Later, Dorfman and Lorincz[52] demonstrated excessive excretion of mucopolysaccharides in the urine of affected patients, and this observation formed the basis for laboratory identification for many years.

During the 1960s, other mucopolysaccharidoses (those of Scheie, Sanfilippo, Morquio, and Maroteaux-Lamy) were described clinically. Van Hoof[191] found that the granules located within hepatic cells of patients with Hurler's syndrome were enlarged lysosomes, thus introducing the concept that the mucopolysaccharidoses are lysosomal storage diseases. Since then, primarily because of the work of Neufeld and coworkers,[135] our understanding of these diseases has changed, and a new classification has been developed (Table 39.1). Using cell culture techniques, several specific factors were identified, which corrected the metabolic abnormalities in the different disorders.[136] Thus, it was found that both Hurler's and Scheie's syndromes, although clinically dissimilar, were missing the same corrective factor, and that Sanfilippo's syndrome included at least three phenotypically similar disorders, identified by cross-correction studies in cell culture.

In the early 1970s specific lysosomal enzyme deficiencies were identified for each of the mucopolysaccharidoses.[121] These enzymatic characterizations (Table 39.1) have led to our present ability to diagnose mucopolysaccharidoses prenatally and also to identify the carrier or heterozygous state of most mucopolysaccharidoses.

In Table 39.1, the various types of mucopolysaccharidoses (MPS) are presented. MPS I exists in three forms, Hurler's (MPS IH), Scheie's (MPS IS) and the Hurler-Scheie syndrome (MPH IH/S), each form being deficient in the same enzyme. The Hurler-Scheie syndrome is believed to be a genetic compound of two allelic mutations.[169] Hunter's syndrome (MPS II) has two distinct clinical forms, each with a different enzyme deficiency. Morquio's syndrome (MPS IV) has at least two forms, each with a different enzyme deficiency and clinical course. Currently, no MPS V exists. Maroteaux-Lamy (MPS VI) has at least two clinical forms, each with the same enzymatic deficiency. Finally, β-glucuronidase deficiency (MPS VII) has a very wide clinical spectrum but the same enzymatic defect.

HURLER'S AND HUNTER'S SYNDROMES

Hurler's syndrome (MPS IH) results from deficiency of the enzyme α-L-iduronidase, while Hunter's syndrome, whether severe (MPS IIA) or mild (MPS IIB), results from sulfoiduronide sulfatase deficiency. Hurler's syndrome is inherited as an autosomal recessive trait, while Hunter's syndrome is inherited as X-linked recessive trait.

Hurler's and Hunter's syndromes share many physical characteristics, although the course and age of development of physical changes and the cardiovascular manifestations are different. Physical characteristics present in both syndromes include progressive coarsening of facial features, hepatosplenomegaly, joint stiffness, kyphosis, dysostosis multiplex, umbilical and inguinal hernias, small stature, enlarged head, and mental retardation. Corneal clouding and lumbar gibbus are present in patients with Hurler's but not Hunter's syndrome. In addition, the mild and severe forms of Hunter's syndrome vary in the severity of the mental retardation. Patients with the mild Hunter form survive until the 3rd decade. Death occurs for Hurler's syndrome and the severe form of Hunter's syndrome (IIa).

Pathology

Because mucopolysaccharides are a major component of connective tissue, their accumulation in the mucopolysaccharidoses is widespread, involving many organs. The material is stored both intra- and intercellularly, the former mainly in lysosomes.[191] The involved cells have large clear vacuoles and have been called "gargoyle cells." Microscopic changes are noted in the connective tissue of each layer of the heart. Collageneous tissue is increased and shows hyaline or mucoid changes.

The most striking changes in the heart occur in the valves and coronary arteries. The mitral valve is most frequently affected (Fig. 39.1), followed by the aortic and tricuspid with

TABLE 39.1 CHARACTERISTICS OF THE MUCOPOLYSACCHARIDOSES

Type	Name	Genetics	Excessive Urinary MPS	Deficient Substance	Cardiovascular	Corneal Clouding	Mental Retardation	Skeletal Changes	Hepatosplenomegaly	Coarse Facies
MPS IH	Hurler syndrome	Autosomal recessive	Dermatan sulfate + heparan sulfate (3:1)	α-L-iduronidase	Systemic hypertension, valve involvement, arterial disease	+	++	Severe	+	+
MPS IS	Scheie syndrome	Autosomal recessive	Dermatan sulfate + heparan sulfate	α-L-iduronidase	Aortic insufficiency	+	−	Mild	−	−
MPS IH/S	Hurler-Scheie compound	Autosomal recessive	Dermatan sulfate + heparan sulfate	α-L-iduronidase	Mitral stenosis	+	+	Severe	+	+
MPS IIA	Hunter syndrome, severe	X-linked recessive	Dermatan sulfate + heparan sulfate (1:1)	Sulfoiduronide sulfatase	Hypertension, valve involvement, arterial disease	−	+	Moderate	+	+
MPS IIB	Hunter syndrome, mild	X-linked recessive	Dermatan sulfate + heparan sulfate	Sulfoiduronide sulfatase	Valve involvement, arterial disease	−	+	Moderate	+	+
MPS IIIA	Sanfilippo syndrome A	Autosomal recessive	Heparan sulfate	Heparan sulfate sulfaminohydrolase	None described	−	++	Mild	+	Mild
MPS IIIB	Sanfilippo syndrome B	Autosomal recessive	Heparan sulfate	N-acetyl-α-D-glucosaminidase	Mitral insufficiency	−	++	Mild	+	Mild
MPS IIIC	Sanfilippo syndrome C	Autosomal recessive	Heparan sulfate	Acetyl CoA:α-glucosaminide N-acetyltransferase	None described	−	++	Mild	+	Mild
MPS IVA	Morquio syndrome, severe	Autosomal recessive	Keratan sulfate	Galactosamine-6-sulfate sulfatase	Aortic insufficiency	+	+	Severe	−	−
MPS IVB	Morquio syndrome, mild	Autosomal recessive	Keratan sulfate	β-galactosidase	None described	+	+	Moderate	−	−
MPS VIA	Maroteaux-Lamy syndrome, classic	Autosomal recessive	Dermatan sulfate	4-sulfo-N-acetylgalactosaminide sulfatase (arylsulfatase B)	Aortic valve disease	+	−	Severe	+	+
MPS VIB	Maroteaux-Lamy syndrome, mild	Autosomal recessive	Dermatan sulfate	Arylsulfatase B	Aortic stenosis	+	−	Moderate	+	+
MPS VII	β-Glucuronidase deficiency (Sly Disease)	Autosomal recessive	Dermatan sulfate + heparan sulfate	β-glucuronidase	Aortic fibromuscular dysplasia, aortic insufficiency	−	+	Moderate	+	±

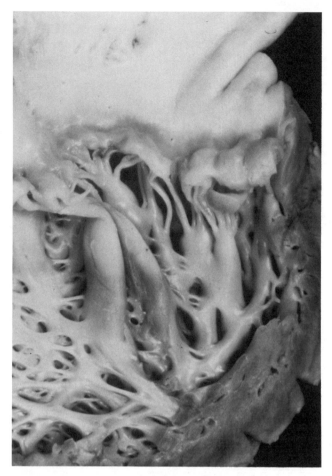

Fig. 39.1 Hurler syndrome in 2-year-old male. Left atrium (*above*) and left ventricle (*below*). Thickening and hooding of mitral valvular leaflets. Thickening of chordae tendineae and endocardium.

nearly equal frequency and the pulmonary valve in a small number of patients.[107] Changes in the mitral valve range from nodular thickening along the free edge of the valve to severe thickening of the entire leaflets with marked thickening and shortening of the chordae tendineae. This causes mitral insufficiency and/or mitral stenosis. The tricuspid valve may show similar changes, but they are not as severe and rarely lead to major hemodynamic alterations. The aortic valve and, less frequently, the pulmonary valve have thickened, rolled, and retracted edges. The valve thickening is due to mucopolysaccharide deposition, excess collagen fibers, and fibroblastic proliferation in the connective tissue.[138]

The endocardium, especially of the left atrium and the left ventricle, may be thickened by accumulated mucopolysaccharides and may show endocardial fibroelastosis or "jet lesions" from turbulent flow through valves. Gross myocardial changes are uncommon, although microscopically the fibers are hypertrophic.[119] The entire heart is usually hypertrophied, the changes most prominent in the left ventricle. Thickening of the pericardium has also been described.

The coronary arteries are often abnormal. For Hurler's syndrome, diffuse and severe coronary arterial narrowing[31] occurs from mucopolysaccharide accumulation, fibrous tissue, and "gargoyle cells." Unlike atherosclerotic heart disease, the coronary arterial narrowing is circumferential. De-

spite these changes, clinical or electrocardiographic evidence of myocardial ischemia is rare. Other arteries, including the aorta and the pulmonary artery, are involved, with the aorta revealing intimal plaques, presumably composed of mucopolysaccharide. Although arterial involvement has been reported in only one-fourth of the patients at postmortem examination,[107] thorough and extensive autopsies should reveal involvement in most patients.

The conduction system of the heart also is abnormal. There is a marked increase in fibrous tissue and collagen fibers infiltrating and surrounding the conduction bundles.[138] In addition, surrounding cells demonstrate the "gargoyle cell" appearance.

Clinical Features

Cardiac involvement occurs in at least 80% of patients, but only one-half show clinical evidence of cardiovascular problems. A cardiac murmur is the most frequent manifestation and is usually heard best at the apex or along the lower left sternal border. The murmur, often representing mitral insufficiency, is high-pitched and radiates to the left axilla. Krovetz and co-workers[107] believe the murmur is usually a vibratory innocent murmur and that organic murmurs are uncommon. Although the murmurs are usually soft, we have heard them at grade 4/6 intensity. Occasionally, a high-pitched early diastolic murmur of aortic insufficiency may be present.

Cardiomegaly may be found without evidence of organic murmur. Systemic hypertension was present in 9 of 15 patients studied by Krovetz and co-workers,[106] and the aortic systolic pressure in one patient was 260 mmHg. These authors also commented on the exaggerated respiratory variation in blood pressure from increased respiratory effort secondary to upper airway obstruction and thoracic cage abnormalities.

If cardiac failure occurs, tachycardia, tachypnea, and moist rales develop. Since hepatosplenomegaly secondary to mucopolysaccharide accumulation is a regular component of Hunter and Hurler syndromes, this valuable indicator of cardiac failure may be difficult to interpret.

Electrocardiographic Features

Electrocardiographic findings vary and range from normal to patterns of right, left, or combined ventricular hypertrophy and atrial enlargement. A pattern of left atrial enlargement and left ventricular hypertrophy usually occurs in patients with mitral insufficiency.

Krovetz and co-workers[107] indicated that the QT interval is prolonged in most patients and an abnormally wide QRST angle is present in one-half.

Radiologic Features

Thoracic roentgenograms reveal the typical skeletal anomalies of broad ribs and anterior beaking of vertebrae. The cardiac silhouette may be normal or may show mild or moderate cardiomegaly. If present, cardiac enlargement is usually generalized, regardless of the type of valvular anomaly, but left atrial enlargement may be more obvious in patients with mitral insufficiency. The pulmonary trunk may be prominent. Pulmonary vascular markings are usually normal, except in the presence of cardiac failure.

Echocardiographic Features

M-mode echocardiograms in patients with Hurler's and Hunter's syndromes have revealed thickening of both the anterior and posterior mitral leaflets and the presence of multiple mitral leaflet echoes.[98] In one patient, a dense band of abnormal echoes obscuring the posterior mitral leaflet ended abruptly in the left atrium and had motion resembling left ventricular endocardium. These characteristics are highly suggestive of mitral annular calcification.[98] Perhaps infiltration of the mitral annulus by mucopolysaccharide is responsible for this pattern, since no calcification was seen on x-ray or fluoroscopy of the patient.

Cardiac Catheterization

The most extensive study of the hemodynamics of these syndromes was reported by Krovetz and co-workers.[106] Among 15 patients, they found a normal cardiac index in 11, a slightly elevated value in 3 others, and a low value in the remaining patient. Systemic and pulmonary arteriolar resistances were increased. Systemic arterial pressures were elevated in nine and normal in six. Right ventricular systolic pressures were usually elevated but not over 42 mm Hg. Right ventricular end-diastolic pressure was elevated in four and left ventricular end-diastolic pressure in five. An unusual notch in the ascending portion of the right ventricular pressure curve was present.

Angiography showed the associated valvular insufficiency and chamber enlargement. The coronary arterial system, visualized angiographically in six patients, appeared normal.[106]

Treatment and Course

Perhaps half the patients die from cardiac disease, either from cardiac failure or suddenly. Cardiac failure results from myocardial involvement, valvular insufficiency, and the myocardial effects of systemic hypertension. Supportive measures directed at respiratory infections and cardiac failure remain the major components of treatment. The prognosis is poor for patients with Hurler's and the severe form of Hunter's syndrome. Early death is the usual outcome.

Currently, no specific treatment has been successful. It was hoped that corrective factors[135] might provide potential for enzymatic replacement by plasma infusions.[50] Long-term benefit has not been derived.

SCHEIE'S AND HURLER-SCHEIE SYNDROMES

Although Scheie's (MPS IS) and the Hurler-Scheie (MPS IH/S) syndromes have different clinical courses, like Hurler's syndrome, they lack alpha-L-iduronidase. Scheie and Hurler gene mutations are allelic, and the Hurler-Scheie syndrome most likely represents a genetic compound of the two abnormal alleles.

Scheie's syndrome is characterized by severe corneal clouding, stiff joints, characteristic claw hands, normal intelligence, and aortic stenosis (AS) and insufficiency (AI). The life-span is usually normal. Early death may result from cardiac complications, although, commonly, the aortic valve disease is mild. A single autopsy study of a patient with Scheie's syndrome revealed gargoyle cells in the endocardium, heart valves and blood vessels similar to those in Hurler's syndrome.[47]

The physical features of the Hurler-Scheie syndrome are intermediate in severity between Hurler's syndrome and Scheie's syndrome. Patients have short stature, severe dysostosis multiplex, corneal clouding, mental retardation, and valvular cardiac lesions. Survival is longer than in Hurler's syndrome, but less than in Scheie's syndrome. Abnormalities of the mitral valve are particularly prominent. Two asymptomatic patients with the Hurler-Scheie syndrome[169] showed auscultatory findings of mitral stenosis: an accentuated first heart sound, opening snap, and a rumbling presystolic murmur. Electrocardiograms showed prolonged PR interval, combined atrial enlargement, and left ventricular hypertrophy. Roentgenograms demonstrated annular calcification of the mitral valve and increased left atrial size. Echocardiographic studies revealed slow early diastolic closing of the mitral valve, multiple echoes from the anterior leaflet, and increased left atrial dimensions.[169]

At autopsy another Hurler-Scheie patient was found to have calcific mitral stenosis and mild calcification of the aortic valve.[187] This patient's affected sibling had cardiac catheterization evidence of moderate mitral stenosis and minimal mitral and aortic insufficiency.

SANFILIPPO'S SYNDROME

Sanfilippo's syndrome exists in three biochemically distinct forms (A, B, and C) each with a different enzyme deficiency (Table 39.1). These patients have severe and progressive mental retardation, mild-to-moderate hepatosplenomegaly, mild dysostosis multiplex, and no corneal clouding. The course is more progressive in type A than in Type B or C.[189]

One patient has been reported with cardiovascular involvement.[86] A 3-year-old child with Type B Sanfilippo's syndrome developed heart failure from severe mitral insufficiency (MI) which required valve replacement. Examination of the excised mitral valve leaflets showed thickened free edges and a cartilaginous consistency. The chordae tendineae were shortened and also had a cartilaginous consistency. Histochemically, the excised leaflets contained large amounts of mucopolysaccharide material.

MORQUIO'S SYNDROME

The Morquio syndrome is characterized by two forms each with a different clinical course and biochemical defect. The severe form of Morquio's syndrome (MPS IV A) results from deficiency of galactosamine-6-sulfate sulfatase. Patients have marked dwarfism, severe truncal shortening, corneal clouding, progressive deafness, normal intelligence, thoracic deformity, and cardiac involvement. Aortic insufficiency has been reported in a number of patients.[119] Autopsy reveals myocardial hypertrophy and thickening of mitral valve leaflets. Histological examination of the cardiac valve leaflets shows "gargoyle cells" and fibrous thickening. Although focal intimal sclerosis occurs in the aorta and coronary arteries, major narrowing is not present. Storage cells, collagenous fibers, and ground substance are responsible for the intimal sclerosis.[60]

Patients with the mild form of Morquio's syndrome (MPS IV B) have a deficiency of a β-galactosidase but have normal galactosamine-6-sulfate sulfatase. They have normal intelligence, mild anterior chest deformity, corneal clouding, and atlantoaxial subluxation. Cardiovascular involvement has not been reported.

MAROTEAUX-LAMY SYNDROME

Maroteaux-Lamy syndrome (MPS VI) results from lysosomal deficiency of arylsulfatase B. There may be three forms, a classic (severe) form, a mild form, and probably an intermediate form.[121] Manifestations include growth retardation, dysostosis multiplex, corneal clouding, coarse facies, hip dysplasia, and cardiac involvement. Patients with the severe form may survive into the 3rd decade. AS and AI are the most frequent cardiac lesions. Occasionally, MI is present.[121]

In an autopsied case, the tricuspid and mitral valves were thickened by large cells containing eosinophilic cytoplasmic granules.[182]

The milder form[148] is characterized by longer life-span, dysostosis multiplex with most serious involvement of hands and hips, corneal clouding and, occasionally, aortic valve disease. Calcific AS has been reported in three brothers[198] with this disease. One of these brothers underwent successful aortic valve replacement. Histological examination revealed marked aortic valve fibrosis and calcification. Cells similar to "Gargoyle cells" were described.

BETA-GLUCURONIDASE DEFICIENCY

There is a marked variation in phenotypic expression of beta-glucuronidase deficiency. Features include unusual facies, hernias, hepatosplenomegaly, corneal clouding, protruberant abdomen, and cardiac disease. Some patients have a cardiac murmur but no evidence of cardiac pathology. One patient had aortic dysplasia.[11] Aortic histology revealed the presence of intercellular and intracellular mucopolysaccharides. A recently identified patient had obstructive cardiomyopathy.[134]

MUCOLIPIDOSES

The mucolipidoses are a group of genetic disorders characterized by widespread storage of mucopolysaccharides, sphingolipids, and glycolipids. In most mucolipidoses, the clinical features of visceromegaly, coarse facies, and skeletal changes resemble the mucopolysaccharidoses. There is, however, no urinary excretion of glycosaminoglycans. Enzymatic deficiencies causing several of these disorders (mucolipidosis I, II, and III) have been described only recently. The metabolic defect for mucolipidosis IV has not been characterized, and cardiac manifestations have not been described. Table 39.2 summarizes major clinical features of the mucolipidoses, including mannosidosis and fucosidosis.

MUCOLIPIDOSIS I

Mucolipidosis I results from deficiency of alpha-N-acetylneuraminidase.[37] There is wide phenotypic variation among patients with this disorder, and some of the variation results from progressive changes with age.[102] In a young child, coarse facies resembling Hurler's syndrome, hepatosplenomegaly, growth retardation, and psychomotor retardation are present. In the older child, cherry-red maculae, degenerative central nervous system disorder, coarse facies, dysostosis multiplex, and corneal clouding are found.

Three cases of mucolipidosis I have been reported with cardiomegaly.[102] Of two with echocardiograms, one had abnormal mitral valve motion suggestive of "myxomatous degeneration." In the second, a 2-year-old infant, echocardio-

graphic evidence of pericardial effusion and thickening of the left ventricular posterior wall was present.

MUCOLIPIDOSIS II

Mucolipidosis II (I-cell disease) is an autosomal recessive disorder characterized by somatic features similar to Hurler's syndrome, that are present at birth. These patients have lysosomal deficiency of a number of hydrolases responsible for metabolism of lipids and mucopolysaccharides. Increased levels of these hydrolases are found in the serum. Recently, the biochemical defect has been identified as deficiency of an enzyme (UDP-N-acetylglucosamine-glycoprotein to N-acetylglucosaminylphosphotransferase ratio) which is responsible for phosphorylation of mannose residues on the hydrolases. This phosphorylation of mannose residues allows binding of hydrolases to membrane receptors for transport into lysosomes.[158]

Major clinical features include coarse facies, severe dysostosis multiplex, hepatomegaly, mental retardation, and joint contractures. Cardiomegaly and cardiac murmurs may be present. The myocardium is infiltrated with storage material, and the valve leaflets and chordae tendineae, especially of the mitral valve, are thickened.[115]

MUCOLIPIDOSIS III

Mucolipidosis III (pseudo-Hurler polydystrophy) has a number of clinical findings similar to Hurler's syndrome, but lacks urinary excretion of mucopolysaccharides and shows a slower progression of skeletal deformities. Major characteristics include stiff joints, claw hand deformity, short stature, hip dysplasia, corneal clouding, and moderate mental retardation.[101]

Biochemically, mucolipidosis III resembles mucolipidosis II. Both conditions have elevated levels of serum hydrolases, lysosomal deficiency of the same hydrolases, and deficiency of the same enzyme required for hydrolase transport into lysosomes.[158]

Although many patients with ML-III have cardiac murmurs or cardiomegaly, cardiovascular disease has not been a serious clinical problem. Mild-to-moderate AI has been the most commonly diagnosed cardiac anomaly in ML-III, but autopsy conformation is unavailable.[121]

MANNOSIDOSIS

Mannosidosis is an autosomal recessive disorder with many clinical similarities to Hurler's syndrome, but mucopolysaccharides are not present in the urine. Instead, the urine contains many mannose-rich oligosaccharides, and mannose-containing compounds are stored in body tissues.

TABLE 39.2   CHARACTERISTICS OF THE MUCOLIPIDOSES

Disease	Enzymatic Defect	Skeletal Changes	Coarse Facies	Hepatosplenomegaly	Mental Retardation	Cardiac Disease	Corneal Clouding
Mucolipidosis I (sialidosis I)	α-N-acetylneuraminidase	Mild	+	+	+	+	±
Mucolipidosis II (I-cell disease)	a	Severe	+	+	++	+	Mild
Mucolipidosis III (pseudo Hurler's polydystrophy)	a	Moderate	±	−	+	+	+
Mucolipidosis IV	Unknown	−	−	−	+	−	+
Mannosidosis	α-mannosidase	+	+	+	+	+	−
Fucosidosis	α-L-fucosidase	+	+	+	+	+	−

a UDP-N-acetylglucosamine:glycoprotein N-acetylglucosaminylphosphotransferase.

The biochemical abnormality results from lysosomal deficiency of the enzyme alpha-mannosidase.

Clinical features include coarsening of facial features, severe deafness, hepatosplenomegaly, mental retardation, and dysostosis multiplex. Autopsy studies of a 3-year-old child revealed accumulation of mannose-containing compounds in cells of the myocardium, endocardium, conduction system, and cardiac valves.[48] Generally, however, cardiac symptoms are minimal. Electrocardiograms may reveal shortened PR intervals.[124] Recently, we have seen a pattern of Wolff-Parkinson-White on the electrocardiogram of a 26-year-old man with mannosidosis.

FUCOSIDOSIS

Fucosidosis is a storage disorder inherited as an autosomal recessive trait with several forms, infantile, juvenile, and adult.[180] In this disorder, the enzyme alpha-L-fucosidase is deficient in lysosomes. Consequently, pathologic examination of the liver of patients with the infantile form has revealed characteristic cytoplasmic inclusions of carbohydrate and lipid material.

Clinical findings include psychomotor retardation, muscular hypotonia, coarse facial features, dysostosis multiplex, progressive neurological deterioration, and recurrent infections. Cardiomegaly, cardiac rhythm disturbances, and electrocardiographic changes have been reported in patients with fucosidosis.[53] Pathological examination has revealed myocardial fiber infiltration by fucose-containing compounds.[53, 54]

SPHINGOLIPIDOSES

The sphingolipidoses are a diverse group of metabolic disorders with abnormal metabolism of sphingolipids. Sphingolipids have a common ceramide core composed of sphingosine (a long chain aminoalcohol) bonded to a long chain fatty acid. Different sphingolipids result from different chemical groups (e.g., galactose) bonded to the hydroxyl group of the sphingosine.

Each of the sphingolipidoses is due to lysosomal deficiency of a distinct enzyme, generally involved in cleavage of different polar groups from the hydroxyl group of sphingosine. The sphingolipidoses include: Farber's disease, Niemann-Pick disease, Krabbe's disease, metachromatic leukodystrophy, Fabry's disease, G_{M1} gangliosidosis, Tay-Sachs disease, and Sandhoff's disease. Except for Fabry's disease, which is X-linked, these conditions have autosomal recessive inheritance. Cardiovascular manifestations have been described in Niemann-Pick, Gaucher's, Fabry's, G_{M1} gangliosidosis, Tay-Sachs, and Sandhoff's diseases.

NIEMANN-PICK DISEASE

Niemann-Pick disease, resulting from lysosomal deficiency of sphingomyelinase, is characterized by accumulation of sphingomyelin in various body tissues, especially liver, spleen, bone marrow, lungs, and central nervous system. Pathological examination has revealed foam cells in many tissues, including the heart. Endocardial fibroelastosis has occurred in at least one patient.[197]

GAUCHER'S DISEASE

Gaucher's disease, the most common sphingolipidosis, results from a deficiency of glucocerebrosidase. Glucocerebrosides accumulate, particularly in cells of reticuloendothelial origin. Characteristic "Gaucher" cells are usually present in bone marrow preparations.

Patients with Gaucher's disease are classified according to clinical course, and physical findings are classified as acute neuropathic (infantile), subacute neuropathic (juvenile), and nonneuropathic (adult). In each type, spleen, liver, and bone marrow contain cells full of glucocerebroside. Most patients have leukopenia, anemia, and bleeding disorders. In the neuropathic forms, glucocerebroside accumulation and neuronal abnormalities contribute to progressive neurological deterioration.

Cardiac involvement in Gaucher's disease occurs as pericardial disease. Constrictive pericarditis and pericardial thickening have been reported.[14, 83] Pulmonary capillaries and pulmonary lymphatics may be filled with glucocerebrosides and may result in pulmonary hypertension.[159]

FABRY'S DISEASE

Fabry's disease is a disorder of glycosphingolipid metabolism caused by deficiency of the enzyme beta-galactosidase A. The disease, inherited in an X-linked fashion, may be expressed in hemiazygous males and heterozygous females (this by selective X-chromosomal inactivation).

The disease is characterized by manifestations of small vessel pathology, including angiokeratomas (typically found between the umbilicus and knees), episodic acroparesthesias, hypohidrosis, and renal failure. Systemic hypertension, cardiac ischemia, and cerebrovascular accidents are commonly associated.

Pathological studies have revealed accumulation of the glycosphingolipid ceramide trihexose in lysosomes of many tissues, including the heart.[12, 61] This material is present in excess in all cardiac tissues, with the greatest concentration present in the mitral valve and left ventricular myocardium.[49] The conduction system is also involved.[12] Glycosphingolipid has also been detected in endothelial, perithelial, and smooth muscle of the vascular system. Progressive accumulation in the vascular system is responsible for many clinical manifestations of Fabry's disease.

Cardiac involvement advances with age. The mitral and aortic valves develop thickening and nodularity. Interchordal hooding of the mitral valve and clinical MI have been described.[12, 20, 49] Coronary arterial involvement and myocardial infarction are commonly present in older patients.

Manifestations of cardiac disease in Fabry patients include anginal chest pain, cardiomegaly, and heart failure. Murmurs of MI or AS may be heard. A short PR interval often is detected on electrocardiograms. Patterns of myocardial infarction, ventricular hypertrophy, or dysrhythmias may also be found.[123]

M-mode echocardiograms reveal that the aortic root dimension increases with age in hemizygous males. There is also thickening of the left ventricular posterior wall.[9] In addition, pansystolic mitral valve prolapse was seen in only one hemizygous male. The lack of abnormal valvular echoes with the M-mode echocardiogram was conspicuous.

G_{M1} GANGLIOSIDOSIS

G_{M1} gangliosidosis is caused by lysosomal deficiency of the enzyme beta-galactosidase and results in accumulation of G_{M1} gangliosides (sphingolipids with at least one sialic acid residue). Several types of G_{M1} gangliosidosis have been described, with classification based on clinical presentation and course. Evidence for cardiovascular involvements has been reported for the infantile generalized form (Type I). Clinical features include coarse facial features, hepatosplenomegaly, cardiomegaly, severe dysostosis multiplex, and progressive mental deterioration. Usually, patients do not survive beyond the 3rd year of life.

Pathological examination has revealed the presence of foamy histiocytes in the myocardium, aortic, and mitral valve leaflets.[109] The hysticocytes are laden with lipid material (gangliosides). The coronary arteries are occluded and narrowed by atheromatous-like material and cells with foamy cytoplasm.[82]

TAY-SACHS DISEASE

The infantile form of G_{M2} gangliosidosis Type 1 (Tay-Sachs disease) is more common than Type II. The disorder, due to deficiency of hexosaminidase A, results in cellular accumulation of gangliosides, particularly in nervous system tissues. Pathological and biochemical studies have revealed chromatographic evidence of a marked increase in gangliosides in cardiac tissues.[160]

Clinical features include cherry red spots in the macula, doll-like facies, progressive neurologic deterioration, and early death. The electrocardiogram can show a prolonged QT interval, abnormal configuration of T waves, and prominent sinus dysrhythmias.[160]

SANDHOFF'S DISEASE

This type of G_{M2} gangliosidosis is caused by deficiency of both hexosaminidase A and B, resulting in accumulation of G_{M2} gangliosides and globosides in many tissues. Clinical findings are similar to those for Tay-Sachs, with early onset of motor deterioration, blindness, cherry red maculae, and

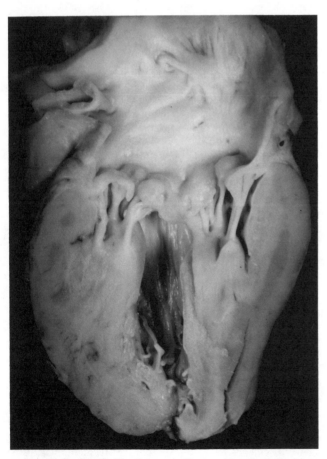

Fig. 39.2 Sandhoff's disease in 2-year-old male. Left atrium (*above*) and left ventricle (*below*). Left ventricular hypertrophy. Thickened and hooded mitral valve. Left atrium shows thickened endocardium. (Reproduced with permission from L. C. Blieden *et al.*[19])

early death. Cardiac involvement is manifested clinically as a cardiomyopathy.[19] G_{M2} gangliosides and globosides can be detected in all cardiac tissues. Thickening of the mitral valve leaflets and chordae tendineae occur (Fig. 39.2). Electron microscopy of mitral valvular tissue and other cardiac tissue reveals laminated lipid material in cytoplasmic organelles. The coronary arteries possess many areas of narrowing of the lumen by intimal proliferation of fibroblasts suspended in foamy fibrocollagenous background.[19, 20]

FRIEDREICH'S ATAXIA

In 1863, Friedreich[65] described six patients manifesting a neurological syndrome with hereditary features. This rare syndrome was subsequently given his name and occurs in approximately 1 in 40,000 births, with sex frequency being equal and parents frequently showing consanguinity. The inheritance pattern is autosomal recessive. The basic neurological disturbance is progressive demyelinization of the spinocerebellar tracts, corticospinal tracts, and posterior columns of the spinal cord. The disease generally becomes manifest in the early childhood years as a gait clumsiness, with the onset insidious. Later findings include gross ataxia, speech disturbances, tremors, nystagmus, pes cavus, and scoliosis, with a characteristic loss of deep tendon reflexes. The disease progresses gradually, with death usually occurring in the early adult years. For unknown reasons, diabetes mellitus develops in almost 10% of cases, more commonly in females, and appears in childhood or early adult life a few years after the onset of neurological dysfunction.[87, 151, 188] Other metabolic abnormalities such as mild hyperbilirubinemia, low serum pyruvate, elevated serum alanine, and elevated urinary alanine and taurine have been reported in some patients, but the significance is unknown.[18]

Five of Friedreich's patients had cardiac abnormalities, but the latter were not considered to be an integral part of the disease. Some years later, Pitt[150] described the clinical and pathologic features of a young adult with Friedreich's ataxia dying in cardiac failure and commented that "... on looking through the records it is astonishing to see how often cardiac failure has been noticed." Since then, cardiac involvement has been regularly emphasized in clinical reports.

Pathology

Typically, there is cardiac hypertrophy of each chamber, especially the left ventricle, and variable atheromatous involvement of the coronary arteries but normal endocardium and valves.[170] Thickening of the left atrial endocardium and mural thrombi (Fig. 39.3) may also occur.[93] Common microscopic findings include: diffuse interstitial fibrosis with compensatory hypertrophy of remaining muscle fibers; large vacuolated hyperchromatic muscle fiber nuclei; separation of Purkinje fibers of node and conducting tissue by a sparse cellular infiltration; and deposition of lipochrome pigment. Muscle fibers appear destroyed by focal coagulation necrosis.[170] Similar findings have subsequently been reported by others[93, 188] including Hewer,[88] who noted hypertrophy of muscle fibers in all 27 cases that he studied. Although the pericardium is usually described as normal, some thickening may occur. Pathological features of idiopathic hypertrophic subaortic stenosis have been reported in Friedreich's ataxia.[67, 179]

No specific metabolic defect has been identified to explain the myocardial changes. One theory suggests that they are secondary to the central nervous system disease and mediated by the sympathetic nervous system. Alternatively, a biochemical defect may independently affect the two organ systems.[29, 188] The suggestion that coronary artery disease

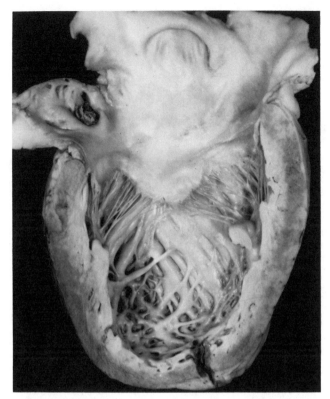

Fig. 39.3 Friedreich's ataxia in a 35-year-old male. Left atrium (*above*) and left ventricle (*below*). Dilated hypertrophied left ventricle. Thrombus in left atrial appendage. Thin, elongate chordae tendineae.

may be responsible for the myocardial changes[130] is supported by James,[96] who attributes the cardiomegaly and death to obliteration of the small coronary arteries. On the other hand, Hewer[88] concludes that the narrowing of arteries is probably a secondary response to cardiac muscle atrophy.

Clinical Features

There are no specific cardiac symptoms. Moreover, because the neurologic disease tends to incapacitate the patient, demands on the heart may progressively decrease, and cardiac disability may not be recognized until a dysrhythmia or heart failure develops.[188] Thoren[188] noted no correlation between the degree of neurologic dysfunction and the degree of cardiac disease, although others have reported parallel development. Exertional dyspnea is the most common complaint, with chest pain noted occasionally. None of 36 patients subject to stress tests by Thoren developed chest pain. Acute rapidly progressive cardiomyopathy has occurred in childhood.[15]

Systolic murmurs occur, but the frequency has varied greatly.[29, 59, 130, 170] Thoren reported systolic murmurs in 16 of 56 patients. Six additonal patients lost previously known murmurs. Murmurs are described as of blowing quality, usually of grade 2 to 3/6 intensity, maximum in midsystole, located in the second left interspace, and are attributed to increased pulmonary blood flow from tachycardia. In some patients, the murmur is related to muscular subaortic stenosis, and its intensity increases following inhalation of amyl nitrate.[190] A loud fourth heart sound may be present, reflecting decreased left ventricular compliance.

Electrocardiographic Features

Abnormalities are very common, particularly T wave changes.[29, 59, 130, 170, 188] Evans and Wright[59] reported the tend-

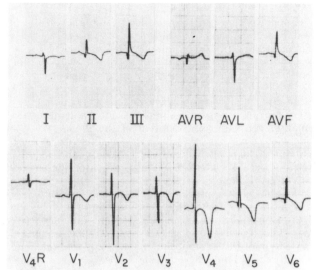

Fig. 39.4 Friedreich's ataxia in a 12-year-old male. Electrocardiogram with QRS axis of +105. Deeply inverted T waves in leads V_4 to V_6, II, III, and AVF.

ency for patients within families to show similar tracings. The diagnostic electrocardiograms may be found in patients not yet showing typical neurologic findings. Of 38 patients,[59] 22 had electrocardiographic abnormalities, although none had murmurs or cardiomegaly. The T wave abnormalities (Fig. 39.4), particularly inversion in the left precordial leads,[29, 59, 170] were observed by Thoren[188] in 92% of his cases. An interesting feature is the tendency for T wave inversion to revert toward normal with time, or briefly after exercise. Ganglionic block produced reversion of T wave abnormalities in 6 of 16 cases, and has been interpreted as evidence of sympathetic nervous system influence. The T wave changes may also be due to hypoxia of cardiac muscle.

Other electrocardiographic abnormalities include sinus tachycardia, supraventricular premature beats, unifocal ventricular premature beats, multifocal premature beats, atrial fibrillation or flutter, left ventricular hypertrophy, right ventricular hypertrophy, right axis deviation, deep Q waves, low voltage QRS complexes, and P wave abnormalities but no ST segment changes or atrioventricular conduction disturbances. Left ventricular hypertrophy tends to occur in younger individuals, and right ventricular hypertrophy tends to occur in older individuals. Electrocardiographic interpretation may be complicated by scoliosis, particularly in older patients.[170, 188]

Vectocardiography may be a more sensitive means of identifying the diffuse and focal myocardial lesions, since grossly irregular QRS loops can be found in patients with normal electrocardiograms.[78] These changes parallel the neurological alterations and tend to be very similar within sibships, just as electrocardiographic findings tend to be similar in siblings.[59, 188]

Radiologic Features

Cardiomegaly may be present[29, 170] but is nonspecific and may regress with time.

Echocardiographic Features

The echocardiogram may be normal, but evidence of cardiomyopathy is found in a third of patients.[177, 190] The interventricular septum is thickened, and the posterior wall may be as well, but the ratio of the septum to posterior wall often exceeds the normal (1.3:1). Systolic anterior motion of the mitral valve may also be present.

Cardiac Catheterization

Thoren[188] found a decreased blood volume especially in disabled patients, and he attributed this to patient inactivity and muscular atrophy. Cardiac catheterization was performed on 17 of his patients with abnormal electrocardiograms, but all had normal rhythm and no signs of cardiac failure. Findings included increased pressure in the right atrium, right ventricle (initial and end-diastolic), pulmonary artery, and pulmonary artery wedge position, and these were found to correlate with duration of the disease. It was concluded that there was decreased compliance of both ventricles. The stroke volume was frequently low.

Soulie and associates[179] found elevated mean pressure in both atria and increased filling pressure in both ventricles in the absence of peripheral signs of cardiac failure. In two of their seven cases, the studies were limited to the right side of the heart. Angiocardiography in two of Thoren's cases showed decreased emptying of the right ventricle, abnormal contraction of the infundibulum of the right ventricle, and hypertrophied, rigid left ventricular walls.

Recent studies show evidence of both right and left ventricular outflow obstruction, which can be provoked or increased with catecholamine infusion or by production of extrasystole.[67, 164, 190] Angiograms show characteristic features of obstructive cardiomyopathy, including small slit-like left ventricular cavity at the end of systole, greatly thickened interventricular septum, and, on lateral view, sharp angulation between the outflow area and apex.

Differential Diagnosis

Patients with Friedreich's ataxia may be erroneously diagnosed as having rheumatic fever, with the ataxia misinterpreted as chorea. Early manifestations may include leg pain,[29] which may also be misinterpreted as rheumatic. Authors point out that a number of their own cases were initially misdiagnosed.[29, 130, 137, 186, 188] If a careful neurological examination is done in all patients with atypical, bizarre, or idiopathic cardiac disease, few cases of Friedreich's ataxia will be missed. The most important clinical step is to check for decreased or absent knee and ankle reflexes.

Heredopathia atactica polyneuritiformis (Refsum's disease), an extremely rare autosomal recessive disease involving retinitis pigmentosa, polyneuropathy with progressive limb paresis, and cerebellar ataxia, often has conduction abnormalities in the electrocardiogram.[111] Cardiac involvement usually does not occur in the other primary neurological diseases of childhood.

Treatment and Course

No specific treatment is available, either for the primary disease or the cardiac involvement. However, dysrhythmias and cardiac failure generally respond to digitalis and other drugs. Occasionally, in a patient with obstructive cardiomyopathy, digitalis may be contraindicated, and propranolol is preferred. The overall clinical picture is that of progressive disability, but death is uncommon in the childhood years.

Symptoms of cardiac disability are also uncommon; they are attributed to the obscuring nature of the progressive neurological disease, which results in decreasing demands on the heart.[29] The primary early cardiac threat is that of dysrhythmia.[29] Pericardial effusion may rarely be seen.[130] Probable myocardial infarction has been reported in a child.[105] A number of patients die in cardiac failure.[29] Of Thoren's 56 patients, 11 died at an average age of 28 years. The causes of death were pulmonary embolism, cerebral embolism, cardiac failure, pulmonary edema, paroxysmal tachycardia, and sarcoma.

MUSCULAR DYSTROPHIES

The term muscular dystrophy has been used to describe several diseases causing degeneration and atrophy of skeletal muscle following genetically determined patterns. In each of these diseases, cardiac involvement may be present. Such involvement was first described by Rinecker in 1859 and confirmed in 1923 by Globus in his review.[73]

Despite biochemical, histological, and other studies, the pathogenesis of the muscular dystrophies remains unknown. Some studies suggest that muscular dystrophies may have systemic membrane defects: increased endogenous erythrocyte membrane phosphorylation in patients with Duchenne muscular dystrophy[161] and abnormalities of lymphocyte capping in a variety of forms of muscular dystrophy. Electron micrographs of erythrocytes have shown membrane surface alterations.[147] At present, however, classification is still based on clinical features, course, distribution of muscular involvement, and genetic patterns.[145, 199] Despite definition of several clinical entities, some patients cannot be classified.

We have attempted to review several categories of muscular dystrophy and their cardiac findings, realizing that our classification is not identical to that of other authors. Cardiac involvement occurs in each type of muscular dystrophy. Of these, the Duchenne type has been the most extensively studied.

DUCHENNE'S PROGRESSIVE MUSCULAR DYSTROPHY

The condition is sex-linked recessive disease in which the initial symptoms develop in the first 5 years of life. The pelvic muscles are involved first leading to lordosis, waddling gait, protuberant abdomen, and difficulty in rising. Pseudohypertrophy of calf muscles develops. Subsequently, the shoulder girdle is involved and then trunk muscles, leading to scoliosis, respiratory insufficiency and pneumonia, immobilization, and death by the 3rd decade of life.

The metabolic abnormality causing this disease is unknown. Studies have shown an elevated serum creatine phosphokinase level in patients with this disorder, even in the neonatal period. Female carriers may show elevated levels, although this is not a uniform finding. Prenatal diagnosis has been made by measurement of greatly elevated creatine phosphokinase activity in fetal blood obtained by placental aspiration,[57, 113] although low fetal levels do not guarantee freedom from the disease. Other enzymes, such as aldolase and various lactic dehydrogenase (LDH) isoenzymes, are elevated in the disease and may even be useful in carrier confirmation.[163] Decreased lymphocyte capping has been demonstrated for affected individuals and female carriers[147] and carriers may also show changes in erythrocyte membrane phosphorylation.[162]

Pathology

In each form of muscular dystrophy, similar microscopic changes in skeletal muscles are found.[143] These include: variation in cross-sectional diameter of muscle fibers, with hypertrophied muscle fibers being adjacent to fibrous areas; interstitial infiltration by mature fatty tissue; increase in interstitial fibrous connective tissue; degenerative changes in the muscle fibers; sarcolemmal nuclear changes; and basophilic staining of single or small clusters of fibers. Severity of cardiac lesions does not correlate with duration or severity of skeletal muscle disease.

Cardiac muscle in Duchenne's dystrophy has similar microscopic changes, though usually less severe. One author found minimal fatty infiltration.[70] Lymphocyte infiltration may be present. Microscopic changes in the atria, ventricles, and the papillary muscles are focal and spotty, with many areas of myocardium appearing normal. The most severe changes are found in the posterobasal part of the left ventricle and the posterior papillary muscle of the mitral valve.[166] The heart may be either of normal size or enlarged. Cardiac hypertrophy and dilatation involving principally the left ventricle can occur. The coronary arteries, cardiac valves, and pericardium are normal. Rarely, the left ventricular endocardium shows fibroelastosis.

James[95] has described degenerative changes in the fibers of the sinus node and unusual noninflammatory degeneration of arteries supplying the sinoatrial and atrioventricular nodes. Less severe but similar changes in other small arteries supplying the myocardium, lungs, and large intestine may be present. Ultrastructural studies show a loss of both thick and thin myofilaments, and alterations of mitochondria and sarcoplasmic reticulum but preservation of nuclear morphology and the transverse tubular system. Again, these changes are most striking in the posterobasal part of the left ventricle.

Clinical Features

Signs or symptoms of cardiovascular disease generally are not evident until long after the appearance of skeletal muscle disease. Despite the frequency of myocardial involvement, usually, little or no evidence of cardiac disease is found clinically.[70] Symptoms of exertional fatigue, dyspnea, and tachycardia may be present, but these often are related to skeletal muscle weakness. Cardiac arrest has occurred during induction of general anesthesia and may be a presenting feature of this disease.[171]

On physical examination, the heart sounds may be of poor quality or the pulmonic component of the second heart sound may be accentuated if pulmonary hypertension develops because of pulmonary disease. Third and fourth heart sounds have been described, suggesting myocardial involvement.[144] Occasionally, systolic murmurs are present. These may be basilar, but more frequently are apical, suggestive of mitral valve prolapse secondary to dystrophic changes in papillary muscles.[144, 167] The murmur may be associated with an apical midsystolic click. Cardiomegaly is usually present in patients with cardiac failure.

Electrocardiographic Features

Electrocardiographic abnormalities occur in 90% of patients with Duchenne type muscular dystrophy. These are the earliest and frequently the only signs of cardiac involvement.[176] Although some have found no correlation of electrocardiographic findings with severity of the disease,[196] others have observed electrocardiographic abnormalities to be more common in disabled patients with long-standing disease.[68, 70]

The major abnormality is an accentuation of the early QRS forces anteriorly and rightward, yielding a tall R wave in Lead V_1 and a deeper than normal Q wave in Lead V_6[68, 70, 144, 192, 196] (Fig. 39.5). The configuration of the QRS complex in Lead V_1 includes RS, Rs, and RSr' patterns. Occasionally, the QRS complexes in Lead V_1 have been interpreted as right bundle branch block or right ventricular hypertrophy,[70, 196] the large Q waves as left ventricular hypertrophy.

The origin of these QRS findings remain unknown, although two views are commonly held: (1) These changes are related to myocardial scarring and indicate a greater loss of posterior forces than anterior forces.[144] This correlates with histologic and ultrastructural alterations occurring predominately in the posterobasal region of the left ventricle.[166] (2)

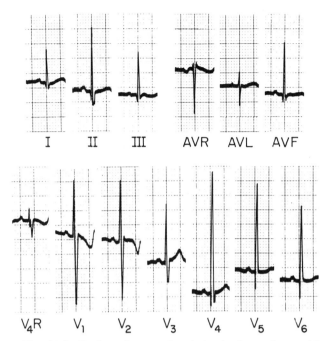

Fig. 39.5 Duchenne's muscular dystrophy in an 8-year-old male. Electrocardiogram shows tall R in lead V_1 and deep Q waves in lead V_6. Pattern of left ventricular hypertrophy. Low voltage T waves.

Because serial electrocardiograms remain similar despite progression of the skeletal muscle disease, others have considered the changes to represent persistence of the neonatal electrocardiogram.[176]

Prolongation of the QT interval has been described, but its significance is unknown. ST segment changes and flat or inverted T waves in the left precordial leads have been found in 30% of the patients.[68, 192]

Vectorcardiographic studies reflect the electrocardiographic findings, and in one study 95% of patients showed at least one abnormality.[62] The most consistent findings were abnormalities in orientation and/or magnitude of planar or spatial ventricular gradient.

Radiologic Features

Roentgenograms frequently show scoliosis as the patients grow older. A prominent pulmonary artery segment may be observed, and cardiomegaly may be observed in patients with cardiac failure.

Echocardiographic Features

Echocardiographic indices of contraction are normal,[2, 74] but reduced diastolic relaxation is found and appears to be a sensitive indicator of early cardiac involvement. In one study,[167] 11 of 20 patients had echocardiographic features of mitral valve prolapse, which correlated with clinical findings in seven. Another study[17] confirmed the high frequency of mitral valve prolapse, including the relatives of affected patients.

Cardiac Catheterization

Cardiac catheterization data have been reported by many authors. In two series, each with 11 patients, right ventricular and pulmonary capillary pressures were normal.[68, 144] Cardiac output varied greatly but was elevated in half the patients. Occasionally, patients have elevated wedge pressures which result from left ventricular failure.

Study of systolic time intervals has shown prolongation of the pre-ejection period and increased isovolumetric contraction period, suggesting an abnormality of myocardial contractility.[128] These changes occurred even in patients with normal electrocardiograms. Pulmonary function studies have shown reduced vital and total lung capacities, impaired maximal breathing capacity, and increased airway passage resistance.[92]

Treatment and Course

No specific therapy is available for the disease. Cardiac complications respond variably to the usual measures. Respiratory complications require vigorous therapy. During anesthesia, hypoxemia should be prevented, depolarizing agents should be avoided, and the patient should be carefully monitored for dysrhythmia.

As already mentioned, in Duchenne's dystrophy there is a progressive increase in symptoms until complete physical incapacitation results. Scoliosis commonly develops. The physical disability seems to lessen cardiac demands, thereby tending to obscure cardiac involvement.[68, 70] Death usually results from intercurrent infection. Less commonly, death results from cardiac dysrhythmias in heart failure.

DUCHENNE'S MUSCULAR DYSTROPHY

In some families with muscular dystrophy, females are also affected, suggesting an autosomal recessive inheritance. Because of its mode of inheritance, this form of muscular dystrophy is the most difficult to define. The clinical features of the myopathy are indistinguishable from the sex-linked recessive form, although it usually progresses less rapidly. Skyring and McKusick[175] encountered four cases which they considered to be this type and were impressed by the absence of QRS abnormalities in Lead V_1, suggesting this absence as a possible differentiating sign.

LIMB-GIRDLE (ERB'S) MUSCULAR DYSTROPHY

The clinical entity limb-girdle muscular dystrophy is probably the composite of several conditions which eventually will be distinguished.[199] In most patients the disease is inherited as an autosomal recessive, although both sporadic and autosomal dominance have been reported.

The clinical picture is less severe than with Duchenne's disease, with the onset of symptoms delayed to late childhood or early adult years.[94] Usually, the muscles of the pelvic girdle and proximal leg are involved first, then those of the shoulder girdle and upper arm. Pseudohypertrophy may occur in the calf muscles in some patients, mimicking Duchenne's disease.

Cardiac involvement is thought to be less severe than in Duchenne's disease, although the findings are similar. There have been three studies of the electrocardiograms in this form,[94, 145, 196] and three-fourths of the patients show abnormalities, including: high voltage QRS complexes in some precordial leads; right ventricular conduction abnormalities; abnormal Q waves; and low voltage T waves. Dysrhythmias are unusual. Symptoms and signs referable to the cardiovascular system are uncommon, although third and/or fourth heart sounds may be heard.[145] Cardiac catheterization data in three patients was normal.[145]

BENIGN DUCHENNE'S DYSTROPHY OR LIMB-GIRDLE DYSTROPHY WITH HYPERTROPHY

This form of muscular dystrophy has an onset after 5 years of age, is slowly progressive, involves the proximal muscle groups, and may have pseudohypertrophy. With these features, classification is difficult, since there are features of both Duchenne's and limb-girdle types. The clinical and laboratory findings are similar to those of Duchenne's,[147] although the electrocardiographic changes are of a lesser degree.

FACIOSCAPULOHUMERAL (LANDOUZY-DEJERINE) MUSCULAR DYSTROPHY

This form shows an autosomal dominant pattern of inheritance, and has a later age of onset, and progresses much more slowly than the previous forms. As the name indicates, it involves the muscles of the face, shoulder, and upper arms. Pseudohypertrophy is not a feature.

Cardiac involvement rarely occurs in this form of dystrophy, and electrocardiographic findings similar to other forms of muscular dystrophy are absent.[196] Cases of atrial paralysis have been described,[8] and this form of muscular dystrophy is the most common cause of that dysrhythmia. Cardiac examination is usually normal. Cardiac catheterization data of patients with this form of muscular dystrophy is essentially normal.[145]

MYOTONIC DYSTROPHY

Although classed with the muscular dystrophies, myotonic dystrophy is a distinct form in which myotonia (increased muscular contractility and decreased muscular relaxation) is combined with muscular weakness. This condition shows three modes of presentation. In infancy, it presents as feeding difficulties due to swallowing abnormalities.[51] In childhood, developmental retardation, poor coordination, and weakness are evident. The facies have a characteristic open mouth and drooling, expressionless, "hatchet" face.[51] Adults with this disease have cataracts, baldness, sterility, personality changes, and cranial hyperostosis.[195] In patients under age 5, the trunk and proximal muscle groups are involved. After age 5 years, the distal muscle groups, facial and neck muscles, are more involved. Cardiac examination is usually normal, although some children show the findings of the late systolic click-murmur syndrome.

Cardiac enlargement and interstitial fibrosis may occur. Histologically, fatty infiltration, variation in myocardial fiber size, and nuclear changes have been observed.[36] In one case, fibrofatty changes were found in the sinus node and atrioventricular conduction system.[103] Electrocardiographic abnormalities occur in up to 90% of the patients.[142, 195] First degree heart block and intraventricular conduction disturbances have been the most common findings.[100] Atrial or ventricular tachyarrhythmias, ST segment and T wave changes, and left axis deviation[95] also occur.

Electrocardiographic findings may precede recognition of neurological changes and are independent of age or severity of the neurologic disease. The frequency of sudden death is high in patients with myotonic dystrophy, because of conduction abnormalities. Electrophysiologic studies[41, 100, 153] have shown abnormal AV nodal conduction, prolonged HV intervals, and occasionally broad His deflections. When studied serially,[153] progression of the conduction abnormality occurred without clinical or electrocardiographic evidence of change. In view of the frequency of conduction abnormalities, patients with symptoms or electrocardiographic evidence of dysrhythmias should be investigated and considered for pacemaker insertion.

JUVENILE RHEUMATOID ARTHRITIS

A disease of unknown etiology, rheumatoid arthritis occurs in all age groups. Its cardiac manifestations likewise may occur at any age, but the type of cardiac involvement in children differs from that in adults. In the past, authors have described the pediatric and adult populations with rheumatoid arthritis separately. This was likely caused by the description by Sir George Still of what he believed to be a separate form of the disease in children, characterized by arthritis (generally involving wrists and knees rather than fingers), lymphadenopathy, splenomegaly, and pericarditis.[183] The pattern of disease described by Still can occur in adults, and the adult pattern of rheumatoid disease can occur in children. Furthermore, perhaps one-third of children with this disease continue to show manifestations as adults.

We will limit our discussions to rheumatoid arthritis in children and not include that in adults, even though they probably represent the same disease and with age-dependent factors modifying the disease manifestations. The disease occurs in approximately one of every 1000 to 2000 children and more frequently in females. Classification of the subgroups of juvenile rheumatoid arthritis (JRA) is based on clinical parameters such as age of onset, extent of joint involvement, sex, and systemic manifestations. The three main groups include systemic disease, polyarthritis, and the pauciarticular forms.

The etiology of JRA is unknown, although infection, autoimmunity, trauma, psychological stress, and genetic factors are under investigation.[38] Recent studies on human leukocyte antigen (HLA) associations in juvenile rheumatoid arthritis populations suggest that there may be a hereditary basis to the pathogenesis. A later onset group, largely male, who are at risk for developing ankylosing spondylitis is associated with HLA-B27.[4, 155] A predominately female group of the pauciarticular group is associated with iritis, antinuclear antibody, and HLA-DRw5.[71]

Pathology

The pathologic findings are more impressive than the clinical findings in regard to cardiac involvement. Unexpected evidence of pericarditis is often found at autopsy (45%) in children who showed no clinical evidence.[112] Pericardial changes, including dense fibrous adhesions, are nonspecific. Constrictive pericarditis is a later complication. Myocarditis and valvular involvement occur rarely. Pirani and Bennett[149] described an 8-year-old child with thickening of the free edges of the mitral and aortic valves and marked infiltration of the aorta by lymphocytes and plasma cells. Others[79] have reported severe cardiac failure secondary to aortic and mitral insufficiency. Laaksonsen[108] described 25 deaths in patients with JRA, five from cardiac complications, including a rheumatic lesion of the aortic valve, rheumatic lesion of the mitral valve, myocarditis, myocardial degeneration, and rheumatic endocarditis, respectively. Autopsy confirmation was provided in only one of these cases. Therefore, unlike the pattern in adults with rheumatoid arthritis, valvular and myocardial changes are uncommon manifestations.

Clinical Features

Juvenile rheumatoid arthritis usually presents one of three modes of onset.[23, 104, 168] In 10 to 20%, an acute systemic illness occurs, with high spiking fever, rash, hepatosplenomegaly, and lymphadenopathy. Arthritic symptoms may be few or absent initially. In another 40 to 50% of patients, a polyarthritic form occurs in which more than five joints may be involved, usually insidiously. Symmetrical joint involvement occurs, resembling the adult form with involvement of knees, ankles, wrists, elbows, and hands. Although the children have fever, weight loss, and anorexia, they are not toxic. The remaining 30 to 40% have the pauciarticular form of the disease. Fewer than five joints are involved. Although systemic symptoms are rare, iridocyclitis is a serious and frequent complication in this form of JRA.[38, 168]

Most cardiac studies of JRA have been retrospective, and the frequency of cardiac involvement has varied greatly, averaging 5%.[112, 122] However, the use of echocardiography may increase the recognition of previously overlooked cardiac involvement.

In children, the cardiovascular manifestations include nonspecific findings. Although transient loud murmurs have been described, murmurs are usually soft, are located along the mid- and upper left sternal borders, and appear to be pulmonary flow murmurs. Tachycardia out of proportion to fever is common. Anemia may play a role in both the tachycardia and murmur.

Pericarditis is the most common type of cardiac involvement, occurring most often in children with the acute systemic form. Although pericarditis is present pathologically in nearly one-half of patients, only 10% show clinical manifestations. Among Still's 19 patients, two had clinical evidence of pericarditis, but three others showed unexpected evidence of pericarditis on postmortem examination.[183]

The largest series of patients with JRA and pericarditis was reported by Lietman and Bywaters.[112] They diagnosed pericarditis clinically in 20 of 285 children with clinical JRA and in 5 of 11 patients at postmortem. Pericarditis occurred more commonly in patients with elevated sedimentation rates, leukocytosis, fever, lymphadenopathy, and rash than those with pulmonary or pleural involvement. Usually, pericarditis followed the development of arthritis (15 patients) but was concurrent in four and preceded it in one patient. Chest pain was present in some. Friction rubs were present, lasted from days to weeks, and were heard often in the presence of pericardial effusion. Clinical signs of pericarditis lasted from 1 to 15 weeks, and several patients had recurrences. Lietman and Bywaters described edema, hepatomegaly, and prominent jugular neck veins, but it is difficult to determine whether these signs of elevated venous pressure occurred as a result of pericardial tamponade or of myocarditis. Cardiac tamponade is a rare complication. In five patients with rheumatoid arthritis and pericarditis, none had paradoxical pulse, but two showed evidence of left heart failure.[131]

Although there is general agreement concerning the occurrence and signs of pericarditis in JRA, there is less unanimity with regard to the occurrence of myocarditis. Clinically, it is difficult to identify myocarditis, whether pericarditis is present or not. Jordan[99] considered evidence of myocarditis to include: persistence of cardiomegaly following pericarditis; cardiomegaly without effusion; electrocardiographic changes; gallop rhythm; and heart failure. Among 30 children with JRA, he found three who fulfilled these criteria, and in two of these pericarditis coexisted. Myocarditis with cardiac failure was reported in 1 of 150 patients from our hospital.[75] There were seven patients with pericarditis in the same group.

Although valvular disease is not considered to occur in JRA, Walsh[193] noted signs of mitral valve disease in 3 of 75 children. The presence of valvular changes in patients with JRA should be considered as possible evidence of coexistent rheumatic fever.

Electrocardiographic Features

Electrocardiographic abnormalities have been reported in 20% of patients. Abnormalities of conduction or of the P wave or QRS complex are rare. ST segment alterations and T wave discordance are the most common changes. T wave changes occur more frequently than ST segment changes and may precede them.[122] Pericarditis may be associated with a normal electrocardiogram.

Radiologic Features

Cardiomegaly may be present, particularly if myocarditis or pericardial effusion is present. In some instances, cardiomegaly may be related to anemia rather than to cardiac disease.

Echocardiographic Features

Echocardiography can detect even small pericardial effusion.[16, 152] Bernstein and co-workers[16] found evidence of pericardial effusion in 20 of 55 patients with JRA. Only four of these 20 patients had pericardial rubs, eight had electrocardiographic abnormalities, and nine had increased cardiac size on roentgenograms. In 11 of their 20 patients, a diagnosis of pericardial effusion could not have been made without echocardiography.

Differential Diagnosis

Differentiation of juvenile rheumatoid arthritis from rheumatic fever may be difficult at times, particularly early in the course of the disease. However, the absence of valvular murmurs, the normal PR interval, and the specific rash are helpful in identification. Greater difficulty may be encountered in the early stages of lupus erythematosus, dermatomyositis, or polyarteritis nodosa, because pericarditis or myocarditis are more common in each. Subsequently established diagnoses on some patients thought to have JRA include psoriasis, ankylosing spondylitis, rheumatic fever, osteochondritis, lupus erythematosus, scleroderma, dermatomyositis, and ulcerative colitis. Rheumatoid spondylitis, Reiter's disease, and psoriatic arthritis are rarely encountered in children but can have cardiac manifestations, particularly in adults.

Treatment and Course

Ordinarily patients with pericarditis require no specific treatment other than the usual for juvenile rheumatoid arthritis.[35] Although corticosteroids have been extensively used, the frequency of serious complications and untoward reactions dictates judicious use of these agents.[35] Corticosteroids probably do not influence the course of the disease, but they reduce the inflammatory aspects. In patients with JRA, few indications for corticosteroids exist, but one is life-threatening carditis. The authors have seen several patients with severe carditis who responded promptly to corticosteroids. In children with pericarditis, Lietman and Bywaters,[112] however, noted no difference in duration, severity, or residua in 11 children receiving corticosteroids, as compared to 13 children receiving none. Similarly, the benefit of digitalis is questionable in patients with carditis. Pericardiocentesis may be indicated in patients with massive pericardial effusion or tamponade, although this situation is uncommon.

The long-term course of the disease results in severe incapacity in one-third of the patients, mild incapacity in one-third, and none in the remaining one-third.[108] Pericarditis and myocarditis usually resolve, although occasionally cardiomegaly persists.

MARFAN'S SYNDROME

The Marfan syndrome is a generalized connective tissue disorder predominantly involving elastic fibers. No specific biochemical etiology has been conclusively established, although the disorder has long been theorized to be due to abnormal collagen or elastin metabolism. Recent evidence indicates that the defect may reside in the production of collagen intermolecular cross-links.[24]

In 1896, Marfan[114] described a 5-year-old girl with long slender extremities which he termed "dolichostenomelia." This patient did not have ophthalmologic or cardiac abnormalities. Subsequently, Achard[1] termed the long thin extremities "arachnodactyly." Later, the eponym Marfan's syndrome was used to describe individuals with long slender extremities and cardiac, and ophthalmologic abnormalities. Ironically, Marfan's original patient very likely had congenital contractural arachnodactyly rather than Marfan's syndrome, and Achard's patient had still a different disease.[84] In spite of this, the term Marfan's syndrome is widely accepted to describe a distinctive phenotype with involvement of the ophthalmologic, cardiovascular and skeletal systems.[120]

The Marfan syndrome encompasses major and minor abnormalities of the skeleton and joints (arachnodactyly, kyphoscoliosis, dolichocephaly, high arched palate, pectus excavatum and other defects of the sternum, dislocated hips, hammer toes, genu recurvatum, pes planus, hyperextensible joints), eyes (subluxation of lens, myopia, iridodonesis, retinal detachment), and cardiovascular system.[120] Inguinal hernias are common and are frequently recurrent. Hypotonia, poor muscular development, and absence of subcutaneous fat may be present. Rudimentary lobes of the lungs, abnormal lobulation, emphysema, cystic disease, and spontaneous pneumothorax have been described.[22, 55] The elastic stroma of alveolar septae is said to show precocious maturation in children, but probably as a secondary phenomenon.[21]

Patients have normal intelligence. The most typical skeletal features include an abnormally low upper to lower body segment ratio, an ability to project the thumb beyond the palm in the closed hand (thumb sign), and overlap of distal phalanges of the 1st and 5th fingers when wrapped around the opposite wrist (wrist sign).[154] In childhood, patients show an acclerated growth in height but not weight, resulting in tall, gangly physiques.

The Marfan syndrome is inherited as an autosomal dominant gene with variable expressivity, resulting in a marked variability in appearance of affected individuals. Although many cases are sporadic, careful examination of relatives decreases the number of such cases to about 15%, with these then attributed to new mutations. Prevalence of the classic Marfan syndrome is 4 to 6/100,000 people. However, since many individuals may not have all the classic manifestations, the prevalence may be much greater.[154]

PATHOLOGY

The first observation of cardiac abnormality is credited to Salle,[165] who, in 1912, described a 2-month-old infant with murmurs, increasing cardiomegaly, attacks of dyspnea, and death.[165] At autopsy, each cardiac chamber was enlarged, and the atrioventricular valve orifices were dilated. The typical aortic changes were first described in 1943 in a 14-year-old girl.[7] A 25-year-old man had similar changes in the aorta and in the pulmonary artery. That same year, a 21-year-old man was described who died suddenly 7 months after an episode of precordial pain, with autopsy revealing aortic insufficiency and rupture of a chronic dissecting aortic aneurysm into the pericardial cavity.[58]

A wide spectrum of cardiac abnormalities is now recognized as an integral part of the Marfan syndrome. These abnormalities represent an abiotrophy (delayed degenerative changes), in contrast to structural defects present at birth (congenital). Nevertheless, major distortions of cardiac structures have been observed in very young infants, indicating that valvular abnormalities can be present at birth. "True" congenital cardiac malformations, though uncommon, occur more often than expected by chance,[89, 146] particularly coarctation of the aorta and atrial septal defect.[110]

By the age of 21 years, clinically evident cardiovascular disease is present in 50% of patients with the Marfan syndrome. All patients probably have histologic changes in blood vessels or cardiac valves by that age. The most common cardiovascular abnormalities include dilatation or aneurysms of the ascending aorta (with or without dissection or rupture), AI, aneurysms of the sinuses of Valsalva, dilatation or aneurysms of the main pulmonary artery (with or without pulmonary valvular insufficiency), and MI, involving dilatation of the mitral annulus, distorted leaflets, or abnormal chordae tendineae.[77, 156] Less common abnormalities are myocardial fibrosis and infarction,[5] rupture of chordae tendineae, rupture of pulmonary arteries, narrowing of coronary ostia, aneurysm of the abdominal aorta, and changes in other valves of the heart. Aortic lesions tend to be the predominant ones in adults,[129] but in children, mitral valvular abnormalities may be more evident.[146] Perhaps this is due to the time course of changes in the aorta.

Microscopic examination of the proximal ascending aorta typically reveals disruption of the elastic media by a metachromatic mucoid material, chondroitin sulfate.[21] This mucoid material and the loss of elastic fibers produces confluent cystic foci in the media tissue, thus giving rise to cystic medial necrosis. The process of cystic medial necrosis results in aneurysmal dilatation of the aortic arch, the sinuses of Valsalva, and the aortic valve annulus, thus predisposing to the development of dissecting aneurysms. Large accumulations of dermatan sulfate or heparan sulfate, and chondroitin sulfate, have also been reported in the media of the aorta.[185] Electron microscopy has shown no abnormality in fine structure of the collagen fibers.[21]

Dilatation of the ascending aorta (Fig. 39.6) begins in the sinuses of Valsalva, the intrapericardial part of the aorta. Aortic insufficiency may result from this dilatation. The coronary arteries, particularly the extramural coronary arteries, show changes of cystic medial necrosis, with an occasional area of incomplete rupture and aneurysmal-like dilatation.[5, 13]

The mitral valve and left atrial endocardium often undergo a fibromyxoid degeneration. The leaflets and endocardium are thickened and distorted by myxoid material, resulting in MI. Prolapse or ballooning (Fig. 39.7) of the mitral valve leaflets, with or without abnormally long chordae tendineae, is common.[25, 80, 156] and fused chordae tendineae may also produce MI.[21] Calcification of the mitral annulus can occur,[76] but the fibrous contractures seen in chronic rheumatic disease are absent.[25]

Similar gross and histologic changes occur in the pulmonary artery, and the myxomatous changes found in the mitral valve may develop in the other cardiac valves. The ventricular myocardium may show hypertrophy, fragmentation, and areas of fibrosis, in part secondary to the valvular lesions. Proliferative and degenerative changes in the arteries supplying the sinoauricular and atrioventricular nodes may be responsible for conduction abnormalities, and similar changes in the smaller coronary arteries may result in myocardial necrosis, fibrosis, and consequent cardiomegaly.[97]

MANIFESTATIONS

Clinical Features

In children and young adults, clinical findings of mitral valvular abnormalities are more frequently noted than aortic lesions.[146] Murmurs of MI are commonly heard due to either

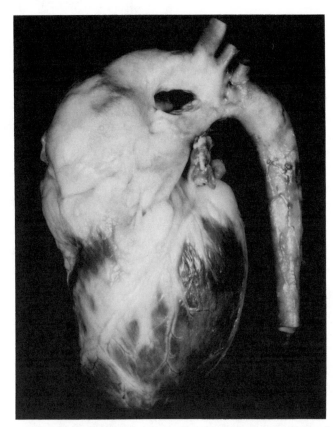

Fig. 39.6 Marfan's syndrome in a 21-year-old male. External appearance of heart and aorta. Greatly dilated ascending aorta. (Reproduced with permission from J. E. Edwards.[56])

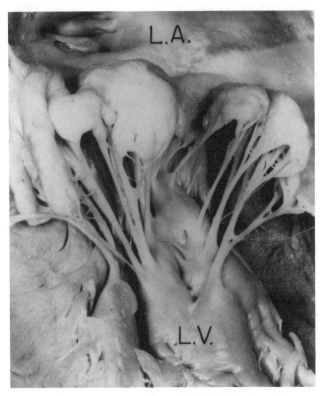

Fig. 39.7 Marfan's syndrome in a 13-year-old male. Left atrium (*L.A.*) and left ventricle (*L.V.*). Elongated chordae tendineae. Marked hooding of mitral valve leaflets. (Reproduced with permission from C. M. Grondin et al.[80])

redundant valve tissue (hemorrhoidal appearance) or elongated chordae tendineae which allows prolapse of the mitral valve.[156, 172] An apical pansystolic murmur may be heard, but often there are findings of the late systolic click-murmur syndrome (mitral valve prolapse or floppy mitral valve syndrome).[118, 141, 146] When the patient is recumbent, there is a late systolic click and soft systolic murmur located at the apex. When the patient stands, the click becomes closer to the first heart sound, and the murmur increases in intensity and duration. The auscultatory finding of a late systolic click and murmur was identified in patients with Marfan's syndrome long before the click syndrome (mitral valve prolapse) was recognized as a common clinical entity.[140, 172] Individuals with Marfan's syndrome may constitute perhaps 5% of all pediatric cases with mitral valve prolapse.

The late systolic murmur almost has a musical quality, and multiple or single clicks in mid to late systole may accompany or initiate the murmur. These clicks and murmur are probably generated by the redundancy and interchordal ballooning of the mitral valvular leaflets.[80, 120]

Aortic insufficiency occurs less frequently in children with Marfan's syndrome. In the 2nd decade of life, aortic dilatation with AI may develop. This is indicated by early aortic diastolic murmurs and aortic systolic ejection clicks. Mitral mid-diastolic murmurs and aortic systolic ejection murmurs may also be present if valvular regurgitation is severe. The presence of aneurysms or dilatation of the aorta may not be evident clinically, but aortic dissection can cause the sudden appearance of systolic and diastolic murmurs. Acute aortic dissection is typically accompanied by severe anterior or posterior chest pain, and cardiovascular collapse.

Accentuation of the pulmonic component of the second heart sound is common in patients with a thin chest wall or dilated pulmonary artery. Exercise intolerance and easy fatigability may appear and progress as the cardiovascular lesions worsen. Cerebral hemorrhage or thrombosis can occur in the childhood years.

Electrocardiographic Features

Although an occasional patient may have a normal electrocardiogram despite significant aortic or mitral valvar abnormalities, signs of left ventricular hypertrophy and first-degree atrioventricular block are usually found. Inversion of T waves in leads II, III, aVF, and V_6 is common,[26, 27] may occur transiently,[146, 172] and may be indicative of papillary muscle dysfunction.[146] Dysrhythmias have been reported, including incomplete or complete atrioventricular block, paroxysmal supraventricular tachycardia, atrial flutter,[40] atrial fibrillation, and the Wolff-Parkinson-White syndrome. A specific electrocardiographic pattern (depressed ST segments with inverted T waves in leads II, III, and aVF) suggestive of posteroinferior myocardial ischemia has been detected in many patients with Marfan's syndrome and systolic click-murmur.[28]

Radiologic Features

Generalized cardiomegaly, left ventricular enlargement, left atrial enlargement, or prominence of the aorta or pulmonary artery may occur, depending upon the type of valvar lesions. Considerable dilatation of the aorta or sinuses of Valsalva, or aneurysms, may be present despite a normal cardiac shadow. Fluoroscopy may fail to clarify aortic size. Interpretation of the cardiac contour may be complicated by the presence of sternal and spinal deformities that commonly develop during the childhood years.

Echocardiographic Features

Echocardiography has become invaluable in the diagnosis and management of cardiovascular disease in patients with Marfan's syndrome. An M-mode echogram of the aorta characteristically shows an increased dimension of the aortic root (Fig. 39.8). At least 60% of Marfan patients have echocardiographic evidence of aortic root dilatation, a finding rarely present in other conditions.[33] With moderate dilatation of the ascending aorta, paradoxical movement of the posterior aortic wall and partial early systolic closure of the aortic cusps may also be detected by echocardiography.[6] Echocardiography is better than roentgenograms for the early detection of aortic root dilatation.[44]

Echocardiography has also detected the presence of mitral valve prolapse in 80 to 90% of Marfan patients, some of whom have no mitral valve murmur.[33, 81] Prolapse of the mitral valve is more commonly recognized for the posterior leaflet and is usually pansystolic (Fig. 39.9). Echocardiography may also diagnose dissection of the aorta[32, 127, 132] by showing two echoes with parallel motion within the aorta.

CARDIAC CATHETERIZATION

Cardiac catheterization and angiocardiography can be performed safely in patients with Marfan's syndrome to provide

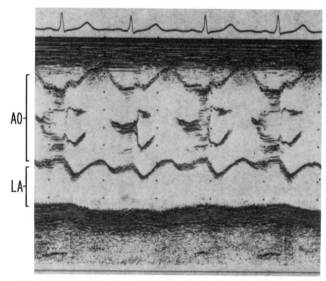

Fig. 39.8 Marfan's syndrome in a 7-year-old female. M mode echocardiogram. Through aorta (*AO*) and left atrium (*LA*). Greatly enlarged aortic root.

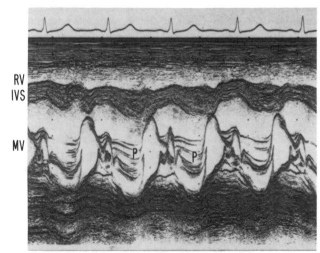

Fig. 39.9 Marfan's syndrome in a 7-year-old female. M mode echocardiogram through mitral valve (*MV*). Pansystolic prolapse (*P*) of posterior leaflet. *IVS*, ventricular septum; *RV*, right ventricle.

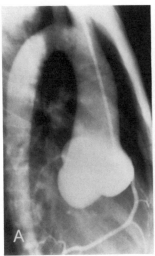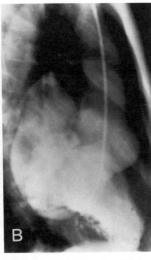

Fig. 39.10 Marfan's syndrome in a 9-year-old female. (*A*) Aortogram. Dilated sinuses of Valsalva and aortic root. (*B*) Left ventriculogram. Lateral view. Prolapse and scalloping of mitral valve with marked mitral insufficiency.

information about cardiac pathology and function. Aortography (Fig. 39.10*A*) typically shows aortic sinuses which may be greatly dilated and symmetrical dilatation of the ascending aorta. Left ventriculography (Fig. 39.10*B*) typically shows prolapse of the mitral valve, which may have a scalloped appearance and may be associated with MI. Although the physique of patients complicates the performance of pulmonary function tests, abnormal relationships have been noted between the inspiratory and expiratory airway resistances and lung volume, but the diffusing surface of the lung is normal.[66]

DIFFERENTIAL DIAGNOSIS

Patients with the classical manifestations of Marfan's syndrome present no problem in diagnosis, nor do those with minimal findings and affected relatives. In the infant, arachnodactyly is the most helpful diagnostic sign and is also a key feature in the older child. However, arachnodactyly can occur in the rubella syndrome, sickle cell anemia, eunuchism, Klinefelter's syndrome, and various muscular disorders. Congenital contractural arachnodactyly can be recognized by the features of multiple congenital joint contractures, arachnodactyly, crumpled ears, and kyphoscoliosis.[10] Heart disease is not usually present. Transmission of contractural arachnodactyly is by autosomal dominant trait, and the prognosis is good for a normal life-span. To complicate classification, an infant has been reported with cardiovascular manifestations of Marfan's syndrome and with joint contractures like congenital contractural arachnodactyly.[81] Perhaps a better classification will develop as more patients with overlapping features are reported. Achard's patient had no cardiac or eye abnormalities and no joint contractures.[1] Other features of Achard's syndrome such as normal length of extremities, brachycephaly, and micrognathia suggest that this entity is different from the Marfan syndrome.

Although the majority of cases of ectopia lentis occur in the Marfan syndrome, this eye disorder is also a common finding in homocystinuria, an autosomal recessive disorder due to deficiency of cystathionine synthetase. Features in common with the Marfan syndrome include long narrow extremities, arachnodactyly, and dislocated lenses. Severe mental retardation is usually present in homocystinuria, not in Marfan's syndrome. Lastly, there is another rare syndrome resembling Marfan's syndrome which consists of arachnodactyly, pigmentary retinal degeneration, cataracts and microcephaly, and probably recessive inheritance.[125]

In several other cardiac disorders (Erdheim's cystic medionecrosis, idiopathic dilatation of the aorta, and prolapsing mitral valve syndrome), the pathologic findings in the aorta and cardiac valves are often indistinguishable from the Marfan syndrome, and some of these cases may represent "forme fruste" variants.[42, 157] Until reliable biochemical tests are available, the diagnosis of Marfan's syndrome continues to be based on clinical examination and cardiac studies, with examination of the family pedigree being an important diagnostic step. The Marfan syndrome should be considered in the differential diagnosis of children with the prolapsing mitral valve syndrome, particularly if skeletal anomalies are also present.

NATURAL HISTORY

The cardiovascular involvement of Marfan's syndrome greatly reduces life expectancy of patients with the disorder. Manifestations of cardiac disease may develop at any age, and may be responsible for death in infancy or old age. Progression of cardiovascular lesions may be rapid or slow, and sudden death may occur in patients with little or no cardiac disability. Mitral insufficiency is a more benign lesion then AI, but rupture of mitral chordae tendineae can constitute a surgical emergency.[173] In a study of 36 children, five deaths occurred, including two after cardiovascular surgery and one during surgery for scoliosis.

Life survival tables based on 257 patients with Marfan's syndrome have been developed. Of 72 deaths, a cardiac cause was found in 52 of the 56 where a cause was known. Thirty-nine deaths occurred from complications of aortic dilatation, and two other deaths were from endocarditis. In the first two decades of life, 10% of females die, and the rate is slightly less for males. The probability of survival dipped to 0.50 by the age of 41 for men and the age of 49 for women.[129] Associated pulmonary abnormalities may predispose patients to pulmonary infections, the most common cause of death prior to the introduction of antibiotics. Likewise, associated kyphoscoliosis can contribute to cardiac disability and death.[194] Endocarditis has been reported in 22 patients, with almost all involving the mitral valve and with but one cure.[178]

TREATMENT

There is no specific treatment for the metabolic disturbance of Marfan's syndrome but the cardiovascular complications generally respond to medical treatment, except for acute aortic dissections. Medical and surgical management of the cardiovascular manifestations is currently oriented toward prevention, in addition to symptomatic treatment. Propranolol has been recommended for patients with aortic dilatation to diminish myocardial contractility and reduce pulsatile flow stress on the aorta. Results of therapy[139] have been inconclusive because propranolol was initially administered after aortic dilatation was already a prominent feature.

Early reports[133, 185] of operative treatment of aortic aneurysms and AI revealed a high operative mortality and low late survival. In a series of 30 patients undergoing operation for aortic aneurysm and AI, six died at surgery, two died after 3 years, and 12 were alive and asymptomatic for 5 or more years postoperatively. Overall, the operative results, particularly for valvar replacement, were disappointing. Some patients with successful valvar replacement continued in cardiac failure, with clinical findings resembling a cardiomyopathy.

Older operative methods[46, 185] have been succeeded by composite replacement of the aortic valve and ascending aorta.[85, 116, 117] This technique requires excision of the aortic valve and interposition of a Dacron composite graft into the dilated ascending aorta. This method decreases the perioperative problems of hemorrhage, acute dissection, and prosthetic valvar leakage.

Earlier operative intervention for patients with aortic root aneurysms and AI has been recommended in effort to improve overall mortality.[117, 154] Elective prophylactic repair of the dilated ascending aorta before cardiac failure or acute aortic dissection is associated with a mortality of less than 10%. The recommendation for elective operation is a maximum aortic root dilatation (5.5 to 6.0 cm) obtained by echocardiography.[117, 154]

Proper management of the Marfan patient depends upon early recognition of the diagnosis and identification of cardiovascular problems. An annual echocardiogram should be obtained to determine aortic dimension. When aortic dilatation becomes prominent (greater than 5.5 cm), consideration should be given to prophylactic composite graft replacement although in children, operation should be delayed until an adequate-size valve can be inserted (with hope of avoiding later reoperation).[154] Since endocarditis occurs in Marfan patients with valvar anomalies, prophylactic antibiotics are recommended.[178]

Patients with the Marfan syndrome and their families must be counseled about the hereditary nature of the disease and the prognosis and changes in life-style that the disease may require. Emotional support is often needed, since the distressing features of the disease can lead to depression, despair, and suicide. The care of patients usually involves several medical specialists, and necessitates close coordination of care. Surgery for scoliosis may be hazardous for patients with cardiovascular involvement. Severe pectus excavatum may present a problem for surgical incisions for cardiac and aortic repair.[126] Contact sports are usually contraindicated, both for ophthalmic (danger of lens displacement and retinal detachment) and cardiac reasons. Activities that elevate blood pressure, such as weight lifting, should be avoided. In addition, there is an increased risk of vascular rupture during pregnancy.

AMYLOIDOSIS

The deposition of amyloid in tissues and organs is termed amyloidosis, and commonly affects the kidney, liver, and heart, although all organ systems can be involved.[34, 43, 72] Amyloid is composed of fibrils with a characteristic appearance under the electron microscope but varies in primary protein composition.[63, 72] Classification remains unsatisfactory, but cases are usually grouped as one of the following five types: primary (often familial, with several distinct genetic types); secondary (to rheumatoid arthritis and other chronic diseases); a tumor-forming type; a form associated with multiple myeloma; and senile type. The primary and senile forms generally involve the heart. The secondary form is the most common type encountered in children, usually in association with rheumatoid arthritis, familial Mediterranean anemia, or suppurative diseases.[184] The frequent involvement of the heart by rheumatoid arthritis itself makes it difficult to diagnose amyloid cardiac complications in such patients without direct pathologic observations. The other forms have rarely been reported in patients under 20 years of age. Andrade[3] described a cluster of primary adult cases in Portugal where the disease commonly developed in the 2nd and 3rd decades of life. Children in affected pedigrees of the primary form have been examined for signs of disease but with negative results.[64]

Cardiac involvement generally manifests itself by signs and symptoms of slowly evolving heart failure with poor response to medical therapy and with death occurring within a few years. Digitalis sensitivity is especially common, particularly in the senile form. Soft nonspecific systolic murmurs are often present, and cardiomegaly may be noted. In some cases, the clinical and cardiac catheterization findings mimic those of constrictive pericarditis.[45] Common electrocardiographic findings include low voltage QRS complexes, prolonged PR interval and other degrees of atrioventricular block, flat or negative T waves, bundle-branch block, left axis deviation, and atrial dysrhythmias.

There is diffuse deposition of amyloid in atrial and ventricular walls, producing an overall firm rubbery consistency. The pericardium, endocardium, and cardiac valves may have grossly visible focal deposits of amyloid, but valvular dysfunction is rare. Microscopic findings include deposition of amyloid in the walls of arteries, particularly the small and medium-size coronary vessels. Amyloid surrounds the muscle fibers, giving a honeycomb structure, and the muscle cells may show atrophy, vacuolization, fragmentation, and even necrosis. There is often involvement of the cardiac conduction tissues, thus providing a partial explanation for the frequent electrocardiographic conduction abnormalities.

Echocardiography has become a useful tool in the identification of cardiac amyloidosis. M mode echograms have demonstrated thickened left ventricular posterior wall, ventricular septum, and right ventricular anterior wall.[69, 174] Additional features which can be identified by 2D echocardiograms include thickened papillary muscles and cardiac valves and a "granular sparkling" appearance, believed to be secondary to amyloid deposit, of thickened cardiac walls.[174]

Amyloidosis is included in the differential diagnosis of myocardiopathies in adults and is a popular subject for clincopathologic conferences.[39] At present, the pediatric cardiologist should include it in his differential diagnosis especially in patients with rheumatoid arthritis.

REFERENCES

1. Achard, M. C. Arachnodactylie. Bull. Mem. Soc. Med. Hosp. Paris 19:834, 1902.
2. Ahmad, M., Sanderson, J. E., Dubowitz, V., and Hallidie-Smith, K. A. Echocardiographic assessment of left ventricular function in Duchenne's muscular dystrophy. Br. Heart J. 40:734, 1978.
3. Andrade, C. A peculiar form of peripheral neuropathy. Brain 75:408, 1952.
4. Ansell, B. M. Spondyloarthropathy in childhood: A review. J. Roy. Soc. Med. 74:205, 1981.
5. Arcilla, R. A., Ow, E. P., Lacina, S., Hamilton, W., and Thilenius, O. G. Paradoxical relation-

ship between mitral valve prolapse and left ventricular function in Marfan's syndrome. Pediatr. Cardiol. 1:223, 1980.
6. Atsuchi, Y., Nagai, Y., Komatsu, Y., Nakamura, K., Shibuya, M., and Hirosawa, K. Echocardiographic manifestations of annuloaortic ectasia: Its "paradoxical" motion of the aorta and premature systolic closure of the aortic valve. Am. Heart J. 93:428, 1977.
7. Baer, R. W., Taussig, H. B., and Oppenheimer, E. H. Congenital aneurysmal dilatation of the aorta associated with arachnodactyly. Bull. Johns Hopkins Hosp. 72:309, 1943.
8. Baldwin, B. J., Talley, R. C., Johnson, C., and

Nutter, D. O. Permanent paralysis of the atrium in a patient with facioscapulohumeral muscular dystrophy. Am. J. Cardiol. 31:649, 1973.
9. Bass, J. L., Shrivastava, S., Grabowski, G., Desnick, R. J., and Moller, J. H. The M-mode echocardiogram in Fabry's disease. Am. Heart J. 100:807, 1980.
10. Beals, R. K., and Hecht, F. Congenital contractural arachnodactyly. A heritable disorder of connective tissue. J. Bone Joint Surg. 53:987, 1971.
11. Beaudet, A. L., DiFerrante, N. M., Ferry, G. D., Nichols, B. L., Jr., and Mullins, C. E.

Variation in the phenotypic expression of β-glucuronidase deficiency. J. Pediatr. 86:388, 1975.

12. Becker, A. E., Schoorl, R., Balk, A. G., and van der Heide, R. M. Cardiac manifestations of Fabry's disease. Report of a case with mitral insufficiency and electrocardiographic evidence of myocardial infarction. Am. J. Cardiol. 36:829, 1975.

13. Becker, A. E., and van Mantgem, J. P. The coronary arteries in Marfan's syndrome: A morphologic study. Am. J. Cardiol. 36:315, 1975.

14. Benbassat, J., Bassan, H., Milwidsky, H., Sacks, M., and Groen, J. J. Constrictive pericarditis in Gaucher's disease. Am. J. Med. 44:647, 1968.

15. Berg, R. A., Kaplan, A. M., Jarrett, P. B., and Molthan, M. E. Friedreich's ataxia with acute cardiomyopathy. Am. J. Dis. Child. 134:390, 1980.

16. Bernstein, B., Takahashi, M., and Hanson, V. Cardiac involvement in juvenile rheumatoid arthritis. J. Pediatr. 85:313, 1974.

17. Biddison, J. H., Dembo, D. H., Spalt, H., Hayes, M. G., and LeDoux, C. W. Familial occurrence of mitral valve prolapse in X-linked muscular dystrophy. Circulation 59:1299, 1979.

18. Blass, J. P., Kark, R. A. P., and Menon, N. K. Low activities of the pyruvate and oxoglutarate dehydrogenase complexes in five patients with Friedreich's ataxia. N. Engl. J. Med. 295:62, 1976.

19. Blieden, L. C., Desnick, R. J., Carter, J. B., Krivit, W., Moller, J. H., and Sharp, H. L. Cardiac involvement in Sandhoff's disease. Inborn error of glycosphingolipid metabolism. Am. J. Cardiol. 34:83, 1974.

20. Blieden, L. C., and Moller, J. H. Cardiac involvement in inherited disorders of metabolism. Prog. Cardiovasc. Dis. 16:615, 1974.

21. Bolande, R. P. The nature of the connective tissue abiotrophy in the Marfan syndrome. Lab. Invest. 12:1087, 1963.

22. Bolande, R. P., and Tucker, A. S. Pulmonary emphysema and other cardiorespiratory lesions as part of the Marfan abiotrophy. Pediatrics 33:356, 1964.

23. Boone, J. E., Baldwin, J., and Levine, C. Juvenile rheumatoid arthritis. Pediatr. Clin. North Am. 21(4):885, 1974.

24. Boucek, R. J., Noble, N. L., Gunja-Smith, Z., and Butler, W. T. The Marfan syndrome: A deficiency in chemically stable collagen crosslinks. N. Engl. J. Med. 305:988, 1981.

25. Bowden, D. H., Favara, B. E., and Donahoe, J. L. Marfan's syndrome: Accelerated course in childhood associated with lesions of mitral valve and pulmonary artery. Am. Heart J. 69:96, 1965.

26. Bowers, D. The electrocardiogram in Marfan's syndrome. Am. J. Cardiol. 7:661, 1961.

27. Bowers, D. An electrocardiographic pattern associated with mitral valve deformity in Marfan's syndrome. Circulation 23:30, 1961.

28. Bowers, D. Primary abnormalities of the mitral valve in Marfan's syndrome: Electrocardiographic findings. Br. Heart J. 31:676, 1969.

29. Boyer, S. H., Chisholm, A. W., and McKusick, V. A. Cardiac aspects of Friedreich's ataxia. Circulation 25:493, 1962.

30. Brante, G. Gargoylism: A mucopolysaccharidosis. Scand. J. Clin. Lab. Invest. 4:43, 1952.

31. Brosius, F. C., and Roberts, W. C. Coronary artery disease in the Hurler syndrome. Qualitative and quantitative analysis of the extent of coronary narrowing at necropsy in six children. Am. J. Cardiol. 47:649, 1981.

32. Brown, O. R., Popp, R. L., and Kloster, F. E. Echocardiographic criteria for aortic root dissection. Am. J. Cardiol. 36:17, 1975.

33. Brown, O. R., DeMots, H., Kloster, F. E., Roberts, A., Menashe, V. D., and Beals, R. K. Aortic root dilatation and mitral valve pro-

lapse in Marfan's syndrome. An echocardiographic study. Circulation 52:651, 1975.

34. Buja, L. M., Khoi, N. B., and Roberts, W. C. Clinically significant cardiac amyloidosis. Am. J. Cardiol. 26:394, 1970.

35. Calabro, J. J., Management of juvenile rheumatoid arthritis. J. Pediatr. 77:355, 1970.

36. Cannon, P. J. The heart and lungs in myotonic muscular dystrophy. Am. J. Med. 32:765, 1962.

37. Cantz, M., Gehler, J., and Spranger, J. Mucolipidosis I: Increased sialic acid content and deficiency of an alpha-N-acetylneuraminidase in cultured fibroblasts. Biochem. Biophys. Res. Commun. 74:732, 1977.

38. Cassidy, J. T. Juvenile rheumatoid arthritis. In Textbook of Rheumatology, edited by W. N. Kelley, E. D. Harris, Jr., S. Ruddy, and C. B. Sledge. W. B. Saunders, Philadelphia, 1981, p. 1279.

39. Castleman, B., Scully, R. E., and McNeely, B. U. Weekly clinicopathological exercise. Case 25-1974. N. Engl. J. Med. 290:1474, 1974.

40. Cipolloni, P. B., Shane, S. R., and Marshall, R. J. Chronic atrial flutter in brothers with the Marfan syndrome. Circulation 31:572, 1965.

41. Clements, S. D., Jr., Colmers, R. A., and Hurst, J. W. Myotonia dystrophica. Ventricular arrhythmias, intraventricular conduction abnormalities, atrioventricular block and Stokes-Adams attacks successfully treated with permanent transvenous pacemaker. Am. J. Cardiol. 37:933, 1976.

42. Cobbs, B. W., Jr. Clinical recognition and medical management of rheumatic heart disease and other acquired valvular disease. In The Heart, Arteries, and Veins, edited by J. W. Hurst, R. B. Logue, R. C. Schant, and N. K. Wenger, ed. 3. McGraw-Hill, New York, 1974, p. 957.

43. Cohen, A. S. Amyloidosis. N. Engl. J. Med. 277:522, 574, 628, 1967.

44. Come, P. C., Bulkley, B. H., McKusick, V. A., and Fortuin, N. J. Echocardiographic recognition of silent aortic root dilatation in Marfan's syndrome. Chest 72:789, 1977.

45. Crockett, L. K., Thompson, M., and Dekker, A. A review of cardiac amyloidosis: Report of a case presenting as constrictive pericarditis. Am. J. Med. Sci. 264:149, 1972.

46. Crosby, I. K., Ashcraft, W. C., and Reed, W. A. Surgery of proximal aorta in Marfan's syndrome. J. Thorac. Cardiovasc. Surg. 66:75, 1973.

47. Dekaban, A. S., Constantopoulos, G., Herman, M. M., and Steusing, J. K. Mucopolysaccharidosis type V (Scheie syndrome). A postmortem study by multidisciplinary techniques with emphasis on the brain. Arch. Pathol. Lab. Med. 100:237, 1976.

48. Desnick, R. J., Sharp, H. L., Grabowski, G. A., Brunning, R. D., Quie, P. G., Sung, J. H., Gorlin, R. J., and Ikonne, J. U. Mannosidosis: Clinical morphologic, immunologic and biochemical studies. Pediatr. Res. 10:985, 1976.

49. Desnick, R. J., Blieden, L. C., Sharp, H. L., Hofschire, P. J., and Moller, J. H. Cardiac valvular anomalies in Fabry disease. Clinical, morphologic and biochemical studies. Circulation 54:818, 1976.

50. DiFerrante, N., Nichols, B. L., Donnelly, P. V., Neri, G., Hrgovcic, R., and Berglund, R. K. Induced degradation of glycosaminoglycans in Hurler's and Hunter's syndromes by plasma infusion. Proc. Natl. Acad. Sci. USA 68:303, 1971.

51. Dodge, P. R., Gamstorp, I., Byers, R. K., and Russell, P. Myotonic dystrophy in infancy and childhood. Pediatrics 35:3, 1965.

52. Dorfman, A., and Lorincz, A. E. Occurrence of urinary acid mucopolysaccharides in the Hurler syndrome. Proc. Natl. Acad. Sci. USA 43:443, 1957.

53. Durand, P., Philippart, M., Barrone, C., and

Della Cella, G. A new glycolipid storage disease. Pediatr. Res. 1:416, 1967.

54. Durand, P., Barrone, C., and Della Cella, G. Fucosidosis. J. Pediatr. 75:665, 1969.

55. Dwyer, E. M., Jr., and Troncale, F. Spontaneous pneumothorax and pulmonary disease in the Marfan syndrome. Ann. Intern. Med. 62:1285, 1965.

56. Edwards, J. E. Lesions causing or simulating aortic insufficiency. Cardiovasc. Clin. 5:128, 1973.

57. Emery, A. E., Burt, D., Dubowitz, V., Rocker, I., Donnai, D., Harris, R., and Donnai, P. Antenatal diagnosis of Duchenne muscular dystrophy. Lancet 1:847, 1979.

58. Etter, L. E., and Glover, L. P. Arachnodactyly complicated by dislocated lens and death from rupture of dissecting aneurysm of the aorta. J.A.M.A. 123:88, 1943.

59. Evans, W., and Wright, G. The electrocardiogram in Friedreich disease. Br. Heart J. 4:91, 1942.

60. Factor, S. M., Biempica, L., and Goldfischer, S. Coronary intimal sclerosis in Morquio's syndrome. Vichows Arch. Pathol. Anat. Histol. 379:1, 1978.

61. Ferrans, V. J., Hibbs, R. G., and Burda, C. D. The heart in Fabry's disease: A histochemical and electron microscopic study. Am. J. Cardiol. 24:95, 1969.

62. Fitch, C. W., and Ainger, L. E. The Frank vectorcardiogram and the electrocardiogram in Duchenne progressive muscular dystrophy. Circulation 35:1124, 1967.

63. Franklin, E. C. The complexity of amyloid. N. Engl. J. Med. 290:512, 1974.

64. Frederiksen, T., Gotzsche, H., Harboe, N., Kiaer, W., and Mellemgaard, K. Familial primary amyloidosis with severe amyloid heart disease. Am. J. Med. 33:328, 1962.

65. Friedreich, N. Uber degenerative atrophie der spinal Hinterstrange. Arch. Pathol. Anat. Physiol. 26:391, 1863.

66. Fuleihan, F. J. D., Suh, S. K., and Shepard, R. H. Some aspects of pulmonary function in the Marfan syndrome. Bull. Johns Hopkins Hosp. 113:320, 1963.

67. Gach, J. V., Andriange, M., and Franck, G. Hypertrophic obstructive cardiomyopathy and Friedreich's ataxia. Report of a case and review of literature. Am. J. Cardiol. 27:436, 1971.

68. Gailani, S., Danowski, T. S., and Fisher, D. S. Muscular dystrophy: Catheterization studies indicating latent congestive heart failure. Circulation 17:583, 1958.

69. Giles, T. D., Leon-Galindo, J., and Burch, G. E. Echocardiographic findings in amyloid cardiomyopathy. South. Med. J. 71:1393, 1978.

70. Gilroy, J., Cahalan, J. L., Berman, R., and Newman, M. Cardiac and pulmonary complications in Duchenne's progressive muscular dystrophy. Circulation 27:484, 1963.

71. Glass, D., Litvin, D., Wallace, K., Chylack, L., Garovoy, M., Carpenter, C. B., and Schur, P. H. Early-onset pauciarticular juvenile rheumatoid arthritis associated with human leukocyte antigen—DRw5, iritis, and antinuclear antibody. J. Clin. Invest. 66:426, 1980.

72. Glenner, G. G., Terry, W. D., and Isersky, C. Amyloidosis: Its nature and pathogenesis. Semin. Hematol. 10:65, 1973.

73. Globus, J. H. The pathologic findings in the heart muscle in progressive muscular dystrophy. Arch. Neurol. Psychiatry 9:59, 1923.

74. Goldberg, S. J., Feldman, L., Reinecke, C., Stern, L. Z., Sahn, D. J., and Allen, H. D. Echocardiographic determination of contraction and relaxation measurements of the left ventricular wall in normal subjects and patients with muscular dystrophy. Circulation 62:1061, 1980.

75. Good, R. A., Venters, H., Page, A. R., and Good, T. A. Diffuse connective tissue diseases

in childhood: With a special comment on connective tissue disease in patients with agammaglobulinemia. J. Lancet 81:192, 1961.

76. Goodman, H. B., and Dorney, E. R. Marfan's syndrome with massive calcification of the mitral annulus at age twenty-six. Am. J. Cardiol. 24:426, 1969.

77. Goyette, E. M., and Palmer, P. W. Cardiovascular lesions in arachnodactyly. Circulation 7:373, 1953.

78. Gregorini, L., Valentini, R., and Libretti, A. The vectorcardiogram in Friedreich's ataxia. Am. Heart J. 87:158, 1974.

79. Grokoest, A. W., Snyder, A. I., and Ragan, C. Some aspects of juvenile rheumatoid arthritis. Bull. Rheum. Dis. 8:147, 1957.

80. Grondin, C. M., Steinberg, C. L., and Edwards, J. E. Dissecting aneurysm complicating Marfan's syndrome (arachnodactyly) in a mother and son. Am. Heart J. 77:301, 1969.

81. Gruber, M. A., Graham, T. P., Jr., Engel, E., and Smith, C. Marfan syndrome with contractural arachnodactyly and severe mitral regurgitation in a premature infant. J. Pediatr. 93:80, 1978.

82. Hadley, R. N., and Hagstrom, J. W. C. Cardiac lesions in a patient with familial neurovisceral lipidosis (generalized gangliosidosis). Am. J. Clin. Pathol. 55:237, 1971.

83. Harvey, P. K. P., Jones, M. C., and Anderson, E. G. Pericardial abnormalities in Gaucher's disease. Br. Heart J. 31:603, 1969.

84. Hecht, F., and Beals, R. K. "New" syndrome of congenital contractural arachnodactyly originally described by Marfan in 1896. Pediatrics 49:574, 1972.

85. Helseth, H. K., Haglin, J. J., Monson, B. K., and Wickstrom, P. H. Results of composite graft replacement for aortic root aneurysms. J. Thorac. Cardiovasc. Surg. 80:754, 1980.

86. Herd, J. K., Subramanian, S., and Robinson, H. Type III mucopolysaccharidois: Report of a case with severe mitral valve involvement. J. Pediatr. 82:101, 1973.

87. Hewer, R. L., and Robinson, N. Diabetes mellitus in Friedreich's ataxia. J. Neurol. Neurosurg. Psychiatry 41:226, 1968.

88. Hewer, R. L. The heart in Friedreich's ataxia. Br. Heart J. 31:5, 1969.

89. Hirst, A. E., Jr., and Gore, I. Marfan's syndrome: A review. Prog. Cardiovasc. Dis. 16:187, 1973.

90. Hunter, C. H. A rare disease in two brothers. Proc. R. Soc Med. 10:104, 1917.

91. Hurler, G. Uber einen typ multipler Abartungen, vorwiegend am Skelettsystem. Z. Kinderheilkd. 24:220, 1919.

92. Inkley, S. R., Oldenberg, F. C., and Vignos, P. J., Jr. Pulmonary function in Duchenne muscular dystrophy related to stage of disease. Am. J. Med. 56:297, 1974.

93. Ivemark, B., and Thoren, C. The pathology of the heart in Friedreich's ataxia. Acta Med. Scand. 175:227, 1964.

94. Jackson, C. E., and Strehler, D. A. Limbgirdle muscular dystrophy: Clinical manifestations and detection of preclinical disease. Pediatrics 41:495, 1968.

95. James, T. N. Observations on the cardiovascular involvement, including the cardiac conduction system, in progressive muscular dystrophy. Am. Heart J. 63:48, 1962.

96. James, T. N. Observations on the cardiovascular involvement in Friedreich's ataxia. Am. Heart J. 66:164, 1963.

97. James, T. N., Frame, B. and Schatz, I. J. Pathology of cardiac conduction system in Marfan's syndrome. Arch. Intern. Med. 114:339, 1964.

98. Johnson, G. L., Vine, D. L., Cottrill, C. M., and Noonan, J. A. Echocardiographic mitral valve deformity in the mucopolysaccharidoses. Pediatrics 67:401, 1981.

99. Jordan, J. D. Cardiopulmonary manifestations of rheumatoid arthritis in childhood.

South. Med. J. 57:1273, 1964.

100. Josephson, M. E., Caracta, A. R., Gallagher, J. J., and Damato, A. N. Site of conduction disturbances in a family with myotonic dystrophy. Am. J. Cardiol. 32:114, 1973.

101. Kelly, T. E., Thomas, G. H., Taylor, H. A., McKusick, V. A., Sly, W. S., Glaser, J. H., Robinow, M., Luzzatti, L., Espiritu, C., Feingold, M., Bull, M. J., Ashenhurst, E. M., and Ives, E. J. Mucolipidosis III (pseudo-Hurler polydystrophy): Clinical and laboratory studies in a series of 12 patients. Johns Hopkins Med. J. 137:156, 1975.

102. Kelly, T. E., Bartoshesky, L., Harris, D. J., McCauley, R. G. K., Feingold, M., and Schott, G. Mucolipidosis I (acid neuraminidase deficiency). Three cases and delineation of the variability of the phenotype. Am. J. Dis. Child. 135:703, 1981.

103. Kennel, A. J., Titus, J. L., and Merideth, J. Pathologic findings in the atrioventricular conduction system in myotonic dystrophy. Mayo Clin. Proc. 49:838, 1974.

104. Kornreich, H. K., and Hanson, V. The rheumatic disease of childhood. Curr. Probl. Pediatr. 4(6):3, 1974.

105. Krongrad, E., and Joos, H. A. Friedreich's ataxia in childhood: Case report with possible myocardial infarction, cerebrovascular thromboembolization, and persistent elevation in cardiac specific LDH. Chest 61:644, 1972.

106. Krovetz, L. J., Lorincz, A. E., and Schiebler, G. L. Cardiovascular manifestations of the Hurler syndrome: Hemodynamic and angiocardiographic observations in 15 patients. Circulation 31:132, 1965.

107. Krovetz, L. J., Lorincz, A. E., and Schiebler, G. L. Cardiovascular manifestations of the Hunter-Hurler syndrome. In Heart Disease in Infants, Children, and Adolescents, edited by A. J. Moss and F. H. Adams. Williams & Wilkins, Baltimore, 1968, p. 916.

108. Laaksonsen, A. L. A prognostic study of juvenile rheumatoid arthritis: Analysis of 544 cases. Acta Paediatr. Scand. (Suppl.) 166:1, 1966.

109. Landing, B. H., Silverman, F. N., Craig, J. M., Jacobi, M. D., Lahey, M. E., and Chadwick, D. L. Familial neurovisceral lipidosis. Am. J. Dis. Child. 108:503, 1964.

110. Leon-Sotomayer, L., and Dietrich, R. A. Marfan syndrome with coarctation and aneurysms of aorta. Texas Med. 62:69, 1966.

111. Lewis, H. D., Jr., White, H. H., and Dunn, M. Refsum's syndrome. A neurological disease with interesting cardiovascular manifestations. Am. J. Cardiol. 17:128, 1966.

112. Lietman, P. S., and Bywaters, E. G. L. Pericarditis in juvenile rheumatoid arthritis. Pediatrics 32:855, 1963.

113. Mahoney, M. J., Haseltine, F. P., Hobbins, J. C., Banker, B. Q., Caskey, C. T., and Golbus, M. S. Prenatal diagnosis of Duchenne's muscular dystrophy. N. Engl. J. Med. 297:968, 1977.

114. Marfan, A. B. Un cas de deformation congenitale des quatre membres plus prononcee aux extremites characterisee par l'allongement des os avec un certain degre d'amincissement. Bull. Mem. Soc. Med. Hosp. Paris 13:220, 1896.

115. Martin, J. J., Leroy, J. G., Farriaux, J. P., Fontaine, G., Desnick, R. J., and Cabello, A. I. Cell disease (mucolipidosis II). A report on its pathology. Acta Neuropathol. 33:285, 1975.

116. Mayer, J. E., Lindsay, W. G., Wang, Y., Jorgensen, C. R., and Nicoloff, D. M. Composite replacement of the aortic valve and ascending aorta. J. Thorac. Cardiovasc. Surg. 76:816, 1978.

117. McDonald, G. R., Schaff, H. V., Pyeritz, R. E., McKusick, V. A., and Gott, V. L. Surgical management of patients with the Marfan syn-

drome and dilatation of the ascending aorta. J. Thorac. Cardiovasc. Surg. 81:180, 1981.

118. McKay, R., and Yacoub, M. H. Clinical and pathological findings in patients with "floppy" valves treated surgically. Circulation (Suppl. III):63, 1973.

119. McKusick, V. A. The mucopolysaccharidoses. In Heritable Disorders of Connective Tissue, ed. 4. C. V. Mosby, St. Louis, 1972, p. 521.

120. McKusick, V. A. The Marfan syndrome. In Heritable Disorders of Connective Tissue, ed. 4. C. V. Mosby, St. Louis, 1972, p. 61.

121. McKusick, V. A., Neufeld, E. F., and Kelly, T. E. The mucopolysaccharide storage diseases. In The Metabolic Basis of Inherited Disease, edited by J. B. Stanbury, J. B. Wyngaarden, and D. S. Frederickson, ed. 4. McGraw-Hill, New York, 1978, p. 1282.

122. McNamara, D. G., and Brewer, E. J., Jr. Carditis with rheumatoid arthritis. In Juvenile Rheumatoid Arthritis, edited by E. J. Brewer, Jr. W. B. Saunders, Philadelphia, 1970, p. 48.

123. Mehta, J., Tuna, N., Moller, J. H., and Desnick, R. J. Electrocardiographic and vectorcardiographic abnormalities in Fabry's disease. Am. Heart J. 93:699, 77.

115. Mehta, J., and Desnick, R. J. Abbreviated PR interval in mannosidosis. J. Pediatr. 92:599, 1978.

125. Mirhosseini, S. A., Holmes, L. B., and Walton, D. S. Syndrome of pigmentary retinal degeneration, cataract, microcephaly and severe mental retardation. J. Med. Genet. 9:193, 1972.

126. Molina, J. E., Northrup, W. F., Olson, F. R., and McBride, J. W. Acute aortic dissection in a patient with Marfan's syndrome and severe pectus excavatum. Minn. Med. 64:411, 1981.

127. Moothart, R. W., Spangler, R. D., and Blount, S. G., Jr. Echocardiography in aortic root dissection and dilatation. Am. J. Cardiol. 36:11, 1975.

128. Morpurgo, M., Finardi, G., Buelcke, G., Casaccia, M., Lissoni, A., and Rampulla, C. L'apparail cardiovasculaire dans la dystrophie musculaire progressive. Arch. Mal. Coeur 66:673, 1972.

129. Murdoch, J. L., Walker, B. A., Halpern, B. L., Kuzma, J. W., and McKusick, V. A. Life expectancy and causes of death in the Marfan syndrome. N. Engl. J. Med. 286:804, 1972.

130. Nadas, A. S., Alimurung, M. M., and Sieracki, L. A. Cardiac manifestations of Friedreich's ataxia. N. Engl. J. Med. 244:239, 1951.

131. Nadas, A. S., and Levy, J. M. Pericarditis in children. Am. J. Cardiol. 7:109, 1961.

132. Nanda, N. C., Gramiak, R., and Shah, P. M. Diagnosis of aortic root dissection by echocardiography. Circulation 48:506, 1973.

133. Nasrallah, A. T., Cooley, D. A., Goussous, Y., Hallman, G. L., Lufschanowski, R., and Leachman, R. D. Surgical experience in patients with Marfan's syndrome, ascending aortic aneurysm and aortic regurgitation. Am. J. Cardiol. 36:338, 1975.

134. Nelson, A. Personal communication.

135. Neufeld, E. F. Mucopolysaccharidoses: The biochemical approach. Hosp. Pract. 7:107, 1972.

136. Neufeld, E. F., and Cantz, M. The mucopolysaccharidoses studied in cell culture. In Lysosomes and Storage Diseases, edited by H. G. Hers and F. Van Hoof. Academic Press, New York, 1973, p. 261.

137. Novick, R., Adams, P., and Anderson, R. C. Cardiac manifestations of Friedreich's ataxia in children. Lancet 75:62, 1955.

138. Okada, R., Rosenthal, I. M., Scaravelli, G., and Lev, M. A histopathologic study of the heart in gargoylism. Arch. Pathol. 84:20, 1967.

139. Ose, L., and McKusick, V. A. Prophylactic use of propranolol in the Marfan syndrome

to prevent aortic dissection. Birth Defects 13:163, 1977.

140. Papaioannou, A. C., Augustsson, M. H., and Gasul, B. M. Early manifestations of the cardiovascular disorders in Marfan syndrome. Pediatrics 27:255, 1961.

141. Papaioannou, A. C., Matsaniotis, N., Cantez, T., and Durst, M. D. Marfan syndrome: Onset and development of cardiovascular lesions in Marfan syndrome. Angiology 21:580, 1970.

142. Payne, C. A., and Greenfield, J. C., Jr. Electrocardiographic abnormalities associated with myotonic dystrophy. Am. Heart J. 65:436, 1963.

143. Pearson, C. M. Muscular dystrophy: Review and recent observations. Am. J. Med. 35:632, 1963.

144. Perloff, J. K., deLeon, A. C., Jr., and O'Doherty, D. The cardiomyopathy of progressive muscular dystrophy. Circulation 33:625, 1966.

145. Perloff, J. K. Cardiomyopathy associated with heredofamilial neuromyopathic disease. Mod. Concepts Cardiovasc. Dis. 40:23, 1971.

146. Phornphutkul, C., Rosenthal, A., and Nadas, A. S. Cardiac manifestations of Marfan syndrome in infancy and childhood. Circulation 47:587, 1973.

147. Pickard, N. A., Gruemer, H. D., Verrill, H. L., Isaacs, E. R., Robinow, M., Nance, W. E., Myers, E. C., and Goldsmith, B. Systemic membrane defect in the proximal muscular dystrophies. N. Engl. J. Med. 299:841, 1978.

148. Pilz, H., vonFigura, K., and Goebel, H. H. Deficiency of arylsulfatase B in 2 brothers aged 40 and 38 years (Maroteaux-Lamy syndrome, type B). Ann. Neurol. 6:315, 1979.

149. Pirani, C. L., and Bennett, G. A., Rheumatoid arthritis: A report of three cases progressing from childhood and emphasizing certain systemic manifestations. Bull. Hosp. Joint Dis. 12:335, 1951.

150. Pitt, G. N. On a case of Friedreich's disease: It's clinical history and postmortem appearances. Guy's Hosp. Rep. 44:369, 1887.

151. Podolsky, S., and Sheremata, W. A. Insulin-dependent diabetes mellitus and Friedreich's ataxia in siblings. Metabolism 19:555, 1970.

152. Prackash, R., Atassi, A., Poske, R., and Rosen, K. M. Prevalence of pericardial effusion and mitral-valve involvement in patients with rheumatoid arthritis without cardiac symptoms: An echocardiographic evaluation. N. Engl. J. Med. 289:597, 1973.

153. Prystowsky, E. N., Pritchett, E. L. C., Roses, A. D., and Gallagher, J. The natural history of conduction system disease in myotonic muscular dystrophy as determined by serial electrophysiologic studies. Circulation 60: 1360, 1979.

154. Pyeritz, R. E., and McKusick, V. A. The Marfan syndrome: Diagnosis and management. N. Engl. J. Med. 300:772, 1979.

155. Rachelefsky, G. S., Terasaki, P. I., Katz, R., and Stiehm, E. R. Increased prevalance of W27 in juvenile rheumatoid arthritis. N. Engl. J. Med. 290:892, 1974.

156. Raghib, G., Jue, K. L., Anderson, R. C., and Edwards, J. E. Marfan's syndrome with mitral insufficiency. Am. J. Cardiol. 16:127, 1965.

157. Read, R. C., Thal, A. P., and Wendt, V. E. Symptomatic valvular myxomatous transformation (the floppy valve syndrome). A possible forme fruste of the Marfan syndrome. Circulation 32:897, 1965.

158. Reitman, M. L., Varki, A., and Kornfeld, S. Fibroblasts from patients with I-cell disease and pseudo-Hurler polydystrophy are deficient in uridine 5'-diphosphate-N-acetylglucosamine: Glycoprotein N-acetylglucosami-

nylphosphotransferase activity. J. Clin. Invest. 67:1574, 1981.

159. Roberts, W. C., and Frederickson, D. S. Gaucher's disease of the lung causing severe pulmonary hypertension with associated acute recurrent pericarditis. Circulation 35:783, 1967.

160. Rodriguez-Torres, R., Schneck, L., and Kleinberg, W. Electrocardiographic and biochemical abnormalities in Tay-Sachs disease. Bull. N.Y. Acad. Med. 47:717, 1971.

161. Roses, A. D., Herbstreith, M. H., and Appel, S. H. Membrane protein kinase alteration in Duchenne muscular dystrophy. Nature 254:350, 1975.

162. Roses, A. D., Roses, M. J., Miller, S. E., Hull, K. L., Jr., and Appel, S. H. Carrier detection in Duchenne muscular dystrophy. N. Engl. J. Med. 294:193, 1976.

163. Roses, A. D., Roses, M. J., Nicholson, G. A., and Roe, C. R. Lactate dehydrogenase isoenzyme 5 in detecting carriers of Duchenne muscular dystrophy. Neurology 27:414, 1977.

164. Ruschampt, D. G., Thilenius, O. G., and Cassels, D. E. Friedreich's ataxia associated with idiopathic subaortic stenosis. Am. Heart J. 84:95, 1972.

165. Salle, V. Uber einen Fall von angeborener abnormer Grosse der Extremitaten mit einen an Akromegalie erinnernden Symptomenkomplex. Jahrb. Kinderheilkd. 75:540, 1912.

166. Sanyal, S. K., Johnson, W. W., Thapar, M. K., and Pitner, S. E. An ultrastructural basis for electrocardiographic alterations associated with Duchenne's progressive muscular dystrophy. Circulation 57:1122, 1978.

167. Sanyal, S. K., Leung, R. F. K., Tierney, R. C., Gilmartin, R., and Pitner, S. Mitral valve prolapse syndrome in children with Duchenne's progressive muscular dystrophy. Pediatrics 63:116, 1979.

168. Schaller, J., and Wedgewood, R. J. Juvenile rheumatoid arthritis: A review. Pediatrics 50:940, 1972.

169. Schieken, R. M., Kerber, R. E., Ionasescu, V. V., and Zellweger, H. Cardiac manifestations of mucopolysaccharidoses. Circulation 52: 700, 1975.

170. Schilero, A. J., Antzis, E., and Dunn, J. Friedreich's ataxia and its cardiac manifestations. Am. Heart J. 44:805, 1952.

171. Seay, A. R., Ziter, F. A., and Thompson, J. A. Cardiac arrest during induction of anesthesia in Duchenne muscular dystrophy. J. Pediatr. 93:88, 1978.

172. Segal, B., Kasparian, H., and Likoff, W. Mitral regurgitation in a patient with Marfan syndrome. Dis. Chest 41:457, 1962.

173. Simpson, J. W., Nora, J. J., and McNamara, D. G. Marfan's syndrome and mitral valve disease. Acute surgical emergencies. Am. Heart J. 77:96, 1969.

174. Siqueira-Filho, A. G., Cunha, C. L. P., Tajik, A. J., Seward, J. B., Schattenberg, T. T., and Giuliani, E. R. M-mode and two-dimensional echocardiographic features in cardiac amyloidosis. Circulation 63:188, 1981.

175. Skyring, A., and McKusick, V. A., Clinical, genetic and electrocardiographic studies in childhood muscular dystrophy. Am. J. Med. Sci. 242:534, 1961.

176. Slucka, C. The electrocardiogram in Duchenne progressive muscular dystrophy. Circulation 38:933, 1968.

177. Smith, E. R., Sangalang, V. E., and Heffernan, L. P. Hypertrophic cardiomyopathy: The heart disease in Friedreich's ataxia. Am. Heart J. 94:428, 1977.

178. Soman, V. R., Breton, G., Hershkowitz, M., and Mark, H. Bacterial endocarditis of mitral valve in Marfan syndrome. Br. Heart J.

36:1247, 1974.

179. Soulie, P., Vernant, P., Gaudeau, S., Calisti, G., Joly, F., Bouchard, F., and Forman, J. Le coeur dans la maladie de Friedreich: Etude hemodynamique droite et gauche. Mal. Cardiovasc. 7:369, 1966.

180. Sovik, O., Lie, S. O., Fluge, G., and Van Hoof, F. Fucosidosis: Severe phenotype with survival to adult age. Eur. J. Pediatr. 135:211, 1980.

181. Spangler, R. D., Nora, J. J., Lortscher, R. H., Wolfe, R. R., and Okin, J. T. Echocardiography in Marfan's syndrome. Chest 69:72, 1976.

182. Spranger, J. W., Koch, F., McKusick, V. A., Natzschka, J. Wiedemann, H. R., and Zellweger, H. Mucopolysaccharidosis VI (Maroteaux-Lamy's disease). Helv. Paediatr. Acta. 25:337, 1970.

183. Still, G. F. On a form of chronic joint disease in children. Med. Chir. Trans. Lond. 80:9, 1897 (reprinted in Arch. Dis. Child. 16:156, 1941).

184. Strauss, R. G., Schubert, W. K., and McAdams, A. J. Amyloidosis in childhood. J. Pediatr. 74:272, 1969.

185. Symbas, P. N., Baldwin, B. J., Silverman, M. E., and Galambos, J. T. Marfan's syndrome with aneurysm of ascending aorta and aortic regurgitation. Surgical treatment and new histochemical observations. Am. J. Cardiol. 25:483, 1970.

186. Thilenius, O. G., and Grossman, B. J. Friedreich's ataxia with heart disease in children. Pediatrics 27:246, 1961.

187. Thompson, J. N., Finley, S. C., Lorincz, A. E., and Finley, W. H. Absence of α-L-iduronidase activity in various tissues from two sibs affected with presumably the Hurler-Scheie syndrome. In Disorders of Connective Tissue, edited by D. Bergsma, Vol. 11. National Foundation, March of Dimes, New York, 1975, p. 341.

188. Thoren, C. Cardiomyopathy in Friedreich's ataxia. Acta Paediatr. 53:1, 1964.

189. VandeKamp, J. J. P. The Sanfilippo syndrome. A clinical and genetical study of 75 patients in the Netherlands Thesis, University of Leiden, 1979.

190. Van der Hauwaert, L. G., and Dumoulin, M. Hypertrophic cardiomyopathy in Friedreich's ataxia. Br. Heart J. 38:1291, 1976.

191. Van Hoof, F. Mucopolysaccharidoses. In Lysosomes and Storage Diseases, edited by H. G. Hers and F. Van Hoof. Academic Press, New York, 1973, p. 218.

192. Wahi, P. L., Bhargava, K. C., and Mohindra, S. Cardiorespiratory changes in progressive muscular dystrophy. Br. Heart J. 33:533, 1971.

193. Walsh, H. Some clinical features of juvenile rheumatoid arthritis. Med. J. Aust. 1:507, 1962.

194. Wanderman, K. L., Goldstein, M. S., and Faber, J. Cor pulmonale secondary to severe kyphoscoliosis in Marfan's syndrome. Chest 67:250, 1975.

195. Welsh, J. D., Hasse, G. R., and Bynum, T. E. Myotonic muscular dystrophy: Systemic manifestations. Arch. Intern. Med. 114:669, 1964.

196. Welsh, J. D., Lynn, T. N., and Hasse, G. R. Cardiac findings in 73 patients with muscular dystrophy. Arch. Intern. Med. 112:199, 1963.

197. Westwood, M. Endocardial fibroelastosis and Niemann-Pick disease. Br. Heart J. 39:1394, 1977.

198. Wilson, C. S., Mankin, H. T., and Pluth, J. R. Aortic stenosis and mucopolysaccharidosis. Ann. Intern. Med. 92:496, 1980.

199. Zundel, W. S., and Tyler, F. H. The muscular dystrophies. N. Engl. J. Med. 273:537, 1965.

40

Atherosclerosis

Guy A. Carter, M.D., and Ronald M. Lauer, M.D.

Arteriosclerosis is a generic term describing disorders resulting in thickening and induration of the arterial wall. Atherosclerosis is one form of arteriosclerosis that underlies most occlusive arterial disease in adults and is the leading cause of death in the United States. The diseases most frequently produced by atherosclerosis are coronary heart disease, stroke, claudication, and renal vascular insufficiency. In a study of 691 autopsies of persons over 20 years of age at death in a community of 30,000, the cause of death was coronary heart disease 32% of the time. This accounted for 40% of all male and 30% of all female deaths.[70] It has also been found that 25% of individuals with atherosclerotic heart disease experiencing their first heart attack will die within 3 hours, often before medical aid may be sought.[42] Although the dramatic symptoms of arterial occlusive disease seldom occur in the childhood years, there are indications that origins of the adult diseases produced by atherosclerosis are developing during the pediatric years. Evidence that atherosclerosis occurs and progresses during childhood comes from autopsy series of children and young men dying of unrelated disease and war injuries.[27, 41, 56] The results of the pathologic study of men killed in the Korean War[27] was significant in its pediatric implications. Of American soldiers who died at an average age of 22 years, 50% had grossly visible atheroma of the aortic wall, and the lumen of at least one coronary artery was reduced by 50% in 10% of those studied. In contrast, no similar lesions were found in the aortas of Chinese or Korean soldiers autopsied at the same time. In similar studies conducted by the Air Forces, 222 autopsies were done on men with an average age of 28 years.[32] Seventy percent had demonstrable coronary atherosclerosis and 21% had actual narrowing of the coronary lumen. These observations that show the disease process so well established in young adults suggest that its origins may develop during the pediatric years, and the pathologic evidence in children supports this view.[74]

PATHOLOGY

This disorder is a nodular type of arteriosclerosis. The early appearance of the atherosclerotic process in childhood has been described by Strong and McGill.[73, 74] Most frequently, the earliest stage described is the fatty streak. This lesion is present in the aorta of some infants, and in many children under the age of 3, and it is found in all children over the age of 3 years. Within the coronary arteries, the fatty streak is rare before age 10 but becomes more frequent after 10 years of age and is nearly always found after the age 20. Aortic fatty streaks are found in nearly all races of children to nearly the same extent and may or may not be important in the later development of atherosclerosis. Coronary lesions, however, show greater variability in populations and tend to parallel the development of raised adult lesions.[55] Typically, the frequency of aortic fatty streaks increases from involvement of 7 to 19% intima at 10 to 14 years to a peak of 20 to 28% of intima involved in most populations between 15 and 29 years, but decreasing thereafter.[30, 67]

The gross appearance of the typical fatty streak is characterized by a diffuse yellow stain in the intima of the artery associated with only slight intimal thickening (Figs. 40.1 and 40.2A). Staining of the vessel with a lipophilic stain facilitates visualization, with the fatty streaks becoming apparent as darkly stained areas of the intima. Microscopically, although some lipid droplets may be found extracellularly in the intima, the vast majority of the lipids will be found intracellularly within foam cells.[30, 31] Focal areas of extracellular lipid droplets have been noted both on light and electron microscopy in areas of grossly normal intima, and may be an early stage in the evolution of the fatty streak. Frequently, some thickening of the intima in association with the presence of the foam cells is seen. The foam cells are characteristically large, rounded cells containing numerous uniform-size lipid droplets. The predominant cell in the fatty streak studied by electron microscopy is a smooth muscle cell or foam cell, containing lipid droplets in small cisternae of agranular endoplasmic reticulum.[30]

The first appearance of a raised atherosclerotic lesion occurs with the development of the fibrous plaque (Fig. 40.2B). In general, the first appearance of the fibrous plaque is at a later age than that of the fatty streak, although the latter can occur at all ages. This lesion also has a better correlation with the later location and development of atherosclerosis than the fatty streak. Unlike the fatty streak, the fibrous plaque shows a marked ethnic and sex variation which parallels the incidence of atherosclerotic heart disease. These first fibrous lesions begin to appear at about 20 to 25 years of age.[74]

On examination of fresh aortas, fibrous plaques appear as firm elevated intimal lesions which are pale grey, glistening, and translucent, often containing an amorphous yellow core. After staining with lipophilic stain they may be partially or completely covered with lipophilic deposits. Microscopic studies of these lesions show the same structures noted in the fatty streaks but in different proportions. The fibrous plaque contains more collagen, with a cap of collagen overlying the lipid-containing cells in the intima. This collagen cap is composed of collagen fibers, small elastic fibers, unidentified fusiform cells, and numerous extracellular bodies. The lipid core in the typical fibrous plaque, however, contains few foam cells. These cells can be seen about the shoulder of the lesion or in the cap of mixed lesions. In early plaques, the lipid may be found as perifibrous droplets. With later development the core breaks up, and the lipid droplets become more pronounced, developing in the late lesions into an amorphous lipid core.[67]

In mid adult life the complicated lesions begin to appear, with the development of intimal ulceration, thrombotic caps, intraplaque hemmorrhages, and calcification (Fig. 40.3). These lesions appear to resemble the late fibrous plaque and result in narrowing or occlusion of the coronary, cerebral, ileofemoral, and renal arteries.

Although it might be assumed that there is a progression of the lesion from the early perifibrous lipid droplets to fatty streaks to fibrous plaque to complicated lesions, analysis of the lipid composition of these different lesions suggests that there may be a different and separate origin of some of these lesions.[19, 67] The cholesterol content of the foam cell lesion is about 21 mg/100 mg of dry tissue, with about 20% of this free cholesterol. There are also about 6 mg/100 mg of dry tissue phospholipid. The fibrous plaque has 40 mg/100 mg of dry tissue of cholesterol with one-third of this as free cholesterol and 10 mg/100 mg of dry tissue of phospholipid. The cholesterol ester fatty acid in the fatty streak lesion was found to be 53% oleic (18:1) and 13% linoleic (18.2), whereas in the fibrous plaque 25% was oleic, and 43% was linoleic. The fatty acid composition of the fatty streak thus varies from the serum composition and occurs with low plasma cholesterol levels, suggesting that there is a local active synthesis of cholesterol, while the composition of the fibrous plaque suggests that the lipid accumulation is related to the lipid infiltration from the circulation.

LIPIDS AND THE ATHEROSCLEROTIC PROCESS

Although development of an atherosclerotic lesion in man and other mammals involves three basic changes (proliferation of smooth muscle cells, the deposition of both intra- and extracellular lipids, especially cholesterol as cholesteryl esters, and the accumulation of an extracellular matrix of collagen, elastin and proteoglycans), the accumulation of cholesterol in the arterial wall is the most impressive and consistent feature of the developing atheroma and appears to play a crucial role in the genesis and continuing development of atherosclerosis. Observations that have supported the role of lipids in atherosclerosis include: no atherosclerosis without the accumulation of lipids in arterial tissue; atherosclerosis that is more common and severe in populations consuming a high cholesterol diet; and the feeding of cholesterol to study animals, which can induce atherosclerosis, which will regress when the cholesterol feeding is discontinued and the plasma cholesterol level falls.[4, 19, 39]

Cholesterol is transported within the blood stream with triglycerides, phospholipids, and the apoproteins as macromolecular complexes identified as lipoproteins. There are

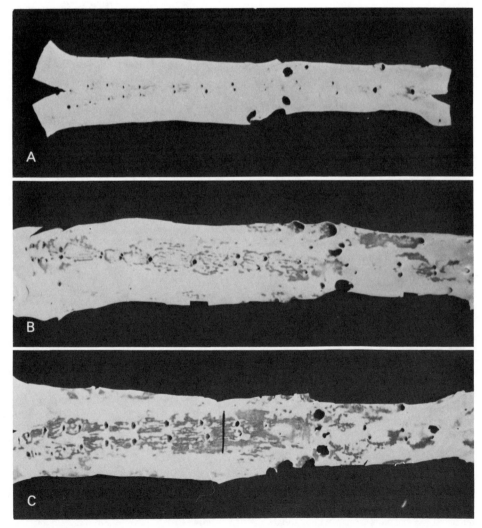

Fig. 40.1 Aortas stained with Sudan IV. (*A*) Thirteen-year-old boy. (*B*) Nineteen-year-old boy and (*C*) Twenty-year-old boy. These represent the average extent of fatty streaking in the 10 to 14, 15 to 20, and 20 to 29 year age groups, respectively (Photographs courtesy of H. C. McGill, M.D., University of Texas, San Antonio, Texas.)

four lipoproteins which can be separated and characterized from those of normal human plasma. These can be named according to their electrophoretic mobility as chylomicrons, beta-, pre-beta-, and alpha-lipoproteins; or they can be identified by their density in graded salt solutions with ultracentrifugation as chylomicrons, very low density (VLDL), low density (LDL), and high density (HDL) lipoproteins (Fig. 40.4). The two systems are interchangeable in that the chylomicrons are identical in both systems. Pre-beta is equivalent to VLDL, beta is equivalent to LDL, and alpha

is equivalent to HDL. Increases in LDL particularly, but also in HDL, VLDL, or chylomicrons alone or in combination, may elevate the total plasma cholesterol levels. Hypertriglyceridemia is most typically the result of elevations in circulating chylomicrons or VLDL, or both. A classification of the hyperlipoproteinemias based on five patterns of elevation of the lipoproteins has been suggested by Fredrickson and Levy[28] and is shown in Figure 40.5.

The basic function of the lipoproteins is the transport of the water-insoluble lipids, most particularly, the energy-rich

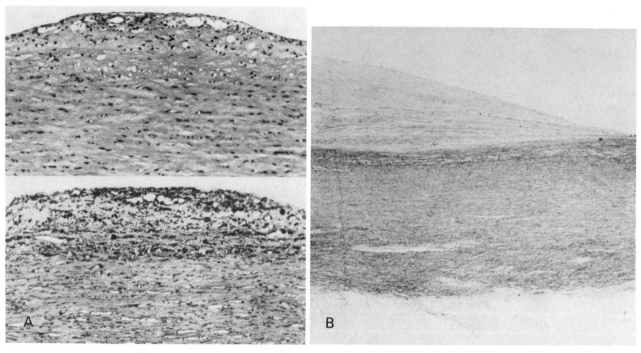

Fig. 40.2   Microscopic sections of a fatty streak and fibrous plaque. (*A*) Fatty streak from aorta in Figure 46.1*C*. (*Top*) Hematoxylin and eosin stain. Large foam cells and fatty vacuoles are indicated by the large empty spaces. (*Bottom*) Oil red O stain of a frozen section adjacent to above. Fat shows as black droplets mostly within cells. (Photographs courtesy of H. C. McGill, M.D., University of Texas, San Antonio, Texas.) (*B*) Hematoxylin and eosin stain of a fibrous plaque. Note the absence of large lipid-containing foam cells as seen in Figure 46.2*A*, and the increased thickness of the collagen cap. (Photograph courtesy of G. C. McMillan, M.D., Atherogenesis Branch, National Heart and Lung Institute (now, National Heart, Lung, and Blood Institute), National Institutes of Health, Bethesda, Md.)

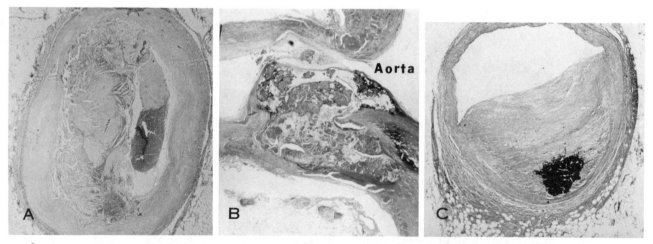

Fig. 40.3   Complex atheromatous plaque in a coronary artery. (*A*) Cross-section of organized ruptured atheroma with platelet and propogated thrombus overlaying lipid atheroma. (*B*) Longitudinal section of organized calcified atheroma occluding the orifice of a coronary artery. (*C*) Cross-section of a densely fibrous plaque with calcification in a coronary artery. (Photographs courtesy of G. C. McMillan, M.D., Atherogenesis Branch, National Heart and Lung Institute (now, National Heart, Lung, and Blood Institute) National Institutes of Health, Bethesda, Md.)

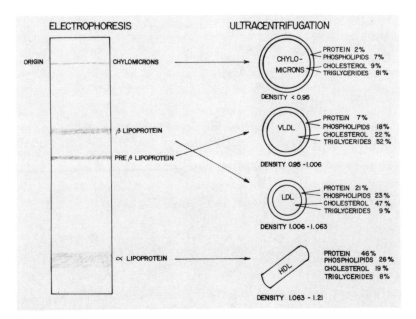

Fig. 40.4 Lipoprotein classification by electrophoresis and density gradients. *VLDL*, very low density lipoproteins; *LDL*, low density lipoproteins; *HDL*, high density lipoproteins.

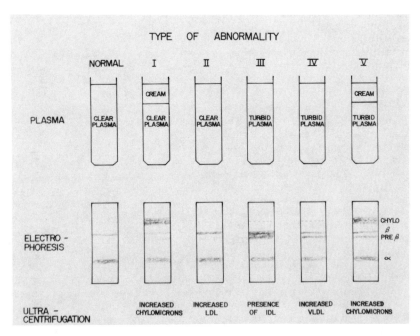

Fig. 40.5 Fredrickson and Levy[28] classification of the hyperlipoproteinemias. *IDL*, intermediate density lipoprotein; other abbreviations as in Figure 40.4.

triglycerides, from sites of synthesis to tissue sites of metabolic use, storage, or catabolism and elimination. In this function, the different lipoproteins subserve differing roles in concert with each other. The chylomicrons are formed within the intestinal mucosa for the transport of dietary (exogenous) triglycerides and thus are generally present in the circulation only following meals. VLDL is synthesized in the liver for the transport of endogenously formed triglycerides and provides one of the major resources of energy in the fasting state. LDL appears to originate as the end product of the catabolism of the VLDL particle and contains the greatest proportion of the circulating plasma cholesterol.

HDL constitutes an entirely different class of lipoproteins which does not have the transport of lipids as their primary role. Rather, HDL contains the peptides necessary for the regulation of major enzymes necessary for the catabolism of the triglyceride-rich lipoproteins, and perhaps is also involved in the transport of tissue cholesterol back to the liver.[61, 68, 69]

As the different lipoprotein classes subserve different functions, it is not unexpected that they would have differing effects in the observed development and progression of atherosclerosis. Of the lipoproteins, LDL particularly and, to a lesser extent, VLDL are the more atherogenic, whereas

TABLE 40.1   THE LIPOPROTEINS

Lipoprotein	Origin	Catabolism	Major Component	Clinical Features of Excess Concentrations in Circulation
Chylomicron	Intestinal mucosal Cells	Peripheral tissue through action of lipoprotein lipase	Exogenous (dietary) triglyceride	Eruptive xanthoma; pancreatitis
VLDL	Liver	Peripheral tissue through action of lipoprotein lipase	Endogenous triglyceride formed from glucose and free fatty acids	Glucose intolerance; eruptive xanthoma; possible early atherosclerosis and strokes
IDL	VLDL	Unclear; possible through action of lipoprotein lipase and/or hepatic lipase	Endogenous triglyceride and cholesterol	Glucose intolerance; early atherosclerosis; tuboeruptive and palmar xanthoma
LDL	VLDL & IDL	Unclear	Cholesterol	Early atherosclerosis; planar, tuberous, and tendinous xanthoma
HDL	Liver, possible GI tract	Unclear	Apoproteins	None

chylomicrons do not appear to be significantly atherogenic (although the chylomicron remnants may be), and HDL appears to serve a protective role[37, 60, 78] (Table 40.1).

In the absence of hypertriglyceridemia, LDL carries the bulk of the plasma cholesterol (70 to 80%), whether the plasma cholesterol is normal or elevated. The origin of tissue cholesterol is believed to be the circulating cholesterol contained in the LDL particle. This is supported by the presence of LDL antigens in tissues and atheromas[39] and the evidence from Brown and Golstein[11] suggesting that peripheral tissues are the major site of LDL catabolism.

Familial Hypercholesterolemia (Familial Hyperlipoproteinemia Type IIa)

This is an autosomal dominant genetic disease characterized by an elevated plasma cholesterol level with a normal plasma triglyceride level. On ultracentrifugation, this presents as an increased concentration of the β-lipoprotein.

It is estimated that one of every 250 to 300 individuals is heterozygous and one of every million individuals is homozygous for this disease. The homozygous form is characterized by profound elevations of plasma cholesterol levels (often in excess of 800 mg/dl), the appearance of tendon and tuberous xanthoma in infancy or early childhood, and rapidly progressive atherosclerotic coronary heart disease. Corneal arcus may occur, and aortic stenosis and mitral insufficiency due to massive lipid accumulations often occur. A polyarthritic syndrome mimicking acute arthritis has been seen and has been diagnosed as acute rheumatic fever when noted in association with mitral insufficiency. The sedimentation rate is elevated probably because of the excess LDL rather than an inflammatory process.[34] In these afflicted children, death usually occurs by the 3rd decade and has occurred at as early as 4 years of age from massive myocardial infarction.

Brown and Goldstein,[11] in studies using skin fibroblast cultures obtained from children with this disorder, have ascribed the manifestations of this disease to a genetically determined abnormality of binding capacity for LDL on the cell surface membrane. This results in a decreased feedback inhibition of the enzyme 3-hydroxy-3-methylglutaryl coenzyme A (HMG CoA) reductase, the rate-controlling enzyme in the cholesterol biosynthetic pathway, which results in increased plasma cholesterol levels by continued oversynthesis of cholesterol by body tissues. On the other hand, sterol balance and turnover studies conducted on afflicted children by Carter et al.[14] have suggested that there is a

TABLE 40.2   PLASMA AND LOW DENSITY LIPOPROTEIN (LDL) LIPID CONCENTRATIONS IN INFANTS[a]

Source	No.	Lipid Levels in mg/dl (Mean ± SD)			
		Birth			One Year
		C	T	LDL	C
Glueck et al.[33]	1800	64 ± 19		37 ± 21	
Darmady et al.[18, b]	302	78 ± 23			191 ± 36
Barnes et al.[8]	747	76 ± 19	52 ± 18		
Greten et al.[38, b]	1323	60 ± 20		35 ± 12	
Kwiterovich et al.[46]	36	74 ± 11	37 ± 15	31 ± 6	
Goldstein et al.[35]	2000	82 ± 20	42 ± 25		
Tsang et al.[76]	56				138 ± 29

[a] C, cholesterol; T, triglyceride; LDL, low density lipoprotein.

[b] Serum levels given. Both plasma and serum can be used for cholesterol determinations; plasma levels are usually lower. Since different laboratories may also use different methods for determining the cholesterol concentration in either plasma or serum, the degree of correspondence between laboratories also depends on the methods used.

defect in the body's ability to eliminate cholesterol. This occurs both as decreased neutral steroid excretion, most profoundly, as decreased acid steroid excretion. In these patients, the observed total body synthesis (from both the sterol balance and from isotopic cholesterol turnover studies) is decreased from normal rather than increased.

The heterozygous form of hyperlipoproteinemia type IIa is less severely afflicting and is frequently asymptomatic during childhood. Tuberous and tendon xanthoma over areas of increased tissue stress and trauma (extensor surfaces of the hands, elbows, feet, and Achilles tendon) may be found in the 2nd or 3rd decades of life. Skin fibroblasts from the heterozygote show a partial defect in the HMG CoA reductase activity.

Cord Blood Studies. There have been several studies directed toward the earliest identification of hyperlipidemia. Since the lipoproteins of the cord blood are fetal in origin, screening of the cord blood has been suggested as a way of detecting those children with type II hyperlipoproteinemia at the earliest age. These mean total cholesterol or LDL cholesterol values are summarized in Tables 40.2 and 40.3.

From these studies, a total plasma cholesterol above 100 mg/dl[33] or LDL cholesterol above 41 mg/dl[46] have been presented as the upper limits of normal. Recent studies indicate that cord blood LDL cholesterol levels are most likely not predictive of the levels these children will have after age 1. Kwiterovich et al.[46] identified 12 children considered to have hyperbetalipoprotein at birth on the basis of their LDL cholesterol level, of which only one was normal at age 1. In a longitudinal study, Darmady et al.[18] reported that only 5 of 30 children who had elevated cord cholesterol levels had elevated levels at age 1 and that the distribution of cholesterol values at age 1 mimicked the distribution of their normal population. In a Cincinnati study,[76] 48 of 56 children with elevated cord cholesterol levels were restudied at age 1 and had normal cholesterol levels. Similarly, in a more recent study of Danish children[3] no significant relationship was found between a child's cord blood LDL cholesterol level and cholesterol level at ages 6 to 10 months or 3 to 4 years. Also, in two children born of homozygous type IIa mothers, the cord plasma and LDL cholesterol levels were normal, even though the mothers' levels were excessively elevated.[15]

Familial Combined Hyperlipidemia (Type IIb)

This is the most common form of hyperlipidemia found in the families of subjects suffering myocardial infarction. Affected family members characteristically have elevated levels of both cholesterol and triglycerides. However, increased cholesterol or increased triglyceride levels alone are frequently observed. This disorder may be the result of the variable expression of a single autosomal dominant gene.[36] It usually does not cause difficulty until the 4th or 5th decade, when coronary artery disease is the most common associated disorder. There are subjects whose serum triglycerides are elevated, or who have hypercholesterolemia with or without hypertriglyceridemia in whom no known mode of inheritance can be documented and who frequently suffer myocardial infarction in early adult life. Hypercholesterolemia may also occur secondarily to other diseases such as nephrosis or hypothyroidism.

Familial Hypertriglyceridemia (Type IV)

This disease is characterized by an increased plasma triglyceride (150 to 1000 mg/dl) level with a lesser increase in the plasma cholesterol level (125 to 350 mg/dl). On plasma ultracentrifugation this presents as an increased VLDL triglyceride level with normal LDL and chylomicrons, and on electrophoresis as an increased concentration of the pre-β-lipoprotein only.

Elevated plasma triglyceride levels may not appear until after the childhood years. The primary metabolic defect in this disorder is a decreased clearance of triglyceride from the VLDL particle by the body tissue. No specific enzymatic defect has been identified.

Type I, III, and V Hyperlipoproteinemia

These are very uncommon disorders.

Type I. This presents in infancy. It causes no increased propensity for vascular disease. The disease is clinically characterized by abdominal pain, pancreatitis, hepatosplenomegaly, eruptive xanthoma, and lipemia retinalis. The blood shows a cream layer over clear plasma on standing. This is the result of a massive accumulation of chylomicrons

TABLE 40.3   PLASMA AND LIPOPROTEIN LIPIDS IN SCHOOLCHILDREN

Source	Age	Lipid Levels in mg/dl (Mean ± SD)[a]							
		Plasma		VLDL		LDL		HDL	
		C	T	C	T	C	T	C	T
Boys									
Morrison et al.[59]	6–11 white	160(25)	55(21)			95(24)		56(11)	
	12–17 white	157(25)	70(33)			96(23)		51(12)	
	6–11 black	167(29)	52(17)			98(26)		62(12)	
	12–17 black	159(30)	60(21)			97(29)		54(12)	
Ellefson et al.[26]	6–10	159(200)	52(96)	6(20)	23(60)	104(140)	15(26)	53(68)	8(13)
	11–14	156(200)	54(115)	10(23)	30(85)	98(141)	15(23)	45(65)	8(13)
	15–18	153(200)	64(139)	15(30)	41(104)	95(136)	15(24)	41(57)	7(11)
Carter[15]	5–8	160(21)	46.7	8(7)	15.7	101(17)	18.4	59(9)	4.2
	9–11	167(28)	47.9	8(5)	16.9	104(25)	17.7	55(11)	5.5
	12–14	157(27)	48.4	7(5)	20.3	97(24)	15.6	52(10)	5.7
	15–17	161(17)	51.2	9(7)	31.2	106(12)	17.2	46(7)	5.9
Girls									
Morrison et al.[59]	6–11 white	161(22)	71(28)			99(20)		51(10)	
	12–17 white	157(24)	72(28)			94(21)		52(11)	
	6–11 black	168(21)	60(27)			102(20)		58(10)	
	12–17 black	164(23)	65(24)			100(24)		56(12)	
Ellefson et al.[26]	6–10	160(208)	57(107)	8(20)	26(78)	107(143)	16(27)	50(66)	8(13)
	11–14	157(207)	67(116)	12(24)	40(85)	98(143)	17(26)	44(63)	9(14)
	15–18	163(215)	58(114)	14(28)	34(84)	101(145)	15(25)	47(64)	8(13)
Carter[15]	5–8	161(29)	48.2	8(6)	16.1	102(30)	19.3	49(11)	4.1
	9–11	166(22)	63.4	11(9)	27.6	105(21)	20.2	50(11)	5.8
	12–14	166(22)	59.4	8(6)	26.8	107(23)	18.6	49(8)	7.2
	15–17	162(23)	56.6	8(8)	25.4	102(20)	17.1	51(10)	6.7

[a] Data from Ellefson et al. presented as median + 95th percentile. Triglyceride data from Carter calculated as geometric mean; thus, SD is not derived. Abbreviations are as previously defined in text and Table 40.2.

in the fasting plasma. Chylomicrons can be identified at the origin of the electrophoretic strip. They are rich in triglycerides and poor in cholesterol, so that their accumulation in substantial quantities in the plasma results in profound hypertriglyceridemia (greater than 1500 mg/dl and usually between 5000 and 10,000 mg/dl) with a much lesser degree of hypercholesterolemia (150 to 500 mg per dl).[50]

Type III Hyperlipoproteinemia. This is characterized by both increased plasma cholesterol and triglyceride levels similar to levels seen in hyperlipoproteinemia type IIb, but presenting as an intermediate density lipoprotein (floating β) which separates on ultracentrifugation at a density of VLDL (0.95 to 1.006) but with cholesterol and triglyceride proportions and electrophoretic mobility more like LDL. On electrophoresis, this presents as a single broad band occupying the areas of both the β and the pre-β-lipoproteins. An association with coronary heart disease has been demonstrated in this disorder.

Type V Hyperlipoproteinemia. This usually does not begin until early adult life. However, several teenagers with the disorder have been found. The mode of inheritance is not established. A family history of diabetes is often obtained. This pattern can be seen in childhood secondary to diabetic acidosis and the nephrotic syndrome. The pattern consists of an increased concentration of VLDL and fasting chylomicronemia which results in lipemic plasma with an upper cream layer. The triglyceride levels are invariably elevated between 500 and 6500 mg/dl with the cholesterol levels between 150 and 1500 mg/dl.[50] This disorder is, to a lesser extent, associated with an increased frequency of coronary artery disease and is associated with chronic pancreatitis.

CORONARY RISK FACTORS

The development of the present concepts of "risk factors" was derived from a number of population studies, including those in Framingham, Massachusetts,[75] and Tecumseh, Michigan.[21] From such studies, a list of factors which are predictive of the development of coronary heart disease have been found. The presence of a particular factor does not imply that it is a causal agent of atherosclerosis, but by its presence or absence, it alters the probability of the development of atherosclerosis, whatever its etiology. Three major risk factors have been delineated (hypercholesterolemia, smoking, and hypertension), and a series of other risk factors less closely correlated with atherosclerosis have also been identified (obesity, physical inactivity, diabetes mellitus, rapid pulse rate, family history of coronary heart disease, and some psychological factors). Some of these risk factors cannot readily be altered or modified but must be recognized, such as: increasing age, male gender, and a positive family history of coronary heart disease. Others, such as: elevated plasma or LDL cholesterol, hypertension, smoking, glucose intolerance (diabetes), and obesity can be altered or modified. Evidence is developing that modification of the risk factors may decrease the risk of coronary events.[45, 64] In addition, the presence of higher levels of HDL cholesterol may be a beneficial risk factor and is associated with a decreased incidence of coronary heart disease.[37, 60, 72, 78]

In combination, these risk factors are additive. For example, the combination of hypercholesterolemia, hypertension, and cigarette smoking increases the incidence of ischemic heart disease eightfold over that of men with none of these factors, fivefold over that for any one factor, and 2½ times greater than with any two factors.[75] Predictive data about the development of atherosclerosis has not been gathered from childhood populations. However, because many of these variables increase with age, the application of adult risk factors to children seems appropriate.

Hypercholesterolemia

Of the risk factors, the plasma cholesterol level is one of the most significant predictors for the development of coronary heart disease. In a comparison of persons over 40 years of age, a three- to fourfold increase in the incidence of coronary heart disease is noted if the cholesterol level is 300 mg/dl rather than 200 mg per dl.[25] The very rapid development of atherosclerotic heart disease in those individuals with the homozygous form of familial hypercholesterolemia who have plasma cholesterol levels of 800 to 1000 mg/dl,[34] also underscores the relative role of the plasma cholesterol level on the development of atherosclerosis. Although hypercholesterolemia may not be a primary etiologic agent in the initiation of atherosclerosis, the presence of cholesterol in the plaque is universal and suggests that this risk factor is the primary factor in the continuing development of the atherosclerotic plaque once initiated.

Of those individuals who constitute the upper ranges of the normal Gaussian distribution curve, the majority do not exhibit elevated plasma cholesterol levels as an expression of an underlying inherited lipid metabolism disorder. Rather, in these instances of sporadic or polygenic hypercholesterolemia, the major determining factor may be the level of dietary cholesterol or the ability to assimilate and metabolize it.

The levels of serum cholesterol and triglyceride in infants and children determined from population studies are shown in Tables 40.2 and 40.3. It is important to note that cholesterol levels in childhood are extremely labile. Of children followed in Muscatine, Iowa, with initial levels exceeding the 95th percentile (230 mg/dl), 70% were less than that level when remeasured approximately 1 year leter without any intervention.[47] This observation indicates the need for repeated measurements of serum cholesterol levels before any child is considered to have hypercholesterolemia.

Therapy for Hyperlipidemia

During childhood, clinical atherosclerotic heart disease is not a manifest problem. Therapy, therefore, is directed toward the prevention rather than the management of this clinical manifestation of the atherosclerotic process. Because dietary cholesterol is not the sole determinate of atherogenesis, it is difficult to recommend that all children follow a diet that is low in cholesterol. However, certain groups of children who are at higher risk for the development of occlusive atheromatous disease during adulthood can be identified. These children, who might benefit by the lowering of their plasma cholesterol, include the progeny of young myocardial infarction victims with hyperlipoproteinemia, children with familial hyperlipoproteinemia, and children with persistent hypercholesterolemia (in excess of 220 mg/dl) found on routine screening.

It has been suggested that because serum cholesterol levels rise throughout the adult years that children with cholesterol levels that are consistently at adult risk levels should be given appropriate dietary and, if necessary, drug therapy. Surgical approaches such as ilial bypass[12] or portocaval shunt[71] to lower plasma cholesterol have been attempted in selected children with homozygous hypercholesterolemia. Whether such interventions in humans can prevent the eventual development of coronary heart disease is at the moment unproved. Experimental studies in animals suggest that lowering of serum cholesterol can result in the regression of atherosclerotic lesions induced by hyperlipidemia.[4, 5, 20]

Diet Therapy. Therapy for hyperlipoproteinemia should emphasize that diet is the treatment of choice and that drugs are an adjunct. Prior to the initiation of drug therapy, considerable effort should be exerted to accomplish dietary alteration appropriate to the lipid abnormality. This fundemental change in life-style often requires that the physician collaborate with a nutritional counselor.

Eating has become a central and predominant part of the American social life-style. Abrupt changes in this part of an individual's life-style can be difficult, if not impossible, to achieve. Better diet adherence may be gained by a more gradual approach, inducing increased restrictions on cholesterol intake until the ultimate goal of no more than 100 mg/day of cholesterol intake is achieved.[16]

The typical American diet provides about 750 mg of cholesterol daily, and 40% of all calories as fat. By encouraging the avoidance of foods high in cholesterol and saturated fat, cholesterol intake can be reduced to 400 to 500 mg with 35% of calories as fat daily. This can be accomplished by deleting egg yolk, butterfat, lard, and organ meat from the diet and substituting margarine for butter, vegetable oils and shortening for lard, and skim milk for whole milk.

Once this is achieved, the next emphasis should be on a transition from using up to 16 ounces of meat per day to no more than 6 to 8 ounces per day. In addition, less fat (margarine, oils, and shortening), milk, and cheeses should be consumed. With these decreases, the total cholesterol intake could be expected to fall to about 250 to 300 mg, and the fat intake to less than 30% of all calories. The final diet should be planned for a meat consumption of no more than 3 to 4 ounces/day, with emphasis on fish and poultry instead of beef and pork. Low cholesterol cheese should be substituted for regular cheese. Increased consumption of whole grains, beans, and legumes should be encouraged during this process. This final diet then represents 100 mg of cholesterol intake, 20% of calories from fat with a polyunsaturated to saturated ratio of approximately 1.5 to 1, 65% of calories from carbohydrates, and 15% of calories from protein. Special recipes for this form of diet have been published by Connor and Connor,[16] Reiter and Bagge,[63] and the American Heart Association.[2]

It has been suggested that the ingestion of moderate amounts of alcohol may result in a decreased incidence of atherosclerotic heart disease, perhaps through an increase in HDL cholesterol levels induced by alcohol.[7] Thus, some speculate that wine consumption has a protective effect in regard to ischemic heart disease,[66] but the data regarding wine or alcohol consumption has not shown a uniform effect on increasing HDL cholesterol or in preventing atherosclerotic heart disease. Thus, we cannot at this time recommend that wine or other alcoholic beverages be added to the diet of children.

Drug Therapy. There will be some patients who will not or cannot reduce their plasma lipid levels to normal by dietary measures alone and will require drug intervention. At present, the drugs most frequently used to reduce the plasma cholesterol level include those which prevent the reabsorption of bile acids (cholestyramine and colestepol) and drugs altering lipoprotein production (probucol, clofibrate, nicotinic acid). Para-aminosalicylic acid-C also has been shown to reduce plasma cholesterol levels, but the method of action has not been defined. Drugs which directly block cholesterol synthesis have to date proved to be too toxic for use. In all cases, the use of drugs, as with diet, must be continued indefinitely to maintain the lowered cholesterol

level. Drug intervention is probably not justified in children whose serum cholesterol is consistently less than 250 mg/dl.

Cholestyramine is provided as a wettable powder in 4-gm packets to be mixed with water before use. It is generally most effective when given in conjunction with meals in order to be available during the time of gallbladder emptying. This resin is not absorbed from the gastrointestinal tract and functions by strongly binding with the bile acids, carrying them into the stool. The usual dose to start is one packet 3 times/day (12 gm/day) for the average school-age child, increasing to two packets three times/day (24 gm) as necessary (250 to 800 gm/kg/day). Occasionally, doses less than 12 gm/day may be effective. The side effects of this drug are few and include constipation and bloating. Malabsorption with increased fecal fat occurs, but no deficiencies of the fat-soluble vitamins have been observed.[49]

A second bile acid binding resin (colestepol) is also available. Colestepol is provided in 5-gm packets, with doses similar to those for cholestyramine. In a study of 2278 hypercholesterolemic subjects randomized to colestepol or placebo and observed over a period of up to 3 years, Dorr et al.[23] observed an average decrease in serum cholesterol of 32 mg/dl at 1 month and 42 mg/dl at 3 years for the treatment group. Placebo changes were 7 mg/dl and 14 mg/dl for the same periods.

Probucol has become available more recently. In a controlled study,[62] probucol produced a mean reduction in plasma cholesterol level of 12% with no consistent effect on triglyceride levels. Available in 500-mg tablets, usual doses are one to two tablets twice/day. Adverse effects include gastrointestinal intolerance, particularly nausea and diarrhea. An apparently species-specific effect of myocardial sensitization with consequent ventricular fibrillation has been observed in the dog.[54]

Clofibrate has proved to be more effective in decreasing the level of the very low density lipoprotein than the low density lipoprotein, and thus has more use in those lipid disorders characterized by high triglyceride levels rather than isolated hypercholesterolemia. The mode of action of this drug is unclear. Adverse effects are uncommon, with nausea being most frequent. Cholelithiasis has, however, been found more frequently in patients on chronic therapy with clofibrate. It is generally used in adults in a dosage of 1 gm twice each day. Its use in children has been limited, thus its long-term effectiveness has yet to be established.

Nicotinic acid is a normal constituent of the diet, but given in doses of 800 to 1500 mg/day in adults, it has been shown to suppress low density lipoprotein levels in the blood. This drug is associated with major side effects, including alteration of liver function and hepatic damage. Many patients complain of peripheral flushing and puritis within 1 or 2 hours after taking each dose. Acanthosis nigricans has been seen, and hyperuricemia is not uncommon. The pediatric use of this drug is generally only in those children with the homozygous form of familial hyperlipoproteinemia in doses of 55 to 85 mg/kg/day.[49]

Para-aminosalicylic acid-C is a purified form of the original para-aminosalicylic acid developed and used for therapy of tuberculosis. It has been shown to have as significant an effect as cholestyramine in lowering serum cholesterol.[9] It has the advantage of being taken as a tablet rather than as a wettable powder. At present, this drug is available only as an investigational drug for the treatment of hypercholesterolemia. Our studies in children suggest an effective dose range of 150 to 200 mg/kg/day. The major side effects observed have been diarrhea, abdominal cramping, increased flatus, and occasional vomiting.

That atherosclerosis may be prevented by alteration of

cholesterol levels has yet to be established. However, intervention begun in childhood and continued into the adult years seems a logical approach.

Smoking

The relationship of smoking to the development of coronary heart disease has been well documented.[24, 75] It has been shown that the habitual consumption of 20 or more cigarettes/day increases the risk of myocardial infarction to three times that of the nonsmoker. This is in part dose related, with lesser consumption being associated with slightly less risk. Smoking operates independently of the other risk factors, but in association with them can appreciably raise the risk, as well as accelerate the changes and contribute to sudden death from coronary heart disease. Fortunately, cessation of smoking is accompanied by a decreased risk comparable to that of the nonsmoker.[40]

Studies in man and animals suggest that cigarette smoking may contribute to the development of atherosclerosis by one or more mechanisms: contributing to the release of catecholamines, increasing the work load of the heart and myocardial oxygen demand; decreasing the coronary oxygen extraction; elevating the blood carboxyhemoglobin levels; and, possibly altering platelet adhesiveness.[40] Of these effects, the first and last appear to be effects of absorbed nicotine, and would appear to be less important than the effects of carbon monoxide absorbed.

The average cigarette contains from 0.5 to 3 mg of nicotine, depending on the brand. The effect of the absorbed nicotine is to increase the heart rate, cardiac output, blood pressure, and coronary blood flow. There is also peripheral vasoconstriction and, when the myocardium has been damaged, some predisposition to dysrhythmia.[10] These effects may be important in the acute manifestation and sudden death of occlusive coronary heart disease but are transient and are of lesser significance in the development of atherosclerosis.

More consistent association of the level of carbon monoxide in the blood and atherosclerosis has been shown.[6, 40] Cigarette smoke may contain from 3 to 6% carbon monoxide and will raise the level of carboxyhemoglobin from less that 1% in the nonsmoker to 4 to 15% in the smoker. The level of carboxyhemoglobin decreases at a rate of 15% per hour, providing for a prolonged elevation in the habitual smoker. These levels in the blood reduce the level of hemoglobin available for oxygen transport creating hypoxemia, shift the oxygen-hemoglobin dissociation curve to the left, decrease coronary oxygen extraction as much as 30%, and may have a direct toxic effect on the arterial endothelial cells. Both carbon monoxide and hypoxemia without carbon monoxide have been shown to produce atherosclerosis in animals.[6]

Among the school age population, smoking appears to be increasing, particularly among girls. There is occasional and moderate smoking in both sexes at all grade levels. By the time children enter 9th grade, 33% may be smoking, many heavily.[29] This trend has been seen in a study of school children in Winnipeg, Canada.[58] In 1960 the numbers of children smoking were 6% of boys and 7% of girls in grades 7 to 9, and 44% of boys and 28% of girls in grades 10 to 12. By 1968 these had increased to 13% of boys and 7% of girls in grades 5 to 6, 31% of boys and 29% of girls in grades 7 to 9, and 46% of boys and 41% of girls in grades 10 to 12.[52] When one considers that the average consumption of cigarettes is now 200 packs/person/year, and the National Tobacco Workers Conference is anticipating a 30% increase by 1985,[57] this trend will produce an increasing number of adults at risk of coronary heart disease from smoking. As the age at which these children start smoking decreases, their exposure to cigarettes in pack years by midadulthood will continue to

increase, with an expected increase in the incidence of coronary heart disease. Every physician who deals with children should indicate this health hazard to both the parents and the children.

Hypertension

The association of hypertension with the development of atherosclerosis and the resulting vascular complications has been underscored by the Veterans Administration Drug Therapy Study which showed that lowering of elevated blood pressure results in a significantly improved morbidity and mortality rate in adult men.[77] Life insurance studies have shown that blood pressure of about 100/60 mm Hg is associated with the longest life expectancy; and with levels between 120/80 to 140/90, the mortality rises progressively. In the Framingham Study the incidence of ischemic heart disease in men 45 to 62 years old with pressures in excess of 160/95 was more than five times that in normotensive men (pressure 140/90 mm Hg or less).

In a school district in Muscatine, Iowa, blood pressures were measured in approximately 4800 school children.[48] If 140 mm Hg systolic and 90 mm Hg diastolic are taken as the upper limits of normal for adult pressure, no children under 9 years of age were found to be hypertensive. However, hypertension occurred commonly in children 14 to 18 years old; 8.9% had systolic hypertension; 12.2% had diastolic hypertension; systolic and diastolic hypertension occurred together in 4.4% and 16.7% had blood pressure elevations of either systolic pressure or diastolic pressure, or both. These pressures were measured on only one occasion.

In evaluating blood pressures in adolescent children, it should be noted that there is marked variability of pressure levels, and one reading does not usually indicate the presence of fixed hypertension. Of the Muscatine children whose initial blood pressures exceeded 140 mm Hg systolic or 90 mm Hg diastolic or were greater than the 95th percentile of systolic or diastolic pressure, less than 1% were found to have persistent hypertension. Of this group with fixed hypertension, half were obese, and of the lean hypertensives a variety of primary causes, including coarctation of the aorta, renal artery stenosis, renal disease, oral contraception, and essential hypertension were found. Thus, fixed essential hypertension was found to be a rare phenomenon in these adolescents. However, the observations in male college students and army officers with transient elevation of blood pressure have indicated that these subjects are more likely to have sustained high pressure in later years.[22, 51]

In children with labile hypertension it would seem prudent to keep them under surveillance. Because of the association of obesity and sodium chloride intake with hypertension, advice about attaining an optimal weight and the avoidance of excessive salt intake should be given to children with hypertension.

Obesity

Numerous studies have shown the relationship of obesity to early mortality from ischemic heart disease.[17, 53] However, obesity is frequently associated with other coronary risk factors, such as hyperlipidemia, hypertension, hyperuricemia, and diabetes. There appears to be no greater risk for ischemic heart disease in those subjects who have isolated obesity.[44]

Obesity can be estimated in many ways. Direct patient observation and clinical judgement is as useful as many more complex methods. Relative weight has been widely used as a coronary risk index in adults; we present it here as a view of childhood obesity, realizing that its importance as a predictor of the development of coronary heart disease in adult life is not established. In the Muscatine, Iowa school district, the heights and weights of 4800 school children were used to compute relative weight for each subject as a percentage above or below the median weight for all subjects with the same height, age, and sex. Thus, those with a relative weight of 100% were at the median weight for height-age-sex category. At all ages, 23% of both boys and girls had relative weights of at least 110%. In the adolescent years a greater number of children were observed to have relative weights in excess of 130%. In the age group 14 to 18 years, 24% of boys and 25% of girls had weights in excess of 110%; 13.1% and 13.6%, respectively, were at least 120%; 7.0% and 8.6%, respectively, were at least 130%. These prevalences would appear to be of importance since reports indicate that obesity has its origins in childhood and persists into adult life.[52] Thus the need for physicians to convince parents and children to become and remain lean is an obvious public health need.

Psychological Factors

Many social and demographic analyses have so far failed to reach any agreement about the relationship of occupation and situational factors and the incidence of ischemic heart disease.[53] In a study carried out by the Western Collaborative Group,[65] men were classified in two groups. "Type A" were compulsive, striving, and deadline conscious and "Type B" were more sluggish and passive. In this prospective study "Type A" men, 39 to 49 years old, had about six times the incidence of new ischemic heart disease as "Type B" men.

Diabetes

Diabetic subjects have a twofold greater incidence of myocardial infarction than nondiabetics. They also have an increased tendency for cerebral thrombosis and infarction but not for cerebral hemorrhage. Occlusive vascular disease results in a marked increase of gangrene in the lower extremities in diabetics. Hypertension is present with twice the frequency in diabetics as for nondiabetics.

There is no consistent lipid abnormality in diabetics, and thus the usual forms of hyperlipidemia are not related to increased risk for ischemic heart disease. Although diabetics respond to low cholesterol low fat diets by lowering their triglyceride and cholesterol levels, the beneficial effect upon the vascular complication of their disease has yet to be established.[1]

Physical Activity

The Framingham study measured the difference of activity level independent of other coronary risk factors and found associations of a higher incidence of ischemic heart disease in more sedentary men. There is also evidence that the more vigorous men have a lower mortality after myocardial infarction than sedentary men.[13, 43] These observations suggest that exercise that enhances cardiopulmonary fitness should become a part of all people's lives. The habits of exercise should be established in childhood and should be maintained through the adult years.

REFERENCES

1. Albrink, M. S.: Dietary and drug treatment of hyperlipidemia in diabetes. Diabetes 23:913, 1974.
2. The American Heart Association Cookbook. American Heart Association. David McKay, New York, 1973.
3. Andersen, G. E., Lifschitz, C., and Friis-Hansen, B.: Dietary habits and serum lipids during the first 4 years of life. Acta Pediatr. Scand. 68:165–170, 1979.
4. Armstrong, M. L.: Evidence of regression of atherosclerosis in primates and man. Postgrad. Med. J. 52:456–461, 1976.
5. Armstrong, M. L., Warner, E. D., and Connor, W. E. Regression of coronary atheromatosis in rhesus monkeys. Circ. Res. 27:59, 1970.
6. Astrup, P., and Kjeldsen, K.: Carbon monoxide, smoking and atherosclerosis. Med. Clin. North Am. 58:323, 1974.
7. Barboriak, J. J., Anderson, A. J., and Hoffman, R. G.: Interrelationship between coronary artery occlusion, high density lipoprotein cholesterol, and alcohol intake. J. Lab. Clin. Med. 94:348, 1979.
8. Barnes, K., Nestel, P. J., Pryke, E. S., and Whyte, H. M. Neonatal plasma lipids. Med. J. Aust. 2:1002, 1972.
9. Barter, P. J., Connor, W. E., Spector, A. A., Armstrong, M. L., Connor, S. L., and Newman, M. A.: Lowering of serum cholesterol and triglycerides by para-aminosalicylic acid in hyperlipoproteinemia. Ann. Intern. Med. 81:619, 1974.
10. Bolazs, T., Ohtake, S., and Cummings, J. R.: Ventricular extrasystoles induced by epinephrine, nicotine, ethanol, vasopressin in dogs with myocardial lesions. Toxicol. Appl. Pharmacol. 15:189, 1969.
11. Brown, M. S., Goldstein, J. L.: Expression of the familial hypercholesterolemia gene in heterozygotes: Mechanism for a dominant disorder in man. Science 185:61, 1974.
12. Buchwald, H., Moore, R. B., and Varco, R. H.: Surgical treatment of hyperlipidemia. Circulation 49 (Suppl. I):1, 1974.
13. Byers, S. O., Friedman, M., Rosenman, R. H., and Freed, S. C.: Excretion of 3-methoxy-4-hydroxymandelic acid in men with behavior pattern associated with high incidence of coronary artery disease. Fed. Proc. 21:99, 1962.
14. Carter, G. A., Connor, W. E., Bhattacharyya, A., and Lin, D.: Cholesterol balance, absorption, and turnover in children with homozygous familial hyperlipoproteinemia type IIa. J. Lipid Res. 20:66–77, 1979.
15. Carter, G. A.: Unpublished data, 1982.
16. Connor, W. E., and Connor, S. L.: The alternative diet book. University of Iowa Press, Iowa City, Iowa, 1976.
17. Chapman, J. M., Coulson, A. H., Clark, V. A., and Borun, E. R.: The differential effect of serum cholesterol, blood pressure and weight on the incidence of myocardial infarction and angina pectoris. J. Chronic Dis. 23:631, 1971.
18. Darmady, J. M., Fosbrooke, A. S., and Lloyd, J. K.: Prospective study of serum cholesterol levels during first year of life. Br. Med. J. 2:685, 1972.
19. Day, A. J., and Walquist, M. L.: Cholesterol ester and phospholipid composition of normal aortas and of atherosclerotic lesions in children. Exp. Mol. Pathol. 13:199, 1970.
20. DePalma, R. G., Klein, L., Bellon, E. M., and Koletsky, S.: Regression of atherosclerotic plaques in rhesus monkeys. Arch. Surg. 115:1268–1278, 1980.
21. Deutscher, S., Ostrander, L. D., and Epstein, F. H.: Familial factors in premature coronary heart disease. Am. J. Epidemiol. 91:233, 1970.
22. Diehl, H. S., and Hesdorffer, M. B.: Changes in blood pressure of young men over 7 year period. Arch. Intern. Med. 52:948, 1933.
23. Dorr, A. E., Gundersen, K., Schneider, Jr., J. C., Spencer, T. W., and Martin, W. B.: Colestepol hydrochloride in hypercholesterolemic patients. Effect on serum cholesterol and mortality. J. Chronic Dis. 31:5, 1978.
24. Doyle, J. T., Dawber, T. R., Kannel, W. B., Kinch, S. H., and Kahn, H. A.: The relationship of cigarette smoking to coronary heart disease. J.A.M.A. 190:108, 1964.
25. Drash, A.: Atherosclerosis, cholesterol and the pediatrician. J. Pediatr. 80:693, 1972.
26. Ellefson, R. D., Elveback, L. R., Hodgson, P. A., and Weidman, W. H.: Cholesterol and triglycerides in serum lipoproteins of young persons in Rochester, Minnesota. Mayo Clin. Proc. 53:307–320, 1978.
27. Enos, W. F., Beyer, J. C., and Holmes, R. H.: Pathogenesis of coronary disease in American soldiers killed in Korea. J.A.M.A. 158:912, 1955.
28. Fredrickson, D. S., and Levy, R. I.: Familial hyperlipoproteinemia. In The Metabolic Basis of Inherited Disease 3rd ed., edited by J. B. Stanbury, J. B. Wyngaarden, and D. S. Fredrickson. McGraw-Hill, New York, 1972, p. 493 ff.
29. Galli, M. A.: A comparative analysis of the attitudes and behaviors of school children (selected grades 4–12) and their parents towards drugs. Doctoral Dissertation, University of Illinois Urbana-Champaign, Ill., 1972.
30. Geer, J. C.: Fine structure of human aortic intimal thickening and fatty streaks. Lab. Invest. 14:1764, 1965.
31. Geer, J. C., McGill, H. C., and Strong, J. P.: The fine structure of human atherosclerotic lesions. Am. J. Pathol. 38:263, 1961.
32. Glantz, W. M., and Sternbridge, V. A.: Coronary artery atherosclerosis as a factor in aircraft accidents and fatalities. J. Aviation Med. 302:75, 1959.
33. Glueck, C. J., Heckman, F., Schoenfeld, M., Steiner, P., and Pearche, W.: Neonatal familial type II hyperlipoproteinemia: Cord blood cholesterol in 1800 births. Metabolism 20:597, 1971.
34. Goldstein, J. L.: The cardiac manifestations of the homozygous and heterozygous forms of familial type II hyperbetalipoproteinemia. Birth Defects 8:202, 1972.

35. Goldstein, J. L., Albers, J. J., Schrott, H. G., Hazzard, W. R., Bierman, E. L., and Motulsky, A. G.: Plasma lipid levels and coronary heart disease in adult relative of newborns with normal elevated cord blood lipids. Am. J. Hum. Genet. 26:727, 1974.

36. Goldstein, J. L., Schrott, H. G., Hazzard, W. R., Bierman, E. L., and Motulsky, A. G.: Genetic analysis of lipid levels in 176 families and delineation of a new inherited disorder, combined hyperlipidemia. J. Clin. Invest. 52:1544, 1973.

37. Gordon, Castelli, W. P., Hjortland, Kannel, W. B., and Dawber, T. R.: High density lipoprotein as a protective factor against coronary heart disease. Am. J. Med. 62:707–714, 1977.

38. Greten, H., Wengeler, H., and Wagner, H.: Early diagnosis of familial type II hyperlipoproteinemia. Nutr. Metab. 15:128, 1973.

39. Hata, Y., and Ishii, T.: The lipids in human atherosclerosis—morphological demonstrations of five forms of atheroma lipids. In Drugs, Lipid Metabolism, and Atherosclerosis, edited by D. Kritchevsky, R. Paoletti, and W. L. Holmes. Plenum Press, New York, 1978, pp. 129–143.

40. The Health Consequences of Smoking: A Report of the Surgeon General. USPHS, Washington, D.C., 1972.

41. Holman, R. L., McGill, H. C., Strong, J. P., and Geer, J. C.: The natural history of atherosclerosis: The early arotic lesions as seen in New Orleans in the middle of the 20th century. Am. J. Pathol. 34:209, 1958.

42. Inter-society commission for heart disease resources. Atherosclerosis study group and epidemiology study group: Primary prevention of atherosclerotic diseases. Circulation 42:A55, 1970.

43. Kannel, W. B.: Physical exercise and lethal atherosclerotic disease. N. Engl. J. Med. 282:1153, 1970.

44. Keys, A., Arvanis, C., Blackburn, H., Van Buchen, F. S. P., Buzina, R., Djordjevic, B. S., Fidanza. F., Karvonen, M. S., Menotti, A., Puddu, V., and Taylor, H. L.: Coronary heart disease: Overweight and obesity as risk factors. Ann. Intern. Med. 77:15, 1972.

45. Kua P. T., Hayase, K., Koster, J. B., and Moreyra A. E.: Use of combined diet and colestepol in long-term (7–7½ years) treatment of patients with type II. Circulation 59:199–211, 1979.

46. Kwiterovich, P. O., Jr., Levy, R. I., and Fredrickson, D. S.: Neonatal diagnosis of familial type II hyperlipoproteinemia. Lancet 1:118, 1973.

47. Lauer, R. M., Clarke, W. R., Reiter, M. A., Connor, W. E.: Spontaneous changes in cholesterol levels in school age children. Circulation 52 (Suppl. II): 43, 1975.

48. Lauer, R. M., Connor, W. E., Leaverton, P. E., Reiter, M. A., Clarke, W. R.: Coronary heart disease risk factors in school children: The Muscatine study. J. Pediatrics 86:697, 1975.

49. Levy, R. I., Fredrickson, D. S., Shulman, R., Bilheimer, D. W., Breslow, J. L., Stone, N. J., Lux, S. E., Sloan, H. R., Krause, R. M., and Herbert, P. N.: Dietary and drug treatment of primary hyperlipoproteinemia. Ann. Intern. Med. 77:267, 1972.

50. Levy, R. I., and Rifkind, B. M.: Diagnosis and management of hyperlipoproteinemia in infants and children. Am. J. Cardiol. 31:547, 1973.

51. Levy, R. L., Hillman, C. C., Stroud, W. D., and White, P. D.: Transient hypertension: Its significances in terms of later development of sustained hypertension and cardiovascular-renal disease. J.A.M.A. 126:829, 1944.

52. Lloyd, J. K., and Wolff, O. H.: Childhood obesity. Br. Med. J. 5245:145, 1961.

53. Marks, H. H.: Influence of obesity on morbidity and mortality. Bull. N.Y. Acad. Med. 36:296, 1960.

54. Marshall, F. N., and Lewis, J. E.: Sensitization to epinephrine induced ventricular fibrillation produced by probucol in dogs. Toxicol. Appl. Pharmacol. 24:594, 1973.

55. McGill, H. C.: Fatty streaks in the coronary arteries and aorta. Lab. Invest. 18:560, 1968.

56. McNamara, J.J., Molot, M. A., Stemple, J. F., and Cutting, R. T.: Coronary artery disease in combat casualties in Viet Nam. J.A.M.A. 216:1185, 1971.

57. Miller, R. H.: Tobacco and tobacco products consumption for 1985. Presented at the 25th National Tobacco Workers Conference, Economics Section, Hamilton, Ontario, Aug. 9, 1973.

58. Morison, J. B.: Report on smoking habits of Winnipeg school children: 1960–1968. Can. Med. Assoc. J. 108:1138, 1973.

59. Morrison, J. A., deGroot, I., Edwards, B. K., Kelly, K. A., Mellier, M. J., Khoury, P., and Glueck, C. J.: Lipids and lipoproteins in 927 schoolchildren, ages 6 to 17 years. Pediatrics 62:990–995, 1978.

60. Nato, H. K., Greenstreet, R. L., David, J. A., Sheldon, W. L., Shirey, E. K., Lewis, R. C., Proudfit, W. L., and Gerrity, R. G.: HDL cholesterol concentration and severity of coronary atherosclerosis determined by cineangiography. Artery 8:101–112, 1980.

61. Osborne, Jr., J. C., and Brewer, Jr., B.: The plasma lipoproteins. Adv. Protein Chem: 253–337, 1977.

62. Polachek, A. A., Katz, H. M., Lack, J., Selig, J., and Littman, M.: Probucol in the long-term treatment of hypercholesterolemia. Curr. Med. Res. Opinion 1:323, 1973.

63. Reiter, M. A., and Bagge, T.: Recipes for heart-

Y appetites. University of Iowa Press, Iowa City, Iowa, 1977.

64. Report from the Committee of Principal Investigators: A cooperative trial in the primary prevention of ischemic heart disease using clofibrate. Br. Heart J. 40:1069–1118, 1978.

65. Rosenman, R. H., Brand, R. J., Jenkins, C. D., Friedman, M., Straus, R., and Wurm, M.: Coronary heart disease in the Western Collaborative Group Study. J.A.M.A. 233:872, 1975. Also: 189–15, 1964; 195:86, 1966.

66. St. Leger, A. S., Cochrane A. L., and Moore, F.: Factors associated with cardiac mortality in developed countries with particular reference to the consumption of wine. Lancet 1:1017, 1979.

67. Smith, E. B., Slater, R. S., and Chu, P. K.: The lipids in raised fatty and fibrous lesions in human aorta. J. Atheroscler. Res. 8:399, 1968.

68. Sodhi, H. S., and Kudchodkar, B. J.: Correlating metabolism of plasma and tissue cholesterol with that of plasma-lipoproteins. Lancet I:513–519, 1973.

69. Sodhi, H. S., and Mason, D. T.: Current concepts in the diagnosis and specific treatment of the hyperlipidemias. In Advances in Heart Disease, vol. 3, edited by D. T. Mason. Grune & Stratton, New York. 1980, pp. 303–329.

70. Spickerman, R. E., Brandenberg, J. T., Acher, R. W. P., and Edward, J. E.: The spectrum of coronary heart disease in a community of 30,000. A clinicopathologic study. Circulation 25:57, 1962.

71. Starzl, T. E., Chase, H. P., Putnam, C. W., and Porter, K. A.: Portocaval shunt in hyperlipoproteinemia. Lancet II: 940, 1973.

72. Streja, D., Steiner, G., and Kwiterovich, Jr. P.O.: Plasma high density lipoproteins and ischemic heart disease. Ann. Intern. Med. 89:871–880, 1978.

73. Strong, J. P., and McGill, H. C.: The natural history of aortic atherosclerosis. Exp. Mol. Pathol. (Suppl.) 1:15, 1963.

74. Strong, J. P., and McGill, H. C., Jr.: The pediatric aspects of atherosclerosis. J. Atheroscler. Res. 9:251, 1969.

75. Truett, J., Cornfield, J., and Kannel, W.: A multivariate analysis of the risk of coronary heart disease in Framingham. J. Chronic Dis. 20:511, 1967.

76. Tsang, R. C., Fallat, R. W., and Glueck, C. J.: Cholesterol at birth and age 1: Comparison of normal and hypercholesterolemic neonates. Pediatrics 53:548, 1974.

77. VA Cooperative Study: Effects of treatment of morbidity in hypertension. I. J.A.M.A. 202:116, 1967; and J.A.M.A. 213(Part II):1143, 1970.

78. Williams, P., Robinson, D., and Bailey, A.: High density lipoprotein and coronary risk factors in normal man. Lancet I:72–74, 1979.

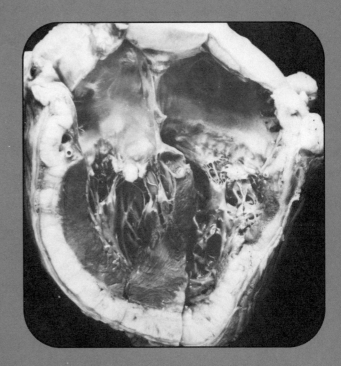

Part 5
SPECIAL
PROBLEMS

41

Heart Disease in the Newborn

Martin H. Lees, M.D., and Cecille O. Sunderland, M.D.

The recognition and identification of serious heart disease in the newborn is a common challenge. Major structural heart disease may closely simulate lung dysfunction and correspondingly, pulmonary disease may mimic heart disease. Quite often, lung and and heart disease coexist, each contributing to the clinical picture.

This chapter is limited to a consideration of the clinical recognition, differential diagnosis, and treatment of *serious* heart disease in the first days of life. The most frequent presenting signs of cyanosis, heart failure, dysrhythmia, and cardiogenic shock are emphasized, although serious cardiovascular disease may also be initially suspected by discovery of dysrhythmia, tachypnea, hepatomegaly, peripheral edema, systemic hypertension, gallop rhythm, or abnormal chest roentgenogram or electrocardiogram.

EXAMINATION OF THE NEONATE SUSPECTED OF HAVING SERIOUS HEART DISEASE

The family history should be reviewed for evidence of congenital heart disease, connective tissue disorder, glycogen storage disease, hypercalcemia, or unusual hereditable disease. Questions relating to the present pregnancy should include inquiries about rubella, Coxsackie virus infection, unusual radiation exposure, maternal diabetes mellitus, or threatened abortion. The birth history should include gestational age and condition of the infant at birth, especially the presence of meconium staining, low Apgar score, and perinatal hypoxemia or acidemia.

Behavior of the Infant

A general appraisal of the infant's spontaneous activity and response to stimuli often provides insight into the seriousness of the disease. A baby with reduced oxygen delivery to the tissues, whether from cyanotic heart disease or heart failure, may show little spontaneous movement, presumably to conserve available oxygen for basal metabolic requirements. In the extreme case, a newborn with severe heart failure from myocarditis, cardiogenic shock, or hypoplastic left heart syndrome may be flaccid and apathetic and show almost no response to external stimuli.

Breathing Patterns

Tachypnea, altered depth of respiration, intercostal retractions, flaring of the alae nasi, grunting, stridor, and apneic spells may all be observed in infants with cardiovascular disease. *Tachypnea* is the least specific sign. A sustained respiratory rate of over 45/minute or over 60/minute in the low birth weight infant is compatible with many types of heart disease, lung disease, or mechanical interference with lung function.

Increased tidal volume is most characteristic of infants with cyanotic heart disease and decreased pulmonary blood flow. Much of the ventilation is wasted because the alveoli are grossly underperfused. Increased depth of respiration is also seen in the newborn with renal agenesis or hypoplasia, persistence of the fetal circulation, multiple pulmonary artery thromboses, alveolar proteinosis, pulmonary oxygen toxicity, and in some infants with bronchopulmonary dysplasia. Decreased tidal volume is found in neonates with severe heart failure, cardiogenic shock, intracerebral hemorrhage, subdural hemorrhage, gross intracranial malformation, meningitis, encephalitis, adrenal failure, and septicemia. Underventilation is usually caused either by stiff, noncompliant lungs or by interference with the normal servomechanisms whereby blood gas abnormalities and cerebrospinal fluid pH regulate respiration.

Intercostal retractions are characteristic of primary lung disease and mechanical interference with lung function. Retractions are also seen in severe heart failure when there is bronchial obstruction caused by alveolar transudate. Intercostal or subcostal retraction implies airway obstruction or noncompliant lungs. In the newborn the sign is most typical of respiratory distress syndrome (RDS) and pneumonia, but it is seen in a wide variety of diseases.

Flaring of the alae nasi is seen most typically in infants with RDS, pneumonia, and heart disease with pulmonary overcirculation complicated by pneumonia. Flaring during inspiration probably represents an attempt by the infant to reduce total airway resistance, much of which is accounted for by the small nasal passages.

Expiratory grunting is typical of primary lung disease, especially RDS and pneumonia. It appears likely that it represents an attempt at prolonging an increased positive pressure in the alveoli.

Stridor suggests mechanical interference with lung function and is suggestive of vascular rings compressing the trachea. It is also observed in tracheomalacia, epiglottitis, Pierre Robin syndrome, cystic hygroma, mucous plugs in the airway, diaphragmatic hernia, pneumothorax, abnormal thoracic cage, bronchogenic cyst, and mediastinal masses. The common denominator is obstruction of the airway during inspiration.

Apneic spells in full-term infants suggest a pathologic condition in the central nervous system or sepsis but also occur in the exhaustion phase of lung and heart disease. Apneic spells are also suggestive of hypocalcemia or hypoglycemia; a number of infants with the hypoplastic left heart syndrome have severe hypoglycemia, and within this group apneic spells are common. Other causes for apneic spells are unrecognized seizures and the congenital central hypoventilation syndrome (Ondine's curse).

Arterial Pulses and Blood Pressure

The radial, posterior tibial, and dorsalis pedis pulses are readily palpable in the normal newborn. Feeling one strong foot pulse that is synchronous with the radial is sufficient to rule out significant adult type postductal coarctation of the aorta (CA). In contrast, it *is* necessary to feel both radial pulses, since supravalvar aortic stenosis, aortic isthmus stenosis, and juxtaductal CA may all lead to an increased pressure in the right arm as compared with pressure in the left. The more common form of CA found in sick neonates is the juxtaductal or preductal form, in which the lower half of the body is perfused with blood originating from the right ventricle. In this situation, the femoral and foot pulses are often normal, and one may be able to observe cyanosis of the feet as compared with the hands. If hyperactive pulses are suspected, as with patent ductus arteriosus (PDA), one may move peripherally and feel the palmar pulses or even the digital pulses which are not normally palpable. Continuous wave Doppler velocimetry is useful in the detection of the retrograde diastolic arterial flow in the descending aorta and femoral arteries that is characteristic of PDA with left to right shunt.[50]

Arm systolic blood pressure can be measured with a 1- to 2-inch cuff and Doppler detection of moving arterial blood. Diastolic pressure may be measured by the Arteriosonde (Roche Medical Products) instrument which detects arterial wall motion as well as blood velocity.

Venous Pressure

In contrast to the examination of arterial pulses in the newborn, assessment of venous pressure is of limited diagnostic aid. The newborn liver appears to act as a readily distensible sponge, giving rise to gross hepatomegaly rather than allowing much rise in central venous pressure. Occasionally, one may observe distended neck veins in the upright infant and, rarely, a prominent "a" wave, suggesting obstruction to right atrial emptying (for example, tricuspid atresia or Ebstein's anomaly of the tricuspid valve).

Liver Size

Ordinarily the liver may be palpable 2 to 3 cm below the right costal margin measured in the nipple-umbilicus line. The size of the liver is a highly reliable index of the severity of right heart failure; in this condition it is frequently 5 or 6 cm below the costal margin.

Peripheral Edema

Occasionally, the back of the hands and dorsum of the feet may show pitting edema as a consequence of heart failure. Rarely, there is more widespread edema, with sacral pitting and puffy eyelids. In general, however, the lack of a major rise in central venous pressure in infants in heart failure appears also to preclude the development of marked edema. An exception is that of fetal hydrops due to intrauterine supraventricular tachycardia (SVT) and heart failure.

Heart Rate

The heart rate in quiet full-term infants averages 130 beats/minute, but the range may vary from 70 to 180 beats/minute during the 1st week of life. A mild sinus dysrhythmia occurs in most newborns and is more pronounced in premature infants. The use of long-term electrocardiographic recordings in full-term newborns has revealed the existence of clinically unsuspected and presumably benign dysrhythmias.

Cardiac Murmurs

Serious heart disease may exist without any heart murmur, and conversely a loud murmur may indicate a benign entity, such as a small ventricular septal defect (VSD).

Radiologic Features

The chest roentgenogram serves two broad purposes: to evaluate the type and severity of heart disease; and to detect some of the many simulators of heart disease, including a wide variety of primary lung diseases and mechanical interference with lung function.

Electrocardiographic Features

The normal newborn electrocardiogram, especially that taken during the first 24 hours of life, shows great variability. The changes probably are secondary to the rapidly changing circulation. Other influences are the infant's gestational age, pH status, and the levels of sodium, potassium, and calcium. Despite the wide variability of the normal newborn electrocardiogram,[26, 27] it is still a useful diagnostic tool. Since it is such a simple noninvasive procedure, it is mandatory in the assessment of any newborn suspected of having cardiovascular disease.

Blood Gases and pH

Estimation of arterial blood gases will aid in assessment of the condition of infants suspected of having heart disease. The effect of breathing 100% O_2 provides some insight into the pathophysiological mechanisms involved. The transcutaneous O_2 electrode ($TcPO_2$) is highly reliable as a reflection of arterial PO_2, and when used in conjunction with breathing 100% O_2 allows detection of significant right to left shunting. Normal infants achieve an abdominal skin $TcPO_2 > 300$ mm Hg, whereas in those with pathologic venous admixture $TcPO_2$ is less than 200 mm Hg.

Hypoglycemia

Initial evaluation should include a screening test for hypoglycemia (Dextrostix); and when the blood glucose level is low, a clinical determination of true blood glucose should be made. Hypoglycemia may simulate congenital heart disease with cardiomegaly[47] and cyanosis. Hypoglycemia also frequently complicates serious newborn heart disease, especially the hypoplastic left heart syndrome.[3] Unexpected hypoglycemia with or without apparent heart disease should prompt a consideration that the infant is "small for dates" or that maternal gestational diabetes mellitus is present. The latter may be diagnosed retrospectively by finding increased hemoglobin A_{1c} levels in the mother for 4 to 8 weeks after delivery.[39] The hypoglycemia should be treated with intravenous glucose while investigation and treatment of the underlying heart disease are proceeding.

Serum Electrolytes

Serum sodium, potassium, and chloride levels should be measured both because electrolyte abnormalities can occur in the infant with serious neonatal cardiovascular disease and because adrenal insufficiency may closely mimic heart disease.[56]

Methemoglobinemia

Congenital or acquired methemoglobinemia may closely simulate cyanotic congenital heart disease. The infant appears a peculiar lavender or slate blue, and blood from a heel prick is chocolate-colored. Blood from an infant with methemoglobinemia fails to become pink when placed on a glass slide and exposed to room air. The diagnosis can be confirmed by spectroscopy with a characteristic absorption peak at 634 μm and by the rapid response to intravenous methylene blue (1 to 2 mg/kg). For long-term medication, ascorbic acid 300 to 500 mg/day administered orally may be preferable but is sometimes less effective.

NEONATAL CYANOSIS

The overwhelming reason for suspecting serious heart disease in the first days of life is cyanosis with or without heart failure. Central cyanosis, due to an abnormally low oxygen saturation of arterial blood is usually recognizable in newborns when 3 gm or more of reduced hemoglobin is present in arterial blood.[32] If the newborn is anemic (8 gm/ 100 ml), the saturation at which cyanosis is visible is very low (63%); whereas if he is polycythemic (24 gm/100 ml) the oxygen saturation may be quite high (88%).

Peripheral cyanosis is defined as blue discoloration or duskiness confined to the skin of the extremities. The arterial blood will be normally saturated. Clearly, there are intermediate conditions in which arterial saturation may be in the range of 90%, and the tongue may appear pink and the extremities cyanotic. Such a baby has peripheral cyanosis resulting from a central disturbance. The clinical distinction of central from peripheral is therefore not always absolute, and elucidation frequently requires the measurement of arterial oxygen saturation or oxygen tension (PaO_2) or transcutaneous PO_2 ($TcPO_2$). Arterial unsaturation (central cyanosis) should be considered to be present if the PaO_2 is below 60 mm Hg at 24 hours of age or if the arterial oxygen saturation is below 94%. This does not infer that a PaO_2 of 60 mm Hg or less necessarily requires investigation, but it means that the infant either has alveolar hypoventilation or has an alveolar-arterial oxygen difference of about 35 mm Hg, possibly due to incomplete lung expansion.

Human fetal hemoglobin has approximately 40% less affinity for 2,3-diphosphoglycerate (2,3-DPG) than adult hemoglobin. This makes fetal hemoglobin behave as if 2,3-DPG levels were low with a shift of the hemoglobin-oxygen dissociation curve to the left and increased oxygen saturation for any given PaO_2. This has the effect of "masking" a serious situation, since a newborn with barely detectable cyanosis may have a PaO_2 of only 35 to 40 mm Hg. Thus, while the relatively high hematocrit of the newborn tends to facilitate recognition of cyanosis, the leftward shift of the Hb-O_2 dissociation curve tends to make recognition more difficult.

Clearly, the measurement of PaO_2 or $TcPO_2$ is more discriminatory than visual inspection or measurement of oxygen saturation. The normal newborn should achieve a PaO_2 of 45 mm Hg by 1 hour of age and 60 mm by 1 day of age. An occasional "normal" infant may have delayed expansion of some alveolar units and take longer than 1 day to achieve a PaO_2 of 60 mm Hg. The infant should not be crying when arterial blood is drawn, since crying can produce both alveolar hypoventilation and right to left atrial shunting. Serial measurements are of great value.

A DIAGNOSTIC APPROACH TO CENTRAL CYANOSIS

Once it is decided that an infant has central cyanosis confirmed by direct measurement of arterial PO_2, it is necessary to determine the cause, since the responsible disease process is rarely self-limiting. Often a definitive diagnosis may be made by clinical observations, chest x-ray, blood-gas values, echocardiogram, and electrocardiogram. Cardiac catheterization and angiocardiography are almost always required for the precise diagnosis of congenital heart disease. An aggressive diagnostic approach is always justified, since in the majority of instances, treatment is available. During the clinical observation, the cyanotic baby should be warm, asleep or quiet, and, if possible, breathing room air.

Respiratory Pattern

Respiration should be observed with regard to frequency, depth, presence of retractions or expiratory grunting, and presence of flaring of the alae nasi.

Spontaneous Movement

Lethargy and lack of adequate spontaneous movement suggest shock, sepsis, or intracranial pathology. However, newborn infants with advanced cyanosis from any cause may become acidotic, hypotonic, and unresponsive to painful stimuli.

Response to 100% Oxygen

It is commonly stated that if an infant becomes pink in oxygen, the hypoxemia is pulmonary in origin, while if he remains blue it is cardiac in origin. Unfortunately, this is an oversimplification. For example, first, there are large intrapulmonary and foramen ovale right to left shunts in many newborns with lung disease (especially RDS), who fail to achieve high arterial PO_2 in 100% O_2. Second, an infant with isolated PDA may be cyanotic from heart failure, alveolar transudate, and obstructed small air passages. He will become pink in 100% O_2 because the mechanism of his hypoxemia is alveolar hypoventilation; yet heart disease is his problem. Finally, if an infant with transposition of the great arteries (TGA) is very cyanotic in room air but becomes less cyanotic in 100% O_2, the explanation is not that the cause of his cyanosis is pulmonary but that 100% O_2 has lowered his pulmonary vascular resistance, allowing better mixing through an existing foramen ovale or PDA, or both. He may clinically appear to become pink, but his arterial PO_2 will never approach 250 mm Hg. Blood gases and the response to 100% O_2 are, therefore, only to be considered as indicative of the disordered physiologic mechanism and the seriousness of the problem rather than as an identification of the problem as pulmonary or cardiac. Nevertheless, if the PaO_2 rises to over 250 mm Hg the infant does not have a major right to left shunt.

Measurement of the arterial pH is also of value because it supplies an estimate of the severity of the problem. When the plasma bicarbonate level and arterial PCO_2 tension are known, rational treatment to return the pH toward normal can be instituted. A slight degree of respiratory acidosis need not be corrected.

Table 41.1 identifies the response of the blood gases in the three common mechanisms for arterial unsaturation. The infant should breath O_2 at an FIO_2 of 0.9 or greater for at least 10 minutes in order to wash out most of the nitrogen from very poorly ventilated areas.

Tolazoline Infusion

Tolazoline (Priscoline) is a potent peripheral vasodilator possessing adrenolytic and cholinergic properties. It acts through the autonomic nervous system and locally to produce dilatation of small blood vessels. Thus, Tolazoline can be given in a dose of 0.5 to 1 mg/kg into the pulmonary artery as a test of pulmonary arteriolar reactivity.[28] The test has been found useful in differentiating lung disease from heart disease when pulmonary hypertension is present. A positive response will be manifested by a lowered pulmonary vascular resistance with a marked increase in PaO_2 in umbilical arterial blood. A positive response is suggestive but not conclusive evidence of a structurally normal heart. For example, a juxtaductal CA with pulmonary hypertension may show a response very similar to the syndrome of "persistence of the fetal circulation." However, with juxtaductal CA the femoral pulses may decrease or disappear as pulmonary artery and right ventricular pressure fall.

Other Laboratory Tests

In addition to measurement of pH, PaO_2 and $PaCO_2$, a Dextrostix test provides a screening test for hypoglycemia

Mechanism	PaO$_2$ room air (mm Hg)	PaCO$_2$ room air (mm Hg)	PaO$_2$ 100% O$_2$ (mm Hg)
Alveolar hypoventilation	Decreased (<60)	Increased (>50)	Normal (>250)
Right to left shunt	Decreased (<60)	Normal (35–45)[b]	Decreased (<150)
Ventilation/perfusion unevenness	Decreased (<60)	Normal (35–45)[b]	Normal (>250)

[a] PaO$_2$ (room air) provides an estimate of the severity of the problem. An increased PaCO$_2$ (room air) implies alveolar hypoventilation, and failure of the PaO$_2$ to increase significantly on 100% O$_2$ implies right to left shunting as the problem.

[b] May rise very slowly with prolonged right to left shunting or ventilation/perfusion unevenness if compensatory hyperventilation is inadequate.

as a contributing factor to central cyanosis. Methemoglobinemia may be suspected by failure of blood to become red when placed on a slide and exposed to room air. Confirmation is obtained by absorption spectrometry. Electrolyte abnormalities may help identify hydration problems, adrenal cortical hyperplasia, and adrenal insufficiency. The latter may closely mimic cyanotic congenital heart disease.[56]

Measurement of hematocrit will allow detection of the hyperviscosity syndrome.[19, 23] The leucocyte count may point towards sepsis.

Radiologic Features

The chest film of the cyanotic baby may reveal a large, small, or abnormally shaped heart. The pulmonary vasculature may be diminished or increased. There may be evidence of pulmonary pathology, abdominal heterotaxia, or other etiologic clues. Such entities as RDS, bronchopulmonary dysplasia, congenital lymphangiectasia, diaphragmatic hernia, lung cysts, hypoplastic and agenetic lung, congenital lobar emphysema, pneumonia, pneumothorax, and chylothorax all give rise to characteristic roentgenographic findings, and all may be associated with cyanosis.[8]

Electrocardiographic Features

The electrocardiogram is frequently disappointing as a diagnostic aid in the newborn period because many of the forms of structural heart disease give rise to little or no cardiac hypertrophy while the infant is in utero, and conversely many respiratory problems are associated with mild right ventricular hypertropy.

In some instances the electrocardiogram is of major diagnostic help. Thus, left axis deviation with left ventricular hypertrophy strongly suggests tricuspid atresia. In other instances the electrocardiogram demonstrates moderate right ventricular hypertrophy, a finding which is consistent with many forms of pulmonary and heart disorders.

Echocardiographic Features

The echocardiogram provides major input into the noninvasive diagnostic process. Single and two-dimensional (2D) recordings can be made without removing the newborn from the incubator. Echocardiographic identification of the hypoplastic left heart syndrome can obviate the need for cardiac catheterization.[38] The echocardiogram may reveal such entities as TGA[11] and such anatomic details as aortic override, chamber size, septal motion, etc.[36]

DISEASES WHICH PRODUCE CENTRAL CYANOSIS

Certain clinical patterns may suggest 1 of 12 diagnostic categories indicated in Table 41.2. However, the clinical and laboratory signs are capricious, and infants sometimes do not manifest typical findings. Cardiac catheterization and angiocardiography are almost always required for the precise

diagnosis of congenital heart disease and sometimes to resolve the pulmonary versus cardiac disease dilemma.

LUNG DISEASES VERSUS HEART DISEASE

The problem of differentiating between lung and heart disease arises frequently in the neonatal period. Certain clinical and laboratory findings favor either primary cardiac or primary pulmonary pathology (Table 41.3); however, the signs are capricious, and sometimes cardiac catheterization and angiography are necessary to resolve the issue.

Particularly difficult is the distinction between "persistence of the fetal circulation" and preductal coarctation of the aorta. There is right to left ductal shunting and pulmonary hypertension with both diagnoses, and distinction frequently requires aortography, since surgery is usually necessary if a juxtaductal CA is present.

PERSISTENCE OF THE FETAL CIRCULATION (PFC SYNDROME)

The term "persistence of the fetal circulation"[20, 21] is applied to the combination of pulmonary hypertension, right to left atrial shunting (through a patent foramen ovale), right to left ductal shunting, and structurally normal heart.

The PFC syndrome may be primary or may be secondary to hyperviscosity of blood,[19, 23] aspiration pneumonia, hypoglycemia or neonatal pulmonary disease. The primary form tends to occur in full-term or postmature infants with no apparent antecedent cause, and it is under these circumstances that its recognition is both difficult and important. The etiology of the primary form is unknown but is quite often associated with perinatal asphyxia, and it is theorized that the condition results when the normal mechanisms that cause a decline in pulmonary vascular resistance and ductus closure fail to occur. Its association with postmaturity suggests the possibility of placental insufficiency as an etiologic component. It is likely that one or more of the prostaglandins may be absent or deficient in PFC syndrome. Prostaglandins are produced by fetal pulmonary vessels.[58] Prostaglandin I$_2$ has been used in the treatment of PFC syndrome[35] and prostaglandin D$_2$ has reduced pulmonary vascular resistance in goat lungs[9] and in lambs.[54]

Newborns with primary PFC syndrome are tachypnic and cyanotic. Right to left ductal shunting results in a higher PaO$_2$ in the right arm than in the legs. This may produce differential cyanosis. The PaCO$_2$ is normal or slightly elevated; the pH is usually depressed because of anaerobic metabolism. The pulmonary closure sound is loud; there is no diagnostically useful murmur. The electrocardiogram shows mild right ventricular hypertrophy, the echocardiogram shows a prolongation of RV preejection period, and the chest roentgenogram may be normal or show moderate cardiac enlargement.

If an infant with a presumptive diagnosis of PFC syndrome can be shown to have improving blood gases, diagnostic catheterization may not be required; however, with a worsen-

TABLE 41.2 DISEASES WHICH PRODUCE CENTRAL CYANOSIS IN THE NEONATE[a]

Category	Examples	Mechanisms of Cyanosis	Major Clinical Signs	Response to 100% Oxygen	Chest X-ray	Arterial pH and PCO2	Useful Laboratory Tests
(1) Congenital heart disease with right to left shunt and *decreased* pulmonary blood flow	Tetralogy of Fallot, Pulmonary atresia, Tricuspid atresia, Tricuspid insufficiency, Extreme pulmonic stenosis, Ebstein's anomaly	Right to left shunting	Deep "sighing" respirations, Heart murmur	No response[b]	Decreased lung vascular markings, Heart may be large or small	pH normal or acidemic, PCO2 normal or low	ECG, echocardiogram, cardiac catheterization, angiography
(2) Congenital heart disease with right to left shunt and *increased* pulmonary blood flow	Transposition of great arteries, Hypoplastic left heart syndrome, Preductal coarctation, Total anomalous pulmonary venous return, Truncus arteriosus, Very large ventricular septal defect	Right to left shunting	Rapid respirations, Heart murmur	No response[b]	Increased lung vascular markings, Large heart except with some cases of total anomalous pulmonary venous return	pH normal or acidemic, PCO2 normal unless heart failure	ECG, echocardiogram, cardiac catheterization, angiography
(3) Congenital or acquired heart disease with left heart failure and alveolar hypoventilation	Atrioventricular canal, Patent ductus arteriosus, Coarctation of aorta, Myocarditis, Paroxysmal atrial tachycardia	Alveolar hypoventilation (alveoli and alveolar ducts partially obstructed with transudate from pulmonary capillaries)	Flaccid and unresponsive with severe heart failure, Rapid shallow respirations, Heart murmur	Good response, PaO2 rises to >250 mm Hg if there is no right to left shunt	Large heart, Prominent lung vascular marking, "Patchy" pneumonia frequent	Acidemia and elevated PCO2	ECG, electrolytes, blood sugar, cardiac catheterization, angiography
(4) Primary lung disease	Respiratory distress syndrome, Atelectasis, Meconium aspiration, Pulmonary hemorrhage, Pneumonia, Bronchopulmonary dysplasia, Lymphangiectasia, Pulmonary agenesis	Alveolar hypoventilation (partially obstructed lung subunits), Right to left shunting (completely obstructed lung subunits), Ventilation/perfusion (V/Q) unevenness	Respiratory "distress" (tachypnea, intercostal retractions, flaring of nostrils, and expiratory grunting)	Good response if hypoventilation or V/Q unevenness is dominant, i.e. PaO2 >250 mm Hg. Poor response if intrapulmonary right to left shunting is present	Diagnostic of specific lung disease	Acidemia and elevated PCO2	Electrolytes, tracheal aspirate, blood culture, tolazoline infusion, and cardiac catheterization.
(5) Mechanical interference with lung function	Diaphragmatic hernia, Pneumothorax, Lobar emphysema, Choanal atresia, Mucous plugs of major bronchi	Compression of normal lung or obstructed airway, Alveolar hypoventilation	Respiratory distress as in category 4, Signs of specific lesions, sometimes but not usually obvious, e.g., bowel sounds in chest	Good response, PaO2 >250 mm Hg	Diagnostic in many instances	Elevated PCO2. In severe instances acidemia is present	Physical signs and chest film usually indicate next step, e.g., operation for diaphragmatic hernia or pleural drainage for tension pneumothorax
(6) "Persistence of the fetal circulation" (PFC) syndrome	Temporary failure of normal vascular responses to birth (primary) or secondary to meconium aspiration group B streptococcal pneumonia, etc.	Pulmonary arterioles remain constricted (as in fetal life), and there is right to left shunting through ductus	Tachypnea, Differential cyanosis, Mimics serious cyanotic heart disease.	Variable	Lung fields show a "ground glass" appearance	Acidemia and elevated PCO2 (many overventilated but underperfused alveoli)	Cardiac catheterization to rule out serious heart disease. Tolazoline responsiveness and spontaneous improvement help establish diagnosis
(7) CNS disease	Intracranial hemorrhage, Seizure disorders	Alveolar hypoventilation	Apneic spells, continuous hypoventilation, or periodic breathing, Seizures or unresponsiveness	Good response, PaO2 >250 mm Hg	Normal, or pneumonia and/or atelectasis may develop	Elevated PCO2 and depressed pH	Lumbar puncture EEG CT scan
(8) Methemoglobinemia	Congenital enzyme deficiency, Acquired (e.g., nitrites)	Abnormal hemoglobin with reduced O2 binding capacity	Very blue but otherwise asymptomatic. Hypoxemia is life-threatening	No response[b]	Normal	Normal or depressed PCO2, Normal pH	Heel-prick blood fails to "pink-up" on exposure to O2. Absorption spectroscopy diagnostic. Infant "pinks-up" dramatically following IV methylene blue (1 mg/kg)

Condition	Causes	Pathophysiology	Clinical findings	O₂ response	Chest x-ray	Blood gas/lab	Diagnostic procedures
			...largement "Jitteriness," apathy, or twitching				...mia, sometimes infusion of glucose IV leads to early improvement. Blood glucose for confirmation; maternal HbA₁c elevated if IDM
	"Small-for-dates" baby	pressure causes right to left atrial shunt		No response		Usually normal	
(10) Hyperviscosity syndrome (high Hgb and Hct)	Twin to twin transfusion Idiopathic, especially in intrauterine growth retardation	High total Hgb (e.g., 25 gm/100 ml) 3-gm reduced Hgb (i.e., saturation 88%), together with increased viscosity and increased arteriovenous O₂ difference produce mild central and marked peripheral cyanosis	Extreme plethora Heart failure	No response	Large heart		Hct over 65%, occasionally up to 85%; venesection plus fluid replacement indicated if CNS or cardiovascular symptoms develop
(11) Shock and sepsis	Septicemia Myocarditis Adrenal failure Perinatal asphyxia	Low cardiac output and "shock lung" lead to alveolar hypoventilation and V/Q unevenness	Apathetic, underresponsive Skin mottled Spleen enlarged Hypotension	Good response, PaO₂ > 250 mm Hg	Large heart with sepsis or myocarditis Heart may be small with adrenal failure	Acidemia and elevated PCO₂	Blood culture (sepsis), ECG, electrolytes (adrenal failure), creatine kinase MB fraction (myocardial damage)
(12) Miscellaneous	Respiratory depression from drugs to mother of neonate Neuromuscular disorders	Hypoventilation	Apathetic, underresponsive	Good response, PaO₂ > 250 mm Hg	Normal or pneumonia	Acidemia and elevated PCO₂	Blood levels of suspected drugs
		Hypoventilation	Muscular hypotonia Werdnig-Hoffman Syndrome	Good response, PaO₂ > 250 mm Hg	Normal or pneumonia	Normal	CNS work-up
	Venoarterial shunts	Right to left shunting	Bruit in lung	No response[b]	Pulmonary AV fistulas usually visible	Normal	Pulmonary arteriography

[a] Modified with permission from M. H. Lees et al.: Southern Medical Journal 67(5), 1974.
[b] Minimal improvement may be seen due to additional physical solution of oxygen in plasma.

TABLE 41.3 CLINICAL AND LABORATORY FINDINGS COMMON WITH PRIMARY HEART DISEASE OR WITH PRIMARY LUNG DISEASE

Clinical and Laboratory Findings	Favors Heart Disease	Favors Lung Disease
Prematurity, postmaturity, or small for gestational age.		X
Fetal distress, especially meconium staining; birth asphyxia; low Apgar scores.		X
Flaccid apathetic infant with little spontaneous movement; apneic spells.	X	X
Tachypnea without other signs of respiratory distress, or deep sighing respirations.	X	
Respiratory distress, i.e., tachypnea with intercostal retractions, grunting, or flaring of alae nasi.	X	X
Marked generalized cyanosis; PaO₂ <25 mm Hg but with normal or reduced PaCO₂.	X	
Generalized cyanosis with PaO₂ <35 mm Hg and PaCO₂ >45 mm Hg.		X
Acidemia, pH <7.2.	X	X
Differential cyanosis	X	X
Cardiomegaly, hepatomegaly, obvious cardiac murmur.	X	
Low PaO₂ on room air; PaO₂ <150 mm Hg on 100% O₂.	X	
Low PaO₂ on room air; PaO₂ >250 mm Hg on 100% O₂.		X
Improvement in pH and PaO₂ following IV tolazoline infusion.		X
Hypoglycemia or high hematocrit (>65).	X	X
Chest x-ray shows clearly ↑ or ↓ pulmonary vascular markings.	X	
Chest x-ray shows snowstorm, reticulogranular pattern.	X	X
Chest x-ray shows blotchy appearance of lung fields consistent with aspiration.		X
Moderate right ventricular hypertrophy on electrocardiogram.	X	X
Gross electrocardiogram abnormality.	X	
Abnormal echocardiogram, e.g., chamber enlargement, abnormal great artery position, or small left ventricle.	X	

ing situation cardiac catheterization and angiocardiography are essential to rule out preductal coarctation of the aorta. An end hole umbilical artery catheter is extremely useful, since an aortogram performed by this route will opacify the entire thoracic aorta.

Spontaneous improvement on the 5th to 7th day of life occurs in 75 to 90% of cases of primary PFC, depending on the diagnostic criteria used. The commonest cause for secondary PFC is the meconium aspiration syndrome where spontaneous recovery is less likely and appears directly related to the volume, viscosity, and distal bronchiolar migration of the meconium aspirated.

Specific measures that have been used to reduce pulmonary vascular resistance include: respiratory alkalosis induced by hyperventilation[12, 45] and pulmonary artery infusion of tolazoline[31] or dopamine.[13] Much attention is currently being directed towards the use of prostaglandin I₂[35] and prostaglandin D₂.[9, 54] At the present, PGI₂ and PGD₂ are not available for human neonatal trial in the U.S. Currently, attempts at PVR reduction in severely affected infants are usually based on ventilator induction of respiratory alkalosis (pH >7.5) or pulmonary artery infusion of dopamine (6 to

20 µg/kg/minute) or pulmonary artery infusion of tolazoline (20 to 50 µg/kg/minute). There is a wide spectrum of response in different infants, and more effective pulmonary vasodilator agents are urgently needed.

HEART FAILURE

The recognition of heart failure during the first days of life is not always straightforward. Heart failure may simulate disease of other organs or systems, and conversely other disease entities may appear with some of the clinical signs of heart failure. Though heart failure is usually the result of structural congenital heart disease or of myocardial disease, it may on occasion be secondary to dysrhythmia, respiratory disease, central nervous system (CNS) disease, anemia, high hematocrit, systemic or pulmonary hypertension, hypoglycemia, or septicemia.

In the newborn, heart failure gives rise to a distinctive clinical syndrome. Common symptoms and signs are feeding difficulties, tachypnea, tachycardia, pulmonary rales and rhonchi, liver enlargement, and cardiomegaly. Less common manifestations include increase in systemic venous pressure, peripheral edema, ascites, pulsus alternans, gallop rhythm, and inappropriate sweating. Pleural and pericardial effusions are exceedingly rare except when the failure has originated in utero. The distinction between left heart failure and right heart failure is less obvious in the newborn than it is in the older child or adult. This difference is caused in part by the fact that many of the lesions producing failure give rise first to left ventricular failure, which in turn causes right ventricular failure. On occasion, one observes "pure" right-sided failure, for example, the newborn with severe isolated pulmonic stenosis, or "pure" left-sided failure, as in the early stages of heart failure associated with aortic stenosis.

Heart failure may progress very rapidly in the first hours and days of life. Delay in transportation, suboptimal environmental temperature, aspiration pneumonia, and other complications may lead to the admission of a near moribund infant in heart failure. Frequently there is no heart murmur, and the clinical picture is more one of advanced cardiogenic shock, with pallor, apathy, minimal spontaneous movement, greatly diminished peripheral pulses, bradycardia, and diminished heart sounds. The respiratory rate may be very rapid with widespread rales, or the infant may have become exhausted with slow respirations or apneic periods. The liver is usually very large, and the spleen may also be enlarged. Sometimes there is peripheral edema.

The clinical picture may closely simulate that of septicemia, meningitis, bronchiolitis, or pneumonia. However, the presence of a very large liver and gross cardiomegaly usually indicate that heart failure is the major problem.

HEART FAILURE WITHOUT STRUCTURAL HEART DISEASE

There are situations in the neonate where heart failure occurs without structural (congenital) heart disease. These include: myocardial damage (due to viruses, asphyxia, protozoa, glycogen, etc); dysrhythmias; PDA complicating respiratory distress syndrome; hypoglycemia; arteriovenous fistula; and severe anemia and polycythemia. Four of the more frequent occurrences are selected for discussion.

PATENT DUCTUS ARTERIOSUS COMPLICATING RESPIRATORY DISTRESS SYNDROME

The importance of the ductus arteriosus as a contributor to the derangements in respiratory distress syndrome (RDS) and bronchopulmonary dysplasia (BPD) has been both long recognized and controversial. It is now recognized[29] that in the very low birth weight (VLBW) infant (<1200 gm), the deficiency in pulmonary arteriolar smooth muscle[61] combined with a large PDA allows a massive left to right shunt because of relatively low pulmonary vascular resistance. Symptomatic PDA, though certainly more common in the VLBW infant, may complicate the recovery of any infant with respiratory disease.

Frequently, the diagnosis of PDA complicating RDS or BPD is straightforward with hyperactive precordium, bounding arterial pulses, and a continuous murmur at 2 LIS. Sometimes, however, the murmur is only systolic, and the diagnosis is less secure. Confirmatory studies include: detection of left atrial and left ventricular enlargement by M mode echocardiography;[53] contrast echocardiography with injection of saline into the aorta and microbubble detection in MPA or RPA[1]; detection of retrograde descending aortic blood flow in diastole using continuous wave Doppler;[50] and aortography. It is important to keep in mind the possibility that the neonate may have coexistent structural heart disease and may be ductus-dependent (e.g., pulmonary atresia).

In the infant who has recovered from RDS and whose illness is complicated by BPD, a PDA may coexist. In this situation it may be difficult to determine the relative contributions of BPD and of PDA to the infant's illness. Measurements which may be useful include the alveolar-arterial difference for CO_2 ($AaDCO_2$),[41] and the detection of descending aortic flow reversal by directional Doppler.[50] Infants with a major BPD component will have a widened $AaDCO_2$ (5 to 25 mm Hg) and a negligible reverse aortic flow, while when PDA is a major contributor to illness, reverse/forward flow ratio exceeds 0.2, and $AaDCO_2$ is less than 10 mm Hg. When respirator dependency or hypercarbia complicate recovery in the presence of even a small PDA, ligation of the PDA may allow recovery.

The treatment of symptomatic PDA in neonates is also controversial. Surgical ligation of a PDA in experienced hands is safe and curative. The use of indomethacin is also safe, provided the infant has no evidence of renal dysfunction or coagulopathy. Indomethacin may be administered by nasogastric tube at a dose of 0.2 mg/kg for up to three times or may be given intravenously as lyophilized indomethacin.[14]

INFANT OF A DIABETIC MOTHER (IDM)

In addition to the increased risk of congenital malformations in the IDM neonate, there are special risks of hypoglycemia,[2] of hypertrophic cardiomyopathy,[60] and of dilated cardiomyopathy.[24] Hypoglycemia in the IDM neonate may be profound, with blood glucose levels less than 10 mg/dl. Glucose appears to be an important energy substrate for the neonatal myocardium, and glucose deficiency is associated both with myocardial failure and cyanosis from right to left atrial shunting. Intravenous glucose administration usually causes rapid improvement.

The hypertrophic cardiomyopathy is usually asymptomatic, transient, and by 10 days begins to show echocardiographic resolution. The echocardiographic features may be quite impressive (Fig. 41.1). In the rare, symptomatic infant, propanolol has been used to produce beta-adrenergic blockade.[51] If there is doubt as to whether the mother had diabetes during pregnancy, the finding of maternal elevation of hemoglobin A_{1c} has been helpful.[39]

PERINATAL ASPHYXIA

Growing recognition of the clinical and laboratory features of "cardiogenic shock" following severe perinatal asphyxia[5, 6] has led to improvements in obstetric care and to early recognition and appropriate treatment of the infant with

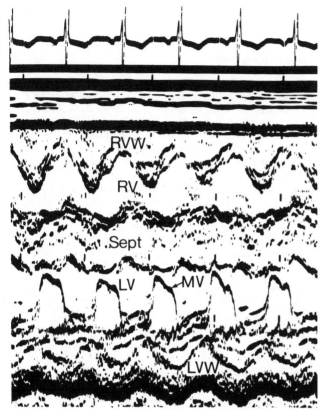

Fig. 41.1 M-mode echocardiogram from a 3-day-old infant of a diabetic mother. There is generalized thickening of the cardiac walls; however, the septum (*Sept*) is thickened to a much greater degree than the left ventricular posterior wall (*LVW*). LV, left ventricle; MV, mitral valve; RV, right ventricle; RVW, right ventricular wall. (Courtesy of Dr. R. Snider and Dr. N. Silverman.)

hypoxemia-related myocardial dysfunction. It appears likely that there exists a clinical spectrum of disorders in the newborn ranging from the least significant, transient tachypnea of the newborn, to the severest, serious combined ventricular failure with systemic hypotension and pulmonary artery hypertension (cardiogenic shock). The following clinical presentations have been described.

Transient Tachypnea of the Newborn

Mild left ventricular dysfunction may produce fluid retention, elevated pulmonary capillary pressure, and reduced lung compliance. Under these circumstances the infant reduces tidal volume and increases respiratory frequency in order to maintain a normal alveolar ventilation.

Tricuspid Valve Insufficiency

This includes RV volume overload and right heart failure. Tricuspid valve dysfunction appears to be secondary to papillary muscle infarction as reflected by elevated serum levels of creatine kinase MB fraction.[4, 42] Sometimes there is also mitral valve dysfunction.[15]

Pulmonary Artery Hypertension

This occurs with a relatively mild prenatal and immediate postnatal course, but with cyanosis, tachypnea, and heart failure developing during the first 24 hours of life. In these infants, it has been postulated that the disorder is one of impaired coronary perfusion to portions of the right and left ventricular myocardium through increased work demands created by unusually severe pulmonary vasoconstriction

from hypoxia.[48] This postulate has been strengthened by electrocardiographic evidence of ischemia and by poor myocardial uptake of thallium 201.[16]

Left Heart Failure with Systemic Hypertension

This presentation appears to follow asphyxia of moderately severe duration and intensity. The elevation of systemic blood pressure is thought to be the result of adrenergic stimulation.[7] The central venous pressure is usually normal.

Left Heart Failure with Systemic Hypotension (Cardiogenic Shock)

It appears likely that the occurrence of systemic hypotension is a time-related phenomenon as demonstrated by Dawes[10] and emphasized by Phibbs.[46] The progression from hypertension to hypotension is consonant with the observations that in the normal lamb fetus endogenous norepinephrine myocardial stores are only one-half of that in the 3-day-old lamb and one-third of that in sheep.[17]

The term cardiogenic shock implies acute primary failure of the heart as a pump. The distinction between cardiogenic shock and severe heart failure is somewhat arbitrary; yet the two appear as different clinical pictures. In the adult, myocardial infarction is overwhelmingly the commonest cause of cardiogenic shock. In the neonate, the clinical picture of cardiogenic shock is encountered infrequently, but it is most common with asphyxial myocardial damage, myocarditis, and with overwhelming septicemia, especially meningococcemia. It is also seen with myocardial infarction secondary to anomalous left coronary artery and with the hypoplastic left heart syndrome.

Use of the word shock implies systemic arterial hypotension—yet many of the less serious and shorter term perinatal hypoxemia episodes are associated with hypertensive or normotensive infants. Myocardial dysfunction associated with systemic hypotension probably represents end-stage dysfunction.

In the typical case of cardiogenic shock in the newborn, the story is that of severe fetal distress, with late and variable decelerations; meconium passage is frequent; and fetal scalp blood pH is in the range of 6.9 to 7.1. Following delivery by emergency cesarian section or by aided vaginal delivery, Apgar scores are typically 1 to 3 at both 1 and 5 minutes. Immediate care includes suctioning, cardiac massage, endotracheal intubation, and the placement of right atrial and aortic catheters by the umbilical vessel route.

At thirty minutes, the preterm infants monitored by Cabal and associates[6] had a normal heart rate, reduced arterial pressure, elevated central venous pressure, and elevated lactic acid. Myocardial dysfunction was manifested during the first 6 hours of life by respiratory distress, hepatomegaly, normal heart rates, gallop rhythm, and markedly decreased heart rate variability. In three infants, the electrocardiograms showed changes suggestive of myocardial ischemia. The chest x-rays showed diffuse parenchymal haziness with pulmonary vascular congestion and cardiac enlargement.

Other asphyxiated infants (full-term) have been described[52] as having mild systemic arterial hypotension with evidence of pulmonary artery hypertension (elevated RPEP/RVET) but without raised central venous pressure. This report suggests that hypoxemia-induced LV dysfunction may have a contributory role in some cases of persistent pulmonary hypertension of the newborn.

Clinical Course

Following restoration of ventilation and normal heart rate, with appropriate attention to correction of hypoglycemia or hypocalcemia, many infants will improve without the use of cardioactive agents. Other infants require single or multiple cardioactive medication, and an occasional infant appears to sustain long-term myocardial damage with a clinical picture of endocardial fibroelastosis.

Treatment

Consideration of systemic artery pressure, pulmonary artery pressure (from RPEP/RVET), and central venous pressure has led to the advocacy of various therapeutic regimens. In addition to routine respirator care, digoxin, and diuretics, attention has been directed to the use of catecholamines and vasodilator agents. Regimens reported to be successful include: for premature infants with hypotension and elevated CVP, Cabal and associates[6] used a continuous infusion of isoproterenol with rapid improvement in 24 to 36 hours; for term infants with hypotension, Leitner et al.[33] used dopamine (2.5 μg/kg/minute) or placebo. Five of seven infants in the dopamine group increased their systolic blood pressure when compared to their predopamine values and the postplacebo values in the control group; for premature infants with systemic hypertension, six received a combination of an inotropic agent (dopamine, 2 to 8 μg/kg/minute) and a short-acting vasodilator (chlorpromazine, 1 to 2 μg/kg/minute).[7] Mean arterial blood pressure fell and skin $TcPCO_2$ decreased; and for term infants with systemic hypertension and elevated CVP, the infants received digitalis and sodium nitroprusside (2 to 6 μg/kg/minute).[52] There was a decrease in arterial and in central venous pressure within 20 minutes. Arterial pH and tissue PO_2 increased, while $TcPCO_2$ decreased.

NEONATAL DYSRHYTHMIAS

There is considerable evidence that after birth there is continued development of the cardiac conduction system, and an increase in the sympathetic innervation of the heart. These factors may account for the observed heart rate variability, and for the frequency of benign dysrhythmias in the newborn. Premature supraventricular and ventricular beats, brief periods of sinus arrest, ectopic atrial rhythms, and wandering atrial pacemaker have all been observed during electrocardiographic monitoring of asymptomatic newborn infants.[40]

Before embarking on the treatment of a tachycardia, bradycardia, or irregular heart beat, one must decide if the dysrhythmia is benign and likely to resolve spontaneously, or if it is potentially serious. Sometimes dysrhythmia indicates underlying extracardiac disease, such as central nervous system disease, sepsis, hypoglycemia, drug toxicity (especially digitalis), severe tissue hypoxia, adrenal insufficiency, electrolyte and acid-base abnormalities. One must also decide if the treatment is likely to be more dangerous than the dysrhythmia. In deciding to treat or not to treat, major consideration should be given to whether the ventricular rate and rhythm are compatible with a normal cardiac output.

Benign Dysrhythmias

Healthy full-term and premature neonates have heart rates which range from 90 to 195 beats/minute. Rates above and below this range that are sustained for 15 seconds or more should have electrocardiographic documentation of the rhythm.

Transient periods of sinus bradycardia may occur during straining, micturition, or during crying. Maternal medications, such as reserpine or propranolol may result in bradycardia in the newborn. Sinus tachycardia occurs with periods of increased activity and crying, and also with fever and hyperthyroidism.

Serious Dysrhythmias

Supraventricular tachycardia (SVT) is the commonest tachydysrhythmia in the newborn. It may be due to dual AV nodal pathways with antegrade conduction down one pathway, and the completion of a circle by retrograde conduction up the other. It may be due to rapid conduction through an accessory bundle, Wolff-Parkinson-White (WPW) syndrome, or due to the existence of an ectopic atrial focus with an automaticity faster than the SA node. There is an increased frequency of the WPW syndrome with SVT in Ebstein's anomaly of the tricuspid valve, and also with corrected transposition of the great arteries.

Intrauterine supraventricular tachycardia, though uncommon, is associated with severe heart failure at birth, and may be lethal. Newburger and Keane[44] described 37 infants with intrauterine SVT; five had preexcitation syndrome (WPW) and 11 had myocarditis or structural heart disease. Twenty-three of the 37 infants had severe heart failure within the first hours of life, and thirteen converted to normal sinus rhythm at delivery or shortly after birth. Four infants were treated prenatally with digoxin administration to the mother and none converted. However, successful conversion with maternally administered propranolol has been reported[59] and successful use of maternal digoxin has now also been reported.[25]

The identification of fetal SVT calls for an aggressive approach. Fetal edema can be assessed by ultrasound, and fetal lung maturity can be defined by the amniotic fluid, lecithin/sphingomyelin ratio (L/S). If the L/S ratio is favorable, and the gestation over 34 weeks (which it usually is), immediate delivery is indicated. If the gestational period and L/S ratio are unfavorable, betamethasone may be administered to induce surfactant production, and conversion with maternally administered propranolol may be tried.

Newborns with SVT are either those in whom the dysrhythmia is discovered during the first few days after birth when they are relatively asymptomatic or are those who are brought to the hospital in heart failure having had the dysrhythmia for several days. The history usually reveals that the infant has become anxious, restless, tachypnic, or "not well." Neonates then usually become "wheezy," and at this stage it is easy for both parent and physician to diagnose a lower respiratory tract infection. As the SVT persists, the infant becomes pale, apathetic, and obviously very sick, with signs of heart failure.

The time taken for an infant to develop heart failure depends mainly on the ventricular rate and the presence or absence of structural heart disease. An infant with serious cyanotic heart disease who develops SVT during the course of cardiac catheterization may worsen in a few minutes, while an infant with a normal heart may tolerate indefinitely a rate of 220 beats/minute.

Treatment. If the infant's condition is critical, DC countershock provides the most immediate method of terminating the attack. In more elective situations, drug therapy can be utilized. Whichever method is chosen, acidosis, electrolyte abnormalities, hypothermia, and hypoxemia should be corrected as far as possible. Vagal stimulation maneuvers are generally unsuccessful and may waste valuable time.

A newborn who has had one attack of SVT has an approximately 20% recurrence risk, and continued maintenance of digoxin for 6 months after the last attack is indicated. Recurrences are more likely in those with underlying Wolff-

Parkinson-White syndrome; and in these patients, continued maintenance of digoxin, sometimes supplemented by quinidine or propranolol may be indicated.

Nadas and associates[40A] have divided infants into prognostically useful clinical groups. The first group consists primarily of male infants under 4 months of age without structural heart disease; the second group is composed of older infants of both sexes with or without heart disease. Recurrences after the age of 1 year are unlikely with the first group; but recurrences are frequent with the second group, particularly if the Wolff-Parkinson-White syndrome is present.

Atrial flutter is infrequent in the neonate, and is likely to be associated with organic heart disease, especially mitral valve disease, endocardial fibroelastosis, Ebstein's anomaly, pulmonary atresia, VSD, CA, and complex heart defects. Atrial flutter has been diagnosed in utero.

Atrial fibrillation is rare in the newborn. It is likely to be associated with serious organic heart disease, especially those conditions associated with left atrial enlargement.

Ventricular tachycardia in neonates most commonly occurs in the presence of organic heart disease, but is rare, except as a complication of cardiac surgery, anesthesia, or cardiac catheterization. Stevens and coworkers[57] reported four cases of ventricular tachycardia in the neonatal period; one case was detected in utero, and all patients survived, two with asymptomatic episodes of ventricular ectopy on long-term follow-up. In their review of 45 cases of ventricular dysrhythmia in the perinatal period, nine were detected in utero, three persisted beyond the perinatal period, and two resulted in death with associated disorders.

Ectopic beats are common in healthy newborn infants, with a frequency of 21 to 31% for healthy prematures and up to 23% for full-term newborns. Supraventricular ectopic beats are more common than ventricular and may arise in the atrium or AV junctional tissue. Occasionally ectopic beats in the newborn may constitute bigeminal rhythm, and we have seen one infant with closely coupled ventricular ectopic beats who had evidence of low output and who responded favorably to oral dilantin.

Sinus node dysfunction is rare in the newborn; however, sometimes pacemaker implantation is necessary because bradycardias become life-threatening. We have seen one newborn with intermittent symptomatic bradydysrhythmia with sinus arrest and paroxysmal tachydysrhythmia (Fig. 41.2). She was treated with prophylactic pacemaker implantation. A previous child in the family had been the victim of sudden infant death syndrome (SIDS).

Atrioventricular block in newborns is unusual, but when it occurs, it is usually asymptomatic. It may be secondary to digitalis administration or viral infections. Some types of congenital heart disease have an increased frequency of AV block. These include corrected transposition of the great arteries, atrial septal defect, Ebstein's anomaly, and complex cyanotic cardiac defects.

The association between congenital complete heart block and maternal connective tissue disorders has been recognized. McCue and coworkers[37] report 22 children with congenital complete heart block, of whom 14 were born to 11 mothers with clinical or laboratory evidence of connective tissue disorder, primarily lupus erythematosus. Pacemaker therapy is sometimes needed if there are symptoms of heart failure, prolonged asystoles, or cerebrovascular insufficiency.

Prolonged QT interval syndrome, when associated with deafness, is known as the Jervell-Lange-Nielsen syndrome and without deafness, the Romano-Ward syndrome. The report by James et al.[30] showing intracardiac neuritis

and neural degeneration in eight patients with long QT syndrome has cast doubt on the hereditary nature, and the possibility of a slow virus has been considered.

The syndrome presents in all grades of severity and may present in the neonatal period as bradycardia or periods of ventricular dysrhythmia. In the example shown (Fig. 41.3), there was a distal 2:1 block, evidently the result of each second P wave being conducted in the prolonged refractory period. Treatment is largely empirical; both high dose propranolol and left stellate ganglion block have been recommended.

CARDIAC CATHETERIZATION AND ANGIOCARDIOGRAPHY

Categorical indications for hemodynamic and angiographic study of the newborn cannot be laid down, but the

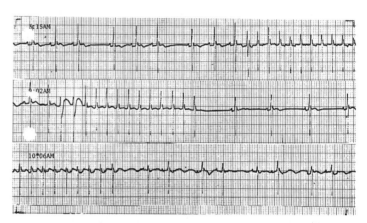

Fig. 41.2 Sinus node dysfunction in a 2-day-old infant. Note periods of sinus bradycardia and periods of supraventricular tachycardia. This child was treated with a pacemaker for periods of sinus bradycardia that were frequent and symptomatic. A sibling had died of SIDS.

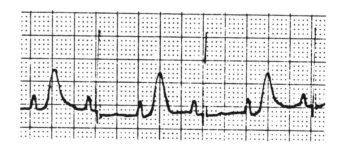

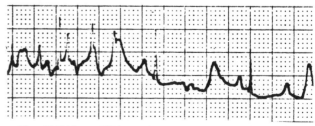

Fig. 41.3 Long QT interval syndrome in a neonate. Note QT interval of 0.7 seconds, with every second P wave blocked probably due to ventricular refractoriness. In the lower strip, note spontaneous termination of ventricular tachycardia.

following are offered as guidelines.

Central cyanosis believed to be of cardiovascular origin and persisting for more than a few hours after birth may be an indication. In some patients there may be cause for procrastination, especially if the infant is cold, acidotic, or anemic, or has other remediable abnormalities, such as hypoglycemia or hyperviscosity. However, most newborns with obvious cardiovascular central cyanosis become steadily worse and should have a firm diagnosis established at the earliest opportunity.

Heart failure is a less common indication than cyanosis. In general, the earlier the onset, the worse the prognosis. Thus, in a 1-day-old newborn, heart failure believed to be caused by structural cardiovascular disease demands urgent investigation, whereas the 28-day-old newborn has already demonstrated viability, and a more elective approach with a trial of intensive medical treatment may be justified.

Various dysrhythmias may be indications for invasive maneuvers; thus, cardiac catheterization may be required for the placement of a temporary transvenous pacemaker in the treatment of complete heart block, digitalis, or other drug toxicity. The recording of an intracardiac electrogram may be necessary for the diagnosis of a specific dysrhythmia.

Certain pulmonary diseases may closely mimic heart disease, and on occasion diagnostic study is the only way of resolving the issue.

Elucidation of the anatomy of a severe vascular ring causing life-threatening airway obstruction is an occasional indication for angiographic study of the neonate. Other uncommon indications include suspicion of pericardial tamponade, pulmonary arteriography, and the instillation of short-acting pharmacologic compounds such as tolazoline directly into the pulmonary artery to lower pulmonary vascular resistance, or of prostaglandin E_1 into the closing ductus arteriosus to increase ductal diameter and increase pulmonary blood flow in critically sick newborns with pulmonary atresia.[49]

DIFFERENTIAL DIAGNOSIS

Despite careful attention to the history, physical examination, electrocardiogram, echocardiogram, and roentgenogram, it is often not possible to make a precise anatomic diagnosis. This is not a reflection of diagnostic inadequacy but is a result of the changing fetal to newborn circulation, the presence of heart failure or pulmonary hypertension, and the nonspecificity of some signs. The usual result is that although one may make an intelligent guess at the structural abnormality, one is left with several conditions with which the signs are compatible. Certain syndrome complexes emerge, based on the presence or absence of major physical signs. Cardiac catheterization combined with selective angiocardiography is essential for accurate diagnosis, except in very rare instances where signs are pathognomonic and the correct treatment is obvious.

PROSTAGLANDIN E₁ IN DUCTUS-DEPENDENT LESIONS

Since the initial report[43] of the use of PGE_1 to dilate the ductus arteriosus in infants with ductus-dependent heart lesions, use and experience has grown, and indications have become firmer. Major indications for the use of PGE_1 as a preoperative intervention include: pulmonary atresia with and without VSD; extreme PS with suprasystemic RV pressure and right heart failure; tricuspid atresia with inadequate pulmonary blood flow; complex cyanotic heart disease with pulmonary atresia; interrupted aortic arch, with PDA supplying descending aorta; severe preductal CA; and transposition of great arteries with inadequate mixing and acidemia.

PGE_1 is most useful when it is used intravenously at a dose of 0.05 to 0.1 μg/kg/minute. The drug begins to act in 10 to 15 minutes, and providing the ductus is not thrombosed, is almost always successful. Typically, arterial PO_2 increases by 15 to 20 mm Hg and allows next day surgery on a metabolically stable infant instead of an acidemic one.

REFERENCES

1. Allen, H. D., Sahn, D. J., and Goldberg, H. T.: New serial contrast technique for assessment of left-to-right shunting PDA in the neonate. Am. J. Cardiol. 41:288, 1978.

2. Amatayakul, O., Cumming, G. R., and Haworth, J. C.: Association of hypoglycemia with cardiac enlargement and heart failure in newborn infants. Arch. Dis. Child. 45:717, 1970.

3. Benzing, G., Schubert, W., Hug, G., and Kaplan, S.: Simultaneous hypoglycemia and acute congestive heart failure. Circulation 40:209, 1969.

4. Bucciarelli, R., Nelson, R. M., Egan, E. A., II, Eitzman, D. V., and Gessner, I. H.: Transient tricuspid insufficiency of the newborn: A form of myocardial dysfunction in stressed newborns, Pediatrics 59:330, 1977.

5. Burnard, E. D., and James, L. S.: Failure of the heart after cardiac asphyxia at birth. Pediatrics 28:545, 1961.

6. Cabal, L. A., Devaskar, U., Siassi, B., Hodgman, J. E., and Emmanoulides, G. C.: Cardiogenic shock associated with perinatal asphyxia in preterm infants. J. Pediatr. 96:705–710, 1980.

7. Cabal, L. A., Plajstek, C. E., Siassi, B., Hodgman, J. E., and Barrenechea, I.: Combined cardiotonic and vasodilator therapy for myocardial dysfunction associated with hypertension in asphyxiated prematures (abstr.). Pediatr. Res. 15:654, 1981.

8. Capitanio, M. A., and Kirkpatrick, J. A.: Roentgen examination in the evaluation of the newborn infant with respiratory distress. J.

Pediatr. 75:896, 1969.

9. Cassin, S., Tod, M., Philips, J., Frisinger, J., Jordan, J., and Gibbs, C.: Effects of prostaglandin D₂ on perinatal circulation. Am. J. Physiol. 240:H755, 1981.

10. Dawes, G. S.: In Foetal and Neonatal Physiology. Chicago, Year Book Publishers, 1968, pp 1–247.

11. Dillon, J. C., Feigenbaum, H., Konecke, L. L., Keutel, J., Hurwitz, R. A., Davis, R. H., and Chang, S.: Echocardiographic manifestations of D-transposition of the great vessels. Am. J. Cardiol. 32(1):74, 1973.

12. Drummond, W. H., Peckham, G. J., and Fox, W. W.: The clinical profile of the newborn with persistent pulmonary hypertension. Clin. Pediatr. 16:335, 1977.

13. Drummond, W. H., Gregory, G. A., Heymann, M. A., and Phibbs, R. A.: The independent effects of hyperventilation, tolazoline, and dopamine on infants with persistent pulmonary hypertension. J. Pediatr. 98:603–611, 1981.

14. Ellison, K., Nadas, A. S., Gersony, W., and Peckham, G.: Patent ductus arteriosus in the premature infant. Diagnosis, clinical course and therapy with indomethacin. Presented at 54th Scientific Sessions. American Heart Association, Dallas, Texas, November 18, 1981.

15. Emmanoulides, G. C., and Baylen, B. G.: Neonatal cardiopulmonary distress without congenital heart disease. Curr. Probl. Pediatr. 9:12, 1979.

16. Finley, J. P., Howman-Giles, R. B., Gilday, D. Z., and Rowe, R. D.: Transient myocardial

ischemia of the newborn infant demonstrated by thallium myocardial imaging. J. Pediatr. 94:263, 1979.

17. Friedman, W. F.: The intrinsic physiologic properties of the developing heart. Prog. Cardiovasc. Dis. 15:87, 1972.

18. Garson, A., Jr., Gillette, P. L., and McNamara, D. G.: Supraventricular tachycardia in children. Clinical features, response to treatment and long term follow-up in 217 patients. Am. J. Cardiol. 45:430, 1980.

19. Gatti, R. A., Muster, A. J., Cole, R. B., and Paul, M. H.: Neonatal polycythemia with transient cyanosis and cardiorespiratory abnormalities. J. Pediatr. 69:1063, 1966.

20. Gersony, W. M.: Persistence of the fetal circulation: A commentary. J. Pediatr. 82:1103, 1973.

21. Gersony, W. M., Duc, G. V., and Sinclair, J. C.: "PFC" syndrome (persistence of the fetal circulation). Circulation 40:111, 1969.

22. Gillette, A. C., Garson, A., Jr., Kugler, J. D., and Cooley, D.: Surgical treatment of supraventricular tachycardia in infants and children. Circulation 60:113, 1979.

23. Gross, G. P., Hathaway, W. E., and McGaughey, H. R.: Hyperviscosity in the neonate. J. Pediatr. 82:1004, 1973.

24. Halliday, H. L.: Hypertrophic cardiomyopathy in infants of poorly-controlled diabetic mothers. Arch. Dis. Child. 56:258–263, 1981.

25. Harrigan, J. T., Kangos, J. J., Sikka, A., Spisso, K. R., Natarajan, N., Rosenfeld, D., Leiman, S., and Korn, D.: Successful treatment of fetal

congestive heart failure secondary to tachycardia. N. Engl. J. Med. 304:1527–1529, 1981.

26. Hastreiter, A. R., and Abella, J. B.: The electrocardiogram in the newborn period. I. The normal infant. J. Pediatr. 78:146, 1971.

27. Hastreiter, A. R., and Abella, J. B.: The electrocardiogram in the newborn period. II. The infant with disease. J. Pediatr. 78:346, 1971.

28. Hoffman, J. I. E.: Differentiation of heart and lung disease in infants In The Heart, Lungs and Circulation of the Fetus and Newborn. Seminar held at University of California, San Francisco, February 10–12, 1975.

29. Jacob, J., Gluck, L., DiSessa, T., Edwards, D., Kulovich, M., Kurlinski, J., Merritt, T. A., and Freidman, W. F.: The contribution of PDA in the neonate with severe RDS. J. Pediatr. 96:79–87, 1980.

30. James, T. N., Froggatt, P., Atkinson, W. J., Jr., Lurie, P. R., McNamara, D. G., Miller, W. W., Schloss, G. T., Carroll, J. R., and North, R. L.: Observations on the pathophysiology of the long QT syndromes with special reference to the neuropathology of the heart. Circulation 57:1221–1231, 1978.

31. Korones, S. B., and Fabien, G. A.: Successful treatment of "persistent fetal circulation" with tolazoline. Pediatr. Res. 9:367, 1975.

32. Lees, M. H.: Cyanosis of the newborn infant. J. Pediatr. 77:484, 1970.

33. Leitner, M., DiSessa, Gluck, L., Coen, R., Ching, C. T., and Friedman, W. F.: Hemodynamic effects of dopamine in neonatal asphyxia (abstr.). Circulation 62:4, Part II, III-25, 1980.

34. Levin, D. L., Mills, L. J., and Weinberg, A. G.: Hemodynamic, pulmonary vascular, and myocardial abnormalities secondary to pharmacologic constriction of the ductus arteriosus. A possible mechanism for persistent pulmonary hypertension and transient tricuspid insufficiency in the newborn infant. Circulation 60:360, 1979.

35. Lock, J. E., Olley, P. M., Coceani, F., Swyer, P. R., and Rowe, R. D.: Use of prostacyclin in persistent fetal circulation. Lancet 1:1343, 1979.

36. Lundstrom, N. R.: Clinical applications of echocardiography in infants and children. Acta Paediatr. Scand. (Suppl.) 243:1–38, 1974.

37. McCue, C. M., Mantakas, M. E., Tingelstad, J. B. and Ruddy, S.: Congenital heart block in newborns of mothers with connective tissue disease. Circulation 56:82–90, 1977.

38. Meyer, R. A., and Kaplan, S.: Noninvasive techniques in pediatric cardiovascular disease. Prog. Cardiovasc. Dis. 15(4):341, 1973.

39. Miller, E., Hare, J. W., Cloherty, J. P., Dunn, P. J., Gleason, R. E., Soeldner, J. S., and Kitzmiller, J. I.: Elevated maternal hemoglobin A₁c in early pregnancy and major congenital anomalies in infants of diabetic mothers. N. Engl. J. Med. 304:1331–1334, 1981.

40. Morgan, B. C., Bloom, R. S., and Guntheroth, W. G.: Cardiac arrhythmias in premature infants. Pediatrics 35:658, 1965.

40a. Nadas, A. S., Daeschner, C. R., Roth, A., and Blumenthal, S. T.: Paroxysmal tachycardia in children. Pediatrics, 9:167, 1950.

41. Neal, W. A., Bessinger, F. B., Hunt, C. E., and Lucas, R. V.: Patent ductus arteriosus complicating respiratory distress syndrome. J. Pediatr. 86:127, 1975.

42. Nelson, R. M., Bucciarelli, R. L., Eitzmann, D. V., Egan, E. A., II., and Gessner, I. H.: Serum creatine phosphokinase MB fraction in newborns with transient tricuspid insufficiency, N. Engl. J. Med. 298:146, 1978.

43. Neutze, J. M., Starling, M. B., Elliott, R. B., and Barratt-Boyes, B. G.: Palliation of cyanotic congenital heart disease in infancy with E-type prostaglandin. Circulation 55:238, 1977.

44. Newburger, J., and Keane, J. F.: Intrauterine supraventricular tachycardia. J. Pediatr. 95:780–786, 1979.

45. Peckham, G. J., and Fox, W. W.: Physiologic factors affecting pulmonary artery pressure in infants with persistent pulmonary hypertension. J. Pediatr. 93:1005-1010, 1978.

46. Phibbs, R. H.: Delivery room management of the newborn. In Neonatology, Pathophysiology and Management of the Newborn, 2nd ed. edited by G. B. Avery. Philadelphia, J. B. Lippincott, 1981, pp. 182–201.

47. Reid, M. M., Reilly, B. J., Murdock, A. I., and Swyer, P. R.: Cardiomegaly in association with neonatal hypoglycemia. Acta Paediatr. Scand. 60:295, 1971.

48. Rowe, R. D., and Hoffmann, T.: Transient myocardial ischemia of the newborn infant: A form of severe cardiorespiratory distress in full-term infants. J. Pediatr. 81:243, 1972.

49. Rudolph, A. M., and Heymann, M. A.: Medical treatment of the ductus arteriosus. Hosp. Pract. 12:57, 1977.

50. Serwer, G. A., Armstrong, B. E., and Anderson, P. A. W.: Non-invasive detection of retrograde descending aortic flow in infants using continuous wave Doppler ultrasonography. J. Pediatr. 97:394, 1980.

51. Shand, D. G., Sell, C. G., and Oates, J. A.: Hypertrophic obstructive cardiomyopathy in an infant: Propranolol therapy for three years. N. Engl. J. Med. 285:843–844, 1971.

52. Siassi, B., Arce, P. H., Cabal, L. A., Sims, M. E. and Pyk, W. U.: Cardiovascular effects of perinatal asphyxia in full term infants (abstr.). Pediatr. Res. 15:472, 1981.

53. Silverman, N. H., Leurs, A. B., Heymann, M. A. and Rudolph, A. M.: Echocardiographic assessment of ductus arteriosus shunt in premature infants. Circulation 50:821, 1974.

54. Soiffer, S. J., Morin, F. C., Roman, C. and Heymann, M. A.: Prostaglandin D₂ (PGD₂) decreases hypoxic pulmonary hypertension in newborn lambs (abstr.). Pediatr. Res. 15:682, 1981.

55. Soler-Soler, J., Sagrista-Sauleda, J., Cabrera, A., Sauleda-Pares, J., Inglesias-Berengue, J., Permanyer-Muralda, G. and Roca-Llop, J.: Effect of verapamil in infants with paroxysmal supraventricular tachycardia. Circulation 59:876–879, 1978.

56. Sommerville, R. J., Nora, J. J., Clayton, G. W., and McNamara, D. G.: Adrenal insufficiency mimicking heart disease in infancy. Pediatrics 42:691, 1968.

57. Stevens, D. C., Schreiner, R. L., Hurwitz, R. A., and Gresham, E. L.: Fetal and neonatal ventricular arrhythmia. Pediatrics 63:771–777, 1979.

58. Terragno, N. A., Terragno, A., and McGiff, J. C.: Role of prostaglandins in blood vessels. Semin. Perinatol. 4:85, 1980.

59. Teuscher, A., Bossi, E., Imhof, P., Erb, E., Stocker, F. P., and Weber, J. W.: Effect of propanolol on fetal tachycardia in diabetic pregnancy. Am. J. Cardiol 42:304–307, 1978.

60. Way, G. L., Ruttenberg, H. D., Eshaghpour, E., Nora, J. J., and Wolfe, R. E.: Hypertrophic obstructive cardiomyopathy in infants of diabetic mothers (abstr.). Circulation 53–54 (Suppl. II):105, 1976.

61. Wagenvoort, C. A., Neufeld, H. N., and Edwards, J. E.: The structure of the pulmonary arterial tree in fetal and early post natal life. Lab. Invest. 10:751, 1961.

42

Pulmonary Hypertension

Marlene Rabinovitch, M.D.

Nothing exists from whose nature some effect does not follow.

Baruch Spinoza

Although it has been called the 'lesser circulation', implying somewhat of a passive role, the response of the pulmonary vascular bed to a variety of conditions and disease states is the major determinant of clinical outcome. This chapter will describe the many ways in which pulmonary hypertension may occur in infancy, childhood, and adolescence (Table 42.1), how its presence can be diagnosed, and how its severity can be assessed. The structural basis for the abnormal hemodynamic state is discussed, and present thinking concerning pathogenesis is outlined. The current approach to treatment is given. Also, the results of recent experimental studies are presented, and speculations are made concerning future directions in research.

DEFECTS WITH INCREASED PULMONARY BLOOD FLOW

The first report of pulmonary hypertension resulting from a congenital heart defect is attributed to Eisenmenger in 1897.[50] He described a 32-year-old man with unexplained

Table 42.1 CAUSES OF PULMONARY HYPERTENSION IN INFANTS, CHILDREN, AND ADOLESCENTS[a]

Cause	Examples
1. Heart disease	With increased pulmonary blood flow
	With increased pulmonary venous pressure
	With decreased pulmonary blood flow
2. Hypoxia	Acute hypoxia
	Chronic hypoxia
	Lung disease: obstructive restrictive
	Upper airway obstruction
	Diminished ventilatory drive
	Disorders of the chest wall
3. Persistent pulmonary hypertension of the newborn	Underdevelopment of the lungs
	Maladaptation of the pulmonary vascular bed
	Maldevelopment of the pulmonary vascular bed
4. Thromboembolic disease	Sickle cell states
	Ventriculovenous shunts for hydrocephalus
5. Portal hypertension	Portal vein thrombosis
	Liver disease
6. Granulomatous disease	Sarcoid
7. Collagen vascular disease	Rheumatoid arthritis
	Lupus erythematosus
8. Drugs	Aminorex
9. Idiopathic	Arterial abnormality
	Venous abnormality

[a] More examples in text and other tables.

exercise intolerance and cyanosis who died in heart failure after an episode of hemoptysis. At postmortem examination, a large ventricular septal defect (VSD) was identified, and there was overriding of the aorta. Many years later, it was observed that the symptoms this man had also occurred in some patients with one of a variety of congenital heart defects in which increased pulmonary blood flow secondary to left to right shunting is followed subsequently by a progressive elevation in pulmonary vascular resistance eventually resulting in reversal of the shunt and cyanosis.[15, 17, 232, 299] The pathologic basis for this clinical entity, which came to be known as the "Eisenmenger syndrome," was thought to be the development of 'endarteritis obliterans' in very small and abnormally muscular peripheral arteries. Hence, the term pulmonary vascular obstructive disease was commonly applied to describe the functional state.[34]

Natural History

Natural history studies reveal that different congenital heart defects vary considerably in the frequency and severity of pulmonary hypertension. The latter is judged by the level of pulmonary vascular resistance, the rate of its progressive elevation, and the potential for its reversibility. For example, in approximately 15% of infants with large unrestrictive VSD, progressive elevation in pulmonary vascular resistance occurs either in late infancy or early childhood.[49, 80, 109] If surgical repair is carried out within the first 2 years of life, the increased pulmonary vascular resistance rarely persists; if correction is delayed longer, the degree of elevation remains at levels observed preoperatively or progressively increases[26, 30, 61] (Fig. 42.1A). In addition, among the group repaired late, those patients who postoperatively have only slightly increased pulmonary artery pressure at rest will usually exhibit an abnormal degree of elevation with exer-

cise[79, 162] (Fig. 42.1B). In patients with a large patent ductus arteriosus (PDA), there are frequency and severity of pulmonary hypertension[216] that are similar to those in patients with a VSD. Patients with a secundum atrial septal defect (ASD) usually have a normal pulmonary artery pressure in childhood, and the 20% that develop progressive elevation do so generally only after the 3rd decade.[14]

Severe pulmonary hypertension will occur in 8% of patients with transposition of the great arteries (TGA) and an intact ventricular septum,[272] but in those who, in addition, have a VSD or PDA, 40% have severe pulmonary hypertension within the first year of life.[194, 286] In fact, by 2 years of age, 75% of this group are thus affected. There have even been case reports of patients with TGA and intact ventricular septum and normal pulmonary artery pressures preoperatively[12, 225] in whom pulmonary hypertension developed after surgical repair.

Virtually all patients with common atrioventricular canal have pulmonary hypertension and develop severe irreversibly increased pulmonary vascular resistance in childhood; the majority will do so by 2 years of age but, in some, this has been observed as early as the first year of life.[196] In all patients with truncus arteriosus and unrestricted pulmonary blood flow, a permanent increase in pulmonary vascular resistance occurs by the second year of life, but the degree of elevation becomes severe by age 7 years.[160] The surgically created systemic to pulmonary artery shunts also may cause pulmonary hypertension; this occurs rarely with a Blalock-Taussig anastomosis, i.e., less than 10% of cases, but is common with a Waterston or Potts shunt where, after 5 years duration, a 30% frequency is reported.[202]

Clinical and Hemodynamic Features

Detecting the patient with a given congenital heart defect who will develop severe pulmonary hypertension or who will do so particularly early in life is difficult. Clinical criteria, i.e., shortening and softening of a heart murmur, accompanied by decreased splitting of the second heart sound and increased intensity of the pulmonic component, may be subtle early on and are not often appreciated except when the condition is advanced. Radiologic features, i.e., an enlarging main pulmonary artery and tortuosity and 'pruning' of the intra-pulmonary arteries, are generally also late manifestations.[116, 291] Electrocardiographic[118] and vectorcardiographic[33] features are useful in detecting early evidence of ventricular hypertrophy but are relatively insensitive as predictors of its severity or of the severity of pulmonary hypertension; the latter is also true for M-mode echocardiographic features, e.g., flattening of the pulmonic 'a' wave,[2] midsystolic closure of the pulmonic valve,[9] prolongation of right ventricular systolic time intervals (pre-ejection period/ejection time > 0.34) or prolongation of right ventricular isovolumic contraction time >25 milliseconds.[174] Radionuclide assessment of right ventricular wall thickness using thallium-201 is largely useful as a screening test to detect pressure overload of the right ventricle (Fig. 42.2A). The use of pulsed Doppler techniques in PDA to detect abbreviated diastolic flow will also predict the presence rather than the severity of pulmonary hypertension (Fig. 42.2B).

Early and frequent cardiac catheterization is the best way to determine and follow the level of pulmonary vascular resistance. Criteria have been suggested to distinguish patients in whom, even after repair, persistent severe elevation in pulmonary vascular resistance is likely[158, 276]: a difference in oxygen saturation between pulmonary arteries and veins of greater than 2.5 volume percent or an absolute level of pulmonary vascular resistance of greater than 10 u/m². Values in the range between 8 and 10 u/m² are considered

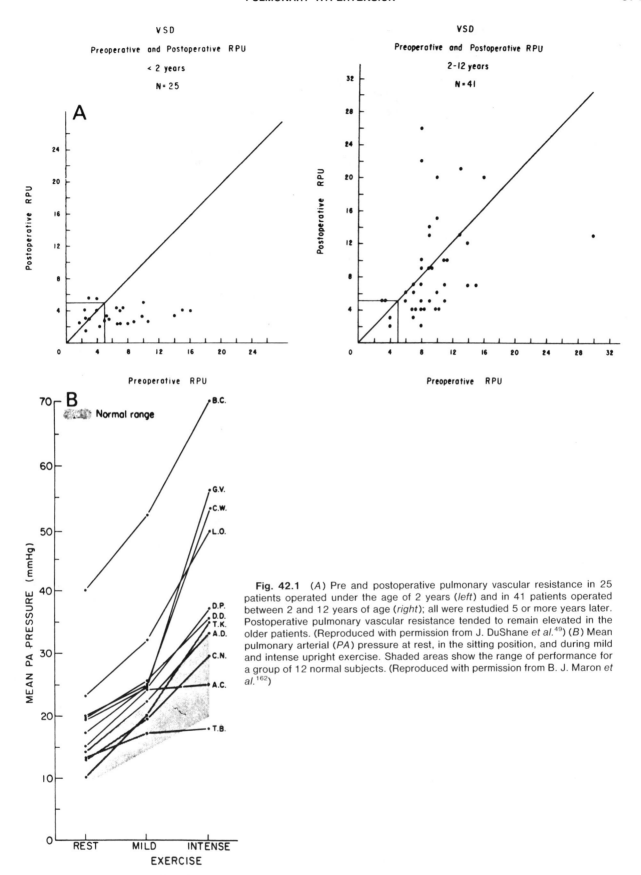

Fig. 42.1 (*A*) Pre and postoperative pulmonary vascular resistance in 25 patients operated under the age of 2 years (*left*) and in 41 patients operated between 2 and 12 years of age (*right*); all were restudied 5 or more years later. Postoperative pulmonary vascular resistance tended to remain elevated in the older patients. (Reproduced with permission from J. DuShane *et al.*[49]) (*B*) Mean pulmonary arterial (*PA*) pressure at rest, in the sitting position, and during mild and intense upright exercise. Shaded areas show the range of performance for a group of 12 normal subjects. (Reproduced with permission from B. J. Maron *et al.*[162])

borderline but very promising if a decrease to 6 u/m² or less can be achieved with the inhalation of 100% oxygen or after the intravenous administration of 1 mg/kg of tolazoline. While the estimation of pulmonary vascular resistance by

the Fick principle is most precise when oxygen consumption is measured,[258] the value obtained reflects the functional state at only one point in time. This measurement is influenced by the degree and type of sedation under which the

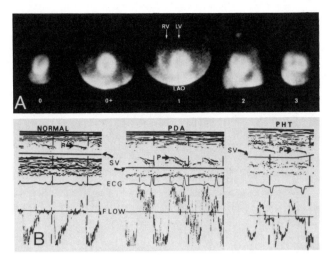

Fig. 42.2 (A) Thallium-201 scintigraphic myocardial images viewed in left anterior oblique projection (LAO). 0 shows a well-defined left ventricular wall (LV) with no right ventricular wall (RV) image; 0+ shows a faint shadow of the RV; 1 shows an RV less dense than the LV; 2 shows equally dense images; and 3 shows a thicker RV, as compared to the LV, image. (Reproduced with permission from M. Rabinovitch et al.[213]) (B) Representative pulsed Doppler echocardiogram of pulmonary artery flow in the normal subject, in the uncomplicated patent ductus arteriosus (PDA), and in the PDA with pulmonary hypertension (PHT). The M-mode echocardiogram shows the pulmonary valve leaflet (P). The sample volume (SV) is also shown. Flow indicates a 0 reference line; in the normal there is no diastolic ductal flow (i.e., above flow line away from transducer). In the PDA with PHT compared to the PDA, diastolic flow is abbreviated. (Reproduced with permission from J. G. Stevenson et al.[257])

patient is examined, e.g., it may be increased during ketamine anesthesia.[265] It is also increased when there is pulmonary disease causing hypoxemia[275] and when there is polycythemia.[227] Pulmonary vascular resistance is often underestimated when there is large flow through systemic collateral vessels, as in patients with TGA and intact ventricular septum.[127] Thus, in certain cases, in addition to the hemodynamic assessment, an evaluation of the structural state of the pulmonary vascular bed can provide useful information.

Structural Features

As early as 1935, Brenner[21] observed different types of pulmonary vascular lesions in patients with congenital heart defects. Heath and Edwards in 1958[95] suggested that there was a progression of structural changes (Grades I through VI) (Fig. 42.3). Grades I and II, medial hypertrophy and intimal hyperplasia, respectively, were considered mild and probably reversible. Grades III and IV were, respectively, lumen occlusion from intimal hyperplasia and early to advanced arterial dilatation. Grade III was thought to be reversible but Grade IV irreversible. Grades V and VI were terminal changes, V being angiomatoid formation and VI fibrinoid necrosis.

The latter changes indicating irreversible disease (Grades IV to VI) seemed to take time to develop and were most frequently identified in older children. Structural changes which correlated with severe and fixed elevation in pulmonary vascular resistance were therefore more difficult to establish in infants and young children.[55, 97, 99] Several investigators tried to quantify the degree of medial hypertrophy, but their measurements did not correlate closely with the preoperative level of pulmonary vascular resistance or with its change postoperatively.[41, 190, 277, 282]

Structural Remodeling and Growth. Beginning in 1965, a new and quantitative method of analysis of the pulmonary vascular bed was developed[44, 51, 107] which was particularly applicable to the study of infants and young children since it considered disturbances in the normal pattern of growth and structural remodeling. The method used the technique of arterial injection of postmortem lung specimen described by Short.[241] A radiopaque barium-gelatin mixture was injected at a constant temperature, and the lung was subsequently inflated with formalin through the bronchial tree. By distending the arteries before fixation, measurement of their diameter and wall thickness was found to be consistent and precise.

It was observed from the postmortem arteriograms that the vessels are prominent in the newborn whereas in the adult they are obscured by a dense background haze produced by the addition of many small intra-acinar arteries not present at birth (Fig. 42.4). On microscopic examination, three features of normal remodeling and growth of the pulmonary vascular bed were established.[107] (1.) With increasing age, muscle is observed in arteries located more peripherally within the acinus. At first nonmuscular arteries become partially muscular and later they become fully muscularized. (2.) At birth, the muscularized arteries are very thick walled, but within a few days, the smallest muscular arteries dilate, and their walls thin to adult levels; by 4 months of age, this process has included the largest muscular pulmonary arteries and is complete. (3.) Arteries grow both in number and size, and they grow most rapidly in infancy. While alveoli also proliferate, the ratio of alveoli to arteries actually decreases from the newborn value of 20:1 to the value of 8:1, which is achieved first in early childhood and which persists (Fig. 42.5).

Morphometric analysis of the lungs from patients who had congenital heart defects revealed disturbed growth and remodeling of the pulmonary vascular bed (Table 42.2). On the postmortem arteriograms from infants with VSD,[91, 106] the axial arteries were dilated at the hilum but narrowed peripherally (Fig. 42.6). On microscopic examination of the pulmonary vascular bed, muscle had extended precociously into normally nonmuscular peripheral arteries, regression of the perinatal musculature had not occurred, and there was additional medial hypertrophy. Also, the peripheral arteries had not grown normally in that they were small in size and few in number. Alveolar differentiation and multiplication, however, were normal. Since there were no regional variations in the lung, in assessment of abnormal muscularity or in evaluation of arterial size or number,[90] application of the morphometric technique to analysis of lung biopsy tissue was feasible.

Lung Biopsy. Lung biopsy studies show that the severity of altered growth and development of the pulmonary vascular bed correlate with the hemodynamic state.[212] Three progressively severe stages are seen. With Grade A there is abnormal extension of muscle into small peripheral arteries or, in addition, there is a mild increase in wall thickness of the normally muscular arteries (less than 1.5 times normal). These patients have increased pulmonary blood flow but normal mean pulmonary artery pressure. Meyrick and Reid[172] have shown from ultrastructural studies of lung biopsy tissue that this change is due to precocious differentiation to mature smooth muscle cells (i.e., the pericyte in the nonmuscular region of the artery and the intermediate cell in the partially muscular region (Fig. 42.7). We can speculate that the stimulus for this change may be 'stretching' of precursor cells due to transmission of a widened pulmonary pulse pressure or that it may be peripheral vasoconstriction; vasoactive mediators may also be involved.

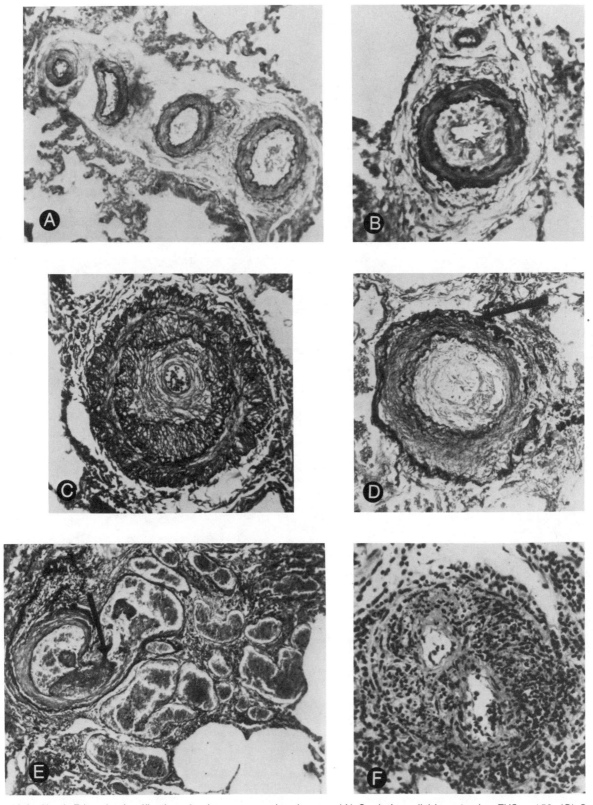

Fig. 42.3 Heath Edwards classification of pulmonary vascular changes. (A) Grade I: medial hypertrophy. *EVG*, ×150. (B) Grade II: cellular intimal proliferation in an abnormally muscular artery. *EVG*, ×250. (C) Grade III: occlusive changes. Media is thickened due to fasciculi of longitudinal muscle, and vessel is all but occluded by fibroelastic tissue. *EVG*, ×150. (D) Grade IV: dilatation. Vessel is dilated, and media is abnormally thin (*arrow*). Lumen is occluded by fibrous tissue. *EVG*, ×150. (E) Grade V: plexiform lesion. There is cellular intimal proliferation (*arrow*); clustered around are numerous thin walled vessels which terminate as capillaries in the alveolar wall. *EVG*, ×95. (F) Grade VI: acute necrotizing arteritis. A severe reactive acute inflammatory exudate is seen through all layers of the vessel. HE, ×250. *EVG*, elastic Van Gieson stain; *HE*, hematoxylin eosin stain. (Reproduced with permission from: C. A. Wagenvoort, D. Heath, and J. E. Edwards: *The Pathology of the Pulmonary Vasculature*. Charles C Thomas, Springfield, Ill., 1964.)

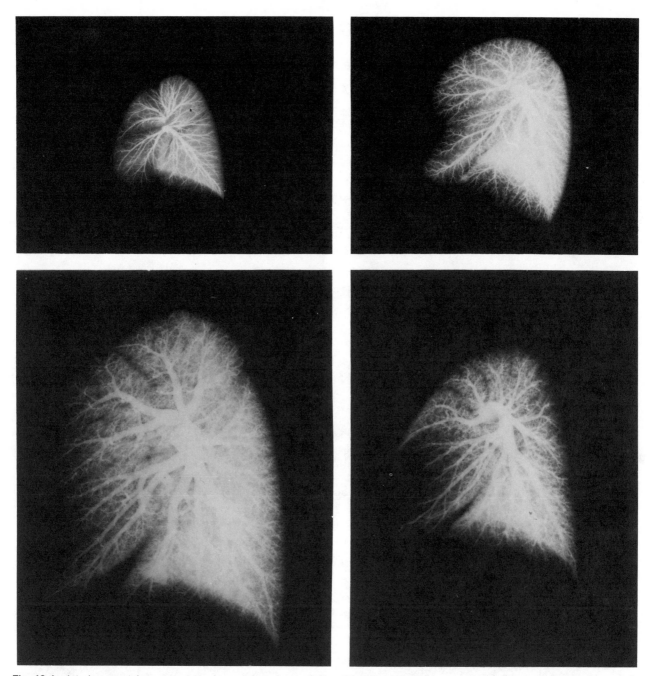

Fig. 42.4 Arteriograms taken postmortem in a newborn (*upper left*), a 3-month-old infant (*upper right*), a 1-year-old infant (*lower right*), and a 10-year-old child (*lower left*). The preacinar artery distribution is complete in the newborn but with increasing age, the background becomes filled in by a dense haze due to the addition and growth of many small intraacinar arteries.

With Grade B, as in Grade A, there is increased extension of muscle but, in addition, there is more severe medial hypertrophy of normally muscular arteries. When medial wall thickness is greater than 1.5 but less than 2 times normal (early Grade B), mild pulmonary hypertension is usually present; when medial wall thickness is more than twice normal (late Grade B), pulmonary hypertension is always present and often with a pressure greater than half that of the systemic level. The medial thickness is due to hypertrophy rather than hyperplasia of pre-existing smooth muscle cells and also to an increase in the intracellular ground substance.[172]

With Grade C, in addition to the findings of 'late Grade B,' arterial concentration is reduced and usually artery size.

Patients with these changes usually have a pulmonary vascular resistance of greater than 3.5 u/m². When the artery number is less than half of normal, pulmonary vascular resistance values are often in excess of 6 u/m². The basis for Grade C is likely the failure of new vessels to grow normally, although some loss of arteries may also occur.

Morphometric Grades A and B are refinements of Heath Edwards Grade I; Grade C is a new feature which appears to be of important functional significance. Grade C may be found with Heath Edwards Grade I, is common with Grade II and is invariable with Grade III; in fact, when Grade III is seen, arterial concentration is generally half of normal or less.

Whether and to what extent abnormal growth and struc-

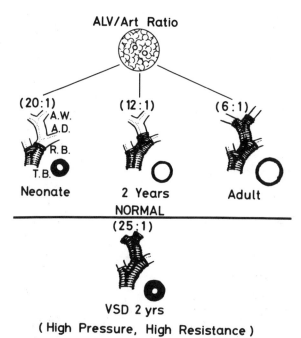

Fig. 42.5 Schema showing peripheral pulmonary arterial development through morphometric changes: extension of muscle into peripheral arteries, percent wall thickness, and artery number (alveolar-arterial ratio), as they relate to age. *Upper panel* shows normal development. *Bottom panel* shows abnormalities in all three features in a 2-year-old child with a hypertensive VSD. *T.B.*, artery accompanying a terminal bronchiolus; *R.B.*, artery accompanying a respiratory bronchiolus; *A.D.*, artery accompanying an alveolar duct; *A.W.*, artery accompanying an alveolar wall; *ALV-Art*, alveolar-arterial ratio. (Reproduced with permission from M. Rabinovitch *et al.*[112])

TABLE 42.2   STRUCTURAL FEATURES QUANTIFIED IN CONGENITAL HEART DEFECTS

Congenital Heart Defect	Artery Size	Artery No.	Extension of Muscle	Medial Wall Thickness
Ventricular septal defect	↓[a]	↓	↑	↑
Hypoplastic left heart	N	↑	↑	↑
Coarctation of the aorta	N	N	↑	↑
Total anomalous pulmonary venous connection	N	N	↑	↑
Tetralogy of Fallot	↓	N or ↑	N	↓ or ↑
Pulmonary atresia	↓	↓	N	↓

[a] ↑, increased, above normal; ↓, decreased, below normal; N, normal.

tural remodeling of the pulmonary vascular bed are permanent and result in persistent pulmonary hypertension can best be determined by correlating these features with postoperative hemodynamic studies. Preliminary investigations show that in patients with Grade B changes, although pulmonary hypertension may be present in the immediate postoperative period, pulmonary pressure 1 year later is usually normal. Patients older than 6 months of age at surgery with Grade C changes have mild persistent elevation in pulmonary vascular resistance at rest (1 year postoperatively) which becomes disproportionately severe under conditions of exercise or alveolar hypoxia.

Quantitative techniques have been successfully applied to the analysis of lung biopsy tissue prepared by frozen section

to help the surgeon decide between a palliative or corrective procedure when preoperative hemodynamic data are borderline or difficult to obtain or to interpret.[210] The ability to predict from biopsy tissue whether even mild elevation in pulmonary vascular resistance will be present postoperatively is of increasing importance in the consideration of patients who require a Fontan procedure.[209] Patients with tricuspid atresia who have had previous systemic to pulmonary artery shunts and those with single ventricle and previous pulmonary artery bands are a particular problem. We currently consider a biopsy showing severe Grade C ($<\frac{1}{2}$ the normal number of arteries) and Grade III or greater changes in 20% of vessels to indicate severe vascular disease which is unlikely to regress postoperatively and may preclude a successful result from closure of a VSD; Grade B (late) medial wall thickness greater than twice normal and/or Grade II changes in any vessels may preclude a favorable result from a Fontan procedure.

Wedge Angiography. Techniques of wedge angiography have been developed to assess preoperatively the structural state of the pulmonary vascular bed. Changes which can be evaluated quantitatively, i.e., sparsity of arborization of the pulmonary tree, abrupt termination, tortuosity and narrowing of small arteries, and reduced background capillary filling, generally reflect advanced changes in the preacinar arteries of at least Heath Edwards Grade III severity.[197] A technique has been described which allows quantitative assessment of abnormalities in a pulmonary wedge angiogram.[208] A balloon catheter is directed to the origin of the axial artery of the posterior basal segment of the right lower lobe; contrast material is injected, and the injection is filmed on biplane cine. The rate of tapering of the arteries is assessed by measuring the length of a segment over which the lumen diameter narrows between 2.5 and 1.5 mm. More abrupt arterial tapering is suggestive of more severe changes in the intraacinar arteries assessed both morphometrically and by the Heath Edwards classification (Table 42.3 and Fig. 42.8).

DEFECTS WITH INCREASED PULMONARY VENOUS PRESSURE

Hemodynamic Features

Heart defects such as mitral stenosis, cor triatriatum, or obstructed total anomalous pulmonary venous connection have in common pulmonary hypertension secondary to elevated pulmonary venous pressure.[36, 155, 292] Following surgical relief of the pulmonary venous hypertension, pulmonary artery pressure generally falls to normal values, but persistent elevation may occur in a small proportion of patients in whom these defects have been successfully corrected.[292] The latter group consists mostly of patients repaired beyond early infancy.

Rheumatic mitral stenosis is uncommon in childhood in the U.S., although large series have been reported from India where the frequency of rheumatic fever is high.[229] Little is known in children, however, of the postoperative pulmonary hemodynamics following mitral valve replacement for rheumatic mitral stenosis. In adult patients, pulmonary artery pressure usually falls dramatically.[289] Pulmonary hypertension also occurs as a result of elevated pulmonary venous pressure in a variety of acquired and congenital cardiomyopathies.[20]

Structural Features

Qualitative Assessment. Collins-Nakai et al.[36] reported greater than Heath Edwards Grade III changes in the ma-

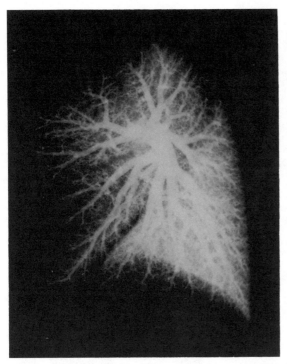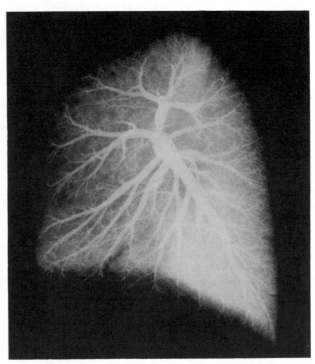

Fig. 42.6 (*Left*) Postmortem arteriogram in a 2-year-old child who died without evidence of cardiorespiratory disease. (*Right*) Postmortem arteriogram in a 2-year-old child with a VSD and elevated pulmonary artery resistance (4 u/m²). Observe how the arteries of the child with the VSD are dilated proximally, appear to taper more abruptly than those of the other child, and stand out prominently against the background. In the other lung, the background is filled in by a dense haze due to the presence of many small peripheral intraacinar arteries.

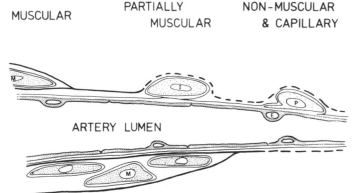

MUSCULAR   PARTIALLY MUSCULAR   NON-MUSCULAR & CAPILLARY

ARTERY LUMEN

Fig. 42.7 Diagrammatic representation of the cells in the wall of the distal part of a pulmonary artery. The smooth muscle cells (*M*) of the medial muscular coat are surrounded by a discrete basement membrane and are situated between both an internal and external elastic lamina (*thick black lines*). In the nonmuscular region of the partially muscular artery, the 'intermediate' cell (*I*) is seen. This cell is surrounded by a basement membrane that fuses, in regions, with that of the endothelial cell (*E*) and is situated internal to the single fragmented internal elastic lamina (*broken dashed lines*). In the wall of the nonmuscular artery and alveolar capillary, the pericyte (*P*) is found. This cell is ensheathed by a basement membrane which is continuous with and thereby shares the basement membrane of the associated artery, and like the 'intermediate'' cell, it is situated internal to the single elastic lamina. (Reproduced with permission from B. Meyrick and L. Reid: Anatomical Records 193:71, 1979.)

jority of patients in their series with congenital mitral stenosis. In patients with total anomalous pulmonary venous connection, abnormal muscularization of the small arteries and veins has been observed from birth, and more severe structural changes (i.e., Heath Edwards Grade III) have been described in infants as young as 1 month of age.[195] In infants with hypoplastic left heart syndrome, there is such severe medial hypertrophy of the small arteries[54, 189, 281] and veins[279] from birth that it must have developed in utero. In both adults and children with rheumatic mitral stenosis, Wagenvoort and Wagenvoort[278] observed increased medial wall thickness of the pulmonary arteries; while in children this is due to hyperplasia of smooth muscle cells, in adults, only hypertrophy is present. This finding may be of important functional significance. The medial hypertrophy described in adults is largely due to edema fluid. After surgical repair, this fluid becomes absorbed, suggesting an explanation as to why pulmonary artery pressure usually falls promptly; in children, however, repression of smooth muscle may be necessary so the fall in pulmonary artery pressure may be more gradual.

Quantitative Assessment. In postmortem arteriograms in infants and children with congenital heart defects with elevated pulmonary venous pressure, the axial pulmonary arteries have a reduced lumen diameter throughout their lengths.[84, 88] The background haze is normal or slightly increased. On microscopic examination of the lung, there is severe extension of muscle into peripheral intra-acinar arteries normally nonmuscular and failure of regression of the fetal musculature of the normally muscular arteries. The vessels, however, appear normal in size and are normal or slightly increased in number.

The presence of pulmonary vascular changes in defects with high pulmonary venous pressure and the capacity for these abnormalities to regress with improvement in hemodynamics may be of relevance, since the newly proposed staged surgical procedure for the treatment of hypoplastic left heart syndrome involves the eventual placement of a right atrial to pulmonary artery conduit.[200]

DEFECTS WITH DECREASED PULMONARY BLOOD FLOW

Hemodynamic Features

Congenital heart defects with decreased pulmonary blood flow such as tetralogy of Fallot or tricuspid atresia have been associated with increased pulmonary vascular resistance even after repair.[129, 156, 209] While pulmonary hypertension is common in patients who have had the creation of large long-standing systemic to pulmonary artery anastomoses, it has also been observed in patients without shunts and in those with pulmonary atresia and large systemic to pulmonary artery collaterals.[156] Evaluating the degree of elevation in pulmonary vascular resistance preoperatively in this group of patients is difficult. Often, the pulmonary artery cannot be entered directly but only through a systemic to pulmo-

nary artery shunt. This may interfere with pulmonary blood flow and give a falsely low calculation of pulmonary vascular resistance. Also, high hematocrit values secondary to polycythemia tend to elevate pulmonary vascular resistance. In patients with large systemic to pulmonary artery collaterals, the presence of peripheral pulmonary artery stenoses or, rarely, obstructive pulmonary vascular disease may cause elevation in pulmonary vascular resistance.[89]

Structural Features

Qualitative Assessment. In patients with congenital heart defects causing low pulmonary blood flow, hypoplasia of the pulmonary arterial musculature is observed,[188, 280] and in those in whom the hematocrit is particularly elevated, thromboembolic changes occur.[92] The creation of systemic to pulmonary artery shunts at first improves the hypoplasia, but secondary to abnormally high flow, medial hypertrophy and intimal hyperplasia soon occur.[40]

Quantitative Assessment. On the postmortem arteriograms, in patients with decreased pulmonary blood flow, the axial arteries are abnormally narrow in lumen diameter.[85, 105, 207] The background haze may also be reduced, as in patients with pulmonary atresia and intact ventricular septum. On microscopic examination of the lung from patients with pulmonary atresia and intact ventricular septum, the intraacinar pulmonary arteries are abnormally thin walled, small in size, and few in number; in patients with tetralogy of Fallot, these vessels are normal or decreased in muscularity, normal in number, and small in size. Alveolar development is impaired in patients with decreased pulmonary blood flow, and this is reflected mostly by reduction in alveolar number. Patients with tetralogy of Fallot and associated pulmonary atresia form a special subgroup in which the relative distribution of central pulmonary arteries and aortopulmonary collaterals determine peripheral pulmonary vascular structure.[87, 266] In patients with tricuspid atresia, the structural state of the pulmonary vascular bed is variable,

TABLE 42.3   CORRELATION OF THE PATHOLOGY, PHYSIOLOGY, AND ANGIOGRAM IN PULMONARY VASCULAR DISEASE

Grade	Pathology	Qp[a]	PPa	Rp	Wedge Angiogram
A	Abnormal extension of muscle into small arteries	↑	N	N	Slow tapering of axial arteries
	± Mild medial hypertrophy	↑	N	N	
B	"A" + severe medial hypertrophy	↑	↑	N	Abrupt tapering
C	"B" + ↓ artery, number, and size	±↑	↑	↑	Very abrupt tapering

*The abbreviations used are: Qp, pulmonary blood flow; P$_{PA}$, mean pulmonary artery pressure; R$_p$, pulmonary vascular resistance; N, normal.

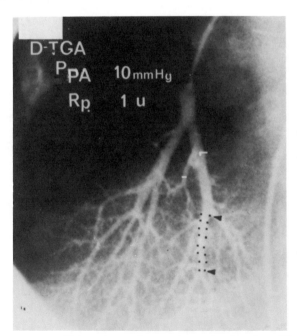 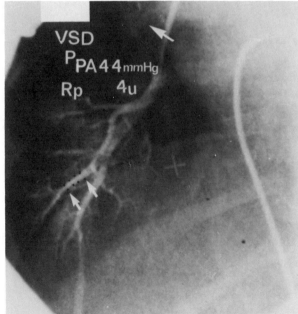

Fig. 42.8 (*Left*) A wedge angiogram shows slow tapering of the axial artery in a child with TGA and normal pulmonary artery pressure (P$_{PA}$) and resistance (R$_p$). Approximate segment length between 2.5 and 1.5-mm internal diameter is marked off (*arrows*). (*Right*) A wedge angiogram in a child with a VSD shows rapid tapering of the artery when there is increased pulmonary artery pressure and resistance. An approximate segment length between 2.5 and 1.5 mm internal diameter is marked off (*arrows*). *Large arrow* denotes takeoff to the right pulmonary artery. (Reproduced with permission from M. Rabinovitch and L. Reid: Cardiovascular Clinics)

depending upon whether pulmonary blood flow is increased or decreased.[209]

TREATMENT OF PULMONARY HYPERTENSION

Surgical Therapy

Surgical correction of congenital heart defects is now possible during the first 2 years of life with low mortality[29, 157, 254] and this will surely impede the development of pulmonary vascular disease. Older patients with TGA and advanced pulmonary vascular disease have undergone palliative Mustard operations, resulting in improved arterial saturation and alleviation of clinical symptoms and severe polycythemia, with the latter a factor which contributes to the progression of advanced pulmonary vascular disease.[13, 253]

Medical Therapy

Vasodilator therapy has been introduced successfully in the treatment of idiopathic pulmonary hypertension and hypertension resulting from chronic obstructive lung disease, but few trials have been given to the treatment of patients with persistent pulmonary hypertension secondary to congenital heart defects. The use of antiplatelet aggregating drugs or anticoagulants may be of value in the polycythemic patient[63] and controlled trials need to be initiated particularly since these patients are at risk for hemoptysis. The use of prophylactic heparin does not appear to alter the high mortality in the immediate postpartum period in women with Eisenmenger's syndrome.[205]

Experimental Studies

That elevation in pulmonary blood flow, pressure, O_2 saturation, venous pressure, or level of hematocrit all contribute to the development of pulmonary vascular changes, as suggested by Nadas and Fyler,[185] seems likely (Table 42.4). What are the neurohumoral mechanisms through which these features operate and first induce ultrastructural, and then structural damage? Is decreased extraction of norepinephrine by the lung important?[247] Why is there so much variation in individual response?[75] What causes the decreased vascular proliferation and precocious differentiation of muscle, and are these changes reversible? The answers to these questions will most likely come first through the study of appropriate animal models, the ground work for which has been laid in the following experiments.

There have been many attempts to simulate the effect of congenital heart defect producing high pulmonary blood flow in an animal model. In adult dogs, it is necessary to anastomose the aorta to a lobe of the pulmonary artery to produce pulmonary hypertension and severe structural changes in the pulmonary vascular bed.[56] Rendas et al.[219] created systemic to pulmonary artery shunts in 4-week-old piglets and demonstrated progressive pulmonary hypertension in association with abnormal extension of muscle into peripheral arteries and medial hypertrophy of normally muscular arteries. Similar hemodynamic and structural features have been produced in the right lung of piglets after ligating the left pulmonary artery in the newborn animal.[86] Pulmonary hypertension also occurred in the right lungs of puppies[231] and minipigs[122] after left pneumonectomy.

Pulmonary venous hypertension has been created experimentally by banding the pulmonary veins[243] or by creating aorta to left atrial shunts.[112] In the latter experiments, analysis of pulmonary artery hydraulic impedance (calculated on the basis of the dynamic relationship between pressure and flow), in addition to pulmonary vascular resistance, suggested that the pulmonary arteries were abnormally stiff and that there was an inability to recruit peripheral vessels during stress.

Levin et al.[139] created coarctation of the aorta in utero in fetal lambs. Although pulmonary venous hypertension did not occur, the excessive intrauterine ductal to pulmonary artery flow was thought responsible for structural changes in the pulmonary arteries. Levin et al.[138] also created low pulmonary blood flow by banding the main pulmonary artery of fetal lambs. The changes in the lung that resulted consisted of diffuse hypoplasia of the musculature of the peripheral pulmonary vessels; those identified were small in caliber and few in number. Haworth et al.[86] ligated the left pulmonary artery in newborn piglets and demonstrated normal development of the intraacinar arteries owing to extensive anastomoses with bronchial arteries, but in the preacinar vessels there was occlusive fibrosis of the lumen.

HYPOXIA

ACUTE HYPOXIA

Clinical Features

The pulmonary hypertension that occurs in response to acute hypoxia is usually mild and rapidly reversible. Hultgren *et al.*[113] demonstrated an 18% increase in pulmonary

TABLE 42.4 FACTORS DETERMINING THE DEVELOPMENT OF PULMONARY VASCULAR DISEASE IN PATIENTS WITH COMMON VARIETIES OF CONGENITAL HEART DISEASE[a]

	Major Factors			Minor Factors				
	↑P_{pa}	↑P_{pv}	↑QPA	↑PO_{2PA}	↓PO_{2SA}	↓PH_{SA}	Hematocrit ↑	PVD
ASD, secundum	−	−	+	+	−	−	−	Unlikely
ASD, primum	−	±	+	+	−	−	−	Possible
TAVC	+	+	+	+	±	±	±	Highly probable
Large VSD	+	±	+	+	−	−	−	Probable
with mitral disease	+	+	+	+	−	−	−	Virtually certain
TF	−	−	−	−	±	+	+	Unlikely till late
with Potts	+	±	+	+	±	−	±	Probable
TGA	±	±	+	+	+	±	+	Virtually certain
with VSD	+	+	+	+	+	±	+	Certain

[a] Adapted from A. S. Nadas, and D. F. Fyler: Pediatric Cardiology, W. B. Saunders, Philadelphia, 1972, p. 684.

[b] The abbreviations used are: PVD, pulmonary vascular disease; P, pressure; PV, pulmonary vein; Q, flow; PA, pulmonary artery; SA, systemic artery; P_{pa} mean pulmonary artery pressure; P_{pv}, mean pulmonary venous pressure; PO_{2PA}, oxygen pressure in pulmonary artery; PO_{2SA}, oxygen pressure in systemic artery; PH_{SA}, PH in systemic artery; QPA, flow in pulmonary artery.

artery pressure in men brought suddenly from sea level to high altitude (7800 feet). There is much variability in individual response to hypoxia; some people hyperventilate and become mildly alkalotic, hardly increasing their pulmonary artery pressure at all, while others develop severe pulmonary hypertension with high altitude pulmonary edema. The mechanism for the latter, which occurs more commonly in children than in adults,[238] is not understood, but several theories have been proposed: endothelial swelling of small arteries occurs in some areas of the lung and causes high resistance—this results in diversion of excessive flow through small vessels causing edema; there is defective fibrinolysis, with formation of microemboli; and there is inadequate diuresis.[71]

Experimental Studies

In animal studies, Tucker et al.[269] observed that the degree of reactivity to hypoxia or the level of pulmonary hypertension varied among the different species in proportion to the amount of smooth muscle in the pulmonary vascular bed. Recent studies by Hales et al.[78] have implicated high levels of circulating dilator prostaglandins to explain the weak responder. It had been recognized by Lloyd[146] that isolated pulmonary arteries will constrict in response to hypoxia, but only if surrounded by a cuff of tissue, which suggested the release of a vasoactive mediator. No unique chemical agent, however, has been found. While angiotensin II is necessary for acute hypoxic pulmonary vasoconstriction, only subpressor doses are required.[11] In fact, Stalcup et al.[251] in endothelial cell culture studies, and Leuenberger et al.,[137] in anesthetized dogs, have shown that during acute hypoxia, angiotensin I converting enzyme is depressed, causing a decrease in angiotensin II and an increase in bradykinin levels. Hypoxic pulmonary vasoconstriction, it is hypothesized, is a response to acute increase in cardiac output associated with bradykinin.

Much debate continues with regard to the role of histamine,[271] serotonin,[125] and catecholamines.[66] There are also advocates of a direct vasoconstrictor effect of hypoxia on smooth muscle involving either calcium,[165] cytochrome P-450,[261] or the rate of oxidative phosphorylation.[228] It is possible, as suggested by the schema of Fishman,[58] that both direct and indirect systems are operative (Fig. 42.9).

We do not know the relationship that exists between acute hypoxic vasoconstriction and the sustained pulmonary hypertension and structural changes in the pulmonary vascular bed induced by chronic hypoxia. Our recent experimental studies of unilaterally banding the pulmonary artery in chronically hypoxic rats would support the hypothesis that some structural changes in hypoxia are influenced by an alteration in the hemodynamics of the pulmonary circulation, and others are more direct effects of hypoxia per se.[211]

CHRONIC HYPOXIA

Clinical Features

In individuals living at high altitudes, there is chronic elevation in pulmonary artery pressure, of which only a small portion is reversible with administration of oxygen. The reversible portion probably constitutes the acute vasoconstrictor component; the irreversible portion is likely due to the structural changes in the pulmonary vascular bed. In a study by Arias-Stella and Saldana,[6] postmortem lung tissue from individuals who had been living at high altitudes was compared with that obtained from sea level dwellers. There were structural changes in the vessels in the 'high altitude' lung specimens; the peripheral arteries were more muscular than normal and had a decreased lumen diameter.

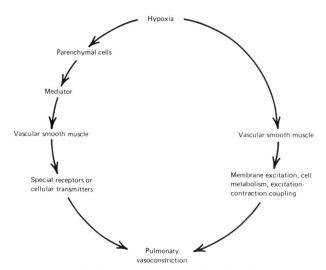

Fig. 42.9 A schema suggesting that hypoxic pulmonary vasoconstriction acts both directly and indirectly through the release of vasoactive mediators. (Reproduced with permission from: A. P. Fishman: Pulmonary Diseases and Disorders. McGraw-Hill, New York, 1980.)

Children living in Denver (elevation 5200 feet) have slightly higher mean pulmonary artery pressures than sea level dwellers, and children living in Moroccocha, Peru (elevation 14,900 feet) have mean pulmonary artery pressures which are twice as high. Moreover, in the high altitude residents, mean pulmonary artery pressure more than doubles with exercise, whereas it only increases by 50% in sea level dwellers (Table 42.5).[274] Grover et al.[73] reported studies in a young girl who, while living in Leadville (10,150 feet), had near systemic level pulmonary artery pressure. After 1 year at sea level, her resting pulmonary artery pressure was normal, but upon exercise it markedly increased, suggesting a structurally abnormal pulmonary vascular bed with limited functional reserve.[73]

Experimental Studies

In the rat, the hemodynamic and structural response of the pulmonary vascular bed to chronic hypoxia has been studied and also the response to chronic intermittent hypoxia.[1, 98, 108, 164, 169, 206, 298] It appears that the total dose of hypoxia determines the response regardless of whether the method of administration is chronic continuous or intermittent.[293] After just 3 days of chronic hypoxia, there is a sustained elevation in pulmonary artery pressure and resistance measured even after the rats have been kept in room air for several hours.[206] This coincides with the time structural changes in the pulmonary vascular bed that are significant, in particular the extension of muscle into peripheral arteries normally nonmuscular. Over the ensuing 2 weeks of hypoxia, mean pulmonary artery pressure progressively rises to double the control values. This increase is accompanied by right ventricular hypertrophy, extension of muscle into peripheral arteries, medial hypertrophy of normally muscular arteries, and reduction in arterial concentration related to alveolar. Ultrastructural studies of the peripheral arteries have shown differentiation of precursor cells into new smooth muscle cells.[169] In the pulmonary artery at the hilum, the adventitia is thickened due to an increase in the number of fibroblasts and ground substance, and the media is also thicker as a result of hypertrophy of smooth muscle cells.[169] The loss of arteries during hypoxia is not understood, but it has been suggested that some of the abnormally muscular

TABLE 42.5 PULMONARY ARTERY PRESSURE AT REST AND DURING EXERCISE IN CHILDREN LIVING AT DIFFERENT ALTITUDES

Place	Altitude (ft)	Barometric pressure (mm Hg)	AO[a] pressure (mm Hg)	Arterial Saturation (%)		Mean PA Pressure (mm Hg)	
				Rest	Exercise	Rest	Exercise
Sea level	0	760	104	97	97	13	21
Denver, Colo.	5,250	625	80	95	94	16	24
Mexico City, Mexico	7,300	580	81	91	–	15	–
Leadville, Colo.	10,150	525	65	92	89	25	54
Morococha, Peru	14,900	445	50	78	69	28	60

[a] The abbreviations used are: PA, pulmonary artery; AO, aortic pressure; –, data not available.

peripheral arteries with their swollen endothelium may become reabsorbed.[236]

The hemodynamic and structural response to one month of hypoxia has been compared in rats of both sexes exposed either during infancy or during adulthood. Females made hypoxic as adults are least responsive, whereas rats of both sexes made hypoxic during infancy are most responsive.[215] The 'hyporesponsiveness' to hypoxia of the female animal has also been observed in other species.[164] Recovery from chronic hypoxia has also been studied in the rat.[98, 108, 167, 215] Mean pulmonary artery pressure returns to near normal level in rats exposed as adults but remains 50% above normal in animals exposed during infancy. In both groups there is incomplete regression of structural changes, but rats exposed during infancy have more severe residual damage.

Ultrastructural studies in the rat have shown that regression of smooth muscle hypertrophy is accompanied by an increase in the amount of elastin and collagen in the vessel wall.[167] Thus, the vessel, while less muscular, is enclosed in a 'tight sheath', and this may interfere with its compliance and its ability to grow. Loss of small arteries is never made up, suggesting that the pulmonary vascular bed after hypoxia may have limited functional reserve.

While the vasoactive mediators of chronic hypoxia are not known, several important associations have been made. Zakheim et al.[301] observed a significant rise in angiotensin II levels on the third day of hypoxic exposure in rabbits (this coincided with the first time we observed significant pulmonary vascular changes in the rat).[206] Angiotensin II levels reached a peak on the 9th day of exposure but returned to normal by day 16. Correlating with the rise in angiotensin II levels, Molteni et al.[177] observed a rise in angiotensin I converting enzyme in mice. Zakheim observed that inhibition of angiotensin I converting enzyme during chronic hypoxia in the rat resulted in a decrease in right ventricular hypertrophy.[300] We also found a reduction in the degree of extension of muscle into peripheral arteries, which correlates with the higher level of bradykinin[214] achieved in response to inhibition of the converting enzyme.

Studies by Kay and Grover[125] and Tucker et al.[270] have suggested that the increased number of mast cells in the lungs of chronically hypoxic animals may indicate a role for histamine or serotonin in initiating the structural changes, but blockers of these compounds have failed to prevent the chronic hypoxic response. Since endothelial injury has been documented in chronic hypoxia, abnormal platelet endothelial interaction and an imbalance favoring the production of the vasoconstrictor thromboxane over the vasodilator prostacyclin[163] may be part of the mechanism of the hemodynamic response, as well as the structural changes.

LUNG DISEASE

Several factors may contribute to the pulmonary hypertension which commonly but not invariably accompanies

severe parenchymal lung disease. These are: level of hypoxia and polycythemia; the degree of endothelial injury and subsequent imbalance in vasoactive mediators; the level of pulmonary venous pressure secondary to dysfunction of the hypoxemic left ventricle; and the nature and severity of the structural damage to the pulmonary arteries. Treatment of the lung disease will decrease the level of pulmonary artery pressure by eliminating the contributing causes and by allowing some regression of the structural changes. The latter, however, ultimately determine the level of pulmonary hypertension and the rate of development of right-sided heart failure (cor pulmonale).

OBSTRUCTIVE LUNG DISEASE

Clinical Features

Unlike in the adult population, in children obstructive lung disorders such as asthma[70] are only rarely associated with the development of pulmonary hypertension. In patients with cystic fibrosis, however, cor pulmonale is common. In studies by Goldring et al.[67] the observation was made that the severity of impaired pulmonary function in patients with cystic fibrosis was not predictive of the level of pulmonary artery pressure; moreover, pulmonary hypertension when present was almost completely reversible with administration of oxygen or tolazoline.[128] It now appears that cor pulmonale is a more frequent late complication.[242] A recent study[256] considered this to be the cause of death in 40% of patients. The prognosis after onset of first symptoms of heart failure is grim, with the median survival 8 months.

Liebman et al.[145] found a good correlation between right ventricular hypertrophy assessed on the vectorcardiogram and decreased vital capacity. An abnormally posterior vector was associated with an increased residual volume. The value of echocardiography in assessing the presence and severity of pulmonary hypertension in cystic fibrosis is still, however, controversial. Due to the shape and hyperaeration of the chest, patients with cystic fibrosis are very difficult to study echocardiographically[297]; when the right ventricle is visualized, an increase in the thickness of its wall and in its cavity size generally reflects advanced disease; when the pulmonary valve is visualized, prolongation of right ventricular systolic time intervals may suggest pulmonary hypertension; finally, left ventricular dysfunction may also be identified echocardiographically.

Structural Features

Ryland and Reid,[234] in their study of the heart and lungs in patients with cystic fibrosis, observed that those with severe lung disease did not always develop right ventricular hypertrophy. When right ventricular hypertrophy was present, however, it generally reflected the degree of abnormal structural remodeling of the pulmonary vascular bed (Fig. 42.10). An increase in the muscularity of small veins was also

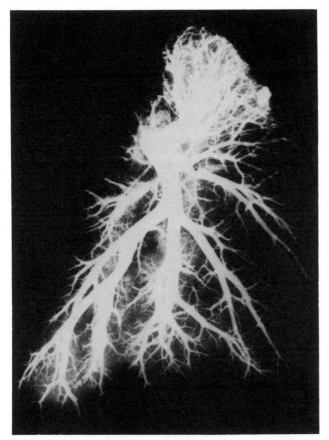

Fig. 42.10 A postmortem arteriogram from a 17-year-old patient with cystic fibrosis and cor pulmonale. The right upper lobe is shrunken and fibrotic, but throughout the lung there is diminished background haze owing to a reduction in the concentration of small peripheral arteries. The abrupt tapering of the axial arteries also suggests pulmonary hypertension.

observed. While the severity of the arterial changes tended to be patchy, reflecting the nature of the lung disease, the venous changes were more uniform, suggesting that they resulted from left atrial hypertension secondary to left ventricular dysfunction.

RESTRICTIVE LUNG DISEASE

Clinical Features

Restrictive lung disease may occur in childhood from a variety of causes, and pulmonary hypertension is a common complication. Examples of such restrictive lung disorders are diffuse interstitial fibrosis (Hamman-Rich),[8] bronchopulmonary dysplasia,[72] radiation fibrosis,[71] chemotherapy toxicity,[249] infiltrative lung tumors,[4] and collagen vascular disease.[224] In the latter, pulmonary vasculitis may be important etiologically, so this will be discussed separately. Reversal of the pulmonary hypertension generally depends upon the ability to affect the course of the interstitial lung disease.

Structural Features

There have been few structural studies in patients with restrictive lung disorders. It has been proposed that, secondary to fibrosis of the alveolar septae, the loss of small alveolar wall arteries results in an increase in pulmonary vascular resistance, and a secondary response to this resistance is likely the hypertrophy of normally muscular arteries. That we have observed the severity of the pulmonary hypertension and the structural changes in the pulmonary arteries

out of proportion to the extent of alveolar fibrosis suggests an additional mechanism of more direct vascular injury.

In a study of the lungs from premature infants in whom bronchopulmonary dysplasia was a complication of severe respiratory distress syndrome, Rendas et al.[218] observed that although the preacinar arteries had dilated appropriately, there was an increase in extension of muscle into normally nonmuscular peripheral arteries which might explain the persistent pulmonary hypertension in these patients. In addition, although the number of peripheral arteries related to alveoli was normal, the marked reduction in alveolar number suggested an absolute decrease in the cross-sectional area of the pulmonary vascular bed.[217]

UPPER AIRWAY OBSTRUCTION

Severe upper airway obstruction from a variety of causes[3, 35, 38, 46, 60, 115, 117, 119, 132, 141, 144, 153, 198, 201, 222, 259] (Fig. 42.11 and Table 42.6) may be complicated by the development of pulmonary hypertension. In each case, the hypertension is not always a direct result of the degree of airway obstruction but seems to depend also on whether there is a central component, i.e., diminished ventilatory drive,[115] or general neuromuscular pharyngeal dysfunction.[259] That pulmonary hypertension seems to result more commonly in patients who, in addition to airway obstruction, have mental retardation[35] has been put forth as supportive evidence. Many paitents with upper airway obstruction have worsening of their symptoms with sleep[259]; this worsening may be mechanical, i.e., having to do with positioning of the head, or it may be the result of a central mechanism.[60] While removal of the airway obstruction often results in prompt return to normal pulmonary artery pressure and resolution of the heart failure,[38] often these symptoms persist for some time. This may be due to slow regression of hypoxia-induced structural changes in the pulmonary vascular bed or persistent impairment of ventilatory drive.[141]

DIMINISHED VENTILATORY DRIVE

Clinical Features

The 'Pickwickian' syndrome described in adults[7, 23] consisting of hypersomnolence and obesity associated with pulmonary hypertension has also been reported in children.[31] The obesity, through increased work of breathing and CO_2 production, stresses the respiratory control system, and depending on its inherent sensitivity,[273] hypoventilation may result, causing further CO_2 retention and hypoxia which contribute to the lethargy and cor pulmonale (Fig. 42.12). Mental retardation is often but not invariably associated with this syndrome. Damage to the respiratory center, either as a primary disorder (Ondine's curse)[57, 166] or secondary to trauma or other neurologic disease,[187] may also result in cor pulmonale due to chronic intermittent hypoxia and hypercarbia.

While the pulmonary hypertension of sleep apnea in adults (Fig. 42.13) is in large part due to airway obstruction, in children it is often the manifestation of an abnormal central mechanism. Shannon et al.[239] found that one third of near miss sudden infant deaths were in children who demonstrated intermittent apnea. Since this periodic apnea, as well as the propensity for sudden infant death, disappears after the first year of life, delayed maturation of the respiratory center seems a hypothetical cause.

Structural Features

Structural studies of the lung at postmortem have been carried out in patients with hypoventilation due to damage

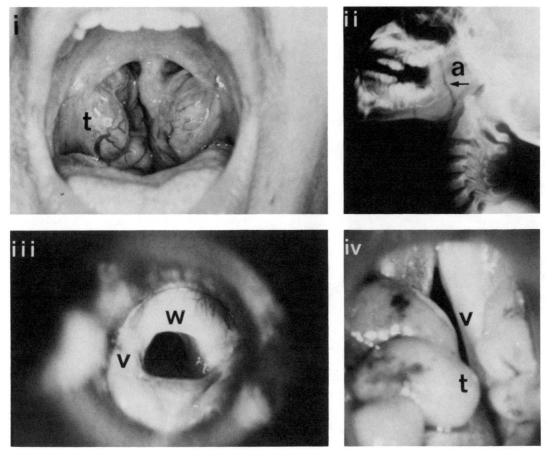

Fig. 42.11 Four different causes of upper airway obstruction. (*i*) Hypertrophied tonsils (*t*). (*ii*) X-ray of head and neck demonstrating compression of nasopharynx (*arrow*) by hypertrophied adenoids (*a*). (*iii*) Glottic web (*w*) adjacent to vocal cord (*v*). (*iv*) Lingual tonsils (*t*).

TABLE 42.6   CAUSES OF UPPER AIRWAY OBSTRUCTION IN CHILDREN

Hypertrophied tonsils and/or adenoids
Laryngotracheomalacia
Subglottic stenosis secondary to congenital web or posttraumatic
Micrognathia with glossoptosis (e.g., Pierre Robin)
Crouzon's disease
Hurler's disease (macroglossia)
Ankylosis of the temperomandibular joint
Craniovertebral anomaly
Laryngeal tumors or cysts
Post cleft palate repair

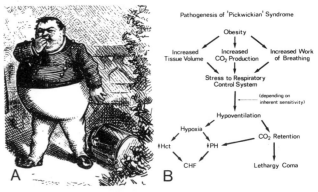

Fig. 42.12 (*A*) Thomas Nast's drawing of the fat boy in "The Pickwick Papers" from an American edition of the Posthumous Papers of the Pickwick Club, London, 1837. New York, 1873. (*B*) A schema of the pathogenesis of pulmonary hypertension in the Pickwickian syndrome. (Modified from J. H. Auchincloss and R. Gilbert.[7])

to the respiratory center[187] and in children with sudden infant death syndrome.[294] In the former, the degree of medial hypertrophy was compatible with hypoxia-induced pulmonary hypertension. In one third of all patients with sudden infant death syndrome[294] and in all 'near miss' infants in whom apnea was documented and who later died suddenly, severe extension of muscle into peripheral arteries was observed.

DISORDERS OF THE CHEST WALL

Neuromuscular disorders affecting the chest wall, such as Duchenne's muscular dystrophy,[65] poliomyelitis,[152] Werdnig-Hoffman disease, and diseases affecting the vertebrae and rib cage, such as scolioses,[10] may so impair ventilation as to cause pulmonary hypertension. In patients with scoliosis,

the heart and lungs have been studied at postmortem using morphometric techniques.[45] Mild right ventricular hypertrophy has been described in association with medial hypertrophy of normally muscular arteries and increased extension of muscle into peripheral arteries and reduced arterial number, changes one ordinarily finds in association with chronic hypoxia-induced pulmonary hypertension. Reduction in arterial number has been found both in lobes with reduced alveolar number as well as in those with normal alveolar number.

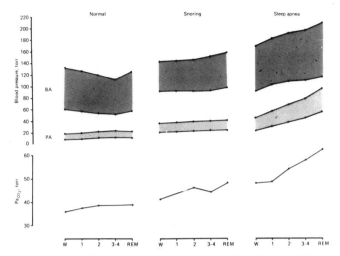

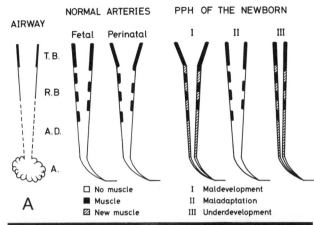

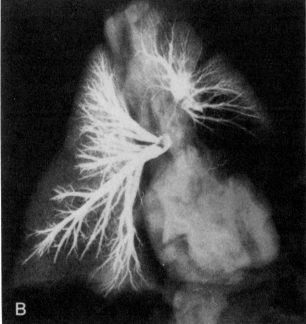

Fig. 42.13 Pulmonary and systemic hypertension associated with hypercarbia in a patient with sleep apnea compared with the normal and snoring individual. (Reproduced with permission from A. P. Fishman: Pulmonary Diseases. McGraw-Hill, New York, 1980.)

PERSISTENT PULMONARY HYPERTENSION OF THE NEWBORN

Persistent pulmonary hypertension of the newborn may result from one of three causes: underdevelopment of the lung and pulmonary vascular bed; maladaptation of the pulmonary vascular bed to extrauterine life as a result of postnatal stress; and maldevelopment of the pulmonary vascular bed in utero from an unknown cause (Fig. 42.14A).

Underdevelopment of the Lung

Hypoplastic or dysplastic lungs may occur as isolated abnormalities[260] or in association with a variety of diseases, e.g., congenital diaphragmatic hernia[104, 130] (Fig. 42.14B), renal agenesis and dysplasia,[103] rhesus isoimmunization,[32] prematurity,[218] absence of the phrenic nerve,[295] and asphyxiating thoracic dystrophy.[68] The derangement and/or hypoplasia of the pulmonary vascular bed will, depending upon its severity, either be incompatible with life or result in reversible or irreversible pulmonary artery hypertension and right to left shunting from birth. In addition to the structural changes in the vessels, the severity of the impaired gas exchanges (hypoxia, hypercarbia) due to abnormalities in the airways no doubt also contributes greatly to the pulmonary hypertension.

Reversal of the pulmonary hypertension postoperatively in infants with congenital diaphragmatic hernia has been achieved with tolazoline[16] and also with the extracorporeal membrane oxygenator.[81] In some cases, however, the hemodynamic abnormality is irreversible.

In lungs studied at postmortem from infants with pulmonary hypoplasia or dysplasia, pulmonary hypertension seems to be associated with a reduced number of arteries appropriate to the reduced number of airways. Often but not always, the arteries are also small but not incompatible with the size of the lung. Also, while the arteries both centrally and peripherally may be more muscular than normal as in congenital diaphragmatic hernia, there may be hypoplasia of the pulmonary musculature as in renal agenesis.

Maladaptation of the Pulmonary Vascular Bed

Infants with perinatal stress from a variety of causes, e.g., hemorrhage, hypoglycemia, aspiration, or hypoxia may fail to demonstrate the normal drop in pulmonary vascular resistance at birth.[147, 184, 220] The normally muscular vessels,

Fig. 42.14 (A) Schema of pulmonary arteries accompanying airways. TB, terminal bronchiolus; RB, respiratory bronchiolus; AD, alveolar duct; A, alveolus. The fetal and perinatal arteries are similar in terms of amount and level of muscularity, but in the latter the smallest fully muscular arteries are dilated. In I, maldevelopment, there is dilatation of muscular arteries, but pulmonary hypertension occurs because there is muscle abnormally peripheral. In II, maladaptation, dilatation of muscular arteries does not take place, and in III, underdevelopment, there is both lack of dilatation and muscle abnormally peripheral; in addition, the pulmonary artery is small in size. (B) Arteriogram showing a small right lung with a distorted and even smaller left lung. Arteries in both lungs are reduced in size and number. (Reproduced with permission from M. Kitagawa et al.[130])

particularly those <200 μm, fail to dilate, and left ventricular dysfunction likely contributes as well.[220] Of all the types of persistent pulmonary hypertension, this in theory should be the most amenable to improvement, following treatment of the pulmonary disorder and general hemodynamic state of the infant with hyperventilation[203] or with vasodilators.[48, 150]

Murphy et al.[184] observed through structural studies of the lung at postmortem in fatal cases of meconium aspiration that the latter, while appearing to be a postnatal stress, is often the manifestation of intrauterine dysfunction. In only 1 of 6 infants was there evidence of failure of normally muscular peripheral arteries to dilate appropriately at birth;

in all the others, the nature and severity of the vascular abnormalities suggested an intrauterine insult.

Maldevelopment of the Pulmonary Vascular Bed

Newborns in whom there is no apparent reason for persistent pulmonary hypertension are the most perplexing of all. Clinical studies have suggested a relationship between maternal ingestion of prostaglandin synthetase inhibitors, either aspirin or indomethacin, and subsequent persistence of pulmonary hypertension in the newborn.[142, 159] In some cases the symptoms were transient, whereas in others they were more severe and with fatal outcome. Considering the large population of women who take aspirin during pregnancy and the low frequency of persistent pulmonary hypertension in their newborn and, conversely, that in the majority of infants with persistent pulmonary hypertension no history of maternal ingestion of these compounds can be documented, it is difficult to be sure of a cause-effect relationship. However, since experimental studies[101, 140] have shown that prostaglandin synthetase inhibitors will constrict the ductus arteriosus in utero and chronic indomethacin treatment in pregnant rats[82] will produce structural changes in the pulmonary vascular bed of the newborn, it seems likely that in an occasional susceptible human fetus there is a relationship.

Murphy et al.[183] have carried out morphometric studies in lungs from fatal cases of persistent pulmonary hypertension of the newborn. The most striking structural feature in the lung is the presence of muscle in arteries, small and peripheral in location, and normally nonmuscular. The muscle cells are surrounded by darkly staining elastic laminae suggesting that they formed several weeks prior to death and, therefore, in utero (Fig. 42.15).[183]

Experimental Studies. The structural changes described in the pulmonary vascular bed of infants with persistent pulmonary hypertension have been reproduced in the offspring of rats that had been treated with indomethacin during pregnancy. There is no animal model to date, however, in which a living newborn has been produced with systemic levels of pulmonary artery pressure and right to left shunting. Recent studies[27, 28, 136, 148, 255] have contributed greatly to our understanding of the response of the fetal and neonatal pulmonary vascular bed to metabolites of arachidonic acid. In fetal and neonatal animals, PGE_1, 6-keto PGE_1, and PGI_2 are potent vasodilators with both pulmonary and systemic effects. $PGF_{2\alpha}$ is a vasoconstrictor, and PGD_2 behaves differently, depending upon the age of the animal.[27] Much is left to be learned about how these and other compounds affect the normal transition of the fetal to neonatal circulation. For example, indomethacin given to a newborn only retards but does not prevent the fall in pulmonary vascular resistance with oxygen.[149] Also to be explored is the interaction between prostaglandins and pulmonary vascular reflexes.[120]

THROMBOEMBOLIC DISEASE

Clinical Features

Diagnosing thromboemboli as a cause of pulmonary hypertension requires a high index of suspicion in patients having disorders in which the former are likely to occur (Table 42.7). For example, thromboemboli frequently occur in children with ventriculoatrial shunts for hydrocephalus[53, 199, 264] due either to clots dislodging from the end of the catheter or to an abnormal fibrinolytic reaction of cerebrospinal fluid within the lung. Children with sickle cell anemia may develop pulmonary thromboses and infarc-

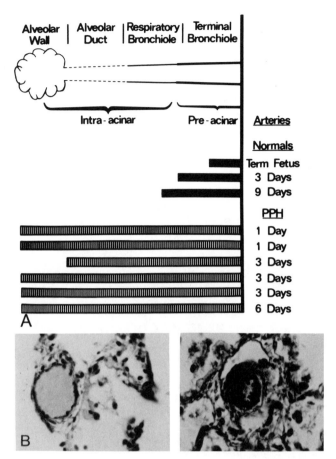

Fig. 42.15 (A) Diagrammatic location of muscle in the walls of the intraacinar arteries. In normal infants less than 1 week of age, no muscular arteries are found within the acinus. All the patients with persistent pulmonary hypertension (PPH) had "extension" of muscle into the small intraacinar arteries. (B) Photomicrographs of alveolar wall arteries distended with the barium gelatin suspension from (left) a 3-day-old infant with normal lungs and (right) a 3-day-old infant with persistent pulmonary hypertension. The normal artery (left) is nonmuscular with a single endothelial cell lining surrounded by a thin layer of connective tissue. The artery wall (right) is comprised of smooth muscle (darkly stained) two cell layers thick surrounded by a thick connective tissue sheath enclosing a dilated lymphatic (located superiorly). Elastin-Van Gieson stain, ×250. (Reproduced with permission from J. D. Murphy et al.[183])

tions.[180] In endogenous areas, ova emboli due to schistosomiasis have been described.[64] Fat emboli may occur secondary to trauma and also in association with collagen vascular disease.[47] Tumor emboli may carry metastatic disease from the kidneys or other abdominal organs, or may be present in association with infiltrative carcinomatous disease of the lung.[161] Right-sided endocarditis and right atrial myxoma may also be sources of emboli.[96, 123, 182] In the newborn and young infant, pulmonary thrombosis may be associated with sepsis and dehydration and portal or renal vein thrombosis.[69]

Diagnosis of the nature and severity of embolic phenomena may be established with chest x-ray and lung scans (Fig. 42.16), though occasionally angiography is necessary.[181] The virtues of thrombolytic versus surgical therapy depend upon the location and distribution of the lesions.[179] There are two factors which probably contribute to the pulmonary hypertension of thromboembolic disease: first, the structural damage and occlusive changes within the large and small arteries; and second, the concomitant release of vasoactive sub-

TABLE 42.7 CAUSES OF THROMBOEMBOLIC DISEASE IN CHILDREN

Ventriculoatrial shunts for hydrocephalus
Fat emboli (post-traumatic or with collagen vascular disease)
Sickle cell anemia
Tumor emboli
Ovaemboli (schistosomiasis)
Thrombosis in other vascular structures (hepatic or renal vein, or deep vein 2° immobilization.)
Sepsis and/or dehydration
Right-sided endocarditis
Right atrial myxoma

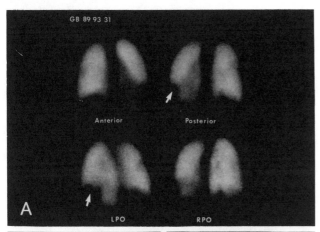

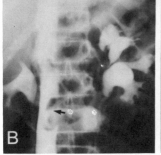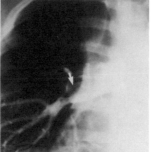

Fig. 42.16 (*A*) Lung perfusion scan performed after injection of technetium-99m macroaggregated albumen in a teenage boy who, after an orthopedic procedure, developed deep vein thromboses and pulmonary emboli. The latter are visualized as filling defects (*arrows*). LPO, left posterior oblique; RPO, right posterior oblique. (*B*) (*Left*) Venous angiogram shows site of tumor (infiltrative reticulum cell sarcoma) in inferior vena cava. (*Right*) Right ventricular cineangiogram demonstrates large embolus from same tumor in right pulmonary artery.

stances, particularly from degenerating platelets, e.g., serotonin and/or thromboxane A_2.[77]

Structural Features

The nature of the pulmonary vascular abnormalities in thromboembolic disorders has not been studied extensively in children, but findings can be expected to be similar to those described in adults. In the postmortem pulmonary arteriograms of adult patients, some vessels show evidence of thrombi (seen as filling defects), and filling of the peripheral distribution of these vessels with contrast material is scant. Other areas of the lung, however, appear normal.[5] Upon microscopic examination of the abnormally filled areas, fibrous intimal hyperplasia is observed, mostly eccentric in nature, in both the preacinar and peripheral intra-

acinar arteries. Some vessels show evidence of having been completely occluded and later recanalized. Microscopic examination of the areas which appear normal on the arteriogram shows peripheral intraacinar pulmonary arteries which are increased both in size and concentration, suggesting compensatory dilatation and recruitment. Throughout the lung there may be medial hypertrophy of muscular arteries, but this probably depends upon the duration of the disease and the severity of pulmonary hypertension.

PORTAL HYPERTENSION

Severe liver disease, producing cirrhosis and intrahepatic portal hypertension, and portal vein thrombosis, producing extrahepatic portal hypertension, have been associated with the development of pulmonary hypertension.[19, 135, 143, 178] The pathogenesis of the latter is not well understood. Severe structural changes occur in the peripheral pulmonary arteries consisting of medial hypertrophy, occlusive cellular intimal hyperplasia, plexiform lesions, and dilatation complexes. It has therefore been postulated that the 'toxic liver' is unable to degrade a certain vasoconstrictor substance which then circulates through the lung in high concentration, causing structural damage to the vessels. In some patients with liver disease, however, there is generalized vasodilatation of the vessels in the lung.[296] In other patients, anastomoses develop between pulmonary and hepatic arteries.[252] Clearly, the pulmonary vascular response (both structural and hemodynamic) in individual patients with liver disease may be very different.

GRANULOMATOUS AND COLLAGEN VASCULAR DISEASES

Pulmonary hypertension may occur either in adults or in children with sarcoidosis. This seems to be due to the presence of obstructive granulomas within the pulmonary arteries.[42, 173, 176]

Pulmonary hypertension may also occur in association with collagen vascular disease, e.g., scleroderma,[37, 186] systemic lupus erythematosis,[121, 192, 235, 237] rheumatoid arthritis,[287] Takayasu's arteritis,[133] polymyositis,[22] and dermatomyositis.[24, 248] There is no one structural basis for the pulmonary hypertension of collegen vascular disease. In some patients there is severe interstitial lung disease with secondary structural changes in the pulmonary arteries, i.e., loss of vessels, and medial hypertrophy. In other patients, there is little parenchymal disease, but a vasculitis is present[263]; in still others, there is severe intimal fibroelastosis in the pulmonary arteries with plexiform formation; and yet in others, thromboembolic phenomena have been described. The pathogeneses of these different pulmonary vascular changes are not understood.

DRUGS

The ingestion of various substances is known to be associated with pulmonary hypertension. Aminorex, which resembles epinephrine in its chemical structure and which suppresses appetite, causes symptoms of right-sided heart failure in 10% of patients within 6 to 12 months of initial administration.[124] The development of pulmonary hypertension is to some extent dose related. On microscopic examination of the lungs from 17 fatal cases, there was severe medial hypertrophy in the small muscular arteries and intimal fibroelastosis, including the presence of plexiform and dilatation lesions.[175]

While there is little direct evidence that oral contraceptives alone, particularly those low in estrogen content will cause the development of pulmonary vascular disease in women, these compounds should be avoided, particularly in susceptible women, e.g., those with congenital heart defects and pulmonary hypertension. Ingestion of pyrrolizidine alkaloids (monocrotaline) e.g. bushtea causes pulmonary hypertension in animals but only veno-occlusive disease of the liver in humans.[124]

Experimental Models

Rats that ingest monocrotaline spectabolis develop pulmonary arterial changes which can be correlated with hemodynamic evidence of progressive pulmonary hypertension and increased pulmonary vascular resistance.[171] Initially, there is an increase in cardiac output which is associated with an increased extension of muscle into peripheral arteries normally nonmuscular. After 2 weeks, when there is an increase in pulmonary artery pressure, medial hypertrophy of normally muscular arteries is apparent and, after 3 weeks, when an increase in pulmonary vascular resistance occurs secondary to both a further rise in pulmonary artery pressure as well as a drop in cardiac output, there is a reduction in the number of peripheral pulmonary arteries, and 'ghost' or disappearing vessels can be seen. Structural changes are similar to those seen in chronic hypoxic exposure but the time course is longer; the sequence of changes and the correlation with progressive hemodynamic disturbance are similar to those observed in patients with congenital heart defects. Ultrastructural studies have shown injury to the vascular endothelium within several hours of monocrotaline injection; inflammatory cells and edema are apparent after 1 week. An imbalance in vasoactive substances can be expected under these circumstances, and this may mediate the structural changes in the pulmonary arteries.

IDIOPATHIC PULMONARY HYPERTENSION

After all known etiologies of pulmonary hypertension have been ruled out, the diagnosis becomes that of 'idiopathic pulmonary hypertension.' This unexplained disease, in which a structural abnormality is always found either in the arteries or in the veins, occurs both in children and adults and, rarely, with a familial tendency.[100, 223] In both groups, it is usually rapidly progressive and invariably fatal, although rare cases of spontaneous regression have been reported.[18, 62] In children there is a 1:1 female-male ratio, but in adults, females are predominantly affected (ratio 4:1).[267] Children are most frequently diagnosed in infancy and die within a year. In general, there is an inverse relationship between the age of onset of symptoms and the duration of illness until death.

The vascular pathology in the 'arterial' form of the disease in infants consists of severe medial hypertrophy of muscular arteries; and we have observed increased extension of muscle and a striking decrease in the concentration of small arteries.[221, 298] In older children, intimal hyperplasia and occlusive changes are found in the pulmonary arteries, as well as plexiform lesions. In adults, in addition to the latter changes, 'ghost' arteries have also been reported. Electron microscopic study by Meyrick et al.[168] performed on a lung biopsy of an adult patient showed severe endothelial injury which they speculated to be the initial site of damage (Fig. 42.17A). In some patients, defective fibrinolysis has been described; in others there has been evidence for an immunologic abnormality, but in most patients studied, these systems have been normal.

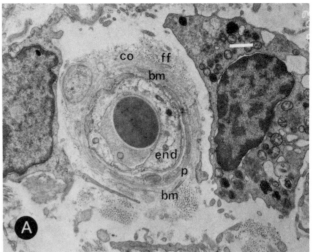

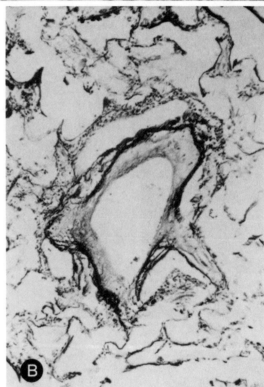

Fig. 42.17 (A) An electron micrograph of an alveolar capillary, 4.2 μm in diameter (measured from basement membranes); the endothelium (end) appears pale and swollen. Around the vessel concentric layers are seen comprised of pericytes (p), basement membranes (bm), fine filaments (ff), and collagen (co). Uranyl acetate and lead citrate, ×5500. (Reproduced with permission from B. Meyrick et al.[168]) (B) Photomicrographs of pulmonary vein with narrowing by loose intimal connective tissue. Elastin-Van Gieson stain, ×125. (Reproduced with permission from A. Rosenthal et al.[226])

In the venous form of idiopathic pulmonary hypertension,[94, 226, 283, 285] the clinical presentation is somewhat different from the arterial in that orthopnea is a characteristic feature and changes suggesting pulmonary edema are apparent on the chest radiograph, despite a normal pulmonary wedge pressure. Structural changes in the lung are most striking in both large and small veins and consist of loose fibrous intimal hyperplasia; the lymphatics are usually quite dilated (Fig. 42.17*B*). There are secondary changes in the arteries of mild medial hypertrophy and intimal hyperplasia. In the youngest patient reported, pulmonary venous changes were described which appear to have occurred in utero.[283]

Various vasodilator agents have been tried in an effort to reduce the level of pulmonary artery pressure, relieve symptoms, and perhaps retard the progression of this disease. The major difficulty lies in the fact that there is no selective pulmonary vasodilator and, so, systemic hypotension usually occurs with a decrease in cardiac output and little change in the pulmonary vascular resistance.

Since idiopathic pulmonary hypertension likely has many etiologies and is diagnosed at different stages, no one agent has been effective either acutely or chronically in all cases studied. Among the most successful agents reported have been isoproterenol,[43, 204, 240] hydralazine,[230] diazoxide,[110, 131, 288] nifedipine,[25, 245] phentolamine,[233] prostacyclin,[76, 290] and long-term oxygen therapy.[191] Verapamil has a very limited effect,[134] as does prostaglandin E[1].[262] Indomethacin has been successful only in conjunction with isoproterenol.[204] The most promising of all these agents seems to be hydralazine. Rubin *et al.*,[230] in a study of adults, reported a decrease in pulmonary artery pressure and in pulmonary vascular resistance which was achieved both at rest and during exercise and which persisted at follow-up 6 months later (Fig. 42.18). Our experience in children, however, has been disappointing.

Studies to determine the mechanism for idiopathic pulmonary hypertension have been aimed mainly at the identification of coagulation disturbances,[52, 59, 114, 268] and thera-

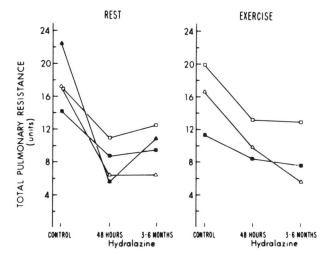

Fig. 42.18 The drop in total pulmonary resistance at 48 hours was significant in all four patients. This response was persistent at 3 to 6 months. (Reproduced with permission from L. J. Rubin and R. M. Peter.[230])

peutic trials with anticoagulants have been reinitiated.[63] Cardiac catheterization is mandatory to diagnose idiopathic pulmonary hypertension, yet this carries risk.[39, 126, 246] Future advances in diagnosis and therapy can best be achieved through the study of lung biopsy tissue.[284]

REFERENCES

1. Abraham, A. S., Kay, J. M., Cole, R. B., and Pincock, A. C.: Hemodynamic and pathological study of the effect of chronic hypoxia and subsequent recovery of the heart and pulmonary vasculature of the rat. Cardiovasc. Res. 5:95, 1971.
2. Acquatella, H., Schiller, N. B., Sharpe, D. N., and Chatterjee, K.: Lack of correlation between echocardiographic pulmonary valve morphology and simultaneous pulmonary arterial pressure. Am. J. Cardiol. 43:946, 1979.
3. Alday, L. E., Vega, P. J., and Heller, A.: Congenital ankylosis of the temporomandibular joint: Resultant upper airway obstruction and cor pulmonale. Chest. 75:384, 1979.
4. Altemus, L. R., and Lee, R. E.: Carcinomatosis of the lung with pulmonary hypertension. Arch. Intern. Med. 119:32, 1967.
5. Anderson, E. G., Simon, G., and Reid, L.: Primary and thromboembolic pulmonary hypertension: A quantitative pathological study. J. Pathol. 110, 1973.
6. Arias-Stella, J., and Saldana, M.: The terminal portion of the pulmonary arterial tree in people native to high altitude. Circulation 28:915, 1963.
7. Auchincloss, J. H., and Gilbert, R.: The cardiorespiratory syndrome related to obesity: Clinical manifestations and pathologic physiology. Prog. Cardiovasc. Dis. 1:413, 1959.
8. Baar, H. S., and Braid, F.: Diffuse interstitial fibrosis of the lungs in childhood. Dis. Child. 32:199, 1957.
9. Bauman, W., Wann, L. S., Childress, R., Weyman, A. E., Feigenbaum, H., and Dillon, J.: Mid systolic notching of the pulmonary valve in the abscence of pulmonary hypertension. Am. J. Cardiol. 43:1049, 1979.
10. Bergofsky, E. J., Turino, G. M., and Fishman, A. P.: Cardiorespiratory failure in kyphoscoliosis. Medicine 38:263, 1959.
11. Berkov, S.: Hypoxic pulmonary vasoconstriction in the rat. The necessary role of angiotensin II. Circ. Res. 35:256, 1974.
12. Berman, W., Jr., Whitman, V., Pierce, W. S.,

and Waldhausen, J. A.: The development of pulmonary vascular obstructive disease after successful Mustard operation in early infancy. Circulation 58:181, 1978.
13. Bernhard, W. F., Dick, M., Sloss, L., Castaneda, A. R., and Nadas, A. S.: The palliative Mustard operation for double outlet right ventricle in transposition. Circulation 54:810, 1976.
14. Besterman, E.: Atrial septal defect with pulmonary hypertension. Br. Heart J. 23:587, 1961.
15. Bing, R. J., Vandam, L. D., and Gray, F. D.: Physiological studies in congenital heart disease. Bull. Johns Hopkins Hosp. 80:323, 1947.
16. Bloss, R. S., Turmen, T., Beardmore, H. E., and Aranda, J. V.: Tolazoline therapy for persistent pulmonary hypertension after congenital diaphragmatic hernia repair. J. Pediatr. 97:984, 1980.
17. Bond, V. F., Jr.: Eisenmenger's complex. Report of two cases and review of cases with autopsy study. Am. Heart J. 42:424, 1951.
18. Bourdillon, P. D., and Oakley, C. M.: Regression of primary pulmonary hypertension. Br. Heart J. 38:264, 1976.
19. Bower, J. S., Dantzker, D. R., and Naylor, B.: Idiopathic pulmonary hypertension associated with nodular pulmonary infiltrates and portal venous thrombosis. Chest 78:111, 1980.
20. Branzi, A., and Magelli, C.: Pulmonary hypertension and acquired cardiopathies. Torace 22:84, 1979.
21. Brenner, O.: Pathology of the vessels of the pulmonary circulation. Part 1. Arch. Intern. Med. 56:211, 1935.
22. Bunch, T. W., Tancredi, R. G., and Lie, J. T.: Pulmonary hypertension in polymyositis. Chest. 79:105, 1981.
23. Burwell, C. S., Robin, E. D., Whaley, R. D., and Bickelmann, A. G.: Extreme obesity associated with alveolar hypoventilation. Am. J. Med. 21:811, 1956.
24. Caldwell, L. W., and Aitchison, J. D.: Pulmonary hypertension in dermatomyositis. Br.

Heart. J. 18:273, 1956.
25. Camerini, F., Alberti, E., Klugman, N., and Salvi, A.: Primary pulmonary hypertension: Effects of nifedipine. Br. Heart J. 44:352, 1980.
26. Cartmill, T. B., DuShane, J. W., McGoon, D. C., and Kirklin, J. W.: Results of repair of ventricular septal defect. J. Thorac. Cardiovasc. Surg. 52:486, 1966.
27. Cassin, S., Todd, M., Philips, J., Frisinger, J., Jordan, J., and Gibbs, C.: Effects of prostaglandin D[2] on perinatal circulation. Am. J. Physiol. 240:H755, 1981.
28. Cassin, S., Tyler, T., and Wallis, R.: The effects of prostaglandin E[1] on fetal pulmonary vascular resistance. Proc. Soc. Exp. Biol. Med. 148:584, 1975.
29. Castaneda, A. R., Lamberti, J., Sade, R. M., Williams, R. G., and Nadas, A. S.: Open heart surgery during the first three months of life. J. Thorac. Cardiovasc. Surg. 68:719, 1974.
30. Castaneda, A. R., Zamora, R., Nicoloff, D. M., Moller, J. H., Hunt, C. E., and Lukas, R. V.: High pressure, high resistance ventricular septal defect: Surgical results of closure through right atrium. Ann. Thorac. Surg. 12:29, 1971.
31. Cayler, G. G., May, S. J., and Riley, H. D.: Cardiorespiratory syndrome of obesity associated with alveolar hypoventilation (Pickwickian syndrome) in children. Pediatrics 27:237, 1961.
32. Chamberlain, D., Hislop, A., Hey, E., and Reid, L.: Pulmonary hypoplasia in babies with severe rhesus isoimmunization: A quantitative study. J. Pathol. 122:43, 1977.
33. Chou, T., Masangkay, M. P., Young, R., Conway, G. F., and Helm, R. A.: Simple quantitative vectorcardiographic criteria for the diagnosis of right ventricular hypertrophy. Circulation 48:1262, 1973.
34. Civin, W. H., and Edwards, J. E.: Pathology of the pulmonary vascular tree. Circulation 2:545, 1950.
35. Cogswell, J. J., and Easton, D. M.: Cor pul-

monale in Pierre Robin syndrome. Arch. Dis. Child. 49:905, 1974.

36. Collins-Nakai, R. L., Rosenthal, A., Castaneda, A. R., Bernhard, W. F., and Nadas, A. S.: Congenital mitral stenosis. A review of 20 years experience. Circulation 56:1039, 1977.

37. Connor, P. K., and Bashour, F. A.: Cardiopulmonary changes in scleroderma. A physiologic study. Am. Heart J. 61:494, 1961.

38. Cox, M. A., Schiebler, G. I., Taylor, W. J., Wheat, M. W., and Krovetz, L. J.: Reversible pulmonary hypertension in a child with respiratory obstruction and cor pulmonale. J. Pediatr. 67:192, 1965.

39. Curti, R. J., Sanches, P. C., Bittencourt, L. A., Nogueira, E. A., Jorge, P. A., Carvalhal, S., and Dos, S.: Primary pulmonary hypertension: Deleterious effects of pulmonary angiography. Report of a case. Arq. Bras. Cardiol. 35:225, 1980.

40. Dammann, J. F., and Ferencz, C.: The pulmonary vascular bed in tetralogy of Fallot. I. Changes associated with pulmonary stenosis. II. Changes following a systemic pulmonary arterial anastomosis. Johns Hopkins Med. J. 106:100, 1960.

41. Dammann, J. F., Ferencz, C.: Malformation in the heart in which both increased pressure and blood flow may act upon the lungs and in which there is common ejectible force. Am. Heart J. 52:210, 1956.

42. Damuth, T. E., Bower, J. S., Cho, K., and Dantzker, D. R.: Major pulmonary artery stenosis causing pulmonary hypertension in sarcoidosis. Chest. 78:888, 1980.

43. Daoud, F. S., Reeves, J. T., and Kelly, D. B.: Isoproterenol as a potential pulmonary vasodilator in primary pulmonary hypertension. Am. J. Cardiol. 42:817, 1978.

44. Davies, G., and Reid, L.: Growth of the alveoli and pulmonary arteries in childhood. Thorax 25:669, 1970.

45. Davies, G., and Reid, L.: Effect of scoliosis on growth of alveoli and pulmonary arteries and on right ventricle. Arch. Dis. Child. 46:623, 1971.

46. Dow, N., and Siggers, D. C.: Cor pulmonale in Crouzon's disease. Arch. Dis. Child. 46:394, 1971.

47. Drummond, D. S., Salter, R. B., and Boone, J.: Fat embolism in children. Can Med. Assoc. J. 101:200, 1969.

48. Drummond, W. H., Gregory, G. A., Heymann, M. A., and Phibbs, R. A.: The independent effects of hyperventilation tolazoline and dopamine on infants with persistent pulmonary hypertension. J. Pediatr. 98:603, 1981.

49. Dushane, J. W., Krongrad, E., Ritter, D. G., and McGoon, D. C.: The fate of raised pulmonary vascular resistance after surgery in ventricular septal defect. In The Child with Congenital Heart Disease after Surgery, edited by R. D. Rowe and B. S. L. Kidd. Futura, Mount Kisco, N. Y., 1976.

50. Eisenmenger, V.: Die angeborenen Defecte der Kammerscheidewand des Herzen. Z. Klin. Med. Suppl. 132:1, 1897.

51. Elliott, F. M., and Reid, L.: Some new facts about the pulmonary artery and its branching pattern. Clin. Radiol. 6:193, 1965.

52. Ellison, C. R., and Brown, J.: Fibrinolysis is pulmonary vascular disease. Lancet 1:786, 1965.

53. Emery, J. L.: Pulmonary embolism in children. Arch. Dis. Child. 37:591, 1962.

54. Ferencz, C., and Dammann, J. F.: The significance of the pulmonary vascular bed in congenital heart disease. V. Lesions of the left side of the heart causing obstruction of the pulmonary venous return. Circulation 16:1046, 1957.

55. Ferencz, C.: Transposition of the great vessels. Pathophysiologic consideration based upon a study of the lungs. Circulation 33:232, 1966.

56. Ferguson, D. J., and Varco, R. L.: The relation of blood pressure and flow to the development and regression of experimentally induced pulmonary hypertension. Circ. Res. 3:152, 1955.

57. Fishman, L. S., Samson, J. H., and Sperling, D. R.: Primary alveolar hypoventilation syndrome (Ondine's curse). Am. J. Dis. Child. 110:155, 1965.

58. Fishman, A. P.: Hypoxia on the pulmonary circulation. How and where it acts. Circ. Res. 38:221, 1976.

59. Franz, R. C., Ziady, F., Coetzee, W. J., and Hugo, N.: A possible causal relationship between defective fibrinolysis and pulmonary hypertension. S. Afr. Med. J. 55:170, 1979.

60. Freeman, M. K., and Manners, J. M.: Cor pulmonale and the Pierre Robin anomaly. Airway management with a nasopharyngeal tube. Anaesthesia 35:282, 1980.

61. Friedli, B., Kidd, B. S., Mustard, W. T., and Keith, J. D.: Ventricular septal defect with increased pulmonary vascular resistance. Am. J. Cardiol. 33:403, 1974.

62. Fujii, A., Rabinovitch, M., and Matthews, E. C.: A case of spontaneous resolution of idiopathic pulmonary hypertension. Br. Heart J., in press, 1982.

63. Fuster, V., Giuliani, E. R., Brandenburg, R. O., Weidman, W. H., and Edwards, W. D.: The natural history of idiopathic pulmonary hypertension (abstr.). Am. J. Cardiol. 47:422, 1981.

64. Garcia-Palmieri, M. R.: Cor pulmonale due to schistosoma mansoni. Am. Heart J. 68:714, 1964.

65. Gilroy, J., Cahalan, J. L., Berman, R., and Newman, M.: Cardiac and pulmonary complications in Duchenne's progressive muscular dystrophy. Circulation 27:484, 1963.

66. Goldring, R. A., Turino, G. M., Cohen, G., Jameson, A. G., Bass, B. G., and Fishman, A. P.: The catecholamines in the pulmonary arterial pressor response to acute hypoxia. J. Clin. Invest. 41:1211, 1964.

67. Goldring, R. M., Fishman, A. P., Turino, G. M., Cohen, H. I., Denning, C. R., and Andersen, D. H.: Pulmonary hypertension and cor pulmonale in cystic fibrosis of the pancreas. J. Pediatr. 65:501, 1964.

68. Goldstein, J. D., and Reid, L. M.: Pulmonary hypoplasia resulting from phrenic nerve agenesis and diaphragmatic amyoplasia. J. Pediatr. 97:282, 1980.

69. Gootman, N., Gross, J., and Mensch, A.: Pulmonary artery thrombosis: A complication occurring with prednisone and chlorothiazide therapy in two nephrotic patients. Pediatrics 34:861, 1964.

70. Griffin, J. T., Kass, L., and Hoffman, M. S.: Cor pulmonale associated with symptoms and signs of asthma in children. Pediatrics 24:54, 1959.

71. Gross, N. J.: Pulmonary effects of radiation therapy. Ann. Intern. Med. 86:81, 1977.

72. Grossman, H., Levin, A. R., Winchester, P. H., and Auld, P. A. M.: Pulmonary hypertension in the Wilson-Mikity syndrome. J. Dis. Child. 114:293, 1972.

73. Grover, R. F., Vogel, J. H. K., Voigt, G. C., and Blount, S. G.: Reversal of high altitude pulmonary hypertension. Am. J. Cardiol. 18:928, 1966.

74. Grover, R. F.: Speculations on the pathogenesis of high-altitude pulmonary edema. Adv. Cardiol. 27:1, 1980.

75. Grover, R. F., Vogel, J. H. K., Averill, K. H., and Blount, S. G. Jr.: Pulmonary hypertension. Individual and species variability relative to vascular reactivity. Am. Heart J. 66:1, 1966.

76. Guadagni, D. N., Ikram, H., and Maslowski, A. H.: Haemodynamic effects of prostacyclin (PG12) in pulmonary hypertension Br. Heart J. 45:385.

77. Gurewich, V., Cohen, M. L., and Thomas, D. P.: Humoral factors in massive pulmonary embolism: An experimental study. Am. Heart J. 76:784, 1968.

78. Hales, C. A., Rouse, E. T., and Slate, J. L.: Influence of aspirin and indomethacin on variability of alveolar hypoxic vasoconstriction. J. Appl. Physiol. 45:33, 1978.

79. Hallidie-Smith, K. A., Wilson, R. S. E., Hart, A., and Ziedifard, E.: Functional status of patients with large ventricular septal defect and pulmonary vascular disease 6–16 years after surgical closure of their defect in childhood. Br. Heart J. 39:1093, 1977.

80. Hallidie-Smith, K. A., Hollman, A. Cleland, W. P., Bentall, H. H., and Goodwin, J. F.: Effects of surgical closure of ventricular septal defects upon pulmonary vascular disease. Br. Heart J. 31:246, 1969.

81. Hardesty, R. L., Griffith, B. P., Debski, R. F., Jeffries, M. R., and Borovetz, H. S.: Extracorporeal membrane oxygenation. Successful treatment of persistent fetal circulation following repair of congenital diaphragmatic hernia. J. Thorac. Cardiovasc. Surg. 81:556, 1981.

82. Harker, L., Kirkpatrick, S. E., Friedman, W. G., and Bloor, C. M.: Effects of indomethacin on the fetal pulmonary circulation. Lab. Invest. 42:121, 1980.

83. Haworth, S. G., and Reid, L.: Persistent fetal circulation: Newly recognized structural features. J. Pediatr. 88:614, 1976.

84. Haworth, S. G., and Reid, L.: Structural study of the pulmonary circulation in total anomalous pulmonary venous return in early infancy. Br. Heart J. 39:80, 1977.

85. Haworth, S. G., and Reid, L.: Quantitative structural study of pulmonary circulation in the newborn with pulmonary atresia. Thorax 32:129, 1977.

86. Haworth, S. G., deLeval, M., and Macartney, F. J.: Hypo and hyperperfusion in the immature lung: Pulmonary arterial development following ligation of the left pulmonary artery in the newborn pig. J. Thorac. Cardiovasc. Surg., in press, 1982.

87. Haworth, S. G., and Macartney, F. J.: Growth and development of the pulmonary circulation in pulmonary atresia with ventricular septal defect and major aortopulmonary collateral arteries. Br. Heart J. 44:14, 1980.

88. Haworth, S. G., and Reid, L.: Quantitative structural study of pulmonary circulation in the newborn with aortic atresia, stenosis or coarctation. Thorax 32:121, 1977.

89. Haworth, S. G., Rees, P. G., Taylor, J. F., Macartney, F. J., deLeval, M., and Stark, J.: Pulmonary atresia with ventricular septal defect and major aortopulmonary collateral arteries: Effect of systemic pulmonary anastomosis. Br. Heart J. 45:133, 1981.

90. Haworth, S. G., and Reid, L: A morphometric study of regional variation in lung structure in infants with pulmonary hypertension and congenital heart defect. A justification of lung biopsy. Br. Heart J. 40:825, 1978.

91. Haworth, S. G., Sauer, U., Buhlmeyer, K., and Reid, L.: The development of the pulmonary circulation in ventricular septal defect: A quantitative structural study. Am. J. Cardiol. 40:781, 1977.

92. Heath, D., DuShane, J. W., Wood, E. H., and Edwards, J. E.: The aetiology of pulmonary thrombosis in cyanotic congenital heart disease and pulmonary stenosis. Thorax 13:213, 1958.

93. Heath, D., and Kay, J. M.: Diet, drugs and pulmonary hypertension. In Progress in Cardiology, Chapter 4, edited by P. M. Yu and J. F. Goodwin. Lea & Febiger, Philadelphia, 1978.

94. Heath, D., Scott, O., and Lynch, J.: Pulmonary venoocclusive disease. Thorax 26:663, 1971.

95. Heath, D., and Edwards, J. E.: The pathology of hypertensive pulmonary vascular disease. Circulation 18:533, 1958.

96. Heath, D., and Mackinnon, J.: Pulmonary hypertension due to myxoma of the right atrium with special reference to the behavior of emboli of myxoma in the lung. Am. Heart J. 68:227, 1964.

97. Heath, D., Swan, H. J. C., DuShane, J. W., and Edwards, J. E.: The relation of medial thickness of small muscular pulmonary arteries to immediate postnatal survival in patients with ventricular septal defect and patent ductus arteriosus. Thorax 13:267, 1958.

98. Heath, D., Edwards, C., Winson, M., and Smith, P.: Effects on the right ventricle, pulmonary vasculature and carotid bodies of the rate of exposure to and recovery from simulated high altitude. Thorax 28:24, 1973.

99. Heath, D., Helmholz, H. F., Burchell, H. B., DuShane, J. W., and Edwards, J. E.: Graded pulmonary vascular changes and hemodynamic findings in cases of atrial and ventricular septal defect and patent ductus arteriosus. Circulation 18:1155, 1958.

100. Hendrix, G. H.: Familial primary pulmonary hypertension. South Med. J. 67:981, 1974.

101. Heymann, M. A., and Rudolph, A. M.: Effects of acetylsalicylic acid on the ductus arteriosus and circulation of fetal lambs in utero. Circ. Res. 38:418, 1976.

102. Hirschfeld, S., Meyer, R., Schwartz, D. C., Korfhagen, J., and Kaplan, S.: The echocardiographic assessment of pulmonary artery pressure and resistance. Circulation 52:642, 1975.

103. Hislop, A., Hey, E., and Reid, L.: The lungs in congenital bilateral renal agenesis and dysplasia. Arch. Dis. Child. 54:32, 1979.

104. Hislop, A., and Reid, L.: Persistent hypoplasia of the lung following repair of congenital diaphragmatic hernia. Thorax 31:450, 1976.

105. Hislop, A., and Reid, L.: Structural changes in the pulmonary arteries and veins in tetralogy of Fallot. Br. Heart J. 35:1178, 1973.

106. Hislop, A., Haworth, S. G., and Reid, L.: Quantitative structural analysis of pulmonary vessels in isolated ventricular septal defects in infancy. Br. Heart J. 37:1014, 1975.

107. Hislop, A., and Reid, L.: Pulmonary arterial development during childhood: Branching pattern and structure. Thorax 28:129, 1973.

108. Hislop, A., and Reid, L.: Changes in the pulmonary arteries of the rat during recovery from hypoxia-induced pulmonary hypertension. Br. J. Exp. Pathol. 58:653, 1977.

109. Hoffman, J. I. E., and Rudolph, A. M.: The natural history of ventricular septal defects in infancy. Am. J. Cardiol. 16:634, 1965.

110. Honey, M., Cotter, L., Davies, N., and Denison, D.: Clinical and haemodynamic effects of diazoxide in primary pulmonary hypertension. Thorax 35:629, 1980.

111. Hopkins, R. A., Hammon, J. W., McHale, P. A., Smith, P. K., and Anderson, R. W.: Pulmonary vascular impedance analysis of adaptation to chronically elevated pulmonary blood flow in the awake dog. Circ. Res. 45:267, 1979.

112. Hopkins, R. A., Hammon, J. W., Jr., McHale, P. A., Smith, P. K., and Anderson, R. W.: An analysis of the pulsatile hemodynamic response of the pulmonary circulation to acute and chronic pulmonary venous hypertension in the awake dog. Circ. Res. 47:902, 1980.

113. Hultgren, H. N., Kelly, J., and Miller, H.: Pulmonary circulation in acclimatized man at high altitude. J. Appl. Physiol. 20:239, 1965.

114. Inglesby, T. V., Singer, J. W., and Gordon, D. S.: Abnormal fibrinolysis in familial pulmonary hypertension. Am. J. Med. 55:5, 1973.

115. Ingram, R. H., and Bishop, J. B.: Ventilatory response to carbon dioxide after removal of chronic upper airway obstruction. Am. Rev. Resp. Dis. 102:645, 1970.

116. Iverson, R. E., Linde, L. E., and Kegel, S.: The diagnosis of progressive pulmonary vascular disease in children with ventricular septal defects. J. Pediatr. 68:594, 1966.

117. Jersaty, R. M., Huszar, R. J., and Basu, S.: Pierre-Robin syndrome: Cause of respiratory obstruction, cor pulmonale and pulmonary edema. Am. J. Dis. Child. 117:710, 1969.

118. Johnson, J. B., Felter, M. L., West, J. R., and Cournand, A.: The relation between electrocardiographic existence of right ventricular hypertrophy and pulmonary arterial pressure in patients with chronic pulmonary disease. Circulation 1:536, 1950.

119. Johnson, G. M., and Todd, D. W.: Cor pulmonale in severe Pierre Robin syndrome. Pediatr. 65:152, 1980.

120. Juratsch, C. E., Emmanouilides, G. C., Thibeault, D. W., Baylen, B. G., Jengo, M. M., and Laks, M. M.: Pulmonary arterial hypertension induced by distention of the main pulmonary artery in conscious newborn, young and adult sheep. Pediatr. Res. 14:133, 1980.

121. Kanemoto, N., Gonda, N., Katsu, M., and Fukada, J.: Two cases of pulmonary hypertension and Raynaud's phenomenon: Primary pulmonary hypertension and systemic lupus erythematosus. Jap. Heart J. 16:354, 1975.

122. Kato, H., Kidd, L., and Olley, P. M.: Effects of hypoxia on pulmonary vascular reactivity in pneumonectomized puppies and minipigs. Circ. Res. 28:397, 1971.

123. Kauffman, S. L., Lynfield, J., and Hennigar, G. R.: Mycotic aneurysms of the intrapulmonary arteries. Circulation 35:90, 1967.

124. Kay, J. M., Smith, P., and Heath, D.: Aminorex and the pulmonary circulation. Thorax 26:262, 1971.

125. Kay, J. M., and Grover, R. F.: Lung mast cells and hypoxic pulmonary hypertension. Prog. Resp. Res. 9:157, 1975.

126. Keane, J. F., Fyler, D. C., and Nadas, A. S.: Hazards of cardiac catheterization in children with primary pulmonary vascular obstruction. Am. Heart J. 96:556, 1978.

127. Keane, J. F., Ellison, R. C., Rudd, M., and Nadas, A. S.: Pulmonary blood flow and left ventricular volumes with transposition of the great arteries and intact ventricular septum. Br. Heart J. 35:521, 1973.

128. Kelminson, L. L., Cotton, E. K., and Vogel, J. H. K.: The reversibility of pulmonary hypertension in patients with cystic fibrosis. Pediatrics 39:24, 1967.

129. Kinsley, R. H., McGoon, D. C., Danielson, G. K., Wallace, R. B., and Mair, D. D.: Pulmonary arterial hypertension after repair of tetralogy of Fallot. J. Thorac Cardiovasc. Surg. 67:110, 1974.

130. Kitagawa, M., Hislop, A., Boyden, E. A., and Reid, L.: Lung hypoplasia in congenital diaphragmatic hernia: A quantitative study of airway, artery and alveolar development. J. Surg. 58:342, 1971.

131. Klinke, W. P., and Gilbert, J. A.: Diazoxide in primary pulmonary hypertension. N. Engl. J. Med. 302:91, 1980.

132. Kreiger, A. J., Rosomoff, H. L., Kuperman, A. S., and Zingesser, L. H.: Occult respiratory dysfunction in craniovertebral anomaly. J. Neurosurg. 31:15, 1969.

133. Lande, A., and Bard, R.: Takayasu's arteritis: An unrecognized cause of pulmonary hypertension. Angiology 27:114, 1976.

134. Landmark, K., Refsum, A. M., Simonsen, S., and Storstein, O.: Verapamil and pulmonary hypertension. Acta. Med. Scand. 204:297, 1978.

135. Lebrec, D., Capron, J. P., Dhumeaux, D., and Benhamou, J. O.: Pulmonary hypertension complicating portal hypertension. Am. Rev. Resp. Dis. 120:849, 1978.

136. Leffler, C. W., Tyler, T. L., and Cassin, S.: Responses of pulmonary and systemic circulations of perinatal goats to prostaglandin E2 Alpha. Can. J. Physiol. Pharmacol. 57:167, 1979.

137. Leuenberger, P. J., Stalcup, S. A., Mellins, R. B., Greenbaum, L. M., and Turino, G. M.: Decrease in angiotensin-1 conversion by acute hypoxia in dogs. Proc. Soc. Exp. Biol. Med. 158:586, 1978.

138. Levin, D. L., Heymann, M. A., and Rudolph, A. M.: Morphological development of the pulmonary vascular bed in experimental pulmonic stenosis. Circulation 59:179, 1979.

139. Levin, D. L., Mills, L. J., and Parkey, M.: Morphological development of the pulmonary vascular bed in experimental coarctaon of the aorta. Circulation 60:349, 1979.

140. Levin, D. L., Mills, L. J., and Weinberg, A. G.: Hemodynamic pulmonary vascular and myocardial abnormalities secondary to pharmacologic constriction of the fetal ductus arteriosus. Circulation 60:360, 1979.

141. Levin, D. L., Muster, A. J., Pachman, L. M., Wessell, W. U., Paul, M. H., and Koshaba, J.: Cor pulmonale secondary to upper airway obstruction. Cardiac catheterization immunologic and psychometric evaluation in nine patients. Chest 68:166, 1975.

142. Levin, D. L., Fixler, D. E., Morriss, F. C., and Tyson, J.: Morphologic analysis of the pulmonary vascular bed in infants exposed in utero to prostaglandin synthetase inhibitors. J. Pediatr. 92:478, 1978.

143. Levine, O. R., Harris, R. C., Blanc, W. A., and Mellins, R. B.: Progressive pulmonary hypertension in children with portal hypertension. J. Pediatr. 83:964, 1973.

144. Levy, A. M., Tabakin, B. S., Hanson, J. S., and Narkewicz, R. M.: Hypertrophied adenoids causing pulmonary hypertension and severe congestive heart failure. N. Engl. J. Med. 277:506, 1967.

145. Liebman, J., Lucas, R. V., Moss, A., and Rosenthal, A.: Cor pulmonale and related cardiovascular effects of cystic fibrosis. In Cystic Fibrosis: Projections into the Future, edited by J. A. Mangos, and R. C. Talamo, Stratten Intercontinental Medical Book Corporation, New York, 1976.

146. Lloyd, T. C., Jr.: Hypoxic pulmonary vasoconstriction: Role of perivascular tissue. J. Appl. Physiol. 25:560, 1968.

147. Lock, J. E., Fuhrman, B. P., Epstein, M. L., Rowe, R. D., and Lucas, R. V.: Pulmonary hypertension following neonatal shock. Pediatr. Cardiol. 1:109, 1979/80.

148. Lock, J. E., Olley, P. M., Coceani, F., Hamilton, F., and Doubilet, G.: Pulmonary and systemic vascular responses to 6-keto-PGE₁ in the conscious lamb. Prostaglandins 18:303, 1979.

149. Lock, J. E., Hamilton, F., Olley, P. M., and Coceani, F.: The effect of alveolar hypoxia on pulmonary vascular responsiveness in the conscious newborn lamb. Can. J. Physiol. Pharmacol. 58:153, 1980.

150. Lock, J. E., Olley, P. M., Coceani, F., Swyer, P. R., and Rowe, R. D.: Use of prostacyclin in persistent fetal circulation (letter). Lancet 1:134, 1979.

151. Luggresi, E., and Coccagna, G.: Sleep, snoring and sleep-apnea syndromes. In Pulmonary Diseases and Disorders, Chapter 33, edited by A. P. Fishman. McGraw-Hill, New York, 1979.

152. Lukas, D. S., and Plum, F.: Pulmonary function in patients convalescing from acute poliomyelitis with respiratory paralysis. Am. J. Med. 12:388, 1952.

153. Luke, M. J., Mehrizi, A., Folger, G. M., and Rowe, R. D.: Chronic nasopharyngeal obstruction as a cause of cardiomegaly, cor pulmonale and pulmonary oedema. Pediatrics 37:762, 1966.

154. Lupi-Herrera, E., Bialostozky, D., and Sob-

rino, A.: The role of isoproterenol in pulmonary artery hypertension of unknown etiology (primary): Short- and long-term evaluation. Chest, 79:292, 1981.

155. Lurie, P. R., and Shumacher, H. B., Jr.: Mitral commissurotomy in childhood. Pediatrics 13:454, 1954.

156. Macartney, F. J., Deverall, P. B., and Scott, O.: Hemodynamic characteristics of systemic arterial blood supply to the lungs. Br. Heart J. 35:28, 1973.

157. Mair, D. D., and McGoon, D. C.: Surgical correction of atrioventricular canal during the first year of life. Am. J. Cardiol. 40:66, 1977.

158. Mair, D. D., Ritter, D. G., Ongley, P. A., and Helmholz, H. F., Jr.: Hemodynamics and evaluation for surgery of patients with complete transposition of the great arteries and ventricular septal defect. Am. J. Cardiol. 28:632, 1971.

159. Manchester, D., Margolis, H. S., and Sheldon, R. E.: Possible association between maternal indomethacin therapy and primary pulmonary hypertension of the newborn. Am. J. Obstet. Gynecol. 126:467, 1976.

160. Marcelletti, C., McGoon, D. C., and Mair, D. D.: The natural history of truncus arteriosus. Circulation 54:108, 1976.

161. Marini, J. J., Bilnoski, W., and Huseby, J. S.: Acute cor pulmonale resulting from tumor microembolism. West. J. Med. 132:77, 1980.

162. Maron, B. J., Redwood, D. R., Hirshfeld, J. W., Jr., Goldstein, R. E., Morrow, A. G., and Epstein, S. E.: Postoperative assessment of patients with ventricular septal defect and pulmonary hypertension. Response to intense and upright exercise. Circulation 48:864, 1973.

163. McGiff, J. C.: Thromboxane and prostacyclin. Implications for function and disease of the vasculature. Adv. Intern. Med. 25:199, 1980.

164. McMurtry, I. F., Frith, C. H., and Will, D. H.: Cardiopulmonary responses of male and female swine to simulated high altitude. J. Appl. Physiol. 35:459, 1973.

165. McMurtry, I. F., Davidson, A. B., Reeves, J. T., and Grover, R. F.: Inhibition of hypoxic pulmonary vasoconstriction by calcium antagonists in isolated rat lungs. Circ. Res. 38:99, 1976.

166. Mellins, R. B., Balfour, H. M., Turino, G. M., and Winters: Failure of automatic control of ventilation (Ondine's curse): Report of an infant with this syndrome and a review of the literature. Medicine 49:487, 1970.

167. Meyrick, B., and Reid, L.: Endothelial and subintimal changes in rat hilar pulmonary artery during recovery from hypoxia: A quantitative ultrastructural study. Lab. Invest. 42:603, 1980.

168. Meyrick, B., Clarke, S. W., Symons, C., Woodgate, D. J., and Reid, L.: Primary pulmonary hypertension. A case report including electronmicroscopic study. Br. J. Dis. Chest 68:11, 1974.

169. Meyrick, B., and Reid, L.: The effect of continued hypoxia on rat pulmonary arterial circulation: An ultrastructural study. Lab. Invest. 38:188, 1978.

170. Meyrick, B., Fujiwara, K., and Reid, L,.: Smooth muscle myosin in precursor and mature smooth muscle cells in normal pulmonary arteries and the effect of hypoxia. Am. J. Anat., in press, 1982.

171. Meyrick, B., Gamble, G., and Reid, L.: Development of crotalaria pulmonary hypertension: Hemodynamic and structural study. Am. J. Physiol. 239:H692, 1980.

172. Meyrick, B., and Reid, L.: Ultrastructural findings in lung biopsy material from children with congenital heart defects. Am. J. Pathol. 101:527, 1980.

173. Michaels, L., Brown, N. J., and Cory-Wright, M.: Arterial changes in pulmonary sarcoidosis. Arch. Pathol. 69:741, 1960.

174. Mills, P., Amara, I., McLaurin, L. P., and Graige, B.: Noninvasive assessment of pulmonary hypertension from right ventricular isovolumic contraction time. Am. J. Cardiol. 46:272, 1980.

175. Mlozoch, J.: Thrombocyte behavior in patients with 'primary pulmonary hypertension.' Pathogenesis of aminorex-induced pulmonary hypertension. Acta Med. Austriaca (Suppl. 1) 7, 1980.

176. Moffat, R. E., Sobonya, R. E., and Chang, C. H.: Childhood sarcoidosis with fatal cor pulmonale. Pediatr. Radiol. 7:180, 1978.

177. Molteni, A., Zakheim, R. M., Mullis, K. B., and Mattioli, L.: The effect of chronic alveolar hypoxia on lung and serum angiotensin I converting enzyme activity. Proc. Soc. Exp. Biol. Med. 147:263, 1974.

178. Morrison, D. B., Gaffney, F. A., Eigenbrodt, E. H., Reynolds, R. C., and Buja, L. M.: Severe pulmonary hypertension associated with macronodular (postnecrotic) cirrhosis and autoimmune phenomena. Am. J. Med. 69:513, 1980.

179. Moser, K. M., and Braunwald, N. S.: Successful surgical intervention in severe chronic thromboembolic pulmonary hypertension. Chest 64:29, 1973.

180. Moser, K. M., and Shea, J. G.: The relationship between pulmonary infarction cor pulmonale and the sickle states. Am. J. Med. 22:561, 1957.

181. Moses, D. C., Silver, T. M., and Bookstein, J. J.: The complementary roles of chest radiography, lung scanning and selective pulmonary angiography in the diagnosis of pulmonary embolism. Circulation 49:179, 1979.

182. Muroff, L. R., and Johnson: Right atrial myxoma presenting as non-resolving pulmonary emboli: Case report. J. Nucl. Med. 70:2996, 1970.

183. Murphy, J. D., Rabinovitch, M., Goldstein, J. D., and Reid, L.: The structural basis of persistent pulmonary hypertension of the newborn infant. J. Pediatr. 98:962, 1981.

184. Murphy, J. D., Rabinovitch, M., and Reid, L.: Pulmonary vascular pathology in fatal neonatal meconium aspiration. Pediatr. Res. 15:673, 1981.

185. Nadas, A. S., and Fyler, D. F.: Pediatric Cardiology. W. B. Saunders, Philadelphia, 1972, p. 684.

186. Naeye, R. L.: Pulmonary vascular lesions in systemic scleroderma. Dis. Chest 44:368, 1963.

187. Naeye, R. L.: Alveolar hypoventilation and cor pulmonale secondary to damage to the respiratory center. Am. J. Cardiol. 8:416, 1961.

188. Naeye, R. L.: Perinatal changes in the pulmonary vascular bed with stenosis and atresia of the pulmonic valve. Am. Heart J. 61:586, 1961.

189. Naeye, R. L.: Perinatal vascular changes associated with underdevelopment of the left heart. Am. J. Pathol. 41:287, 1962.

190. Naeye, R. L.: Pulmonary arterial bed in ventricular septal defect: A quantitative study of anatomic features in early childhood. Circulation 34:962, 1966.

191. Nagasaka, Y., Akutsu, H., Lee, Y. S., Fujimoto, S., and Chikamori, J.: Long-term favorable effect of oxygen administration on a patient with primary pulmonary hypertension. Chest 74:299, 1978.

192. Nair, S. S., Askari, A. D., Popelka, C. G., and Kleinerman, J. F.: Pulmonary hypertension and systemic lupus erythematosus. Arch. Intern. Med. 140:109, 1980.

193. Nayar, H. S., Mathur, R. M., and Ranade, V. V.: The role of serotonin (5-hydroxytryptamine) in the pulmonary arterial pressor response during acute hypoxia. Indian J. Med. Res. 60:1665, 1972.

194. Newfeld, E. A., Paul, M. H., Muster, A. J., and Idriss, F. S.: Pulmonary vascular disease in complete transposition of the great arteries: A study of 200 patients. Am. J. Cardiol. 34:75, 1974.

195. Newfeld, E. A., Wilson, A., Paul, M. H., and Reisch, J. S.: Pulmonary vascular disease in total anomalous pulmonary venous drainage. Circulation 61:103, 1980.

196. Newfeld, E. A., Sher, M., Paul, M. H., and Higashi, N.: Pulmonary vascular disease in complete atrioventricular canal defect. Am. J. Cardiol. 39:721, 1977.

197. Nihill, M. R., and McNamara, D. G.: Magnification pulmonary wedge angiography in the evaluation of children with congenital heart disease and pulmonary hypertension. Circulation 58:1094, 1978.

198. Noonan, J. A.: Reversible cor pulmonale due to hypertrophied tonsils and adenoids: Studies in two cases. Circulation 32:164 (Suppl. 11) 1965.

199. Noonan, J. A., and Ehmke, D. A.: Complications of ventriculovenous shunts for control of hydrocephalus. Report of three cases with thromboemboli to the lungs. N. Engl. J. Med. 269:70, 1963.

200. Norwood, W. I., Jr., Kirklin, J. K., and Sanders, S. P.: Hypoplastic left heart syndrome experience with palliative surgery. Am. J. Cardiol. 45:87, 1980.

201. Paparo, G. P., and Symchych, P. S.: Postintubation subglottic stenosis and cor pulmonale. J. Pediatr. 90:97, 1977.

202. Paul, M. H., Miller, R. A., and Potts, W. J.: Long-term results of aortic pulmonary anastomosis in tetralogy of Fallot: An analysis of the first 100 cases eleven to thirteen years after operation. Circulation. 23:525, 1961.

203. Peckham, G. J., and Fox, W. W.: Physiologic factors affecting pulmonary artery pressure in infants with persistent pulmonary hypertension. 93:1005, 1978.

204. Person, B., and Proctor, R. J.: Primary pulmonary hypertension. Responses to indomethacin, terbutaline and isoproterenol. Chest 76:601, 1979.

205. Pitts, J. A., Crosby, W. M., and Basta, L. L.: Eisenmenger's syndrome in pregnancy: Does heparin prophylaxis improve maternal mortality rate? Am. Heart J. 93:321, 1977.

206. Rabinovitch, M., Gamble, W., Nadas, A. S., Miettinen, O. S., and Reid, L.: Rat pulmonary circulation after chronic hypoxia: Hemodynamic and structural features. Am. J. Physiol. 236:H818, 1979.

207. Rabinovitch, M., DeLeon, V. H., Castaneda, A. R., and Reid, L.: The pulmonary vascular bed in patients with tetralogy of Fallot with and without pulmonary atresia. Circulation, in press, 1982.

208. Rabinovitch, M., Keane, J. F., Fellows, K. E., Castaneda, A. R., and Reid, L.: Quantitative analysis of the pulmonary wedge angiogram in congenital heart defects. Correlation with hemodynamic data and morphometric findings in lung biopsy tissue. Circulation 63:152, 1981.

209. Rabinovitch, M., Sanders, S. P., Castaneda, A. R., and Reid, L.: Morphometric analysis of lung biopsy tissue in candidates for Fontan-type surgical procedures (abstr.) Am. J. Cardiol. 47:947, 1981.

210. Rabinovitch, M., Castaneda, A. R., and Reid, L.: Lung biopsy with frozen section as a diagnostic aid in patients with congenital heart defects. Am. J. Cardiol. 47:77, 1981.

211. Rabinovitch, M., Konstam, M. A., Gamble, W. J., Papanicolaou, N., Treves, S., and Reid, L.: Changes in pulmonary blood flow influence the structural response of the rat lung to chronic hypoxia (abstr.). Am. Rev. Resp. Dis. 123:129, 1981.

212. Rabinovitch, M., Haworth, S. G., Castaneda, A. R., Nadas, A. S., and Reid, L.: Lung biopsy

in congenital heart disease: A morphometric approach to pulmonary vascular disease. Circulation 58:1107, 1978.

213. Rabinovitch, M., Fischer, K. C., and Treves, S.: Quantitative thallium-201 myocardial imaging in assessing right ventricular pressure in patients with congenital heart defects. Br. Heart J. 45:198, 1981.

214. Rabinovitch, M., Gamble, W. J., Williams, G. H., and Reid, L.: SQ 14,225 converting enzyme inhibitor diminishes pulmonary artery hypertension secondary to chronic hypoxia in rat (abstr.). Fed. Proc. 39:765, 1980.

215. Rabinovitch, M., Gamble, W. J., Miettinen, O. S., and Reid, L.: Age and sex influence on pulmonary hypertension on chronic hypoxia and on recovery. Am. J. Physiol. 240:H62, 1981.

216. Reid, J. M., Stevenson, J. G., Coleman, E. N., Barclay, R. S., Welsh, T. M., Fyfe, W. M., and Inal, J. A.: Moderate to severe pulmonary hypertension accompanying patent ductus arteriosus. Br. Heart J. 26:600, 1964.

217. Reid, L.: Bronchopulmonary dysplasia—Pathology. J. Pediatr. 95:836, 1979.

218. Rendas, A., Brown, E. R., Avery, M. E., and Reid, L. M.: Prematurity, hypoplasia of the pulmonary vascular bed and hypertension: Fatal outcome in a ten month old infant. Am. Rev. Resp. Dis. 121:873, 1980.

219. Rendas, A., Lennox, S., and Reid, L.: Aortopulmonary shunts in growing pigs. J. Thorac. Cardiovasc. Surg. 77:109, 1979.

220. Riemenschneider, T. A., Neilsen, H. C., Ruttenberg, H. D., and Jaffe, R. B.: Disturbances of the transitional circulation: Spectrum of pulmonary hypertension and myocardial dysfunction. Pediatrics 89:622, 1976.

221. Robertson, B.: Idiopathic pulmonary hypertension in infancy and childhood. Acta. Pathol. Microbiol. Scand. 79:217, 1971.

222. Robson, M. C., Stankiewicz, J. A., and Mendelsohn, J. S.: Cor pulmonale secondary to cleft palate repair. Plast. Reconstr. Surg. 59:754, 1977.

223. Rogge, J. D., Mishkin, M. E., and Genovese, P. D.: Familial occurrence of primary pulmonary hypertension. Ann. Intern. Med. 65:672, 1966.

224. Rosenberg, A. M., Petty, R. E., Cumming, G. R., and Koehler, B. E.: Pulmonary hypertension in a child with mixed connective tissue disorder. J. Rheumatol. 6:700, 1979.

225. Rosengart, R., Fishbein, M., and Emmanouilides, G. C.: Progressive pulmonary vascular disease after surgical correction (Mustard procedure) of transposition of the great arteries with intact ventricular septum. Am. J. Cardiol. 35:107, 1975.

226. Rosenthal, A., Vawter, G., and Wagenvoort, C. A.: Intrapulmonary venoocclusive disease. Am. J. Cardiol. 31:78, 1973.

227. Rosenthal, A., Nathan, D. G., Marty, A. T., Button, L. N., Miettinen, O. S., and Nadas, A. S.: Acute hemodynamic effects of red cell volume reduction in polycythemia of cyanotic congenital heart disease. Circulation 42:297, 1970.

228. Rounds, S., and McMurtry, I. F.: Inhibitors of oxidative ATP production cause transient vasoconstriction and block subsequent pressor responses in rat lungs. Circ. Res. 48:393, 1981.

229. Roy, S. B., Bhatia, M. L., Lazaro, E. J., and Ramalingaswami, V.: Juvenile mitral stenosis in India. Lancet 2:1193, 1963.

230. Rubin, L. J., and Peter, R. H.: Oral hydralazine therapy for primary pulmonary hypertension. N. Engl. J. Med. 302:69, 1980.

231. Rudolph, A. M., Neuhauser, E. B. D., Golinko, R. J., and Auld, P. A. N.: Effects of pneumonectomy on pulmonary circulation in adult and young animals. Circ. Res. 9:856, 1961.

232. Rudolph, A. M., and Nadas, A. S.: The pulmonary circulation and congenital heart disease. Considerations of the role of the pulmonary circulation in certain systemic-pulmonary communications. N. Engl. J. Med. 267:96 and 1022, 1962.

233. Ruskin, J. N., and Hutter, A. M., Jr.: Primary pulmonary hypertension treated with oral phentolamine. Ann. Intern. Med. 90:772, 1979.

234. Ryland, D., and Reid, L.: The pulmonary circulation in cystic fibrosis. Thorax 30:285, 1975.

235. Sack, K. E., Bekheit, S., Fadem, S. Z., and Bedrossian, C. W. M.: Severe pulmonary vascular disease in systemic lupus erythematosus. South. Med. J. 72:1016, 1979.

236. Sandison, J. C.: Observations in the growth of blood vessels as seen in the transparent chamber introduced into the rabbit's ear. Am. J. Anat. 41:475, 1928.

237. Santini, D., Fox, D., Kloner, R. A., Konstamm, M., Rude, R. E., and Lorell, B. H.: Pulmonary hypertension in systemic lupus erythematosus: Hemodynamics and effects of vasodilator therapy. Clin. Cardiol. 3:406, 1980.

238. Scoggin, C. H., Hyers, T. M., Reeves, J. T., and Grover, R. F.: High altitude pulmonary edema in children and young adults of Leadville, Colorado. N. Engl. J. Med. 297:1269, 1977.

239. Shannon, D. C., Kelly, D. H., and O'Connell, K.: Abnormal regulation of ventilation in sudden infant death syndrome. N. Engl. J. Med. 297:747, 1977.

240. Shettigar, U. R., Hultgren, H. N., Specter, M., Martin, R., and Davies, D. M.: Primary pulmonary hypertension. Favorable effect of isoproterenol. N. Engl. J. Med. 295:1414, 1976.

241. Short, D. S.: The application of arteriography to the pathological study of pulmonary hypertension. In Pulmonary Circulation, edited by W. R. Adams and I. Veith. Grune & Stratton, New York, 1959, pp. 233–242.

242. Siassi, B., Moss, A. J., and Dooley, R. R.: Clinical recognition of cor pulmonale in cystic fibrosis. J. Pediatr. 78:794, 1971.

243. Silove, E. D., Tavernor, W. D., and Berry, C. L.: Reactive pulmonary arterial hypertension after pulmonary venous constriction in the calf. Cardiovasc. Res. 6:36, 1972.

244. Silverman, N. H., Snider, A. R., and Rudolph, A. M.: Evaluation of pulmonary hypertension by M-mode echocardiography in children with ventricular septal defect. Circulation 61:1125, 1980.

245. Simonneau, G., Escourrou, P., Duroux, P., and Lockhart, A.: Inhibition of hypoxic pulmonary vasoconstriction by nifedipine. N. Engl. J. Med. 304:1582, 1981.

246. Snider, G. L., Ferris, E., Gaensler, E. A., Messer, J. V., Hayes, J. A., Gersten, M. M., and Coutu, R. E.: Primary pulmonary hypertension: A fatality during pulmonary angiography. Chest 64:628, 1973.

247. Sole, M. J., Drobac, M., Schwartz, L., Hussain, M. N., and Vaughan-Neil, E. F.: The extraction of circulating catecholamines by the lungs in normal man and in patients with pulmonary hypertension. Circulation 60:160, 1979.

248. Solov'eva, A. P.: Lesions of the respiratory system in dermatomyositis. Ter. Arkh. 51:88, 1979.

249. Sostman, H. D., Matthay, R. A., and Putnam, C. E.: Cytotoxic drug-induced disease. Am. J. Med. 62:608, 1977.

250. Spooner, E. W., Perry, B. L., Stern, A. M., and Sigmann, J. M.: Estimation of pulmonary/systemic resistance ratios from echocardiographic systolic time intervals in young patients with congenital or acquired heart disease. Am. J. Cardiol. 42:810, 1978.

251. Stalcup, S. A., Lipset, J. S., Woan, J. M.,

Leuenberger, P. J., and Mellins, R. B.: Inhibition of angiotensin converting enzyme activity in cultured endothelial cells by hypoxia. J. Clin. Invest. 63:966, 1979.

252. Stanley, N. N., Williams, A. J., and Dewar, C. A.: Hypoxia and hydrothoraces in a case of liver cirrhosis: Correlation of physiological, scintographic and pathological findings. Thorax 32:457, 1977.

253. Stark, J., DeLeval, M. R., and Taylor, J. F. N.: Mustard operation and creation of ventricular septal defect in two patients with transposition of the great arteries, intact ventricular septum, and pulmonary vascular disease. Am. J. Cardiol. 38:524, 1976.

254. Stark, J., DeLeval, M. R., Waterston, D. J., Grahm, G. R., and Bonham-Carter, R. E.: Corrective surgery of transposition of the great arteries in the first year of life. Results in 63 infants. J. Thorac. Cardiovasc. Surg. 67:673, 1974.

255. Starling, M. B., Neutze, J. M., and Elliott, R. L.: Control of elevated pulmonary vascular resistance in neonatal swine with prostacyclin (PG$_{12}$). Prostaglandins Med. 3:103, 1979.

256. Stern, R. C., Borkat, G., Hirschfeld, S. S., Boat, T. F., Matthews, L. W., Liebman, J., and Doershuk, C. F.: Heart failure in cystic fibrosis. Treatment and prognosis of cor pulmonale with failure of the right side of the heart. Am. J. Dis. Child. 134:267, 1980.

257. Stevenson, G., Kawabori, I., and Guntheroth, W. G.: Noninvasive detection of pulmonary hypertension in patent ductus arteriosus by pulsed Doppler echocardiography. Circulation 60:355, 1979.

258. Stocker, F. P., Wilkoss, W., Miettinen, O. S., and Nadas, A. S.: Oxygen consumption in infants with heart disease. J. Pediatr. 80:43, 1972.

259. Suckerman, S., and Healy, G. B.: Sleep apnea syndrome associated with upper airway obstruction. Laryngoscope 89:878, 1979.

260. Swischuk, L. E., Richardson, C. J., Nichols, M. M., and Ingman, M. J.: Primary pulmonary hypoplasia in the neonate. J. Pediatr. 95:573, 1979.

261. Sylvester, J. T., and McGowan, C.: The effects of agents that bind to cytochrome P-450 on hypoxic pulmonary vasoconstriction. Circ. Res. 43:429, 1978.

262. Szczerlik, J., Dubiel, J. S., Mysik, M., Pyzik, Z., Krol, R., and Horzela, T.: Effects of prostaglandin E$_1$ on pulmonary circulation in patients with pulmonary hypertension. Br. Heart J. 40:1397, 1978.

263. Takiainen, P., Taskinen, E., Vuopio, P., Kekomaki, R., and Wager, O.: Autoimmune haemolytic anaemia and pulmonary vasculitis associated with circulating immune complexes. J. Clin. Lab. Immunol. 3:139, 1980.

264. Talner, N. S., Lin, H. Y., Oberman, H. A., and Schmidt, R. W.: Thromboembolism complicating Holter valve shunt. A clinico-pathologic study of two patients treated with this procedure for hydrocephalus. Am. J. Dis. Child. 101:602, 1961.

265. Tarnow, J., and Hess, W.: Pulmonary hypertension and pulmonary edema caused by intravenous ketamine. Anesthetist 27:486, 1978.

266. Thiene, G., Frescura, C., Bini, R. M., Valente, M., and Gallucci, V.: Histology of pulmonary arterial supply in pulmonary atresia with ventricular septal defect. Circulation 60:1066, 1979.

267. Thilenius, O. G., Nadas, A. S., and Jocklin, H.: Primary pulmonary vascular obstruction in children. Pediatrics 36:75, 1965.

268. Tubbs, R. R., Levin, R. D., Shirey, E. K., and Hoffman, G. C.: Fibrinolysis in familial pulmonary hypertension. Am. J. Clin. Pathol. 71:384, 1979.

269. Tucker, A., McMurtry, I. F., Reeves, J. T., Alexander, A. F., Will, D. H., and Grover, R. F.: Lung vascular smooth muscle as a deter-

minant of pulmonary hypertension at high altitude. Am. J. Physiol. 228:762, 1975.

270. Tucker, A., McMurtry, I. F., Alexander, A. F., Reeves, J. T., and Grover, R. F.: Lung mast cell density and distribution in chronically hypoxic animals. J. Appl. Physiol. 42:174, 1977.

271. Tucker, A., Weir, E. K., Reeves, J. T., and Grover, R. C.: Histamine H_1 and H_2 receptors in pulmonary and systemic vasculature of the dog. Am. J. Physiol. 229:1008, 1975.

272. Viles, P. M., Ongley, P. A., and Titus, J. L.: The spectrum of pulmonary vascular disease in transposition of the great arteries. Circulation 40:31, 1969.

273. Vogel, J. H. K., Hartley, H. L., Jamieson, G., and Grover, R. F.: Impairment of ventilatory response to hypoxia in individuals with obesity and hypoventilation: A concept of the Pickwickian syndrome. Circulation 36 (II):258, 1967.

274. Vogel, J. H. K., Pryor, R., and Blount, S. G., Jr.: The cardiovascular system in children from high altitude. J. Pediatr. 64:315, 1964.

275. Vogel, J. H. K., McNamara, D. C., and Blount, S. G., Jr.: Role of hypoxia in determining pulmonary vascular resistance in infants with ventricular septal defect. Am. J. Cardiol. 20:346, 1967.

276. Vogel, J. H. K., Grover, R. F., Jamieson, G., and Blount, S. G., Jr.: Longterm physiologic observation in patients with ventricular septal defect and increased pulmonary vascular resistance. Adv. Cardiol. 11:108, 1974.

277. Wagenvoort, C. A., Neufeld, H. N., and Edwards, J. E.: Percentage arterial wall thickness. Lab. Invest. 10:751, 1961.

278. Wagenvoort, C. A., and Wagenvoort, N.: Smooth muscle content of pulmonary arterial media in pulmonary venous hypertension as compared to other forms of pulmonary hypertension. Chest, in Press, 1982.

279. Wagenvoort, C. A.: Morphologic changes in the pulmonary veins. Hum. Pathol. 1:205, 1970.

280. Wagenvoort, C. A., and Edwards, J. E.: The pulmonary arterial tree in pulmonic atresia. Arch. Pathol. 71:646, 1961.

281. Wagenvoort, C. A., and Edwards, J. E.: The pulmonary arterial tree in aortic atresia with intact ventricular septum. Lab. Invest. 10:924, 1961.

282. Wagenvoort, C. A.: Vasoconstriction and medial hypertrophy in pulmonary hypertension. J. Pathol. Bacteriol. 78:503, 1960.

283. Wagenvoort, C. A., Losekoot, G., and Mulder, E.: Pulmonary veno-occlusive disease of presumably intrauterine origin. Thorax 26:429, 1971.

284. Wagenvoort, C. A.: Lung biopsy specimens in the evaluation of pulmonary vascular disease. Chest 77:614, 1980.

285. Wagenvoort, C. A., and Wagenvoort, N.: Primary pulmonary hypertension. Circulation 42:1163, 1970.

286. Waldman, J. D., Paul, M. H., Newfeld, E. A., Muster, A. J., and Idriss, F. S.: Transposition of the great arteries with intact ventricular septum and patent ductus arteriosus. Am. J. Cardiol. 39:232, 1977.

287. Walker, W. C., and Wright, V.: Pulmonary lesions and rheumatoid arthritis. Medicine 47:501, 1968.

288. Wang, S. W. S., Pohl, J. E. F., Rowlands, D. J., and Wade, E. G.: Diazoxide in treatment of primary pulmonary hypertension. Br. Heart J. 40:572, 1978.

289. Ward, C., and Hancock, B. W.: Extreme pulmonary hypertension caused by mitral valve disease. Natural history and results of surgery. Br. Heart J. 37:74, 1975.

290. Watkins, W. D., Peterson, M. B., Crone, R. K., Shannon, D. C., and Levine, L.: Prostacyclin and prostaglandin E1 for severe idiopathic pulmonary artery hypertension (letter). Lancet 1:1083, 1980.

291. Weidman, W. H., DuShane, J. W., and Kincaid, O. W.: Observations concerning progressive pulmonary vascular obstruction in children with ventricular septal defects. Am.

Heart J. 65:148, 1963.

292. Whight, C. M., Barratt-Boyes, B. G., Calder, A. L., Neutze, J. M., and Brandt, P. W. T.: Total anomalous pulmonary venous connection: Long term results following repair in infancy. J. Thorac. Cardiovasc. Surg. 75:52, 1978.

293. Widimsky, J., Urbanova, D., Resl, J., Ostadal, B., Peluch, V., and Prochazka, J.: Effect of intermittent altitude hypoxia on the myocardium and lesser circulation in the rat. Cardiovasc. Res. 7:798, 1973.

294. Williams, A., Vawter, G., and Reid, L.: Increased muscularity of the pulmonary circulation in victims of sudden infant death syndrome. Pediatrics 63:18, 1979.

295. Williams, A.: Personal communication.

296. Williams, A., Trewby, P., Williams, R., and Reid, L.: Structural alterations to the pulmonary circulation in fulminant hepatic failure. Thorax 34:447, 1975.

297. Williams, R. G., and Tucker, C. R.: Pulmonary artery hypertension. In Echocardiographic Diagnosis of Congenital Heart Disease, Chap. 20. Little, Brown and Company, Boston, 1977, p. 165.

298. Wolman, M.: Hypertrophy of the branches of the pulmonary artery and its possible relationship with the so-called primary pulmonary arteriosclerosis in 2 infants with hypertrophy of the right heart. Am. J. Med. Sci. 220:133, 1950.

299. Wood, P.: The Eisenmenger syndrome of pulmonary hypertension with reversed central shunt. Br. Med. J. 2:701, 755, 1958.

300. Zakheim, R. M., Mattioli, L., Molteni, A., Mullis, K. B., and Bartley, J.: Prevention of pulmonary vascular changes of chronic alveolar hypoxia by inhibition of angiotensin I converting enzyme in the rat. Lab. Invest. 33:57, 1975.

301. Zakheim, R. M., Molteni, A., Mattioli, L., and Park, H.: Plasma angiotensin II levels in hypoxic and hypovolemic stress in unanesthetized rabbits. J. Appl. Physiol. 41:462, 1976.

43

Systemic Hypertension

Jennifer M. H. Loggie, M.D.

Atherosclerosis and one of its major risk factors, primary hypertension, are recognized as serious public health problems throughout the western world. In the past two decades, attention has begun to focus on the likelihood that both have their origins in childhood and that both genetic and environmental factors contribute to their development.

Zinner et al.[132] showed that the familial aggregation of blood pressure, known to exist by adult life, was already present in childhood. This finding has since been confirmed and extended, and it appears that correlations may already exist between the blood pressures of newborn infants and their mothers, although the data are inconsistent.[15, 47, 69] In 1971, Londe et al.[79] published their observation that in apparently normal children, with blood pressure levels persistently at or just outside the normal blood pressure distribution curve for age, no identifiable cause for "hypertension" had been found in over 90% of patients. The concept that adult levels of blood pressure should not be used to define hypertension in children of various ages had not previously been addressed by pediatricians. Furthermore, the concept

that primary or essential hypertension was common in the young was not widely held and was not borne out by data from referral centers where predominantly secondary forms of hypertension were identified. The differences in the populations studied likely contributed to the discrepancy. The subjects reported by Londe et al.[79] were asymptomatic youngsters being found on routine office examination to have top normal or minimal elevations in blood pressure. The children seen in referral centers were usually moderately or severely hypertensive by any standards and were sometimes symptomatic. With the referral of more asymptomatic children and adolescents to our clinic, by the mid 1970s, we too were finding that the majority of the teenagers had no underlying cause for their elevated blood pressure. Like Londe et al.[79] and Levine et al.,[70] we found that a large number of these youngsters were overweight (63%), and many (70%) had first degree relatives with hypertension, although the family history was not complete for all patients.

Through the decade of the seventies, in Muscatine, Iowa, and Bogalusa, Louisiana, large scale epidemiologic studies of coronary artery risk factors in children were initiated and are continuing. Among other things, blood pressure distribution curves have been developed from cross-sectional data for children of various ages.[93, 121] Furthermore, it has become apparent from longitudinal data generated in these populations and others[12, 133] that in the young, tracking of blood pressure occurs over time. The correlation between blood pressure measurements made at two points in time for children is, however, not as strong as for adults.

Progress is, thus, finally being made toward understanding the etiology and pathogenesis of hypertensive and atherosclerotic cardiovascular disease by studying the young. If it is true that environmental factors interact with genetic predispositions to produce these disorders that have reached epidemic proportions in our society, it may be possible to develop strategies to eliminate or ameliorate the former.

REGULATION OF BLOOD PRESSURE

Blood pressure is a function of cardiac output and total peripheral resistance; for it to rise, output, resistance, or both must increase. Lund-Johansen[84] has reported that initially, in early essential hypertension, cardiac output is increased while peripheral resistance is normal. The level of resistance is, however, probably abnormally high for the increased level of cardiac output. Later in established essential hypertension, the same investigator found that cardiac output returned to normal and peripheral resistance rose. Dustan and Tarazi[20] in other hemodynamic studies of young individuals with hypertension have not found the same consistency in the relationships between cardiac output, peripheral resistance, and duration of hypertension. This area is being further studied by several workers.

The basis for an initial increase in cardiac output when it occurs early in the course of some forms of human and animal hypertension is not clearly understood. It has been attributed to venoconstriction and/or an expansion of extracellular fluid volume. Increased vascular resistance probably relates in part to the viscosity of blood as well as resulting from both structural and functional changes in arteriolar smooth muscle. These changes are thought to be due to an interaction of wall stress, neurohumoral influences, and genetic factors.

The kidney in its regulatory capacity of salt and water excretion probably plays a major role in the development and maintenance of most forms of hypertension. Renin secretion by the kidney is regulated by a variety of factors, including circulating catecholamines and increased activity of the noradrenergic renal sympathetic nerves. Renin release results in activation of the angiotensin-aldosterone system. The angiotensin II that is derived from conversion of angiotensin I in the lungs produces vasoconstriction via its effect on vascular smooth muscle. It also regulates the secretion of aldosterone. In addition, angiotensin II acts centrally to increase sympathetic discharge, vasopressin secretion, and water intake. It also potentiates the release of norepinephrine at vasoconstrictor nerve endings and appears to interact with both the prostaglandin and kallikrein systems. Although the role of the prostaglandins in blood pressure control has not yet been elucidated, they apparently affect regulation of the renin-angiotensin system, renal sodium and water excretion, and tone of vascular smooth muscle. Likewise, the role of the kinin peptides in blood pressure regulation is not yet clear but may be important. They are released by kallikreins from kininogen substrate and are highly effective vasodilators.

It has already been intimated that via angiotensin II, for example, the brain is involved in the control of arterial pressure. In some forms of hypertension, the central nervous system may, in fact, play a critical role through regulating the amount and pattern of autonomic discharge, and by controlling the release of various hormones that affect blood volume. The central nervous system and the peripheral autonomic nervous system are integrated into a functional unit with afferent and efferent pathways. The afferent pathways and sensory receptors that may be involved in hypertension in some way include arterial and cardiopulmonary baroreceptors and receptors in skeletal muscle, skin, and viscera.

As many have pointed out, the control of blood pressure is extremely complex, and hypertension is probably multifactorial in origin.

METHODS OF BLOOD PRESSURE MEASUREMENT

Auscultation

In practice, blood pressure is most frequently measured indirectly using an auscultatory technique. It is usually recommended that, as a rule of thumb, the bladder inside the cuff should be wide enough to cover two-thirds of the upper arm without the lower edge impinging on the antecubital space. It is also recommended that the bladder should be long enough to encircle the arm, in order to evenly occlude the tissues overlying the brachial artery, but should not overlap on itself. This second recommendation is not, however, based on firm data. Voors[123] has shown that cuff bladders that encircle 90% of the entire arm circumference (with a fixed bladder width) eliminate the effect of arm circumference. Unfortunately, he did not study the interaction of cuff bladder width with bladder length. However, in their survey, Prineas et al.[104] used cuff bladders that encircled at least 90% of the upper arm and, in 88% of subjects, the length of the cuff bladder was ≥120% of the inner length of the upper arm. More than 70% of their measurements had to be made with a specially designed cuff bladder measuring 9 × 30 cm, and this has led them to recommend that longer cuff bladders, with more variable cuff widths, should be commercially available for measuring blood pressure in children.

In pediatric practice the three groups of children in whom cuff size may be difficult to decide on with confidence include young infants, obese or large teenagers, and youngsters with thin but long arms. These last are usually in the 6- to 7-year age group or are youngsters with malnutrition, such as individuals with cystic fibrosis or anorexia nervosa. The 2.5-cm wide cuff, available for newborn babies, is probably only adequate for some premature infants. For obese children and adolescents, the 14 × 40 cm large adult cuff is widely used, but the validity of readings made with it probably needs verification. Similarly, cuff size in those individuals with long, very thin arms bears further evaluation.

Indirect measurement of blood pressure is at best imprecise, and a number of factors, other than cuff size, may affect the accuracy of the readings obtained. Cuffs with aneroid manometers, although conveniently portable, need regular calibration against mercury manometers, since the aneroid is subject to hysteresis. The mercury manometer itself, though accurate, has to be periodically inspected in order to ensure that the column is intact and that there has not been oxidation of mercury.[92]

Observer error may be minimized by having the subject of the blood pressure measurement in a quiet room. If a mercury manometer is to be used, the meniscus should be at the level of the eye, and the cuff should be deflated smoothly at about 2 to 5 mm Hg/second. Clearly anyone with a hearing deficit may have a problem in correctly noting the Korotkoff sounds and may need to use an amplifying stethoscope.

Presently, it is recommended that, in children, the fourth

Korotkoff phase should be regarded as the diastolic blood pressure, although the disappearance of sounds should also be recorded. In adults, the fifth Korotkoff phase is still considered more representative of diastolic blood pressure. It is useful in recording blood pressure if the limb and cuff size used, patient position and disposition, are all recorded. In crying or agitated children or those with, for example, decerebrate posturing, any single blood pressure reading may be elevated beyond the patient's normal average pressure. Likewise, a bladder distended with urine is said to increase blood pressure.[92]

Of some interest are the findings that blood pressure in children varies with time of day and with room temperature.[104] In one study, blood pressure has been found to be lower in normal children in the morning than in the afternoon. Clinically, we have also found this to be true in hypertensive children. It has also been reported that systolic blood pressure is inversely related to room temperature, decreasing with increasing temperature, while the fourth Korotkoff phase diastolic blood pressure increases with room temperature.

Prineas et al.[104] have commented that despite the use of protocols carefully designed to eliminate most sources of methodologic observation bias, the effects of season, temperature, and individual observers remain statistically significant determinants of blood pressure that are independent of many other factors. They have concluded that the magnitude of these effects is large enough to have both clinical and epidemiological consequences. Since data relevant to all of these points are rarely reported, the selection of appropriate normal blood pressure standards is made difficult for practitioners. In general, the best that one can do is to select a set of standards and try to adhere, as closely as possible, to the methodology used by the investigators who established them. Clearly, standards obtained in seated children may not be appropriate for evaluating readings obtained in supine youngsters. In this regard, Londe and Gollub[81] recommend measuring blood pressure in the supine position so that the arm is at heart level. This is based on the observation that artifactually high blood pressure readings may be obtained if the arm is dependent when the blood pressure is measured in the seated position.[81]

Ultrasound

In infants and small children it is often difficult to accurately auscultate blood pressure. In this age group it has become widespread hospital practice to measure blood pressure with machines that use ultrasound. The indirect measurement of systolic blood pressure utilizing the Doppler principle was first described in 1968,[127] and has since been evaluated and found reliable in the young.[10, 21, 38] Accurate diastolic blood pressures are not as easily achieved with this method of measurement.

The Doppler technique is based on the principle that when ultrasound waves are directed towards an immobile structure, such as an occluded artery, they are reflected back without any change in frequency. However, when ultrasound waves are directed toward a moving structure, such as a pulsating artery, the frequency of the reflected waves is altered (Doppler effect). The alteration in frequency and, therefore, the pitch of the audible sounds varies with the velocity of blood flow. The altered frequency of reflected sounds can be amplified to produce an audible and/or visual signal.

A cuff, to which a transducer is attached, is positioned with the transducer overlying the brachial artery. As when blood pressure is to be auscultated, the cuff is then inflated to occlude the artery. Until the artery reopens with deflation of cuff pressure, ultrasound waves are reflected back with no change in frequency. With the onset of arterial pulsation and

blood flow, there is a change in the frequency of the reflected waves that is audible. The onset of high frequency signals is read as the systolic blood pressure, and these signals continue until the pressure in the cuff is lower than that in the artery. Thereafter, the artery remains open throughout systole and diastole, and the ultrasonic signal becomes muffled. The muffling of sound is taken to represent diastolic blood pressure but is not always a clear endpoint.

Blood pressure varies in babies, depending on their degree of alertness, and tends to be higher when they are fully awake. In addition, sucking may further elevate the blood pressure. Careful attention must be paid to placing the transducer over the brachial artery, and also in selecting appropriate cuff for limb size.[16] In practice this is not always done. Also, other variables are introduced in the clinical setting (such as measuring popliteal pressure) that may affect the validity or interpretation of the readings obtained.

At present, the cost of blood pressure equipment that uses the Doppler principle precludes its use outside the hospital setting.

Flush Method

This method of measuring blood pressure in infants was introduced in 1952[13, 43] but has been less frequently practiced in the past decade. It is still a useful method for determining mean arterial pressure but is cumbersome and, for best results, requires two observers. Unfortunately, as with all other forms of blood pressure measurement, inaccurate technique results in errors in measurement. In addition, severe anemia, peripheral edema, or the presence of marked hypothermia, all affect the end point. Unlike other methods, however, cuff size within the range of 5 to 9.5 cm does not affect the readings.[91]

A cuff is applied to either the wrist or ankle, with the infant in a recumbent position. The limb used for the measurement is then elevated, and the extremity, distal to the cuff, is compressed by firmly wrapping it with an elastic bandage or soft rubber drain. These maneuvers are intended to drain the hand or foot of blood and cannot be adequately substituted for by simple compression with the observer's hand. This results in incomplete drainage.

When the extremity has been wrapped to the lower edge of the cuff, this is inflated to 200 mm Hg, and the limb is placed horizontally. With a deflation rate of 5 mm Hg/second, a point is reached at which flushing of the blanched distal portion of the extremity occurs. This point approximates mean arterial pressure.

If coarctation of the aorta is suspected, simultaneous measurements can be made in an arm and leg by three observers. Since one is trying to evaluate for the presence of a gradient, it is unnecessary for the baby to be quiet during the measurement.

Palpation

This method is still sometimes used for estimating systolic blood pressure, particularly in young children. The radial pulse is located, the blood pressure cuff is inflated to about 200 mm Hg and then deflated, with the observer's fingers remaining over the artery. The first palpable beat is recorded as systolic blood pressure but is probably actually 5 to 10 mm Hg lower than that which one would record by auscultation.

Oscillometry

Visual oscillometry was introduced at the turn of the century but has had little application in clinical medicine until recently.[131] The oscillations produced by the arterial pulse are transmitted to a mercury column. As cuff pressure is lowered, the points at which oscillations appear and disappear are recorded as systolic and diastolic blood pressure. The point at which maximal oscillation occurs represents mean arterial pressure (MAP). An instrument that automatically determines MAP using this technique is now commercially available. It has been used both in humans[59] and in animals.[89]

BLOOD PRESSURE AT VARIOUS AGES

Blood pressure distribution curves have been developed by measuring blood pressure levels in a variety of populations of children and adolescents in the United States[26, 44, 93] and elsewhere.[3] Those published in the Report of the Task Force on Blood Pressure Control in Children[93] have been the most publicized. For teenagers from early adolescence on, they show ninety-fifth percentiles for both systolic and diastolic blood pressure that tend to be higher than those reported by others[26, 44] and that also exceed the ordinarily accepted cutoff point (140/90 mm Hg) used to define hypertension in younger adults. Differences in the data obtained from various surveys may be due to sample size, methodological differences that introduce bias, or actual differences in the populations surveyed.[27, 28]

Blood pressure has not been measured in large numbers of infants and children under the age of 4 years using various methods. Some data are, however, available[16, 21]; the more recent studies have been performed utilizing the Doppler technique. Under the conditions of a research study, this method gives reproducible results, but in practice, where less care may be taken in obtaining readings, caution is needed in interpreting them.

Confounding the study of blood pressure in the young are the variables of growth and maturation. Voors et al.[124] reported on height and body mass as determinants of blood pressure in children. They and others[110, 114] have recommended that blood pressure should be related to height or body mass rather than age. Katz et al.[57] have also proposed that variations in growth and maturity within age groups in childhood and adolescence have a significant effect on both systolic and diastolic blood pressure. They suggest, based on their data (that include skeletal age), that standards that take these factors into account should be developed and used clinically. Their hypothesis is that if the blood pressure increase that is seen during adolescence is largely associated with an increase in body size, then those teenagers who mature earlier will attain their adult blood pressure level at an earlier age than those who mature later. Two children or teenagers may not, therefore, be comparable at a given blood pressure level, at a given age, since growth and maturation have not been put into the equation. A less mature small individual whose blood pressure is in the higher "normal" ranges for age may be more at risk for developing clearly elevated blood pressure after he has gone through a growth spurt that rapidly increases his body mass, than a more mature, larger individual of the same age who has the same level of blood pressure but who has already gone through his growth spurt.

DEFINITION OF HYPERTENSION

Considering the infancy of the area under study, it is hardly surprising that what constitutes early hypertension in the young remains debated. Uniformity in defining degrees of hypertension in childhood and adolescence is also lacking.[78] It follows that the prevalence of both fixed and borderline hypertension in teenagers and children is uncertain, since definitions and methodology vary from survey to survey.[76]

The Task Force on Blood Pressure Control in Children[93] has recommended that if a youngster is found to have a seated systolic or diastolic blood pressure at or above the 95th percentile for age on three or more occasions, he should be considered hypertensive. Others[58] believe that blood pressure trends over time, the presence of symptoms and the hemodynamic characteristics, better define the hypertensive state than blood pressure readings alone. This allows the concept that individuals who initially have blood pressure readings in the lower strata of the normal blood pressure distribution curve and who later have blood pressure levels persistently in the upper strata may, in fact, have hypertension, albeit their levels remain within the "normal blood pressure distribution for age." Our long-term clinical experience suggests that three blood pressure readings are insufficient for diagnosing hypertension when only top normal/borderline values are initially found. Multiple readings over several months are more helpful in defining trends in such individuals.

Adams and Landaw[1] have recently questioned "What are healthy blood pressures for children?" They contend that the aging process *need not* be associated with increasing blood pressure as we have been led to believe. As evidence, they cite the well known fact that many adults in the U.S. have the same blood pressure they had as infants—100/60 mm Hg. They also point out that in many primitive societies, the blood pressure does not increase with age.

Adams and Landaw[1] are also particularly critical of the widespread use by clinicians of the National Heart, Lung and Blood Institute's published percentile graphs of blood pressure against age.[93] These graphs show a continual rise of blood pressure with age beginning at 6 years. They[1] argue that data which are essentially a description of an *unhealthy* population should not be used to set norms for health. They also suggest that cross-sectional screening studies should not be used to construct blood pressure distribution curves that are later used for longitudinal follow-up of individual children.*

The question of standards is made more difficult if it is, indeed, better to evaluate blood pressure in terms of height, body mass, or maturation. A consensus will be reached eventually, perhaps on this issue. To reiterate, if one takes care of children and adolescents, it is presently common practice to select one of the available sets of standards and to adhere to the methodology that was used to establish the curves. In clinical practice, we prefer to obtain blood pressure measurements from patients both supine and after a few minutes of being seated, since many of our youngsters with borderline blood pressures have higher diastolic blood pressure readings in the latter position.

One of the difficulties in managing children and adolescents who are found to have blood pressures at the top of the normal distribution curve for age is that their outcome is presently not known. Several studies of pediatric populations have demonstrated significant correlations between blood pressure measurements made at two points in time, but more longitudinal data are necessary in order to firmly establish that tracking continues into adult life. Certainly, in individual children and adolescents, blood pressure variability from visit to visit makes predictability of outcome difficult. One fact seems fairly certain from several studies[65, 114, 128] and that is that weight or other measures of ponderosity are positively correlated with blood pressure in both adolescence and early life. Moreover, the increase in blood pressure over time has been shown to be related to the actual weight gained.

CAUSES OF HYPERTENSION

Most of the known causes of persistent hypertension and of acute transient hypertension in children and adolescents

_____

* Their "healthy" standards are: systolic, 108 ± 9 mm Hg and diastolic, 70 ± 8 mm Hg.

TABLE 43.1   CONDITIONS ASSOCIATED WITH TRANSIENT OR INTERMITTENT HYPERTENSION

Renal
 Acute glomerulonephritis
 Anaphylactoid purpura
 Hemolytic-uremic syndrome
 Transfusion to patients with renal disease
 Acute ureteric occlusion
Drugs—Toxins
 Therapy with corticosteroids
 Reserpine overdose
 Amphetamine overdose
 Birth control pills
 Mercury poisoning
 Topical sympathomimetic agents
Miscellaneous
 Licorice ingestion (candy or chewing tobacco)
 Burns
 Intra- and postoperative

Neurogenic
 Increased intracranial pressure
 Central dysautonomia (e.g., after brain trauma or surgery)
 Limb or cervical traction
 Familial dysautonomia
 Guillain-Barré syndrome
 Other cord lesions
Metabolic/endocrine
 Hypercalcemia
 Hypernatremia
 Congenital adrenal hyperplasia
 Prolonged bedrest/immobilization
 Acute intermittent porphyria

TABLE 43.2   CAUSES OF SECONDARY CHRONIC HYPERTENSION

Renal
 Chronic glomerulonephritis (any form)
 Congenital defects (hypoplasia, polycystic kidneys)
 Pyelonephritis
 Bilateral or unilateral hydronephrosis
 After renal transplantation (rejection, original disease, arterial stenosis)
 Renal infarction
 Perirenal hematoma
 Tumors (Wilm's, hemangiopericytoma)
Vascular
 Coarctation of the aorta
 Hypoplasia of the aorta
 Diffuse arteritis
 Renal artery disease (stenosis, fistula, thrombosis, aneurysm, compression)
 Renal vein thrombosis

Endocrine
 Pheochromocytoma
 Neuroblastoma
 Cushing's syndrome
 Hydroxylase deficiencies
 Primary aldosteronism (hyperplasia or adenoma)
 Dexamethasone—suppressible aldosteronism
 Adrenal carcinoma
 Ovarian tumors
 Hyperparathyroidism
Metabolic
 Diabetes mellitus with renal disease
 Gouty nephropathy
 Tyrosinosis

are listed in Tables 43.1 and 43.2. Although a large variety of forms of hypertension exist, little has been done to study the mechanisms involved in their causation. In fact, not a great deal is presently known about the development of the systems involved in blood pressure control, such as the renin-angiotensin-aldosterone system and the autonomic nervous system.[122] It is known that plasma renin activity (PRA) and concentration, as well as renin substrate, are higher in newborn infants than in adults and that they gradually decrease during childhood,[50, 62, 111, 117] There are, however, no longitudinal studies describing the development of the renin-angiotensin system nor of other systems that interact with it. Plasma aldosterone is also elevated in the newborn infant and correlates with PRA but not with blood pressure, gestational age, birth weight, or sex.[8, 17, 113] The

postnatal changes that occur in plasma aldosterone are controversial, and there are few studies of aldosterone secretion or excretion in infants.[11, 87, 129]

The documented lability of pulse rate, temperature, and respiratory rate in young infants all suggest autonomic immaturity, and it remains uncertain when, in postnatal life, this system becomes mature.[73] Similarly, renal function is not fully developed in the newborn baby and glomerular filtration rate, renal blood flow, and tubular function reach mature values by 1 to 2 years of age. There is a reduced ability to excrete sodium in response to a saline load in the neonatal period, and the significance of postnatal changes in intrarenal blood flow are still unclear. Likewise, the mechanisms of body water regulation and the relationships of blood volume and blood pressure are poorly understood in the young. Clearly, with little information available about the normal development of those systems and organs involved in blood pressure control, our understanding of abnormalities that lead to hypertension in childhood is quite rudimentary.

PRIMARY HYPERTENSION

While it seems likely that genetic and environmental factors interact to produce primary or essential hypertension, one or another mechanism may dominate to produce different forms of the disorder. To date, it appears that polygeneic inheritance accounts in part for the tendency to develop an elevated blood pressure. A number of recent studies have addressed the genetic influences affecting blood pressure. For example, Grim et al.[46] have described genetic influences on the renin-angiotensin-aldosterone system, the renal excretion of electrolytes, and plasma and urinary norepinephrine.[86] In other studies, Ward et al.[126] have looked at the effects of migration on the familial aggregation of blood pressure. They have concluded that, in their population, genetic factors did play an important role in determining the blood pressure distribution but stress that "genetic heritability" should not be equated with causation. Studies by Feinleib et al.[24] in adult twins and those of Biron et al.[9] in adopted children also strongly suggest that there are genetic determinants of blood pressure.

Gillum[41] has recently reviewed the pathophysiology of hypertension in blacks and whites, examining those factors known to affect blood pressure. Since hypertension is more severe in and affects more blacks than whites, an understanding of the mechanisms involved in its development in different races is important. In cross-sectional studies of children aged 5 to 14 years in a biracial community, Berenson et al.[7] have shown an increase in PRA over blood pressure strata in whites but not in blacks. In black children, those in the highest stratum of blood pressure had the lowest PRA, and PRA also decreased slightly with age. Mean serum dopamine-β-hydroxylase (DβH) concentrations were also consistently lower in blacks, and when plotted against levels for PRA, marked racial differences were noted. There was an absence of black children in the high renin high DβH group, a relationship opposite to that found in white children. White children (but not blacks) also showed increased resting heart rates in the high blood pressure stratum. These findings suggested to the investigators that sympathomimetic influences on blood pressure and heart rate might be greater in whites and might play a greater role in the development of early hypertension.

Voors et al.[125] have also reported a positive correlation between 24-hour urinary sodium excretion as measured the same day in black children in their high blood pressure strata, as well as a decrease in urinary potassium excretion. In the same population it has also been found that by the age of 10 or 11 years, black females have a higher sodium intake than other sex-race groups.[31] It is of note that black children in the high blood pressure strata had somewhat lower creatinine clearances than those in the low blood pressure strata.

These findings in children are of particular interest since Luft and his co-workers[82, 83] have reported that black adults had higher blood pressures following saline infusions than their matched white counterparts. They also showed a blunted natriuretic response[83] to saline loads, as well as values for PRA that were lower than those of whites. While no specific intrinsic renal defect was demonstrated in blacks, it was observed that glomerular filtration rate decreased faster with age in whites. Based on their findings, they speculated that blacks might have a relatively diminished glomerular ultrafiltration coefficient compared to whites and that this might lead to sodium retention and a higher blood pressure. Initially this might manifest as a blunted natriuretic response and suppression of PRA, with later development of frank hypertension. Clearly, if differences in autonomic and hormonal influences on blood pressure exist between blacks and whites, approaches to both the prevention and treatment of essential hypertension may differ for the two races. It has, for example, been noted that most blacks with essential hypertension respond to a diuretic with a fall in blood pressure, while only about 20% of whites show a similar response. Conversely, most white individuals with essential hypertension respond favorably to use of only a beta-blocker, while most blacks do not.

The association of hypertension and obesity in adults has been well documented. Likewise, there appears to be a real relationship between being overweight and having an elevated blood pressure in childhood and adolescence.[22, 114, 128] Whether it is only those who are genetically prone to hypertension who develop it when they become overweight is unclear. It has also been questioned whether in obese individuals the increased salt intake that may accompany an increased caloric intake may actually be responsible for causing hypertension in those susceptible to it. Recent studies by a number of investigators[22, 114, 128] have begun to address these complex interrelationships in adolescents. The methodology for studying obesity and sodium balance in free-living populations is, however, not yet well developed, and this may account for the difference in the results that have been obtained. It has been found that a small number of overnight urine collections provide a poor index of current sodium excretion as does a single 24-hour urine collection. This is because a large salt load, ingested on one day, may be excreted over the next several days.

Ellison et al.[22] have reported that in 248 "normal" adolescents, aged 16 to 17 years, heavier and more obese individuals ingested large amounts of sodium. This was attributed to an increased saltiness of the diet rather than to a higher consumption of calories. These workers found no association between sodium excretion in three overnight urine specimens and level of systolic blood pressure. Similarly, in young adults, Kotchen et al.[61] did not demonstrate an association between blood pressure and urinary sodium excretion based on one overnight urine collection. Siervogel et al.,[114] on the other hand, found equivocal evidence of a relationship between fourth phase diastolic blood pressure and urinary electrolyte excretion in 154 white children, aged 8 to 18 years, after adjusting for differences in body size. Similarly, Watson et al.[128] found a weak but discernible association between systolic blood pressure and the urinary excretion of sodium and potassium in black and white female adolescents and young adults. Like Voors et al.,[125] Watson et al.[128] found that blacks excreted more sodium and less potassium than whites. This suggested to them that the intake of sodium and potassium might play a role in producing the increased prevalence of hypertension found in blacks. Unlike Berenson

et al.,[7] Kotchen et al.[61] have not found a decreased creatinine clearance across blood pressure strata in young adults, but their data are presented by sex rather than by race. Clearly, a great deal more work needs to be done if we are to understand the roles of obesity, sodium, and potassium in the pathogenesis of primary hypertension.

The role of stress and personality in the development of early primary hypertension also remains poorly understood, and few studies have been undertaken in the young. As previously mentioned, some evidence[84] indicates that initially, in early primary hypertension, cardiac output increases while peripheral resistance remains normal. There are those who suggest that the hemodynamic changes of early hypertension are related to stress-mediated overactivity of the sympathetic nervous system.[35, 56]

Markers for Primary Hypertension

From both an epidemiologic and clinical point of view, it would be useful to have markers that identified those young individuals at risk for the development of later primary hypertension. Presently, from tracking correlations, it appears that a child's blood pressure is the single best predictor of his later blood pressure level. According to Higgins et al.,[49] fatness and a knowledge of parental blood pressure in children add little to predictiveness of risk because a given child's blood pressure level is correlated with his weight and his parents' blood pressure. Nonetheless, accuracy of prediction of outcome based on one or a few blood pressure readings is presently not great for individual children. Fixler and his associates[27] have also reported that blood pressure response to exercise testing is no more predictive of later blood pressure level in high school students than blood pressure readings themselves.

An interesting study by Falkner et al.[23] showed quite striking differences in heart rate and blood pressure response to arithmetic stress in three groups of adolescents. One group was, however, genetically prone (by family history) to the development of hypertension; the other was not. Whether the differences in response to a standard stress of this type will remain constant over time and have predictive value remains to be seen.

In the same vein, in our clinical experience young individuals are found periodically to have hypertension in association with the stress of a fracture or with anesthesia for nonrenal surgery. Those with fractures to whom I refer are not children who are also in traction where other factors may be operant.[72, 120] Observing these youngsters, we find that their blood pressure usually returns to top normal or to borderline values and that the majority have positive family histories for essential hypertension. We speculate that their abnormal cardiovascular response to stress may be a clue that hypertension will develop later. These individuals, as well as those who develop hypertension with thermal injury,[101] are worthy of prolonged follow-up to see what their outcome will be with respect to blood pressure.

Interest in biochemical markers has recently been heightened by the reports of Garay and Meyer[36] and Garay et al.[37] In 1979,[36] it was reported that a new and simple test had been developed for measuring net sodium (Na^+) and potassium (K^+) fluxes in Na^+-loaded K^+-depleted human erythrocytes. In adults with essential hypertension, there was a constant increase in net K^+ influx, and it was theorized that this was due to higher Na^+, K^+ pump activity. In patients with more severe essential hypertension, it was found that Na^+ efflux from erythrocytes dropped so that in all patients with essential hypertension, the ratio of Na^+ to K^+ net fluxes was reduced. In patients with hypertension of renal origin, Na^+ and K^+ fluxes were not found to be perturbed. Of particular interest was the finding that in young normotensive individuals born to normotensive parents, erythrocyte K^+ influx was normal. In five of eight normotensive individuals born to parents with essential hypertension, K^+ influx was, however, increased. These findings have since been extended by the same workers in a larger group of subjects.[37] They do, however, caution that severe renal failure reduces the flux ratio and distorts the result of the test. Erythrocyte Na^+ and K^+ fluxes need to be investigated across the distribution of blood pressure in children and, particularly, in the offspring of parents with essential hypertension in order to evaluate their validity as markers.

Another possible biochemical marker may be urinary kallikrein concentration. Zinner et al.[134] have shown not only that there is familial aggregation of blood pressure in childhood but also that there is familial aggregation of this enzyme that is involved in the production of vasodilator peptides. Urinary kallikrein concentration was found to be lower in black than in white children and was inversely related to blood pressure. Furthermore, the relationship was relatively stable on two examinations over a 3- to 4-year time interval. The kallikrein-kinin system possesses hypotensive and natriuretic properties, and there are conflicting reports of its activity in adults with essential hypertension, as well as its relationship to the renin-angiotensin-aldosterone system.[51, 67, 68, 71] Further studies in children and adolescents of this system and its relationship to other systems involved in blood pressure control are needed.

SECONDARY HYPERTENSION

It remains uncertain how prevalent persistent hypertension is in the pediatric population because most of the screening studies that have been undertaken have involved blood pressure measurement on only one occasion. In addition, many investigators have used different definitions for identifying those with an elevated blood pressure. Levine et al.[70] screened a high school population and found that less than 2% had persistent hypertension. Rames et al.[105] also reported that less than 1% of the children that they screened had persistent elevations in blood pressure. These data suggest that general screening programs for children and adolescents are not cost-effective for case finding. If screening programs are to be undertaken in young populations, they should have as their target high risk groups, such as inner city black youths in their mid- and late teens. Blood pressure should, however, be measured annually as a routine in clinics and doctors' offices. This will identify those young individuals with high normal or borderline blood pressures and also those with clearly elevated blood pressures who have not yet become symptomatic. As in adults, so in youngsters, hypertension is usually asymptomatic until considerable vascular damage has occurred. We have seen children with diastolic blood pressure readings of 140 to 160 mm Hg who have had no complaints and who have had underlying renal or renovascular disease probably of long standing. These children, if undetected, develop encephalopathy, heart and renal failure, and even cerebrovascular accidents. To not detect them at an earlier stage is a tragedy.

Not surprisingly, the prevalence in children and adolescents of primary and secondary forms of hypertension also remains to be clarified. Again, because of a lack of standardization of populations and of definitions, various investigators have arrived at conclusions that are often at odds. Londe et al.[79] found that over 90% of their patients had no identifiable organic cause for hypertension. Rames et al.[105] found that of 41 children with persistent hypertension, 23 had weights in excess of 120%, 13 lean subjects had primary hypertension, and only 5 had secondary forms of elevated

blood pressure. Likewise, Levine et al.[70] found that none of 28 hypertensive high school children had organic disease, but 64% were obese. The populations in all three studies were relatively similar in that they consisted of asymptomatic youngsters, identified as having high blood pressure on routine testing either in the office[79] or in the field setting.

In general, data based on surveys of hospitalized children and adolescents with persistent hypertension suggest that primary hypertension is uncommon, while renal disorders are the leading cause of elevated blood pressure in juveniles.[122] For example, in Toronto,[106] 73% of patients reportedly had renal disease, 16% essential hypertension, and 9% endocrine causes for elevated blood pressure. In London,[40] 78% of children had renal hypertension, 15% coarctation of the aorta, 1% essential hypertension, and 1% hypertension secondary to obesity. Figures from the New York Hospital — Cornell Medical Center also support the notion that renal diseases and coarctation of the aorta are responsible for most elevated blood pressure in the young.[122] It seems likely that in the populations described, children who required hospitalization probably had moderate or severe hypertension. This, in all likelihood, accounts for the distribution of causes found in them.

By 1974, we had found that the majority of the teenagers seen by us had no identifiable organic cause for their hypertension.[74] As mentioned earlier, many were overweight, and the majority had first degree relatives with hypertension. Particularly in black teenagers and white male adolescents, primary hypertension is the commonest diagnosis in our clinic. This is, of course, not to say that any form of hypertension cannot exist in any child or teenager of either sex and any race. It can and does. Conversely, primary hypertension can occur and has been diagnosed in white female adolescents, although in them we more often find an underlying disease to account for their high blood pressure.

Ours is a mixed population of individuals with mild to severe hypertension. The majority of them have been asymptomatic and are identified on routine examination in doctors' offices or clinics. The majority of them have not required hospitalization for evaluation so that a review of hospital medical records for a discharge diagnosis of hypertension would not identify this group as a part of the hypertensive pediatric population. The more severe the hypertension, the more likely are our patients to be admitted for study and treatment. In this group of patients, we, like others, often find underlying pathology, particularly renal or renovascular disease. The skew in our patient population is that we do not see youngsters with coarctation of the aorta and the glomerulonephritides.

Renal Disorders

Renal disorders are the commonest cause of severe hypertension seen at referral centers.[80] In series from both London and New York, just over 50% of young individuals with renal disease and hypertension had glomerulonephritis of some type.[122] Twenty-five percent had nephropathy secondary to obstructive uropathy, 14 to 16% had congenital renal malformation, and 8% in both series had renovascular disease. This last figure is similar to our own,[75] and most of these children had fibromuscular dysplasia. In some cases, this is diffuse (involving both the systemic and pulmonary circulations) and progressive.[16] Children with neurofibromatosis may also have involvement of their renal arteries with stenosis and hypertension.

No concerted or systematic attempts have been made to define the mechanisms responsible for hypertension in the various renal disorders of childhood. It is thought that some are primarily renin-dependent, others volume-dependent, or mixed. In children with Wilm's tumor or hemangiopericytoma, some evidence suggests that a pressor substance, akin to angiotensin, may be produced in excess to account for the hypertension.[90, 108] For Wilm's tumor, it has also been theorized that a cellophane-wrap phenomenon and/or distortion of the renal artery by tumor mass may contribute to the elevation in blood pressure that sometimes occurs.

While surgical repair of renal artery stenosis can be curative of hypertension in young individuals, it is often technically difficult. The place of percutaneous transluminal renal artery angioplasty remains to be evaluated in the pediatric population.

Coarctation of the Aorta

Coarctation of the thoracic aorta is one of the commonest causes of an elevated blood pressure in infants and young children. Abdominal coarctation is, on the other hand, quite rare.[112] Both are frequently anatomically correctable by surgery. It has, however, now become clear that hypertension frequently persists or recurs after correction of thoracic coarctation.[130] The reasons for this remain speculative.[30]

The mechanisms involved in the development of hypertension in patients with coarctation of the aorta and in the paradoxical hypertension that sometimes develops early after surgical repair are not yet clearly delineated. Recent work with volume depletion and administration of the angiotensin antagonist, saralasin, suggests that the renin-angiotensin-aldosterone system is involved.[99] It has been postulated that initially renin release leads to volume expansion through angiotensin-induced stimulation of aldosterone secretion. The volume expansion eventually leads to suppression of PRA, and this may account for why, in older studies, PRA was not found to be increased. Volume contraction through salt restriction or diuresis is now used as a tool to unmask the role played by the renin-angiotensin sysem.

Endocrine Disorders

The endocrine disorders of mineralocorticoid excess that may result in the development of hypertension include: II β-hydroxylase deficiency; 17 hydroxylase deficiency; primary aldosteronism; dexamethasone suppressible aldosteronism; and Cushing's syndrome. With the exception of the last, these are all characterized by a low peripheral PRA.[95, 96] In Cushing's syndrome, PRA may be normal or increased, but this condition should be suspected on clinical grounds.

In the experience of most investigators, hypertension due to these disorders is quite uncommon in the pediatric population. Primary aldosteronism seems to be especially rare and, when it occurs, it is more often due to adrenal hyperplasia than to the presence of an adenoma.

Pheochromocytoma, another hormone-secreting tumor that may cause hypertension,[116] is also quite uncommon in childhood, although it is not as rare as adrenal adenoma. It generally declares itself through its clinical presentation, and the diagnosis can usually be confirmed by measuring increased amounts of catecholamines in plasma or urine. The metabolites of the free amines (vanillylmandelic acid and metanephrines) may also be increased in the urine.

Pheochromocytomas may occur anywhere where sympathetic tissue has occurred during prenatal development, and in children these tumors are frequently either extraadrenal in site or multiple in origin. Children with neurofibromatosis are said to have an increased frequency of pheochromocytoma. In other patients there may be a family history of pheochromocytoma in association with multiple endocrine adenopathy (thyroid, parathyroid tumors), type II. Malignant pheochromocytoma is quite rare, but these rumors may be large and spread widely. They respond poorly to chemotherapy and radiation.

Neonatal Disorders

A word should be said about hypertension in the neonatal period, since an increased frequency of renovascular disease has been described in some centers.[2] Previously, coarctation of the aorta or renal parenchymal disease would have been considered the most likely causes of severe hypertension in very young infants. Renal artery thrombosis in babies who have had indwelling umbilical catheters is now recognized with increased frequency. With closure of a patent ductus arteriosus, embolization to the renal artery with subsequent hypertension has also been described.[19, 29] Adelman[2] has suggested that many infants with renovascular hypertension eventually become normotensive if managed medically. This is in contrast to children with muscular dysplasia of the renal arteries who often become severely hypertensive and refractory to drug therapy.

DIAGNOSTIC EVALUATION

If a young person presents with a blood pressure that is abnormal even by adult standards, particularly if the individual is symptomatic, evaluation should proceed promptly. In those who have a top normal or mildly elevated blood pressure reading, multiple further readings and the blood pressure trend over time will determine the need for diagnostic evaluation. The studies that are performed in any child or adolescent presenting with either persistent borderline or definite hypertension should be determined by that individual's clinical presentation. A careful personal history, family history, and physical examination are all mandatory. The family history should explore not only the presence of hypertension in family members but also the occurrence of early myocardial infarction, stroke, renal disease and/or failure, diabetes mellitus, thyroid and other endocrine diseases, and tumors causing an increased blood pressure. If first degree relatives have not had their blood pressure measured within a year, it may be helpful to measure it in each of them. This is especially important if the patient has a twin. Urinalysis is a relatively cheap and simple screen for those diseases, like the nephritides, that present with hematuria and/or proteinuria.

Guidelines for what laboratory studies should be undertaken are at present based largely on anecdotal clinical experience. Centers with a longer experience and with more accumulated negative test results tend to be more conservative in their approach. It is our practice, when borderline blood pressure readings persist over 6 to 12 months, to measure the serum chemistries: blood urea nitrogen, creatinine, cholesterol (and its fractions), fasting glucose and triglycerides, as well as uric acid. An electrocardiogram and a roentgenogram of the chest are also obtained. Our intent with these studies is to determine if target organ damage has developed and if coronary artery risk factors other than hypertension are also present. Kotchen et al.[61] have recently shown a clustering of risk factors in young adults. They also showed that serum cholesterol, triglyceride, uric acid, and glucose concentrations were related to body weight as well as to blood pressure.

Eventually it may be unequivocally shown that echocardiography is a more sensitive method for detecting left ventricular hypertrophy (LVH) than use of the ECG in hypertensive youths.[63] Based on the high frequency of findings suggestive of LVH in a young, mildly hypertensive population studied echocardiographically, Cutilletta[14] has proposed that the hypertrophy is not evidence of target organ damage but rather reflects that the heart is pathologically involved in the earliest stages of essential hypertension. It remains to be proven if, with adequate lowering of blood pressure, the electrocardiographic and roentgenologic evidence of LVH is observed to regress.

Our routine measurement of serum uric acid is based on the observation that in half of the young males whom we see with borderline blood pressure values, the level is elevated. Prebis et al.[102] have found that 42% of youngsters with primary hypertension have elevated serum uric acid while on an unrestricted sodium intake. The significance of the finding is not clear, although it is speculated that hyperuricemia indicates that early hypertensive renal damage already exists. When diuretics are used to treat youngsters with mild hypertension, hyperuricemia may be markedly accentuated.

In nonobese young individuals with persistent hypertension, it remains our practice to obtain an excretory urogram. Our yield of abnormal studies among asymptomatic adolescents with a strong family history of essential hypertension has been, however, quite low.

It was earlier noted that not a great deal is known about the development of the human renin-angiotensin-aldosterone system. Values for PRA tend to be higher in infancy than by midchildhood,[50, 111, 117] and to use this tool effectively, one needs to have age-adjusted reference values. Because of our lack of general information in this area, it seems unreasonable to recommend the measurement of peripheral PRA as a general diagnostic screening test. At present, when children or adolescents are admitted for evaluation of moderately severe hypertension (children, supine diastolic blood pressure $\geq$100 mm Hg; adolescents, $\geq$110 mm Hg), we obtain plasma for peripheral PRA after at least 1 hour in the supine position. We prefer to obtain the blood under standardized conditions similar to those described for adults, but if there is some urgent need to start drug therapy, we forego 8 hours of bedrest and 3 to 4 hours of ambulation. In our experience, the primary value of measuring peripheral PRA has been as a screening test for those rare low renin forms of hypertension that are associated with mineralocorticoid excess. Others[109] have found it useful for screening for renal forms of hypertension.

Robson[109] and Loggie et al.[78] have reviewed their recommendations for renal angiography, for obtaining renal venous blood for the measurement of PRA, and for renal biopsy. This is an area where recommendations are based on clinical experience rather than on well documented evidence. The presence of unexplained moderately severe persistent diastolic hypertension, the presence of unexplained hematuria with persistent hypertension, or the presence of a well-defined, persistent epigastric bruit with moderately severe chronic hypertension, all probably indicate the need to pursue rapidly abdominal angiography. The presence of an epigastric bruit does not, however, mean that renal artery stenosis will be found. Conversely, the absence of a bruit does not preclude the existence of renal artery pathology. Arteriography should also be undertaken in a child with more than mild unexplained hypertension before that individual is labeled as having primary hypertension.[60, 64] Our yield of positive angiograms has, however, been lower in teenagers than in children[77] and quite low in the presence of mild degrees of hypertension.

The usefulness in the young hypertensive of radionuclide studies is not clear.[109] Conclusions seem to be based primarily on adult experience. It is our impression that these studies have limited value in the evaluation of hypertensive children but may have some value in following children with repaired renovascular lesions.

The predictive value, for surgical cure of hypertension in children, of renal vein renin ratios has not been extensively evaluated.[42] Measurement of PRA at the time of angiography seems a reasonable recommendation. Whether one can interpret the values based on adult data is open to question.[18, 29] In our experience a renal vein renin ratio in excess of 1.5:1 can occur in children in whom no structural lesion is demonstrable radiographically. Conversely, if an operable renal artery lesion is demonstrated in a hypertensive child with a renal vein renin ratio <1.5:1, we would still recommend surgical repair. This is clearly another area that needs extensive evaluation in the field of juvenile hypertension. Similarly, the diagnostic use of angiotensin blocking agents in children with hypertension needs exploration.

Finally, accumulated negative information suggests to us that routine measurements of urinary catecholamines and their metabolites are not warranted. Similarly, we do not routinely measure aldosterone, cortisol, urinary 17 keto- or 17 hydroxy-steroids unless some clue that an adrenocortical form of hypertension exists. If abnormalities are found they should be pursued with appropriate hormonal studies.

MANAGEMENT

There is some evidence that increased levels of systolic blood pressure in the late teenage years are associated with an increased cardiovascular morbidity.[98] Likewise, there is some evidence that hypertensive diastolic blood pressure levels found on a single occasion in late adolescence or in early adult life, are also associated with an increased cardiovascular morbidity and mortality.[48, 55] The natural history for young individuals found to have systolic or diastolic blood pressure levels at or just above the 95th percentile for age is not yet adequately described. This poses a problem in terms of intervention, particularly if drug therapy is being contemplated. Although not well described, the published pharmacology[88, 115] of the antihypertensive drugs suggests that, in the short term, these agents are as effective in lowering blood pressure in hypertensive children as they are in adults. Their side effects on acute administration, and even with chronic administration over a few years, seem also to be similar to those seen in adults. Their long-term effects, given chronically to growing, maturing humans, are, however, not clear. On the one hand, by lowering blood pressure, one wonders if the complications of elevated blood pressure will be prevented or, on the other hand, one wonders if the drugs will interfere in subtle ways with the growth and development or cause such perturbations in other coronary artery risk factors (for example, serum cholesterol) that their beneficial effects will be negated. It is clearly too soon to say and it is, therefore, difficult to make recommendations about when drugs should be started in the management of mild hypertension in the young. New evidence in adults suggests that those with diastolic blood pressure readings persistently $\geq$90 mm Hg are hypertensive and benefit from drug treatment.[52, 53]

Figures 43.1 and 43.2 show the trends of blood pressure over time in two black male adolescents, both of whom had one parent with primary hypertension. One developed LVH by ECG; the other became "normotensive" and has always had a normal ECG. If both had been drug-treated early, at similar levels of blood pressure, one might not have developed LVH, and the other might have been exposed unnecessarily to several years of therapy. It seems reasonable, when making a decision about introducing hypotensive agents, to assess young individuals for family history of serious hypertensive complications, as well as evaluating them for other coronary artery risk factors and evidence of target organ damage. Freis[32] has suggested that these factors, as well as race and sex, should be taken into account when a decision is being made to treat adults with drugs with diastolic blood pressure levels between 90 to 95 mm Hg. Similar consideration may have to be given to these factors in managing young hypertensive patients.

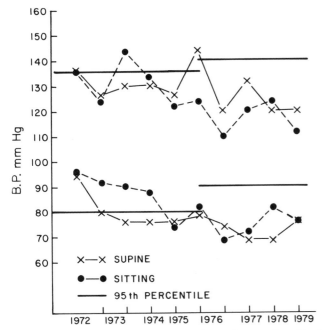

Fig. 43.1 Blood pressure measured over 7 years in a black teenage male with one parent with hypertension. Presently asymptomatic, normotensive, and without evidence of target organ damage.

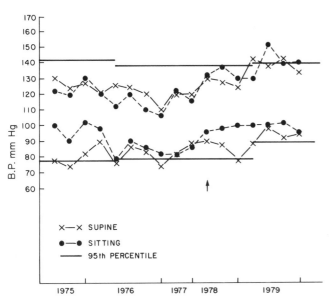

Fig. 43.2 Blood pressure measured over 5 years in a black adolescent male with one parent with hypertension. Left ventricular hypertrophy (*arrow*) has developed.

NONPHARMACOLOGIC CONSIDERATIONS

Diet

Ponderosity in adolescence appears to be related to increased levels of blood pressure.[22, 114, 128] Kotchen et al.[61] have also shown a relationship between weight and other coronary artery risk factors in young adults, aged 19 to 24 years. It seems reasonable, therefore, to recommend weight reduction as a first step in the control of mild hypertension in children and adolescents who are obese. Unfortunately, in free living youngsters, it is not often possible to obtain salutary results. A variety of strategies, including behavior modification and organized exercise programs, can be employed, but the treat-

ment of juvenile obesity is both time-consuming and often disappointing.

Lauer and Clarke[66] have reported the normalization of blood pressure in 10 youngsters, aged 6 to 18 years, who were able to lose weight. In our experience, only hospitalized children and adolescents have been able to lose significant amounts of weight. The normalization of their blood pressure in this setting may have been as much due to the environment as to the weight loss. It has been noted that in the mildly hypertensive young, as in adults, blood pressure often decreases when they are hospitalized. Furthermore, our patients who have lost weight in the hospital have also been on salt restriction.

The evidence that sodium chloride plays a role in the development of human essential hypertension is largely circumstantial.[119] Most physicians, however, recommend that salt intake should be reduced in individuals with mild hypertension, as well as in those with more severe hypertension who are drug-treated. In the former group of patients, it is hoped that a reduction in salt will result in a lowering of blood pressure that will obviate the need for drug therapy. In the latter group, by maintaining salt restriction, one hopes to prevent excessive loss of potassium in the urine in diuretic-treated patients. This may prevent the need to give potassium supplements that are poorly accepted by all age groups.

Presently, there are no data that show the effect of sodium restriction on the blood pressures of hypertensive youths. Nor is it presently known what amount of salt is allowable at various ages.[103] Sensitivity to salt may be highly individual in its effect on blood pressure and, as more is learned about it, more selective restriction of sodium chloride may be possible when dealing with hypertensive individuals.

Other Nonpharmacologic Interventions

The place of aerobic exercise, biofeedback, and other relaxation techniques, is still being evaluated in adults with hypertension. Reported results are contradictory, and no evidence for their efficacy has yet been reported in the pediatric population. Their attractiveness to pediatricians as therapeutic tools lies in the fact that, if effective, they would obviate the need to use potentially harmful drugs.

There are those who recommend that hypertensive youngsters avoid weight lifting and other nonstatic exercise. This is based on the finding that large increases in systolic blood pressure occur when young individuals with borderline or high blood pressure are exercised on the bicycle ergometer. The detriment to their health from this has not yet been established.

Contraception

In the United States, hypertension induced by the oral contraceptives is said to be the commonest form of secondary hypertension among adult females. Finnerty[25] has reported that 7.5% of previously normotensive women developed high blood pressure while taking oral contraceptives, whereas there was aggravation of previously existing hypertension also in 7.5% of his female population.

Since more adolescent females are sexually active and at a younger age than heretofore, the physician caring for hypertensive teenagers should be alert to their special problems with respect to both contraception and pregnancy. Use of oral contraceptives is not completely contraindicated in females with hypertension, particularly if the risk of pregnancy outweighs the risk of some exacerbation of hypertension. While use of intrauterine devices has been considered a preferable choice for sexually active hypertensive adolescents, these too have a number of important adverse effects. It is helpful when managing such patients to work in cooperation with a gynecologist.

If pregnancy occurs, the risks and need for careful supervision need to be discussed. Many individuals with mild hypertension do well when pregnant, and elevated blood pressure alone is not, therefore, a contraindication to pregnancy. Of primary concern in managing hypertensive pregnant females is the fact that most of the antihypertensive drugs and diuretics cross the placenta and have the potential to affect the fetus.

Compliance

Compliance in returning for medical care, adhering to diets, and in taking prescribed medications continue to be major problems in the management of asymptomatic adults with high blood pressure. In adolescents with hypertension, this too presents a problem.

Strategies that have been used for improving adherence to treatment in adults include education and reeducation about high blood pressure, evaluation of and improvement in patient-health care provider relations, and improving appointment scheduling. In addition, drug regimens should be kept as simple as possible, with once or twice daily dosing being used as often as is feasible. Blood pressure self-measurements at home have also been incorporated into the care plans of many patients with a view to improving compliance. By allowing individuals to see for themselves how they are responding, it is believed that they may take greater responsibility for their own treatment.

While compliance is also a problem with teenagers with hypertension, none of the strategies just mentioned have been studied for their impact in this age group. Furthermore, most of the educational literature that is available for hypertensive patients is directed toward adults. To a 14- or 15-year-old, the threat of a stroke at 40 or 50 has no particular relevance.

DRUGS

When mild hypertension has failed to respond to non-pharmacologic management or when moderate and persistently elevated blood pressure is present, drug therapy is usually begun. As in adults, the approach in the young has been one of the stepped use of the various classes of drugs. Treatment is usually initiated with a diuretic, an adrenergically active agent is then added if necessary and, if blood pressure is still not controlled, a vasodilator or prazosin is also added (Table 43.3). If the level of blood pressure is still suboptimal, a second adrenergically active drug may be prescribed or the converting enzyme inhibitor, captopril, may be substituted for the three-drug regimen. Use of this agent in the young has, however, been more limited than in adults.[33, 97]

Diuretics

Chlorothiazide has had widespread use in children both as a diuretic and in the treatment of hypertension. When used to treat high blood pressure, it initially causes depletion of sodium and water, but its later effect seems to be due to an incompletely understood action on vascular smooth muscle. There are no published dose-response curves for its hypotensive effect in the young, and the doses used to treat hypertension are, therefore, the same as those recommended for use in producing diuresis. The major adverse effects are due to depletion of volume and electrolytes. Hyperuricemia may also be induced. In diabetes mellitus, type one, the thiazides may exacerbate any tendency towards hypokalemia, but they do not aggravate hyperglycemia. In type two diabetes mellitus, the thiazides may, however, make it harder to regulate blood sugar.

Furosemide has been used extensively to treat hypertension in young patients with renal failure in whom the thiazide diuretics are ineffective. In individuals with normal or mildly impaired renal function, there is no advantage to using this agent. Ethacrynic acid, also a loop diuretic, is used less frequently in pediatric practice than furosemide. We have, however, prescribed it on occasions for patients allergic to the sulfa derivatives, such as the thiazides and furosemide. Metolazone is another diuretic that has been found to be effective as an antihypertensive agent in adults. Its use in children and adolescents for this purpose has been limited.

Spironolactone is needed infrequently in the management of juvenile hypertension, since primary aldosteronism is quite rare. It can, however, be used for its potassium-sparing effects in those who develop hypokalemia with the thiazides and furosemide, and who tolerate oral potassium supplements poorly. In males, it causes gynecomastia that can be quite prominent. It may also have other endocrine effects, and it is expensive. Triamterene is an alternative to spironolactone if primarily a potassium-sparing effect is required.

Except for the beta-blockers, all of the adrenergically active drugs and also the vasodilators cause occult salt and water retention that leads to pseudotolerance to their effect. For this reason, a diuretic is usually needed when one or more of these agents is used.

Neurally Active Agents

The beta-blockers, methyldopa, clonidine hydrochloride, reserpine, and guanethidine, comprise the more commonly used agents in this group, although the last two are now infrequently prescribed. The beta-blockers include propranolol, metoprolol, and nadolol. Of the three, propranolol has had the most pediatric usage.

In children and adolescents who do not have asthma or diabetes mellitus, we prefer to use propranolol as the first agent of choice in the neurally active class of drugs. It is our experience that it produces fewer side effects than methyldopa, although fatigue and impaired exercise tolerance occur. It can be given twice a day, as can metroprolol. Only nadolol, a nonspecific beta-blocker like propranolol, is recommended once a day. Metoprolol is said, at lower doses, to be more selective for beta-1 receptors than the other two drugs. In the higher doses that are often required to treat hypertension, this selectivity tends to be lost. The blood pressure-lowering mechanism of action of these agents is probably complex. For example, propranolol decreases cardiac output, depresses peripheral PRA, and also has central nervous system effects. It is a particularly useful drug for the treatment of hypertension secondary to renal disease. It may also be useful for treating patients with hypertension who also have either migraine headaches or symptomatic mitral valve prolapse. In addition, we have used it as a first step agent (bypassing the diuretics) in youngsters with early primary hypertension and evidence of a hyperkinetic circulation.[34]

Methyldopa remains our first choice of the neurally active agents for youngsters with hypertension who have asthma, diabetes mellitus, or severe allergic rhinitis. In this last group of patients, we have, on occasion, precipitated acute bronchospasm by use of either propranolol or metoprolol. Methyldopa has been free of this side effect and also does not seem to interact adversely with the drugs needed to treat or prevent asthma. However, it produces sedation, fatigue, and depression in a number of patients, and those taking it need to be monitored carefully for these effects. Hemolytic anemia and hepatotoxicity are unusual complications of therapy. In

TABLE 43.3   ORAL DRUGS USED TO TREAT HYPERTENSION

Class	Drug Name	Usual Starting Dose	Common Side Effects	Available Oral Dosage Forms
Diuretics	Chlorothiazide	10–20 mg/kg/day	Hypokalemia, hyperuricemia	Tablets, 250, 500 mg Suspension, 250 mg/5 ml
	Furosemide	1–2 mg/kg/day	Hypokalemia, hyperuricemia	Tablets, 20, 40 mg Liquid, 10 mg/ml
	Spironolactone	1 mg/kg/day	Hyperkalemia, gynecomastia	Tablets, 25 mg
Neurally active agents	Propranolol	1 mg/kg/day	Bradycardia, fatigue	Tablets, 10, 20, 40, 80 mg
	Metoprolol	Undetermined	Bradycardia, fatigue	Tablets, 50, 100 mg
	Nadolol	Undetermined	Bradycardia, fatigue	Tablets, 40 mg
	Methyldopa	10 mg/kg/day	Fatigue, depression, postural hypotension	Tablets, 125, 250, 500 mg Suspension, 250 mg/5 ml
	Clonidine HCl	Undetermined	Bradycardia, dry mouth Overshoot with abrupt cessation of treatment	Tablets, 0.1, 0.2 mg
	Reserpine	0.02 mg/kg/day (maximum 0.5)	Nasal stuffiness, depression	Tablets, 0.1, 0.25 mg
	Guanethidine	0.2–0.5 mg/kg/day	Postural and exertional hypotension, bradycardia, retrograde ejaculation	Tablets, 10, 25 mg
Vasodilators	Hyralazine	0.75–1 mg/kg/day	Tachycardia, headache, nausea	Tablets, 10, 25, 50 mg
	Minoxidil	0.2 mg/kg/day	Tachycardia, salt and water retention, hypertrichosis	Tablets, 2.5, 10 mg
	Prazosin	Undetermined	Tachycardia, postural hypotension, "first dose" phenomenon	Capsules, 1, 2, 5 mg
Other	Captopril	Dosage, on a weight basis, comparable to that used for adults who start at 25 mg t.i.d.	Rash, loss of taste, fever[a]	Tablets, 25, 50, 100 mg

[a] Uncommon but more serious: neutropenia, renal failure, proteinuria.

patients with mild or moderate hypertension, methyldopa can be used successfully in a twice daily dosage regimen.

Clonidine hydrochloride, like methyldopa, appears to act centrally. It has, as its main mechanism of action, central alpha-adrenergic stimulation that results in a decreased sympathetic outflow from the brain. Its efficacy and cardiovascular effects are similar to those of methyldopa. Its major side effects are dry mouth and bradycardia. In a small number of adults in whom clonidine has been abruptly terminated, a severe overshoot in blood pressure has occurred. This phenomenon has not been described in children. Reserpine, although cheap and often effective in controlling blood pressure smoothly with once daily dosing, has largely been replaced by the beta-blockers. In adults, and also in teenagers, it use has frequently been associated with depression. In younger children, its major adverse effect appears to be marked nasal congestion. Reports of a potential association between the administration of reserpine and the development of breast cancer[4] also contribute to a decline in its use in the treatment of hypertension.

Similarly, with the advent of more effective agents with fewer side effects, the use of guanethidine has declined. This drug is usually most effective in the upright position. Its major adverse effects include postural hypotension, sometimes marked and resulting in syncope, as well as exercise-induced fainting. This latter effect is of particular concern in active youngsters.

Phenoxybenzamine and phentolamine are both alpha-adrenergic blocking agents that are used, almost exclusively, for the treatment of hypertension due to catecholamine-secreting tumors. The former is long-acting and produces smoother control of blood pressure than the latter to which, also, tachyphylaxis may develop. In patients with tumors who are refractory to the alpha-blocking drugs, alpha-methyl-paratyrosine may be a useful alternative.

Vasodilators

Hydralazine and minoxidil are the two direct vasodilators that are available for oral use in the management of hypertension. The latter is reserved for the treatment of severe refractory hypertension because of its serious side effects. It causes marked retention of sodium and water, as well as unsightly hypertrichosis in the majority of patients. Hydralazine, too, may cause salt and water retention but usually not of the degree seen with minoxidil. Both drugs may cause tachycardia and palpitations, as well as headache, if given in the absence of a neurally active agent.

In adults given hydralazine at dosages in excess of 200 mg/day, a syndrome resembling lupus erythematosus may be induced. Arthralgia, fever, rash, and malaise, characterize the illness and renal and central nervous system involvement are quite rare.[100] It is usually reversible with discontinuation of the hydralazine but, in some individuals, may have a protracted course. Case reports in children[54] have been uncommon, and we have seen only one probable case in 15 years.

Prazosin was initially released as a direct vasodilator. It is now considered also to have postsynaptic alpha-blocking capability and has been used successfully in the management of hypertension due to pheochromocytoma. Its pediatric clinical pharmacology is poorly characterized, but we have found that it is well tolerated with relatively few side effects, other than mild tachycardia. We have used it primarily in the management of young people with asthma, who have tolerated methyldopa poorly, and in those with renal disease. Since dose-response curves have not been developed for

TABLE 43.4   PARENTERAL DRUGS USED TO TREAT HYPTERTENSION

Class	Drug Name	Route	Usual Starting Dose	Common Side Effects
Diuretics	Furosemide	IV	1 mg/kg/dose	Volume and electrolyte depletion
Neurally active agents[b]	Methyldopa	IV	5–10 mg/kg/dose[c]	Sedation, bradycardia
	Reserpine	IM	Patients <25 kg: 0.02 mg/kg/dose Patients >25 kg: 0.5–1 mg total dose	Flushing, sedation, bradycardia, increased output of gastric acid
Vasodilators	Hydralazine	IV, IM	0.15 mg/kg/dose	Tachycardia, headache, nausea and vomiting
	Diazoxide	IV	3–5 mg/kg/dose	Transient tachycardia, salt and water retention
	Sodium nitroprusside	IV	0.5 μg/kg/min	Hypotension, tachycardia

[a] Hypotension may occur with any antihypertensive drug.

[b] The role of IV propranolol in children with hypertension has not been determined.

[c] This should be diluted in 5% dextrose-water and infused over 30 to 60 minutes.

children, the so-called "first dose phenomenon" is always of concern if too high a dosage is used initially. In adults exhibiting the "first dose phenomenon," hypotension and tachycardia develop within the first few hours after starting treatment, particularly in ambulatory patients. It is, therefore, recommended that the first dose, as well as subsequent increases in dose, should be made at bedtime. In children, we have preferred to initiate treatment in an in-patient setting.

Other Drugs

In its passage through the lung, angiotensin I is converted to angiotensin II by a converting enzyme, peptidyldipeptide carboxy hydrolase. An inhibitor of this enzyme, captopril, is now available for the management of refractory hypertension. Angiotensin-converting enzyme is identical to bradykininase, and it has been suggested that captopril may also interfere with the degradation of bradykinin. With interruption of the renin-angiotensin system, PRA tends to rise, and aldosterone to decrease. In some patients, this results in a significant rise in serum potassium. Pediatric experience[33, 97] has been limited, but captopril certainly has a place in the management of children with severe hypertension mediated through the renin-angiotensin system. Drug fever, rash, loss of taste, renal failure, proteinuria, and neutropenia have all been described as adverse effects in adults. Their frequency in the young is not yet known.

Saralasin, an angiotensin-blocking agent, as well as the calcium channel-blocking drugs may, eventually, become available for the management of high blood pressure.

HYPERTENSIVE EMERGENCIES

As blood pressure has become more routinely measured in pediatric practice, fewer children present with encephalopathy due to chronic, undiagnosed hypertension. Seizures related to elevated blood pressure remain, however, the commonest form of pediatric hypertensive emergency. The high blood pressure may be of acute onset as, for example, in children with burns, or it may be secondary to some long-standing underlying disease, such as hypoplastic kidneys.

Acute left ventricular failure and cerebrovascular accidents infrequently complicate juvenile hypertension. If they occur, however, they require emergency management.

For reasons that remain unclear, young individuals infrequently develop retinal hemorrhages and exudates. Similarly, hypertensive encephalopathy may occur in the absence of papilledema. It is, therefore, difficult to determine at what level of diastolic blood pressure aggressive therapy with parenteral antihypertensive drugs should be instituted. In making a decision one has to consider the cause of the hypertension, its likely duration, evidence for the presence of target organ damage, the patient's symptoms, and, if known, the usual course of hypertension in the condition being treated. To arbitrarily pick a number for the institution of parenteral drug therapy is probably a simplistic approach.

In treating hypertensive encephalopathy in the young or for managing severe hypertension of renal origin, intravenous diazoxide is often the drug of choice.[5] Experience has shown this agent to be both effective and relatively safe.[85] In children with an unstable cardiovascular system (e.g., following a cerebrovascular accident) and hypertension, in those with heart failure, or in youngsters with severe hypertension considered possibly due to catecholamine excess, intravenous sodium nitroprusside is probably a safer choice. With this drug, reduction of the blood pressure can be titrated at a controlled rate.[45] If diazoxide is given rapidly intravenously, a precipitous fall in blood pressure occurs within a few minutes of administration of an effective dose.

Methyldopa, reserpine, and hydralazine are all available for administration by the parenteral route (Table 43.4). The first two both produce unwanted sedation and may take several hours to produce an adequate hypotensive effect. Hydralazine, given in the absence of a drug like propranolol, tends to cause unacceptable tachycardia, nausea, vomiting, and headache. Its onset of action, when effective, is, however, rapid, i.e., within a few minutes if given intravenously and within 30 minutes if given intramuscularly. Finally, intravenous furosemide is a useful adjunctive emergency drug for the management of volume overload in the presence of hypertension.

PROGNOSIS IN HYPERTENSION

Children and adolescents who have persistently and unequivocally high levels of blood pressure develop hypertensive target organ damage. The time course for the development of these complications, as well as that for their regression, is poorly documented. It has also been noted that, even with severe hypertension, retinal arteriolar changes rarely are as extensive as those seen in adults.

Given that the complications of chronic hypertension eventually develop and that life is thereby shortened for both children and adolescents who have it, the need for drug

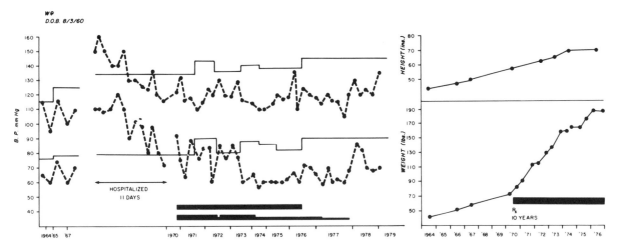

Fig. 43.3 On the *left*, blood pressure measurements in a white female, aged 7 at presentation, who was found to have underlying renal disease. Drug therapy was reduced in a stepwise fashion (*black bars*) and then discontinued. She remains normotensive. On the *right*, a rapid gain in weight began coincidentally with the start of antihypertensive drugs. This phenomenon has been noted in other hypertensive children.

therapy is not a debatable issue in youngsters with unequivocal hypertension. Still and Cottom[118] showed that the average duration of life for such individuals was 14 months from the time of referral if the diastolic blood pressure was ≥120 mm Hg and the ECG showed LVH. In similar children, and with more effective hypotensive agents available to us, we have shown that the blood pressure can be effectively lowered and life prolonged.[77] The patient that we have followed the longest presented at age 7 years with LVH and diastolic blood pressure levels of 120 mm Hg. On drug therapy, 15 years later, she remains under good control with respect to her hypertension.

It is not yet clear, however, how long drug therapy is necessary. Figure 43.3 shows the blood pressure response to treatment in a young girl with moderately severe hypertension thought to be secondary to dysplastic kidneys. After a period of drug-induced normotension, it was possible to stop her antihypertensive drugs and she has since remained normotensive.

PRIMARY PREVENTION OF HYPERTENSION

Primary hypertension is a major public health problem among adults throughout the western world. It is also being identified with increasing frequency among adolescents. There is little that can be done from a public health point of view about the genetic aspects of blood pressure. The thrust for prevention, therefore, has to be directed toward altering environmental factors that contribute to the development of essential hypertension. At present, obesity and high intake of dietary salt are thought to be two of the factors.

Efforts are now being made to educate the public about the sodium chloride content of foodstuffs available in the markeplace.[103] These efforts should be intensified through better food labeling and by improved nutritional education for both the lay and the medical public. Within the school systems, emphasis should be placed on good cardiovascular health habits and nutrition. In this regard, the help of educators, school nutritionists, school nurses, physical fitness teachers, and team coaches should be enlisted.

Major changes in any national life-style are generally effected gradually. It is, therefore, important that within their practices, physicians should also be encouraged to try to identify young patients who are at increased risk for high blood pressure. Good histories of adult cardiovascular disease within families are still not routinely recorded by pediatricians or others who care for children and adolescents. There is a need to know not only whether first and second degree relatives have hypertension but also at what age it was diagnosed and what complications have arisen. Furthermore, the practitioner is in an ideal position to identify overweight children and their families. He can then try to intervene before obesity has become established and intractable.[94]

REFERENCES

1. Adams, F. H., and Landaw, E. M.: What are healthy blood pressures for children? Pediatrics 68:268, 1981.
2. Adelman, R. D.: Neonatal hypertension. Pediatr. Clin. North Am. 25:99, 1978.
3. Antonini, A. C., and Dal Palu, C.: Pressione arteriosa sistolica. In Pordenone Study on the Precursors of Atherosclerosis in Childhood, edited by A. C. Antonini and C. Dal Palu, 1980, p. 109.
4. Armstrong, B., Skegg, D., White, G., and Doll, R.: Rauwolfia derivatives and breast cancer in hypertensive women. Lancet 2:8, 1976.
5. Balfe, J. W., and Rance, C. P.: Recognition and management of hypertensive crises in childhood. Pediatr. Clin. North Am. 25:159, 1978.
6. Becu, L.: Personal communication, Hospital de Ninos, Buenos Aires, 1979.

7. Berenson, G. A., Voors, A. W., Dalferes, E. R., et al.: Creatinine clearance, electrolytes and plasma renin activity related to the blood pressure of white and black children. J. Lab. Clin. Med. 93:535, 1979.
8. Beitins, I. Z., Baynard, F., Levitsky, L., et al.: Plasma, aldosterone concentration at delivery and during newborn period. J. Clin. Invest. 51:386, 1972.
9. Biron, P., Mongeau, J. C., and Bertrand, C.: Familial aggregation of blood pressure in 558 adopted children. Can. Med. Assoc. J. 115:773, 1976.
10. Black, I. F. S., Kotrapu, N., and Massie, H.: Application of Doppler ultrasound to blood pressure measurement in small infants. J. Pediatr. 81:932, 1972.
11. Blizzard, R. M., Liddle, G. W., Migeon, C. J., et al.: Aldosterone excretion in virilizing ad-

renal hyperplasia. Clin. Invest. 38:1442, 1959.
12. Buck, C. W.: The persistence of elevated blood pressure first observed at age 5. J. Chronic Dis. 26:101, 1973.
13. Cappe, B. E., and Pallin, I. M.: Systolic blood pressure determination in the newborn and infant. Anesthesiology 13:648, 1952.
14. Cutilletta, A. F.: Cardiovascular-hemodynamics role. In Hypertension in the Young (symposium). Johns Hopkins Medical Institution, Baltimore, 1980.
15. deSwiet, M., and Shinebourne, E. A.: Blood pressure in infancy (editorial). Am. Heart J. 94:399, 1977.
16. deSwiet, M., Fayers, P., and Shinebourne, E. A.: Systolic blood pressure in a population of infants in the first year of life: The Brompton Study. Pediatrics 65:1028, 1980.
17. Dillon, M. J., Gillin, M. E. A., Ryness, J. M.,

et al.: Plasma renin activity and aldosterone concentration in the human newborn. Arch. Dis. Child. 51:537, 1976.

18. Dillon, M. J., Shah, V., and Barratt, T. M.: Renal vein renin measurements in children with hypertension. Br. Med. J. 2:168, 1978.

19. Durante, D., Jones, D., and Spitzer, R.: Neonatal renal arterial embolism syndrome. J. Pediatr. 89:978, 1976.

20. Dustan, H. P., and Tarazi, R. C.: Hemodynamic abnormalities of adolescent hypertension. In Juvenile Hypertension, edited by M. I. New and L. S. Levine. Raven Press, New York, 1977, p. 181.

21. Dweck, H. S., and Cassady, G.: Indirect blood pressure measurement in newborns. Am. J. Dis. Child. 127:492, 1974.

22. Ellison, R. C., Senko, J. R., Harper, G. P., et al.: Obesity, sodium intake and blood pressure in adolescence. Hypertension, Part 2, 2:78, 1980.

23. Falkner, B., Onesti, G., Angelakos, et al.: Cardiovascular responses to mental stress in normal adolescents with hypertensive parents. Hemodynamics and mental stress in adolescents. Hypertension, Part 1, 1:23, 1979.

24. Feinleib, M., Garrison, R. J., Fabsitz, R., et al.: The National Heart, Lung and Blood Institute Twin Study of Cardiovascular Disease Risk Factors. Methodology and summary of results (Abstr.). Am. J. Epidemiol. 106:248, 1977.

25. Finnerty, F. A., Jr.: Contraception and pregnancy in the young female hypertensive patient. Pediatr. Clin. North Am. 25:119, 1978.

26. Fixler, D. E., Laird, W. P., Fitzgerald, V., et al.: Hypertension screening in schools: Results of the Dallas study. Pediatrics 63:32, 1979.

27. Fixler, D. E., Kautz, J. A., and Dana, K.: Systolic blood pressure differences among pediatric epidemiological studies. Hypertension, Part 2, 2:3, 1980.

28. Fixler, D. E., Laird, W. P., and Dana, K.: Prognostic value of exercise testing in hypertensive adolescents. Proceedings of the World Congress of Paediatric Cardiology, London, 1980.

29. Ford, K. T., Teplick, S. K., and Clarke, R. E.: Renal artery embolism causing neonatal hypertension. Radiology 113:169, 1974.

30. Fox, S., Pierce, W. S., and Waldhausen, J. A.: Pathogenesis of paradoxical hypertension after coarctation repair. Ann. Thorac. Surg. 29:135, 1980.

31. Frank, G. C., Berenson, G. S., and Webber, L. S.: Dietary studies and the relationship of cardiovascular disease in 10 year old children. Bogalusa Heart Study. Am. J. Clin. Nutr. 31:328, 1978.

32. Freis, E. D.: The treatment of hypertension—why, when and how. In "Hypertension Manual," edited by J. H. Laragh. Dun-Donnelley Publishing Corp., New York, 1974, p. 743.

33. Friedman, A., Chesney, R. W., Ball, D., et al.: Effective use of captopril (angiotensin I converting enzyme inhibitor) in severe childhood hypertension. J. Pediatr. 97:664, 1980.

34. Frolich, E. D., Tarazi, R. C., and Dustan, H. P.: Hyperdynamic beta-adrenergic circulatory state. Arch. Intern. Med. 123:1, 1969.

35. Frolich, E. D.: The adrenergic nervous system and hypertension: State of the art. Mayo Clin. Proc. 52:361, 1977.

36. Garay, R. P., and Meyer, P.: A new test showing abnormal net Na+ and K+ fluxes in erythrocytes of essential hypertension patients. Lancet 1:349, 1979.

37. Garay, R. P., Elghozi, J. L., Dagher, et al.: Laboratory distinction between essential and secondary hypertension by measurement of erythrocyte cation fluxes. N. Engl. J. Med. 302:769, 1980.

38. George, C. F., Lewis, P. J., and Petrie, A.: Clinical experience with use of ultrasound sphygmomanometer. Br. Heart J. 37:804, 1975.

39. Gerdts, K-G., Shah, V., Savage, J. M., et al.: Renal vein renin measurements in normotensive children. J. Pediatr. 95:953, 1979.

40. Gill, D. G., DaCosta, B. M., Cameron, J. S., et al.: Analysis of 100 children with severe and persistent hypertension. Arch. Dis. Child. 51:951, 1976.

41. Gillum, R. F.: Pathophysiology of hypertension in blacks and whites: A review of the basis of racial blood pressure differences. Hypertension 1:468, 1979.

42. Godard, C.: Predictive value of renal vein renin measurements in children with various forms of renal hypertension: An international study. Helv. Paediatr. Acta 32:49, 1977.

43. Goldring, D., and Wohltmann, H.: Flush method of blood pressure determinations in newborn infants. J. Pediatr. 40:285, 1952.

44. Goldring, D., Londe, S., Sivakoff, M., et al.: Blood pressure in a high school population. J. Pediatr. 91:884, 1977.

45. Gordillo-Paniagna, G., Velasquez-Jones, L., Martini, R., and Valdez-Bolanos: Sodium nitroprusside treatment of severe arterial hypertension in children. J. Pediatr. 87:799, 1975.

46. Grim, C. E., Miller, J. Z., Luft, F. C., et al.: Genetic influences on renin, aldosterone, and the renal excretion of sodium and potassium following volume expansion and contraction in normal man. Hypertension, Part 1, 1:583, 1979.

47. Hennekens, C. H., Jesse, M. J., Klein, B. E., et al.: Aggregation of blood pressure in infants and their siblings. Am. J. Epidemiol. 103:457, 1976.

48. Heyden, S., Bartel, A. G., Hames, C. G., et al.: Elevated blood pressure levels in adolescents. J.A.M.A. 209:1683, 1969.

49. Higgins, M. W., Keller, J. B., Metzner, H. L., et al.: Studies of blood pressure in Tecumseh, Mich. 2. Antecedents in children and of hypertension in young adults. Hypertension, Part 2, 2:117, 1980.

50. Hiner, L. B., Gruskin, A. B., Baluarte, H. J., et al.: Plasma renin activity in normal children. J. Pediatr. 89:258, 1976.

51. Holland, O. B., Chud, J. M., and Braunstein, H.: Urine kallikrein excretion in essential and mineralocorticoid hypertension. J. Clin. Invest. 65:347, 1980.

52. Hypertension Detection and Follow-Up Program Cooperative Group: Five year findings. I. Reduction in mortality of persons with high blood pressure, including mild hypertension. J.A.M.A. 242:2562, 1979.

53. Hypertension Detection and Follow-Up Program Cooperative Group: Five year findings. II. Mortality by race-sex and age. J.A.M.A. 242:2572, 1979.

54. Irias, J. J.: Hydralazine-induced lupus erythematous like syndrome. Am. J. Dis. Child. 129:862, 1975.

55. Julius, S.: Clinical and physiological significance of borderline hypertension at youth. Pediatr. Clin. North Am. 25:35, 1978.

56. Kaplan, N. M.: The sympathetic nervous system and hypertension. J. Hum. Stress 4:29, 1978.

57. Katz, S. H., Hediger, M. L., Schall, J. I., et al.: Blood pressure, growth and maturation from childhood through adolescence: Mixed longitudinal analyses of the Philadelphia blood pressure project. Hypertension, Part 2, 2:55, 1980.

58. Kilcoyne, M. M.: The developing phase of primary hypertension. I. Identification of the problem. Mod. Concepts Cardiovasc. Dis. 49:19, 1980.

59. Kimble, K. J., Darnall, R. A., Jr., Yelderman, M., Ariagno, R., and Ream, A. K.: An automated oscillometric technique for estimating mean arterial pressure in critically ill newborns. Anesthesiology 54:423, 1981.

60. Korobkin, M., Perloff, D. L., and Palubinskas, A. J.: Renal arteriography in the evaluation of unexplained hypertension in children and adolescents. J. Pediatr. 88:388, 1976.

61. Kotchen, J. M., Kotchen, T. A., and Guthrie, G. P., Jr.: Correlates of adolescent blood pressure at 5 year follow-up. Hypertension, Part 2, 2:124, 1980.

62. Kotchen, T. A., Strickland, A. L., Rice, T. W., et al.: A study of the renin-angiotensin system in newborn infants. J. Pediatr. 80:938, 1972.

63. Laird, W. P., and Fixler, D. E.: Left ventricular hypertrophy in adolescents with elevated blood pressure: Assessment by chest roentgenography, electrocardiography and echocardiography. Pediatrics 67:255, 1981.

64. Lanning, P., and Uhari, M.: The radiological evaluation of children with hypertension. Eur. J. Pediatr. 132:147, 1979.

65. Lauer, R. M., Connor, W. E., Leaverton, P. E., et al.: Coronary heart disease risk factors in school children: The Muscatine study. J. Pediatr. 86:697, 1975.

66. Lauer, R. M., and Clarke, W. R.: Immediate and long-term prognostic significance of childhood blood pressure levels. In Childhood Prevention of Atherosclerosis and Hypertension, edited by R. M. Lauer and R. B. Shekelle. Raven Press, New York, 1980, p. 281.

67. Lawton, W. J., and Fitz, A. E.: Urinary kallikrein in normal renin essential hypertension. Circulation 56:856, 1977.

68. Lawton, W. J., and Fitz, A. E.: Abnormality in kallikrein in hypertension is not related to aldosterone or plasma renin activity. Hypertension, Part 2, 2:787, 1980.

69. Lee, Y. H., Rosner, B., and Gould, J. B.: Familial aggregation in blood pressure of newborn infants and their mothers. Pediatrics 58:722, 1976.

70. Levine, L. S., Lewy, J. E., and New, M. I.: Hypertension in high school students: Evaluation in New York City. N.Y. State J. Med. 76:40, 1976.

71. Levy, S. B., Lilley, J. J., Frigon, R. P., et al.: Urinary kallikrein and plasma renin activity as determinants of renal blood flow. J. Clin. Invest. 60:129, 1977.

72. Linshaw, M. A., Stapleton, F. B., Gruskin, A. B., et al.: Traction related hypertension in children. J. Pediatr. 95:994, 1979.

73. Loggie, J. M. H.: Development of the autonomic nervous system. In Scientific Foundations of Paediatrics, edited by J. A. Davis and J. Dobbing, 2nd ed. William Heinemann Medical Books, London, 1974, pp. 640–648.

74. Loggie, J.: Essential hypertension in adolescents. Postgrad. Med. 56:133, 1974.

75. Loggie, J. M. H.: Juvenile hypertension. Compr. Ther. 3:47, 1977.

76. Loggie, J.: Prevalence of hypertension and distribution of causes. In Juvenile Hypertension, edited by M. New and M. S. Levine. Raven Press, New York, 1977, p. 1.

77. Loggie, J. M. H.: Systemic hypertension. In Heart Disease in Infants, Children and Adolescents, edited by A. Moss, F. Adams, and G. Emmanouilides. Williams & Wilkins, Baltimore, 1977, p. 645.

78. Loggie, J., New, M. I., and Robson, A.: Hypertension in the pediatric patient: A reappraisal. J. Pediatr. 94:685, 1979.

79. Londe, S., Bourgoignie, J. J., Robson, A. M., et al.: Hypertension in apparently normal children. J. Pediatr. 78:569, 1971.

80. Londe, S.: Causes of hypertension in the young. Pediatr. Clin. North Am. 25:41, 1978.

81. Londe, S., and Gollub, S. W.: Arm position and blood pressure. J. Pediatr. 94:617, 1979.

82. Luft, F. C., Grim, C. E., Higgins, J. T., Jr., et al.: Differences in responses to sodium administration in normotensive white and black subjects. J. Lab. Clin. Med. 90:555, 1977.

83. Luft, F. C., Grim, C. E., Fineberg, N., et al.:

Effects of volume expansion and contraction in normotensive whites, blacks and subjects of different ages. Circulation 59:643, 1979.

84. Lund-Johansen, P.: Hemodynamics in early essential hypertension. Acta Med. Scand. (Suppl.) 482:1, 1967.

85. McCrory, W. W., Kohaut, E. C., Lewy, J. E., et al.: The safety of intravenous diazoxide in children with severe hypertension. Clin. Pediatr. 18:661, 1979.

86. Miller, J. Z., Luft, F. C., Grim, C. E., et al.: Genetic influences on plasma and urinary norepinephrine after volume expansion and contraction in normal men. J. Clin. Endocrinol. Metab. 50:219, 1980.

87. Minick, M. C., and Conn, J. W.: Aldosterone excretion from infancy to adult life. Metabolism 13:681, 1964.

88. Mirkin, B. L., and Sinaiko, A.: Clinical pharmacology and therapeutic utilization of antihypertensive agents in children. In Juvenile Hypertension, edited by M. I. New and L. S. Levine. Raven Press, New York, 1977, p. 195.

89. Mitchell, D. S., Peel, H. H. Wigodsky, H. S., et al.: Non-invasive oscillometric measurement of blood pressure in baboons (papio cynocephalus). Lab. Anim. Sci. 30:666, 1980.

90. Mitchell, J. D., Baxter, T. J., Blair-West, J. R., et al.: Renin levels in nephroblastoma (Wilm's tumor). Report of a renin secreting tumor. Arch. Dis. Child. 45:376, 1970.

91. Moss, A. J., Liebling, W., Austin, W. O., et al.: An evaluation of the flush method for determining blood pressure in infants. Pediatrics 20:53, 1957.

92. Moss, A. J.: Indirect methods of blood pressure measurement. Pediatr. Clin. North Am. 25:3, 1978.

93. National Heart, Lung and Blood Institute: Report of the Task Force on Blood Pressure Control in Children. Pediatrics 59(Suppl.):797, 1977.

94. Neumann, C. G.: Prevention of obesity in infancy and childhood. In Childhood Prevention of Atherosclerosis and Hypertension, edited by R. M. Lauer and R. B. Shekelle. Raven Press, New York, 1980, p. 367.

95. New, M. I., and Levine, L. S.: An unidentified ACTH-stimulable adrenal steroid in childhood hypertension. In Juvenile Hypertension, edited by M. I. New and L. S. Levine. Raven Press, New York, 1977, p. 143.

96. New, M. I., and Levine, L. S.: Adrenocortical hypertension. Pediatr. Clin. North Am. 25:67, 1978.

97. Oberfield, S. E., Case, D. B., Levine, L. S., et al.: Use of the oral angiotensin I converting enzyme inhibitor (captopril) in childhood malignant hypertension. J. Pediatr. 95:641, 1979.

98. Paffenbarger, R. S., Jr., Thorne, M. C., and Wing, S. L.: Chronic disease in former college students. VIII. Characteristics in youth predisposing to hypertension in later years. Am. J. Epidemiol. 88:25, 1968.

99. Parker, F. B., Jr., Farrell, B., Streeten, D. P. H., et al.: Hypertensive mechanisms and coarctation of the aorta. J. Thorac. Cardiovasc. Surg. 80:568, 1980.

100. Perry, H. M.: Late toxicity of hydralazine resembling systemic lupus erythematosus or rheumatoid arthritis. Am. J. Med. 54:58, 1973.

101. Popp, M. B., Friedberg, B. L., and McMillan, B. G.: Clinical characteristics of hypertension in burned children. Ann. Surg. 191:483, 1980.

102. Prebis, J. W., Gruskin, A. B., Polinsky, M. S., et al.: Uric acid in childhood essential hypertension. J. Pediatr. 98:702, 1981.

103. Prineas, R. J., Gillum, R. F., and Blackburn, H.: Possibilities for primary prevention of hypertension. In Childhood Prevention of Atherosclerosis and Hypertension, edited by R. M. Lauer and R. B. Shekelle. Raven Press, New York, 1980, p. 357.

104. Prineas, R. J., Gillum, R. F., Horibe, H., et al.: The Minneapolis children's blood pressure study. Part I. Standards of measurements for children's blood pressure. Hypertension, Part 2, 2:18, 1980.

105. Rames, L. K., Clarke, W. R., Connor, W. E., et al.: Normal blood pressure and the evaluation of sustained blood pressure elevation in childhood: The Muscatine Study. Pediatrics 61:245, 1978.

106. Rance, C. P., Arbus, G. S., Balfe, J. W., et al.: Persistent systemic hypertension in infants and children. Pediatr. Clin. North Am. 21:801, 1974.

107. Reisin, E., Abel, R., Modan, M., et al.: Effect of weight loss without salt restriction on the reduction of blood pressure in overweight hypertensive patients. N. Engl. J. Med. 298:1, 1978.

108. Robertson, P. W., Klidjian, A., Harding, L. K., et al.: Hypertension due to renin-secreting renal tumour. Am. J. Med. 43:963, 1967.

109. Robson, A. M.: Special diagnostic studies for the detection of renal and renovascular forms of hypertension. Pediatr. Clin. North Am. 25:83, 1978.

110. Rosner, B., Hennekens, C. H., Kass, E. H., et al.: Age-specific correlation analyses of longitudinal blood pressure data. Am. J. Epidemiol. 106:306, 1977.

111. Sassard, J., Sann, L., Vincent, R., et al.: Plasma renin activity in normal subjects from infancy to puberty. J. Clin. Endocrinol. Metab. 40:524, 1975.

112. Scott, H. W., Jr., Dean, R. H., Boerth, R., et al.: Coarctation of the abdominal aorta: Pathophysiological and therapeutic considerations. Ann. Surg. 189:746, 1979.

113. Siegel, S., Fisher, D. A., Oh, W., et al.: Serum aldosterone concentrations related to sodium balance in the newborn infant. Pediatrics 53:410, 1974.

114. Siervogel, R. N., Frey, M. A. B., Kezdi, P., et al.: Blood pressure, electrolytes and body size: Their relationship. Hypertension, Part 2, 2:83, 1980.

115. Sinaiko, A. R., and Mirkin, B. L.: Clinical pharmacology of antihypertensive drugs in children. Pediatr. Clin. North Am. 25:137, 1978.

116. Stackpole, R. H., Melicow, M., and Uson, A. C.: Pheochromocytoma in children: Report of 9 cases and review of first 100 published cases with follow-up studies. J. Pediatr. 63:314, 1963.

117. Stalker, H. P., Holland, N. H., Kotchen, J. M., et al.: Plasma renin activity in healthy children. J. Pediatr. 89:256, 1976.

118. Still, J. L., and Cottom, D.: Severe hypertension in children. Arch. Dis. Child. 42:34, 1967.

119. Tobian, L.: The relationship of salt to hypertension. Am. J. Clin. Nutr. 32:2739, 1979.

120. Turner, M. C., Ruley, E. J., Buckley, K. M., et al.: Blood pressure elevation in children with orthopedic immobilization. J. Pediatr. 95:989, 1979.

121. U.S. Government Printing Office: Cardiovascular profile of 15,000 children of school age in 3 communities. DHEW Publication No. (N.I.H.) 78:1472, 1978.

122. U.S. Government Printing Office: Report of the Hypertension Task Force, Vol. 6—Current Research and Recommendations from the Task Force subgroups on Pediatrics-Genetics. DH Publication No. (N.I.H.) 79:1628, 1979.

123. Voors, A. W.: Cuff bladder size in a blood pressure survey of children. Am. J. Epidemiol. 101:489, 1975.

124. Voors, A. W., Webber, L. S., Frerichs, R. R., et al.: Body height and body mass as determinants of basal blood pressure in children—The Bogalusa Heart Study. Am. J. Epidemiol. 106:101, 1977.

125. Voors, A. W., Berenson, G. S., Dalferes, E. R., et al.: Racial differences in blood pressure control. Science 204:1091, 1979.

126. Ward, R. H., Chinn, P. G., and Pryor, I. A. M.: Tokelau Island migrant study effect of migration on the familial aggregation of blood pressure. Hypertension, Part 2, 2:43, 1980.

127. Ware, R. W., Laenger, C. J., Sr., and Heath, C. A.: Development of indirect blood pressure sensing technique for aerospace vehicle and simulator use. Volume III. Design, characteristics and operating instruction, AM RL - TR - 67 - 201 (II), Wright Patterson AFB, Ohio, Aerospace Medical Research Laboratories, August, 1968.

128. Watson, R. L., Langford, H. G., Abernethy, J. D., et al.: Urinary electrolytes, body weight, blood pressure, pooled cross-sectional results among four groups of adolescent females. Hypertension, Part 2, 2:93, 1980.

129. Weldon, V., Kowarski, A., and Migeon, C. J.: Aldosterone secretion rates in normal subjects from infancy to adulthood. Pediatrics 39:713, 1967.

130. Williams, W. S., Shindo, G., Trusler, G. A., et al.: Results of repair of coarctation of the aorta during infancy. J. Thorac. Cardiovasc. Surg. 79:603, 1980.

131. Yelderman, M., and Ream, A. K.: Indirect measurement of mean blood pressure in the anesthetized patient. Anesthesiology 50:253, 1979.

132. Zinner, S. H., Levy, P. S., and Kass, E. H.: Familial aggregation of blood pressure in childhood. N. Engl. J. Med. 284:401, 1971.

133. Zinner, S. H., Martin, L. F., Sacks, F., et al.: Longitudinal study of blood pressure in childhood. Am. J. Epidemiol. 100:437, 1974.

134. Zinner, S. H., Margolius, H. S., Rosner, B. R., et al.: Stability of blood pressure rank and urinary kallikrein concentration in childhood: An 8 year follow-up. Circulation 58:908, 1978.

44

Heart Failure

Norman S. Talner, M.D.

Heart failure in infancy and childhood represents a clinical syndrome which reflects the inability of the myocardium to meet the metabolic requirements of the body including those needs incurred by the growth process. This state may arise as a consequence of: excessive work load imposed on cardiac muscle usually by structural defects (mechanical factors); intrinsic alterations in myocardial performance as with inflammatory disease (myocardial factors); or from a combination of mechanical and myocardial elements. The sequelae of these factors are manifest clinically by signs of pulmonary and systemic venous congestion, and the operation of adaptive mechanisms, particularly those associated with increased adrenergic activity.

This syndrome is encountered frequently in the pediatric age group, especially in infancy, and has been the subject of several reviews.[36, 46, 54, 64, 65] The major aims of this chapter are: to present the physiologic mechanisms of heart failure, particularly as they apply to the younger age groups; to correlate the clinical expression of heart failure in the infant and child with physiologic derangements; and to provide a rational basis for diagnosis and treatment. Within this framework, the subject will be reviewed in terms of etiology, physiology, clinical manifestations, treatment, and prognosis.

ETIOLOGY

Congenital cardiac defects are usually responsible for the occurrence of heart failure in infancy and childhood, although the frequency is difficult to assess. In the New England Regional Infant Cardiac Program, where approximately 350 to 450 high-risk infants are admitted each year, upwards of 80% will have heart failure as a major component of their clinical presentation. After infancy, the frequency of heart failure strikingly diminishes.

The leading causes of heart failure in infancy relate to congenital cardiac defects and include: the hypoplastic left heart syndrome; coarctation of the aorta; ventricular septal defect; patent ductus arteriosus; atrioventricular canal; anomalous pulmonary venous connection; and transposition of the great arteries. Primary myocardial disease, particularly myocarditis, may evoke heart failure at any time, including the newborn period. Endocardial fibroelastosis, which had been listed as the leading cause of cardiac failure after the first 3 months of life in the first edition of this text, has continued to diminish in frequency. There is increasing evidence, however, that endocardial fibroelastosis in many instances represents a later stage in the evolution of a pathologic process which began as an acute myocarditis.[30, 56]

A variety of conditions, usually acquired, may produce cardiac decompensation in patients over the age of 1 year. Rheumatic heart disease, endocarditis, endomyocardial disease, and severe cardiac dysrhythmias now assume the leading roles in the etiology of cardiac failure. In addition, heart failure may occur as a complication of open heart surgical procedures. Myopericardial diseases, which may lead to cardiac failure, are usually of viral etiology, although bacterial infection, parasitic infestations, drug idiosyncrasies, and nutritional deficiencies have been incriminated. In many instances, a specific etiologic agent cannot be isolated, and a diagnosis of endomyocardial disease is listed as the cause of cardiac failure.

Heart failure may also appear as a consequence of changes in blood gas tensions and pH following severe neonatal asphyxia or obstructive disease of the upper or lower airway, such as: massively enlarged tonsils and adenoids; laryngomalacia; and cystic fibrosis. In these conditions, signs of cardiac decompensation reflect the effects of lowered PaO_2 and pH on the myocardium and pulmonary and systemic vasculature. In the newborn period, persistence of the fetal circulation with increased pulmonary vascular resistance can be associated with signs of right-sided heart failure. Asphyxial events during the delivery have also resulted in myocardial ischemia and have led to papillary muscle dysfunction and a low cardiac output.[6]

Other infrequently encountered causes of myocardial failure include severe anemia, glycogen storage disease, vasculitis (Kawasaki disease), mucopolysaccharide defects, Friedreich's ataxia, muscular dystrophy, cardiac tumors, and various metabolic diseases. In addition, heart failure may be provoked iatrogenically by the rapid infusion of fluids, especially blood and serum albumin.

The causes of heart failure in infancy and childhood may be classified on the basis of the fundamental disturbance in myocardial performance. These would include alterations in work load imposed on essentially normal cardiac muscle or primary disturbances in cardiac muscle function. Excessive work load can arise from volume overloading of the ventricles as might occur with large left to right shunts, valvular insufficiency, and systemic arteriovenous fistulae, or from pressure overloading of the ventricles, as might take place with obstruction to outflow, as seen in aortic stenosis, pulmonary stenosis, or coarctation of the aorta, or to inflow, as seen with mitral stenosis, cor triatriatum, or tricuspid stenosis.

Primary disorders affecting the inotropic state of cardiac muscle arise from inflammatory disease, electrolyte disturbances, endocrine problems, and coronary artery lesions. Myocardial performance may also be impaired by alterations in the chronotropic state of the heart as observed with tachydysrhythmias or severe forms of heart block.

The time of onset of symptoms of cardiac failure with congenital heart defects may provide a clue as to etiology of the impairment present. This is of interest from the standpoint of alterations in fetal hemodynamics, including changes in fetal flow pathways and pulmonary and systemic vascular resistances. Heart failure occurring at the time of birth signifies compromise of fetal circulatory function. Reisman et al.[52] have indicated that volume overloading of the right heart from tricuspid or pulmonary insufficiency or a systemic arteriovenous fistula, hypoplasia of the left heart, including premature closure of the foramen ovale with pulmonary venous obstruction, and birth asphyxia are the main causes of heart failure within the first few hours of life.

The hypoplastic left heart syndrome, principally aortic atresia, usually presents during the first week of life with signs of low systemic perfusion secondary to constriction of the ductus arteriosus and a falling pulmonary vascular resistance. These infants may tolerate their severe defect for 1 to 2 days, while the ductus remains widely patent, with the systemic circular bed perfused in retrograde fashion from the pulmonary artery with blood of relatively low oxygen tension. When the ductus arteriosus constricts, pulses diminish and a severe metabolic acidemia develops. With low systemic perfusion, it is noteworthy that the systemic arterial oxygen tension usually rises, reflecting an increase in the pulmonary-to-systemic blood flow ratio.

Coarctation of the aorta (CA) as a solitary lesion or in association with other cardiac defects usually presents with low systemic perfusion toward the end of the first or second week of life. The fetal flow pathway, the ductus arteriosus, provides the mechanism that leads to the development of heart failure, as in the hypoplastic left heart syndrome. During the fetal state, blood flow may pass through the aortic isthmus to the descending aorta via the aortic mouth of the ductus arteriosus in an unobstructed fashion, even though the basic pathologic lesion of coarctation, the posterior aortic shelf, is present in utero. Postnatally, as the ductus arteriosus undergoes constriction, the ventricle then faces an acute increase in afterload, and signs of cardiac failure rapidly ensue.[27, 55, 66]

In patients with total anomalous pulmonary venous connection, the signs of heart failure may be delayed if fetal flow channels remain patent, providing an escape mechanism for the obstructed pulmonary circuit. When the fetal channels become obliterated, signs of heart failure follow in the wake of pulmonary venous obstruction.

The presence of a patent ductus arteriosus (PDA) and the early development of heart failure in the small premature infant constitute an important clinical problem, particularly as there is an increasing survival of premature infants with idiopathic respiratory distress syndrome. The physiologic basis for this relates to a very rapid fall in pulmonary vascular resistance after birth in premature infants, permitting a large left to right shunt through the ductus arteriosus. Of equal importance in the preterm and newborn infant is the high resting cardiac output which limits the ability of the myocardium to handle a volume overload imposed by a left to right shunt. Other factors to be considered, however, include an increasing tendency toward transudation (leaky capillaries) in the more immature infants and intrinsic mechanical differences between fetal and adult cardiac muscle.

The timing of onset of heart failure in term infants with large left to right shunt at the ventricular or great artery level relates to the rapidity of postnatal fall in pulmonary vascular resistance. In addition to the postnatal alteration in the pulmonary vascular bed, the decrease in hemoglobin concentration after birth by diminishing viscosity, contributes to the fall in pulmonary vascular resistance.[32] Recent experience indicates that these infants manifest signs of interstitial pulmonary edema by 2 weeks of age, although the full-blown picture of cardiac failure may not be readily apparent before 6 weeks of age. Delays in the postnatal fall in pulmonary vascular resistance occur in infants born at altitude as compared to sea level patients.[70] Similarly, infants with pulmonary disease and diminished alveolar PO_2 and

elevated PCO_2 may also demonstrate a delay in the maturation of the pulmonary bed.[53]

PHYSIOLOGY

Determinants of Myocardial Performance

The performance of the heart as a muscle-pump system is dependent on its mechanical properties, in particular its shortening characteristics. The latter, in turn, reflects the summated and integrated working of the basic contractile element, the sarcomere.

The intrinsic properties of developing normal cardiac muscle have been extensively studied by Friedman et al.[22] Fetal myocardium develops a considerably greater resting tension for any degree of stretch than does adult myocardium, probably due to the lesser number of sarcomeres and greater water content of fetal muscle. When stimulated to contract, fetal myocardium develops less tension at any resting length than that of the adult. It should be noted, however, that, when corrections are made for noncontractile mass, the fetal cardiac muscle performs as well as adult cardiac muscle. Therefore, while the intrinsic strength of the sarcomeres appears to be similar at both ages, adult ventricular muscle generates more force per unit area.

There are four major determinants of myocardial performance which may occupy roles in the development of heart failure in infants and children.[28] The first of these, preload, relates to ventricular filling and can be estimated by end-diastolic volume. Augmentation of venous return increases preload with the heart responding via the Frank-Starling mechanism with an increase in the rate and extent of ventricular emptying. The volume-loaded ventricle is accompanied by an increase in ejection fraction, cardiac output, and peak dp/dt.

The second determinant is the force opposing myocardial fiber shortening or ejection load and is analogous to the afterload of the isolated muscle preparation. In the pressure-loaded ventricle encountered in infants under 2 weeks of age with coarctation of the aorta, there is a severe depression of left ventricular ejection fraction and output associated with normal left ventricular size. These alterations appear to be largely afterload related.[27] Infants who presented between 1 month and 8 months had less impairment of left heart function attributable to the development of compensatory left ventricular hypertrophy.

The third determinant is the contractile or inotropic state and is defined as the rate and force of contraction from a given preload and afterload. A decrease in contractile state is accompanied by a diminution in dp/dt, ejection fraction, and cardiac output from an increased or unchanged end-diastolic volume or systemic pressure.

Heart rate is the fourth major determinant, with increasing frequency of contraction producing a diminution in end-diastolic volume as diastolic filling is compromised. In general, tachydysrhythmias produce a fall in ejection fraction and cardiac output, while peak dp/dt increases.

In heart failure, isolated alterations in any one of these determinants would be unusual without changes in the other components.

ADAPTIVE MECHANISMS

It is now appropriate to review the fundamental adaptive mechanisms involved in modulation of the performance of the heart noted in heart failure as they pertain to infants and children. These include: altered ventricular mechanics associated with dilatation and hypertrophy; changes in the biochemistry of the cardiac muscle cell, including excitation-contraction coupling; alterations in fluid movement within the lung; intrinsic changes in red blood cell function related to oxygen transport; and disturbed autonomic control of myocardial performance and circulatory function.

Mechanical Factors

Ventricular Dilatation. One of the basic responses of the heart to the increased stress imposed by volume or pressure overloads is utilization of the Frank-Starling mechanism. An increase in end-diastolic volume of the ventricle permits the ejection of a larger stroke volume, even in the presence of diminished fiber shortening. However, because of geometric factors, the maintenance of systolic ventricular pressure in the presence of a dilated chamber is associated with an increase in wall tension and augmented myocardial oxygen requirement.

The adaptation to a volume overload is limited in the infant. This is due to the relatively high resting cardiac output, which therefore encroaches on diastolic reserve.[36] In addition, factors such as the development of anemia and febrile episodes will further compromise the ability of an infant to handle a volume overload.

Ventricular Hypertrophy. When an abnormal load is imposed on a ventricle, the development of myocardial hypertrophy provides the heart with another compensatory mechanism. When the load is extremely high, as with severe aortic or pulmonary stenosis, this compensation may no longer be adequate to permit the pumping mechanism to satisfy tissue oxygen requirements. The contractile state of the hypertrophied but nonfailing myocardium secondary to pressure loading is intermediate between that of normal and cardiac muscle with cardiac failure. With depression of each unit of the myocardium, the absolute increase in mass maintains an intermediary level of compensation.[62] The subendocardial region may become underperfused in relation to its oxygen needs with severe obstructive lesions, and signs of subendocardial ischemia become evident.

The hypertrophic response represents an attempt to maintain wall stress within the normal range. Wall stress as such is the force operative within a cross-sectional area of myocardium and takes into consideration wall thickness. With cardiac failure and chamber distension which is greater than the increase in wall thickness, wall stress will be greater than normal.

The translation of mechanical stress as might be imposed by volume and pressure overloads into an alteration of growth (hypertrophy) within the cell is a biologic process currently under investigation. There appear to be initial changes in the cell surface in the vicinity of the nucleus with increased wall tension that are reflected in altered amino acid transport, glucose uptake, and heightened RNA polymerase activity.[20] Increased RNA synthesis is stimulated early in the hypertrophic process, with muscle growth resulting primarily from enlargement of cell size rather than cellular hyperplasia.[26]

Contractility and energetics are normal in volume overload states as contrasted with the observations seen with pressure-induced hypertrophy where contractility is diminished.[10] Thus, hypertrophy is not the common denominator for the abnormalities in myocardial function and energetics, but rather the type of stress initiating the hypertrophy appears to be the factor which may be detrimental to myocardial contractility.

Also of interest is the observation that pressure-induced hypertrophy and abnormalities of contractility and cell energetics are reversible following removal of the afterload.[11] Alterations in connective tissue elements which accompany an increment in ventricular mass may not resolve, particularly if the process has been of long duration.

Dilatation and hypertrophy can be viewed as early manifestations of compromised cardiac performance, since, once they are evident, the heart has a diminished capability to handle further increases in mechanical load or decreases in myocardial contractility.

Biochemical Factors

Data suggest that the processes of energy production are sufficient to meet energy demands and may be normal.[51] Myocardial energy stores may be depressed with heart failure which is related to creatinine metabolism and not causally related to cardiac failure. The heart is able to convert chemical energy to mechanical work, although the rate may be reduced as indicated by a decrease in myofibrillar ATPase activity.[2] The fetal and newborn heart uses carbohydrates as its major energy source and has enzymatic deficiencies in relation to its ability to utilize fatty acids to meet energy requirements.[72] Of interest is the observation that carbohydrate stores have been noted to be diminished in infants with severe cardiac failure.[5]

Cardiac energy metabolism in the developing fetus and newborn has been reviewed by Friedman.[63] Mitochondria are the main source of the production of myocardial ATP, and the heart is dependent primarily on aerobic metabolism as in the adult. Oxidative phosphorylation in mitochondria from fetal and newborn sheep also show no age-related differences. Mitochondria from fetal and newborn lambs demonstrate increased oxygen consumption per milligram of protein in the presence of ADP when compared to the adult. Respiratory control ratios, a measure of the dependence of respiratory rate of ADP, are increased significantly in the fetus and newborn. Oxygen consumption in mitochondria uncoupled from ADP is higher in the fetus and newborn than in the adult, a reflection of increased electron transport. This increase in aerobic capacity of mitochondria may contribute toward meeting the additional energy requirements related to growth. Furthermore, age-dependent differences in mitochondrial oxidative phosphorylation may improve tolerance to hypoxia and represent a mechanism which is additive to the well-known increased anaerobic capacity of developing mammals.

Schwartz et al.[57] have reported increased State III respiration of mitochondria from the pressure-loaded hypertrophied but nonfailing rabbit myocardium. There is, in addition, an increase in State IV respiration (nonphosphorylating oxygen consumption) of mitochondria from pressure-loaded hypertrophic myocardium without cardiac failure.

Excitation-Contraction Coupling

The mobilization of calcium from extracellular and/or intracellular sites to the contractile elements begins with the excitation of the sarcolemma and terminates when calcium is bound to the modulatory protein, troponin. This is the excitation-contraction coupling process.[1, 34, 35] In cardiac muscle, the chain of events is as follows: with depolarization of the sarcolemma and T-system (tubules) by the cardiac action potential, calcium flux takes place, which results in an increase in calcium ion concentration within the cardiac cell. Calcium moves from the outside to the inside of the cell along a concentration gradient associated with an increased permeability of the sarcolemma to calcium and possibly the mobilization of calcium from the sarcolemma itself. Activation of myofilaments is achieved by release of intracellular stores of bound calcium from the sarcoplasmic reticulum plus the calcium derived from extracellular and sarcolemma sources. When calcium ion concentration rises above 10^{-7}M in the region of the myofilaments, calcium is then bound to troponin which initiates a chain of reactions which leads to the formation of actomyosin and muscle contraction. The development of tension is proportional to calcium release and activation of cross-bridges. Relaxation occurs when the calcium ion concentration surrounding the myofilaments falls, probably secondary to uptake by the sarcoplasmic reticulum.

The role of c-AMP-dependent phosphorylation in the regulation of myocardial function has been intensively studied.[9] In the cardiac muscle cell, regulatory substrates for modulating myocardial contractility are the myofibrillar proteins, sarcoplasmic reticulum, and the sarcolemma membrane. Phosphorylation of troponin I by cyclic AMP-dependent protein kinase may play a role in the regulation of myofibrillar ATPase sensitivity to calcium, and thereby alter contractility.[36] Recently, the phosphorylation of myosin light chains has also been associated with interventions which alter the inotropic state of cardiac muscle. The sarcoplasmic reticulum and sarcolemma may be other sites where cyclic AMP-dependent phosphorylation formation may be involved in the modulation of muscle function.

All of these sites that relate to the regulation of calcium movement and the contraction of cardiac muscle may be the loci for the altered cardiac performance seen with heart failure.

Adrenergic Mechanisms

An important mechanism in the regulation of cardiac performance pertains to the activity of the autonomic nervous system, particularly adrenergic function. The influence of the neurotransmitter substance, norepinephrine, on myocardial performance (beta receptor function) includes augmentation of heart rate, reduction in cardiac dimensions, increase in velocity of ejection and rate of tension development. Alpha receptor function relates to the control of peripheral vascular beds with the potential for altering regional perfusion.

Cholinergic effects on the myocardium relate to a decrease in the duration of the action potential and subsequent cellular influx of ionized calcium. Acetylcholine, the cholinergic substance, reduces adenyl cyclase activity which may be followed by decreased ventricular contractility.

In the adult with cardiac failure, cardiac norepinephrine stores are decreased with a depression of uptake, release, and subcellular distribution of norepinephrine as well. A loss of adrenergic nerves may take place with cardiac failure, and there is a reduction of tyrosine hydroxylase (the rate limiting enzyme in norepinephrine synthesis) in dogs with experimental heart failure as well as in specimens of cardiac muscle obtained at the time of cardiac surgery. The prolonged increase in sympathetic activity that accompanies heart failure may be the major factor responsible for the decrease in tyrosine hydroxylase activity. Catecholamine metabolite excretion has been found to be increased in infants with heart failure.[39]

The failing heart is limited in its response to nerve stimulation and dependent on circulating catecholamines of adrenal origin to maintain function. Dogs with cardiac failure show a decreased response to sympathetic stimulation, and beta receptor blockade with propranolol accentuates the signs of heart failure.[12]

Possibly related are the investigations by Friedman[22], in fetal and newborn mammals. Dynamic changes in the ana-

tomic, biochemical, and physiologic distribution of cardiac catecholamines take place in the perinatal period with age-dependent differences in the pharmacologic responsiveness of ventricular myocardium to norepinephrine. The hearts of fetal and newborn lambs at term are suprasensitive to norepinephrine. Histochemical studies have demonstrated that these hearts are only partially innervated at birth, with much of the norepinephrine residing in preterminal nerve trunks rather than in terminal nerve endings. Beta receptor sensitivity in fetal, newborn, and adult hearts are similar, so that the receptor sites appear to be fully functional prior to complete development of innervation. Tyrosine hydroxylase activity is decreased along with a diminished norepinephrine concentration in the myocardium. The adrenal glands, on the other hand, show abundant catecholamine stores. This has raised the suggestion that during the perinatal period the interaction between a suprasensitive myocardium and adrenal release of catecholamines occupy a compensatory role to maintain myocardial contractility. Thus, there are many similarities between adrenergic function in the fetal and newborn heart and the autonomic status observed in adults with heart failure. The small norepinephrine stores in the heart of the fetus and newborn, however, may be a functional pool which is capable of responding to adrenergic stimulation.[17] The magnitude and duration of stimulation required to deplete this source must still be defined.

Erythrocyte Oxygen Transport

In heart failure, delivery of oxygen to the tissues is compromised. A compensatory mechanism, which permits improvement of tissue oxygenation by increased oxygen-unloading capacity, resides in the red blood cell. This is accomplished by a rightward shift of the oxyhemoglobin dissociation curve via the 2,3-diphosphoglycerate mechanism and will be accompanied by an increase in the P50 value (oxygen tension at 50% saturation). This has been demonstrated in infants with cardiac failure, as well as in cyanotic states such as transposition of the great arteries and pulmonary atresia.[43] The increase in oxygen unloading is proportional to the degree of cyanosis or reduction in cardiac output. Following correction of lesions associated with cardiac failure, the rightward shift of the oxyhemoglobin dissociation curve returns to normal.

Pulmonary Dynamics

The pathogenesis of pulmonary edema has been more precisely characterized as the result of physiologic and ultrastructural investigations.[21, 62] Lung edema can be defined as an imbalance between the forces that move water into the extravascular spaces and the biologic devices for its removal. Under normal circumstances, any increase in water in the pulmonary interstitial space is associated with an increase in lymph flow and maintenance of the alveolar space free of protein. Should the excess rate of formation persist or increase, lung edema becomes manifest first as interstitial edema, with alveolar and airway edema representing later states in the process of fluid transudation. The clinical picture is dependent on the site of accumulation of lung water. Interstitial edema is manifest by an alteration in breathing pattern (tachypnea), possibly as a consequence of stimulation of juxtacapillary receptors (J receptors) localized in the pulmonary interstitial space[49] (Fig. 44.1). At this point, gas exchange function is maintained close to normal, as alveolar edema is not present. There will also be no auscultatory evidence of pulmonary edema at this time. This is the situation encountered in most infants with signs of cardiac failure. As fluid accumulates in the alveolar space, gas ex-

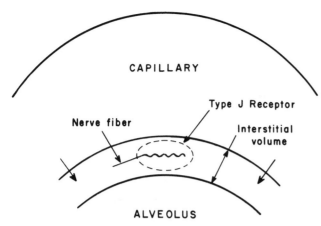

Fig. 44.1. Schematic representation of alveolar-pulmonary capillary relationship showing sites for fluid accumulation and critical location of the J receptors in the pulmonary interstitial space. (Modified from A. S. Paintal.[49]).

change function becomes impaired, first with a further decrease in arterial PaO_2, and finally by an increase in $PaCO_2$.[68] At this stage, rales and expiratory wheezing may be heard. The latter findings reflect fluid accumulation in the alveolar and peribronchiolar spaces.

Renal Mechanisms

The kidney occupies a crucial role in helping to restore adequate systemic blood flow in the presence of those pathologic states associated with heart failure. Through salt and water retention, the kidney provides a means for increasing the venous return and end-diastolic volume of the ventricle. This can potentially augment stroke volume via the Frank-Starling relationship and increase cardiac output.

The renal response to heart failure is physiologically similar to that of hypovolemia.[7] Both of these states share the common factor of a diminished cardiac output and diminished renal plasma flow. The retention of salt and water occurs as an attempt to restore intravascular volume and renal perfusion. The sequence of events that leads to enhanced sodium and water reabsorption begins with a decline in renal plasma flow secondary to the fall in cardiac output and a redistribution of systemic blood flow. With the fall in cardiac output there is constriction of the efferent glomerular arteriole and increased renal vascular resistance due to increased alpha adrenergic activity. This rise in efferent resistance allows a greater fraction of the plasma to be filtered, thus glomerular filtration rate is near the normal range while renal plasma flow is reduced. The increased filtration fraction will lower the postglomerular capillary hydrostatic pressure and increase the concentration of protein in the postglomerular peritubular capillaries. The combination of an increase in capillary oncotic pressure and decreased hydrostatic pressure both serve to enhance peritubular capillary uptake of proximal tubular fluid and, thus, increase the quantity of sodium reabsorbed in the proximal portion of the nephron.

In addition to the enhanced proximal tubular reabsorption, there is an increase in sodium reabsorption in the distal tubule and collecting duct. This takes place via the action of aldosterone in response to circulating angiotensin II.[14] Renin is secreted into the circulation from the juxtaglomerular cells surrounding renal afferent arterioles. The circulating substrate for renin is angiotensinogin. The trigger for renal release of renin is multifactorial: baroreceptor stimulation of the afferent arterioles due to decreased stretch secondary to

the fall in renal perfusion; stimulation of the macula densa by increased sodium or chloride in distal renal tubule; and stimulation of juxtaglomerular cells by adrenergic nerves and increased circulating norepinephrine. In the patient with heart failure, the first and third mechanisms seem more likely, since the solute concentration in the distal tubule at the macula densa would be expected to be decreased.

In plasma, renin acts on angiotensinogin to produce angiotensin I. During circulation to the lungs a converting enzyme cleaves two amino acids from angiotensin I to form angiotensin II. This potent vasoconstrictor serves as the principal stimulus for the release of aldosterone from the adrenal gland. Aldosterone catabolism is suppressed by decreased hepatic blood flow which contributes to the increased quantities of circulating aldosterone present in cardiac failure. Hyperaldosteronism has been documented in infants with heart failure.[3] Furthermore, urinary excretion of aldosterone has been shown to be increased in infants with circulatory failure.[64]

Other Regional Circulations

Changes in regional blood flow take place secondary to a fall in cardiac output. The effects of elevated venous pressure and low blood flow in the kidney have been discussed. Patients with low cardiac output at rest maintain their arterial blood pressure at a normal level by reflex vasoconstriction, probably initiated by baroreceptor stimulation. This is essential to maintain adequate perfusion of the central nervous system and the myocardium. This vasoconstriction is not generalized but regional, with a selective reduction in blood flow to the less vital organs of the body. The blood flow to the skin is diminished at a relatively early stage, and this has been confirmed by the plethysmography (Fig. 44.2). Skin and muscle blood flow is increased following the administration of digitalis. The peripheral cyanosis and cold skin of patients with heart failure, as well as the diminution in urinary output and alterations in regional blood flow, represent clinical evidence of peripheral vasoconstriction.

Body Metabolism

The striking degree of malnutrition that may accompany chronic heart failure has been noted by many and seems to parallel the severity of the disorder. The primary systemic event resulting from cardiac failure is cellular hypoxia. Closely related are a voluntary or imposed reduction in food

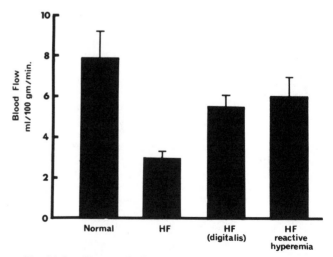

Fig. 44.2. Changes in the peripheral circulation in normal infants and infants with heart failure (HF).

intake and a relative or absolute degree of hypermetabolism. The latter has been documented in infants with cardiac failure by Lees et al.[40] who has shown that oxygen consumption in relation to body weight is increased. In infants with low perfusion states or severe hypoxemia, however, VO_2 has been shown to be decreased.

Other mechanisms which may also account for wasting with cardiac failure include protein-losing enteropathy, fat malabsorption, and digitalis intoxication. Correction of the cardiac defects affords the optimal avenue of therapeutic approach by removing tissue hypoxia as the primary inciting cause.

CLINICAL MANIFESTATIONS

While the signs and symptoms of heart failure in children are similar to those encountered in adults, the more subtle manifestations of heart failure in the infant constitute a major diagnostic challenge. The findings associated with cardiac failure will be discussed from the standpoint of alterations in circulatory physiology and as such fall into three general categories: direct alterations of myocardial performance, and the operation of adaptive mechanisms; pulmonary congestion; and systemic venous congestion.

SIGNS OF IMPAIRED MYOCARDIAL PERFORMANCE

Cardiac Enlargement

The presence of an enlarged cardiac silhouette on roentgen examination is the most consistent sign of impaired cardiac function and represents ventricular dilatation and/or hypertrophy. Cardiac size may be normal, however, with compromised function in the early stages of myocarditis, tachydysrhythmias, obstruction to pulmonary venous return, and pericardial constriction. The x-ray examination will also permit an assessment of the presence of pulmonary congestion and the association of inflammatory disease. A distinction between arterial and venous markings is difficult to make, especially in the small infant.

Tachycardia

An increase in heart rate above 160 per minute in infants and above 100 per minute in older children is commonly seen with cardiac failure. Tachycardia represents an adaptive mechanism to provide oxygen delivery to the tissues in the presence of lowered systemic perfusion. The increase in heart rate is an indicator of increased activity of the autonomic nervous system. Rates in excess of 230 per minute would raise the possibility of paroxysmal supraventricular tachycardia, which may have provoked the bout of cardiac failure. In older patients, a faster than normal cardiac rate with exercise with a delay in return to resting levels may be seen with early heart failure, even though the rate in the resting state might be normal.

Gallop Rhythm

A triple rhythm may be heard on auscultation in infants and children with myocardial failure, disappearing as failure is controlled. While this finding may represent an increase in flow across the atrioventricular valves in the presence of a large left to right shunt, a protodiastolic gallop coming at the time of rapid passive ventricular filling should raise the possibility of impaired ventricular function.

Peripheral Arterial Pulsations

Cold extremities, weakly palpable peripheral pulses, and lowered blood pressure are commonly seen when systemic blood flow is diminished. There may also be mottling of the extremities as further evidence of impaired tissue perfusion. When such infants respond to digitalis therapy or other inotropic intervention, it may be noted that arterial pulsations improve, the level of systolic blood pressure rises, and pulse pressure increases. Arterial pulsations may be bounding with an increased pulse pressure, even in the presence of severe cardiac failure, if a high output state exists, such as that associated with a large systemic arteriovenous fistula, or when there is a large runoff from the aorta into the pulmonary circulation. This may also be seen in states in which the hemoglobin content is less than 5 gm/dl.

Pulsus Paradoxus

This occurs frequently in children with large left to right shunts and is readily detected during auscultation for blood pressure determination. As the pressure in the cuff falls, one hears the systolic sound at first during expiration only, then at lower pressures during both expiration and inspiration. A similar phenomenon has been noted in older children with primary myocardial disease, as well as more classically in the accumulation of fluid in the pericardial sac. This represents variations in ventricular filling and output secondary to marked swings in intrapulmonary pressures.

Pulses Alternans

A change in peak systolic pressure, such that every second beat is of lower pressure, may be associated with myocardial disease and diminished ventricular performance. Palpation of the arterial pulse can detect this alteration in pressure from beat to beat, as well as changes in the rate of rise of the pressure pulse.

Growth Failure

Infants with cardiac failure are undernourished as a reflection of decreased systemic blood flow with impaired tissue perfusion. When the circulation is severely compromised, VO_2 falls, curtailing the infant's ability to grow. Respiratory difficulties contribute to a deficit in caloric intake, while, at the same time, hypermetabolism may raise energy requirements.

Sweating

Increased sweating has been noted in infants with cardiac failure, and this probably represents increased activity of the autonomic nervous system in the presence of impaired myocardial performance.

SIGNS OF PULMONARY CONGESTION

The major presenting manifestations of cardiac failure in infants relate to signs of altered respiratory function. These occur with left ventricular failure or pulmonary venous obstruction and are usually present prior to signs of systemic venous congestion.

Tachypnea

An increase in respiratory frequency with a decrease in tidal volume represents the clinical manifestation of interstitial pulmonary edema. At this point, respiratory effort may appear to be only minimally increased. As heart failure becomes more severe with the development of alveolar and bronchiolar edema, ventilatory function is significantly compromised, and air hunger may be evidenced by intercostal retractions, grunting, and labored respirations.

Wheezing

Rudolph[53] has called attention to the occurrence of wheezing as a sign of left ventricular failure in infancy. This picture may be easily confused with bronchiolitis, bronchopneumonia, and bronchial asthma. Obstructive phenomena may result from compression of the airway by distended pulmonary vasculature or an enlarged left atrium. Small airway edema may be the consequence of severe accumulation of water in the lung.

Rales

Rales are not usually heard until a considerable amount of fluid has entered alveoli, and their absence does not necessarily indicate that there is no pulmonary edema. If present, however, it implies that the process is severe and that not only has the interstitial space been involved but the alveolar space as well.

Cyanosis

With alveolar edema, cyanosis may be present even if the heart defect is not associated with intracardiac right to left shunting, thus supporting the presence of impaired gas exchange consequent to fluid accumulation in the lung. If there is an underlying lesion associated with decreased arterial oxygen tension, such as transposition of the great arteries, truncus arteriosus, and anomalous pulmonary venous connection, pulmonary congestion will further depress the level of PaO_2.

Dyspnea

Dyspnea with effort and paroxysmal nocturnal dyspnea are more characteristic of the older patient in cardiac failure and, when present, signify the presence of lesions compromising left ventricular performance or pulmonary blood flow. Infants, when challenged by feeding, will require a longer period of time to finish their formula, and this may be the infantile equivalent of dyspnea with exertion.

Cough

A chronic, hacking cough may also be present in children secondary to congestion of bronchial mucosa. Pulmonary infections should always be considered where coughing is a prominent symptom or if there is an elevation of temperature.

SIGNS OF SYSTEMIC VENOUS CONGESTION

Hepatomegaly

Enlargement of the liver is the most consistent sign of systemic venous congestion. This usually occurs following defects producing left heart failure, but pure right ventricular decompensation may be seen with pulmonary vascular obstructive disease and isolated pulmonary valve stenosis. Hepatic enlargement may also be associated with tricuspid valve disease, pericardial constriction, and anomalous pulmonary venous connection. Congestion of the liver reflects an increase in blood volume and venomotor tone. Tenderness of the liver and the absence of a firm, discrete edge can usually be elicited in older children with cardiac failure. Systolic pulsations of the liver may also occur with failure of the right heart and denotes insufficiency of the right atrioventricular valve. Presystolic pulsations indicate augmented atrial contractions secondary to either impaired right ventricular filling or increased resistance to blood flow across the foramen ovale. Specific timing of pulsations is difficult in the infant but can be elicited by simultaneous palpation of the liver edge and auscultation of the heart. In infancy, jaundice may occur in association with hepatic congestion and reflects the inability of the congested liver to handle bilirubin adequately.

Neck Vein Distention

Further evidence of elevation of systemic venous pressure may be seen in older children with cardiac failure by noting distention of neck veins but, because of their short neck, this is a sign that is difficult to assess in infants. Prominence of the veins on the back of the hand is a useful sign in small children. These veins should empty if the hand is held at or just above the sternal notch with the infant at an angle of 45°. Venous distention should be associated with other signs of systemic venous congestion.

Peripheral Edema

This is a rare finding with cardiac failure in infants and, when present, it usually signifies a poor outlook. Edema occurs when capillary pressure has risen above its normal level and fluid flows into the tissue spaces. The rate of edema development depends on the height of the capillary pressure and the resistance of tissues to stretch. Facial edema is more common in children than peripheral edema, while ascites and generalized anasarca are rare, except in older children with restrictive pericardial disease or severely compromised myocardial function.

Radiologic Findings

The importance of the x-ray examination in assessing cardiac size and pulmonary congestion has been discussed. Examples of chest x-rays obtained in infants with heart failure are shown in Figure 44.3. Any roentgenologic study performed on severely ill infants should be carried out as expeditiously as possible. We avoid barium instillation in these infants because of the dangers of aspiration. Fluoroscopy offers no additional information and prolongs the examination. If a pericardial effusion is a consideration, echocardiographic imaging should be performed.

Electrocardiographic Findings

The electrocardiogram is of little aid in the diagnosis of heart failure. Nonspecific T wave changes and alterations in the ST segment occur, as well as an increase in the height of the P wave. Low voltages with T wave abnormalities are frequently seen with myocarditis. The electrocardiogram may be helpful, however, in diagnosing dysrhythmias which may have precipitated cardiac failure.

Echocardiography

Ultrasound techniques have been introduced to assess myocardial function with measurement of right and left ventricular dimensions, circumferential fiber shortening rate, and ejection fraction, as well as systolic time intervals.[45, 60] Refinement of this technique in infants and young children permits a noninvasive method for assessing ventricular performance and is of use in following responses to therapeutic interventions.

Systolic Time Intervals

Another noninvasive approach to estimate ventricular function in heart failure is the determination of systolic time intervals using the electrocardiogram, phonocardiogram, and an arterial pulse tracing (axillary or carotid)[41] or appropriate echocardiographic images. Systolic time intervals were reviewed in 10 newborns and infants with cardiac failure before and after the administration of digoxin. Small doses of digoxin (30 µg/kg) produced shortening of the preejection period (PEP), while larger doses (80 µg/kg) usually elicited no further changes in PEP. The systolic ejection period was unaltered in this study. Park, Dimich, and Steinfeld[50] measured systolic time intervals in 150 normal infants and 15

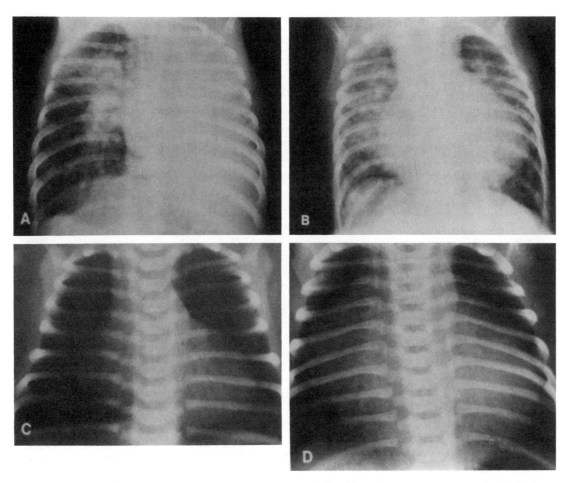

Fig. 44.3. Roentgenograms in infants presenting with cardiac failure. (*A*) Large volume left to right shunt with atelectasis of the left lower lung. (*B*) Large volume left to right shunt with pulmonary edema. (*C*) Cardiac enlargement (RA and RV) in an infant with critical pulmonary valve stenosis and signs of right heart failure. Striking diminution in pulmonary vascular markings can be seen. (*D*) Massive cardiomegaly in a 6-hour-old infant with congenital tricuspid insufficiency and systemic venous congestion.

babies with signs of left heart failure.[50] Systolic time intervals in infants with heart failure were found to be different from those reported in adults. Babies with large VSDs or CA had prolonged ejection times with respect to heart rate, while PEP was normal.

Blood Gases and pH

Certain patterns of blood gas and pH alterations have been observed in association with varying hemodynamic states that are accompanied by heart failure (Fig. 44.4).[67, 69] Volume overloading situations with severe pulmonary venous congestion are characterized by a slight diminution in PaO_2 levels due to intrapulmonary right to left shunting and ventilation-perfusion abnormalities. This is accompanied by a mild respiratory acidemia in those infants with severe heart failure and signifies that alveolar edema is present. Infants with milder symptoms of cardiac failure tend to show a respiratory alkalosis coinciding with interstitial rather than alveolar pulmonary edema. When pulmonary venous obstruction is the major hemodynamic problem, respiratory acidemia is commonly observed. The level of arterial oxygen tension is lower than with the volume overload group because of obligatory right to left shunting.

When infants with severe compromise of systemic perfusion were studied, a metabolic acidemia was found, the results of the accumulation of acid metabolites. Paradoxically, as pH falls, PaO_2 rises as a consequence of increasing pulmonary blood flow and diminished systemic output.

When the arterial oxygen tension is extremely low, as would be encountered in obstruction to pulmonary blood flow or TGA arteries with limited mixing, a metabolic acidemia also develops as a consequence of increased anaerobic metabolism. Under these circumstances, systemic blood flow is augmented but, despite this, the amount of oxygen delivered is insufficient to meet tissue demands.

Several characteristic changes in serum electrolytes have been observed in infants with cardiac failure.[64] These observations include the finding of hyponatremia (<120 mEq/liter). This probably reflects an increase in water retention in relation to sodium rather than a negative sodium balance. Hyponatremia has also been noted in adult patients with heart failure even when total body sodium was abnormally increased. When water-loading studies were performed, these patients failed to excrete the load normally. Overproduction or diminished inactivation of antidiuretic hormone was originally postulated as the mechanism leading to hyponatremia. Studies suggest that exaggerated proximal renal tubular reabsorption of glomerular filtrate, rather than antidiuretic hormone activity, may limit formation of free water in some patients with cardiac failure.[4]

Hypochloremia and an increase in bicarbonate represent compensatory responses to respiratory acidemia involving renal as well as blood and tissue buffer mechanisms.

Potassium levels may be elevated probably as a result of the release of intracellular cation with impaired tissue perfusion. Further evidence of tissue hypoxia relates to a rise of lactic acid in infants with cardiac failure.

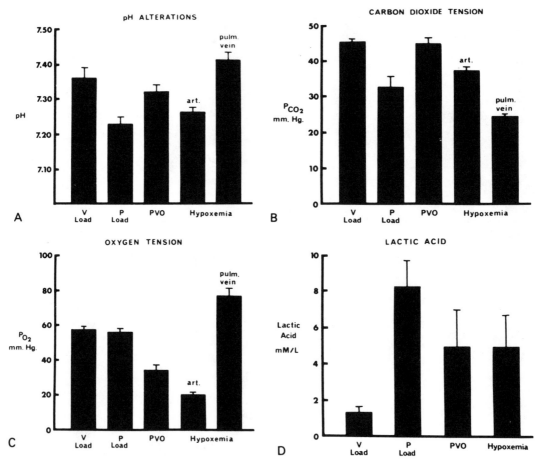

Fig. 44.4. pH, Pa_{CO2}, Pa_{O2}, and lactic alterations with volume (*V*) loading, pressure (*P*) loading, pulmonary venous obstruction (*PVO*), and hypoxemic states associated with heart failure.

Hemoglobin and Red Blood Count

A decrease in hemoglobin concentration and red blood cell count, indicating the presence of severe anemia, may initiate circulatory changes by either suddenly depleting blood volume with vascular collapse or, in a more chronic situation, by decreasing oxygen-carrying capacity and producing tissue hypoxia. Long-standing anemia is characterized by an elevated cardiac output and decreased peripheral resistance. An anemia may also accentuate the circulatory abnormalities associated with any primary cardiac problem. In the newborn period, a placental transfusion or twin-to-twin transfusion can produce volume overloading and heart failure. Under these circumstances, the hemoglobin and hematocrit will be elevated.

White Blood Count

An elevation of white blood count may be seen with cardiac failure and need not necessarily signify infection. Leukopenia has been noted in infants and children with viral myocarditis.

Sedimentation Rate

The significance of the sedimentation rate in a child with rheumatic fever and cardiac failure has been the subject of controversy. Spagnuolo and Feinstein[61] have proposed that a rheumatic fever patient with heart failure and a normal sedimentation rate has developed decompensation on the basis of a structural abnormality, e.g., severe mitral insufficiency. On the other hand, if the sedimentation rate is elevated, there is usually an active inflammatory process present.

Urinary Findings

Patients with heart failure may have albuminuria, urine of high specific gravity, and microscopic hematuria. Urinary output will be low in the presence of severe failure, and an increase in output can be used as a sign of improved myocardial function and a favorable response to anticongestive agents.

Blood Glucose and Calcium

Benzing et al.[5] reported the occurrence of severe hypoglycemia as a complication of heart failure in infants with congenital cardiac defects. Improvement of their clinical state followed the administration of glucose. Depletion of hepatic glycogen stores was documented by liver biopsy. The determination blood glucose should be carried out in any infant in heart failure, as treatment of hypoglycemia may afford considerable clinical improvement. In addition to blood glucose, serum calcium values may be low, as in infants of diabetic mothers. Cardiac function has, on occasion, dramatically improved following correction of hypocalcemia.

Hemodynamic Studies

The few hemodynamic investigations that have been carried out, while infants have been in manifest cardiac failure, have uncovered several interesting findings. Moss and Duffie[44] studied the levels of right atrial and systemic venous pressure in 22 infants during right heart catheterization at a time when they were thought to be in cardiac decompensation. Contrary to findings in adults, their data suggest that elevation of right atrial pressures appeared only as a terminal event. This observation may be explained by increased distensibility of the venous compartment in infants which will allow volume changes without significant pressure changes (increased compliance). Another consideration, however, concerns the effects of intrathoracic pressure on atrial dynamics in infants with failure so that the effective atrial pressures (atrial less intrathoracic) must be determined rather than the absolute level.

We have studied a number of infants with left ventricular failure secondary to left ventricular outflow obstruction or large left to right shunts, and these have shown, in most instances, the expected elevations of left ventricular end-diastolic, left atrial mean, and pulmonary venous pressures. In addition, arteriovenous oxygen content differences have been increased, indicating that systemic blood flow is diminished with increased oxygen extraction. We have also observed evidence of left to right shunting at the atrial level in infants in failure with either a large PDA or VSD. These infants were subsequently shown not to have an ASD. Left to right shunting via an incompetent foramen ovale may be a mechanism to maintain a lower pressure in the pulmonary veins while transferring a volume load to the right side of the circulation, although lowered filling pressures of the left ventricle may compromise left ventricular output.

Studies on older children with primary myocardial disease have shown abnormalities of their ventricular and atrial pressure tracings. Analysis of the ventricular pressure pulse revealed an early diastolic dip followed by plateauing, whereas right atrial pressure curves demonstrated prominence of an early diastolic depression coincident with the diastolic dip of the right ventricle. A marked fall in right atrial pressure occurred with ventricular ejection and, together with the early diastolic fall, produced an M-shaped or W-shaped atrial trace. The mean atrial pressures were elevated, and an impaired "x" descent or systolic plateau was observed on a few occasions. The latter may signify tricuspid insufficiency. Findings similar to these have also been seen in children and adults with pericardial disease.

Patient assessment can now include estimation of blood flow, pressure, chamber size, and volumes. From these variables and their derivatives, information related to myocardial distensibility and muscle mechanisms has been obtained. For each of the four major determinants of myocardial performance, alterations in end-diastolic volume, ejection fraction, peak dp/dt, and cardiac output have been measured (see section on Mechanical Factors). Moreover, muscle function can be characterized independently of pre- and afterload by the evaluation of the end-systolic pressure-volume relationship.[73]

DIFFERENTIAL DIAGNOSIS

The diagnosis of heart failure in older children is readily accomplished from the clinical manifestations. In infancy, however, the differential diagnosis usually rests between respiratory distress arising from cardiac disease and that associated with primary pulmonary disorders or alterations in the pulmonary circulation. The problems in differentiating pulmonary and cardiac causes of respiratory distress have been reviewed by Rudolph.[53]

Difficulties in recognizing cardiac failure in infants arise because typical cardiac findings are absent or obscured or because similar signs may exist with either cardiac or pulmonary conditions. Characteristic murmurs with certain defects, which are easily detectable at a later age, may not be present initially. Furthermore, breathing may be noisy and interfere with adequate auscultation of the heart.

The detection of rales or rhonchi on examination of the chest may not be especially helpful since these may be present with either cardiac or pulmonary disease. This is also true of hepatosplenomegaly as the liver and spleen may appear enlarged to palpation due to downward displacement of the diaphragm in patients with obstructive bronchopulmonary disease.

Cyanosis in association with pulmonary or cardiac disease may be only mild or moderate in degree. Marked cyanosis usually means a cardiac problem. The administration of oxygen to note improvement in oxygen saturation or the concomitant use of positive airway pressure may permit a differentiation between cardiac and pulmonary disease, particularly if there is an element of atelectasis. It should be pointed out, however, that infants with severe pulmonary lesions or a constricted pulmonary vascular bed with shunting through fetal pathways may not show an improvement in color with oxygen administration, and a decrease in cyanosis may be noted in the presence of a large left to right shunt with associated pulmonary insufficiency. The use of continuous positive airway pressure has been suggested as an added means to differentiate cardiac from respiratory problems.[58] If atelectasis constitutes a major factor responsible for lowering arterial oxygen tension, then the use of continuous positive airway pressure will effect a rise in the level of oxygenation. If cardiac disease with fixed right to left shunting is present, however, the PaO_2 may fall with continuous positive airway pressure.

An enlarged heart on x-ray examination should indicate the likelihood of a cardiac problem. It is important to reemphasize, nevertheless, that with some cardiac lesions the heart may appear normal in size. This is characteristic of obstructed pulmonary venous connection, where a considerable amount of blood is trapped in the pulmonary and systemic circulations. Under these circumstances, pulmonary congestion is represented by a typical radiologic pattern consisting of a diffuse, hazy, ground-glass appearance of the lung fields. In other conditions, the character of the lung fields may not be particularly helpful, since increased vascular markings, arterial or venous, may be difficult to distinguish from diffuse bronchopneumonia. Furthermore, pulmonary disease of an obstructive nature associated with a fall in arterial PaO_2 and a rise in $PaCO_2$ can induce depression of myocardial performance.

Recognition of the respiratory signs of left ventricular failure and pulmonary venous obstruction should result in a correct diagnosis by clinical and radiologic means in most instances. It should be stressed that a clear-cut differentiation at times may be extremely difficult. Infants with primary cardiac disease may have superimposed pulmonary problems while, in other situations, severe respiratory disease may be accompanied by signs of impaired myocardial function. The use of nuclear imaging and echocardiography provides additional means whereby cardiac disease may be more precisely defined.

TREATMENT

The treatment of heart failure must focus on measures which will improve myocardial performance. Careful attention to the clinical state is necessary with accurate recordings of heart rate, rhythm, respiratory frequency, pulse volume, weight, liver size, neck vein distension, pulmonary findings, degree of peripheral edema, and the presence or absence of cyanosis. Frequent clinical reappraisal is important in evaluating response to therapy.

DIGITALIS

Digitalis glycosides remain the drugs of choice in the treatment of heart failure in infants and children. During the past few years, important contributions concerning the mode of action of these medications have been made which have served to improve our understanding of their remarkable therapeutic qualities.

Cellular Basis for Action

The mechanism of action of digitalis in improving ventricular performance appears to reside in the control of ionic fluxes that accompany and mediate cardiac contraction. Langer[37] has been unable to demonstrate an increase in force development without demonstrating the inhibitory effects on active sodium pumping, and this process has been localized to the sarcolemma. Digitalis appears to interfere with the ATPase necessary for the removal of sodium from the cell by an active transport mechanism. Inhibition of the sodium pump would permit sodium to accumulate at the inner surface of the cell membrane. This accumulation would then allow for the influx of calcium into the area of the myofilament with each excitation, thus potentiating contractility.

Movement of potassium ions secondary to the sodium inhibition also takes place. As sodium increases in the cell, potassium is depleted in order to maintain an isoosmotic state. This probably has importance in relation to the toxic effects of digitalis with the production of dysrhythmias and heart block. Decreased potassium at the external surface of the cardiac muscle cell increases sensitivity of glycoside. This could also occur as a consequence of potent kaliuretic agents, such as ethacrynic acid and furosemide.

The appropriateness of digitalis in the treatment of the large volume left to right shunt has been open to question. When myocardial performance has been assessed using echocardiographic techniques to estimate the velocity of circumferential fiber shortening rate and ejection fraction, all of the values have been normal or supranormal. These findings reflect to some extent a decreased afterload and increased preload, present in left to right shunts, which would enhance the ability of the ventricles to eject large volumes of blood even if contractility was depressed. White and Lietman[74] have suggested that digitalis is of little value in infants with large left to right shunts in the face of these normal indices of ventricular contractility. While these lesions produce circulatory congestion, true myocardial failure does not appear to be present. On this basis they suggest a search for alternative forms of therapy. In this regard, our experience with afterload-reducing agents, such as sodium nitroprusside and hydralazine, have thus far been unrewarding, although alpha-adrenergic blockade with phentolamine has been shown to reduce the shunt size in experimentally produced ventricular septal defects.[63] We have been able, however, to diminish the magnitude of the left to right shunt in patients with large ventricular defects with the use of isovolemic exchange transfusion while maintaining systemic oxygen transport.[32]

The favorable response to digitalis observed in infants with left to right shunts suggests that the hemodynamic state is altered by the intervention. We speculate that digitalis may support myocardial function while adrenergic stimulation is withdrawn. This has been documented in the experimental animal where the administration of a rapidly acting digitalis glycoside diminishes sympathetic stimulation of the heart and peripheral circulation.[25] The decrease in heart rate, slowing of the respirations, and decrease in oxygen consumption which we have observed following the administration of digoxin would support the beneficial clinical response and would be in line with sympathetic withdrawal as glycoside therapy is instituted. Thus, we may substitute the local digitalis effect on myocardial contractility while removing the generalized increased adrenergic support which would be responsible for increasing body metabolism, tachycardia, and sweating.

Hemodynamic Effects

The principal hemodynamic effect of digitalis is its ability to increase the force of ventricular contraction. All other cardiovascular responses are considered secondary to this inotropic effect. When digitalis improves ventricular contractility, the ventricle empties more completely during systole, and the cardiac chambers are filled at a lower pressure. This initiates a series of responses which result in a rise in cardiac output, a decrease in cardiac enlargement, reduction in elevated venous pressure, and a slowing of heart rate.

Digitalis has also been shown to augment the force of contraction of the nonfailing heart, giving rise to the suggestion that it may exert a protective effect on myocardial function, when an unusual load or the hazard of depressed function is anticipated, such as in open heart surgery.

The effects of digitalis on the peripheral circulation occur secondary to improvement in myocardial function. With better cardiac performance, an increase in forearm blood flow and a decrease in vascular resistance and venomotor tone indicate a diminution in reflex arteriolar and venular constriction.

Effects on Conduction

The electrocardiographic effects of therapeutic doses of digitalis, such as depression or coving of the T waves, are manifestations of altered repolarization. Depression of the ST segment may also be evidence, while prolongation of the PR interval occurs with higher doses. Toxic doses may evoke extrasystoles, atrial dysrhythmias with block, and ventricular fibrillation.

Most of the effects of digitalis on conduction are only apparent when toxic ranges are reached. The refractory period of the AV node and His bundle is lengthened, while the refractory phase of the atria and ventricles is shortened. The latter may account for the increased irritability with larger doses of the medication. Slowing of cardiac rate probably reflects antiadrenergic activity, as myocardial performance is improved.

Metabolism, Distribution, and Excretion

The availability of labelled glycosides has afforded the opportunity to study distribution of these drugs. Serum levels following the administration of tritiated digoxin to patients with cardiac failure decrease along three exponential curves.[15, 16, 48] The first curve corresponds to distribution of the drug in blood, the second to dispersal in tissues, and the third to metabolism and excretion. Tritiated digoxin, when given orally, is 80% absorbed with a peak in the serum at 30 to 60 minutes following ingestion. When given intravenously, the serum peak is reached in 15 to 20 minutes.

The more rapid rate of renal excretion of digoxin when

compared to digitoxin is related to its breakdown into polar metabolites which are readily excreted. Sixty percent of administered C^{14} labeled digitoxin can be recovered in the urine as a combination of the drug and various metabolites.[48] Seventeen percent of the glycoside is lost in the feces.

The use of cardiopulmonary bypass has raised several questions related to the distribution and excretion of digitalis. The effect of bypass on digitalis disposition has been studied by several groups. In some of these investigations, concentrations of the drug in the myocardium did not appear to be altered, while others have found small decreases in radioactivity in cardiac muscle, with some glycoside appearing in the heart lung machine.[16]

Preparations and Dose

Regardless of the preparation used, the guiding principles for management remain the same. The particular glycoside chosen will ultimately depend on the experience of the physician prescribing the medication but, in general, one need only be familiar with a preparation that can be administered by the oral and parenteral routes.

Digoxin has been the most widely used digitalis glycoside in infants and children and is available in oral and parenteral forms. Absorption is variable from the gastrointestinal tract, and the parenteral dose is calculated at 75% of the oral dose. Advantages of digoxin for infants include a rapid excretion rate, allowing adjustment of dosage to meet individual needs, and ease of administration via a calibrated dropper. Rapidity of excretion may also be a disadvantage, for if the medication is stopped, digitalis effect is lost quickly, and signs of cardiac failure may reappear.

Engle[19] has championed the use of digitoxin for the treatment of cardiac failure, feeling that more stable control is achieved. This is a longer-acting digitalis glycoside which can be administered orally and parenterally. Absorption is complete from the gastrointestinal tract, so that the oral and parenteral doses are equal. Fears concerning prolonged toxicity with this preparation have not been realized.

All who have written on the use of digitalis in infants and children have cautioned about individual variations in response to the drug and the necessity for adjusting the dosage of the medication according to the patient's response. This is particularly true in treating children with inflammatory disease of the myocardium or in the postoperative state where enhanced sensitivity to digitalis is common.

When digitalis is prescribed, explicit instructions must be given to avoid potential errors which may result in a fatal outcome. The type of preparation to be used, e.g., digoxin or digitoxin, and its route of administration should be carefully set forth. The total digitalizing dose must be listed along with the basis (μg/kg) for arriving at this figure. Each dose in micrograms must be written out clearly, and the number of cubic centimeters of the preparation containing this amount shown. Calculations should be checked independently by another physician, if at all possible. In this way, decimal point errors may be picked up. Another precautionary point concerns the oral and parenteral preparations of digoxin. The oral preparation contains 50 μg/ml while the parenteral medication has 100 μg/ml or 250 μg/ml if the adult preparation is used. Therefore, these preparations cannot be used interchangeably.

Dosage schedules for digoxin are listed in Table 44.1. Over the past few years, we have utilized the intravenous route for acute severe heart failure more frequently, while for the less seriously ill infant or child we have administered the medication orally. In many instances, when early signs of heart failure are present, the maintenance dosage can be begun without a priming dose, and full digitalization will be achieved over 4 or 5 days. This approach requires only one calculation (maintenance dose) and lessens the chance for errors.

Parents should be shown how to use the calibrated dropper and must be instructed on signs of digitalis intoxication. They should report immediately if vomiting or changes in cardiac rate occur. The preparation should be stored out of reach of other siblings, as the accidental ingestion of digitalis has become a problem in its own right.

Neill[47] has called attention to the voluminous literature on the initial uses of digitalis for the control of cardiac failure but there is a paucity of reports on its continuance and discontinuance. After control of cardiac failure in the infant has been established, these infants are usually allowed to "outgrow the medication" sometime during the second year. Hastreiter and Miller[30] and Manning et al.[42] have stressed the need for prolonged administration of digitalis to patients with endocardial fibroelastosis and myocarditis. They recommend that the drug be given for at least 2 years after the onset of symptoms and that it be discontinued only if the cardiothoracic ratio is less than 55%, the child is asymptomatic, and there are no T wave changes in the left precordial leads.

Infants who have had a bout of paroxysmal supraventricular tachycardia during the first 3 months of life, who do not have underlying heart disease, should receive digitalis for at least 1 year.

Toxicity

While digitalis remains unchallenged as the most important single drug used for the treatment of cardiac failure, a relatively narrow gap exists between the optimum therapeutic dose of the agent and the dose that is toxic. The use of digitalis may require monitoring of the serum digoxin concentration, so that therapeutic levels of the drug are obtained and toxicity avoided. Close checks of serum electrolytes and frequent electrocardiographic monitoring are also required, particularly if myocarditis is the major problem. Serum digoxin levels have been shown to be in the range of 2.8 ± 1.9 ng/ml for infants, a level greater than obtained in older children or adults where 1.3 ± 0.4 ng/ml or 1.3 ± 0.6 ng/ml were encountered.[31] Infants with similar dose schedules show a higher serum concentration when digoxin is administered intravenously rather than orally. Sixty-five percent of infants on standard doses achieve levels greater than 2.0 ng/ml, which would be a level of toxicity in adults. The toxic range for infants seems to be in the range of 4 to 5 ng/ml, while in children it is in the range of 3 ng/ml. The value of a serum digoxin level relates to its usefulness in the diagnosis of digitalis toxicity and in the evaluation of patients in whom accidental ingestion has taken place. It also permits an assessment of the adequacy of digitalization and is of aid in the management of patients where renal problems exist.

TABLE 44.1   DIGOXIN PREPARATIONS AND DOSAGES

Oral	Parenteral	Digitalization (TDD[a])	Maintenance
Elixir 50 μg/ml	100 μg/ml	Prematures 20 μg/kg	5 μg/kg in divided doses
Unscored tablets 125 μg	250 μg/ml	<2 years 50 μg/kg	10–15 μg/kg in divided doses
Scored tablets 250 μg		>2 years 25–50 μg/kg	5–10 μg/kg in divided doses

[a] TDD, Total digitalizing dose, oral or IV.

Digitoxin concentrations have also been assessed in infants and children, and these studies confirm that infants tolerate a higher serum digitoxin concentration without toxicity than adults.[24] The assay has been used as a guide to the recognition of toxicity in infants, with a fair margin existing between toxic levels of 71 ng/ml as compared to therapeutic levels in the range of 30 ng/ml. The possible advantage of the digitoxin relates to its hepatic rather than renal clearance, which would be of benefit in situations where renal function is compromised. It has the additional advantage of requiring only a single daily dose to achieve steady serum concentrations.

The gap between therapeutic and toxic levels may be narrowed by many factors which must be taken into consideration when treating the patient. These include variations in individual susceptibility, age, electrolyte composition, and the presence of inflammatory myocardial disease. Interference with the normal dissipation of the drug may result from renal or hepatic disease. This problem may be further accentuated by intracellular potassium depletion which has followed the long continued administration of potent diuretic agents and may not necessarily be reflected in the serum level. The recognition of potassium depletion as one of the most common predisposing causes for digitalis intoxication is clearly desirable in order to initiate appropriate therapy. If the serum level is under 3.0 mEq/liter, there is strong evidence of potassium loss.

In the infant and child, digitalis intoxication may be associated with nonspecific constitutional disturbances. These include weakness and apathy, nausea and vomiting, and occasionally worsening of heart failure. Digitalis usually produces changes in electrocardiogram, and these consist of shortened QT intervals, sagging or depression of the ST segments, and flattening or inversion of the T waves. These alterations do not indicate toxicity, nor are they a measure of therapeutic effect. They are simply evidence of digitalis administration. Digitalis intoxication as manifest in the electrocardiogram in the infant or child may provide a spectrum of disorders of cardiac rhythm. It is often said that digitalis excess may result in almost any of the known cardiac dysrhythmias.

The key to the successful treatment of digitalis intoxication is early recognition of the problem and prompt withdrawal of the medication. This will usually result in disappearance of the dysrhythmias. Electrocardiographic monitoring of the patient is essential. Disturbances in cardiac rhythm which impair cardiac output do, however, require acute interventions. Sinus bradycardia, sinoatrial arrest, and second and third degree heart block may respond to atropine but may, on occasion, require electrical pacing. Phenytoin and lidocaine are useful agents in the treatment of ectopic dysrhythmias. The intravenous dose of phenytoin is 1 to 5 mg/kg in divided doses over 1 hour. Lidocaine may be administered as a bolus injection of 1 mg/kg followed by a continuous infusion of 1 mg/kg/hour.

The use of intravenous potassium supplementation is recommended when hypokalemia is present but should be used with caution and under close electrocardiographic monitoring. Propranolol has also achieved some success for digoxin-induced dysrhythmias. With this medication, undesirable effects include bradycardia and decreased myocardial contractility.

For immediate life-threatening dysrhythmias refractory to other modes of therapy, DC countershock can be utilized, although it may itself produce severe rhythm disturbances. When used, the energy to achieve conversion should be started at lower levels in order to possibly avoid this problem.

The use of cardiac glycoside-specific antibodies for the treatment of digitalis intoxication has been introduced.[59] Antiserum from animals previously immunized with digoxin-albumin conjugates has reversed digitalis intoxication in the animal model. Fab fragments of digoxin-specific antibodies have been obtained and have certain advantages over purified intact antibodies. The smaller size of the Fab molecule permits it to pass through the glomerulus and be excreted in the urine. Digoxin-bound Fab fragments are then rapidly excreted. Plans are under way to have the Fab fragments available at centers for the treatment of patients with life-threatening digitalis intoxication which has failed to respond to the standard methods of therapy.

OTHER INOTROPIC DRUGS

The beta receptor agonists, isoproterenol, dopamine, or dobutamine have been utilized in infants and children with severe heart failure. The majority of experience has been with isoproterenol which will improve tissue perfusion by its positive inotropic effects, although its chronotropic action and dysrhythmia production have on occasion limited the usefulness of this agent. Isoproterenol also produces a peripheral vasodilatation, diminishing peripheral vascular resistance with augmentation of cutaneous and skeletal blood flow.[33]

Dopamine, a naturally occurring catecholamine that is the precursor of norepinephrine, is another positive inotropic agent. This medication does not appear to produce marked chronotropic changes, while regional perfusion, particularly to the kidney, is enhanced.[18, 33]

Dobutamine is a synthetic sympathomimetic amine that stimulates beta 1-, beta 2-, and alpha-adrenergic receptors.[52a] When compared to isoproterenol at equivalent inotropic effects, this agent exerts a weaker beta 2-adrenergic action. Dobutamine is also a weaker alpha-adrenergic agent than dopamine. In contrast to dopamine, however, dobutamine does not alter renal blood flow but does alter the redistribution of cardiac output in favor of the coronary and skeletal muscle circulations. In doses up to 10 μg/kg/minute cardiac output increases while systemic and pulmonary vascular resistances decrease, as compared to dopamine where at slightly lower doses the systemic and pulmonary vascular resistances increase.

All of the sympathomimetic amines can induce serious cardiac dysrhythmias, and therefore the electrocardiogram must be observed carefully during the administration of these agents. They also may be used in conjunction with vasodilator therapy but require constant measurement of cardiac output and filling pressures in order to avoid hypovolemia and compromised systemic perfusion.

The dosage schedules for isoproterenol, dopamine, and dobutamine are listed in Table 44.2. These drugs should be administered via an infusion pump with monitoring of cen-

TABLE 44.2   INOTROPIC DRUGS

Agent	Dosage Form	Dose[a]
Isoproterenol	250 μg/ml	0.05–0.5 μg/kg/min; usual dose, 0.1 μ/kg/min
Dopamine	40 mg/ml	5–10 μg/kg/min; up to 50 μg/kg/min
Dobutamine	25 mg/ml when diluted	5–10 μg/kg/min

[a] Given in 5% glucose and water.

tral venous and wedge pressure, arterial pressure, electro-cardiogram, and urinary output. Careful attention should be paid to avoiding excessive fluid loads and the production of hyperosmolar states. The latter may develop as a consequence of injudicious use of sodium bicarbonate to correct the metabolic acidemia.

VASODILATOR THERAPY

Alterations in the resistance and capacitance of the peripheral vascular bed can affect the performance of the heart as a pump. An increase in systemic vascular resistance at a constant preload and inotropic state will result in a decrease in cardiac output. This has led to the use of vasodilator therapy in order to relax vascular smooth muscle and thereby alter loading conditions on the heart and modify cardiac performance.[8, 9a] When the major effect is to relax arteriolar smooth muscle, afterload is reduced, and this may augment cardiac output. Venodilatation, on the other hand, exerts its effects on preload by increasing the capacitance of the systemic vascular bed and lowering filling volumes. This will diminish pulmonary and systemic venous congestion. When these agents are used, close monitoring of filling pressures and arterial blood pressure must be carried out, otherwise it is possible for the clinical status to deteriorate because of a fall in filling pressure and of the development of systemic hypotension, both of which may decrease cardiac output. The specific choice of a dilator agent is then dependent on whether the clinician desires to alter preload or afterload or both.

A pure venodilator would be expected to be beneficial for those patients with increased end-diastolic volumes but would be contraindicated when filling pressures are normal, as might occur following diuretic therapy. Afterload-reducing agents would be expected to be most beneficial when systemic vascular resistance is increased and cardiac output has fallen. Under these conditions arteriolar dilators are capable of producing an increase in stroke volume and cardiac output and thereby reducing symptoms that arise from compromised systemic perfusion.

There are a number of vasodilators that have been used in infants and children, particularly in the management of the low output states that may occur following the repair of congenital cardiac defects. They have also been used in the treatment of the refractory heart failure seen with cardiomyopathies. Sodium nitroprusside is probably the most widely used vasodilator. This agent must be administered intravenously. It is a smooth muscle dilator on both arterioles and veins and acts to decrease filling pressure and lower systemic vascular resistance. When used, the patient's blood pressure must be monitored closely, as hypotension can occur. This can be reversed with volume infusion or the use of a vasoconstrictor. Sodium nitroprusside is converted to thiocyanate in the presence of thiosulfate. Thiocyanate is excreted by the kidney. When renal function is impaired the use of nitroprusside may lead to thiocyanate toxicity with central nervous system symptomatology, hypothyroidism, abdominal pain, and muscular twitching. Serum levels of thiocyanate should be measured and the drug discontinued if the levels are greater than 6 mg/dl.

The agent phentolamine has also been used in heart failure. The principal modes of action of this drug are: to block alpha-adrenergic receptors, primarily of arterioles; to directly relax vascular smooth muscle; and to increase norepinephrine release and thus achieve chronotropic and inotropic effects. In a similar fashion to nitroprusside, this drug must be administered intravenously, is short acting, and requires titration in order to achieve the desired therapeutic effect.

Agents that act primarily on capacitance vessels include the nitrates. They may be administered via various routes, which makes them available for long-term usage. The side effects of all nitrates include headache and postural hypotension.

Hydralazine is an effective oral vasodilator which acts directly on arteriolar smooth muscle. The action on the resistance vessels results in an increase in cardiac output with little effect on ventricular filling. Side effects of this medication include headache, nausea and vomiting, drug-induced fever, and rash. A systemic lupus erythematosis-like syndrome has been described in 15% of patients who are usually on high dose therapy. Since relatively high doses of hydralazine are required, this may represent a significant complication.

Prazosin is a potent alpha-adrenergic blocking agent but not at presynaptic sites. It has direct action on vascular smooth muscle. The medication can be used orally and has effects similar to nitroprusside. Side effects include arthralgias, headache, urinary incontinence, rashes, and a dry mouth. There are many reports of "first dose" phenomenon in which transient faintness, dizziness, palpitation, and occasionally syncope may occur.

Another group of agents that inhibit the renin-angiotensin system have been recently introduced. A competetive antagonist of angiotensin II, saralasin, has increased cardiac output and reduced systemic and end-diastolic pressures. This had led to the development of other agents, captopril and teprotide, which block the conversion of angiotensin I to angiotensin II.[14a] Few adverse side effects have been reported, although there have been reports of the development of the nephrotic syndrome following the use of captapril.

The vasodilator agents that have been used clinically are listed in Table 44.3. The bulk of the pediatric experience has been with sodium nitroprusside, hydralazine, phentolamine, and the nitrates.[14b]

DIURETICS

Physiologic Basis for Diuretic Therapy

Diminished perfusion of the kidneys is the result of failure of the pumping mechanism. This reduction in renal blood flow is then associated with a signal to the kidney to conserve sodium, the factor which underlies fluid retention. Diuretics occupy a key role in the treatment of the congestive element of cardiac failure, but it should be kept in mind that the primary aims of therapy are to improve myocardial performance and decrease pulmonary and systemic venous congestion.[29, 38]

The major diuretic drugs available for the treatment of heart failure include: the thiazides, the loop diuretics, and the aldosterone antagonists.

TABLE 44.3 VASODILATOR DRUGS

Agent	Route	Dose
Sodium nitroprusside	IV	0.5–2.0 μg/kg/min[a]
Phentolamine	IV	1–5 μg/kg/min[a]
Trimethaphan	IV	3–5 μg/kg/min[a]
Isosorbide dinitrate	Oral	5 mg q6h[a]
Nitroglycerin ointment	Topical	0.5–3.0 inch tapes
Hydralazine	IV	0.5–1.0 mg/kg
	Oral	1.0–5.0 mg/kg
Prazosin	Oral	25 μg/kg/q6h

[a] Dose must be titrated.

Drugs

Thiazides. The sites of action of chlorothiazide and hydrothiazide are in the proximal tubule and in the diluting segment of the distal tubule. These drugs do not interfere with urinary concentration. This results in an inhibition of free water formation and an excretion of sodium, water, chloride, potassium, and other ions. The kaliuretic effect contributes one of the problems in usage.

Loop Diuretics. Ethcrynic acid and furosemide exert a quantitatively greater effect than thiazides by interfering with diluting mechanisms in the distal cortical tubules. In addition, they block sodium transport in the loop of Henle and early ascending limb and, therefore, slow the process of urinary concentration, as well as affecting diluting function. Their major utilization is in the acute treatment of heart failure. Their chronic usage requires vigorous attention to the problems of hypoosmolarity and potassium loss.

Aldosterone Antagonists. Aldosterone promotes sodium retention and potassium excretion. Consequently, their antagonists assume a role in diuretic therapy. Of the pharmacologic agents available, spironolactone is the most widely used. These drugs act by competing for receptor sites at the distal renal tubule where aldosterone-catalyzed exchange between sodium and potassium ions takes place. These drugs have value in correcting the potassium loss produced by thiazides or ethacrynic acid and furosemide. Preparations and dosage schedules for patients requiring diuretic therapy are outlined in Table 44.4.

Problems with Diuretic Therapy

The use of diuretic drugs may produce alterations in electrolyte composition, and their administration demands frequent checks of acid-base equilibrium. Walker and Cooke[71] have reviewed the electrolyte abnormalities associated with the use of diuretic agents in adults with cardiac failure. These are summarized in the following paragraphs.

Dilutional Hyponatremia. A lowered serum sodium concentration usually reflects retention of greater quantities of water than sodium rather than salt depletion from diuretic therapy.[4] We have not been impressed with related symptomatology occurring in infants with hyponatremia, although in adults signs of mental aberration, somnolence progressing to coma, and convulsions have been observed. Treatment of this condition relates to the improvement of myocardial function coupled with water restriction. When myocardial function improves, sodium and water balance will usually return to normal.

Hypokalemia. Potassium loss is enhanced by thiazide, furosemide, and ethacrynic acid diuretics which may deplete body potassium stores. This occurs because these drugs increase the quantity of sodium that reaches the distal tubule, and here the sodium-for-potassium exchange results in considerably greater potassium excretion. The effect of hypokalemia on digitalis sensitivity has already been discussed.

Hyperkalemia. This hazard arises in patients with severe cardiac failure who are receiving diuretics that inhibit potassium secretion (spironolactone) or in patients who fail to respond to diuretics. In the latter situation, giving potassium supplements may result in dangerous elevation of serum potassium.

Disturbances in Hydrogen Ion Concentration. Hypochloremic alkalosis may be seen in older children as a result of depression of the sodium and chloride transport mechanism. No manifestations are usually associated with these alterations. The sequence of events following the administration of diuretic agents, which evoke a sodium diuresis, involves depression of sodium chloride reabsorption and a tendency of the kidney to compensate for sodium loss. This results in a greater excretion of chloride than sodium. As this continues, hypochloremia develops. The anion deficit is repaired by elevating bicarbonate concentration, and thus the overall effect is the production of hypochloremic alkalosis.

Acute Sodium Depletion. One of the more common complications of diuretic therapy is acute sodium depletion. The symptoms involve lethargy and somnolence following a massive diuresis induced by vigorous decongestive measures. This is associated with complete disappearance of edema and possible reduction in skin turgor. In extreme cases, there may be a substantial drop in blood pressure. In general, however, this complication is usually not very severe and, if recognized, can be reversed by liberalizing sodium intake. Salt depletion can nearly always be avoided, if diuretic therapy is initiated cautiously in relatively low doses and 2 to 3 days are allowed between injections to permit an evaluation of the patient's response to therapy.

OTHER THERAPEUTIC MEASURES

Position

The use of a modified cardiac chair seems to improve pulmonary function in infants with cardiac failure. This can be achieved by elevation of the head and shoulders to at least a 45° angle by placing a pillow behind the back and a small blanket roll beneath the knees or by the use of an infant seat. It is important to maintain the lower extremities dependent to permit peripheral pooling, thus lessening the load on the pulmonary circulation. For older children, the head of the bed should be elevated to ease respirations and allow for peripheral rather than pulmonary pooling.

Oxygen

Oxygen tensions are diminished in infants with cardiac failure, further depriving the tissues of their oxygen supply. When infants are placed in an oxygen environment with increased humidity, they usually improve. Adequate humidification is necessary to loosen secretions, and this can be achieved by the use of a conventional oxygen tent with the oxygen bubbled through a nebulizer. Adequate temperature control should be achieved in the tent so that the infant's body temperature can be maintained within the neutral range and extreme fluctuations are avoided.

Bed Rest

In attempting to decrease the load on the compromised myocardium, bed rest is usually advised, particularly for the

TABLE 44.4   DIURETIC DRUGS[a]

Agent	Route	Dose
Thiazide		
Chlorothiazide	Oral	20–40 mg/kg/day
Hydrochlorothiazide	Oral	2–5 mg/kg/day
Loop diuretics		
Ethacrynic acid	IV	1 mg/kg/dose
	Oral	2–3 mg/kg/day
Furosemide	IV	1–3 mg/kg/dose
	Oral	2–5 mg/kg/day
Aldosterone antagonists		
Spironolactone	Oral	1–2 mg/kg/day

[a] Intermittent therapy is recommended on a long-term basis to prevent electrolyte complications.

older child with acquired cardiac disease. This takes the form of adherence to a prescribed bed rest regimen when the child is ill, with increasing activity as he responds favorably to therapy. Television has afforded youngsters considerable distraction while they are being treated and perhaps provides the proper environment for carrying out a bed rest program. Nadas and Fyler[46] have stressed a flexible program of imposed bed rest which takes into consideration the child's reaction to his disease.

Diet

In most instances, cardiac failure can be controlled by the use of digitalis and diuretic agents without altering dietary composition. During the initial attempts at management of the critically ill infant, we give clear liquid feedings of 10% glucose and water to avoid the problems associated with the aspiration of formula. As the infant responds to treatment, formulae are prescribed that provide adequate calories to meet growth requirements and absence of diarrhea and vomiting. Excessive concentration of the formula and high protein feeding should be avoided, as these increase the osmotic load on the kidney while failing to supply adequate amounts of water.

We have used simulated breast milk preparations in feeding infants with heart failure because of the low solute load and protein content. Low sodium formulae are available, but many are not palatable, provide too little sodium to satisfy growth requirements, and may be associated with electrolyte disturbances.

In children with signs of systemic venous congestion and peripheral edema, a diet with no added salt is prescribed. Dietary management has to be modified, however, depending on the child's reaction to salt restriction. A happy child whose excess salt and water are controlled with medications is obviously preferred to a miserable patient who, feeling deprived of his rights to enjoy food, refuses to eat.

Steroids

The utilization of corticosteroids in conjunction with digitalis and diuretic therapy has diminished the mortality from heart failure seen with rheumatic carditis and viral myocarditis.[54] If these patients evidence cardiac failure, prednisone therapy is begun at a dosage of 2 mg/kg/day. When signs of decompensation come under control, usually within a week, we taper the steroid over a 5- to 7-day period, switching to salicylates in those patients with rheumatic carditis.

Mechanical Ventilation

In infants with severe pulmonary edema and accompanying respiratory failure ($PaCO_2$ >50 mm Hg), controlled ventilation is indicated with endotracheal intubation, muscle relaxants, and a volume-controlled positive pressure respirator. The addition of positive-end expiratory pressure is also beneficial. This has been accomplished in a few infants with large volume left to right shunts in severe cardiac failure and has allowed us to proceed with diagnostic studies and palliative or corrective surgery under conditions in which blood gas tensions and pH values more closely approximate normal.

Antibiotics

It is difficult to rule out the presence of infection in infants or older children with cardiac failure. Indeed, infection may frequently precipitate a bout of cardiac failure. We routinely obtain nasopharyngeal and blood cultures in all infants with cardiac decompensation and administer antibiotics in the presence of a likely infection. Temperature elevation should be controlled with antipyretics to decrease oxygen demands.

Sedation

With pulmonary edema, morphine sulfate, 0.05 mg/kg, can be given subcutaneously, if the infants are carefully observed. Patients with pulmonary congestion seem to breathe more easily, and gas exchange improves. This therapeutic approach is usually only necessary as one attempts to bring failure under control.

Treatment of Underlying Condition

It should be emphasized that control of heart failure is only a preliminary to establish a diagnosis. Many corrective procedures are now available for the seriously ill infant with congenital heart disease that may result in improvement in cardiac function. In many situations, diagnostic studies may have to be carried out in the face of frank failure in the hope that a procedure may be offered which will improve oxygen supply to the tissues or diminish overloading of the pulmonary circulation.

In other conditions, specific therapy, such as antibiotics for infections, packed cell transfusions for anemia, conversion of cardiac dysrhythmias with drugs or electrical countershock, reduction of blood pressure with antihypertensive agents, and substitution therapy for metabolic disease may improve myocardial performance. The use of steroids may be lifesaving in acute fulminating cardiac failure associated with rheumatic fever and myopericarditis. Aids to respiration may also improve pulmonary function in patients with cystic fibrosis or severe pulmonary disease. Adenoidectomy will reverse the sequence of events leading to cardiac failure in young patients with massive tonsillar and adenoidal hypertrophy. In managing these problems, an increase in oxygen tension and pH and a fall in carbon dioxide tension will exert a favorable effect on the pulmonary circulation and myocardium.

Counseling

The approach to the parents of infants and children with heart failure should include a frank discussion of specific cardiac problems, genetic implications, and treatment. Experience gained from conferences with a number of parent groups indicates that the term "failure" connotes a terminal condition or heart stoppage and should be avoided. We have utilized such expressions as "lung congestion," "liver congestion," "impaired pumping ability" and so forth to depict the clinical status, and these seem to be accepted more readily.

PROGNOSIS

The prognosis of heart failure is dependent on the severity of the underlying disease process. This is particularly true of the first 6 months of life where the highest mortality exists, a consequence of severe structural malformations of the heart. Most deaths occur during the first week, with a stepwise decrease in mortality with each succeeding week. After the first year of life, a variety of conditions, usually acquired, produce decompensation, but they represent only 10% of the total number of pediatric patients with cardiac failure.

The poor prognosis for the infant with a congenital heart defect and cardiac failure has been improved somewhat by a more vigorous approach toward early diagnosis and surgical treatment. It should be stressed that a newborn infant, who is in heart failure from a cardiac anomaly, should be regarded as both a medical emergency and a potential surgical candidate. Such an infant should be transferred to a center where all facilities and personnel are available for a complete investigation and possible surgical intervention. This institution should be equipped to carry out cardiac catheterization and angiocardiography on critically ill infants. After a short period of aggressive medical management, one should be prepared to follow the diagnostic studies with surgical intervention if indicated. At present, earlier recognition and prompt medical treatment, as well as the introduction of corrective surgical procedures, have improved the outlook for patients with large volume left to right shunts, coarctation of the aorta, and anomalous pulmonary venous connection. Balloon atrial septostomy and utilization of the Mustard operation have strikingly altered mortality rates for infants with transposition of the great arteries. With severe outflow obstruction to the left or right side, surgical intervention has also been life-saving.

REFERENCES

1. Adams, R. J., and Schwartz, A.: Comparative mechanisms for contraction of cardiac and skeletal muscle. Chest 78:123, 1981.
2. Alpert, N. R., and Gordon, M. S.: Myofibrillar adenosine triphosphatase activity in congestive heart failure. Am. J. Physiol. 202:940, 1962.
3. Baylen, B. G., Johnson, G., Tsang, R., et al.: The occurrence of hyperaldosteronism in infants with congestive heart failure. Am. J. Cardiol. 45:305, 1980.
4. Bell, N. H., Schedl, H. P., and Bartter, F. C.: An explanation for abnormal water retention and hypoosmolarity in congestive heart failure. Am. J. Med. 36:351, 1964.
5. Benzing, G., III, Schubert, W., Hug, G., and Kaplan, S.: Simultaneous hypoglycemia and acute congestive heart failure. Circulation 40:209, 1969.
6. Bucciarelli, R. L., Nelson, R. M., Egan, E. A., Eitzman, D., and Gessner, I. H.: Transient tricuspid insufficiency of the newborn. A form of myocardial dysfunction in stressed newborns. Pediatrics 59:330, 1977.
7. Cannon, P. J.: The kidney in heart failure. N. Engl. J. Med. 296:25, 1977.
8. Chatterjee, K., and Parmley, W. W.: The role of vasodilator therapy in heart failure. Prog. Cardiovasc. Dis. 19:301, 1977.
9. Chidsey, C. A., Braunwald, E., and Morrow, A. G.: Catecholamine excretion of cardiac stores of norepinephrine in congestive heart failure. Am. J. Med. 39:442, 1965.
9a. Cohn, J. N., and Franciosa, J. A.: Vasodilator therapy of cardiac failure. N. Engl. J. Med. 294:27, 254, 1977.
9b. Conti, M. A., and Adelstein, R. S.: Phosphorylation of cyclic adenosine 3'5'-monophosphate-dependent protein kinase regulates myosin light chain kinase. Fed. Proc. 39:1569, 1980.
10. Cooper, G., IV, Puga, F. J., Zujko, K. J., Harrison, C. E., and Coleman, H. N., III: Normal myocardial function and energetics in volume-overloaded hypertrophy in the cat. Circ. Res. 32:140, 1973.
11. Cooper, G., IV, Satava, R. M., Harrison, C. E., and Coleman, H. N., III: Normal myocardial function and energetics after reversing pressure-overload hypertrophy. Am. J. Physiol. 225:1158, 1974.
12. Covell, J. W., Chidsey, C. A., and Braunwald, E.: Reduction of the cardiac response to postganglionic sympathetic nerve stimulation in experimental heart failure. Circ. Res. 19:51, 1966.
13. Danilowicz, D., Rudolph, A. M., and Hoffman, J. I. E.: Delayed closure of the ductus arteriosus in premature infants. Pediatrics 37:74, 1965.
14. Davis, J. O., Hartroft, P. M., Titus, E. O., Carpenter, C. J., Ayers, C. R., and Spiegel, H. E.: The role of the renin-angiotensin system in the control of aldosterone secretion. J. Clin. Invest. 41:378, 1962.
14a. Davis, R., Ribner, H. S., Keung, E., LeJemtel, T. H., and Sonnenblick, E. H.: Treatment of chronic congestive heart failure with captopril, an oral inhibitor of angiotensin-converting enzyme. N. Engl. J. Med. 301:177, 1979.

14b. Dillon, T. R., Meyer, R. A., and Kaplan, S.: Vasodilator therapy for congestive heart failure. J. Pediatr. 96:623, 1980.
15. Doherty, J. E., deSoyza, N., Kane, J. J., Bissett, J. K., and Murphy, M.: Clinical pharmokinetics of digitalis glycosides. Prog. Cardiovasc. Dis. 21:141, 1978.
16. Doherty, J. E., and Perkins, W. H.: Studies with tritiated digoxin in human subjects after intravenous administration. Am. Heart J. 63:528, 1962.
17. Downing, S. E., Talner, N. S., Campbell, A. G. M., Halloran, K. H., and Wax, H. B.: Influence of cardiac sympathetic nerve stimulation on ventricular function in the newborn lamb. Circ. Res. 25:417, 1969.
18. Driscoll, D. J., Gillette, P. C., and McNamara, D. G.: The use of dopamine in children. J. Pediatr. 92:309, 1978.
19. Engle, M. A.: Treatment of the failing heart. Pediatr. Clin. North Am. 11:247, 1964.
20. Fanburg, B. L.: Experimental cardiac hypertrophy. N. Engl. J. Med. 282:723, 1970.
21. Fishman, A. P.: Pulmonary edema. The water-exchanging function of the lung. Circulation 46:390, 1972.
22. Friedman, W. F.: The intrinsic physiologic properties of the developing heart. In Neonatal Heart Disease, edited by W. F. Friedman, M. Lesch, and E. H. Sonnenblick. Grune & Stratton, New York, 1973, p. 21.
23. Friedman, W. F., Pool, P. E., Jacobowitz, D., Seagren, S. C., and Braunwald, E.: Sympathetic innervation of the developing rabbit heart. Biochemical and histochemical comparisons of fetal, neonatal and adult myocardium. Circ. Res. 23:25, 1968.
24. Giardina, A. C. V., Ehlers, K. H., Morrison, J. B., and Engle, M. A.: Serum digitoxin concentrations in infants and children. Circulation 51:713, 1975.
25. Gillis, R. A.: Cardiac sympathetic nerve activity: Changes induced by ouebain and propranolol. Science 166:508, 1969.
26. Gluck, L., Talner, N. S., Stern, H., Gardner, T. H., and Kulovich, M. V.: Experimental cardiac hypertrophy: Concentrations of RNA in the ventricles. Science 144:1244, 1964.
27. Graham, T. P., Atwood, G. F., Boerth, R. C., Roucek, R. J., and Smith, C. W.: Right and left heart size and function in infants with symptomatic coarctation. Circulation 56:641, 1977.
28. Graham, T. P., and Jarmakani, J. M.: Hemodynamic investigation of congenital heart disease in infancy and childhood. In Neonatal Heart Disease, edited by W. F. Friedman, M. Lesch, and E. H. Sonnenblick. Grune & Stratton, New York, 1973, p. 127.
29. Grantham, J. J., and Chonko, A. M.: The physiologic basis and clinical use of diuretics. In Sodium and Water Homeostasis, edited by B. M. Brenner and J. H. Stein, Vol. I. Churchill Livingstone, New York, 1978, p. 179.
30. Hastreiter, A. R., and Miller, R. A.: Management of primary endomyocardial disease. The myocarditis-endocardial fibroelastosis syndrome. Pediatr. Clin. North Am. 11:401, 1964.
31. Hayes, C. J., Butler, V. P., Jr., and Gersony, W. M.: Serum digoxin studies in infants and

children. Pediatrics 52:561, 1973.
32. Hellenbrand, W. E., Lister, G., Kleinman, C. S., and Talner, N. S.: Effects of exchange (ExTx) on the pulmonary and systemic circulations in left-to-right shunts ($Q_{L,R}$). Pediatr. Res. 15:464, 1981.
33. Holloway, E. L., Stinson, E. B., Derby, G. C., and Harrison, D. C.: Action of drugs in patients early after cardiac surgery. 1. Comparison of isoproterenol and dopamine. Am. J. Cardiol. 35:656, 1975.
34. Ito, Y., and Chidsey, C. A.: Intracellular calcium and myocardial contractility. IV. Distribution of calcium in the failing heart. J. Mol. Cell Cardiol. 4:507, 1972.
35. Katz, A. M.: Contractile proteins of the heart. Physiol. Rev. 50:63, 1970.
36. Keith, J. D., Rowe, R. D., and Vlad, P.: Congestive heart failure. In Heart Disease in Infancy and Childhood, 3rd ed. Macmillan, New York, 1978, p. 163.
36a. Kerrick, W. G. L., Hoar, P. E., and Cassidy: Calcium-activated tension: The role of myosin light chain phosphorylation. Fed. Proc. 39:1558, 1980.
36b. Klopfenstein, H. S., and Rudolph, A. M.: Postnatal changes in the circulation and responses to volume loading in sheep. Circ. Res. 42:839, 1978.
37. Langer, G. A.: Effects of digitalis on myocardial ionic exchange. Circulation 46:180, 1972.
38. Laragh, J. H.: Diagnosis and treatment: The proper use of newer diuretics. Ann. Intern. Med. 67:606, 1967.
39. Lees, M. H.: Catecholamine metabolite excretion of infants with heart failure. J. Pediatr. 69:259, 1966.
40. Lees, M. H., Bristow, J. D., Griswold, H. E., and Olmsted, R. W.: Relative hypermetabolism in infants with congenital heart disease and undernutrition. Pediatrics 36:183, 1965.
41. Levy, A. M., Leaman, D. M., and Hanson, J. S.: Effects of digoxin on systolic time intervals of neonates and infants. Circulation 46:816, 1972.
42. Manning, J. A., Sellers, F. J., Bynum, R. S., and Keith, J. D.: The medical management of clinical endocardial fibroelastosis. Circulation 29:60, 1964.
43. Miller, W. W., Oski, F. A., and Delivoria-Papadopoulas, M.: Increased oxygen release in hypoxemia and heart failure (abstr.). Pediatr. Res. 4:444, 1970.
44. Moss, A. J., and Duffie, E. R., Jr.: Congestive heart failure in infancy. Significance of the venous pressure. J. Pediatr. 60:346, 1962.
45. Murray, J. A., Johnston, W., and Reid, J. M.: Echocardiographic determination of left ventricular dimensions, volumes and performance. Am. J. Cardiol. 30:252, 1972.
46. Nadas, A. S., and Fyler, D. C.: Congestive failure. In Pediatric Cardiology, 3rd ed. Part II, Chap. 12. W. B. Saunders, Philadelphia, 1972, p. 262.
47. Neill, C. A.: The use of digitalis in infants and children. Prog. Cardiovasc. Dis. 7:399, 1965.
48. Okita, G. T.: Metabolism of radioactive cardiac glycosides. Pharmacologist 6:45, 1964.
49. Paintal, A. S.: The mechanism of excitation of type J receptors, and the J reflex. In Breath-

ing: Hering-Breuer Centenary Symposium, edited by R. Porter. J & A Churchill, London, 1970, p. 59.

50. Park, S., Dimich, I., and Steinfeld, L.: Systolic time intervals in infants with heart failure. Circulation 42 (Suppl. 3):31, 1970.

51. Pool, P. E.: Confestive heart failure: Biochemical and physiologic observations. Am. J. Med. Sci. 258:328, 1969.

52. Reisman, M., Hipona, F. A., Bloor, C. M., and Talner, N. S.: Congenital tricuspid insufficiency. A cause of massive cardiomegaly and heart failure in the neonate. J. Pediatr. 66:869, 1965.

52a. Robie, N. W., and Goldberg, L. I.: Comparative systemic and regional hemodynamic effects of dopamine and dobutamine. Am. Heart J. 90:340, 1975.

53. Rudolph, A. M.: Diagnosis and treatment: Respiratory distress and cardiac disease in infancy. Pediatrics 35:999, 1965.

54. Rudolph A. M.: Cardiac failure in children: A hemodynamic overview. In The Myocardium: Failure and Infarction, edited by E. Braunwald, Section III, Chap. 10. H. P. Publishing Co., New York, 1974, p. 102.

55. Rudolph, A. M., Heymann, M. A., and Spitznas, U.: Hemodynamic considerations in the development of narrowing of the aorta. Am. J. Cardiol. 30:514, 1972.

56. St. Geme, J. W., Peralta, H., Farias, E., Davis, C. W. C., and Noren, G. R.: Experimental gestational mumps virus infection and endocardial fibroelastosis. Pediatrics 48:821, 1971.

57. Schwartz, A., Sordahl, C. A., and McCollum, W. B.: Studies on mitochondria and the muscle relaxing system. In Myocardiology: Recent Advances in Studies on Cardiac Structure and Metabolism, edited by E. Bajusz and G. Rona, Vol. 1. University Park Press, Baltimore, 1972, p. 12.

58. Shannon, D. C., Lusser, M., Goldblatt, A., and Bunnell, J. B.: The cyanotic infant—Heart disease or lung disease. N. Engl. J. Med. 287:951, 1972.

59. Smith, T. W., Haber, E., Yeatman, L., and Butler, V. P., Jr.: Reversal of advanced digoxin intoxication with Fab fragments of digoxin-specific antibodies. N. Engl. J. Med. 294:797, 1976.

60. Sonnenblick, E. H., and Strobeck, J. E.: Derived indexes of ventricular and myocardial function. N. Engl. J. Med. 296:978, 1977.

61. Spagnuolo, M., and Feinstein, A. R.: Congestive heart failure and rheumatic activity in young patients with rheumatic heart disease. Pediatrics 33:653, 1964.

62. Spann, J. F., Jr., Buccino, R. A., Sonnenblick, E. H., and Braunwald, E.: Contractile state of cardiac muscle obtained from cats with experimentally produced ventricular hypertrophy and cardiac failure. Circ. Res. 21:341, 1967.

62a. Staub, N. C.: Pulmonary edema. Physiol. Rev. 54:678, 1974.

63. Su, J. Y., and Friedman, W. F.: Comparison of the responses of fetal and adult cardiac muscle to hypoxia. Am. J. Physiol. 224:1249, 1973.

63a. Synhorst, D. P., Lauer, R. M., Coty, D. B., and Brady, M. J.: Hemodynamic effects of vasodilator agents in dogs with experimental ventricular septal defects. Circulation 54:472, 1976.

64. Talner, N. S.: Pathophysiology of cardiac failure in the newborn. In Pathophysiology of Congenital Heart Disease, edited by F. H. Adams, H. J. C. Swan, and V. E. Hall. University of California Press, Berkeley, UCLA Forum in Medical Sciences No. 10, 1970, p. 119.

65. Talner, N. S.: Congestive heart failure in the infant: A functional approach. Pediatr. Clin. North. Am. 18:1011, 1971.

66. Talner, N. S., and Berman, M. A.: Postnatal development of coarctation of the aorta: The role of the ductus arteriosus. Pediatrics 56:562, 1975.

67. Talner, N. S., and Campbell, A. G. M.: Recognition and management of cardiologic problems in the newborn infant. In Neonatal Heart Disease, edited by W. F. Friedman, M. Lesch, and E. H. Sonnenblick. Grune & Stratton, New York, 1973, p. 95.

68. Talner, N. S., Sanyal, S. K., Halloran, K. H., Garner, T. H., and Ordway, N. K.: Congestive heart failure in infancy. 1. Abnormalities in blood gases and acid-base equilibrium. Pediatrics 35:20, 1965.

69. Talner, N. S., and Lister, G.: Oxygen transport in congenital heart disease. In Pediatric Cardiovascular Disease, edited by M. A. Engle, Vol. 11, Chap. 7. F. A. Davis, Philadelphia, 1980, p. 129.

70. Vogel, J. H. K., McNamara, D. G., and Blount, S. G., Jr.: Role of hypoxia in determining pulmonary vascular resistance in infants with ventricular septal defects. Am. J. Cardiol. 20:346, 1967.

71. Walker, W. G., and Cooke, C. R.: Diuretics and electrolyte abnormalities in congestive heart failure. III. Electrolyte disturbance in congestive heart failure. Mod. Concepts Cardiovasc. Dis. 34:17, 1965.

72. Warshaw, J. B.: Cellular metabolism during fetal development. IV. Fatty acid activation, acyl transfer and fatty acid oxidation during development of the check and rat. Dev. Biol. 28:537, 1972.

73. Weber, K. T., and Janicki, J. S.: The heart as a muscle-pump system and the concept of heart failure. Am. Heart J. 98:376, 1979.

74. White, R. D., and Lietman, P. S.: Commentary: A reappraisal of digitalis for infants with left-to-right shunts and "heart failure." J. Pediatr. 92:867, 1978.

45

Dysrhythmias

Paul C. Gillette, M.D., Arthur Garson, Jr., M.D., Co-burn J. Porter, M.D., and Dan G. McNamara, M.D.

We have chosen the term dysrhythmia, rather than arrhythmia, because we feel the prefix "dys" indicates abnormal, which is the meaning we intend. Arrhythmia indicates a complete absence of rhythm, which is only the case in fibrillation or, perhaps, sinus arrhythmia.

Cardiac dysrhythmias are being recognized with increasing frequency in infants and children. There are three reasons for this: pediatricians and pediatric cardiologists have become more aware of dysrhythmias; techniques for detection of dysrhythmias, including fetal echocardiography and fetal cardiac monitoring, have resulted in earlier and more accurate detection of dysrhythmias in this age group; and there has been a real increase in the number of dysrhythmias in children because they occur frequently after cardiac operations. It is likely that the number of such dysrhythmias will continue to increase as the number and complexity of operations increase. Specific techniques to prevent dysrhythmias offer hope for a decrease in their number in the future.

The tools used to diagnose and treat dysrhythmias have markedly improved in the last several years. In addition to history, physical examination, and standard electrocardiography, physicians who care for children with dysrhythmias have available very small 24-hour ambulatory tape recorders, telemetry, transtelephonic monitoring, and treadmill or bicycle exercise electrocardiography. Body surface mapping techniques may be useful in some situations. Hospitalized patients may be monitored either in intensive care units or by telemetry while they are ambulatory in the hospital. Intracardiac electrophysiologic studies performed in the catheterization laboratory are used in complex dysrhythmias of all types which require definitive diagnosis.

CLASSIFICATION OF DYSRHYTHMIAS

Dysrhythmias may be classified according to etiology as: (a) developmental (congenital complete AV block, reciprocating tachycardia due to Wolff-Parkinson-White syndrome (WPW), congenital prolonged QT interval); (b) secondary to other cardiac disease (atrial flutter in a patient with stretched atria due to tricuspid atresia, Ebstein's anomaly, or rheumatic valvular disease); (c) secondary to noncardiac diseases (central nervous system (CNS), endocrine, or metabolic disorders, infectious diseases, collagen vascular diseases, infiltrative disease); (d) surgically acquired (sick sinus, complete AV block); or (e) primary dysrhythmias (AV node reentry tachycardia, premature ventricular contractions in a patient with a normal heart). The classification of dysrhythmias according to etiology is useful in reminding one that the best treatment is removal of the etiology. Unfortunately, this is rarely possible, as in the case of infectious or endocrine etiology. This concept, however, has been expanded in the surgical treatment of dysrhythmias involving division of Kent bundles or destruction of automatic foci.

Although there is now considerable information on the cellular basis of dysrhythmias[1] and an understanding of these principles helps in understanding the mechanisms of dysrhythmias, they are not critical to the understanding and treatment of dysrhythmias. We thus will not use the usual classification of disorders of impulse formation versus impulse conduction. Rather, we will use a classification based on the clinical presentation of patients with dysrhythmias. First, we will present an approach to the surface ECG which we have found useful in the diagnosis of cardiac dysrhythmias.

INTERPRETATION OF DYSRHYTHMIAS

Certain principles are helpful in the analysis of the cardiac rhythm in children. We have developed a deductive method of diagnosis which, while not including every possible dysrhythmia, will place most rhythm disorders in a single category.[2] In analyzing the ECG, certain questions must be answered sequentially (Fig. 45.1).

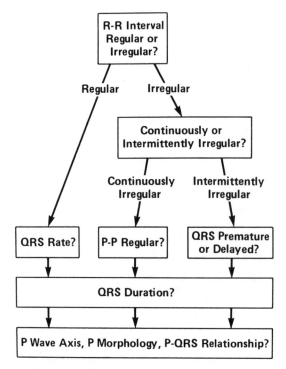

Fig. 45.1 Flow diagram for use in the systemic interpretation of dysrhythmias from the surface electrocardiogram.

1. Is the RR interval regular? We consider a rhythm to be regular if the RR intervals vary by less than 0.08 seconds. If the RR interval (ventricular rate) is regular, the answers to three further questions will categorize the rhythm.

2. Is the ventricular rate normal, decreased, or increased for the patient's age and clinical condition? The range of normal sinus rates vary with age and can be found in Table 45.1. For a newborn baby, a rate of 95/minute is bradycardia, and for a 17-year-old adolescent, the same rate is tachycardia.

3. Is the QRS duration normal or prolonged? The range of normal QRS durations vary with age and can be found elsewhere in this volume. A QRS duration longer than 0.09 seconds is prolonged at any age. If the QRS duration is prolonged, the specific morphology must be determined: complete right bundle branch block (terminal conduction delay directed towards the right and anteriorly—positive in V_1); complete left bundle branch block (conduction delay throughout the QRS complex directed leftward and posteriorly—positive in V_6); Wolff-Parkinson-White syndrome (short PR interval and a slow initial deflection or "delta wave"); and diffuse intraventricular conduction delay (conduction delay throughout the QRS complex with a nonspecific pattern).

4. What is the atrial activity? When the atria depolarize, one of three patterns is observed on the electrocardiogram: Are there P waves, flutter waves, or fibrillation? If P waves are visible, the P wave axis must be determined. Normal sinus P waves have an axis of 0 to 90°, i.e., originating from the high right atrium. A P wave originating from the left atrium has an axis between 91 and 269°, i.e., negative in lead I. Finally, the relationship of atrial depolarizations to the QRS complexes must be determined. If the atrial depolarizations are not related in a regular way to the QRS complexes, atrioventricular (AV) dissociation is diagnosed. AV dissociation occurs in several dysrhythmias with entirely different mechanisms. Therefore, AV dissociation should never be the only diagnosis in the interpretation of an electrocardiogram. There are three causes for AV dissociation: *slowing of sinus or atrial rhythm* with junctional rhythm occurring at a normal junctional rate; *an accelerated junctional or ventricular tachycardia* without retrograde conduction results in an abnormally rapid ventricular rate with a normal atrial rate; and *complete AV block* is the best example of AV dissociation because, by definition, the atria and ventricles are unrelated.

If the RR intervals are irregular, they can be either irregularly irregular or continuously irregular, or there can be a basic, regular RR interval into which an irregular RR interval is intermittently introduced. If the RR interval varies continuously, the next question to be answered is whether the P to P intervals are regular or irregular. In pediatrics, the most common example of a continuously irregular RR interval is sinus arrhythmia: the P to P intervals also are irregular, and there is a P wave preceding each QRS complex. The other example of a continuously varying RR interval is atrial fibrillation. If the RR intervals vary continuously but the P to P interval is regular, the most likely diagnosis is second degree AV block. In typical type I second degree AV block (Wenckebach), the PR intervals progressively lengthen, and RR intervals progressively shorten until an atrial depolarization occurs without a subsequent QRS complex, and the cycle begins again. In type II second degree AV block, the PR intervals of conducted beats remain constant, but the RR intervals may vary if the number of conducted atrial depolarizations varies.

If there is a basic regular RR interval which is interrupted intermittently, the initial question is whether the first irregular RR interval is shorter or longer than the basic regular RR interval. If the QRS is premature (by at least 0.04 seconds), the QRS duration is determined next. If the QRS duration is normal, the premature QRS can result from either: intermittent conduction of a sinus beat into a predominant junctional rhythm—a so-called "sinus capture" beat; premature atrial contraction; or premature junctional contraction. If the premature QRS has a prolonged duration, the possibilities are either: sinus capture with aberration; premature atrial contraction with aberration; or premature ventricular contraction. Since it is impossible on a surface electrocardiogram to differentiate a premature junctional contraction with aberration from a premature ventricular contraction, we have chosen to classify all wide premature QRS complexes without preceding P waves as premature ventricular contractions.

If the QRS complex is not premature but rather delayed (by 0.04 seconds or more), the QRS duration is determined next. If the QRS is normal in duration, the answers to three further questions will clarify the rhythm. The first refers to the basic supraventricular rhythm: in second degree AV block, the supraventricular rhythm continues uninterrupted; in a nonconducted premature atrial contraction, a different morphology P wave is introduced prematurely; and with a "pause" in the supraventricular rhythm, no atrial activity is observed.

Secondly, what is the RR interval preceding in the delayed QRS? In type II second degree AV block, the preceding RR interval is twice the basic RR interval; in a nonconducted premature atrial contraction, the preceding RR interval is less than the basic RR interval. In a "pause," the preceding RR interval can be of any duration but is always longer than the basic RR interval.

The third question concerns the atrial activity immediately preceding the delayed QRS complex. In AV block, or a nonconducted premature atrial contraction, the delayed QRS is preceded by a regular supraventricular P wave. In a pause with an atrial escape beat, the delayed QRS is preceded by a P wave with a different axis and morphology from the regular P wave. In a pause with a junctional escape beat, the delayed QRS is not preceded by a P wave.

If the QRS complex is delayed and the QRS duration is prolonged, the most common rhythm is a pause with a ventricular escape beat.

Using this method of analysis, dysrhythmias can be grouped into one of 14 categories. Assignment into a category depends upon the regularity of the RR interval, the QRS rate, and the QRS duration. This method has been explained in detail in a recent publication.[2]

INTRACARDIAC ELECTROPHYSIOLOGIC EVALUATION

Since intracardiac electrophysiologic (EP) studies have assumed such importance in the evaluation of cardiac dysrhythmias in recent years, our technique will be described briefly. It is more fully described in Chapter 3 of Pediatric Cardiac Dysrhythmias.[3] The indication for EP studies is a dysrhythmia or suspected dysrhythmia in which an important question exists which is likely to be answered by such a study and cannot be answered by noninvasive tests. An example of such a question is: Does a patient with recurrent supraventricular tachycardia who does not have WPW on his ECG have a concealed Kent bundle? The indications for EP study will vary from center to center according to the experience of the physicians.

To perform an EP study, most children must be sedated. We use meperidine (2 mg/kg) and promethazine (1 mg/kg) intramuscularly 30 minutes prior to study. If additional sedation is necessary, we usually use additional meperidine and promethazine (1/2 mg/kg) and (1/4 mg/kg IV). This mixture probably enhances sinus node automaticity and in rare cases may make SVT difficult to induce, but we have found no better sedative.

Electrode catheters are introduced by standard percutaneous technique and positioned using fluoroscopy. A standard 6 French tripolar catheter is used for recording the His bundle potential. The catheter is advanced into the right ventricle until only a ventricular electrogram is recorded. It is then withdrawn with strong clockwise torque until nearly equal atrial and ventricular electrograms are recorded with a sharp discrete potential between them. A potential recorded with large ventricular depolarization and small or absent atrial depolarization is likely to be the right bundle branch potential.

The conduction times through the AV node (LSRA-H) and from the bundle of His to the ventricle (H-V) are measured from the beginning of one deflection to the beginning of the next (Fig. 45.2). A second catheter should be inserted percutaneously through the same or opposite femoral vein if additional conduction times or pacing are needed. A special order 5 French quadrapolar catheter (Elecath) with 3- to 5-mm interelectrode distance is useful in this

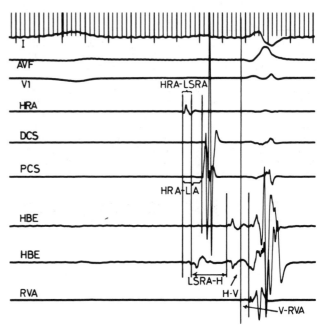

Fig. 45.2 Method for measurement of intracardiac conduction intervals. *Vertical lines* are drawn through the site of earliest activation of the intracardiac electrograms to be measured. High right atrium to low septal right atrium is measured from the beginning of the high right atrial electrogram to the beginning of the low septal right atrial electrogram. This encompasses conduction through the atrial muscle from the sinus node to the atrioventricular node. Low septal right atrium to His interval is measured from the beginning of the respective electrograms. This includes atrioventricular nodal conduction time. His to ventricular interval includes conduction through the bundle of His and the bundle branches in the Purkinje system. The ventricular to right ventricular apex conduction time is conduction through the right bundle branch. The high right atrium to left atrium conduction time indicates the time it takes for conduction through the atrial muscle from the sinus node to the place of the left atrium measured at the coronary sinus.

situation. Internodal (intraatrial) conduction times may be measured from the high right atrium (HRA) to the atrial deflection (LSRA) on the His bundle tracing.

Sinus node function is evaluated by two techniques.[4] Sinus node automaticity is evaluated by pacing the atrium near the sinus node at several rates faster than the sinus rate for 30 seconds and recording the time interval from the last pacing stimulus to the first sinus beat (the sinus node recovery time). This can be corrected by subtracting the prepacing sinus cycle length (CSNRT) (Fig. 45.3).[5, 6] Sinoatrial conduction time is evaluated by introducing single premature atrial stimuli into sinus rhythm using a programmable stimulator.[7, 8] The approximate time it takes the impulse to conduct into and out of the sinus node can then be calculated. Both

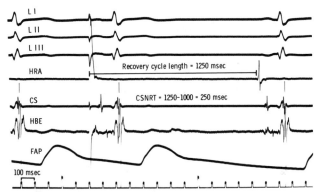

Fig. 45.3 Technique for determining a corrected sinus node recovery time. Shown are surface ECG leads I, II, and III, recorded simultaneously with intracardiac leads, high right atrium, coronary sinus, His bundle, and femoral artery pressure with 100-millisecond time lines. The first two QRS complexes are in response to high right atrial pacing. Pacing is then stopped, and the recovery sinus cycle length is measured from the last pacing spike to the first sinus depolarization on the high right atrial electrogram. This value measures 1250 milliseconds. To obtain the corrected sinus node recovery time, the preceding sinus cycle length, 1000 milliseconds in this case, is subtracted from the 1250 milliseconds to obtain a 250-millisecond corrected sinus node recovery time (*CSNRT*).

of these methods should be used in each patient because abnormalities of one may mask those of the other.

The function of the atrioventricular conduction system is evaluated partially during the same studies which evaluate sinus node function. The pacing rate at which type I (Wenckebach) second degree AV block occurs is an index of AV node function (Fig. 45.4).[9] The degree of prematurity at which a premature atrial contraction (PAC) blocks in the AV node or His-Purkinje system, i.e., the refractory period of these structures, is also a useful index of their function.[10-12] Conduction blocks within and below the bundle of His occur frequently during stimulation studies.[13] Retrograde conduction properties are evaluated by ventricular pacing and premature stimulation. Twenty-five percent of patients will manifest reentry within the His-Purkinje system during ventricular stimulation studies (Fig. 45.5).

The propensity of patients to develop supraventricular or ventricular tachycardia, as well as the mechanism of their tachycardia, may also be evaluated by the above-mentioned stimulation studies.[14-17] Reentrant tachydysrhythmias are usually inducible by stimulation studies while those due to automatic foci are not. The presence or absence and the location of accessory conduction pathways are determined by the atrial activation sequence during supraventricular tachycardia (SVT). For this type of study, four electrode catheters are used to record from the high right atrium, low septal right atrium, left atrium (coronary sinus), and right ventricle.[18, 19] The refractory periods of accessory connections may be determined using the same techniques as for the normal conduction system.

ABNORMALLY SLOW HEART RATE (BRADYDYSRHYTHMIA)

The definition of heart rate which is abnormally slow depends on the patient's age, clinical state, and physical training. Results of 24-hour ambulatory electrocardiograms (ECGs) are gradually defining the range of normal resting heart rates in children. Sleeping and resting heart rates are found to be much lower than those published previously;

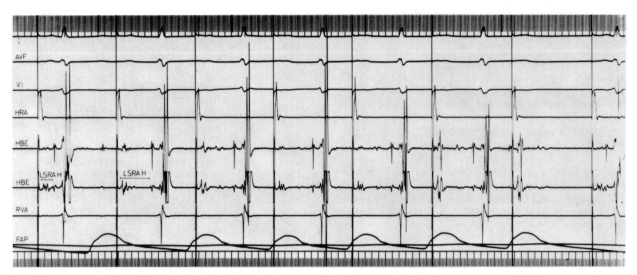

Fig. 45.4 Demonstration of Wenckebach periodicity in response to high right atrial pacing. Shown are surface ECG leads *I*, *AVF*, and *V₁*, recorded together with high right atrium (*HRA*), two His bundle electrograms (*HBE*) and a right ventricular apex (*RVA*) electrogram, and femoral artery pressure (*FAP*). The high right atrium is being paced. The PR interval progressively lengthens from the first paced beat to the seventh paced beat which is blocked above the His bundle depolarization. Prolongation of the PR interval is due totally to prolongation of the *LSRA* to *H* interval. Wenckebach periodicity is normal in response to high right atrial pacing but occurs at an abnormally slow pacing rate in this patient.

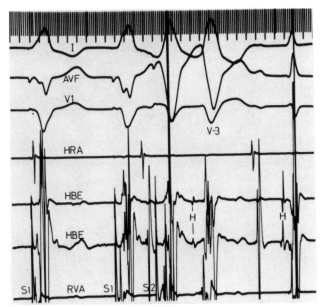

Fig. 45.5 Demonstration of reentry within the His-Purkinje system in response to a premature ventricular stimulus. Shown are surface ECG leads *I*, *AVF*, and V1, together with a high right atrium (*HRA*), two His bundle electrograms (*HBEs*), and a right ventricular apex (*RVA*) electrogram, together with femoral artery pressure and time lines. The first two beats (S1) are in response to ventricular pacing. The third beat is a premature ventricular stimulus (S2). Between the third beat and the fourth beat, a clear His bundle depolarization can be seen. The fourth QRS has exactly the same morphology as the third QRS. Thus, this beat labeled V3 has all the criteria of a His-Purkinje reentrant beat. These are a normal phenomena during ventricular extrastimulation studies in adults and children and do not represent a propensity to ventricular tachydysrhythmias.

resting rates evidently had been taken from children who were nervous about having ECGs.[20]

Table 45.1 shows our current standards of normal heart rates for infants and children. There is marked beat-to-beat variation in infants' and young children's heart rates, most of which is explained by sinus arrhythmia.

The most common cause of bradycardia in newborn infants and children is *complete atrioventricular* (AV) block (3° AV block)—either congenital or acquired. The acquired subgroup may be further subdivided into surgical and nonsurgically acquired complete AV block. Nonsurgical etiologies include infectious processes, muscle diseases, and idiopathic.

Congenital Complete AV Block

Complete AV block is defined as complete absence of conduction of atrial impulses to the ventricle (Fig. 45.6). Congenital complete AV block is often diagnosed antenatally. As obstetricians become more aware of this problem, fewer babies with congenital complete AV block are delivered by needless emergency cesarean sections for "fetal distress".[21] Two-dimensional echocardiography may be used to distinguish complete AV block from sinus bradycardia antenatally by observing the mitral valve (MV) motion and ventricular contractions. Echocardiography is also useful in looking for fetal edema (hydrops) which may indicate that the fetus is distressed by the chronic low heart rate. The fetal heart rate does not always correlate with the postnatal heart rate, so delivery should take place in a unit where urgent temporary cardiac pacing may be performed. The

decision as to whether or not to employ cardiac pacing in a baby may be a difficult one. Any baby who manifests heart failure (HF) should be paced. In the unfortunate combination of events where congenital complete AV block coexists with some other neonatal stress, such as the respiratory distress syndrome, pacing (at least temporarily) may be necessary to save the baby.

A baby who does not have HF or a neonatal stress situation may be evaluated by the criteria of Michaelsson and Engle.[22] These authors found that infants with a ventricular rate persistently below 55 beats/minute and an atrial rate persistently over 140 beats/minute were much more likely to die in the first year of life. Infants with associated congenital heart defects were also more likely to die. We tend to place less importance on the atrial rate because we have noted babies with associated sinus bradycardia who clearly needed pacemakers. Patients with a wide QRS are almost certainly at higher risk of death.

The majority of deaths from congenital complete AV block occur in the first year of life so that careful frequent observation must be accomplished during this period. After the first year of life, although deaths are uncommon, symptoms continue to appear. The most serious of these is syncope. We recently evaluated several clinical factors thought to be useful in predicting syncope in 24 patients who had had their site of block determined by His bundle electrography.[23] As expected, the majority of patients had block between the atrium and AV node, while a few had block in the bundle of His or in the distal conduction system. Localization of the site of block to the AV node was not protective from syncopal episodes. The response of the escape pacemaker to overdrive pacing also was not predictive as to the

TABLE 45.1 NORMAL HEART RATES FOR INFANTS AND CHILDREN

Age	Heart Rate (beats/min)		
	Resting (Awake)	Resting (Sleeping)	Exercise (Fever)
Newborn	100–180	80–160	Up to 220
1 wk to 3 mo	100–220	80–200	Up to 220
3 mo to 2 yr	80–150	70–120	Up to 200
2 yr to 10 yr	70–110	60–90	Up to 200
10 yr to adult	55–90	50–90	Up to 200

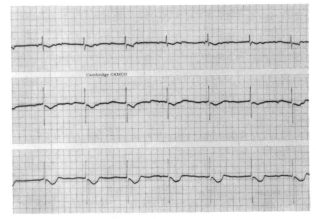

Fig. 45.6 Congenital complete atrioventricular block. Shown are simultaneously recorded surface ECG leads V1, V2, and V3. There is complete dissociation between the QRSs with a rate of approximately 45 beats/minute and the P waves with a rate of 80 beats/minute. The QRSs are narrow and normal in morphology.

occurrence of syncope. The best predictor of syncopal episodes was a resting awake ventricular rate less than 50 beats/minute. Many of these patients, including those with syncope, could increase their rate during exercise to greater than 100 beats/minute.

A decreased exercise tolerance is an often overlooked symptom in patients with congenital complete AV block. Many patients report a great subjective improvement in their exercise tolerance after pacemaker implantation for other indications such as syncope.

Ventricular ectopy is recognized as an important associated finding in patients with complete AV block.[24, 25] Although it is not yet clearly established, it is likely that some syncopal episodes and deaths in older patients with congenital complete AV block are due to ventricular tachydysrhythmias rather than severe bradycardia.

Each patient with congenital complete AV block should be thoroughly evaluated for associated congenital heart defects. This should include physical examination, ECG, chest roentgenogram, and echocardiography. Cardiac catheterization is usually not necessary. Each patient should have an initial 24-hour ECG to evaluate the degree of bradycardia as well as to search for ventricular ectopy.[24, 26] Follow-up 24-hour ECG at 3- to 5-year intervals should also be performed.

At the age of 4 to 5 years an exercise test should be performed and repeated every 3 to 5 years. This will evaluate the patient's exercise tolerance as well as evaluate for ventricular ectopy.

Intracardiac electrophysiologic studies are not necessary in each patient but should be reserved for the patient about whom a clear decision with regard to pacing cannot be made. Electrophysiological studies are also helpful in choosing the type of pacemaker to be implanted.

Based on our studies and those in the literature, we have developed the following set of criteria for permanent pacing in infants and children with congenital complete AV block. All of these are not based on firm scientific information, but some represent compromises based on the best available data.

Patients who are symptomatic from syncope or heart failure should have implantation of a permanent pacemaker. Patients with block below the bundle of His should be paced. This includes the majority of patients with wide QRS escape rhythms (Fig. 45.7). Infants with ventricular rates consistently less than 55 beats/minute should be paced. Older children with ventricular rates less than 50 beats/minute should also be paced. Infants with moderate or severe associated congenital heart defects should probably be paced if their rate is less than 65 to 70 beats/minute or, if they have mild heart failure, since their mortality rate is high. Frequent or complex ventricular dysrhythmias may be an indication for pacing, particularly if there is cardiomegaly. Moderate or severe exercise intolerance is also an indication for pacing.

Surgically Acquired Complete AV Block

Complete AV block is still one of the most serious complications of surgical correction of congenital cardiac defects. Improvements in the surgeons' knowledge of the anatomy of the conduction system as well as intraoperative mapping have decreased frequency in the simpler lesions. In more complex congenital heart defects, however, even an absolute knowledge of the location of the conduction system does not always prevent surgical complete AV block.

Surgical AV block may be either transient or permanent. Transient block is treated with temporary pacing wires placed at the time of surgery. We have proposed a method of managing patients with persistent surgical complete AV

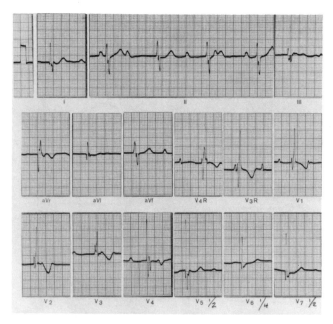

Fig. 45.7 Congenital complete atrioventricular block with abnormally wide QRS complexes. Shown is a 15-lead ECG from a 4-year-old girl. Although the rhythm appears to be fixed 2:1 atrioventricular block in the rhythm strip in lead II, examination of other leads, such as lead V1 and V3R shows that the rhythm is instead complete atrioventricular block. There is right bundle branch block morphology of the QRS. Ventricular rate is 72/minute. Intracardiac electrophysiologic study showed a block below the His bundle potential. The parents of this patient refused pacemaker implantation, and she experienced sudden death at home.

block.[27] These patients are paced with temporary pacing wires for a period of 10 to 14 days. At this point, if they still are not able to maintain an adequate ventricular rate without pacing to produce a satisfactory cardiac output a permanent pacemaker is implanted. Patients who are able to maintain a ventricular rate of greater than 50 and who have no symptoms of heart failure or syncope are investigated by intracardiac electrophysiologic study.

The site of block is localized by recording the His bundle potential. The response of the escape pacemaker is tested by overdrive pacing at several rates for 30 to 60 seconds. If the block is within the AV node, a permanent pacemaker is not recommended; if block is within or below the bundle of His, permanent pacing is recommended. The hemodynamic responses to ventricular pacing, as well as atrial synchronous ventricular pacing and AV sequential pacing, are evaluated and used to help determine the type of pacemaker to be implanted. If an atrial synchronous ventricular pacemaker may be implanted, sinus node studies are also mandatory.

In patients in whom it is chosen not to implant a pacemaker, careful follow-up studies are performed using, in addition to a physical examination, surface electrocardiography, radiography, echocardiography, 24-hour ambulatory electrocardiography, and exercise electrocardiography to determine the patient's continuing lack of need for pacemaker over the years. A few of these patients may develop increasingly severe hemodynamic abnormalities which require pacing in the next few years after surgery.

Patients who develop transient surgical complete AV block, as well as right bundle branch block with left axis deviation, or right bundle branch block with first degree AV block, or right bundle branch block with left axis deviation with first degree AV block, are also studied by intracardiac electrophysiologic studies to try to determine the integrity of their distal conduction system. The site of block in these patients is variable, and not all patients with bifascicular block or with bifascicular block plus first degree AV block have prolonged conduction in the distal conduction system. We do not currently use these data for an immediate clinical decision, but rather include this in our decision as to the frequency and intensity of the patients further long-term follow-up.

Nonsurgically Acquired Complete Atrioventricular Block

Nonsurgically acquired complete AV block is infrequent in children. Infectious processes are the most common etiology, but a few cases of idiopathic fibrous degeneration of the conduction system and tumors in the conduction system are seen in the pediatric age range. Patients with cardiomyopathies of various types are also subject to degeneration of the conduction system. The prognosis in these patients depends on not only the site of block and the current ventricular escape rate, as in congenital and surgically acquired complete AV block, but also on the reversibility or progression of their disease process. These factors are taken into consideration when deciding upon the need for pacemaker implantation. For example, patients with certain congenital opthalmologic lesions and first and second degree atrioventricular block can be counted on to progress to third degree AV block and should be considered as pacemaker candidates.[28] For patients in whom an infectious etiology is found, temporary pacing may suffice until the infectious process is controlled.[29] Some of these patients, however, have permanent lesions of their conduction system and require permanent pacing.

Sinus Bradycardia

Sinus bradycardia is another cause of a slow heart rate in infants and children. Congenital isolated sinus bradycardia in young infants is very rare. Sinus bradycardia is, however, a common transient finding in severe systemic disease, particularly hypoxemia, acidosis, and increased intracranial pressure in young infants.

The most common permanent cause of sinus bradycardia in children is surgical damage to the sinus node, most frequently seen after Mustard's operation (Fig. 45.8).[30] This may occur either immediately after operation or years later. The AV junctional escape focus frequently results in an adequate ventricular rate, but in some cases the junctional automaticity also appears to be depressed. Tachydysrhythmias also are often associated and will be discussed in a later section.

Infants and children with known or suspected sinus brady-

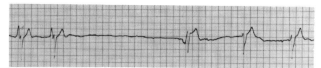

Fig. 45.8 Marked sinus bradycardia in a patient after the Fontan operation for tricuspid atresia. Shown is a strip from a 24-hour ambulatory electrocardiogram. The first two beats represent sinus rhythm at a rate of 60. No sinus beats are then seen for 4200 milliseconds. The sinus P wave and a QRS complex are then seen to occur simultaneously, and a junctional rhythm at a rate of slightly less than 40 beats/minute takes over. Electrophysiologic study confirmed severe sinus node dysfunction, and a permanent pacemaker was implanted.

cardia should have at least one 24-hour ambulatory ECG. Additional dysrhythmias are frequently found, including atrial tachycardia and premature ventricular contractions. The exact degree of bradycardia during activities and sleep may also be documented. A stress ECG is useful in children older than 5 years of age, as it will test for sinoatrial incompetence by showing that the heart rate cannot increase by the normal amount. Invasive testing is also warranted if symptoms are present or suspected.

Sinus node automaticity may be tested by pacing the atria at several rates faster than the sinus rate and recording the sinus node recovery time, which may then be "corrected" by subtracting the resting sinus cycle length (CSNRT). This interval has been found to be abnormal in adults with sinus node disease, as well as in many children after Mustard's operation.[30] A variant of this interval, the corrected "pacemaker" recovery time (CPRT), measures the escape interval if the sinus node is not the first to escape.[31] A prolonged CPRT has been shown to be associated with the development of late dysrhythmias after Mustard's operation.[32]

The time of conduction of the sinoatrial impulse to the atrial muscle (SACT) may now also be estimated indirectly and, more recently, directly measured in man. The technique of Strauss of inducing single premature atrial stimuli with a programmable pacemaker has been adapted to children by Kugler and coworkers.[33] A high frequency of abnormalities of this index of sinoatrial node function was also found in children with abnormal sinus node automaticity. It is important to use both the CSNRT and SACT indices, since they compliment each other. For example, a very prolonged sinoatrial conduction time (SACT) would not allow the paced impulses to reset the sinus node and might lead to a falsely normal value of the corrected sinus node recovery time (CSNRT). If only a CSNRT is measured in such a patient, he may be thought to have normal sinoatrial node function when, in reality, both are abnormal.

During electrophysiologic evaluation of a patient with sinus node dysfunction, the function of the atrial muscle and atrioventricular conduction system should also be evaluated. If a pacemaker is to be inserted, it is important to know the function of the AV node and His-Purkinje system. If these are normal, an atrial demand pacemaker is preferable, since it preserves normal synchrony of the heart's depolarization and contractile sequence and will also help prevent tachydysrhythmias. We have found that in patients with sick sinus syndrome (SSS) due to the Mustard operation or repair of a secundum atrial septal defect, the AV conduction system is usually normal, whereas other intracardiac operations, such as repair of ostium primum atrial septal defect or common atrium, often damage the AV conduction system. In this situation, we usually use AV sequential demand pacing.

The Bradycardia-Tachycardia Syndrome

Our current plan in patients with bradycardia-tachycardia syndrome is to attempt to prevent tachydysrhythmias with digoxin while carefully observing the sinus or junctional rate. If symptomatic dysrhythmias recur, then insertion of a permanent atrial or sequential pacemaker is performed as outlined in the previous section. In some instances, this prevents the need for pharmacologic treatment of the tachydysrhythmia, while in others, drugs are still necessary. We do not use propranolol or quinidine-like drugs in patients with abnormal sinus node function without a pacemaker because of the high risk of worsening bradycardia and sudden death.

IMPLANTABLE PACEMAKERS

Major advances have been made in the last several years in pacemaker and pacemaker lead technology.[34] Pacemakers are now commercially available which are small enough to be implanted successfully in virtually any size baby. All pacemakers now rely on lithium batteries, giving them a lifespan of between 5 and 10 years. We have already noted a decrease in the frequency of hospitalization of our pacemaker patients. Prior to lithium batteries, patients required hospitalization on the average of once every 18 months; whereas now, it is possible to avoid hospitalization for greater than 4 years in most patients.

Pacing leads have also improved greatly in the last several years. Epicardial screw-in leads have virtually replaced the stab-in type and have made it possible to use different epicardial implant techniques which do not require a thoracotomy. The frequency of lead fractures has decreased markedly due to improvements in design and material of the leads. Transvenous leads have undergone an even more marked improvement, and they are now a real consideration in the pediatric population. Polyurethane is replacing silastic as the catheter material, allowing for smaller catheters with a lower coefficient of friction and less thrombogenicity. Active and passive fixation devices have almost eliminated the problems of early and late lead dislodgement. The tined or screw-in atrial J lead makes atrial pacing as easy to achieve and as reliable as ventricular pacing, even in patients who have had previous heart surgery.

The physiology of the pacing system to be implanted in the pediatric patient has become an important decision.[35] The choices include atrial demand pacemakers for sick sinus syndrome and ventricular demand and AV sequential or atrial sensing pacemakers for patients with AV block. If a transvenous lead can be implanted to avoid a thoracotomy, then an atrial system offers several advantages (Fig. 45.9). First, it allows normal AV synchrony and normal ventricular excitation, which will result in a better cardiac output. Ventricular pacing with 1:1 retrograde conduction to the atrium may decrease cardiac output by emptying the atrium if it contracts soon after the ventricle. Atrial pacing also may decrease the frequency of atrial tachydysrhythmias by pre-

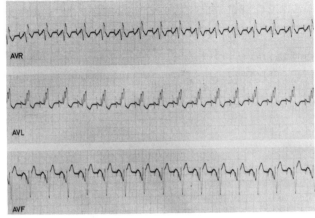

Fig. 45.10 Electrocardiogram from a patient with an implanted atrioventricular sequential pacemaker. Shown are surface ECG leads AVR, AVL, and AVF recorded simultaneously. Pacemaker spikes can be seen capturing both the atrium and the ventricle. As can be seen in lead AVL, it is sometimes difficult to determine whether the atrium is being captured in any single electrocardiographic lead.

vention of atrial bradycardia and premature beats. In patients with both sick sinus syndrome and atrioventricular conduction defects, AV sequential pacemakers are useful (Fig. 45.10). In patients with complete atrioventricular block, atrial sensing ventricular-inhibited pacemakers are now the unit of choice.

Programmability is available in most pacemakers. Programmable features include: rate, output (pulse width, voltage, or current), sensitivity, mode (demand versus fixed rate), sensing refractory period, and hysteresis. Rate programmability is the most useful programmable parameter. We have also had occasion to program output, sensitivity, refractory period, and hysteresis.

A formal follow-up system for each pacemaker patient is imperative. The system should be based in the medical center where the pacemaker is implanted. Both transtelephonic and clinical evaluations are necessary. The clinical evaluations can be performed once a year whereas transtelephonic evaluation is performed once a month for the first year and once every 3 months thereafter (Fig. 45.11).

Due to these advances in pacemakers, leads, implant techniques, and our understanding of pacemakers, we no longer fear the implantation of a pacemaker but look on it as a useful therapeutic maneuver.

SUPRAVENTRICULAR TACHYCARDIA

Supraventricular tachycardia (SVT), a rapid normal QRS tachycardia, is a common dysrhythmia in children.[36] It usually presents in one of three ways: supraventricular tachycardia in the infant, supraventricular tachycardia in the older child, and chronic supraventricular tachycardia.

SVT in the Infant

The most frequent presentation is that of an infant, often under 4 months old, who is taken to the physician because of poor feeding or extreme fussiness. Rarely do the parents note the rapid breathing or ashen color which is frequently present. The heart rate is rapid, 200 to 300 beats/min, and is usually regular. The infant will often have signs of heart failure. Occasionally, frank circulatory shock will be present.

Acute Treatment. This is a true medical emergency! Vagal maneuvers are hardly ever effective. Pharmacologic

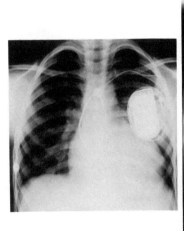
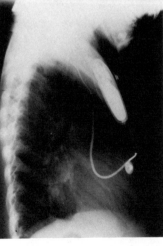

Fig. 45.9 Transvenous atrial J lead implanted in a 5-year-old child with severe sick sinus syndrome, hypertrophic cardiomyopathy, and cardiac arrest. This lead was implanted by cephalic cutdown; a pacemaker was implanted infraclavicularly with complete control of the patient's rhythm and symptoms.

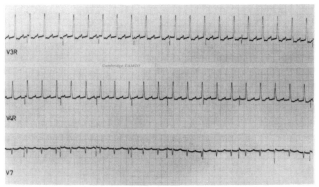

Fig. 45.11 Electrocardiogram from a patient with a broken pacemaker lead. Shown are simultaneously recorded surface ECG leads V3R, V4R, and V7. The patient, postoperative for the Mustard operation, is in supraventricular tachycardia at a rate of 140 beats/minute. There is a 1:1 atrioventricular conduction. The pacemaker is neither sensing nor capturing the ventricle, as evidenced by the fact that it continues to pace at a rate of 50/minute, which was its set rate, but does not interrupt the ventricular rate. This malfunction was picked up during a routine transtelephonic check. The patient had had a bicycle accident 1 week previously, at which time the handlebar had jabbed into his left upper quadrant where the pacemaker was implanted. Fortunately, at the time of the fracture he was in supraventricular tachycardia and remained asymptomatic until his routine transtelephonic checkup detected the malfunction.

measures are too slow and may not be successful. Direct current (DC) synchronized cardioversion is the treatment of choice. We have found 1/4 watt-second/pound to be usually effective. This is in contradistinction to the 1 watt-second/pound recommended for ventricular dysrhythmias. Synchronization of the discharge to the peak of the QRS complex is imperative, since discharge on the T wave may lead to ventricular fibrillation. The fibrillation can be rapidly converted by a second unsynchronized DC shock but should be avoided nonetheless. Intravenous digitalization should be carried out immediately after conversion, giving one-half the loading dose and following with two subsequent doses (each at 1/4 the loading dose) at 8-hour intervals to prevent recurrence. Digitalization is not carried out before cardioversion, as it may increase the risk of ventricular fibrillation.

If the infant is seen before heart failure or shock becomes evident, rapid treatment is indicated nonetheless. Vagal maneuvers, including neosynephrine, also are very unlikely to work, even in the less severely ill infant. The diving reflex, however, is frequently successful in infants who are not in severe heart failure or shock, and it should be tried. The safest and easiest way to do this involves filling a small plastic bag with ice and covering the infant's face with the plastic bag.[37] This seems safer than dunking the infant's face in ice water, as has been previously suggested. The percentage of infants in whom this technique works has not yet been determined. For those in whom it does not work, some would advocate intravenous digitalization. We favor electrocardioversion because it rapidly restores circulation to normal, and it is almost always effective.

In the rare infant in whom DC cardioversion is ineffective, overdrive pacing and further therapy should be carried out in the electrophysiology catheterization laboratory if the infant is seriously ill. Failure of cardioversion often indicates that the mechanism of the SVT is automatic rather than reentry. In this case, overdrive pacing will also be ineffective. The next pharmacologic treatment would be intravenous propranolol (0.01 to 0.1 mg/kg). Because this drug can cause sinus bradycardia, a small pacing catheter should be placed in the right ventricle for emergency pacing.

Reserpine has been reported to be successful in treating the automatic focus type of tachycardia; however, verapamil has been completely ineffective in our experience. One patient who transiently stopped having tachycardia developed sinus bradycardia requiring pacing after a second dose of verapamil. Verapamil resulted in severe hypotension and increased the rate of tachycardia in two patients with junctional automatic ectopic focus tachycardia in our series (Fig. 45.12). Animal investigation has indicated that verapamil may have a more depressant effect on the neonatal myocardium than the adult myocardium. Therefore, we recommend, caution in using verapamil in infants with supraventricular tachycardia.

If the infant is critically ill, pacing the atrium at a rate faster than the tachycardia will often result in 2:1 AV block with marked hemodynamic improvement. In some instances, paired ventricular pacing, may be lifesaving. This would be particularly true in the case of a junctional automatic ectopic tachycardia.

It should be emphasized that the majority of infants under 4 months of age convert easily with DC cardioversion and, if digitalized, have few recurrences. Frequently digitalis may be withdrawn at 1 year of age without further problems.

Chronic Treatment. Of the infants in this group, 25 to 50% will manifest the Wolff-Parkinson-White syndrome (WPW) on their ECG after conversion to sinus rhythm (Fig. 45.13).[38] Currently, a controversy exists with regard to prophylactic treatment of this group. SVT in patients with WPW is usually due to antegrade conduction over the AV node and retrograde conduction over the accessory connection (Fig. 45.14). Digoxin may prevent SVT by slowing conduction in the AV node. It has been shown in adults and a small number of children that digitalis may shorten the antegrade refractory period of the accessory connection (AC) responsible for WPW. This shortening of the antegrade refractory period makes these patients more susceptible to ventricular fibrillation if they develop atrial fibrillation, atrial flutter, or a very early premature atrial depolarization (Fig. 45.15). That this rarely happens in pediatric patients is attested to by the frequent usage of digitalis with no unto-

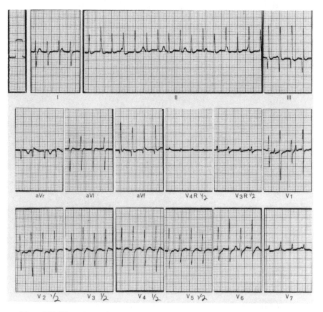

Fig. 45.12 Junctional automatic ectopic tachycardia. As can be seen best in lead II, there is a narrow QRS rate faster than the atrial rate. The variation in QRS size is due to respiratory variation in this severely distressed patient.

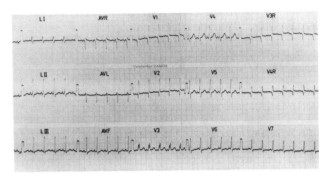

Fig. 45.13 Fifteen-lead electrocardiogram demonstrating Wolff-Parkinson-White syndrome. The delta wave and abnormally short PR interval can be best seen in leads V6 and V7. Square calibration pulses can be seen preceding lead I and in between each additional set of simultaneously recorded leads. This tracing demonstrates nicely the fact that the delta wave may be virtually invisible in some leads such as lead III, and may be negative in some leads, such as V1.

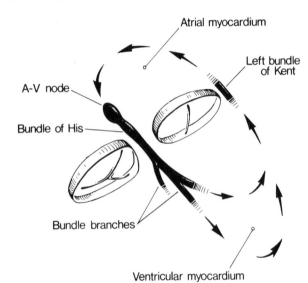

Fig. 45.14 Diagramatic representation of the reentry circuit in patients with either concealed or manifest Wolff-Parkinson-White syndrome. The reentry circuit involves antegrade conduction through the AV node, the bundle of His, the bundle branch system, ventricular myocardium, retrograde through the accessory connection (bundle of Kent) through the atrial myocardium and back to the AV node.

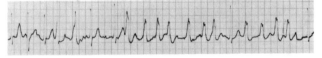

Fig. 45.15 Surface electrocardiographic pattern of atrial fibrillation in a patient with Wolff-Parkinson-White syndrome. The irregular disorganized atrial activity can best be seen just to the left of center. Beats conducted through both the normal and the accessory pathways can be seen. The normal beats are represented by the narrow QRS complexes, and the beats through the accessory connection are represented by the wide QRS complexes.

ward effects in this situation. There are instances, however, of sudden death in children with WPW taking digoxin.

We currently perform intracardiac electrophysiologic studies on patients over 1 year of age with WPW and SVT who need treatment to determine which may safely take digitalis (Fig. 45.16).[18, 39] We establish the antegrade refrac-

tory period of the AC before and after ouabain as well as the response of the AC to induced atrial fibrillation or flutter. If the accessory connection's refractory period is less than 220 msec before or after ouabain, consideration should be given to alternate therapy. Our preliminary results indicate that this is an unusual occurrence in the pediatric age range.

In the rare infant without WPW on surface ECG in whom long-term control of SVT is not possible with digoxin, an electrophysiologic study is indicated. Many of these patients will be found to have concealed WPW, i.e., an AC which conducts only in the retrograde direction.[19] This type of AC makes up the same part of the reentry loop as AC in the manifest WPW.

SVT in the Older Child

The second type of presentation of SVT is the older child with his first episode. This patient is more likely to have manifest or concealed Wolff-Parkinson-White syndrome. This group of patients does not present in heart failure or shock as frequently as the younger patient because: the rate is often slower; the children often recognize the tachycardia and report it to their parents; or even if the children do not recognize the tachycardia, they feel bad and are taken to the physician.

In these patients, a somewhat different initial treatment is used. Vagal maneuvers may be effective. Initially, we try a modified Valsalva maneuver in which the child is in a supine position and is asked to "make a big stomach and hold it." Pressure is then applied to the abdomen, being

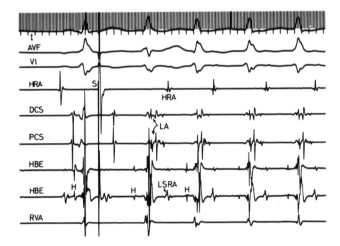

Fig. 45.16 Intracardiac recordings in a patient with Wolff-Parkinson-White syndrome due to a left-side accessory connection, both during sinus rhythm and induced paroxysmal supraventricular tachycardia. Shown are surface ECG leads I, AVF, and V1 recorded simultaneously with a high right atrial, distal coronary sinus, proximal coronary sinus, two His bundle electrograms, RV apex electrograms, femoral artery pressure, and time lines. In sinus rhythm, the atrial activation precedes normally from the high right atrium to the low septal right atrium, followed by the left atrium manifested on the coronary sinus electrograms. An abnormally short time can be seen between left atrial and left ventricular depolarization on the coronary sinus electrogram. His bundle depolarization occurs almost simultaneously with the left ventricular depolarization. After an induced PAC in the high right atrium, there is delayed conduction through the AV node; the H to V interval normalizes, as does the QRS. On the coronary sinus electrogram immediately after ventricular depolarization, the left atrium can be seen to be reactivated followed by the low septal right atrium, high right atrium, bundle of His and, again, the ventricles. This is repeated, and a supraventricular tachycardia is initiated. The reentry circuit in this example of supraventricular tachycardia is exactly as depicted in Figure 45.14.

careful not to be so forceful as to injure an intraabdominal organ. This pressure on the child by the physician is held for 20 or 30 seconds and then released immediately.

We have had no experience with the chest thump for supraventricular tachycardia, but it has been reported to be successful. The diving reflex using either the ice bag or facial immersion in ice cold water is also frequently successful in this age group. We feel that eyeball pressure carries a greater risk than the likely benefit because of the possibility of retinal detachment. Intravenous phenylephrine (0.01 to 0.1 mg/kg) may be successful even if other vagal maneuvers have failed. We begin with a dose of 0.01 mg/kg as an intravenous bolus and gradually increase the dose until the patient's blood pressure is doubled. If the dose of phenylephrine which doubles the blood pressure is not effective, higher doses are not likely to be effective and may be dangerous. Tensilon (0.2 mg/kg) may also be used to enhance vagal tone. Atropine should always be immediately available to administer as an antidote to excessive bradycardia in response to Tensilon or Neo-synephrine.

Intravenous verapamil, which has just become commercially available, is likely to become the treatment of choice for supraventricular tachycardia in the older child who does not respond to vagal maneuvers and who is not in acute heart failure.[40] Verapamil may be administered at a dose of 0.1 mg/kg intravenously over a 30-second period. It usually stops reentrant tachycardias less than a minute after administration. The dose may be repeated once, 5 minutes after initial administration, if the patient is still in tachycardia and has not developed hypotension. Atropine, isoproterenol, and calcium chloride should be readily available for acute intravenous administration to reverse either the bradycardic or hypotensive effects of verapamil. These are rarely encountered, but the physician must be ready to counteract them. Verapamil is contraindicated in the patient who has received propranolol or other beta-blockers within the past 48 hours and may be contraindicated in patients who have received quinidine or disopyramide. We also recommend caution in using verapamil in the patient who is likely to have sick sinus syndrome. Verapamil rarely converts atrial flutter or fibrillation to sinus rhythm but can be used to slow the ventricular response. Verapamil could also be used to slow the ventricular response to an atrial automatic focus tachycardia, although it will not convert the tachycardia to sinus rhythm. Because of our experience with intravenous verapamil in two patients with junctional automatic tachycardia, we feel that it is contraindicated in this type of tachycardia.[40] For patients in whom verapamil is ineffective, DC cardioversion is also likely to be ineffective but may be tried in a dose of 1/4 watt-second/pound. If DC cardioversion fails, then the same regimen as recommended for infants can be followed. Alternatively, if the patient is clinically stable and has a relatively slow tachycardia, chronic digitalization may be begun in an effort to slow the tachycardia and improve the mechanical function of the heart.

Chronic SVT

The third type of presentation is that of a chronic tachycardia that persists for weeks to years. This is in contradistinction to the previous two groups with paroxysmal tachycardia. Characteristically, chronic SVT is usually slower, longer lasting, less symptom-producing, and more influenced by the autonomic nervous system. Many of these patients have evidence of myocardial dysfunction which may be secondary to the tachycardia or may reflect some previous insult which caused both. Electrophysiologic studies in these patients have revealed three common mechanisms: an automatic etopic focus located in the atrium or bundle of His (AV junction)[41, 42]; a concealed AC (unidirectional retrograde accessory pathway (URAP)), often right anterior[43, 19]; or AV node reentry with the fast pathway as the antegrade limb and the slow pathway as the retrograde limb (Fig. 45.17).[44, 45]

The treatment of chronic SVT is based on a knowledge of the mechanism of the tachycardia, the rate of the tachycardia, and the degree of myocardial dysfunction evidenced by chest roentgenograms, echocardiography, and symptoms noted by the patient. The patient should be treated with digoxin to improve myocardial performance. Digoxin may slow the rate of tachycardia and, in an occasional case, may convert a patient with a concealed accessory connection or AV node reentry to sinus rhythm. If digoxin does not convert the patient to sinus rhythm, a decision must be made as to whether further treatment is indicated. If the patient is symptomatic or if there is evidence of significant myocardial dysfunction, further treatment should be undertaken. We have not found a medical treatment plan which is consistently successful in converting atrial automatic focus tachycardias to sinus rhythm, or which consistently reduces the rate of the tachycardia to an acceptable level in the majority of patients.

Although these patients may be asymptomatic for years, if the tachycardia rate is consistently above 150 in the infant or 120 in the teenager, myocardial dysfunction almost invariably occurs. In symptomatic patients or patients with myocardial dysfunction, we have found surgical removal or cryodestruction of the automatic focus to be the most successful treatment.[46] To date, we have only performed this operation in seven patients, but each of the patients is now

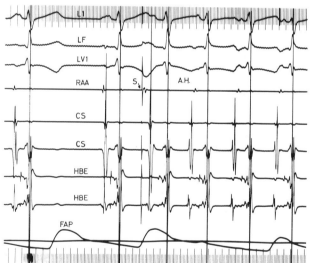

Fig. 45.17 Induction of AV node reentry tachycardia is shown on surface ECG leads I, AVF, and V1 recorded simultaneously with a right atrial appendage, two coronary sinuses, two His bundle electrograms with phasic and mean femoral artery pressure, and time lines. The first two beats are sinus with nearly equal activation of the low septal right atrium, proximal coronary sinus, and right atrial appendage followed by a distal coronary sinus. An induced PAT, results in lengthening of the A to H interval and immediately after ventricular depolarization, the low septal right atrium is again activated resulting in a run of supraventricular tachycardia. As can be seen in this case, the most frequent type of AV node reentry supraventricular tachycardia seen in pediatric patients involves a short conduction time in the antegrade direction and a long conduction time in the retrograde direction. The retrograde activation sequence from the low septal right atrium to coronary sinus and the right atrial appendage can be correlated with a negative P wave in lead AVF, a positive P wave in lead I.

asymptomatic with sinus rhythm. If long-term follow-up confirms these good results, then this form of treatment may be offered to patients who are less symptomatic or have only the beginnings of myocardial dysfunction.

The chronic SVT caused by concealed accessory connections may be treated somewhat more successfully medically. The addition of propranolol or quinidine to digoxin will convert some patients to sinus rhythm. The decision must then be made as to whether long-term treatment with depressive drugs, is preferable to surgical division of the accessory connection. We have tended to favor the surgical alternative in these patients in recent years.[47]

Chronic atrioventricular nodal reentry tachycardia occasionally may be successfully treated with digoxin or the combination of digoxin and propranolol. In our experience, however, this is rarely the case. Oral verapamil, together with digoxin, has been successful in controlling virtually every patient with chronic atrioventricular nodal reentry tachycardia.

Surgical Treatment of SVT

Surgical treatment is necessary for SVT in only a small percentage of infants and children. Occasionally, however, a patient is found who does not respond to medical treatment, or in whom the side effects of medical treatment outweigh the small risk of surgery. Each type of SVT is now amenable to surgical treatment.

Surgical treatment can be divided into the indirect and direct forms. Indirect treatment would include pacing to prevent bradycardic induction of supraventricular tachycardia, whether it is demand atrial or ventricular pacing. Another indirect treatment is implantation of an automatic or externally controlled overdrive pacemaker. Examples of each of these have been used successfully in infants and children. The most promising is the implantable completely automatic multiprogrammable overdrive pacemaker produced by Intermedics (Cybertach Intermedics Inc., Freeport, Texas), which has a large variety of overdrive rates and durations (Fig. 45.18).[48] Miniaturization of this pacemaker will make it more acceptable in infants and children. Another indirect form of surgical treatment of SVT would be surgical destruction of the bundle of His in a patient with an atrial automatic focus tachycardia, atrial flutter, or fibrillation with implantation of a ventricular demand pacemaker.[48] Currently, this would be used only if more direct forms had failed.

Direct surgical treatment of SVT began with surgical division of accessory connections in the Wolff-Parkinson-White syndrome.[49, 50] This treatment is now so successful that some physicians recommend surgical division of the accessory connection in preference to lifelong medical treatment. The success rate for this type of treatment in our institution in infants and children is approximately 90% (Fig. 45.19). More recently, direct surgical treatment of SVT has been expanded to automatic ectopic focus tachycardias in which the automatic focus can be ablated by cryothermic treatment. Cryothermia has also been used in our institution in one case of junctional automatic focus tachycardia in which the junctional automatic focus was ablated and a permanent ventricular pacemaker was installed successfully.

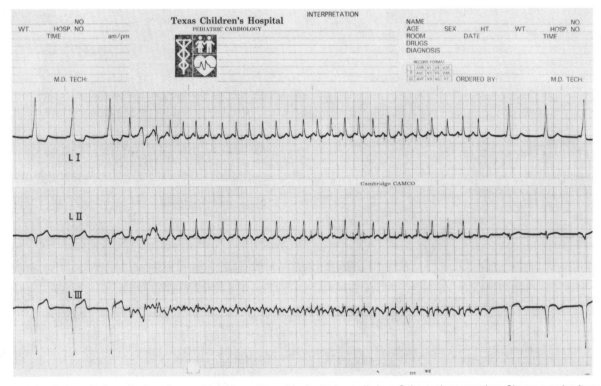

Fig. 45.18 Demonstration of automatic overdrive of a supraventricular tachycardia by a Cybertach pacemaker. Shown are simultaneously recorded surface leads I, II, and III in a patient with the WPW syndrome. After the third QRS complex, a magnet is applied to the pacemaker to place it in fixed rate mode. The first pacing spike seen in the ST segment of the third QRS captures the atrium and induces a narrow QRS supraventricular tachycardia. The magnet is removed until after two more fixed rate beats. Eight beats after the magnet is removed, the pacemaker starts to pace in an overdrive mode and on cessation results in sinus rhythm with WPW conduction. In a patient with WPW syndrome, the benefits of such a pacemaker must weigh against the possibility of inducing a rapid ventricular rhythm, and only patients with relatively long refractory periods of the accessory pathway should be considered for chronic implantation of such a device.

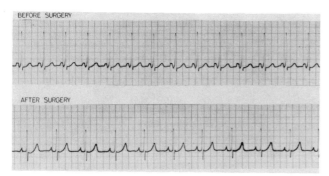

Fig. 45.19 Pre- and postoperative electrocardiograms in a patient who underwent surgical division of accessory connection for Wolff-Parkinson-White syndrome with supraventricular tachycardia. In the *top tracing* taken before surgery, the delta wave and short PR interval are clearly visible. In the *bottom tracing*, taken shortly after surgery, the QRS has normalized, as has the PR interval.

THE WOLFF-PARKINSON-WHITE SYNDROME

The Wolff-Parkinson-White (WPW) syndrome is due to the presence of an accessory connection (AC) which usually conducts electrical activity faster than the AV node. This AC, however, may conduct so slowly or fail to conduct in the antegrade direction that it is concealed on the surface ECG. These "concealed" unidirectional retrograde accessory pathways (URAP) may nonetheless form a part of a tachycardia reentry circuit and may be detected by intracardiac electrophysiological study. Accessory connections which conduct only in the antegrade direction may also participate in dysrhythmias by conducting the impulses of atrial flutter or fibrillation to the ventricles.

The natural history of the WPW syndrome has been a subject of interest. In our review of this subject, we found that 26% of our patients with WPW ceased having the syndrome on their ECG during follow-up. Only part of these patients stopped having episodes of tachycardia, perhaps indicating that their AC continued to function in the retrograde direction only. The clinical course most frequently followed by patients who do not lose their WPW is of frequent tachycardias during infancy, followed by a period during childhood with much less frequent or no dysrhythmias. Puberty often is associated with a second period of increasingly frequent tachycardias which may decrease again in the 3rd decade. Some patients will again develop worsening tachydysrhythmias in later adulthood as coronary and hypertensive heart disease begin to interact with the WPW. There is another group of patients who do not have dysrhythmias in the pediatric age range but who have onset of severe, sometimes life-threatening, episodes of atrial flutter or fibrillation in adulthood. In our experience, these patients usually have extremely short antegrade refractory periods of their AC.

In addition to being the underlying cause of many cases of SVT, WPW frequently complicates the diagnosis of congenital heart defects by making the ECG inaccurate in detecting ventricular hypertrophy. Patients with congenital heart disease are at greater risk of atrial flutter or atrial fibrillation than patients with WPW and otherwise normal hearts and, thus, require special consideration with regard to treatment with digitalis, as mentioned before. Determination of the antegrade refractory period (ARP) of the AC before and after ouabain is indicated in these patients if digitalis is needed in their treatment. Quinidine may be needed to lengthen the ARP of the AC. Division of the AC should be considered during repair of associated congenital heart defects, since postoperative dysrhythmias may be extremely severe in patients with WPW.

VENTRICULAR TACHYCARDIA

Ventricular tachycardia is defined as three or more premature ventricular contractions in a row[51] (Fig. 45.20). These, of course, would be wide QRS complexes and, if a His bundle catheter were recorded, would not have a His depolarization preceding onset of the QRS complexes. Atrioventricular dissociation with a slower atrial rate than ventricular rate is frequently but not always present. Sinus captures and fusion beats are another indication of ventricular tachycardia but are not necessary for this diagnosis. This dysrhythmia is being recognized with increasing frequency in children, particularly in patients after operations for congenital heart disease.[52-54]

Ventricular tachycardia should be differentiated from ventricular escape rhythm, which is a wide QRS rhythm at a slower rate than the preceding sinus rate. It should also be differentiated from accelerated ventricular rhythm, which is a ventricular rhythm at approximately the same rate or slightly faster than the underlying sinus rate.

Ventricular tachycardia is a rather uncommon dysrhythmia in children who have not undergone intracardiac surgery. In many cases a specific cause can be found, such as an intramyocardial tumor, metabolic disturbance, cardiomyopathy, drug ingestion, or drug toxicity from a prior prescribed antidysrhythmic medication. The long QT interval syndrome is another cause of ventricular tachycardia and fibrillation (Fig. 45.21).[55, 56] This ECG diagnosis should be searched for in each patient with ventricular dysrhythmias and in each patient with unexplained syncope or near syncope. Patients with ventricular tachycardia associated with a specific etiology, as mentioned above, are frequently symptomatic. On the other hand, patients with idiopathic ventricular tachycardia usually have no symptoms. Reasons for this are not fully understood, but the slower rate may be a partial explanation, as well as the patient's excellent overall myocardial function.

Patients who are postoperative for congenital heart defects do not tolerate ventricular tachycardia well and are subject to sudden death. In a review of 207 patients who survived intracardiac repair of tetralogy of Fallot, 21 were found to have premature ventricular contractions (PVCs) on a routine resting electrocardiogram. Eight of these 21 died a mean of 3.4 years after surgery. Each of these eight patients had a right ventricular peak systolic pressure of 70 mm Hg or more. None had left arterior hemiblock. Two of these pa-

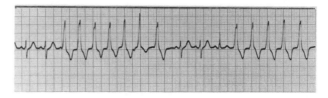

Fig. 45.20 Electrocardiographic tracing of paroxysmal ventricular tachycardia. The first two beats are sinus beats followed by a run of ventricular tachycardia. The first beat of ventricular tachycardia starts after the sinus P wave. The sixth beat of ventricular tachycardia is a fusion beat partially activated by the ventricular tachycardia and partially activated by the low atrial depolarization just preceding it. After two sinus beats, the ventricular tachycardia resumes with another fusion beat which is mostly sinus and only partially originates from the ventricular tachycardia.

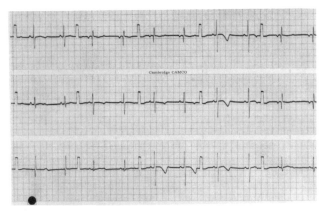

Fig. 45.21 Electrocardiogram from an infant with the prolonged QT interval syndrome who had multiple episodes of ventricular fibrillation. The prolonged QT interval, as well as the bizarre T wave morphology, is most pronounced in V5 and V6.

tients were known to have had ventricular tachycardias (VTs) before death. It is, therefore, clear that the association of PVCs and residual sequelae after correlation of tetralogy of Fallot carries a serious prognosis. Other series have also found a high frequency of ventricular tachydysrhythmias in postoperative tetralogies and an association with sudden death. A greater percentage will be found to have PVCs if a treadmill test is performed.[57] The significance of these PVCs is not known but we consider them essentially the same as resting PVCs. Suppression of PVCs by exercise in a patient postoperative for tetralogy of Fallot has been found not to be indicative of a good prognosis. This is in contrast to patients with a normal heart in whom exercise suppression of PVCs has been found to correlate with an excellent prognosis.

The induction of either sustained or nonsustained ventricular tachycardia by electrical stimulation of the heart during cardiac catheterization has been found to correlate with symptomatic ventricular dysrhythmias in the postoperative tetralogy of Fallot group. It is not possible to induce VT or ventricular fibrillation (VF) in the normal heart by programmed stimulation of the ventricles. It usually is possible in adults with VT. This is also true in postoperative pediatric patients who have clinical VT but not those who are clinically dysrhythmia free. During electrical stimulation of the heart in children with idiopathic VT, it has not been routinely possible to induce VT. Since most reentrant dysrhythmias can be induced by programmed stimulation, this may be an indication that this type of VT is due to enhanced automaticity.

A new anatomic substrate has been reported by Frank and Fontaine.[58] They coined the term arrhythmogenic right ventricular dysplasia (ARVD) for a VT originating in the RV in cases with isolated RV cardiomyopathy. We have found this disease also in the pediatric population. A retrospective review of angiography in our patients with VT and left bundle branch block (LBBB) pattern during VT found four of 9 to have abnormal right ventricular morphology.[59]

Treatment

In our experience, it has rarely been possible to completely control asymptomatic ventricular tachycardia in pediatric patients with an otherwise normal heart. For this reason and because these patients appear to have an excellent prognosis, our policy is not to treat such patients.

In patients with abnormal hemodynamics, vigorous treatment is undertaken. We have found phenytoin an effective

treatment for patients in this category.[60] Greater than 90% of patients with severely abnormal hemodynamics had complete control of their ventricular dysrhythmia by phenytoin. In those with moderately abnormal hemodynamics, the results are slightly less good, but phenytoin remains the drug of choice. In this group, when the ventricular dysrhythmia is controlled, no patient has experienced sudden death. Phenytoin has not been effective in patients with mitral valve prolapse and thus we prefer instead to use propranolol.

In patients in whom medical treatment is ineffective in controlling severely symptomatic ventricular dysrhythmias, surgery may be considered.[61] If a patient has an intramyocardial tumor, removal of the tumor frequently results in disappearance of the ventricular tachycardia. In patients with a reentrant mechanism for their ventricular tachycardia documented by the electrophysiology study, incision through the reentry circuit is frequently successful in stopping the dysrhythmia. This has been shown particularly in patients after repair of tetralogy of Fallot as well as in patients with arrhythmogenic RV dysplasia.

ATRIAL FLUTTER AND FIBRILLATION

Atrial flutter and atrial fibrillation are tachydysrhythmias which originate above the bifurcation of the bundle of His. They could, therefore, be classified as supraventricular tachycardias. We have chosen to separate these dysrhythmias because of their different presentation, clinical course, electrocardiographic pattern, and response to treatment.

Atrial flutter is defined as a rapid atrial tachycardia with characteristic flutter waves (Fig. 45.22).[61] The flutter waves will not be seen in each electrocardiographic lead but are often seen best in 2, 3, AVF and V1. The rate of atrial flutter is most frequently 300 beats/minute, but in infants, the rate of atrial flutter may range as high as 400 to 450 beats/minute. Atrial rates much less than 280 beats/minute are usually not considered to be atrial flutter. The ventricular response to atrial flutter can range from 1:1 conduction to various degrees of second degree AV block.

Atrial flutter is most commonly seen in two groups of pediatric patients. The first group are those with large stretched atria due to congenital or acquired heart disease; the three most common lesions are: tricuspid atresia, Ebstein's anomaly, and rheumatic mitral valve disease. The second group frequently seen is neonates, often with otherwise normal hearts. Both groups of patients frequently develop heart failure if the atrial flutter is not converted.

Treatment is always indicated in a patient with atrial flutter. Direct current cardioversion is the most frequently successful and the most rapid method of restoring a normal heart rhythm. This is almost always successful in the neo-

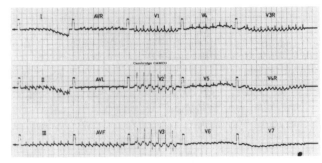

Fig. 45.22 Atrial flutter with 2:1 block in an infant. The flutter waves are best seen in the right chest leads and in the inferior limb leads.

natal group and frequently is successful in the group with stretched atria. We usually perform DC cardioversion immediately upon diagnosis in neonates but usually treat the older patient with stretched atria with digitalis and quinidine before conversion. This is because the older patient with stretched atria is more likely to rapidly revert to atrial flutter after initially successful cardioversion. After conversion, neonates are always treated with digoxin and, if this proves ineffective in controlling the atrial flutter, propranolol is added as the second drug of choice. Occasionally, quinidine may be needed as a replacement for propranolol. Neonates are treated for 1 year if they have no recurrence, following which the medication can usually be stopped without a recurrence of the flutter. Older patients may benefit from a surgical procedure to improve their hemodynamic status, and only in this situation can the medical treatment be safely withdrawn.

Atrial fibrillation is a less common dysrhythmia in infants and children. In atrial fibrillation, there is a fine or slightly more coarse variation in the base line and a completely irregular ventricular response. Atrial fibrillation occurs in the same group of patients with stretched atria that was described in atrial flutter. Atrial fibrillation is also known to occur in the Wolff-Parkinson-White syndrome, in which case there may be very rapid conduction to the ventricles. An irregular wide QRS tachydysrhythmia should always be suspected to be atrial fibrillation with Wolff-Parkinson-White syndrome in atrial fibrillation or atrial flutter, digitalis is contraindicated. This is because of the propensity for digitalis to increase the rapidity of conduction over the Kent bundle. In patients without Wolff-Parkinson-White, digoxin is very useful in slowing atrioventricular conduction over the normal conduction system. Propranolol may be added to digoxin to further slow conduction. Each patient with atrial fibrillation should be converted in order to see if medication will maintain sinus rhythm. Persistent atrial fibrillation may be an indication for surgery in patients with stretched atria.

IRREGULARITY OF HEART RATE WITHOUT TACHYCARDIA

Conduction disturbances are infrequently seen in children, except those with underlying heart disease. These conduction disturbances include first degree AV block, second degree AV block, and bundle branch blocks. The significance of these conduction disturbances is determined by their severity, their location in the conduction system, and their associated heart disease.

First Degree AV Block

First degree AV block is almost never of any clinical significance by itself. It is frequently seen as an isolated finding or in association with acute rheumatic fever. In these situations the block is in the AV node when studied by intracardiac electrophysiology. First degree AV block is also often seen in association with congenital heart disease. Intracardiac electrophysiologic studies have localized these blocks to all parts of the conduction system, from the atrial muscle to the bundle branch system. Postoperative first degree AV blocks may also be found in any part of the conduction system and are usually of little significance.

Disturbances in the Trifascicular Intraventricular Conduction System

Conduction disturbances in the trifascicular intraventricular conduction system are most commonly seen after cardiac surgery.[62, 63] They are of more varied prognostic signif-

icance. Isolated right bundle branch block is of little or no importance and does not imply heart disease in the patient with an otherwise normal heart. In the postoperative patient it is also of little significance, in the short term, whether it is due to a distal or proximal lesion. In the long run (40 to 50 years), these patients may have an increased frequency of complete AV block, since adults may develop left bundle branch block.

Bifascicular block pattern is an ECG diagnosis frequently made but poorly understood. The pattern most often seen in children is right bundle branch block and left anterior hemiblock. In most instances there probably is not true complete block in either fascicle, but rather the pattern is due to abnormal development of the conduction system. This is particularly true in primum atrial septal defect. Only in patients in whom bifascicular block develops after surgery is it likely to be a true conduction block. The prognosis of these patients has not yet been determined but may be little different from that of other postoperative patients.

Left bundle branch block can be considered a special form of bifascicular block since two of the three fascicles are nonfunctional. Since the right bundle branch is the most likely fascicle to suffer later damage, these patients may be at risk for complete AV block. Complete left bundle block is a rare postoperative lesion, but patients with this diagnosis should always be considered for permanent pacing. An exception might be the patient who develops left bundle branch block after resection of a subaortic stenosis, since they do not appear to be at high risk of developing complete AV block later. The prognosis of children with left bundle branch block and an otherwise normal heart is unknown.

Trifascicular block is very rare in children. The diagnosis of trifascicular conduction delay can best be made using intracardiac electrophysiology. The surface ECG diagnosis of bifascicular block pattern plus first degree AV block is *not* synonymous with trifascicular block. This may often be due to proximal block in one fascicle, distal or proximal block in another, and first degree block in the AV node. Only rarely is this pattern due to actual conduction delay in all three fascicles.

Second Degree AV Block

Second degree AV block is uncommonly seen in pediatric patients.[64] Wenckebach (Mobitz type I) second degree AV block is found occasionally in an otherwise normal heart and is usually of little significance. One case has been reported which progressed to symptomatic complete AV block.[64] We have found this type of second degree AV block to be in the AV node when studied by intracardiac electrophysiology. Mobitz type II second degree AV block is more serious and is usually due to block in the distal AV conduction system (Fig. 45.23).

Premature Contractions

Premature atrial, junctional, and ventricular contractions are also of concern in some situations. When they occur in

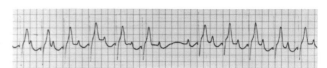

Fig. 45.23 Second degree AV block type II, shown as an ambulatory electrocardiographic tracing of a patient with first degree AV. The degree of first degree AV block is stable, and a P wave is suddenly dropped. The ensuing PR interval is essentially the same as the preceding PR interval.

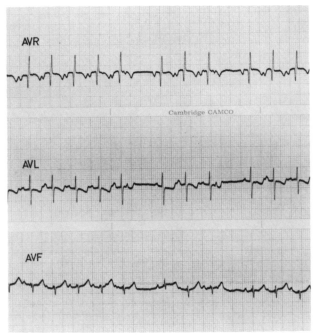

Fig. 45.24 Blocked premature atrial beats in a neonate. Shown are leads AVR, AVL, and AVF. After the fifth QRS complex, a P wave can be seen deforming the ST segment. This P wave does not conduct the ventricles, and sinus rhythm resumes for three more beats before another blocked premature atrial contraction occurs.

the child with a normal heart, they are often benign. Premature ventricular contractions (PVCs) which disappear with exercise have been found to be benign in children with normal hearts. Premature atrial contractions (PACs) and premature junctional contractions which behave in a like manner almost certainly are also benign.

Premature atrial contractions in infants under 1 year of age are a special circumstance. If the contractions are frequent and early, they often lead to atrial flutter or supraventricular tachycardia. Our plan has been to observe the baby in the hospital for 1 week to search for signs of myocarditis, hyperthyroidism, etc, and to determine if the PACs decrease in frequency or disappear. If they do not then, we institute therapy with digoxin. If digoxin is ineffective, we add propranolol. Even if atrial flutter or SVT occur while the infant is taking these two drugs, the ventricular rate will likely be slower, and HF will not develop.

PACs in infants also often conduct aberrantly or block completely in the AV conduction system. Aberrantly conducted PACs may be mistaken for PVCs. A careful search of the preceding T wave will often reveal the premature P wave. Blocked PACs may be confused with sinus bradycardia (Fig. 45.24). If the premature P waves are seen, digitalis or digitalis and propranolol often stop the PACs and increase the ventricular rate.

Multiform PVCs, those which occur in runs of three or more and those which occur in children with associated heart disease, are more serious.

Our plan for investigation and treatment of postoperative PVCs is presented in the section on ventricular tachycardia. This plan is valid for other postoperative patients and for those with other serious heart disease. Occasionally, a child with a normal heart will require treatment for PVCs, and these are then treated as ventricular tachycardia.

Premature atrial and junctional contractions rarely require treatment unless they cause symptoms or SVT.

There are many variations of normal rhythm which should not be mistaken for abnormalities. These include sinus arrhythmia, wandering atrial pacemaker, and sinus arrhythmia with junctional escape. Each are seen with increasing frequency with the use of 24-hour ambulatory ECGs. We consider each of these to be benign.

REFERENCES

1. Reder, R. F., and Rosen, M. R.: Basic electrophysiologic principles: Application to treatment of dysrhythmias. In Pediatric Cardiac Dysrhythmias, edited by P. C. Gillette and A. Garson, Jr. Grune & Stratton, New York, 1981, pp. 121–143.
2. Garson, A. Jr., Gillette, P. C., and McNamara, D. G.: A Guide in Cardiac Dysrhythmias in Children. Grune & Stratton, New York, 1980.
3. Gillette, P. C., and Garson, A., Jr.: Intracardiac electrophysiologic studies: Use in determining the site and mechanisms of dysrhythmias. In: Pediatric Cardiac Dysrhythmias, edited by P. C. Gillette and A. Garson, Jr. Grune & Stratton, New York, 1981, pp. 77–120.
4. Kugler, J. D.: Sinoatrial node dysfunction. In: Pediatric Cardiac Dysrhythmias, edited by P. C. Gillette and A. Garson, Jr. Grune & Stratton, New York, 1981, pp. 265–293.
5. Narula, O. S., Samet, P., and Javier, R. P.: Significance of the sinus node recovery time. Circulation 45:140–152, 1972.
6. Gutgesell, H. P., Gillette, P. C., and McNamara, D. G.: The response of the sinoatrial node to rapid atrial stimulation (abstr.). Pediatr. Res. 8:350, 1974.
7. Strauss, H. C., Saroff, A. L., Bigger, J. T., et al.: Premature atrial stimulation as a key to the understanding of sinoatrial conduction in man. Circulation 47:86–93, 1973.
8. Kugler, J. D., Gillette, P. C., Mullins, C. E., et al.: Sinoatrial conduction in children: An index of sinoatrial node function. Circulation 59:1266–1276, 1979.
9. Gillette, P. C., Mullins, C. E., and McNamara, D. G.: Functional properties of the atrioventricular node in infants and children (abstr.). Pediatr. Res. 9:53, 1975.
10. Wit, A. L., Weiss, M. B., Berkowitz, W. D., et al.: Patterns of A-V conduction in the human heart. Circ. Res. 27:345–352, 1970.
11. Denes, P., Wu, D., Dhingra, R., et al.: The effect of cycle length on cardiac refractory periods in man. Circulation 49:32–38, 1974.
12. DuBrow, I. W., Fisher, E. Q., Amat-y-Leon, F., et al.: Comparison of cardiac refractory periods in children and adults. Circulation 51:485–496, 1975.
13. Wolff, G. S., Mehta, A., Tamer, D., Garcia, O. L., Pichoff, A. S., Costa, A., Fener, P. L., Sung, R., and Gelband, H.: His-Purkinje responses and refractory periods during atrial extrastimulation in children with heart defects. Circulation 63:1383–1391, 1981.
14. Goldreyer, B. N., and Bigger, J. T.: Site of reentry in paroxysmal supraventricular tachycardia in man. Circulation 43:15–23, 1971.
15. Goldreyer, B. N., Gallagher, J. J., and Damato, A. N.: The electrophysiologic demonstration of atrial ectopic tachycardia in man. Am Heart J 85:205–211, 1973.
16. Gillette, P. C.: The mechanisms of supraventricular tachycardia in children. Circulation 54:133–139, 1976.
17. Gillette, P. C., and Garson, A.: Electrophysiologic and pharmacologic characteristics of automatic ectopic atrial tachycardia. Circulation 56:571–575, 1977.
18. Gillette, P. C., Garson, A., and Kugler, J. D.: WPW in children: Electrophysiologic and pharmacologic characteristics. Circulation 60:1487–1495, 1979.
19. Gillette, P. C.: Concealed anomalous cardiac conduction pathways: A frequent cause of supraventricular tachycardia. Am. J. Cardiol. 40:848–852, 1977.
20. Southall, D. P., Johnston, F., Shinebourne, E. A., and Johnston, P. G.: 24-hour electrocardiographic study of heart rate and rhythm patterns in population of healthy children. Br. Heart J. 45:281–291, 1981.
21. Kleinman, C. S., Hobbins, J. C., Jaffe, C. C., et al.: Echocardiographic studies of the human fetus: Prenatal diagnosis of congenital heart disease and cardiac dysrhythmias. Pediatrics 65:1059–1066, 1980.
22. Michaelsson, M., and Engle, M. A.: Congenital complete heart block: An internation study of the natural history. In Cardiovascular Clinics, edited by A. N. Brest and M. A. Engle. F. A. Davis, Philadelphia, 1972, p. 85.
23. Karpawich, P. P., Garson, A., Gillette, P. C., Hesslein, P. S., Porter, C. J., and McNamara, D. G.: Congenital complete atrioventricular block: Clinical and electrophysiologic prediction of need for pacemaker insertion. Am. J. Cardiol. 48:1098–1102, 1982.
24. Levy, A. M., Camm, A. J., and Keane, J. F.: Multiple arrhythmias detected during nocturnal monitoring in patients with congenital complete heart block. Circulation 55:247–253, 1977.
25. Winkler, R. B., Freed, M. D., and Nadas, A. S.: Exercise induced ventricular ectopy in children and young adults with complete heart

block. Am. Heart J. 9:87–92, 1980.
26. Porter, C. J., Gillette, P. C., and McNamara, D. G.: 24-hour ambulatory ECGs in the detection and management of cardiac dysrhythmias in infants and children. Pediatr. Cardiol. 1:203–208, 1980.
27. Driscoll, D. J., Gillette, P. C., and Hallman, G. L., et al.: Management of surgical complete atrioventricular block in children. Am. J. Cardiol. 43:1175–1180, 1979.
28. Morriss, J. H., Eugster, G. S., Nora, J. J., et al.: His bundle recordings in progressive external ophthalmoplegia. J. Pediatr. 81:1167–1170, 1972.
29. Morriss, J. H., Gillette, P. C., and Barrett, F. F.: Atrioventricular block complicating meningitis: Treatment with emergency cardiac pacing. Pediatrics 58:866–869, 1976.
30. Gillette, P. C., Kugler, J. D., A. Garson, Jr., Gutgesell, H. P., Duff, D. F., and McNamara, D. G.: The mechanisms of cardiac dysrhythmias after the Mustard operation for transposition of the great arteries. Am. J. Cardiol. 45:1225–1230, 1980.
31. Gillette, P. C., El-Said, G. M., Sivarajan, N., et al.: Electrophysiological abnormalities after Mustard's operation for transposition of the great arteries. Br. Heart J. 36:186–191, 1974.
32. El-Said, G. M., Gillette, P. C., Mullins, C. E., et al.: Significance of pacemaker recovery time after the Mustard operation for transposition of the great arteries. Am. J. Cardiol. 30:526–532, 1972.
33. Kugler, J. D., Gillette, P. C., Mullins, C. E., et al.: Sinoatrial conduction in children: An index of sinoatrial node function. Circulation 59:1266–1276, 1979.
34. Yabek, S. M., Jarmakani, J. M., and Roberts, N. K.: Sinus node function in children: Factors influencing its evaluation. Circulation 53:28–32, 1976.
35. Morriss, J. H., Ott, D. A., Cooley, D. A., Gillette, P. C.: Pacemakers—indications, implantations, and follow-up. In Pediatric Cardiac Dysrhythmias, edited by P. C. Gillette and A. Garson, Jr. Grune & Stratton, New York, 1981, pp. 421–436.
36. Garson, A., and Gillette, P. C.: Supraventricular tachycardia. In Pediatric Cardiac Dysrhythmias, edited by P. C. Gillette and A. Garson, Jr. Grune & Stratton, New York, 1981, pp. 177–253.
37. Bisset, G. S., Gaum, W. E., and Kaplan, S.: The ice bag: A new technique for interruption of supraventricular tachycardia. J. Pediatr.

97:593–595, 1980.
38. Wolff, G. S., Han, J., and Curran, J: Wolff-Parkinson-White syndrome in the neonate. Am. J. Cardiol. 41:559–563, 1978.
39. Gillette, P. C.: The preexcitation syndromes. In Pediatric Cardiac Dysrhythmias, edited by P. C. Gillette and A. Garson, Jr. Grune & Stratton, New York, 1981, pp. 153–176.
40. Porter, C. J., Gillette, P. C., Garson, A., Hesslein, P. S., Karpawich, P. P., and McNamara, D. G.: The effects of verapamil on supraventricular tachycardia in children. Am. J. Cardiol. 48:487–491, 1981.
41. Gillette, P. C., and Garson, A.: Electrophysiologic and pharmacologic characteristics of automatic ectopic atrial tachycardia. Circulation 56:571–575, 1977.
42. Garson, A., and Gillette, P. C.: Junctional ectopic tachycardia in children: Electrocardiography, electrophysiology and pharmacologic response. Am. J. Cardiol. 44:298–302, 1979.
43. Orzan, F., and Gillette, P. C.: Reciprocating tachycardia due to a right-sided unidirectional retrograde anomalous pathway. PACE 1:306–312, 1978.
44. Wolff, G. S., Sung, R. J., Pickoff, A., et al: The fast-slow form of atrioventricular nodal reentrant tachycardia in children. Am. J. Cardiol. 43:1181–1188, 1979.
45. Gillette, P. C.: The mechanisms of supraventricular tachycardia in children. Circulation 54:133–139, 1976.
46. Gillette, P. C., Garson, A., Hesslein, P. S., et al.: Successful surgical treatment of atrial, junctional and ventricular tachycardia in infants and children. Am. Heart J., in press, 1982.
47. Gallagher, J. J., Pritchett, E. L. C., Sealy, W. C., et al.: The preexcitation syndromes. Prog. Cardiovasc. Dis. 20:285, 1978.
48. Gillette, P. C.: Advances in the diagnosis and treatment of tachydysrhythmias in children. Am. Heart. J. 102:111–120, 1981.
49. Gallagher, J. J., Gilbert, M., Svenson, R. H., et al.: Wolff-Parkinson-White syndrome, the problem, evaluation, and surgical correction. Circulation 51:767–785, 1975.
50. Kugler, J. D., Gillette, P. C., Duff, D. F., et al.: Elective mapping and surgical division of the bundle of Kent in a patient with Ebstein's anomaly who required tricuspid valve replacement. Am. J. Cardiol. 41:602–605, 1978.
51. Garson, A.: Ventricular dysrhythmias. In Pediatric Cardiac Dysrhythmias, edited by P. C. Gillette and A. Garson, Jr. Grune & Stratton,

New York, 1981, pp. 295–360.
52. Pedersen, D., Zipes, D. P., Foster, P. R., et al.: Ventricular tachycardia and ventricular fibrillation in a young population. Circulation 60:988–997, 1979.
53. Vetter, V. L., Horowitz, L. N., and Josephson, M. E.: Recurrent sustained ventricular tachycardia in pediatric patients. Circulation 57/58:196, 1978.
54. Garson, A., Jr., Nihill, M. R., McNamara, D. G., et al.: Status of the adult and adolescent after repair of tetralogy of Fallot. Circulation 59:1232–1240, 1979.
55. Romano, C., Gemme, G., and Pongiglione, R.: Aritmie cardiache rare dell'eta' pediatrica. II. Assessi sincopali per fibrillazione ventricolare parossistica. Clin. Pediatr. 45:656–683, 1963.
56. Ward, O. C.: A new familial cardiac syndrome in children. J. Irish Med. Assoc. 54:103–106, 1964.
57. Garson, A., Gillette, P. C., Gutgesell, H. P., et al.: Stress-induced ventricular arrhythmias after tetralogy of Fallot repair. Am. J. Cardiol. 46:1006–1012, 1980.
58. Garson, A.: Ventricular dysrhythmias. Cardiovasc. Rev., in press, 1982.
59. Dungan, W. T., Garson, A., and Gillette, P. C.: Arrhythmogenic right ventricular dysplasia: A cause of ventricular tachycardia in children with apparently normal hearts. Am. Heart. J., in press, 1982.
60. Garson, A., Kugler, J. D., Gillette, P. C., et al.: Control of late postoperative ventricular arrhythmias with phenytoin in young patients. Am. J. Cardiol. 46:260–294, 1980.
61. Shih, J. Y., Gillette, P. C., and Garson, A.: Atrial flutter and fibrillation. In Pediatric Cardiac Dysrhythmias, edited by P. C. Gillette and A. Garson, Jr. Grune & Stratton, New York, 1981, pp. 255–263.
62. Krongrad, E.: Prognosis for patients with congenital heart disease and postoperative intraventricular conduction defects. Circulation 57:867–870, 1978.
63. Stegg, C. N., Krongrad, E., Davachi, F., et al.: Postoperative left anterior hemiblock and right bundle branch block following repair of tetralogy of Fallot: Clinical and etiologic considerations. Circulation 51:1026–1029, 1975.
64. Young, D., Eisenberg, R., Fish, B., et al.: Wenckebach arterioventricular block (Mobitz type I) in children and adolescents. Am. J. Cardiol. 40:393–399, 1977.

46

Cardiac Tumors

Jesse E. Edwards, M.D.

Cardiac tumors collectively are rare in infancy and childhood. The manifestations vary considerably, depending, in part, upon the histologic type, but mainly upon the location of the tumor. Involvement of the conduction tissue may be manifested clinically as a dysrhythmia. Intracavitary neoplasms, because of their space-occupying feature, may be responsible for inflow obstruction into the chamber harboring the tumor. As such tumors may concomitantly obstruct

a valve, murmurs may vary in nature from time to time or may be intermittently present and absent. Fragmentation of intracavitary tumors may lead to embolism, either pulmonary or systemic, depending upon the location of the tumor.

Involvement of the myocardium may lead to myocardial failure and to signs of localized lesions in electrocardiograms and echocardiograms. Pericardial involvement, which usually is caused by a malignant tumor, is manifested chiefly as cardiac compression, and this may be associated with other features simulating infectious pericarditis.

With the foregoing as a background, cardiac neoplasms will be discussed primarily according to the types found in the study of McAllister and Fenoglio[18] and listed in Tables 46.1 and 46.2.

In his comprehensive treatise on cardiac tumors, McAllister[17] summarized the highlights regarding the most common tumors found in infants and children. According to this author, in the young the most common cardiac tumor is the rhabdomyoma. Moreover, in infants under 1 year old, more than three-quarters of tumors are rhabdomyomas and teratomas. In subjects from 1 to 15 years of age, 80% of cardiac tumors are accounted for by rhabdomyomas, fibromas, and myxomas.

BENIGN TUMORS

RHABDOMYOMA

Rhabdomyoma classically involves the myocardium in numerous areas. One or several of the lesions may appear as a gross mass, often larger than a ventricular cavity. Commonly, the major mass lies in the ventricular septum, but it may appear in the wall of any of the chambers or in the atrial septum. Smaller lesions are common and may be recognized grossly as pale nodules. Some may be observed only as tiny, microscopic-sized nodules. The individual masses are discrete, pale, and homogeneous (Fig. 46.1).

Histologically, the cells are uniformly swollen to gross proportions, as they are distended with glycogen. In preparations from which this substance has been washed out, the cells are highly vacuolated and appear in remarkable contrast to the surrounding unaffected myocardial fibers. Metastases do not occur, and cardiac disability results either from the obstructive effects of a large mass and/or from multifocal replacement of the myocardium by the lesion.

Cerebral lesions of tuberous sclerosis are observed in somewhat over one-third of cases,[17] and cutaneous lesions in the form of adenomas of the sebaceous glands may be associated in cases of congenital rhabdomyoma of the heart.

The nature of the myocardial lesion was thoroughly reviewed by Hudson.[13] According to this author, three views are held: the tumor is a hamartoma of the myocardium; the tumor represents a maldevelopment of the Purkinje fibers;

TABLE 46.1   TUMORS AND CYSTS IN THE HEART AND PERICARDIUM IN INFANTS[a]

Type	No.	%
Benign		
Rhabdomyoma	28[b]	58.3
Teratoma	9	18.8
Fibroma	6	12.5
Hemangioma	1	2.1
Mesothelioma of the AV node	1	2.1
Subtotal	45	93.7
Bronchogenic cyst	1	2.1
Subtotal	1	2.1
Malignant		
Fibrosarcoma	1	2.1
Rhabdomyosarcoma	1	2.1
Subtotal	2	4.2
Total	48	100.0

[a] From H. A. McAllister and J. J. Fenoglio[18] and the Armed Forces Institute of Pathology.

[b] Includes three stillborn infants.

TABLE 46.2   TUMORS AND CYSTS OF THE HEART AND PERICARDIUM IN CHILDREN[a]

Type	No.	%
Benign		
Rhabdomyoma	35	39.3
Fibroma	12	13.5
Myxoma	12	13.5
Teratoma	11	12.4
Hemangioma	4	4.5
Mesothelioma of the AV node	3	3.4
Neurofibroma	1	1.1
Subtotal	78	87.6
Pericardial cyst	2	2.2
Bronchogenic cyst	1	1.1
Subtotal	3	3.4
Malignant		
Malignant teratoma	4	4.5
Rhabdomyosarcoma	2	2.2
Neurogenic sarcoma	1	1.1
Fibrosarcoma	1	1.1
Subtotal	8	9.0
Total	89	100.0

[a] From H. A. McAllister and J. J. Fenoglio[18] and the Armed Forces Institute of Pathology.

or the lesion represents a localized form of cardiac glycogenosis.

Ultrastructural studies by Fenoglio and associates[7] favor the view that the tumor cell is an embryonic myoblast.

Among patients who are symptomatic in infancy, symptoms are usually of cardiac origin, while in those individuals who live to childhood or adult life, the effects of associated cerebral tuberous sclerosis in the form of mental retardation dominate the clinical picture. Suspicion of a rhabdomyoma may result from electrocardiographic signs of a localized loss of electrical activity or of dysrhythmias and from the presence of a space-occupying mass in a cavity of the heart, as seen by angiocardiographic or echocardiographic study.[1] In the case of Neal and associates[19] a mass obstructing the tricuspid orifice yielded a clinical picture suggesting tricuspid atresia.

In a case reported by Shrivastava and associates,[24] a 13-year-old boy who had been apparently healthy died after an acute illness. The massively enlarged heart harbored widely distributed myocardial fibers having the histologic characteristics of rhabdomyoma cells. Since there were no discrete tumor nodules, and in view of the widespread distribution of abnormal cells, the case was considered to conform to a rare condition previously named rhabdomyomatosis.

TERATOMA

Benign teratoma is the designation generally given to multiloculated cystic lesions which arise over the intrapericardial portions of the great arteries and in which elements of the three germ layers are represented upon histologic examination. Among subjects harboring these uncommon tumors there is a strong tendency for the female sex to be represented. According to Bigelow and associates,[4] of the five reported cases, three were found in infants or children. Beck[3] removed a massive tumor of this type from a 22-year-old man.

FIBROMA

Benign solid tumors of fibroblastic origin may occur in the wall of any of the chambers, such as near the apical region

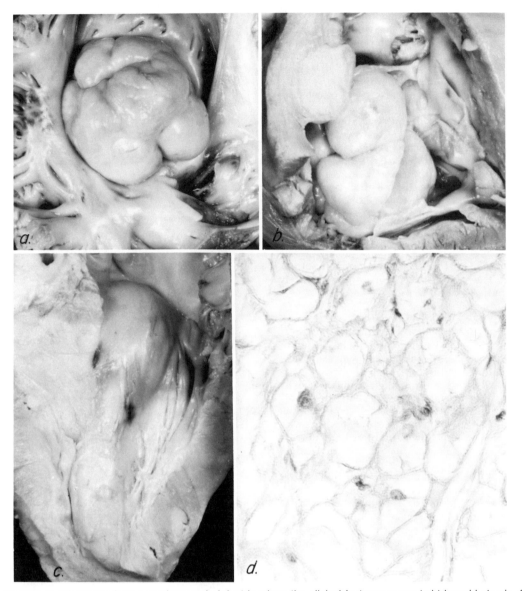

Fig. 46.1 Cardiac rhabdomyoma from a newborn male infant in whom the clinical features suggested tricuspid atresia. (*a.*) Interior of right atrium viewed from above. The tricuspid orifice is obstructed by a rhabdomyoma. (*b.*) Interior of right ventricle. The mass seen in *a* has partially protruded through the tricuspid orifice. Smaller nodules are present in the right ventricular wall. (*c.*) Left ventricle. In addition to small intramural nodules, there is a prominent mass in the subaortic area. (*d.*) Photomicrograph of tumor obstructing the tricuspid orifice. Large clear cells characteristic of congenital rhabdomyoma. H & E, ×340.

of the left ventricle, but most commonly they occur in the ventricular septum. Symptoms depend upon location and size of the tumors. Those in the ventricular septum may cause interference with conduction. Most tumors that occur in a ventricular wall cause no symptoms.

Symptoms result from herniation of the tumor into the cavity of the involved chamber. Among the few reported cases of this condition which were reviewed by Prichard,[22] calcification is common.

In their review of the literature, Geha and associates[11] found that of 36 cases, 31 were children. McAllister[17] observed that the fibroma was the second most common cardiac tumor among children. Although the tumor does not possess a capsule, it may be sufficiently discrete as to be removable in some cases.[11, 20] In others, its periphery intermingles with myocardial tissue to the degree that resection cannot be accomplished.[27]

Extension from the main mass into surrounding myocar-

dial tissue resembles the invasive character of benign fibroblastic tumors that occur in extracardiac locations.

In the case of Bigelow and associates,[4] which involved a 3-day-old female infant, the histologic features of the tumor were those of fibromatous tissue, among which were cardiac muscle fibers. Because of the tendency for so-called fibromas to be associated with elements other than those of fibroblastic origin, Prichard[22] preferred to include fibromas under a broad heading of hamartoma.

In subjects with neurofibromatosis (von Recklinghausen's disease), a rare example of neurofibroma involving the wall of either ventricle may be observed.[17]

HAMARTOMA AND ANGIOMA

Solid solitary benign tumors containing various elements, including fibroblasts, fat cells, endothelial formations, and cardiac muscle, may be termed hamartomas. As indicated, there is some justification for grouping lesions of this type with those in which only fibroblastic elements are identifiable. In the views of Anbe and Fine,[2] such tumors are usually lymphangiomas and, less commonly, take on appearances that justify their being considered as arterial or venous malformations, so-called vascular hamartomas.

Rare examples of lymphangioma have been reviewed by Bigelow and associates.[4] These authors refer to the case of Lymburner which involved a 10-month-old boy with a lymphangioma in the superficial aspect of the right atrial wall. In that case, a cystic hygroma of the neck and mediastinum was also present. In the review cited, there is mention of the case of Armstrong and Monckeburg, in which a lymphangioma occurred in the bundle of His in a 5 1/2-year-old boy with heart block.

In the newborn it is common to observe on the tricuspid and mitral valves several cavernous, blood-filled spaces which grossly present as tiny purple spots on the atrial aspects of the leaflets. These formations should not be considered tumors and are to be viewed as normal structures of the newborn. They tend to regress, as they are rarely observed beyond the newborn period.

INTRACAVITARY MYXOMA

The reviews of Mahaim[16] and Prichard[22] indicate that of all primary cardiac tumors the intracavitary myxoma constitutes about one-half the cases.

As with nearly all cardiac tumors, the myxoma is usually identified either clinically or at necropsy in adult subjects.[5, 23] Yet, it occurs in children and therefore needs consideration in this book. In McAllister's[17] series, 9% of 130 patients with cardiac myxomas were under 15 years of age. Myxoma is more common in the female than male by a ratio of about 2:1.[23]

Differding and associates[6] consider that the earliest age at which unquestioned intracavitary myxomas have been observed is 3 years. In their analysis of 38 reported examples of surgically treated cases (including two of their own), there were three children 8, 12, and 14 years old, respectively. The case of Goldberg and associates[12] involved a 3-year-old boy who suffered cerebral and cutaneous embolism from a left atrial myxoma.

Except for the rare involvement of the left or right ventricle, the intracavitary myxomas are characteristically atrial in origin. Of the latter, about 75% are primary in the left atrium and the balance are in the right.[5, 17, 23] Characteristically, the tumor is intracavitary and solitary. Multiple myxomas were observed in 5% of McAllister's cases.[17]

The gross appearance of the intracavitary myxoma is that of a pedunculated tumor, with the peduncle characteristically attached to the atrial septum by a pedicle of varying size (Fig. 46.2). There is a peculiar predilection for the pedicle to be attached in the region of the foramen ovale. On the right side, the site of attachment is most often to the rim of the foramen ovale, while on the left side the pedicle usually attaches near the position of interatrial ostium secundum. St. John Sutton and associates[23] observed that the sites of atrial septal attachments may uncommonly vary from the classic. The tumor may vary in size from about 1 cm in diameter to a large mass that may all but fill the chamber in which it lies. The surface, in some cases, is smooth, while in others it is grossly papillary, resembling a bunch of grapes.

The fundamental nature of the tumor is for it to be pale, tan, translucent, and gelatinous but, since surface erosion and deposit of blood clot may occur, the tumor may appear brown to purple in color.

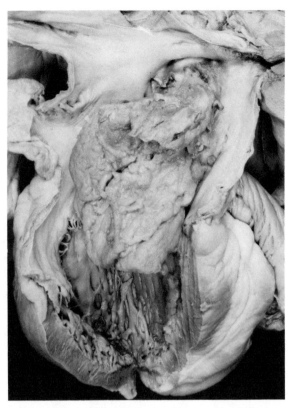

Fig. 46.2   Left atrial myxoma from a 13-year-old girl. The tumor, the attachment of which is to the atrial septum, has occupied considerable space of the left atrium and has extended through the mitral orifice. (Reproduced with permission from L. P. Sterns *et al.*: Br. Heart J. 26:75, 1966.)

Although there is still debate as to whether this lesion is a thrombus or an entity other than thrombus, an ever broadening experience strongly favors the view of Prichard[22] that it is a specific entity different from an organized thrombus. This view is based upon a number of factors. Classically, there is no valvular or other cardiac disease, a feature in striking contrast to that when true atrial thrombi are present. While thrombi of the atrial septum have a strong tendency to involve the atrial appendage, myxomas characteristically do not arise from these structures. Atrial fibrillation, commonly present in cases of atrial thrombosis, is classically absent in instances of atrial myxoma. Organized thrombosis with deposits of hemosiderin may occur in some parts of myxomas. These are to be viewed as the result of fragmentation of the tumor with denudation of the surface. Electron microscopic studies support the myxoma as a distinct entity.

The histologic appearance of the intracavitary myxoma varies somewhat, but a fundamental phenomenon is that it is composed primarily of a homogeneous mucoid basophilic material (Fig. 46.3). Within this, cords of cells, two cells thick, frequently ramify. In some areas, fibroblast-like cells may be arranged in palisade formation. Reference has been made to the presence, in some cases, of areas resembling reaction to secondary thrombosis.

The symptoms of intracavitary myxomas depend upon two phenomena: fragmentation with embolism[25] and occupation of cavitary space. Pulmonary embolism, in the form of either large masses or of multiple small particles, is possible. In the latter event, a picture of obstructive pulmonary hypertension may result. Those tumors which involve the left side of the heart may lead to embolic occlusion of

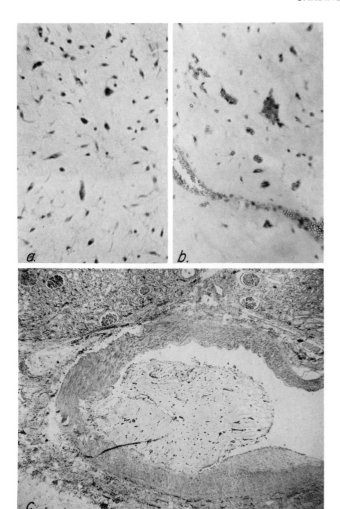

Fig. 46.3 Photomicrographs of left atrial myxoma from the 13-year-old girl whose heart is illustrated in Figure 46.2. (*a.*) A highly cellular area of the tumor. H & E, ×200. (*b.*) The interstitial tissue is more abundant than in *a*. The individual cells are less fusiform in shape. A blood vessel is present in this portion of the tumor. Hematoxylin and eosin, ×200. (*c.*) Photomicrograph of a renal artery. An embolus of myxomatous tissue is attached to the wall and partially obstructs the lumen of the artery. Focal renal infarction was present. H & E, ×57. (Reproduced with permission from L. P. Sterns *et al.*: Br. Heart J. 26:75, 1966.)

any of the systemic arteries, including the aorta,[15, 31] and of those of the brain. Depending upon the size of embolic particles, the result of embolism may be manifested clinically as localized involvement of one or a limited number of organs (Fig. 46.3c), or disseminated involvement of skin, muscle, and internal organs. The latter type of process may be confused clinically with polyarteritis nodosa. Histologic examination of an embolus removed from a systemic artery may, in an occasional case, be the first sign of a left atrial myxoma.[5, 8]

The manifestations of involvement of cavitary space are dependent upon the chamber involved. When the tumor originates in the right atrium, its clinical manifestations are those of obstruction to the inflow of blood into the right side of the heart with features of edema, albuminuria, and elevation of systemic venous pressure. The differential diagnosis includes constrictive pericarditis and tricuspid stenosis. In those cases wherein tricuspid stenosis is suspected, an important point is absence of involvement of the mitral

valve, since in acquired rheumatic stenosis of the tricuspid valve it is almost universal that the mitral valve is also involved. Ebstein's anomaly of the tricuspid valve may also be simulated by a right atrial myxoma.

When the myxoma involves the left atrium, features of mitral valvular disease are commonly duplicated. These include pulmonary hypertension, right ventricular hypertrophy and structural changes in the pulmonary vascular bed. Even a murmur considered characteristic of mitral stenosis or insufficiency may be observed. In the presence of signs of mitral valvular disease, a left atrial myxoma may be suspected under certain circumstances. These include: a normal-sized left atrium, changing character of the murmur, embolic phenomena, and fainting spells. In the young child, rheumatic mitral stenosis is rare. In this age group, therefore, signs of mitral stenosis should be suspect of left atrial myxoma.

Physiologic studies have indicated certain differences in left atrial pressure pulse characteristics between mitral stenosis and left atrial myxoma.[10] These include an abnormally high V wave in the presence of other features that favor mitral stenosis. Reliable methods of making the clinical diagnosis of an atrial myxoma are by angiocardiography and echocardiography.[21, 23, 29] In such studies a filling defect or mass created by the tumor is usually diagnostic.

Differing and associates[6] gave a historical review of the surgical treatment of atrial myxoma. Before the era of open heart surgery, varying degrees of success were obtained by other surgeons in the management of this problem. In some cases, closed methods of removal of myxomas were aided by induced hypothermia of the patient. With the use of pump oxygenator systems, removal of intracavitary myxomas has achieved a position of a standard procedure with predictable results. It is to be emphasized that all of the pedicle of the tumor should be removed; otherwise, recurrence is possible. To effect complete removal, it is usually advisable to resect that part of the atrial septum to which the pedicle is attached.

MESOTHELIOMA OF AV NODE

A benign tumor of mesothelial origin,[9] variously designated as mesothelioma, lymphangioendothelioma, or collothelioma, may involve the atrioventricular (AV) node and adjacent atrial septal tissue. Often so small as not to be detected by gross examination, this tumor, containing epithelial-like inclusions, is important as a cause of interference with AV conduction, including complete heart block (Fig. 46.4), and so is to be numbered among conditions causing sudden and unexpected death. More common in the female than in the male, the tumor may be observed at any age. Among McAllister's[17] 12 cases, the ages ranged from 11 months to 71 years. Ibarra-Perez and associates[14] observed that of reported cases, 16 were under 30 years of age. Their case involved a 17-year-old girl with two ventricular septal defects and first degree AV dissociation.

PERICARDIAL CYSTS

As a pericardial cyst may be confused with a cardiac tumor, particularly one of pericardial origin, it is appropriate to consider this subject.

The cyst usually is solitary, lobulated, unilocular, and filled with colorless fluid. Calcification of the fibrous wall may occur. It lies against the parietal pericardium and rarely communicates with the pericardial sac. McAllister and Fenoglio[18] found that the most common locations are the costophrenic angles and more commonly on the right than the

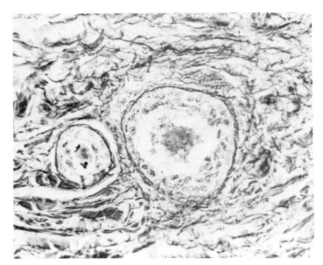

Fig. 46.4 Photomicrograph of mesothelioma of atrioventricular node. Epithelial-like structures form a characteristic feature of the tumor. H & E, ×240. (Reproduced with permission from C. Ibarra-Perez et al.[14])

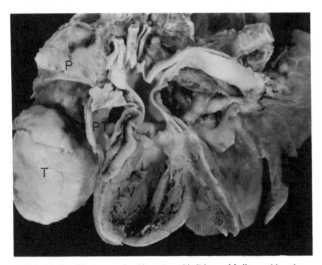

Fig. 46.5 Photograph of heart and left lung. Malignant teratoma in a 2-year-old girl. Malignant teratoma (T) arises from the pericardium near the pulmonary trunk (PT). P, reflected parietal pericardium; LV, left ventricle.

left. Uncommonly, the cyst may lie in the anterior-superior mediastinum or the posterior mediastinum.

The pericardial cyst is probably a congenital anomaly. As these are usually not a cause of symptoms, they are most commonly discovered in thoracic roentgenograms taken for unrelated circumstances.

Not only are the pericardial cysts to be distinguished from solid pericardial tumors, but also from defects of the pericardium through which cardiac herniation has occurred. Also, localized aneurysms or diverticula of the left or right atrial appendages enter into the differential diagnosis.

PRIMARY MALIGNANT TUMORS

Fortunately, primary malignant tumors of the heart are rare in infants and children.[28] In the review of McAllister,[17] the most commonly recognized types in this age group were malignant teratoma and rhabdomyosarcoma. Less commonly, fibrosarcoma and neurogenic sarcoma were repre-

sented. The malignant teratoma is more common in the female than in the male. As with the benign form of teratoma, the tumors tend to be primary in relation to the pericardium at the base of the heart (Figs. 46.5 to 46.7). While evidence of pericardial disease is dominant in such

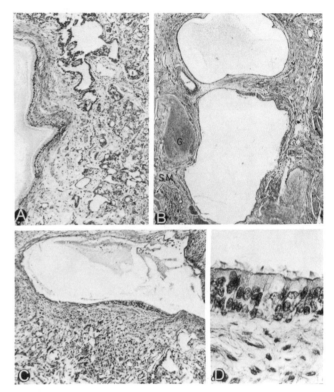

Fig. 46.6 Photomicrographs of malignant teratoma in a 2-year-old girl, the gross specimen of which is illustrated in Figure 46.5. H & E, ×48. (A) Cyst lined by intestinal-type epithelium and surrounded by carcinomatous tissue. (B) Two spaces lined principally by bronchial type epithelium and surrounded by a focus of glial tissue (G). At the periphery, smooth muscle bundles are evident (SM). H & E, ×7. (C) Cyst lined in part by bronchial epithelium and surrounded by carcinomatous tissue. H & E, ×25. (D) Ciliated bronchial epithelium from lining of cyst shown in C. H & E, ×470.

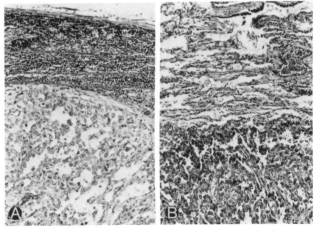

Fig. 46.7 Carcinomatous metastases of teratoma in the case of a girl 2 years old, photographs of which are shown in Figures 46.5 and 46.6. (A) Lymph node partly replaced by carcinoma. H& E, ×90. (B) Metastatic carcinoma in lung. H & E, ×90.

tumors, invasion of cardiac structures may lead to conduction disturbances and to ventricular outflow obstruction.

The other types of malignant tumors tend to be primary in the myocardium, with the right-sided chambers being slightly more commonly involved than the left. Some may be primary in the atrial septum.

Those malignant tumors arising in the myocardium have tendencies to extend into its cavity of primary involvement and also into the pericardial cavity. The clinical manifestations are dependent upon these phenomena, commonly yielding features of occupation of space of a cavity and of pericardial disease, including effusion and cardiac constriction. Also, nonspecific features of loss of weight, fever, and malaise may dominate the clinical picture.

METASTATIC TUMORS

As malignant tumors are relatively uncommon in infants and children, so is it infrequent to observe metastatic tumors of the heart.[30] The most common type of tumor involving the heart secondarily in children is either the malignant lymphoma or sarcomatous manifestations in leukemia. When such involvement occurs, the lesion either may be functionally insignificant, or it may give rise to symptoms. If symptoms occur, they may become apparent after the primary tumor has been discovered, or they may constitute the basis for the presenting complaint.

Symptoms of metastatic tumors of the heart depend upon the site or sites of metastases. When metastases to the myocardium occur, there may be interference with conduction on the basis of involvement of the major conduction pathways. In a rare case, a myocardial or an endocardial metastasis may be sufficiently large as to occupy cavitary space and may be responsible for signs of obstruction to the flow of blood.

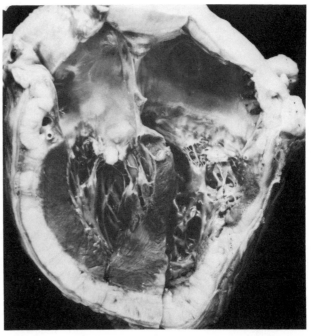

Fig. 46.8 Heart viewed from behind. The epicardium over each of the four chambers is grossly thickened by pale tissue. The latter represents focal leukemic infiltration in an adult patient with chronic myeloid leukemia. (Reproduced with permission from J. E. Edwards: An Atlas of Acquired Diseases of the Heart and Great Vessels. W. B. Saunders, Philadelphia, 1961.)

Pericardial involvement (Fig. 46.8) may give rise to signs of cardiac compression either from effusion associated with metastases to this region or from solid tumor encasing the heart.[26]

REFERENCES

1. Allen, H. D., Blieden, L. C., Stone, F. M., Bessinger, F. B., and Lucas, R. V.: Echocardiographic demonstration of a right ventricular tumor in a neonate. J. Pediatr. 84:854, 1974.
2. Anbe, D. T., and Fine, G.: Cardiac lymphangioma and lipoma. Report of a case of simultaneous occurrence in association with lipomatous infiltration of the myocardium and cardiac arrhythmia. Am. Heart J. 86:227, 1973.
3. Beck, C. S.: An interpericardial teratoma and a tumor of the heart: Both removed operatively. Ann. Surg. 116:161, 1942.
4. Bigelow, N. H., Klinger, S., and Wright, A. W.: Primary tumors of the heart in infancy and early childhood. Cancer 7:549, 1954.
5. Bulkley, B. H., and Hutchins, G. M.: Atrial myxoma: A fifty year review. Am. Heart J. 97:639, 1979.
6. Differding, J. T., Gardner, R. E., and Roe, B. B.: Intracardiac myxomas with report of two unusual cases and successful removal. Circulation 23:929, 1961.
7. Fenoglio, J. J., Jr., Diana, D. J., Bowen, T. E., McAllister, H. A., and Ferrans, V. J.: Ultrastructure of a cardiac rhabdomyoma. Hum. Pathol. 8:700, 1977.
8. Fine, G.: Embolism: Pulmonary and systemic. Cardiovasc. Clin. 4:115, 1972.
9. Fine, G.: Primary tumors of the pericardium and heart. Cardiovasc. Clin. 5:208, 1973.
10. Fish, R. G., Takaro, T., and Crymes, T.: Left atrial pressure pulses in the presence of myxoma. Circulation 20:413, 1959.

11. Geha, A. S., Wiedman, W. H., Soule, E. H., and McGoon, D. C.: Intramural ventricular cardiac fibroma: Successful removal in two cases and review of literature. Circulation 36:427, 1967.
12. Goldberg, H. P., Glenn, F., Dotter, C. T., and Steinberg, I.: Myxoma of the left atrium: Diagnosis made during life with operative and postmortem findings. Circulation 6:762, 1952.
13. Hudson, R. E. B.: Cardiovascular Pathology. Williams & Wilkins, Baltimore, 1965.
14. Ibarra-Perez, C., Korns, M. E., and Edwards, J. E.: Mesothelioma of the atrioventricular node. Chest 63:824, 1973.
15. Kay, J. H., Anderson, R. M., Meihaus, J., Lewis, R., Magidson, O., Bernstein, S., and Griffith, G. C.: Surgical removal of an intracavitary left ventricular myxoma. Circulation 20:881, 1959.
16. Mahaim, I.: Les Tumeurs et les Polypes du Coeur: Etude Anatomoclinique. Masson et Cie, Paris, 1945.
17. McAllister, H. A., Jr.: Primary tumors and cysts of the heart and pericardium. Curr. Prob. Cardiol. 4 (2):1979.
18. McAllister, H. A., and Fenoglio, J. J.: Tumors of the cardiovascular system. In: Atlas of Tumor Pathology. Armed Forces Institute of Pathology, Washington, D. C., 1978.
19. Neal, W. A., Knight, L., Blieden, L. C., Bessinger, F. B., Jr., and Edwards, J. E.: Congenital rhabdomyoma of heart simulating tricuspid atresia. Am. Heart J. 89:514, 1975.

20. Parks, F. R., Jr., Adams, F., and Longmire, W. P., Jr.: Successful excision of a left ventricular hamartoma. Report of a case. Circulation 26:1316, 1962.
21. Petsas, A. A., Gottlieb, S., Kingsley, B., Segal, B. L., and Myerburg, R. J.: Echocardiographic diagnosis of left atrial myxoma. Usefulness of suprasternal approach. Br. Heart J. 38:627, 1976.
22. Prichard, R. W.: Tumors of the heart: Review of the subject and report of one hundred and fifty cases. Arch. Pathol. 51:98, 1951.
23. St. John Sutton, M. G., Mercier, L-A., Giuliani, E. R., and Lie, J. T.: Atrial myxomas. A review of clinical experience in 40 patients. Proc. Mayo Clin. 55:371, 1980.
24. Shrivastava, S., Jacks, J. J., White, R. S., and Edwards, J. E.: Diffuse rhabdomyomatosis of the heart. Arch. Pathol. 101:78, 1977.
25. Silverman, J., Olwin, J. S., and Graettinger, J. S.: Cardiac myxomas with systemic embolization. Review of the literature and report of a case. Circulation 26:99, 1962.
26. Thurber, D. L., Edwards, J. E., and Achor, R. W. P.: Secondary malignant tumors of the pericardium. Circulation 26:228, 1962.
27. Van der Hauwaert, L. G., Corbeel, L., and Maldagne, P.: Fibroma of the right ventricle producing severe tricuspid stenosis. Circulation 32:451, 1965.
28. Whorton, C. M.: Primary malignant tumors of the heart. Report of a case. Cancer 2:245, 1949.
29. Wolfe, S. B., Popp, R. L., and Feigenbaum, H.:

Diagnosis of atrial tumors by ultrasound. Circulation 39:615, 1969.
30. Yater, W. M.: Tumors of the heart and pericardium. Pathology, symptomatology, and re-

port of nine cases. Arch. Intern. Med. 48:627, 1931.
31. Young, R. D., and Hunter, W. C.: Primary

myxoma of the left ventricle with embolic occlusion of the abdominal aorta and renal arteries. Arch. Pathol. 43:86, 1947.

47

Postoperative Problems

Mary Allen Engle, M.D.

Cardiac surgery, which corrects or ameliorates abnormalities, can relieve disability and/or prevent future difficulty. For these real and often spectacular benefits, some patients pay a higher price than others when they undergo the discomfort and illness associated with the postoperative syndromes or other postoperative complications. All the syndromes followed an advance in surgical technic: resection of coarctation of the aorta, operation within the pericardium, the use of extracorporeal circulation, or the insertion of prostheses in or near abnormal valves.

The syndromes share several common features. They are more easily described than explained. The setting in which they occur can be defined, but the reason the syndrome develops in one patient and not in others is not clear. For some conditions it has been suggested that autoantibodies may play a role in pathogenesis. The manifestations, which vary in severity and in duration, are self-limited so that it is difficult to judge effects of therapy. Antibiotics commonly used after cardiac surgery have no role in elimination nor in treatment of the syndromes. For each, mild cases may go unrecognized; so the true frequency is probably higher than that reported. Fever is a feature of each. Therefore, diagnosis rests not only on recognizing the characteristics of that syndrome but also on excluding other causes of febrile illness in postoperative patients with heart disease. In particular, infective endocarditis must be ruled out since the prognosis and treatment are quite different. Fortunately, bacterial or fungal endocarditis in the early and in the remote postoperative period is a rarity.

POSTCOARCTECTOMY SYNDROME

Severe, intermittent abdominal pain, beginning 4 to 8 days after resection of coarctation of the aorta (CA), heralds the onset of this syndrome. Fever, leukocytosis, melena, ascites, abdominal distension, and signs of intestinal obstruction are manifestations which when severe can lead to abdominal exploration and resection of necrotic small bowel. Death followed in four of the first seven patients reported with gangrenous bowel at exploration.[6, 29, 37, 48] If early resection is not carried out, some may show later effects of malabsorption and obstruction due to multiple stenoses and fistulas between loops of bowel involved in the inflammatory process.[19, 30]

Clagett and Jampolis[7] in 1951 were the first to comment on the occurrence of severe abdominal pain after resection of CA. It was Sealy[44] who first described the findings of infarcted bowel and an extensive panarteritis of vessels below the level of the coarctation. Ring and Lewis[41] analyzed a group of these patients and called the condition a syndrome. Groves and Effler[19] and later Mays and Sergeant[30] described the late sequelae with malabsorption and intestinal fibrosis and fistulas.

Frequency is difficult to judge. Mays and Sergeant[30] gave the frequency as 20% of those immediately surviving resection. This is far higher than our experience wherein only 1 to 2% manifested abdominal pain, distension, and fever. These subsided completely after a few days and did not become severe enough to warrant laparotomy. Schuster and Gross[43] reviewed their experience in 505 patients operated upon for CA and did not mention the occurrence of the syndrome. Groves and Effler found it in 5%, whereas Ring and Lewis[41] recognized it in 28% of patients. I believe it is becoming rare.

The sex predilection for males and the age range have been that of patients undergoing resection of CA. Groves and Effler[19] reported on a 5-month-old infant and Lober and Lillehei[29] on a 46-year-old adult with the syndrome. The syndrome seems, however, to occur chiefly in children under the age of 5 years.

The pathogenesis has been described as an arteritis resulting from postoperative changes in circulatory dynamics of pressure and flow after relief of the obstruction in the aorta.[6, 44, 45] Why only a few of the patients with equally complete relief of CA have the syndrome is not understood. Necroses in the arteries and arterioles below the level of coarctation involve chiefly the media but frequently the entire wall, with occlusion of terminal portions. Lober and Lillehei[29] noted the similarity of the lesions to those of periarteritis nodosa. Symptomatically the superior mesenteric system is the main one affected, although involvement of renal vessels may account for reactive hypertension,[45] and in one patient the arteritis caused damage to the spinal cord as well as the gastrointestinal tract.[48] Infarction of the small intestine and portions of proximal colon with multiple ulcerations were found in the acute stage. Months later the end stage of the syndrome consists not of arteritis but of intestinal ulcerations, fistulas, segments of stenosis, and complete dissolution of continuity of the bowel.[19, 30] In the early stages, the condition resembles acute necrotizing enterocolitis such as occurs in some critically ill premature infants and in some babies undergoing cardiac surgery utilizing profound hypothermia.

The diagnosis is based on an awareness of the condition when a patient in the 1st postoperative week has abdominal pain and signs that suggest mesenteric thrombosis. It is to be differentiated from other causes of abdominal pain, for instance, rupture of an infarcted spleen.[19]

Treatment is expectant, with close observation, intravenous feeding, and avoidance of laparotomy unless necessary. Resection of infarcted bowel may be extensive.[29] The deaths reported have been in patients undergoing abdominal surgery,[6, 29, 37, 48] but these were also the most seriously affected. There may be complications if extensively involved bowel is not resected.[19, 30] Sealy and co-workers[45] noted that the syndrome tended to occur in patients with reactive hypertension and recommended the use of sympathicolytic drugs. They reported on the reduction of hypertension, relief of abdominal pain, and eventual recovery in two patients so treated.

Steroids were of little benefit to a child in whom the associated symptom of arthralgia was relieved, but not the abdominal pain. The child required operation 2 months later for resection of ileum that was involved in an inflammatory mass.[19] No other sequelae and no late occurrence or recurrence has been reported.

A second postoperative event that has been more common in our experience than the above syndrome has been hyperreactive hypertension in the 1st week or two after resection of CA. Just as with the former syndrome, it is not possible to predict prior to surgery which patients will have a rise in the blood pressure in the arms higher than that observed preoperatively, but it tends to occur more in young children. The mechanism is unknown. Blood pressure is also elevated in the legs, attesting to the fact that the problem is not inadequate resection of the CA and destruction of collaterals. Strong et al.[51] found no elevation of plasma renin activity in their 12 patients studied prior to and following coarctectomy. In the two children with this complication, the peripheral renin was no different than in the other 10.[51]

These patients show no edema or evidence of renal impairment. It seems to us that the combination of an underdeveloped systemic vascular bed distal to the coarctation and a hyperkinetic cardiac status early postoperatively may be responsible. Untreated, the hypertension may result in a cerebrovascular accident. We recommend antihypertensive agents if the blood pressure in the arms of a child exceeds 150/90 mm Hg. If the pressure is markedly elevated, intravenous diazoxide in a dose of 5 mg/kg can drop the pressure to a nearly normal level within 2 or 3 minutes. Agents such as nitroprusside, hydralazine, or reserpine can control the hypertension. The medication can usually be tapered and discontinued after a few days to a few weeks. Restriction of salt intake together with limitation of fluids and the use of diuretics are helpful as adjuncts, and in mildly hypertensive children these may be all that is needed.

THE POSTPERICARDIOTOMY SYNDROME

A febrile illness with pericardial and pleural reaction and effusion, and sometimes pulmonary parenchymal involvement following surgery in which the pericardium is opened constitutes the postpericardiotomy syndrome (PPS).[13, 15, 16, 23] There is usually only a single period of illness, but recurrences may take place months or years later. Sometimes the fever merges with that of the 1st days or week following operation. Somewhat less often, there is an afebrile period before the fever appears or reappears 2 to 3 weeks postoperatively. It is unusual for the fever and other signs of the syndrome to be more delayed than this. The fever may be sustained or spiking. Generally the peak is between 38 and 39°C, but spikes as high as 40°C may occur. It usually subsides within 2 to 3 weeks.

Accompanying the fever, as nonspecific signs of inflammation, are leukocytosis and elevated sedimentation rate. Malaise is variable. The appetite may be poor. Some patients do not appear ill; other children are merely irritable; but a few are desperately sick, especially if the fever is high or there is cardiac tamponade. The symptoms and the radiologic evidence of enlarged "cardiac" silhouette of the child with early signs of tamponade may be mistaken for cardiac failure. The distinction is important, since each requires prompt therapy that differs for the two conditions. Echocardiography is helpful in differential diagnosis.[17, 22] Emergency pericardiocentesis may be required. The fluid withdrawn may be serosanguinous if early in the course or simply serous later on. It is sterile for bacteria.

Signs of pericardial involvement include electrocardiographic and radiologic changes (Figs. 47.1 and 47.2) as well

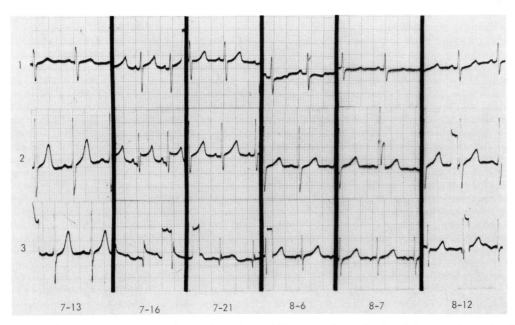

Fig. 47.1 Serial limb leads of the electrocardiogram in a 5-year-old in whom the postpericardiotomy syndrome developed following closure of a ventricular septal defect on July 14 (7-14). Two days later the expected sinus tachycardia and elevation of ST segments in leads 2 and 3 are consistent with surgical pericarditis. Although the electrocardiogram 1 week later appears normal, those taken 3 weeks postoperatively on 8-6 and 8-7 when evidence of postpericardiotomy syndrome was present show abnormality of T waves with inversion of T1 and then the beginning of return to normal, which was achieved after 1 more week.

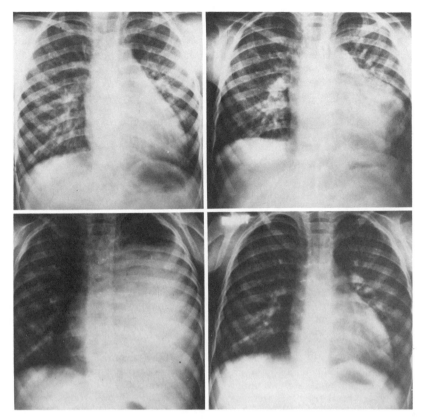

Fig. 47.2 Preoperative and postoperative roentgenogram of a 3-year-old who underwent closure of a large ventricular septal defect. In *upper left* photograph is seen the preoperative film which shows moderate cardiomegaly and increased pulmonary vascularity. On *upper right* is a film in 3rd postoperative week which shows some pericardial effusion. At *lower left* there is massive pericardial effusion and a left pleural effusion. The syndrome persisted for 2 months and he required several pericardiocenteses before the condition subsided. Film on *bottom right* 3 months postoperatively shows resolution of effusions.

as other signs, depending on the age and condition of the patient. Chest pain characteristic of pericardial irritation is precordial, radiates to the left shoulder, and worsens with inspiration and in the supine position. The pain may be sharp and stabbing or a persistent, dull ache. Its disappearance can mean improvement or alternatively, worsening when accumulation of fluid separates the pericardial surfaces. A pericardial friction rub can be heard at some time during the syndrome in most patients, but it may come and go even on the same day, and it usually does not last as long as the electrocardiographic or radiologic signs. Disappearance of the rub may mean healing or effusion. The rub may be so soft that it is confused with a murmur; usually it sounds scratchy and superficial in systole and diastole.

In all patients with pericardiotomy, it is common for the electrocardiogram to show elevation of ST segment followed by minor changes in T waves as evidence of surgical pericarditis in the first 2 or 3 days postoperatively. In those who have no evidence of the PPS, these findings disappear within a week, whereas in those with the syndrome abnormalities persist. The T waves in limb leads and usually in left precordial leads become flat or inverted and gradually return to normal. These electrocardiographic changes (Fig. 47.1) take longer to resolve than do the other signs of the syndrome. Digitalis or the presence of right bundle branch block may interfere with interpretation of these changes. Only with large pericardial effusion does voltage of QRS decrease appreciably.

Evidence of pericardial involvement radiologically consists of changes due to collection of fluid within the sac.[12, 14] The "cardiac" shadow (actually the pericardial sac) enlarges (Fig.

47.2). A sign of slight change is the filling in of the area on the left heart border beneath and alongside the convexity of the main pulmonary artery. The margins of the silhouette may be irregular but usually are smooth. With marked effusion, a radiolucent vertical line in lateral view may be seen separating the density that is pericardial shadow anteriorly from that of epicardium.

Echocardiography[17, 22] has proven useful in confirming the presence of pericardial effusion and in evaluating its size (Fig. 47.3). It has replaced angiocardiography, which can also confirm the presence of pericardial effusion by demonstrating opacified cardiac chambers within the fluid-distended pericardial sac. Instillation of air as contrast agent at the time of pericardiocentesis can also delineate the stretched parietal pericardium and its degree of thickening, but rarely is either of these procedures indicated for diagnosis or management.

Signs of pleural involvement are common, especially on the left. Pleural effusions and friction rubs rarely are found except in this syndrome, for chest catheters inserted at the end of the operation drain fluid that forms in decreasing amounts in the first 2 or 3 days. Pulmonary parenchymal changes are less common than pleural reaction.

In those patients with the syndrome whose pericardium has been reopened later for a second operation, the old, fibrous thickening of the pericardium has appeared no different from the healed surgical pericarditis of other patients at reoperation who did not have the syndrome. Constrictive pericarditis has not occurred in our patients.

This syndrome was first noted in 1952 with the advent of surgery for mitral stenosis,[25, 50] and there was concern that it

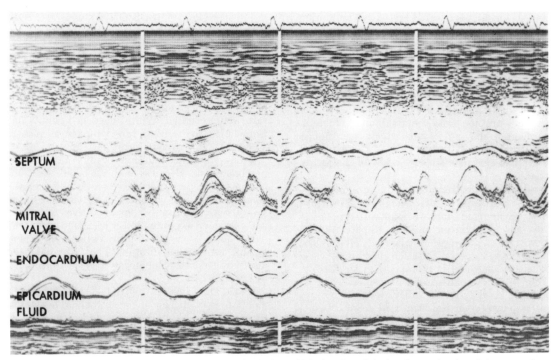

Fig. 47.3 Echocardiogram demonstrates large pericardial effusion which developed during the postpericardiotomy syndrome in an 11-year-old operated upon because of severe hypertrophic subaortic stenosis. In addition to the pericardial effusion, indicated by the large clear space outside the epicardium, this echocardiogram demonstrates the abnormal systolic anterior motion of the mitral valve and the hypertrophy of the left ventricular wall and septum, characteristic features of the condition of hypertrophic obstructive cardiomyopathy.

represented reactivation of rheumatic fever. In 1958, we reported on the syndrome in patients with congenital heart disease and pointed out that the common denominator in patients with congenital and acquired heart disease in whom the syndrome developed was wide incision of the pericardial sac.[23] Since the condition occurred in this setting, and irrespective of any other surgical procedure (cardiotomy, valvotomy, arteriotomy, or exploration), the designation "postpericardiotomy syndrome" was suggested. An apparently identical syndrome follows myocardial infarction[9] and as a consequence of traumatic hemopericardium, even when the chest trauma is nonpenetrating.[18, 52] Features common to all three situations are damage of myocardium and blood in the pericardial sac.[23] The syndrome also resembles benign, idiopathic, or viral pericarditis.

The frequency is about 25 to 30% of patients undergoing pericardiotomy, and after traumatic hemopericardium it is 30%. The reasons why some individuals respond with manifestations of the syndrome while most do not is still not clarified. Possible explanations include viral infection[10, 13, 23, 33] and an autoimmune reaction.[13, 23] In a prospective, triple-blind study of 400 survivors of intrapericardial surgery, we found that development of antiheart antibodies in high titre correlated with clinical signs of the syndrome, which occurred in 27% of the patients. In addition, in 280 of these patients whose sera were analyzed for antibody against adenovirus, coxsackie B1-6 and cytomegalovirus, a fourfold or greater rise in titre occurred in 70% of those with the syndrome and with heart-reactive antibody, but in only 5% of those with no antiheart antibody or syndrome.[15, 16] These findings suggest that the syndrome is an autoimmune response in association with a recent or remote viral infection.

Recurrences are uncommon, but they may take place months or years later. Usually they are mild, but they may be associated with pericardial effusion again. One child required pericardiectomy because of chronic, recurrent pericardial effusions.[31]

The age range is that of patients undergoing cardiac surgery. However, infants under the age of 2 years are unlikely to develop the syndrome. Only four babies out of 112 had PPS, whereas 36% of the older age groups had the complication.[15, 16] One of the advantages to early open heart surgery in infants is their relative freedom from the postpericardiotomy syndrome.

Diagnosis is based on awareness of this possibility in a patient whose pericardium has been opened. The condition is recognized by the findings just described. Detection of antiheart antibody in high titre is a confirmatory diagnostic test.[15] At the same time, other causes for fever should be excluded, especially endocarditis. Cardiac failure may be suggested by the radiologic findings of cardiac enlargement, pericardial and pleural effusion, and by symptoms of cardiac tamponade. It is also to be differentiated from the febrile illness that occurs about the 6th week following surgery with perfusion on the heart-lung machine, which is associated with lymphocytosis and hepatosplenomegaly (see below). Both postoperative complications can develop in the same person, with the onset of the postperfusion syndrome usually occurring after resolution of the postpericardiotomy syndrome.

The illness is self-limited, lasting 2 to 3 weeks. More cases are mild than are severe. Both factors make it difficult to judge effects of therapy in a condition such as this where etiology is unknown. Antibiotics have had no effect in preventing or treating the condition. Diuretics may be helpful for those with effusions. One of the most important measures in treatment when pericardial effusion is moderate or large is rest in bed until fever has disappeared and radiologic and electrocardiographic abnormalities are clearing or have disappeared. Like McGuinness and Taussig,[33] we have observed worsening of the condition when ambulation is begun before the signs abate. Some have required an emergency pericardiocentesis for cardiac tamponade that developed within a few days of discharge. Treatment that can be life-saving is pericardiocentesis for tamponade.[14] While early ambulation may enhance the production of pericardial effusion, rest in bed does not prevent it. One must be alert to the possibility of tamponade when a child becomes listless, anorectic, irritable, and pale, with grunting respirations, tenderness over an enlarging liver, and a preference for an upright position. Tachycardia, tachypnea, rising venous pressure, and falling arterial pressure with a paradoxical pulse complete the picture. Heart sounds are not always muffled, and voltage in the electrocardiogram may not be abnormally low, though it is less than usual for that patient. Use of the exploring electrocardiographic electrode adds to safety of the procedure (Fig. 47.4).[14]

For severe illness, corticosteroids cause a prompt disappearance of fever and lessening of discomfort. In our prospective study of the syndrome, we followed the clinical course and response of antiheart antibody in patients with severe syndrome, six of whom received steroids for 3 weeks, with the dose being reduced by half each succeeding week. Six others received salicylates in therapeutic doses for several weeks (Fig. 47.5). In comparison to those receiving no specific medication and those on salicylates, we found a more prompt response in clinical signs and drop in heart-reactive antibody in the steroid-treated group.[16]

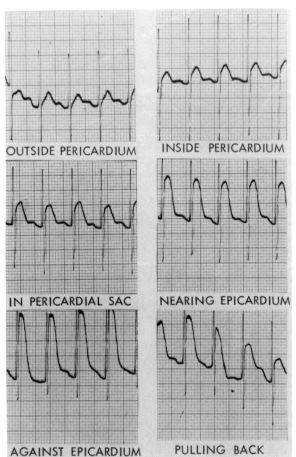

Fig. 47.4 Selected strips obtained at continuous electrocardiographic monitoring during pericardiocentesis. ST segment becomes elevated as pericardium is entered and rises increasingly as needle approaches and touches epicardium as the fluid is withdrawn and the pericardial surfaces approximate. The needle should promptly be pulled back if such contact is made. The ST segments immediately return to an appropriate level of elevation.

POSTPERFUSION SYNDROME OF LYMPHOCYTOSIS AND HEPATOSPLENOMEGALY

The appearance of fever, splenomegaly, and atypical lymphocytes about 3 to 6 weeks after cardiac surgery employing extracorporeal circulation constitutes the postperfusion syndrome. In addition to splenomegaly the liver may be enlarged and the lymph nodes readily palpable. A transient rash may be noted. White blood cell counts have ranged from 5 to 15 thousand and the lymphocytic percentage from 40 to 82% with 7 to 34% atypical.

It resembles the conditions of infectious lymphocytosis or mononucleosis. Because of the delayed onset, most of the patients have been discharged from the hospital before the condition appears. In some, it is found in the absence of symptoms on a routine postoperative visit. Others notice malaise, poor appetite, and a lowgrade fever with evening elevation to 38 or 39° C. Most patients have not been sick enough for rehospitalization. The fever has been of short duration. Hepatosplenomegaly has lasted from a few weeks to 3 to 4 months.

Battle and Hewlett[4] and Kreel et al.[28] were the first to mention splenomegaly and atypical lymphocytes after extracorporeal circulation. Wheeler and associates[53] recognized that it was a new syndrome which occurred only after open heart operation utilizing a pump oxygenator. Others reported similar findings.[1, 3, 21, 49]

The frequency of the syndrome initially was probably higher than reported, since in many instances it is so mild that the patient recognizes no illness, and it usually occurs after he has left the hospital. Prior to present modifications of perfusion techniques, the frequency was around 5 to 10% of the survivors of extracorporeal circulation. Seaman and Starr[46] observed it in 11 of 280 survivors (4%); Smith[49] in 9 of 173 (5%); Holswade et al.[21] in 14 of 170 (8%); and Wheeler and associates[53] in 6 of 54 patients (11%). It occurs in children and adults following perfusion for open repair of congenital and acquired heart disease. There is no sex predilection. No recurrences have been reported.

Originally the etiology was unknown, but the syndrome resembled a viral illness.[21, 53] Then cytomegalovirus was demonstrated to be the causative agent.[36] Use of freshly drawn blood permitted transfer of an inapparent viremia of healthy donors. The syndrome has almost disappeared since the hemodilution technique, with blood drawn a day or more before operation, has become widespread.

The diagnosis is based on the setting in which the illness occurs, on the findings in the peripheral blood, and on the demonstration of cytomegalovirus in the urine or of a changing titre in the serum to cytomegalovirus. The importance of this benign syndrome, aside from the temporary inconvenience of fever and malaise, is that it be differentiated from endocarditis. It is also to be distinguished from the postpericardiotomy syndrome with fever, and pericardial and pleural involvement. Atypical lymphocytes do not occur in increased numbers in the latter condition. Furthermore, the postpericardiotomy syndrome occurs earlier and tends to recur. We have seen patients who have had both syndromes, but only one instance of postperfusion syndrome was encountered in the last 400 survivors of cardiopulmonary bypass in our ongoing study of the postpericardiotomy syndrome (see above).

MECHANICAL HEMOLYTIC ANEMIA SYNDROME

Intravascular hemolytic anemia of mechanical origin has occurred in rare instances after open heart surgery for ostium

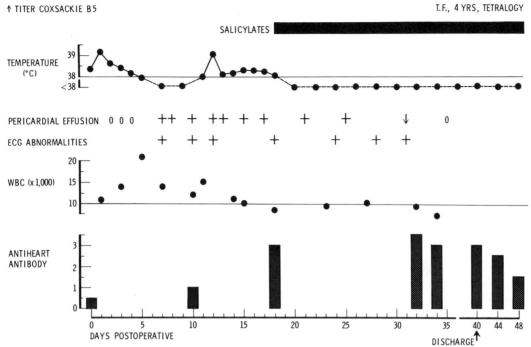

Fig. 47.5 Course of postpericardiotomy syndrome in a 4-year-old who underwent repair of tetralogy of Fallot. The days postoperative are shown on the baseline, with the date of discharge indicated by an *arrow* on the 40th day. The early postoperative fever subsided by the end of the 1st week, but returned in the 2nd week and persisted until salicylates were begun on the 18th day. The leukocytosis declined as the fever dropped, but the other signs of the postperiocardiotomy syndrome persisted until the 30th day, when improvement began and was maintained. At the *bottom* is shown the level of antiheart antibody. Initially negative, it began to rise on the 10th day, exceeded 2+ through the 44th day, and began to decline at 48 days. *ECG,* electrocardiogram; *WBC,* white blood cells.

primum defects with cleft mitral valve[35, 42, 47] and for aortic and mitral valve replacement.[5, 24, 34, 39] It is believed to be due to unusual intracardiac turbulence with fragmentation of red cells. Secondarily, iron deficiency anemia is superimposed.

This situation was brought to attention by Sayed *et al.*,[42] who pursued the cause of a severe, persistent hemolytic anemia and then corrected it by identifying and removing the cause of the trauma to the erythrocytes. Their patient was a 25-year-old man who underwent surgery for an ostium primum defect with slight mitral insufficiency. A Teflon patch was used to close the defect; the cleft mitral valve was not repaired. On the 18th day, signs of hemolytic anemia appeared: pallor, jaundice, dark urine, fever, with a hemoglobin of 6.5 gm/100 ml, abnormally crenated and fragmented red blood cells (RBC) on smear, and a reticulocyte response of 7.7%. Only the red cells were affected. There was free hemoglobin and methemalbumin in the serum, and hemosiderin in the urine. The mean life span of Cr^{51}-labeled RBC was reduced to 6 to 9 days. Their studies led to the conclusion that the anemia was due not to an immune mechanism nor an abnormality of the patient's cells but instead, to intravascular hemolysis. Prednisone had no effect. Over a 6-month period he received 60 blood transfusions and then was reoperated. A small cul-de-sac of bare Teflon was found on the left atrial side of the patch adjacent to the abnormal aortic cusp of the mitral valve. They reasoned that cells in the regurgitant jet of blood were traumatized when they hit the bare felt. The endocardium was sutured over the area, and the patient's anemia was cured.

Sigler *et al.*[47] reported on three additional cases, each with Teflon patch for repair of an atrioventricular canal defect and with suture of a cleft of the mitral valve. Within the first 2 weeks after surgery, fever, severe anemia, and splenomegaly appeared. Two had, in addition, petechiae, splinter hemorrhages, and erythematous swelling of the fingertips, features that strongly suggested endocarditis. Blood cultures were negative, however, and hematologic findings of hemoglobinemia, methemalbuminemia, and hemosiderinuria led to the conclusion that there was intravascular hemolysis from unusual turbulence within the heart. An additional component of iron deficiency developed in association with excessive loss of iron in the urine as the mechanical hemolysis continued. Two patients were reoperated upon, but no lack of endothelialization of the patch was found. Instead, the mitral valve had become detached from the patch. The mitral cleft was again repaired. One patient survived; the murmur of mitral insufficiency disappeared and so did the anemia. The third patient's anemia could be controlled with iron therapy.

Subsequently others reported patients who had severe hemolytic anemia beginning within days or weeks of the operation, not only after surgery for ostium primum with cleft mitral valve[35] but also after replacement of the mitral or the aortic valve because of insufficiency or obstruction.[5, 24, 34, 39] In all these situations, the jetting occurred at high pressure from the left ventricle.

The frequency of this syndrome is not known. Most reports of surgery for atrioventricular canal defects do not mention anemia. Since it can occur in severe form, it is likely that there are milder cases in whom reticulocyte response is adequate to compensate for the increased mechanical destruction of red cells, and in whom urinary loss of iron is not enough to cause iron deficiency. Response to treatment of the hemolytic anemia depends on its severity and on the presence of secondarily acquired iron deficiency. If the anemia can be controlled medically, this is preferable to reoperation. In our experience, oral iron therapy has been all that is needed.

POSTOPERATIVE RESPIRATORY DISTRESS SYNDROME

A serious respiratory complication is that of widespread, diffuse hemorrhagic atelectasis, sometimes referred to as "pump lungs" or the postperfusion pulmonary congestion syndrome, or the adult respiratory distress syndrome.[38] There are gradations in severity and in recoverability, but in its severe form it is lethal; the lungs lose the capacity for gas exchange. At autopsy they are dark red, heavy, collapsed, and they show pulmonary alveolar and parenchymal hemorrhage and atelectasis. The cause is not clear. One can speculate that a vital substance essential for lung integrity, such as surfactant, is washed out and/or that the pulmonary capillary bed becomes so distended with blood that the pulmonary microcirculation is compromised and vessels rupture. Cyanosis, respiratory acidosis, low cardiac output with metabolic acidosis, oliguria or anuria, loss of consciousness, and death can occur. If the lungs are not too seriously damaged, use of the respirator and appropriate supportive measures may modify the changes in pH, PO_2, and PCO_2 and tide the patient over until lung function is restored. Use of positive end-expiratory pressure, continuously or intermittently, has been utilized with benefit.[32]

OTHER POSTOPERATIVE COMPLICATIONS

Following cardiac surgery other complications may develop which are not syndromes but contribute to postoperative morbidity and mortality. Some of them must be differentiated from the syndromes just described. Williams *et al.*,[54] in a prospective study of complications in adults, found that of 150 survivors of cardiac surgery, 107 patients had 187 medical complications.

A pediatric perspective on postoperative illnesses follows. Certain complications tend to occur in situations in which anticipation of the event may result in prevention or in early treatment before manifestations become severe. In general, the younger the individual and the sicker the patient, the more meticulous the anesthetic, surgical, pediatric, cardiologic, and nursing care must be in order to prevent or to treat promptly these complications.

CARDIAC

Low cardiac output is manifest by hypotension, vasoconstriction, acrocyanosis, oliguria, and metabolic acidosis. If this problem occurs, it is usually in the first hours or days after surgery, and in the patient with a serious cardiac problem relieved only incompletely or after prolonged cardiac bypass. Careful monitoring and correction of abnormalities of the patient's arterial pressure, venous pressure, cardiac rate and rhythm, respiratory exchange, pH and blood gases, and blood, fluid, and electrolyte balance may bring him through this period. Digitalis, dopamine, and furosemide may help. Two conditions which can cause similar symptoms and which require prompt recognition are inadequate replacement of blood and cardiac tamponade from bleeding into the pericardial sac.

Cardiac failure which appears for the first time after cardiac surgery is usually the result of a new cardiac burden imposed by the operation or is the result of circulatory overload. The symptoms and signs of cardiac failure may be simulated by the postpericardiotomy syndrome if there is enlargement of the cardiac silhouette by pericardial fluid and there are pleural effusions. Tachypnea and respiratory distress along with congestion of the liver and venous engorgement occur with cardiac tamponade as well as with failure. Cardiac failure treated prior to surgery may require treatment only for the early postoperative period or not at all, if the cause for the failure has been completely corrected or greatly improved by the operation.

Dysrhythmias after operation are uncommon in the pediatric age group. Supraventricular tachyrhythmias and the "sick sinus syndrome" occur in a few patients, especially following closure of sinus venosus type of atrial septal defects and performance of the intraatrial venous rerouting operation for transposition of the great arteries (the Mustard procedure). When care is taken at surgery so as not to damage the region of the sinus node near the superior vena cava and to do as little harm as possible to intraatrial conducting pathways, especially near the coronary sinus, the serious tachyrhythmias and unstable rhythm have been to a great extent prevented.[11] Paroxysmal supraventricular tachycardia or atrial flutter usually responds to digitalis or to DC conversion. If it is recurrent, we maintain such patients on digitalis for a few months in an attempt to prevent recurrence of the dysrhythmia. Other supraventricular dysrhythmias, such as atrial premature contractions, shifting pacemaker, interference dissociation, and atrioventricular (AV) junctional rhythm at a suitable rate usually require no treatment, but the patient should be observed closely for worsening of the disturbance.

Ventricular dysrhythmias are unusual. Those encountered early while the patient is in the intensive care unit usually respond to intravenous lidocaine or to DC conversion. Those which unexpectedly occur late postoperatively may be associated with sudden death. Quinidine or propranolol may be needed for a prolonged period to control paroxysms of ventricular tachycardia.

Atrioventricular conduction disturbances were a great problem in the early days of surgery to close ventricular septal defects or atrioventricular canal defects, but fortunately heart block occurs now only rarely. This improvement is due to better understanding of the anatomy of the conduction system so that sutures can be placed properly to avoid damage to the region of atrioventricular conduction located between the junctional tissue near the coronary sinus and the point of takeoff of the right bundle branch.

Despite precautions at the time of the operation, including the use of intracardiac mapping of the conduction system in complex anomalies,[27] AV block may still develop at or after surgery. It may be temporary or permanent. If it appears while the patient is in the operating room, pacemaker wires should be sutured into the myocardium so that, until normal conduction returns, the heart can be paced at an appropriate rate for the demands of the early postoperative period. Partial or complete heart block which appears after the patient has left the operating room or in the late postoperative period is unusual.

Postoperative complete heart block that persists has a poor prognosis. Sudden death has occurred months or years later. Although there are drawbacks to implanted pacemakers in the growing infant and child, we believe that surgically induced complete heart block is an indication for a permanent pacemaker.

Right bundle branch block occurs regularly when ventricular defects are closed, but it seems to have no harmful physiologic consequences unless possibly when it is associated with left axis deviation as left anterior hemiblock. There may under this circumstance be an increased risk of sudden complete heart block or sudden death.

GASTROINTESTINAL

Except for the occasional abdominal distension that occurs if oral feedings are given too fast, complications referable to the gastrointestinal tract are rare. A "stress" ulcer of the duodenum with hemorrhage necessitated resection in two babies we treated. An infrequent, distressing, and sometimes lethal occurrence that has come to attention with the use of profound hypothermia has been that of necrotizing enterocolitis.

GENITOURINARY

Some patients with congenital heart disease have abnormalities of the urinary tract as well, and if these are recognized in advance, postoperative complications may be anticipated and minimized. In patients who have preoperative diagnostic studies that include injection of contrast medium, we obtain a film of the kidneys, ureters, and bladder at the same time for such screening.[40]

Urinary output is one of the physiologic variables monitored in the early postoperative period. After cardiopulmonary bypass, there is customarily a diuresis for the first few hours. Thereafter, declining urinary flow inappropriate for the intravenous fluids administered, may be the first evidence of a decreasing cardiac output or of renal impairment. In situations when oliguria or anuria occur, strict regulation of intravenous fluids to match the urinary output plus insensible water loss and attention to electrolyte balance may help the patient to survive. Rarely, peritoneal or hemodialysis may be necessary.

HEMATOLOGIC

Excessive postoperative bleeding can be a real problem after open heart surgery, especially in polycythemic patients with tetralogy of Fallot and much collateral circulation. The surgeon must decide whether postoperative changes in blood volume and blood pressure may have caused small vessels to open and bleed so that exploration of the chest is needed, or whether the anticoagulant used during cardiac bypass was not properly neutralized, or whether there has been damage during extracorporeal circulation to some component of the clotting mechanism or to vessel walls or tissues. Determination in the surgical intensive care unit of prothrombin time, partial thromboplastin time, and platelet count can help settle the question, so that if a specific deficiency exists, it can be further delineated and corrected with the appropriate agent. Restraint is urged in the use of products prepared from pooled plasma such as are used for correction of deficiencies in factors II, VII, IX, and XI, since there is then a risk of hepatitis with jaundice.

INFECTIONS

Fever is common in the postoperative syndromes, and infection must be ruled out before the fever can be ascribed to a syndrome. The most serious infections are sepsis and endocarditis.[26] These are diagnosed on the basis of a high index of suspicion and by repeated blood cultures in a patient with sustained or spiking fever. In the early postoperative period, no other symptom may be present. If the infection occurs later, the signs that one associates with endocarditis may be found, such as splenomegaly, petechiae, hematuria, emboli, anemia, and debility. Characteristic of blood stream infection in the early postoperative period is that the organisms tend to be unusual and resistant to commonly employed antibiotics. *Staphylococcus aureus, Micrococcus, Aerobacter aerogenes, Pseudomonas aeruginosa*, and fungi are among the offenders.

Prophylactically, we give antibiotics in therapeutic doses beginning the night before surgery and continuing for the first 4 to 5 days, when all tubes have been removed. Thereafter, antibiotics are administered only on indication. There is strict adherence to aseptic technique, not only in the operating room but also in the surgical intensive care unit. The frequency of endocarditis in our experience has been less than 1% over the years.

Other infections include wound infections, urinary tract infections, pneumonia, and hepatitis. The risk of hepatitis when blood transfusion is given has been minimized by screening donors for Australia antigen, but a risk remains whenever a pooled plasma product is used postoperatively to correct a deficiency of factors.

NEUROLOGIC

Though care is taken to identify the left recurrent laryngeal nerve and not to cut it, injury sometimes occurs when the nerve is stretched or displaced during surgery for a patent ductus arteriosus or coarctation of the aorta. The change in voice rarely lasts more than a few weeks, for the left vocal cord either regains its strength or the right cord compensates for the weakness. Horner's syndrome with ptosis of the lid and a small pupil on that side follows injury to the sympathetic nerves during dissection of the subclavian artery for anastomosis to the pulmonary artery. Paralysis of the diaphragm with elevation and paradoxical motion occurs if the phrenic nerve is damaged or as a result of postoperative changes in adjacent tissues. Injury to the spinal cord may follow cross-clamping of the aorta for resection of coarctation of the aorta.

An uncommon but serious neurologic complication is that of vascular thrombosis and hemiplegia. Those especially at risk are the anemic, hypoxemic infant and the intensely polycythemic, cyanotic older patient. Close attention to fluid and blood balance should help to prevent this complication. After open heart surgery a patient may not regain consciousness promptly because of inadequate cerebral perfusion during cardiac bypass or because of embolism of air which had been trapped in the left side of the heart. Meticulous operative technic has practically eliminated this complication. Under anesthesia or in the early postoperative period, episodes of hypoxemia or hypotension may leave residual brain damage.

RESPIRATORY

Proper respiratory management is one of the most critical features of successful perioperative care.[32, 38] Small infants are especially likely candidates for early postoperative laryngeal edema, airway obstruction, or atelectasis. Skillful anesthesia and intensive nursing care are important in prevention or amelioration of these problems. Children complain little of chest pain related to the incision. They can usually be encouraged to breathe deeply and cough effectively. The use of chest drainage tubes prevents the occurrence of pleural effusion in the early postoperative period. If pleural effusion develops later, it is usually in association with the postpericardiotomy syndrome or with chylothorax, which is rare and usually subsides spontaneously. Surgery to identify the leak should be undertaken only if there are no signs of clearing after a reasonable waiting period.[20] Some children with the Noonan syndrome have an abnormality of lymphatic channels that makes them at risk for chylothorax.[2] Pneumothorax occasionally occurs. Only if it is large does it need to be aspirated. Paralysis of the diaphragm occurs sometimes when dissection about the phrenic nerve stretches or injures it. In the early postoperative period this may impose a handicap because it interferes with effective cough and ventilation. In some instances, after a few weeks or months, the elevated diaphragm which moves paradoxically functions normally again.

VASCULAR

Except for the hypoxemic and anemic or polycythemic patient, who may be a candidate for thrombosis of cerebral vessels or for excessive bleeding, infants and children are relatively free from vascular complications postoperatively. Sacrifice of the subclavian artery is well tolerated, though that extremity is cooler than its mate and may grow less well.[8] Following femoral arteriotomy for aortic perfusion on cardiac bypass, the pulse in that leg may be small or impalpable, due to spasm or thrombosis, but surgery to remove a clot is rarely needed. Even though the pulse continues to be less well felt than before surgery, collateral pathways are adequate and claudication is rare. Thrombophlebitis is a risk if indwelling catheters are kept in place for more than a few days. An infrequent occurrence is the "anterior compartment syndrome" in which the lower part of the limb on the side that has been cannulated for cardiopulmonary bypass becomes swollen, tense, pale, and intensely painful. Venous outflow and arterial inflow become obstructed. Muscular and neurologic impairment can result if the swelling of the tense anterior compartment is not relieved by incisions in the skin. We have seen four instances of this rare complication. Use of aortotomy rather than femoral arteriotomy for arterial inflow from the pump-oxygenator may be preventive.

In general, infants and children tolerate cardiac surgery and convalescence remarkably well and emerge as psychologically secure as on admission and more physically sound. Realization that there are complications of surgery should serve continually to improve the perioperative period through constant attention to details that might prevent a complication and by prompt recognition and treatment of those that occur.

REFERENCES

1. Anderson, R., and Larson, O.: Fever, splenomegaly and atypical lymphocytes after open-heart surgery. Lancet 2:947, 1963.
2. Baltaxe, H. A., Lee, J. G., Ehlers, K. H., and Engle, M. A.: Pulmonary lymphangiectasia demonstrated by lymphangiography in 2 patients with Noonan's syndrome. Radiology 115:149, 1975.
3. Bastin, R., Lapresle, C., and Dufrene, F.: Syndrome fébrile avec réaction sanguine mononucleosique après chirurgie thoracique. Presse Med. 73:63, 1965.
4. Battle, J. D., Jr., and Hewlett, J. S.: Hematologic changes observed after extracorporeal circulation during open-heart operations. Cleveland Clin. Q. 25:112, 1958.
5. Bell, R. E., Petuoglu, S., and Fraser, R. S.: Chronic haemolysis occurring in patients following cardiac surgery. Br. Heart J. 29:327, 1967.
6. Benson, W. R., and Sealy, W. C.: Arterial necrosis following resection of coarctation of the aorta. Lab. Invest. 5:359, 1956.
7. Clagett, O. T., and Jampolis, R. W.: Coarctation of the aorta: A study of seventy cases in which surgical exploration was performed. Arch. Surg. 63:337, 1951.
8. Currarino, G., and Engle, M. A.: The effects of ligation of the subclavian artery on the bones and soft tissues of the arm. J. Pediatr. 67:808, 1965.
9. Dressler, W.: Post-myocardial-infarction syndrome: Preliminary report of complication resembling idiopathic, recurrent, benign pericarditis. J.A.M.A. 160:1379, 1956.
10. Drusin, L. M., Engle, M. A., Hagstrom, J. W. C., and Schwartz, M. S.: The postpericardiotomy syndrome. A six-year epidemiologic study. N. Engl. J. Med. 272:597, 1965.
11. Ebert, P. A., Gay, W. A., Jr., and Engle, M. A.: Correction of transposition of the great arteries: Relationship of the coronary sinus and postoperative arrhythmias. Ann. Surg. 140:433, 1974.
12. Ellis, K., Malm, J. R., Bowman, O. B., Jr., and King, D. L.: Roentgenographic findings after pericardial surgery. Radiol. Clin. North Am. 9:327, 1971.
13. Engle, M. A., and Ito, T.: The postpericardiotomy syndrome. Am. J. Cardiol. 7:73, 1961.
14. Engle, M. A., and Marx, N. R.: The postpericardiotomy and postperfusion syndromes. Heart Bull. 14:33, 1965.
15. Engle, M. A., Zabriskie, J. B., Senterfit, L. B., Gay, W. A., Jr., O'Loughlin, J. E., and Ehlers, K. H.: Viral illness and the postpericardiotomy syndrome. A prospective study in children. Circulation 62:1151–1158, 1980.
16. Engle, M. A., Zabriskie, J. B., Senterfit, L. B.,

Tay, D. J., and Ebert, P. A.: Immunologic and virologic studies in the postpericardiotomy syndrome. J. Pediatr. 87:1103, 1975.
17. Feigenbaum, H., Waldhausen, J. A., and Hyde, L. P.: Ultrasound diagnosis of pericardial effusion. J.A.M.A. 191:711, 1965.
18. Goodkind, M. J., Bloomer, W. E., and Goodyer, V. N.: Recurrent pericardial effusion after nonpenetrating chest trauma. Report of two cases treated with adrenocortical steroids. N. Engl. J. Med. 263:874, 1960.
19. Groves, L. K., and Effler, D. B.: Problems in surgical management of coarctation of the aorta. J. Thorac. Cardiovasc. Surg. 39:60, 1960.
20. Higgins, C. B., and Mulder, D. G.: Chylothorax after surgery for congenital heart disease. J. Thorac. Cardiovasc. Surg. 61:411, 1971.
21. Holswade, G. R., Engle, M. A., Redo, S. F., Goldsmith, E. I., and Barondess, J. A.: Development of viral disease and a viral disease-like syndrome after extra-corporeal circulation. Circulation 27:812, 1963.
22. Horowitz, M. S., Schultz, C. S., Stinson, E. B., Harrison, D. C. and Popp, R. L.: Echocardiography in pericardial effusion. Circulation 50:239, 1974.
23. Ito, T., Engle, M. A., and Goldberg, H. P.: Postpericardiotomy syndrome following surgery for nonrheumatic heart disease. Circulation 17:549, 1958.
24. Jacobson, R. J., Rath, C. E., and Perloff, J. K.: Intravascular haemolysis and thrombocytopenia in left ventricular outflow obstruction. Br. Heart J. 35:849, 1973.
25. Janton, O. H., Glover, R. P., O'Neil, T. J. E., Gregory, J. E., and Froio, G. R.: Results of the surgical treatment of mitral stenosis. Circulation 6:321, 1952.
26. Johnson, D. H., Rosenthal, A., and Nadas, A. S.: A forty-year review of bacterial endocarditis in infancy and childhood. Circulation 51:581, 1975.
27. Kaiser, G. A., Waldo, A. L., Beach, P. M., Bowman, J. O., Hoffman, B. F., and Malm, J. R.: Specialized cardiac conduction system: Improved electrophysiologic identification techniques at surgery. Arch. Surg. 101:673, 1970.
28. Kreel, I., Zaroff, L. I., Cantor, J. C., Krasna, I., and Baronofsky, I. D.: A syndrome following total body perfusion. Surg. Gynecol. Obstet. 111:321, 1960.
29. Lober, P. H., and Lillehei, C. W.: Necrotizing panarteritis following repair of coarctation of aorta: Report of two cases. Surgery 35:950, 1954.
30. Mays, E. T., and Sergeant, C. K.: Postcoarctectomy syndrome. Arch. Surg. 91:58, 1965.
31. McCabe, J. C., Engle, M. A., and Ebert, P. A.: Chronic pericardial effusion requiring pericar-

diectomy in the postpericardiotomy syndrome. J. Thorac. Cardiovasc. Surg. 67:814, 1974.
32. McConnell, D. H., Maloney, J. V., and Buckberg, G. D.: Postoperative intermittent positive-pressure breathing treatments: Physiological considerations. J. Thorac. Cardiovasc. Surg. 68:944, 1974.
33. McGuinness, J. B., and Taussig, H. B.: The postpericardiotomy syndrome: Its relationship to ambulation in the presence of "benign" pericardial and pleural reaction. Circulation 26:500, 1962.
34. Miller, B. L., Pearson, H. A., Sheta, M. W., Jr., White, A. W., Jr., and Schiebler, G. L.: Delayed onset of hemolytic anemia in a child: An indicator of ball variance of aortic valve prosthesis. Circulation 40:55, 1969.
35. Neill, C. A.: Editorial: Postoperative hemolytic anemia in endocardial cushion defects. Circulation 30:801, 1964.
36. Paloheimo, J. A., van Essen, R., Klemola, E., Kaarainen, L., and Siltanen, P.: Subclinical cytomegalo-virus infections and cytomegalovirus mononucleosis after open heart surgery. Am. J. Cardiol. 22:624, 1968.
37. Perez-Alvarez, J. J., and Oudkerk, S.: Necrotizing arteriolitis of the abdominal organs as a postoperative complication following correction of coarctation of the aorta: A case report. Surgery 37:833, 1955.
38. Petty, T. L., and Hudson, L. D.: Acute pulmonary injury and repair (the adult respiratory distress syndrome): The 16th Aspen lung conference. Chest, 65, April and July supplements, 1974.
39. Pirofsky, B., Sutherland, D. W., Starr, A., and Griswold, H. E.: Hemolytic anemia complicating aortic-valve surgery. N. Engl. J. Med. 272:235, 1965.
40. Rao, S., Engle, M. A., and Levin, A. R.: Silent anomalies of the urinary tract and congenital heart disease. Chest 67:685, 1975.
41. Ring, D. M., and Lewis, F. J.: Abdominal pain following surgical correction of coarctation of aorta: A syndrome. J. Thorac. Cardiovasc. Surg. 31:718, 1956.
42. Sayed, H. N., Dacie, J. V., Handley, D. A., Lewisk, S. M., and Cleland, W. P.: Haemolytic anaemia of mechanical origin after open heart surgery. Thorax 16:356, 1961.
43. Schuster, S. R., and Gross, R. E.: Surgery for coarctation of aorta: Review of 500 cases. J. Thorac. Cardiovasc. Surg. 43:54, 1962.
44. Sealy, W. C.: Indications for surgical treatment of coarctation of aorta. Surg. Gynecol. Obstet. 97:301, 1953.
45. Sealy, W. C., Harris, J. S., Young, W. G., and Callaway, H. A.: Paradoxical hypertension fol-

lowing resection of coarctation of aorta. Surgery 42:135, 1957.
46. Seaman, A. J., and Starr, A.: Febrile postcardiotomy lymphocytic splenomegaly. Ann. Surg. 156:956, 1962.
47. Sigler, A. I., Forman, E. N., Zinkham, W. H., and Neill, C. A.: Severe intravascular hemolysis following surgical repair of endocardial cushion defects. Am. J. Med. 35:467, 1963.
48. Singleton, A. O., McGinnis, L. S., and Eason, H. R.: Arteritis following correction of coarc-

tation of the aorta. Surgery 45:665, 1959.
49. Smith, D. R.: A syndrome resembling infectious mononucleosis after open-heart surgery. Br. Med. J. 1:945, 1964.
50. Soloff, L. A., Zatuchni, J., Janton, O. H., O'Neil, T. J. E., and Glover, R. P.: Reactivation of rheumatic fever following mitral commissurotomy. Circulation 8:481, 1953.
51. Strong, W. B., Botti, R. E., Silbert, D. R., and Liebman, J.: Peripheral and renal vein plasma renin activity in coarctation of the aorta. Pe-

diatrics 45:254, 1974.
52. Tabatznik, B., and Isaacs, J. P.: Postpericardiotomy syndrome following traumatic hemopericardium. Am. J. Cardiol. 7:83, 1961.
53. Wheeler, E. C., Turner, J. D., and Scannell, J. G.: Fever, splenomegaly and atypical lymphocytes. N. Engl. J. Med. 266:454, 1962.
54. Williams, J. F., Jr., Morrow, A. G., and Braunwald, E.: The incidence and management of "medical" complications following cardiac operations. Circulation 32:608, 1965.

48

Cardiomyopathies

Barry J. Maron, M.D.

Cardiomyopathies, or diseases of the myocardium, are not uncommonly encountered in infants and children. However, our understanding of this diverse group of diseases is constantly evolving with regard to clinical identification, natural history, and therapy.

Cardiomyopathies may be considered to be either *primary* when no associated cardiovascular or systemic disease is present or *secondary* when the myocardial abnormality is thought to be related to an associated disease. In addition, cardiomyopathies have been classified with regard to their anatomic and functional features: hypertrophic; congestive or dilated; obliterative; and restrictive.[35] This chapter will discuss principally those primary forms of myocardial disease which affect infants and children.

HYPERTROPHIC CARDIOMYOPATHY

Hypertrophic cardiomyopathy is a primary disease of cardiac muscle that is probably congenital, is often genetically transmitted, and is characterized by a hypertrophied but nondilated left ventricle in the absence of another cardiac or systemic disease capable of producing left ventricular hypertrophy. Hypertrophic cardiomyopathy is a complex clinical and pathologic entity and has often been the subject of controversy. In 1958, Teare[110] presented the first systematic report of this disease, which he believed to be characterized by "asymmetrical hypertrophy of the heart" and nondilated ventricular cavities. Subsequent investigations have led to a dramatic evolution of the concepts concerning the clinical and physiologic spectrum of hypertrophic cardiomyopathy which, in the process, had acquired no fewer than 58 names (Fig. 48.1).

The majority of terms used to describe hypertrophic cardiomyopathy emphasize left ventricular outflow obstruction, a finding that has been thought to be highly characteristic of this disease. Thus, the names idiopathic hypertrophic subaortic stenosis, hypertrophic obstructive cardiomyopathy, muscular subaortic stenosis became widely used. However, the application of echocardiography to cardiac diagnosis in the early 1970s demonstrated that a large proportion of patients with hypertrophic cardiomyopathy either have no or mild obstruction to left ventricular outflow under basal conditions.[1, 116] Echocardiography also identified the asymmetric distribution of hypertrophy characteristic of hypertrophic cardiomyopathy, leading to the creation of the

term asymmetric septal hypertrophy (acronym ASH) to describe this disease entity.[42] However, because asymmetric septal hypertrophy is not an invariable feature of hypertrophic cardiomyopathy and because asymmetric ventricular wall thickening commonly occurs as a consequence of other cardiac lesions, asymmetric septal hypertrophy has not found wide acceptance as a suitable name for this disease.

PATHOLOGY

Our concepts of the anatomic structure of hearts with hypertrophic cardiomyopathy are derived from observations made at necropsy[78, 93, 118] and by echocardiography.[1, 19, 34, 42–45, 70] Gross examination of the heart at necropsy shows that the most characteristic feature of this disease is a hypertrophied nondilated left ventricle. At necropsy such hearts often weigh more than 600 gm (range 350 to 1200 gm; normal < 400). An unique feature of the pattern of hypertrophy in this disease is its asymmetric distribution (Fig. 48.2). In the vast majority of patients (about 90%), the ventricular septum is disproportionately thickened relative to the left ventricular free wall. In addition, the left and right atrial cavities are usually dilated at necropsy, although many living patients with hypertrophic cardiomyopathy have normal atrial size, as determined by echocardiography.

The aortic, pulmonic, and tricuspid valves are normal. However, patients often show thickening of the anterior mitral leaflet associated with localized endocardial thickening on the ventricular septum in the left ventricular outflow tract adjacent to the anterior leaflet. This endocardial plaque (which is observed in patients with and without subaortic obstruction) probably results from contact of the anterior leaflet with the septum during systole as well as diastole.

Focal scarring of the myocardium and subendocardium is frequently present in the ventricular septum, left ventricular free wall, and papillary muscles of adults with hypertrophic cardiomyopathy. About 10% of patients with hypertrophic cardiomyopathy observed at necropsy have substantial transmural scarring of the ventricular wall in the absence of major atherosclerosis of the extramural coronary arteries.[64] Such patients may also show dilatation of the left ventricle, although it is often possible to document that a nondilated left ventricle was present earlier in the clinical course.

In the majority of patients with hypertrophic cardiomyopathy studied at necropsy, the extramural coronary arteries

Fig. 48.1 Terms that have been used to describe hypertrophic cardiomyopathy.

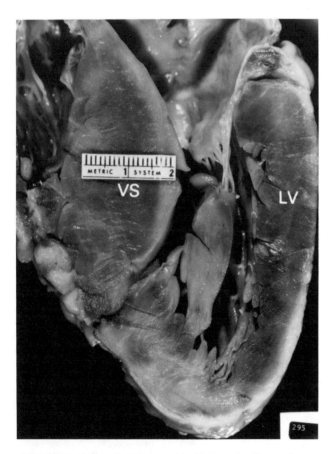

Fig. 48.2 Heart of a 12-year-old with hypertrophic cardiomyopathy. Ventricular septum (*VS*) is markedly thickened and bulges into the left ventricular outflow tract and cavity. The septum is disproportionately thickened with respect to the left ventricular free wall (*LV*).

appear widely patent. However, these patients are not protected against the development of coronary atherosclerosis. It seems that the frequency and extent of coronary atherosclerosis in patients with hypertrophic cardiomyopathy is what might be expected in patients of similar age and sex without that disease. However, abnormalities of the *intramural* coronary arteries are frequently present. These vessels commonly show thickening of the wall and narrowing of the lumen. The cause and significance of this finding is unclear.

The unique architecture of the myocardium in patients with hypertrophic cardiomyopathy has been emphasized in a number of reports.[23, 65, 67, 69, 110] Cardiac muscle cells in both the ventricular septum and left ventricular free wall show an increased transverse diameter; these hypertrophied cells may have bizarre shapes and may maintain intercellular connections with several adjacent cells (Fig. 48.3). In addition, many myocardial cells are not arranged in normal parallel alignment but are oriented at oblique and perpendicular angles to each other (Fig. 48.4).

Disorganization of cardiac muscle cells occurs in 95% of patients with hypertrophic cardiomyopathy and usually occupies substantial portions of ventricular septal myocardium (an average of about 33% of the septum).[65] Left ventricular free wall disorganization may also be substantial (involving about 25% of the free wall), indicating that disorganized myocardial architecture is diffuse and not limited to the septum.[69] The finding of marked septal disorganization in symptomatic infants with hypertrophic cardiomyopathy suggests that this histologic abnormality can be congenital.[58, 72] However, the presence of disorganized cells is not pathognomonic of hypertrophic cardiomyopathy. Small foci of disorganized cells may be found occasionally in the ventricular septum of infants, children, and adults with acquired or congenital heart diseases other than hypertrophic cardiomyopathy.[65, 67]

While marked ventricular septal and free wall disorganization is a reliable histologic marker of hypertrophic cardio-

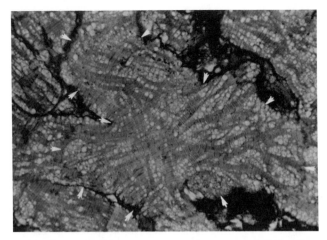

Fig. 48.3 Light micrograph of section of ventricular septum from a patient with hypertrophic cardiomyopathy. A hypertrophied and stellate-shaped muscle cell containing obliquely and transversely oriented myofibrils is shown in the center. Cell outline is indicated by *arrowheads*. This cardiac muscle cell maintains intercellular connections with several adjacent cells. Alkaline toluidine blue, ×1200.

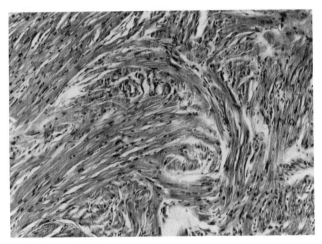

Fig. 48.4 Histologic section of ventricular septum from infant with hypertrophic cardiomyopathy. Some cardiac muscle cells have lost their normal parallel alignment and are arranged perpendicularly and obliquely to each other. Hematoxylin and eosin, ×200.

myopathy, the clinical relevance of this abnormality remains unclear. It is possible that disorganized myocardial cells may impair the transmission of normal electrophysiologic impulses and thereby serve as a nidus for primary fatal ventricular dysrhythmias.

PHYSIOLOGY

In many patients with hypertrophic cardiomyopathy, obstruction to left ventricular outflow is present at rest or with provocative maneuvers. Left ventricular outflow obstruction usually occurs as a result of an abnormal forward movement of the anterior leaflet of the mitral valve during systole and apposition of the leaflet with the hypertrophied ventricular septum.[43, 44, 101, 102, 105] It has been proposed that the systolic anterior motion is due to traction on the mitral valve by papillary muscles malaligned by the massively hypertrophied septum. Perhaps more likely, the anterior mitral leaf-

let is sucked forward by a high velocity jet through a narrowed outflow tract, i.e., a Venturi effect. The presence of substantial septal hypertrophy at the cardiac base adjacent to the mitral valve and the anterior position of the mitral valve within the left ventricular cavity at the onset of systole seem to be important determinants in the creation of a narrowed left ventricular outflow tract and obstruction to outflow.

The left ventricular outflow tract can be localized as the site of obstruction by the demonstration of a pressure gradient between the left ventricular cavity and the subvalvar area by left heart catheterization (Fig. 48.5). The zone of elevated intraventricular pressure includes the inflow tract of the left ventricle and extends from the ventricular apex to the leaflets of the mitral valve.

Differences in the systolic pressure gradient among patients with hypertrophic cardiomyopathy has led to the following hemodynamic classification: (1) *obstructive*, if a pressure gradient of at least 30 mm Hg is present under basal conditions; (2) *provocable*, if a gradient of at least 30 mm Hg is not present under basal conditions and can be elicited only by an intervention such as Valsalva maneuver, isoproterenol infusion, or amyl nitrite inhalation; and (3) *nonobstructive*, if a gradient of more than 30 mm Hg is not present under basal conditions and cannot be elicited with provocative interventions. However, it should be emphasized that due to relatively mild fluctuations in the magnitude of gradient, some patients may change from one of these groups to another. In addition, some patients have been identified in whom obstruction to left ventricular outflow has either disappeared[13, 86] or developed spontaneously[119] during a period of prolonged clinical observation.

Studies of aortic flow in patients with obstructive hypertrophic cardiomyopathy reveal that a large fraction of the stroke volume, approximately 80%, is ejected during the first one-half of ventricular systole.[11] The pressure gradient is absent or very small during the period of rapid ejection in very early systole; during the second half of systole, a significant gradient rapidly develops. A phase in late systole can be observed when the pressure gradient persists while little flow can be measured. Of interest, patients without obstruction to outflow similarly show ventricular ejection that is completed early in systole.[83]

In addition to obstruction to left ventricular outflow, patients with hypertrophic cardiomyopathy also manifest what Goodwin et al.[35, 36] have termed left ventricular "inflow ob-

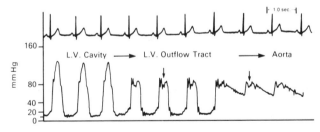

Fig. 48.5 Pressure tracing recorded continuously as the catheter was withdrawn from the left ventricular cavity through the left ventricular outflow tract and into the ascending aorta. Note that the pressure gradient occurs within the left ventricle. There is a notch on the upstroke of the left ventricular pressure pulse at approximately 100 mm Hg corresponding to the value of the peak systolic pressure distal to the obstruction. In the left ventricular outflow tract, the pressure pulse exhibits a midsystolic dip (*arrow*) and a secondary elevation late in systole. A similar contour during systole is present in the aortic pressure pulse.

struction." In such circumstances the left ventricle is stiffened, resulting in abnormally low ventricular compliance and impedance to filling.[118] Therefore, in patients with hypertrophic cardiomyopathy, systolic function may be normal or even supranormal while diastolic filling may be impaired and may contribute importantly to functional limitation.[8, 38, 107] Abnormal diastolic filling may contribute to the hemodynamic and symptomatic burden in certain patients with obstruction to left ventricular outflow but may also constitute the primary physiologic abnormality in those patients without obstruction. Hence, there is ample evidence that both outflow and inflow obstruction are important in hypertrophic cardiomyopathy.

ETIOLOGY

Hypertrophic cardiomyopathy is unique in that it is one of the few primary cardiac disorders to commonly demonstrate Mendelian genetic transmission.[16] In about 60% of families, at least one first degree relative of the index case can be shown to have hypertrophic cardiomyopathy by clinical or echocardiographic studies. The pattern of genetic transmission in such families is usually most consistent with an autosomal dominant transmission. While the frequency with which hypertrophic cardiomyopathy is transmitted to relatives may vary among families, the overall percentage of affected relatives in a group of families is only about 20%. Furthermore, only about one-third of affected first degree relatives appear to have important clinical or symptomatic manifestations of their condition. The remainder appear to have a "subclinical" manifestation of the disease detectable only by echocardiographic studies. For these reasons it is unclear whether routine screening is indicated for all asymptomatic relatives of patients with hypertrophic cardiomyopathy. However, a family history of premature cardiac death should necessitate echocardiographic evaluation of surviving relatives since the clinical expression of this disease may be particularly virulent and result in frequent premature deaths in certain families (e.g., "malignant" hypertrophic cardiomyopathy).

In about 40% of families, a genetic etiology cannot be documented. It is not known whether such "sporadic" occurrences represent genetic mutations or whether they are due to nongenetic factors which have yet to be defined.

In addition, hypertrophic cardiomyopathy has been described in patients with a number of noncardiac diseases such as neuroectodermal anomalies[108] (pheochromocytoma, tuberous sclerosis, neurofibromatosis, and lentiginosis), Friedreich ataxia,[67] Turner[85] and Noonan syndromes,[21] and hyperthyroidism.[67] It is not clear whether such relatively infrequent associations imply an etiologic relationship or whether they represent the sporadic association of two diseases. There have also been instances in which certain manifestations of hypertrophic cardiomyopathy are acquired (e.g., after pulmonary artery banding[29] or aortic valve replacement[112]).

MANIFESTATIONS

Clinical Features

The findings on physical examination in patients with hypertrophic cardiomyopathy are variable and related in large measure to hemodynamic state.[11] In patients with obstruction to outflow (i.e., typical idiopathic hypertrophic subaortic stenosis), a double or triple left ventricular apical impulse may be palpable. These impulses include the usual systolic outward thrust, a presystolic and occasionally an early diastolic expansion. In addition, patients with obstruction have a medium-pitch systolic ejection murmur that varies in intensity depending on the magnitude of the subvalvular gradient (Fig. 48.6). Patients with loud systolic murmurs of at least grade 3/6 intensity usually have peak systolic gradients greater than 50 mm Hg. Softer murmurs are usually associated with gradients of less than 50 mm Hg. The murmur is most prominent along the lower left sternal border in two-thirds of patients and loudest at the apex in one-third. When the systolic murmur is loud, there may be transmission to the axilla and base of the heart but only rarely is it heard well over the carotid vessels.

Physiologic maneuvers or pharmacologic interventions at the bedside may alter the murmur and may prove useful in the evaluation of a patient with hypertrophic cardiomyopathy.[11] For example, the systolic murmur is accentuated by amyl nitrite inhalation, with standing, or during the Valsalva maneuver, and it is diminished by squatting or isometric handgrip. In contrast, the systolic ejection murmur is decreased in intensity during Valsalva maneuver in patients with valvular aortic stenosis (AS) and decreased with amyl nitrite inhalation in patients with rheumatic mitral insufficiency (MI) or ventricular septal defect (VSD).

The systolic murmur tends to be holosystolic at the apex, and for this reason patients with hypertrophic cardiomyopathy may be incorrectly diagnosed as having rheumatic MI. An apical diastolic rumbling murmur is occasionally heard in patients with obstructive or nonobstructive hypertrophic cardiomyopathy. The genesis of this murmur is unclear, although it is probably related to left ventricular "inflow obstruction."

Splitting of the second heart sound is physiological in most patients but may be paradoxical, particularly in individuals with substantial gradients at rest. Systolic ejection sounds are rare in hypertrophic cardiomyopathy, and their origin is unclear.

The carotid and brachial pulses are unusually sharp and fast rising (Fig. 48.6) with a distinct bisferiens contour.[11] Indirect carotid pulse recordings usually demonstrate a bifid pulse contour, a shortened upstroke time, and a normal or slightly increased ejection period.[11]

Physical findings in patients *without* outflow obstruction may be subtle and often do not suggest the presence of

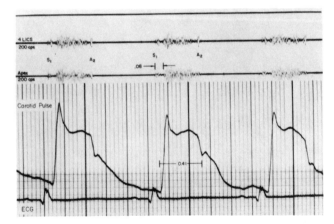

Fig. 48.6 Recording obtained from a patient with obstructive hypertrophic cardiomyopathy. Apical systolic murmur begins 0.08 second after the first heart sound (S_1) and continues to the aortic component of the second sound (A_2). Carotid pulse tracings show a rapid early peak characteristic of a dynamic type of left ventricular outflow obstruction. Ejection time is prolonged.

underlying heart disease. The left ventricular impulse may be single and not prominent, and the systolic murmur may be soft or even absent. For this reason, the diagnosis of nonobstructive hypertrophic cardiomyopathy may be difficult to confirm without echocardiographic studies.

Most commonly, in infants and children, hypertrophic cardiomyopathy is first identified or suspected clinically because of a cardiac murmur. The onset of symptoms usually occurs later, between 20 and 40 years of age, although symptoms may be evident at any age. For example, infants may incur severe progressive heart failure,[72] while in other patients the onset of symptoms may not occur until the 6th or 7th decades of life. Although the overall frequency of cardiac symptoms is lower in patients with the nonobstructive form of hypertrophic cardiomyopathy, the severity of symptoms may be similar in those patients with obstruction and those patients without obstruction to outflow. In patients with outflow obstruction, no correlation exists between the frequency and severity of symptoms and the magnitude of obstruction.

In about 75% of symptomatic patients, functional limitation due to dyspnea and/or fatigue is the predominant complaint. Such patients may also commonly experience chest pain, dizziness (particularly when assuming an erect position), syncope, paroxysmal nocturnal dyspnea, or palpitations. In the minority of patients, chest pain or syncope may be the predominant or only symptom. Chest pain may appear as typical angina pectoris in some older children and adults with hypertrophic cardiomyopathy and may have features atypical of angina in others. In the latter patients, chest pain may have a sharp or aching quality, may often last for hours, is not associated with ischemic electrocardiographic changes, and may be worse after administration of sublingual nitroglycerin. The cause of chest pain in patients with hypertrophic cardiomyopathy is poorly understood but most likely results from an imbalance in myocardial oxygen supply and demand relationships.

Atrial fibrillation is an unfavorable complication in hypertrophic cardiomyopathy, but is very rarely seen in patients less than 21 years of age. It is usually poorly tolerated and associated with left atrial dilatation,[45] clinical deterioration, and advanced disease because it further impairs the filling of an already poorly compliant left ventricle. Hypertrophic cardiomyopathy occurs more commonly in males; the sex distribution is usually about 65% males and 35% females.[11] Reports from diverse geographical areas suggest that hypertrophic cardiomyopathy is not limited to any particular locality.

Assessment of the natural history of patients with hypertrophic cardiomyopathy has become difficult because of the widespread use of propranolol, verapamil, and operative intervention. Nevertheless, judging from available data, the clinical course of patients with hypertrophic cardiomyopathy is best described as *variable*[3, 28, 39, 103]; meaningful generalizations concerning prognosis are, at present, difficult to make. Although some patients progressively deteriorate or die prematurely, most remain stable for many years; only rarely will a patient manifest spontaneous improvement. Premature cardiac death is not uncommon in patients with hypertrophic cardiomyopathy, and the annual mortality rate has been reported to be 4%. Such deaths are usually sudden and unexpected (in about 85%), although death may also occur in the setting of chronic progressive heart failure.

Of those patients identified as having hypertrophic cardiomyopathy in infancy or childhood, about one-half have either died from their disease or experienced clinical deterioration early in life (Fig. 48.7).[25, 59, 72] The onset of heart

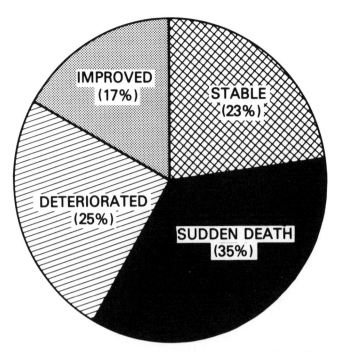

Fig. 48.7 Clinical course of patients with hypertrophic cardiomyopathy identified during childhood at the National Heart, Lung, and Blood Institute.

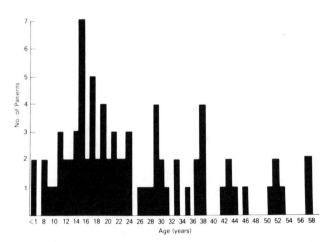

Fig. 48.8 Age distribution for 78 patients who died suddenly with hypertrophic cardiomyopathy and were evaluated at the National Heart, Lung, and Blood Institute.

failure in the first year of life appears to be a particularly unfavorable prognostic sign, with such patients rarely surviving the first year of life.

Certain clinical findings help to describe the profile of the patient who is at risk for sudden death.[73, 76] First, sudden death is particularly common in young patients between 12 and 30 years of age (Fig. 48.8). About one-half have previously been asymptomatic, with sudden death the initial clinical manifestation of hypertrophic cardiomyopathy[62]; fully one-third die while participating in strenuous physical activities.[73] Furthermore, hypertrophic cardiomyopathy is a particularly common cause of sudden death in highly conditioned young athletes. Secondly, genetic influences may predispose certain individuals to premature cardiac death. In some families with hypertrophic cardiomyopathy, sudden death is frequent, occurring in two or more first degree relatives ("malignant" hypertrophic cardiomyopathy) (Fig. 48.9).[61] Third, the finding of ventricular tachycardia on 24-hour ambulatory electrocardiogram appears to identify a risk factor associated with sudden death and is an indication for antidysrhythmic therapy.[71] It has been suggested that the occurrence of syncope is associated with an increased risk for sudden death[76]; others do not regard syncope as a particularly ominous prognostic sign.[73] Sudden death shows no particular predilection for patients either with or without obstruction to left ventricular outflow.[59, 73, 76]

The mechanism of sudden death in patients with hypertrophic cardiomyopathy has not been definitively defined, and indeed it may not be the same in each patient with hypertrophic cardiomyopathy. Initially, it was believed that sudden death occurred after an acute increase in obstruction to left ventricular outflow. However, perhaps more likely, sudden death results from a ventricular dysrhythmia.[71, 75] Accessory atrioventricular connections have been identified in some patients, suggesting that dysrhythmia complicating preexcitation could be responsible for sudden death.[51]

Electrocardiographic Features

The electrocardiogram is abnormal in about 90% of patients with hypertrophic cardiomyopathy and may show a wide variety of patterns (Fig. 48.10).[98] It is common for the abnormalities to be so marked that the tracing takes on a "bizarre" appearance, but no particular pattern is characteristic of the majority of patients with hypertrophic cardiomyopathy. Furthermore, the pattern does not discriminate those patients with or without obstruction to left ventricular outflow[98] or patients at risk for sudden death.[73]

The most common ECG abnormalities are left ventricular hypertrophy, ST segment and T wave changes, left atrial enlargement, abnormal Q waves, and diminished or absent R waves in the lateral precordial leads ("pseudoinfarct" pattern). Infants with this disease often have the paradoxic finding of right ventricular hypertrophy, which is usually associated with obstruction to right ventricular outflow.[72] It has been proposed that Q waves in patients with hypertrophic cardiomyopathy emanate from depolarization of the thickened septum; however, most patients with a markedly thickened septum do not show Q waves, and many patients with Q waves do not have marked septal hypertrophy.

In about 10% of patients the ECG is normal. Such patients usually have the nonobstructive form of the disease, with hypertrophy confined to a small portion of the ventricular septum.

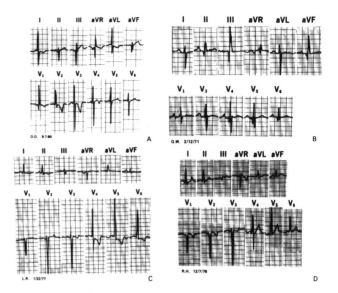

Fig. 48.10 Electrocardiograms obtained in four infants or children with hypertrophic cardiomyopathy showing a variety of patterns. (*A*) Right ventricular hypertrophy with predominant R waves in leads V₁ and V₂: left axis deviation and left atrial enlargement are also present. (*B*) Probable right ventricular hypertrophy and wide Q waves in leads II, III, AVF, and V₄ to V₆ and intraventricular conduction defect. (*C*) Left ventricular hypertrophy with ST segment and T wave abnormalities ("strain" pattern) and small R waves and deep S waves in right precordial leads. (*D*) Suggestive of left ventricular hypertrophy with deep S waves and absent or small R waves in leads V₁ to V₃.

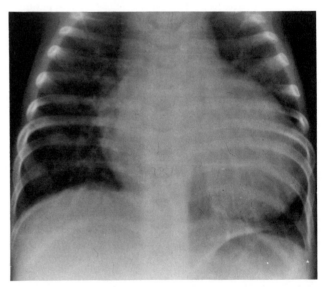

Fig. 48.11 Radiograph from a 5-month-old infant with hypertrophic cardiomyopathy showing marked cardiac enlargement.

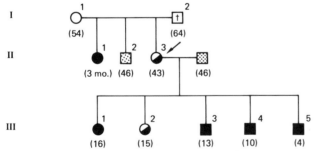

Fig. 48.9 Pedigree of family with unusual number of premature sudden deaths ("malignant" hypertrophic cardiomyopathy). Four of the five offspring of the propositus (*arrow*) have died suddenly before 17 years of age (● and ■); ◑, alive with hypertrophic cardiomyopathy; ○, no data available; ▨, alive without evidence of hypertrophic cardiomyopathy; ⊞, death from noncardiac cause; *round symbols* = female; *square symbols*, male. Patient ages are shown in *parentheses* below symbols.

Radiographic Features

In recent years, with the advent of echocardiography, examination of the heart by chest X-ray has been of diminished diagnostic usefulness. Cardiac size on chest roentgenogram is increased in two-thirds of patients with hypertrophic cardiomyopathy[11] and particularly in infants with this disease (Fig. 48.11).[72] Increased cardiac silhouette is usually due to increased cardiac mass and left atrial enlargement but rarely to left ventricular cavity dilatation. However, the presence or degree of cardiomegaly does not correlate with the clinical course or any other important clinical parameter.

There is marked variability in the qualitative appearance of the cardiac silhouette, although generally the heart appears more globular than in patients with aortic valvular stenosis. Increased pulmonary vascular markings are present in about 10% of patients, usually those with elevated pulmonary venous pressures. The aorta is normal sized. Other less common radiographic features include right atrial enlargement, mitral annular calcification in older patients, and small pericardial effusion.

Echocardiographic Features

The finding of an absolute increase in ventricular septal thickness and a ventricular septal to left ventricular free wall thickness ratio of 1.3 or greater in a patient with a nondilated left ventricle is an important diagnostic marker of hypertrophic cardiomyopathy (Fig. 48.12).[1, 42] The thickened ventricular septum often appears hypocontractile due to its diminished systolic thickening, excursion, or both.[17, 96] However, two important points require emphasis here. First, a number of other congenital or acquired heart diseases may secondarily produce septal hypertrophy and, thereby, an increase in the septal-free wall thickness ratio.[67] Such malformations include those producing right ventricular hypertension, as well as lesions affecting the left side of the heart.

Second, the septal-free wall ratio "cutoff" of ≥1.3 is not entirely reliable in evaluating infants and young children, in whom ventricular wall thicknesses are not greatly increased in absolute terms. Small differences in septal or free wall

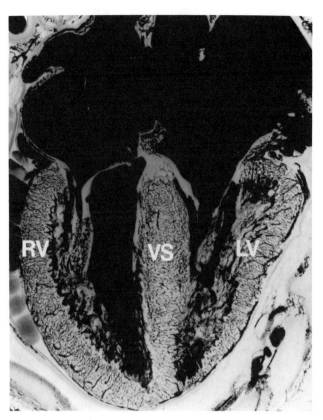

Fig. 48.13 Frontally sectioned heart of a fetus of 10 weeks gestation showing a ventricular septum (VS) which is disproportionately thicker than the left ventricular free wall (LV). Ventricular cavities are filled with India ink that was injected into the umbilical vein at the time of preparation of the specimen. RV, right ventricle.

thickness in such patients may produce exaggerated alterations in the resultant ratio and an incorrect diagnosis of hypertrophic cardiomyopathy.[66] For example, an abnormal septal-free wall ratio has been reported in as many as 20% of infants with other congenital heart malformations.[66] Also, serial echocardiographic studies have shown that disproportionate thickening of the septum in infants with congenital heart disease may be transient and may disappear by 2 years of age, due to continued thickening of the posterior left ventricular wall.[53] Therefore, young patients suspected of having hypertrophic cardiomyopathy based on an abnormal septal-free wall ratio should also show: marked absolute ventricular septal thickening and persistence of an abnormal septal-free wall ratio (i.e., ≥1.3) after 2 years of age.

Asymmetric left ventricular hypertrophy, characteristic of the heart of patients with hypertrophic cardiomyopathy, has been shown to be present at birth and very early in life and, hence, is probably congenital.[58, 72] However, further thickening of the septum and free wall probably occurs with aging and growth through the first 2 decades of life. It is of interest that, while the morphologic expression of hypertrophic cardiomyopathy is congenital, patients with this disease usually do not develop symptoms until much later in life. Furthermore, there is no evidence that increased symptomatology is accompanied by progression of hypertrophy or by any other change in cardiac structure. Of note, disproportionate thickening of the ventricular septum is also a characteristic anatomic feature of the normal embryonic and fetal human heart (Fig. 48.13).[63] Therefore, it is possible that asymmetric septal hypertrophy in patients with hypertrophic cardio-

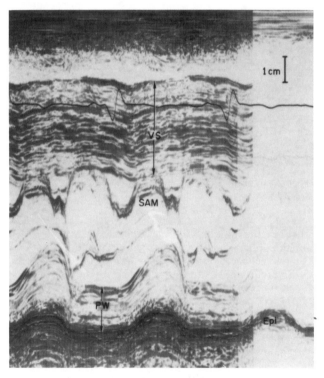

Fig. 48.12 M-mode echocardiogram from a patient with obstructive hypertrophic cardiomyopathy. The ventricular septum (VS) is markedly hypertrophied and is 2.2 times the thickness of the posterobasal left ventricular free wall (PW). Marked systolic anterior motion of the anterior mitral leaflet (SAM) is present.

myopathy represents postnatal persistence of a normal anatomic feature of the developing heart.

Systolic anterior motion of the anterior mitral leaflet (SAM) is well visualized with M-mode echocardiography.[43, 44, 101, 102] Abrupt anterior motion of the anterior leaflet toward the ventricular septum occurs in early systole with the onset of ejection and reaches its peak at the end of the first third of systole, when the leaflet either approaches or comes into contact with the ventricular septum (Fig. 48.12). The anterior leaflet may reach a plateau through the second one-third of systole and then moves posteriorly away from the septum during the last portion of systole. SAM results in narrowing of the left ventricular outflow tract during midsystole, at a time corresponding to the peak of the systolic murmur, the dip in the arterial pressure pulse contour, premature systolic aortic valve closure, and the presence of the subvalvular gradient. SAM is not a particularly sensitive marker for hypertrophic cardiomyopathy because of the high prevalence of patients with this disease who do not have outflow obstruction. SAM is, however, very uncommon in other cardiac diseases and, hence, the specificity of this finding is extremely high (i.e., 97%).[67]

A reasonably accurate assessment of the hemodynamic state in patients with hypertrophic cardiomyopathy can be made from M-mode echocardiography,[43, 101, 102] often obviating the necessity of monitoring the magnitude of left ventricular outflow obstruction by performing serial cardiac catheterizations. The magnitude and duration of systolic anterior motion of the anterior mitral leaflet on M-mode echocardiogram is directly related to the magnitude of the left ventricular outflow gradient.[43] For example, prolonged contact of the anterior mitral leaflet with the ventricular septal endocardium throughout midsystole is indicative of marked subaortic obstruction. On the other hand, a mild or trivial degree of systolic anterior motion will not produce a gradient.

Patients with outflow gradients at rest usually also show premature systolic closure of the aortic valve.[50] This abnormality appears as an abrupt posterior motion of the anterior (right coronary) leaflet associated with anterior motion of the noncoronary leaflet, producing partial closure of the leaflets in midsystole. This pattern of aortic leaflet separation is probably a reflection of the aortic flow velocity alterations characteristic of hypertrophic cardiomyopathy, i.e., a sharp early peak in flow followed by an abrupt decrease in midsystole and a second slower peak in late systole.[10] The "spike and dome" contour of the aortic pressure pulse recorded directly at cardiac catheterization[11] is probably also a manifestation of these flow velocity patterns.

In addition, the M-mode echocardiogram may be normal and therefore not diagnostic of hypertrophic cardiomyopathy in about 10% of patients with this disease.[70] In these patients the asymmetric pattern of hypertrophy involves regions of the left ventricle which are not accessible to the M-mode beam, e.g., the anterolateral free wall, posterior portion of ventricular septum, or apical portions of the left ventricle ("apical hypertrophic cardiomyopathy"), but which can be visualized only with 2D echocardiography (Fig. 48.14).[70] Such patients with hypertrophic cardiomyopathy and a normal M-mode echocardiogram usually have an abnormal electrocardiogram and a family history of hypertrophic cardiomyopathy. Occasionally, patients with hypertrophic cardiomyopathy show concentric (symmetric) left ventricular hypertrophy on the M-mode echocardiogram with a septal-free wall ratio of 1.0–1.2. However, 2D echocardiography almost invariably demonstrates "asymmetric" hypertrophy in regions of the left ventricular wall inaccessible to the M-mode beam.

Two-dimensional echocardiography has also produced

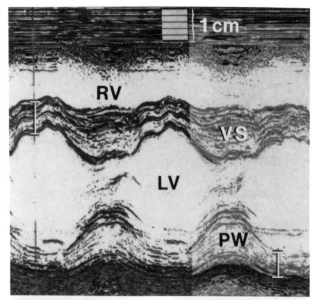

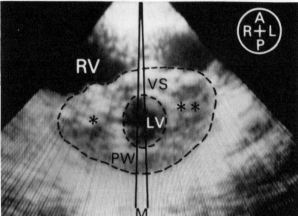

Fig. 48.14 M-mode echocardiogram (*top*) and stop-frame of 2D echocardiogram (*bottom*) from a 14-year-old child with hypertrophic cardiomyopathy. M-mode echocardiogram shows no thickening of the ventricular septum (*VS*) or posterior free wall (*PW*) and is not diagnostic of hypertrophic cardiomyopathy. 2D echocardiogram shows hypertrophy primarily in the posterior portion of ventricular septum (*) and anterolateral free wall (**), regions of the left ventricle not accessible to the M-mode beam (*M*). The inner and outer limits of the left ventricular wall are indicated by the *dashed line* for clarity. *LV*, left ventricular cavity; *RV*, right ventricle, *A*, anterior; *P*, posterior; *L*, left; *R*, right.

other insights into the wide morphologic spectrum of hypertrophic cardiomyopathy, even in those patients in whom the M-mode echocardiogram is diagnostic of the disease (Fig. 48.15). For example, the majority of patients (55%) with this disease have substantial hypertrophy involving the anterolateral left ventricular free wall as well as the ventricular septum while 20% show hypertrophy of the entire ventricular septum (with normal left ventricular free wall thickness); about 10% have hypertrophy confined to only the anterior portion of ventricular septum.[70] These patterns of distribution of left ventricular hypertrophy appear to have clinical relevance. Patients with the most diffuse distribution of hypertrophy, involving the septum and free wall, more commonly show substantial functional limitation, obstruction to left ventricular outflow at rest, and left ventricular hypertrophy on ECG. Genetic transmission of hypertrophic cardiomyopathy may occur with each of the morphologic types of the disease.

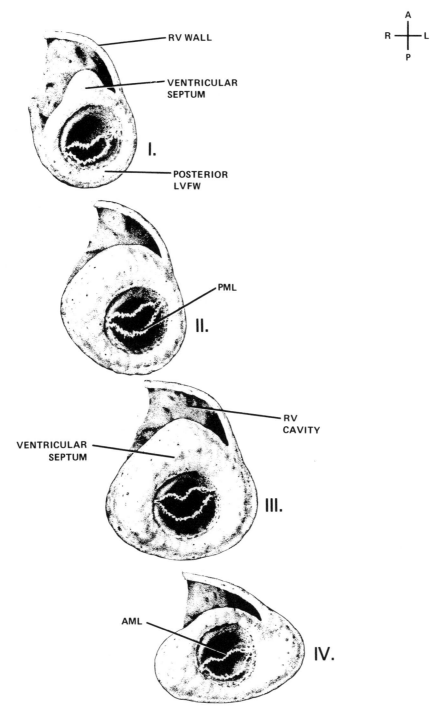

A
R ─┼─ L
P

Fig. 48.15 Artistic representation of the four patterns of hypertrophy identified by wide angle two-dimensional echocardiography in patients with hypertrophic cardiomyopathy. Only cross-sectional planes at the level of the mitral valve are shown. Hypertrophy is confined to the anterior portion of ventricular septum in Type I, involves the entire septum in Type II, and involves substantial portions of the septum and anterolateral left ventricular free wall in Type III. In patients with Type IV, hypertrophy involves regions of the left ventricle other than the basal anterior septum, and therefore the M-mode echocardiogram may be normal. *AML*, anterior mitral leaflet; *LVFW*, left ventricular free wall; *PML*, posterior mitral leaflet; *RV*, right ventricle.

CARDIAC CATHETERIZATION

The left ventricular outflow tract gradient in patients with hypertrophic cardiomyopathy is most easily measured with a freely mobile catheter in the body of the left ventricle and a simultaneous reference catheter in a systemic artery. Confirmation of the intraventricular nature of the pressure gradient may be accomplished by retrograde arterial catheteri-

zation, by recording intraventricular pressure continuously as the catheter is slowly withdrawn from the left ventricular apex into the subvalvular chamber. The fall in ventricular systolic pressure usually occurs abruptly when the tip of the catheter is 2 to 4 cm below the aortic valve. This is in contrast to patients with fixed "discrete" forms of congenital subaortic stenosis where the site of obstruction is closer to the aortic valve. Commonly, there is a distinct notch on the upstroke of the left ventricular pressure pulse at approximately the same level as the peak pressure distal to the obstruction (Fig. 48.5). The magnitude of the outflow gradient in a population of patients with this disease may vary from trivial to severe, with the average gradient about 50–60 mm Hg and marked gradients of >100 mm Hg common.

In infants and young children, obstruction to right ventricular outflow is common and is usually found in association with left ventricular outflow obstruction. In one series, right ventricular outflow obstruction occurred in over 60% of infants; often, the magnitude of subpulmonic obstruction was equal to or greater than that of subaortic obstruction (Fig. 48.16).[72] Right ventricular outflow obstruction in young patients is probably due to bulging of the asymmetrically

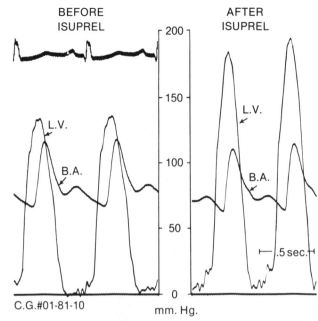

Fig. 48.17   Effects of an infusion of isoproterenol in a patient with hypertrophic cardiomyopathy and mild obstruction to left ventricular outflow in the basal state.

hypertrophied ventricular septum into the relatively small outflow tract.

A unique aspect of hypertrophic cardiomyopathy is the dynamic nature of this systolic pressure gradient. The magnitude of the gradient may vary during the course of a single hemodynamic study, at sequential cardiac catheterizations, or even from moment to moment.[11] At catheterization the gradient between the left ventricle and aorta can be reduced or augmented by several different interventions; whether the gradient increases or decreases seems to correlate with the capacity of the intervention to alter either arterial pressure, myocardial contractility, or ventricular volume. Thus, outflow gradient is reduced or abolished by interventions that increase arterial pressure, decrease myocardial contractility, or increase left ventricular volume (i.e., propranolol, phenylephrine, squatting, elevation of the legs, or handgrip). On the other hand, the gradient is augmented by interventions that decrease arterial pressure, increase contractility, or decrease ventricular volume (i.e., nitroglycerine, amyl nitrite, Valsalva maneuver, premature ventricular contraction, isoproterenol, or digitalis) (Fig. 48.17). These marked variations in the severity of obstruction that occur in obstructive hypertrophic cardiomyopathy distinguish such patients from those with heart diseases producing "fixed" obstruction to left ventricular outflow.

Lability of obstruction is exemplified by a distinctive response to premature ventricular contraction (the Brockenbrough phenomenon).[11] In normal individuals, or in patients with "fixed" obstruction to left ventricular outflow, the augmented force of contraction accompanying the premature contraction results in an increased systemic arterial pulse pressure of the postextrasystolic beat. In contrast, in 80% of patients with obstructive hypertrophic cardiomyopathy, the arterial pressure of the beat following the premature contraction fails to exceed that of the control beat.

Intraventricular pressure differences can be recorded in the absence of obstruction when the left ventricle empties rapidly and completely and the catheter tip lies within the obliterated portions of left ventricular cavity. The catheter

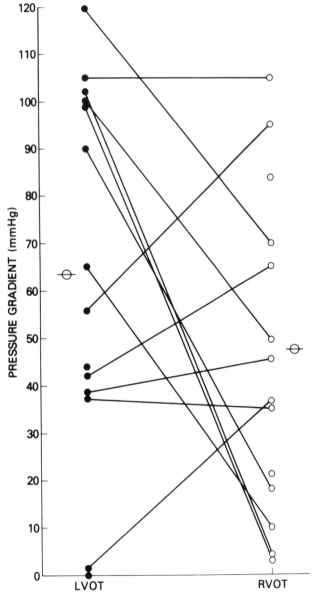

Fig. 48.16   Left ventricular outflow tract (LVOT) and right ventricular outflow tract (RVOT) peak systolic pressure gradients in 16 infants with hypertrophic cardiomyopathy. Data for each of the patients in whom both left and right ventricular outflow gradients were measured are connected by a line. Θ, mean values.

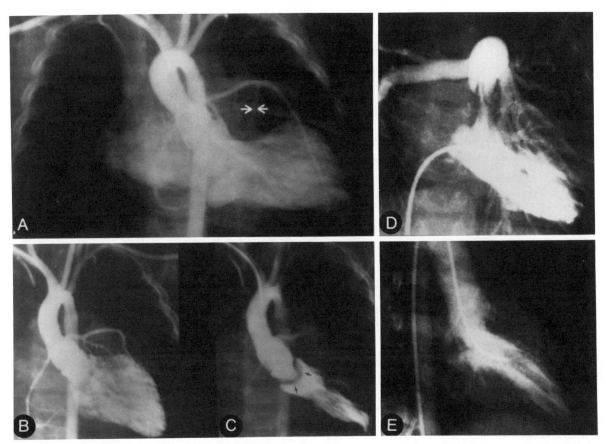

Fig. 48.18 Angiocardiograms obtained in the posteroanterior projection in four infants with hypertrophic cardiomyopathy showing a variety of diastolic and systolic abnormalities. (*A*) Frontal projection showing abnormal diastolic left ventricular contour in which superior indentation of the cavity is produced by marked hypertrophy of the ventricular septum. Septal coronary artery (*arrows*) arises from the left anterior descending coronary artery. Opacification of the left atrium indicates mitral regurgitation. Diastolic (*B*) and systolic (*C*) frames from another patient showing a hypercontractile left ventricle and marked systolic anterior motion of the anterior mitral leaflet (*arrows*). (*D*) Right ventricular angiocardiogram during systole from an infant with a right ventricular outflow tract gradient of 95 mm Hg showing narrowing of the outflow tract. (*E*) Angiocardiogram in the lateral projection at end systole showing marked emptying of the left ventricle, obliteration of the apex, and a "ballerina slipper" configuration.

may record the left ventricular wall tension, which can lead to the spurious diagnosis of intraventricular obstruction. Various hemodynamic maneuvers have been employed to differentiate patients with "cavity obliteration" from those with true obstruction; the most reliable of these is simultaneous measurement of left ventricular inflow pressure and aortic pressure.[94]

ANGIOCARDIOGRAPHY

When visualized by angiography, the left ventricle demonstrates altered ventricular morphology and may also identify the region of outflow obstruction (Fig. 48.18). The width of the left ventricular cavity during diastole is usually decreased, the ventricular wall is thickened, and the shape of the cavity is distorted. In the frontal projection, during diastole, the left ventricular outflow tract appears indented superiorly (just lateral to the aortic valve) where ventricular septal hypertrophy is substantial; the inferomedial aspect of the ventricle is also indented due to hypertrophy of the posteromedial papillary muscle and posterior ventricular septum.

The mechanism of left ventricular outflow obstruction may be best visualized in the lateral or left anterior oblique projections in systole utilizing cineangiography. The ventric-

ular septum projects into the left ventricular outflow tract; most importantly, the leading edge of the anterior mitral leaflet can be seen to be held in the outflow tract and to come into contact with the hypertrophied septum during midsystole, creating a radiolucent shelf-like projection in the outflow tract about 2 cm below the aortic annulus (Fig. 48.18*C*).

In the majority of patients, the left ventricle exhibits increased contractility associated with apical cavity obliteration. In such ventricles, emptying of the left ventricle at end systole is often so complete that all that can be seen of the apical portion of the ventricle is just a ribbon of contrast material between the two papillary muscles. In diastole, the configuration of the hypercontractile ventricle (in the frontal plane) has been likened to a "ballerina slipper" (Fig. 48.18*E*). Left ventricular apical cavity obliteration is, however, not pathognomonic for hypertrophic cardiomyopathy and may occasionally be observed in patients with systemic hypertension or valvular aortic stenosis.[90] In some patients with hypertrophic cardiomyopathy, the left ventricle assumes an "hourglass configuration" in which the area of most marked cavity obliteration is located in the midcavity region, distal to the mitral leaflet tips, rather than at the apex. Some of the latter patients may actually have left ventricular outflow obstruction at the level of the muscular midcavity constriction.[22] In a minority of patients, the left ventricle is not greatly distorted, and contractility appears normal. Any of these angiographic patterns may be present in patients either with or without outflow obstruction at rest.

The angiographic appearance of the ventricular septum in hypertrophic cardiomyopathy is best demonstrated by biventricular cineangiography performed in the left anterior oblique projection.[91] This technique permits identification of the left and right surfaces of ventricular septum and qualitative and quantitative assessments of the contour and thickness of the septum.

The asymmetrically hypertrophied ventricular septum may also impinge on the outflow tract of the right ventricle (Fig. 48.18D). The septal "bulge" appears as a large muscular band separating the right ventricular inflow from outflow tract and angiographically resembles an anomalous muscle bundle of the right ventricle. This abnormality may be responsible for the right ventricular outflow tract gradients present in infants and young children with hypertrophic cardiomyopathy.[72]

Mitral insufficiency is commonly demonstrable by angiography[11, 117] and has been reported to occur in 40 to 100% of patients with outflow obstruction at rest. Some degree of MI is probably present in virtually all patients with outflow obstruction, although it is usually mild to moderate and rarely severe. Pharmacologic interventions which abolish the outflow tract gradient also ameliorate MI, suggesting that the MI is secondary to systolic anterior motion of the anterior mitral leaflet and outflow obstruction.[117]

DIFFERENTIAL DIAGNOSIS

Hypertrophic cardiomyopathy has been termed the "great masquerader" because of its propensity to mimic and be confused diagnostically with several other cardiac diseases; hence, a high index of suspicion is often required, particularly in infants and young children. Hypertrophic cardiomyopathy in infants may present with a variety of clinical manifestations, including heart failure, enlarged cardiac silhouette on chest x-ray, loud systolic murmur heard best at the lower left sternal border or apex, right ventricular hypertrophy on ECG and cyanosis, presumably due to right to left shunting across a patent foramen ovale in the presence of right ventricular hypertension. For these reasons, hypertrophic cardiomyopathy in the young may easily be confused with other congenital cardiac malformations. In children with no or minimal outflow tract obstruction at rest, a soft systolic ejection murmur may be thought to be "innocent." In adults, hypertrophic cardiomyopathy may mimic coronary heart disease when chest pain is typical of angina pectoris. The majority of these diagnostic ambiguities are resolved by echocardiographic studies which will demonstrate the typical structural features of hypertrophic cardiomyopathy.

Hypertrophic cardiomyopathy in infants must also be distinguished from a transient nonfamilial condition that occurs in infants of diabetic mothers. These latter infants characteristically manifest disproportionate thickening of the ventricular septum, systolic anterior motion of the anterior mitral leaflet (associated with a left ventricular outflow gradient) and heart failure. Such infants of diabetic mothers, unlike those with "true" hypertrophic cardiomyopathy, usually show symptomatic improvement (either spontaneously, with the termination of digitalis treatment, or with propranolol therapy), loss of outflow obstruction, and regression of septal hypertrophy within the first few months of life.[37, 115]

TREATMENT

Circumstances which cause an increase in left ventricular outflow tract obstruction may result in symptomatic or hemodynamic deterioration. Therefore, excessive use of diuretics or the administration of preload or afterload reducing agents, beta-agonist drugs, or digitalis glycosides should be restricted in the treatment of hypertrophic cardiomyopathy since they each tend to increase subaortic obstruction.

The treatment of patients with hypertrophic cardiomyopathy centers about two central issues: alleviation of cardiac symptoms and prevention of sudden death. In symptomatic patients, the mainstay of medical treatment has been beta-adrenergic blocking agents, particularly propranolol. A broad-based experience with this drug over 15 years indicates that it is useful in relieving symptoms and improving exercise capacity in many patients.[2, 109]

The mechanisms by which beta-adrenergic blockers exert beneficial effects are complex. Symptoms such as dyspnea and syncope or presyncope may be improved by propranolol because a decrease in heart rate and myocardial contractility have the effect of reducing obstruction to left ventricular outflow when sympathetic activity is increased. Improvement in angina pectoris with propranolol is thought to be related to a diminution in myocardial oxygen requirements. Propranolol reduces heart rate, myocardial contractility, and transmural wall tension, all of which contribute to a decrease in myocardial oxygen demands. Propranolol, also, has antidysrhythmic properties and theoretically may reduce the frequency of syncope, dizziness, or even sudden death by preventing ventricular dysrhythmias. However, some investigators have shown the occurrence of potentially life-threatening ventricular dysrhythmias not to be altered substantially by propranolol administration.[75]

While propranolol is an effective agent for treatment of symptoms, it is unclear at this time whether this drug consistently alters the natural history of symptomatic patients with hypertrophic cardiomyopathy or diminishes the likelihood of sudden death. Some investigators have urged the aggressive treatment of symptoms as well as all high-grade ventricular dysrhythmias with "complete" beta-adrenergic blockade (average propranolol dose of 460 mg/day) alone or in combination with other antidysrhythmic drugs.[12, 27] However, the chronic administration of propranolol is commonly accompanied by fatigue and tiredness, which themselves may constitute a substantial functional limitation to some patients.

The therapeutic strategy for the *asymptomatic* patient with hypertrophic cardiomyopathy is controversial, and no definitive answers are currently available. However, propranolol has been administered prophylactically to asymptomatic or mildly symptomatic patients in the hope of preventing progression of the disease process or the occurrence of sudden death. Goodwin and Oakley[35] have recommended the use of beta-adrenergic blockers for all patients as soon as the diagnosis is made and regardless of the degree of symptomatic limitation or the magnitude of outflow obstruction. Others[61, 62] would limit the prophylactic use of propranolol to asymptomatic patients with a family history of premature sudden death and to patients who demonstrate marked ventricular septal thickening by echocardiography and a distinctly abnormal electrocardiogram. It should be emphasized, however, that propranolol does not convey absolute protection against sudden death; about 25% of those patients who die suddenly have taken apparently adequate doses of propranolol during the period just prior to death.[73] Because sudden death commonly occurs during severe exertion, asymptomatic children should be advised against participation in competitive athletics or particularly strenuous physical activities.

More recently, calcium channel blockers such as verapamil have proven useful in improving exercise capacity and symptomatic status of patients with hypertrophic cardiomyopathy.[48] To date, verapamil has been administered primarily to severely symptomatic patients who have failed to benefit from beta-adrenergic blocking agents. About one-half of the patients who do not improve on propranolol report functional improvement with verapamil.[90] Verapamil appears to exert its major beneficial effects by improving left ventricular filling,[8] although reduction in left ventricular outflow gradient has been demonstrated after the acute administration of verapamil.[90]

If paroxysmal atrial fibrillation occurs, quinidine or digitalis should be administered to control this dysrhythmia. In addition, because of the risk of systemic embolization, an anticoagulant should be given. If digitalis glycosides are administered to such patients, they should be given cautiously because of their tendency to intensify obstruction to left ventricular outflow.

The medical treatment of patients with hypertrophic cardiomyopathy and marked heart failure represents a difficult problem. Occasionally, patients progress to an "end stage" of their disease, characterized by severe cardiac failure in association with supraventricular dysrhythmias, absence of outflow obstruction, dilated ventricular cavities, and impaired systolic function.[64] At necropsy, such patients often show widespread transmural scarring of the left ventricle unassociated with major coronary atherosclerosis. Patients with "end stage" hypertrophic cardiomyopathy may respond transiently to digitalis and diuretics. Infants may also manifest severe heart failure in the presence of normal systolic function and obstruction to left ventricular outflow. Measures directed at reducing outflow obstruction are indicated in this situation, including judicious use of propranolol and diuretic agents.

Two other considerations in managing patients with hypertrophic cardiomyopathy which may impact on daily lifestyle concern recommendations for antimicrobial prophylaxis and pregnancy. Although the risk of endocarditis appears to be small, vegetations have been reported to occur on the aortic or mitral valves or on the septal endocardium at the site of the contact plaque.[54] Therefore, patients with hypertrophic cardiomyopathy, particularly those with outflow obstruction, should receive antibiotics prior to dental or surgical procedures in a fashion similar to that of patients with valvular or congenital heart disease. Patients with hypertrophic cardiomyopathy tolerate pregnancy well, although treatment with propranolol is often utilized.[87] Vaginal delivery is not contraindicated, although it may be preferable to deliver by cesarean section patients with marked obstruction to left ventricular outflow.

Operation is usually recommended for those patients with severe symptoms refractory to treatment with propranolol or verapamil who also have obstruction to left ventricular outflow under basal conditions or with provocation (gradient ≥ 50 mm Hg). Operation is *not* recommended for asymptomatic or mildly symptomatic patients with obstruction, since the risk of operation is not trivial (operative mortality of 5 to 10%), the course of the disease in such patients is not well defined, and no evidence exists indicating that prophylactic relief of obstruction will prolong survival. A number of operative procedures have been proposed, but the most successful has been the transaortic ventricular septal myotomy-myectomy (Morrow procedure) (Fig. 48.19).[82] Results from several medical centers utilizing this operation over the past 20 years have been excellent, i.e., the vast majority of patients have shown symptomatic and hemodynamic benefit after operation (Fig. 48.20). Of the 240 patients operated on at the National Heart, Lung and Blood Institute, 70% experienced marked symptomatic benefit 1 to 20 years (average 5 years) after operation.[60] In addition, 98% of patients showed reduction or abolition of the outflow gradient under basal

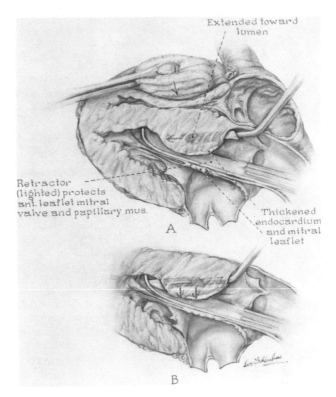

Fig. 48.19 Operation for obstructive hypertrophic cardiomyopathy (ventricular septal myotomy-myectomy). The first myotomy is made with an angled knife just to the right of the center of the right coronary leaflet. The blade is inserted into the septum in the long axis of the ventricle for a distance of about 4 cm. (*A*). The knife edge incises the septum with a sawing motion directed toward the ventricular lumen (*B*). Subsequently (but not shown here), a second vertical myotomy is made to the left of and parallel to the first myotomy. A transverse incision is then made connecting the myotomies at the base of the right coronary leaflet. The bar of muscle between the vertical myotomies is then detached from the septum.

conditions,[60] which was accompanied by reduction or abolition of systolic anterior motion of the anterior mitral leaflet[102]. Long-term postoperative follow-up studies have demonstrated that outflow obstruction at rest does not reoccur, although a mild to moderate gradient may often be elicited by provocative pharmacologic intervention.

Operation and relief of outflow obstruction do not entirely prevent progression of symptoms or fatal events or abolish atrial fibrillation.[60] Nine percent of patients have had persistent or recurrent severe functional limitation postoperatively, and 7% died late after operation of causes related to hypertrophic cardiomyopathy. Late postoperative deaths are either sudden (presumably related to a ventricular dysrhythmia) or due to chronic heart failure. Hence, the underlying cardiomyopathic process inherent in all patients with hypertrophic cardiomyopathy is one of the critical factors in determining prognosis.

Since left ventricular outflow obstruction in this condition results from abnormal forward motion of the anterior mitral leaflet during systole, excision and prosthetic replacement of the mitral valve have been recommended as an operative procedure.[18] While mitral valve replacement appears to abolish the outflow gradient, it nevertheless conveys all the potential complications related to placement of a prosthesis within a small left ventricular cavity. Therefore, mitral valve

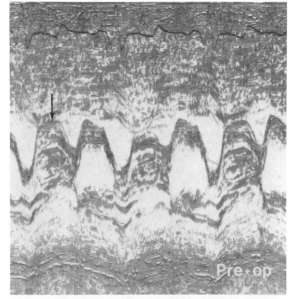

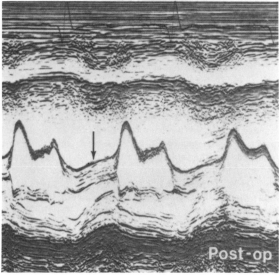

Fig. 48.20 M-mode echocardiograms recorded before and after ventricular septal myotomy-myectomy in a 12-year-old with obstructive hypertrophic cardiomyopathy demonstrating abolition of left ventricular outflow tract obstruction by operation. The preoperative echocardiogram (*above*) shows marked systolic anterior motion of the anterior mitral leaflet and prolonged contact between the anterior leaflet and ventricular septum (*arrow*) which was responsible for marked left ventricular outflow tract obstruction. Echocardiogram obtained 5 years after operation (*below*) shows loss of systolic anterior motion (*arrow*); at this time the patient had no left ventricular outflow gradient at rest.

replacement would not seem to be indicated in patients with hypertrophic cardiomyopathy.

The right ventricular outflow gradient often present in infants may be relieved by operative resection of hypertrophied muscle in the outflow tract. However, it is unclear at this time whether such a procedure is necessary in the first few years of life.

ENDOCARDIAL FIBROELASTOSIS

Focal thickening of the mural endocardium or cardiac valves is commonly present in a wide variety of heart dis-

eases. However, particularly marked and diffuse thickening of the endocardium is often observed in infants and children with signs and symptoms of cardiovascular disease.

Endocardial fibroelastosis (EFE) has been classified into two types: a primary form which produces a distinct clinical syndrome in infancy characterized by cardiac enlargement, heart failure, and absence of significant cardiac murmur; and a secondary form in which diffuse endocardial thickening presumably results from increased wall stress in a heterogeneous group of congenital cardiac malformations producing left ventricular overload. This secondary form of EFE occurs in AS, CA, discrete or tunnel subaortic stenosis, MI or MS, aberrant origin of the left coronary artery from the pulmonary artery, PDA, and in the diminutive left ventricle associated with aortic valve atresia.

The remainder of this discussion will deal with the primary type of EFE, which involves the left ventricle in the absence of other major cardiac malformations. Primary EFE has been subdivided into the more common type associated with left ventricular dilatation and a rare "contracted type" which occurs in about 5% of patients with EFE.

Patients with primary EFE have been noted previously to comprise about 2 to 4% of all cases of congenital heart disease and occur once in about 5000 live births.[80] EFE has been described as the most common cause of heart failure and death in children with heart disease between the ages of 2 months and 1 year. However, an apparent decline in the occurrence of EFE has been noted in the United States in recent years. There are no consistent regional or seasonal influences on the prevalence of EFE. The disease also occurs equally in either sex, and there does not appear to be a selective racial distribution.

ETIOLOGY

Although an etiology for EFE has never been definitively substantiated, a number of mechanisms have been proposed for the pathogenesis of this disease,[7, 49, 99] including: viral infection; congenital developmental defect of endocardium; subendocardial hypoxia; genetic and impaired lymphatic drainage of the heart.

Perhaps the postulate for which the most circumstantial evidence has been accumulated is that which suggests that primary EFE may be of viral etiology and may be a sequel to interstitial myocarditis.[30, 47] This evidence is based on: (1) clinical and electrocardiographic findings in EFE, which are often indistinguishable from those of chronic myocarditis; (2) frequent postmortem histologic findings of myocarditis or myocardial fibrosis in patients with EFE and characterization of the histologic evolution from interstitial myocarditis to EFE; (3) a spontaneous animal model, "round heart disease" in turkeys, has many of the clinical and pathological features of primary EFE in patients; surviving birds show the transition of myocarditis to EFE, and virus particles have been detected in the avian hearts with electron microscopy; (4) certain epidemiologic data which correlate the occurrence of EFE with Coxsackie B epidemics and increased frequency of deaths due to EFE following such epidemics of viral disease; (5) isolation of Coxsackie B virus from myocardial tissue in some infants with EFE; (6) the known high susceptibility of embryonic heart tissue to several viruses such as Coxsackie B, mumps, and other paramyxoviruses; and (7) experimental production of EFE in animals by inoculation with various viruses.

The mechanism by which myocarditis may serve as a precursor for primary EFE is not known, although it has been proposed that diffuse interstitial myocarditis produces marked ventricular dilatation.[47] Continuation of the myocarditis and development of relative MI due to left ventricular dilatation increases the functional burden on the ventricle. After the myocarditis has largely subsided, marked dilatation persists, resulting in increased ventricular wall tension and thereby stimulating the process of endocardial thickening.

A relationship between mumps virus and primary EFE was suggested by the discovery of positive skin reactions to inactivated mumps viral antigen among infants with this disease.[106] However, the lack of serologically detectable antibody to mumps virus in such cases, the failure of some investigators to find positive skin tests in known instances of the disease, and the absence of EFE in infants born to mothers suffering from mumps during pregnancy make any etiological relationship dubious.[32]

The majority of cases of endocardial fibroelastosis occur sporadically. However, in a minority of families, the multiple occurrences of endocardial fibroelastosis suggests that this abnormality occasionally may be genetically transmitted. In one epidemiologic analysis of 119 pedigrees of children with EFE,[15] an affected sibling with this disease was identified in 9% of the families. In contrast to other types of congenital heart disease, in which affected siblings show concordance as well as discordance, in families with EFE the lesion was completely concordant (i.e., there were no other forms of congenital heart disease). No single pattern of inheritance appears to apply to such familial occurrences of EFE, although x-linked recessive, autosomal dominant with incomplete penetrance, and autosomal recessive have been reported.[116]

PATHOLOGY

In the common dilated variety, the heart is usually markedly increased in size, attaining about two to four times its normal weight due primarily to enlargement of the left ventricle and left atrium. In most cases, the heart has a globular shape. The left ventricle is greatly dilated, but the left ventricular wall is normal or near normal in thickness. The right ventricle becomes displaced to the right and anteriorly, and its cavity is usually flattened. The pulmonary artery may be moderately enlarged. The aorta and coronary vessels appear grossly normal.

The endocardium of the left ventricle has an opaque, glistening, "milky-white" appearance that is reminiscent of porcelain and may be more obvious in the fixed than in the fresh state (Figs. 48.21 and 48.22). The endocardial thickening is diffuse, although it is most prominent in the left ventricular outflow tract. The thickness of the endocardium ranges from less than a millimeter to several millimeters (Fig. 48.21). The trabeculae carnae are flattened, adding to the smooth appearance of the lining of the left ventricular cavity. The chordae tendinae are shortened and thickened, and the mitral leaflets appear smaller than normal. The papillary muscles are partially incorporated in the fibrotic process so that they are flattened at their bases and hypoplastic.

The left ventricle is primarily affected, although cavity dilatation and endocardial thickening may be found in the left atrium of two-thirds of the patients. Less frequently, and usually terminally, the right ventricle and right atrium become involved. Occasionally, the disease may preferentially involve the left atrium,[6] even the right ventricle. The extent of chamber dilatation increases with age, as does the degree of endocardial thickening. In approximately 50% of cases, there is involvement of the mitral and aortic valves (most commonly the mitral), although the pulmonary and tricuspid valves are rarely affected. In those patients in whom exten-

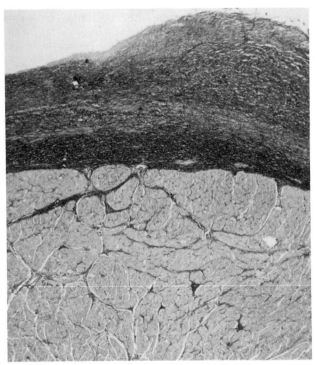

Fig. 48.21 Section of the left ventricle from an infant with primary endocardial fibroelastosis. Endocardium is markedly thickened, and the adjacent myocardium is uninvolved. Courtesy of Dr. William C. Roberts, Pathology Section, National Heart, Lung, and Blood Institute.

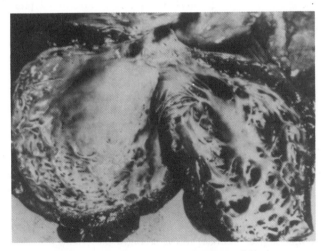

Fig. 48.22 Typical appearance of the left ventricle at necropsy in an infant with primary endocardial fibroelastosis. The left ventricular cavity is dilated; the thickened endocardium presents a smooth "milky-white" appearance.

sive aortic or mitral valvular involvement occurs, the valves may be markedly deformed, producing valvular incompetence or stenosis.

Histologically, the pathologic abnormalities are confined primarily to the endocardium. There is a marked hyperplasia of the constituents of the endocardium, particularly collagenous elastic fibers. Hence, the basic abnormality in EFE appears to be the synthesis of abnormally large amounts of elastic and collagenous fibers, rather than a qualitative change in the structure of the elastic fibers.[26] However, the average size of elastic fibers in the thickened endocardium appears to be larger in primary EFE than in the secondary variety present in patients with other cardiac malformations.[26] Surface deposits of fibrin have been detected by electron microscopy by some investigators. The underlying myocardium generally appears normal, although vacuolization of muscle fibers may occur in the subendocardium as well as in the papillary muscles and trabeculae carnae associated with foci of fibrosis and calcification. Analysis of tissue obtained by transvascular endomyocardial biopsy has been proposed as a method of identifying EFE during life,[31] but as yet has not gained widespread acceptance.

MANIFESTATIONS

Clinical Features

Neither the clinical nor hemodynamic findings of EFE are pathognomonic for this disease and, hence, a certain diagnosis can only be made at necropsy. However, based on available clinicopathologic information, the disease is typically manifested by cardiac decompensation of relatively rapid onset in a previously healthy infant.[40, 52, 100] Symptoms initially occur in the first year of life in about 80% of patients and in the first 3 months in one-third of patients. Infants exhibit classical findings of left heart failure manifested by tachypnea or fatigue with feedings, grunting respirations with subcostal and intercostal retractions, and sometimes fine expiratory wheezes or fine rales in the lung bases. Pallor, increased perspiration, or peripheral cyanosis may be observed. Fever, leukocytosis, anemia, and skin rash may also be present at the time of admission to the hospital. About one-fifth of the cases have a history of frequent or recent respiratory tract infections. In older children, dyspnea on exertion, orthopnea, chest discomfort or abdominal pain, persistent and dry cough, irritability, lethargy, anorexia, vomiting, and, sometimes, diarrhea occur. In rare cases, the onset of heart failure is so acute as to produce cardiogenic shock or even sudden death. Thrombi, which have formed and become adherent to the wall of the dilated left ventricle or other cardiac chambers, may embolize to the lungs, coronary arteries, or cerebral arteries and may result in death. Primary EFE has also been reported occasionally in adolescents and adults,[5] including one patient who lived until 46 years of age. When the disease occurs in this age group, it appears to be similar morphologically to that which is seen in infants and young children.

On physical examination, the heart is enlarged with the apical impulse displaced to the anterior or midaxillary line in the 5th or 6th left interspace. Tachycardia is present; the first and second heart sounds are usually normal but may be muffled. In older patients with pulmonary hypertension, the pulmonary component of the second heart sound is accentuated. A loud third heart sound is an almost constant finding during cardiac failure and produces a gallop rhythm. Cardiac murmurs are usually absent, but there may be a soft systolic murmur along the left sternal border in about 40% of patients. An apical systolic murmur reflecting MI may appear later in over one-half the patients.[81] Diastolic murmurs are rare. The blood pressure is either normal or low. With the onset of heart failure, the liver and spleen enlarge.

Peripheral edema, pleural effusion, and pericardial effusion are rare, although in older children, evidence of increased venous pressure may cause distention of the jugular veins. The peripheral pulses are usually normal, except in patients with a very acute course in which these pulses may be weak or imperceptible. Growth retardation is pronounced in patients with a prolonged clinical course. In about one-third of those patients who die, body weight is below the 3rd percentile.

The clinical course of patients with EFE is variable.[40, 41, 52] Perhaps most commonly the disease is characterized by acute onset of cardiac failure, which is then relentlessly progressive and terminates in death within weeks, usually between 2 and 6 months of age. Vigorous anticongestive therapy with digitalis and diuretic agents may meet with some initial response and remission of cardiac failure, but the downhill course is resumed shortly thereafter.

A more chronic course is commonly observed in patients who survive for periods of a few months up to several years.[40, 41, 52] In such patients a good response to treatment is initially obtained, with disappearance of symptoms and signs of cardiac failure. Subsequently, a variable cyclical clinical course occurs with recurrences of heart failure related to cessation or inadequate dosage of digitalis, to respiratory or other intercurrent infection, or to progression of the disease; remissions may be obtained during periods of hospitalization with intensification of medical therapy. Eventually, a stage of chronic cardiac failure is established and continues until a terminal episode intervenes.

Electrocardiographic Features

After the newborn period, the electrocardiogram shows left ventricular hypertrophy in 70 to 95% of cases.[114] Tall R waves are most often present in the left precordial leads, frequently in association with deep Q waves and marked inversion or flattening of T waves in those leads. Tall R waves may also occur in leads I, II, and AVF with inverted or flattened T waves in one or more of these leads. The QRS axis is usually normal. Combined ventricular hypertrophy may develop in patients with relatively long survival as the effects of pulmonary hypertension and right ventricular enlargement are added to the preexisting left ventricular overload. Right ventricular hypertrophy with tall R waves in the right precordial leads and right axis deviation are sometimes evident in the first few weeks of life with acute cardiac failure, particularly in newborns with the "contracted" form.

Patterns of left, right, or combined atrial enlargement are common, occurring in 35 to 60% of cases. Conduction or rhythm abnormalities occur in 20% of patients, including Wolff-Parkinson-White syndrome, left bundle branch block, and complete heart block, as well as a variety of supraventricular and ventricular dysrhythmias; atrial flutter or fibrillation are observed primarily in chronic cases with an enlarged left atrium.

Radiologic Features

Cardiac enlargement is present in 95% of patients and is usually marked; the cardiothoracic ratio is greater than 0.65 in 50% of patients (Fig. 48.23). In some patients cardiac enlargement is present since birth; in others, heart size is normal in the first few weeks or months of life, and cardiac enlargement develops subsequently.

The shape of the heart is variable, although there are two common contours: with the left border of the heart extending laterally and downward, indicative of predominant left ventricular enlargement, and globular shape with round right and left heart borders, indicative of marked dilatation of all cardiac chambers.

Echocardiographic Features

The echocardiogram shows normal or slightly increased ventricular septal and posterior left ventricular free wall thicknesses. The left ventricular end-diastolic and end-systolic transverse dimensions are increased. Left ventricular transverse dimension changes little between systole and diastole and, hence, the ejection fraction and percent fractional shortening are diminished.[33] Left atrial size is also

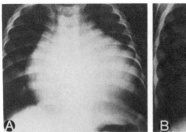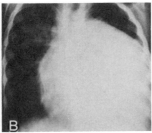

Fig. 48.23 Chest x-ray obtained in the frontal view from two patients with primary endocardial fibroelastosis. (*A*) Typical enlarged globular heart. (*b*) Massive cardiomegaly in terminally ill infant.

increased. The thickened endocardium is usually not identifiable on the echocardiogram. When the clinical condition improves after therapy with digitalis and diuretic agents, echocardiograms may show an increase in percent shortening fraction, and velocity of fiber shortening, and a decrease in left ventricular and left atrial dimension.[33]

CARDIAC CATHETERIZATION

Hemodynamic findings in infants with EFE include variable degrees of elevation in left ventricular end-diastolic pressure, as well as left atrial and pulmonary arterial wedge pressures.[56, 77] Pulmonary hypertension occurs in about one-fourth of the patients but only rarely is the systolic pulmonary arterial pressure more than one-half the value of systemic pressure. Marked pulmonary hypertension is usually present in older children with this condition. Arteriovenous oxygen difference is wide. Cardiac output and left ventricular stroke volume are usually normal,[77] despite the relatively poor left ventricular contractility evidenced by angiocardiography.

ANGIOCARDIOGRAPHY

The angiocardiographic findings, although not specific, may be very suggestive of EFE. Prominent features consist of marked dilatation of the left ventricular cavity with relatively mild thickening of the venticular wall. The left ventricular chamber has a globular or spherical shape. Left ventricular end-diastolic and end-systolic volumes are greatly increased, and there is little change in left ventricular chamber size from diastole to systole, resulting in a low ejection fraction (Fig. 48.24).[79] Left ventricular contraction may have a dyskinetic or akinetic pattern in rare cases. The left atrium is frequently enlarged, and its contractions are often vigorous by comparison with the left ventricle. If MI exists, contrast medium is observed in the left atrium with selective left ventricular angiography.[77] The right ventricle is usually normal in size but may be enlarged in more severely affected cases.

PROGNOSIS

Definitive information regarding the prognosis of children with isolated EFE is difficult to obtain because in clinically studied living populations of patients suspected of having EFE, there usually is no anatomic documentation of the disease. However, even when these limitations are taken into account, prognosis appears poor, although not so universally fatal as it was once thought to be.[40, 41, 52] It has been estimated that when proper treatment is instituted, approximately one-

third of patients diagnosed clinically as having EFE die of progressive heart failure, one-third survive but experience persistent symptoms or show residual electrocardiographic abnormalities and radiographic evidence of cardiac enlargement, and the remaining one-third exhibit complete recovery.[40, 41] On the other hand, some clinicians doubt that the anatomic or functional abnormalities of EFE are reversible and maintain that those patients thought to have EFE clinically who made an apparently complete recovery actually had other forms of endomyocardial disease.[84]

Those factors which appear to favorably influence the prognosis of children with EFE are[41, 57]: early recognition and institution of medical care and prompt and prolonged administration of digitalis therapy for a minimum period of 2 years, resulting in clinical improvement and reversion of the electrocardiogram and chest x-ray to normal.

Poor prognostic signs include presentation with heart failure in the newborn period, and recurrence of episodes of heart failure despite adequate treatment, particularly if these episodes occur more than 6 months after the initial onset of symptoms.[41, 57] Only about 10% of patients with three or more episodes of cardiac decompensation recover completely while about one-half with only a single episode of heart failure recover completely. In addition, it is rare to encounter a patient with EFE presenting in the newborn period who survives the first month of life.

DIFFERENTIAL DIAGNOSIS

Clinical differentiation between primary EFE and *myocarditis* in infants and young children may be particularly difficult. In patients with EFE, the electrocardiogram shows left ventricular hypertrophy or tall QRS voltages in about 90% of patients. Conversely, the electrocardiogram in myocarditis shows a pattern consistent with left ventricular hypertrophy in only about 10% of cases and usually demonstrates QRS voltages that are decreased in magnitude.

Cases of myocarditis with a subacute or chronic course are particularly difficult to distinguish from isolated EFE. Substantial evidence suggests the existence of a viral and, perhaps, a common etiology for EFE and myocarditis; hence, myocarditis and EFE may not be two distinct clinical entities, but rather different stages of the same disease. The echocardiogram has not proven useful in differentiating my- differentiating myocarditis and EFE.

Anomalous origin of the left coronary artery from the pulmonary trunk also may produce marked left heart failure.

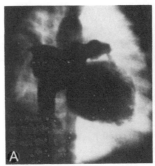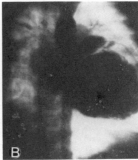

Fig. 48.24 Left ventricular angiocardiogram obtained in the frontal view during systole (*A*) and diastole (*B*) from a patient with primary endocardial fibroelastosis. The left ventricle is markedly dilated and has a globular appearance. There is little volume change from systole to diastole.

However, this disease generally has electrocardiographic signs of anterolateral myocardial infarction. Angiocardiography is diagnostic, since injection of contrast material into the aorta will demonstrate absence of the origin of the left coronary artery from the aorta and its filling retrograde via a tortuous right coronary artery. Of note, some patients with anomalous origin of the coronary artery may show secondary EFE with MI.

Glycogen-storage disease of the heart is a uniformly fatal disease of infancy in which death usually occurs during the first 8 months of life due to progressive heart failure. The electrocardiogram may show left ventricular hypertrophy with "strain." However, the majority of these children have generalized muscular weakness and macroglossia which distinguishes them from patients with EFE. A biopsy of involved muscle will confirm the diagnosis.

Hypertrophic cardiomyopathy in infants may be incorrectly diagnosed as EFE because of the presence of cardiac enlargement and heart failure. When obstruction to outflow is not present in infants with hypertrophic cardiomyopathy, a loud murmur will not be present, adding to the difficulty in making the clinical distinction between EFE and hypertrophic cardiomyopathy. However, almost without exception, echocardiography will resolve this diagnostic dilemma by demonstrating the marked (usually asymmetric) left ventricular hypertrophy and nondilated left ventricular cavity characteristic of hypertrophic cardiomyopathy. In addition, angiographic and echocardiographic studies will show normal or hypercontractile left ventricular systolic function in hypertrophic cardiomyopathy, in contrast to the impairment of ventricular function that is characteristic of EFE.

It is difficult to distinguish clinically those relatively rare instances of *idiopathic congestive (dilated) cardiomyopathy* occurring in infancy from EFE; definitive confirmation of the diagnosis may be obtained only at necropsy.

Calcification of the coronary arteries in infancy is part of a widespread disease process involving calcification of the arteries throughout the body. This disease is uniformly fatal and does not respond to digitalis therapy. In the majority of instances, these infants die because of the general arterial involvement, rather than because of a specific effect on the heart. Heart failure may occur and produce findings similar to that found in EFE. Radiographic studies of various organs may reveal calcification of arteries and lead to the correct diagnosis.

TREATMENT

Optimal treatment of primary EFE is early, adequate, and prolonged therapy with digitalis.[41, 57] There is no general agreement as to the length of time digitalis should be administered. It has been recommended that digitalis be continued for a minimum of 2 to 3 years and then be gradually discontinued, but only if symptoms are absent, heart size is normal, and the ECG has reverted to normal. Premature withdrawal of digitalis, or its administration in inadequate dosage, often leads to the reappearance of symptoms and cardiac failure.

Diuretic agents have been useful in the treatment of severe heart failure. It is rarely necessary to limit sodium intake in infants. In the acute stage of heart failure, oxygen is often necessary to treat hypoxemia secondary to pulmonary edema. Morphine may be useful in treating pulmonary edema and extreme anxiety. Intercurrent infections must be treated promptly with appropriate antibiotics; respiratory infections are especially prone to precipitate or complicate episodes of cardiac failure.

Operative treatments such as pericardial poudrage and mitral valve replacement have been attempted but often lack therapeutic rationale, incur high mortality rates, and have not been particularly successful in altering the clinical course.[89] For these reasons, operative therapy for EFE has not gained general acceptance.

LEFT VENTRICULAR ENDOCARDIAL FIBROELASTOSIS OF THE CONTRACTED TYPE

In this very rare lesion, the left ventricle may be small or normal in size. The left ventricular cavity is lined by a diffusely thickened endocardium, but the left ventricular wall is distinctly thicker than in the dilated type of EFE. The right ventricle is markedly dilated and hypertrophied. Both left and right atria are also greatly dilated, and the mitral orifice is small.

EFE is often of the contracted type in the newborn infant, a period in life during which death is uncommon from the dilated form of EFE. Signs and symptoms simulate those of mitral stenosis with severe pulmonary venous and arterial hypertension and chronic right-sided heart failure. Cardiac decompensation occurs early in life and is progressive. Marked cardiomegaly on chest x-ray, generalized edema, and hepatomegaly are often prominent. There is usually a precordial bulge and a marked ventricular heave at the lower left sternal border. No significant murmurs are heard. The second heart sound is normally or narrowly split and has a loud pulmonic component. Third and fourth heart sounds may be heard. The electrocardiogram usually shows right ventricular hypertrophy with ST segment and T wave changes in the precordial leads and left atrial or combined atrial enlargement.[111]

Hemodynamics resemble left ventricular "inflow" obstruction with impaired left ventricular filling. Left atrial pressure is high, a diastolic gradient is present across the mitral valve, and pulmonary arterial pressure is at systemic level. The contracted form of EFE may be differentiated from other forms of pulmonary venous obstruction by elevation of the left ventricular end-diastolic pressure and absence of a diastolic pressure gradient distal to the pulmonary veins.

Angiocardiography shows a normal or small left ventricle with a thickened wall. Left ventricular contractility is distinctly better than in the dilated type but may still be impaired. The end-systolic volume is increased, the left atrium is enlarged, and there may be some dilatation of the pulmonary arteries. The contracted form of EFE almost always occurs sporadically. Only occasionally has a familial predilection been reported.

IDIOPATHIC CONGESTIVE (DILATED) CARDIOMYOPATHY

Idiopathic congestive cardiomyopathy is a primary disease of the myocardium which does not result from valvular, hypertensive, pulmonary, infiltrative, or coronary artery disease. At necropsy, congestive cardiomyopathy is characterized by dilatation of both ventricular cavities, increased myocardial mass, and absence of inflammatory cells in the myocardial wall (Fig. 48.25).[68] Despite the increased heart weight, the maximal thickness of the left ventricular free wall and of the ventricular septum is usually not more than expected for age. Ventricular dilatation is associated with reduced ejection fraction and increased end-systolic volume (Fig. 48.26), as well as left atrial dilatation.[33] The size of the left ventricular cavity is probably proportional to the severity and duration of heart failure. These hearts may be distinguished from those with primary EFE by the absence of diffuse endocardial thickening, and from hypertrophic

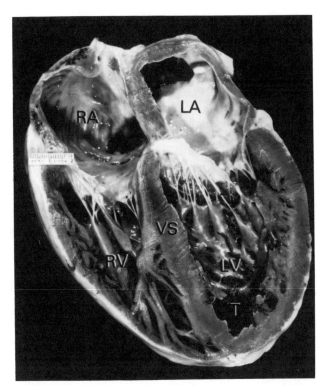

Fig. 48.25 Heart of an adolescent girl with idiopathic congestive cardiomyopathy. Heart weight of 540 gm is twice normal, and the ventricular cavities (particularly the left) are dilated. However, ventricular wall thicknesses are normal. Thrombus (*T*) is present at the apex of the left ventricle (*LV*). RA, right atrium; *RV*, right ventricle; *LA*, left atrium; *VS*, ventricular septum. (Courtesy of Dr. William C. Roberts, Pathology Section, National Heart, Lung and Blood Institute.)

dilatation of the tubules of the sarcoplasmic reticulum and the T system; myofibrillar damage; a variety of mitochondrial alterations; and the absence of viral particles. In general, the extent of the degenerative changes in myocardial cells correlates with the duration and severity of cardiac dysfunction, suggesting that the progression of degenerative changes in cardiac muscle may be responsible for the clinical deterioration and therapeutic unresponsiveness.

Patients with idiopathic congestive cardiomyopathy demonstrate marked enlargement of the cardiac silhouette on chest x-ray (Fig. 48.27) and physical signs of heart failure with hepatomegaly, evidence of pulmonary congestion, and a prominent third heart sound. These patients usually have no murmur or only a soft systolic ejection murmur along the left sternal border, although a murmur typical of MI may be present at the apex. Electrocardiogram usually shows nonspecific ST segment and T wave abnormalities, left and/or right atrial enlargement, or a pattern suggesting a healed anterior wall infarction (without evidence of anterior infarct at necropsy) (Fig. 48.28).

It should be emphasized that it is difficult to establish the clinical course and prognosis for patients with idiopathic congestive cardiomyopathy. Patients with this disease who improve and survive do not provide an anatomic basis for a definitive diagnosis, since it is often difficult to distinguish clinically the primary myocardial diseases of infancy and childhood associated with ventricular dilatation, i.e., myocarditis, endocardial fibroelastosis, and idiopathic congestive cardiomyopathy. Furthermore, most clinical studies of cardiomyopathy in children tend to group a number of primary endomyocardial disorders together for analysis, making it as

cardiomyopathy by the ventricular dilatation and lack of substantial ventricular wall thickening.

In congestive cardiomyopathy, increased end-systolic ventricular volume leads to relative stasis of blood in the apical portions of the ventricular cavities, and this often results in intracavitary thrombosis. About 75% of patients with congestive cardiomyopathy have left ventricular thrombi at necropsy.[68] Thrombi are also frequently present in one or both atrial appendages, presumably the consequence of poor atrial emptying and relative stasis of blood in the appendages. In addition, intracardiac thrombi may give rise to pulmonary and systemic emboli.

Left ventricular scarring is observed by gross inspection in less than 25% of the patients, and it is usually limited to the papillary muscles and subendocardium.[64, 68, 93] Thus, impaired myocardial contractility in patients with congestive cardiomyopathy cannot be explained on the basis of ventricular scarring alone. Valvular regurgitation appears to be due to papillary muscle dysfunction, since the tricuspid and mitral valvular annuli are usually only mildly dilated.

Histologic studies of the myocardial walls in patients with congestive cardiomyopathy disclose nonspecific changes. Many myocardial cells appear hypertrophied; others appear atrophied. The amount of fibrous tissue between myocardial cells usually is increased to a varying degree. Inflammatory cells are absent. The intramural coronary arteries are normal. Ultrastructural studies have demonstrated other nonspecific changes, including: intracellular edema, increased numbers of lipid droplets, lysosomes, and lipofuscin granules;

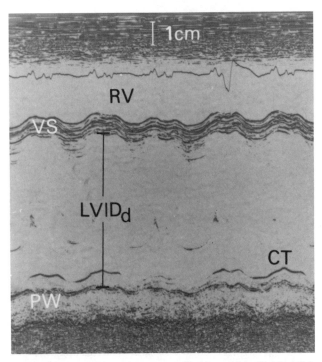

Fig. 48.26 Echocardiogram recorded in a child with idiopathic congestive cardiomyopathy. The left ventricular cavity is markedly dilated (transverse diastolic dimension of 64 mm); the posterior free wall (*PW*) thickens little in systole, and ejection fraction is greatly diminished. There is paradoxical ventricular septal motion. The ventricular septum (*VS*) and PW are of normal thickness. The right ventricular (*RV*) cavity is also mildly dilated. *LVID*d, left ventricular internal dimension in diastole; *CT*, chordae tendineae.

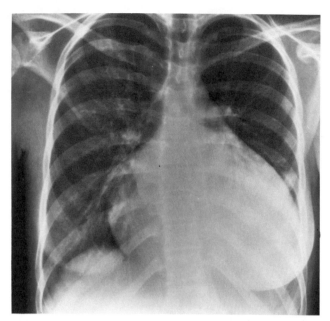

Fig. 48.27 Chest roentgenogram in a 15-year-old patient with idiopathic dilated cardiomyopathy showing marked enlargement of the cardiac silhouette.

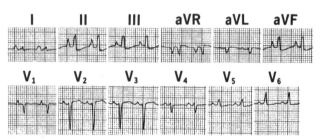

Fig. 48.28 Electrocardiogram recorded 1 day before death in a 15-year-old girl with idiopathic dilated (congestive) cardomyopathy showing sinus tachycardia, right atrial enlargement, and absent or small R waves in the right precordial leads suggesting anterior wall infarction. (At necropsy, the left ventricular wall was free of necrosis and fibrosis.)

difficult to assess the natural history of each clinical entity separately.

Nevertheless, it has been documented that idiopathic congestive cardiomyopathy may be present in infancy as an acute illness with a rapid course in the setting of severe progressive heart failure.[68] Since patients may die within a few days or weeks of the onset of their illness, a viral infection is usually suspected as the etiology. More commonly, the disease occurs in children and adolescents where the clinical course of nonsurvivors may be more prolonged, up to 5 years.

Treatment has traditionally consisted of aggressive administration of digitalis and diuretic agents. Symptomatic improvement is usually accompanied by an increase in ejection fraction as well as by reduced left ventricular diastolic dimension and left atrial size, as assessed by echocardiography. However, one or more indices of left ventricular function may remain abnormal despite resolution of symptoms and reduction in heart size on the chest x-ray.

The occurrence of congestive cardiomyopathy in infants and children is usually sporadic. However, in some families, the disease appears to be genetically transmitted.[4, 95]

HISTIOCYTOID CARDIOMYOPATHY OF INFANCY

A number of terms have been used to describe a cardiomypathy of infancy characterized by histiocytoid changes in the cardiac muscle cells, e.g., isolated cardiac lipidosis, lipid histiocytosis, focal myocardial degeneration, focal lipid cardiomyopathy, and oncocytic cardiomyopathy. This rare syndrome occurs in infants 6 months to 2 years of age and is manifested by intractable supraventricular or ventricular tachydysrhythmias which may occur as early as the second day of life and may eventually lead to death within days or up to 2 months.[24] An occasional patient may present with sudden death as the first manifestation of the disease. Pathologically, this disease is characterized by cardiac hypertrophy and a distinctive type of myocardial cell degeneration. Cardiac muscle cells are transformed into enlarged round cells with a foamy, granular cytoplasm which resembles histiocytes. The degenerated cells are distributed within multiple foci throughout the myocardium, including conducting tissue, and appear grossly as a yellow-white discoloration. Ultrastructurally, these cells demonstrate virtual absence of contractile elements and greatly increased numbers of mitochondria (Fig. 48.29).[24] In addition, small nodules containing cells similar in appearance are commonly present on or near the cardiac valves. The etiology of histiocytoid cardiomyopathy is unknown, but it has been suggested that the myocardial damage characteristic of this disease is produced by an intrauterine viral infection. Of note, some patients have been noted to have severe malformations of the eyes similar to those observed in the congenital rubella syndrome.[104]

CARDIOMYOPATHY IN INFANTS OF DIABETIC MOTHERS

Infants of diabetic mothers are large for gestational age, have generalized organomegaly, and are subject to hypogly-

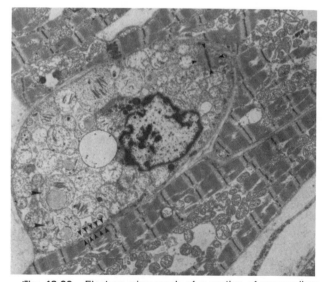

Fig. 48.29 Electron micrograph of a portion of myocardium from an infant with histiocytoid cardiomyopathy. Cardiac muscle cells with normal contractile elements surround a small histiocyte-like cell that contains only one fragment of a myofibril (*small arrowheads, upper right*) but is filled with closely packed mitochondria (*large arrowheads, lower left side*). A desmosome (*paired arrowheads, lower left*) still connects this cell to an adjacent muscle cell. ×9000. Courtesy of Dr. Victor J. Ferrans, Pathology Branch, National Heart, Lung, and Blood Institute.

cemia and hypocalcemia. Respiratory distress commonly occurs shortly after birth. Cardiac mass is increased in an estimated 15% of such infants and is due to hypertrophy of cardiac muscle cells, rather than to myocardial glycogen deposition, as initially thought.[37] While mild cardiac hypertrophy may be identified by echocardiography in asymptomatic infants of diabetic mothers, more substantial hypertrophy is present in symptomatic infants.

In particular, some infants of diabetic mothers show morphologic and functional[37, 115] abnormalities on echocardiographic study that resemble hypertrophic cardiomyopathy. These infants have marked asymmetric thickening of the ventricular septum relative to the left ventricular free wall. Systolic anterior motion of the anterior mitral leaflet (associated with left ventricular outflow obstruction) may be present. The left ventricular cavity is normal or decreased in size, and systolic function is normal or increased.

Infants of diabetic mothers may have large hearts on chest x-ray, regardless of whether cardiomyopathy is present. However, cardiac enlargement is almost always present in those symptomatic infants of diabetic mothers with asymmetric thickening of the ventricular septum. Electrocardiogram may show right, left, or combined ventricular hypertrophy.

Unlike hypertrophic cardiomyopathy, the cardiomyopathy of infants of diabetic mothers resolves during the first 6 months of life. Cardiorespiratory distress improves, outflow obstruction disappears, and septal thickening regresses for the most part.[37] In addition, echocardiographic studies of family members suggest that the cardiomyopathy is not genetically transmitted. Hence, although the cardiomyopathy of infants of diabetic mothers and "true" hypertrophic cardiomyopathy in infants have similar clinical and morphologic features, the transient and nonfamilial nature of the cardiomyopathy of infants of diabetic mothers suggests that it is a separate disease entity and is probably a manifestation of the generalized organomegaly present in these infants.

Recommended therapy consists of providing maintenance fluids intravenously, ventilatory assistance if needed, and correcting hypoglycemia and hypocalcemia.[37] Propranolol therapy may be helpful but usually is not necessary.

GLYCOGEN STORAGE DISEASE OF THE HEART

A deficiency of one or more of the enzymes involved in the biosynthesis and degradation of glycogen produces glycogen storage disease, of which at least eight types have been described. Most cases of glycogen storage disease producing cardiac involvement belong to Type II (Pompe's disease) caused by a deficiency of alpha-1,4-glucosidase, a lysosomal enzyme that hydrolyzes glycogen to glucose. The glycogen within the cardiac muscle cells is biochemically and morphologically normal but is present in excessive amounts both within lysosomes and free in the cytoplasm. Infants with glycogen storage disease characteristically demonstrate hypotonia, macroglossia, poor reflexes, and assume the "frog position." A weak cry, inability to nurse or suck, and choking are also prominent symptoms in the newborn period.

Cardiac mass is markedly increased, with heart weight 3 to 6 times normal.[20, 92] The left ventricular wall thickens considerably, and the left ventricular cavity is normal sized or small. The ventricular septum and left ventricular free wall may be thickened symmetrically (concentric left ventricular hypertrophy) or asymmetrically with either the septum or free wall thickest.[20, 92] Endocardial fibroelastosis of the left ventricle may also be present.

Ventricular outflow tract obstruction associated with a loud systolic murmur may occur and, hence, patients with glycogen storage disease of the heart may mimic clinically patients with obstructive hypertrophic cardiomyopathy. Obstruction may be subaortic and associated with systolic anterior motion of the mitral valve,[92] or may be combined subaortic and subpulmonic. Infusion of isoproterenol may produce a left ventricular outflow gradient, not present under basal conditions.

The electrocardiogram usually shows left ventricular hypertrophy (usually with "strain" pattern and Q waves in the lateral precordial leads), left axis deviation, and short PR interval. Chest x-ray demonstrates marked enlargement of the cardiac silhouette.

Patients with glycogen storage disease of the heart develop marked heart failure for which there is no effective therapy. Death usually occurs within the first 6 months of life, but survival for up to 3 years has been reported.

AMYLOIDOSIS

Amyloid involvement of the heart is not a common problem in childhood and is usually observed only in patients over the age of 21.[93] Amyloidosis may primarily involve the heart, although patients with cardiac amyloidoses often have other systemic diseases such as multiple myeloma. Pathologically, deposits of amyloid are present between cardiac muscle cells. Cardiac mass is increased, the ventricular walls are symmetrically thickened, and the ventricular cavities are nondilated. The myocardium is characteristically firm, rubbery, and noncompliant. Clinically, patients with amyloidosis show heart failure which is poorly responsive to digitalis. Of note, the electrocardiogram characteristically shows low voltages, as well as conduction disturbances, or a pattern simulating healed anterior myocardial infarction.

MYOCARDIAL IRON DEPOSITION

The deposition of iron within myocardial cells may produce cardiac dysfunction with congestive cardiomyopathy.[93] Significant myocardial iron deposition may be observed occasionally in children with primary hemosiderosis, but iron overload is more commonly evident in patients with chronic anemia (usually beta-thalassemia), requiring multiple blood transfusions. Iron deposition most often involves the ventricles and less commonly the atria and conducting system. Electrocardiographic abnormalities usually include conduction abnormalities and dysrhythmias.

Early in the course of their disease, these patients show by echocardiography symmetrically increased left ventricular wall thicknesses (concentric left ventricular hypertrophy) in the presence of normal-sized ventricular cavities and normal systolic function (i.e., ejection fraction).[46] Subsequently, when myocardial iron overload is severe, such patients may demonstrate marked left ventricular dilatation, left atrial enlargement, and decreased ejection fraction, thereby resembling patients with congestive cardiomyopathy.

HYPEREOSINOPHILIC SYNDROME

A form of endomyocardial disease has been described as part of a distinct syndrome characterized by blood eosinophilia without identifiable cause (i.e., exclusive of parasitic, allergic, or autoimmune disease). This disease, known as hypereosinophilic syndrome, is characterized by bone marrow eosinophilia, as well as by tissue infiltration by eosinophils. Almost any organ may be affected, but the heart is most commonly involved. Because of its wide clinical spectrum, with involvement of many organs, hypereosinophilic syndrome has been given many names which indicate a particular characteristic of the disease process (e.g., eosinophilic leukemia, idiopathic eosinophilia, Löffler's fibroplastic endocarditis, disseminated eosinophilic collagen vascular disease, and endomyocardial disease with eosinophilia). This disease also appears to be related morphologically to a form of endomyocardial fibrosis described in parts of Africa which apparently is not associated with eosinophilia but does occur in children.

In hypereosinophilic syndrome, the heart shows symmetric left ventricular wall thickening and nondilated ventricular cavities.[93] While systolic function is normal, there is some evidence to suggest the presence of a restrictive cardiomyopathy involving impairment to left ventricular filling. Mural thrombi not uncommonly form in the ventricular cavities and may be the source of emboli and subsequent cerebrovascular accident.

In addition, a distinctive abnormality of the mitral valve may lead to major MI. This mitral valve alteration is characterized by scarring of the posterior mitral leaflet, such that it becomes adhered to the posterobasal left ventricular wall, immobile and regurgitant. The origin of this scarring process is not definitively known, although it may emanate from organization of mural thrombus located in that region of the left ventricle.

Hypereosinophilic syndrome is a serious disorder that often demonstrates a progressive course associated with high morbidity and mortality. It usually occurs in adulthood but has occasionally been observed in adolescents. Therapy has been reserved for patients with major, progressive organ system involvement and dysfunction. Recently, patients treated with corticosteroids and/or hydroxyurea have shown improved survival (only 4% mortality, 3 years after the onset of their disease.)[88] A few patients with severe MI have undergone mitral valve replacement.

ACROMEGALY

Some patients with acromegaly show evidence of myocardial disease, even in the absence of systemic hypertension, coronary artery disease, valvular heart disease, or diabetes. This entity, which has been termed "acromegalic cardiomyopathy," usually occurs in adults but occasionally is the cause of morbidity and mortality in adolescents.[74] Echocardiographic and necropsy studies have shown that the structural abnormality in this disease is a symmetrically thickened left ventricular wall associated with a nondilated ventricular cavity.[97] The wall thickening and increased heart weight are, however, not massive.[55] Heart weight is seldom as much as twice the expected weight relative to body size, and increased cardiac weight disproportionate to that of the liver, spleen, and kidneys is uncommon. Clinically, the condition is manifested by electrocardiographic abnormalities (usually dysrhythmias and conduction abnormalities) and heart failure that often responds poorly to treatment with digitalis and diuretics. The progression of the cardiomyopathy does not correlate well with plasma growth hormone concentration. Therefore, there is little evidence at this time to implicate growth hormone as the cause of "acromegalic cardiomyopathy."

The prevalence of cardiomyopathy in the acromegalic population is not known because many patients in the various published reports were referred for evaluation *because of* evidence of cardiac disease. Hence, most studies probably overestimate the occurrence of cardiomyopathy in a hospital-based population of patients with acromegaly.

REFERENCES

1. Abbasi, A. S., MacAlpin, R. N., Eber, L. M., and Pearce, M. L.: Echocardiographic diagnosis of idiopathic hypertrophic cardiomyopathy without outflow obstruction. Circulation 46:897, 1972.
2. Adelman, A. G., Shah, P. M., Gramiak, R., and Wigle, E. D.: Long-term propranolol therapy in muscular subaortic stenosis. Br. Heart J. 32:804, 1970.
3. Adelman, A. G., Wigle, E. D., Ranganathan, N., Webb, G. D., Kidd, B. S. L., Bigelow, W. G., and Silver, M. D.: The clinical course in muscular subaortic stenosis. A retrospective and prospective study of 60 hemodynamically proved cases. Ann. Intern. Med. 77:515, 1972.
4. Anselmi, A., Suarez, J. A., Anselmi, G., Moleiro, F., de Suarez, C., and Ruesta, V.: Primary cardiomyopathy in identical twins. Am. J. Cardiol. 35:97, 1975.
5. Auld, W. H. R., and Watson, H.: Fibro-elastosis of the heart in adolescence. Br. Heart J. 19:186, 1957.
6. Björkhem, G., Lundström, N.-R., Wallentin, I., and Carlgren, L.-E.: Endocardial fibroelastosis with predominant involvement of left atrium. Possibility of diagnosis by non-invasive methods. Br. Heart J. 46:331, 1981.
7. Black-Schaffer, B.: Infantile endocardial fibroelastosis. A suggested etiology. Arch. Pathol. 63:281, 1957.
8. Bonow, R. O., Rosing, D. R., Bacharach, S. L., Green, M. V., Kent, K. M., Lipson, L. C., Maron, B. J., Leon, M. B., and Epstein, S. E.: Effects of verapamil on left ventricular systolic function and diastolic filling in patients with hypertrophic cardiomyopathy. Assessment with radionuclide cineangiography. Circulation 64:787, 1981.
9. Borer, J. S., Henry, W. L., and Epstein, S. E.: Echocardiographic observations in patients with systemic infiltrative disease involving the heart. Am. J. Cardiol. 39:184, 1977.
10. Boughner, D. R., Shuid, R. L., and Persaud, D. A.: Hypertrophic obstructive cardiomyopathy: Assessment by echocardiographic and Doppler ultrasound techniques. Br. Heart J. 37:917, 1975.
11. Braunwald, E., Lambrew, C. T., Rockoff, S. D., Ross, J., Jr., and Morrow, A. G.: Idiopathic hypertrophic subaortic stenosis. I. A description of the disease based upon an analysis of 64 patients. Circulation 30 (Suppl. IV):3, 1964.
12. Canedo, M. I., Frank, M. J., and Abdulla, A. M.: Rhythm disturbances in hypertrophic cardiomyopathy: Prevalence, relation to symptoms and management. Am. J. Cardiol. 45:848, 1980.
13. Carter, W. H., Whalen, R. E., and McIntosh, H. D.: Reversal of hemodynamic and phonocardiographic abnormalities in idiopathic hypertrophic subaortic stenosis. Am. J. Cardiol. 28:722, 1971.
14. Chahine, R. A., Raizner, A. E., Ishimori, T., and Montero, A. C.: Echocardiographic, haemodynamic and angiographic correlations in hypertrophic cardiomyopathy. Br. Heart J. 39:945, 1977.
15. Chen, S., Thompson, M. W., and Rose, V.: Endocardial fibroelastosis: Family studies with special reference to counseling. J. Pediatr. 79:385, 1971.
16. Clark, C. E., Henry, W. L., and Epstein, S. E.: Familial prevalence and genetic transmission of idiopathic hypertrophic subaortic stenosis. N. Engl. J. Med. 289:709, 1973.
17. Cohen, M. V., Cooperman, L. B., and Rosenblum, R.: Regional myocardial function in idiopathic hypertrophic subaortic stenosis. Circulation 52:842, 1975.
18. Cooley, D. A., Leachman, R. D., and Wukasch, D. C.: Diffuse muscular subaortic stenosis: Surgical treatment. Am. J. Card. 31:1, 1973.
19. Doi, V. L., McKenna, W. J., Gehrke, J., Oakley, C. M., and Goodwin, J. F.: M-mode echocardiography in hypertrophic cardiomyopathy: Diagnostic criteria and prediction of obstruction. Am. J. Cardiol. 45:6, 1980.
20. Ehlers, K. H., Hagstron, J. W. C., Lukas, D. S., Redo, S. F., and Engle, M. A.: Glycogen-storage disease of the myocardium with obstruction to left ventricular outflow. Circulation 25:96, 1962.
21. Ehlers, K. H., Engle, M. A., Levin, A. R., and Deely, W. J.: Eccentric ventricular hypertrophy in familial and sporadic instances of 46XX, XY Turner phenotype. Circulation 45:639, 1972.
22. Falicov, R. E., and Resnekov, L.: Mid ventricular obstruction in hypertrophic obstructive cardiomyopathy. Br. Heart J. 39:701,

1977.

23. Ferrans, V. J., Morrow, A. G., and Roberts, W. C.: Myocardial ultrastructure in idiopathic hypertrophic subaortic stenosis. A study of operatively excised left ventricular outflow tract muscle in 14 patients. Circulation 45:769, 1972.

24. Ferrans, V. J., McAllister, H. A., Jr., and Haese, W. H.: Infantile cardiomyopathy with histiocytoid change in cardiac muscle cells. Report of six patients. Circulation 53:708, 1976.

25. Fiddler, G. L., Tajik, A. J., Weidman, W. H., McGoon, D. C., Ritter, D. G., and Giuliani, E. R.: Idiopathic hypertrophic subaortic stenosis in the young. Am. J. Cardiol. 42:793, 1978.

26. Fishbein, M. C., Ferrans, V. J., and Roberts, W. C.: Histologic and ultrastructural features of primary and secondary endocardial fibroelastosis. Arch. Pathol. Lab. Med. 101:49, 1977.

27. Frank, M. J., Abdulla, A. M., Canedo, M. I., and Saylors, R. E.: Long-term medical management of hypertrophic obstructive cardiomyopathy. Am. J. Cardiol. 42:993, 1978.

28. Frank, S., and Braunwald, E.: Idiopathic hypertrophic subaortic stenosis. Clinical analysis of 126 patients with emphasis on the natural history. Circulation 37:759, 1968.

29. Freed, M. D., Rosenthal, A., Plauth, W. H., Jr., and Nadas, A. S.: Development of subaortic stenosis after pulmonary artery banding. Circulation 47-48 (Suppl. III):7, 1973.

30. Fruhling, L., Korn, R., Lavillaureix, J., Surjus, A., and Foussereau, S.: La myo-endocardite chronique fibroélastique du nouveau-né et du nourrisson fibro-elastose. Ann. Anat. Pathol. 7:227, 1962.

31. Fujita, M., Neustein, H. B., and Lurie, P. R.: Transvascular endomyocardial biopsy in infants and small children. Myocardial findings in 10 cases of cardiomyopathy. Hum. Pathol. 10:15, 1979.

32. Gersony, W. M., Katz, S. L., and Nadas, A. S.: Endocardial fibroelastosis and mumps virus. Pediatrics 37:430, 1966.

33. Ghafour, A. S., and Gutgesell, H. P.: Echocardiographic evaluation of left ventricular function in children with congestive cardiomyopathy. Am. J. Cardiol. 44:1332, 1979.

34. Gilbert, B. W., Pollick, C., Adelman, A. G., and Wigle, E. D.: Hypertrophic cardiomyopathy: Subclassification by M-mode echocardiography. Am. J. Cardiol. 45:861, 1980.

35. Goodwin, J. F., and Oakley, C. M.: The cardiomyopathies. Br. Heart J. 34:545, 1972.

36. Goodwin, J. F., Hollman, A., Cleland, W. P., and Teare, R. D.: Obstructive cardiomyopathy simulating aortic stenosis. Br. Heart J. 22:403, 1960.

37. Gutgesell, H. P., Speer, M., and Rosenberg, H. S.: Further characterization of the hypertrophic cardiomyopathy of infants of diabetic mothers. Circulation 61:441, 1980.

38. Hanrath, P., Mathey, D. G., Siegert, R., and Bleifeld, W.: Left ventricular relaxation and filling pattern in different forms of left ventricular hypertrophy: An echocardiographic study. Am. J. Cardiol. 45:15, 1980.

39. Hardarson, T., De la Calzada, C. S., Curiel, R., and Goodwin, J. F.: Prognosis and mortality of hypertrophic obstructive cardiomyopathy. Lancet 2:1462, 1973.

40. Harris, L. C., and Nghiem, Q. X.: Cardiomyopathies in infants and children. Prog. Cardiovasc. Dis. 15:255, 1972.

41. Hastreiter, A. R., and Miller, R. A.: Management of primary endomyocardial disease. The myocarditis-endocardial fibroelastosis syndrome. Pediatr. Clin. North Am. 11:401, 1964.

42. Henry, W. L., Clark, C. E., and Epstein, S. E.: Asymmetric septal hypertrophy (ASH): Echocardiographic identification of the pathognomonic anatomic abnormality of IHSS. Circulation 47:225, 1973.

43. Henry, W. L., Clark, C. E., Glancy, D. L., and Epstein, S. E.: Echocardiographic measurement of the left ventricular outflow gradient in idiopathic hypertrophic subaortic stenosis. N. Engl. J. Med. 288:989, 1973.

44. Henry, W. L., Clark, C. E., Griffith, J. M., and Epstein, S. E.: Mechanism of left ventricular outflow obstruction in patients with obstructive asymmetric septal hypertrophy (idiopathic hypertrophic subaortic stenosis). Am. J. Cardiol. 35:337, 1975.

45. Henry, W. L., Morganroth, J., Pearlman, A. S., Clark, C. E., Redwood, D. R., Itscoitz, S. B., and Epstein, S. E.: Relation between echocardiographically determined left atrial size and atrial fibrillation. Circulation 53:273, 1976.

46. Henry, W. L., Nienhuis, A. W., Wiener, M., Miller, D. R., Canale, V. C., and Piomelli, S.: Echocardiographic abnormalities in patients with transfusion—dependent anemia and secondary myocardial iron deposition. Am. J. Med. 64:547, 1978.

47. Hutchins, G. M., and Vie, S. A.: The progression of interstitial myocarditis to idiopathic endocardial fibroelastosis. Am. J. Pathol. 66:483, 1972.

48. Kaltenbach, M., Hopf, R., Kober, G., Bussmann, W. D., Keller, M., and Peterson, D. Y.: Treatment of hypertrophic obstructive cardiomyopathy with verapamil. Br. Heart J. 42:35, 1979.

49. Kline, I. K., Miller, A. J., Pick, R., Katz, L. N.: Relationship between human endocardial fibroelastosis and obstruction of cardiac lymphatics. Circulation 30:728, 1964.

50. Krajcer, Z., Orzan, F., Pechacek, L. W., Garcia, E., and Leachman, R. O.: Early systolic closure of the aortic valve in patients with hypertrophic subaortic stenosis and discrete subaortic stenosis. Correlation with preoperative and postoperative hemodynamics. Am. J. Cardiol. 41:823, 1978.

51. Krikler, D. M., Davies, M. J., Rowland, E., Goodwin, J. F., Evans, R. C., and Shaw, D. B.: Sudden death in hypertrophic cardiomyopathy: Associated accessory atrioventricular pathways. Br. Heart J. 43:245, 1980.

52. Lambert, E. D., and Vlad, P.: Primary endomyocardial disease. Pediatr. Clin. North Am. 5:1057, 1958.

53. Larter, W. E., Allen, H. D., Sahn, D. J., and Goldberg, S. J.: The asymmetrically hypertrophied septum. Further differentiation of its causes. Circulation 53:19, 1976.

54. LeJemtel, T. H., Factor, S. M., Koenigsberg, M., O'Reilly, M., Frater, R., and Sonnenblick, E. H.: Mural vegetations at the site of endocardial trauma in infective endocarditis complicating idiopathic hypertrophic subaortic stenosis. Am. J. Cardiol. 44:569, 1979.

55. Lie, J. T., and Grossman, S. J.: Pathology of the heart in acromegaly: Anatomic findings in 27 autopsied patients. Am. Heart J. 100:41, 1980.

56. Lynfield, J., Gasul, B. M., Luan, L. L., and Dillon, R. F.: Right and left heart catheterization and angiocardiographic findings in idiopathic cardiac hypertrophy with endocardial fibroelastosis. Circulation 21:386, 1960.

57. Manning, J. A., Sellers, F. J., Bynum, R. S., and Keith, J. D.: The medical management of clinical endocardial fibroelastosis. Circulation 29:60, 1964.

58. Maron, B. J., Edwards, J. E., Henry, W. L., Clark, C. E., Bingle, G. J., and Epstein, S. E.: Asymmetric septal hypertrophy (ASH) in infancy. Circulation 50:809, 1974.

59. Maron, B. J., Henry, W. L., Clark, C. E., Redwood, D. R., Roberts, W. C., and Epstein, S. E.: Asymmetric septal hypertrophy in childhood. Circulation 53:9, 1976.

60. Maron, B. J., Merrill, W. H., Freier, P. A., Kent, K. M., Epstein, S. E., and Morrow, A. G.: Long-term clinical course and symptomatic status of patients after operation for hypertrophic subaortic stenosis. Circulation 57:1205, 1978.

61. Maron, B. J., Lipson, L. C., Roberts, W. C., Savage, D. D., and Epstein, S. E.: "Malignant" hypertrophic cardiomyopathy: Identification of a subgroup of families with unusually frequent premature death. Am. J. Cardiol. 41:1133, 1978.

62. Maron, B. J., Roberts, W. C., Edwards, J. E., McAllister, H. A., Foley, D. D., and Epstein, S. E.: Sudden death in patients with hypertrophic cardiomyopathy: Characterization of 26 patients without functional limitation. Am. J. Cardiol. 41:803, 1978.

63. Maron, B. J., Verter, J., and Kapur, S.: Disproportionate ventricular septal thickening in the developing normal human heart. Circulation 57:520, 1978.

64. Maron, B. J., Epstein, S. E., and Roberts, W. C.: Hypertrophic cardiomyopathy and transmural myocardial infarction without significant atherosclerosis of the extramural coronary arteries. Am. J. Cardiol. 43:1086, 1979.

65. Maron, B. J., and Roberts, W. C.: Quantitative analysis of cardiac muscle cell disorganization in the ventricular septum of patients with hypertrophic cardiomyopathy. Circulation 59:689, 1979.

66. Maron, B. J., Edwards, J. E., Moller, J., and Epstein, S. E.: Prevalence and characteristics of disproportionate ventricular septal thickening in infants with congenital heart disease. Circulation 59:126, 1979.

67. Maron, B. J., and Epstein, S. E.: Hypertrophic cardiomyopathy. Recent observations regarding the specificity of three hallmarks of the disease: Asymmetric septal hypertrophy, septal disorganization, and systolic anterior motion of the anterior mitral leaflet. Am. J. Cardiol. 45:141, 1980.

68. Maron, B. J., and Roberts, W. C.: Cardiomyopathies in the first two decades of life. In Pediatric Cardiovascular Disease, Cardiovasc. Clin., edited by M. A. Engle. F. A. Davis Co., Philadelphia, 1981, p. 35.

69. Maron, B. J., Anan, T. J., and Roberts, W. C.: Quantitative analysis of the distribution of cardiac muscle cell disorganization in the left ventricular wall of patients with hypertrophic cardiomyopathy. Circulation 63:882, 1981.

70. Maron, B. J., Gottdiener, J. S., and Epstein, S. E.: Patterns and significance of the distribution of left ventricular hypertrophy in hypertrophic cardiomyopathy: A wide-angle, two-dimensional echocardiographic study of 125 patients. Am. J. Cardiol. 48:418, 1981.

71. Maron, B. J., Savage, D. D., Wolfson, J. K., and Epstein, S. E.: Prognostic significance of 24-hour ambulatory electrocardiographic monitoring in patients with hypertrophic cardiomyopathy: A prospective study. Am. J. Cardiol. 48:252, 1981.

72. Maron, B. J., Tajik, A. J., Ruttenberg, H. D., Graham, T. P., Atwood, G. F., Victorica, B. E., Lie, J. T., and Roberts, W. C.: Hypertrophic cardiomyopathy in infants: Clinical features and natural history. Circulation 65:1388, 1982.

73. Maron, B. J., Roberts, W. C., and Epstein, S. E.: Sudden death in hypertrophic cardiomyopathy: Profile of 78 patients. Circulation, in press, 1982.

74. McGuffin, W. L., Sherman, B. M., Roth, J., Gorden, P., Kahn, C. R., Roberts, W. C., and Frommer, P. L.: Acromegaly and cardiovascular disorders. A prospective study. Ann. Intern. Med. 81:11, 1974.

75. McKenna, W. J., Chetty, S., Oakley, C. M.,

and Goodwin, J. F.: Arrhythmia in hypertrophic cardiomyopathy: Exercise and 48-hour ambulatory electrocardiographic assessment with and without beta adrenergic blocking therapy. Am. J. Cardiol. 45:1, 1980.

76. McKenna, W., Deanfield, J., Faruqui, A., England, D., Oakley, C., and Goodwin, J.: Prognosis in hypertrophic cardiomyopathy: Role of age and clinical, electrocardiographic and hemodynamic features. Am. J. Cardiol. 47:532, 1981.

77. McLoughlin, T. G., Schiebler, G. L., and Krovetz, L. J.: Hemodynamic findings in children with endocardial fibroelastosis. Am. Heart J. 75:162, 1968.

78. Menges, H., Brandenburg, R. O., and Brown, A. L.: The clinical, hemodynamic and pathologic diagnosis of muscular subvalvular aortic stenosis. Circulation 24:1126, 1961.

79. Miller, G. A. H., Rahimtoola, S. H., Ongley, P. A., and Swan, H. J. C.: Left ventricular volume and volume change in endocardial fibroelastosis. Am. J. Cardiol. 15:631, 1965.

80. Mitchell, S. C., Froehlich, L. A., Banas, J. S., and Gilkeson, M. R.: An epidemiologic assessment of primary endocardial fibroblastosis. Am. J. Cardiol. 18:859, 1966.

81. Moller, J. H., Lucas, R. V., Adams, P., Jr., Anderson, R. C., Jorgens, J., and Edwards, J. E.: Endocardial fibroelastosis. A clinical and anatomic study of 47 patients with emphasis on the relationship to mitral insufficiency. Circulation 30:759, 1964.

82. Morrow, A. G.: Hypertrophic subaortic stenosis. Operative methods utilized to relieve left ventricular outflow obstruction. J. Thorac. Cardiovasc. Surg. 76:423, 1978.

83. Murgo, J. P., Alter, B. R., Dorethy, J. F., Altobelli, S. A., and McGranahan, G. M.: Dynamics of left ventricular ejection in obstructive and nonobstructive hypertrophic cardiomyopathy. J. Clin. Invest. 66:1369, 1980.

84. Nadas, A. S., and Fyler, D. C.: *Pediatric Cardiology*, 3rd edition. W. B. Saunders, Philadelphia, 1972, p. 233.

85. Nghiem, Q. X., Toledo, J. R., Schreiber, M. H., Harris, L. C., Lockhart, L. L., Tyson, K. R.: Congenital idiopathic hypertrophic subaortic stenosis associated with a phenotypic Turner's syndrome. Am. J. Cardiol. 30:683, 1972.

86. Oakley, C.: Ventricular hypertrophy in cardiomyopathy. Br. Heart J. 33:179, 1971.

87. Oakley, G. D. G., McGarry, K., Limb, D. G., and Oakley, C. M.: Management of pregnancy in patients with hypertrophic cardiomyopathy. Br. Med. J. 1:1749, 1979.

88. Parrillo, J. E., Fauci, A. S., and Wolff, S. M.: Therapy of the hypereosinophilic syndrome. Ann. Intern. Med. 89:167, 1978.

89. Paul, R. N., and Robbins, S. G.: Surgical treatment for endocardial fibroelastosis or anomalous left coronary artery: Four years experience with poudrage. Am. J. Cardiol. 1:694, 1958.

90. Rosing, D. R., Kent, K. M., Maron, B. J., and Epstein, S. E.: Verapamil therapy: A new approach to the pharmacologic treatment of hypertrophic cardiomyopathy. II. Effects on exercise capacity and symptomatic status. Circulation 60:1208, 1979.

91. Redwood, D. R., Scherer, J. L., and Epstein, S. E.: Biventricular cineangiography in the evaluation of patients with asymmetric septal hypertrophy. Circulation 49:1116, 1974.

92. Rees, A., Elbl, F., Minhas, K., and Solinger, R.: Echocardiographic evidence of outflow tract obstruction in Pompe's disease (glycogen storage disease of the heart). Am. J. Cardiol. 37:1103, 1976.

93. Roberts, W. C., and Ferrans, V. J.: The pathologic anatomy of the cardiomyopathies. Idiopathic dilated and hypertrophic types, infiltrative types, and endomyocardial disease with and without eosinophilia. Hum. Pathol. 6:287, 1975.

94. Ross, J., Braunwald, E., Gault, J. H., Mason, D. T., and Morrow, A. G.: The mechanism of the intraventricular pressure gradient in idiopathic hypertrophic subaortic stenosis. Circulation 34:558, 1966.

95. Ross, R. S., Bulkley, B. H., Hutchins, G. M., Harshey, J. S., Jones, R. A., Kraus, H., Liebman, J., Thorne, C. M., Weinberg, S. B., Weech, A. A., and Weech, A. A., Jr.: Idiopathic familial myocardiopathy in three generations: A clinical and pathologic study. Am. Heart J. 96:170, 1978.

96. Rossen, R. M., Goodman, D. J., Ingham, E. R., and Popp, R. L.: Ventricular systolic septal thickening and excursion in idiopathic hypertrophic subaortic stenosis. N. Engl. J. Med. 291:1317, 1974.

97. Savage, D. D., Henry, W. L., Eastman, R. C., Borer, J. S., and Gorden, P.: Echocardiographic assessment of cardiac anatomy and function in acromegalic patients. Am. J. Med. 67:823, 1979.

98. Savage, D. D., Seides, S. F., Clark, C. E., Henry, W. L., Maron, B. J., Robinson, F. C., and Epstein, S. E.: Electrocardiographic findings in patients with obstructive and nonobstructive hypertrophic cardiomyopathy. Circulation 58:402, 1978.

99. Schryer, M. J., and Karnauchow, P. N.: Endocardial fibroelastosis: Etiologic and pathogenetic considerations in children. Am. Heart J. 88:557, 1974.

100. Sellers, F. J., Keith, J. D., and Manning, J. A.: The diagnosis of primary endocardial fibroelastosis. Circulation 29:49, 1964.

101. Shah, P. M., Gramiak, R., and Kramer, D. H.: Ultrasound localization of left ventricular outflow obstruction in hypertrophic obstructive cardiomyopathy. Circulation 40:3, 1969.

102. Shah, P. M., Gramiak, R., Adelman, A. G., and Wigle, E. D.: Echocardiographic assessment of the effects of surgery and propranolol on the dynamics of outflow obstruction in hypertrophic subaortic stenosis. Circulation 45:516, 1972.

103. Shah, P. M., Adelman, A. G., Wigle, E. D., Gobel, F. L., Burchell, H. B., Hardarson, T., Curiel, R., De la Calzada C., Oakley, C. M., and Goodwin, J. F.: The natural (and unnatural) course of hypertrophic obstructive cardiomyopathy. A multicenter study. Circ. Res. 34 and 35 (Suppl. II):II-179, 1973.

104. Silver, M. M., Burns, J. E., Sethi, R. K., and Rowe, R. D.: Oncocytic cardiomyopathy in an infant with oncocytosis in exocrine and endocrine glands. Hum. Pathol. 11:598, 1980.

105. Simon, A. L., Ross, J., and Gault, J. H.: Angiographic anatomy of the left ventricle and mitral valve in idiopathic hypertrophic subaortic stenosis. Circulation 36:852, 1967.

106. St. Geme, J. W., Jr., Noren, G. R., and Adams, P., Jr.: Proposed embryopathic relation between mumps virus and primary endocardial fibroelastosis. N. Engl. J. Med. 275:339, 1966.

107. St. John Sutton, M. G., Tajik, A. J., Gibson, D. G., Brown, D. J., Seward, J. B., and Giuliani, E. R.: Echocardiographic assessment of left ventricular filling and septal and posterior wall dynamics in idiopathic hypertrophic subaortic stenosis. Circulation 57:512, 1978.

108. St. John Sutton, M. G., Tajik, A. J., Giuliani, E. R., Gordon, H., and Su, W. P. D.: Hypertrophic obstructive cardiomyopathy and lentiginosis: A little known neural ectodermal syndrome. Am. J. Cardiol. 47:214, 1981.

109. Stenson, R. E., Flamm, M. D., Harrison, D. C., and Hancock, E. W.: Hypertrophic subaortic stenosis. Clinical and hemodynamic effects of long-term propranolol therapy. Am. J. Cardiol. 31:763, 1973.

110. Teare, D.: Asymmetrical hypertrophy of the heart in young patients. Br. Heart J. 20:1, 1958.

111. Tingelstad, J. B., Shiel, F. O. M., and McCue, C. M.: The electrocardiogram in the contracted type of primary endocardial fibroelastosis. Am. J. Cardiol. 27:304, 1971.

112. Thompson, R., Ahmed, M., Pridie, R., and Yacoub, M.: Hypertrophic cardiomyopathy after aortic valve replacement. Am. J. Cardiol. 45:33, 1980.

113. van Buchem, F. S. P., Arends, A., and Schröeder, E. A.: Endocardial fibroelastosis in adolescents and young adults. Br. Heart J. 21:229, 1959.

114. Vlad, P., Rowe, R. D., and Keith, J. D.: The electrocardiogram in primary endocardial fibroelastosis. Br. Heart J. 17:189, 1955.

115. Way, G. L., Wolfe, R. R., Eshaghpour, E., Bender, R. L., Jaffe, R. B., and Ruttenberg, H. D.: The natural history of hypertrophic cardiomyopathy in infants of diabetic mothers. J. Pediatr. 95:1020, 1979.

116. Westwood, M., Harris, R., Burn, J. L., and Barson, A. J.: Heredity in primary endocardial fibroelastosis. Br. Heart J. 37:1077, 1975.

117. Wigle, D. E., Adelman, A. G., Auger, P., and Marquis, Y.: Mitral regurgitation in muscular subaortic stenosis. Am. J. Cardiol. 24:698, 1969.

118. Wigle, E. D., Heimbecker, R. O., and Gunton, R. W.: Idiopathic ventricular septal hypertrophy causing muscular subaortic stenosis. Circulation 26:325, 1962.

119. Williams, R. G., Ellison, R. C., and Nadas, A. S.: Development of left ventricular outflow obstruction in idiopathic hypertrophic subaortic stenosis. Report of a case. N. Engl. J. Med. 288:868, 1973.

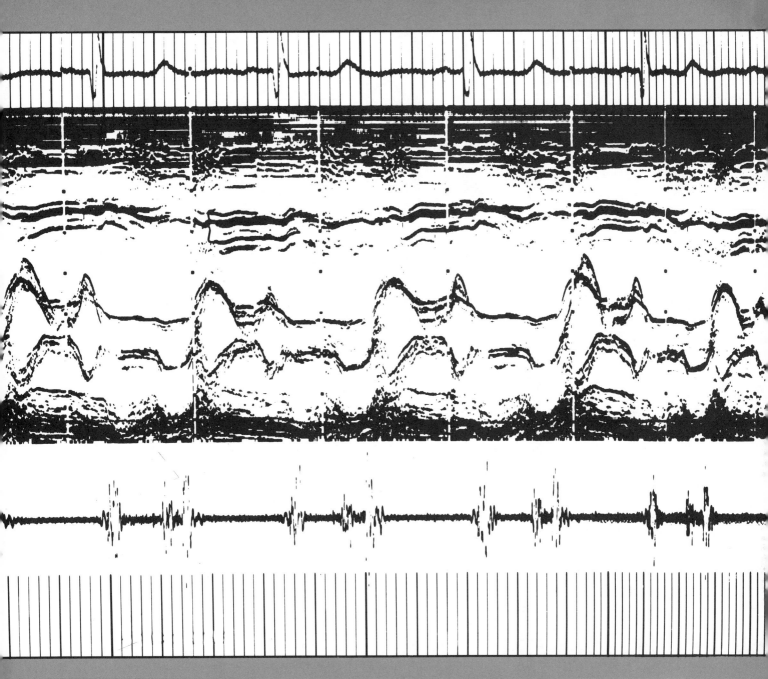

Part 6
APPENDIX

Appendix: Drugs and Dosages in Pediatrics

Roger A. Hurwitz, M.D.

A. Digitalis[a]

Drug	Route	Digitalization	Maintenance	Onset Action	Maximal Action	Duration	Supplied
Digoxin (Lanoxin)	p.o.	Premature: 0.025 mg/kg Newborn: 0.04 mg/kg <2 yr: 0.04–0.06 mg/kg >2 yr: 0.02–0.04 mg/kg	25–33% of T.D.D. divided into 2 doses/day	1–2 hr	4–8 hr	4–7 days	Amp: 0.1, 0.25 mg/ml Elixir: 0.05 mg/ml Tab: 0.125, 0.25, 0.5 mg
	IM	75–80% of p.o. dose		15–60 min	2–5 hr	4–7 days	
	IV	75–80% of p.o. dose		5–30 min	2–5 hr	4–7 days	
Digitoxin (Crystodigin, Digitaline Nativelle, Purodigin)	p.o.	Premature and newborn: 0.02–0.03 mg/kg <2 yr: 0.035 mg/kg >2 yr: 0.025 mg/kg	10–20% of T.D.D. as 1 dose/day	2–4 hr	8–24 hr	2–3 wk	Amp: 0.2 mg/ml Elixir: Digitaline Nativelle, 0.05 mg/ml Tab: 0.05, 0.1 mg
	IM	Same as p.o.		1–2 hr	4–12 hr	2–3 wk	
	IV			30 min–2 hr			

[a] Abbreviations used are: Amp, ampule; tab, tablet; T.D.D., total digitalizing dose.

B. *Diuretic*

Drug	Route	Dose	Onset Action	Mechanism of Action	Precautions and Complications	Supplied
Chlorothiazide (Diuril)	p.o.	20–40 mg/kg/day in 2 doses	1–2 hr	Inhibits renal tubular reabsorption	Electrolyte problems; need K^+ supplements	Tab: 250, 500 mg; Syrup: 250 mg/5 ml
Chlorthalidone* (Hygroton)	p.o.	0.2–0.5 mg/kg/day	2–4 hrs; prolonged effect (48 hr)	Cortical diluting segment, ascending limb of Henle loop	Severe renal disease; may precipitate azotemia	Tab: 25, 50, 100 mg
Ethacrynic acid (Edecrin)	IV	0.4–0.6 mg/kg/day	10–20 min	Blocks loop of Henle Na^+ reabsorption	Metabolic alkalosis.	Vial: 50 mg each
	p.o.	10–20 mg/kg/day in 4 doses	1 hr		Hypokalemia	Tab: 25, 50 mg
Furosemide (Lasix)	IV, IM	1–2 mg/kg/dose	5–15 min	Inhibits renal tubular and Henle loop Na^+ reabsorption	Metabolic alkalosis + hypokalemia	Amp: 10 mg/ml; Tab: 20, 40 mg; Syrup: 10 mg/ml
	p.o.	1–4 mg/kg/day	30–60 min			
Hydrochlorothiazide (Hydrodiuril)	p.o.	2.0–3.5 mg/kg/day in 2 doses	1–2 hr	Same as Diuril	Electrolyte imbalance; need K^+ supplement	Tab: 25, 50 mg
Spironolactone (Aldactone)	p.o.	1.5–3.0 mg/kg/day in 2–3 doses	Alone, 4–5/day for good response	Aldosterone blocker	K^+ retention	Tab: 25 mg

* Asterisk indicates throughout Appendix a drug not yet approved or with enough information to provide pediatric dosage or a commercially available agent.

C. *Cardiotonic*

Drug	Route	Dose	Onset Action	Mechanism of Action	Precautions and Complications	Supplied
Amrinone*	IV	0.5–1.0 mg/kg q15–30 min	Minutes	Inotropism other than via catecholamines	Dysrhythmia Thrombocytopenia	
	p.o.	1–3 mg/kg q8h	Hours			
Dobutamine (Dobutrex)	IV	2–10 μg/kg/min	Minutes	Inotropism via beta receptors	Hypertrophic cardiomyopathy Ventricular ectopy; tachycardia; hypertension	Vial: 20 ml, 12 mg/ml
Dopamine (Intropin)	IV (inactive in alkali)	5–25 μg/kg/min	Minutes	Inotropism Selective vasodilation (renal)	Potentiate pheochromocytoma; tachyarrhythmias; tissue necrosis	Amp: 5 ml, 40, 80 mg/ml
Epinephrine (adrenaline)	IV	0.5–1.0 ml in 10 ml saline slowly IV or 0.5 mg (0.5 ml) in 100 ml drip; or 1 μg/kg/min	Seconds to 1 min.	Chronotropic and inotropic effects	Severe tachycardia	Amp: 1 ml (1:1000); Vials: 30 ml (1:1000)
Isoproterenol (Isuprel)	IV	Arrest: 1 mg/250 ml 5% glucose; slow drip till effect; 0.05–0.4 μg/kg/min	30–60 sec	Chronotropic and inotropic; vasodilator	Ventricular excitability	Amp: 1 ml = 0.2 mg (1:5000)
	Sublingual	5–20 mg q3–4h	Minutes			Glossets 5, 10, 15 mg
	Rectal	2.5–15 mg q4–6h	Minutes			
Levarterenol (Levophed, norepinephrine)	IV	1 ml in 250 ml solution slow drip; start at 0.1 μg/kg/min	Seconds	Pressor agent	Hypertension; severe slough if not into vein	Amp: 0.2%: 4 ml with 1000 ml diluent = 4 μg base/ml

D. Antihypertensive, Vasodilatory, Afterload Reduction

Drug	Route	Dose	Onset Action	Mechanism of Action	Precautions and Complications	Supplied
Chlorothiazide		See Diuretic agents				
Ethacrynic acid		See Diuretic agents				
Furosemide		See Diuretic agents				
Diazoxide (Hyperstat)	IV	3–5 mg/kg/dose as bolus; may repeat q4–12h	1–2 min	Vasodilator	Hypotension Hyperglycemia	Amp: 15 mg/ml
Dipyridamole* (Persantine)	p.o.	25–50 mg 1–3 times/day, 1 hr before meals	Days	Coronary vasodilator?	Hypotension	Tab: 25, 75 mg
Hydrochlorothiazide		See Diuretic agents				
Hydralazine (Apresoline)	IV	0.8–3.0 mg/kg/day in 4–6 doses over 30 min	10–30 min	Peripheral vasodilation	Hypotension Tachycardia Lupus-like syndrome	Amp: 20 mg/ml Tab: 10, 25, 50 mg
	p.o.	Initial: 0.75 mg/kg/day in 3–4 doses May increase 2–5 × amount over next 4 weeks	Hours–days may have to await titrated effect			
Methyldopa (Aldomet)	IV	10–40 mg/kg/day in 4 doses	2–4 hr	Decarboxylase inhibitor	Liver damage Anemia	Solution: 50 mg/ml Tab: 125, 250 mg
	p.o.	10–50 mg/kg/day in 2–3 doses	6–12 hr			
Metoprolol* (Lopressor)	p.o.	25–100 mg q8–12h	1–2 hr	Beta adrenergic receptor blockade; beta₁ at lower dosage	Similar to Inderal but less bronchospasm	Tab: 50, 100 mg
Nifedipine*	IV	0.01–0.02 mg/kg,	Minutes	Calcium antagonist; primary vasodilation	Hypotension	Cap: 10 mg
	p.o.	1–2 mg/kg/day in 4 doses	1–2 hr			

Table D—continued

Drug	Route	Dose	Onset Action	Mechanism of Action	Precautions and Complications	Supplied
Nitroprusside (Nipride)	IV	0.5–1.5 µg/kg/min in IV drip	Minutes	Peripheral vasodilation; afterload reduction	Hypotension Cyanide toxicity	Vial: 5 ml, 10 mg/ml
Phentolamine (Regitine)	IV	0.1 mg/kg/dose	2–10 min	Adrenergic blockade	Hypotension	Amp: 5 mg Tab: 50 mg
	p.o.	5 mg/kg/day in 4 doses				
Prazosin* (Minipres)	p.o.	2–10 mg/day in 2–3 doses	1–3 hr	Vasodilator; blockade alpha-adrenergic receptors	Hypotension; Syncope	Cap: 1, 2 mg
Propranolol	See antidysrhythmics	Note higher dose for hypertension, 1–7 mg/kg/day				
Reserpine (Serpasil)	IM	0.07 mg/kg every 12–24 hr (works well with hydralazine)	Hours	Central	Hypotension Depression	Amp and Vial: 2.5 mg/ml Tab: 0.1, 0.25, 0.5, 1.0–5.0 mg Elixir: 0.25 mg/5 ml
Tolazoline (Priscoline)	IV	1–2 mg/kg slow push; Maint[a]: 2.0 mg/kg/hr	Minutes	Vasorelaxation?	Hyper or hypotension Gastric ulcer	Vial: 10 ml, 25 mg/ml

[a] Maint, maintenance.

E. Analgesia and Sedation

Drug	Route	Dose	Onset Action	Mechanism	Precautions and Complications	Supplied
Chlorpromazine (Thorazine)	IM	1–2 mg/kg/day in 3–4 doses	Minutes	Tranquilization	Hypotension Hepatotoxicity Agranulocytosis	Amp and Vials: 25 mg/ml Tab: 10, 25, 50, 100, 200 mg Syrup: 10 mg/5 ml Suppos: 25 mg each
	p.o.	2–3 mg/kg/day in 4 doses	30–60 min			
	Rectal	3–4 mg/kg/day in 3–4 doses	Slightly faster than p.o.			
Diazepam (Valium)	IV	0.1–0.25 mg/kg/dose slowly; may repeat 30–60 min	Minutes	Limbic system to induce calming	Apnea, somnolence	Amp: 2 ml Vial: 10 ml Both: 5 mg/ml
	p.o.	3–6 mg/day in 3 doses	30–60 min	Adjunct in status epilepticus		
Hydroxyzine Pamoate (Vistaril)	IM	0.5–1.5 mg/kg/dose	Minutes	Ataraxic	Potentiates narcotics	Vial: 25, 50 mg/ml Tab: 25, 50, 100 mg Syrup: 25 mg/5 ml
	p.o.	1–2 mg/kg/day in 2–4 doses	30–60 min			
Ketamine (Ketalar)	IV	1–4 mg/kg initial, smaller doses q30min p.r.n.	1 min	Somatic sensory blockade	Emergence reactions Respiratory depression Increase in pulmonary resistance	Vial: 20, 25, 50 mg 10 mg/ml
Meperidine (Demerol)	IV, IM	5–7 mg/kg/day in 4–6 doses	Parenteral: 2–5 min	Narcotic analgesia	Respiratory and CNS depression Tachycardia	Vials: 50, 100 mg/ml Amp: 25 mg/0.5 ml, 50 mg/1ml Tab: 50, 100 mg Elixir: 50 mg/5 ml
	p.o.	Same	5–30 min			
Morphine sulfate	SC	0.1–0.2 mg/kg qh	4–6 minutes	Strongest narcotic analgesic Nonspecific aid in congestive failure, pulmonary edema, anoxic spells	Respiratory and CNS depression	Amp: 10, 15 mg/ml
Promethazine (Phenergan)	IM	0.5–1 mg/kg q4–6 h	Minutes	Antihistaminic Antiemetic	CNS depression	Amp: 25 mg/ml Vials: 50 mg/ml Tab: 12.5, 25, 50 mg Syrup: 6.25 mg/5 ml Suppos: 25, 50 mg
	p.o.	1–2 mg/kg/day in 3–4 doses	30–60 min			
	Rectal	As p.o.	30–60 min			

F. Antidysrhythmic

Drug	Route	Dose	Onset Action	Mechanism	Precautions and Complications	Supplied
Amiodarone*	IV	3–6 mg/kg	5–10 min	Smooth muscle relaxant; inhibits aupha- and beta-adrenergic receptors	Hypotension Heart block	
	p.o.	5–7 mg/kg/day for wk; then 2–4 mg/kg/day	4–6 hr	Prolongs action potential	Thyroid dysfunction; corneal deposits	
Aprindine*	IV	2–4 mg/kg slow infusion over 1 hr	5–10 min	Prolongs conduction	CNS-tremors Agranulocytosis	
	p.o.	Load 1–3 mg/kg/day for 2–3 doses for 2–3 days; Maint: 0.5–1.5 mg/kg/day in 3 doses	2–3 hr (long half-life)	Increases effective refractory period of atria and ventricles		
Atropine sulfate	IV SC p.o.	0.01–0.03 mg/kg q4–6 h, max: 0.4 mg/dose	Seconds Minutes About 1 hr	Parasympathetic block	Tachycardia	Vials: 0.4 mg/ml 0.5 mg/ml Tab: 0.3, 0.4, 0.6 mg
Bretylium* tosylate* (Bretylol)	IV	5 mg/kg as bolus, 5 mg/kg q6h, p.r.n.-up to 48 hr	Minutes	Inhibits norepinephrine release	Hypotension Aggravates digitalis toxicity	Amp: 10 ml, 50 mg/ml
Digitalis		See Cardiotonics				
Diphenylhydantoin (Dilantin)	IV	Initial: 3–5 mg/kg in 5 min	5–10 min	Controversial	Bradycardia Blood dyscrasia	Vial: 50 mg/ml Tab: 50 mg Caps: 30, 100 mg Susp: 125 mg/5 ml
	p.o.	2–5 mg/kg/day in 2–3 doses	2–4 hr			
Disopyramide* (Norpace)	IV	1.5–2.5 mg/kg as slow bolus	Minutes	Quinidine-like direct, depressant on myocardium	Heart failure	Cap: 100, 150 mg
	p.o.	2–6 mg/kg/day in 4 doses	1 hr	Anticholinergic activity	Anticholinergic response	
Edrophonium (Tensilon)	IV	0.1–0.2 mg/kg in single dose (not more than 10 mg/dose)	Seconds to 1 min	Inhibits cholinesterase and cholinergic effect	Severe cholinergic reaction	Amp: 10 mg/ml
Encainide*	IV	0.5–1.0 mg/kg/dose	Minutes	Prolongs His-Purkinje system conduction	Postural hypotension	
	p.o.	1–3 mg/kg/day in 4 doses	1 hr approx.	As above; also lengthens atrial and ventricular refractoriness	Dysrhythmia	
Ephedrine sulfate	IV IM p.o.	50 mg in 100 ml 5% D/W in slow drip 0.8–1.6 mg/kg/day in 4 doses	Seconds to minutes Minutes to 1 hr	Sympathomimetic		Amp: 25, 50 mg/ml Tab: 25, 50 mg Syrup: 16 mg/4 ml
Isoproterenol (Isuprel)		See Cardiotonics				
Lidocaine (Xylocaine)	IV	0.5–1.0 mg/kg q 20–60 min p.r.n.	15–90 sec	Local anesthetic Depresses myocardial irritability	Dysrhythmia	Vials: 0.5, 1.0, 2.0% Amp: 1.0, 2.0%

Table F—continued

Drug	Route	Dose	Onset Action	Mechanism	Precautions and Complications	Supplied
Phenylephrine (Neo-Synephrine)	IV	0.005–0.01 mg/kg/dose	Seconds	Vasoconstriction	Hypertension Dysrhythmia	Amp: 10 mg/ml
	IM or SC	0.01–0.1 mg/kg q1–2 h				
Procaine amide (Pronestyl)	IV	10–100 mg diluted as slow 5 min drip q10–30 min p.r.n.	1–5 min	Depresses myocardial excitability and conduction	Hypotension Blood dyscrasia Lupus-like syndrome	Vials: 100 mg/ml, 500 mg/ml
	IM	5–8 mg/kg q6h may try 50–100 q2h (with 50 mg increments)	5–30 min			Caps: 250, 375, 500 mg
	p.o.	40–60 mg/kg/day in 4–6 doses	30–60 min			
Propranolol (Inderal)	IV	0.01–0.15 mg/kg over 10 min, q6–8h p.r.n.	2–5 min	Beta-adrenergic blockade	Decreased cardiac output Dysrhythmias Hypoglycemia Asthma	Vials: 1 mg/ml Tab: 10 mg, 50 mg
	p.o.	0.5–1.0 mg/kg dose q6h	30–60 min			
Quinidine gluconate	IM	2–10 mg/kg q3–6h p.r.n. (usual 100–500 mg/dose)	5–15 min	Depresses atrial and ventricular excitability Vagolytic	Cardiac arrest Depresses contractility Blood dyscrasia	Amp: 80 mg/ml Dura-tab: 330 mg
	p.o.	10–30 mg/kg/day (usual 160–660 mg q12h)	4–8 hr			
	IV	About 0.5 mg/kg as slow drip with 800 mg/100 ml glucose				
Quinidine sulfate	p.o.	Start with 3–6 mg/kg q2–3 h, × 5; may increase to 12 mg/kg q2–3 h × 5; maintenance as determined by above	1 hr	As above	As above	Tabs: 100, 200, 300 mg
Verapamil (Isoptin, Calan)	IV	0.1–0.2 mg/kg over 1 min; may repeat in 30 min	Minutes	Calcium antagonist	Heart failure Hypotension Atrial fibrillation WPW[a] Have CaCl ready	Amp: 2 ml, 2.5 mg/ml
	p.o.	3–6 mg/kg/day in 3 doses				

[a]WPW, Wolff-Parkinson-White syndrome.

G. Anticoagulant

Drug	Route	Dose	Onset Action	Mechanism	Precautions and Complications	Supplied
Bishydroxycoumarin (Dicumarol)	p.o.	Keep prothrombin time 15–25% of normal Initial: 50–100 mg Maint: 10–50 mg/day	12–24 hr	Inhibits prothrombin synthesis	Bleeding (Vitamin K is antidote)	Tab: 25, 50, 100 mg
Heparin	IV	Initial: 50–100 units/kg Maint: 100 units/kg q4h Keep clotting time 2–3 × normal	1–5 min	Multiple actions on blood clotting	Bleeding (Protamine sulfate is antidote)	1 mg ≅ 100 units Amp and Vial: 1000, 5000, 10,000 and 20,000 units/ml
Warfarin (Coumadin)	IV p.o.	Initial: 10–30 mg/day Maint: 1–5 mg/day		As Dicumarol	As Dicumarol	Vial and Amp: 25 mg/ml Tab: 2, 2.5, 5, 10 mg

H. Lipid and Cholesterol Lowering

Drug	Route	Dose	Onset Action	Mechanism	Precautions and Complications	Supplied
Cholestyramine (Questran)	p.o.	250–1500 mg/kg/day in 2–4 doses	Min–hr	Absorbs bile acid Decreases synthesis	Fat soluble vitamin deficiency Bleeding Constipation Hyperchloremic acidosis	Packets: each has 4 gm active ingredient
Colestipol	p.o.			Similar to cholestyramine		Pack: 5 gm active
Clofibrate (Atromid-S)	p.o.	0.5–1.5 mg/day in 2–3 doses	Weeks to months before effect noted	Decreases synthesis of some lipoproteins	Blood dyscrasia Hepatic dysfunction Myositis; tumors Dysrhythmia	Caps: 500 mg
Neomycin sulfate	p.o.	20–40 mg/kg/day in 4 doses	Hours	Changes bowel flora and absorption	Ototoxicity Bacterial overgrowth Renal toxicity	Tab: 500 mg
Nicotinic acid	p.o.	25–75 mg/kg day in 2–3 doses with meals	Hours to days	Decreases synthesis Reduces fatty acid turnover	Hepatic dysfunction Flushing, nausea, diarrhea	Tab: 100, 500, 1000 mg

I. *Acid-Base, Electrolytes*

Drug	Route	Dose	Onset Action	Mechanism	Precautions and Complications	Supplied
Ammonium chloride	p.o.	75 mg/kg/day in 4 doses	Often use 3 days before mercurials	Supports mercurial action	Acidosis if usage prolonged	Tab: 300 mg
Calcium chloride	IV	1–4 ml of 10% solution; can give 300 mg/kg/day in 4 doses	Minutes	Strengthens myocardium	Causes slough if given subcutaneously; Bradycardia	Amp: 10% (100 mg/ml)
Calcium gluconate	IV	2–6 ml of 10% solution	Minutes	Strengthens myocardium	May cause slough if given subcutaneously; Bradycardia	Amp: 10% (100 mg/ml)
	p.o.	500 mg/kg/day in 4 doses	1–2 hr			
Potassium chloride		Daily K^+ requirement is 1–2 mEq/kg/day		Cellular metabolism	Dysrhythmia	Sol. for IV: (15% KCl) 20 ml = 40 mEq; Tabs: 300, 500 mg
	IV	0.5 mEq/kg/hr (Do not exceed 2 mEq/kg); slow drip of 40–80 mEq KCl/1000 ml 5% D/W^a	Minutes	Useful in digitalis toxicity	ECG: monitor for IV use	
	p.o.	1–1.5 mEq/kg/day 75–125 mg/kg/day (1–4 gm/day)	Hours			
Potassium triplex	p.o.	As above	Hours			Solution: 15 mEq K^+/5 ml
Potassium gluconate (Kaon)	p.o.	As above	Hours			Elixir: 7 mEq K^+/5 ml
Sodium bicarbonate	IV	0.058 gm raises PCO_2 ~ 1 mEq/kg	Seconds	Produces metabolic alkalosis	Alkalosis increases Na^+; Fast infusion may cause cerebral edema	Amp: 50 ml = 3.75 gm, = 44.6 mEq

^{a} D/W, dextrose in water.

J. *Ductal Specific*

Drug	Route	Dose	Onset Action	Mechanism	Precautions and Complications	Supplied
Indomethacin (Indocin)	IV	0.2 mg/kg then	Minutes	Antiinflammatory Prostaglandin inhibition	Gastrointestinal or other bleeding; Infection, renal impairment	Cap: 25 mg
	p.o.	0.1 mg/kg q12h for 2 doses p.r.n.	30–60 min			
Prostaglandin E_1 (Alprostadil, Prostin VR)	IV	0.01–0.1 µg/kg/min	Minutes	Smooth muscle relaxation, especially ductal	Apnea, fever, hypotension	Amp: 500 µg/ml

INDEX